deWit's

Medical-Surgical Nursing

Concepts and Practice

EDITION

4

deWit's
Medical-Surgical Nursing
Concepts and Practice

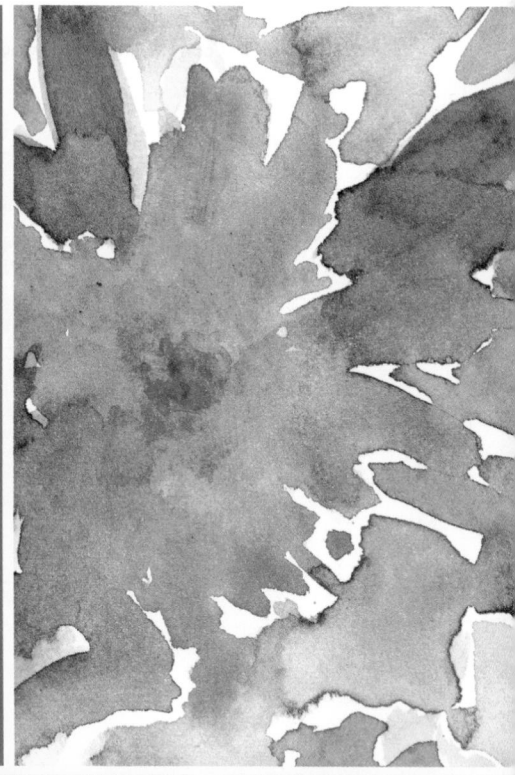

Holly K. Stromberg, RN, BSN, MSN, PHN, Alumnus CCRN
Professor Emeritus of Nursing
Allan Hancock College;
Clinical Educator
Marian Regional Medical Center
Santa Maria, California

ELSEVIER

3251 Riverport Lane
St. Louis, Missouri 63043

DEWIT'S MEDICAL-SURGICAL NURSING: CONCEPTS AND PRACTICE, FOURTH EDITION

ISBN: 978-0-323-60844-2

Library of Congress Control Number: 2019951917

Senior Content Strategist: Nancy O'Brien
Senior Content Development Manager: Lisa Newton
Senior Content Development Specialist: Laura Selkirk
Publishing Services Manager: Julie Eddy
Senior Project Manager: Tracey Schriefer
Design Direction: Renee Duenow

Printed in Canada

Last digit is the print number: 9 8 7 6 5 4 3 2

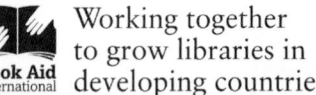

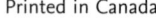

To my husband, who has been the "wind beneath my wings"
for this project and my biggest supporter in this journey called life.

To the rest of my family for their love and support,
especially to Aunt Kay, the prayer warrior.

To the students and colleagues who taught me through example and questioning,
thank you for enhancing my practice and enriching my life.

Contributors

Nicole Heimgartner, RN, DNP, COI
Adjunct Faculty, Nursing
American Sentinel University
Aurora, Colorado
Vice President and Nursing Consultant
Connect: RN2ED
Beavercreek, Ohio

Stephen McGhee, RN, DNP, MSc, PGCE, RNT, VR
Director of Global Affairs, College of Nursing
University of South Florida
Tampa, Florida

Cherie R. Rebar, RN, PhD, MBA, COI
Professor of Nursing
Wittenberg University
Springfield, Ohio
Adjunct Faculty, Nursing
Mercy College
Toledo, Ohio
Affiliate Faculty, Nursing
Indiana Wesleyan University
Marion, Indiana

Constance Visovsky, RN, PhD, ACNP, FAAN
Professor, College of Nursing
University of South Florida
Tampa, Florida

Cheryl Zambroski, RN, PhD
Associate Professor, College of Nursing
University of South Florida
Tampa, Florida

Reviewers

Kimberly Ann Amos, RN, MS(N), PhD, CNE
Director of Nursing
Isothermal Community College
Spindale, North Carolina

Sheryl Buckner, RN, PhD, ANEF
Assistant Professor, College of Nursing
University of Oklahoma
Oklahoma City, Oklahoma

Natasha Fontaine, RN, BN, PIDP
Health Services, Practical Nursing Department
College of the Rockies
Cranbrook, British Columbia, Canada

Linda Gambill, RN, MSN/Ed
Practical Nursing Program Director
Southwest Virginia Community College
Cedar Bluff, Virginia

Odelia Garcia, RN, BSN, MS, MSN
Registered Nurse, Vocational Nursing Program
Texas State Technical College—Harlingen
Harlingen, Texas

Melanie Gray, RN, PhD
Faculty Associate Degree Nursing Program
Milwaukee Area Technical College
Milwaukee, Wisconsin

Alice M. Hupp, RN, BS
Lead Instructor, Vocational Nursing
North Central Texas College
Gainesville, Texas

Lorraine Kelley, RN, MSN, BSHA/HIS
Faculty, Department of Nursing and Emergency Medical Services
Pensacola State College
Pensacola, Florida

Mischelle Monagle, RN, MSN, MBA
Dean of College of Nursing & Health Professions
Carl Sandburg College
Galesburg, Illinois

Victoria Plagenz, BSN, MSN, PhD
Associate Professor
University of Providence
Great Falls, Montana

Misty Stone, RN, MSN
Clinical Assistant Professor, Nursing
The University of North Carolina at Pembroke
Pembroke, North Carolina

Magan Swilley, RN, MSN
Associate of Science in Nursing Faculty
Regional Technical College
Thomasville, Georgia

Rebecca Toothaker, RN, MSN/Ed, PhD
Assistant Professor of Nursing
Bloomsburg University
Bloomsburg, Pennsylvania

LPN Advisory Board

Nancy Bohnarczyk, MA
Adjunct Instructor
College of Mount St. Vincent
New York, New York

Nicola Contreras, BN, RN
Faculty
Galen College
San Antonio, Texas

Dolores Cotton, MSN, RN
Practical Nursing Coordinator
Meridian Technology Center
Stillwater, Oklahoma

Patricia Donovan, MSN, RN
Director of Practical Nursing and Curriculum Chair
Porter and Chester Institute
Rocky Hill, Connecticut

Nancy Haughton, MSN, RN
Practical Nursing Program Faculty
Chester County Intermediate Unit
Downingtown, Pennsylvania

Dawn Johnson, DNP, RN, Ed
Practical Nurse Educator
Reno, Nevada

Mary E. Johnson, RN, MSN
Director of Nursing
Dorsey Schools
Roseville, Michigan

Bonnie Kehm, PhD, RN
Faculty Program Director
Excelsior College
Albany, New York

Tawnya S. Lawson, MS, RN
Dean, Practical Nursing Program
Hondros College
Westerville, Ohio

Kristin Madigan, MS, RN
Nursing Faculty
Pine Technical and Community College
Pine City, Minnesota

Hana Malik, DNP, FNP-BC
Academic Director
Illinois College of Nursing
Lombard, Illinois

Mary Lee Pollard, PhD, RN, CNE
Dean, School of Nursing
Excelsior College
Albany, New York

Barbara Ratliff, MSN, RN
Program Director, Practical Nursing
Cincinnati State
Cincinnati, Ohio

Mary Ruiz-Nuve, RN, MSN
Director of Practical Nursing Program
St. Louis College of Health Careers
St. Louis, Missouri

Renee Sheehan, RN, MSN/Ed
Director of Nursing, Vocational Nursing
Nursing Assistant Programs
Summit College
Colton, California

Faye Silverman, RN, MSN/ED, WOCN, PHN
Nursing Education Consultant
Online Nursing Instructor
Lancaster, California

Fleur de Liza S. Tobias-Cuyco, BSc, CPhT
Dean, Director of Student Affairs, and Instructor
Preferred College of Nursing
Los Angeles, California

To the Instructor

ABOUT THE TEXT

Medical-Surgical Nursing: Concepts and Practice is written specifically for the licensed practical/vocational nurse (LPN/LVN) student, who must be educated to work within various settings, including hospitals, long-term care facilities, rehabilitation institutes, ambulatory clinics, psychiatric agencies, health care providers' offices, and home care agencies. All of the most common adult medical-surgical disorders are covered, but particular attention is devoted to disorders most prevalent in our society. Special consideration is given to the older adult population, those with chronic illnesses, and others in long-term care settings.

This text builds on—but does not repeat—the concepts and skills presented in a fundamentals of nursing course. Many states are expanding LPN/LVN scope of practice, via certification, to include administration of intravenous (IV) fluids and medications, but others do not. Information on IV therapy is included within this text so that schools in states where such certification is possible will have the necessary educational materials.

With the expanding and changing role of the LPN/LVN there is an even greater need for **critical thinking** and the development of **clinical judgment.** These crucial skills are stressed throughout the clinical chapters and again in the *Study Guide.* **Evidence-based practice** is designated with a special icon so that students come to understand that the foundation of nursing care is in research. **Best practices** are highlighted throughout the narrative with an icon to emphasize cutting-edge information related to interventions.

The nursing process and its application to nursing care is an organizing principle throughout, and patients' needs are presented as the focus of nursing care. There is an emphasis on practical **assessment—including data collection**—to determine problems, monitor for the onset of complications, and evaluate the effectiveness of care. Data collection from the geriatric patient requires greater ability to elicit pertinent information from the patient and family, and the achievement of this skill is a major focus of this text. The text emphasizes the role of LPN/LVNs in data collection to assist the registered nurse (RN) in choosing appropriate **nursing diagnoses** or formulating problem statements for each patient. Many health care agencies are not using NANDA-I nursing diagnoses and are using problem statements instead. Agencies that use a collaborative care plan do not use nursing diagnoses at all. The NCLEX-PN® Examination no longer uses NANDA-I nursing diagnoses. For these reasons, this text provides problem statements on the inside back cover. NANDA-I nursing diagnoses are discussed but not listed in the text.

Planning holistic care must include consideration of the patient's cultural background and its impact on perception of health, illness, and health practices. **Implementation of nursing actions** is the heart of patient care and LPN/LVN practice. The nursing actions presented are specific, comprehensive, and organized by common care problems to decrease repetition of information within a chapter. This helps the student master concepts rather than memorize facts. The concepts covered are listed at the beginning of the chapter. Further interventions are discussed with each disorder as appropriate, and ***safe practice*** is emphasized throughout the text. Additional focal points are using **expected outcomes** and **evaluating** nursing care to ensure that those outcomes and goals have been met.

Patient teaching for health promotion and self-care is a basic function of the LPN/LVN. Each clinical chapter points out ways in which nurses can teach the public how to prevent many of the problems discussed.

LPN/LVN nurse practice acts do not encompass **delegation** as a function. With a few exceptions, only RNs can delegate, although in many situations LPN/LVNs can **assign** tasks. Collaboration with other health care workers and the use of basic management skills to provide coordinated, cost-effective patient care is essential. In this text we particularly speak to the LPN/LVN management role in working with nursing assistants and assigning tasks appropriately.

PEDAGOGICAL FEATURES

Special pedagogical features throughout the text help you teach your students to understand the chapter content and apply it in practice:

- The text has been thoroughly updated with the new **NCLEX-PN® Test Plan** in mind.
- Overreaching **concepts** that are addressed in the chapter are listed at the beginning of each chapter. These concepts help fit together ideas and information to aid in formation of a holistic understanding of the patient situation.
- Competencies identified through the **Quality and Safety Education for Nurses (QSEN) initiative**—and the associated knowledge, skills, and attitudes (KSAs)—have been integrated into the content and

were a continual focus during the writing of this text and its ancillaries.

- The Joint Commission's **National Patient Safety Goals** are highlighted to help students integrate safety measures and quality controls into their practice, and **Safety Alerts** remind students of specific safety concerns.
- The Joint Commission's **National Quality Core Measures** and the Institute for Healthcare Improvement's (IHI) **bundles** are described as additional measures for providing safe, effective, and quality care.
- The purpose of ***Healthy People 2030*** as a nationwide health improvement agenda is explained. Goals related to specific patient problems are available on the healthypeople.gov website. Other **Health Promotion** boxes throughout the text also emphasize the importance of health promotion, disease prevention, and reduction of health care costs.
- **Evidence-based practice** is designated with a special icon so that the student will see the thrust of nursing toward a foundation based in research.
- **Overview of Anatomy and Physiology** at the beginning of each system introduction chapter provides basic information for understanding the body system and its disorders. Normal physiologic changes associated with aging are presented for each body system.
- **The Nursing Process** provides a consistent framework for the disorders chapters.
- Separate **Theory** and **Clinical Practice objectives** highlight the chapter's main learning goals.
- **Concept Maps** found in disorders chapters are designed to help students visualize difficult material and to illustrate how a disorder's multiple symptoms, treatments, and side effects relate to each other.
- End-of-chapter **Review Questions for the NCLEX® Examination** include **multiple-choice and alternate-format questions,** and an extensive set of Interactive Review questions for the NCLEX® Examination is located on the Evolve website for students.
- The easily understandable **writing style** is aimed at gaining and retaining student attention to reading assignments.
- The term *patient* rather than *client* is used because that is the term still used in hospitals. *Resident* is used for those in long-term care facilities.
- A section in each chapter of the *Study Guide* has been designed to assist the student to more easily master the chapter content and to enhance English skills.
- **Bolded text** throughout the narrative emphasizes key concepts and practice.

ORGANIZATION OF THE TEXT

Unit I addresses medical-surgical nursing settings, nursing roles and issues, health care trends, assignment considerations, the nursing process, measures related to safe and effective care, and critical thinking. **Unit II** covers key medical-surgical nursing topics, including fluids and electrolytes, surgical patient care, infections, pain, cancer, and palliative care, and contains a separate chapter on chronic illness, rehabilitation, and the interdisciplinary health care team. **Units III through XIV** cover all of the body systems and their most common disorders, each unit beginning with a system overview, followed by specific disorders chapters. **Unit XV** addresses emergency and disaster management—including bioterrorism—as well as trauma and shock. **Unit XVI** is entirely devoted to mental health nursing and includes information on anxiety and mood disorders, eating disorders, cognitive disorders, thought and personality disorders, and substance use disorders.

Content on legal and ethical issues, nutrition considerations, care of the older adult, communication, cultural diversity, complementary and alternative therapies, patient teaching, home care, health promotion, and assignment and delegation has been integrated as appropriate rather than including individual chapters on these subjects. End-of-life issues and palliative care are presented at the end of Chapter 8: *Care of Patients With Cancer.* **Chronic illness** and **rehabilitation care** are growing areas, and Chapter 9 addresses the differences in care approaches and nursing care for these individuals as well as the interaction of the interdisciplinary health care team. Based on reviewer feedback, multiple sections of content have been resequenced to provide a better flow of information. Care of the LGBTQIA+ patient has been added to Chapter 38: *The Reproductive System.*

LPN THREADS

The fourth edition of *Medical-Surgical Nursing: Concepts and Practice* shares some features and design elements with other Elsevier LPN/LVN textbooks. The purpose of these *LPN Threads* is to make it easier for students and instructors to use the various books required by the relatively brief and demanding LPN/LVN curriculum. The following features are included in the *LPN Threads*.

- The **full-color design, cover, photos,** and **illustrations** are visually appealing and pedagogically useful.
- **Objectives** (numbered) begin each chapter, provide a framework for content, and are especially important in providing the structure for the TEACH Lesson Plans for the textbook.
- **Key Terms** with phonetic pronunciations and page number references are listed at the beginning of each chapter. Key terms appear in color in the chapter and are defined briefly, with full definitions in the **Glossary.** The goal is to help the student reader with limited proficiency in English to develop a greater command of the pronunciation of scientific and nonscientific English terminology.
- A wide variety of **special features** relate to critical thinking, clinical practice, health promotion, safety,

patient teaching, complementary and alternative therapies, communication, home health care, delegation and assignment, and more. The Student section of this introduction shows the icons used and descriptions of the features.

- **Critical Thinking Questions** presented at the end of each chapter and with Nursing Care Plans give students opportunities to practice critical thinking and clinical decision-making skills with realistic patient scenarios. Answers are provided in the Student Resources section on the Evolve website.
- **Key Points** at the end of each chapter correlate to the objectives and serve as a useful chapter review.
- A full suite of **Instructor Resources** is available, including TEACH Lesson Plans and Pre-Tests, PowerPoint Slides and Student Handouts, Test Bank, Image Collection, and the Answer Key to the *Study Guide*.
- In addition to consistent content, design, and support resources, these textbooks benefit from the advice and input of the **Elsevier LPN/LVN Advisory Board** (see p. viii)

FOR THE INSTRUCTOR

The comprehensive and free Evolve Instructor Resources with TEACH Instructor Resource include the following:

- **Test Bank** with approximately 1400 multiple-choice and alternate-format questions with correct answer, rationale, textbook page reference, topic, step of the nursing process, objective, cognitive level, and NCLEX® category of client needs
- **TEACH Instructor Resource** with Lesson Plans, Pre-Tests, PowerPoint Slides, and Student Handouts
- **Image Collection** that contains all illustrations and photographs in the textbook and some supplemental images
- **Answer Key** for the *Study Guide*
- **Suggestions for Working With English as a Second Language (ESL) Students**

FOR THE STUDENT

The Evolve Student Resources include the following assets:

- **Animations** depicting anatomy, physiology, and pathophysiology
- **Answers and Rationales** for end-of-chapter Review Questions for the NCLEX® Examination
- **Answer Guidelines** for Think Critically boxes, Nursing Care Plan Critical Thinking Questions, and the end-of-chapter Critical Thinking Questions
- **Audio Clips** of heart and lung sounds
- **Audio Glossary** with pronunciations in English and Spanish
- **Calculators** for determining body mass index (BMI), body surface area, fluid deficit, Glasgow Coma Scale score, IV dosages, and conversion of units
- **Clinical References,** including forms, checklists, and assessment tools
- **Fluids and Electrolytes Tutorial**
- **Helpful Phrases for Communicating in Spanish**
- **Interactive Review Questions for the NCLEX® Examination**
- **Video clips** of patient assessment

The ***Study Guide*** (sold separately) is a valuable supplement to help students understand and apply the textbook content. There is an emphasis on **priority setting and decision making** throughout the chapters. Varied question and activity types provide students with learning tools for reinforcement and exploration of text material. Terminology, short-answer, multiple-choice, and alternate-format Review Questions for the NCLEX® Examination; Critical Thinking Activities; and a special section called *Steps Toward Better Communication*—written by an ESL specialist—appear in most chapters. Other activity types include Completion, Identification, Review of Structure and Function, Priority Setting, and Application of Nursing Process. The *Study Guide* Answer Key is provided for instructors on the Evolve website.

To the Student

READING AND REVIEW TOOLS

- **Objectives** introduce the chapter topics.
- **Key Terms** are listed with page number references, and difficult medical, nursing, or scientific terms are accompanied by simple phonetic pronunciations. Key terms are considered essential to understanding chapter content and are defined within the chapter. Key terms are in color the first time they appear in the narrative and are briefly defined in the text, with complete definitions in the Glossary.
- Each chapter ends with a ***Get Ready for the NCLEX® Examination!* section,** which includes (1) **Key Points** that reiterate the chapter objectives and serve as a useful review of concepts; (2) a list of **Additional Resources,** including the *Study Guide* and Evolve Resources; (3) an extensive set of **Review Questions for the NCLEX® Examination,** with Answers and Rationales on Evolve; and (4) **Critical Thinking Questions,** with Answer Guidelines on Evolve.
- **References** in the back of the text cite evidence-based information. A **Bibliography** in the back of the text provides resources for enhancing knowledge.

CHAPTER FEATURES

Assignment Considerations address situations in which the RN delegates tasks to the LPN/LVN or when the LPN/LVN assigns tasks to nurse assistants as allowed by each state's nurse practice act.

Clinical Cues provide guidance and advice related to the application of nursing care.

Communication boxes provide guidance in therapeutic communication skills in realistic patient care situations.

Complementary and Alternative Therapies boxes contain information on how nontraditional treatments for medical-surgical conditions may be used to complement traditional treatment.

Cultural Considerations explore select specific cultural preferences and how to address the needs of culturally diverse patients and families.

Focused Assessment boxes are located in each body system overview chapter and include history taking and psychosocial assessment, physical assessment, and guidance on how to collect data and information for specific disorders.

Health Promotion boxes emphasize healthy lifestyle choices, preventive behaviors, and screening tests.

Home Care Considerations focus on postdischarge adaptations of medical-surgical nursing care to the home environment.

Legal and Ethical Considerations present pertinent information about the legal issues and ethical dilemmas that may face the practicing nurse.

Medication tables provide quick access to information about medications commonly used in medical-surgical nursing care.

Nursing Care Plans, developed around specific case studies, include nursing diagnoses with an emphasis on patient goals and outcomes and questions to promote **critical thinking.** Additional nursing care plans are available on the Evolve site.

Nutrition Considerations related to nursing care for specific disorders address the need for holistic care.

Older Adult Care Points address the unique medical-surgical care issues that affect older adults and provide suggestions for assessment (data collection) and particular interventions for the long-term and home care patient.

Patient Teaching boxes include step-by-step instructions and self-care guidelines.

Safety Alerts emphasize the importance of maintaining safety in patient care to protect patients, family, health care providers, and the public from accidents, spread of disease, and medication-related issues.

Think Critically boxes encourage students to synthesize information and apply concepts beyond the scope of the chapter.

Animations depicting anatomy, physiology, and pathophysiology and available on Evolve are referenced with icons in the margins where applicable.

Best Practice icons highlight current information related to interventions.

Evidence-Based Practice icons highlight current references to research in nursing and medical practice.

Video clips of patient assessment available on Evolve are referenced with icons in the margins where applicable.

Acknowledgments

This textbook would not exist without the efforts of Susan C. deWit, author, educator, and mentor. Her tenacity and insight developed the *Medical Surgical Textbook* as well as the *Fundamentals* text that have become a solid foundation for LPN/LVN nursing programs. Her vision and clarity in writing have been a pleasure to build on.

Multiple writers have been contributors to or coauthors of the previous three editions. Their foundational work is appreciated.

The work of the contributors and reviewers for this edition is also greatly appreciated. Their assistance has made this edition a better product than it would have been without their contributions.

In previous editions of the work, Thomas Sadowski has done a phenomenal job with the ESL review and suggestions. He also evaluated every chapter in the text and Study Guide and provided recommendations for making information more understandable for the ESL students. Likewise, Southwestern Washington Medical Center graciously allowed photography within their facility. Their patients, staff, and administration were so willing to help with whatever they could for the education of nursing students. Jack Sanders was a talented, creative, professional photographer whose beautiful photos continue to be seen throughout this book. Ginger Navarro was a wonderful and efficient photo coordinator and her help was invaluable.

Marian Regional Medical Center welcomed the use of their facility for real world photographs to help illustrate concepts and equipment in the 4th edition of the book. Their cooperation and collaboration are very much appreciated.

Thanks to the following people for their hard work and dedication to preparing a great ancillary package with the textbook. Thank you to Joanna Cain for revising the NCLEX review questions and to Tiffany Jakubowski for updating the Test Bank. Also, thanks to Sara Hardin, Content Development Specialst, for her work on the *Study Guide* and to Charla Hollin for the PowerPoints and TEACH materials.

Thank you to Susan Broadhurst for excellent copyediting and to the proofreaders that helped keep things consistent and correct. Thanks also to the behind-the-scenes people who keep things moving but never have their names appear in publications.

Thanks to Nancy O'Brien, Senior Content Strategist; Laura Selkirk, Senior Content Development Specialist; and Tracey Schriefer, Senior Project Manager at Elsevier, who have brought this project to fruition. Their dedication, professionalism, and collegiality have kept the project on track. Their continued encouragement, direction, and expertise have greatly improved the work. Thank you.

Teaching nursing has been one of the most exciting and gratifying phases of my career. I hope this textbook and its ancillaries make your job as an instructor easier and your class preparation more time efficient. May your students find excitement and joy in learning and applying the classroom knowledge to clinical practice, touching and changing lives.

Holly K. Stromberg

Contents

Caring for Medical-Surgical Patients

1

http://evolve.elsevier.com/deWit/medsurg

Objectives

Theory

1. Compare the roles and functions of the licensed practical/vocational nurse (LPN/LVN) with those of the registered nurse (RN).
2. Identify sites of employment for LPN/LVNs in medical-surgical nursing.
3. Correlate the nurse practice act (NPA) and the standards of practice for the LPN/LVN that guide the practice of each nurse.
4. Relate how Quality and Safety Education for Nurses (QSEN) applies to LPN/LVN practice.
5. Demonstrate knowledge of how evidence-based practice is formulated.
6. Explain the importance of National Patient Safety Goals and how they relate to patient safety.
7. Predict how *Healthy People 2030* can help decrease health care costs.
8. Determine how the current health care system attempts to provide health care for all.
9. Describe how hospitals are reimbursed under the diagnosis-related group (DRG) system of Medicare, including care excluded from reimbursement.

Clinical Practice

10. Demonstrate ways to provide holistic care.
11. Take part in delegation of tasks to unlicensed assistive personnel (UAP).

Key Terms

active listening (ĂK-tĭv LĬ-sĕn-ĭng, p. 2)
acuity (ă-KŪ-ĭ-tē, p. 4)
advocate (ĂD-vō-kăt, p. 2)
capitation (kă-pĭ-TĀ-shŭn, p. 9)
coinsurance (kō-ĭn-SHŪ-rĕnz, p. 7)
complementary and alternative medicine (CAM) (KŎM-plĕ-MĔN-tĕ-rē ănd ăl-TŬR-nă-tĭv MĔD-ĭ-sĭn, p. 6)
copayment (kō-PĀY-mĕnt, p. 7)
cost containment (kŏst kŏn-TĀN-mĕnt, p. 7)
deductible (dē-DŬK-tĭ-bŭl, p. 7)
delegation (DĔL-ĭ-GĀ-shŭn, p. 3)
dependent (dĕ-PĔN-dĕnt, p. 10)
diagnosis-related groups (DRGs) (dī-ăg-NŌ-sĭs rē-LĀ-tĕd grūpz, p. 8)
empathy (ĔM-pă-thē, p. 10)
fee-for-service (fē fŏr SĔR-vĭs, p. 7)
health maintenance organizations (HMOs) (hĕlth MĀN-tĕ-nĕnz ōr-gă-nĭ-ZĀ-shŭnz, p. 9)
Healthy People 2030 (HĔLTH-ē PĒ-pl, p. 7)
holistic care (hō-LĬS-tĭk kār, p. 6)
managed care (MĂN-ăjd kār, p. 7)
Medicaid (mĕd-ĭ-KĀD, p. 7)
Medicare (mĕd-ĭ-KĀR, p. 7)
nonjudgmental (NŎN-jŭj-MĔN-tăl, p. 11)
nurse practice acts (NPAs) (nŭrz PRĂK-tĭs ăkts, p. 3)
preferred provider organizations (PPOs) (prĕ-FŬRD prō-vī-dĕr ōr-gă-nĭ-ZĀ-shŭnz, p. 9)
prospective payment system (PPS) (prŏs-PĔK-tĭv pā-mĕnt sĭs-tĕm, p. 8)
provider (prō-VĪ-dĕr, p. 2)
stereotypes (STĔR-ē-ō-tīps, p. 11)
unlicensed assistive personnel (UAP) (un-LĪ-sĕnst ă-SĬS-tĭv pĕr-sŏ-NĔL, p. 3)

Concepts Covered in This Chapter

- Professional Identity
- Safety
- Health Care Quality
- Health Care Economics
- Health Care Law
- Communication
- Culture
- Spirituality

CARING FOR MEDICAL-SURGICAL PATIENTS

Licensed practical/vocational nurses (LPN/LVNs), along with other health care team members, promote and maintain health, prevent disease and disability, care for individuals during rehabilitation, and assist dying patients to maintain the best quality of life possible. Patients can have a single diagnosis of a medical or surgical condition or a combination of medical and/or surgical diagnoses (comorbidity). The nursing process is used to plan and deliver safe, competent care to patients (or clients). LPN/LVNs carry out prescribed therapeutic regimens and protocols by acting in various roles.

ROLES OF THE LPN/LVN

Today you have an exciting, evolving role as an LPN/LVN. Roles include caregiver, educator, collaborator, **advocate**, leader, and delegator. As a caregiver, you perform treatments, give medications, and provide care to meet patients' basic needs. You gather data to assist in planning and evaluating care. You assist patients with exercise and help them obtain sufficient rest, all while keeping their environment neat, clean, and orderly. Therapeutic communication and **active listening** (listening with concentration and focused energy) are incorporated into your care. You give objective and thorough end-of-shift reports and document objectively about the care given and the status of patients.

Clinical Cues

If a patient declines morning care (bath, brushing teeth, etc.), you can be flexible and fit it in elsewhere in your day, as time allows. Leaving care to be performed by the next shift is not acceptable practice because it burdens the oncoming staff. Listen to the patient's reasons for not wanting care. If it appears that care really is being refused for a complete day, talk with the staff nurse or charge nurse about it. Although the patient does have the right to refuse care, you can often gain the patient's cooperation if the benefits of care are explained. Conferring with more experienced team members can help a new nurse determine when the routine can be altered in the patient's best interests.

As an educator, you provide health teaching to patients and their significant others to maintain wellness or promote healing. An important aspect of nursing care is to show patients and families how to care for themselves or for loved ones to prevent complications, restore health, and prevent further illness. You teach basic hygiene and nutrition to promote good health. Examples of teaching include reinforcing what the registered nurse (RN) or **provider** advises regarding scheduled diagnostic tests, upcoming surgery, how to treat a wound, or how to change a dressing, while also addressing the patient's questions and concerns. Other teaching activities concern how to take prescribed medication, what side effects to report, and the self-care activities and lifestyle changes required to promote rehabilitation and independence. You contribute to the discharge plan by reinforcing discharge instructions and providing information to patients about community resources and self-help groups.

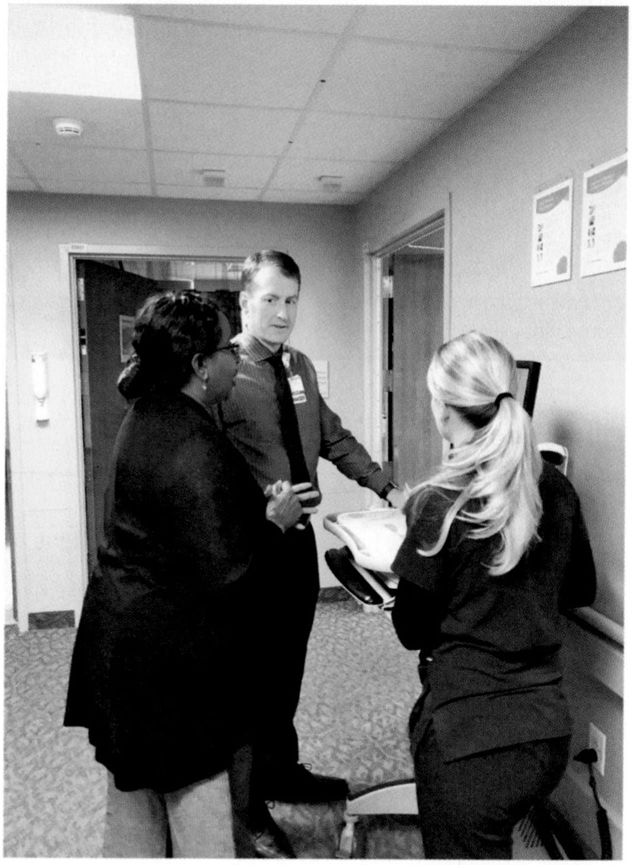

Fig. 1.1 A nurse, social worker, and nurse manager collaborate on finding resources for a patient.

Think Critically

How could you reinforce dietary teaching for a patient newly diagnosed with diabetes?

As a collaborator, you interact with other members of the health care team to provide the patient with an integrated, comprehensive plan of care (Fig. 1.1). You work closely with the RNs and nursing assistants to ensure that all aspects of the patient's basic needs are met. When you share information with the team members, the team can best use the expertise and experience of the various team members. You assist in recognizing when a patient is experiencing complications and intervene to maintain patient safety. You assist with the discharge plan and deliver discharge instructions and teaching.

Facility and unit routine can lead to an impersonal health care system that loses its focus on patients' rights. The American Hospital Association (AHA) published *The Patient Care Partnership: Understanding Expectations, Rights and Responsibilities* in 2003, and this is still the document in use. As an advocate, you stand up for patients' rights and ensure that their needs are met. Advocating for a patient could be as simple as arranging for special food or meals at times other than those within the facility's routine, or it may entail informing the health care provider of a patient concern.

Think Critically

Can you think of other situations in which you might be an advocate for your patient?

The most common leadership role for the LPN/LVN is in a long-term care facility (nursing home). In this setting, the LPN/LVN commonly assumes the role of charge nurse. Many **nurse practice acts (NPAs)** specifically state that the LPN/LVN charge nurse in a nursing home functions under the general supervision of an RN, who is either on site or available by phone.

Think Critically

What (if any) restrictions does your state's NPA place on the charge nurse position?

As a leader and delegator, you must know when and which tasks to delegate and which to assign to nursing assistants when acting as the charge nurse (Fig. 1.2). The charge nurse assigns tasks within the job description and capability of **unlicensed assistive personnel (UAP)** to distribute the workload among available staff. To **delegate** is to transfer authority. In the LPN/LVN leadership context, **delegation** involves transferring to qualified UAP the responsibility to perform a selected nursing task or activity in a selected patient situation that is within the job description of the one delegating. You must be knowledgeable about the skills and judgment capabilities of those to whom you delegate. Not all state NPAs include delegation of nursing tasks or activities as an LPN/LVN role, and state NPAs vary greatly on protocol for delegation (Box 1.1). Appropriate tasks to delegate include the following:

- Those that frequently reoccur in the daily care of patients
- Those that do not require the UAP to exercise nursing judgment

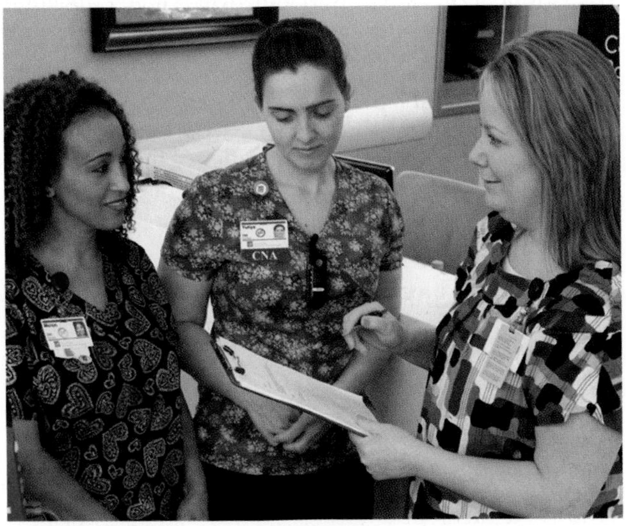

Fig. 1.2 A charge nurse is assigning tasks to nursing assistants.

- Those that do not require complex application of the nursing process
- Those for which results are predictable and potential risk is minimal
- Those for which a standard procedure is to be used

Clinical Cues

The LPN/LVN always works under the supervision of an RN or a licensed health care provider.

Because a patient's condition can change so rapidly, judgment must be developed through experience as to what and when it is wise to delegate. The position paper of the National Council of State Boards of Nursing (NCSBN), originally published in 2006 and updated in 2016, titled *ANA and NCSBN Joint Statement on Delegation* provides a decision-making algorithm to be used by licensed individuals in clinical settings as a guide for delegating nursing duties. The position statement identifies "Five Rights" to ensure when delegating:

1. **Right Task:** The task can legally be delegated for a specific patient.
2. **Right Circumstances:** The patient is stable, independent nursing judgment is not required for the task, and resources to perform the task are available.

Box 1.1 Comparison of Assigning and Delegating by the LPN/LVN Charge Nurse

Ask yourself the following questions:

1. Are the tasks or activities within a nursing assistant's job description?
   - **When assigning:** Yes.
   - **When delegating:** No. The tasks or activities delegated are in the job description of the LPN/LVN. Specific tasks and activities are not listed. Permitted delegated tasks or activities depend on the NPA, patient situation, and documented expertise of the nursing assistant.
2. May the nursing assistant refuse the nursing task or activity?
   - **When assigning:** No, unless staff person thinks they are unqualified for the task or activity assignment.
   - **When delegating:** Yes. In addition, the nursing assistant must voluntarily accept the task or activity.
3. Who holds accountability for the nursing task or activity?
   - **When assigning:** The nursing assistant is accountable for completing the task or activity and doing so in a safe manner.
   - **When delegating:** The LPN/LVN is accountable for delegating the right task or activity to the right person.

Adapted from Knecht P: *Success in practical/vocational nursing: from student to leader,* ed 8, Philadelphia, 2017, Elsevier.

3. **Right Person:** The person asked to perform the task is competent and qualified to do so.
4. **Right Direction and Communication:** The objective and specifically what should be done and when, what to report to the delegating nurse, and when to make the report are explained.
5. **Right Supervision and Evaluation:** The delegating nurse needs to monitor the performance of the task, to intervene when needed, to evaluate the results of the task, to ensure proper documentation, and to provide feedback to the unlicensed person.

Working with others in this supervisory capacity requires tact and effective communication skills. Therapeutic communication should be used when communicating with staff, especially when making requests. Address staff by name to gain their attention and explain the purpose of the communication. Explain the requirements of a request and offer a timeline for completion. Obtain feedback that the request was understood and again when it is carried out, and express appreciation for cooperation and the work completed. You are responsible for care given by others to whom you have delegated. Tasks assigned must be verified to have been completed and to have been accomplished properly, and the care given must be documented.

? Think Critically

What is your role as a member of the team when in the clinical area? List three examples. To whom on staff do you communicate the care you give? To whom do you go with questions? What is your instructor's role?

EMPLOYMENT OPPORTUNITIES

In today's medical atmosphere, hospital care involves high-**acuity** patients (very ill patients with complex needs) who require a high level of nursing care. Hospitals are using more and more RNs because of the complexity of care. Employment opportunities for LPN/LVNs vary considerably geographically, but most graduates of practical/vocational nursing programs are employed in long-term care, extended care, or community-based settings. Some sites of employment are listed in Box 1.2.

? Think Critically

What are the current medical-surgical opportunities for employment where you live? List two agencies you can contact for this information.

Box 1.2 Sites of Possible Employment for LPN/LVNs

AREAS WITHIN A HOSPITAL
- General patient units
- Outpatient surgery
- Intermediate care unit (step-down unit)
- Intravenous (IV) therapy team[a]
- Emergency department

ADDITIONAL SITES FOR EMPLOYMENT OPPORTUNITIES
- Long-term care facility (nursing home)
- Ambulatory care (clinics and health care provider offices)
- Rehabilitation services (extended care, postacute care, subacute care)
- Hospice care
- Adult group homes
- Assisted living facilities
- Homes for individuals with developmental disabilities
- Home health care
- Hospice care agency
- Military service
- Jails and prisons

[a]Requires postgraduate education and certification.

ETHICAL AND LEGAL PRACTICE

Each state's NPA defines the role and scope of practice of LPN/LVNs. It is always your responsibility to be aware of the scope of the practice act of the state in which you are employed. Ethical practice means that the LPN/LVN abides by the *Code for Nurses* learned in the Fundamentals of Nursing course, adheres to the National Patient Safety Goals, and honors privacy according to the Health Insurance Portability and Accountability Act (HIPAA). National Patient Safety Goals evolve from year to year (Table 1.1).

? Think Critically

Nurse practice acts vary considerably from state to state. Where can you obtain a copy of your state's NPA?

Follow your institution's guidelines and policies. The facility might more strictly limit the LPN/LVN's role than does the state's NPA, but **no employer can give nurses permission to do more than their license allows.** The National Association for Practical Nurse Education and Service (NAPNES) and the National Federation of Licensed Practical Nurses (NFLPN) are practical/vocational nursing organizations that provide standards to guide the role of the LPN/LVN. These standards of practice echo the values and priorities of the profession, provide guidelines for safe and competent nursing care, and may also be used as legal standards in court.

QUALITY AND SAFETY

In *Health Professions Education: A Bridge to Quality,* the Institute of Medicine (IOM, 2003) identified the following five competencies:

1. Provide patient-centered care.
2. Collaborate with the interdisciplinary health care team.
3. Implement evidence-based practice.

4. Use quality improvement in patient care.
5. Use informatics in patient care.

Multiple interdisciplinary agencies published *Core Competencies for Interprofessional Collaborative Practice* (Interprofessional Education Collaborative Expert Panel, 2011), which further developed these five competencies. The Leapfrog Hospital Safety Grade (2017) organization states, "As many as 440,000 people die every year from hospital errors, injuries, accidents and infections."

Table 1.1 **National Patient Safety Goals 2019 (Hospital)**

Identify patients correctly	Use two ways to identify patients. This is done to ensure that each patient gets the correct medication or treatment. Make sure that the correct patient gets the correct blood when they get a blood transfusion.
Improve staff communication	Get important test results and data to the right staff person in a timely manner.
Use medicines safely	Before a procedure, label medicines that are not labeled. Do this in the area where medicines and supplies are set up. Be very careful with anticoagulant medications. Do a medication reconciliation for each patient as they are admitted, after surgery, and when being discharged. Explain to the patient the importance of taking a medication list to each health care provider visit.
Use alarms safely	Ensure that alarms on medical equipment are heard and responded to on time.
Prevent infection	Use hand-cleaning guidelines from the Centers for Disease Control and Prevention (CDC) or the World Health Organization (WHO). Use proven guidelines to prevent infections that are difficult to treat, of the blood from central lines, after surgery, and of the urinary tract caused by catheters.
Identify patient safety risks	Identify patients at risk for suicide. Applies to nonpsychiatric settings in the patient population being treated for emotional or behavioral disorders.
Prevent mistakes in surgery	Make certain that the correct surgery is done on the correct patient and at the correct site on the patient's body. Mark the correct place where surgery is to be done. Pause before the surgery to make certain that a mistake is not being made.

The Quality and Safety Education for Nurses (QSEN) initiative added *safety* as a separate competency to the IOM set. Specific knowledge, skills, and attitudes have been identified to assist with the development of the competencies incorporated into nursing curriculum.

Patient-centered care means that the patient is a full partner in decisions about their care. Compassionate and coordinated care should be planned and delivered with respect and consideration for the patient's preferences, values, and needs. Collaboration with the interdisciplinary (ID) team requires open communication, mutual respect, and shared decision making. An important member of the ID team is the care manager, who may be a designated nurse or a social worker within the hospital. The case manager strives to work with the ID team to provide quality and cost-effective services and resources so that positive patient outcomes are achieved.

EVIDENCE-BASED PRACTICE (EBP)

Evidence-based practice uses the best current evidence from research findings to make decisions about patient care. Evidence data are drawn from quality improvement (QI) practices, management initiatives such as those from The Joint Commission (TJC), and professional organization standards. Formulation of guidelines involves reviewing current research (evidence), testing the findings in clinical settings, distributing the guidelines, and then keeping them current. Nurses are expected to provide care based on scientific studies to ensure best practice. Nurses must continually seek scientific evidence that supports best patient outcomes.

QUALITY IMPROVEMENT

Nurses use data from completed interventions to monitor the outcomes of the care delivered by various processes and then use the resulting data to design methods of quality improvement. Each accredited health care agency has a QI program in place that sets standards for care (Fig. 1.3). These standards are based on standards for nursing practice set by the American Nurses Association, the AHA, and TJC. Various models may be used for monitoring and improving quality, including total quality management (TQM), continuous quality improvement (CQI), and Focus, Analyze, Develop, Execute (FADE). Nursing units may have a QI committee or delegate nursing staff to do periodic audits of charts to determine whether standards of care are being upheld and to what extent compliance is occurring. The goal is to find discrepancies and continually improve the safety and quality of patient care systems (QSEN Competencies, 2018). Medical-surgical nurses are expected to do the following:

- Identify indicators to monitor the quality and effectiveness of care delivered.
- Gather and evaluate data to monitor the effectiveness of care.

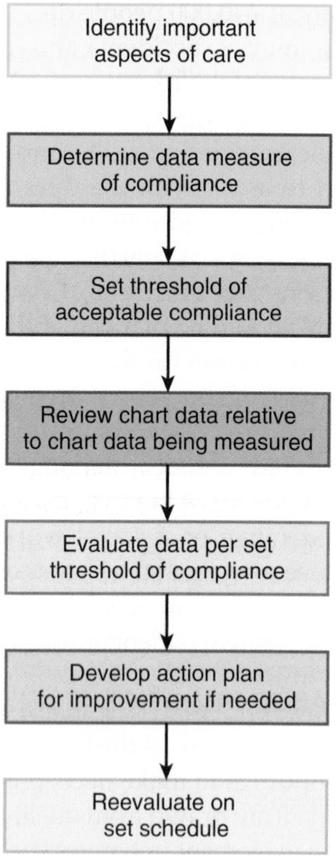

Fig. 1.3 Continuous quality improvement process.

- Recommend ways to improve care.
- Implement activities to improve care.

INFORMATICS

Using information and technology to communicate, manage knowledge, prevent or mitigate error, and support decision making comprises informatics (QSEN Competencies, 2018). The key components of informatics are communication, documentation, electronic data access, and data use. The electronic health record (EHR), or electronic medical record (EMR), is at the heart of informatics. The EHR is central to documenting nursing and interdisciplinary care and patient health data.

Central hospital or agency computers store all data and connect to the internet to allow searches for information on disease processes, medications, diagnostic tests, current care guidelines, and evidence-based practice research. Mobile devices are also used by health care professionals for data access and team communication through text or email. Many health professionals use tablets or smartphones to access data and to communicate with other team members. Devices used for communication of patient information must be approved by the facility to ensure secure data transfer.

SAFETY

Every nurse should consider safety during every patient interaction. Patients are vulnerable to injury when they are ill or incapacitated in the hospital. The NCSBN has identified areas in which nursing practice can improve safety. Clear communication of patient data and clinical assessments is one area. Using the SBAR (Situation, Background, Assessment, and Recommendation) technique when communicating with other members of the team is one way to promote clarity and safety. The Joint Commission has several suggested techniques to improve hand-off communication, which has been identified as a major point of miscommunication that may result in harm to the patient (TJC, 2017).

Be attentive to the National Patient Safety Goals (see Table 1.1). It is vital that you prepare medications in a quiet atmosphere and use the Six Rights of Medication Administration and nursing responsibilities when administering medications to patients. You must know the purpose, action, side effects, and nursing implications of each medication to be given. Evaluation of the medication's effect is often given insufficient attention. Always check orders carefully before performing a procedure. To ensure patient safety as well as your own, rigorously adhere to infection control guidelines at all times and use proper equipment and methods to lift and turn patients to avoid injuries. Always check electrical equipment before use. Report unsafe practices and self-report errors to promote a safer environment. Follow core measures that are in place to prevent infection to promote better patient outcomes.

HEALTH CARE TODAY

BIOMEDICINE

Biomedicine is the dominant health system in the United States and focuses on symptoms. The goal of biomedicine is to find the cause of disease and to eliminate or correct the problem; it does not emphasize prevention. However, many Americans use methods that focus on the whole body—and not exclusively on symptoms—when treating disease. Holistic medicine, or **holistic care**, incorporates a variety of measures and techniques to treat the whole person including the mind, not just the body.

COMPLEMENTARY AND ALTERNATIVE MEDICINE (CAM)

Complementary (used in conjunction with biomedical treatments) **and alternative** (substituted for biomedical medicine) **medicine (CAM)** focuses on assisting the body's own healing powers and restoring body balance. The National Center for Complementary and Integrative Health (NCCIH) of the National Institutes of Health (NIH) researches and evaluates the effectiveness and safety of CAM therapies. Natural medicines often have not undergone scientific studies to determine correct doses, side effects, or risk of interactions with other medicines or foods. Patients need to be reminded that all herbals and supplements need to be included when they are asked for a list of drugs taken.

HEALTHY PEOPLE 2030

Healthy People 2030 is a health promotion and disease prevention initiative by the U.S. Department of Health and Human Services (HHS) aimed at improving the health of people in the United States by promoting longer, healthier lives. The four overarching goals are as follows:

1. Attain high-quality, longer lives free of preventable disease, disability, injury, and premature death.
2. Achieve health equity, eliminate disparities, and improve the health of all groups.
3. Create social and physical environments that promote good health for all.
4. Promote quality of life, healthy development, and healthy behaviors across all life stages.

Individuals, groups, and organizations must work together to incorporate the goals of *Healthy People 2030* into current programs, education, special events, publications, and meetings. Every LPN/LVN has the responsibility to educate patients about healthy lifestyles and to work with their communities through education for health promotion. You can also model healthier lifestyles for your patients by not smoking, maintaining healthy eating habits, and exercising.

FINANCING OF HEALTH CARE

HEALTH INSURANCE: GOVERNMENT AND PRIVATE FUNDING

It is helpful to understand a little about payment methods because it is important to keep **cost containment** in mind when delivering nursing care. Health insurance, like any type of insurance, spreads risk among a group of insured individuals. The young and the healthy generally do not have claims for as many health care services as older adults. When the fee structure is equivalent for all, the young and healthy subsidize (support) the sick and older people covered by the insurance provider. Most full-time employees can obtain private health insurance through their employers. People of working age who are healthy enough to continue full-time employment are not the biggest consumers of health care dollars. Retirees with chronic health problems and younger people not able to work traditionally had difficulty obtaining health insurance, so in 1965 Medicare and Medicaid were created by the federal government to cover the needs of these groups. Today, Medicare and Medicaid fund the care for 58% of hospitalized patients.

At the time of this writing, the federal government is again making changes to the health care financing laws and options.

The traditional method of financing health care services, **fee-for-service**, involves direct reimbursement by an insurance company to a provider (a licensed health care professional such as a health care provider, dentist, or nurse practitioner) whose health care services are covered by a health insurance plan. To improve coverage of costs, insurance providers charge a **deductible** (the yearly amount an insured person must spend out-of-pocket for health care services *before* the insurance provider will begin to pay for services), a **copayment** (the amount an insured person must pay at the time of an office visit, for a prescription, or for hospital service), and **coinsurance** (once a deductible is met, the percentage of the total bill the insured person must pay). The insurance company subtracts the amount the patient must pay from the total bill and then pays the remainder to the provider.

Medicare is a federal public insurance program that helps to partially finance health care for everyone older than 65 years (and their spouses) who have at least a 10-year (40 quarters) record in Medicare-covered employment and who are citizens or permanent residents of the United States. Coverage is also given to people younger than 65 years who have end-stage renal disease or are permanently and totally disabled. Those eligible because of age or disability are entitled, by law, to the benefits of Medicare programs. In November 2003, Congress passed the Medicare Prescription Drug, Improvement, and Modernization Act, the largest expansion of Medicare since it was enacted in 1965 (Box 1.3). Medicare A covers hospital and durable medical equipment expenses. Part B of Medicare covers out-of-hospital expenses. Medicare Part C involves **managed care** providers. Part D is the Medicare drug program that covers a portion of prescription expenses. There are monthly premiums for Parts B, C, and D, as well as deductibles and copayment amounts. Many patients with Medicare purchase a private supplemental health insurance policy to help pay for expenses not covered by Medicare.

The **Medicaid** program, which is funded jointly by the federal and state governments, provides medical assistance for eligible families and individuals with low incomes and few resources. Each state establishes its own program services and requirements, including eligibility. Proportionally, Medicaid is the second largest item in state budgets (Box 1.4). The program is meant to cover the population of people considered to be living under the federal poverty level (FPL). Many people just above the FPL are working families who do not have insurance.

The federal government has been attempting to set up a system of insurance that will allow health care coverage for all. The role of the government in health care and the components of the plan have been the topics of much discussion and disagreement. The Affordable Care Act (ACA) was implemented in 2010 by the Obama administration, and the American Health Care Act (AHCA) was proposed by the Trump administration in 2017, passing in the House but not the Senate. The goal is to have a mechanism for affordable insurance for those not covered by employers or not able to purchase private insurance due to health circumstances or income. The HHS has identified multiple strategic goals, the first being to strengthen health care (Box 1.5).

Box 1.3 Basic Components of Medicare

MEDICARE PART A
- Is available without cost to those eligible for the program.
- Helps pay for inpatient hospital care, including drugs, supplies, laboratory tests, radiology, and the intensive care unit.
- Covers 20 days after hospitalization at a skilled nursing facility for rehabilitation services, home health care services under certain conditions, and hospice care.
- Does not pay for nursing home custodial services (e.g., patients needing help only with activities of daily living or feeding), private rooms, telephones, or televisions provided by hospitals or skilled nursing facilities.

MEDICARE PART B
- Is similar to a major medical insurance plan and is funded by monthly premiums based on income.
- Requires a deductible and pays 80% of most covered charges. The remaining 20% of charges are the patient's responsibility.
- Helps pay for medically necessary providers' services; outpatient hospital services (including emergency department visits); ambulance transportation; diagnostic tests, including laboratory services and mammography and Pap smear screenings; and physical therapy, occupational therapy, and speech therapy in a hospital outpatient department or Medicare-certified rehabilitation agency.
- Does not pay for most prescription drugs, routine physicals, services not related to treatment of illness or injury, dental care, dentures, cosmetic surgery, routine foot care, hearing aids, eye examinations, or glasses.

MEDICARE PART C
- Refers to Medicare Advantage plans, such as HMOs or regional PPOs.
- Provides Parts A, B, and D benefits to people who elect this type of coverage instead of the original fee-for-service program.

MEDICARE PART D
- Refers to the outpatient prescription drug benefit.
- Is available to all Medicare enrollees in the original fee-for-service program for an additional monthly fee.

Box 1.4 The Medicaid Program

- Medicaid is the second largest item in state budgets and covers more than 50 million low-income children and individuals, many in working families.
- Medicaid is the largest source of health insurance for children in the United States. The Children's Health Insurance Program (CHIP) supplements Medicaid in some states by providing coverage for children from lower income families who do not qualify for Medicaid.
- Medicaid is the primary source of health and long-term care coverage for low-income individuals with disabilities or chronic illnesses and those who need mental health services and substance abuse treatment.
- Medicaid covers services that Medicare does not cover for low-income Medicare beneficiaries, including long-term care and vision and dental care. Medicare beneficiaries who are also enrolled in Medicaid are known as *dual eligibles*.

Box 1.5 HHS Strategic Goal: Strengthen Health Care

- Make coverage more secure for those who have insurance, and extend affordable coverage to the uninsured.
- Improve health care quality and patient safety.
- Emphasize primary and preventive care, linked with community prevention services.
- Reduce the growth of health care costs while promoting high-value, effective care.
- Ensure access to quality, culturally competent care, including long-term services and supports, for vulnerable populations.
- Improve health care and population health through meaningful use of health information technology.

COST CONTAINMENT

The driving force today in all health care facilities is cost containment (holding costs to within fixed limits while remaining competitive in the health care marketplace). Health care agencies are interested in improving their "bottom line" with business principles that reduce waste and inefficiency. Consumers want the cost of health care to be reduced while high-quality care and service are maintained. Service, quality, and cost control are attributes of health care that need to be understood and considered in all clinical situations (Box 1.6).

The federal government was the first group to try to stop the skyrocketing cost of health care. In 1983 the Health Care Financing Administration (now the Centers for Medicare and Medicaid Services [CMS]) adopted a system called **diagnosis-related groups (DRGs)**, or illness groups. This system pays hospitals a flat rate for Medicare services, and hospitals know in advance how much they will be reimbursed by this **prospective payment system (PPS)**. Under the DRG system, the fee the government will pay for hospitalization depends on the DRG category (illness). Hospitals receive a flat fee for each patient's DRG category, **regardless of length of stay in the hospital;** thus hospitals have an incentive to treat patients and discharge them as quickly as possible. If the hospital keeps the patient longer than the government's fee will cover, and the patient cannot be reclassified in the DRG system, the hospital must absorb the difference in costs. However, if the acute care facility can treat the patient for less than the guaranteed reimbursement amount, **the facility can keep the difference in payment as profit.** Because Medicare patients, like all patients, are discharged sooner from hospitals than

Box 1.6 LPN/LVN Role in Containing Health Care Costs in the Work Setting

1. Only take linens and supplies that will be used immediately into the patient's room. Supplies not used for the patient must be put in the trash and unused linens must be rewashed.
2. Follow facility policy for documenting all patient care for reimbursement.
3. Organize patient care for effective and efficient use of time. It is less expensive to do something right the first time.
4. Implement nursing care to help prevent complications and catch signs of complications.

Box 1.7 Health Care–Associated Conditions Not Paid for by Medicare or Medicaid

The conditions listed are those that are acquired during hospitalization and considered preventable.

- Foreign object left in the patient after surgery
- Air embolism
- Blood incompatibility
- Stages III and IV pressure ulcers
- Falls and trauma (fractures, dislocations, intracranial injuries, crushing injuries, burns, electrical shocks)
- Poor glycemic control (diabetic ketoacidosis, hyperosmolar hyperglycemic state, hypoglycemic coma, secondary diabetes with ketoacidosis, secondary diabetes with hyperosmolarity)
- Catheter-related urinary tract infection
- Vascular catheter–associated infection
- Surgical site infection after coronary artery bypass graft, particularly mediastinitis (infection in the chest), or after bariatric surgery, gastroenterostomy, laparoscopic gastric restrictive surgery, or orthopedic procedures
- Deep vein thrombosis or pulmonary embolism after total knee replacement or hip replacement
- Surgical site infection after cardiac implantable electronic device insertion
- Iatrogenic pneumothorax with venous catheterization

Data from Centers for Medicare and Medicaid Services (CMS): Medicare program: general information, 2018. Retrieved from http://www.cms.gov/Medicare/Medicare-General-Information/MedicareGenInfo/index.html.

they were in the past, extended care units or skilled care facilities and home care are commonly used to continue convalescence. With the goal of improving quality of care and saving millions of taxpayer dollars each year, Medicare will not cover specific *preventable* conditions of hospitalized patients (Box 1.7). To prevent premature discharge, Medicare will either not cover the hospitalization or levy a fine if readmission occurs within a defined period.

When Medicare and Medicaid adopted DRGs, the private insurance companies followed their lead. The organization that is the largest health care insurance system thereby provides the most funding to health care providers and sets the standards for reimbursement. Guidelines and methods used by Medicare and Medicaid have become the standard for insurance payment to health care facilities and providers.

? Think Critically

Should Medicare pay for new, expensive technological procedures developed to treat common medical problems of older adults? Should cost-effectiveness be a factor in treating Medicare patients? Explain the reasoning behind your answer.

Another measure aimed at cost containment is **capitation**, an alternative to fee-for-service payment. It involves a set monthly fee charged by the provider of health care services for each member of the insurance group for a specific set of health care services. If services cost more than the monthly fee, the provider absorbs the cost of those services. At the end of the year, if any money is left over from the unused portions of monthly fees, the health care provider keeps this remainder as a profit.

Managed care is a type of group health insurance developed to provide quality health care with cost and care use controls. This is accomplished by paying providers to care for groups of patients for a set capitation fee and by limiting services. Medical necessity and the appropriateness of health care services are monitored by a use review system. Types of managed care systems include **health maintenance organizations (HMOs)** and **preferred provider organizations (PPOs)**. This option is used by both Medicare and private insurance companies.

PROVIDING HOLISTIC CARE

Holistic nursing care involves being aware of and attending to the physiologic, psychological, social, cultural, and spiritual needs of patients. Data for many of these needs can be collected and interventions carried out while care and treatments are administered. Assisting with bathing, feeding, ambulating, and other physical care provides an opportunity to find out about dimensions of the patient's life beyond physical problems. Use time with the patient constructively. Data gathering guidelines are presented in Chapter 2.

PROMOTING A THERAPEUTIC NURSE-PATIENT RELATIONSHIP

The focus of the nurse-patient relationship is on the patient's problems and needs. The relationship is therapeutic because it provides the patient with the help needed for healing or for a return to wellness. In comparison, a social relationship lacks goals, exists primarily for pleasure, and meets the needs of each person in the relationship. You need to maintain a therapeutic relationship when working with patients and avoid using patient contact to meet personal needs (e.g., the need to be liked, for friendship, or for approval).

Develop awareness of your own personal needs and separate them from the patient's needs. A therapeutic nurse-patient relationship ends when the patient has completed treatment or therapy.

A patient who is physically ill is also affected emotionally by the illness or injury. It is not unusual for patients to display behavior that is not their usual manner. Patients' emotional needs and the resulting behaviors are usually temporary and related to the stresses of illness. Occasionally patient behavior is related to underlying disorders that will benefit from a psychiatric consultation or treatment (see Chapters 46 to 49). Even patients whose primary illness is physical rather than psychological can sometimes express emotional discomfort through **dependent** (inability or unwillingness to do tasks for oneself), withdrawn, hostile, or manipulative behavior. They may act in ways that are confusing and uncomfortable for a nurse who is not prepared to act therapeutically. It is important to not take statements or behaviors personally but to objectively consider why the patient may be responding in this manner (see the Evolve website for Nursing Interventions for Patients with Difficult Behaviors). It is particularly important to note if this is a change in behavior and may signal a change in condition.

It is easier to deal with patients' behavior if their responses to particular situations are understood. Your task is to recognize that patients' behavior results from their current situation. Appropriate nursing responses require kindness, understanding, and sometimes firmness. People may become childlike and fearful when they are ill, or they may act as if they are unaffected by their illness. Patients appreciate having someone available to guide them through their ordeal in a therapeutic manner.

> **? Think Critically**
>
> When assigned to a patient recuperating from major surgery who is displaying very dependent behavior, how can you help promote a return to independence?

Inability to assume personal responsibilities can be a source of worry for patients and may interfere with a positive outcome after illness or surgery. Some patients are caring for aging parents; are grandparents who play an active, daily role in caring for grandchildren; or are single parents with young children. If a patient lives alone, pet care may be a concern. Patients who are employed may have used up available sick leave, may not have health insurance, or may have a high insurance deductible that is a concern. Patients enrolled in an educational program might be concerned about having to drop a course or leave a program because of time lost to hospitalization, diagnostic tests, or restrictions such as not being able to drive. Conversing with these patients in a therapeutic manner may help them identify their concerns and begin problem solving.

> **? Think Critically**
>
> What effect would your admission today for an emergency appendectomy have on your life? How could you resolve your concerns? Who could help you in this situation?

Establishing Trust

To develop a therapeutic relationship, trust needs to be established between the patient and the nurse. In today's health care system, time with patients is limited and each patient contact must be used efficiently. Knock before entering the room, give your name, identify yourself as a nursing student or LPN/LVN student, and give the reason for your visit. Explain how long you will be on duty, inform the patient when to expect meals to arrive and the approximate time health care providers may visit, and so on. Explain what care will be given on the shift and when it will be offered. Many older patients are not accustomed to the informality of having strangers address them by their given (first) name. Clarify how the patient would like to be addressed. Put the patient at ease with a pleasant, unhurried approach.

Using Empathy

An important part of the nurse-patient relationship is your ability to demonstrate empathy. No one can know or feel what another experiences. **Empathy** involves accurately perceiving the patient's feelings and understanding their meanings, even though you cannot experience the same emotional effect of these feelings, and displaying appreciation for what the other person is feeling.

An empathetic nurse conveys the interpretation of the patient's feelings back to the patient, for validation of accuracy. In this way, the patient's feelings are valued and accepted as legitimate. An example of an empathetic statement is "You appear to be upset about your surgery tomorrow." In contrast, sympathy involves entering into feelings with patients and is displayed by showing sorrow and pity. An example of a sympathetic statement is "You poor thing. I had that surgery." Patients judge their health care experiences by the nature of the help they receive.

Using Therapeutic Communication

Communicate at the level of the patient's understanding. Active listening helps the patient express needs and feelings. Ask patients what they think and actively listen to their answers, concerns, and fears by rephrasing the message when the patient is finished to verify that you understand. Avoid judging the message or the patient. Make sure that the patient's and your verbal and nonverbal communication are congruent. Avoid forming a response while the patient is speaking. Answer all of the patient's questions, when possible. Admit when you do not know the answer to a question and find out and deliver the answer as soon as possible. The focus needs to be on the physical and mental well-being of patients. Thank the patient for cooperation and attention as appropriate.

Maintaining Patients' Self-Esteem

A major problem for patients of any age during illness or debilitation is the loss of self-esteem. Avoid referring to a patient by the illness or diagnosis; instead refer to the patient by name. Identify the strengths of patients and find a way to support those strengths and thereby sustain their self-esteem. Allowing patients to perform what self-care they can manage and praising them for any effort with activities of daily living or rehabilitation exercises helps rebuild self-esteem. Nurses and providers are especially important in providing encouragement.

Think Critically

Have you observed a patient being treated in a less-than-respectful manner? How did it make you feel? How would you have treated the patient to preserve or build self-esteem?

Ensuring Pain Control

Many nursing actions help decrease patient stress, but pain control is an especially important action. Anticipate patients' pain control needs before they are expressed—for example, administer prescribed pain medication before painful procedures. After surgery, regularly assess for pain and medicate as needed per orders. Patients with chronic disease often need regular medication for pain relief. Assess the need for further pain medication before the next dose is due and determine whether the medication is effective. If the pain medicine is not doing its job, approach the health care provider and ask for an order change. Use adjunctive measures such as distraction for pain control. Provide whatever comfort measures you can, such as a straightened bed or a massage for added relief. Touch can be reassuring, calming, and encouraging to patients. In this era of awareness of sexual harassment, some nurses may be afraid to touch patients. Ask if touch is okay or touch an arm or a hand and watch the patient's reaction to see if this gesture is acceptable. Be aware of cultural taboos about being touched. Touch that is therapeutic can range from a friendly touch on the shoulder to massage or exercise of joints. Touch has been shown to effectively help manage pain in patients experiencing illness or disease.

MEETING CULTURAL NEEDS

Health care must accommodate patients of many cultural backgrounds. Patients may think and behave differently because of social class, religion, ethnic background, minority group status, marital status, or sexual preference. Avoid making judgments about people who are culturally different from you. You should be open-minded and **nonjudgmental**, take differences at face value, accept people as they are, and give high-quality care. **Transcultural nursing** involves recognizing cultural diversity and delivering nursing care that is sensitive to the particular needs of the patient and family. To do this you must develop cultural competence through knowledge of various cultures and by being sensitive to issues and preferences related to culture, race, gender, sexual orientation, social class, and economic situation. Cultural competence requires examining your own values, attitudes, beliefs, and prejudices; keeping an open mind; and attempting to look at the world through the perspectives of diverse cultures.

Older Adult Care Points

- Treat older adults with respect. Do not assume a mental impairment is present unless one is stated by the health care provider in the chart. Speak at a normal volume, with a medium to low pitch, and enunciate clearly.
- Be certain eyeglasses and/or hearing aids are in place before beginning an interaction.
- Display patience and plan extra time because it may take older adults longer to accomplish usual tasks or to formulate answers to questions.
- Give information slowly and ask for feedback to evaluate understanding. Supply printed material when possible.
- Have the patient answer questions rather than allowing other family members or friends to answer.
- Include the older adult in decision making and care planning.

Think Critically

Can you give examples of judgmental behaviors you observed in staff members during your clinical rotation?

The philosophy of **individual worth** is the belief in the uniqueness and value of each human being. Nurses need to realize that individuals have the right to live according to personal beliefs and values **as long as those beliefs and values do not interfere with the rights of others and are within the law.** Applying information to all individuals in a group can lead to assumptions, which are called **stereotypes**. A stereotype is a generic simplification used to describe all members of a group, without exception. Stereotyping is an element of profiling and provides an expectation that all individuals in a group will act in a particular way in a given situation. Profiling ignores individual differences. Members of any group or culture may not wholly observe the values and practices of their culture. Information about cultural groups can help explain—but cannot predict—individual behavior.

MEETING SPIRITUAL NEEDS

Spirituality incorporates the beliefs and values that provide strength and hope, awareness of self (including

Cultural Considerations

Examples of Cultural Preferences

- People from the Philippines are very courteous and are hesitant to say "no" or disagree, particularly with someone they hold in esteem. This may result in an individual giving the impression that they understand instructions from the health care provider or nurse when in fact they do not. They may make little direct eye contact since it is considered rude and confrontational. Avoiding eye contact is considered a sign of respect. Family is important, and a family member should be allowed at the bedside at all times. Due to modesty, the patient may be reluctant to venture out of the room to ambulate.
- Many Cambodians believe that the soul resides in the head, and it is inappropriate to touch their heads without permission. Ask before touching the head when changing head dressings or administering eye drops. Lowering the eyes or looking downward when being spoken to or instructed by someone deemed superior or older is a sign of respect.
- Hmong from Southeast Asia do not traditionally shake hands. Greetings are delivered verbally. Information giving and decision making should be accomplished through the head of the household. Physical marks that are related to home treatments may be seen on the body.
- When disease strikes, people may blame pathogens (germs), spirits, or an imbalance in the body. Some cultural groups have folk medicine rituals or special procedures to address maladies (e.g., rubbing the skin with the edge of a coin to release the toxins causing illness). Some groups have special individuals who are charged with curing disease (health care provider, herbalist, shaman, or curandero). Some groups believe that special foods, food combinations ("cold" foods for "hot" illness), or herbs (echinacea, feverfew) can prevent or cure illnesses. Others see no relationship between the diet and health. Some patients consider the prevention of illness as an attempt to control the future; they may wonder about the need to see a health care provider for preventive care (e.g., immunizations). Different beliefs of patients need to be respected.

inner strengths), and understanding of life's meaning and purpose. Patients have a spiritual self with spiritual needs and may use spiritual practices to meet those needs. Examples of personal spiritual practices may include gardening, reading inspirational books, listening to music, meditating, praying, communing with nature, practicing breathing techniques, volunteering, expressing gratitude, and counting blessings.

Spirituality and *religion* are related terms, but they do not have the same meaning. Religion attempts to formalize and ritualize spiritual beliefs. Some patients fulfill spiritual needs by belonging to a religious denomination. Concrete symbols, such as books, pictures, icons, herb packets, beads, statues, jewelry, and other objects, can affirm patients' connection with their belief in a higher power. The value of patients' rituals and religious practices is determined by their faith and is not subject to scientific evidence. Spirituality, on the other hand, does not necessarily include religion.

Crisis situations often surface in acute health care situations. Patients' beliefs and values can profoundly affect their response to these crises, attitude toward treatment, and rate of recovery. The need for spiritual care for patients and families may be intensified by hospitalization, pain experiences, chronic or incurable disease, terminal illness, or the death of a loved one. The pastoral care team allies with nurses in providing spiritual care for patients. Follow agency policy for arranging visits of patients' clergy or spiritual advisors, when such visits are desired, and provide private time for spiritual or religious practices.

Treating each patient as a unique individual requires you to consider all aspects of the patient's humanity—physiologic, psychological, spiritual, and cultural—and incorporate this understanding in delivering individualized care.

Get Ready for the NCLEX® Examination!

Key Points

- Medical-surgical nursing is a vast nursing specialty that involves several roles for LPN/LVNs.
- Qualities and skills needed by LPN/LVNs for medical-surgical nursing include upholding clinical practice standards, providing safe patient care, teaching patients, communicating effectively, working as a collaborative member of the health care team, advocating for the patient, and displaying leadership.
- Assignment involves allocating tasks to unlicensed personnel—when those tasks are within their job descriptions.
- Delegation involves designating to unlicensed personnel duties that are in the job description of the LPN/LVN, are within the boundaries of the NPA, and are advisable considering the patient situation.
- The most common site of employment for LPN/LVNs as a charge nurse is a nursing home or long-term care facility.
- Each state's NPA defines what the LPN/LVN legally can and cannot do in practice, including delegating from the position of charge nurse. LPN/LVNs use evidence-based practice, quality improvement measures, informatics, and safety practices to enhance the quality and safety of nursing care.

- Health care today includes biomedicine, complementary and alternative medicine practices, and the *Healthy People 2030* initiative.
- The ACA, Medicare, and Medicaid are examples of government-sponsored health insurance in the United States.
- To help curb rising health care costs, the federal government adopted the payment system of DRGs as part of Medicare.
- In another measure to cut costs, preventable hospital-acquired problems will not be reimbursed by Medicare.
- Holistic care includes awareness of the physical, psychological, social, cultural, and spiritual needs of patients when planning and delivering care.

Additional Learning Resources

SG Go to your Study Guide for additional learning activities to help you master this chapter content.

Go to your Evolve website (http://evolve.elsevier.com/deWit/medsurg) for the following FREE learning resources:
- Animations, audio, and video
- Answers and rationales for questions and activities
- Glossary with pronunciations in English and Spanish
- Interactive Review Questions and more!

Review Questions for the NCLEX® Examination

1. Which of the following is (are) within the role of the LPN/LVN? *(Select all that apply.)*
  1. Admitting a patient on a medical-surgical unit
  2. Changing a dressing on a postoperative patient
  3. Assessing a patient whose condition has deteriorated
  4. Collaborating with the physical therapist on how to motivate the patient to ambulate
  5. Advocating for a patient with a health care provider when prescribed pain medication is insufficient
  6. Teaching the patient about the side effects of a new medication
  NCLEX Client Need: Safe and Effective Care Environment: Coordinated Care

2. What should be the *first* thing considered before delegating a specific task? *(Priority setting.)*
  1. Know whether the task is within the scope of practice of the LPN/LVN.
  2. Be aware of the nursing assistant's competency and experience.
  3. Seek approval from the facility administration.
  4. Provide adequate explanation and oversight of the task.
  NCLEX Client Need: Safe and Effective Care Environment: Coordinated Care

3. In caring for patients with pressure injuries, which task would be most appropriate to assign to the nursing assistant?
  1. Providing assistance in making dietary choices, including fluids
  2. Participating in determining the appropriate type of wound care
  3. Repositioning the patient every 2 hours
  4. Describing the condition of the wound and any drainage
  NCLEX Client Need: Safe and Effective Care Environment: Coordinated Care

4. Which cultural custom would be important to understand when being introduced to a Hmong patient?
  1. Eye lowering is a sign of respect.
  2. Touching the head is considered honoring.
  3. Verbal greetings, not handshakes, are given.
  4. Out of courtesy, they may agree and nod.
  NCLEX Client Need: Psychosocial Integrity

5. QSEN prepares you to: *(Select all that apply.)*
  1. carry out nursing tasks efficiently for a group of patients.
  2. consider safety factors at all times when delivering care.
  3. apply evidence-based practice to the care of patients.
  4. use informatics to collaborate and communicate with the health care team.
  5. note ways that quality of care might be improved.
  6. assign tasks to UAP on the team in a timely manner.
  NCLEX Client Need: Safe and Effective Care Environment: Safety and Infection Control

6. In the process of developing evidence-based practice, after reviewing current research studies, the next step is to:
  1. validate the findings in practice.
  2. use data to improve safety.
  3. evaluate outcomes based on evidence.
  4. search for and collect sources of evidence.
  NCLEX Client Need: Safe and Effective Care Environment: Safety and Infection Control

7. One way in which nurses apply National Patient Safety Goals to patients is to:
  1. report signs of infection in a patient's wound immediately.
  2. use two methods to identify patients each time before administering a medication.
  3. educate patients about the purpose and side effects of each medication.
  4. use lift equipment to get patients out of bed and into a chair.
  NCLEX Client Need: Physiological Integrity: Reduction of Risk Potential

8. The reason that Medicare will not pay for care for a deep vein thrombosis on a patient in the hospital after knee replacement is:
   1. the patient was considered at risk for this problem.
   2. the deep vein thrombosis is considered preventable.
   3. Medicare is working hard to lower costs of the program.
   4. the patient's private insurance will cover the costs.

   NCLEX Client Need: Safe and Effective Care Environment: Coordinated Care
9. Which statement, made by an LPN/LVN during a patient interaction, indicates a therapeutic response?
   1. "I am sorry for your loss. I just lost my mother last year."
   2. "Try putting on some ointment before dressing the wound."
   3. "Are you saying that your cast is uncomfortable? Tell me more about your discomfort."
   4. "I understand. I do not like surgery either."

   NCLEX Client Need: Psychosocial Integrity
10. You find a confused patient with a history of falls attempting to get out of bed. To maintain the patient's self-esteem and safety, your intervention should be to:
    1. apply physical restraints to keep the patient in bed.
    2. administer sedatives per the health care provider's order.
    3. activate a bed alarm to notify staff.
    4. ascertain what the patient is searching for.

    NCLEX Client Need: Safe and Effective Care Environment: Safety and Infection Control

Critical Thinking Questions

Scenario A

Rosa, a student, is about to graduate as an LPN/LVN. She wants to begin searching for a job within her community. In looking at local advertisements, she notices that some are for RNs and some are for LPN/LVNs.

1. What type of employment and duties require an RN rather than a new LPN/LVN?
2. When seeking employment in a long-term care facility or a rehabilitation facility, what type of positions might be available for LPN/LVNs?
3. What is the overall requirement for an LPN/LVN no matter where they work?

Scenario B

Hector Pulido, age 75, who has pneumonia, was surprised at the aloofness of the admission clerk as she "entered" him into the electronic system during his first hospital experience. Two personnel who assisted him to his assigned room called him "Hector." Neither introduced themselves or indicated the role they played in his admission. While he was wearing a patient gown that did not fit his large frame and waiting for a nurse to interview him, people kept coming into his room without knocking. One asked his wife if he drank coffee or tea with his meals. That night, the sound of televisions, the click and beep of machines, and staff talking in the halls prevented him from getting a good night's sleep.

1. List the things that went wrong with Mr. Pulido's admission-day experience.
2. Describe how you would have made his admission day a better experience.
3. Explain the reasons for the things you chose to do differently.

Scenario C

The United States federal government is faced with budget problems resulting in large deficits and the need to reduce spending. Congress suggests reducing spending by making cuts in the Medicare and Medicaid programs. The congressional representative for your district asks for your opinion and your rationale in response to each of the following questions.

1. Should Medicare pay the cost of coronary bypass surgery for an active 85-year-old person?
2. Should Medicaid pay for care in an extended care facility for an 88-year-old person who has had a stroke and is long-term comatose?
3. Should Medicare or Medicaid pay for lifestyle prescription drugs (e.g., Viagra) for men who are eligible for these programs?

Critical Thinking and the Nursing Process

2

http://evolve.elsevier.com/deWit/medsurg

Objectives

Theory

1. Illustrate how critical thinking affects clinical judgment.
2. Explain what characteristics are necessary to think critically.
3. Explain how problem solving and decision making are a part of critical thinking.
4. Discuss the licensed practical/vocational nurse (LPN/LVN) standards for medical-surgical nursing practice.
5. Explain three fundamental beliefs about human life that are the basis for the nursing process.
6. Distinguish how critical thinking, clinical reasoning, and clinical judgment are applied to the nursing process.

Clinical Practice

7. Identify factors that influence critical thinking during patient care.
8. Provide a clinical example of how the nursing process is used in the care of medical-surgical patients.
9. Demonstrate each of the following techniques of physical examination: inspection and observation, olfaction, auscultation, and percussion.
10. Include the patient in formulation of the nursing care plan.
11. Use clinical reasoning to prioritize care for a specific patient.
12. Prepare a prioritized list for beginning-of-shift assessment of a specific patient.

Key Terms

auscultation (ăw-skŭl-TĀ-shŭn, p. 21)
clinical judgment (KLĬN-ĭ-kăl JŬJ-mĕnt, p. 15)
congruent (kŏn-GRŪ-ĕnt, p. 20)
critical thinking (KRĬ-tĭ-căl THĬNG-kĭng, p. 15)
data collection (DĀ-tă, p. 18)
evaluation (ĭh-văl-ū-Ā-shŭn, p. 26)
expected outcomes (ĕk-SPĔCT-ĕd ŎWt-kŭmz, p. 25)
focused assessment (FŌ-kŭsed ŭ-SĔS-mĕnt, p. 21)
goals (gōlz, p. 25)
implementation (ĭm-plĭ-mĕn-TĀ-shŭn, p. 17)
inspection (ĭn-SPĔK-shŭn, p. 20)
interdisciplinary (collaborative) care plans (kŏ-LĂB-ĕr-ă-tĭv plănz, p. 26)
NANDA-I (NĂN-dă-Ī, p. 23)
nursing diagnosis (NŬRZ-ĭng dī-ĭg-NŌ-sēs, p. 23)
nursing interventions (NŬRZ-ĭng ĭn-tĕr-VĔN-shŭnz, p. 25)
nursing process (NŬRZ-ĭng PRŎ-sĕs, p. 17)
objective data (ŏb-JĔK-tĭv DĀ-tă, p. 18)
observation (ŏb-sĕr-VĀ-shŭn, p. 20)
olfaction (ōl-FĂK-shŭn, p. 20)
palpation (păl-PĀ-shŭn, p. 21)
percussion (pĕr-KŬ-shŭn, p. 21)
planning (PLĂN-ĭng, p. 17)
polypharmacy (PŎL-ē-făr'mă-sē, p. 18)
priority setting (prī-ŌR-ĕ-tē SĔt-ĭng, p. 24)
subjective data (sŭb-JĔK-tĭv DĀ-tă, p. 18)

Concepts Covered in This Chapter

- Clinical Judgment
- Communication
- Collaboration

CRITICAL THINKING AND CLINICAL JUDGMENT

Critical thinking is a method for solving problems. It is directed, purposeful mental activity by which you evaluate ideas, construct plans, and determine desired outcomes. *Reasoning* is a synonym used for critical thinking. In nursing practice, critical thinking incorporates the scientific method and uses clinical reasoning to make reliable observations and to draw sound conclusions from obtained data. Developing critical thinking skills is a lifelong process and improves over time with experience. **Clinical judgment** is the result of critical thinking applied to clinical situations.

Critical thinking applied to clinical judgment in practical/vocational nursing can be described as the following:

- Purposeful, informed, and outcome focused (results oriented), requiring careful identification of patient problems, issues, and risks and making accurate

Box 2.1 Characteristics of the Critical Thinker

- Maintains an open mind and a questioning attitude
- Recognizes own biases and limitations
- Is persistent in seeking solutions
- Separates relevant information from irrelevant information
- Recognizes inconsistencies in data gathered
- Identifies missing information
- Considers all possibilities
- Assumes an empathetic attitude
- Uses an organized and systematic approach to problems
- Verifies accuracy and reliability of data
- Considers all possible solutions before making a decision
- Admits what they do not know
- Reasons logically
- Strives for excellence and improvement
- Draws valid conclusions from the evidence or data
- Sets priorities and makes carefully considered decisions
- Is flexible, realistic, creative, humble, honest, curious, and insightful

decisions about what is happening, what needs to be done, and what the priorities are for patient care
- Driven by patient, family, and community health care needs
- Based on principles of the nursing process (Box 2.1) and the scientific method
- Focused on using both logic and intuition and based on knowledge, skills, and the professional experience of the licensed practical/vocational nurse (LPN/LVN)
- Guided by standards and ethical codes of the following organizations:
  - National Association for Practical Nurse Education and Service (NAPNES) *Standards of Practice for Licensed Practical/Vocational Nurses* and *Code of Ethics*
  - National Federation of Licensed Practical Nurses (NFLPN) *Nursing Practice Standards for the Licensed Practical/Vocational Nurse* and *The Code for Licensed Practical/Vocational Nurses*
- Interested in strategies that make the most of human potential (e.g., using individual strengths) and compensate for problems created by human nature (e.g., overcoming the powerful influence of personal beliefs, values, and prejudices)
- Committed to constantly reevaluating, self-correcting, and striving to improve (e.g., practicing skills, learning new skills, attending classes and workshops, and reading nursing journals) (Alfaro-Lefevre, 2017; Knecht, 2017)

? Think Critically

List three examples in which you might use critical thinking in the classroom.

Critical thinking is most effective when the brain is purposefully engaged—for example, when attentively listening to a report at the beginning of the shift and thinking about how you will apply the information you have gained. Observe the critical thinking activities that take place among the nurses during the report as they collaborate in solving a patient-related problem. Observe the same elements later in the shift as nurses make decisions about patient care issues or about when to notify the health care provider of a problem or a need for a change of orders. Consider the following when receiving a report:
- What will I be expected to do for my assigned patients?
- What are the priorities of nursing care for each patient?
- What areas need further clarification?
- What procedures can be done independently, and which require supervision?

Examine your thinking and the thinking of others and apply the knowledge to patient care. Critical thinking is based on science and scientific principles and includes the following:
- Collecting data in an organized way
- Verifying data
- Looking for gaps in information
- Analyzing the data

As a nurse, you must access, understand, recall, and use information as the basis for critical thinking in the clinical area. A sound knowledge base is essential to critical thinking, and that base will grow throughout your nursing education and practice. Critical thinking allows you to apply learned knowledge and principles to different patient care situations.

FACTORS THAT INFLUENCE CRITICAL THINKING AND NURSING CARE

Attitude

A major factor in learning to apply critical thinking is attitude. The critical thinker is humble and recognizes that they do not have all the answers; they also recognize that their perceptions may be clouded by personal values and beliefs. The critical thinker makes an effort to consider evidence that is presented objectively.

Communication Skills

The critical thinker communicates effectively both orally and in writing. Thoughts are reflected on before speaking, and information is presented in a clear, concise manner. The critical thinker listens attentively. Documentation clearly conveys to other health team members what was planned, the patient's reaction to any care offered or provided, and whether expected outcomes were met (Box 2.2).

It is helpful to identify a nurse who is skilled at thinking critically and who can communicate clearly both verbally and through charting. This person can serve as a mentor as you learn to apply critical thinking

Box 2.2 Actual Examples of Student Charting (Unclear Communication)

- Vaginal packing out. Dr. Heffle in.
- Dr. Jones in. Had large, formed brown stool.
- On the second day the knee was better, and on the third day it disappeared.
- She is numb from the toes down.
- Patient was alert and nonresponsive.

and knowledge. The most effective mentor will be one who coaches by asking questions, rather than someone who merely provides answers.

Many other factors influence your critical thinking, such as your personality, age or maturity, prejudices and biases, past experiences, and situational factors such as anxiety, stress, and fatigue.

? Think Critically

When listening to the report on a patient, what constitutes attentive listening? How does critical thinking help you obtain all the data you need to care for the patient?

Problem Solving and Decision Making

The ability to problem solve and make decisions is integral to critical thinking. Incorporating scientific knowledge and research into nursing requires a consistent, logical method to solve problems. Using the scientific method, one first defines the problem, then gathers information, analyzes the information, and develops solutions (Box 2.3). Next a decision is made about which solution to use; then **implementation** of the solution occurs. Evidence-based research findings are considered when choosing actions to implement the solution.

INTEGRATING CRITICAL THINKING AND THE NURSING PROCESS

Critical thinking, clinical reasoning, and clinical judgment are integral to the nursing process. It is essential to know the boundaries of the role of the LPN/LVN in your state. If in doubt about the role of the LPN/LVN in the nursing process, direct your questions to your state's board of nursing. According to National Council of State Boards of Nursing (NCSBN) research, all U.S. states and territories identify a scope of practice for either LPNs or LVNs. However, the scope of practice allowed varies widely. Most LPN/LVN scopes of practice stipulate a directed role under the supervision of a registered nurse (RN), but scopes of practice differ from state to state in the areas of care **planning**, assessment, intravenous therapy, teaching, and delegation (Knecht, 2017).

The NCSBN has clearly defined the LPN/LVN role in the nursing process. What does your state's nurse practice act (NPA) indicate about the role of the LPN/LVN?

Box 2.3 Steps in the Problem-Solving Process

1. Define the problem clearly.
2. Consider all possible alternatives as solutions to the problem.
3. Consider the possible outcomes, both positive and negative, for each alternative.
4. Predict the likelihood of each outcome occurring.
5. Choose the alternative with the best chance of success and least chance of undesirable outcomes.

Adapted from Williams P: *deWit's fundamental concepts and skills for nursing*, ed 5, St. Louis, 2018, Elsevier.

Box 2.4 Four Phases of the Nursing Process for LPN/LVNs

1. **Data collection:** Assist the RN by systematically gathering and reviewing information about the patient and communicating it to appropriate members of the health care team.
2. **Planning:** Assist the RN in the development of expected outcomes and interventions for a patient's plan of care.
3. **Implementation:** Provide planned nursing care to accomplish expected outcomes.
4. **Evaluation:** Compare actual outcomes of nursing care to expected outcomes and assist with updating the nursing care plan.

? Think Critically

What questions do you have regarding clarification of your state's nurse practice act?

Nursing process is critical thinking, clinical reasoning, and clinical judgment in the language of nursing. It is an orderly way to assess a patient's response to current health status and to plan, implement, and evaluate the patient's response to nursing care (see the Evolve website for Nursing Care Plan Form). It is a way to communicate to all nursing personnel what is to be done and who is to do it, during all shifts. The nursing process provides a way to make changes in the patient's plan of care if progress is not being made. It builds on a patient's strengths and creates a partnership between the nurse and patient whenever possible. The goal of the nursing process is to alleviate, minimize, or prevent real or potential health problems (Box 2.4).

APPLYING LPN/LVN STANDARDS IN MEDICAL-SURGICAL NURSING

The five basic steps of the nursing process are (1) assessment (data collection), (2) nursing diagnosis/problem identification, (3) planning, (4) implementation, and (5) evaluation. The LPN/LVN assists the RN with steps 1, 3, 4, and 5. The RN is responsible for formulating the problem statements in step 2 from the assessment data obtained from all sources.

ASSESSMENT (DATA COLLECTION)

The purpose of **data collection** is to have a relevant database from which patient problems and potential problems may be identified. Data collection provides the basis for developing a problem list, from which problem statements or nursing diagnoses will be developed. The RN is responsible for the initial admission assessment, but the LPN/LVN may be asked to assist with parts of it. The LPN/LVN is responsible for ongoing assessment for assigned patients.

The LPN/LVN acts in a more independent role when participating in data collection (assessment) and during the implementation phase of the nursing process (see the Evolve website for Admission Data Collection Form and Physical Assessment Form). LPN/LVNs systematically gather and review data about the patient and communicate their findings to appropriate members of the health care team. A complete database includes a thorough health history, physical assessment, psychosocial assessment, and cultural and spiritual assessments. Many sources are used to compile a complete database for the patient. Most health care facilities use a standardized form for the **admission assessment**. Both **subjective data** (data that the patient gives that cannot be seen or felt by another, such as pain) and **objective data** (data that can be verified by sight, smell, touch, or sound) are included.

If there is an immediate life-threatening problem, determine immediately what action must be taken and whether additional expertise is needed to address the problem. Once the patient's physical condition is stabilized, a formal care plan can be developed (Nursing Care Plan 2.1).

Sources of Information for the Database

Admission forms, history, and physical. An admission form is completed if paper charting is used (see the Evolve website for Admission Data Collection Form and Physical Assessment Form). The admission form covers basic information such as the reason for admission, allergies, home medications, and other important information. If the patient has been hospitalized in the past, previous records may be sent to the unit or may be available electronically. The medical diagnosis will guide you in collecting assessment data and in identifying patient problems. Check to see if results of preliminary laboratory work, imaging studies, or other test results have been completed. If available, read the current information before entering the patient's room; knowing current information will enhance your critical thinking and observation skills during your initial patient contact (and will keep you from repeating obvious questions).

Think Critically

How many sources can you identify that would provide information for a nursing database on a patient who has been admitted to a long-term care facility?

Box 2.5 Interview Suggestions

- Introduce yourself to the patient by name and as an LPN/LVN student.
- Be respectful.
- A patient is entitled to be addressed by their surname. Do so, unless the patient asks you to address them differently.
- Pull up a chair so that the patient can see you at eye level and can hear you clearly.
- Speak slowly and clearly.
- Ask your questions without dropping your voice at the end of the sentence. Be alert to any hearing difficulty the patient may have.
- Give time for the patient to respond.
- Attempt to resolve incongruence between body language and responses.
- Ask for clarification if you are unsure what the patient means by a particular statement or response.
- Summarize for the patient what you think you heard during the interview.
- Ask the patient for any corrections or additions.

Interview. Ask the patient what they think is their major problem or "chief complaint." Other questions concern the present level of pain, when the last bowel movement occurred, problems with urination or appetite, difficulty sleeping, and whether they have any additional concerns or complaints. The patient is the primary source of current information and knows more about the problem than anyone else.

If for some reason the patient is incapacitated, secondary sources of information are useful (e.g., spouse, significant other, relative, friend, or patient advocate). The secondary source can also help verify information that was provided by the patient. Box 2.5 provides suggestions for interviewing. The remainder of the admission form is filled out and includes the status of advance directives, assessments for fall risk, pain level, pressure injury risk, suicide risk, nutrition requirements, and ability to perform activities of daily living. Psychosocial, cultural, and spiritual assessment data are gathered as well.

Older Adult Care Points

Plan extra time for an interview with a patient who is older. An older person who is ill may think and speak more slowly than expected, may have a hearing loss, and often has a longer health history to relate than does a younger person.

After obtaining a list of current medications from the patient or transferring facility, a medication reconciliation form to identify and prevent **polypharmacy** (multiple drugs prescribed for the same condition by different health care providers) is filled out (see the Evolve website for Medication Reconciliation Form). Some acute care facilities have pharmacy staff compile this information on paper or in the electronic health record (EHR). Medication reconciliation also reduces the risk of medication order

Nursing Care Plan 2.1 Care of the Patient With Imbalanced Nutrition

SCENARIO

Mr. Nielson, age 82, was admitted because of dizziness and weakness. He is a frail-looking man who walks slowly and with hesitation. The patient has experienced loss of appetite, loss of weight, and loss of energy since his right lung lobectomy 3 years ago.

PROBLEM STATEMENT/NURSING DIAGNOSIS

Altered nutrition/Imbalanced nutrition: less than body requirements related to loss of appetite and weakness and weight loss.

SUPPORTING ASSESSMENT DATA

Objective: Height 5′9″, weight 128 lb, loss of 35 lb

Goals/Expected Outcomes	Nursing Interventions	Selected Rationale	Evaluation
Goal: No further weight loss Outcomes Patient will eat 1500 calories of soft diet and drink 2000 mL of liquids each 24-h period.	Serve six small meals at 8 A.M., 10 A.M., noon, 2 P.M., 4 P.M., and 6 P.M.	Small, attractively arranged soft diet of favorite foods will entice patient to eat without feeling too full.	Encouraged to eat until he felt full.
	Assist patient to chair using minimal assistance.	Sitting up encourages proper digestion.	Sitting up for all meals.
	Encourage self-feeding. Assist only if needed. Assess preferred diet.	Encourages independence. Patients eat more when presented with food they prefer.	Feeding self. Prefers chicken, mashed potatoes, gravy, creamed peas, and lemon pie.
	Set up tray for easy reach.	Preserves strength and helps patient overcome weakness.	Trays set up. Continue plan.
By day 2, patient will drink 1000 mL during 24-h period.	Offer 240 mL of liquids at 6 A.M., 9 A.M., 11 A.M., 3 P.M., 5 P.M., 7 P.M., and 9 P.M. Vary choices with apple juice, orange juice, lemon-lime drink, tea, ice cream, water, and gelatin.	A variety of favorite liquids in small amounts, alternating between meals, will be easier to consume.	Intake: 500 mL this shift.
	Record time, amount, and liquids taken.	Verifies amount of liquid consumed.	
By day 4, patient will be able to remove lids and cut most of meat.	Day 1: Open packages and milk carton. Cut meat. Encourage patient to remove lids. Day 2: Open milk carton and cut meat. Day 3: Cut meat	Helps conserve energy. Progressive increase in activity will build strength.	Continue plan.
Patient will verbalize increased energy and spend more time awake during the day.	Collect data on amount of hours patient is awake and the length and number of naps.	Provides objective data as a baseline.	Patient states that he feels more energetic and will decrease the length of morning and afternoon nap times to 30 min each.
	Group activities to allow for rest periods.	Allows for uninterrupted rest.	

CRITICAL THINKING QUESTIONS

1. What practical methods can you use to entice the patient to eat, without actually feeding him?
2. What measures can you use to encourage activity, without tiring the patient excessively?

errors and adverse interactions between drugs. Patient allergies and medications—prescription, over-the-counter, and herbal preparations and supplements—are included on the form, which is reviewed by both the provider and the pharmacist. Patients need to know that the information gathered will be recorded and used in planning their care. It also helps prevent neglecting to continue an important home medication that may not be directly related to the reason for admission. Many medications require maintenance of adequate blood levels to be therapeutic.

Physical assessment. Physical data collection usually begins with measuring the patient's blood pressure, pulse, respiration, pulse oximetry, temperature, weight, and height. **Accuracy is essential.** Data collection correlates current readings with the baseline data, with trends of past readings, with the patient's current clinical status, and with any medical care that has been provided. Such data yield significant information about the patient's condition and response to medication and other treatments. Complete assessments are performed daily.

Focused Assessment

General Interview Guide

SOCIAL ASSESSMENT

- What is your living situation?
- Who lives with you?
- Who may the health care team discuss your condition with in addition to you?
- What kind of work do you do?
- Do you have spiritual beliefs that we can help support?
- Do you have concerns regarding finances related to this hospitalization?
- How are things at home if you are not there while in the hospital?
- Are there any medical problems that are common in your family?
- Have you had previous surgeries or serious injuries?
- In your life now, who is helpful to you?
- What prescription drugs do you take? What over-the-counter medicines or supplements?
- Do you smoke? How much? What do you smoke?
- Do you drink alcohol? How often do you drink and how much?
- Do you use any other drugs?
- Are you allergic to any drugs? Foods? Other substances? What kind of reaction do you have?
- Are you on a special diet at home?

PHYSICAL ASSESSMENT

- Why were you admitted here?
- What health problems do you have?
- Do you routinely see doctors? If so, for what?

REVIEW OF SYSTEMS (ASK QUESTIONS ABOUT THE FOLLOWING)

Head and Neck

Frequent headaches; dizziness, ringing of the ears, hearing problems; visual problems, glaucoma, cataracts, glasses or contact lenses; surgery of the brain, eyes, or ears; frequent colds; nasal allergies; sinus infections; frequent sore throats; hoarseness; trouble swallowing; swollen glands; mouth sores; date of last dental examination; history of thyroid problems; use of a hearing aid; difficulty sleeping, napping

Chest

Male and female: Cough, sputum production; asthma, wheezing, frequent bronchitis; history of pneumonia; tuberculosis, exposure to tuberculosis; exposure to occupational respiratory hazards; palpitations, chest pain; shortness of breath; history of heart problems, murmurs, hypertension; anemia; surgery

Female: Frequency of breast examinations; date of last mammogram; nipple discharge; breast lumps

Abdomen (Gastrointestinal Tract)

Indigestion; pain; nausea; vomiting; excessive thirst or hunger; frequency of bowel movements; change in bowel movements; rectal bleeding; black or tarry stools; constipation; diarrhea; excessive gas; hemorrhoids; history of gallbladder or liver problems

Genitourinary (Inquire With Cultural Sensitivity)

Male and female: Problems with urination; up at night to urinate; dribbling of urine; history of urinary tract infection; stones

Female: Sexual activity; sexual problems; menstrual cycle and any problems; last menstrual period; bleeding between periods or after menopause; vaginal discharge; date of last Pap smear; history of sexually transmitted infections or vaginal disorders

Male: Sexual activity; genital problems; penile discharge; history of sexually transmitted infections; sexual problems

Extremities and Musculoskeletal System

Joint pain or stiffness; back problems; muscle pain; limited range of motion; vascular problems in legs or arms; easy bruising; skin lesions; history of phlebitis; thrombophlebitis; gout, osteoarthritis, rheumatoid arthritis, fractures, injury

PSYCHOLOGICAL ASSESSMENT

- Are you experiencing anxiety? Depression?
- Do you have unusual memory problems?
- Do you have difficulty thinking?
- Are you ever confused?

Inspection and observation. **Inspection** (looking) and **observation** (looking and noting) are important aspects of nursing assessment. Use your eyes to pick up clues about the patient's physical and mental condition. Note the patient's facial expression, posture, grimaces, and movements and whether answers are **congruent** (match the feeling tone of what is said verbally). Inspect the hair, skin, nails, and oral mucous membranes for data about hydration and dental hygiene. Observe the patient's state of personal care. Is the hair combed, and are the nails clean and reasonably trimmed? Is there anything in the room that gives evidence of support systems, family, or friends?

Olfaction. **Olfaction** (smelling) can provide data about a patient's personal hygiene, as well as clues to possible illness. The sweet, fruity odor of acetone can be indicative of diabetic acidosis. The smell of newly mown clover can be present with hepatic coma. The smell of alcohol indicates that the patient has been drinking. Sometimes patients with acute alcoholism may smell like aftershave, mouthwash, vanilla, Sterno, or other substances that contain a high percentage of alcohol. Foul or metallic mouth odors usually indicate poor oral hygiene or periodontal disease. Odor from the nose may be indicative of chronic sinusitis with postnasal drip or an obstruction in the nasal passages.

Patients who have anemia, an endocrine problem, or a central nervous system abnormality may try to cover up unpleasant body odor with bath powder or heavy perfume. An unpleasant genital odor may indicate an infection, poor hygiene, or insufficient fluid intake (commonly found in female patients in long-term care facilities). Without additional attention, body areas that are unattended may become reddened, irritated, and sometimes infected.

Palpation. Palpate (touch) the patient's skin to determine whether it feels healthy or is coarse, dry, swollen, cold, or clammy. Dryness may be related to dehydration, and swelling may indicate edema (fluid in the tissues). If you depress the skin with your fingers and your touch leaves pitting (indentation) on the skin, edema is present. Measure and record the depth of pitting and the length of time the tissue remains indented (see Chapter 3, Fig. 3.5). **Palpation** of the skin can provide additional information. Cold extremities may indicate poor circulation. Hot tissue may result from localized inflammation, and you will want to examine the area more carefully. Use your fingertips, not your thumb, to palpate the pulses. Use the flat of the hand to palpate the abdomen to determine whether it is soft or hard and whether there are any tender areas. Palpate the breasts for abnormal growths. Premenopausal women may have masses in their breasts, making it difficult to determine which lumps are significant (this is a good time to ask for assistance from your instructor, the staff RN, or the clinical nurse specialist).

Auscultation. **Auscultation** (listening) is an important skill in gathering data. Listen to the sounds of the patient's breathing—with a stethoscope and without a stethoscope. You may hear wheezing from constricted bronchi or stridor caused by a partial airway obstruction. Listening to the quality of a patient's cough will determine whether it is dry or moist. With the stethoscope, the sounds are amplified, and you can auscultate normal, abnormal, or adventitious breath sounds (Fig. 2.1). Listen to the apical pulse at the apex of the heart and on the abdomen for bowel sounds; listen carefully in each quadrant (Fig. 2.2).

Percussion. **Percussion** consists of using light, quick tapping on different surfaces of the body to tell the size, location, and density of different organs, especially in the chest, abdomen, and kidney areas. Percussion of the abdomen will reveal areas of excessive gas in the bowel.

Daily Focused Assessment (Data Collection)

A daily **focused assessment**, usually performed at the beginning of the shift, is directed to areas in which the patient is experiencing health problems. This assessment augments the admission assessment of the patient and is based on the identified problems, data from the report, and medical diagnoses and treatment. Many hospitals have standardized assessment forms for collecting head-to-toe data on the patient. Information from the patient's chart and care plan is used to identify areas in which focused assessment data should be collected. Ask for a demonstration of an appropriate head-to-toe assessment.

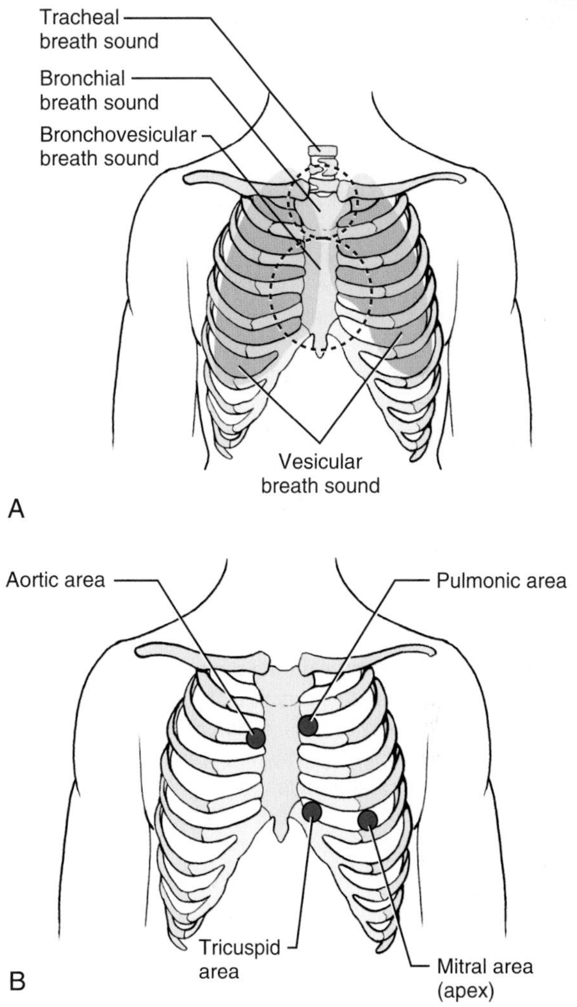

Fig. 2.1 **A,** Locations of normal lung sounds. **B,** Place the stethoscope at the apex of the heart (5th intercostal space) to listen to the apical pulse.

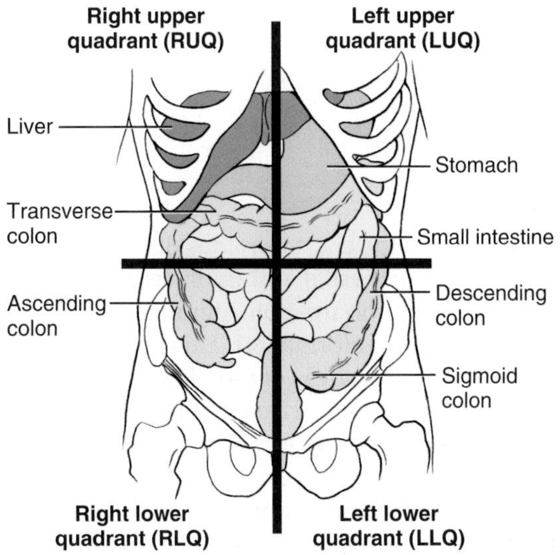

Fig. 2.2 Listen for bowel sounds in all four quadrants of the abdomen.

Focused Assessment

Beginning-of-Shift Assessment

PHYSICAL REVIEW*

- Assess the patient's level of consciousness (LOC), including their ability to respond quickly and appropriately and their orientation to person, place, and time. Refer to the Glasgow Coma Scale in Chapter 21 for patients with neurologic problems.
- Check the patient's ability to think (mentate) by asking questions within their capacity (e.g., Who is the president?).
- Observe the skin color and texture and degree of moisture.
- Note the appearance of the eyes.
- Measure the vital signs (temperature, pulse, respiration, pulse oximetry, and blood pressure). Note the rhythm and strength of the pulse, rhythm and depth of respiration, and respiratory effort.
- Ask the patient to describe any pain. Determine the location, severity, quality, and precipitating and alleviating factors.
- Auscultate the chest using the stethoscope. Listen for breath sounds, noting normal, abnormal, and adventitious breath sounds. Listen at the apex of the heart, checking for regularity of rhythm. Auscultate the apical pulse for 60 seconds to count the rate and note the rhythm of the heartbeat. It is difficult for a new nurse to pick up extra heart sounds, but you can determine whether there is an increase or decrease in the heart rate.
- Assess the skin turgor (elasticity) by gently lifting the skin on the upper chest with your thumb and forefinger and observing the speed with which it snaps back when you let go.
- Observe the contour of the abdomen (e.g., flat, round, distended).
- When the patient is in a supine position or low Fowler position, auscultate bowel sounds in all four quadrants.
- Gently palpate the abdomen with the palm side of the fingers, noting whether the abdomen is soft or firm. Also ask the patient whether they are experiencing any pain or discomfort, indicating areas of tenderness. Inquire about appetite and weight changes.
- Assess the patient's bowel and bladder status. Note the time of their last bowel movement (from the chart or by asking the patient) and whether flatus is being passed. Review the intake and output (I&O) for the past 24 hours. Observe and palpate the pubic area to assess bladder distention, especially if there is a discrepancy between the current and previous I&O. If urinary retention is suspected, a bladder scanner may be available for verification. If the patient has an indwelling catheter, observe the characteristics of the urine in the drainage tube and the rate of drainage.
- Ask the patient to move each extremity. Observe their ability to actively move the joints through the range of motion and the coordination of the movements. If the patient is unable to actively move any joints, assist them with passive motion and note the degree of flexibility. Ask the patient to move their extremities against resistance, to determine extremity strength. You can also determine the patient's level of cooperation and ability to follow directions during the exercises.
- Compare the peripheral pulses bilaterally.
- Note the presence of any edema.

TUBES AND EQUIPMENT STATUS

- **Intravenous catheter:** Condition of site; fluid in progress, rate, additives; time next fluid is to be hung
- **Nasogastric tube:** Suction setting; amount and character of drainage; patency of tube; security of tube; confirm that tube markings are correct to ensure that the tube has not moved since insertion
- **Urinary catheter:** Character and quantity of drainage; tubing not positioned underneath patient; properly secured
- **Dressings:** Location; drains in place; wound suction devices; amount and character of wound drainage; condition of dressing
- **Patient-controlled analgesia pump:** Properly functioning; correct medication infusing; amount of solution remaining; end-tidal carbon dioxide (CO_2) monitoring in place (if part of protocol)
- **Oxygen:** Type of delivery device, rate of flow
- **Equipment:** Applied properly; functioning as ordered

*The physical review may include a head-to-toe assessment based on the patient's needs.

Chart Review

The face sheet of the chart provides demographic data such as address, marital status, insurance coverage, age, date of birth, occupation, significant others, and emergency contact information. This information may be located in various areas of the EHR. The health care provider's history, physical examination, progress notes, and results of diagnostic tests give an overview of the patient's total health status and provide a summary of current health problems and progress toward resolving them. Allergy information should be identified as part of the admission information and displayed prominently on the front of the chart, on the header of the EHR page, and in other locations as required by the facility's policies and procedures. The current provider's orders provide a clue as to the plan for that day (tests or treatments).

The medication profile sheets, screens, or medication administration record (MAR) lists the routine and as-needed (PRN) medications and provides documentation of medication administration. Consultation notes or nursing documentation includes narrative notes and flow sheets that describe care provided to the patient and the patient's response to that care.

Older Adult Care Points

You walk into your assigned patient's room and find that Mr. Nethers, age 72, has a sitter because he pulled out his oxygen tube, intravenous (IV) line, and urinary catheter earlier that morning. He has also attempted to get out of bed several times. Yesterday he was alert and had a lucid conversation with you. Mr. Nethers had surgery yesterday after you left the unit to go to class, and you see in the documentation that he has been receiving hydrocodone-acetaminophen for pain. You recall that this medication could have a severe behavioral side effect, especially for an older patient. You inform the medication nurse of your observations and ask that the health care provider be consulted before giving additional doses.

Diagnostic Test Results

Review laboratory and test data to identify general concerns and to confirm assessment findings. Particularly note test data related to the patient's problems that indicate improvement or a complication.

Other Resources

Course textbooks are a primary resource; other texts, journal articles, and the internet can provide a wealth of information. Handheld devices with downloaded electronic resources (e.g., medical-surgical, drug, and laboratory texts) and apps provide instant access to clinical resources. Because there is no control over information placed on the internet, resources should be evaluated carefully. Your instructor, pharmacists, dietitians, social workers, occupational therapists, physical therapists, physicians, and other specialists can provide valuable information about specific aspects of the patient. Work to gain a comprehensive picture of the patient's situation, diagnoses, medications, and potential actions for care.

ANALYSIS AND NURSING DIAGNOSIS

The LPN/LVN reports data collection findings to the RN and assists in verifying, categorizing, and grouping the collected data in a logical order. The LPN/LVN also assists in analyzing the data to determine significant relationships among data, patient needs, and problems. A *prioritized* list of patient problems is developed. The focus is on actual and potential patient problems that can be addressed with independent nursing interventions. From the analysis, the RN chooses problem statements or uses nursing diagnoses from the **NANDA-I** list. Many facilities do not use NANDA-I nursing diagnoses. They use problem statements on care plans, or they use interdisciplinary care plans with the medical diagnosis listed.

Nursing care is based on the *priority* of patient problems. High-priority problems are dealt with first, and lower priority problems are dealt with as time permits. The problem statements or nursing diagnoses are based on all available patient data, including—but not limited to—the nursing assessment (subjective and objective) data, the diagnostic test data, and the medical diagnosis. Placing a problem statement or nursing diagnosis in the care plan means that the nurse is accepting accountability for the accuracy of the statement. Permitting a problem to continue without designating a problem statement can lead to patient harm (Alfaro-Lefevre, 2017).

Think Critically

What is important in choosing the correct problem statement for a care plan? How would you determine that a problem statement or nursing diagnosis on a facility care plan is appropriate for the patient?

It is important to differentiate between a problem statement or **nursing diagnosis** and a medical diagnosis. The health care provider is concerned with health problems that can be treated with surgery, medications, and other forms of therapy provided or prescribed by them. Problem statements or nursing diagnoses identify the patient's response to an illness or a health condition. Nursing practice addresses physical, psychological, social, cultural, and spiritual comfort and well-being; the prevention of complications; and patient education. Nursing care focuses on preventing, minimizing, and alleviating specific health problems. Although the provider is responsible for managing medical problems, the RN uses clues from the medical diagnosis to identify patient problems and to develop accurate nursing problem statements or nursing diagnoses.

When using NANDA-I diagnoses, NANDA-I–approved stems are based on an analysis of available data. These approved stems label the patient problems that can be treated independently using nursing interventions. Other components of a NANDA-I nursing diagnosis make statements specific to the patient's situation and direct the planning and implementation phases of the nursing process. A complete NANDA-I nursing diagnosis includes the problem (NANDA-I stem), the etiology (related causes of the problem), and the signs and symptoms (evidence of the problem).

The etiology component describes the known or suspected cause or causes of a problem (e.g., a patient's altered breathing patterns could be related to etiologies of reduced lung capacity, anxiety, or pain). The signs and symptoms of the problem describe the subjective and objective evidence of the problem (i.e., the diagnosis is supported [evidenced] by the assessment data). To follow our example, a patient's altered breathing pattern might be evidenced by a statement of shortness of breath or by observation of dyspnea (difficulty breathing), changes in respiratory rate or rhythm, or decreased oxygen saturation levels. The problem statement would be: Altered breathing pattern related to pneumonia as evidenced by patient complaint of shortness of breath, observed use of accessory muscles, O_2 saturation of 89% on room air.

Actual problems are problems that the patient currently exhibits, and documentation should include all three components of the diagnosis statement (problem,

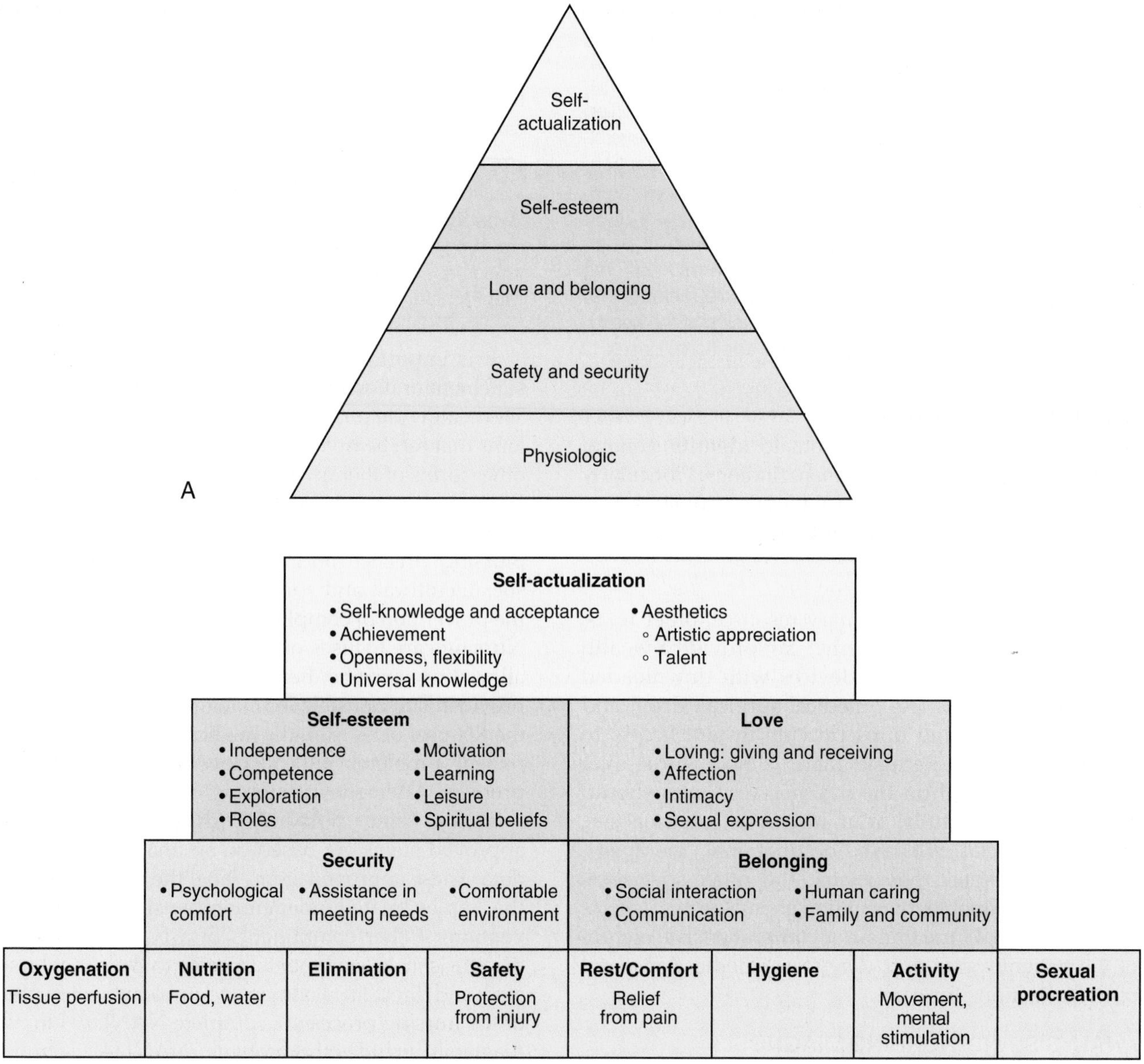

Fig. 2.3 **A,** Maslow's hierarchy of needs. **B,** Evolving hierarchy of needs adapted by nursing to help determine priorities of care. (From Williams P: *deWit's fundamental concepts and skills for nursing*, ed 5, St. Louis, 2018, Elsevier.)

etiology, signs and symptoms). Sometimes the patient does not currently exhibit evidence of actual problems, but the data demonstrate that a problem could occur; these situations describe potential problems. An example of a potential problem is: *Potential for Fluid deficit related to vomiting and diarrhea.* In this example, the patient is not currently showing signs of dehydration but is at risk because of the fluid loss associated with vomiting and diarrhea. Potential problems alert you to take preventive measures rather than wait for a problem to materialize before taking action. Even though many facilities do not use NANDA-I nursing diagnoses, the LPN/LVN may be expected to be familiar with the NANDA-I list of nursing diagnoses.

Setting Priorities of Care

Priority setting is a method of handling problems and tasks according to the importance (priority) of the patient's problems. Maslow's hierarchy of needs is one way to prioritize patient problems and nursing care (Fig. 2.3). Other factors to consider are safety and involvement of the patient (see Chapter 1). Problem statements or nursing diagnoses are listed on the care plan in order of priority. The need to sustain life, such as an airway and breathing, must be attended to immediately, even before a formal care plan is developed. All possible patient problems might not be included in the initial plan. As problem statements or nursing diagnoses are dealt with successfully, they are modified or discontinued. Other problems are added to the plan as they arise.

PLANNING

LPN/LVN standards of care indicate that the LPN/LVN will use the nursing process in planning nursing care and will assist the RN in the identification of health goals, outcomes, and interventions for a patient's plan of care. For a care plan to be effective, the patient should be involved in determining which problems are most important. Data regarding what the patient is willing and able to do to improve the situation and what education is needed are also gathered for the care plan. Sometimes, something you might consider minor is very important to the patient.

Goals and Expected Outcomes

All goals or expected outcomes, set together by the patient and the nurse, must be patient centered, be realistically achievable, be measurable, and include a time frame within which they will be met. Goals and expected outcomes relate to (1) restoring health when there is a health problem and (2) promoting health when the patient's resources can and should be directed at regaining or maintaining health. For example, the patient is eager to learn how to live with the diagnosis of diabetes. The patient needs to be instructed about the illness, how to monitor the glucose level, what action is needed to stabilize the glucose level, how to administer insulin or oral medication, how to maintain a therapeutic diet, what kinds and what frequency of exercise are appropriate, how to prevent infections, and when to seek additional medical help.

Goals state a general intent about what the patient will achieve. **Expected outcomes** describe a specific result expected at a certain point in time. The terms are used interchangeably in some agencies. *Outcome* generally is used to describe what the patient, not the nurse, will do. An outcome is written as *"The patient will ..."* Patient input is important to establish motivation to accomplish the outcome. Outcome statements are derived from the signs and symptoms included in the problem statements. The word *patient* is used as the subject of the statement. The outcome statements are written with a subject, an action verb, conditions or modifiers, and the criterion (standard) for desired performance. Expected outcomes should include the following:

- Patient activity that can be observed or patient knowledge that can be assessed. Consider how "the patient will select *[action verb, which can be measured or observed]* low-sodium foods from a list" provides a better indicator of knowledge than "the patient will understand *[passive verb]* a low-sodium diet."
- A description of how the patient's behavior will be measured, including the accuracy and quality of performance and the time frame within which the objective is to be met.

Nursing Interventions

Nursing interventions are nursing actions and patient activities chosen to achieve the goals and expected outcomes. Evidence-based practice research is considered to locate best practices for the types of interventions that are appropriate for each problem statement or nursing diagnosis. Independent nursing interventions can be initiated and implemented without a health care provider's order. Dependent actions are ordered by the provider. Chosen interventions are listed on the nursing care plan.

Prioritizing Delivery of Care

Prioritizing care is the most important step in planning competent, timely patient care. Prioritizing of care includes when to give medications, measure vital signs, monitor blood glucose, change dressings, check IVs, and so on. Prioritizing also includes identifying which tasks are urgent and which tasks can wait. An urgent task would be administering medication on schedule, whereas a nonurgent task would be ambulating the patient.

Nursing students often have only one or two patients assigned to them for clinical care. After graduation, the norm is four to six patients. During times of low staffing, expect the number of assigned patients to increase. Once you receive your assignments:

- Review the patient's chart, computer printout, or whichever system is used for patient information.
- Look up required drug information for each routine and PRN drug listed, including IV solutions and additives.
- List focused assessments you will make and data you will collect, both at intervals and before you go off duty.
- List procedures that will be performed and a list of equipment for each.
- Attend report, make additional notes, and question what you do not understand.
- Make rounds on all your assigned patients (unless a bedside report was given). Seeing the patient alerts you to changes that need immediate attention.
- Consider a plan for your shift, including when the patient might be out of the unit for a test, when medications are due, when meals are served, when health care providers usually make rounds, what time physical therapy or respiratory therapy might be working with the patient, treatments that are ordered, and when a spouse might arrive to visit. Consider when patient teaching might be worked in and when you might chart and revise the care plan if needed.

Priority setting is a skill that must be developed to work efficiently and safely. During prioritizing, it should become apparent if there is a need to assign some tasks to others.

IMPLEMENTATION

LPN/LVN standards require that you provide care within the scope of practice to accomplish established goals. Standardized care plans are frequently found on medical-surgical units and include generic nursing care for commonly encountered patient problems. The standardized plan is not individualized for a specific patient. However, problems and interventions can be added or deleted if they are not appropriate for the patient. An individualized plan of care is more thorough because it is developed for a specific patient.

Distinguish which activities you need to carry out and which activities the patient must learn to do to gain independence. Sometimes when you are very busy, it seems faster to do an activity for the patient (e.g., feeding a patient who needs to learn to feed themselves). The interventions listed in the care plan should indicate that the caregiver is to sit beside the patient and encourage them verbally, as needed. In this way the patient will gain independence by eventually feeding themselves.

Staff Communication Regarding Care

Communication among staff members occurs in numerous ways throughout the day. Sometimes staff communication must be immediate to communicate urgent and relevant data that were discovered during an assessment of the patient. Urgent data are usually communicated verbally and may require immediate action. Use the SBAR format (**S**ituation, **B**ackground, **A**ssessment, **R**ecommendation) for communicating information.

Charting occurs on nurses' notes, treatment flow sheets, MARs, and activity flow sheets. Nurses also might chart on common charting forms with other health care providers. Health care facilities are moving to electronic documentation and records management. Most acute care facilities have transitioned to electronic records and many long-term care facilities use computerized charting. An EHR is a computerized comprehensive record of a patient's history and care across all facilities and admissions (Williams, 2018). Security of information is extremely important whether located on paper or a computer.

Think critically about what needs to be documented and be succinct in recording the information. Follow agency policy for the method of documentation to be used (e.g., problem-oriented record, focus charting, or charting by exception).

Legal and Ethical Considerations

Privacy and Protected Health Information

Other clinicians, such as the dietitian, respiratory therapist, and social worker, contribute to the documentation in the patient's chart. Information provided by these clinicians completes the comprehensive picture of the patient.

Any protected health information in a patient's chart must be carefully guarded to avoid violating the confidentiality component of the Health Insurance Portability and Accountability Act (HIPAA). Information retained by a student for educational purposes must be devoid of identifying information. Student preparation paperwork that contains protected health information must be destroyed before leaving the facility according to the policies and procedures of the facility.

Report is conducted at the change of shifts according to facility protocol to ensure continuity of care for patients. On some medical-surgical units, all staff members listen to report on all patients, the advantage of which is that all nurses and nursing assistants are aware of the needs of every patient. Other units use an individualized report system in which a nurse receives report on assigned patients only. Walking rounds are another method for change-of-shift report in which nurses go to patients' rooms and the departing nurse and the patient describe what happened during the previous shift. They discuss what the departing nurse and the patient see as priorities for the next shift. This is more time consuming than other methods, but walking rounds provide a sense of partnering for the patient, and the arriving nurse has an opportunity to see and hear the patient before beginning care. Having appropriate information available during report facilitates discussion of identified patient priorities.

Think Critically

What information is needed to effectively receive and give report? What are the items to which you will pay greatest attention or that you will emphasize?

EVALUATION

The LPN/LVN standards require comparison of *actual* outcomes of patient care to the *expected* outcomes. This comparison is known as **evaluation**. Evaluation begins as soon as a nursing plan is implemented. To make the comparisons needed for evaluation, collect data with every patient contact, think critically about how the patient is progressing in response to nursing actions, and determine whether there is a way to improve care. Daily evaluation is part of the natural flow of the nursing process, regardless of the time frame established for patient outcomes. The collected and documented data demonstrate a patient's progress toward meeting the expected outcomes. If the data show a lack of progress toward meeting the expected outcomes with planned interventions, the interventions should be reviewed and revised.

INTERDISCIPLINARY (COLLABORATIVE) CARE PLANS

Interdisciplinary (collaborative) care plans require input from all health team members involved in patient care (see the Evolve website for Interdisciplinary [Collaborative] Care Plan). The collaborative care plan is developed using the interdisciplinary focus of each professional (e.g., nurse, social worker, occupational therapist, recreational therapist). A separate care plan for each profession is considered repetitious. The focus of interdisciplinary planning is patient problems rather than nursing diagnoses, making the language used in the plan common to all professions. Interdisciplinary care plans have the following characteristics:

- The patient's medical diagnosis is used, rather than a problem statement or nursing diagnosis.

- Observations (data collected) are shared among all providers involved in the care of the patient.
- A problem list is developed and prioritized. The patient's statement of problems that led to admission is considered. **Priority is given to lifesaving or physiologic needs.**
- A shared care plan is created, identifying specific and shared responsibilities for all professions represented.
- The plan is discussed with the patient (when possible) or patient advocate. The team plays a supportive role during implementation of the plan.
- Documentation of progress is usually made on a common form or computer record to allow easy access for all team members involved with the patient.
- Evaluation is ongoing, with periodic in-depth evaluation by the team on agreed-on dates. Interventions are deleted, added, and changed as needed.

Get Ready for the NCLEX® Examination!

Key Points

- Critical thinking generates new ideas and judges the worth of those ideas. Critical thinking prompts the LPN/LVN to ask what could be improved and what measures would prevent further harm to the patient.
- Clinical judgment is a proactive reasoning skill that uses critical thinking in the clinical area to determine the appropriate actions to take in specific situations.
- Factors that influence critical thinking and the decisions about nursing care include our culture, personal motivation, attitude, and verbal and written communication ability.
- The nursing process is an advanced problem-solving method used to collect and analyze data to plan, implement, and evaluate patient care in an orderly way.
- Goals and expected outcomes are patient centered and describe what the patient will achieve.
- Receiving a patient assignment and preparing a preliminary care plan before beginning patient care is considered safe practice for student nurses.
- Techniques of physical examination used by the LPN/LVN include inspection and observation, olfaction, palpation, percussion, and auscultation. Nurses need to be aware of common laboratory and other diagnostic tests and their relationship to common illness. Laboratory and diagnostic tests also provide a way to track the effectiveness of treatments and the emergence of side effects of medications.
- Staff communication takes place both verbally and by charting. Urgent communication is done verbally and as soon as possible.
- Interdisciplinary (collaborative) care plans are used in health facilities where one plan for all disciplines works best.

Additional Learning Resources

SG Go to your Study Guide for additional learning activities to help you master this chapter content.

Go to your Evolve website (http://evolve.elsevier.com/deWit/medsurg) for the following FREE learning resources:

- Animations, audio, and video
- Answers and rationales for questions and activities
- Glossary with pronunciations in English and Spanish
- Interactive Review Questions and more!

Review Questions for the NCLEX® Examination

1. Which critical thinking skill is important to apply when formulating a nursing care plan?
   1. Having the nursing assistant help with assessment.
   2. Reading the history and physical in the chart.
   3. Analyzing the data to determine appropriate nursing diagnoses.
   4. Including the patient in formulating the care plan.

   NCLEX Client Need: Safe and Effective Care Environment: Coordinated Care
2. Critical thinking is important in the nursing process because it:
   1. can provide a better outcome for the patient.
   2. simplifies the planning process for the nurse.
   3. allows the patient to have input on the plan.
   4. directly communicates the plan to others.

   NCLEX Client Need: Safe and Effective Care Environment: Coordinated Care
3. The assessment technique of percussion is used by the nurse to:
   1. determine whether lung sounds are normal.
   2. assess for air in the intestine.
   3. check for abdominal rigidity.
   4. assess the degree of abdominal pain.

   NCLEX Client Need: Physiological Integrity: Physiologic Adaptation
4. Assessing a patient's sleep patterns should include which aspect(s)? *(Select all that apply.)*
   1. Family history of sleep disorders
   2. Rituals associated with sleep
   3. Feelings of restfulness
   4. Diet choices
   5. Urinary habits

   NCLEX Client Need: Physiologic Integrity: Basic Care and Comfort
5. When caring for an older woman who developed a 5-cm pressure ulcer on her sacrum because of being immobilized and incontinent, an appropriate expected outcome for the problem of altered skin integrity would be:
   1. "Patient will be able to ambulate to the bathroom with minimal assistance."
   2. "Turning and repositioning schedules will be provided for the staff."
   3. "Patient will demonstrate a decrease in size of the ulcer within 1 week."
   4. "Family will be able to provide protein-rich foods during the hospital stay."

   NCLEX Client Need: Safe and Effective Care Environment: Coordinated Care

6. Risk for falls would be considered a high priority for a patient with which of these problems? (*Select all that apply*)
   1. Altered skin integrity due to repair of umbilical hernia
   2. Altered mobility due to knee arthritis
   3. Altered nutrition due to weight of 265 lb
   4. Altered self-care due to extreme weakness
   5. Altered swallowing ability due to esophageal stricture
   6. Altered cardiac output decreased due to cardiomyopathy

   NCLEX Client Need: Safe and Effective Care Environment: Safety and Infection Control
7. You are collecting data from an older patient with a history of fractures who has just had gallbladder surgery. Along with a focused assessment, you should include:
   1. determining orientation to person, place, and time.
   2. auscultating for a heart murmur.
   3. checking peripheral pulses.
   4. testing passive and active range of motion.

   NCLEX Client Need: Physiological Integrity: Reduction of Risk Potential
8. When evaluating patient understanding regarding the use of an incentive spirometer, which statement confirms a need for more teaching?
   1. "I will inhale as deeply as possible each time I use the spirometer."
   2. "I need to tilt the incentive spirometer slightly to reduce effort."
   3. "To monitor progress, I will record the top volume achieved."
   4. "I need to seal my lips around the mouthpiece."

   NCLEX Client Need: Physiological Integrity: Reduction of Risk Potential
9. Using critical thinking, choose the nursing actions that should be implemented when addressing the needs of an older patient with the problem diagnosis of *Altered nutrition due to poor dentition. (Select all that apply.)*
   1. Encourage more fluid intake of fluids with food value if not contraindicated by the medical condition.
   2. Inspect the oral cavity and the condition of mucous membranes and teeth.
   3. Assist with swallowing.
   4. Initiate a speech therapy consult.
   5. Monitor daily caloric intake and weekly weights.
   6. Provide mouth care every 2 hours while awake.

   NCLEX Client Need: Safe and Effective Care Environment: Coordinated Care
10. When evaluating for side effects of the action of "administer anticoagulant," which patient statement(s) would strongly correlate with a side effect problem? *(Select all that apply.)*
    1. "I have noticed some blood streaking in my bowel movements."
    2. "I have been embarrassed by frequent, uncontrollable gassiness."
    3. "My urine has been cloudy, with an odd aroma."
    4. "I readily bruise whenever I bump into anything."
    5. "I notice some blood when I floss my teeth."

    NCLEX Client Need: Physiological Integrity: Pharmacological Therapies

Critical Thinking Questions

Scenario A

Review the section "Critical Thinking and Clinical Judgment." Consider how the critical thinking points discussed have helped you learn clinical judgment.

1. Describe an example from personal experience explaining how you used critical thinking and clinical judgment in a situation involving a patient, a patient's family member, or a friend.
2. Is there more you could have done, or could what you did have been done in a better way?
3. Did your action prevent harm to the person?

Scenario B

Mr. Nash is 68 years old and describes himself as a tough guy. He is currently on bed rest after surgery for a right femur fracture. He fell from his roof while adjusting the satellite dish. His main theme is "What do I have to do to get out of here?" Although grumpy, Mr. Nash's positive attribute is that he will do whatever will get him released from the hospital: "I've got to smell my own air and I want my evening beer!" The problem statement in his chart is *Altered mobility due to right leg surgery.*

1. Write an example of a patient-centered expected outcome for Mr. Nash that is realistic, time referenced, and measurable.
2. Plan nursing interventions to meet the expected outcome you have written.

Scenario C

Because no jobs are currently available in the medical-surgical unit at the local hospital, you have applied for work at the mental health facility. You know that your medical-surgical observation skills will be useful in data collection (assessment). The mental health facility uses interdisciplinary care plans.

1. Explain the major differences between a nursing process–focused plan and an interdisciplinary plan.
2. What is the responsibility of each medical specialist for developing and carrying out the interdisciplinary plan?

Scenario D

You are assigned to a mixed medical-surgical nursing unit for your student assignment. You have arrived half an hour early (at 6:30 A.M.) to begin preparation for patient care on the medical-surgical unit at the local hospital. Your assignment involves the following four patients:

Patient 1: Scheduled for abdominal surgery at 10 A.M.; arrives during report and says she was held up in traffic

Patient 2: Newly diagnosed with diabetes, requiring blood glucose readings before each meal with nutritional insulin dosing

Patient 3: Total knee replacement 2 days ago; is scheduled for physical therapy (PT) at 10 A.M.

Patient 4: Has pneumonia; admitted during the night; oxygen at 4 L/min via nasal cannula; has an oxygen saturation monitor

1. Which tasks are priorities?
2. How soon before surgery should the preoperative preparation start?
3. What time is glucose monitoring performed, and does the patient receive insulin based on the glucose reading?
4. When are IVs assessed?
5. What is required for preparation for PT?
6. Which patients need a full assessment, and which need a focused assessment?
7. Does Patient 3 require a dressing change and, if so, when?

3 Fluids, Electrolytes, Acid-Base Balance, and Intravenous Therapy

http://evolve.elsevier.com/deWit/medsurg

Objectives

Theory

1. Explain the various functions that fluid performs in the body.
2. Describe the body's mechanisms for fluid regulation.
3. List three ways in which body fluids are continually being distributed among the body's fluid compartments.
4. Distinguish the signs and symptoms of various electrolyte imbalances.
5. Discuss why older adults have more problems with fluid and electrolyte imbalances.
6. Describe the disorders that cause specific fluid and electrolyte imbalances.
7. Compare the major causes of acid-base imbalances.
8. Apply interventions to correct an acid-base imbalance.
9. Discuss the steps in managing an intravenous infusion.
10. Explain the measures used to prevent the complications of intravenous therapy.
11. Identify intravenous fluids that are isotonic and when they are used.
12. Interpret the principles of intravenous therapy.

Clinical Practice

13. Assess patients for signs of dehydration.
14. Correctly assess for and identify edema and signs of overhydration.
15. Apply knowledge of normal laboratory values to recognize electrolyte imbalances.
16. Perform interventions to correct an electrolyte imbalance.
17. Determine whether a patient has an acid-base imbalance.
18. Implement measures to prevent the complications of intravenous therapy.
19. Compare interventions for the care of a patient receiving total parenteral nutrition with those for a patient undergoing intravenous therapy.

Key Terms

acidosis (ăh-sĭ-DŌ-sĭs, p. 46)
active transport (ĂK-tĭv, p. 34)
aldosterone (ăl-DŎS-tĕr-ōn, p. 32)
alkalosis (ăl-kă-LŌ-sĭs, p. 45)
anion gap (ĂN-ī-ŏn găp, p. 46)
anions (ĂN-ī-ŏnz, p. 41)
antidiuretic hormone (ADH) (ăn-tĭ-dī-ū-RĔT-ĭk HŎR-mōn, p. 32)
ascites (ăh-SĪ-tēz, p. 41)
atrial natriuretic peptide (ANP) (Ā-trē-ăl nā-trē-yū-RĔT-ĭk PĔP-tīd, p. 32)
brain or B-type natriuretic peptide (BNP) (Brān or Bē-tīp nā-trē-yū-RĔT-ĭk PĔP-tīd, p. 32)
carpopedal spasm (KĂR-pō-PĔD-ăl spăzm, p. 45)
cations (KĂT-ī-ŏnz, p. 41)
dehydration (dē-hī-DRĀ-shŭn, p. 35)
diffusion (dĭ-FŪ-zhŭn, p. 32)
edema (ĕh-DĒ-mă, p. 40)
electrolytes (ĕh-LĔK-trō-līts, p. 41)
extracellular (ĕks-tră-SĔL-ū-lăr, p. 31)
filtration (fĭl-TRĀ-shŭn, p. 34)
hydrostatic pressure (hī-drō-STĂ-tĭk PRĔ-shŭr, p. 34)
hypercalcemia (hī-pĕr-kăl-SĒ-mē-ăh, p. 45)
hyperchloremia (hī-pĕr-klŏr-Ē-mē-ăh, p. 46)
hyperkalemia (hī-pĕr-kă-LĒ-mē-ăh, p. 45)
hypermagnesemia (hī-pĕr-măg-nĕ-SĒ-mē-ăh, p. 46)
hypernatremia (hī-pĕr-nā-TRĒ-mē-ăh, p. 41)
hyperphosphatemia (hī-pĕr-fŏs-fă-TĒ-mē-ăh, p. 46)
hypertonic (hī-pĕr-TŎN-ĭk, p. 34)
hyperventilation (hī-pĕr-vĕn-tĭ-LĀ-shŭn, p. 47)
hypervolemia (hī-pĕr-vō-LĒ-mē-ăh, p. 39)
hypocalcemia (hī-pō-kăl-SĒ-mē-ăh, p. 45)
hypochloremia (hī-pō-klŏr-Ē-mē-ăh, p. 46)
hypodermoclysis (hī-pō-dĕrm-ōk-LĪ-sĭs, p. 52)
hypokalemia (hī-pō-kă-LĒ-mē-ăh, p. 44)
hypomagnesemia (hī-pō-măg-nĕ-SĒ-mē-ăh, p. 46)
hyponatremia (hī-pō-nă-TRĒ-mē-ăh, p. 41)
hypophosphatemia (hī-pō-fŏs-făw-TĒ-mē-ăh, p. 46)
hypotonic (hī-pō-TŎN-ĭk, p. 34)
hypoventilation (hī-pō-vĕn-tĭ-LĀ-shŭn, p. 47)
hypovolemia (hī-pō-vō-LĒ-mē-ăh, p. 40)
hypoxemia (hī-pŏk-SĒ-mē-ăh, p. 50)
insensible (ĭn-sen(t)-sĕ-bĕl, p. 34)
interstitial (ĭn-tĕr-STĬSH-ăl, p. 32)
intracellular (ĭn-tră-SĔL-ū-lăr, p. 31)
intravascular (ĭn-tră-VĂS-cū-lăr, p. 32)

ions (ī-ŏnz, p. 32)
isotonic (ī-sō-TŎN-ĭk, p. 34)
ketoacidosis (kē-tō-ă-sĭ-DŌ-sĭs, p. 49)
osmolality (ŏz-mō-LĂ-lĭ-tē, p. 32)
osmosis (ŏz-MŌ-sĭs, p. 34)
stridor (STRĪ-dŏr, p. 50)
tetany (TĔT-ă-nē, p. 45)
transcellular (trăns-SĔ-lū-lăr, p. 32)
turgor (TŬR-gŏr, p. 35)

Concepts Covered in This Chapter

- Fluids and Electrolytes
- Acid-Base Balance

More than half of the human body's weight is water. Throughout life there is a gradual decline in the amount of body water. An infant's body is approximately 77% water, and an older adult's body is about 45% water. Women's bodies have less water than men's. **The older adult and the very young are more likely to experience severe consequences with even minor changes in their fluid balance.** Fatty tissue does not contain as much water as other tissues; thus the greater the amount of fat in the body, the less the percentage of body water. Maintaining a healthy weight is important in regulating the body's percentage of water. Keeping body fluids within a normal range is especially necessary because for every cell of every organ, life processes take place within fluid. The nutrients needed for life, reproduction, and the normal functioning of a cell must be dissolved or suspended in water, and the largest part of each cell is fluid. For all of the cell's life processes to take place, there must be a continuous exchange of water, glucose, oxygen, nutrients, electrolytes, and waste products. Water in the body has four main functions:

1. Be a vehicle for the transportation of substances to and from the cells
2. Aid heat regulation by providing perspiration, which evaporates and cools the body
3. Assist in the maintenance of hydrogen (H^+) balance in the body
4. Serve as a medium for the enzymatic action of digestion

Table 3.1 shows sources of water and avenues of a body's water loss.

DISTRIBUTION AND REGULATION OF BODY FLUIDS

PATHOPHYSIOLOGY

Body fluids are continually in motion, moving in and out of the blood and lymph vessels, through the spaces surrounding the cells, and through the bodies of the cells themselves. Fluid within the cell is considered to be in one compartment (**intracellular**) and fluid outside the cell in another (**extracellular**) (Fig. 3.1). The three types of extracellular fluid (ECF) and body fluid distribution

Table 3.1 Sources of Water and Avenues of Water Loss

SOURCE	24 HOURS (AVERAGE INTAKE)	AVENUE OF LOSS	AMOUNT OF LOSS (AVERAGE OUTPUT)
Oral fluids	1500 mL	Urine	1500 mL
Food	800 mL	Perspiration	400 mL
Metabolism	200 mL	Feces	200 mL
		Expired air	400 mL
Total	**2500 mL**		**2500 mL**

Modified from Williams P: *deWit's fundamental concepts and skills for nursing*, ed 5, Philadelphia, 2018, Elsevier.

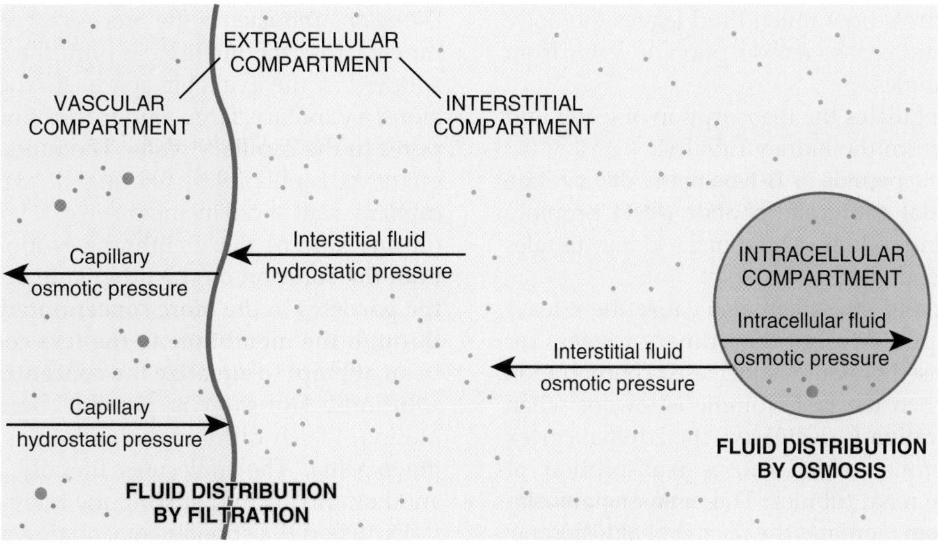

Fig. 3.1 Factors that influence body fluid distribution.

Box 3.1 Body Fluid Distribution

EXTRACELLULAR FLUID (OUTSIDE OF CELLS)
- Approximately one third of total body water
- Transports water, nutrients, oxygen, waste, etc., to and from the cells
- Regulated by renal, metabolic, and neurologic factors
- High in sodium (Na^+) content

Intravascular Fluid
- Fluid within the blood vessels
- Consists of plasma and fluid within blood cells
- Contains large amounts of protein and electrolytes

Interstitial Fluid
- Fluid in the spaces surrounding the cells
- High in Na^+ content

Transcellular Fluid
- Includes aqueous humor; saliva; cerebrospinal, pleural, peritoneal, synovial, and pericardial fluids; gastrointestinal secretions; and fluid in the urinary system and lymphatics

INTRACELLULAR FLUID (WITHIN CELLS)
- About two thirds of total body fluid
- Fluid contained within the cell walls; most cell walls are permeable to water
- High in potassium (K^+) content

Modified from Williams P: *Fundamental concepts and skills for nursing,* ed 5, Philadelphia, 2018, Elsevier.

are shown in Box 3.1. Excretion of the body's fluid is achieved mainly through the kidney, with some loss in stool. Control of fluid balance is managed by the following:

- **Osmoreceptors** in the hypothalamus sense the internal environment (ratio of fluid to solutes) and promote the intake of fluid (thirst mechanism) when needed.
- **Baroreceptors** in the carotid sinus and aortic arch detect pressure changes that indicate an increase or decrease in blood volume and stimulate the sympathetic or parasympathetic nervous system to return the pressure to normal.
- **Antidiuretic hormone (ADH)**, released by the posterior pituitary, controls how much fluid leaves the body in the urine and causes reabsorption of water from the kidney tubules.
- **Aldosterone** regulates the reabsorption of water and sodium ions from the kidney tubules.
- **Brain natriuretic peptide** or **B-type natriuretic peptide (BNP)** and **atrial natriuretic peptide (ANP)** promote loss of water and sodium ions from the kidney tubules and cause vasodilatation.

Pain, nausea, and stress can also cause the release of ADH by the pituitary, but the primary triggers for release are decreased pressure or increased concentration of the blood. When the ECF volume is low, or when sodium concentration is decreased, the adrenal cortex releases aldosterone, which causes reabsorption of sodium from the renal tubules. The **renin-angiotensin-aldosterone system** regulates the release of aldosterone. Renin is released when there is decreased blood flow to the kidney. Baroreceptors in the atrium of the heart detect fluid overload and stimulate the myocardium to release ANP. ANP helps protect the body from fluid overload by increasing sodium excretion. Where sodium goes, water follows. If the ventricles are stretched with volume, BNP is released and is a stronger diuretic than ANP.

To be normally distributed within the body, water and the substances suspended or dissolved in water must move from compartment to compartment. As blood flows through the capillaries, fluid and solutes can move into the **interstitial** spaces, where the cells of the body can exchange nutrients and wastes. Several processes accomplish the movement of fluids, electrolytes, nutrients, and waste products back and forth across the cell membranes (Fig. 3.2). Assessment of fluid balance is primarily achieved through monitoring of the **intravascular** space and external signs and symptoms of too much or too little fluid. Labs are drawn and blood pressure is assessed in the vasculature. Intracellular, interstitial, and **transcellular** fluids are not accessible for testing or measuring, which is why weight is used to monitor total body water.

OSMOLALITY

Nonelectrolyte solutes include protein, urea, glucose, creatinine, and bilirubin. Along with the electrolytes, these solutes contribute to the **osmolality** (concentration of the solution determined by the number of solutes in it) of the body fluid. Osmolality controls water movement and the body fluid distribution in the intracellular and extracellular compartments. Potassium maintains the osmolality of the intracellular fluid (ICF). Sodium controls the osmolality of the ECF. Normal osmolality of body fluids is 280 to 294 milliosmoles per kilogram (mOsm/kg) (Fig. 3.3).

MOVEMENT OF FLUID AND ELECTROLYTES

Passive Transport

Diffusion. **Diffusion** is the process by which substances move across the membrane until they are evenly distributed in the available space. As the plasma moves along a capillary, large amounts of fluid filter through pores in the capillary walls. The fluid moves into and out of the capillaries by filtering through the permeable capillary wall or cell membrane walls. **When the solution on one side of the membrane is more concentrated than the solution on the other side of the membrane, the particles in the more concentrated solution travel through the membrane to the less concentrated side in an attempt to equalize the concentration of the two solutions.** Diffusion is possible because of **kinetic** motion, which diffuses the molecules in the ICF and the plasma. The molecules literally bounce off one another, mixing and stirring the body fluids.

Diffusion is a spontaneous mixing and moving that allows the exchange of molecules, **ions** (electrically

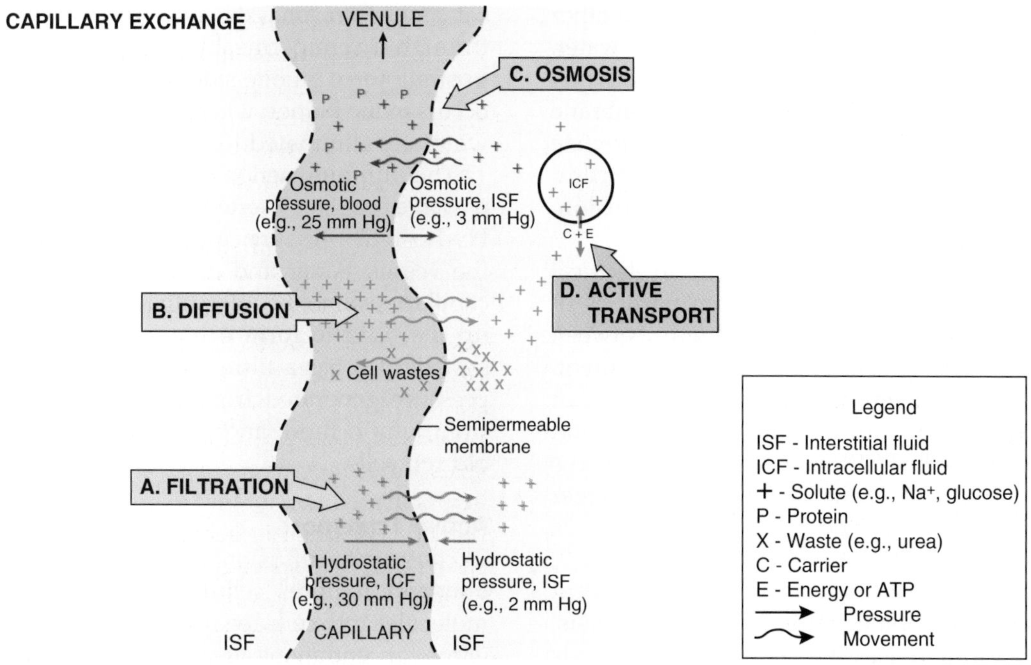

Fig. 3.2 Movement of water and electrolytes between compartments. (From Hubert RJ, VanMeter KC: *Gould's pathophysiology for health professions,* ed 6, St. Louis, 2018, Elsevier.)

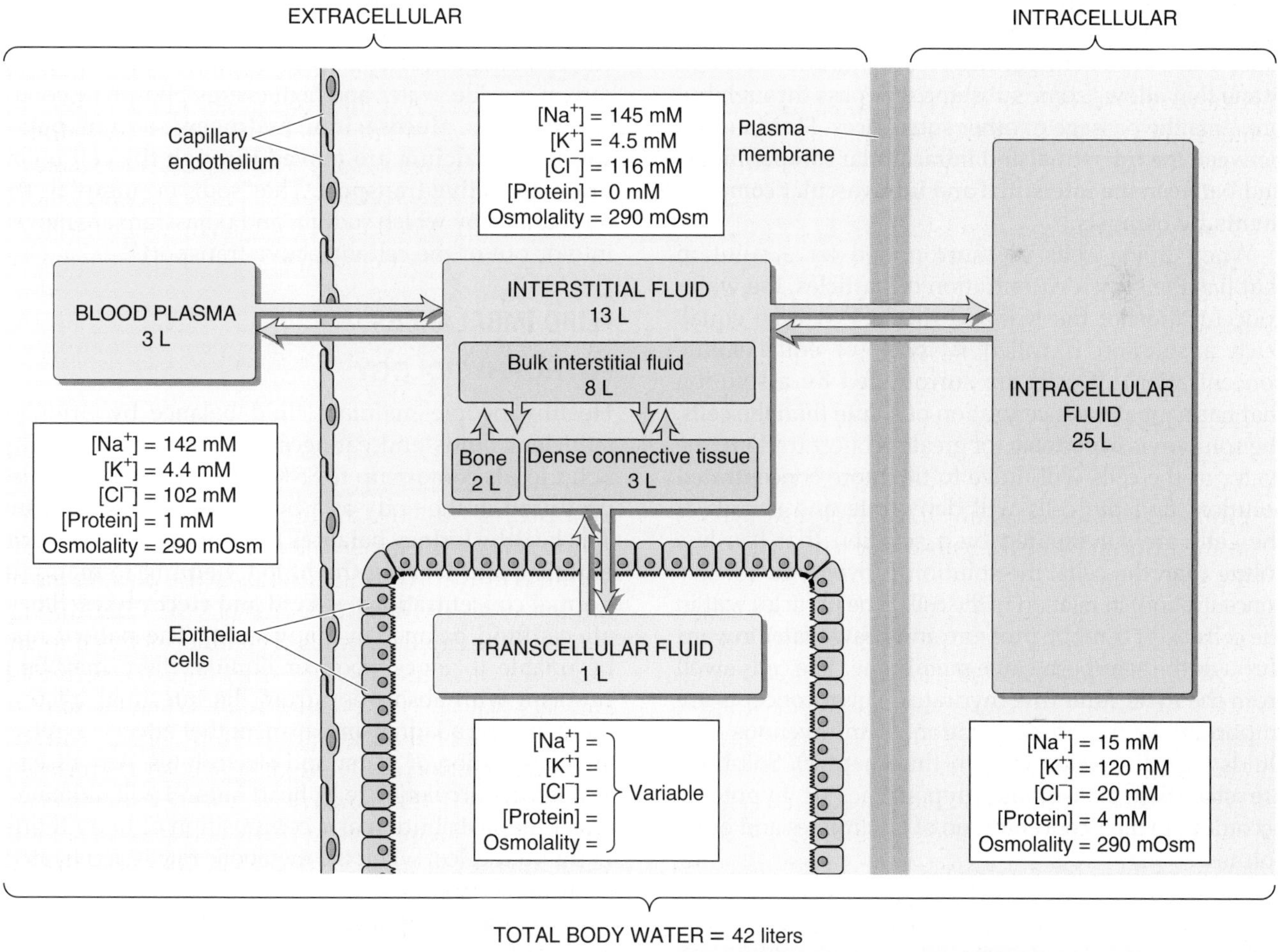

Fig. 3.3 The fluid compartments of a prototypic adult human weighing 70 kg. Total body water is divided into four major compartments: intracellular fluid (green), interstitial fluid (blue), blood plasma (red), and transcellular water such as synovial fluid (tan). Color codes for each of these compartments are maintained throughout this book. (From Boron WF, Boulpaep EL: *Medical physiology*, ed 3, Philadelphia, 2017, Elsevier.)

charged particles), cellular nutrients, wastes, and other substances dissolved or suspended in body water. Substances will move from a high to a low concentration until the concentration on both sides of the membrane is equal. This is called *movement down a concentration gradient.* **Glucose, oxygen, carbon dioxide, water, and other small ions and molecules move by diffusion, which is a process of equalization.**

Diffusion may occur by movement along an electrical gradient as well. The attraction between particles of opposite charge and the repellent action between particles of like charge create an electrical gradient. Many intracellular proteins have a negative charge that tends to attract the positively charged sodium and potassium ions from the ECF. The ions will diffuse across the membrane until there is a balance of electrical charges on each side of the membrane.

Osmosis. **Osmosis** is the movement of pure solvent (liquid) across a membrane. **Water moves by osmosis.** When there are differences in concentration of fluids in the various compartments, osmotic pressure (what holds fluid in the vascular space) will move water from the area of lesser concentration of solutes to the area of greater concentration until the solutions in the compartments are of equal concentration. The process takes place via a **semipermeable membrane**—a membrane that allows some substances to pass through but prevents the passage of other substances. **Fluid moves between the interstitial and intracellular compartments and between the interstitial and intravascular compartments by osmosis.**

When living cells are surrounded by a solution that has the same concentration of particles, the water concentration of the ICF and the ECF will be equal. Such a solution is called **isotonic** (of equal solute concentration). If cells are surrounded by a solution that has a greater concentration of solute than the cells, the solution is **hypertonic** (of greater concentration), the water in the cells will move to the more concentrated solution, and the cells will dehydrate and shrink. If the cells are surrounded by a solution that has less solute than the cells, the solution is **hypotonic** (of less concentration) in relation to the cells. The particles within the cells exert osmotic pressure and draw water inward through the semipermeable membrane. The cells swell from the extra fluid (overhydrate). These concepts are important to the administration of intravenous (IV) fluids (see discussion later in this chapter). Solutions are classified as isotonic, hypertonic, or hypotonic according to their concentration of electrolytes and other solutes.

? Think Critically

Describe to a classmate the difference between osmosis and diffusion.

Filtration. **Filtration** is the movement of water and solutes through a semipermeable membrane as a result of a pushing force on one side of the membrane. Filtration occurs in the kidney, where waste substances and excess water are eliminated.

The pumping action of the heart creates **hydrostatic pressure** (pressure exerted by fluid) within the capillaries. Hydrostatic pressure causes fluid to press outward on the vessel. Water and electrolytes move through the capillary wall to the interstitial fluid. The nephrons pick up the fluid to form urine for excretion. The lymph system also has a filtration role using the hydrostatic pressure generated from the heart. It filters bacteria from lymph fluid, and the spleen filters the blood of old red cells.

Active Transport

In contrast to diffusion, osmosis, and filtration, **active transport** requires cellular energy, which can move molecules into cells regardless of their electrical charge or the concentrations already in the cell. **Active transport may move substances from an area of lower concentration to an area of higher concentration.** The energy source for the process is adenosine triphosphate (ATP). ATP is produced during the complex metabolic processes in the body's cells. Enzyme reactions metabolize carbon chains of sugars, fatty acids, and amino acids, yielding carbon dioxide, water, and high-energy phosphate bonds. **Amino acids, glucose, iron, hydrogen, sodium, potassium, and calcium are moved through the cell membrane by active transport.** The "sodium pump" is the mechanism by which sodium and potassium are moved into or out of the cell via active transport.

FLUID IMBALANCES

PATHOPHYSIOLOGY

Healthy people maintain fluid balance by drinking sufficient fluids and eating a balanced diet each day. Solid foods contain up to 85% water, and water is also produced in the body as a by-product of metabolism. **The healthy kidney balances the amount of substances entering and leaving the blood, helping to maintain normal concentrations of fluid and electrolytes.** Illness affects fluid balance in many ways. The patient may be unable to ingest food or liquids, there may be a problem with absorption from the intestinal tract, or there may be a kidney impairment that affects excretion or reabsorption of water and electrolytes. Any disease that affects circulation (e.g., heart failure) will ultimately affect the distribution and composition of body fluids. Extra fluid is lost when the metabolic rate is accelerated, such as occurs in fever, thyroid crisis, burns, severe trauma, and states of extreme stress. Perspiration can account for a fluid loss of up to 2 L/h in an adult. For every degree of fever on the Celsius scale, an **insensible** (unaware of) water loss of 10% may occur. Perspiration and water lost in respiration are insensible losses. When the weather is hot and dry, water loss from the body is greater. Patients on mechanical ventilators, those with rapid respirations, and those with severe diarrhea or excessive amounts of fistula drainage also lose greater quantities of water. **Any seriously ill patient is at risk for a fluid and electrolyte imbalance.**

A fluid imbalance exists when there is an excess (too much) or a deficit (too little) of water in the body. When this occurs, there will be an accompanying imbalance in the substances dissolved in body water. When considering sodium imbalances, **it is important to remember that water follows sodium in the body, through osmosis.** The sodium concentration causes an osmotic pull, and water will go to where the sodium concentration is highest.

Think Critically

Give an example of active transport taking place within the body.

DEFICIENT FLUID VOLUME

Patients at risk for deficient fluid volume are those who are unable to take in sufficient quantities of fluid because of impaired swallowing, extreme weakness, disorientation or coma, or the unavailability of water and those who lose excessive amounts of fluid through prolonged vomiting, diarrhea, hemorrhage, diaphoresis (sweating), excessive wound drainage, or diuretic therapy.

When a fluid deficit occurs, water moves from the cells into the interstitial and intravascular spaces. This movement of water out of the cells causes **dehydration** of the cells. Dehydration is treated by administering fluid orally, intravenously, or through feeding or gastrectomy tubes. For patients who will be unable to take in fluids or food on their own for an extended period, a feeding tube must be placed or total parenteral nutrition (TPN) started (see Chapter 29). Signs and symptoms of dehydration are presented in Box 3.2. **Turgor** (degree of elasticity) is checked by gently pinching up the skin over the abdomen, forearm, sternum, forehead, clavicle, or thigh (Fig. 3.4). In a person with normal fluid balance, the pinched skin will immediately fall back to normal when released. If a fluid deficit is present, the skin may remain elevated or tented for several seconds. However, because pinching the skin to measure fluid deficit also measures skin elasticity, this test is not a valid indicator of fluid status in older adults, whose skin is often inelastic and routinely tents when pinched. In infants, dehydration is evident by sunken fontanels.

Clinical Cues

The most accurate measure of fluid gain or loss for any age group is weight change. A weight gain or loss of 2.2 lb (1 kg) in 24 hours indicates a gain or loss of 1 L of fluid.

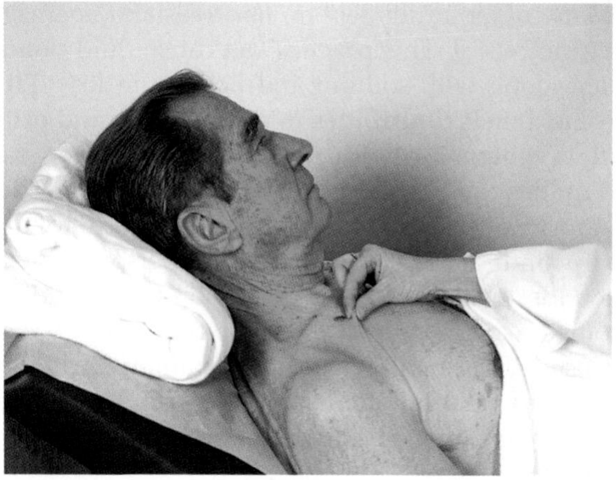

Fig. 3.4 Testing tissue turgor. (From Jarvis C: *Physical examination and health assessment*, ed 7, St. Louis, 2016, Elsevier.)

Box 3.2 Signs and Symptoms of Dehydration and Overhydration

SIGNS AND SYMPTOMS OF DEHYDRATION

- Thirst
- Poor skin turgor
- Weight loss
- Weakness
- Complaints of dizziness
- Postural hypotension
- Decreased urine production
- Dark, concentrated urine
- Dry, cracked lips and tongue
- Dry mucous membranes
- Sunken, soft eyeballs
- Thick saliva
- Dry, scaly skin
- Flat neck veins when lying down
- Rapid, weak, thready pulse
- Elevated temperature ≥100.6° F (38.1° C)
- Increased hematocrit
- High urine specific gravity with low volume

SIGNS AND SYMPTOMS OF OVERHYDRATION

- Weight gain
- Slow, bounding pulse
- Elevated blood pressure
- Firm subcutaneous tissues
- Possibly edema
- Possibly crackles in lungs on auscultation
- Lethargy, possibly seizures
- Possibly visible neck veins when lying down
- Decreased serum sodium
- Decreased hematocrit from hemodilution
- Low urine specific gravity with high volume

Older Adult Care Points

Fluid volume deficit is a common problem in older adults. There is an age-related decline in total body water and a decrease in thirst sensation and taste that causes older adults to become dehydrated more easily. If urinary incontinence is a problem, the person becomes reluctant to drink extra fluids. Thirst is a late sign of dehydration in older adults.

Many older adults rely on laxatives and enemas to clear the bowel. This practice can cause fluid volume deficit along with sodium and potassium loss. **Fluid volume deficit contributes to constipation and orthostatic hypotension with related dizziness and falls and makes the person more susceptible to infection.**

A furrowed, dry tongue that is not the result of drug therapy indicates a fluid deficit. If the person has fever, this adds to the fluid loss. Because of the fluid and accompanying electrolyte losses, the person may become confused. Offering the patient small amounts of liquid and electrolyte solution frequently—if fluid can be kept down—helps prevent additional problems.

Clinical Cues

Measure the blood pressure and pulse in the lying, sitting, and standing positions. A systolic blood pressure drop of 20 mm Hg accompanied by a pulse rate increase of 10 beats per minute (bpm) at 1 minute after the position change suggests a fluid volume deficit. This is called *orthostatic* or *postural hypotension.*

Nursing Management

Provide an adequate fluid intake for those who are unable to do this for themselves. Include the patient's preferences for liquids on the plan of care. The patient should receive fruit juices, bouillon, and any other nutritious liquid tolerated (Nursing Care Plan 3.1).

A common cause of excessive fluid loss is abnormally rapid excretion of intestinal fluids, such as occurs from vomiting and diarrhea.

Assignment Considerations

Increasing Fluid Intake

If a nursing assistant or unlicensed assistive personnel (UAP) is available to assist, *assign* the task of increasing a patient's fluid intake to that person. Work out a timed plan to help the patient with regular, periodic intake of fluids by mouth. Ask that the patient drink 4 oz of fluid every hour. Advise of any safety precautions regarding difficulty swallowing or need for assistance.

Think Critically

Why is it important to the body's function to administer fluid and electrolytes during a fever?

NAUSEA AND VOMITING

Nausea is a feeling of discomfort or an unpleasant sensation vaguely felt in the epigastrium and abdomen. It is a symptom of illness and is often accompanied by vomiting. Nausea is experienced when nerve endings in the stomach and other parts of the body are irritated. Irritated nerve endings in the stomach send messages to the part of the brain that controls the vomiting reflex; however, nerve cells in other parts of the body can trigger the same response. Pain can trigger the nausea-vomiting mechanism. Nausea and vomiting are automatic responses of the involuntary autonomic nervous system to unpleasant stimuli.

Complementary and Alternative Therapies

Preventing Nausea

Sea bands (acupressure wristbands) are very helpful to many people who suffer from nausea and vomiting. They are available at most drugstores. Ginger tea and ginger ale are other alternative therapies that have proven helpful, as are small pieces of ginger candy.

Nausea and vomiting may occur from gastrointestinal (GI) irritation from foods, viruses, radiation of the mucosa, and some drugs and other chemicals. Certain types of anesthetics may trigger nausea, as may pregnancy.

The patient may complain of nausea or feeling "sick to my stomach," queasiness, abdominal pain, epigastric discomfort or burning, and vomiting. The patient may also exhibit pallor; mild diaphoresis; cold, clammy skin; or excessive salivation and may attempt to remain quiet and motionless. **If vomiting occurs, the vomitus should be observed for odor, color, contents (e.g., undigested food), and amount.** Noting and recording vomiting patterns, conditions that trigger vomiting, and quality of nausea as described by the patient can be helpful in planning treatment.

Medical treatment for nausea consists of administering one of the antiemetic drugs (Table 3.2). Antihistamines, sedatives and hypnotics, anticholinergics, phenothiazines, and other drugs are used to control nausea and vomiting. The patient is given nothing by mouth (kept NPO) until vomiting has stopped; afterward, the patient is allowed clear liquids, progressing slowly to a regular diet. Ice chips or sips of carbonated drinks at first are usually tolerated well.

Nursing Management

Have the patient lie down and turn the head to one side, or have the patient sit and lower the head between their legs so that vomitus is not aspirated into the respiratory tract. Hold an emesis basin or bag close to the side of the face. Use a cool, damp washcloth to wipe the patient's face and the back of the neck. Have the patient breathe through the mouth. Provide mouth care after the episode. Sucking on ice chips helps reduce nausea in some patients. A quiet, cool, odor-free environment helps calm nausea. If nausea and vomiting persist, observe for dehydration. Any fluid loss through the GI tract—vomiting or diarrhea—can cause hypokalemia and hyponatremia.

Nursing Care Plan 3.1 Care of the Patient With Deficient Fluid Volume

SCENARIO

Mrs. Cabot, age 78, is admitted to the hospital after 3 days of vomiting and diarrhea. She is confused, disoriented, dehydrated, and very weak.

PROBLEM STATEMENT/NURSING DIAGNOSIS

Fluid volume deficit related to fluid loss and inability to take in sufficient fluids.

SUPPORTING ASSESSMENT DATA

Subjective: Hx of vomiting and diarrhea for 3 days; unable to keep anything in stomach. Had eaten food at a church picnic on a hot day.

Objective: Furrowed tongue, tenting of skin on sternum, thick saliva, and dry mucous membranes; 3-lb weight loss from normal. Urine sp. gr. 1.030; scant urine; temp. 101.4° F (40° C). Na^+ = 160 mEq/L

Goals/Expected Outcomes	Nursing Interventions	Selected Rationale	Evaluation*
Diarrhea and vomiting will stop within 24 h.	Medicate with antiemetic and antidiarrheal as ordered.	Antiemetic should stop vomiting and antidiarrheal should limit fluid loss through stool.	Ondansetron (Zofran) 4 mg is given IV. Has not vomited in last hour.
	Reduce odors in room to decrease nausea.	Odors contribute to nausea.	No odor in room.
	Offer mouth care after vomiting and at least q2h.	Mouth care promotes comfort and reduces nausea.	Mouth care provided.
	When vomiting stops, administer medication for diarrhea as ordered.	Medication will slow or stop the diarrhea. Antidiarrheals are given orally.	Took diphenoxylate/atropine tab with a sip of Gatorade.
No skin breakdown due to frequent stooling.	Keep patient clean and dry.	Prevents skin breakdown.	No open skin areas.
	Provide assistance to bathroom as needed.	Assistance helps prevent falls in weak patients.	Assistance provided ×4.
	Protect perianal skin with ointment as ordered.	A barrier cream or ointment will protect the perianal skin from excoriation from diarrhea.	Perianal skin slightly reddened.
Fluid balance will be reestablished within 72 h.	Monitor IV site and fluid every hour. Initiate IV therapy as ordered.	IV therapy will replenish fluids and electrolytes in the body.	IV fluids infusing. Site clean, dry without redness.
	Initiate I&O recording.	I&O record provides data to determine degree of fluid imbalance.	Two liquid stools. Continue plan.
	When able to take PO fluids, offer sips of electrolyte solution, and progress to a clear liquid diet.	Small sips of fluid are easier to keep in the stomach. Electrolyte solution replenishes low electrolytes.	Taking sips of a sports drink designed to replenish carbohydrates and electrolytes.
	Monitor mucous membrane status and skin turgor.	Provides data about rehydration status.	Mucous membranes more moist.
	Weigh daily.	Weight is the most accurate measurement of total body water.	Same weight as on admission.
	Monitor electrolyte values.	Provides data about electrolyte imbalances.	Laboratory results not back yet. Continue plan.

CRITICAL THINKING QUESTIONS

1. What would be other concerns that should be addressed in her care plan?
2. What do you think is the cause of her confusion and disorientation?

*Evaluation data must be documented in the medical record.
Hx, History; *I&O,* intake and output; *IV,* intravenous; *PO,* oral; *q2h,* every 2 hours; *sp. gr.,* specific gravity; *temp.,* temperature.

Table 3.2 Drugs Commonly Prescribed to Treat Vomiting and Diarrhea

CLASSIFICATION	ACTION	NURSING IMPLICATIONS	PATIENT TEACHING
Antiemetics			
Hydroxyzine (Vistaril, Atarax) Promethazine (Phenergan)	Antihistamine-antiemetic used to stop nausea and vomiting Depresses the central nervous system (CNS)	Give by Z-track injection. Never give IV (except promethazine) or subcutaneously. Monitor vital signs. Check compatibility before mixing with other drugs. Monitor for dizziness and hypotension. Observe for urinary retention.	Avoid concurrent alcohol ingestion or other CNS depressants. Avoid activities that require alertness. Raise patient slowly to prevent dizziness. Avoid prolonged sunlight.
Prochlorperazine maleate (Compazine)	Blocks chemoreceptor trigger zone, which in turn acts on vomiting center Stops nausea and vomiting	Monitor vital signs and for respiratory depression, especially in older adults. Check compatibilities before mixing with other drugs. Watch for seizures, muscle stiffness, and other negative reactions.	Avoid hazardous activities; avoid alcohol and other CNS depressants. Advise urine may be pink to reddish brown. Avoid the sun or use sunscreen and protective clothing. Report bleeding, rash, bruising, blurred vision, or clay-colored stools.
Ondansetron (Zofran)	Blocks serotonin peripherally, centrally, and in the small intestine	Monitor for extrapyramidal signs (shuffling gait, tremors, grimacing, rigidity). Observe for rash or bronchospasm.	Report diarrhea, constipation, rash, change in respiration, or discomfort at IV insertion site.
Metoclopramide (Reglan, Metozolv)	Decreases reflux, stimulates stomach emptying, and raises threshold of chemoreceptor trigger zone	Monitor for extrapyramidal symptoms with IV administration. Assess for rash. Monitor renal function, blood pressure, and heart rate.	Report involuntary eye, facial, or limb movements. Avoid alcohol.
Antidiarrheals			
Diphenoxylate atropine (Lomotil)	Slows intestinal motility. Slows or stops diarrhea.	Assess bowel pattern and monitor for constipation. Discontinue if not effective after 2 days of treatment.	Do not use alcohol or CNS depressants. Do not exceed the prescribed dosage. May be habit forming. Avoid hazardous activities.
Loperamide HCl (Imodium)	Works on intestinal muscles to decrease peristalsis; reduces volume and increases stool bulk Slows or stops diarrhea	Monitor stools and for electrolyte imbalances. Monitor for dehydration. Discontinue if not effective after 2 days of treatment.	Drowsiness may occur; do not operate machinery. Do not take other over-the-counter preparations.
Kaolin-pectin (Kaopectate)	Decreases gastric motility and water content of stool; acts as absorbent and demulcent	Monitor bowel pattern. Monitor for dehydration and electrolyte imbalances.	Do not exceed recommended dosage. Shake suspension well. Take other medications 2 h before or after administration.
Bismuth subsalicylate (Pepto-Bismol)	Inhibits prostaglandin synthesis responsible for gastrointestinal hypermotility; stimulates absorption of fluid and electrolytes Prevents or stops diarrhea	Monitor bowel pattern. Do not give to children younger than 3 yr.	Shake liquid before using. The tongue may darken and stools may turn black. Do not take other salicylates along with this medication. Stop taking if diarrhea has not stopped in 2 days.
Camphorated opium tincture (paregoric)	Opiate that acts to decrease intestinal motility	Controlled substance. Addictive with long-term use. Monitor bowel function. May cause nausea and vomiting.	Do not exceed prescribed dosage. Causes CNS depression; do not operate machinery.

Older Adult Care Points

Older patients must be rehydrated cautiously. Any patient who has a cardiac problem is at risk for fluid overload from IV infusions. If fluid is infused too fast, it can cause the patient to go into heart failure. **If an IV infusion falls behind, do not make up for lost time by infusing fluid at a rate faster than ordered.**

DIARRHEA

Diarrhea is defined as the rapid movement of fecal matter through the intestine. Frequent, watery bowel movements; abdominal cramping; and general weakness characterize diarrhea. Diarrheic watery stools often contain mucus and are blood streaked. It is the consistency rather than the number of stools per day that is the hallmark of diarrhea. In some cases the number can be as high as 15 to 20 liquid stools. If the condition is chronic, the patient can suffer from dehydration, malnutrition, and anemia. During diarrhea, patients absorb nutrients poorly and lose water and electrolytes. These electrolytic substances—especially the potassium needed by the body to prevent alkalosis—are lost in large amounts by patients with diarrhea.

Most diarrhea is related to local irritation of the intestinal mucosa, especially irritation caused by infectious agents such as *Salmonella, Clostridium difficile,* and *Escherichia coli*. Other irritants include chemicals and foods. Chronic and prolonged diarrhea is typical of such disorders as ulcerative colitis, irritable bowel syndrome, allergies, lactose intolerance, and nontropical sprue. Gluten intolerance is recognized to cause GI disorders, and sensitivity to gluten includes alternate bouts of diarrhea and constipation in its list of symptoms. Obstruction to the flow of intestinal contents, such as from a tumor or a fecal impaction, also can produce diarrhea when only the liquid components can pass the obstruction.

To rest the intestines and stomach of a patient with acute diarrhea, limit the intake of foods. Once oral feedings are allowed, begin clear liquids and progress to bland liquids and then solid foods of increased calories and high-protein, high-carbohydrate content. Give rehydrating solutions containing glucose and electrolytes first. **Avoid iced fluids, carbonated drinks, whole milk, roughage, raw fruits, and highly seasoned foods.**

Medications prescribed for diarrhea depend on the cause of the disorder and the length of time the condition has been present (see Table 3.2). Mild cases usually respond well to over-the-counter medications such as kaolin and bismuth preparations (e.g., Kaopectate), which coat the intestinal tract and make the stools firmer. Bismuth subsalicylate (e.g., Pepto-Bismol) is the recommended treatment for "traveler's diarrhea"; when given in advance of travel, bismuth subsalicylate may prevent this type of diarrhea. Diarrhea caused by infections may be treated with drugs that are specific for the causative organism. Depending on the organism responsible, it is sometimes advisable to allow the toxins to be eliminated naturally from the body, so drugs may not be given initially. Bowel sounds are likely to be gurgling and tinkling sounds that come in waves and are hyperactive. Note and record the bowel sounds and number of stools during the shift and the characteristics of each stool and any associated pain.

Think Critically

If a patient has food poisoning and suffers from vomiting and diarrhea, what type of fluid and electrolyte imbalance may the patient develop?

Nursing Management

Nursing measures for diarrhea aim to provide physical and mental rest, prevent unnecessary loss of water and nutrients, protect the rectal mucosa, and eventually replace lost fluids. Diarrhea can be associated with nervous tension and anxiety. The patient often is embarrassed by the condition and inconvenienced by frequent trips to the bathroom or the need to request a bedpan. This emotional stress only serves to make the condition worse. Help the patient's anxiety by maintaining a calm and dignified manner, accepting and understanding the patient's behavior, and providing privacy and a restful environment for the patient.

Think Critically

How would you assess a patient with diarrhea for signs of dehydration?

EXCESS FLUID VOLUME

An excessive amount of body water usually occurs first in the extracellular compartment because this is where water enters and leaves the body. When people become ill, they may receive more water than they excrete, which can happen if they receive IV fluid too quickly or are persuaded to drink more fluids than they can eliminate. These situations lead to fluid volume excess, and the patient is likely to develop **water intoxication.**

Impaired elimination, such as occurs in renal failure, is a major cause of fluid volume excess (see Box 3.2). An objective measure of water excess and circulatory overload is the hematocrit. The hematocrit measures the percentage of red blood cells in a volume of whole blood. When fluid volume excess occurs, **hypervolemia** (excessive blood volume) may also occur. Hypervolemia elevates blood pressure.

Clinical Cues

Normal hematocrit values range from 35 to 54 mL of red blood cells per 100 mL of whole blood, depending on age and sex. If there is an excess of water, the proportion of red blood cells to milliliters of blood will be lower, and the hematocrit will be below the normal values because of dilution by the water.

Urine concentration provides another clue to the fluid status. Urine concentration is commonly measured by specific gravity and compared with the specific gravity of distilled water, which is 1.000. Urine contains urea, electrolytes, and other substances, so its specific gravity will exceed 1.000 and ranges between 1.003 and 1.030. The average range is 1.010 to 1.025.

Edema

Edema is associated with the retention of water, sodium, and chloride and is defined as an accumulation of freely moving interstitial fluid (fluid surrounding cells). Look for puffy eyelids and swollen hands. Edema also can occur in body cavities, as in the peritoneal cavity (ascites) and the cranial cavity. The accumulation of body fluids can affect almost all tissue spaces (*generalized edema*). Alternatively, fluid accumulation can affect a limited area (*localized edema*). Generalized edema occurs when the body's mechanisms for eliminating excess sodium fail or there is a decrease in substances in the bloodstream that normally would hold fluid in the vascular space. Edema becomes life-threatening when accumulated fluids overload the circulatory system, as in congestive heart failure, and when fluids accumulate in the lungs, as in pulmonary edema.

Four general causes of edema are (1) an increase in capillary hydrostatic pressure, (2) a loss of plasma proteins, (3) an obstruction of lymphatic circulation, and (4) an increase in capillary permeability.

Increased hydrostatic pressure causes pulmonary edema. A loss of plasma proteins decreases osmotic pressure in the vascular system, causing fluid to leak from the vessels, leading to edema. A tumor or infection can damage a lymph node, or lymph nodes may be removed during cancer surgery. Lymph nodes can also be nonfunctional related to congenital causes. Regardless of the reason for lymph node dysfunction or absence, lymph may accumulate in the tissues, resulting in **lymphedema**.

When an inflammatory response or infection occurs, histamine and other chemical mediators are released from the cells involved in the tissue injury. These chemicals cause increased capillary permeability, and more fluid moves into the interstitial spaces. Proteins leak into the interstitial spaces also, decreasing the osmotic pressure in the capillaries. Protein in the interstitial spaces holds fluid there rather than moving that fluid back into the capillaries. When fluid shifts from the vascular space (from the plasma) to the interstitial space, dehydration and **hypovolemia** (too little blood volume) can occur. The volume responsible for blood pressure and circulation is the fluid in the vascular space. When fluid shifts occur from the vascular space to the interstitial space, tissue edema may be present, but the actual circulating volume may be deficient. The shift of fluid is called *third spacing* and may occur with extensive trauma, burns, peritonitis, intestinal obstruction, nephrosis, sepsis, or cirrhosis of the liver in which there is an increase in capillary hydrostatic pressure or increased capillary membrane permeability.

? Think Critically

What characteristics would you expect to find in a urine specimen from a patient who is dehydrated? How would it differ from a urine specimen from a patient who has a fluid volume excess?

Localized edema often occurs with inflammation. Localized edema usually is nonpitting, does not come and go, and is characterized by tight, shiny skin that is stretched over a hard and red area. Causes of localized edema include trauma, allergies, burns, obstruction of lymph flow, cellulitis, and deep vein thrombosis (DVT).

Dependent edema is noted in the feet, ankles, and lower legs or in the sacral region of patients confined to the bed or chair. Dependent edema is an effect of gravity and therefore can be somewhat relieved by elevating the affected body part 18 inches (or above heart level when possible) and by repositioning the patient frequently. Pitting edema is common in patients with dependent edema. The name is derived from the fact that pressing a fingertip against the swollen tissue can create a pit or depression. **To check for pitting edema, press your thumb into the patient's skin at a bony prominence, such as the tibia or malleolus, and hold for 5 seconds.** If the depression, or "pit," remains for a while after the pressure is released, the patient has pitting edema. Assessing the severity and progress of pitting edema in the feet and ankles (pedal edema) can be done more accurately by rating the findings and comparing assessments from one shift to another (Fig. 3.5).

The scale used for rating pitting edema is:

- 1+ Mild pitting—slight indentation with no perceptible swelling of the leg
- 2+ Moderate pitting—indentation subsides quickly, foot is perceived as mildly swollen
- 3+ Deep pitting—indentation remains for a short time and leg looks swollen
- 4+ Very deep pitting—indentation lasts for a long time and leg is very swollen

Treatment. Treatment of a fluid imbalance involves correcting the underlying cause and assisting the body to rebalance fluid content. For conditions of edema, fluid may be restricted or diuretic drugs may be administered to facilitate excretion of the excess fluid. A diuretic is a drug that prompts the kidneys to increase the excretion of fluid. Bed rest may be ordered to facilitate fluid excretion because the kidneys function best when the body is supine.

A low-sodium diet is initiated. Elastic stockings or sequential compression devices are ordered for foot and leg edema. Intake and output (I&O) recording is requested.

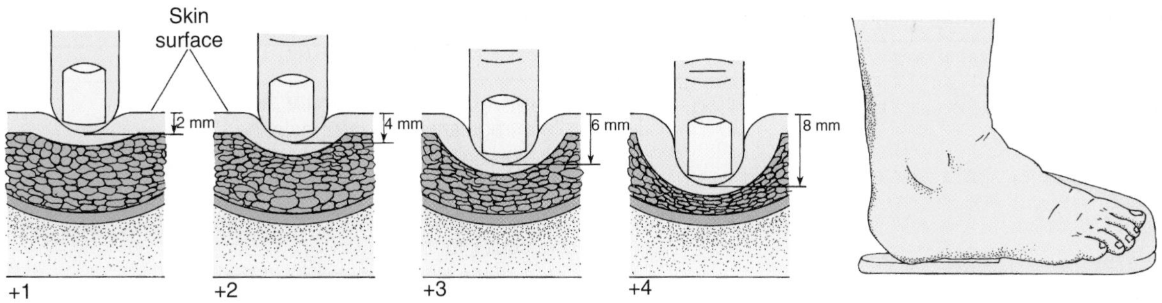

Fig. 3.5 Measuring pedal edema.

> **Think Critically**
>
> Describe the assessments you would make to determine whether your 68-year-old patient is experiencing edema.

HOME CARE

It is important to teach patients with a fluid deficit and their family how to measure fluid I&O and how to keep a log of the amounts. The patient should be encouraged to take small amounts of liquid every hour while awake. If the patient has been vomiting, it is better to let carbonated beverages go flat before drinking them, to decrease stomach distention.

If an older adult has been vomiting considerably for several hours or has had constant diarrhea without fluid intake, a visit to the emergency department is necessary so that IV fluids can be given to prevent serious dehydration.

A patient with fluid excess should be weighed daily and a chart kept. The patient and family should be taught how to assess edema and to record findings. If edema is worsening or weight is increasing, the health care provider should be notified.

> **Think Critically**
>
> Why should you watch for signs of fluid imbalance in any patient who has a serious infection or who has suffered considerable physical trauma?

ELECTROLYTES

Some molecules, when placed in solution, undergo a separation of their atoms into electrically charged ions. These molecules are called **electrolytes** because their atomic particles can conduct an electrical current. The molecules of electrolytes break up into atomic particles that are either negatively charged (**anions**) or positively charged (**cations**). For example, when sodium chloride (table salt) is dissolved in body water, its molecules separate into sodium ions, which are positively charged (Na^+), and chloride ions, which are negatively charged (Cl^-).

Because electrolytes are electrically charged, they are chemically active. This chemical activity allows for the creation of an electrical impulse across the cell membrane, making possible the transmission of nerve impulses, contraction of muscles, and excretion of hormones and other substances from glandular cells. Thus electrolytes are essential to the normal functioning of the body.

ELECTROLYTE IMBALANCES

Electrolytes have many functions in the body. To determine whether there is an electrolyte imbalance, you must know the normal range for each electrolyte (Table 3.3). Many disorders can cause a shift in electrolytes and thus an imbalance—with too much or too little of an electrolyte circulating in the bloodstream or inside the cells of the body.

Sodium Imbalances

Hyponatremia. **Hyponatremia**, a deficit of sodium in the blood (Na^+ <135 mEq/L), is the most common electrolyte imbalance. Hyponatremia can occur from a sodium loss, an inadequate intake of dietary sodium, or an excess of water. Decreased secretion of aldosterone results in sodium loss. Congestive heart failure, liver disease with **ascites** (abnormal accumulation of fluid within the peritoneal cavity), and chronic renal failure result in excessive water retention—without concurrent sodium retention—and this results in hypervolemia combined with hyponatremia. Decreased osmotic pressure in the extracellular compartment may cause a fluid shift into the cells. A decrease in blood pressure may occur. The average intake of sodium is 4 to 5 g/day. The consequence of hyponatremia is impaired nerve conduction. Table 3.4 presents the signs and symptoms, risk factors, and nursing interventions for hyponatremia.

Hypernatremia. **Hypernatremia** occurs when the sodium level rises above 145 mEq/L. Water loss from fever, respiratory infection, or watery diarrhea can cause hypernatremia, but usually impaired thirst or restricted access to water are primary causes. The body tries to correct the situation by conserving water through reabsorption in the renal tubules. Good tissue turgor and firm subcutaneous tissues can be observed during hypernatremia. Hypernatremia causes an osmotic shift of fluid from the cells to the interstitial spaces, causing a cellular dehydration and interruption of normal cell processes. **Sodium intake is restricted for patients with hypernatremia** (see Table 3.4).

Table 3.3 Normal Ranges and Functions of Major Electrolytes

ELECTROLYTE	NORMAL RANGE	SI[a] UNIT	FUNCTION
Sodium (Na^+)	135–145 mEq/L	135–145 mmol/L	**Major cation of the extracellular fluid** Major role in regulation of water balance Regulates extracellular fluid volume through osmotic pressure **Water follows sodium concentration in the body** Essential to the transmission of nerve impulses and helps maintain neuromuscular function Important in controlling contractility of the heart Helps maintain acid-base balance Aids in maintenance of electroneutrality
Potassium (K^+)	3.5–5.0 mEq/L	3.5–5.0 mmol/L	**Major intracellular cation** Important to nerve transmission and muscle contraction Helps maintain normal heart rhythm Helps maintain plasma acid-base balance
Calcium (Ca^{2+})	8.4–10.6 mg/dL	2.10–2.65 mmol/L	Involved in formation of bones and teeth Necessary for blood coagulation Essential for normal nerve and muscle activity
Magnesium (Mg^{2+})	1.3–2.1 mg/dL	0.65–1.05 mmol/L	Necessary for building bones and teeth Necessary for nerve transmission and involved in muscle contraction Plays an important role in many metabolic reactions, where it acts as a cofactor to cellular enzymes
Phosphate (PO_4^-)	3.0–4.5 mg/dL	1.0–1.5 mmol/L	Necessary for formation of adenosine triphosphate (ATP) Cofactor in carbohydrate, protein, and lipid metabolism Activates B-complex vitamins
Chloride (Cl^-)	96–106 mEq/L	96–106 mmol/L	Helps maintain acid-base balance Important to formation of hydrochloric acid for secretion to the stomach Aids in maintaining plasma electroneutrality
Bicarbonate (HCO_3^-)	22–26 mEq/L	23–29 mmol/L	A buffer that neutralizes excess acids in the body Helps regulate acid-base balance Is usually obtained with an arterial blood gas but can be measured in a venous blood gas.

Modified from Williams P: *deWit's fundamental concepts and skills for nursing*, ed 5, Philadelphia, 2018, Elsevier.
[a]International System of Units.

Table 3.4 Electrolyte Imbalances and Nursing Interventions

SERUM VALUE	SIGNS AND SYMPTOMS	CAUSES AND RISK FACTORS	NURSING INTERVENTIONS
Sodium (Normal Range: 135–145 mEq/L)			
Hyponatremia <135 mEq/L	Central nervous system and neuromuscular changes resulting from failure of swollen cells to transmit electrical impulses Fatigue, lethargy, headache, mental confusion, altered level of consciousness, anxiety, coma, anorexia, nausea, vomiting, muscle cramps, seizures, decreased sensation, decreased blood pressure (BP)	Inadequate sodium intake, as in patients on low-sodium diets Excessive intake or retention of water (kidney failure and heart failure) Loss of bile, which is rich in sodium, as a result of fistulas, drainage, gastrointestinal surgery, nausea and vomiting, and suction Loss of sodium through burn wounds Administration of intravenous (IV) fluids that do not contain electrolytes	Restrict water intake as ordered for patients with congestive heart failure, kidney failure, and inadequate antidiuretic hormone production. Liberalize a low-sodium diet. Closely monitor patient receiving IV solutions to correct hyponatremia. Replace water loss with fluids containing sodium.
Hypernatremia >145 mEq/L	Dry mucous membranes, taut skin turgor, intense thirst, flushed skin, oliguria, possibly elevated temperature Weakness, lethargy, irritability, twitching, seizures, coma, intracranial bleeding Low-grade fever	High-sodium diet, inadequate water intake as in a comatose, mentally confused, or debilitated patient Excessive sweating, diarrhea, failure of kidney to reabsorb water from urine Administration of high-protein, hyperosmotic tube feedings and osmotic diuretics	Encourage increased fluid intake. Measure intake and output (I&O). Give water between tube feedings. Restrict sodium intake. Monitor temperature.

Table 3.4 Electrolyte Imbalances and Nursing Interventions—cont'd

SERUM VALUE	SIGNS AND SYMPTOMS	CAUSES AND RISK FACTORS	NURSING INTERVENTIONS
Potassium (Normal Range: 3.5–5.0 mEq/L)			
Hypokalemia <3.5 mEq/L	Abdominal pain, paralytic ileus, gaseous distention of intestines Cardiac dysrhythmias, muscle weakness, decreased reflexes, paralysis, urinary retention, increased urinary pH, lethargy, confusion, electrocardiogram (ECG) changes	Inadequate intake of potassium-rich foods Loss of potassium in urine when kidneys do not reabsorb the mineral Loss of potassium from intestinal tract as a result of diarrhea or vomiting, drainage from fistulas, or overuse of gastric suction Improper use of diuretics	Instruct patients (especially those taking diuretics) about foods high in potassium content; encourage intake. Observe closely for signs of digitalis toxicity in patients taking this drug. Teach patients to watch for signs of hypokalemia. Administer potassium chloride supplement as ordered. Monitor I&O and cardiac rhythm.
Hyperkalemia >5.0 mEq/L	Muscle weakness, fatigue, hypotension, nausea, paresthesias, paralysis, cardiac dysrhythmias, ECG changes	Kidney failure, decreased kidney function Intestinal obstruction that prevents elimination of potassium in the feces Addison disease, digitalis toxicity, uncontrolled diabetes mellitus, insulin deficit, crushing injuries, and burns Overuse of potassium-containing salt substitute or overuse of potassium-sparing diuretic	Decrease intake of foods high in potassium. Increase fluid intake to enhance urinary excretion of potassium; provide adequate carbohydrate intake to prevent use of body proteins for energy. Carefully administer proper dose of insulin to diabetic patients. Instruct patient in proper use of salt substitutes containing potassium.
Calcium (Normal Range: 8.4–10.6 mg/dL)			
Hypocalcemia <8.4 mg/dL	Paresthesias, abdominal cramps, weak pulse, decreased BP, seizures, muscle spasms, tetany, hand spasm, positive Chvostek sign, positive Trousseau sign, cardiac dysrhythmia, wheezing, dyspnea, difficulty swallowing, colic, cardiac failure, excessive blood transfusions	Metastatic cancer Inadequate dietary intake of calcium and vitamin D Impaired absorption of calcium from intestinal tract, as in diarrhea, sprue, or overuse of laxatives and enemas containing phosphates (phosphorus tends to be more readily absorbed from the intestinal tract than calcium and suppresses calcium retention in the body) Hyposecretion of parathyroid hormone (the parathyroid regulates calcium and phosphorus levels) Chronic kidney disease (retention of phosphorus decreases calcium levels)	Encourage adults to consume sufficient calcium from cheese, broccoli, shrimp, and other dietary sources. Be prepared to administer calcium gluconate to a patient having thyroidectomy in case of surgical damage to the parathyroid glands. Give all oral medicines containing calcium 30 min before meals to facilitate absorption.
Hypercalcemia >10.6 mg/dL	Anorexia, nausea, abdominal pain, constipation, muscle weakness, oliguria, confusion Renal calculi, pathologic fractures, dysrhythmias, cardiac arrest	Excess intake of calcium, as in patient taking antacids indiscriminately Excess intake of vitamin D Conditions that cause movement of calcium out of bones and into extracellular fluid (e.g., bone tumor, multiple fractures) Tumors of the lung, stomach, and kidney and multiple myeloma Immobility and osteoporosis Hyperparathyroidism	Administer diuretics as prescribed to increase urinary output and calcium excretion. Monitor I&O; encourage high fluid intake (3000–4000 mL/day).

Continued

Table 3.4 Electrolyte Imbalances and Nursing Interventions—cont'd

SERUM VALUE	SIGNS AND SYMPTOMS	CAUSES AND RISK FACTORS	NURSING INTERVENTIONS
Magnesium (Normal Range: 1.3–2.1 mEq/L)			
Hypomagnesemia <1.3 mEq/L	Insomnia, hyperactive reflexes, leg and foot cramps, twitching, tremors Seizures, cardiac dysrhythmias, positive Chvostek sign, positive Trousseau sign, vertigo, hypocalcemia, hypokalemia	Chronic malnutrition, chronic diarrhea Bowel resection with ileostomy or colostomy Chronic alcoholism Thiazide diuretic use Prolonged gastric suction Acute pancreatitis Biliary or intestinal fistula Osmotic diuretic therapy Diabetic ketoacidosis	Provide diet counseling to help at-risk patients increase their level of magnesium (e.g., milk and cereals). Monitor IV infusions of magnesium closely. Monitor I&O.
Hypermagnesemia >2.1 mEq/L	Hypotension, sweating and flushing, nausea and vomiting Muscle weakness, paralysis, respiratory depression Cardiac dysrhythmias	Overuse of antacids and cathartics containing magnesium Aspiration of seawater, as in near-drowning Chronic kidney disease	Teach patients to avoid abuse of laxatives and antacids; instruct patients with renal problems to avoid over-the-counter drugs that contain magnesium. Encourage fluid intake to increase urinary excretion of magnesium if not contraindicated. Monitor I&O. Administer diuretics as ordered.
Phosphate (Normal Range: 3.0–4.5 mg/dL)			
Hypophosphatemia <3.0 mg/dL	Confusion, seizures, numbness, weakness, possible coma Chronic state: rickets and osteomalacia	Vitamin D deficiency or hyperparathyroidism Use of aluminum-containing antacids	Assess for vitamin D deficiency, hyperparathyroidism, or overuse of aluminum-containing antacids.
Hyperphosphatemia >4.5 mg/dL	Anorexia, nausea, vomiting	Renal insufficiency	Assess for restlessness, confusion, chest pain, and cyanosis. Monitor respirations. Check all electrolyte levels.

Modified from Williams P: *deWit's fundamental concepts and skills for nursing,* ed 5, Philadelphia, 2018, Elsevier.

Nutrition Considerations

Foods High in Sodium*

- Buttermilk
- Canned meats or fish
- Canned soups
- Canned vegetables
- Casserole and pasta mixes
- Catsup
- Cheese (all kinds)
- Delicatessen meats
- Dried fruits
- Dried soup mixes
- Foods containing monosodium glutamate (MSG)
- Frozen vegetables with sauces
- Gravy mixes
- Ham
- Hot dogs
- Olives
- Pickles
- Prepared mustard
- Preserved meats
- Processed foods
- Salted nuts
- Salted popcorn
- Salted snack foods
- Softened water
- Soy sauce
- Tomato or vegetable juice

*Check all packaged food labels for sodium content.

Potassium Imbalances

Hypokalemia. **Hypokalemia** occurs when the potassium (K^+) level falls below 3.5 mEq/L and has a variety of causes. Hypokalemia can cause serious problems. See Table 3.4 for risk factors, signs and symptoms, and interventions for hypokalemia.

It is important to teach patients taking diuretics that are not potassium sparing to increase potassium in the diet, take potassium supplements as prescribed, and watch for signs of hypokalemia.

Severe hypokalemia (K^+ <2.5 mEq/L) may cause cardiac arrest. Extra potassium must be given to help correct an imbalance.

Nutrition Considerations

Common Foods High in Potassium

- Apricots
- Avocado
- Baked potato with skin (small)
- Banana (1 medium)
- Cantaloupe (¼ medium)
- Dates, chopped
- Figs
- Honeydew melon (¼ medium)
- Mango
- Orange juice
- Orange (1 medium)
- Pinto beans (½ cup)
- Prune juice (½ cup)
- Prunes
- Raisins, seedless
- Spinach
- Tomatoes
- Winter squash

Safety Alert

Intravenous Potassium

Adequate renal function must be present before IV potassium is administered. Intravenous potassium must always be diluted before administration and is never given as a "push" (rapid, undiluted) injection.

Hyperkalemia. **Hyperkalemia** occurs when the serum potassium level rises above 5.0 mEq/L. The most common reason for increased potassium levels is decreased excretion by the kidneys due to either renal insufficiency or drug effects. The mechanical disruption of cell membranes causes a shift of potassium from the ICF to the ECF. This shift happens when extensive tissue damage occurs from burns or crush injuries, resulting in increased serum potassium. **Hyperkalemia can cause life-threatening cardiac dysrhythmia.**

Calcium Imbalances

Hypocalcemia. **Hypocalcemia** occurs when the calcium level drops below 8.4 mg/dL. Hypocalcemia results from disorders in which there is a shift of calcium into the bone. Removal or injury of the parathyroid glands during thyroidectomy causes parathyroid hormone deficiency and consequent hypocalcemia. Conditions that cause **alkalosis** (excess of alkaline or decrease of acid substances in the blood and body fluids) may cause hypocalcemia. Hypocalcemia in renal failure results from retention of phosphate ions, which causes a loss of calcium ions. In addition, during renal failure vitamin D is not activated, causing the loss of absorption of calcium from the intestinal tract.

Calcium ions are needed for a variety of metabolic processes and enzyme reactions, including for blood clotting. Calcium deficit upsets the stability of nerve membranes, causing abnormalities in nerve conduction and muscle contractions. **Carpopedal spasm** (also called Trousseau sign), hyperactive reflexes, Chvostek sign, and **tetany** (skeletal muscle spasm in which the muscles are in sustained contraction and cause spasm) may occur. Laryngospasm may occur if the deficit is severe (see Table 3.4).

Check for Trousseau and Chvostek signs when calcium or magnesium deficit is a possibility. To test for Trousseau sign, place a blood pressure cuff on the arm, inflate above systolic pressure, and hold for 3 minutes; if a spasm of the hand occurs, the reaction is positive (Fig. 3.6). Tapping the facial nerve about an inch in front of the earlobe assesses Chvostek sign. A unilateral twitching of the face is a positive response (Fig. 3.7). Test deep tendon reflexes by tapping a partially stretched muscle tendon with a percussion hammer. The extent of the reflex is scored from 0 to 4+, with 0 representing no response, 2+ a normal response, and 4+ a hyperactive response.

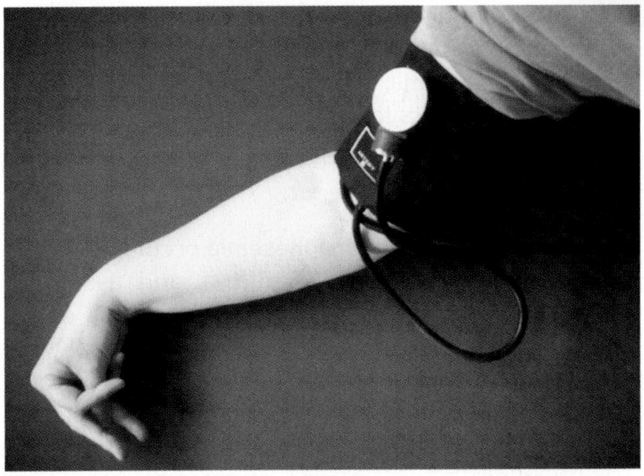

Fig. 3.6 Palmar flexion (carpopedal spasm) indicating positive Trousseau sign in hypocalcemia. (From Ignatavicius DD, Workman ML, Rebar CR: *Medical-Surgical Nursing: Concepts for Interprofessional Collaborative Care*, ed 9, St. Louis, 2018, Elsevier.)

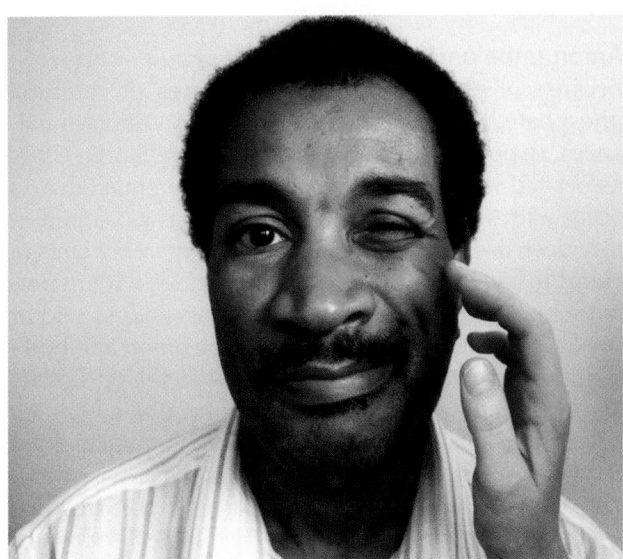

Fig. 3.7 Facial muscle response indicating positive Chvostek sign in hypocalcemia. (From Ignatavicius DD, Workman ML, Rebar CR: *Medical-Surgical Nursing: Concepts for Interprofessional Collaborative Care*, ed 9, St. Louis, 2018, Elsevier.)

Hypercalcemia. **Hypercalcemia** occurs when the serum calcium level is above 10.6 mg/dL. This can occur during periods of lengthy immobilization, when calcium is mobilized from the bone, or when an excess of calcium or vitamin D is taken into the body. See Table 3.4 for signs and symptoms, risk factors, and interventions. Administer diuretics to increase calcium excretion and encourage high fluid intake.

Magnesium Imbalances

Hypomagnesemia. **Hypomagnesemia** occurs when the serum level drops below 1.3 mEq/L and usually is present when hypokalemia and hypocalcemia occur. Magnesium is important in deoxyribonucleic acid (DNA) and protein synthesis and in many enzyme reactions. Magnesium imbalances are rare but can be caused by a variety of factors (see Table 3.4).

Hypermagnesemia. **Hypermagnesemia** is present when the serum level is above 2.1 mEq/L. It can occur in the presence of renal failure or from overuse of magnesium-containing antacids and cathartics. Hypermagnesemia is rare.

Anion Imbalances

Because of electroneutrality, imbalances of chloride, phosphate, and bicarbonate accompany cation imbalances. **Hypochloremia** (a chloride level <95 mEq/L) is associated with hyponatremia. Hypochloremia can also occur with severe vomiting and is seen as a compensatory decrease in acid-base disorders. **Hyperchloremia** (a chloride level >103 mEq/L) that coincides with hypernatremia is a form of metabolic **acidosis** (excess acid or depletion of alkaline substances in the blood and body tissues). **Hypophosphatemia** occurs when the phosphate level falls below 3.0 mg/dL. Hypophosphatemia may result from use of aluminum-containing antacids that bind phosphate, vitamin D deficiency, or hyperparathyroidism. **Hyperphosphatemia** (a level >4.5 mg/dL) commonly occurs in renal failure. See Table 3.4 for signs and symptoms of phosphate imbalance.

The difference between the primary measured cations and the primary measured anions is called the **anion gap**. The cations measured include sodium and potassium and the anions include chloride and bicarbonate. The normal value is 3 to 11 mEq/L. It is used to help identify acid-base disturbances. High anion gap numbers may indicate an acidotic state.

ACID-BASE SYSTEM

PHYSIOLOGY

It is crucial to maintain acid-base balance because cell enzymes function within a very narrow pH range (7.35 to 7.45). To understand the concept of acid-base balance and how it is maintained in the body fluids, you should be familiar with some basic facts about biochemistry and the terms commonly used in discussions of hydrogen ion concentration (Box 3.3).

Nutrients in the blood diffuse into the cells, where various metabolic processes take place. Metabolic wastes, including acids, from those cellular processes diffuse back from the cells to the blood. The following three mechanisms control or try to rebalance pH:

- Buffer pairs—groups of chemicals that absorb excess acids or excess bases—circulating in the blood respond to pH changes quickly. The bicarbonate–carbonic acid buffer system is responsible for more than half of the buffering. Three other buffer systems in the body include the phosphate, hemoglobin, and protein systems.
- The respiratory system alters breathing rate and depth. Because carbon dioxide (CO_2) dissolves in the blood and combines with water to form carbonic acid, retaining or blowing off CO_2 helps retain or eliminate acids from the body.
- The kidneys change the excretion rate of acids and the production and absorption of bicarbonate ion. The kidneys are slow to compensate but are the most effective compensating mechanism (Fig. 3.8).

The bicarbonate–carbonic acid buffer system links an acid (CO_2) with water and a base (bicarbonate ion). A buffer is a substance that increases the amount of acid or alkali in the solution to produce a unit change in pH. The balance of the bicarbonate ions and carbonic acid ions is controlled by the respiratory system and by the kidneys. The CO_2 produced by cell metabolism diffuses into the blood. There CO_2 reacts with water

Box 3.3 Some Chemistry Facts Related to Acid-Base Balance

- An *acid* is a substance capable of giving up a hydrogen ion during chemical exchange.
- A *base* is a substance capable of accepting a hydrogen ion during chemical exchange.
- Acids react with bases to form water and a salt.
- **A reaction of an acid and a base to form water and a salt is a *neutralization* reaction because *both the acid and the base are neutralized.***
- Acids react with carbonates and bicarbonates to form carbon dioxide gas.
- The term *pH* refers to the concentration of hydrogen (H) in a solution. The "p" represents a *negative* logarithm, which is an inverse proportion. This means that **the higher the concentration of hydrogen ions in a solution, the lower the pH.** A higher pH indicates the opposite—that is, a lower concentration of hydrogen ions.
- A chemically neutral solution has a pH of 7.0.
- **The pH of the body's fluids is normally somewhat alkaline (between 7.35 and 7.45).**
- A pH below 7.25 or above 7.55 is considered life-threatening.
- A pH below 6.8 (*acidosis*) or above 7.8 (*alkalosis*) usually is fatal.
- A blood pH of 7.4 indicates a ratio of 1 part carbonic acid to 20 parts bicarbonate (base).
- Acidosis is the result of either a loss of base or an accumulation of acid.

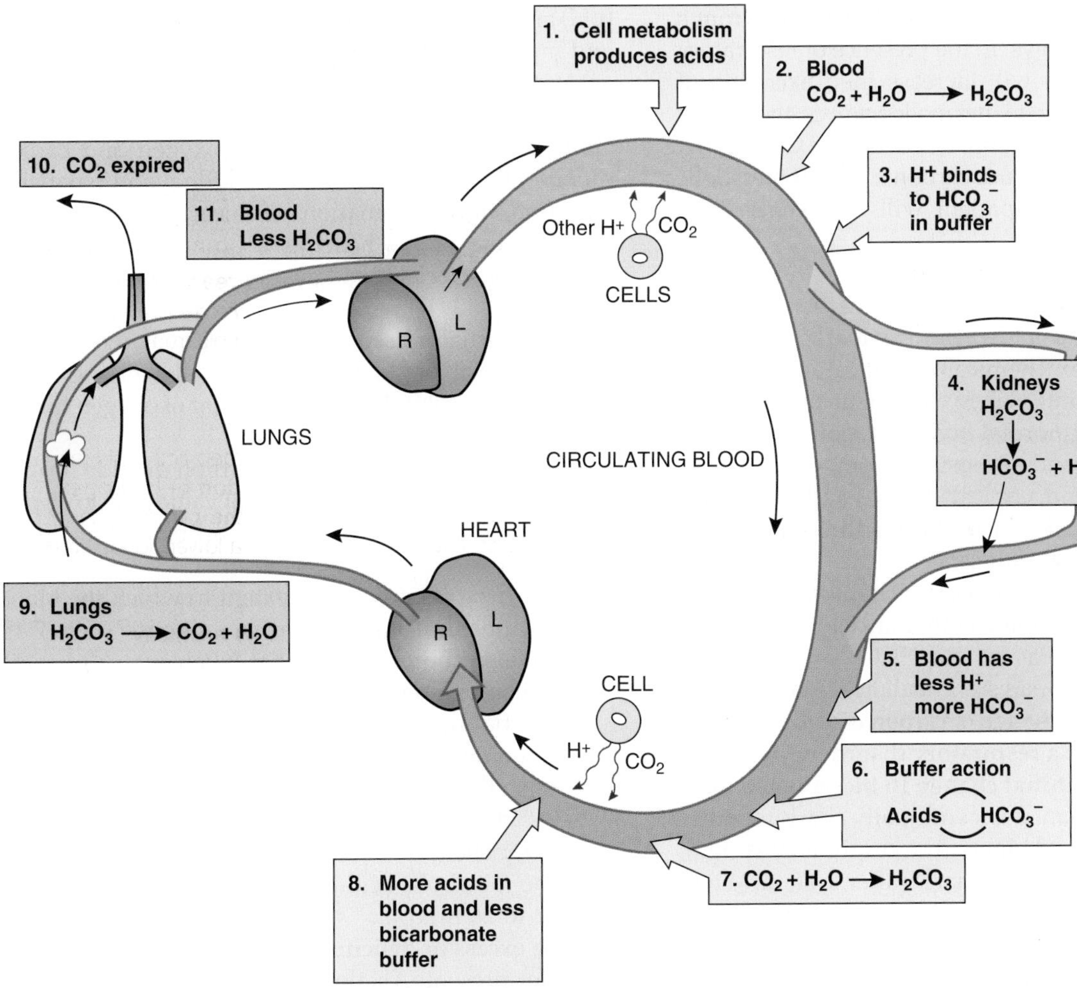

Fig. 3.8 Regulation of acid-base balance by chemical buffers, respiratory system, and renal system. (From William P: *deWit's fundamental concepts and skills for nursing,* ed 5, St. Louis, 2018, Elsevier.)

and forms carbonic acid. The carbonic acid dissociates (separates) to form hydrogen ions and bicarbonate ions, as needed. The process can be reversed in the lungs, freeing up CO_2 so it can be expired along with water, thereby reducing the total acid in the body.

Enzymes in the kidney promote the formation of hydrogen ions, which are excreted in the urine while the bicarbonate ions are returned to the blood. The kidneys, through the influence of aldosterone, can exchange hydrogen ions for sodium ions. Acids can be removed in the kidney by combining them with ammonia and other basic chemicals. Urine pH can vary from 4.5 to 8.0 as kidney compensation occurs.

ACID-BASE IMBALANCES

PATHOPHYSIOLOGY

Most of the body's metabolic activities produce CO_2 gas, which moves from the tissues into the blood, where it combines with water to form carbonic acid ($CO_2 + H_2O = H_2CO_3$). The body deals with this constant manufacture of acid in a number of ways so that the correct ratio of carbonic acid to bicarbonate can be maintained and an alkaline environment provided for normal cellular activities. If the ratio is not maintained, the acid-base balance is upset. Either the pH will fall below the normal range and acidosis will occur or the pH will rise above normal range and alkalosis will be present. As long as the ratio of carbonic acid to bicarbonate is maintained at 1:20, the pH remains within normal limits. In a respiratory imbalance, the lungs retain or "blow off" (excrete) CO_2. In **hypoventilation** the lungs do not eliminate enough CO_2, and CO_2 remains in the body, unites with water, and forms carbonic acid. The opposite is **hyperventilation**, in which too much CO_2 may be blown off.

The kidneys are the principal organs of control in maintaining a normal pH during metabolic activities because they either reabsorb or excrete bicarbonate. If they eliminate too much bicarbonate, acidosis will develop. Conversely, if they fail to eliminate enough bicarbonate and allow it to be reabsorbed into the bloodstream, alkalosis will develop.

In the presence of respiratory acidosis, the kidneys will retain and manufacture more bicarbonate than normal so that it is available to neutralize the excess acid. However, this is a slow process that takes from a few hours to several days. In the presence of respiratory alkalosis, the kidneys will increase their excretion of bicarbonate. In response to metabolic acidosis, the patient will involuntarily hyperventilate to remove CO_2 so that it is not available to produce carbonic acid. If metabolic alkalosis develops, the patient will hypoventilate to retain the supply of CO_2.

The foregoing information on acid-base balance, hydrogen ion concentration, and the carbon dioxide–bicarbonate ratio does not represent an in-depth explanation. Many complex chemical activities are involved in maintaining an internal environment that must be slightly alkaline for normal body function.

Because acidosis and alkalosis are common to a great variety of medical and surgical illnesses and conditions, the chapters on specific illnesses will address associated problems of acid-base imbalance.

The four types of acid-base imbalances are shown in Table 3.5. To determine whether an acid-base imbalance exists, the pH, $Paco_2$, and HCO_3^- are measured by arterial blood gas analysis. Imbalances may be acute or chronic. **An initial change in carbon dioxide is nearly always the result of a respiratory disorder. Metabolic disorders show an initial change in bicarbonate ions.** Three control mechanisms continually work together to maintain acid-base balance: the respiratory system, the kidneys, and the bicarbonate buffer system. When an imbalance occurs, the lungs and kidneys try to compensate by working to bring the pH back toward normal limits.

ARTERIAL BLOOD GAS ANALYSIS

Studies of the percentages of gases (oxygen and carbon dioxide) in the blood and the hydrogen ion concentration (pH) are useful in assessing the status of both respiratory and metabolic acid-base imbalances. Blood gas studies are valuable indicators of a patient's progress toward recovery, or lack of it. Blood gas analyses reflect the ability of the lungs to exchange oxygen and carbon dioxide, the effectiveness of the kidneys in balancing retention and elimination of bicarbonate, and the effectiveness of the heart as a pump. The results of analyses of arterial blood gases (ABGs) are reported as follows:

- **Pao_2:** Partial pressure (P) exerted by oxygen (o_2) in the arterial blood (a). The normal value is 80 to 100 mm Hg; it indicates the amount of oxygen carried in the blood.
- **$Paco_2$:** Partial pressure (P) of carbon dioxide (co_2) in the arterial blood (a). The normal value is 35 to 45 mm Hg; it indicates the amount of carbon dioxide in the blood.
- **pH:** An expression of the extent to which the blood is alkaline or acid. The normal value is 7.35 to 7.45.
- **Sao_2** (also abbreviated **O_2 Sat.**): Percentage of available hemoglobin that is saturated (Sa) with oxygen (o_2)—that is, the ratio of the amount of oxygen that is combined with hemoglobin to the total amount of oxygen the hemoglobin can carry. The normal value is 94% to 100%.
- **HCO_3^-:** The level of plasma bicarbonate; an indicator of the metabolic acid-base status. The normal value is 22 to 26 mEq/L.
- **Base excess or deficit:** Indicates the amount of blood buffer present. Alkalosis is present when this value is abnormally high. Abnormally low values indicate acidosis. Alkalosis is measured in "+" or "–" values.

Table 3.5 The Four Acid-Base Imbalances

IMBALANCE	CAUSES	BLOOD GAS VALUES
Respiratory acidosis	Slow, shallow respirations Respiratory congestion or obstruction	pH <7.35 $Paco_2$ >45 mm Hg
Metabolic acidosis	Shock (poor circulation) Diabetic ketoacidosis Renal failure Diarrhea	pH <7.35 HCO_3^- <22 mEq/L
Respiratory alkalosis	Hyperventilation	pH >7.45 $Paco_2$ <35 mm Hg
Metabolic alkalosis	Vomiting Excessive antacid intake Hypokalemia	pH >7.45 HCO_3^- >26 mEq/L

From Williams P: *deWit's fundamental concepts and skills for nursing*, ed 5, Philadelphia, 2018, Elsevier.

RESPIRATORY ACIDOSIS

An increase in carbon dioxide levels occurs in a variety of disorders. It is seen in the following conditions:

- Acute problems such as airway obstruction, pneumonia, asthma, chest injuries, or pulmonary edema
- Chronic obstructive pulmonary disease (COPD), such as emphysema
- With opiate use that depresses the respiratory rate

? Think Critically

What could you do to help prevent respiratory acidosis in a home care patient who has pneumonia?

A patient with COPD is most likely to develop acute acidosis when an infection of the respiratory tract further impairs breathing capacity and the removal of carbon dioxide. Signs and symptoms of respiratory acidosis include complaints of increasing difficulty in breathing, a history of respiratory obstruction (acute or chronic), dyspnea, weakness, dizziness, restlessness, sleepiness, and change in mental alertness.

The treatment for respiratory acidosis is establishment or maintenance of an airway. Use of noninvasive positive pressure ventilation or the insertion of an endotracheal tube may be necessary. Oxygen administration may be needed, and the assistance of a mechanical ventilator may be required. Conservative treatment includes deep-breathing exercises with use of an incentive spirometer, bronchodilators, and antibiotics if indicated. Care must be taken when administering certain drugs that depress the respiratory center, including narcotics, hypnotics, and tranquilizers.

The patient must be watched closely for respiratory and cardiac arrest. Should either occur, it will be necessary to maintain respiration and circulation artificially through cardiopulmonary resuscitation.

Clinical Cues

In patients with COPD, the respiratory drive mechanism is altered, and oxygen can act as a respiratory depressant. Oxygen should be administered with great care to these patients (no more than 2 to 3 L/min) because it can cause respiratory arrest.

If a patient's history is unknown, oxygen is begun at a rate of 2 to 3 L/min until it is determined that a higher flow rate can be tolerated.

METABOLIC ACIDOSIS

An excessive loss of bicarbonate ions or an increased production or retention of hydrogen ions leads to metabolic acidosis. The main causes of metabolic acidosis include:

- Excessive loss of bicarbonate ions from diarrhea
- Renal failure
- Diabetic ketoacidosis (DKA)
- Hyperkalemia
- Sepsis

In diabetes mellitus, insulin insufficiency leads to excessive burning of fats, and the end product is fatty acids. When more energy than usual is expended, as in athletic competition, lactic acid builds up in the body as oxygenation of tissue falls. In kidney disease there is decreased excretion of acids and decreased production of bicarbonate. The increased buildup of acids causes metabolic acidosis.

The symptoms of metabolic acidosis include weakness, lethargy, headache, and confusion (Concept Map 3.1). If the acidosis is not relieved, these symptoms progress to stupor, unconsciousness, coma, and death. The breath of the patient with DKA may have a fruity odor from the ketone bodies (**ketoacidosis**). Vomiting

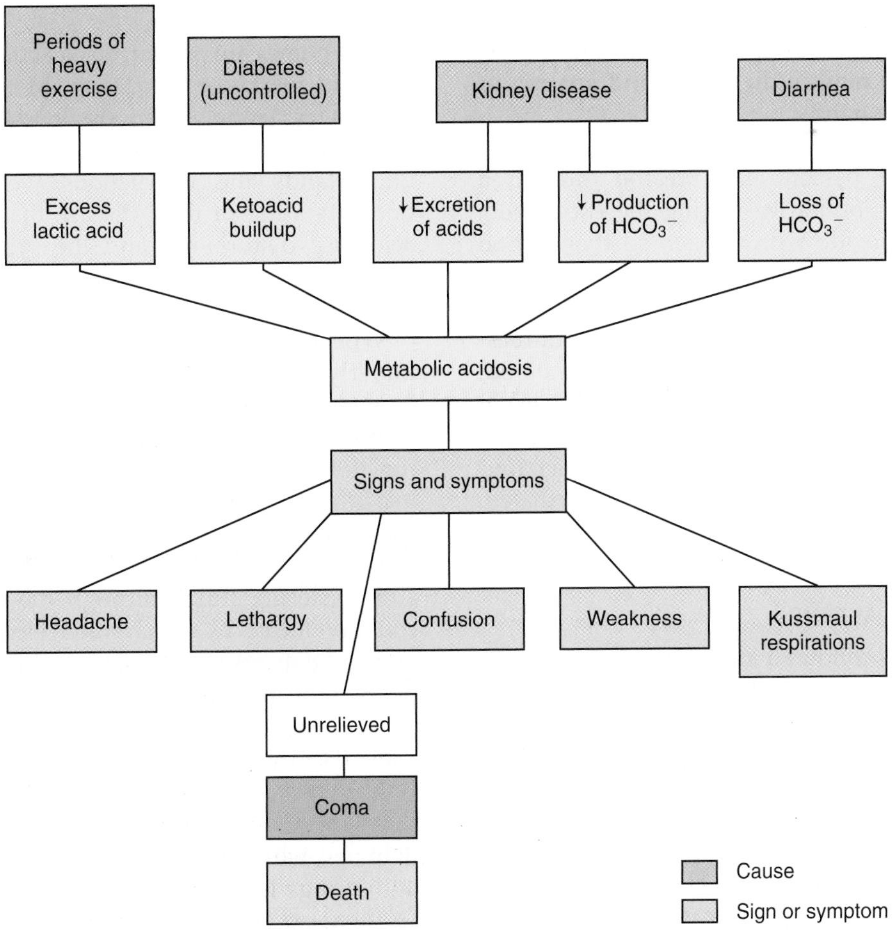

Concept Map 3.1 Causes, signs, and symptoms of metabolic acidosis.

and diarrhea may occur and aggravate the metabolic imbalance because of the loss of fluids and electrolytes, which are essential to restoring the acid-base balance. When compensatory mechanisms are working to correct metabolic acidosis, the patient may have deep, rapid breathing (Kussmaul respirations) and may secrete urine with a low pH.

Treatment of metabolic acidosis is aimed at the underlying cause. Insulin is administered if the patient is in diabetic ketoacidosis. Dialysis may be necessary to correct the problem in a patient with kidney failure. **Immediate treatment of severe metabolic acidosis requires treating the underlying cause and administration of IV bicarbonate.**

RESPIRATORY ALKALOSIS

Alkalosis is less common than acidosis. Hyperventilation (a rapid respiratory rate) results in respiratory alkalosis. Hyperventilation is usually caused by:

- Anxiety
- High fever
- An overdose of aspirin

Patients hyperventilate for a variety of reasons, including **hypoxemia** (insufficient oxygen, which triggers an automatic increase in respiration), reactions to certain drugs, pain, and panic. The overzealous use of mechanical ventilation also can cause hyperventilation when too much CO_2 is blown off. Head injuries may also lead to hyperventilation. **Symptoms of respiratory alkalosis include deep, rapid breathing; tingling of the fingers; pallor around the mouth; dizziness; and spasms of the muscles of the hands.**

Treatment for hyperventilation addresses the underlying disorder. The person may breathe through a rebreather mask temporarily, mixing the excessively exhaled carbon dioxide with oxygen so that carbon dioxide is reinhaled. If the underlying cause of respiratory alkalosis is panic, treatment is aimed at preventing further hyperventilation and helping the patient reestablish a normal level of carbon dioxide in the blood. Sedatives may be given to calm the patient. To aid in the retention of carbon dioxide, the patient may be instructed to hold the breath or to breathe into a paper sack and then rebreathe the carbon dioxide just exhaled. This recycling of carbon dioxide can eventually restore normal carbonic acid levels in the blood.

METABOLIC ALKALOSIS

Metabolic alkalosis follows a loss of hydrochloric acid from the stomach. Causes include:

- Vomiting
- Extensive GI suction
- Hypokalemia
- Excessive use of antacids with bicarbonate

Hypokalemia causes metabolic alkalosis because the kidney retains K^+ while excreting H^+.

Other causes include drainage from intestinal fistula; diuresis resulting from potent diuretics that increase potassium loss in the urine; and steroid therapy, which causes retention of sodium and chloride and loss of potassium and hydrogen.

Symptoms of metabolic alkalosis include such neurologic signs as irritability, disorientation, lethargy, muscle twitching, tingling and numbness of the fingers, and convulsions and respiratory manifestations such as slow, shallow respirations; decreased chest movements; and cyanosis. In addition, there may be symptoms of potassium and calcium depletion. If alkalosis progresses, tetany will occur, with resulting seizures and coma. Tetany is characterized by severe muscle cramps, carpopedal spasms, laryngeal spasms, and **stridor** (a shrill, harsh sound on inspiration).

Treatment is directed at correcting the underlying cause and attempting to restore the body fluids to a less alkaline state. Fluids and electrolytes are replaced orally and parenterally as needed. Emergency measures include the administration of an acidifying solution, such as ammonium chloride. Fig. 3.9 compares the causes, physiologic effects, and compensatory mechanisms for acidosis and alkalosis.

? Think Critically

Identify the type of imbalance that might result from (1) rapid respiratory rate, (2) out-of-control diabetes, (3) renal failure, and (4) excessive use of antacids for a nervous stomach.

HOME CARE

For the home care patient, teach about the requirements for fluid intake or restriction. Monitor adherence to sodium restriction by periodically checking the patient's food intake. Obtain feedback to be certain the patient understands the instructions. Verify the patient's understanding of their disease that could lead to an acid-base disturbance and the symptoms to report. Collaborate with the patient on the plan of care to obtain patient compliance.

When acid-base imbalance occurs, control of the underlying disorder is a priority. Blood gases are monitored, and oxygen and electrolytes are administered as needed. Nursing measures to improve pulmonary function are instituted as appropriate.

INTRAVENOUS FLUID THERAPY

Administering fluids through the veins is the most common means by which water, electrolytes, nutrients, and some drugs may be given when oral intake is not possible or must be supplemented. Multiple methods of infusing fluids and medications are available. See Table 3.6. Intravenous therapy is often used when a fluid deficit is present or when there are electrolyte imbalances. Intravenous fluids may also be used to help reestablish acid-base balance. Medications are administered in an IV solution when rapid action is required. TPN is used for administering nutrients to patients with GI problems who cannot take in nutrients in any other way.

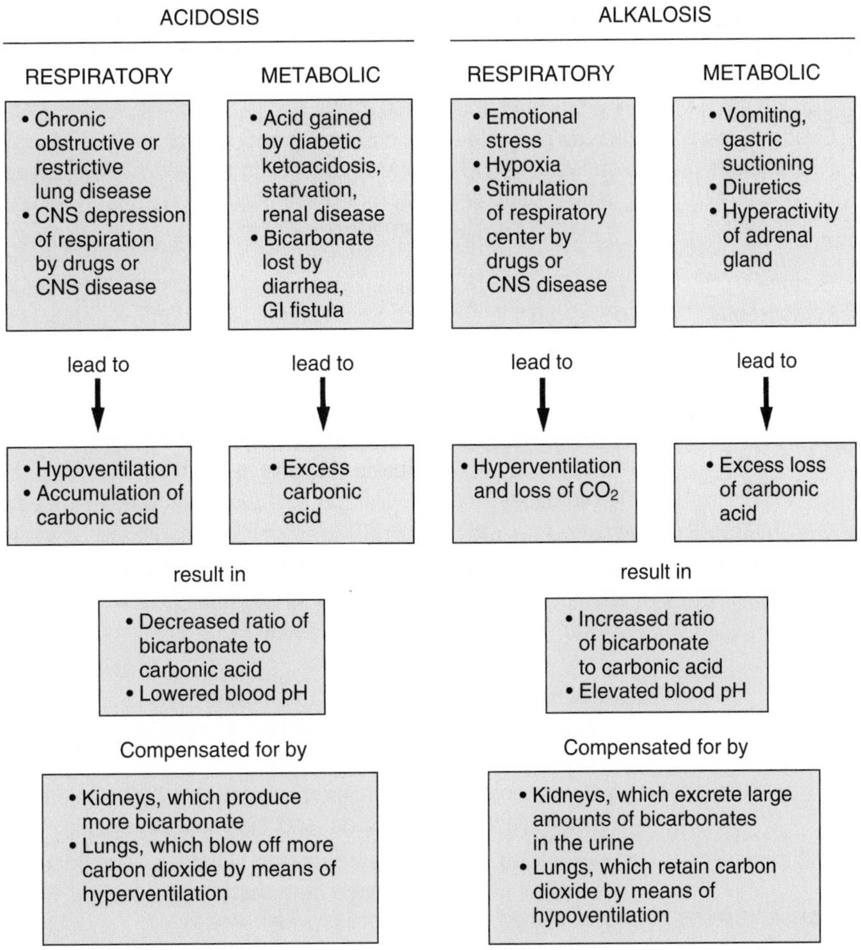

Fig. 3.9 Comparison of causes, physiologic effects, and compensatory mechanisms for acidosis and alkalosis. *CNS*, Central nervous system; *GI*, gastrointestinal. (From Williams P: *deWit's fundamental concepts and skills for nursing*, ed 5, St. Louis, 2018, Elsevier.)

Some terms related to the concentration of an IV fluid and its effect on cells include:

- *Isotonic:* A solution that has the same osmotic pressure as ICF. Body cells can be bathed in an isotonic solution without net flow of water across the cell membrane.
- *Hypotonic:* A solution that has a lower osmotic pressure (is less concentrated) than that of body fluids. Cells bathed in a hypotonic solution will swell as water passes from the less concentrated solution across the cell membrane and into the cell. **Note: Sterile distilled water is hypotonic and is never added to an IV solution.**
- *Hypertonic:* A solution that has a higher osmotic pressure than that of body fluids. Cells bathed in a hypertonic solution will shrink as water passes out of the cell into the fluid surrounding it.

An example of an isotonic solution is 0.9% normal saline. Hypotonic solutions are those with less than 5% glucose or with anions less than 150 mEq/L. Fluids commonly used in IV therapy are presented in Table 3.7.

Blood-related fluids that are given IV include whole blood; packed cells from which the plasma has been removed, leaving only the red blood cells; platelets; and plasma. Whole blood is rarely given. Even with hemorrhage, blood components are usually given for replacement. Packed cells may be administered to patients with anemia or some other blood disorder. Plasma is stored in the frozen state, so the order will be for fresh frozen plasma (FFP). Plasma is given primarily to replace coagulation factors but may also be used to increase blood volume (as in shock) and to provide protein. Protein can also be supplemented by use of human albumin.

In the treatment of shock, **plasma expanders** are administered to increase the volume of plasma. Examples of plasma expanders are low-molecular-weight dextran, albumin, Hespan, and Plasmanate. Blood disorders and blood product administration are further presented in Chapter 16.

NURSING RESPONSIBILITIES IN ADMINISTERING INTRAVENOUS FLUIDS

Responsibility for the safe and effective administration of IV fluids rests with every member of the nursing staff.

Table 3.6 Access Methods for Fluids and Medications

		CONSIDERATIONS/USES	DWELL TIME
Peripheral Venous			
Short (<3 in)	Over-the-needle IV catheter	Bedside procedure. RN scope of practice in all states, LVN/LPN scope of practice in some states. Used for infusion of blood, fluids, and medications. Fluid osmolarity <900 mOsm/L.	Based on daily assessment; should not be replaced more frequently than q72–96h unless there is a complication
	Butterfly	Used for blood draw only.	Minutes
	Intraosseous	Special training required. Some states allow both RNs and LPN/LVNs to insert. Used for fluids and medications.	No more than 24 h
Midline (3–8 in)		Special training required. Usually inserted with ultrasound guidance. Most states allow only RNs to insert. Used for infusion of blood, fluids, and medications.	6–8 wk
Central Venous			
Multilumen nontunneled percutaneous catheter		Health care providers. Specialized training for advanced practice RNs. Used for infusion of blood, TPN, fluids, and medications.	3–5 days
PICC		Special training for RNs. Some states allow LVN/LPNs to insert with training. Used for infusion of blood, TPN, fluids, and medications.	Up to a year
Implanted port		Usually implanted by health care provider. Used for infusion of blood, TPN, fluids, and medications.	Years
Tunneled	IV access	Usually placed by health care provider. Used for infusion of blood, TPN, fluids, and medications.	Months to years
	Dialysis catheter	Usually placed by health care provider. Accessed only by dialysis staff.	Months to years
Nonvascular			
Hypodermoclysis		Small subcutaneous needle infuses fluids slowly into the tissues. Placed by RNs and LVN/LPNs.	3–7 days
Subcutaneous infusion		Subcutaneous needle placement by RNs and LVN/LPNs for medication administration.	7 days
Epidural		Catheter placed by health care provider, pain medication infusion monitored by RN.	24–48 h

IV, Intravenous; *LVN/LPN*, licensed vocational/practical nurse; *PICC*, peripherally inserted central catheter; *RN*, registered nurse; *TPN*, total parenteral nutrition.

Legal and Ethical Considerations

Intravenous Therapy Guidelines

Check your state's nurse practice act to determine what aspects of IV therapy, if any, your state allows the LPN/LVN to perform. With the continuation of the nursing shortage, a few states have expanded their LPN/LVN practice act to allow licensed LPN/LVNs to perform a variety of IV therapy functions. Other states are considering expanding their practice acts accordingly.

As with any therapeutic measure, IV therapy is not without its hazards to the patient. Many complications can be avoided through careful handling of equipment and meticulous monitoring of the patient's reaction to the fluids being administered. Maintaining sterility is paramount. IV access devices provide a direct route to the bloodstream for organisms when aseptic technique is compromised.

Safety Alert

Intravenous Line Connection Safety

When connecting an IV solution or disconnecting a line, always trace the line to where it connects to the patient to make certain that it is an IV line and connects to an IV device. Many mistakes have been made when IV fluids have been connected to the wrong device.

The four goals of nursing care for a patient receiving an IV infusion are to (1) prevent infection, (2) minimize physical injury to the veins and surrounding tissues,

Table 3.7 Commonly Prescribed IV Solutions

SOLUTION	TONICITY	MOSM/KG	GLUCOSE (G/L)	INDICATIONS AND CONSIDERATIONS
Dextrose in Water				
5%	Isotonic	278	50	Provides free water necessary for renal excretion of solutes Used to replace water losses and treat hypernatremia Provides 170 calories/L Does not provide any electrolytes
10%	Hypertonic	556	100	Provides free water only, no electrolytes Provides 340 calories/L
Saline				
0.45%	Hypotonic	154	0	Provides free water in addition to Na^+ and Cl^- Used to replace hypotonic fluid losses Used as maintenance solution, although it does not replace daily losses of other electrolytes Provides no calories
0.9%	Isotonic	308	0	Used to expand intravascular volume and replace extracellular fluid losses Only solution that may be administered with blood products Contains Na^+ and Cl^- in excess of plasma levels Does not provide free water, calories, other electrolytes May cause intravascular overload or hyperchloremic acidosis
3.0%	Hypertonic	1026	0	Used to treat symptomatic hyponatremia Must be administered slowly and with extreme caution because it may cause dangerous intravascular volume overload and pulmonary edema
Dextrose in Saline				
5% in 0.225%	Isotonic	355	50	Provides Na^+, Cl^-, and free water Used to replace hypotonic losses and treat hypernatremia Provides 170 calories/L
5% in 0.45%	Hypertonic	432	50	Provides Na^+ and Cl^- and is used as a maintenance solution Provides 170 calories/L
5% in 0.9%	Hypertonic	586	50	Used to treat hyponatremia and metabolic acidosis Provides 170 calories/L
Multiple Electrolyte Solutions				
Ringer solution	Isotonic	309	0	Similar in composition to plasma except that it has excess Cl^-, no Mg^{2+}, and no HCO_3^- Does not provide free water or calories Used to expand the intravascular volume and replace extracellular fluid losses
Lactated Ringer (Hartmann) solution	Isotonic	273	0	Similar in composition to normal plasma except that it does not contain Mg^{2+} Used to treat losses from burns and lower gastrointestinal tract May be used to treat mild metabolic acidosis but should not be used to treat lactic acidosis Does not provide free water or calories

Modified from Lewis SM, Bucher, L, Heitkemper MM, et al.: *Medical-surgical nursing: assessment and management of clinical problems,* ed 10, St. Louis, 2017, Elsevier.

(3) administer the correct fluid at the prescribed time and at a safe rate of flow, and (4) observe the patient's reaction to the fluid and medications being administered (Box 3.4).

All equipment and fluids used for IV therapy must be sterile and safe for administration. **Before any plastic bag or bottle of solution is added to an IV set, it must be checked for leaks and possible contamination.**

Safety Alert

Intravenous Solution Safety

A plastic bag of solution may be squeezed to check for leaks. Any solution that is discolored or has small particles, a white cloud, or film in it should not be used. If there is no vacuum in a bottle when it is opened, the solution may be contaminated. Gently invert the bag or bottle and hold it up to the light so you can see if there are any particles floating in it.

Box 3.4 The Six Rights Applied to Intravenous Therapy

Be sure you have:

1. The right solution with or without additives as ordered and/or the correct solution to follow what has been infusing
2. The right dose (amount) of solution and additive as ordered
3. The right route (peripheral intravenous [IV] or central line)
4. The right time (to infuse)
5. The right patient as identified with two identifiers
6. The right documentation

In addition:

- Teach the patient the reason for administration of the fluid and/or drug and the signs and symptoms of problems to report to you.
- Check for drug allergies.
- Be aware of potential interactions with IV medications or irrigating solutions.
- Maintain sterility of all solutions, tubing, and connections.

When a new bottle of fluid or additional medication is added to an IV infusion already in progress, strict surgical asepsis must be observed because there is a danger of introducing bacteria into the patient's blood system. Because of the danger of incompatibility, it is essential to check each drug and each solution to be certain they can be mixed. Various online resources are available, and your pharmacist is a good resource to consult. **Always wash your hands just before handling IV fluids and equipment. The port on the IV tubing into which the administration set of a piggyback medication is to be attached must be carefully and thoroughly wiped with a fresh alcohol swab, scrubbing thoroughly for 15 seconds, before the tubing is attached to the container. If a protective alcohol cap is in use, follow the manufacturer's recommendations for sanitizing.**

There should be a clear occlusive (airtight) dressing over the IV insertion site. The edges of the dressing should adhere to the skin on all sides. Tubing should be secured so that accidental pulling on the tubing will not affect the IV cannula. Dressings are changed according to agency protocol; current guidelines recommend changing dressings every 5 to 7 days. If a dressing becomes loose, soiled, or contaminated, it should be removed and a new dressing applied (Box 3.5). Label tubing and dressings with the date.

The site of venipuncture should be watched closely for signs of inflammation. Redness, swelling, and heat in the area should be reported because these are possible signs of phlebitis. Chills and elevated body temperature may indicate a bacterial infection. Table 3.8 presents the potential complications of IV therapy.

When an IV infusion is discontinued, the tubing is clamped, all tape is removed, and the needle or catheter is gently but quickly withdrawn using Standard Precautions (see Chapter 6). Check to be sure that the catheter has been completely removed and the tip is intact. A dry, sterile gauze is held on the site with enough pressure to control the leakage of blood and avoid the formation of a hematoma. If possible, raise the patient's limb for a minute or two to drain blood from the site of insertion and help prevent leakage of blood from the punctured vein. If the patient is taking antiplatelet or anticoagulant medications, be prepared to hold pressure for an extended time.

A safety goal of The Joint Commission requires that at least two patient identifiers (neither identifier being the patient's room number) must be used whenever IV

Box 3.5 Intravenous Therapy Guidelines

- **Keep intravenous (IV) fluid sterile.** Make sure that everything that comes in contact with the solution is sterile, including the inside surface of the cannula hub and all connecting points between the bag and the drip chamber and between the tubing and the needle.
- **Protect the cannula site from contamination to prevent possible infection.** An airtight, transparent dressing is used over the cannula site.
- **Keep tubing free of air.** Clear tubing of air before connecting to the cannula. Do not allow the current bag to run dry before changing to the next one.
- **Hang fluids at the correct height.** Fluids flow through the tubing by the force of gravity. If there is negative pressure in the IV line, blood will flow back into the tubing. IV bags hung above the pump flow into the pump by gravity.
- **Carefully regulate the rate of flow.** If the IV infusion is behind schedule, do not open the clamp and run in a large amount of fluid at one time to catch up. Rather, recalculate either (1) the span of time for the infusion or (2) the rate of drops per minute for the fluid to run at the ordered rate. Make sure an infusion pump is programed correctly.
- **Track intake and output when a patient is receiving IV fluids or blood.** Keep accurate intake and output records and compare intake with output over 24 hours.
- **The solution to run in first should be hung the highest.** When a second bag is attached piggyback to a primary IV line, lower the primary bag without clamping the tubing so that it will begin to flow when the piggyback has run in. Attach the piggyback beneath the roller clamp on the primary tubing.
- **Assess the site frequently for signs of complications.** Infiltration, swelling at the IV site, irritation of the vein, formation of a clot stopping the flow, or systemic reaction should be identified quickly. Signs of infiltration are pain or discomfort at the site caused by dislodgement of the needle or puncture of the vein. Vital signs should be taken several times a day to detect early signs of infection or adverse reaction.

Table 3.8 Complications of Intravenous Therapy and Nursing Interventions

COMPLICATION	SIGNS AND SYMPTOMS	NURSING INTERVENTIONS
Local		
Infiltration (infusion of IV fluids into tissues)	Arm swollen, tender, cool to touch; IV catheter may or may not have blood return	Remove IV catheter and restart IV infusion in the other extremity.
Extravasation (infusion of medications or chemicals into tissues that can cause injury)	Pain at insertion site, tender and cool to touch, IV flow slows, edema, burning, blanching, fluid leaking around catheter Tissue sloughing may occur in 1–4 wk	Stop infusion immediately. If drug is involved, aspirate from short cannula. Then remove the IV catheter after injecting an antidote through the IV catheter if one is available and restart in the other extremity. Apply cold compresses if not contraindicated. Photograph site. Monitor site for 24 h. Provide written instructions for patient and family.
Phlebitis (inflammation of the vein caused by chemicals, trauma, or infection)	Vein hard with skin red, swollen, tender, warm Blood return present IV infusion may or may not be sluggish	Remove IV catheter and document; apply warm, moist pack to the IV site. Restart IV infusion in other extremity. Monitor frequently.
Thrombophlebitis (inflammation of the vein caused by a clot)	Site red, tender, warm IV infusion sluggish	Never irrigate the IV catheter; remove the IV catheter, notify the provider, and restart IV infusion in opposite extremity. Apply cool compresses initially, followed by warm compresses.
IV site skin infection (usually caused by inadequate skin prep)	Site hot, red, and painful but not hard or swollen Discharge at IV site IV infusion sluggish	Remove IV catheter, restart in opposite extremity, and change entire administration system. Clean site with alcohol. Apply warm compresses.
Venous spasm (usually secondary to rapid infusion of cold fluids)	Slowing of infusion rate Cramping or pain at or above the insertion site Numbness in the area Inability to withdraw peripherally inserted central catheter (PICC) or midline catheter	Slow infusion rate and apply warm compresses. Do not apply tension to catheter or forcibly remove it. Encourage consumption of warm liquids. Keep extremity covered and dry.
Nerve damage (usually secondary to improper insertion technique)	Tingling, "pins and needles" feeling, or numbness at or below the catheter insertion site	Immediately stop the cannula insertion if patient complains of severe pain. If sensations do not go away once the catheter is secured, remove the catheter.
Catheter embolus (usually caused by reinsertion of the needle into the cannula that has already been advanced off the needle)	Decrease in blood pressure (BP); pain along vein; weak, rapid pulse; cyanosis of nail beds; loss of consciousness	Remove IV catheter and inspect, place a tourniquet high on limb of IV site, notify provider, obtain x-ray, and prepare for surgery to remove pieces.
Systemic		
Infection (systemic infection is sepsis)	Fever, chills, general malaise, increased white blood cells (WBCs)	Change the infusion system, notify the provider, and obtain cultures as ordered.
Speed shock (caused by too-rapid infusion of medications)	Light-headedness or dizziness, flushed face, irregular pulse, decreased BP, loss of consciousness, cardiac arrest	Stop the infusion, notify the provider, and monitor vital signs frequently. Run dextrose 5% in water at a keep-vein-open rate.
Circulatory overload (caused by excessive [for the individual patient] administration of IV fluids)	Shortness of breath, tachypnea, increased BP, moist cough, crackles, puffiness around eyes and dependent edema	Elevate head of the bed, assess lung sounds, keep patient warm, assess for edema, and slow the infusion rate; notify the provider. Administer oxygen and diuretic as ordered.

fluid is administered. You should check the patient's armband against the medication administration record (MAR) for the correct name and the correct agency identification number and then ask the patient to state their name.

Safety Alert

Six Rights for Intravenous Therapy

The IV administration of fluids requires the same safety precautions as any other medication. Follow the Six Rights and the additional rules for drug administration (see Box 3.4). The label must be read and compared with the order or the MAR three times to ensure that the correct solution is being given to the correct patient. The patient's ID band must be checked each time a solution is administered, and the bar code on the bag must be scanned if using an electronic MAR.

CALCULATING AND REGULATING THE RATE OF FLOW

Rate of flow is an important factor in safe and effective IV therapy. Intravenous setups should be checked once every hour to be certain that the fluid is running correctly and that there are no problems. When possible, use an IV pump that is set for the specific rate of flow to administer IV fluids. Intravenous pumps, although not infallible, keep IV fluids flowing at the desired rate and act as safeguards should a problem arise. **Even when an IV pump is used, you must check to see that it is delivering the solution accurately, as prescribed.** Principles that affect the rate of flow for IV infusions *not* administered by a pump are as follows:

- The higher the container is placed above the level of the patient's heart, the faster the rate of flow because gravity affects flow.
- The fuller the container, the faster the rate of flow.
- The more viscous (thicker) the fluid, the slower the flow; for example, packed red cells will flow more slowly than 5% dextrose in water.
- The larger the diameter of the needle and tubing, the faster the flow.
- The higher the pressure within the vein, the slower the flow. As an infusion progresses and the veins become fuller, the IV solution may drip more slowly.
- Fluid will pass through a straight tube faster than through one that is coiled or hanging below the level of the cannula.

There usually is a chart available to determine the number of drops that should be given per minute to administer a given amount of fluid in a specified time. The IV tubing package will contain information about the number of drops the set will deliver per milliliter. If a chart is not available, calculate the number of drops per minute to be infused. To check the rate of flow, you must know how many drops should pass through the drip chamber in **1 minute.**

Once the number of drops per minute has been set and the IV infusion is flowing, the IV setup must be checked at 30- to 60-minute intervals to be sure that it continues to flow at the prescribed rate. As explained in the list of principles that affect the rate of flow, a number of factors can speed up or slow down the infusion.

If the IV infusion slows down and has not been checked and readjusted for some time, **no attempt should be made to "catch up"** by speeding up the rate of flow beyond that ordered. This can lead to circulatory overload and a volume excess that may produce pulmonary edema in susceptible patients. Table 3.9 presents points to check when an IV solution will not run at the prescribed rate.

Think Critically

How would you calculate the rate of flow for an order for "1000 mL of D_5W (dextrose 5% in water) over 8 hours" using a drip set that delivers 15 drops (gtt)/mL? How would the rate differ if the drip set delivers 20 gtt/mL? How would you calculate the flow rate for an order for "250 mL NS [normal saline] at 50 mL/h" using a microdrip set (60 gtt/mL)?

Table 3.9 Troubleshooting Intravenous Infusion Flow

CHECK	RATIONALE
Height of infusion container	Patient may have changed position. The container should be at least 36 inches above the heart. Most pump manufacturers recommend 12 inches above the pump.
System vent	The air vent, required for infusing with glass bottles, may be absent or occluded, which will prevent the flow.
Position of tubing	Tubing may be kinked, obstructing flow. Check the full length of the tubing, including above the pump.
Position of the extremity where the site is located	Flexion of the extremity may have compressed the vein, slowing the flow.
Any possible obstruction to flow	A protective device on the limb may be too tight. Tape may be compressing the circumference of the extremity. The most common obstruction is an unopened clamp.
Position of the cannula within the vessel	The cannula may be lying against the vessel wall, obstructing flow. Slightly turning the cannula to reposition the tip may cure the problem. Re-taping may also help.
If other measures have not opened the line, attempt to aspirate blood from the cannula	A small clot may be obstructing the cannula. Aspiration may withdraw the clot.

Intravenous Intake

IV infusion pumps track the amount of fluid infused through them. At the end of the shift the count is zeroed and the volume infused is recorded in the medical record. Some pumps interface with the electronic health record (EHR) and upload the information to the electronic chart. If a pump is not used, the total amount of IV fluid infused during the shift is calculated at the end of the shift. For example, if the beginning count is 350 mL (in the container at the beginning of the shift), that 350 mL is infused during the shift, then a new solution of 1000 mL is added (during the same shift), and some additional infusion takes place, we calculate the amount infused as follows:

	COUNT	INFUSED
Count at beginning of shift	350 mL	
New solution added at 11:30	1000 mL	350 mL
Count at end of shift	525 mL	475 mL
Total amount of IV intake for shift		825 mL

> **Safety Alert**
>
> **No Margin for Error**
>
> Intravenous therapy may become such a commonplace procedure to nurses that they are tempted to be complacent about it. However, it should never be thought of as a routine procedure that requires little attention. Any fluid or medication that enters a vein has an immediate effect. There is no margin for error in its administration.

Flushing As-Needed Locks or Central Intravenous Lines

Flushing the catheter or line prevents contact and reactions between the fluid that was last infused and incompatible drugs. Flushing the catheter or line maintains patency of the lumen. Either normal saline alone or normal saline followed by a heparin solution is used.

Before using an as-needed (PRN) lock, flush the catheter according to agency policy to determine patency (openness) of the lumen and to flush out any heparinized solution. The procedure will depend on the type of valved catheter or positive fluid-displacement needleless device in place. The flushing procedure always begins with gentle aspiration to see if a blood return is obtained. Do not pull back blood into the syringe; a small amount of blood in the tubing attached to the IV cannula is adequate to verify placement and patency. When flushing the catheter, apply slow, gentle pressure to the syringe plunger. **If you feel any resistance, stop the procedure immediately.** Proceeding may force a clot into the venous circulation that will become an embolus that could cause severe damage to the patient. Depending on the length of the catheter in place, 3 to 10 mL of normal saline is used.

> **Safety Alert**
>
> **Flushing Intravenous Catheters**
>
> Do not use more than 30 mL of bacteriostatic normal saline within a 24-hour period to flush the catheter. Always use single-dose vials or syringes of solution for flushing. **Do not use a multiple-dose vial for this purpose because it may be contaminated and could cause infection.**

PRN locks and catheters should be flushed immediately after use or whenever an IV piggyback medication infusion is completed. Delay in disconnecting the intermittent infusion administration set and flushing the lock could allow blood backflow into the catheter lumen because the infusion pressure drops lower than the venous pressure when the infusion is complete. In such a case, a clot can form, occluding the lumen. The catheter can also clot off if the infusion pump is stopped without disconnecting the IV tubing and flushing the PRN lock. **Be aware of when an intermittent infusion should be completed, and at the appropriate time be at the bedside prepared to remove the piggyback infusion setup and to flush the PRN lock. IV pumps will alarm when complete so that the IV site may be appropriately managed.**

Providing Central Line Care

If a gauze dressing is in place, provide site care every 24 to 48 hours per agency protocol. Transparent dressings require site care every 5 to 7 days. Every central line dressing should be examined once each shift, and the dressing should be changed if it is soiled. Central line dressing change and site care are sterile procedures. The old dressing is removed using exam gloves. A Central Line Bundle (a series of interventions) has been developed by the Institute for Healthcare Improvement (IHI) to prevent infection from central lines. It has five components: optimal site selection, chlorhexidine skin antisepsis, hand hygiene, maximal barrier precautions, and daily review of line necessity with prompt removal if it is not needed (IHI, 2013).

Blood drawing. Drawing blood from a central line is performed using strict aseptic technique. Blood is withdrawn for discard, then the sample is obtained. Follow agency protocols for flushing after the blood draw and timing of caps changes.

Partial or total parenteral nutrition. Many patients with fluid and electrolyte imbalances are nutritionally depleted. Partial parenteral nutrition (PPN) is given when a patient cannot maintain an adequate nutritional status with oral intake. PPN is given through a large

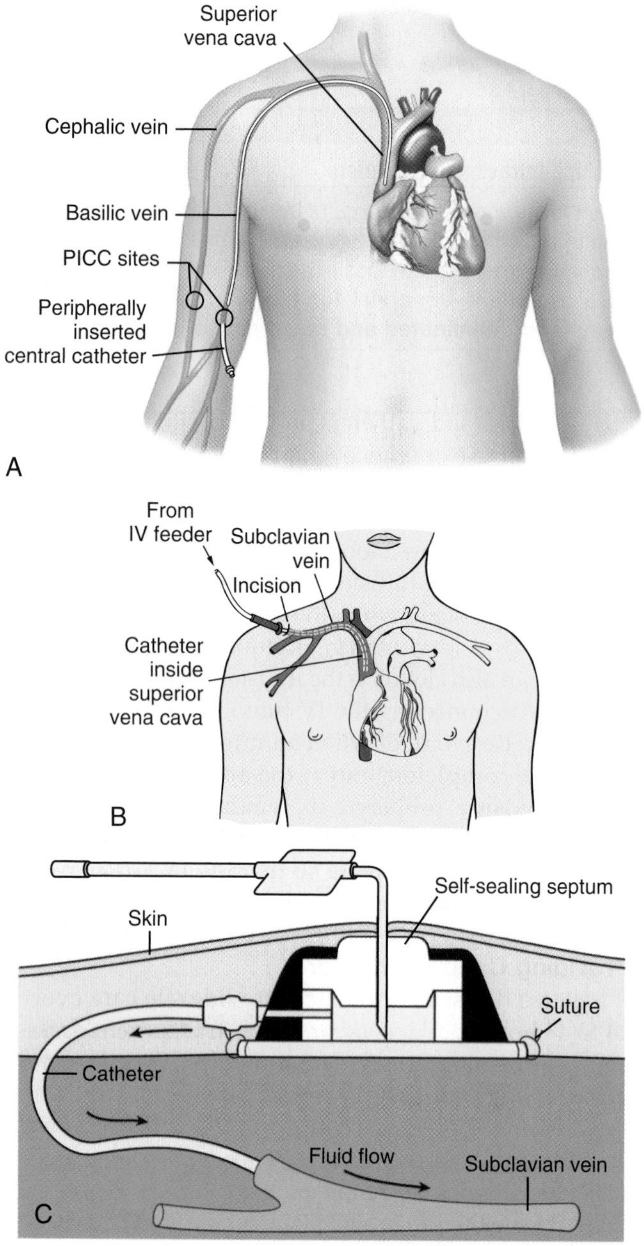

Fig. 3.10 **A,** Placement of a peripherally inserted central catheter *(PICC)* through the antecubital fossa. **B,** Placement of a central venous catheter inserted into the subclavian vein. **C,** Implanted port for infusion of fluids and medications and for blood sampling. *IV,* Intravenous. (**A** from Lewis SL, Bucher L, Heitkemper MM, et al.: *Medical-surgical nursing: assessment and management of clinical problems,* ed 10, St. Louis, 2017, Elsevier. **B** from Elkin MK, Perry AG, Potter AG: *Nursing interventions and clinical skills,* ed 3, St. Louis, 2004, Mosby.)

peripheral vein in the arm. If sufficient nutrition cannot be delivered by oral intake and PPN or by enteral feedings, TPN is begun (see Chapter 28). Fig. 3.10 shows placement of a peripherally inserted central catheter (PICC), a central venous catheter, and an implanted port for infusion of fluids and medications and for blood sampling.

Focused Assessment

Data Collection for Problems of Fluid, Electrolyte, and Acid-Base Imbalance

Assess the following:

Current Illness

Head

- Alertness, orientation, dizziness, signs of confusion, irritability, restlessness
- Appearance of eyes and eyelids
- Condition of oral mucous membranes, tongue, thickness of saliva

Skin and Extremities

- Color, moisture, temperature, areas of discoloration
- Turgor
- Tightness of rings
- Evidence and degree of edema
- Strength of hand grip
- Cramping of muscles
- Reflexes
- Chvostek sign
- Trousseau sign

Laboratory and Diagnostic Tests

- Hematocrit changes
- Urine amount, color, odor, and specific gravity
- Electrolyte values
- Blood gas values
- Electrocardiogram T-wave changes

Vital Signs

- Blood pressure changes
- Pulse rate, rhythm, and character
- Temperature
- Respirations
- Change in weight

Lungs

- Breath sounds (any crackles?)

Intake and Output

Known Disease Conditions

Medications

NURSING MANAGEMENT

ASSESSMENT (DATA COLLECTION)

First, assess the patient for *risk* of fluid, electrolyte, or acid-base imbalance, then assess for actual signs and symptoms of fluid, electrolyte, and acid-base imbalance. Question the patient about subjective signs and symptoms.

Older Adult Care Points

Remember that checking for tenting is not an accurate way to assess dehydration in older adults because their skin loses elasticity with aging and will tent with normal hydration. It is better to check for dry mucous membranes, concentrated urine, and other signs and symptoms in these patients.

NURSING DIAGNOSIS

Analyze the assessment data, identify problem areas, and choose problem statements or nursing diagnoses.

Common problem statements for patients with fluid, electrolyte, or acid-base imbalances include:

- Fluid volume deficit
- Fluid volume overload
- Potential for electrolyte imbalance
- Altered tissue perfusion
- Altered cardiac output
- Altered gas exchange
- Altered breathing pattern

Other problem statements may be appropriate as a result of the fluid, electrolyte, or acid-base imbalance or may be related to the cause of the imbalance—for example, diarrhea.

◆ PLANNING

The goal is to restore the patient's fluid, electrolyte, or acid-base balance. Write the individual expected outcomes. Expected outcomes might be one or more of the following:

- Patient will exhibit normal skin turgor.
- Patient's weight will stabilize at normal baseline.
- Intake and output will be balanced.
- Blood gases will return to normal.
- Breath sounds will be clear to auscultation.
- There will be no evidence of edema.
- Electrolyte values will be within normal limits.
- Patient will not experience complications of IV therapy.

See Nursing Care Plan 3.1 for examples of expected outcomes with nursing interventions.

◆ IMPLEMENTATION

When patients are unable to take in sufficient fluids on their own, work with the health care provider to provide adequate fluid and electrolytes. If patients can swallow and retain fluid, assist patients to frequently take small amounts of fluid. Establish a plan for assisting with both hot and cold liquid consumption. With conscientious care, the need for IV feeding can be avoided. It is helpful to assess what the patient prefers. In addition to water, offer the patient fruit juices, bouillon, ice pops, soft drinks, or gelatin.

Think Critically

What type of fluid and electrolyte imbalance is a patient who has gastroenteritis and is suffering from both vomiting and diarrhea likely to have?

A patient with fluid volume excess may have an order for fluid restriction. This means that the patient may take in only a certain amount of fluid over a 24-hour period. Verify if the restriction includes IV fluids. Work out a schedule of fluid intake so that liquids are spaced evenly and the patient does not receive all the allotted liquids in a short time. A typical schedule would be: day, 600 mL; evening, 400 mL; night, 200 mL. If not prohibited, sugarless hard candies and chewing gum can help relieve thirst. Frequent oral care is essential.

Diuretics may be prescribed, particularly if there is a potential for congestive heart failure or pulmonary edema. For patients at such risk, daily weight and electrolyte status must be monitored, along with I&O.

Assignment Considerations

Obtaining a Daily Weight

When assigning the daily weighing of patients to a certified nursing assistant (CNA) or UAP, remind the person that weight should be measured before breakfast, with the patient in essentially the same amount of clothing as at the last measurement, and after voiding. The same scale should be used each day to ensure reliable data for comparison. Any gain of 2 lb or more over 2 days should be reported to you immediately.

Skin care is particularly important in preventing a breakdown over an edematous area. The stretched skin is extremely fragile, has a decreased blood supply, and is no longer flexible. Keep bed linens dry and smooth and turn the patient frequently to relieve pressure over bony prominences. **Be very gentle in repositioning and turning the patient; to avoid friction on the skin, use a turning sheet. A break in edematous skin can quickly form a pressure ulcer.**

When acid-base imbalance occurs, institute control of the underlying disorder. Monitor blood gases and administer oxygen and electrolytes as needed. Apply nursing measures to improve pulmonary function, as appropriate.

Think Critically

Your patient has a PaO_2 of 94, pH of 7.32, $PaCO_2$ of 48, and HCO_3^- of 26. What type of acid-base imbalance does the patient have?

◆ EVALUATION

Every 24 hours, perform evaluations to determine whether nursing interventions are assisting the patient to meet expected outcomes. If the patient is not progressing toward achievement of the outcomes, problem solve and think critically to determine why, then alter the plan of care appropriately. When a specific outcome is met, discontinue that portion of the plan.

COMMUNITY CARE

Nurses in long-term care facilities deal every day with the problems of delicate fluid balance in their older adult patients. These patients often are taking multiple drugs that can affect their fluid and electrolyte status. Diuretics in particular can upset fluid and electrolyte status. It is especially important that the long-term care and home care nurse be vigilant for the signs of hypokalemia (see Table 3.4). Potassium imbalances are particularly dangerous for heart patients. Hypokalemia alters the way digitalis is metabolized in the body and predisposes the patient to digitalis toxicity. Signs of digitalis toxicity are fatigue, anorexia, headache, blurred vision, yellow-green halos around lights, nausea, diarrhea, and cardiac dysrhythmias.

Clinical Cues

Any patient in a long-term care facility or at home who is taking digitalis and is experiencing nausea, vomiting, diarrhea, or fluid and electrolyte alterations should be questioned daily about symptoms of hypokalemia and digitalis toxicity.

Dehydration and hyponatremia from infection account for many of the hospital admissions of patients from long-term care facilities and home situations. It takes a caring, skillful nurse to see that long-term care and home care patients take in enough fluids without interfering with their nutritional intake.

The home care nurse must collaborate with the infusion company nurse when the patient is receiving IV fluids at home or is on TPN. Clear instructions must be given to the patient and family regarding the IV therapy. An older adult patient who has a fluid volume excess from congestive heart failure may already have a diminished appetite. In this instance restricting sodium in the diet may do more harm than good. You, along with the health care provider, must make individual judgments about the patient's priority needs.

Patient Teaching

Home Care Intravenous Therapy

Call me when:

- Swelling, redness, or pain occurs at the IV site or along the vessel.
- The solution will not flow even after you have checked that the clamps are open.
- The solution leaks at the catheter site and you have checked to see that the tubing is firmly attached to the catheter.
- The patient's temperature rises above 100° F (38° C).

Telephone number ____________

Get Ready for the NCLEX® Examination!

Key Points

- Fluid balance is essential because the life processes of every cell take place within fluid.
- Infants and older adults are at greatest risk for fluid imbalance.
- Water has four main functions in the body.
- Body fluids are distributed in intracellular compartments and extracellular compartments.
- Control of fluid balance is managed by hormones and by the thirst mechanism.
- Fluids and solutes move within the body by diffusion, filtration, osmosis, and active transport.
- Tonicity refers to the amount of solutes in relation to the amount of fluid.
- Filtration occurs through a semipermeable membrane.
- Hydrostatic pressure causes filtration of fluid out of the intravascular system into the interstitial spaces.
- Water diffuses by osmosis.
- Diffusion moves water from the interstitial spaces into the cells.
- The kidney is a major factor in the regulation of fluid and electrolyte balance in the body.
- Fluid volume deficit may result from fluid losses or because of lack of fluid intake (see Table 3.1).
- A fluid deficit causes dehydration. Checking skin turgor is one way to assess for dehydration.
- Check the tongue and mucous membranes of older adults to assess for dehydration.
- Weight change is the most accurate measure of fluid gain or loss.
- Fluid deficit is a common problem in older adults.
- Electrolytes need to be replaced along with fluid when there has been a fluid deficit.
- Prolonged vomiting leads to sodium and potassium deficits and metabolic alkalosis.
- Position the vomiting patient so that aspiration of vomitus does not occur.
- Rehydrate the dehydrated older adult patient cautiously so that overhydration does not occur.
- Medications can be administered to help stop vomiting and diarrhea (see Table 3.2).
- Fluid volume excess leads to hypervolemia, edema, and possibly pulmonary edema.
- Assessment will reveal elevated blood pressure and a full, bounding pulse.
- Edema may be localized or general; pitting edema may occur.
- Loss of plasma proteins may cause edema.
- When fluid shifts from the intravascular space to the interstitial spaces, hypovolemia may occur.
- With fluid excess, sensorium may be clouded.
- Edema may be treated with diuretic medications, a low-sodium diet, and elastic stockings or sequential compression devices.
- Electrolytes are responsible for the transmission of nerve impulses, contraction of muscles, and excretion of hormones (see Table 3.3).
- Urine output must be at least 30 mL/h before IV potassium is given.
- Intravenous potassium is always diluted and never given as a bolus injection.
- Acid-base imbalances upset the normal function of the body's systems.

- The kidneys are the principal organ in controlling a normal pH; the lungs also assist.
- Too much carbonic acid in the body causes acidosis; too much bicarbonate in the body causes alkalosis.
- Changes in carbon dioxide are usually respiratory; changes in bicarbonate are usually metabolic.
- Diabetic ketoacidosis causes metabolic acidosis and can be life-threatening.
- Arterial blood gases are analyzed to determine whether there is an acid-base imbalance and what type of imbalance is present.
- Each acid-base imbalance has its own signs and symptoms and probable treatments.
- Every ill patient should be assessed for a fluid, electrolyte, and acid-base imbalance.
- Intravenous therapy can provide the patient with fluid, electrolytes, and nutrients.
- Intravenous fluids are isotonic, hypotonic, or hypertonic (see Table 3.7).
- Intravenous therapy must be administered in a strict aseptic manner.
- The Six Rights should be used when administering any IV fluid or drug (see Box 3.4).
- Monitoring for complications of IV therapy is a top priority (see Table 3.8).
- Rate of IV flow must be monitored closely; never rely solely on an IV pump.
- Older adults can become fluid overloaded very quickly.
- Subcutaneous infusion is mostly used for pain control.
- TPN is used when a patient cannot obtain adequate nutrition by other means.

Additional Learning Resources

SG Go to your Study Guide for additional learning activities to help you master this chapter content.

Go to your Evolve website (http://evolve.elsevier.com/deWit/medsurg) for the following FREE learning resources:

- Animations, audio, and video
- Answers and rationales for questions and activities
- Glossary with pronunciations in English and Spanish
- Interactive Review Questions and more!

Review Questions for the NCLEX® Examination

1. What should nurses monitor when a patient is receiving a diuretic regularly? (*Select all that apply.*)
   1. Skin turgor and integrity
   2. Daily weight
   3. Electrolyte status
   4. Mentation

   NCLEX Client Need: Physiological Integrity: Reduction of Risk Potential

2. Which patient(s) can be considered at high risk for fluid and electrolyte imbalance? *(Select all that apply.)*
   1. A 45-year-old woman with thyroid crisis
   2. A 35-year-old trauma victim on a ventilator
   3. A 60-year-old woman with temperature of 99.6° F (37° C)
   4. A 70-year-old man on anticoagulant therapy
   5. A 30-year-old woman complaining of persistent diarrhea

   NCLEX Client Need: Physiological Integrity: Reduction of Risk Potential

3. An older adult man is admitted for severe disorientation, confusion, and general weakness. His spouse reports that he is not able to tolerate any food or fluids and has had several episodes of vomiting and diarrhea. Which imbalance(s) is/are the patient most likely experiencing? (*Select all that apply*)
   1. Hypokalemia
   2. Metabolic acidosis
   3. Hyponatremia
   4. Respiratory alkalosis
   5. Hypochloremia

   NCLEX Client Need: Physiological Integrity: Physiological Adaptation

4. In planning care for a patient with congestive heart failure, you choose the problem statement: fluid volume overload due to altered cardiac output. The problem statement would most likely be supported by which sign or symptom?
   1. Temperature of 101.5° F (38.6° C)
   2. Hematocrit 35%
   3. Fine crackles in the lung sounds
   4. Clear, yellow urine

   NCLEX Client Need: Physiological Integrity: Physiological Adaptation

5. A patient who has congestive heart failure has a fluid excess with a weight gain of 1.5 pounds since yesterday and edematous ankles. Which health care provider's order has the highest priority?
   1. Maintain accurate intake and output.
   2. Monitor skin for signs of breakdown.
   3. Administer furosemide 40 mg PO (by mouth) once daily.
   4. Obtain daily weight.

   NCLEX Client Need: Physiological Integrity: Physiological Adaptation

6. A new patient on the floor has been diagnosed with gastroenteritis. What would be the most critical level to assess?
   1. Blood glucose
   2. Potassium
   3. Calcium
   4. Sodium

   NCLEX Client Need: Physiological Integrity: Physiological Adaptation

7. You appropriately elicit a sign of hypocalcemia by:
   1. tapping the face about 1 inch from the ear.
   2. palpating a partially stretched tendon.
   3. inspecting facial symmetry.
   4. applying pressure on the radial pulse.

   NCLEX Client Need: Physiological Integrity: Reduction in Risk Potential
8. At the beginning of shift, there is 400 mL of fluid in the IV bag. A piggyback medication containing 100 mL is hung at 12:00 noon to run over 30 minutes. You hang a new bag of 1000 mL at 1:00 P.M. to run at 125 mL/h. At the end of shift there is 250 mL left in the bag. The count for the total amount of fluid infused during your shift ending at 7:00 P.M. is:
   1. 1250 mL.
   2. 1285 mL.
   3. 1300 mL.
   4. 1520 mL.

   NCLEX Client Need: Physiological Integrity: Pharmacological Therapies
9. Which would be the most accurate way to assess for dehydration in an older adult patient?
   1. Skin turgor
   2. Urine output
   3. Respirations
   4. Thirst levels

   NCLEX Client Need: Physiological Integrity: Physiological Adaptation
10. You respond to a patient complaining of pain, swelling, and wetness over the peripheral IV site. On assessment, you find that the IV insertion site is tender and cool to touch. These are signs and symptoms of:
    1. phlebitis.
    2. infiltration.
    3. infection.
    4. venous spasm.

    NCLEX Client Need: Safe and Effective Care Environment: Safety and Infection Control

Critical Thinking Questions

Scenario A

Mrs. Thompson, age 64, is admitted to the hospital for congestive heart failure. She is very edematous. She is slightly confused on admission, and although she is not on absolute bed rest, she tells you she is too weak to get out of bed.

1. What type of diet would you expect the health care provider to order for Mrs. Thompson? Why?
2. Why are daily weights ordered for Mrs. Thompson? Why are those data important?
3. Mrs. Thompson is on fluid restrictions. How would you schedule her fluid intake?

Scenario B

Mr. Mendez, age 76, is admitted with dehydration and diarrhea. He is confused and listless.

1. What parameters would you assess to see if his fluid balance is improving?
2. What electrolyte imbalances would you expect to find?
3. Why would you need to keep a close eye on the IV infusion that is ordered?
4. What acid-base imbalance is he likely to be experiencing?
5. What assessment data would tell you that the plan of care is working to rebalance his fluid and electrolytes?

Care of Preoperative and Intraoperative Surgical Patients

4

http://evolve.elsevier.com/deWit/medsurg

Objectives

Theory

1. Discuss the advantages of current technological advances in surgery.
2. Explain the physical, emotional, and psychosocial preparation of patients for surgical procedures.
3. Identify the types of patients most at risk for surgical complications and state why each patient is at risk.
4. Plan and implement patient and family teaching to prevent postoperative complications.
5. Compare the roles of the scrub nurse and the circulating nurse.
6. Analyze the differences in the various types of anesthesia and list the advantages and disadvantages of each to the health care team and the patient.

Clinical Practice

7. Perform a thorough nursing assessment for a preoperative patient.
8. Teach a patient postoperative exercises during the preoperative period.
9. Prepare a patient for surgery using a preoperative checklist.
10. Document preoperative care and assessment data.
11. Observe during a patient's surgery.

Key Terms

anesthesia (ăn-ĕs-THĒ-zē-ă, p. 78)
atelectasis (ă-tĕ-LĔK-tă-sĭs, p. 69)
autologous (ăw-TŎL-ŏ-gŭs, p. 65)
capnography (kăp-NŎG-ră-fē, p. 79)
dehiscence (dē-HĬS-ĕntz, p. 69)
palliative (PĂL-ē-ŭ-tĭv, p. 64)
perioperative (pĕr-ē-ŎP-ĕr-ă-tĭv, p. 65)
pneumonia (nū-MŌ-nē-ă, p. 69)
prosthesis (prŏs-THĒ-sĭs, p. 67)
robotics (rō-bŏ-tĭks, p. 65)
stasis (STĀ-sĭs, p. 72)
thrombophlebitis (thrŏm-bō-flĕ-BĪ-tĭs, p. 72)

Concepts Covered in This Chapter

- Infection
- Mobility
- Tissue Integrity
- Pain
- Patient Education
- Communication
- Collaboration
- Safety

SURGERY

Surgery is performed for a variety of reasons (Table 4.1). For the patient, any type of surgery is a serious event. Knowing terminology specific to surgical procedures helps you envision the procedure so that you may better prepare patients for surgery and care for them afterward (Box 4.1). Surgery may be elective, urgent, or performed as an emergency.

In a hospital, surgery may be performed as a same-day or outpatient procedure or as an inpatient procedure. Many surgeries are done in a freestanding surgery center. Minor surgery is often performed in a health care provider's office; licensed practical/vocational nurses (LPN/LVNs) assist more often with surgery in this setting. For any surgery, preparation usually begins before admission. The patient undergoes diagnostic tests and is taught preoperative and postoperative care in the days just before the scheduled surgery. The ability to deliver and reinforce teaching for postoperative and home care is crucial to the well-being and quick recovery of patients.

TECHNOLOGICAL ADVANCES IN SURGERY

Laparoscopic and endoscopic procedures have replaced many "open" surgeries (in which a large incision is necessary). Minimally invasive laparoscopic surgery (done through small openings in the abdomen) can be performed more quickly. This results in less trauma to

Table 4.1 Selected Categories of Surgical Procedures

CATEGORY	DESCRIPTION	CONDITION OR SURGICAL PROCEDURE
Reasons for Surgery		
Diagnostic	Performed to determine the origin and cause of a disorder or the cell type for cancer	Breast biopsy Exploratory laparotomy Arthroscopy
Curative	Performed to resolve a health problem by repairing or removing the cause	Laparoscopic cholecystectomy Mastectomy Hysterectomy
Restorative	Performed to improve a patient's functional ability	Total knee replacement Finger reimplantation
Palliative	Performed to relieve symptoms of a disease process, but does not cure	Colostomy Nerve root resection Tumor debulking Ileostomy
Cosmetic	Performed primarily to alter or enhance personal appearance	Liposuction Revision of scars Rhinoplasty Blepharoplasty
Urgency of Surgery		
Elective	Planned for correction of a nonacute problem	Cataract removal Hernia repair Hemorrhoidectomy Total joint replacement
Urgent	Requires prompt intervention; may be life-threatening if treatment is delayed more than 24–48 h	Intestinal obstruction Bladder obstruction Kidney or ureteral stones Bone fracture Eye injury Acute cholecystitis
Emergent	Requires immediate intervention to prevent life-threatening consequences	Gunshot or stab wound Severe bleeding Abdominal aortic aneurysm Compound fracture Appendectomy
Degree of Risk of Surgery		
Minor	Procedure without significant risk; often done with local anesthesia	Incision and drainage (I&D) Implantation of a venous access device (VAD) Muscle biopsy
Major	Procedure of greater risk, usually longer and more extensive than a minor procedure	Mitral valve replacement Pancreas transplant Lymph node dissection
Extent of Surgery		
Simple	Only the most overtly affected areas are involved in the surgery	Simple/partial mastectomy
Radical	Extensive surgery beyond the area obviously involved; is directed at finding a root cause	Radical prostatectomy Radical hysterectomy
Minimally invasive surgery (MIS)	Surgery performed in a body cavity or body area through one or more endoscopes; can correct problems, remove organs, take tissue for biopsy, re-route blood vessels and drainage systems; is a fast-growing and ever-changing type of surgery	Arthroscopy Tubal ligation Hysterectomy Lung lobectomy Coronary artery bypass Cholecystectomy

From Ignatavicius DD, Workman ML, Blair M, et al.: *Medical-surgical nursing: concepts for interprofessional collaborative care,* ed 9, St. Louis, 2018, Elsevier.

Box 4.1 Terminology Used for Surgical Procedures

Suffixes are often attached to a stem word to describe a surgical procedure. For example, *appendectomy* means cutting out the appendix.

-ectomy: Cutting out or off (colectomy: cutting out a part of the colon)

-lysis: Removal or destruction of (neurolysis: freeing a nerve from adhesions)

-oma: Tumor (excision of a fibroma: removal of a connective tissue tumor)

-ostomy: To furnish with an outlet (colostomy: creating an outlet for the colon from the body)

-otomy: Cutting into (thoracotomy: cutting into the chest cavity)

-plasty: Revision, molding, or repair of tissue (mammoplasty: revision of the breast)

-pexy: Fixation, anchoring in place (orchiopexy: fixation of an undescended testicle in the scrotum)

tissue, less inflammatory response, and therefore less pain and a faster recovery. For example, laparoscopic cholecystectomy for gallbladder removal has reduced a patient's recovery time from 6 weeks to approximately 1 week. Endoscopic surgery (in which fiberoptic technologies are used to visualize interior structures of the body), operating microscopes, and lasers are commonplace in the surgical suite.

Medical **robotics** (design of computerized, mechanical instruments) provides a key to less invasive, less traumatic surgeries. A medical robot is operated from a nearby computer while the surgeon views magnified three-dimensional images of the surgical field on the computer's screen. The robot's tiny camera has multiple lenses that allow magnification up to 12 times that of normal vision. There are assistants and a second surgeon next to the patient, but the primary surgeon at the computer uses the robot to perform the surgery. Remote-controlled instruments are inserted through small incisions. An advantage of using the robot is that it has "rock-steady" hands, providing precision that is beyond human dexterity. Because only small incisions are needed, the patient has less pain postoperatively and requires less time to heal. With robotic surgical techniques, the patient experiences less scarring (because incisions are smaller), and the small surgical wounds heal faster. Surgeries can be transmitted via videoconferencing to locations around the world to enhance the skill levels of surgeons everywhere.

AUTOLOGOUS BLOOD FOR TRANSFUSION

Since the mid-1980s, patients undergoing elective surgery have had the option of banking their own blood before surgery in case a transfusion is needed. The patient's blood is withdrawn at the blood bank several weeks before the surgery, prepared, and stored. The blood is prepared for **autologous** (related to self) transfusion. Cell savers can be used to collect and salvage blood during and after surgery, so that the patient's own blood can be reinfused if the patient needs it. Access to autologous procedures has greatly decreased the anxiety of patients who fear infection with a bloodborne virus, such as human immunodeficiency virus (HIV) or hepatitis B or C.

BLOODLESS SURGERY

Some patients opt for bloodless surgery to avoid completely the risk inherent in a blood transfusion. Bloodless surgery uses a combination of techniques to minimize blood loss and maximize blood volume and function. Epoetin alfa (Epogen, Procrit) may be given before surgery to stimulate red blood cell production, and hemostatic agents may be given before or during surgery to promote clotting (Crookston, 2016). During surgery, the surgeon may request induced hypotension or hypothermia to decrease oxygen demand.

Another bloodless surgical technique is hemodilution, in which several units of the patient's blood are removed and replaced with crystalloids or colloids to expand vascular volume. Hemodilution decreases blood viscosity, improves oxygen transport, and—if bleeding occurs during surgery—minimizes the loss of red blood cells. The removed blood may or may not be returned at the end of the procedure based on the patient's preference.

Cultural Considerations

Jehovah's Witness Patients and Blood Transfusions

Followers of Jehovah's Witness will not accept a blood transfusion from another person because of their religious beliefs. They believe that there are eternal consequences from receiving blood not their own. In the past, this precluded them from having certain major surgeries. Now bloodless surgery is one option for them because of management techniques.

❖ PERIOPERATIVE NURSING MANAGEMENT

Perioperative nursing refers to care of the patient before, during, and after surgery. You play a key role during the perioperative period.

◆ ASSESSMENT (DATA COLLECTION)

Before surgery, the patient should be in the best possible physical condition. In emergencies, of course, physical condition cannot be controlled, but planned surgery may be postponed until the patient is physically able to withstand the stress of anesthesia and major surgery. To determine the patient's readiness for surgery, a thorough health assessment is conducted and risk factors are considered. In addition to the admission assessment data that are gathered when the patient is first admitted (see Chapter 2), the perioperative nurse gathers data specific to the surgical procedure and postoperative course. Thorough assessment facilitates planning of care during and after surgery.

Older Adult Care Points

Patients older than 75 years have surgical complication rates three times higher than those of younger adults. An older adult patient is less able to adjust and compensate for the stress of surgery, because physiologic reserves (cardiac, respiratory, renal) have already declined with age. Older adult patients are more likely to have impaired renal, hepatic, respiratory, and cardiac functions that alter their metabolism and excretion of drugs and anesthesia. The presence of chronic diseases causes vulnerability to fluid and electrolyte imbalances during and after surgery.

When assessing the presurgical patient, any significant deviations from normal range should be brought to the attention of the surgeon. For example, an elevated temperature might indicate an infection that would need to be brought under control before surgery.

Think Critically

If your 76-year-old patient seems confused the morning after a hip replacement, what would you check in their chart to see if there has been an alteration?

Knowing the patient's usual blood pressure reading is necessary for comparison after surgery to determine if the patient is stable. Height and weight are measured and charted before surgery so the anesthesiologist can accurately calculate anesthetic dosages. Allergies must be identified and noted clearly in the medical record and on an allergy bracelet worn on the patient's arm.

Assessment for particular risk factors for surgical site infection includes preexisting infection or medical condition, nasal bacterial colonization, malnutrition, advancing age, diabetes mellitus, nicotine use, immunosuppression, and obesity.

Focused Assessment

Preoperative Data Collection

HEALTH HISTORY AND PSYCHOSOCIAL ASSESSMENT

- Have you previously had surgery? What was your experience?
- What is the reason for this surgery?
- How do you feel about having this surgery?
- What do you know about this surgery and the before and after care?
- What are your expectations of this surgery?
- Have you or any family members ever experienced any problems with surgery or anesthesia?
- Will this surgery create any problems in your usual roles or relationships?
- Do you have any chronic illnesses?
- Have you gained or lost considerable weight recently?
- Do you have any allergies to medications, iodine, shellfish, adhesive tape, or latex?
- What medications, over-the-counter preparations, vitamins, herbs, and supplements do you take?
- Do you smoke? How much and for how many years?
- What is your usual use of alcohol?
- When was your last bowel movement?
- Do you have any problems with urination?
- Do you currently have an upper respiratory tract infection?
- Do you have any musculoskeletal problems that need to be addressed during positioning for surgery?
- Do you have health insurance?
- What people will be able to help you during your recovery?
- Will you be able to cope with inconveniences during your recovery without additional help?
- How do you usually cope with pain?
- Are there particular concerns or fears you have regarding the surgery now?

CULTURAL ASSESSMENT

- What is your primary language?
- Do you have any cultural or spiritual practices that you would like to observe during this period of surgery and recovery?
- What are your cultural customs regarding privacy, blood transfusions, and disposal of body parts?

SPIRITUAL ASSESSMENT

- Do you have spiritual or religious beliefs?
- Do you wish to talk with or see your spiritual or religious advisor?
- Is there any conflict between your value or belief system and this planned surgery?

PHYSICAL ASSESSMENT

- Measure height and weight.
- Measure vital signs.
- Auscultate the lungs and heart.
- Listen for bowel sounds.
- Check pulses and compare bilaterally.
- Gather basic neurologic data: level of consciousness; orientation to time, place, and person; ability to think, answer questions, and follow instructions.
- Assess skin status, integrity, moisture, and temperature.
- Assess for recent tattoos, piercings, and body jewelry.
- Assess for limitations in joint range of motion.
- Assess for muscle weakness.
- Assess for loose teeth, dentures, bridges, contact lenses, hearing aids, and other prostheses.

LABORATORY AND DIAGNOSTIC TEST DATA

- Verify that test results are in the chart.
- Note any abnormal findings.

Safety Alert

Latex Allergy

A patient who is allergic to latex is at high risk of exposure during surgery when unconscious and unable to monitor the environment. Contact and airborne precautions are necessary. The perioperative nurse must be constantly vigilant to keep anything with latex on it out of the patient's environment. Even rubber stoppers on medication bottles or intravenous (IV) supply containers can be a problem. The operating room must be prepared to be "latex free." A "latex-free" crash cart is kept at hand in case of emergency.

Think Critically

Why would a localized infection be a contraindication for surgery in some instances?

It is particularly important to know if a patient is taking a corticosteroid, which can delay wound healing, alter fluid and electrolyte balance, and affect several metabolic functions in the body—factors that increase surgical risk. Patients should be questioned about medicines and eye drops that may contain a corticosteroid. Corticosteroids should be tapered slowly before surgery but never stopped abruptly. Many patients are on routine antiplatelet or anticoagulant medications for various cardiovascular disorders. This information is extremely important to share with the health care team. Vitamin E, aspirin and other nonsteroidal antiinflammatory drugs (NSAIDs), and anticoagulants have a continuing effect on blood clotting for several days; these supplements and medicines are usually discontinued 7 to 14 days before surgery. If the surgery is urgent or emergent, these medications will contribute to intraoperative and postoperative bleeding

Complementary and Alternative Therapies

Herbals and Supplements

Most anesthesiologists will ask patients to discontinue taking herbal supplements 2 to 3 weeks before surgery because many herbal supplements interact with anesthetic agents or interfere with blood clotting. If doing without a supplement is not possible, the herbal supplement container should be brought to the anesthesiologist. Black cohosh, St. John's wort, feverfew, valerian, goldenseal, licorice, and kava can have interactions with other medications and anesthetics and should be stopped 2 to 3 weeks before surgery. Ginger, feverfew, garlic, ginseng, and ginkgo biloba all can have adverse effects on clotting mechanisms. It is best to stop all herbal supplements several days before surgery. After surgery, the patient should ask the health care provider when each herb can be restarted.

Nutritional status and body weight are significant factors in healing and repair of the surgical site. Obesity presents problems for such routine procedures as venipuncture and intubation for general anesthesia, and **obesity causes prolonged uptake of anesthetic drugs.**

The operating room personnel are notified if the patient has a hearing impairment, is essentially blind when glasses are not in place, or has a **prosthesis** (artificial body part).

The news that surgery is needed usually comes as an emotional shock to patients and their families. Surgery causes changes in the routine of their lives that could result in personal and financial burdens. Surgery will alter the lives of some patients permanently and possibly may leave them physically impaired. Others might expect to be greatly helped by the surgical procedure. In any event, there will be fears and misgivings about the prospect of undergoing anesthesia and surgery.

Cultural Considerations

Beliefs Regarding Surgery

Cultural beliefs and values regarding surgery must be taken into consideration. If a female patient's culture has strict rules for female attire, she needs assurance of sufficient privacy and protection of modesty to allay any fears she might have. Such issues and interventions must be conveyed to the surgical team. If there are cultural taboos regarding an aspect of the surgery, the surgical team needs to know them and plan a way to achieve a good outcome without violating such taboos. It is especially important to know whether the patient will accept a blood transfusion.

Older Adult Care Points

Older patients who are experiencing serious depression are at high risk for complications of surgery because their motivation for recovery often is very low.

Determine whether the patient will have adequate help at home when discharged from the hospital. Many older people live alone and, although self-sufficient before surgery, may have difficulty preparing meals, bathing, or performing wound care while recovering from surgery. Some patients benefit from a short stay at an acute rehabilitation facility to regain strength and independence before returning to their home.

Some people are concerned about whether they will "wake up" or survive the anesthesia and surgical procedure. Some patients have a strong spiritual belief that helps them cope independently with sickness, suffering, and death. Others may need help in finding the spiritual support they need. Still others do not want to discuss this facet of their lives. Allow time with clergy or a spiritual advisor before the surgical procedure according to the patient's desire.

Laboratory and Diagnostic Test Data

Box 4.2 lists the tests most frequently required before surgery. A chest radiograph is usually obtained, and an electrocardiogram is ordered for many patients older than 40 years. If the patient has lung disease, pulmonary function tests may be ordered. If the laboratory reports indicate any abnormal values, surgery may be

Box 4.2 Commonly Ordered Preoperative Tests

Laboratory
Complete blood cell count (CBC)
Urinalysis (UA)
- Prothrombin time (PT)/INR
- Partial thromboplastin time (PTT)
- Blood type and crossmatch
- Pregnancy test for women of childbearing age

Metabolic panel
- Liver function tests (AST, ALT, bilirubin)[a]
- Renal function tests (BUN, creatinine)[a]

Blood glucose
Electrolytes
Other tests
- ECG
- Chest x-ray

[a]May be ordered as part of a metabolic panel or sequential multiple assay (SMA)–6 or SMA-12.
ALT, Alanine aminotransferase; *AST*, aspartate aminotransferase; *BUN*, blood urea nitrogen; *ECG*, electrocardiogram; *INR*, international normalized ratio.

postponed. Most surgeons prefer to delay surgery if a patient's hemoglobin level is below 10 g/dL.

Think Critically

Why would anemia make a patient a poor surgical candidate?

Surgery puts a strain on the cardiovascular, renal, and respiratory systems. Liver function is important because the liver is involved in synthesizing clotting factors, producing albumin, and metabolizing and detoxifying drugs. Although requesting preoperative diagnostic tests is the responsibility of the health care provider, you will need to explain to the patient why these tests have been ordered and report to the provider any significant abnormalities.

Surgical Risk Factors

Carefully assess the patient before surgery for risk of complications (Table 4.2). Infants and older adults are at higher risk for complications of surgery due to either immature body systems or a decline in function of various body systems. Maintaining core body temperature is one concern when caring for these patients. Although smoking (or vaping) is a risk factor, research has shown that quitting smoking and alcohol intake 3 to 8 weeks before surgery will reduce the incidence of serious postoperative complications (American Association of Nurse Anesthetists, 2017). Smoking is not allowed within the hospital. Make sure to obtain a nicotine patch for the patient when appropriate.

Think Critically

What points would you make when explaining how smoking is harmful to the patient having surgery?

Learning Needs

General information should be provided to the surgical patient about what will happen immediately before, during, and after surgery, as well as specific preventive measures (see Implementation). If members of the family or supportive friends are expected to assist the patient during the postoperative period, they need to be instructed during teaching sessions.

Patient and Family Teaching

General Preoperative Teaching

Whenever possible, one or more family members should be included in teaching sessions. All surgical patients should receive information related to:

- **Preoperative procedures:** Skin preparation, care of belongings, restriction of food and liquid intake, and administration of bedtime sedatives if ordered and preoperative medication; if any routine medications are to be taken; time to come to the hospital
- **Technical information:** Anticipated surgical procedure; location of incisions; dressings, tubes, drains, catheters, or other equipment that is expected
- **Day of surgery:** Time surgery is scheduled, time to arrive at the hospital, or time patient will leave their room; probable length of procedure; effects of preoperative medications; where family will wait, when and where family can see the patient after surgery; pain control and postoperative routine
- **Postanesthesia care unit (PACU):** General environment (noise, lights, equipment); frequent taking of vital signs and pulse oximetry, and administration of oxygen
- **Hospital room location:** Location of the unit; expected length of stay; visiting privileges

◆ NURSING DIAGNOSIS

The LPN/LVN assists in gathering data so that based on the total assessment data, the registered nurse (RN) can formulate problem statements in the preoperative stage that include both actual and potential problems. Common preoperative problem statements include:

- Anxiety due to the surgical experience and outcome
- Fear due to the potential for death, effects of impending surgery, or loss of control due to anesthesia
- Potential for grief due to impending loss of a body function or body part
- Insufficient knowledge of preoperative and postoperative routines
- Insomnia due to stress or unfamiliar environment
- Limited coping ability due to lack of problem-solving skills or adequate support
- Altered role performance due to inability to perform job duties or to care for children during hospitalization

Each problem is supported by data obtained during the nursing assessment.

◆ PLANNING

Specific expected outcomes are written for each problem (Nursing Care Plan 4.1). However, there are general

Table 4.2 Surgical Risk Factors

FACTOR	KEY POINTS
Diabetes mellitus and other chronic diseases	Stress of surgery may cause swings in blood glucose levels that are difficult to control, even for patients without diabetes. Patients may receive intravenous insulin during and after surgery. Wound healing tends to be delayed in patients with diabetes, making the risk of **dehiscence** (wound separation) greater. The incidence of infection in surgical wounds is also higher. Liver and kidney disease makes it more difficult to metabolize and eliminate anesthesia and waste products.
Advanced age with inactivity	Healing is slower in older adults. The risk of disuse syndrome, hypostatic **pneumonia** (inflammation and consolidation in the lungs), and thrombus formation is higher in inactive older adults.
Very young person	Infants have difficulty with temperature control and in maintaining normal circulatory blood volume; they are at risk of dehydration.
Malnutrition	Inadequate nutritional stores lead to infection, poor wound healing, and skin breakdown.
Dehydration	Reduced circulating volume reduces kidney perfusion and predisposes the patient to a reduced urine output and thrombus formation. Dehydration also alters electrolyte values. A dehydrated patient is more at risk for problems with pressure areas during surgery.
Obesity	An extremely heavy patient does not breathe as deeply and is at risk of hypostatic pneumonia. Excessive fatty tissue also is a factor in poor wound healing.
Cardiovascular problems	Patients with hypertension, left ventricular hypertrophy, cardiac dysrhythmias, or a history of congestive heart failure are at a higher risk for myocardial infarction from the stresses of surgery and anesthesia.
Peripheral vascular disease	Poor circulation in the extremities predisposes the patient to possible thrombus formation and pressure sores on the lower legs and feet. Antiembolism stockings or devices are generally prescribed for use during and after surgery.
Liver disease	Interferes with normal blood clotting; liver cannot properly detoxify anesthetics and other drugs.
Respiratory disease	Inhaled anesthetics may irritate the respiratory mucosa, creating more secretions. With immobility there is greater probability of accumulated secretions and inflammation of the lungs and bronchial tree. Impaired oxygen–carbon dioxide exchange may cause acid-base imbalance.
Substance abuse or alcohol dependence	May alter reaction to anesthetic agents. Alcohol dependence may cause withdrawal symptoms if the use of alcohol is discontinued abruptly.
Smoking	Causes increased lung secretions from anesthesia and predisposes the patient to **atelectasis** (collapsed alveoli) and pneumonia postoperatively. Smokers are more prone to thrombus formation.
Regular use of certain drugs	Aspirin, nonsteroidal antiinflammatory drugs, and anticoagulants make the patient more prone to excessive bleeding. Corticosteroids reduce the body's response to infection and delay the healing process.
Excessive fear	Stimulates the sympathetic nervous system and causes the release of hormones, causing swings in the body's chemistry and vital signs. Increased muscle tension makes surgery more difficult. Physical manifestations of fear can interfere with achieving the desired state of anesthesia.

Adapted from Williams P: *deWit's fundamental concepts and skills for nursing,* ed 5, St. Louis, 2018, Elsevier.

nursing goals for all preoperative patients. The expectation is that the patient will be:

- Prepared for surgery physically and emotionally
- Able to demonstrate deep-breathing, coughing, and leg exercises
- Able to verbalize understanding of the procedure and the expectations for the postoperative period
- Able to maintain fluid and electrolyte balance throughout the perioperative period

When preoperative patients are assigned, you must plan your work for the shift carefully to have the patients ready for surgery without neglecting the needs of other assigned patients.

Clinical Cues

At the beginning of the shift, check to see that any ordered preoperative medications are on hand. Often IV medications are sent with the patient to the surgical holding area, where further preparation of the patient is performed. Check the surgery schedule and estimate the time needed to prepare the patient for surgery.

Nursing Care Plan 4.1 Care of a Patient Scheduled for a Simple Mastectomy

SCENARIO

Mrs. Talbot, a married 38-year-old woman and the mother of two children ages 16 and 14 years, is scheduled for a simple mastectomy as treatment for a localized malignant tumor that was detected by self-examination of her breasts.

PROBLEM STATEMENT/NURSING DIAGNOSIS

Fear related to cancer, disfigurement, and possible death.

SUPPORTING ASSESSMENT DATA

Subjective: Grandmother died of breast cancer.

Objective: Malignant tumor by biopsy; crying at intervals; states is worried about husband's reaction to the loss of the breast.

Goals/Expected Outcomes	Nursing Interventions	Selected Rationale	Evaluation
Patient will discuss fears openly by discharge.	Establish rapport and trust.	Establishing trust helps patient express fears and concerns.	Spent time with patient answering questions.
Patient will look at incisional area before discharge.	Encourage her to discuss fears with nurse and family.	Expressing fears decreases anxiety.	
Patient will identify spiritual or emotional support before discharge.	Encourage her to think of cancer as a challenge.	A positive perspective empowers the patient.	
Patient will talk about having cancer by discharge.	Help her to identify specific fears and deal with each one separately.	Identifying fears decreases the fear of the unknown. Dispelling fear and anxiety makes learning easier.	Stated is afraid of chemotherapy. Is now using the word "cancer" when discussing her surgery. Discussed ways to meet the challenges of chemotherapy.
	Teach relaxation exercises to decrease anxiety.	Relaxation exercises help decrease anxiety.	Expressed willingness to learn a relaxation exercise. Tried relaxation exercises twice.
Patient will join support group for cancer patients after discharge. Patient will use community resources after discharge.	Advise of community resources available to her.		Expressed appreciation for information about a support group.

PROBLEM STATEMENT/NURSING DIAGNOSIS

Insufficient knowledge about preoperative routine and postoperative care.

SUPPORTING ASSESSMENT DATA

Subjective: States, "I've never had surgery before. What will I need to do?"

Objective: Puzzled expression on face; no history of surgical procedures.

Goals/Expected Outcomes	Nursing Interventions	Selected Rationale	Evaluation
Patient will verbalize understanding of preoperative procedures and requirements before surgery.	Do preoperative teaching for patient and family: routine procedures; NPO status; expected tubes and drains; equipment to expect in room; probable length of surgery; where family will wait; pain-relief measures; handling of arm on operative side; coughing, deep-breathing, and leg exercises; ambulation; diet; daily postoperative routine.	Knowledge reduces fear of the unknown and anxiety.	Performed return demonstrations and verbalized understanding of routine and procedures.
Family will express understanding of what will happen preoperatively, where they will stay during surgery, and what to expect after surgery by end of teaching session			Family verbalized understanding of what to expect.

Nursing Care Plan 4.1 Care of a Patient Scheduled for a Simple Mastectomy—cont'd

Goals/Expected Outcomes	Nursing Interventions	Selected Rationale	Evaluation
	Call pastor or chaplain if patient desires a visit.	Clergy can be a positive support in time of stress.	A pastoral visit is scheduled for this afternoon.
	Provide private time for patient and husband and patient and family.	Private time is necessary for serious discussions.	Will have private talk with husband and one with children later today.

CRITICAL THINKING QUESTIONS

1. How would you specifically assess this patient's learning needs?
2. How could you assess for any cultural factors that would affect the patient's learning or your teaching?

◆ IMPLEMENTATION

Preoperatively, your time is divided between preparing the patient for surgery and teaching the patient about what will happen and how to hasten recovery. The same-day surgery patient receives teaching from the health care provider's office nurse or from a surgical intake nurse. Teaching sessions may be scheduled when the patient comes for diagnostic testing. Sending written instructions home with the patient reinforces what has been taught. Before entering the hospital for surgery, the patient should be given a phone number to call for answers to questions that may arise. In a same-day surgery or outpatient surgery setting, teaching is reinforced as the patient is being prepared for their procedure. Protocols may differ from one facility to another.

Older Adult Care Points

It is particularly important to reinforce instruction and information given to older adult patients. It is best to have a family member present during teaching. The anxiety of surgery, unfamiliar surroundings, diminished hearing and vision, and forgetfulness make learning more difficult and may decrease retention of information. Seek specific feedback periodically on points that are important for the patient to remember. Treat all patients with respect and dignity.

Consent for Surgery

Before the surgeon can perform an operation, written permission signed by the patient, guardian, or whoever holds power of attorney must be obtained (see the Evolve website for a Consent for Surgery form). This written consent protects the surgeon against claims of unauthorized surgery and provides the patient an opportunity to exercise the right of **informed consent**. In most hospitals, the "consent" is a printed form that the patient signs before surgery. The correct surgical procedure is identified on the consent form. The surgeon explains the procedure, risks, and benefits. The patient must be mentally competent and give consent freely and without coercion. Your signature confirms that the patient understands the procedure they are consenting to and have had their questions answered. The consent form is attached to the patient's chart and is sent to the operating room (OR) with the patient. **You must always check that a consent form has been signed before giving the preoperative medication.** Many facilities using an electronic health record (EHR) still use paper consent forms. Many hospitals require that a signed "Power of Attorney for Health Care" declaring a health care proxy be in the chart before surgery. In an emergency situation, if a patient is not capable of giving consent due to their condition, a relative cannot be reached, and delaying surgical intervention would put the patient in jeopardy, surgery may proceed without a signed consent.

Legal and Ethical Considerations

Giving Surgical Consent

Mrs. Jones, age 66, was slightly confused as a result of dehydration when she was brought to the hospital. She has signed a surgical consent for a hip replacement, but her daughter feels her mother was confused when she signed the form and questions its validity. What will you do? How would the surgeon verify that Mrs. Jones was not confused when she signed the form?

Clinical Cues

Patients have the right to change their minds and revoke consent until the time of surgery. If a patient tells you the surgery is not wanted, delay preoperative preparations and explore the issue with the patient. If it appears the consent for surgery really is being revoked, notify the charge nurse and the surgeon.

Think Critically

Why should the consent be signed before giving any preoperative medication? What happens if a patient has been given the preoperative medication and then it is discovered that the surgical consent form has not been signed?

Food and Fluids

Food and fluids will often be restricted for 8 hours before surgery, and the patient is placed on NPO (*nil per os,* which means "nothing by mouth") status. A light meal such as toast and clear fluids may be allowed up to 6 hours before surgery. Clear liquids such as black coffee, tea, apple juice, or carbonated beverages may be consumed up to 2 hours before surgery in elective cases (American Society of Anesthesiologists, 2017). Often the surgeon or anesthesiologist will allow an oral blood pressure medication, heart medication, or anticonvulsant to be taken with a sip of water on the morning of surgery. Always check the health care provider's order before giving anything by mouth in the immediate preoperative period. The purpose of oral restriction is to prevent nausea, vomiting, and aspiration. NPO status also may be implemented with regional or local anesthesia, in case general anesthesia has to be used. **Confirm with the patient that the NPO order has been heeded.** Insulin may or may not be given; check the orders.

Elimination

If the patient is having abdominal or colon surgery, a colon lavage solution or enemas may be ordered to clear the intestines of fecal matter. The patient may be placed on a special soft or liquid diet for the 3 days before surgery to decrease the content of the bowel.

When completing the preoperative checklist, ask the patient to empty the bladder (unless a catheter is in place). If the bladder is not empty, relaxation induced by medications and anesthesia causes the urge to urinate. The bladder should be emptied before any sedating medication is given.

Tubes and Equipment

If a nasogastric (NG) tube will be inserted during surgery for postoperative use, explain its purpose, its care, and what it will feel like to the patient. Give an estimate of how long the tube will remain in the stomach. The tube is usually removed when bowel sounds return and nausea has passed. If surgery has occurred in the stomach or intestinal tract, the tube may remain in place longer. Explain the function of other tubes such as drains, an IV line, oxygen delivery and monitoring devices, a chest tube, and a urinary catheter, as well as their care and probable duration of use.

? Think Critically

If a patient has an NG tube in place, what necessary assessments must you make?

Rest and Sedation

It is desirable for the patient to be as well rested as possible before surgery so that the body is not compromised in meeting the stresses of anesthesia and the surgical procedure. A sedative may be ordered for the patient the night before surgery, but the inpatient often must ask for it. Check on the inpatient frequently during the night. If the patient awakens and is restless, sit and listen and try to dispel fears, offer a soothing back rub, or give backup sedation as ordered. A patient scheduled for same-day surgery should take the sedative at home and retire early the night before because it will be necessary to arise early to enter the hospital.

Pain Control

Many surgeons order a patient-controlled analgesia (PCA) pump for their patients postoperatively. If a PCA pump is ordered, patients should receive instruction before surgery about the pump and how to operate it. If patients will be receiving injections for pain control, explain that this type of medication is ordered on an as-needed basis every 3 to 4 hours and that patients must ask for it. Oral pain medication is usually ordered every 4 to 6 hours as needed. Explain that asking for the pain medication before the pain becomes severe makes it easier to control the pain level. **It is your responsibility to gather data regarding the patient's pain throughout the shift and to offer interventions for relief.** Teach the patient about the pain scale that is used at the facility (see Chapter 7).

Skin Preparation

The night or morning before surgery, the patient may be asked to shower with a special antibacterial cleanser or just soap and water to remove as many microorganisms from the skin as possible. On the morning of the surgery, hair may be removed from the operative site—this is done either in the surgical holding area or in the OR. Only hair that may interfere with the surgery is removed. As a Core Measure for reducing surgical site infection, use hair clippers only for hair removal before surgery (The Joint Commission [TJC], 2009). Explain to the patient the hair removal area to be prepared, the hair removal process, and the timing for hair removal. Nail polish is removed so that the pulse oximeter can function correctly when attached to the finger. Makeup is removed; note the presence of permanent makeup on the preoperative checklist. Ask about contact lenses and have them removed as well. Skin piercing jewelry should be removed. If electrosurgery is used, the metal can heat up, causing burns. Oral piercings can interfere with airway management. Decorative dermal implants may need removal by the implanter, surgeon, or primary care physician. Management of piercings should be determined when planning for the surgical procedure.

Preoperative Teaching

Teaching the patient correct breathing, coughing, turning, and leg exercises is a high priority during the preoperative period. It is helpful to have a relative or close friend present for these teaching sessions so that this person can later coach and give encouragement to the patient. Instruct the patient about what to expect before, during, and after surgery. Help same-day surgery patients devise a schedule for doing the necessary exercises.

Venous return is often hampered during the surgical procedure due to the position assumed on the operating table and pooling of blood in the lower extremities. **Stasis** (slowing of flow) of blood places the patient at risk for **thrombophlebitis** (blood clot and inflammation of a vessel). Specific leg exercises help prevent this complication (Fig. 4.1). Explain the importance of doing the exercises, show the patient how to do each one, and

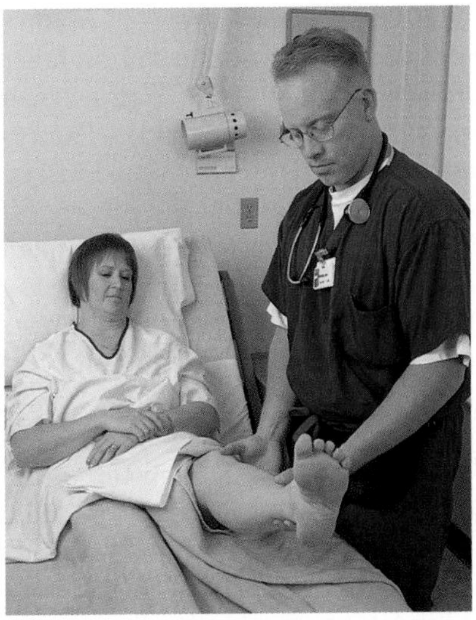

Fig. 4.1 Teaching foot and leg exercises. (From Williams P: *deWit's fundamental concepts and skills for nursing,* ed 5, St. Louis, 2018, Elsevier.)

ask for a return demonstration. One way to remind patients to do the exercises is to have them exercise whenever a commercial comes on, if they watch TV. The exercises should be done after surgery at least 5 to 10 times every hour while awake, until the patient is up and moving around normally. During the surgical procedure when the patient is completely immobile, pneumatic antiembolic stockings (PAS) are used to help prevent deep vein thrombosis (DVT). The stockings are also called intermittent pneumatic compression (IPC) devices. These stockings may remain on until the patient is fully ambulatory. Use of PAS, leg exercises, and low-dose heparin therapy are used for DVT prophylaxis in bedbound patients.

Patient and Family Teaching

Postoperative Foot and Leg Exercises

Whenever possible, one or more family members should be included in teaching sessions.

- Flex and extend the right foot, moving the toes upward and downward, four or five times.
- Repeat with the left foot.
- Trace circles to the right with the right foot five times; repeat with circles to the left.
- Trace circles to the right with the left foot five times; repeat with circles to the left.
- Bend the right leg at the knee, sliding the foot back toward the buttocks as far as possible; raise the bent leg off the bed, extend the leg, and dorsiflex the foot; extend the foot and lower the leg to the bed.
- Bend the left leg at the knee, sliding the foot back toward the buttocks as far as possible; raise the bent leg off the bed, extend the leg, and dorsiflex the foot; extend the foot and lower the leg to the bed.
- Tighten the buttocks muscles for a count of 10 and release to exercise the quadriceps muscles.
- Repeat each exercise four more times.

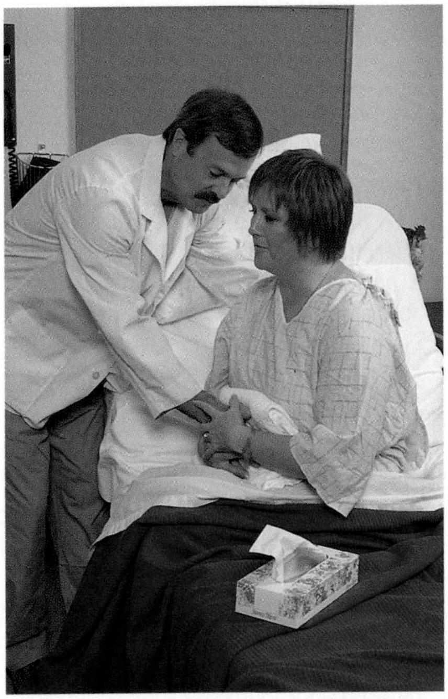

Fig. 4.2 Teaching deep breathing and coughing while splinting the incision. (From Williams P: *deWit's fundamental concepts and skills for nursing,* ed 5, St. Louis, 2018, Elsevier.)

Deep Breathing and Coughing

For deep breathing and coughing, it is preferable for the patient to sit up, with the back away from the mattress or chair. This allows for full lung expansion and clearing of excretions. The surgical chest or abdominal incision should be splinted with a pillow (Fig. 4.2).

Clinical Cues

A small, firm "coughing pillow" can be made by folding a bath towel or a light blanket and securing it inside a pillowcase with the ends tucked inside over the towel or blanket.

The surgeon may order use of an incentive spirometer. Instruct the patient in its use and supervise until the patient has mastered the technique.

Turning

Show the patient how to turn in bed by flexing the legs to relax the abdominal muscles, placing a pillow between the legs, grabbing on to the side of the bed, and slowly turning to the side. This maneuver is also used for getting out of bed. A trapeze bar for orthopedic patients is very helpful for turning and repositioning.

Family Instructions

Advise the family to come to the hospital 1 to 1.5 hours before surgery. The family should be told about the usual routines, where to wait, the approximate time before the patient may be expected to return, and what to anticipate in the way of tubes, equipment, and patient appearance after surgery. This knowledge keeps the family from thinking the patient has "taken a turn for

Patient and Family Teaching

Lung Exercises

Whenever possible, one or more family members should be included in patient teaching.

DEEP BREATHING

- Sit up away from the mattress.
- Take a deep breath in through the nose, hold for a few seconds, and slowly exhale.
- Repeat four more times.
- Perform every 2 hours during the day and when awakened at night for vital signs.

FORCED EXHALATION COUGHING

- Sit up away from the mattress.
- Splint the abdominal or chest incision:
  - Take a deep breath through the nose and cough as you exhale with the mouth open but covered with a tissue.
  - If you cannot move secretions with your cough, use a forced exhalation cough.
  - Take a deep breath through the nose and forcibly quickly exhale, producing a "huff" cough.
  - Repeat the process using three short "huffs" as you exhale to bring the secretions to the mouth, where they can be expectorated. Repeat until no secretions are audible in the lungs, resting between attempts.
  - Perform every 2 hours during the day and when awakened at night for vital signs.

USING AN INCENTIVE SPIROMETER

- Sit up away from the mattress.
- Insert the mouthpiece, covering it completely with the lips.
- Take a slow, deep breath and hold it for at least 3 seconds.
- Remove the device and exhale slowly, keeping the lips puckered.
- Breathe normally for a few breaths.
- Try to increase the inspired volume by at least 100 mL with each breath on the spirometer.
- Once maximal volume is achieved, attempt to inspire this volume 10 times, resting for a few breaths between each attempt.
- Clean the mouthpiece of the spirometer when finished.
- During the first 3 postoperative days, try to do this every hour.

Safety Alert

Coughing

With most eye, ear, nose, or throat surgeries as well as spinal and intracranial surgeries, coughing is contraindicated. Deep breathing is encouraged, but make sure that coughing is appropriate for the type of procedure performed.

the worse" when they see the extra equipment for suction, oxygen, or IV therapy in use after surgery. A warning about the occasional delays in starting surgery can keep the family from becoming excessively anxious if the patient is not back at the expected time.

Immediate Preoperative Care

The patient is usually dressed in a clean hospital gown, without underwear, for the OR. Hair is covered with a surgical paper cap. Long hair should be fixed to minimize tangling, and all hairpins and barrettes must be removed. Ask about body piercings and the presence of piercing jewelry, including in the tongue and genital areas. Explain why *all* jewelry must be removed for safety because of the electrocautery used during surgery and the danger of an electrical burn from conduction of electricity through metal.

Jewelry, along with money and credit cards, is given to a family member or relative to keep or is secured in a valuables envelope and placed in a safe, according to facility policy. If a wedding band is to be worn to surgery, tape the ring to the finger without restricting circulation and tape a cotton ball over the stone to prevent loss when the tape is removed. Dentures are removed, placed in a labeled cup, and kept in a designated place, according to hospital policy. Sometimes the anesthesiologist will order the dentures left in place to facilitate the administration of anesthesia by mask. If a hearing aid is left in place, a very visible note should be placed on the front of the chart, and placement of the hearing aid should be noted on the preoperative checklist sheet.

Verify that the identification bracelet matches the chart to avoid any error or mix-up of patients in the OR. Verify that the procedure site indicated on the surgical consent form is the same as what the patient states. The procedure site will be verified and marked on the patient before transport to surgery or in the preoperative holding area if not done previously. Make sure that all diagnostic tests have been completed and results are available, reporting any significant abnormalities. Verify that a history and physical have been completed and are available in the medical record.

Clinical Cues

Attend to all items on the preoperative checklist that can be handled ahead of time (Fig. 4.3). This prevents hurrying, which can increase mistakes, and prevents delaying administration of any preoperative medication while the list is completed. Many facilities use an online form.

Medications may be given in the surgical holding area or in the outpatient unit. Most preoperative medications are given by the anesthesiologist immediately before surgery. A medication to inhibit gastric acid secretion may be administered intravenously. You may need to send any IV piggyback antibiotic or other medication ordered to the OR with the patient.

Preoperative medications may be given to:

- Reduce anxiety and promote a restful state
- Decrease secretion of mucus and other body fluids
- Counteract nausea and reduce emesis
- Enhance the effects of the anesthetic

PREOP/PREPROCEDURE CHECKLIST/REPORT FORM

PATIENT LABEL

1SURG

Date	Time	
Surgery/procedure		YES
Correct patient ID band on		☐
	On chart	☐
	Dictated	☐

History and Physical
H&P 24 hours to 30 days: update with "No Pertinent Change in History & Physical" stamp
H&P 31-180 days: H&P update form #2396
OB H&P Update for Surgery/Procedures form #2543

	YES	N/A
Initiate Anesthesia Preop order 101.S09. As appropriate initiate OB Anesthesia Order 144.P11	☐	
Include at least one page of patient ID stickers	☐	
Procedural consent: Signed/On Chart	☐	
Procedural site verified with patient/guardian	☐	
Procedural site marked when laterality (including internal laterality), multiple structures (fingers, toes, lesions) or multiple levels (spine). Specify site: ________	☐	☐
Preop antibiotic given	☐	☐
Interpreter if needed	☐	☐
HBOC transfer report on chart (when applicable)	☐	☐
Acuscan MAR-LOS custom report on chart (when applicable)	☐	☐

OB ☐ The Department of Social and Health Services consent for sterilization completed and on chart dated ≥ than 30 days prior to procedure (*unless meets exception criteria, listed in Standards of Care Notebook)
☐ Notify anesthesia provider

Diagnostic ☐ Labs on chart ☐ X-rays with patient (when appropriate) ☐ When applicable Glucose: ________/time ______
☐ Type and screen ☐ ECG (when applicable) Blood units available: # ____________

Medications/IV ☐ MAR on chart ☐ IV/Saline lock in place ☐ If TPN running, start second peripheral IV site

Belongings	Labeled	With Patient/Family	To OR
Contacts			
Glasses			
Hearing aids R L Both			
Dentures ☐ Upper ☐ Lower ☐ Partial			

Prep ☐ Personal clothing removed ☐ Prep completed
☐ Snap gown ☐ Voided, time: ____________ ☐ Foley
☐ Jewelry/body piercings: ☐ None ☐ Taped ☐ Family ☐ Patient registration safe
☐ Preop teaching done Last oral/fluid intake: ____________ Time: ____________

Unit based or bedside procedures: FINAL VERIFICATION
☐ Correct patient ☐ Correct side/site ☐ Correct position
☐ Correct procedure ☐ Correct equipment/trays

REPORT USING SBAR: Provide an opportunity to ask and answer questions. Include significant history/special needs.

INITIALS/OR SIGNATURE IF SIGNATURE PAGE NOT USED

Fig. 4.3 Preoperative checklist. (From Williams P: *deWit's fundamental concepts and skills for nursing,* ed 5, St. Louis, 2018, Elsevier. Courtesy Peace Health Southwest Medical Center, Vancouver, Wash.)

Assist in transferring the patient to the stretcher when the transport person comes to take the patient to surgery. Compare the patient's identification bracelet name and numbers with the transport request sheet for accuracy. Check the medical record to make certain that everything ordered has been done and complete final documentation.

Safety Alert

Preventing Falls

If the patient has received a sedative preoperatively, remember to put up the side rails of the bed per facility protocol and to lower the bed. Place the call light button within reach and remind the patient not to get up without assistance. These are important patient safety measures after administering sedatives.

Cultural Considerations

Differences in Drug Metabolism

Asian people, and particularly Chinese patients, metabolize psychotropic drugs differently from people of other ethnic groups. Valium causes greater sedation with normal doses. Atropine is also metabolized differently and can greatly accelerate the heart rate. Asian patients should be monitored closely when receiving these drugs.

Older Adult Care Points

Because of decreasing liver and kidney function that occurs with age, older adult patients, especially those older than 75 years, will need reduced dosages of preoperative narcotics and sedatives. Observe for signs of toxicity.

Think Critically

How would you handle a situation in which a patient scheduled for an abdominal procedure has put back on underwear or jewelry after you finished doing the preoperative checklist?

Preparation of the Patient Unit

While patients are in surgery, prepare the room for their return. Make the bed with fresh linens; include a drawsheet between the shoulder and the knee areas that can be used as a lift sheet to reposition the patient. For abdominal or perineal surgery, place an underpad at the hip area to catch excess drainage. Fan-fold the top covers to the far side of the bed or to the bottom of the bed. Raise the bed to the height of the stretcher that will return the patient and arrange furniture so that the stretcher can be pulled up alongside the bed. Many facilities retrieve the bed and place the patient directly on it from the OR table. Having the bed ready is helpful to the transport process. Place the IV pole or pump at the head of the bed.

Gather an emesis basin or bag, tissues, a frequent vital signs sheet or postoperative record, an intake and output (I&O) sheet (for paper charting), and a small towel and washcloth and place them on the bedside table or console (Fig. 4.4). Obtain a mobile workstation if an EHR is used. Connect oxygen and suction equipment if their need is anticipated. A thermometer, sphygmomanometer, pulse oximeter, and stethoscope should be close at hand on the patient's return to the unit. If a PCA pump, sequential pneumatic compression devices, or a passive range-of-motion machine will be needed, see that it is obtained and ready. Communication with the PACU nurses is helpful in identifying the devices that have been implemented in the OR or PACU and those that need to be available in the receiving unit.

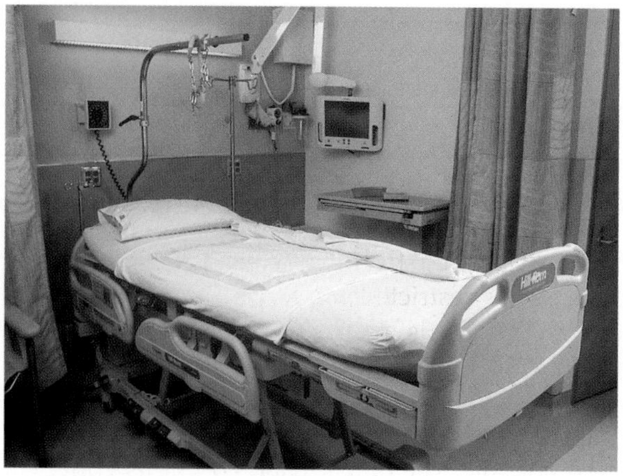

Fig. 4.4 Room prepared for surgical patient's return.

◆ Evaluation

Evaluation is accomplished by determining whether the nursing goals have been met. If the patient is properly prepared for surgery, kept NPO, and is reasonably calm and knowledgeable about the procedure and what is expected, the general goals have been met. If the preoperative medications were not given on time or the patient was not ready for transport at the appointed time, review your steps to see where improvement can occur. Data are gathered to determine if expected outcomes written for individual problem statements are being met (see Nursing Care Plan 4.1).

THE SURGICAL TEAM

The surgical team consists of the surgeon, assistant to the surgeon, anesthesia care provider, circulating nurse, and scrub person or scrub technician. The surgeon is the head of the surgical team and may be a physician (MD), oral surgeon (DDS or DMD), osteopath (OD), or podiatrist (DPM). The first surgical assistant is another physician, a physician's assistant, a surgical resident, or a specially trained and authorized RN or surgical technician. Other assistants may be RNs or LPN/LVNs. The surgeon, physician's assistant(s), and scrub nurse or scrub technician are sterile members who work within the sterile field maintaining asepsis with sterile surgical attire of sterile gowns and gloves. The circulating nurse and anesthesiologist or anesthetist do not work within the sterile field and do not wear sterile gowns and gloves. However, OR scrubs, hair covering, and face mask are required in the OR.

THE SURGICAL SUITE

ORs are removed from other areas of the hospital, and access is restricted to OR personnel and surgical patients. The OR is maintained as a positive pressure environment to reduce the entrance of microbes that might cause infection. The surgical suite is divided into three distinct areas to help keep the ORs as microbe free as possible. The unrestricted zone is essentially the control desk area. Street clothes may be permitted here. Semirestricted zones include the hallways and outer regions of the ORs. The circulating nurse and anesthesia care providers work in these areas. Clean scrub clothes and caps are required. The restricted zone is the area surrounding the operating table and instrument trays and table. Personnel wear scrub clothes, sterile gowns, caps, masks, and sterile gloves within this area. Asepsis is the responsibility of all surgical personnel.

The temperature in the OR is kept at 66° to 70° F (18.9° to 21.1° C) to discourage microbial growth and to keep the surgical team comfortable under the bright lights and in the layers of surgical clothing. Cabinets, instrument tables, instrument trays, and disposal buckets are usually made of stainless steel that can be easily cleaned and disinfected. The restricted area is scrubbed down with disinfectant after each procedure. The entire room is kept scrupulously clean.

THE SURGICAL HOLDING AREA

The patient is transported to the holding area in the surgical suite. The holding area nurse, often the circulating nurse, greets the patient and verifies the patient's identification (Fig. 4.5). Review of the medical record verifies that all preoperative orders have been accomplished, the signed surgical consent form is present, the risk assessment is documented, and the preoperative checklist is complete. The correct surgical site markings are checked. The Universal Protocol to prevent wrong-site surgery is followed in the holding area and in the OR (TJC, 2009). You should offer emotional support and answer any questions. The anesthesiologist may greet the patient, start an IV line if one has not been established, administer preoperative medications, and prepare the patient for anesthesia. When the OR is ready, the patient is transferred to the operating table. Patient identification is verified again by the circulating nurse.

ROLES OF THE CIRCULATING NURSE AND THE SCRUB PERSON

A surgical technician or a specially trained nurse (LPN/LVN or RN) may be the scrub person. This person functions within the sterile area of the operating room (Box 4.3, Fig. 4.6). **Sterile technique is maintained at**

Box 4.3 Major Functions of the Scrub Nurse or Technician

- Gathers all equipment for the procedure
- Prepares all sterile supplies and instruments using sterile technique
- Gowns and gloves surgeons on entry into operating room
- Assists with sterile draping of the patient
- Maintains sterility within the sterile field during surgery
- Hands instruments and supplies to the operating team during surgery, anticipating what is needed
- Maintains a neat instrument table
- Labels and handles surgical specimens correctly
- Maintains an accurate count of sponges, sharps, and instruments on the sterile field; verifies counts with the circulating nurse before and after surgery
- Monitors for breaks in sterile technique and points them out
- Cleans up after the surgery is over

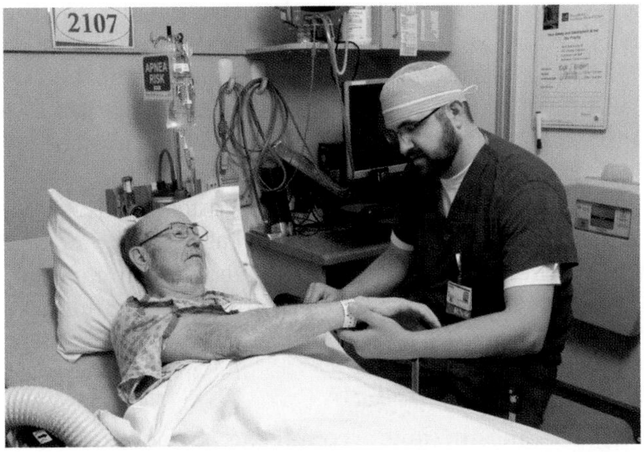

Fig. 4.5 Patient in the surgical holding area.

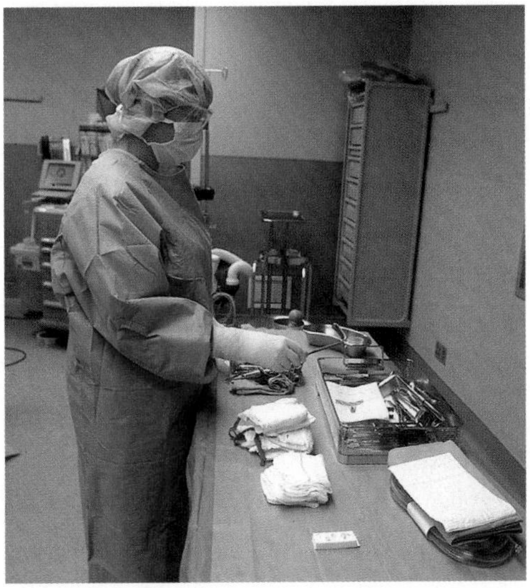

Fig. 4.6 Scrub nurse setting up the instrument table in the operating room.

all times. Any break in sterile technique should be pointed out immediately by the circulating nurse or any member of the OR team and remedied.

The circulating nurse is responsible, along with the anesthesia care provider, for maintaining the safety and dignity of the patient and bringing needed items to the operating team, as well as for many other duties (Box 4.4). The circulating nurse is the communication link between the OR and those outside the surgical suite.

Box 4.4 Major Functions of the Circulating Nurse

- Coordinates care, oversees the environment, and cares for the patient in the operating room
- Greets the patient and performs patient assessment
- Verifies that consent is signed and accurate and that surgical site is correctly marked
- Checks medical record and preoperative forms for completeness
- Sets up the operating room; adjusts lights, stools, and discard buckets; and ensures that supplies and diagnostic support are available
- Gathers, counts, and checks all equipment and supplies that are anticipated to be used, ensuring its safe function
- Opens sterile supplies for the scrub nurse
- Provides needed padding and warming or cooling devices for the operating table
- Assists with the transfer of the patient to the operating table and positions the patient
- Places the electrocautery ground pad on the patient if electrocautery is to be used
- Assists the anesthesia provider
- May prep the patient's skin before sterile draping occurs
- May insert a Foley catheter
- Initiates the procedural time-out
- Handles labeling and disposition of specimens
- Coordinates activities with radiology and pathology departments
- Monitors urine and blood loss during surgery and reports findings to the surgeon
- Supplies, monitors, and documents the infusion of ordered fluids
- Observes for breaks in sterile technique and announces them to the team
- Monitors traffic and noise within the operating room
- Communicates information on the surgery's progress to family during long procedures
- Documents care, events, interventions, drugs, fluids, and findings
- Assists the scrub person with final count of sponges, sharps, and instruments
- Helps transfer the patient to the gurney and accompanies the patient to the recovery area, providing a report of the surgery and patient condition to the recovery nurse in collaboration with the anesthesia provider
- Verifies that the count of equipment is the same after surgery as before

! Safety Alert

Time-Out

Before surgery begins, while all members of the team are present, a "time-out" occurs during which a final verification of the correct patient, procedure, site, and implants (if applicable) is performed. Any questions or concerns must be resolved before the procedure begins.

The patient is positioned with padding to prevent injury to nerves and to minimize pressure over bony prominences. Serious injury and pressure ulcers can develop from improper positioning or lack of padding for a surgical procedure (see Chapter 42). Safety straps are secured to safeguard the patient.

ANESTHESIA

Anesthesia (the loss of sensory perception) has been in use for surgical procedures since the 1840s. Newer anesthetics and techniques make anesthesia safer than ever, but **there is still a risk any time a patient is anesthetized.** The goals of anesthesia administration are to (1) prevent pain; (2) achieve adequate muscle relaxation; (3) calm fears and ease anxiety; and (4) induce forgetfulness of an unpleasant experience. Anesthetics are administered in a number of ways to achieve these goals (Table 4.3). Patients are classified according to their age, physical condition, and risk status and are assigned a risk potential. The choice of anesthesia depends on the type of surgical procedure to be performed and the risk potential. The anesthetic to be used is chosen by the anesthesia care provider, although it is discussed with the patient. The anesthesia care provider may be an anesthesiologist, another physician, or a certified registered nurse anesthetist (CRNA) who is supervised by an anesthesiologist.

GENERAL ANESTHESIA

General anesthesia is induced by the administration of an inhalant gas or by medication introduced intravenously. During general anesthesia, the patient is in a deep sleep state with muscle relaxation and is not aware of the surroundings. The deep muscle relaxation includes the neck and throat, which means the patient can no longer maintain their own airway. An endotracheal tube or laryngeal mask may be placed to maintain and protect the airway. There are three stages of general anesthesia:

1. **Induction:** Unconsciousness is induced.
2. **Maintenance:** Period during which the surgical procedure is performed.
3. **Emergence:** Surgery is completed, and the patient is prepared to return to consciousness; neuromuscular blocking agents are reversed.

REGIONAL ANESTHESIA

Regional anesthesia is accomplished by administering a nerve block. It is often more economical than general

Table 4.3 Types of Anesthesia

TYPE	USE	ADVANTAGE
General		
Inhalation	Extensive surgery for which it is desirable for patient to be unconscious with relaxed muscles	Well controlled with assisted ventilation; few side effects
Intravenous	Shorter surgery; rapid induction	Little postoperative nausea or vomiting
Regional		
Spinal	Surgery in lower half of body; for patients unable to undergo general anesthesia	Patient can be conscious; does not require fasting No nausea or vomiting from anesthesia
Epidural	For gynecologic procedures and childbirth	No diet restrictions postoperatively
Nerve block	Foot surgery and some orthopedic surgeries	Patient is conscious; can cooperate with instructions
Local	Minor surgical procedures	Can produce good pain control for many hours postoperatively; patient may remain conscious Numbs an area for a short period of time
Procedural/Conscious Sedation, also called Procedural Sedation and Analgesia (PSA)		
	Surgery of short duration for which unconsciousness is undesirable May be used in combination with local, spinal, or nerve blocks to enhance patient comfort	Reversal is rapid Patient is unaware but can breathe without assistance Little if any nausea or vomiting Amnesia of surgery
Other		
Hypnosis	Surgery for patients who are unable to have general anesthesia and where regional anesthesia is inappropriate	No drug side effects
Cryothermia	Surgery for patient who cannot tolerate other anesthesia, such as in life-threatening trauma	Provides decrease in pain

Older Adult Care Points

The physiologic changes that occur with aging affect the way drugs are taken up, used, and excreted. Obtaining an accurate height and weight of older adult patients is very important for calculation of anesthetic agents and medication dosages. Adverse drug responses are increased in the older adult population. In general, smaller dosages of drugs are required, and fat-soluble drugs in particular have a longer duration of action and a slower elimination period.

anesthesia. Regional anesthesia may be accomplished by injecting the spinal, epidural, caudal, or peripheral nerve area. The block anesthetizes the local area or the area distal to the block. Spinal or epidural blocks are typically used for high-risk patients undergoing pelvic or lower extremity surgery; epidural blocks are widely used in obstetric procedures.

PROCEDURAL OR CONSCIOUS SEDATION ANESTHESIA (MODERATE SEDATION)

A local anesthetic agent or regional anesthesia to numb the area plus IV sedation is used to provide systemic analgesia and sedation during a surgical procedure. The combination can be used for any procedure that can be done with local or regional anesthesia and is becoming increasingly common. The patient is monitored closely for blood pressure changes, oxygen saturation levels, carbon dioxide levels, and heart activity. Carbon dioxide levels must be monitored by **capnography** (measurement of inhaled and exhaled carbon dioxide) for any procedural or higher level of sedation (American Society of Anesthesiologists, 2015). Capnography provides a graphic representation of exhaled carbon dioxide. Carbon dioxide monitoring can be done without intubation with a nasal cannula–like device.

Complementary and Alternative Therapies

Music's Effects

Music that the patient likes is known to have a calming effect on preoperative patients. Research studying the use of music delivered by earphones to a patient during surgery has shown that music may reduce the amount of anesthesia and analgesia needed (Flanagan & Kerin, 2017). The patient appears to become more relaxed and less anxious. Before and after surgery, listening to a CD with preferred music or with no recording on it through earphones appears to lower anxiety and pain, probably because the earphones decrease outside sensory stimulation.

LOCAL ANESTHESIA

Local anesthesia is used for minor procedures such as superficial tissue biopsies, surface cyst excision, insertion of a pacemaker, and insertion of vascular access devices. Procedural sedation may also be given for some procedures in addition to the local. A patient who has had local anesthesia is transferred directly to the nursing unit and does not need care in the PACU (also called the postanesthesia recovery room [PAR or PARR] or postanesthesia recovery unit [PARU]) (see Chapter 5).

POTENTIAL INTRAOPERATIVE COMPLICATIONS

Potential intraoperative complications of surgery include:
- Hemorrhage
- Infection
- Fluid volume excess or deficit
- Hypothermia
- Malignant hyperthermia
- Injury related to positioning

No surgical personnel with an active infection should be in the OR. Surgical asepsis is practiced with great care to prevent contamination of the surgical site. Counts of sponges, needles, and instruments are performed to verify that no equipment has been left in a wound, where it might cause a postoperative infection or complication.

Many associations and agencies have banded together to promote a program to decrease surgical infections and complications. Core Measures and National Patient Safety Goals include proper hair removal, timely antibiotic administration, blood glucose control, prevention of thromboembolic events, and prevention of adverse cardiac events (Bratzler, 2009).

Intravenous fluids are carefully regulated by the anesthesia care provider and the surgeon. The cool atmosphere, cool IV fluids, inhalation of cool anesthetic gases, and exposure of body surfaces will lower a patient's normal body temperature. Body temperature is monitored during surgery to ensure that it does not become dangerously low. Sometimes hypothermia is desirable for certain lengthy procedures to decrease the metabolic needs of the body. However, if the patient's temperature drops too low, warmed IV fluids may be administered or a body warming device may be used. Unless contraindicated, body temperature of surgical patients is maintained with forced air warming blankets during surgery. Hypothermia can adversely affect cardiac function and may make the body more susceptible to infection as well as increase bleeding and delay wound healing. Keeping the body at a normal temperature has been found to decrease postoperative wound infection (Berrios-Torres, Umscheid, & Bratzler, 2017). Prophylactic antibiotics work best when given within 1 hour prior to the surgical incision (Anderson & Sexton, 2018).

Malignant hyperthermia is an inherited disorder. In patients with malignant hyperthermia, muscle metabolism and heat production increase rapidly and uncontrollably in response to the stress of surgery and some anesthetic agents. Fever, tachycardia, cyanosis, tachypnea, muscle rigidity, diaphoresis, hypotension, and irregular heart rate develop. If not treated quickly, cardiac arrest can occur. The circulating nurse monitors the patient's temperature along with the anesthesia care provider. If the temperature begins to rise rapidly, anesthesia is discontinued and the surgical team takes measures to correct the physiologic problems.

During a surgical procedure, the patient is placed in one position for an extended period. Such positioning places the patient at risk for injury, such as problems of immobility and pressure damage to the skin and underlying tissue. A variety of materials are used for padding pressure areas and stabilizing the patient's body. The circulating nurse must understand the risk factors for each surgical position and must pad joints and pressure areas accordingly. Joint problems and pressure ulcers can develop days after surgery from damage that occurred during the surgical procedure.

Get Ready for the NCLEX® Examination!

Key Points

- Surgical procedures vary in reason, urgency, degree of risk, and extent (see Table 4.1).
- The use of lasers, fiberoptic endoscopes with high-resolution video cameras, operating microscopes, and robotic technology has revolutionized surgery.
- Autologous transfusion or bloodless surgery techniques are reducing problems that can be caused by blood transfusions from outside donors.
- A thorough assessment is performed, during which any risk factors for surgery are identified (see Focused Assessment).
- Older adult patients are at much greater risk from surgery and anesthesia than are younger adults.
- Cultural factors and preferences should always be assessed and considered.
- An appropriate individual nursing care plan is formulated for the preoperative period.
- The surgeon must obtain informed consent from the patient before surgery is performed.
- Preoperative procedures are performed in a timely manner.
- The method to be used for postoperative pain control is explained and discussed with the patient.
- Preoperative teaching of exercises to be performed postoperatively is very important; the patient is taught turning, leg, deep-breathing, and coughing exercises.
- Immediate preoperative care includes checking to see that all jewelry and metal objects have been removed from the patient.
- A signed surgical consent form is checked before preoperative medication is administered.

- Once preoperative sedation (if ordered) is administered, the patient is cautioned to stay in bed to prevent falls.
- The patient's identity and the correct surgical site are carefully checked and marked before the patient is transported to surgery.
- The Universal Protocol is followed to prevent wrong-site surgery.
- Several measures are instituted to prevent surgical site infection and other complications.
- The OR is kept as microbe-free as possible.
- Surgical asepsis is the responsibility of the entire OR staff.
- A "time-out" occurs just before the start of the surgical procedure to recheck the patient's identity, the surgical procedure to be performed, and the site of the surgery.
- The scrub person and the circulating nurse, along with the surgeon and anesthesiologist or CRNA, provide care for the patient while in the OR.
- The circulating nurse and the scrub person have distinctly different roles.
- Anesthesia is used to prevent pain; to achieve adequate muscle relaxation; and to calm fear, allay anxiety, and induce amnesia of an unpleasant experience.
- Inhalant gases and IV medications are used to induce general anesthesia, and the patient progresses through stages of induction to total anesthesia.
- Regional anesthesia, procedural (moderate) sedation, or local anesthesia is used for many surgical procedures.
- There is a risk of several complications during the intraoperative period.
- Patients are positioned carefully, and pressure points and joints are padded to prevent injury.
- The circulating nurse, anesthesia care provider, and surgeon observe for symptoms of complications, and measures are taken immediately to avert a problem.

Additional Learning Resources

SG Go to your Study Guide for additional learning activities to help you master this chapter content.

Go to your Evolve website (http://evolve.elsevier.com/deWit/medsurg) for the following FREE learning resources:

- Animations, audio, and video
- Answers and rationales for questions and activities
- Glossary with pronunciations in English and Spanish
- Interactive Review Questions and more!

Review Questions for the NCLEX® Examination

1. An advantage of robotic surgery is that the surgeon has:
   1. an assistant at the computer guiding instruments.
   2. an unobstructed view of the operative site.
   3. use of a laser to perform the operation.
   4. the ability to make precise movements of the instruments.

   NCLEX Client Need: Physiological Integrity: Reduction of Risk Potential

2. Surgical risk factors include: *(Select all that apply.)*
   1. obesity
   2. malnutrition
   3. age of 51 years
   4. diabetes mellitus
   5. dehydration
   6. osteoarthritis
   7. smoking or excessive alcohol use
   8. cardiovascular or respiratory problems

   NCLEX Client Need: Physiological Integrity: Reduction of Risk Potential

3. Regarding informed consent for a surgical procedure, the nurse is responsible for which aspect(s)? *(Select all that apply.)*
   1. Verifying that the consent has been signed and witnessed before sending the patient to surgery
   2. Explaining the risks and benefits of the procedure
   3. Determining the mental capacity of the patient
   4. Administering any preoperative medications after verification that the consent has been signed
   5. Verifying that the patient understands the procedure they signed the consent for

   NCLEX Client Need: Safe and Effective Care Environment: Coordinated Care

4. In discussing options for fluid resuscitation during major surgery, the health care provider indicated the availability of bloodless surgery. Bloodless surgery may include which intervention(s)? *(Select all that apply.)*
   1. Administration of Epogen
   2. Administration of volume expanders
   3. Induction of hypothermia
   4. Banking blood before surgery
   5. Autologous transfusion

   NCLEX Client Need: Physiological Integrity: Reduction of Risk Potential

5. While reviewing the morning vital signs of a preoperative patient, which patient information warrants immediate notification of the surgeon?
   1. Temperature 99.5° F (37.5° C)
   2. Serum potassium 3.2 mEq/L
   3. Bronchovesicular breath sounds
   4. Blood pressure 135/80 mm Hg

   NCLEX Client Need: Safe and Effective Care: Coordinated Care

6. The nurse reinforces the importance of turning, coughing, and deep breathing to a preoperative patient. Which patient statement indicates a need for further instruction?
   1. "I could place a pillow to brace my abdominal incision to reduce pain with coughing."
   2. "I would lie still in bed to reduce the risk of injuring my surgical wound."
   3. "Coughing would help reduce pneumonia."
   4. "Immediately getting out of bed speeds up recuperation."

   NCLEX Client Need: Health Promotion and Maintenance

7. Your patient has been diagnosed with acute appendicitis and is going to surgery. The surgeon has explained the procedure to the patient and family and writes the following orders. Place them in the order in which you would carry them out. *(Priority setting.)*
   1. Consent for laparoscopic appendectomy with possible open appendectomy.
   2. Ancef 1 g IVPB now.
   3. Nothing by mouth (NPO).
   4. Morphine sulfate 4 mg IVP every 3 hours as needed for pain.
   5. CBC, metabolic panel.
   6. IV normal saline 150 cc/h.

   NCLEX Client Need: Safe and Effective Care Environment: Coordinated Care

8. When teaching a patient to use an incentive spirometer, you determine that the patient's technique is correct if the patient is:
   1. exhaling forcibly after holding the breath for 30 seconds.
   2. using the spirometer for 5 breaths every hour.
   3. taking slow, deep breaths and holding each for at least 3 seconds.
   4. exhaling forcibly into the spirometer.

   NCLEX Client Need: Physiological Integrity: Reduction of Risk Potential

9. While transferring from the preoperative area to the surgical suite, the patient asks, "Am I going to make it?" An appropriate response by you would be:
   1. "Everything will be all right."
   2. "Didn't your surgeon discuss the possible adverse outcomes of the procedure?"
   3. "You seem anxious. Tell me more about how you are feeling."
   4. "Your surgeon has performed the procedure several times."

   NCLEX Client Need: Psychosocial Integrity

10. During major surgery, the patient is considered at risk for:
    1. injury related to placement in one position for an extended period.
    2. altered nutrition because of prolonged fasting.
    3. hypervolemia from irrigation and IV fluids used in surgery.
    4. hypertension because of continuous infusion of fluids.

    NCLEX Client Need: Physiological Integrity: Reduction of Risk Potential

11. After same-day surgery, the patient is ready to go home when:
    1. an adult is there to drive the patient home.
    2. the patient is alert, ambulatory, and able to empty the bladder.
    3. pain is controlled with oral analgesia.
    4. nausea has passed and the patient is taking fluids.

    NCLEX Client Need: Safe and Effective Care Environment: Safety and Infection Control

12. Cefazolin (Ancef) 1 g IV is ordered to infuse over 30 minutes during surgery. It has been mixed in a 50-mL piggyback bag. If the tubing delivers 15 gtt/mL, how many drops per minute should be infused?

    ____

    NCLEX Client Need: Physiological Integrity: Pharmacological Therapies

Critical Thinking Questions

Scenario A

Your patient is scheduled for abdominal surgery this morning. You are assigned two other patients to care for as well. One of these patients is stable and will be going home. The other patient is going for a computed tomography (CT) scan at 9:30 A.M.

1. Describe in detail how you would plan your morning care for these three patients.
2. Your surgical patient shares with you that they are having second thoughts about having this surgery. How would you handle the situation?
3. You notice that the patient scheduled for surgery is wearing a St. Christopher medal under the gown as they return from emptying their bladder. You had told the patient to remove it earlier. How would you handle this situation?

Scenario B

On your first day on the surgical unit, you are assigned a patient who is scheduled for surgery at 10:00 A.M. The following preoperative medications are ordered: Lotensin 10 mg PO with sip of water and cefazolin 250 mg IV 1 hour before incision.

1. What would you check in the patient's chart as part of preoperative preparation?
2. What steps would you take to complete the preoperative checklist and charting for this patient? When would you start the preoperative preparation?
3. When would you give the dose of Lotensin? How would you handle the dose of cefazolin?

Scenario C

A patient is scheduled for right hip surgery. You have been asked to have them sign the surgical consent form because the surgeon forgot to have the patient do it the previous evening.

1. What should you do before asking the patient to sign the consent form?
2. The patient asks when and how they will be "prepped for surgery." What would you tell them?
3. The patient inquires as to when they will be able to see their family after surgery. What would you tell them?

Care of Postoperative Surgical Patients

5

http://evolve.elsevier.com/deWit/medsurg

Objectives

Theory

1. Describe the care of a patient in the postanesthesia care unit (PACU).
2. Compare differences in the care of a patient undergoing general anesthesia and one having spinal anesthesia.
3. Formulate a complete plan of care for a postoperative patient returning from the PACU.
4. Discuss measures to prevent postoperative infection.
5. Prioritize measures to promote safety for postoperative patients.

Clinical Practice

6. Identify how to promote adequate ventilation of the lungs during recovery from anesthesia in the PACU.
7. Perform an immediate postoperative assessment when a patient returns to the nursing unit.
8. Apply interventions to prevent postoperative complications.
9. Assess for postoperative pain and provide comfort measures and pain relief.
10. Promote early ambulation and return to independence in activities of daily living.
11. Perform discharge teaching necessary for postoperative home self-care.

Key Terms

anaphylaxis (ă-nă-fă-LĂK-sĭs, p. 95)
atelectasis (ă-tĕ-LĔK-tă-sĭs, p. 86)
dehiscence (dĕ-HĬS-ĕntz, p. 93)
embolus (ĔM-bō-lŭs, p. 90)
evisceration (ē-vĭs-ĕr-Ā-shŭn, p. 93)
hematoma (hē-mă-TŌ-mă, p. 91)
malignant hyperthermia (MH) (mă-LĬG-nănt hī-pĕr-THĔR-mē-ă, p. 95)
paralytic ileus (păr-ă-LĬT-ĭk ĬL-ē-ŭs, p. 89)
pneumonia (nū-MŌ-nē-ă, p. 88)
purulence (PŪ-rū-lĕns, p. 91)
seroma (sĕ-RŌ-mă, p. 91)
thrombophlebitis (thrŏm-bō-flĕ-BĪ-tĭs, p. 87)
thrombosis (thrŏm-BŌ-sĭs, p. 87)

Concepts Covered in This Chapter

- Gas Exchange
- Infection
- Tissue Integrity
- Mobility
- Pain
- Patient Education

IMMEDIATE POSTOPERATIVE CARE

POSTANESTHESIA CARE UNIT

When surgery with general anesthesia is completed, the patient is usually transferred to the postanesthesia care unit (PACU) adjacent to the surgical suites (Fig. 5.1). Patients who have had spinal anesthesia for a major procedure also go to the PACU. Very critically ill patients, such as those recovering from open heart surgery, are often taken directly to the intensive care unit for anesthesia recovery. Surgical patients who had procedural sedation or a local or regional anesthetic usually recover in the ambulatory surgery area. The PACU nurse receives a verbal report from the anesthesia care provider about the procedure, blood loss, anesthesia administered, fluids infused, medications administered, and any problems encountered.

The patient is immediately attached to the cardiac and pulse oximeter monitors, and oxygen is usually administered if the patient had general anesthesia. Oxygen helps eliminate the anesthetic gases and helps meet the increased metabolic demand for oxygen caused by surgery. Any respiratory problems are immediately addressed because maintenance of airway and adequate ventilation take priority. An oral airway, laryngeal mask airway, or endotracheal tube may still be in place because the anesthesia medications often relax the tongue enough to occlude the airway and the patient may not be awake enough for removal of the airway device. Alternatively,

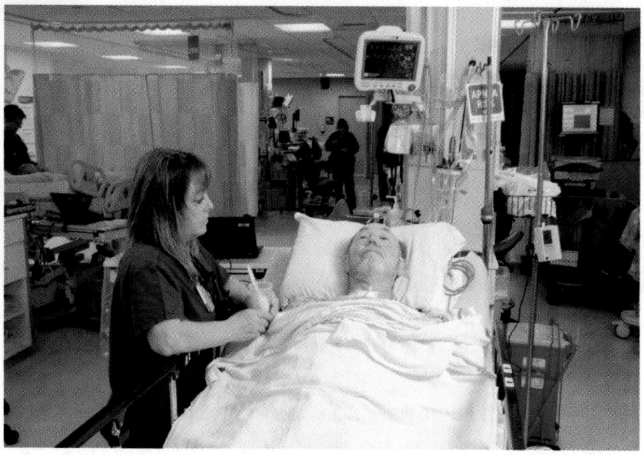

Fig. 5.1 A nurse caring for a patient in the postanesthesia care unit.

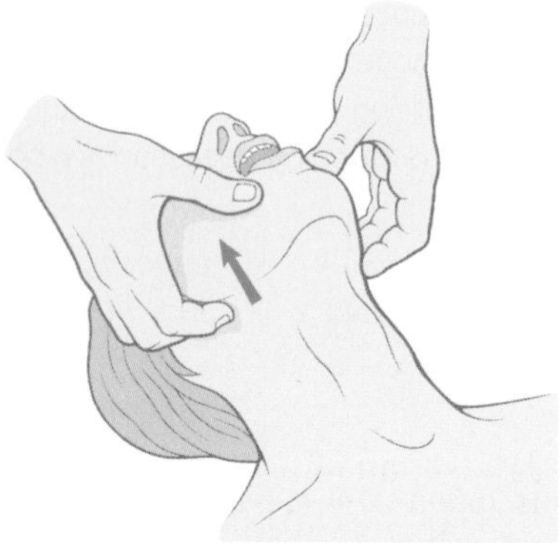

Fig. 5.2 The head tilt–jaw thrust maneuver provides a patent upper airway by tensing the muscles attached to the tongue, thus pulling the tongue away from the posterior pharynx. Forward displacement of the mandible is accomplished by grasping the angles of the mandible and lifting with both hands, which serves to displace the mandible forward while tilting the head backward. (From Pardo Jr M, Miller RD: *Basics of anesthesia*, ed 7, Philadelphia, 2018, Elsevier.)

the airway can be opened by moving the jaw forward (Fig. 5.2). Suction is turned on and is readily available to clear secretions. If needed, mechanical ventilation is provided. Warm blankets are placed over the patient, vital signs are assessed and compared with baseline readings, and a full neurologic assessment is performed. Neurologic assessment includes level of consciousness; orientation; sensory and motor status; and size, equality, and reactivity of the pupils. The patient may be asleep, drowsy but arousable, or awake.

Determine intake and output (I&O) to assess the function of the urinary system. Closely monitor urinary output. Check all intravenous (IV) lines for patency, verify that the solutions and the flow rate are correct, and inspect wound drains and evacuation devices for proper function. Assess dressings for unexpected drainage.

Surgical recovery can take from 1 to 6 hours. Time of stay in the PACU is determined by the operative procedure and the type of anesthesia used. Assess for return of the gag reflex by determining whether the patient can swallow their secretions.

Box 5.1 Postanesthesia Care Unit Report to Nursing Unit Nurse

GENERAL INFORMATION

- Patient's name and age
- Diagnosis
- Allergies
- Stability level

SURGICAL DATA

- Surgeon's name
- Surgical procedure performed
- Length of surgery time
- Unexpected surgical events
- Vital sign trends during surgery
- Anesthetic administered
- Medications administered during surgery and recovery
- Amount of blood loss and replacement

POSTANESTHESIA CARE COURSE

- Vital signs and oxygen saturation
- Urine output
- Intravenous solutions and blood products administered, with amounts
- Tubes, drains, and equipment in use
- Results of any intraoperative laboratory or diagnostic tests (note whether patient or family has been told pathology results)
- Pain status and time of last dose of analgesia
- Any problems encountered

The patient may wake up confused and may need reorientation and reassurance that the surgery is over, that they are in the recovery room, and that their family member or contact person has been notified. Once the patient is awake, family members are sometimes allowed to visit for a few minutes so that they are assured that their loved one is all right and recovering. Assessments are performed at least every 15 minutes or according to the status of the patient. Assessment for complications of the surgery and anesthesia are ongoing. The patient remains in the PACU until the vital signs are stable and the patient is awake and able to respond to stimuli. A form of the Aldrete scoring system or other system is used to determine readiness for transfer. Activity, respiration, circulation, consciousness, skin color, and oxygen saturation are each given a score. A patient with a score of 9 or 10 is ready for transfer to the nursing unit. Report is given to the staff nurse (Box 5.1).

? Think Critically

What is the number-one priority of care for a patient in the PACU?

For many procedures the patient may be transferred from the operating room (OR) directly back to the same-day surgery unit. You monitor the patient's respirations, circulation, vital signs, neurologic status, fluid balance, wound drainage and dressings, and comfort level. When the vital signs are stable, the patient is allowed to sit up and then is ambulated. If discharge criteria are met, the patient may be discharged when able to ambulate unassisted, take fluids without nausea, and empty the bladder. Recovery time in the same-day surgery unit is usually 1 to 3 hours. Discharge teaching begins before the surgery and continues once the patient is again alert. Written instructions are always sent home with the patient. If the patient has undergone sedation, another adult must provide transportation home after same-day surgery. Advise surgery patients who have received anesthesia or procedural sedation not to resume normal activities or make important decisions for at least 24 hours after surgery. The contact information of the surgeon and the signs and symptoms to report are written on the postoperative instruction sheet.

? Think Critically

How would you assess a patient to determine whether the gag (swallowing) reflex has returned sufficiently after sedation to allow them to have a few ice chips?

NURSING MANAGEMENT

ASSESSMENT (DATA COLLECTION)

After the patient is transferred from recovery, check their identity, settle them in bed, and perform an initial postoperative assessment. **Airway, breathing, and circulation are always the top priorities.** This provides a baseline against which frequent postoperative assessment data can be compared to prevent or quickly detect signs of complications. Vital signs are taken more frequently if they are unstable; this is a nursing judgment.

Monitoring for signs of the various surgical complications that may occur is a major nursing responsibility. The first 72 hours after surgery require frequent observations to detect signs of postoperative complications.

NURSING DIAGNOSIS

Problem statements commonly used for postoperative patients who have undergone general anesthesia include the following:

- Altered gas exchange due to the effect of anesthesia on the lungs

Focused Assessment

Postoperative Assessment

AREA	ASSESSMENT	SCHEDULE
Airway	Lung sounds, depth and quality of air movement Respiratory rate	Auscultate lungs initially; respiratory rate every 15 min until easily arousable, then assess quality of respirations with vital signs assessment
	Oxygen saturation	Note per vital signs schedule and whenever in room
	Oxygen delivery at rate ordered and patency of system	Check oxygen delivery system with initial assessment and each shift
	End-tidal carbon dioxide (CO_2) monitoring if patient-controlled analgesia (PCA) used or otherwise ordered	Check with oxygen saturation
Circulation	Auscultate heart; check peripheral pulses and sensation, especially distal to surgical site; assess skin color	Initially every 4 h × 2, then with vital signs; if surgery was on an extremity, assess each time vital signs are measured
Mental status	Level of consciousness and orientation	Initially and then with full vital signs
Vital signs	Temperature	Check initially, then every 8 h once stable
	Blood pressure, pulse, and respirations	Check every 15 min × 1 h, every 30 min × 4, every 1 h × 4, every 4 h × 24–48 h; or per agency protocol
Fluid status and hydration	Intravenous infusion site and flow rate	Check initially and when in room
	Intake and output	Check each shift
	Skin turgor; oral membranes	Check initially and each shift
Surgical site	Check for bleeding; mark boundaries of drainage on dressing with the time; assess wound drainage in containers	Initially and every 1 h × 4, then with vital signs
Gastrointestinal	Auscultate bowel sounds; assess abdomen	Initially, then every 8 h
	Check nasogastric drainage color, character, amount	Check drainage whenever in room
Tubes	Check for patency and function of each	Initially, then with vital signs and after turning
Kidney function	Assess urine output from Foley catheter; must void within 8 h if no Foley in place	Initially and every 1 h × 4; then if >30 mL/h, every 4 h
Pain	Use a pain scale and observation of nonverbal behaviors	Initially and with vital signs; assess at least every 3 h
Skin	Pressure areas over bony prominences	Initially and every 2 h
Safety	All equipment is intact and safely functioning	Initially and each shift

Assignment Considerations

Postoperative Vital Signs

Because postoperative patients need close vigilance in the early postoperative period, it is best not to assign the taking of frequent vital signs to an unlicensed assistive personnel (UAP) for the first couple of hours. Other parameters besides the measurement of vital signs need to be checked on a frequent schedule. After the first couple of hours, the task of vital sign measurement can be assigned to a UAP proficient in obtaining accurate measurements. Remind the UAP of exactly what to report: temperature elevation above 99.8° F (37.1° C), blood pressure (BP) alteration of a specific amount down or up from the baseline, tachycardia, and respiratory rate above or below normal range.

- Altered breathing pattern due to analgesia and pain
- Altered skin integrity due to surgical incision
- Potential for infection due to surgical wound
- Potential for injury due to sedation, decreased level of consciousness, or excessive blood loss
- Acute pain due to disruption of tissue
- Alteration in airway clearance due to inability to breathe deeply and cough without discomfort
- Fluid volume deficit due to fluid loss and nothing by mouth (NPO) status
- Potential for constipation due to opioid analgesics, decreased mobility, and decreased peristalsis
- Altered self-care ability due to decreased mobility, use of tubes, and presence of dressings
- Potential for altered myocardial tissue perfusion due to surgery, anesthesia, and positioning in the OR
- Altered coping ability due to loss of body part or change in body image
- Altered urinary elimination due to effects of anesthesia or presence of catheter

For patients who have undergone spinal anesthesia, problem statements also include:

- Altered mobility due to effects of spinal anesthesia
- Potential for injury due to decreased sensation and movement in lower extremities

◆ PLANNING

The expected outcomes depend on the specific problem statements. General nursing goals include:

- Maintain patent airway and adequate respiratory exchange.
- Maintain adequate tissue perfusion.
- Promote normal physiologic body function.
- Prevent injury.
- Promote comfort and rest.
- Promote wound healing.
- Promote psychological adjustment to lifestyle or body image changes.
- Prevent postoperative complications.

When planning your work for the shift, allow time for frequent postoperative assessments. Careful planning is essential so that proper care for the early postoperative patient does not override the needs of other patients.

◆ IMPLEMENTATION

Maintain Oxygenation and Ventilation

Postoperative patients are at risk for respiratory problems from the effects of anesthesia on the lungs, being in one position for the duration of surgery, and limited mobility in the immediate postoperative period. **Maintaining a patent airway is a priority measure to promote oxygenation and ventilation.** Unless contraindicated, the patient must be positioned on the side or with the head turned to the side to prevent aspiration until fully recovered and alert and the gag reflex is intact. Monitor oxygen saturation closely, and administer oxygen as ordered to maintain appropriate levels of oxygenation. Ventilation is the movement of gases in and out of the lungs and is measured by CO_2. Monitor end-tidal CO_2 if indicated to assess for adequate ventilation.

Older Adult Care Points

Providing adequate pain control for older adult patients has been shown to prevent respiratory complications because patients whose incisional pain is controlled will breathe more deeply and are more able to follow instructions for respiratory care.

Some degree of **atelectasis** (collapse of alveoli in the lungs) exists after anesthesia. A mild hypoxia is usually present for about 48 hours after surgery. A large percentage of all patients who have had either abdominal or thoracic surgery suffer from increasing atelectasis and pneumonitis. **If any area of the lung remains atelectatic for more than 72 hours, hypostatic pneumonia from retained secretions is likely to occur.** A low-grade fever in the first 24 to 48 hours often indicates atelectasis.

Hypostatic pneumonia results when lack of movement or of position change causes stasis of secretions, which become a breeding ground for bacteria. Auscultate the lungs carefully for abnormal sounds indicating retained secretions, assess the rate and depth of breathing, and encourage the patient to deep-breathe and cough every 2 hours to promote airway clearance. Coughing to remove secretions may be contraindicated for patients who have had a hernia repair or eye, ear, brain, jaw, or plastic surgery. Check the surgeon's orders. If the patient cannot cough effectively, instruct him to "huff" cough (see Chapter 4). If the patient is too weak to remove secretions, tracheal suctioning is indicated.

Ensure that the patient turns every 2 hours, which changes the distribution of gas and blood flow in the lungs and helps move secretions. Early ambulation is ordered to promote ventilation.

The use of an incentive spirometer is especially helpful to prevent atelectasis and hypoventilation (see Chapter 4). It should be used every hour while the patient is awake for the first 24 hours after surgery and every 2 hours thereafter. Older adult patients may need extra coaching to master the spirometer technique.

Older Adult Care Points

The risk of hypoventilation is greater in older adults because lung expansion may be hampered by calcification of costal cartilage and weakened respiratory muscles. End-tidal CO_2 monitoring is effective in identifying hypoventilation in at-risk patients.

A pulse oximeter may be used to determine blood oxygenation. Monitor oxygen readings periodically and report oxygen saturation (Sao_2) readings below 95%.

Maintain Circulation and Tissue Perfusion

When considerable blood is lost during surgery, a blood transfusion may be ordered. Autologous blood may be transfused if the patient donated blood several weeks before surgery or if the patient's blood was collected as it was lost during surgery. This blood is filtered and returned to the patient. Be vigilant for signs of shock and check for visible hemorrhage by measuring the amount of blood on dressings. (See Prevent Postoperative Complications and Chapter 5.)

If surgery involves an extremity (arm, leg, foot, or hand) or if a procedure has been performed on any major blood vessel (aorta, femoral artery), the distal or peripheral pulse is checked during each full assessment. Swelling at the surgical site can compress vessels and decrease blood flow distal to the surgical site. The skin distal to the surgical site should be warm to the touch, and there should be brisk capillary refill in the fingers or toes. Color, movement, and sensation of the fingers and toes should be checked to detect nerve or blood vessel compression from swelling and edema.

BP and pulse should be compared with preoperative values to determine whether there are significant changes. An increase in pulse may indicate that internal bleeding is occurring, but it can also signify incomplete pain control. BP that falls below the patient's normal baseline level may indicate major bleeding.

Core Measures (The Joint Commission [TJC], 2017) require antithrombosis therapy after many surgeries. The use of sequential compression devices (SCDs) on the legs is recommended. SCDs alternately compress and release, squeezing the legs and propelling blood along the vessels, increasing venous return from the legs and helping prevent stasis of blood in the lower extremities (Fig. 5.3). The SCDs should be checked frequently to ensure proper fit and function. They should be removed at least once per shift to allow air circulation to the skin or for bathing and full skin inspection (Gould et al., 2012). As danger of **thrombosis** decreases, compression stockings may take the place of the SCDs. The stockings must be fitted correctly and should be checked frequently to ensure that they fit smoothly. Orders for ambulation are implemented as soon as the patient is up and walking.

Low-molecular-weight subcutaneous heparin injections may be ordered as a general precaution and for any patient who has a history of **thrombophlebitis** (clot and inflammation in a blood vessel) or is at high risk for thrombosis. Question the patient about pain, swelling, or tenderness in the legs. If the patient complains of leg pain, gently assess the skin for increased warmth and notify the surgeon.

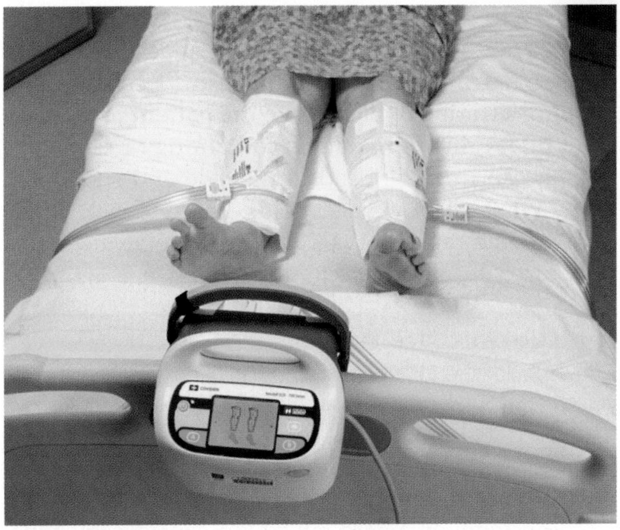

Fig. 5.3 Sequential compression devices in place to prevent thrombus formation.

Think Critically

The initial vital sign readings for your patient on return from surgery were BP 138/86, pulse 76, respirations 14, temperature 97.7° F (36.5° C). An hour later they were BP 126/74, pulse 80, respirations 14, temperature 98.0° F (36.7° C). What action, if any, should you take?

Prevent Injury

Safety is a primary concern until the patient is fully recovered from anesthesia. Always leave the bed in the low position after administering care. Remind the patient to call for assistance as needed and be certain the call bell is within reach. Core Measures (TJC, 2017) require the use of interventions to prevent falls. Remember that you are the patient's advocate while they are recovering from surgery and anesthesia or under the influence of narcotic analgesia. Be certain that all appropriate safety measures are implemented and listed on the patient's care plan.

Reassure patients who have had spinal anesthesia that it is normal for the legs to feel numb and heavy and that feeling will soon return to normal. Maintain a flat position with only a pillow until feeling returns. Sense of position in space will return to the legs first, followed by sensation to deep pressure, voluntary movement, and finally feeling of superficial pain and temperature. A feeling of "pins and needles" in the legs is common. The patient is susceptible to hypotension until all effects of the spinal anesthesia are gone. Lying flat for 6 to 8 hours may decrease the chance of post–spinal anesthesia headache. If a headache develops, staying flat in bed reduces the pain. Keep IV fluid running as ordered. **Encourage the patient to increase fluid intake, including fluids containing caffeine.** The patient can turn the head to the side and sip from a straw while someone else holds the container. Fluids and caffeine raise the vascular pressure at the spinal puncture site and help seal the hole.

? Think Critically

How would care for a patient who has had spinal anesthesia differ from care for a patient who has had general anesthesia?

Many surgical procedures last several hours, which means that the patient has been lying motionless, in a fixed position, on a hard table for a considerable time. Check pressure points related to the position the patient was in during surgery and provide padding and appropriate positioning for areas that are painful (see Chapter 4).

? Think Critically

Your postoperative patient was placed in a right side-lying position during surgery. Which specific places should you check for signs of pressure problems? How would you position a patient who is complaining of pain in the right hip as well as pain in the left flank where the surgery occurred?

Older Adult Care Points

Because skin is fragile and older adults have less subcutaneous tissue, check bony prominences carefully for signs of breakdown. Joint strains can occur from the positioning necessary for certain types of surgery; perform position changes slowly and gently.

Prevent Infection

Use aseptic technique when caring for postoperative patients. Good hand hygiene is the primary means of preventing infection. Dressing changes are performed with strict sterile technique while the patient is in the hospital; the patient may use clean technique at home. Encouraging fluid intake to flush the bladder will help prevent a bladder infection in patients who were catheterized or have an indwelling catheter. Turning, coughing, deep breathing, and ambulation will assist in preventing **pneumonia** (inflammation and accumulation of exudate in the lung) from retained secretions and lack of movement. Aseptically handling drains and aseptically emptying wound drainage devices prevent the entry of microorganisms.

Core Measures (TJC, 2017) state that if the patient is receiving a prophylactic antibiotic, it must be discontinued within 24 hours after surgery. Assess the surgical wound area each shift and assess for signs of infection (e.g., local pain, increased tenderness, warmth, redness, or drainage of purulent material). Monitor the blood count for increasing leukocytes (white blood cells [WBCs]) and the body temperature for an unexpected increase. Keeping blood glucose within normal limits helps prevent wound infection (Anderson & Sexton, 2017).

Maintain Fluid Balance and Elimination

Urine output is closely monitored after surgery. If the patient has an indwelling catheter, observe the urine in the bag every hour in the early postoperative period. Report a urine flow of less than 30 mL/h to the charge nurse. Check the catheter to ensure that it is not kinked and that the connecting tubing is not lying beneath the patient. A patient without a catheter in place must void within 4 to 8 hours depending on the type of surgery and the anesthesia used. If the patient is unable to empty the bladder spontaneously, obtain a bladder scan and, if needed, an order for catheterization. **If flow is less than 60 mL over a 2-hour period, the surgeon must be notified.**

Assignment Considerations

Urinary Output

When a UAP is assigned to turn the patient every 2 hours, remind the UAP to check that the tubing of any indwelling catheter is not under the patient or crimped. If the UAP is assigned the task of emptying the Foley catheter bag at the end of the shift, ask that you be notified if there is less than 30 mL/h of urine for the shift in the output. Verify that the UAP knows to maintain sterility of the urinary catheter system and to wipe the spout with an alcohol sponge after emptying the urine bag.

Patients usually return from surgery with an IV infusion running. Depending on the type of surgery, IV fluids may be continued for a few days or discontinued after the fluid has infused. Check orders to see that the correct solution is running. **No potassium additive should be given until the urine flow is at least 30 mL/h.** Potassium may cause hyperkalemia if kidney function is not adequate. Assess the IV site each hour for patency, flow rate, and complications. Document all IV fluids administered as intake on the I&O record.

As soon as the patient is conscious and the gag reflex has returned, offer a few ice chips or sips of water unless there is an order to maintain NPO status. Document all oral intake as well as IV fluids administered. At the end of each shift, calculate and document the difference between intake and output. Because fluids were lost during surgery, the body will initially retain fluid. Postoperatively, the output will slowly increase until it is more than the intake; after 2 to 3 days, fluids should again be balanced.

Clinical Cues

A cup of ice equals ½ cup of water.

Anesthesia may cause nausea and vomiting. Keep the emesis basin or bag close by, and position the patient on the side to prevent aspiration. Check the orders to determine on which side the patient can be positioned. The surgeon usually writes an order for medication in the event of excessive nausea or vomiting. **To prevent stress on the incision and sutures, it is best to medicate the patient before actual vomiting occurs.**

Apply a cool cloth to the forehead and back of the neck, rinse the mouth, rid the room of odors, and provide a quiet environment to help reduce nausea. After emesis, mouth care should be provided. If vomiting is uncontrolled with medication, a nasogastric (NG) tube that suctions stomach contents may need to be inserted.

Promote Gastrointestinal Function and Nutrition

Surgeons often keep the patient NPO after open abdominal procedures because handling of the gastrointestinal (GI) tract and general anesthesia cause peristalsis to halt, which means that secretions will not flow through the system properly. If abdominal distention occurs, an NG tube may be placed to remove gathering secretions. When an NG tube is in place, check that it is positioned and functioning properly and that the suction is set according to orders. Assess the amount of drainage produced every 1 to 2 hours. If the drainage turns dark brown and grainy, it should be checked for blood using a special reagent. Report the presence of blood to the surgeon.

A healthy surgical patient may be kept on nothing but IV fluids for several days without developing a serious nutritional problem. If extensive tissue repair is required for healing or the patient was malnourished preoperatively, supplemental nutrition by enteral or parenteral feeding may be started (see Chapters 3 and 27 for details of enteral and total parenteral nutrition). A patient who is NPO and kept on IV fluids will lose some weight because there are insufficient calories in the IV fluids to meet total daily requirements. A liter of 5% dextrose in water contains only 200 calories.

After surgery that required general anesthesia, the patient will not be allowed to eat solid foods until bowel sounds have returned because of the risk of developing **paralytic ileus** (failure of forward movement of bowel contents). Ice chips and clear liquids offered in the early postoperative period may stimulate peristalsis and help promote the return of normal bowel function.

> **Clinical Cues**
>
> When permitted by the surgeon, chewing sugarless gum can speed bowel recovery after abdominal surgery. Gum chewing has also been shown to be effective for recovery from paralytic ileus (Kalff, Wehner, & Litkouhi, 2017).

At least once per shift, or according to hospital policy, listen for bowel sounds in all four quadrants. Once they are heard and the patient is tolerating ice chips and clear liquids, a regular diet may be implemented. The patient may be allowed to eat right away after spinal anesthesia. The surgeon may order that the diet be advanced based on the nursing assessment.

Discomfort from abdominal distention and considerable flatus may occur after general anesthesia because of decreased or absent peristalsis. Taking only small amounts of liquid or food at a time, drinking only tepid liquids, and refraining from drinking with a straw helps keep flatus to a minimum, and ambulating helps move and evacuate gas. If permitted and the patient cannot ambulate, the patient can try resting in a slight Trendelenburg position, with the legs and rectum higher than the stomach, which may assist in evacuation of flatus.

Once the patient is eating again, a bowel movement should occur within 2 to 3 days. If this does not occur, an order for a suppository or laxative may be needed to stimulate a bowel movement. Patients receiving narcotic analgesics may become constipated and require stool softeners or laxatives to produce normal bowel movements. Length of stay after an operative procedure may be only 2 to 3 days. Make sure information about constipation is covered in the discharge teaching.

> **Think Critically**
>
> Name four specific interventions to prevent constipation in a postoperative patient who is receiving narcotic analgesics for pain.

Promote Comfort

Pain and discomfort interfere with rest and inhibit the processes of healing and repair. Although analgesic drugs are almost always prescribed for postoperative patients, comfort measures also should be used. Nonsteroidal antiinflammatory drugs (NSAIDs) and nonnarcotic analgesics work on both the peripheral nervous system and the central nervous system (CNS) to control pain and may be used to augment opioids. Opioids tend to depress respirations and the cough reflex and therefore may contribute to the development of pulmonary problems. Opioids also can increase the possibility of nausea and vomiting. Using other drugs in combination with opioids helps control pain with the fewest side effects.

Pain must be reduced so that the patient will rest, turn, cough, deep-breathe frequently, and ambulate as soon as possible. Medication should be given consistently for the first 24 to 48 hours postoperatively. **Assess pain level and effectiveness of analgesia using a pain scale at least every 2 to 3 hours.** Remind the patient to request medication before the pain becomes severe, such as when at 3 to 4 on the pain scale.

If the patient complains of pain on transfer to the unit, refer to the notes from the recovery unit nurse. Note any medications administered both preoperatively and postoperatively. If respirations are within normal limits and there is no contraindication to doing so, medicate the patient promptly with the ordered analgesic. If it is too soon to give more analgesia, reposition the patient, be sure that the bladder is not distended and causing discomfort, check that the patient is warm enough, and use other comfort measures such as distraction and imagery to relieve the pain. Note when analgesia is due and have it ready to administer at the appointed time.

Teach relaxation techniques that can help decrease the patient's discomfort (see Chapter 7). Pain medication may be administered by subcutaneous or intramuscular injection, intravenously, epidurally, or by intermittent administration of local anesthetic into the tissues with a catheter. Three methods commonly used for pain control are the PCA pump, the epidural catheter, and the continuous peripheral nerve block for extremity pain. Pain, methods of pain control, and pain medications and their administration are discussed in greater detail in Chapter 7.

Maintain Temperature

Operating rooms are kept very cool so that the staff members working under the bright lights do not become overheated and the growth of organisms is inhibited. The patient's temperature in this environment often decreases, especially during prolonged abdominal surgery in which the peritoneal cavity has been open for a long period. Warming during surgery is recommended, and the Core Measures specifically state the importance of warming the patient who is undergoing colon surgery (Institute for Healthcare Improvement [IHI], 2013a; TJC, 2017). Postoperatively, the patient may feel cold and should be kept warm with extra blankets or warmed bath blankets applied under the top covers. Placing socks on the patient's feet may help. Some anesthetic agents may cause tremors as they are metabolized. This usually occurs in the PACU phase of care. If uncontrollable shivering occurs, contact the surgeon for medication orders.

Dressings on extremities should be checked to be certain that they are not so tight that circulation is impaired. Check the pulse, skin temperature, sensation, and movement distal to the surgical site to evaluate circulation (neurovascular assessment). You should be able to slip your little finger between a dressing and the extremity. Dressings that are too tight cause pain.

Occasionally, continuous hiccoughs occur after surgery, making the patient quite uncomfortable. Having the patient breathe into a paper bag will often relieve the hiccoughs, and sedatives and tranquilizers are sometimes prescribed to promote relaxation and reduce irritation of the phrenic nerve. Severe, persistent cases of hiccoughs may require surgical interruption (at a later time) of impulses along the nerve pathways to remove the cause of the spasms of the diaphragm.

Complementary and Alternative Therapies

Stopping Hiccoughs

An alternative treatment for hiccoughs is to massage the earlobes. Massage activates the acupressure points, interrupting the hiccough reflex. Other commonly used remedies include the following:
- Stick a finger in each ear and hold your breath.
- Drink from a glass that someone else is holding for you.
- Breathe deeply into a paper bag 20 times.
- Place a teaspoon of sugar or peanut butter on the tongue and let it slowly dissolve; the hiccoughs will be gone when the sugar or peanut butter has dissolved.
- Acupuncture.
- Hypnosis.

Promote Rest and Activity

Patients need sleep after surgery. Keep the room quiet and group nursing activities to prevent waking the patient more often than necessary. At least every 2 hours, the patient must do leg exercises and change position. Orders for ambulation may begin within several hours after surgery. Raise the head of the bed first and let the body adjust to the position change. Then sit the patient on the side of the bed, allowing the legs to dangle over the side with the feet on the floor or a foot stool. After a few minutes, slowly assist the patient to stand. Assist the patient to walk around the room or for at least a few steps. Use a gait belt and have someone assist you if the patient is very weak. Pain medication can be timed to decrease pain during ambulation if it does not make the patient too groggy.

Emphasize that exercise is vital to prevent circulatory problems and offer praise for all efforts. Keeping blood from pooling in the extremities helps prevent thrombus formation and **embolus** (a thrombus or clot that travels and lodges elsewhere in the body). Continue to ambulate, in the hospital or at home, on a set schedule until the patient can do so independently. In many hospitals, physical therapy orders are written and the physical therapist is responsible for ambulating the patient and overseeing range-of-motion exercises.

If the patient is on strict bed rest, range-of-motion exercises must be performed at least four times a day. The patient may do active range of motion on most joints, but passive range of motion must be done on joints the patient is unable to exercise unless physical therapy visits have been ordered. Family members also may help with these exercises.

Promote Wound Healing

Surgical incisions most often heal by primary, or first, intention (Table 5.1). Adequate rest, sufficient blood supply, and proper nutrition all promote wound healing (see the Evolve website for Phases of Wound Healing). Rest decreases the metabolic rate and allows nutrients to be used for healing rather than activity. Proteins provide the amino acids that are the building blocks of tissue and are vital to the healing process. Blood transports amino

Table 5.1 Phases of Primary Intention Wound Healing[a]

PHASE	ACTIVITY
Phase I	
Acute inflammatory reaction (3–4 days)	Process of hemostasis. Constriction of blood vessels, platelet aggregation and the formation of fibrin, and epithelial cell migration. Phagocytosis occurs. Scab forms.
Phase II	
Proliferation and granulation (day 3 or 4 to 2–3 wk)	Macrophages clear debris, fibroblasts synthesize collagen, capillary networks are built, and granulation tissue is formed. Closure by contracture begins.
Phase III	
Scar maturation and contracture (3–6 wk)	Remodeling with collagen lysis and synthesis; scar tissue thins and becomes paler but stronger.

[a]A surgical incision most often heals by primary intention. Many accidental wounds and some infected wounds heal by secondary or tertiary intention.

acids and other elements needed for rebuilding tissue and is essential to healing. Good circulation ensures that blood reaches the wound. Vitamin C is necessary for collagen production, the formation of capillaries that bring blood to the healing tissues, and resistance to infection. The minerals zinc, copper, and iron also assist in the formation of collagen.

Nutrition Considerations

Foods High in Vitamin C and Protein

FOODS HIGH IN VITAMIN C	FOODS HIGH IN PROTEIN
• Citrus fruits and juices	• Meats: chicken, beef, pork, lamb[a]
• Strawberries	• Cottage cheese
• Cantaloupe	• Milk[a]
• Tomatoes	• Cheese
• Bell peppers	• Peanut butter
• Cabbage	• Beans
• Turnip or collard greens	• Eggs
• Broccoli	• Ice cream
• Mangos	• Grain products: breads, pasta
• Peaches	• Tofu; soy products
• Pineapple	
• Potatoes	

[a]Meats and milk products contain the highest amounts of protein.

Factors interfering with wound healing. Mechanical injury from friction, pressure, or abrasion—such as can occur when tape is removed—disrupts the healing tissue and prolongs wound healing. Physical injury destroys granulation tissue, which is the framework on which new cells grow and mature to form a covering for the wound. Handle all wounds gently and shield them from injury. When dressings are removed from a wound, take care not to dislodge granulation tissue. **Smoking decreases the amount of hemoglobin available to carry oxygen to the healing tissues and prolongs healing time.**

The presence of pathogenic organisms in a wound prolongs the inflammatory process and delays healing. Antiinfective drugs are sometimes given postoperatively to prevent wound infection and should be administered as ordered to maintain appropriate blood levels of the drugs. Corticosteroids taken for a chronic condition will slow the healing process because they suppress the immune and inflammatory responses.

Excessive stress, apprehension, and emotional disturbances seem to make the body more vulnerable to invasion by foreign organisms by depressing the immune system. When under excessive stress, the body also is less able to mobilize the elements and cells that promote healing.

Older Adult Care Points

- Older adults often have chronic diseases that interfere with oxygenation, transport of nutrients to the cells, and removal of waste from the cells.
- Vitamin and mineral deficiencies are common in older adults and contribute to poor wound healing.
- Regeneration of tissue takes more time in older adults, partially because of the slower metabolic rate that occurs with age.

Interventions for wound care. The surgical wound should be inspected during dressing changes or at least once a day. Assessment includes observing the incision line for signs of excessive swelling, formation of a **hematoma** (blood-filled swelling), formation of a **seroma** (serum-filled swelling), redness, or tearing of the skin or other signs of separation of the edges of skin that have been sutured or stapled together. Normally a surgical wound is sealed within hours, and little drainage is expected. The surgical incision is usually kept covered with the dressing placed in the OR for a minimum of 24 hours. After the wound edges are sealed, the wound may be left open to air or a light protective dressing applied. Report and document evidence of bleeding, **purulence** (pus), or any other sign that the wound is not healing properly. Document the appearance of any drainage. Drainage may be serous (clear or very light yellow), serosanguineous (reddish yellow), or sanguineous (blood red). If a significant amount of drainage is expected, a wound drain is placed when closing the incision. Documentation should include whether sutures or staples are intact and the wound edges are well approximated.

The best way to prevent hospital-acquired infection of a surgical wound is always to wash your hands before doing wound care or touching the patient, to use aseptic technique and Standard Precautions for dressing changes, and to change the dressings as ordered. Additional factors that may slow wound healing in a postoperative abdominal surgery patient include vomiting, abdominal distention, and strenuous respiratory efforts, such as coughing and forcefully exhaling breaths of air without proper splinting of the incision. The wound should be properly splinted for coughing to prevent dehiscence of the incision (see Chapter 4, Fig. 4.2).

Dressings. **Surgical dressings should be checked each time vital signs are taken for the first 24 hours after surgery, every 4 hours during the next 24 hours, and then at least every 8 hours for as long as the surgical wound is covered with a dressing.** If a wound is not expected to drain but drainage is evident, the surgeon should be notified. If drainage is outlined and the time and date are noted, you can tell if the wound is draining more than it should over a period of hours. The surgeon usually does the first dressing change. If the dressing becomes saturated before that dressing change, it should be reinforced by placing more dressing material over the area. If it is within the orders, remove outer dressings—leaving those in direct contact with the wound—and secure new outer dressings in place. When there is excessive drainage, the dressing probably will require reinforcing every 4 hours. Changing the dressing more often than once a shift is not recommended because of the dangers of introducing infectious agents, of traumatizing the wound, and of interfering with tissue regeneration.

Each time the dressing is changed as ordered, the amount and characteristics of drainage on the dressing should be noted and documented. If the wound is infected, the odor of the drainage can give a clue as to the kind of organism causing the infection. A musty odor is characteristic of aerobic organisms. An acrid (sharp, stinging) or putrid (foul) odor is characteristic of anaerobes. Anaerobic infections are commonly seen after colorectal and vaginal surgery. An infected wound should be cultured to see what organism is causing the infection.

Drains. Drains are used to (1) prevent accumulation of fluids or air at the operative site; (2) protect suture lines; and (3) remove specific fluids, such as bile, cerebrospinal fluid, or drainage from an abscess. Drains not attached to a suction device are attached to a drainage bag or have dressings placed to catch the fluid. An example of a drain is the *Penrose,* which is inserted into the abdominal cavity or any other area where an abscess, fistula, or other condition requires drainage (Fig. 5.4). A T-tube drain may be placed in the common bile duct after surgery on the gallbladder or liver.

Some drains are connected to an apparatus that creates continuous suction to facilitate removal of fluid and gas. If a drain is kinked, the accumulated fluid and gas can cause pain, create dead air space (which delays healing), damage the healing tissue at the suture lines, and delay healing by compressing surrounding capillaries and cutting off oxygen supply to the cells.

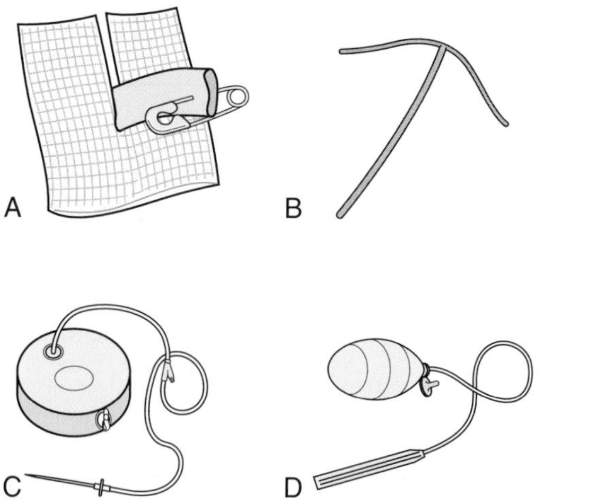

Fig. 5.4 Wound drains. **A,** Penrose drain. **B,** T-tube drain. **C,** Closed wound suction device (Hemovac). **D,** Bulb reservoir (Jackson-Pratt).

One kind of drain system is the closed wound suction device (e.g., Hemovac). The drainage catheter is connected to a spring-loaded drum and is collapsed at least once each shift to create the desired suction, which pulls fluid into a collection area of the device (see Fig. 5.4, *C* and Fig. 5.5, *A*).

Bulb reservoir suction devices are about the size of the bulb on a BP cuff and have a valve on top (e.g., Jackson-Pratt). The valve is opened to allow removal of fluid and to collapse the bulb; the valve is then closed to create negative pressure, which provides the suction. As drainage accumulates in the bulb, it is emptied and recompressed (see Fig. 5.4, *D* and Fig. 5.5, *B*). This procedure should be done to suction devices at least once per shift.

Negative pressure drainage systems consist of a semiocclusive dressing that has tubing connected to the vacuum device. The technique is also called vacuum-assisted wound closure. The negative pressure dressing and system promote wound healing by direct and indirect effects. The closed system maintains a warm, moist environment while removing wound edema, directly enhancing wound healing. The indirect effects of negative pressure include increased blood flow, decreased inflammatory response, and changes in cellular metabolism promoting wound closure (Gestring, 2018).

Removing sutures and staples. When an order is written to remove sutures or staples, check the order, gather the proper equipment, inform the patient about the procedure, correctly identify the patient, wash hands, don gloves, and inspect the incision carefully. For a long incision or an incision over a joint, remove every other suture or staple first (Fig. 5.6). If the edges of the incision do not pull apart, remove the rest of the sutures

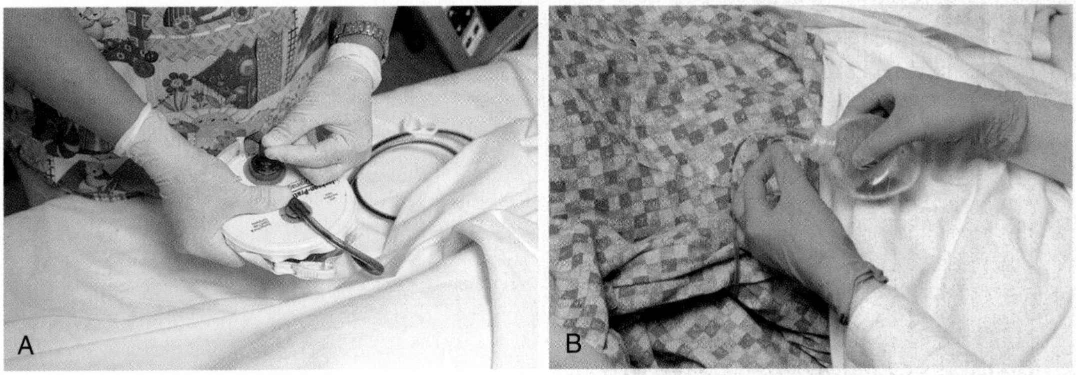

Fig. 5.5 Reactivating surgical wound suction devices by compressing the suction device after emptying the reservoir. **A,** Closed wound suction device. **B,** Bulb reservoir. (From Williams P: *deWit's fundamental concepts and skills for nursing,* ed 5, Philadelphia, 2018, Elsevier.)

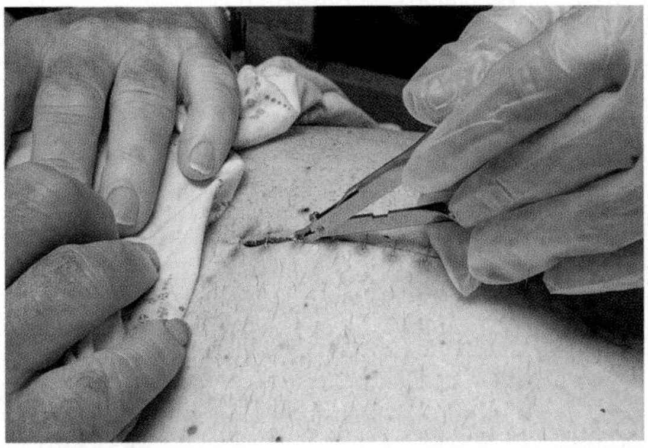

Fig. 5.6 Surgical staples are removed with a special implement.

or staples. Often **Steri-Strips** (small, reinforced strips of adhesive) are applied to hold the incision together until healing is complete.

Prevent Postoperative Complications

Table 5.2 summarizes the major postoperative complications and the nursing interventions to prevent them. Some complications are immediately life-threatening.

Wound infection. Infection of a wound can occur after any surgical procedure, but it is more common in wounds caused by accidental injury and in wounds that were already infected at the time of surgery. A prophylactic antibiotic after surgery may be ordered to prevent a wound infection. **If an infection is going to develop, it usually becomes apparent 2 to 7 days postoperatively.** Most patients will already be at home when postoperative infection becomes evident.

> **Clinical Cues**
>
> *Subjective* complaints that may indicate infection include fatigue, loss of appetite, headache, nausea, or general malaise or pain. *Objective* signs may include pain, redness, swelling and induration in the area, purulent drainage, fever, increased pulse rate, elevated WBC count, and swollen lymph nodes in adjacent areas.

If an infection occurs, cultures are obtained, and appropriate antibiotics are given for a specific length of time. Wound irrigations may be ordered for an open infected wound. Sterile normal saline is the most common solution used for this purpose. The wound may be packed with dressings moistened with the sterile saline solution.

A noninfected wound should not be cleaned or irrigated with anything but sterile normal saline; other substances irritate the tissue and slow healing. Transmission-based isolation precautions or contact precautions are instituted when a wound is infected (see Chapter 6). Gowns and gloves are worn when performing dressing changes or when irrigating infected wounds. If splattering is likely, protective eyewear and masks are also worn. Soiled dressings and supplies are bagged in plastic barrier bags to be deposited in a biohazard trash receptacle. **Dressings from an infected wound should never be placed in the patient's room trash container.**

Dehiscence and evisceration. When caring for a patient who has undergone abdominal surgery, you must be alert for possible disruption or separation of some or all layers of the surgical wound. This is called **dehiscence** (Fig. 5.7). If the wound completely separates and the contents of the abdominal cavity (viscera) protrude through the incision, the condition is called **evisceration** (see Fig. 5.7).

> **Clinical Cues**
>
> Dehiscence can occur at any time during the postoperative period, but it most commonly occurs between the fifth and twelfth postoperative days—when the patient is feeling stronger and more active, but healing is not complete, or when infection has occurred. When checking an abdominal surgical wound, be particularly aware of any drainage. There is often a noticeable increase in the amount of serosanguineous drainage before the separation of the wound layers becomes apparent. Subjectively, the patient may not notice any symptoms until there is a feeling of "giving way" in the wound.

Table 5.2 Postoperative Complications

PROBLEM	SIGNS AND SYMPTOMS	PREVENTIVE INTERVENTIONS
Atelectasis	Decreased breath sounds over areas not aerating; dyspnea	Deep breathing and coughing; use of incentive spirometer; early ambulation; teach to cough properly.
Pneumonia: hypostatic, aspiration, or bacterial	Fever, malaise, increased sputum, purulent sputum, cough, flushed skin, dyspnea, pain on inspiration; abnormal breath sounds, crackles, rhonchi	Deep breathing, coughing, and frequent turning; early ambulation; incentive spirometer use; range-of-motion exercises if unable to ambulate; medication if bacterial.
Paralytic (adynamic) ileus	No bowel sounds 24–36 h after surgery or fewer than 5 sounds/min	Monitor bowel sounds; encourage early ambulation; clear fluids as tolerated. Use nonopioid medications for pain control when possible.
Thrombophlebitis	Pain or warmth in calf of leg, swollen leg, area on leg warm to touch; possible temperature elevation	Encourage leg exercises; keep the patient well hydrated; encourage ambulation; use antiembolic stockings or devices. Low-dose anticoagulation as ordered.
Urinary retention	Distended bladder; inability to void spontaneously	Palpate bladder or use bladder scanner; encourage voiding, if unable to void within 8 h obtain an order for catheterization; medicate to increase urinary sphincter tone as ordered.
Urinary tract infection	Dysuria, frequency, foul-smelling urine	Force fluids when allowed; encourage frequent voiding; teach proper perineal cleanliness; keep catheter clean and patent; use aseptic technique to empty drainage bag.
Hypoventilation	Decreased rate and depth of breathing, decreased O_2 saturation and increased CO_2 levels. Decreased level of consciousness.	Rouse patient frequently until the anesthesia medications have cleared the system. Monitor pulse oximetry and end-tidal CO_2. Give opioid medications cautiously. Encourage fluids and movement.
Wound infection	Redness, swelling, pain, warmth, drainage, fever, increased leukocytes, rapid pulse and respirations (fever 72 h after surgery indicates infection in some system or in the wound)	Assess wound characteristics and drainage. Monitor white blood cell count and temperature. Use aseptic technique for wound care; encourage adequate nutrition and fluids; encourage activity. Antibiotics as ordered.
Pulmonary embolus	Shortness of breath, anxiety, chest pain, rapid pulse and respirations, cyanosis, cough, bloody sputum, decreased oxygen saturation.	Prevention: Antiembolism stockings, adequate fluid intake, frequent turning or ambulation, preventive anticoagulant as ordered; leg exercises. Treatment: Oxygen to maintain ordered O_2 saturation. Therapeutic anticoagulation.
Hemorrhage and shock	Evidence of copious bleeding; decreased blood pressure, elevated pulse, cold clammy skin, decreased urinary output	Give blood or volume expander; stop bleeding. Place in shock position with feet and legs elevated and head flat; administer ordered medications to raise blood pressure; administer oxygen; measure vital signs frequently.
Wound dehiscence	Discharge of serosanguineous drainage from wound and sensation that "something gave"; separation of wound edges	Teach to splint properly for coughing with abdominal incisions. Assess wound edge approximation with each wound assessment. Monitor any drainage after wound edges are closed. Protect exposed tissue and report.
Evisceration	Intestines visible through abdominal incision	Place patient supine with knees flexed; cover wound with sterile saline-soaked gauze or towels; return to operating room for repair; monitor for shock.
Fluid imbalance	Signs of overhydration: crackles in lungs, edema, weight gain Signs of dehydration: weight loss, diminished pulse, dry mucous membranes, decreased tissue turgor	Control intravenous flow rate. Monitor intake and output; correct imbalances. Output will be less than intake for first 72 h after surgery with general anesthesia. Auscultate lungs each shift. Monitor weight; check for edema.
Malignant hyperthermia	High temperature, cardiac dysrhythmias, muscle rigidity, hypotension, tachypnea, and dark cola-colored urine	Genetic predisposition; can only monitor and treat symptoms; apply cooling blanket and ice packs. Give dantrolene as ordered.

Modified from Williams P: *deWit's fundamental concepts and skills for nursing,* ed 5, Philadelphia, 2018, Elsevier.

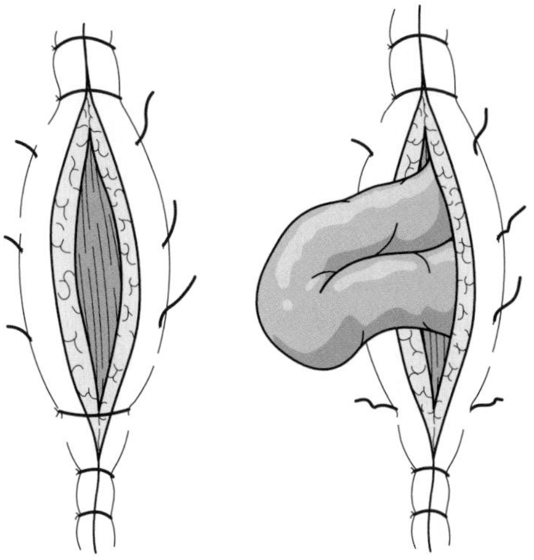

Fig. 5.7 Complications of wound healing: dehiscence and evisceration. (From Williams P: *deWit's fundamental concepts and skills for nursing,* ed 5, Philadelphia, 2018, Elsevier.)

Wound separation or disruption usually is brought on by a sudden strain or stress on the suture lines (e.g., when the patient sneezes, coughs, or has an episode of retching and vomiting). **Patients most at risk for dehiscence and evisceration are those who are diabetic, obese, malnourished, or dehydrated; have a malignancy; have experienced multiple traumas to the abdomen; or have an infected wound.** Abdominal distention and broken sutures or disrupted staples are other factors in wound disruption. Wound dehiscence may be partial or complete. The amount of wound disruption will determine treatment. Most wound dehiscence is secondary to infection, so treatment will commonly include antibiotics. A wound anywhere on the body can dehisce, but evisceration can occur only in abdominal wounds. Evisceration creates an emergency that requires immediate surgery and is a very serious complication. The immediate treatment for evisceration before reparative surgery includes having the patient lie supine with the knees flexed. The wound should be covered with a sterile towel or sterile dressings moistened with sterile normal saline. Positioning with the knees flexed prevents abdominal muscle strain. Keep the patient calm while waiting for the arrival of emergency medical services.

Home Care Considerations

In Case of Dehiscence or Evisceration

If evisceration occurs at home, moisten sterile gauze with sterile water (or fresh water if sterile is unavailable) and place it over the exposed bowel to keep the bowel membrane moist. Immediately notify the home care agency or the surgeon, call someone to help, and have the patient lie supine with the knees flexed and the moistened dressings in place. If wound dehiscence occurs, notify the health care provider and follow the instructions given.

Think Critically

Identify seven assessment findings that together would indicate a wound infection.

Immediate postoperative complications. The most common complication of anesthesia medications is respiratory depression compounded by administration of opioid pain medications. Frequent assessment of the patient is needed in the immediate postoperative period to identify hypoxia or hypercapnia (monitored by end-tidal CO_2; see Chapter 12). In addition to the respiratory assessment, vital signs will indicate if hypotension is present. Shock, which can quickly develop into a life-threatening emergency, presents the most immediate danger to the patient. Shock disrupts normal physiologic function and can result from failure of the heart to function as a pump (**cardiogenic shock**), such as in cardiac arrest (see Chapter 20); a low volume of blood (**hypovolemic shock**), such as in hemorrhage; or dilation of the blood vessels as a result of faulty nervous system regulation (**distributive shock**; see Chapter 45). Distributive shock includes **anaphylaxis** (severe allergic reaction), such as in hypersensitivity to a drug or other allergen (see Chapter 11). Shock can also result from sepsis, which occurs when toxins from bacteria relax and dilate blood vessels, resulting in a drop in blood pressure (see Chapters 6 and 45). Early identification and treatment of hypotension can prevent patient deterioration.

Clinical Cues

Early signs of impending hypovolemic shock from hemorrhage are thirst, restlessness, tachycardia, and tachypnea. Changes in the vital signs may be the only warning sign of shock.

As shock progresses, BP begins to drop and pulse rate increases. Pulse may be bounding at first but becomes thready and indistinct as circulatory collapse occurs. Skin becomes cold and clammy, and pallor becomes evident. There may be air hunger with cyanosis of the lips and nail beds as a result of tissue hypoxia. As shock deepens, blood pressure continues to fall, and the patient loses consciousness, eventually becoming comatose. Untreated shock is fatal.

Both general and local anesthesia can bring about circulatory collapse. If there is evidence of shock, the patient should be placed in the supine position with the lower extremities elevated to add blood volume to the vital organs. Pain contributes to the progression of shock; however, administering narcotics can decrease blood pressure further. Fluids are given and the health care provider notified.

See Chapter 45 for specific treatments for shock.

Malignant hyperthermia. **Malignant hyperthermia (MH)** is a rare but life-threatening complication of general anesthetic agents, including halothane, isoflurane, enflurane, and succinylcholine. MH occurs from a biochemical reaction in genetically predisposed persons. Most MH occurs during the surgical procedure in the OR. Signs of MH include high temperature, cardiac dysrhythmia, rigidity of the jaw or other muscles, hypotension, tachypnea, and dark cola-colored urine. A late sign of MH is an extremely high temperature of up to 111.2° F (44.0° C). Notify the anesthesiologist and surgeon immediately if any of these signs occur. If it is not treated swiftly and effectively, MH can be fatal. Dantrolene is the drug of choice to treat this condition. The patient is immediately cooled, and cardiac and respiratory support is given as needed (Litman, 2018).

Promote Psychological Adjustment

When surgery alters physical appearance, the patient may not only be concerned about the ability to perform self-care postoperatively but also have considerable changes in body image, particularly if there is extensive scarring. If part of an extremity, an organ, or part of a breast has been surgically removed, the necessary psychological adjustment is considerable and takes a long time.

Communication

Recovering From Abdominal Surgery

Mrs. Wilson, age 74, is recovering from abdominal surgery. Although her body language tells her nurse that she is experiencing pain, she has denied any need for pain medication since she administered her PCA dose 3 hours earlier.

Nurse: "Mrs. Wilson, I would like to see you able to cough more vigorously, move about in bed more, and walk around more frequently. I think that if you would use your pain pump more often, you would be more comfortable doing your exercises and coughing."

Mrs. Wilson: "I'm not that uncomfortable, and those medications always cause problems for me."

Nurse: "Problems?"

Mrs. Wilson: "Yes, I get really constipated."

Nurse: "The doctor has a stool softener ordered for you to help prevent constipation, and by increasing fluids, we should be able to control that. Do you have other problems with the pain medication?"

Mrs. Wilson: "Yes, it makes me light-headed and unsteady on my feet."

Nurse: "If the pain medication makes you light-headed, we can switch you to a different medication, and one of us will stay with you when you are out of bed to see that you do not fall."

Mrs. Wilson: "I'm very afraid of falling, breaking a hip, and adding to my troubles."

Nurse: "By taking the medication and being more comfortable, you'll feel more like doing your exercises. That's how you can help prevent postoperative complications such as pneumonia or blood clots."

Mrs. Wilson: "I certainly don't want pneumonia or a blood clot!"

Nurse: "Moving about more will also increase circulation and help your wound to heal faster."

Mrs. Wilson: "Okay, I'll take the pain medication if it will help me prevent complications."

Assess the patient for signs of ineffective coping, including withdrawn, depressed behavior; less attention to grooming than before; and poor communication efforts. If these signs occur, work with the patient to identify areas of concern and collaborate with other health team members to develop a plan of assistance. Help the patient by encouraging discussion of feelings regarding what has been removed and the effect it might have on the patient's life. Be an active listener; gradually focus the patient on the positives in life rather than on the loss incurred. It helps to refer the patient to a support group of people who have undergone a similar experience and are also learning to cope.

◆ EVALUATION

Evaluative statements regarding previously stated goals and expected outcomes might include:

- Lungs clear to auscultation; respirations 18
- Pulse 82, BP 136/86, peripheral pulses present
- Pain controlled for 4 hours with analgesia; states pain medication controls pain for about 4 hours
- Incision clean, dry, and without redness
- Patient expresses gladness that periods of pain and malaise will be gone
- No signs of thrombophlebitis or infection

Each nursing care plan is evaluated on whether the individual specific outcomes have been met. Further examples of evaluation are in Nursing Care Plan 5.1.

DISCHARGE PLANNING

With same-day surgery and early release from the hospital after inpatient surgery, it is vital that discharge planning be started at admission or several days before the surgery. Assess the need for home care. Will the patient need assistance with bathing, meals, or dressing changes? It may be necessary to arrange home health care with an aide to assist with bathing and with a nurse to assess the patient's condition and provide wound care. Equipment, such as oxygen, suction, or an IV pump, may need to be ordered before discharge so that the transition to home goes smoothly.

Cultural Considerations

Performing Wound Care

Although not overly modest, traditional Chinese people may hesitate in touching their own bodies, so it is important to assess who will perform wound care and change dressings at home. A home health nurse may need to be accessed, or teaching of another family member may be important.

Family or relatives must be included in discharge planning and teaching. Often it is a family member who will do the dressing changes, monitor for side effects of medication, alert the surgeon to signs of complications, and provide general support to the patient during recovery.

Nursing Care Plan 5.1 Care of a Patient Who Has Had a Simple Mastectomy

SCENARIO

Mrs. Talbot, a married 38-year-old woman and the mother of two children ages 16 and 14 years, underwent a simple mastectomy with sentinel node biopsy as treatment for a 4.5-cm malignant tumor.

PROBLEM STATEMENT/NURSING DIAGNOSIS

Altered skin integrity related to surgical wound.

SUPPORTING ASSESSMENT DATA

Objective: Right mastectomy; dressing on right chest.

Goals/Expected Outcomes	Nursing Interventions	Selected Rationale	Evaluation
Wound will be free of signs of infection at discharge.	Keep bulb suction drain functioning properly.	Suction is needed to pull drainage from operative site.	No signs of infection. Incision clean, dry, and without reddening.
Wound will heal completely within 6 weeks.	Note character and amount of drainage; document.	Helps detect excessive bleeding.	Draining small amounts of serosanguineous fluid.
	Reinforce dressing as needed.		No need for dressing reinforcement.
	Assess for excessive bleeding q1h for 4 h, then q2h for first 24 h.		Small amount of serosanguineous drainage in drain.
	Assess swelling and pulses in arm q2h to detect excessive swelling in arm.	Swelling in arm can cause nerve damage.	Minimal swelling in arm; pulses are 2+.
	Monitor temperature and white blood cell (WBC) count.	Temperature and WBC count trends will show if infection is developing.	No increase in temperature or WBC count.
	Assess wound for signs of infection with each dressing change.	Sterile dressing helps prevent infection.	Wound clean and dry without signs of infection.
	Change dressing q8–24h as needed.		Surgeon changed dressing this afternoon. Continue plan.

PROBLEM STATEMENT/NURSING DIAGNOSIS

Acute pain related to surgical incision.

SUPPORTING ASSESSMENT DATA

Subjective: Complains of incisional pain and discomfort.
Objective: Right mastectomy; rates pain at 6 on pain scale.

Goals/Expected Outcomes	Nursing Interventions	Selected Rationale	Evaluation
Pain will be controlled to a level of 4 or less	Instruct on use of patient-controlled analgesia (PCA).	Knowledge is needed to use PCA effectively.	Using PCA appropriately.
	Assess pain level q2 h.	Assessing pain level will show whether pain is adequately controlled.	Pain level consistently below 4.
	Provide comfort measures.	Comfort measures increase effect of analgesia.	Straightened bed; brought warmed blanket.
Pain is controlled by oral analgesia by discharge.	Administer analgesics as ordered.		Continue plan.

PROBLEM STATEMENT/NURSING DIAGNOSIS

Potential for altered gas exchange related to anesthesia and pain medications.

SUPPORTING ASSESSMENT DATA

Subjective: "I don't like using the incentive spirometer. Do I have to cough? It hurts."
Objective: Had general anesthesia. Restricted mobility. Receiving opioids for pain.

Goals/Expected Outcomes	Nursing Interventions	Selected Rationale	Evaluation
Lung sounds will remain clear and oxygen saturation greater than 94%.	Have patient use incentive spirometer q1h while awake.	Incentive spirometer use opens alveoli, decreasing atelectasis.	Using incentive spirometer; barely diminished breath sounds in lung bases.

Continued

Nursing Care Plan 5.1 Care of a Patient Who Has Had a Simple Mastectomy—cont'd

Goals/Expected Outcomes	Nursing Interventions	Selected Rationale	Evaluation
	Have patient cough q2h.	Coughing clears secretions from lung irritation caused by anesthesia.	Coughed secretions are clear.
	Auscultate lungs q4h.	Auscultation determines status of breath sounds.	Lungs clear.
	Encourage ambulation.		Ambulated ×2.
	Monitor temperature, respirations, and oxygen saturation.		Continue plan.

PROBLEM STATEMENT/NURSING DIAGNOSIS

Potential for grieving related to loss of body part and perception of femininity.

SUPPORTING ASSESSMENT DATA

Subjective: Expresses concern about husband's reaction to surgery.
Objective: Right mastectomy.

Goals/Expected Outcomes	Nursing Interventions	Selected Rationale	Evaluation
Patient will verbalize feelings of self-worth and confidence.	Have patient list her strengths and positive attributes.	Focusing on strengths can help counter feelings of loss.	Is patient verbalizing feelings of confidence and self-worth? Not yet.
Patient will discuss sadness over loss of breast.	Encourage sharing of sad feelings and fears with husband.	Talking openly with husband may provide reassurance.	Expressed sadness over breast loss to husband.
	Talk with husband privately about his feelings.	Involvement will show her he still cares for her.	Husband reluctant to speak about the surgery or his feelings so far.
	Involve husband in patient's care.		
	Encourage children to discuss their feelings and fears with patient.		Children have not been in yet today.
	Encourage independence in patient.	Independence increases self-confidence.	Brushed her teeth. Continue plan.

CRITICAL THINKING QUESTIONS

1. You auscultate the patient's lungs on the evening after surgery, and sounds are diminished in the bases. What do you think it means?
2. What would you do if the radial pulse in the arm on the same side as the breast surgery becomes weaker and harder to detect?

When the patient is discharged, review specific instructions regarding care at home, including care of the incision or wound, diet requirements, activity level allowed, medications, and signs and symptoms of complications to report to the health care provider. Make certain the patient understands when to see the provider for follow-up. Send home sufficient supplies of items needed for dressing changes, and tell the patient and family where more items can be obtained. Make every attempt to ensure that the patient does not go home with unanswered questions.

Patient Teaching

Discharge Instructions for a Same-Day Surgery Patient

DIET

- Type of diet and importance of proper nutrition for healing
- Dietary restrictions, if any
- Avoiding alcohol for first 24 hours after anesthesia
- Special dietary recommendations
- Recommended fluid intake

ACTIVITY

- Recommended exercise and frequency
- Instructions for special equipment: crutches, walker, cane, splint, etc.
- Schedule for deep-breathing, coughing, and leg exercises; how long to continue these activities; splinting the incision when coughing and getting out of bed

Patient Teaching

Discharge Instructions for a Same-Day Surgery Patient—cont'd

- Recommended rest periods
- Activity restrictions (i.e., driving, intercourse, and lifting)
- Application, use, and care of antiembolism stockings

WOUND CARE
- Hand hygiene
- Dressing changes and frequency
- Cleansing of wound; irrigations
- Drainage observations
- Signs to report
- Use of heat or cold packs for discomfort
- Supplies and where to obtain them

TEMPERATURE MONITORING
- Record time and temperature
- Report temperature greater than 100° F (38° C)

BATHING
- Type of bath
- Frequency

MEDICATIONS
- Analgesics
- Antibiotics
- Sedatives
- Vitamin supplements
- Other medications

PRECAUTIONS RELATED TO ANESTHESIA OR SIDE EFFECTS OF MEDICATION
- Caution regarding using machinery
- Caution regarding making decisions for 24 hours
- Drug interactions
- Potential for constipation
- Potential for urinary retention

SIGNS AND SYMPTOMS TO REPORT
- Elevated temperature
- Increasing malaise
- Severe pain or swelling
- Bleeding through bandage
- Decreased sensation below surgical site
- Severe nausea and vomiting
- Failure to urinate within 8 hours

OTHER
- Scheduled follow-up appointment with the surgeon
- Expectation for return to usual activities
- Expectation for return to feeling normal

Think Critically

An older adult patient who has had a hip replacement and who has chronic lung disease is being discharged home to the care of a 78-year-old spouse. Which health care professionals would you collaborate with to plan appropriate continuing care for the patient?

COMMUNITY CARE

The patient may be given follow-up care at an outpatient clinic, health care provider's office, subacute care unit, rehabilitation unit, or extended care unit or at the patient's home. The nurse case manager will coordinate the care of the whole team, collaborating with the social worker, physical therapist, respiratory therapist, nurse's aide, dietitian, pharmacist, physician, and other health care professionals. You assess the patient's condition and progress, perform treatments and procedures such as wound care, and reinforce teaching about the signs and symptoms of complications. The quality of nursing care delivered postoperatively often is the factor that prevents complications and rehospitalization.

Even patients who are ambulatory and normally self-sufficient usually need assistance or reassurance with anything more than a simple dressing change, which is particularly true if the patient lives alone. You must verify that the patient can adequately perform self-care and collaborate with the patient, health care provider, social worker, and community agencies to secure the assistance the patient needs.

Home Care Considerations

General Points for Home Care for Postsurgical Patients

- Knows about each medication to be taken, when to take it, and what side effects to watch for and is able to obtain the medications
- Understands the diet, any restrictions, and guidelines for fluid intake
- Understands that alcohol must be avoided for 24 hours after surgery and while taking opioids for pain management
- Verbalizes restrictions on activity and instructions for use of any special equipment such as crutches, splint, walker, and so forth
- Understands not to drive or make important decisions for 24 hours after anesthesia
- Verbalizes the type of bath permitted and how to protect the wound
- Can demonstrate cleansing and dressing of the wound; verbalizes where to obtain supplies
- Verbalizes signs and symptoms to report to the surgeon
- Understands how to schedule a follow-up appointment with the surgeon
- Understands written instructions for all essential points of care and consultation

Get Ready for the NCLEX® Examination!

Key Points

- Nurses in the recovery unit monitor patients very closely until they have stable vital signs and are arousable from anesthesia.
- Maintaining a patent airway is the highest priority.
- You are vigilant for signs of complications and perform frequent assessments during the postoperative period.
- Nursing interventions are aimed at providing pain control, comfort, and fluid balance; protecting the patient from injury; maintaining vital functions; and preventing infection.
- You try to prevent or intervene in the many potential complications from surgery.
- Discharge planning begins at admission and covers all areas of basic needs, wound care, and activity restrictions.
- Written instructions regarding all aspects of postoperative care should be sent home with the patient.

Additional Learning Resources

SG Go to your Study Guide for additional learning activities to help you master this chapter content.

Go to your Evolve website (http://evolve.elsevier.com/deWit/medsurg) for the following FREE learning resources:

- Animations, audio, and video
- Answers and rationales for questions and activities
- Glossary with pronunciations in English and Spanish
- Interactive Review Questions and more!

Review Questions for the NCLEX® Examination

1. When prioritizing safety measures for a postoperative patient in the PACU, you would: (*Place in order of priority.*)
   1. observe for urine flow of at least 30 mL per hour.
   2. position the unconscious patient on the side to prevent aspiration.
   3. check for a patent airway and the rate and depth of respiration.
   4. check infusing IV fluids for the correct fluid and flow rate.
   5. observe the dressing for any blood saturation.
   6. monitor drains for excessive fluid drainage.

   NCLEX Client Need: Physiological Integrity: Reduction of Risk Potential
2. While performing an assessment of a newly postoperative patient, you note the following: temperature 104.9° F (40.5° C), BP 90/60, pulse 58, respirations 30, rigidity of the jaw muscles, and dark urine. The priority nursing action would be to:
   1. instruct the patient to relax and take deep breaths.
   2. notify the surgeon immediately.
   3. administer pain medications.
   4. give a tepid sponge bath.

   NCLEX Client Need: Physiological Integrity: Physiological Adaptation
3. On arrival from the PACU, the patient complains of severe thirst. You find that the patient is increasingly restless, tachypneic, and tachycardic. Considering these findings, what would you likely suspect?
   1. Hypovolemia
   2. Cardiogenic shock
   3. Normal response to anesthesia
   4. Pain medication overdose

   NCLEX Client Need: Physiological Integrity: Reduction of Risk Potential
4. You know that care for the patient having spinal anesthesia differs from that of the patient undergoing general anesthesia in that during recovery: (*Select all that apply.*)
   1. the patient will be unresponsive immediately after surgery.
   2. muscles in the lower part of the body will be flaccid immediately after surgery.
   3. the patient will be able to eat immediately upon return to the nursing unit.
   4. monitoring for a patent airway is a top priority in the PACU.
   5. the patient will be alert upon entry to the PACU.
   6. nausea may be a problem during recovery from anesthesia.

   NCLEX Client Need: Safe and Effective Care Environment: Coordinated Care
5. You know that an older adult patient who had open reduction and internal fixation of the right femur is at risk for infection because of the surgical incision and repair and lessened immunity that occurs in older age. A desired result of interventions for this risk would be that the:
   1. patient will not develop a temperature greater than 102.2° F (39.0° C).
   2. patient will report the signs and symptoms of redness, drainage, and swelling.
   3. patient will verbalize understanding of aseptic technique before discharge.
   4. patient will not develop a wound infection before discharge.

   NCLEX Client Need: Safe and Effective Care Environment: Safety and Infection Control
6. To promote wound healing, you instruct the postoperative patient to eat foods high in protein. Which food choice by the patient warrants further patient teaching?
   1. Caesar salad with French bread
   2. Tuna sandwich, carrot strips, and watermelon chunks
   3. Broccoli cheese soup, crackers, and an orange
   4. Broiled chicken breast, steamed broccoli, and mashed potatoes

   NCLEX Client Need: Health Promotion and Maintenance

7. One measure you can take to promote early patient ambulation and a return to independence in activities of daily living is to:
   1. open cartons and items on the food tray while the patient has an IV infusing.
   2. provide a bedside commode for toileting in the initial postoperative period.
   3. encourage visitors to play cards or board games with the patient.
   4. assist the patient to walk to a chair in front of the sink to bathe areas easily reached.

   NCLEX Client Need: Health Promotion and Maintenance
8. While caring for the postoperative patient, you must reinforce which measure(s) to reduce the incidence of complications? *(Select all that apply.)*
   1. Use the incentive spirometer every hour while awake.
   2. Ambulate the designated distance six times a day.
   3. After deep breathing, cough effectively every 4 hours.
   4. Turn or change position at least every 2 hours.
   5. Assess for pain and provide prompt relief.

   NCLEX Client Need: Physiological Integrity: Reduction of Risk Potential
9. What action(s) would be appropriate when caring for a postoperative patient with a bulb suction wound drain? *(Select all that apply.)*
   1. Assess the wound drain for patency.
   2. Measure the amount of drainage.
   3. Compress the bulb to reestablish pressure.
   4. Rinse the bulb with sterile water after emptying it.
   5. Notify the surgeon when there is no drainage.

   NCLEX Client Need: Physiological Integrity: Reduction of Risk Potential
10. The patient is prescribed antiembolism stockings before discharge. The patient asks you, "Why do I need these stockings?" The best response would be:
    1. "Your surgeon ordered these stockings."
    2. "These help prevent formation of clots in the legs."
    3. "These massage your legs to make you feel better."
    4. "You sound upset. Do these stockings bother you?"

    NCLEX Client Need: Health Promotion and Maintenance
11. Which patient statement indicates a need for further teaching regarding the use of a patient-controlled analgesia (PCA) pump?
    1. "I control my pain medication by pressing the button."
    2. "To a certain extent, I control the amount of pain medication I can have."
    3. "I need to tell a nurse if the pain is not controlled well."
    4. "I need to call a nurse when I need pain medication."

    NCLEX Client Need: Physiological Integrity: Pharmacological Therapies
12. A 38-year-old woman who has undergone bilateral radical mastectomy is withdrawn and quiet. She is afebrile with no apparent complaints of pain. Her dressings are dry and intact. Pulses are full on both upper extremities. Considering the data, the major problem at this time would be:
    1. pain in the surgical area.
    2. potential surgical site infection
    3. distress over the loss of her breasts.
    4. concern about her children at home.

    NCLEX Client Need: Psychosocial Integrity
13. After a surgical procedure, a priority point to emphasize to the patient when performing discharge teaching for self-care is:
    1. eating sufficient protein and vitamin C to promote healing.
    2. always washing the hands before starting a dressing change.
    3. ambulating on a set schedule each day, extending the distance a little each day.
    4. obtaining at least 8 hours of sleep each night.

    NCLEX Client Need: Health Promotion and Maintenance

Critical Thinking Questions

Scenario A

Ms. Simpson just had a laparoscopic colon resection for a tumor, and you are assisting with her care in the PACU. She is waking up but still groggy, and her breathing is somewhat shallow.

1. What would you do to improve her respiratory status?
2. Describe the method used to ensure an open airway.

Scenario B

You are assigned to care for a 37-year-old man who just had a same-day surgical repair of a ventral hernia with spinal anesthesia.

1. How does the care of this patient differ from that of a patient who had inhalation or general anesthesia?
2. If this patient has difficulty voiding after surgery, how could you assist him?
3. If he develops a spinal headache, what measures could be taken to decrease his discomfort?

Scenario C

Mrs. Saunders is a 58-year-old woman who underwent an abdominal hysterectomy and exploration for cancer of the uterus. She returned to the nursing unit from surgery 1 hour ago and has an IV infusion running into the right forearm. Her BP has gradually fallen from 138/88 to 102/62. She is restless, complains of thirst, and is anxious.

1. What assessments would you make?
2. What actions would you take? In what order would you perform these actions?

Scenario D

Mr. Jackson is a 68-year-old man with a history of asthma and frequent respiratory infections. He is recovering from chest surgery.

1. What are his increased risks for hypostatic pneumonia?
2. What nursing actions would you implement to help prevent this complication?
3. What signs and symptoms would indicate that he might have hypostatic pneumonia?

6 Infection Prevention and Control

http://evolve.elsevier.com/deWit/medsurg

Objectives

Theory

1. Examine the factors that increase the risk of infection.
2. Discuss how the body uses its natural defensive mechanisms to protect against infection.
3. Explain how fever plays a role in the prevention of infection.
4. Describe the classic signs of infection.
5. Distinguish situations that require the use of Transmission-Based Precautions.
6. List the types of personal protective equipment and analyze situations for whether they should be used.
7. Describe factors that make older adults more susceptible to infections.
8. Analyze factors that may impair the process of healing and repair of damaged tissue.

Clinical Practice

9. Care for a patient whose condition requires Transmission-Based Precautions.
10. From a day's patient assignment, determine the risk factors for infection for each patient.

Key Terms

acquired (ăk-KWĪ-ĕrd, p. 106)
agent (Ā-gĕnt, p. 102)
communicable (kŏ-MŪ-nĭ-kă-bŭl, p. 102)
disease (dĭ-ZĒZ, p. 102)
exudate (ĔKS-ū-dāt, p. 107)
hand hygiene (HĪ-gēn, p. 111)
health care–associated infection (HAI) (hĕlth kār ĕ-SŌ-shē-ā-tĕd ĭn-FĔK-shŭn, p. 115)
host (hōst, p. 103)
immunity (ĭ-MŪ-nĭ-tē, p. 106)
infection (ĭn-FĔK-shŭn, p. 102)
inflammation (ĭn-flă-MĀ-shŭn, p. 109)
innate (ĭ-NĀT, p. 106)
macrophages (MĂK-rō-făj-ĕz, p. 107)
medical asepsis (MĔD-ĭ-kăl ă-SĔP-sĭs, p. 117)
multidrug-resistant organism (MDRO) (MŬL-tĭ-drŭg rē-ZĬS-tĕnt ŌR-găn-ĭz-ĕm, p. 116)
normal flora (NŌR-măl FLŌR-ă, p. 102)
pathogen (PĂTH-ō-gĕn, p. 103)
personal protective equipment (PPE) (PĔR-sŭn-ŭl prō-TĔK-shŭn ē-KWĬP-mĕnt, p. 112)
phagocytosis (făg-ō-sī-TŌ-sĭs, p. 104)
sepsis (SĔP-sĭs, p. 117)
shedding (shĕd-ĭng, p. 102)
Standard Precautions (STĂN-dĕrd prĕ-KĂW-shŭnz, p. 111)
surgical asepsis (SŬR-jĭ-kăl ă-SĔP-sĭs, p. 117)
susceptible (sŭs-SĔP-tĭ-bŭl, p. 102)
Transmission-Based Precautions (trans-MĬSH-ŭn bāst prē-KĂW-shŭnz, p. 111)
vectors (VĔK-tĕrz, p. 110)

Concepts Covered in This Chapter

- Immunity
- Inflammation
- Infection
- Caregiving
- Health Care Economics

THE INFECTIOUS PROCESS AND DISEASE

Normal flora (microorganisms that normally exist in the body and provide natural immunity against certain infections) are most often found on or in body systems that have some form of contact with the outside environment (Table 6.1). Normal flora prevent the most harmful microorganisms from colonizing the body. Understanding how the body defends itself against infection, and how to prevent further exposure to **pathogenic** (disease-producing) microorganisms, is crucial to provide safe and effective nursing care.

An **infection** is the presence and growth of pathogenic microorganisms in a **susceptible** (lacking resistance) host. Infection can be **communicable** (passed from one person to another directly through touch or indirectly by using a contaminated object) or noncommunicable. **Disease** is one possible outcome of an infection. Once an infection has occurred, the person is considered communicable until the organism is no longer **shedding** (to lose by natural process) from the body. This period of communicability varies by the type of pathogen involved and the host's ability to fight off the infecting **agent** (any substance capable of producing an effect, whether

Table 6.1 Normal Flora of the Body[a]

SITE	NORMAL FLORA
Eye	*Corynebacterium* species *Neisseria* species *Staphylococcus aureus* *Staphylococcus epidermidis* *Streptococcus* species
Upper respiratory tract (nose, mouth, throat)	*Corynebacterium* species *Enterobacter* species *Haemophilus* species *Klebsiella* species *Lactobacillus* species *Neisseria* species *Staphylococcus* species *Streptococcus viridans* Various types of anaerobes
Skin	*Corynebacterium* species *Staphylococcus aureus* *Staphylococcus epidermidis* *Streptococcus* species Yeasts such as candida and pityrosporum
Small bowel and colon	*Bacteroides* species *Clostridium perfringens* *Enterobacter* species (i.e., coliform) *Escherichia coli* *Streptococcus faecalis*
Vagina	*Corynebacterium* species *Klebsiella* species *Lactobacillus* species *Proteus* species *Pseudomonas* species *Staphylococcus* species *Streptococcus* species

Modified from Williams P: *deWit's fundamental concepts and skills for nursing,* ed 5, St. Louis, 2018, Elsevier.
[a]The central nervous system, lower respiratory tract, and upper and lower urinary tracts are normally sterile. This table lists only those organisms most commonly found in various body systems. They can also cause illness or infection if they are able to invade another system within the body.

Box 6.1 Factors That Influence Infection and Disease

HOST

Intrinsic (born with it)
- Age, sex, race
- Genetic factors
- Chronic diseases (e.g., cystic fibrosis)

Extrinsic (environmental)
- Personal behaviors (e.g., drugs, alcohol, hygiene, sexual practices)
- Occupation
- Socioeconomic status
- Chronic diseases (e.g., chronic obstructive pulmonary disease [COPD], type 2 diabetes)

AGENT

Virulence: The degree to which the organism can infect or damage the host
- Bacterial, fungal, viral, and protozoal microbes can be involved; each has a different virulence and mode of transmission.
- Organic and inorganic chemicals, pesticides, and pharmaceuticals can help or hinder growth of microbes.
- Ionizing radiation, cold, heat, electricity, and noise can increase or decrease microbe growth.

ENVIRONMENT[a]

Coexisting chronic disease (e.g., hypertension, diabetes mellitus)
Overcrowded living environment (e.g., dormitory or prison setting)
Travel to countries or regions with endemic diseases (e.g., tuberculosis, coccidioidomycosis)
Vectors (e.g., mosquitoes, flies, ticks, fleas)
Water supply
Climate

[a]Environment includes not only the body, but also where an individual lives and works.

physical, chemical, or biological). For example, after entering the body, bacteria must find a way to attach to a **host** (an organism in which another, usually parasitic, organism is nourished and harbored) cell to multiply. Once the organisms have found a place to multiply, they can spread through the body via the circulatory or lymphatic system. **The development of an infection is dependent on the interrelationship among the host, the agent, and the environment** (Box 6.1).

FACTORS THAT INFLUENCE INFECTIOUS DISEASE

Many factors concerning the host determine the type of response the body will have to an invading pathogen. Risk of exposure is influenced by the lifestyle, occupation, and socioeconomic status of the host. The underlying disease state, as well as the immunologic and nutritional status of the host, influences the degree of resistance or susceptibility the body will have to the pathogen. Environmental factors can also increase the likelihood of developing an infection (Fig. 6.1).

DISEASE-PRODUCING PATHOGENS

Any microorganism capable of producing disease is known as a **pathogen**. Once pathogens have entered the body, many are able to adapt to their new environment, enhancing survival and increasing their likelihood of causing illness or disease. Pathogens can be transmitted from one person to another through one of three routes: *airborne, contact,* or *droplet.* Hand hygiene is the primary way to prevent the spread or transmission of pathogenic microorganisms. Following respiratory etiquette by covering your cough or sneeze and performing hand hygiene afterward help prevent the spread of infection.

Categories of Microorganisms

Six categories of microorganisms are known to cause infection in humans: bacteria (including *Rickettsia,*

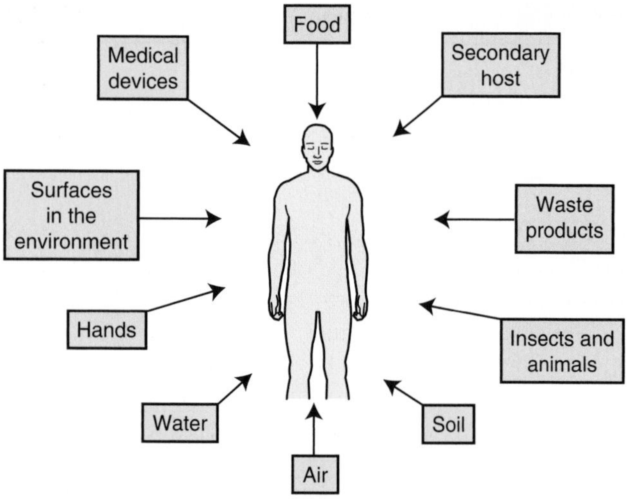

Fig. 6.1 The environment and the spread of infection. (Redrawn from Sattar SA, Springthorpe VS. In Rutala WA, editor: *Disinfection, sterilization and antisepsis*, Washington, D.C., 2010, Association for Professionals in Infection Control and Epidemiology.)

Chlamydia, and *Mycoplasma*), viruses, protozoa, fungi, helminths, and prions.

Bacteria. Bacteria are classified into three major categories according to their shape, gram-staining properties, and requirements for oxygen. Round or spherical bacteria are referred to as *cocci,* rod-shaped bacteria are referred to as *bacilli,* and spiral or corkscrew-shaped bacteria are referred to as *spirochetes.* Some bacteria grow in chains (streptococci), some grow in pairs (diplococci), and some grow in clusters (staphylococci).

Bacteria that require oxygen to live and reproduce are *aerobic;* those that cannot tolerate the presence of oxygen are *anaerobic.* When bacteria enter the body, they trigger the immune system to produce **antibodies** (proteins that fight and destroy antigens). Some bacteria produce poisonous substances called **endotoxins** (toxins found within the bacteria that are released when the cell breaks apart); others produce **exotoxins** (excreted by both gram-negative and gram-positive bacteria).

Different bacteria thrive under different environmental conditions. Some form **spores** (a protective covering over the original cell) to protect themselves against destruction from heat, cold, lack of water, toxic chemicals, and radiation. Examples of spore-forming infectious diseases are anthrax and botulism. Other bacteria thrive best in water, such as *Pseudomonas* species or *Legionella.* The bacterium that causes tuberculosis can survive for years in many environments. Some bacteria, such as *Staphylococcus aureus,* can survive in very high temperatures.

Mycoplasmas, once believed to be a virus, are very small bacteria that do not have a cell wall. They are more like an extracellular parasite because they attach themselves to epithelial cells that line the body cavities and outer surfaces, such as the skin. They tend to be slow growing. For example, *Mycoplasma pneumoniae* can take up to 3 weeks to incubate before signs or symptoms begin to appear.

Rickettsia are small, round, or rod-shaped bacteria that are often transmitted by the bites of body lice, ticks, and fleas. Chlamydia is also a bacterium and is typically transmitted via close contact, especially sexual contact. Both are dependent on a living host.

Different methods can prevent infection and its spread. A physiologic response can stimulate the immune system to produce a fever and trigger the body's immune response to destroy the invading pathogenic microorganism through **phagocytosis** (ingestion and digestion of bacteria). Cleaning, sterilizing, or boiling inanimate objects, such as a glass or surgical instruments, can prevent the spread of infection after the items are used by or on a patient. The correct antimicrobial agent must be given, and the entire dose regimen must be completed as prescribed to prevent the risk for developing infection with a multidrug-resistant organism (MDRO).

Viruses. Viruses are not cells. They inject themselves into existing cells to reproduce. They do not have cell walls and cannot be treated with antibiotics or antifungals. They are composed of either deoxyribonucleic acid (DNA) or ribonucleic acid (RNA), have an outside coating made of protein, and are dependent on the cell they have invaded to survive and reproduce. Some viruses use the cytoplasm from the cell they have attacked to develop an "envelope" that makes it harder for the body's immune system to destroy them. Viruses can keep changing their protein markers, called *antigens,* making it difficult for the virus to be neutralized or killed by white blood cells (WBCs). Once viruses have established themselves in the body, they can trigger an immune response that is harmful to the cells. They can also damage cells by preventing protein synthesis from occurring. New viral elements can be released into the circulation either by the virus breaking down the wall of the cell it has invaded and releasing copies of its genetic material or by small offshoots bursting, thereby infecting other cells.

Viruses are classified as one of three types: (1) latent, which can reside in the body for years without producing symptoms and then suddenly cause an acute flare-up of symptoms (e.g., herpes simplex); (2) **oncogenic** (cancer causing), which can alter the cell walls to the point where the cells become malignant; and (3) active, which enter the body, invade a number of cells, and infect the body (e.g., influenza and severe acute respiratory syndrome, which are discussed in Chapter 14).

Viruses and bacteria vary in their resistance to destruction by chemical disinfectants, but most are easily inactivated or destroyed by heat. However, some of the hepatitis viruses must be boiled for as long as 30 minutes at a temperature at or above 185° F (85° C) before they can be considered nonpathogenic. It is important to note that antibiotics do not help fight a viral infection, but antiviral agents, such as acyclovir, can help limit the virulence of a viral infection if taken at the first signs of illness.

Protozoa. Protozoa are one-celled parasitic organisms that have the ability to move. There are four main types, named by their method of travel within their environment. They are called amoebas, ciliates, flagellates, or sporozoa. These microorganisms are typically found in water and soil. Many protozoa species can lie dormant. Although thousands of species exist, only a few are pathogenic to humans. To cause disease, some protozoans must be ingested, whereas others are introduced into the body through the bite of a vector (a carrier), such as a mosquito.

Fungi. Fungi are very small, primitive organisms that grow on living plants, animals, and other decaying organic material. They thrive in warm, moist environments. Fungal infections in humans are called *mycoses* and are classified into three main types: (1) cutaneous mycoses, which grow in the outer layer of the skin; (2) subcutaneous mycoses, which involve the deeper layers of the skin, subcutaneous tissues, and sometimes bone; and (3) systemic or deep mycoses, which involve internal organs.

Fungal infections are difficult to eradicate once they have invaded a host because fungi tend to form spores that are resistant to ordinary antimicrobial agents. Antifungal agents can be given topically or systemically but can be toxic to the liver and the nervous system; therefore the course of treatment must be carried out cautiously and over a long period.

Fungal infections commonly found in immune-competent hosts include coccidioidomycosis (caused by *Coccidioides immitis*), histoplasmosis (caused by *Histoplasma capsulatum*), and blastomycosis (caused by *Blastomyces dermatitidis*). They are all systemic mycoses caused by inhalation of airborne spores. Once in the lung, the spores take root and then can spread to any part of the body. However, most fungal infections are self-limited and do not cause clinical disease.

Opportunistic fungal infections (infections that occur in a person with a depressed immune system) are more typically found in patients who have some form of immune compromise and typically include species from *Candida,* part of the normal body flora; *Cryptococcus,* found in soil usually associated with bird droppings, which can infect any organ in the body, including the brain and the meninges; and *Aspergillus,* found in soil, dust, and decomposing organic material. Inhaled spores are the usual mode of transmission.

Other Infectious Agents

Helminths. Helminths are worms (round, flat, or hook-like) and flukes. All are parasitic and are typically spread via the fecal-oral route. Pinworms are most commonly found in children and cause significant itching in the perianal area because the eggs are laid outside the rectum. Flatworms, such as a tapeworm, can grow up to 50 feet long and live in the intestines. Hookworm and fluke infestations can easily penetrate the skin, are found in the blood, and invade organs such as the liver and lungs. Flatworms and flukes can cause significant weight loss and debilitation.

Prions. Transmissible spongiform encephalopathies (TSEs) are thought to be caused by prions, an abnormally folded protein. It is not fully understood how they form, are transmitted, and cause disease. TSEs include Creutzfeldt-Jakob disease and bovine spongiform encephalopathy, also known as "mad cow disease." Since prions are a protein and not technically a living organism, there is no chemical that can "kill" them. Researchers are actively seeking answers to the questions of prion formation, transmission, and treatment.

THE BODY'S DEFENSE AGAINST INFECTION

The four primary lines of defense the body has against infection are (1) the skin and mucous membranes, (2) normal flora, (3) the inflammatory response, and (4) the immune response.

> **? Think Critically**
>
> In the work environment, where do you think you are most likely to come in contact with pathogens that might cause infection? What precautions can you take to prevent or decrease your risk of exposure?

SKIN

Mechanical and Chemical Barriers to Infection

Mechanical barriers. Mechanical barriers are intact skin and mucous membranes. They are the primary defense the body has against invading microorganisms and infection. Skin, being the largest organ of the body, serves as a first line of defense against harmful agents in the environment. It functions as a protective covering for the more delicate and vulnerable underlying tissues and organs.

The portals of exit and entry provide the means by which pathogens move in and out of the body. For example, pathogens typically exit or enter the body where the skin and mucous membranes meet, such as through the mouth, nose, and gastrointestinal or genitourinary tracts, as well as through a cut in the skin.

Chemical barriers. Chemical barriers assist the skin and mucous membranes in fighting off invasive organisms by the secretion of tears, saliva, and mucus. Lactic and fatty acids, which inhibit the growth of bacteria, are excreted via sweat and the sebaceous glands. Secretions from the mucous membranes lining the respiratory, gastrointestinal, and reproductive tracts contain an abundance of a bactericidal enzyme called *lysozyme.* This same enzyme is found in tears and saliva. Stomach acid and digestive enzymes kill off most swallowed microorganisms. Mucus produced by the respiratory tract helps capture a variety of inhaled particles. *Cilia* (tiny hairs) line the respiratory tract, trap organisms and debris with the help of mucus, and then propel them up and out of the body with a wavelike action.

> **? Think Critically**
>
> What effect might medications such as esomeprazole (Nexium) and omeprazole (Prilosec), which are proton pump inhibitors and reduce stomach acid, have on a person's general health? How will this affect a patient's ability to fight off pathogenic microorganisms that may be swallowed?

Protective and Defensive Mechanisms Against Infection

Our bodies have two forms of **immunity** (the body's ability to be unaffected by a particular disease or condition) against infections. They are **innate** (born with, or natural) and **acquired** (develops throughout life) (Table 6.2). See Chapter 10 for more detail. When the body's defense mechanisms are stressed or exhausted, it is more susceptible to infection. Heredity, the degree of natural resistance, and one's own immune status are the greatest determinants of infection, but personal habits and behaviors are also factors to consider. General health, state of nutrition, hormone balance, immune status, and the presence of a chronic disease, such as diabetes mellitus, may influence the degree of susceptibility a person has to infection.

Fever. Fever is one of the primary mechanisms the body uses to prevent infection from an invading microorganism. Once the immune system has determined that an invasion is being attempted, it signals the hypothalamus in the brain to raise the body temperature to fight off the infection. The increased metabolic and oxygen demand at the cellular level that results from the increased body temperature causes increased heart and respiratory rates. Shivering occurs to increase the core body temperature, blood is shunted away from the skin to reduce heat loss, and the patient may complain of "freezing to death." It is at this point in the inflammatory response that fever is noticeably increased. In an attempt to decrease the body temperature through evaporation, **diaphoresis** (sweating) occurs. This increased heat in the body creates a hostile environment to the microorganisms, and an intact immune system can destroy them efficiently. Fever up to 102.0° F (38.9° C) in adults is not usually treated unless the patient is uncomfortable. Once the threat of infection is no longer present, the immune system again signals the hypothalamus, and the body can start cooling down on its own.

> **? Think Critically**
>
> A patient asks you to explain what causes a person to have an increased temperature. Would the age of the patient be a factor you should consider in your teaching?

Nutrition. Poor nutrition predisposes a person to develop an infection because the body may not have sufficient protein stores to generate enough antibodies to help fight off an infection. The very young and older adults have less efficient immune systems, which is why it is important to ensure that these age groups have received the appropriate vaccinations and immunizations. Excessive stress also influences a person's immune status.

Table 6.2 Innate and Adaptive Immunity

	Innate Immunity	Adaptive Immunity
Names	Nonspecific immunity, native immunity, genetic immunity, natural immunity, inborn immunity	Specific immunity, acquired immunity
Characteristics		
Specificity	Not specific: recognizes variety of different groups of foreign cells or particles	Specific: recognizes specific antigens on specific cells or particles
Speed of reaction	Rapid: immediate up to several hours	Slower: several hours to several days
Memory	No enhanced response to repeated exposures to the same antigen	Enhanced responses to repeated exposures to the same antigen
Reaction to "self"	Normally does not react to self and prevents injury to the individual's own cells	Normally does not react to self and prevents injury to the individual's own cells
Components		
Barriers to prevent entry of harmful particles	Skin, mucosa, antimicrobial chemicals	Lymphocytes in epithelia, antibodies released at epithelial surfaces
Blood proteins	Complement, interferon (IFN), others	Antibodies
White blood cells involved	Phagocytes (macrophages, neutrophils), natural killer (NK) cells	Lymphocytes (B cells and T cells)

Adapted from Patton K: *Anatomy and physiology*, ed 10, St. Louis, 2019, Elsevier.

Table 6.3 Types of Antibodies

ANTIBODY	DESCRIPTION
IgM	• Because of its large size, tends to stay in the blood vessels • Binds to the antigen and works to clear the pathogen from the body
IgG	• Most abundant immunoglobulin found in the body • Crosses the placental barrier, reaching the developing fetus • Provides passive immunity until the fetus's own immune system can defend itself
IgA	• Found in tears, mucus, saliva, gastric fluid, colostrum, and sweat • Prevents pathogens from attaching to or penetrating epithelial cells, such as the skin
IgE	• Binds to mast cells and basophils and releases histamine and heparin • Stimulates a hypersensitive reaction, as seen in bronchial asthma or systemic anaphylaxis
IgD	• Works together with IgM • Among other functions, stimulates certain cells in the immune system; overall role in the immune response is unclear

Stress can increase blood cortisol levels, which will decrease the antiinflammatory response of the body.

Antigens. An antigen is a form of protein found on the outside of cells that allows the body to identify it as "self" (native) or "nonself" (foreign). Antigens can stimulate the immune response to wipe out microorganisms.

Antibodies. Antibodies, also known as immunoglobulins (Ig), are one part of acquired immunity. They have many functions, such as neutralizing toxins and killing invading pathogens. There are five types of antibodies: IgM, IgG, IgA, IgE, and IgD (Table 6.3). IgE can bind to mast cells and basophils and release histamine and heparin. This in turn stimulates a hypersensitive reaction, as seen in bronchial asthma or systemic anaphylaxis.

Bone marrow. The bone marrow is a major component of the body's defense system. Bone marrow plays an important role in manufacturing blood products that help the body defend itself against infection. These products are called *leukocytes,* which include *neutrophils, macrophages,* and *lymphocytes.*

Leukocytosis. Leukocytosis is an increased number of **leukocytes** (WBCs), usually seen at the beginning of an infection when the person's immune system has not been overly stressed. Leukocytosis is seen more often with bacterial than viral infections. When infection does occur, the bone marrow is stimulated to produce and release more leukocytes to help the body fight infection. The WBC count on the complete blood cell count (CBC) is used to identify elevations.

Phagocytosis. The process of *phagocytosis* is a form of innate immunity. This is the body's first line of defense at the cellular level. Within the first few hours of the onset of the inflammatory process, the monocytes swell up (becoming macrophages) and migrate to the site of inflammation. Neutrophils, which are a type of leukocyte, are also released and can kill both aerobic and anaerobic organisms. After the macrophages and neutrophils engulf and destroy bacteria and other foreign matter, they die, producing an **exudate** (discharge) that is composed of tissue, fluid, dead cells, and their by-products. This exudate, usually yellow or green in color, is commonly known as *pus* and is a sign of infection.

Macrophages. **Macrophages** are *monocytes* (large leukocytes) that have left the bloodstream and migrated into the tissues. They ingest and destroy pathogens and clear away the cellular debris and dead neutrophils in the latter stages of an infection. Macrophages cleanse the lymphatic fluid as it passes through the lymph nodes and perform a similar action on the blood as it passes through the liver and spleen.

Liver cells. As part of the innate immune system, about 50% of all macrophage cells can be found in the liver's Kupffer cells. These macrophages act either to prevent invasion by pathogens mechanically or to neutralize the pathogen chemically (through the pH of body secretions). Macrophages also destroy bacteria that have found their way into the blood circulation through the liver's portal system. The body's defense mechanisms against pathogens are summarized in Table 6.4.

NORMAL FLORA

The flora that are normally present on the skin and in the mucous membranes, gastrointestinal tract, and vagina coexist with the body and control the growth of harmful pathogens. When the amount of the normal flora is diminished, other pathogens may cause infection. When the body's immune system is suppressed for any reason, normal flora may grow out of control and cause infection. For example, *Candida albicans* commonly causes a yeast infection (thrush) after treatment with antibiotics because the normal flora have been destroyed, allowing the *Candida* to flourish. *Clostridium difficile (C. diff)* is prevalent in the environment and part of the normal flora of the bowel. Administration of antibiotics disrupts the normal balance of bowel flora, allowing the *C. diff* to cause colitis. *C. diff* produces a spore that is not destroyed by alcohol-based hand hygiene products. Soap and water must be used for hand cleansing and bleach used for equipment. Table 6.5 shows changes in the natural defense mechanisms that occur with age and cause older adults to become more susceptible to infection.

Table 6.4 The Body's Mechanism of Defense Against Infection

MECHANISM	FACTORS INVOLVED IN PROTECTION
Adaptive immunity	**Includes humoral and cell-mediated immune responses.**
Antibody-mediated (humoral) immune response (antigen-antibody; B lymphocytes)	Antibodies are produced against invading pathogens and inactivate or destroy them.
Cell-mediated immune response (T lymphocytes)	Sensitized T cells kill or inactivate antigens by chemical release or secretion of substances that destroy the antigen.
Innate (natural) immunity	**Determined by age, ethnicity, and genetics. Increases resistance to disease.**
Intact skin	Skin is the first defense; slightly acid pH and normal flora present an unfavorable environment for colonization of pathogens.
Normal flora	Present on skin and in mucous membranes of oral cavity, gastrointestinal tract, and vagina. Help prevent excessive growth of pathogens.
Mucous membranes	Mucous membranes, with their mucociliary action, provide mechanical protection against invasion of pathogens. Mucus secretions contain enzymes that inhibit many microorganisms. The respiratory system clears about 90% of introduced pathogens.
Gastrointestinal tract	Peristaltic action empties the gastrointestinal tract of pathogenic organisms. Acidic pH of stomach secretions, bile, pancreatic enzymes, and mucus protects against invasion by harmful pathogens.
Genitourinary tract	Flushing of urine through the system washes out microorganisms. The acidic pH of urine helps maintain a sterile environment in the system.
Inflammation	Cells damaged by pathogens release enzymes, and leukocytes are attracted to the area; the damaged area is "walled off," and phagocytosis disposes of the microorganisms and dead tissue.
Phagocytosis by white blood cells	Leukocytes, neutrophils, and macrophages (large monocytes) engulf, ingest, kill, and dispose of invading microorganisms.
Fever	Fever may not always occur with an infection, especially with immunocompromised or debilitated patients or patients who have been on long-term corticosteroid therapy. Surface blood vessels constrict, which leads to shivering to hold heat in the body (to kill the invading organisms). Increases metabolic rate, which can be problematic for patients with cardiorespiratory problems because of increased workload on the heart and circulatory system. Fever stops once the antiinflammatory agents have helped restore homeostasis.

Table 6.5 Changes in Natural Defense Mechanisms That Occur With Age

CHANGE	CONSEQUENCE
Decreased skin turgor and greater skin friability	Skin is more susceptible to friction damage and tearing.
Decreased elasticity and atherosclerosis of peripheral vessels	Decreased blood flow to extremities produces slower wound healing.
Calcification of heart valves	Provides a location for bacteria to attach and cause endocarditis.
Stiffness of thorax from arthritis or aging changes, weakened respiratory muscles, decreased ciliary action from smoking or exposure to air pollution	Decreased ability to maintain good oxygenation leads to less respiratory reserve; a greater tendency to retain secretions occurs because cilia cannot move foreign substances and secretions as easily; cough reflex and effort are diminished.
Decreased gastrointestinal tract motility as muscles weaken; decreased acid production	Acid is insufficient to inhibit growth of pathogens; decreased motility allows organisms to remain in the gastrointestinal tract and multiply.
Prostate changes, bladder prolapse, and urethral strictures	The bladder is not completely emptied at each voiding, which allows for stagnation and provides a medium for growth of pathogens.
Decreased immune response because bone marrow does not produce new blood cells as rapidly	Mobilization of body defenses to fight infection and heal wounds is slower.

THE INFLAMMATORY RESPONSE

Inflammation is an immediate, localized, protective response of the body to any kind of injury or damage to its cells or tissues. It is considered the second line of defense to infection at the cellular level (Fig. 6.2). Three basic purposes of the inflammatory response are to (1) neutralize and destroy harmful agents, (2) limit their spread to other tissues in the body by walling off the organisms, and (3) prepare the damaged tissues for repair. The inflammatory response is also triggered when microbes or other "nonself" components are identified. Current research is identifying stress as an activator of inflammation leading to stress-related diseases (Liu, Wang, & Jiang, 2017).

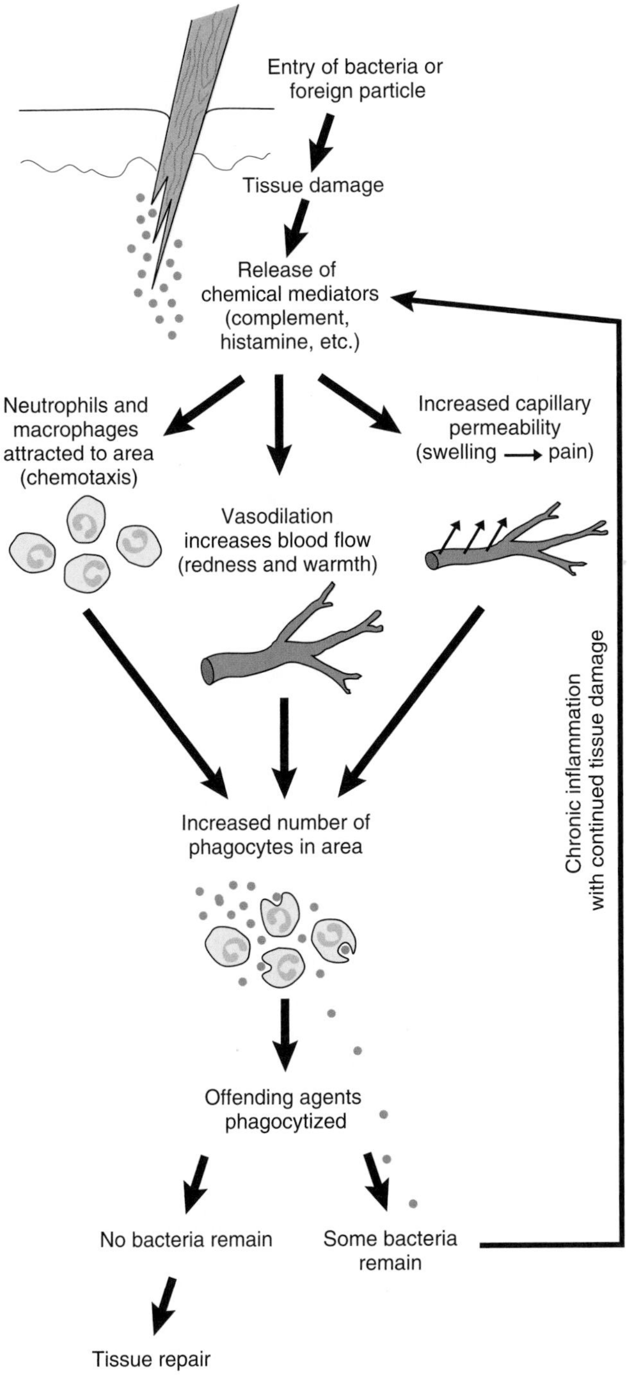

Fig. 6.2 Steps in the inflammatory process. (From Applegate E: *The anatomy and physiology learning system,* ed 4, Philadelphia, 2010, Saunders.)

Inflammatory Changes

Changes that are part of the inflammatory response can occur locally, at the site of injury, and systemically. These changes involve (1) the cells of the damaged tissues and adjacent connective tissues; (2) the blood vessels in and near the site of injury, activating the clotting mechanism; (3) the blood cells, particularly the leukocytes; (4) the macrophages and phagocyte activity; (5) the immune system; and (6) the hormonal system. An inadequate inflammatory response may cause active, systemic infection.

> **Clinical Cues**
>
> The five local signs and symptoms of inflammation are heat, redness, swelling, pain, and limitation or loss of function. Not all inflammation means infection. A sprained ankle will result in all of these symptoms, without resulting in an infection.

Signs and Symptoms of Inflammation

Local reactions. *Redness* and *heat* are caused by the increased blood flow to the affected area. *Swelling* is the result of the increased permeability of the capillaries and the leakage of fluid from the blood into the tissue spaces around the cells. Blockage of lymphatic drainage from the site also contributes to the local swelling. *Pain,* the result of irritated nerve endings, is caused by the chemicals released by the defensive cells and the accumulation of fluid in the area.

Systemic reactions. Systemic reactions to inflammation are familiar to anyone who has had the flu or another generalized infection. Headache, **myalgia** (muscle aches), fever, diaphoresis, chills, **anorexia** (loss of appetite), and **malaise** (weakness) are some of the more common signs and symptoms experienced with a systemic infection. (Note: An inflammatory response can occur in the absence of an infection, such as with rheumatoid arthritis or a histamine response triggered by an insect bite.)

Nursing care for patients who have a systemic infection includes providing for a balanced fluid intake and output, pain relief, and temperature control. Measures to ensure adequate nutrition and rest are used. If there is an inadequate inflammatory response to a systemic infection, bacterial infections may spread elsewhere in the body and delay tissue repair and wound healing.

Chemical Release and Vascular Changes

The complement system is a group of proteins that lie dormant in the body until they have been activated through an encounter with a foreign substance. The activation of these proteins enhances phagocytosis and the inflammatory process. This process is measured by the laboratory test C-reactive protein (CRP). If viral invasion has occurred, the chemical interferon is released to protect the cells against further viral invasion. As soon as damage occurs, the blood vessels in the injured area briefly constrict and, as histamine and serotonin are released, then dilate so that more blood is brought to the damaged cells. The walls of the capillaries become more permeable (i.e., their pores enlarge) so that water, proteins, and defensive cells such as neutrophils and macrophages can seep into the fluid surrounding the damaged cells to remove pathogens through the process of phagocytosis. One of the classic outward signs of inflammation is leakage of fluid into the spaces around the cells, producing a localized swelling, or *edema*. This results in a "walling off" of the area and delays the spread of pathogens, toxins, and other harmful agents to the rest of the body.

THE IMMUNE RESPONSE

The third line of defense is the immune response, which attempts to defend and protect the body through a series of complex chemical and mechanical activities. These activities involve (1) the detection of entry by foreign agents as soon as they gain access to the body's cells; (2) immediate recognition of the agents as foreign or alien; and (3) the ability to distinguish one kind of foreign agent from another and to "remember" that particular agent if it appears again years later. The specific antibodies and antitoxins produced by the immune response are transported by the circulatory system to the tissue spaces that surround the site of inflammation. They attack the foreign cells and neutralize the toxins those cells produce. The immune response is discussed more fully in Chapter 10.

Hormonal Response

Some hormones, such as cortisol, a glucocorticoid produced in the adrenal cortex, have an *antiinflammatory* action that limits inflammation to the locally damaged tissues. Other hormones, such as aldosterone, a mineralocorticoid also produced in the adrenal cortex, are *proinflammatory,* which means that they stimulate the body's protective inflammatory response. Thus the hormones have a regulatory effect on the inflammatory process so that the response is well balanced and provides maximum benefit.

The Chain of Infection

For an infectious disease to be spread from one person to another, certain conditions must be met. Infection occurs through a cyclical interrelated process like links in a chain (Fig. 6.3). Prevention or control of infection is aimed at interrupting the chain of infection. This can include the performance of hand hygiene or the wearing of gloves to protect the hands or a cover gown to protect one's clothing.

The mechanism of transmission of a pathogenic agent within the environment or to another person is by either direct or indirect contact. **Vectors** such as mosquitoes, fleas, ticks, and flies can transmit pathogens through their bites or stings.

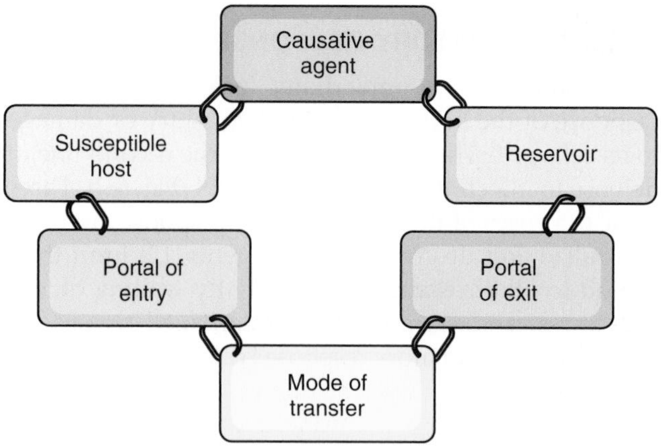

Fig. 6.3 The cyclical process of infection. Each link of the infection cycle must be present and occur in the proper sequence to produce disease. (From Williams P: *deWit's fundamental concepts and skills for nursing*, ed 5, St. Louis, 2018, Elsevier.)

Box 6.2 Human Reservoirs

CARRIER OR COLONIZED

The person is colonized with or carries the actual infection but does not show any obvious signs or symptoms. Because the individual does not feel ill, they typically do not take precautions to prevent the spread of infection and can transmit it to others.

INFECTIOUS (SYMPTOMATIC)

The person has obvious signs and symptoms of infection; they are less likely to spread infection because precautions are usually taken.

The three most important aspects in the infection chain are the interaction of the *agent*, the *host*, and the *mode of transmission*.

A reservoir is any place a pathogen is normally found (Box 6.2). The reservoir can be *animate* (living), such as people, animals, and insects, or it can be *inanimate* (nonliving), as found in soil, in water, and on surfaces of objects such as a cup or bed rails. The body can be a reservoir because pathogenic organisms can grow and multiply *(colonize)* on the skin or inside the body without causing a specific immune response or an infection. Infectious agents can also be found in body excretions or secretions such as saliva, sputum, urine, feces, and wound drainage. Individuals who have become colonized with a specific pathogen, such as methicillin-resistant *Staphylococcus aureus* (MRSA) or vancomycin-resistant enterococci (VRE), can be asymptomatic carriers *(reservoirs)* and unknowingly spread the infection to others because they are not aware that they have been exposed and are now colonized with an organism that is known to be multidrug resistant. In the home or community, contaminated or improperly cooked food, stagnant water, or sewage can also be sources of infection.

INFECTION PREVENTION AND CONTROL

PREVENTING AND CONTROLLING THE SPREAD OF INFECTION

Hand Hygiene

Hand hygiene is the primary intervention any health care provider can use to control the spread of infection. Hand hygiene can be performed with soap and water, if hands are visibly soiled, or with an alcohol-based hand sanitizing solution for routine decontamination. It is important to note that hand hygiene must be performed *regardless* of whether gloves were used or not. Artificial fingernails, extenders, or gels are not recommended for health care providers who have direct patient contact because pathogens can be found beneath the nails.

Clinical Cues

Remove any rings or other forms of jewelry before washing hands with soap and water. Hand hygiene should be performed with an approved soap under warm running water, using friction, for at least 15 to 30 seconds. Ensure that the areas between fingers and the dorsal and palmar aspects of both hands are thoroughly rubbed.

PRECAUTION CATEGORIES FOR INFECTION PREVENTION AND CONTROL

Standard Precautions

Standard Precautions were mandated by the Centers for Disease Control and Prevention (CDC) in the 1980s (Box 6.3; also see Appendix B). These precautions are designed to prevent the transmission of microorganisms from one patient to another, as well as to protect the health care worker from unnecessary exposure to infection. Standard Precautions are to be used on all patients because their potential for being colonized, or already infectious, is not always known. Barrier precautions, such as gloves or isolation techniques that include the proper handling and disposal of secretions, excretions, and exudates, can prevent the transmission of pathogens from one person or object to another. The most current CDC Guidelines and Recommendations related to infection prevention and control in a variety of health care settings can be found at https://www.cdc.gov/infectioncontrol/guidelines/index.html.

Clinical Cues

Personal protective equipment (PPE) is used to protect the one providing care from exposure to pathogens. When wearing gloves, keep in mind that they are a protective barrier for you; they do not protect the patient from whatever might be on the gloves. Do not touch anything with a dirty glove that you would not touch with a dirty hand. Change gloves frequently and perform hand hygiene as per protocol.

Box 6.3 Standard Precautions

1. Use barrier precautions, such as gloves, gown, face mask, and protective eyewear, to prevent exposure of skin or mucous membranes to a patient's blood, body fluid, or other potentially infectious materials while providing care or assisting with a procedure for your patient.
   a. Change gloves between contact with one body part and another (e.g., respiratory and urinary).
   b. Discard used gloves in the appropriate waste container; do not wash or reuse them.
   c. Perform hand hygiene immediately after removing gloves.
2. Prevent injury by needle stick or cuts from sharp instruments.
   a. Be cautious and attentive any time you are handling a needle or sharp instrument.
   b. Do not recap a used needle by hand; scoop the cap onto the needle on a flat surface or deploy the safety device attached to the needle.
   c. Immediately dispose of a used needle or other sharp instrument in the puncture-resistant container provided for that purpose in the room.
   d. Replace puncture-resistant containers when they are three-quarters full and as needed; do not attempt to push needles into a container that is too full.
3. Prevent possible self-contamination or exposure through broken skin.
   a. If you have open lesions or weeping dermatitis, do not give direct patient care or handle patient care equipment until the condition has resolved.
4. Prevent possible self-contamination during cardiopulmonary resuscitation.
   a. Use a disposable barrier device or resuscitation bag for emergency mouth-to-mouth breathing.
   b. Wear the appropriate personal protective equipment (PPE) whenever possible.

Transmission-Based Precautions

Transmission-Based Precautions incorporate Standard Precaution techniques with additional protective actions specific to the organism and how it is spread. These safety measures should be implemented for patients with a suspected or confirmed infection or who are known to be colonized with a highly transmissible organism such as tuberculosis or Ebola. These additional precautions are known as airborne, contact, and droplet precautions. Precautions for patients with Ebola infections are different from the other transmission-based procedures and are listed in Table 6.6. Health care facilities usually place information cards on the door to the patient's room to ensure that everyone who enters the room is aware of the safety precautions and the personal protective equipment (PPE) that must be used before entry. Depending on the microorganism involved, you verify which types of Transmission-Based Precautions should be used. If unsure as to what is required, contact the facility's infection preventionist for guidance. The effectiveness of Standard

Table 6.6 Isolation Precautions (Transmission-Based Precautions and Expanded Precautions for Ebola)

PRIVATE ROOM[a]	MASKS	GOWNS	GLOVES	COMMON DISEASES PLACED IN ISOLATION CATEGORY
Airborne Infection Isolation				
Always; door to room must be kept closed at all times	Must wear a fit-tested NIOSH-approved N95 respirator	No, unless draining wounds	No, unless draining wounds	Pulmonary or laryngeal tuberculosis or draining tuberculosis skin lesions; smallpox, viral hemorrhagic fever, severe acute respiratory syndrome (SARS); measles; varicella, disseminated zoster
Contact Precautions				
Preferred; cohorting of patients with same type of infection is acceptable	Situation dependent	Always; if patients are cohorted, staff must perform hand hygiene and change PPE *between* patients	Always; if patients are cohorted, staff must perform hand hygiene and change PPE *between* patients	Open or draining wounds; history of MRSA, VRE, ESBL positive; diarrhea; MDRO infections
Droplet Precautions				
Preferred; cohorting of patients with same type of infection is acceptable	Wear a surgical mask when entering room; patient should wear mask during transport and observe cough etiquette	Not usually	When helping with cough-inducing procedures or discarding used tissues	Pneumonia, influenza, rubella, pertussis, streptococcal pharyngitis, meningitis caused by *Neisseria meningitidis* or *Haemophilus influenzae* type B
Ebola Precautions[a]				
Requires "buddy" to assist with donning and doffing PPE. Note: Information in this table is not in exact order of donning PPE.				
Mandatory	Must wear N95 respiratory mask, full-face shield, cover hair	[a]Change into hospital-issued scrubs or disposable scrubs, then don impervious cover gown and hood that cover all of the neck and chest If activities performed in the patient's room are likely to dislodge cuff of gown, secure cuff with Coban or tape	Don first pair before donning impervious shoe and leg covers, don cover gown Second pair is donned after face mask, hair cover, and hood are donned	Airborne and contact precautions with "buddy" observing all aspects of care being provided to ensure that no exposure or contamination has occurred to the nurse in the room caring for a patient with Ebola

[a]In most cases, patients infected with the same organism may share a room. For any patient in airborne isolation or expanded precautions, such as with Ebola, limit the time the patient is out of the room; notify the receiving unit or department that the patient is in isolation so that appropriate measures can be taken before the arrival of the patient. For a patient infected with Ebola, a two-nurse team is required: one to care for the patient, the other to observe the first nurse to ensure that Transmission-Based Precautions, hand hygiene, etc., have not been compromised.

ESBL, Extended-spectrum beta-lactamase; *MDRO,* multidrug-resistant organism; *MRSA,* methicillin-resistant *Staphylococcus aureus; NIOSH,* National Institute of Occupational Safety and Health; *PPE,* personal protective equipment; *VRE,* vancomycin-resistant enterococci.

Precautions and Transmission-Based Precautions depends on rigorous compliance with the infection prevention and control precautions.

Personal Protective Equipment

Personal protective equipment (PPE) involves the use of a barrier to protect a person from exposure to bloodborne pathogens, body fluids, or other potentially infectious

? Think Critically

What type of Transmission-Based Precautions would be necessary for a patient who is admitted with complications of Ebola? What PPE would you need to assist this patient with activities of daily living? How must it be donned and doffed? See the CDC website (https://www.cdc.gov/vhf/ebola/hcp/ppe-training/index.html) for Ebola PPE Donning Instructions for more detailed information and pictorial description.

materials. These barriers include but are not limited to gloves, cover gowns, face masks, eye protection, face shields, and respirator masks. Ebola is a virus that is extremely lethal but is transmitted only through direct contact with blood or body fluids. When it comes to caring for a patient with Ebola, the CDC (2015) states: "To protect healthcare workers during care of a patient with EVD, healthcare facilities must provide onsite management and oversight on the safe use of PPE and implement administrative and environmental controls with continuous safety checks through direct observation of healthcare workers during the PPE donning and doffing processes." Current guidelines for correct use of PPE when caring for patients with Ebola can be found on the CDC website (https://www.cdc.gov/vhf/ebola/hcp/ppe-training/index.html). By law, health care facilities are required to provide PPE at no expense to the staff (Occupational Safety and Health Administration Bloodborne Pathogens Standards, 1910.132[h][1]). If you suspect you have a latex allergy, contact your Occupational/Employee Health Services department so that a more detailed assessment can be made. If it is determined that a latex allergy does exist, your facility is required to provide you with the appropriate PPE. Fig. 6.4 shows methods for donning and removing PPE.

Clinical Cues

Remember, when you are using PPE, you cannot retrieve common items from your uniform pocket (e.g., pen, alcohol pad, or stethoscope). You must plan ahead and obtain the necessary supplies and equipment before entering the patient's room.

DONNING AND REMOVING PPE

Donning Personal Protective Equipment (PPE)

The type of PPE will vary based on the level of precautions required, such as Standard and Contact, Droplet, or Airborne Isolation Precautions.

Gown
- Fully cover torso from neck to knees, arms to end of wrist, and wrap around the back
- Fasten in back at neck and waist

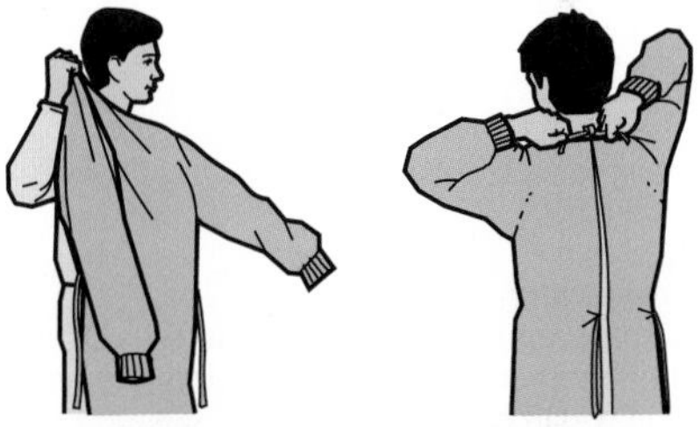

Mask or respirator
- Secure ties or elastic band at middle of head and neck
- Fit flexible band to nose bridge
- Fit snug to face and below chin
- Fit-check respirator

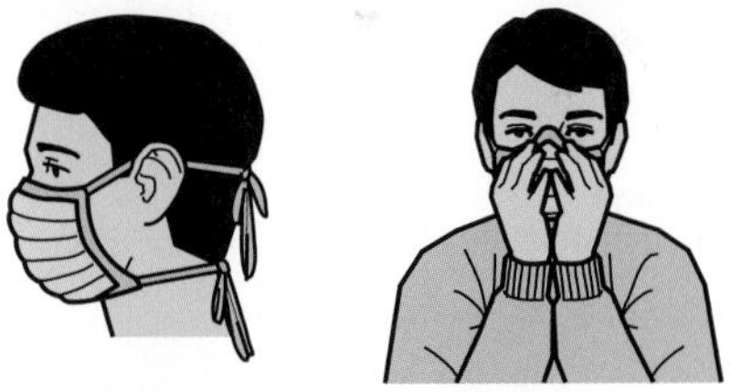

Goggles or face shield
- Put over face and eyes and adjust to fit

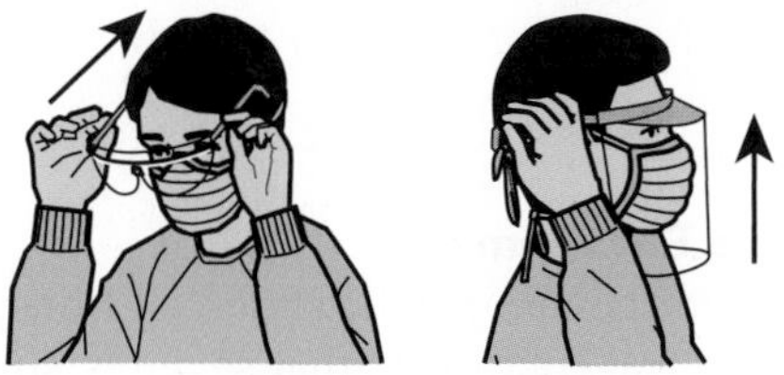

Gloves
- Extend to cover wrist of isolation gown

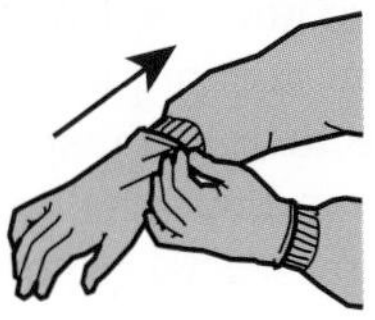

SAFE WORK PRACTICES
- Keep hands away from face
- Limit surfaces touched
- Change gown and gloves when torn or heavily contaminated
- Perform hand hygiene

A

Fig. 6.4 A, Donning personal protective equipment (PPE).

Continued

Removing Personal Protective Equipment (PPE)

Remove PPE at doorway before leaving patient room, or in anteroom; remove respirator outside of room.

Gloves
- Outside of gloves are contaminated!
- Grasp outside of glove with opposite gloved hand; peel off
- Hold removed glove in gloved hand
- Slide fingers of ungloved hand under remaining glove at wrist

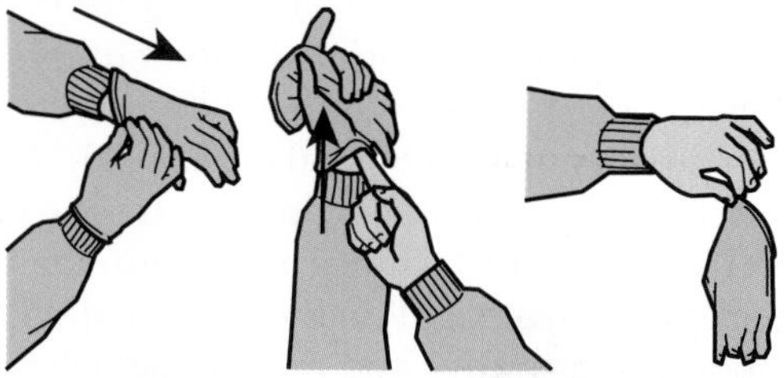

Goggles or face shield
- Outside of goggles or face shield is contaminated!
- To remove, handle by "clean" head band or ear pieces
- Place in designated receptacle for reprocessing or in waste container

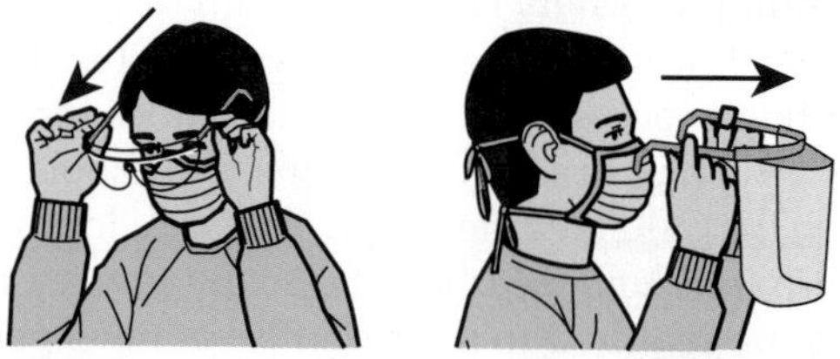

Gown
- Gown front and sleeves are contaminated!
- Unfasten neck, undo the waist ties
- Remove gown using a peeling motion; pull gown from each shoulder toward the same hand
- Gown will turn inside out
- Hold removed gown away from body, roll into a bundle, and discard into waste or linen receptacle

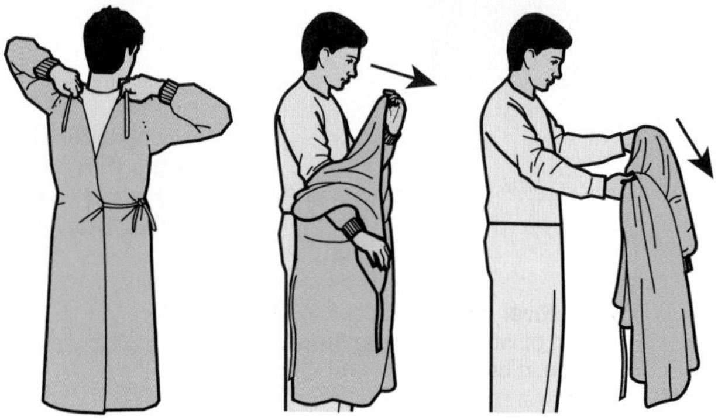

Mask or respirator
- Front of mask/respirator is contaminated—DO NOT TOUCH!
- Grasp bottom then top ties/elastics and remove
- Discard in waste container

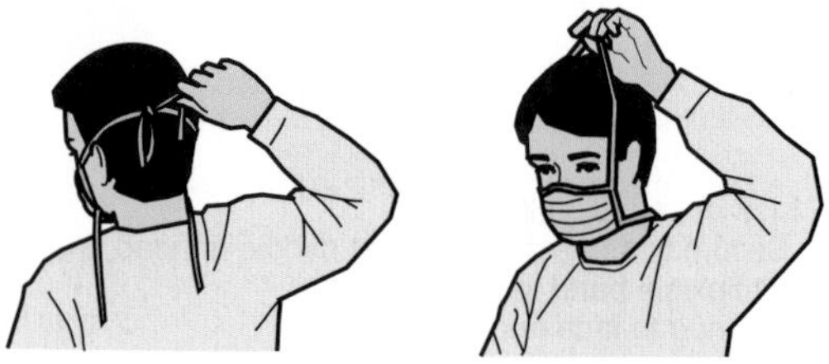

Hand hygiene
- Perform immediately after removing all PPE!

B

Fig. 6.4, cont'd B, Removing PPE.

Protective Environment

Patients with hematopoietic stem cell transplantation or other clinical conditions that severely suppress the immune system require highly specialized forms of expanded isolation techniques. Nurses and all staff who provide care to the transplant recipient receive detailed education and training on the appropriate care. Interventions include special airflow and filtration rooms with positive air pressure, smooth surfaces to aid in disinfection, and minimizing the length of time the patient is outside the protective environment. Staff must be free from signs and symptoms of illness. For additional information, refer to the facility's policy and procedure manuals or the CDC's website at www.cdc.gov.

Respiratory Hygiene and Cough Etiquette

Two methods of preventing droplets from spreading to others are teaching people to cover their mouth when sneezing or coughing and turning the head away to prevent coughing into someone else's face (Fig. 6.5). In addition, educating patients and families to dispose of soiled tissues in waste containers and to perform hand hygiene after contact with actual or potentially contaminated items is important. To prevent the transmission of pathogenic microorganisms to a patient, instruct the patient to avoid contact with others who may have an infection.

Transmission of an infectious organism can be interrupted at the portal of entry by using only clean or sterile items when caring for patients. Use of effective hand hygiene techniques by health care workers, visitors, and patients is key in the prevention of infection. Immunization and measures to boost immunity through proper nutrition and a healthy lifestyle also increase a person's resistance to infection. One of the *Healthy People 2030* objectives is to increase the proportion of adults who are immunized for influenza and pneumococcal disease. Table 6.7 lists factors that can make a host more susceptible to pathogens.

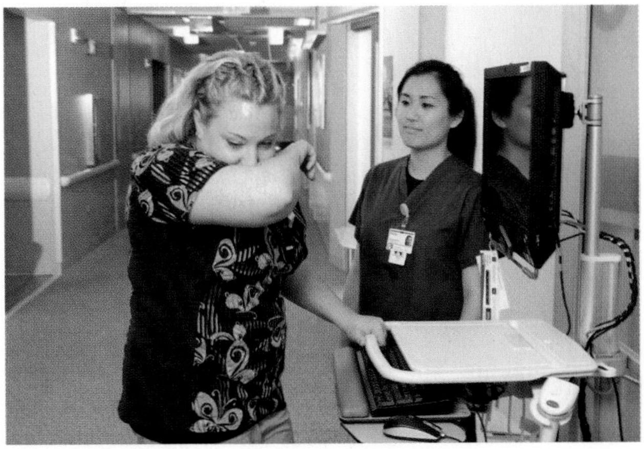

Fig. 6.5 Cover your cough to help prevent the spread of infection.

HEALTH CARE–ASSOCIATED INFECTIONS

A **health care–associated infection (HAI)** occurs when a patient is cared for in any kind of health care setting and acquires an infection. There are specific criteria for the infection to be classified as an HAI, such as length of time in the facility before the onset or appearance of the infection. Because health services are provided in a wide variety of locations, such as acute care facilities, outpatient surgery or dialysis centers, homes, and mobile clinics, it is sometimes difficult to determine where the patient became infected. Detailed documentation is essential in determining whether an infection the patient has was community or health care acquired.

Although inanimate objects such as needles, contaminated surgical instruments, and linens are major sources of infection in these settings, every patient is

Table 6.7 Risk Factors for Increased Susceptibility to Infection

RISK FACTOR	CONSEQUENCE
Altered defense mechanisms	Body damage from trauma; breaks in the skin or mucous membranes; fractures.
Lower than normal leukocyte (white blood cell) count	Bone marrow suppression from chemotherapy or toxic agents; genetic or acquired agranulocytosis, such as that seen with chemotherapy drugs.
Age	Older adult patients and the very young are more susceptible to infection, probably because of declining or immature immune function.
Excessive stress or fatigue	These states seem to interfere with the body's normal defense mechanisms.
Malnutrition	Poor nutrition interferes with cell growth and replacement, which contributes to decreased immune function.
Alcoholism	Inhibits the immune system.
Preexisting chronic illnesses, such as diabetes mellitus, adrenal insufficiency, renal failure, or liver disease; serious illness such as pneumonia, peritonitis, etc.	These disease states upset the normal homeostatic balance within the body, impairing the normal defense mechanisms. Serious illness taxes the immune system, causing greater susceptibility to other pathogens.
Immunosuppressive treatment, chemotherapy, or corticosteroid treatment	These treatments depress the immune system or harm the bone marrow, decreasing the number of leukocytes. Corticosteroids depress the inflammatory response, inhibiting one of the body's defense mechanisms.
Invasive equipment or indwelling tubes	Endotracheal or tracheostomy tubes, intravenous cannulas, wound drains, feeding tubes, and urinary catheters provide a potential route of entry for pathogens.
Smoking or inhalation of toxic chemicals	Inhibits ciliary action of the respiratory tract. Toxic chemicals may damage bone marrow, inhibiting the production of leukocytes.
Intravenous drug abuse	Allows introduction of microorganisms into the bloodstream from contaminated needles or from lack of aseptic technique.
Unsafe sexual practices (not knowing history or health status of sexual partner, not using condoms)	Allows entry of pathogenic organisms through the genital mucosal tissue.
Unsafe handling of needles and sharps	Potential for breaks in the skin through which pathogens may enter.

Adapted from Ignatavicius DD, Workman ML, Rebar C, et al.: *Medical-surgical nursing: patient centered collaborative care*, ed 9, St. Louis, 2018, Elsevier.

Table 6.8 Preventing and Controlling Health Care–Associated Infections

MOST COMMON SITES	NURSING INTERVENTIONS
Urinary tract	Catheterize only when absolutely necessary. Observe sterile technique when catheterizing. Keep drainage system for indwelling catheter closed, off the floor, and below bladder level at all times to prevent urine reflux. Empty urine drainage bag into a clean container, without contaminating the spout. Wipe the spout with an alcohol pad before securing it. Remove indwelling catheters as soon as possible to decrease risk of infection.
Surgical wounds	Administer prophylactic antimicrobials as ordered. Change soiled dressings and linens promptly and dispose of them in the correct container. Ensure that the patient has adequate nutrition and sufficient fluid intake.
Respiratory tract	Encourage the patient to cough, deep-breathe, use incentive spirometer, and move. Perform suctioning, tracheostomy care, and other procedures under aseptic technique. Protect the patient from others with colds or other signs of infection.
Bloodstream (bacteremia)	Maintain meticulous aseptic technique in the administration of intravenous (IV) fluids. Use aseptic technique when accessing IV ports. Follow the recommended procedure for care of the insertion site (including the dressing) and IV tubing and catheters. Assess the site for increased redness, pain, or infiltration. Remove and insert new IV sets per facility policy and when indicated.

directly and indirectly in contact with large numbers of health care workers, each of whom could be the source of infection. Therefore it is important to ensure that appropriate precautions, such as hand hygiene and Transmission-Based Precaution techniques, are followed at all times. Table 6.8 presents HAI risk factors. The Joint Commission (TJC) announced that any observation by surveyors of "individual" failure to perform hand hygiene in the process of direct patient care will be cited as a deficiency starting January 2018 (TJC, 2017).

MULTIDRUG RESISTANT ORGANISMS (MDRO)

Organisms that are resistant to more than one antibiotic are called **multidrug resistant organisms (MDROs)**. A list of organisms and guidelines for preventing and treating MDROs can be found on the CDC website. Overuse of antibiotics has led to mutations of the organisms, making them resistant to the antibiotics that were previously effective.

THE COST OF HEALTH CARE–ASSOCIATED INFECTIONS

Human suffering, prolonged hospital stays, and time lost from work are some of the concerns with HAIs. The annual cost of HAIs is estimated to be $9.8 billion. Central line–associated bloodstream infections are the most costly, followed by ventilator-associated pneumonia and surgical site infections. Other infections included in the top five are *C. diff* and catheter-associated urinary tract infections. The Joint Commission, CDC, Agency for Healthcare Research and Quality (AHRQ), and Institute for Healthcare Improvement are among some of the agencies working to decrease the incidence of HAIs. More than 650,000 patients per year develop an HAI. Increased training and surveillance are being implemented to prevent infections and monitor them when they occur. Insurance reimbursement may be denied or limited for increased length of stay and treatment costs for infections that were considered preventable (AHRQ, 2017).

NURSING INTERVENTIONS TO PREVENT HEALTH CARE–ASSOCIATED INFECTIONS

The primary way to break the chain of infection is careful attention to hand hygiene before and after any direct patient contact, before and after any invasive or sterile procedure, after contact with infectious materials (e.g., wound drainage, feces, urine, or sputum), and before contact with immunocompromised patients. However, for hand hygiene to be effective, you need to know what cleansing product to use. For example, if the patient has an *S. aureus* infection, the health care worker can use either soap and water or an alcohol-based hand sanitizer to cleanse the hands. However, if the patient has a *C. diff* or *C. albicans* infection, the health care worker must use only soap and water to cleanse the hands. The alcohol in alcohol-based sanitizers only makes the spores for these organisms "sticky"; it does not kill them. In addition, if a patient with *C. diff* is discharged, the housekeeping staff needs to know that the patient had this type of infection so that the appropriate cleaning agents will be used. Reducing catheter-related infections is one of TJC's 2019 National Patient Safety Goals and a *Healthy People 2030* objective. Interventions for this important goal include hand hygiene, use of a standardized kit for dressing changes, and chlorhexidine-based antiseptic for skin preparation.

Clinical Cues

In accordance with National Patient Safety Goals (TJC, 2019), compliance with guidelines for hand hygiene is one of the primary issues for reducing HAIs. Make a point of performing hand hygiene in view of the patient and the family; this increases their confidence in your ability as a caregiver and demonstrates your attention to preventing infection.

Used or contaminated items should not be placed on the floor or remain in an uncovered disposal container in the patient's room. Disposing of infectious materials, such as soiled dressings, full suction containers, and contaminated equipment, in covered, moisture-resistant biohazard containers helps contain microorganisms as well as odors. Protecting patients from others with respiratory infections and from visitors with other communicable diseases is also appropriate. Table 6.8 reviews the major sites of HAIs, the infectious agents most often responsible, and some of the interventions nurses may take to prevent or control the spread of infection.

Clinical Cues

There may be times when you are not quite sure where to dispose of materials used in the treatment of a patient. If the item has blood or body fluids on or in it where you can squeeze, sling, fling, or flick it from or off the material, it should be disposed of in the biohazard waste container.

Along with preventive interventions and appropriate treatments, you must continuously assess the patient to identify early signs of infection or its spread. It is also helpful to review and document each patient's immunization status against such infections as tetanus, pertussis, influenza, hepatitis B, pneumococcal pneumonia, and varicella.

INFECTION SURVEILLANCE AND REPORTING

Surveillance requires that nurses be alert for signs or symptoms of infection in patients under their care. Monitor laboratory results for an elevation in the WBC count. You should routinely assess patients for unexpected elevation of temperature; malaise; cough; loss of appetite; foul-smelling urine; new-onset diarrhea; and wounds that are red, swollen, painful, or have a foul-smelling discharge. It is important to note the color of the purulent drainage; this is helpful in identifying the kind of organism that may be causing an infection (e.g., *S. aureus* produces a golden discharge, *Pseudomonas aeruginosa* has bluish-green discharge).

Pay particular attention to patients who are more susceptible to infection. These patients include those who (1) are weakened by severe illness or injury; (2) have drainage tubes, intravenous catheters, or other invasive devices for monitoring or treatment; (3) are very young or very old; (4) have had recent surgery; or (5) are immunocompromised. When an infection is suspected, report this to the patient's health care provider. In certain situations, Transmission-Based Precautions may need to be instituted even before culture results are available. If there is a question as to what type of precautions to initiate, contact the facility's infection prevention and control department.

MEDICAL ASEPSIS AND SURGICAL ASEPSIS

Medical Asepsis

Medical asepsis (the goal of which is to reduce microorganisms) includes hand hygiene, separation or isolation of the patient, use of appropriate precautions for the handling and disposing of contaminated articles, and other techniques devised to contain and destroy infectious agents, such as cleansing and disinfection.

Surgical Asepsis

Surgical asepsis (the goal of which is to eliminate microorganisms completely) involves the sterilizing of instruments, skin, and other articles that will be used to perform surgery or other types of sterile procedures. Surgical procedure typically requires that the first line of defense (i.e., the skin) be compromised in some way. Surgical asepsis must also be used when placing an intravenous catheter into a vein, when inserting a Foley catheter into the urinary bladder, during the placement of internal monitoring devices, or during other invasive procedures such as a cardiac angiogram. Hand hygiene for surgical asepsis is more vigorous and must be performed according to the facility's policy and procedure. In a surgically aseptic environment, surgical gowns, face masks, and sterile gloves are necessary and must be put on and removed in a specific way. Procedures being performed at the bedside that require surgical asepsis, such as a central line placement, require that all persons in the room wear a face mask and head cover. The person performing the procedure must also wear sterile gloves and a sterile cover gown. The patient must be covered with sterile drapes, and only sterile equipment and supplies are to be used. The door to the room must be closed throughout the procedure (Marschall et al., 2014).

SEPSIS AND SEPTIC SHOCK

If a patient's HAI or community-acquired infection is not adequately treated, the pathogen may enter the bloodstream, causing a bacteremia and **sepsis** with a systemic inflammatory response. When microorganisms enter the bloodstream, they are carried throughout the body and may invade any tissue or body system. Symptoms of the inflammatory and immune response include but are not limited to tachycardia, **tachypnea** (rapid breathing), fever, and an elevated WBC count. These clinical findings are known as the systemic inflammatory response syndrome (SIRS) criteria. An altered level of consciousness may also occur. If the infection is identified and treated in the early stages, full recovery is possible. Sepsis (caused by circulating pathogens) is most commonly associated with bacterial invasion from gram-negative bacteria, such as *Pseudomonas aeruginosa, Escherichia coli,* and *Klebsiella pneumoniae,* or gram-positive bacteria, such as *Staphylococcus aureus* and *Streptococcus pneumoniae.* The toxins secreted into the blood from these pathogens react with the blood vessels and cell membranes, stimulating a massive inflammatory and immune response. Increased capillary permeability with loss of fluid from the vascular space, cellular injury, and greatly increased cellular metabolic rates can result in septic shock and damage to end organs (Napolitano, 2018). Refer to Chapter 45 for further information on SIRS and septic shock.

NURSING INTERVENTIONS FOR PATIENTS WITH SEPSIS

Patients who are at risk for sepsis must be identified and then closely monitored for changes from the baseline assessment, such as a change in mental status, tachycardia, tachypnea, changes in blood pressure, and decreased urine output. The temperature may be normal or elevated, depending on the organism or organisms that are causing the sepsis. Pneumonia and postsurgical wound infections are two conditions that can lead to sepsis if not quickly identified and treated, and some patients, often older adults, experience **hypothermia** (below normal temperature) when septic.

Sepsis is diagnosed from the clinical presentation of the patient and the results of laboratory tests, such as elevated leukocyte count, elevated lactate levels, and serial blood cultures that may be positive for invading microorganisms. Antimicrobial sensitivities are performed on these pathogens to determine which drugs would be most appropriate to treat the infection. Ensuring that the correct antimicrobial agents are prescribed in a timely manner decreases the risk of the patient developing a multidrug-resistant infection and eliminates the pathogens as quickly as possible.

NURSING MANAGEMENT

ASSESSMENT (DATA COLLECTION)

Detecting infection in a patient requires a thorough nursing assessment. Subjective data can be obtained by asking the patient to describe symptoms and time of onset. Questions should also include whether the patient is having or has had pain, headache, stiff neck, fever, or chills. The interview is based on the patient's complaints; for example, if the patient states that it hurts to go to the bathroom, ask if there is also urgency or burning when trying to empty the bladder. With some signs and symptoms, it may be appropriate to ask if patients have traveled outside the country recently (e.g., amoebic dysentery); if they were bitten by any insects before the onset of symptoms (e.g., West Nile virus); or if they have a compromised immune system, either from disease or from drug exposure (i.e., chemotherapy agents).

> **Clinical Cues**
>
> Subjective complaints that may indicate infection include fatigue, loss of appetite, headache, nausea, general malaise, and pain.

Objective data often point to the specific body system affected by the infection but may also include systemic signs such as fever, tachycardia, or tachypnea. Data collection includes assessing vital signs; auscultating the lungs to check for abnormal breath sounds; inspecting the skin for lesions or rashes; and checking the urine for cloudiness, discoloration, abnormal odor, and increased specific gravity. Bowel sounds are auscultated in all four quadrants, and then the abdomen is gently palpated for signs of tenderness. In addition, look for signs of local infection such as redness, swelling, pain or tenderness on palpation or movement, heat in the affected area, and possibly loss of function of the affected body part.

> **Older Adult Care Points**
>
> Many older adults, especially those older than 80 years, have a low baseline body temperature. Because of decreased inflammatory and immune response, their temperature may rise very little in the presence of infection. Small increases in temperature in these patients may be quite significant. Signs of inflammation may not be present or may be milder than what is typically seen in a younger person. A decrease in mental alertness, increased fatigue, or sudden onset of confusion, irritability, or apathy may be a clue that an infection is present.

Diagnostic Tests

Laboratory data that may indicate infection include an elevated WBC count, changes in the distribution and number of the various types of leukocytes, elevated CRP, and microbiology cultures that test positive for microorganisms.

Bacteriologic tests are performed by culturing specimens of blood, body fluids, or waste products such as feces. When obtaining a culture, be careful to (1) use aseptic technique, where indicated and with sterile equipment; (2) only collect fresh material from the suspected site, avoiding contamination by microbes from nearby tissues and fluids; and (3) use the appropriate container for the sample, making sure the container is correctly labeled and tightly covered to avoid spilling and contamination during transport to the laboratory. Also note on the laboratory requisition form whether the patient was given any antimicrobial agents before the specimen was collected. This is because some microorganisms may have responded to the administered drug and thus be in such low quantities at the time of collection, they may not grow in the culture media.

Ideally specimens are collected before antimicrobials are initiated, but if there is difficulty obtaining a sample, drug therapy should not be delayed.

Sensitivity tests are done in conjunction with microbiology cultures to determine which antimicrobials can most effectively destroy or inhibit the multiplication and growth of the specific infecting microbe. Once this has been determined, verify that the antimicrobial medications being given are effective for eliminating the identified organism. Inadequate dosages or delays in administration can lead to a genetic mutation of the pathogen involved or the development of a multidrug-resistant organism (MDRO).

With some infectious diseases, such as tuberculosis and coccidioidomycosis, blood tests may be done to look for antigens or antibodies. Radiography (x-rays), computed tomography (CT), or magnetic resonance imaging (MRI) may be used to detect changes in the tissues or organs and to locate abscesses anywhere within the body.

◆ NURSING DIAGNOSIS

The specific type of infection and the problem it presents determine the correct problem statement. For example, if the patient has a urinary tract infection, the more specific problem statement would be *Altered urinary function*. In some cases, collaboration with other health team members helps establish the correct problem statement. Any patient entering the hospital for surgery or an invasive procedure is at risk for an HAI. Therefore *Potential for infection* should be listed as a problem statement or nursing diagnosis on the patient's care plan. The problem statements *Insufficient knowledge* due to lack of information and understanding about the disease and the problems of infection prevention and *Altered ability for self-care* should always be considered (Nursing Care Plan 6.1).

◆ PLANNING

The planning phase of the nursing process should take into account the physical strength of the patient and the need for rest. Every effort should be made to maintain the integrity of the skin and mucous membranes so that they continue to serve as effective barriers to infectious agents. Good skin care, oral hygiene, and personal cleanliness are essential. The psychological effect of Transmission-Based Precautions must be addressed; some patients may feel "dirty" or that people are avoiding them because they have an infectious disease.

Cultural Considerations

Hot and Cold Foods

In some Asian cultures there is a belief that a balance of hot and cold foods should be eaten when a fever or infection is present. Cold foods, such as watermelon or white radish soup, are thought to help the body fight off the infection and regain its balance.

Many Hispanic cultures have a belief that "hot" and "cold" forces are thrown out of balance during an illness. Cold foods, such as dairy products, honey, or fresh vegetables, may be preferred by the Hispanic patient with an infection.

Nursing Care Plan 6.1 Care of a Patient With an Infected Abdominal Wound

SCENARIO

Mr. Collins is a 28-year-old man who has been diagnosed with a lower abdominal wound infection that is culture positive for methicillin-resistant *Staphylococcus aureus* (MRSA). He is going to be discharged in 2 days.

PROBLEM STATEMENT/NURSING DIAGNOSIS

Altered skin integrity related to infected abdominal wound.

SUPPORTING ASSESSMENT DATA

Objective: Wound is open and draining purulent fluid. Drainage from abdominal wound is culture positive for MRSA, a multidrug-resistant organism (MDRO).

Goals/Expected Outcomes	Nursing Interventions	Selected Rationale	Evaluation
Infection will be controlled and not spread.	Place under contact precautions and explain purpose and requirement to patient and visitors.	To prevent the spread of infection to other patients and staff	No evidence of spread of infection
	Assist patient with bath to ensure skin has been cleaned.	Enables the nurse to do a thorough skin assessment	Bathed
	Change wound dressing as ordered and as needed.	Ensures that the wound is assessed at least daily and the nurse can track progression of wound treatment	Dressing changed; less drainage and redness
	Monitor vital signs, complete blood cell count, microbiology cultures.	Indicates progress in resolving the infection	Vital signs stable WBCs normalizing Outcomes met

Continued

Nursing Care Plan 6.1 Care of a Patient With an Infected Abdominal Wound—cont'd

PROBLEM STATEMENT/NURSING DIAGNOSIS

Insufficient knowledge related to proper wound care at home.

SUPPORTING ASSESSMENT DATA

Subjective: States, "I don't know how to change the dressing."

Goals/Expected Outcomes	Nursing Interventions	Selected Rationale	Evaluation
Before discharge, the patient and family member will be able to: Demonstrate proper hand hygiene techniques.	Demonstrate proper hand hygiene techniques and observe patient and family member perform this task.	Providing opportunities for education and training throughout the hospital stay increases the knowledge base the patient or family member can build on.	Patient verbalizes reasons for contact precautions; patient and family member demonstrate proper hand hygiene, wound cleansing, and dressing change techniques using medical asepsis; patient and family member verbalize signs and symptoms to report to health care provider; and patient states that he knows how to take medication and why he must finish the prescription.
State reasons for using contact precautions for dressing change.	Discuss reasons for contact precautions with patient and caregiver and provide supplemental written or audiovisual materials.	Addresses different learning styles of the adult patient/learner.	Patient and family member state they understand the need for contact precautions.
Demonstrate dressing change, maintaining medical asepsis before discharge.	Demonstrate dressing change and wound cleansing procedure; obtain return demonstration from patient and family member before discharge.	Providing hands-on training increases the understanding of wound healing and need for appropriate wound care.	Demonstrated dressing change with correct technique. Will observe practice and return demonstration before discharge.
List signs and symptoms that should be reported to provider.	Instruct patient and family to watch for elevated temperature, increased redness, swelling, pain, or purulent discharge from wound, and to report any such findings to provider.	Knowing what to look for and report decreases the risk of adverse outcomes.	Explained signs and symptoms to watch for and left printed sheet. Will seek feedback before discharge.
State why it is important to complete the course of antimicrobial therapy exactly as directed.	Explain importance of taking medication exactly as prescribed and of finishing entire prescription.	Taking antimicrobials as prescribed decreases the risk of the patient developing an MDRO infection.	Obtained feedback from patient; he states rationale correctly.

CRITICAL THINKING QUESTIONS

1. What other nursing methods that promote healing could you implement?
2. How would you recommend the patient's linens be laundered at home?

◆ IMPLEMENTATION

Providing a quiet environment with uninterrupted rest periods is important in the recovery process. Relieving the discomforts of fever and muscle aches is accomplished by tepid sponge baths, ice bags placed in the axilla or groin, antipyretics, and massage. Warm compresses and the application of heat, as appropriate, can also promote healing. Mild physical exercise promotes circulation and helps some patients relax. It can also increase blood circulation to an infected area. This ultimately will help remove the metabolic wastes that were produced from the body.

Provide patient and family teaching regarding the infection, including:

- The purposes of diagnostic tests, treatments, and special precautions
- Why the family must help maintain medical asepsis to prevent the spread of infection to themselves and others

Administering Antimicrobial Agents

Administer antimicrobial drugs on time to maintain effective blood levels. In addition, monitor the patient for drug side effects and evaluate the progress of the patient to determine whether the drug is effective in eradicating the infection. General nursing actions for the administration of antimicrobial medications are shown in Table 6.9.

Before administering the prescribed drug, be familiar with the different antimicrobial agent classifications: antibacterial, antiviral, antifungal, and anthelmintic (Box 6.4).

Clinical Cues

Patients who frequently receive antibiotic treatment are at risk for *Clostridium difficile infection (CDI)*, an HAI that causes severe colitis and diarrhea. *C. diff* colonizes the gut when the normal flora have been disrupted due to antibiotic therapy. Patients being treated for a third episode of CDI are recommended to have fecal microbiota transplantation (FMT). Stool collected from a healthy donor is instilled into the patient with recurrent CDI. With more than two treatments given, FMT was 90% effective (Kelly, Lamont, & Bakken, 2018).

There are two primary categories of antibacterial agents: narrow spectrum and broad spectrum. Both kinds inhibit replication and growth of bacterial organisms. The most common side effects are nausea, vomiting, and diarrhea. The narrow-spectrum agents primarily work on a select type of microorganism, such as a gram-positive organism that is susceptible to penicillin. A broad-spectrum antibiotic can attack a larger group of organisms. However, these agents can also cause superinfections because they kill off many of the "good bacteria" in the body. A narrow-spectrum antibiotic is the preferred choice for treatment over a broad-spectrum agent because it primarily destroys the pathogenic organism and also reduces the risk of developing an MDRO infection.

Antiviral agents interfere with the DNA or RNA synthesis required for the virus to duplicate itself. The most common side effects are headache, nausea, vomiting, anorexia, and diarrhea; more severe side effects include acute renal failure, encephalopathy, and bleeding disorders.

Antifungal agents increase permeability of the cell membrane by binding with certain components, leading to decreased nutrient availability to the cell. The most common side effects are headache, fever, chills, nausea, vomiting, and anorexia; more severe side effects include acute kidney and/or liver failure and hemorrhagic gastroenteritis.

Anthelmintic agents cause paralysis of the invading parasite, and common side effects include dizziness, headache, fever, nausea, vomiting, anorexia, diarrhea, and rash.

Box 6.4 Antimicrobial Drug Classifications[a]

ANTIBACTERIAL AGENTS

Narrow Spectrum

Gram-Positive Cocci and Gram-Positive Bacilli

Penicillins G and V
Penicillinase-resistant penicillins: oxacillin, nafcillin
Vancomycin
Erythromycin
Clindamycin

Gram-Negative Aerobes

Aminoglycosides: gentamicin, tobramycin, neomycin, azithromycin
Cephalosporins
- First generation (e.g., cefazolin [Ancef], cephalexin [Keflex])
- Second generation (e.g., cefaclor [Ceclor], cefotetan [Cefotan], cefuroxime [Zinacef])

Mycobacterium Tuberculosis

Ethambutol
Isoniazid
Pyrazinamide
Rifampin

Broad Spectrum

Gram-Positive Cocci and Gram-Negative Bacilli

Broad-spectrum penicillins (e.g., ampicillin)
Cephalosporins
- Third generation (e.g., cefepime [Maxipime], cefixime [Suprax], cefotaxime [Claforan], ceftriaxone [Rocephin])

Tetracyclines (e.g., doxycycline, minocycline)
Carbapenems (e.g., imipenem, meropenem)
Sulfonamides (e.g., sulfasalazine, sulfisoxazole)
Fluoroquinolones: ciprofloxacin

ANTIVIRAL AGENTS

Acyclovir
Amantadine
Azidothymidine
Oseltamivir phosphate
Peramivir
Saquinavir
Zanamivir

ANTIFUNGAL AGENTS

Amphotericin B
Ketoconazole
Itraconazole

ANTHELMINTIC AGENTS

Pyrantel

[a]As with any drug, it is important to know what the drug is and what it is being given for and to provide close nursing observation, especially if the patient has never received the drug in the past. Teaching the patient signs and symptoms to report is also an important part of providing safe and effective nursing care.

Adapted from Burchum J, Rosenthal L: *Lehne's pharmacology for nursing care*, ed 10, St. Louis, 2019, Elsevier.

Supporting Coping Mechanisms

Stress makes the body more vulnerable to invasion by foreign organisms by depressing the immune system. When under excessive stress, the body also is less able to mobilize the elements and cells that promote healing. Nurses should realize that the attitude shown toward

Table 6.9 General Nursing Implications for the Administration of Antimicrobial Drugs

NURSING IMPLICATIONS	RATIONALE
Before Giving the Antimicrobial Drug	
Check all drugs the patient is receiving for drug interactions with the antimicrobial prescribed.	To prevent toxicity or lack of absorption
Know the reason why the patient is to receive an antimicrobial drug (question the health care provider if the drug does not seem appropriate for the patient).	To help prevent drug administration errors
Check that the dosage of the antimicrobial drug is appropriate for the patient who may have decreased kidney or liver function.	To ensure drug levels do not build up to a toxic level
Verify allergies with the patient before administering an antimicrobial drug.	To prevent allergic reaction or adverse outcomes
Ensure cultures have been obtained before administering the antimicrobial agent. If culture and sensitivity results are available, verify that the drug that was ordered is one to which the organism is sensitive. If it is not, clarify the order with the health care provider.	To ensure medication being given is appropriate for the microorganism involved
Check precautions for administration of the antimicrobial drug, especially when the patient is pregnant or lactating.	To prevent harm to the developing fetus or infant
When Giving an Antimicrobial Drug	
Follow the "Six Rights" of medication administration.	To prevent errors and injury to the patient
Give each dose of an antimicrobial drug as close to the scheduled time as possible.	To maintain a consistent blood level of the drug
Check to see if serum drug levels have been ordered. Ensure that they are drawn as specified by the provider.	To ensure drug dosage is effective and to ensure toxicity will not occur
Possible Side/Adverse Effects	
Know and monitor for the possible side effects of the antimicrobial drug. The most common general side effects are gastrointestinal upset, anorexia, nausea, diarrhea, rash, and photosensitivity.	To aid the nurse in effectively teaching the patient about what to observe for and report to the provider
Monitor patient for signs of allergic reaction, such as rash, hives, itching, drug fever, swelling of the mucous membranes, difficulty breathing, or anaphylaxis.	To ensure appropriate interventions are instituted quickly and to prevent more severe outcomes, including death
Check for signs of superinfection in patients taking high doses of an antimicrobial drug for an extended period (e.g., oral thrush, vaginal itching or discharge, diarrhea).	To ensure appropriate countermeasures can be instituted in a timely manner
Patient Teaching	
"Take the medication with a full glass of water."	To aid with absorption
"Take all of an antimicrobial drug prescription, regardless of whether you feel better and have no obvious signs or symptoms of infection."	To prevent the development of multidrug-resistant microorganisms
"Take the medication in relationship to meals." (Different drugs vary in this respect; some need to be taken with food and some should be taken on an empty stomach.)	For best absorption of the drug with minimal gastrointestinal side effects
"Discontinue the drug and notify the health care provider if an allergic reaction occurs."	To ensure treatment is instituted quickly and to prevent more severe outcomes, including death; may require an alternate type of antibiotic to be prescribed
"Use a sunblock and protective clothing when sun exposure is unavoidable when taking an antimicrobial agent that is known to cause photosensitivity."	To decrease the risk of sunburn
Unless contraindicated, "Increase fluid intake to 2500–3000 mL/day, especially when taking a sulfa-type drug."	To prevent crystallization in the kidneys and promote drug excretion

a patient and the ways in which you strive to meet the patient's needs could reduce stress and promote healing.

If an illness is lengthy, concerns about work and home responsibilities may cause anxiety or increase the patient's stress levels. Therefore collaboration with a social worker or case manager for solutions to such problems may be needed.

Patient Teaching for Preventing and Controlling Infection

Appropriate teaching is essential so that the patient and the patient's family will understand why specific precautions are necessary. Before beginning teaching, find out how much the patient or family knows about the patient's condition and the problems that may arise. Nurses have an obligation to teach patients and/or their family how to care for themselves and how to prevent infection through good personal hygiene.

Patient Teaching

How to Prevent and Control Infection

Teach the patient and family:
- The ways in which the infection is transmitted
- How to perform proper hand hygiene
- Correct techniques for wound care
- The approved method for disinfecting or sanitizing equipment, supplies, and linens
- The correct method for proper handling and disposal of contaminated articles
- Any specific precautions for the type of infection the patient has

A patient taking antimicrobial medications at home must be taught how to take them as prescribed and not to discontinue taking any antimicrobial medication, even if symptoms are gone, until all medication has been taken. Explain to the patient and the family that stopping before the full amount of medication has been taken can lead to a superinfection and possibly readmission to the hospital.

◆ EVALUATION

Evaluation of the success of interventions includes data indicating the following:
- Temperature, pulse, and respirations are within normal range.
- WBC count is within normal limits, and cultures are negative.
- Patient is able to rest comfortably.
- Pain and discomfort are absent or decreased in severity.
- Fluid and nutritional needs are being met.

COMMUNITY CARE

As more nurses work in community settings, opportunities to educate the public about preventing the spread of infection become even more important. Controlling the spread of infectious diseases within the community is accomplished in conjunction with public health officials. Their major goals, and those of nurses who work with them, are to (1) promote sanitary standards in communities, (2) identify persons who are highly susceptible to infection and reduce their chances of developing an infectious disease, and (3) provide immunization programs to protect people against certain communicable diseases.

HOME CARE

The home care nurse must educate the patient and family members to help prevent infection. All people living in the home should be instructed to wash their hands as soon as they return home from being out in a public place. Microorganisms are picked up on the hands from a variety of items, such as shopping cart handles, elevator buttons, door handles, and cellphones. Hand sanitizer is available in many public places and can easily be carried in travel-size containers when out in public. The incidence of colds and flu might be decreased if, during influenza season, people who are at increased risk for infection stay away from crowded stores and theaters where pathogens are likely to be airborne.

The home care nurse must teach the techniques of medical asepsis to patients and family members to prevent cross-infection from one person to another or the spread of infection in the patient. Hand hygiene is stressed, and family members are taught not to share personal items, especially toothbrushes or razors that might be contaminated by blood. Dishes and eating utensils are washed with soap and hot water or in the dishwasher. The patient's soiled linens, clothing, and towels should be washed as soon as possible or stored in closed plastic bags until washed. Surfaces contaminated with traces of blood, urine, feces, or vomitus should be sanitized using a clean cloth, soap, and hot water and then recleaned with a 1:10 solution of chlorine bleach and hot water. Within the home, the patient and family are taught to contain infectious wastes such as dressings and soiled tissues in a sealed, impermeable plastic bag, to minimize odors. The bags can then be disposed of in the garbage cans outside the home.

Maintaining a healthy lifestyle that promotes an intact immune system increases a person's resistance to infection. Obtaining adequate sleep, eating properly, and exercising regularly contribute to increased resistance to illness or infection. Adopting effective stress reduction techniques and using them regularly can also be beneficial.

LONG-TERM CARE

Older adults in long-term care or assisted living facilities often have chronic illnesses that add to their susceptibility. Many older adults have low-grade infections of

Health Promotion

What You Can Do to Prevent Infections at Home

- Wash your hands often.
  - **When:** Before eating; before, during, and after handling or preparing food; before dressing a wound, giving or taking medicine, or inserting contact lenses; after contact with body fluids or blood; after changing a diaper; after using the bathroom; after handling animals or their toys, leashes, or waste; after handling anything contaminated, such as trash, drainage, soil, etc.
  - **How:** Wet hands and apply soap, briskly rub hands together for 20 seconds, rinse thoroughly with warm water, and dry with a clean towel.
- Routinely clean surfaces.
  - **In kitchen:** Clean counters, cutting boards, and all other surfaces before, during, and after preparing food, especially meat and poultry. Use hot, soapy water and scrub cutting boards well. Avoid wooden cutting boards because they tend to hold more bacteria.
  - **In bathroom:** Clean and disinfect all surfaces routinely.
- Handle and prepare food safely.
  - **Clean:** Clean hands and work surfaces often.
  - **Separate:** Do not cross-contaminate one food with another; use separate cutting boards for meat and fresh produce and keep food separate in the refrigerator.
  - **Cook:** Cook foods to proper temperatures; use a food thermometer. Find recommended food cooking temperatures at www.isitdoneyet.gov.
  - **Chill:** Refrigerate foods promptly. Do not thaw frozen foods on the countertop.
- Get immunized.
  - Make sure you and your loved ones get the necessary shots suggested by your health care provider at the proper time, and maintain immunization records for the family. Ask your provider about special programs that provide free shots for your child or older adult parent.
- Use antimicrobials appropriately.
  - Take antimicrobials exactly as prescribed by your health care provider. Antibiotics do not work against viruses such as colds or flu.
- Be careful with pets.
  - Follow the immunization schedule for your pets as recommended by the vet.
  - Clean litter boxes daily and perform hand hygiene immediately afterward.
  - Make sure your child does not put any object or hands in his or her mouth after touching animals.
  - Wash hands thoroughly after contact with animals, especially after visiting farms, petting zoos, and fairs.
  - Use flea and tick prevention treatment on cats and dogs.
- Avoid contact with wild animals.
  - Do not leave food around and keep garbage cans sealed around your home.
  - Clear brush, grass, and debris around your home.
  - Seal any entrance holes to animal dens, if any are found inside or outside your home.
  - Use insect repellent to prevent ticks.

the urinary, respiratory, or gastrointestinal tract that can be easily passed on to others if hand hygiene is not consistently practiced. Help residents wash their hands before meals and after toileting, before and after being in community rooms such as the dining room or social activities lounge, and any time their hands become soiled. Cleaning incontinent patients promptly and maintaining skin integrity are essential nursing functions.

Get Ready for the NCLEX® Examination!

Key Points

- Normal flora are needed to help prevent harmful microorganisms from colonizing or infecting the body.
- An infection is the presence and growth of pathogenic microorganisms in a susceptible host to the extent that tissue damage occurs.
- The relationship among the host, the agent, and the environment is what determines whether an infection will occur.
- A pathogen is any organism that, if allowed to grow, can cause infection or disease.
- Multiple types of antimicrobial drugs can be used to fight infection: antibiotics for bacterial infections, antivirals for viral infections, and antifungals for fungal infections.
- The body has mechanical barriers, such as the skin and mucous membranes, and chemical barriers, such as tears or saliva, that help fight against infection.
- Fever is one of the primary immune responses to fighting off invading microorganisms.
- Hand hygiene is the number-one way to prevent the spread of infection.
- There are three types of Transmission-Based Precautions: airborne, contact, and droplet. Each requires different PPE and isolation protocols.
- A patient with suspected or confirmed Ebola virus infection requires that PPE be donned and doffed so that no skin or mucus membranes are exposed to the patient's blood or body fluids at any time during the provision of nursing care.

- Using respiratory hygiene and cough etiquette helps prevent the spread of infection.
- Blood or other body fluid specimens for culture must be collected before the start of any antimicrobial agent.
- Assess how much the patient already knows about preventing the spread of infection and teach about hand hygiene, the correct use of antimicrobial agents, cleaning of wounds, and keeping the home environment clean.
- You must model scrupulous hand hygiene compliance for patients and family members.

Additional Learning Resources

SG Go to your Study Guide for additional learning activities to help you master this chapter content.

Go to your Evolve website (http://evolve.elsevier.com/deWit/medsurg) for the following FREE learning resources:

- Animations, audio, and video
- Answers and rationales for questions and activities
- Glossary with pronunciations in English and Spanish
- Interactive Review Questions and more!

Review Questions for the NCLEX® Examination

1. You are admitting a patient with an infected abdominal wound. Wound cultures are positive for methicillin-resistant *Staphylococcus aureus.* Appropriate nursing care for this patient includes:
  1. monitoring temperature and white blood cell count.
  2. placing the patient on strict intake and output.
  3. instituting respiratory precautions.
  4. encouraging ambulation along the hallways.

NCLEX Client Need: Safe and Effective Care Environment: Safety and Infection Control

2. During an assessment, you note fever, fatigue, general weakness, cold and clammy skin, nausea, vomiting, and diarrhea. You recognize that the body is fighting infection by what means?
  1. Antigen-antibody reaction
  2. The inflammatory response
  3. Chemical release of interferon
  4. The acquired immune response

NCLEX Client Need: Physiological Integrity: Physiological Adaptation

3. Which patient instruction is most critical to a patient being discharged on antibiotic therapy?
  1. "Wash your hands."
  2. "Increase fluid intake."
  3. "Reduce stress."
  4. "Take all the antibiotics as prescribed."

NCLEX Client Need: Physiological Integrity: Pharmacological Therapies

4. You are observing a nursing student who must perform a dressing change for a patient. You would intervene if the student:
  1. gathers all needed supplies prior to entering the patient room.
  2. identifies the patient using two identifiers.
  3. performs hand hygiene before donning clean gloves to remove the old dressing.
  4. prepares supplies, dons sterile gloves, and removes the old dressing.

NCLEX Client Need: Safe and Effective Care Environment: Safety and Infection Control

5. When administering an ordered antimicrobial for an infection, you should check the laboratory results for:
  1. elevated white blood cells.
  2. culture and sensitivity.
  3. C-reactive protein.
  4. kidney and liver function.

NCLEX Client Need: Physiological Integrity: Pharmacological Therapies

6. You assume the care of a patient with active pulmonary tuberculosis. You know that appropriate management of the patient includes: (*Select all that apply*)
  1. placement of the patient in a room with special air handling.
  2. use of a face shield and gown for patient contact.
  3. use of Standard Precautions with airborne precautions.
  4. administration of ordered antimicrobials.
  5. use of fit tested N95 masks or respirators.

NCLEX Client Need: Safe and Effective Care Environment: Safety and Infection Control

7. The need for protective isolation and its parameters are being explained to the patient. She wails, "How can I hug my children when I am locked up in this room?" An appropriate response would be:
  1. "They can see you through the glass door."
  2. "You can communicate through the intercom system or via your cellphone."
  3. "All people carry microorganisms, and your immune system cannot fight off any infection right now."
  4. "It won't be long before you can hug them again, and we need to keep you safe from infection."

NCLEX Client Need: Safe and Effective Care Environment: Safety and Infection Control

8. Which intervention would you implement for a patient with active pulmonary tuberculosis who is socially isolated related to imposed airborne precautions?
  1. Limit the number of visitors to immediate family.
  2. Suggest alternative means of contact, such as email and phone calls.
  3. Arrange for a nursing assistant to sit with the patient.
  4. Reinforce the rationale for airborne precautions.

NCLEX Client Need: Psychosocial Integrity

9. You are caring for an older adult patient and note a change in mental status. The skin is flushed, warm, and dry. There is a full, bounding pulse and decreased urine output. In order of priority, which actions should you take? *(Place in order of priority.)*
   1. Notify the charge nurse of your findings.
   2. Draw the patient's blood as ordered by the health care provider for blood cultures.
   3. Take a full set of vital signs and compare them to the baseline.
   4. Check the patient's history to determine risk for sepsis.

   NCLEX Client Need: Physiological Integrity: Reduction of Risk Potential
10. Cross-infection among members of the household who care for a relative with a severe infection can be prevented by which behavior(s)? *(Select all that apply.)*
    1. Sharing personal items
    2. Practicing good hand hygiene
    3. Using a diluted bleach to clean surfaces
    4. Sealing used dressings in impermeable bags
    5. Washing soiled linens weekly

    NCLEX Client Need: Safe and Effective Care Environment: Safety and Infection Control

Critical Thinking Questions

Scenario A

Mrs. Compton, age 44, is admitted to the hospital for a hysterectomy. During the admission assessment procedure, you notice a large, draining abscess in her axillary region. She also has a temperature of 100° F (37.7° C), and she tells you that she has not felt well for the past few days.

1. What would be your course of action after this assessment?

Scenario B

Mr. Lopez, age 18, has been admitted to the orthopedic unit after an automobile accident. He sustained an open fracture of the femur which has been surgically repaired.

1. What are some expected signs and symptoms of inflammation that he might experience?
2. What specific problems might his care present for you?

Scenario C

Mrs. Kay is an older adult woman who comes to the clinic for treatment of an abrasion on her arm that she sustained "while picking up my cat." She is alert, oriented, and very cheerful and talkative. You notice that she is slightly underweight and that her clothes are not very clean.

1. What additional assessment might you make about the wound and the injury because she mentioned the cat?
2. What changes related to aging are likely to affect Mrs. Kay's natural defense mechanisms to fight infection?
3. Based on the scenario, identify issues that will affect wound healing and self-care for Mrs. Kay.
4. Explain why older adults may have a normal or even subnormal temperature in the presence of infection.

Care of Patients With Pain

7

http://evolve.elsevier.com/deWit/medsurg

Objectives

Theory

1. Review the gate control theory of pain and its relationship to nursing care.
2. Discuss how the neuromatrix and central sensitivity theories help explain types of pain other than those arising from tissue injury.
3. Demonstrate an understanding of the current view of pain as a specific entity requiring appropriate intervention.
4. Compare nociceptive and neuropathic pain and nursing care for each.
5. Explain how pain perception is affected by personal situations and cultural backgrounds.
6. Analyze the major differences between acute and chronic pain and their management.
7. Give examples of the different pharmacologic approaches to pain that include the use of adjunctive measures.

Clinical Practice

8. Demonstrate the use of appropriate pain evaluation tools and measures for a variety of patients.
9. Recognize common side effects of analgesics and describe techniques for addressing them.
10. Employ nonpharmacologic approaches to pain management with a variety of patients.
11. Demonstrate the use of the nursing process when caring for patients experiencing pain.

Key Terms

acute pain (ă-KŪT pān, p. 130)
adjuvant (ĂJ-ŭ-vănt, p. 130)
buccal mucosa (BŪK-ăl mū-CŌ-să, p. 139)
chronic pain (KRŎN-ĭk pān, p. 130)
endorphins (ĕn-DŎR-fĭnz, p. 128)
epidural (ĕ-pĭ-DŬ-rŭl, p. 139)
intractable pain (ĭn-TRĂK-tĭ-bŭl pān, p. 140)
modulation (mŏd-ū-LĀ-shŭn, p. 129)
neuropathic pain (nū-rō-PĂTH-ĭk pān, p. 130)
nociceptive pain (nō-sē-SĔP-tĭv pān, p. 128)
pain threshold (pān THRĔSH-ōld, p. 130)
pain tolerance (pān TŎL-ŭr-ĕnz, p. 130)
perception (pĕr-CĔP-shŭn, p. 129)
phantom pain (FĂN-tŭm pān, p. 128)
placebos (plă-SĒ-bōz, p. 137)
referred pain (rĭ-FŬRD pān, p. 134)
transduction (trănz-DŬK-shŭn, p. 128)
transmission (trănz-MĬ-shŭn, p. 129)

Concepts Covered in This Chapter

- Pain
- Fatigue
- Stress
- Patient Education
- Safety
- Care Coordination

THEORIES OF PAIN

Pain is considered not just a symptom, but also a specific problem that needs to be treated. *Pain* is defined as a neurologic response to unpleasant stimuli. Pain receptors are distributed abundantly throughout the skin and in many deeper structures of the body. Receptors for pain do not become dulled with repeated stimulation, and under some conditions repeated stimulation results in an increase in the acuteness of the pain sensation.

Several theoretical models are used to describe the experience of pain. It is important to understand that the way in which pain is believed to be generated guides treatment choices. Research is demonstrating that the mechanism of pain is much more complex than previously thought and that early pain theories inadequately address nonspecific pain such as fibromyalgia and non–tissue-related conditions such as phantom pain. One theory explains that pain is initiated when various chemicals are released from damaged cells. It may be helpful to think of pain as being controlled by a "gate" in the central nervous system (Fig. 7.1). When the gate is open, the pain sensation is allowed through. When the gate is closed, the pain sensation is blocked. The **gate control theory** recognizes that stimuli other than pain pass through the same gate. When a large volume of nonpainful stimuli are competing for the gate, pain impulses may be blocked. A high volume of pain, however, may override other stimuli and pass

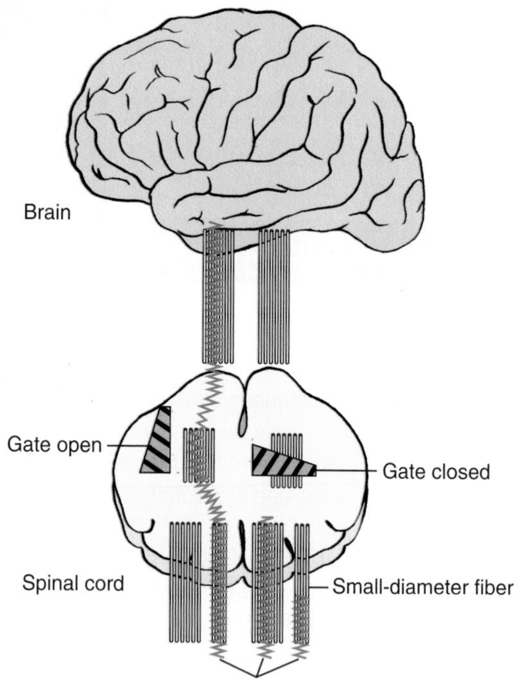

Fig. 7.1 The gate control theory of pain. (From Williams P: *deWit's fundamental concepts and skills for nursing*, ed 5, St. Louis, 2018, Elsevier.)

through the gate, causing the individual to perceive the pain.

Aspects of this theory relate to nursing practice in several ways:

- Two types of nerve fibers—small-diameter and large-diameter nerve fibers—carry pain stimuli.
- Activity in the small-diameter nerve fibers seems to open the gate, and activity in the large-diameter nerve fibers seems to close it.
- Massage and vibration produce activity in the large-diameter nerve fibers.
- High levels of sensory input create brainstem impulses that seem to close the gate. Distraction in the form of activity or social interaction produces these brainstem impulses.
- An increase in anxiety seems to open the gate, and a decrease in anxiety seems to close it. The fear that pain will not be controlled may increase pain intensity, and knowing that pain can be or is being controlled may reduce pain.

Another way of looking at pain and its management is the idea of *pieces of pain*. The more intense the pain, the greater the number of pieces, and therefore a greater number of pieces of treatment will be required to control the pain. This idea indicates that inadequate analgesia results in leftover pieces of pain, and so total relief or control has not been achieved. The pieces of pain are a complex bundle of physiologic nerve and tissue responses as well as personal experience, cultural, and social influences. To be effective, pain management requires a holistic approach.

The human body produces substances called **endorphins** (endogenous opiates) that attach to receptor sites and block pain sensation. It is unknown how endorphins work, but their properties appear to modify and inhibit unpleasant stimuli, reduce anxiety, and relieve pain. Endorphins may produce feelings of euphoria and well-being. For example, the "runner's high" may occur because endorphins are released after physical exercise. Endorphins also are associated with states of pleasure such as laughter, appetizing food, love, and sex (Chaudhry & Bhimji, 2018).

Another theory of pain is that there is a *neuromatrix* where pain is a multidimensional experience in which stimuli are influenced by such things as past experience, cultural learning, personality variables, and influences from various body systems. This theory links pain to the central nervous system. Multiple types of pain are not fully explained by the idea that traumatized tissue sends signals to the brain, where pain is processed. Centralizing the pain experience to the central nervous system explains **phantom pain**, which occurs where no actual tissue is involved but real pain exists (Turk & Gatchel, 2018). Another term that has a similar application is *central sensitivity syndrome*. This terminology is used to explain general pain conditions such as fibromyalgia (Czarnecki & Turner, 2018).

CLASSIFICATION OF PAIN

Pain can be classified as one of three types: (1) acute pain, such as from trauma or surgery; (2) cancer pain; and (3) noncancer pain (e.g., postherpetic neuralgia, diabetic neuropathy, arthritis). There are two pathophysiologic classifications of pain: *nociceptive* and *neuropathic*. Some pain researchers are proposing an "other" category for pain not explained by tissue or nerve irritation. If not all pain is from a nociceptive or neuropathic source, different treatments are needed to address the "other" types of pain.

NOCICEPTIVE PAIN

Nociceptive pain is associated with pain stimuli from either *somatic* (body tissue) or *visceral* (organ) structures. Somatic nociceptive pain arises from injury to tissue where pain receptors called *nociceptors* are located. These nociceptors may be found in skin, connective tissue, bones, joints, or muscles. Trauma, burns, or surgery may cause injuries that trigger somatic nociceptive pain. Visceral nociceptive pain arises from pathophysiologic conditions in visceral organs, such as the organs of the gastrointestinal tract. Pathologic conditions that trigger visceral nociceptive pain include tumors and obstructions of the organs (Table 7.1).

Four pain processes are associated with nociceptive pain (Fig. 7.2; Lewis et al., 2017):

1. **Transduction** begins when tissue damage causes the release of substances that stimulate the nociceptors and initiate the sensation of pain.

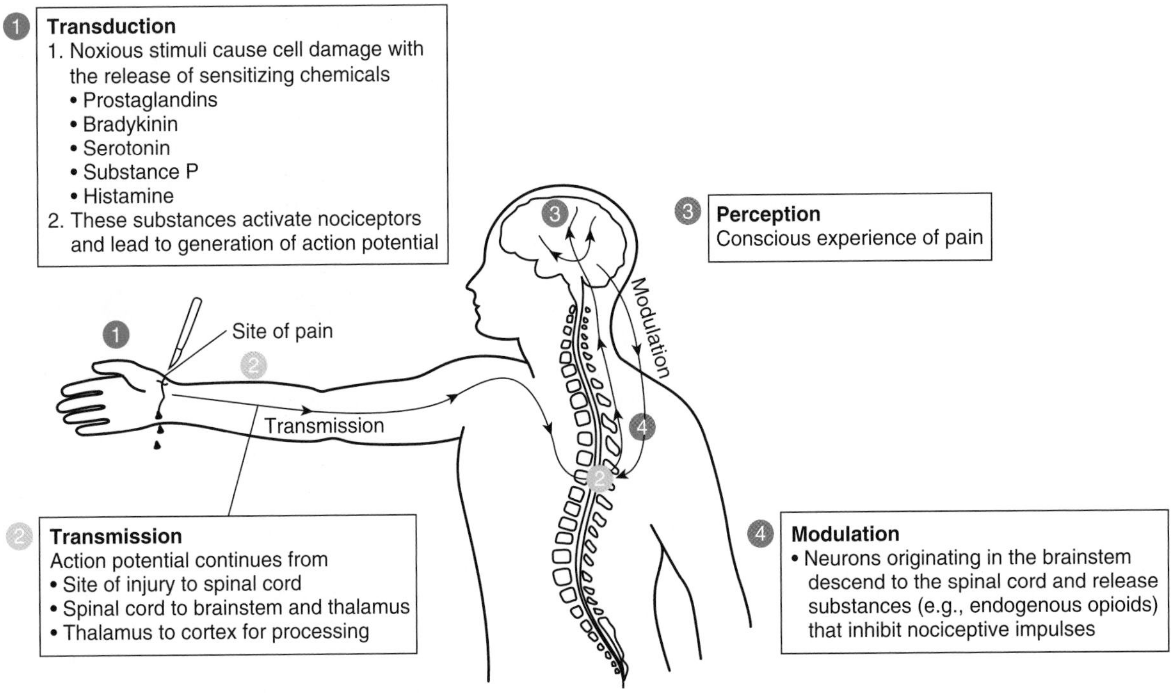

1 Transduction
1. Noxious stimuli cause cell damage with the release of sensitizing chemicals
• Prostaglandins
• Bradykinin
• Serotonin
• Substance P
• Histamine
2. These substances activate nociceptors and lead to generation of action potential
3 Perception
Conscious experience of pain
Modulation
Site of pain
Transmission
2 Transmission
Action potential continues from
• Site of injury to spinal cord
• Spinal cord to brainstem and thalamus
• Thalamus to cortex for processing
4 Modulation
• Neurons originating in the brainstem descend to the spinal cord and release substances (e.g., endogenous opioids) that inhibit nociceptive impulses

Fig. 7.2 Nociceptive pain originates when tissue is injured. *1,* Transduction. *2,* Transmission. *3,* Perception. *4,* Modulation. (From Lewis SL, Bucher L, Heitkemper MM, et al.: *Medical-surgical nursing: assessment and management of clinical problems,* ed 10, St. Louis, 2017, Elsevier.)

Table 7.1 Physiologic Sources of Pain

PHYSIOLOGIC STRUCTURE	CHARACTERISTICS OF PAIN	SOURCES OF ACUTE POSTOPERATIVE PAIN	SOURCES OF CHRONIC PAIN SYNDROMES
Nociceptive Pain			
Somatic Pain Cutaneous or superficial: skin and subcutaneous tissues Deep somatic: bone, muscle, blood vessels, connective tissues	Sharp, burning, dull, aching, cramping	Incisional pain, pain at insertion sites of tubes and drains, wound complications, orthopedic procedures, skeletal muscle tissue	Bony metastases, osteoarthritis and rheumatoid arthritis, low back pain, peripheral vascular diseases
Visceral Pain Organs and the linings of the body cavities	Poorly localized Diffuse, deep cramping or splitting, sharp, stabbing	Chest tubes, abdominal tubes and drains, bladder distention or spasms, intestinal distention	Pancreatitis, liver metastases, colitis, appendicitis
Neuropathic Pain			
Peripheral and central nerve fibers, spinal cord, and central nervous system	Poorly localized Shooting, burning, fiery, shocklike, sharp, painful numbness	Postmastectomy pain, nerve compression or injury caused by a surgical procedure	HIV-related pain, diabetic neuropathy, postherpetic neuralgia, chemotherapy-induced neuropathies, multiple sclerosis

Adapted from Ignatavicius DD, Workman ML, Rebar CR, et al.: *Medical-surgical nursing: critical thinking for collaborative care,* ed 9, St. Louis, 2018, Elsevier.
HIV, Human immunodeficiency virus.

2. **Transmission** involves movement of the pain sensation to the spinal cord.
3. **Perception** occurs when impulses reach the brain and the pain is recognized.
4. **Modulation** occurs when neurons in the brain send signals back down the spinal cord by release of neurotransmitters.

Aspects of nociceptive pain relate to nursing practice in several ways:

- Treatment of nociceptive pain may be directed toward one or all of the four phases.
- Nonsteroidal antiinflammatory drugs (NSAIDs) work by blocking the production of the substances that trigger the nociceptors in the transduction phase.

- Opioids interfere with the transmission phase.
- Nonpharmacologic treatments, such as distraction and guided imagery, may be effective during the perception phase.
- Drugs that block neurotransmitter uptake work in the modulation stage.

NEUROPATHIC PAIN

Neuropathic pain is associated with a dysfunction of the nervous system that involves an abnormality in the processing of sensations. These dysfunctions in the nervous system are often associated with medical conditions rather than with tissue damage. The dysfunction may occur in the peripheral or central nervous system. In peripheral nervous system neuropathic pain, it is believed that pain receptors become sensitive to stimuli and send pain signals more easily. Nerve endings grow additional branches that send stronger pain signals to the brain. Neuropathic pain may be the result of damage to nerve roots, such as compression or entrapment.

Aspects of neuropathic pain relate to nursing practice in several ways:

- Analgesics and opioids usually do not relieve neuropathic pain.
- **Adjuvant** medications such as NSAIDs, tricyclic antidepressants, anticonvulsants, and corticosteroids relieve neuropathic pain.

> **Think Critically**
>
> What type of pain do you think a patient with an acute gallbladder attack might be experiencing?

PERCEPTION OF PAIN

Pain is a subjective experience. Only the patient knows the location of the pain, its degree of intensity, and which treatment regimen works and how long it is effective. **This is why the patient must be asked about pain.** (See Focused Assessment.) Reactions to pain can vary widely from person to person and in the same individual under different circumstances.

Pain threshold is the point at which pain is perceived. Relaxation and distraction strategies can alter the perception of pain. **Pain tolerance** is the length of time or the intensity of pain a person will endure before outwardly responding to it. Tolerance varies among people and is influenced by culture, pain experience, expectations, and role behaviors. People with **acute pain** (of recent onset, lasting less than 6 months) may have physiologic symptoms such as increased pulse and respiratory rates, increased blood pressure, diaphoresis, and increased muscle tension. They may also experience nausea and vomiting. People with **chronic pain** (lasting months or years) may have learned adaptive methods that allow them to have some control over their pain. Symptoms associated with chronic pain include irritability, depression, withdrawal, and insomnia. Coping with any pain takes a lot of energy, and patients who are debilitated are less able to withstand pain than are people with healthy energy levels. Fatigue caused by pain can lead to an increase in pain perception. Pain causes a variety of physiologic responses, and while the presence of any of these factors may indicate pain, their absence does not prove the absence of pain.

> **Clinical Cues**
>
> Patients who have a substance abuse problem are not to be denied pain medication when they experience acute pain. Patients who are being treated for long-term chronic pain often require higher doses of pain medication after surgery or trauma.

A person's cultural background influences feelings about pain. In much of Western culture it is considered desirable to have a high pain tolerance, particularly among men. Other cultures promote the idea that to endure pain is natural or honorable. Your role as the nurse is to develop a therapeutic relationship with the patient that allows them to express their thoughts, fears, and beliefs regarding pain. This then helps you guide appropriate pain-relief approaches. You must make the values and beliefs of the patient central to the plan of care even when you do not share those values. **Learning to accept without judgment the various ways of coping with and expressing pain is a necessary process for nurses.**

ACUTE VERSUS CHRONIC PAIN

ACUTE PAIN

Acute pain usually has a known cause: a surgical procedure, minor burn, sprained ankle, or other injury causing tissue trauma. The pain sensation may be brief or last for several weeks to months. Pain extending beyond 6 months is considered chronic pain. Table 7.2 compares acute and chronic pain. Concept Map 7.1 shows the various types and causes of pain.

CHRONIC PAIN

Chronic pain may have a known cause or be a result of central sensitivity syndrome or neuromatrix causes. Because of the physiologic mechanisms and psychosocial factors, using nonpharmacological interventions to treat chronic pain can be effective. Behavioral and psychological interventions may alter how the patient experiences the pain by affecting the patient's emotional state and cognitive process, thereby altering the pain experience. Control of chronic pain is very difficult and many times inadequate. Patients become discouraged with less than optimal pain control, which makes it difficult to live life in a meaningful way. Pain is a stressor to the body and takes energy to manage. For these reasons chronic pain is often associated with depression and fatigue.

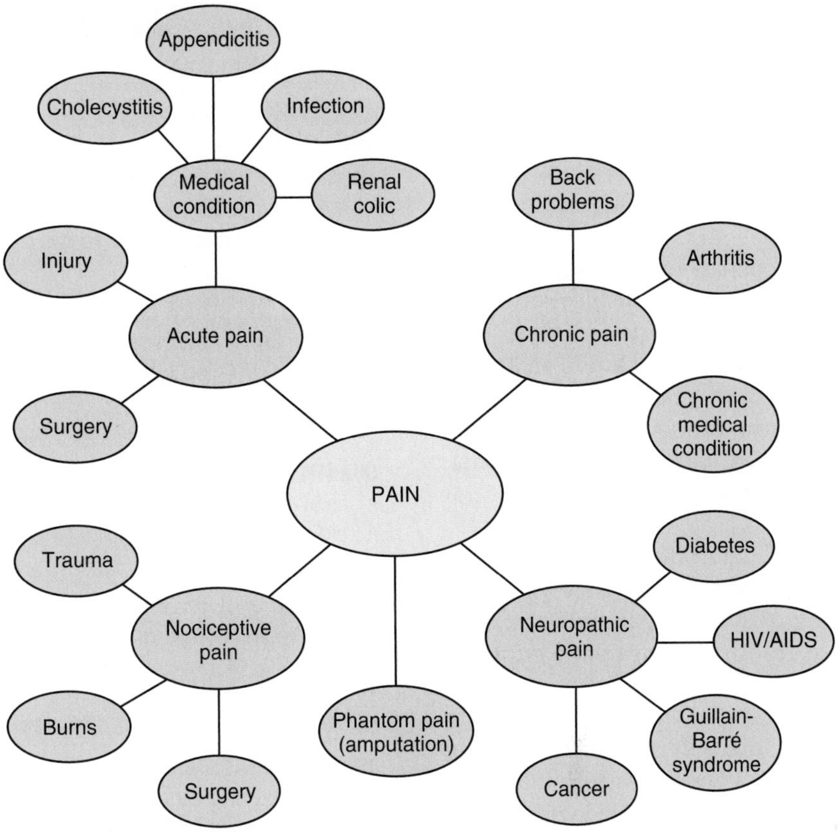

Concept Map 7.1 The various types and causes of pain. *AIDS,* Acquired immunodeficiency syndrome; *HIV,* human immunodeficiency virus.

Table 7.2 Acute Versus Chronic Pain

	ACUTE PAIN	CHRONIC PAIN
Duration	Hours to days.	Months to years.
Prognosis for relief	Good; may resolve spontaneously or in response to analgesic therapy.	Poor unless complicating factors are removed; spontaneous relief is unusual.
Cause	Relatively easy to identify.	Sometimes the cause is known, but diagnosis may be complex or undetermined.
Psychosocial effects	Usually transient or none. May temporarily disrupt normal activities or routine.	Can affect ability to earn a living, enjoy social activities, or maintain self-esteem.
Effect of therapy	Medication is usually beneficial; surgery is often helpful.	Medications may be helpful, but patient may become dependent. Multiple-medication regimen may be used. Surgery may help but also may worsen the problem.

Older Adult Care Points

Between 60% and 75% of older adults have chronic pain. The most common conditions that cause pain in this age group are joint problems from osteoarthritis, degenerative disk disease, osteoporosis, low back pain, and pain from previous fracture sites. The pain may be combined with other chronic diseases and cause debilitation. If chronic pain is adequately controlled, quality of life is improved (Murphy, Karlin-Zysman, & Anandan, 2018).

NURSING MANAGEMENT

ASSESSMENT (DATA COLLECTION)

Because no technology can accurately and objectively measure pain, you must use a combination of evaluation methods, including observation, rating scales, and the patient's self-report of pain. The patient is the only one with firsthand knowledge of the pain. Their report of pain needs to be used for management decisions, as do all other pain data. **Pain is to be assessed every time vital signs are taken (or more frequently if**

indicated) by asking the patient to rate any pain and describe its characteristics.

Observation

Appearance. The patient's face may look tense, drawn, or pale. There may be a grimace or even a look of fear. The body may be in a rigid, nonmoving position.

Behavior. A normally verbal patient may become quiet or withdrawn. One who is normally pleasant may become irritable, demanding, or argumentative. The individual may protect or "cradle" the painful area with the hands or arms or assume a fetal position with the legs drawn up. Tears, refusal of food or drink, or any behavior that is out of the ordinary for the individual may be an indication of pain.

Activity level. A person in pain often reduces activity to a minimum. Staying in bed, creeping slowly from place to place, stooping over during ambulation, and stopping frequently to rest or lean against a support can all indicate pain.

Verbalization. Many individuals in pain may verbalize their discomfort, but it is not always easy to interpret the degree of pain from what is said. Limited vocabulary, lack of experience in verbalizing abstract concepts, fear of disbelief or disapproval, cultural stoicism, and fear of medication side effects or of becoming addicted to analgesics all can impair the person's ability to communicate the degree of pain.

Physiologic clues. Physiologic clues to pain include rapid, shallow, or guarded respirations; pallor; diaphoresis; increased pulse; elevated blood pressure; dilated pupils; and tenseness of the skeletal muscles. Other problems can also cause these physiologic clues to occur. All physiologic changes must be fully assessed to determine the cause.

Clinical Cues

When questioning a patient's comfort level, use words other than *pain*. For some individuals pain does not include soreness, discomfort, aching, or other milder forms of pain. Find out how the patient labels their discomfort and then use that term when reassessing their pain.

Pain Rating Scales

Several rating scales have been developed to evaluate pain. When using a pain rating scale, it is important that the nursing staff use it consistently and that the patient fully understands how to use it. The type of scale being used and any pertinent information about how the patient uses the scale must be communicated to the health care team.

Numbered scale. Numbered scales ask the patient to rate the degree of pain as a number from 0 to 5 or 0 to 10, with 0 indicating no pain and the highest number indicating the greatest amount of pain imaginable. The numbers in between show graduated levels of pain. The scale may be verbal or drawn on a piece of paper so that the person can mark or point to the degree of pain. Numbered scales can be used very effectively with people who have a good understanding of the numerical concept. They are not appropriate for young children, anyone who has difficulty with numbers, or anyone who is confused or disoriented.

Visual scale. Some visual scales use photographs or simple drawings of faces that progress through a series of expressions showing a pain-free state (happy and smiling) and then increased discomfort. The final image shows a face either crying or with an intense grimace (Fig. 7.3).

Focused Assessment

The Patient With Pain

Ask the following questions while assessing a patient with pain.

LOCATION

- Where is your pain?
- Would you please point to the pain?

CHARACTERISTICS

- Would you please describe your pain?
- What words would you use to describe the pain? (Aching, burning, gnawing, sharp, stabbing, shooting, etc.)
- Is the pain constant or does it come and go?

QUANTITY

- How strong or intense is your pain?
- How strong is your pain on this scale?

PATTERN

- How long have you had this pain?
- Did the pain begin during activity, before eating, after eating?
- Did the pain start suddenly?
- Has the pain increased over time?

ASSOCIATED FACTORS

- Have you had other symptoms such as nausea and vomiting, shortness of breath, rapid heart rate, sweating?
- What do your family members usually do when they are in pain?
- Do you have any chronic problems that cause pain?

ALLEVIATING FACTORS

- What have you tried to relieve the pain? (Medication, certain position, application of heat or cold, distraction, etc.)
- Did it work?

AGGRAVATING FACTORS

- What, if anything, makes the pain increase?

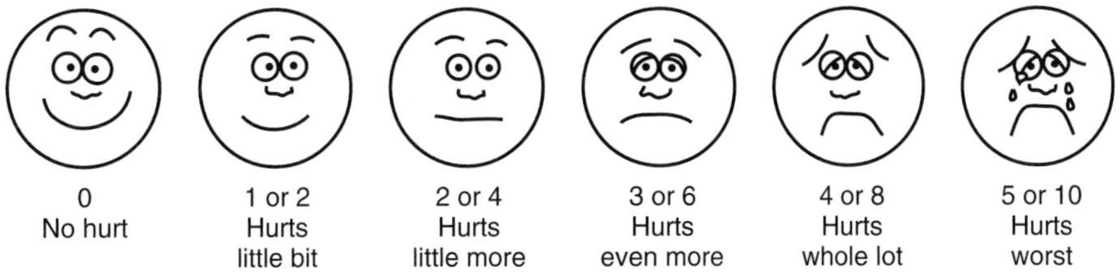

Fig. 7.3 Wong-Baker FACES pain rating scale. For coding purposes, numbers 0, 2, 4, 6, 8, and 10 can be substituted for the 0-to-5 system to accommodate a 0-to-10 system. (From Hockenberry MJ, Wilson D, Rodgers CC: *Wong's essentials of pediatric nursing,* ed 10, St. Louis, 2017, Elsevier.)

Face	0 No particular expression or smile	1 Occasional grimace or frown, withdrawn, disinterested	2 Frequent to constant frown, clenched jaw, quivering chin
Legs	0 Normal position or relaxed	1 Uneasy, restless, tense	2 Kicking, or legs drawn up
Activity	0 Lying quietly, normal position, moves easily	1 Squirming, shifting back and forth, tense	2 Arched, rigid, or jerking
Cry	0 No cry (awake or asleep)	1 Moans or whimpers, occasional complaint	2 Cries steadily, screams or sobs, frequent complaints
Consolability	0 Content, relaxed	1 Reassured by occasional touching, hugging, or talking to; distractible	2 Difficult to console or comfort

Fig. 7.4 Face, legs, activity, cry, and consolability (FLACC) scale used to assess pain in cognitively impaired people. (Copyright 2002, reprinted with permission from The Regents of the University of Michigan.)

Color scale. A color scale allows the patient to select colors that represent varying degrees of pain. Colored pieces of paper or plastic (e.g., poker chips), crayons, or markers can be used. The patient selects a color that represents no pain, a color that represents severe pain, and then one, two, or three other colors for pain levels in between. This scale is often used with children, but very young children cannot understand more than three or four possible choices.

Pieces of pain scale. A pieces of pain scale uses five poker chips or other identical, plain objects that represent "pieces" of pain. The patient indicates the degree of pain by selecting the number of chips that equals the intensity of pain being experienced.

Behavioral pain (face, legs, activity, cry, consolability [FLACC]) scale. A behavioral pain scale is used with patients who are cognitively impaired or who cannot speak. You assess the patient's behavior in categories such as facial expression, limb movement, and activity level (Fig. 7.4). A score from 0 to 2 is obtained for each category, and the category scores are added together to arrive at a pain score total of 0 to 10. This type of scale is useful when assessing the pain of confused or nonverbal adults, infants, and young children.

? Think Critically

Explain the difference between acute and chronic pain.

Data Collection Difficulties

Much of the data gathered when assessing a patient's pain comes from conversations with the patient. Concepts of the true meaning of words in a common language may vary greatly from person to person. It is important to discuss the common words used to describe pain and to agree on their meaning (Table 7.3). It is important for documentation to include the patient's exact words.

Having to communicate through an interpreter or to deal with language difficulties when you and the patient do not speak the same language compounds the problem of communicating pain. Whenever possible, use a medical professional (rather than a family member) with a good knowledge of both languages as an interpreter. Most hospitals have a list of approved interpreters to assist in these situations. Patients may hide personal, embarrassing, or painful information if the interpreter is a family member or friend. All acute care facilities are required to have translation services available. The translators may be available in person or by telephone. Fully use the services available so that accurate pain assessments are performed.

Table 7.3 Common Terms to Help Patients Describe Pain

Degree of pain (from least to most severe)	Absent, minimal, mild, moderate, fairly severe, severe, very or extremely severe, excruciating
Quality of pain	Crushing, tingling, itching, throbbing, pulsating, twisting, pulling, burning, searing, stabbing, tearing, biting, blinding, nauseating, debilitating
Frequency of pain	Constant, intermittent, occasional, related to something specific (e.g., only when coughing)

Describing the location of pain can be made difficult by the phenomenon of **referred pain** (pain felt in a part of the body that is different from where the pain originates) (Fig. 7.5). Heart pain may be felt in the jaw or radiating down the arm. Gastric pain may center in the area of the heart rather than in the stomach. There also is a tendency not to believe an individual's statement of pain if there is no outward appearance of pain. For example, a patient watching an exciting football game with a friend may enjoy the game even if their surgical incision is quite painful. The lack of a grimace or of physiologic changes indicative of pain may be viewed as an absence of pain, when in fact the patient is using distraction as a way of coping with the presence of pain. People may fall asleep even though pain is severe, particularly if uncontrolled pain has left them in a state of exhaustion.

? Think Critically

Which pain scale would you use for a 24-year-old patient? Why? Which one would you use for a patient who is cognitively impaired? Why?

Cultural Considerations

Cultural, Social, and Faith-Based Beliefs and Pain

There is extreme variation in how individuals perceive pain. This perception of pain is influenced by multiple factors, including genetics and culture. Culture includes shared beliefs and values from racial, religious, or social groups. Social groups include individual families. With the current diversity in the United States, it is very difficult to assume shared beliefs based on ethnicity, religion, or affiliation with a group. You must consider the patient's individual values and beliefs regarding pain, understanding that a mix of beliefs and expressions may be held by the same individual.

	PREFERENCES AND ACTION
CULTURAL/SOCIAL FACTORS	
Stoic/denies pain: may not admit to having pain and may continue with regular activities.	May have many reasons for not admitting to pain: lack of understanding of pain control methods, fear of addiction, family expectations.
Open expression of pain: very vocal and descriptive.	Be accepting of the patient's expression of pain and obtain the necessary assessment to guide adequate pain relief.
Controlling: pain is something to be controlled, and this must be done promptly.	Wants immediate actions taken. Involve the patient in the pain management plan, so they understand what is being done and the timing.
Not to be tolerated: pain is unacceptable and must be eliminated.	May be in denial about their medical condition. Will need information on what pain is expected, how the health care team will manage their pain, and how they can help.
Inevitable: life is painful, and pain is something to be endured.	May need to be informed about options to make them more comfortable.
FAITH-BASED BELIEFS	
It is God's will: God is in control.	May ask for God's intercession through prayer. May wish for clergy visit.
Punishment: consequence of actions.	May not want pain medication, believing that they deserve the pain.
Means of attaining greater reward: enduring pain gains rewards in the afterlife.	May not wish relief from the pain so that greater rewards will be earned.
Imbalance in the universe: pain indicates that imbalance exists.	May prefer cultural treatments. Pain is spiritual.
Spirits cause sickness/pain: external forces are causing pain.	May want a spiritual leader to perform rituals.
Atonement: making amends for wrong actions.	May be hesitant to take pain medications.

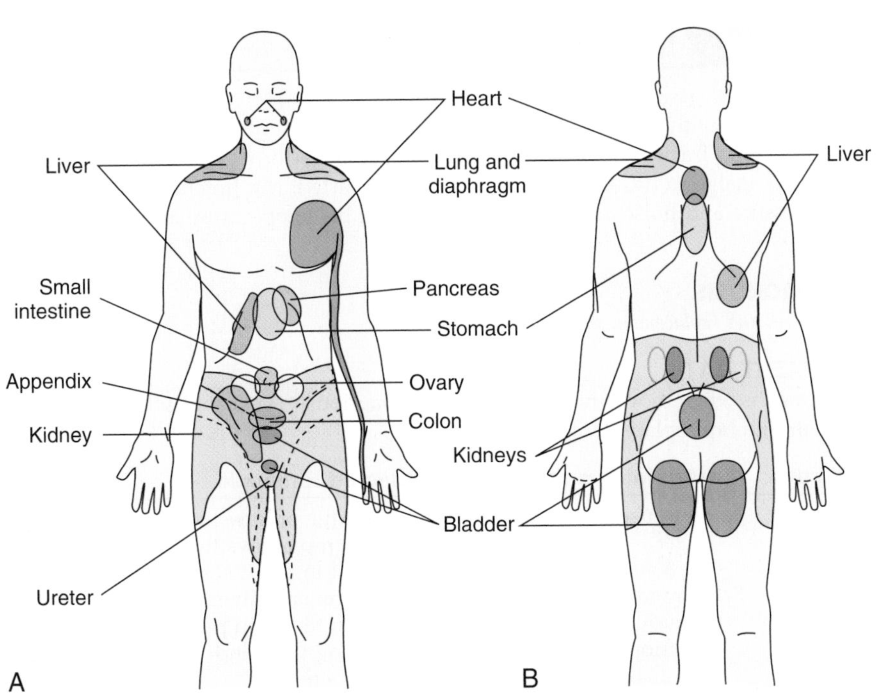

Fig. 7.5 Usual sites of referred pain. **A,** Front. **B,** Back. (From Lewis SL, Bucher L, Heitkemper MM, et al.: *Medical-surgical nursing: assessment and management of clinical problems*, ed 10, St. Louis, 2017, Elsevier.)

◆ NURSING DIAGNOSIS

The nursing problem statement is pain, either acute or chronic. The pain is usually linked with a medical condition, and the patient has symptoms that are addressed in the plan of care. Other conditions or pain treatment may require additional nursing problem statements, such as altered activity tolerance, altered breathing pattern, constipation, fall risk, fatigue, altered role performance, or potential for social isolation.

◆ PLANNING

The overall goal is *relief* of pain. If that is impossible to achieve, the goal is *control* of pain. Plan goals of nursing care that are realistic, measurable, and achievable. Planning should be a team effort that includes the patient and relies on both pharmacologic and nonpharmacologic interventions. Include input on pain management from pharmacists, therapists, and other health care professionals. The type of medication, method of delivery, and comfort measures will change as the patient's needs change. Planning must address all areas that affect the patient's pain management needs, including family situation, cultural influences, financial constraints, and whether pain is acute or chronic (Nursing Care Plan 7.1).

◆ IMPLEMENTATION

Reassess all patients for pain at the beginning of each shift (and intermittently throughout the shift), clinic appointment, or home visit and revise interventions based on the findings. Appropriate interventions include providing analgesics as ordered, using nonpharmacologic measures such as repositioning or massage (adjunctive measures), and reporting to the health care provider when measures are not effective or have unwanted side effects. Implementation also includes teaching the patient and family how to monitor the effects of treatment. False perceptions of pain may need to be addressed (Table 7.4).

Preventing complications from medications is an important aspect of implementation. Specific actions include:

- Documentation of any known drug allergies
- Accurate recording of pertinent information obtained during the initial assessment phase, such as current medications and previous experience with pain, analgesics, and adjuncts to pain relief
- Patient and family teaching regarding dose, frequency, the need to first consult with the health care provider or nurse before taking any other medications to avoid dangerous interactions, possible side effects, and what to report
- Appropriate monitoring of effects of any medications given and prompt notification of the provider should medications fail to relieve pain or problems occur
- Measures to prevent constipation when taking an opioid medication
- Accurate and complete documentation of any adverse reactions to treatment and communication of that information to other health care providers, to the patient, and to appropriate family members

◆ EVALUATION

Ask the patient about the effectiveness of the pain control measures. How quickly did relief occur?

Nursing Care Plan 7.1 Care of the Patient With Pain

SCENARIO

Mr. Jimenez, a 63-year-old patient with a history of a construction work accident, has been admitted through the emergency department after a fall and left hip fracture. A total hip replacement was performed this morning. Orders include morphine sulfate via patient-controlled analgesia (PCA), which has just been started. Mr. Jimenez has complained of pain at 7 on a 0-to-10 scale. His blood pressure and pulse are slightly elevated, but his temperature and respirations are normal. He has been restless and moaning.

PROBLEM/NURSING DIAGNOSIS

Pain related to surgical incision and replacement of hip.

SUPPORTING ASSESSMENT DATA

Subjective: Grimaces and moans when moves in bed; moves very cautiously; states muscles feel sore.

Objective: Incision at left hip; hip replacement this morning.

Goals/Expected Outcomes	Nursing Interventions	Selected Rationale	Evaluation
Patient will report pain at 4 or less on a 0-to-10 scale within 2 h.	Teach to use the PCA pump.	Knowledge of how to use the pump allows the patient to use it correctly.	Using pump correctly but without good relief.
	Encourage relaxation techniques, provide diversionary activities such as television and electronic games.	Relaxation and diversion are known to lessen pain by focusing the mind elsewhere.	Taught relaxation exercise. Does not wish to watch TV at present. Will use electronic poker game.
	Assess for anxiety and concern about job and ability to keep working.	Anxiety and fear can increase the perception of pain.	Expresses concern about being out of work and what will happen to his family.
	Encourage use of the PCA before ambulation, exercise, or repositioning.	Medicating before activity reduces pain from the activity.	Medicated before physical therapy visit.
	Position in good body alignment.	When the body is in correct alignment, joints hurt less.	Repositioned in correct alignment with abduction pillow q2h.
	Apply cold packs to reduce swelling over large bruise on lower thigh.	Cold reduces swelling by vasoconstriction and dulls the perception of pain.	Cold pack over thigh for 20 min every hour × 8 h.
	Observe frequently for pain relief and side effects of medication.	If pain is inadequately relieved, other measures to relieve it can be used. Knowing if side effects are occurring allows measures to be taken to alleviate or prevent them.	No side effects noted other than drowsiness. Pain at 3.
	Keep abduction wedge in place when supine.	Keeping leg abducted prevents dislocation of the hip and reduces pain.	Wedge in place when in bed.

CRITICAL THINKING QUESTIONS

1. If the PCA pump medication is not controlling the pain adequately, what would you do?
2. Considering the age of the patient and the type of surgery, which possible side effects of the analgesia would be of greatest concern? What interventions would you use to try to counter the side effects and prevent problems?

How long did it last? To what degree was the pain controlled? Were there any unpleasant side effects? Whenever possible, use patient verbalization as the primary evaluation tool. For evaluation, use a pain assessment tool with the patient before the pain is treated and again after treatment to compare the patient's response.

If the patient is unable to verbalize, evaluate the objective signs. For instance, an aphasic stroke patient might thrash, moan, and look fearful when in pain, and evaluation of effective analgesia might include the following: "Mr. Jones lying quietly, free of facial tension, watching the activity around him. He did not moan when repositioned 1 hour after analgesic given."

Clinical Cues

Evaluation of the effectiveness of the pain control medication used should be based on the route of administration. Medications given by mouth may take 30 to 45 minutes to be effective. Injections are effective within 30 to 45 minutes. Intravenous (IV) medications are effective within 5 to 15 minutes.

Table 7.4 False Perceptions of Pain

FALSE PERCEPTION	FACT
If pain is present, there must be a demonstrable cause.	Pain can be present even though no cause can be found. Although damage to the cells does lead to the release of chemicals that stimulate the pain receptors, in many cases pain may be present even if no cellular abnormality can be found. A patient with a migraine headache may or may not suffer less than a patient with a brain tumor. We cannot say that just because the brain tumor can be shown on a brain scan and the headache cannot, the person with the brain tumor has greater pain than the person with the migraine headache.
A person who has a low tolerance for pain has no self-control and probably is emotionally immature or childish.	Pain tolerance is a physiologic response to pain that is made more complex by psychosocial factors, many of which can be beyond the control of the patient. Tolerance of pain is defined as that duration or intensity of pain the person is willing to endure without seeking relief. Pain tolerance varies greatly from one individual to another and varies in the same individual from time to time. Nurses often place a high value on a patient's ability to feel pain without complaining or asking for relief. Those who value a high pain tolerance usually impose their own values on their patients by ignoring or belittling patient reports of pain. The person who should decide how willing they ought to be to tolerate pain is the one who is suffering pain.
Neonates are too neurologically immature to perceive or remember pain, so analgesia is unnecessary in this age group.	Neonates do perceive and maintain memory of pain. They cry and pull away from procedures such as heelstick blood tests. Male infants cry and struggle when they are circumcised. Neonates with medical conditions that require repeated blood tests begin to cry and pull away as soon as someone grasps the foot as if to perform a blood test, indicating a memory of pain from previous heel sticks. Analgesia for neonates is appropriate during procedures or situations that would be known to cause pain in more mature patients.
Older adult patients have a decreased ability to perceive pain, and pain medicines are dangerous for them because of their age.	Ability to express pain may be impaired by decreased cognitive function, but acute pain is still perceived. Advanced age combined with physical impairments, such as decreased kidney or liver function, may reduce tolerance for various medications, but with appropriate dosing and monitoring older patients can have good pain management without severe side effects. Untreated pain will interfere with sleep, nutrition, healing, and general well-being.
Reactions to acute pain and chronic pain are the same.	In general, acute pain is more often associated with anxiety and chronic pain is more often associated with depression. Emotional reactions such as anxiety and depression do not cause pain, but they can intensify pain. The management of acute and chronic pain is not the same, as discussed in the chapter text.
Addiction to pain-relieving drugs is always a hazard, and for the sake of the patient, nurses often must withhold a drug even though the patient asks for it.	A very small percentage of patients (probably less than 1% and no more than 3%) become addicted to drugs administered for the purpose of relieving acute pain. Although addiction is an increasing problem in the United States, acute pain managed properly is not the reason for the increase in opioid addiction. Patients need adequate pain relief.
Placebos (substances prescribed that contain no medication, such as sterile saline or sugar pills) are very useful in assessing whether a patient has pain.	There is no basis for believing that a patient who finds relief from pain after receiving a placebo has been pretending to have pain. Sufficient study of this subject shows that actual pain is sometimes well relieved by placebos.

◆ DOCUMENTATION

All measures to control pain must be documented accurately:

- Initial pain assessment (location, intensity, duration of the pain, and the method used to assess [e.g., pain scale, patient verbalization]; document aggravating and alleviating factors)
- Measures taken (e.g., analgesic medication, adjunctive measures)
- Evaluation of effectiveness of measures
- Provider notification of problems or concerns and provider response, if applicable
- Related patient or family education provided

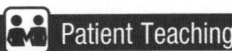

Patient Teaching

Managing Pain

Take medication before pain is severe and take the medication regularly until the pain is well controlled before lengthening the time between doses. Use distraction, imagery, or relaxation exercises to augment the effect of the pain medication.

Example of Pain Documentation

Paper charting – 01100. States pain level after physical therapy at 7 on a 0-to-10 scale. Hydrocodone/acetaminophen 5/325 mg given PO. 45 minutes after administration, states pain level is now 2 to 3. Pulse 72, respirations 16, moving freely in bed. Discussed pain-relief needs; suggested that he request pain medication before next therapy session (Signature).

The electronic health record (EHR) will prompt inclusion of the pain scale rating and the response of the patient to the medication.

Think Critically

What do you think is the most difficult aspect of evaluating someone's pain?

MANAGEMENT OF PAIN

Effective pain management is not just a matter of giving the right medicine at the right time. It is a combination of a stepped approach of pharmacologic measures coordinated with nonpharmacologic approaches that together give the individual the greatest possible degree of comfort for the longest possible time.

Home Care Considerations

Maintain a Medication Record

To prevent overdosage and toxicity, jot down the time pain medication is taken at home or make a note on an electronic device. It is easy to forget just when a medication has been taken.

PHARMACOLOGIC APPROACHES

Analgesics and Routes of Administration

Table 7.5 lists common analgesics by category and action.

Oral analgesics. An oral analgesic is any substance taken by mouth for the control of pain and is the most common route of administration. Oral analgesics include over-the-counter (OTC) medications such as acetaminophen (Tylenol), aspirin (Bayer), and ibuprofen (Advil, Motrin)

Table 7.5 Drugs Commonly Used to Treat Pain

TYPE OF DRUG	PRIMARY USE	EXAMPLES AND ROUTES OF ADMINISTRATION	NURSING IMPLICATIONS
Nonopioid analgesics, including nonsteroidal antiinflammatory drugs (NSAIDs)	Block pain at the peripheral nervous system level by decreasing inflammation	aspirin[a] (PO, chewable, topical), acetaminophen[a] (PO, IV), ibuprofen[a] (PO) ketoprofen[a] (PO), naproxen[a] (PO). indomethacin (PO), ketorolac (may be given PO, IM, or IV). Other NSAIDs are available as topical creams, gels, rubs, solutions, or sprays.	Educate patients not to use in combination with over-the-counter (OTC) dosage of same medication. Some have antiplatelet action and can increase the risk of bleeding. For localized pain, consider topical preparations.
Opioids[b]	Block pain at the central nervous system level	Morphine (PO, subcut, IM, IV transdermal patch, PCA), meperidine (PO, IV, IM), hydromorphone (PO, IV, subcut, IM, rectal, PCA) hydrocodone (PO), codeine (PO, IM), fentanyl (IV, transdermal, intranasal, PCA), tramadol (PO, IV, IM), buprenorphine (sublingual, intranasal, transdermal, subcut). Methadone is also available but is not routinely used for pain control.	Constipation common, can be severe. Can cause respiratory depression; antidote is naloxone (IM, IV, subcut, sublingual, intranasal; Narcan).
Medications with nonanalgesic primary actions used as adjuncts to pain control	Various mechanisms of action	Antidepressants: amitriptyline (PO), imipramine (PO, IM), trazodone hydrochloride (PO) Anticonvulsants: phenytoin (PO, IV), carbamazepine (PO, IV), gabapentin (PO), pregabalin (PO) Stimulants: caffeine (PO, IV), dextroamphetamine (PO) Muscle relaxants: carisoprodol (PO), baclofen (PO, transdermal, intrathecal) Chemotherapeutic agents: methotrexate (PO, IV, IM, subcut)	Varied because of different mechanisms of action. Always be aware of side effects and possible adverse reactions.

[a]Come in OTC and prescription doses.
[b]Combination drugs are often used. These may combine two forms of analgesic (e.g., acetaminophen and codeine) or an analgesic with another type of medication, such as an antihistamine. It is important to be aware of the ingredients contained in combination drugs to avoid administering excessive amounts of one of the components. The patient should receive no more than a total daily dose of 4000 mg of acetaminophen.
IM, Intramuscular; *IV,* intravenous; *PCA,* patient-controlled analgesia; *PO,* oral.

and prescription medications such as codeine and morphine. Oral analgesics are available in extended-release forms that can provide 12 to 24 hours of pain relief. Prescription analgesics include opioids such as hydrocodone and hydromorphone (Dilaudid). Hydrocodone is usually combined with acetaminophen (Vicodan, Norco), so care needs to be taken to ensure that any OTC medications containing acetaminophen taken with prescription medications do not exceed the recommended limit for acetaminophen.

Safety Alert

Preventing Acetaminophen Overdose

When administering acetaminophen, check all other medications and OTC drugs the patient is receiving. Many OTC drugs combine acetaminophen with other drugs. Toxicity may occur if more than the total recommended safe dosage of 4000 mg/day for an adult without liver impairment is ingested.

Injectable analgesics. Many analgesics are given through various forms of injections, including intramuscular (IM), subcutaneous (SC), and intravenous (IV). IM injections are not the mode of choice when there is an ongoing need for analgesics. This mode is usually used for one or two doses when other routes of administration are not indicated. Infusions of medications can be given via the IV and SC routes in addition to individual doses.

Topical analgesics. Topical analgesics are medications placed in a specific area on the skin to be absorbed by the vascular system or local tissues. These topical preparations may be lotions, gels, creams, or patches. Lidocaine for local pain may be given via patch. In addition, transdermal patches are used for sustained release of medications. Opioids are available in patches and are absorbed systemically from the skin. Some analgesics can be administered through the **buccal mucosa** (mucous membrane lining the inside of the mouth). This route is helpful for patients with a decreased level of consciousness or swallowing difficulty. The medication is absorbed by the mouth tissues, and there is no need to swallow the medication. Nasal instillation is another possible route to put medications in contact with mucous membranes for absorption.

Safety Alert

Pain Patch

Fentanyl patches used for severe pain can cause death from overdose. Oxycontin patches may cause overdose as well. Overdose is most likely to occur when old patches are not removed and multiple patches are present. Signs of overdose are difficulty breathing; shallow breathing; extreme sleepiness; and inability to think, talk, or walk normally. Faintness, dizziness, and confusion are other signs.

Clinical Cues

Always remove the old transdermal patch before applying a new one; cleanse the skin where the old patch has been. The patch must be removed before the patient undergoes magnetic resonance imaging (MRI) to prevent a burn from the foil in the patch.

Patient-controlled analgesia. Patient-controlled analgesia (PCA) is an infusion device controlled by the patient that injects the prescribed dose of analgesia. The PCA machine is programmed so that the patient can decide when a dose is given but cannot exceed the maximum dose or minimum time interval ordered by the health care provider. PCA is usually given IV, but it may also be administered SC. Subcutaneous infusion is rarely used in acute care but may be used in the home setting. Morphine and hydromorphone (Dilaudid) are most commonly used for PCA. The PCA device can be programmed to deliver a continuous infusion, a patient-initiated dose, or both. The intent of the PCA device is to put the patient in control of when they receive doses of medication. If a patient is not capable of knowing when and how to push the button, they are not a candidate for this type of pain medication delivery. Continuous infusions may be used in situations where patients are not capable of participating. The Institute for Safe Medication Practices (ISMP) warns against the policy of "PCA by proxy," which occurs when a person other than the patient is put in control of delivering medication doses through the PCA device (ISMP, 2016).

Even with appropriate programming, the level of opioid given may depress respirations. In 2014 the Centers for Medicare & Medicaid Services (CMS) updated its medication administration policy to include the mandate that any patient receiving PCA opioids be monitored for hypoxia and hypoventilation. These are clinically monitored via pulse oximetry and end-tidal carbon dioxide (CO_2) measurements in addition to physical assessment. Physical assessment includes use of a sedation scale (CMS, 2014). See Fig. 7.6 for an example of an infusion device with end-tidal CO_2 monitoring capability.

Epidural analgesic. An epidural analgesic is medication infused directly into the **epidural** space near the base of the spine using a programmable pump. An anesthesiologist inserts the infusion catheter. Patients receiving epidural analgesia such as morphine need to be monitored for possible delayed respiratory suppression or apnea, bradycardia, hypotension, urinary retention, nausea and vomiting, and allergic reactions such as itching or hives. Report adverse symptoms to the anesthesiologist immediately, and observe the insertion site for signs of infection, localized allergic reaction, and leaking. Usually a registered nurse (RN) is responsible for pump management and patient assessment.

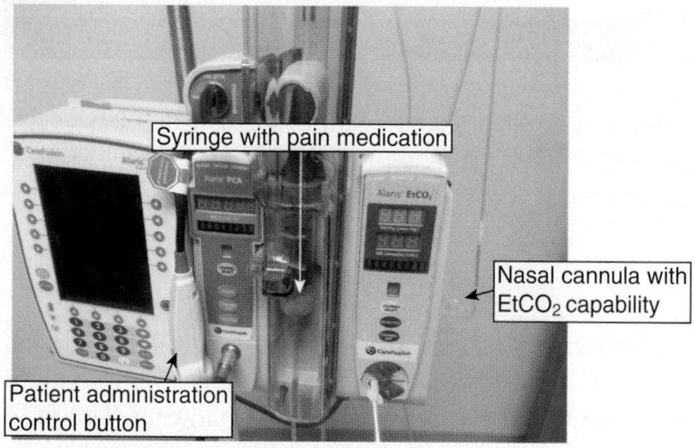

Fig. 7.6 Patient-controlled analgesia (PCA) pump with end-tidal carbon dioxide (CO_2) monitoring.

Peripheral nerve catheter. A small catheter is placed to deliver local anesthetic to the sheath of a peripheral nerve. These catheters are typically used postoperatively for patients who have had orthopedic procedures such as total joint replacement. A recent study showed that this technique of analgesia was also effective for patients with burns on the extremities (Kovac et al., 2018).

Nonanalgesic Medications Used for Pain Control

Antidepressants. A number of antidepressant medications are effective in controlling specific types of pain, such as nerve root pain. Medications such as amitriptyline, imipramine, clomipramine, and nortriptyline are being used as first-line treatments for neuropathic pain. They may be given alone or in combination with other analgesic medications.

Immunosuppressants. Occasionally drugs such as methotrexate (Rheumatrex) are used for **intractable pain** or to prevent further inflammation and joint damage in rheumatoid conditions by modifying the immune response. Steroids are used to decrease the inflammatory response in conditions where the inflammation is the primary cause of pain.

Anticonvulsants. Anticonvulsants, such as gabapentin (Neurontin), are routinely used for treatment of neuropathic pain. Pregabalin (Lyrica) has been approved for the pain of fibromyalgia. Some patients experience side effects of grogginess and slowed reactions.

Muscle relaxants. Muscle relaxants, such as baclofen, are often used adjunctively to ease spasm in patients with back pain, multiple sclerosis, and other neurologic and muscular disorders.

Marijuana. When patients have limited relief from medication, adjuvants, and other nonpharmacologic methods, the health care provider may prescribe medical marijuana in states where its use is legal. There are multiple biologically active components called cannabinoids in marijuana. The human body produces cannabinoids and has receptor sites in the brain, peripheral nervous tissue, and the immune and blood-producing systems (Halawa et al., 2018). Use of cannabinoids derived from plants can affect these sites, producing pain relief, decreasing nausea, reducing seizures, decreasing stress, and promoting sleep.

The controversy surrounding the use of medical marijuana continues, and its legality varies from state to state. The U.S. Food and Drug Administration (FDA) defines medical marijuana as use of the whole plant or its extracts to treat conditions. The FDA has not approved the marijuana plant as medicine. Two FDA-approved cannabinoid medications are currently available in pill form. Clinical studies have found that cannabinoids are less effective for acute pain, inflammatory, and nociceptive states but work well for multiple sclerosis pain (Halawa et al., 2018).

Special Considerations in Pain Management

Pharmacologic analgesics, including OTC drugs, may be administered to patients in a health care facility only under a health care provider's order, to prevent unwanted interactions with other prescribed medications. For example, aspirin, commonly taken for occasional headache and arthritis pain, is a powerful anticoagulant. Aspirin can lead to dangerous complications for someone with a bleeding disorder or who is taking another anticoagulant medication. Acetaminophen in high doses is toxic to the liver and may be contraindicated in patients with a liver disorder. Alerting patients that OTC drugs can have serious interactions with their prescribed drugs is an important part of patient education.

Patients who chronically use opioids often experience acute pain from surgery or trauma and are undermedicated. The regular use of opioids repeatedly stimulates the opioid receptors, producing an increased sensitivity to pain. Chronic use also produces a physiologic tolerance that requires increased dosing to produce the same result. Providers are reluctant to order high doses of opioids due to fear of causing an overdose, increased regulations on prescribing, and inadequate knowledge of the needs of the opioid-tolerant patient (Arnold & Childers, 2018). You should advocate for adequate pain control for all patients, including those who may require higher dosing of opioids. Addiction assessments should be done, and appropriate referrals should be made. An acute pain episode requiring analgesics is not the optimal time to initiate addiction withdrawal treatment.

Nurses' Responsibilities

In addition to following the "Six Rights" (right patient, right drug, right dose, right route, right time, right documentation), you have a variety of responsibilities when giving analgesic medications (Box 7.1).

Side Effects and Complications of Pain Medications

Probably the most common—and one of the most distressing—side effect of pain medication is constipation.

Box 7.1 Nursing Responsibilities When Administering Analgesics

1. Document the drug, dose, route, time of administration (including location of injection site for intramuscular or subcutaneous injections), and reason for drug administration.
2. Monitor the effectiveness of pain relief after 15 to 30 minutes and at 1- to 2-hour intervals. Document the degree and duration of pain relief in the patient record.
3. If the analgesic is ineffective, determine whether a stronger analgesic is available to the patient and administer it per health care provider order. If no other analgesic is available, notify the provider that the medication is not effective. Also notify the provider if the medication is initially effective but the duration of effect is too short to maintain patient comfort until the next dose may be given.
4. If the analgesic results in unwanted side effects (e.g., depressed vital signs, vomiting, altered level of consciousness), monitor the patient closely and notify the provider before administering another dose.

Analgesics such as morphine, meperidine, and codeine slow peristalsis. Fecal material becomes compacted and dry because of the extended time needed for passage through the intestines. Measures to prevent constipation should begin with the first dose of the medication.

Patients receiving these medications for any length of time should be monitored carefully for regular, normal bowel movements. **Oral fluids must be increased if possible.** Stool softeners and fiber-based laxatives, such as psyllium (Metamucil), can be helpful if approved by the health care provider. Miralax also has proven very effective for opioid-induced constipation. Prescription medications are also available when OTC remedies are ineffective.

Older Adult Care Points

Help prevent constipation in older adult patients who are receiving opioid analgesics by encouraging the increased intake of fluids and fiber; administering an ordered stool softener; suggesting prunes or prune juice; and monitoring for bloating, discomfort, and lack of daily bowel movement.

Some side effects of opioids, such as drowsiness and euphoria, generally last only for the first few days and then spontaneously disappear. Allergic reactions, such as itching and hives, must be reported immediately. Discontinue the medication and obtain an alternative order. The patient may need an antihistamine such as diphenhydramine (Benadryl) for relief of itching.

Opioid analgesics can depress the respiratory system to the point of apnea (no respiration). Should this occur, resuscitation must begin immediately. In the hospital setting, provide respiratory support and call the code or Rapid Response Team. In the home, provider's office, or clinic, provide respiratory support and call 911. The standard treatment for respiratory suppression from an opioid is naloxone (Narcan), an effective opioid antagonist that can be given IM or IV.

Legal and Ethical Considerations

Pain Control at the End of Life

Patients and their families often worry that treating the terminally ill with medication at a level sufficient to control pain may hasten death. "In truth, opioids are unlikely to hasten death if used in an appropriate manner by a skilled clinician" (Jackson & Nabati, 2018). Health care providers have a moral obligation to adequately treat pain even at the very end of life. Opioids are administered for the purpose of relieving pain, not to hasten death.

Opioid Epidemic

According to the Centers for Disease Control and Prevention (CDC), 115 Americans die daily from an overdose of opioids (CDC, 2017). The drugs involved include prescription medications, illegal substances, and illegally manufactured substances. In April 2017 the Department of Health and Human Services (HHS) announced priorities for combating the opioid crisis: (1) improving access to treatment and recovery services, (2) promoting use of overdose-reversing drugs, (3) strengthening our understanding of the epidemic through better public health surveillance, (4) providing support for cutting-edge research on pain and addiction, and (5) advancing better practices for pain management. These strategies can be seen in the increased availability of naloxone (Narcan) for use by first responders, friends, and family members. Most states have changed the process for prescription opioids to help limit abuse. There are multiple opinions on how the epidemic started, how to intervene, and who is responsible, but there is no debate that opioid addiction and overdose are major health issues in the United States.

NONPHARMACOLOGIC APPROACHES

A variety of methods exist for relieving pain without or in addition to medications. Using adjuncts can increase the effectiveness of pain medication and may decrease the frequency at which it is needed.

Sleep

Adequate sleep and rest are major factors in healing. **Rest increases pain tolerance and improves response to analgesia.** Allow adequate time between treatments for naps, and plan care to keep sleep interruptions to a minimum. For instance, take vital signs when the patient is awake to use the bathroom or requests pain medication. It is important to remember that exhaustion will cause a patient to sleep, even while experiencing severe pain, but such sleep is not as therapeutic. Appropriate analgesia combined with adequate rest and other comfort measures promotes healing. Smoothing bedclothes, plumping pillows, adjusting lighting, and repositioning all increase comfort.

Heat

Gentle heat is very soothing for many types of pain. Heat promotes vasodilation of the area, which promotes increased blood supply and movement of nutrients to the affected area. Sources include warm blankets, heating devices, whirlpools, tub baths, heat lamps, and chemical self-heating packs. Always check the temperature before applying heat, and monitor the patient closely for tolerance. To prevent injury to the skin, never apply a heating device directly to the surface of the skin. The very young and the very old are particularly sensitive to heat. Anyone with an altered level of consciousness or loss of normal sensation may not realize something is too hot, and those with loss of movement may not be able to move away from the heat source when necessary.

Older Adult Care Points

The skin of older adults is thin and burns more easily. Stroke patients and those with diabetic neuropathy commonly have areas of lost or diminished sensation, and patients with senile dementia may not recognize that something is too hot. Even an alert and oriented older adult may fall asleep and be burned. Monitor any heat application very carefully. **Do not apply heat to any areas where nerve damage or decreased sensation has occurred.**

Menthol. When applied to the skin, menthol causes warming, which may have an analgesic effect. Mentholated products are usually massaged into the skin, giving the individual the benefit of both massage and warmth. They are available OTC but require a health care provider's order in a hospital or clinic setting. Do not use menthol with external heating devices to avoid overheating the skin surface. Caution the patient to wash their hands well after applying menthol to prevent contact of the menthol with the eyes or mucous membranes.

Cold

Cold is particularly helpful in reducing swelling through vasoconstriction. It also can be effective in relieving muscle spasms and some types of joint pain. Cold decreases metabolic rate and nerve conduction velocity, decreasing pain sensations. Some individuals are very sensitive to cold. If cold applications cause shivering, tensing of the muscles, or an increase in pain or spasm, discontinue their use.

Clinical Cues

The effectiveness of cold is maximized in 15 to 20 minutes. Remove the source after that time.

Distraction

Any activity that takes a person's attention away from pain is called a *distraction.* This includes watching television, talking with friends, using an electronic device, or playing a game. People have an innate ability to distract themselves from their surroundings or situation. Health care workers may mistakenly interpret patients' ability to distract themselves as proof that there is no pain. Distracting activities can take the patient's mind off the pain momentarily, but distractions do not stop pain. Distraction can be helpful in bridging the time gap between giving an analgesic and the onset of pain relief.

Relaxation

Relaxation, also called "tension release," involves the conscious relaxation of muscle groups. Tension release is typically done as a progression, beginning at the feet and moving up the body, ending with the neck and facial muscles. Initially you can guide the patient verbally, slowly directing their attention to the next muscle group to be relaxed. After one or two sessions, many patients can effectively provide their own relaxation sequence (see the Evolve website for Relaxation Exercise).

Guided Imagery

Guided imagery involves assisting patients to form mental images of a pleasant environment where they are comfortable and happy. For some, the experience is visual; in their minds they "see" a beautiful place. For others, it is a process of achieving a feeling of comfort and peace. Either is highly effective in giving the patient a brief mental break from pain.

Meditation

Meditation involves the use of a focus point, which may be a sound, a repeated phrase (sometimes called a *mantra*), the sound of the breath as it moves in and out of the body, or a visual image. The visual image may be a picture or object the patient gazes at, or it may be an imagined image (e.g., a candle's flame, a leaf moving with the breeze, beach waves). Meditation works best when practiced daily.

Hypnosis

Hypnosis, or therapeutic suggestion, should be done by a trained practitioner. It involves the use of focusing and relaxation to induce a trancelike state during which a patient receives suggestions that may be helpful after returning to a normal level of consciousness. Hypnosis has strong objective evidence that shows it is effective in the treatment of chronic pain (Bonshtein, 2018).

Biofeedback

Biofeedback involves the use of a machine that uses electrodes attached to the skin to measure the degree of muscular tension. The machine has colored lights and an audible tone that changes in pitch from higher to lower as the patient relaxes. The patient receives visual and auditory confirmation of self-induced relaxation. This technique is particularly effective with people who are highly competitive because it rewards success and allows them to "win" the game.

Music

Music used alone can be highly effective in bringing about relaxation and can be used as a focal point for meditation or to enhance other distracting activities. Nature sounds, including the ocean, running streams, breezes, rain, and birds singing, also can induce relaxation.

Binders

Binders are helpful for strains, sprains, and wounds or surgical incisions that are packed. They support the tissues during movement, such as ambulation or coughing, which reduces the pain. Temporary support using a pillow, folded bath blanket, or other semi-firm surface can also help splint an abdominal or chest incision when coughing or moving.

Massage

The use of long, firm strokes; short, soft, circular strokes; and occasionally gentle pounding with the sides of the hands stimulates circulation, relaxes muscles, and increases the general sense of well-being. When the painful area has inflammation or consists of a wound or an incision, massaging another area of the body with gentle but firm pressure helps the patient direct attention away from the pain. Always be guided by the patient's sense of comfort. Use only the degree of pressure that is pleasant and relaxing.

Simple massage can be done by a family member with just a little instruction, giving them an opportunity to assist in the care in a positive and loving way. Massage should not be used on any area that has been reddened by pressure. This tissue is already compromised, and massage can cause further damage through **shearing**, the traumatic pulling of tissue layers away from one another.

Acupuncture and Acupressure

Acupuncture originated centuries ago in China and involves the use of tiny needles inserted into the skin at specific points along lines called *meridians*, a concept similar to that of nerve pathways. Research has shown that acupuncture helps relieve knee pain from osteoarthritis and back and headache pain (Ahn, 2018). Acupressure involves the use of external finger pressure at the meridian points to achieve similar effects. Both acupuncture and acupressure require extensive training for proper use and should be done only by someone fully trained in these procedures.

> **Complementary and Alternative Therapies**
>
> **Pain Relief**
>
> Complementary and alternative therapies are used more for pain relief than for anything else. Therapies include relaxation, meditation, biofeedback, yoga, hypnosis, imagery, chiropractic, acupuncture, acupressure, massage, aromatherapy, and herbal preparations and supplements.

Electrostimulation Devices

Transcutaneous electrical nerve stimulation (TENS) uses a small electrical stimulator attached to the skin with electrodes placed around the area of pain. A low current running between the electrodes acts to block pain sensation. The degree of stimulation can be controlled by the patient using dials on the stimulator. The application of TENS requires specific training and must be ordered by a health care provider (Fig. 7.7). Some patients find TENS unpleasant rather than helpful. In such cases, the provider should be notified and an alternative method of pain control selected. **Scrambler therapy** involves an electrical stimulus delivered through the skin like TENS. Skin electrodes are placed above and below the site of pain. The device is designed to "scramble" the pain signals and replace them with a nonpainful stimulus.

Spinal Cord Stimulator

A spinal cord stimulator can be implanted under the skin, with a wire placed in the epidural space adjacent to nerves that innervate the affected body area. The electric current produced masks the pain signals. This device is used for patients with chronic pain who have not responded to medications or other methods of pain management.

Invasive treatments. An epidural injection may be used to ease nerve pain. The medication dosage given directly to the epidural space is less than the oral dose, so patients suffer no central nervous system side effects. They can work and drive while being relieved of severe pain.

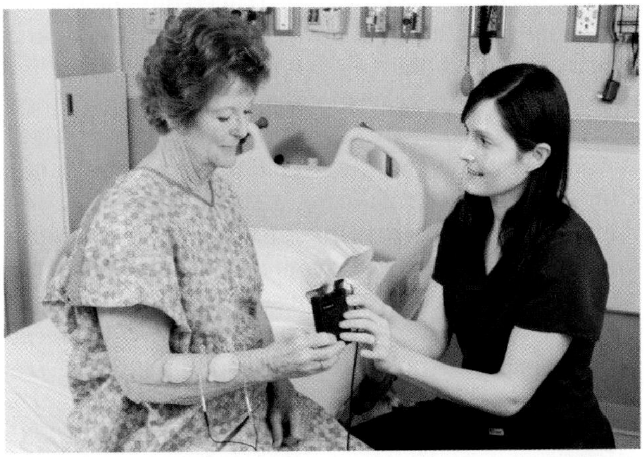

Fig. 7.7 Instructing the patient on how to use a transcutaneous electrical nerve stimulation (TENS) unit.

Epidural injection is recommended no more than two to three times a year, and there is some evidence that these injections make the patient more prone to fracture. Intrathecal (into the subarachnoid space) injections may also be given. When intrathecal or epidural delivery is successful and needs to be ongoing, a surgically implanted refillable pain pump and catheter can be placed. The medications delivered are usually an opioid with a local anesthetic (bupivacaine).

Think Critically

What types of nonpharmacologic methods would you use for a patient who is complaining of shoulder muscle pain after an automobile accident?

COMMUNITY CARE

Community care for pain can take place in a variety of settings, with varying levels of training among direct caregivers. Nurses may need to work with the social worker before discharge to put in place all necessary measures to control pain for the patient who is going home. Nurses in the community should help educate people about the complementary and alternative resources available to treat chronic pain.

EXTENDED CARE

Extended care facilities may provide rehabilitative services, long-term care services, or both. Each type of care may include specific pain management needs. Patients undergoing rehabilitation often have acute pain related to therapy, particularly in the early phases. It is important that therapy be scheduled to allow for adequate rest and recovery time. It also is important that analgesic medication be given on a schedule that provides the patient with the greatest pain relief during therapy sessions. This assists the patient to cooperate with therapy, which in turn encourages a more rapid recovery. When planning, always include the patient, who knows best which medication and time schedule provides the most effective pain relief.

Long-term care facilities—also called nursing homes, skilled nursing facilities, transitional care units, and board and care homes—often have patients who live there for the last weeks, months, or even years of their lives. In such settings, the term *resident* rather than *patient* is used. Residents may have pain resulting from a fall, after dental work, or during a period of illness, and they may have chronic pain from arthritis, degenerative disorders, or cancer. Residents may be mentally alert and oriented, be alert but confused, or have a decreased level of consciousness. Each of these individuals can perceive pain and should be given appropriate analgesics when pain exists.

Nurses can be of great assistance to health care providers in ordering analgesia by providing accurate information about the type of pain, the frequency, the intensity, and precipitating factors. For instance, a resident with degenerative arthritis and chronic joint pain may benefit from a routine oral analgesic such as acetaminophen or ibuprofen. Those with more severe chronic problems, such as cancer, may benefit from routine time-released medications such as MS Contin (oral morphine sulfate in a time-released tablet). As pain increases, an increased dosage of opioid may be needed to gain relief, but remember that older adults and debilitated individuals may be more drug sensitive. Monitor all medications carefully and work with the provider to ensure that the resident's pain is being appropriately addressed. Ideally the resident is comfortable, alert, and able to participate in activities of their choice. Nurses in the long-term care setting must make pain assessment and management a priority.

HOME CARE

The number of individuals receiving skilled and professional nursing care at home is increasing rapidly. The average length of stay in an acute care facility is less than 5 days. Patients may go home from the hospital with peripheral or central IV lines providing analgesia. You provide patient and family education on pain management in the home setting, which includes verbal and written instructions about the medication and any equipment used to dispense it. Telephone numbers that give the patient and family access to 24-hour assistance should be prominently displayed.

Just as in an inpatient setting, home care patients must be evaluated for the continued safety and effectiveness of the analgesic medication. Contact the health care provider any time the medication orders need to be adjusted. Adjuncts to pain management, such as simple massage, relaxation techniques, and the use of pillows, warmth, repositioning, or soft music, are taught to patients and families for use in the home care setting.

Current guidelines for home care by agencies such as Medicare require that case management be done by a licensed professional. This usually is an RN, although a registered physical therapist may fill this role for patients whose only acute need is continued restorative therapy. The role of the licensed practical/vocational nurse (LPN/LVN) is that of direct patient care under the guidance of the case manager. The LPN/LVN may monitor an ongoing infusion and discontinue the infusion as needed but must report any difficulties immediately to the case manager for intervention. Some states offer IV therapy certification for LPN/LVNs, which allows them to infuse medications.

Always be alert to an increase in pain resulting from changes in the disease process. The provider needs to be notified of the change so that appropriate measures, including adjusting or changing the medications, can take place.

Get Ready for the NCLEX® Examination!

Key Points

- Only the patient knows where the pain is and its degree of intensity.
- Pain is a neurologic response to unpleasant stimuli.
- Pain tolerance varies from one individual to another.
- Pain threshold is the point at which pain is perceived.
- Endorphins can block pain sensation.
- The gate control theory states that when the gate is open, pain sensation is allowed through; when the gate is closed, pain is blocked.
- The neuromatrix theory states that pain is a multidimensional experience influenced by past experience, cultural learning, personality variables, and influences from various body systems.
- The two pathophysiologic classifications of pain are nociceptive and neuropathic.
- Nociceptive pain derives from stimulation of somatic or visceral structures.
- There are four phases of nociceptive pain: transduction, transmission, perception, and modulation.
- Neuropathic pain derives from dysfunction of the nervous system.
- The patient should be asked to use an appropriate pain scale.
- Cultural factors and beliefs affect each person's perception of pain.
- Pain assessment and data collection include the areas of appearance, behavior, activity level, verbalization, and physiologic clues.
- An interpreter may be required to gather correct data about a patient's pain.
- Goals of care are (1) relief of pain and (2) control of pain.
- Pharmacologic and nonpharmacologic methods are used to treat pain.
- Neuropathic pain is relieved with NSAIDs, tricyclic antidepressants, anticonvulsants, and corticosteroids.
- False perceptions about pain may affect care (see Table 7.4).
- Evaluating the effectiveness of measures used to relieve pain is a primary nursing responsibility.
- Always follow the "Six Rights" when administering pain medication.
- Ask the patient about pain level and pain relief from medication at regular intervals.
- It is important to be knowledgeable about the commonly used analgesics (see Table 7.5).
- Constipation is a common side effect of opioid analgesia, and preventive measures should be used as soon as an opioid is begun.
- Adequate sleep assists in controlling pain.
- Acupuncture and biofeedback have been proven to be effective for many people for various types of pain.
- Chronic pain is common among older adults in long-term care facilities.

Additional Learning Resources

SG Go to your Study Guide for additional learning activities to help you master this chapter content.

Go to your Evolve website (http://evolve.elsevier.com/deWit/medsurg) for the following FREE learning resources:

- Animations, audio, and video
- Answers and rationales for questions and activities
- Glossary with pronunciations in English and Spanish
- Interactive Review Questions and more!

Review Questions for the NCLEX® Examination

1. You administer ketorolac (Toradol) 30 mg IM to a 30-year-old male patient. The gate control theory indicates that the next nursing action to assist in pain control would be to:
   1. recap the needle.
   2. massage the area.
   3. check for pain relief in 45 minutes.
   4. encourage an activity that will provide distraction.

   NCLEX Client Need: Physiological Integrity: Pharmacological Therapies
2. In determining the patient's perception of pain, which question(s) would be useful in assessing pain? *(Select all that apply.)*
   1. "Where are you hurting?"
   2. "What pain control measures have worked in the past?"
   3. "How would you describe your pain?"
   4. "What were you doing before the onset of the pain?"
   5. "Are you sleeping adequately?"

   NCLEX Client Need: Physiological Integrity: Basic Care and Comfort
3. You know that acute and chronic pain may be handled differently. Which of the following is correct?
   1. Hypnotherapy is effective in acute pain states.
   2. Chronic pain is best treated by PCA.
   3. Acute pain is difficult to manage in the postoperative patient.
   4. Chronic pain is best managed by a holistic approach to ensure that good long-term pain control is possible for the patient.

   NCLEX Client Need: Physiological Integrity: Basic Care and Comfort

4. A patient who has osteoarthritis is experiencing right knee pain daily. You know that this type of pain usually has the best result if treated by:
   1. oxycodone.
   2. ibuprofen.
   3. Lyrica.
   4. prednisone.

   NCLEX Client Need: Physiological Integrity: Pharmacological Therapies
5. A 25-year-old woman who was in a minor automobile accident along with her 5-year-old son has a minor laceration on her arm that does not require stitches. Her son is being examined in the next room. The woman is moaning about the pain in her arm. You understand that her expression of pain is possibly influenced by: *(Select all that apply.)*
   1. blood on her skirt and blouse from the arm laceration.
   2. her family and societal culture of being vocal about pain.
   3. relief that another driver was not hurt in the accident and the car has minor damage.
   4. worry about her son possibly sustaining a severe injury in the accident.

   NCLEX Client Need: Psychosocial Integrity
6. An appropriate short-term outcome written for a patient with acute pain after surgery would be:
   1. the patient will demonstrate use of a PCA pump.
   2. the nurse will assess for adequate pain relief.
   3. the incision will heal without infection.
   4. pain will be adequately controlled with a PCA pump.

   NCLEX Client Need: Safe and Effective Care Environment: Coordinated Care
7. A patient with chronic pain requiring further measures to decrease the pain asks you, "What is a TENS unit?" What is the best nursing response?
   1. "It is an implant in the epidural space adjacent to nerves that innervate the affected body area."
   2. "It provides a small electrical stimulus to the skin around the area of pain."
   3. "It involves the use of external finger pressure at the meridian points."
   4. "It supports the tissues during movement."

   NCLEX Client Need: Integrated Processes: Teaching and Learning
8. A patient is discharged with a prescription for oral oxycodone with acetaminophen tablets (5 mg/325 mg), two tablets every 6 hours as needed. The patient takes Tylenol Extra Strength (500 mg) twice a day for headaches. If the patient takes the medication as ordered (every 6 hours) and the supplemental Tylenol, how many milligrams of acetaminophen will be ingested in 24 hours? ____________________. *(Fill in the blank.)*

   NCLEX Client Need: Physiological Integrity: Pharmacological Therapies
9. Before you administer an opioid analgesic to a patient, the *most* important nursing action is to:
   1. check the blood pressure.
   2. provide other comfort measures first.
   3. assess for possible constipation.
   4. assess the rate and depth of respirations.

   NCLEX Client Need: Physiological Integrity: Pharmacological Therapies
10. A 25-year-old patient complains of moderate pain at their incision site. Morphine sulfate is administered IV. The most appropriate nursing action after the injection would be to:
    1. evaluate the effectiveness of the pain medication in 2 hours.
    2. encourage the patient to close their eyes and rest.
    3. suggest that the patient play solitaire or watch something interesting on TV.
    4. administer ordered ibuprofen orally.

    NCLEX Client Need: Physiological Integrity: Pharmacological Therapies
11. You are assigned to care for a patient with an epidural infusion for analgesia. Which sign or symptom related to this treatment would require immediate health care provider notification?
    1. Blood pressure 80/60 mm Hg
    2. Temperature 99.5° F (37.5° C)
    3. Respirations 12/min
    4. Urinary output less than 30 mL/h

    NCLEX Client Need: Physiological Integrity: Pharmacological Therapies
12. A long-term care nurse is caring for an older adult male patient who appears to be withdrawn and quiet. He grimaces whenever he is touched. The *most* appropriate nursing action would be to:
    1. administer pain medication.
    2. assess for underlying causes of the patient's behavior.
    3. reposition the patient and check him again in 2 hours.
    4. notify the health care provider.

    NCLEX Client Need: Health Promotion and Maintenance

Critical Thinking Questions

Scenario A

Jo Ann Patterson, age 56, has suffered shoulder pain from an old, healed fracture for several years. When the pain is too severe to be controlled with acetaminophen, her health care provider recommends that she use a prescribed oral opioid analgesic. However, Jo Ann does not want to continue taking drugs that she "might become addicted to."

1. How would you respond to Jo Ann's statement regarding fear of addiction to the pain medication?
2. What other measures could you suggest for management of Jo Ann's pain?

Scenario B

Tom Johnson, a 30-year-old construction worker, had a bowel resection 3 days ago. He is determined to get back to work quickly and is cooperative about ambulation. He refuses pain medication, stating, "I don't need it." You note that he stops frequently to lean against the wall, walks stooped over, and grimaces when no one is looking.

1. Why might Tom be refusing pain medication?
2. What information might you share regarding pain control and getting well after major surgery?
3. What suggestions might you make to Tom regarding his comfort?

Scenario C

Jim Tolliver, age 32, sprained his left ankle while playing football with his friends this morning. He consults his neighbor (who is a nurse) about what to do because his ankle is hurting a lot.

1. What should his nurse neighbor do first?
2. What should be suggested to Jim regarding home treatment?
3. What precautions should the neighbor take regarding further treatment?

8 Care of Patients With Cancer

http://evolve.elsevier.com/deWit/medsurg

Objectives

Theory

1. Identify the differences between normal cells and cancer cells.
2. Understand the process of cancer metastasis.
3. Understand the genetic, chemical, physical, and infectious processes associated with cancer development.
4. Understand the implications of cultural and individual factors and race to cancer development.
5. Understand the various classifications of tumors and the TNM staging system.
6. Apply principles of cancer prevention in the care of well populations.
7. Understand the use of different tests in the diagnosis of cancer.
8. Apply knowledge of the stages of the grieving process experienced by a patient dying of cancer to the patient's coping level.

Clinical Practice

9. Devise an individualized plan of care for a patient receiving radiation or chemotherapy for cancer treatment.
10. Implement a teaching plan for a patient who has bone marrow suppression from cancer treatment.
11. Evaluate nursing interventions to help a patient cope with the common problems of cancer and its treatment.
12. Apply appropriate nursing interventions to help patients and families cope with the psychological and psychosocial effects of cancer and its treatment.
13. Apply nursing interventions to help cancer patients cope with death and dying.

Key Terms

apoptosis (ăp-ŏp-TŌ-sĭs, p. 149)
biopsy (BĪ-ŏp-sē, p. 160)
brachytherapy (bra-kē-thĕr-ĕ-pē, p. 167)
carcinogens (kăr-SĬN-ō-jĕnz, p. 152)
carcinoma (kăr-sĭ-NŌ-mă, p. 155)
cytology (sī-TŎL-ō-jē, p. 156)
cytotoxic (sī-tō-TŎK-sĭk, p. 169)
deoxyribonucleic acid (DNA) (dē-ŏks-ē-rī-bō-nū-KLĀ-ĭk ĂS-ĭd, p. 150)
extravasation (ĕks-trăv-ă-SĀ-shŭn, p. 171)
gene (jēn, p. 150)
incidence (ĬN-sĕ-dĕns, p. 149)
leukemia (lū-KĒ-mē-ă, p. 155)
lymphoma (lĭm-FŌ-mă, p. 155)
malignant (mă-LĬG-nănt, p. 150)
melanoma (mĕl-ă-NŌ-mă, p. 155)
metastasis (mĕ-TĂS-tă-sĭs, p. 150)
mitosis (mī-TŌ-sĭs, p. 149)
mortality (mōr-TĂL-ĭ-tē, p. 149)
mutation (mū-TĀ-shŭn, p. 151)
neoplasm (NĒ-ō-plăzm, p. 149)
occult blood (ŏ-KŬLT blŭd, p. 156)
oncogene (ŎNGK-ō-jēn, p. 151)
palliative care (PĂL-ē-ă-tĭv kār, p. 179)
prognosis (prŏg-NŌ-sĭs, p. 150)
promoters (prō-MŌ-tĕrz, p. 153)
sarcoma (săr-kŌ-mă, p. 155)
TNM staging (tē ĕn ĕm STĀ-jĭng, p. 155)
transformation (trănz-fĕr-MĀ-shŭn, p. 153)
tumor (TŪ-mŏr, p. 150)
tumor markers (TŪ-mŏr MĂR-kĕrz, p. 161)
vesicants (VĔ-si-kĕntz, p. 171)

Concepts Covered in This Chapter

- Homeostasis and Regulation
- Protection and Movement
- Resilience
- Mood and Cognition
- Nursing Attributes and Roles
- Care Competencies
- Health Care Delivery

THE IMPACT OF CANCER

***Cancer* is the term given to a collection of related diseases that are characterized by uncontrolled, abnormal cell growth and spread into surrounding tissues** (National Cancer Institute, 2015). New treatments have greatly improved the survival of patients with cancer, with 68% of patients living 5 years or longer. Cancer is now considered a chronic disease that can worsen and improve again over the course of a patient's

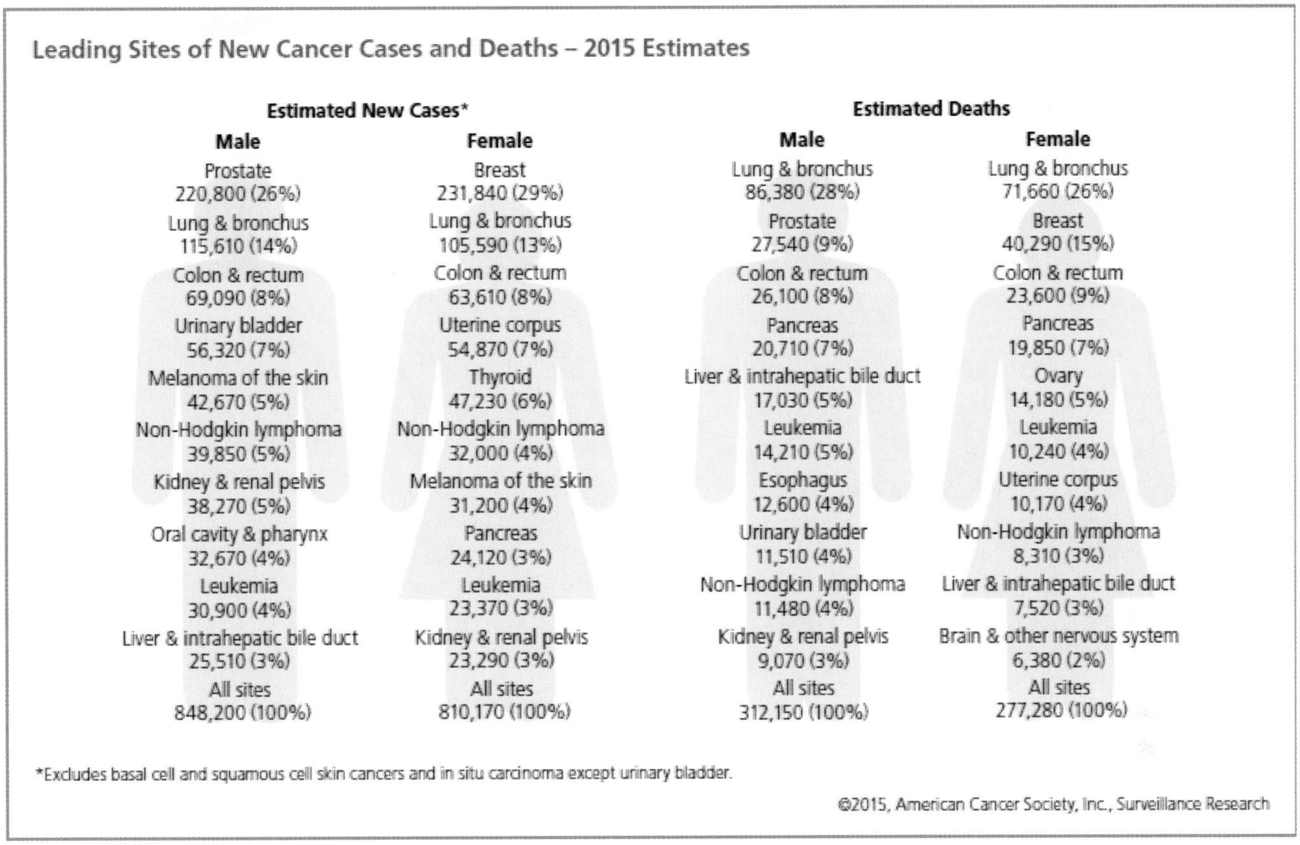

Leading Sites of New Cancer Cases and Deaths – 2015 Estimates
Estimated New Cases*
Male
Prostate
220,800 (26%)
Lung & bronchus
115,610 (14%)
Colon & rectum
69,090 (8%)
Urinary bladder
56,320 (7%)
Melanoma of the skin
42,670 (5%)
Non-Hodgkin lymphoma
39,850 (5%)
Kidney & renal pelvis
38,270 (5%)
Oral cavity & pharynx
32,670 (4%)
Leukemia
30,900 (4%)
Liver & intrahepatic bile duct
25,510 (3%)
All sites
848,200 (100%)
Female
Breast
231,840 (29%)
Lung & bronchus
105,590 (13%)
Colon & rectum
63,610 (8%)
Uterine corpus
54,870 (7%)
Thyroid
47,230 (6%)
Non-Hodgkin lymphoma
32,000 (4%)
Melanoma of the skin
31,200 (4%)
Pancreas
24,120 (3%)
Leukemia
23,370 (3%)
Kidney & renal pelvis
23,290 (3%)
All sites
810,170 (100%)
Estimated Deaths
Male
Lung & bronchus
86,380 (28%)
Prostate
27,540 (9%)
Colon & rectum
26,100 (8%)
Pancreas
20,710 (7%)
Liver & intrahepatic bile duct
17,030 (5%)
Leukemia
14,210 (5%)
Esophagus
12,600 (4%)
Urinary bladder
11,510 (4%)
Non-Hodgkin lymphoma
11,480 (4%)
Kidney & renal pelvis
9,070 (3%)
All sites
312,150 (100%)
Female
Lung & bronchus
71,660 (26%)
Breast
40,290 (15%)
Colon & rectum
23,600 (9%)
Pancreas
19,850 (7%)
Ovary
14,180 (5%)
Leukemia
10,240 (4%)
Uterine corpus
10,170 (4%)
Non-Hodgkin lymphoma
8,310 (3%)
Liver & intrahepatic bile duct
7,520 (3%)
Brain & other nervous system
6,380 (2%)
All sites
277,280 (100%)
*Excludes basal cell and squamous cell skin cancers and in situ carcinoma except urinary bladder.
©2015, American Cancer Society, Inc., Surveillance Research

Fig. 8.1 Leading sites of new cancer cases and deaths. (American Cancer Society. Cancer Facts and Figures 2015. Atlanta: American Cancer Society, Inc.)

life. In 2017 approximately 688,780 new cancer cases were diagnosed, and 600,920 cancer deaths occurred in the United States. The prostate, breast, lung and bronchus, and colon and rectum are the leading sites for new cancers and cancer deaths (American Cancer Society [ACS], 2017).

The current **incidence** of all cancers is about 20% higher in each racial or ethnic population of men. For males, the incidence of prostate, lung, and colorectal cancers has generally declined over time, but the incidence of liver, melanoma, and thyroid cancers is increasing. For females, the incidence of breast cancer has increased slightly for nonwhite women over the last 10 years. Lung and colorectal cancers have been declining in women. As in men, increased incidence of thyroid and liver cancers has been observed in women. However, cancer incidence rates for all cancers are higher among black men and white women.

Cancer death rates have been declining since the 1990s, with the combined death rate for men and women dropping 25% from 1991 to 2014. Lung cancer remains the leading cause of cancer **mortality** (death) among men, followed by colorectal and prostate cancers; deaths from liver and pancreatic cancers have been increasing slightly. Among women, lung, breast, and colorectal cancers are the leading causes of cancer deaths. Deaths from cancer of the uterus have been increasing since 2000.

Fig. 8.1 shows the leading sites of new cancer cases and deaths.

PATHOPHYSIOLOGY OF CANCER

NORMAL CELLS

To understand how cancer cells develop and behave, it is first important to understand normal cells. Normal cells are designed for a purpose in the human body, making proteins or producing products that help the body to function normally. Normal growth of cells and tissues occurs during infancy and childhood. Once adulthood is reached, most of the body's normal cells only grow and reproduce through **mitosis** (a type of cell division that results in two cells having the same number and type of chromosomes) to replace damaged or dead cells following illness or injury. For example, when you fall and skin your knee, normal skin cells will reproduce to replace the lost skin. Once the missing area is filled, the reproduction of skin cells stops. With the exception of blood cells traveling through the body's vessels, normal cells remain in place and do not travel or invade neighboring tissue. Normal cells die when damaged or diseased by undergoing a process called **apoptosis**, or programmed cell death. An abnormal replication of cells results in a **neoplasm**, a new growth of a benign or cancerous tissue or tumor.

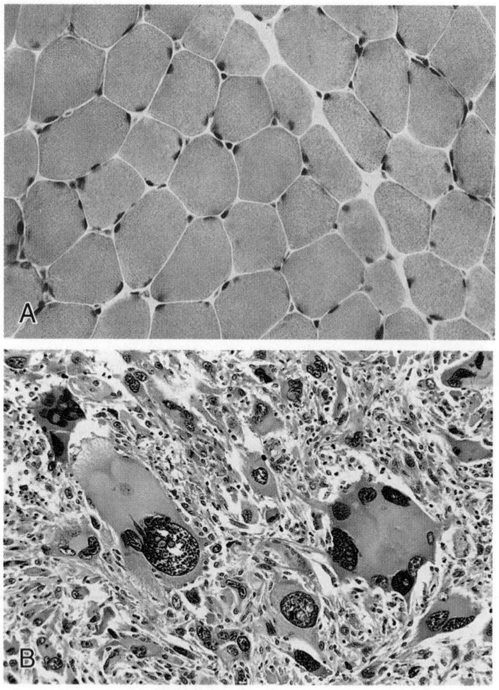

Fig. 8.2 Normal and malignant skeletal muscle cells. **A,** Normal skeletal muscle cells. Note that cells are well differentiated and similar in appearance. **B,** Malignant tumor cells in skeletal muscle (rhabdomyosarcoma). (**A,** From Damjanov I, Linder J, editors: *Anderson's pathology*, ed 10, St. Louis, 1996, Mosby. **B,** From Kumar V, Abbas AK, Aster JC: *Robbins and Cotran pathologic basis of disease*, ed 9, Philadelphia, 2015, Elsevier; courtesy Dr. Trace Worrell, Department of Pathology, University of Texas Southwestern Medical School, Dallas.)

CANCER CELLS

Cancer cells do not behave like normal cells. Cancer development begins when damage to the **genes** of a normal cell lead to continuous cell division. **Cancer cells are called malignant cells because damage to the cells' deoxyribonucleic acid (DNA) causes the cells to reproduce in an uncontrolled way and then invade other tissues and organs.** Malignant cells do not seem to "know" when to stop multiplying. Cancer cells multiply continuously in great numbers in a disorganized way, growing on top of each other, forming a mass or **tumor**. They continue to grow and expand locally and then can break off and travel through the bloodstream or lymph tissues to other parts of the body. This process is called **metastasis**. Cancer cells' demand for nutrients depletes the supply of nourishment available for normal cells. Cancer cells take on new characteristics, so that they do not resemble the cells of the original tissue. The gene damage that led to cancer in the first place takes on new damage or mutations that allow cancer cells to avoid programmed cell death (apoptosis) (Fig. 8.2).

METASTASIS

As stated earlier, metastasis refers to the movement of malignant cells from the original site of the cancer to another part of the body (Table 8.1). Malignant cells can metastasize by breaking off from the primary tumor

Table 8.1 Common Sites of Metastasis for Different Cancer Types

CANCER TYPE	SITES OF METASTASIS
Breast cancer	Bone[a] Lung[a] Liver Brain
Lung cancer	Brain[a] Bone Liver Lymph nodes Pancreas
Colorectal cancer	Liver[a] Lymph nodes Adjacent structures
Prostate cancer	Bone (especially spine and legs)[a] Pelvic nodes
Melanoma	Gastrointestinal tract Lymph nodes Lung Brain
Primary brain cancer	Central nervous system

From Ignatavicius DD, Workman ML, Rebar CR, et al.: *Medical-surgical nursing: patient-centered collaborative care*, ed 9, St. Louis, 2018, Elsevier.
[a]Most common site of metastasis for the specific malignant neoplasm.

and traveling to other sites in the body through the blood and lymph, similar to the way bacterial cells spread during an infection. Malignant cells also can be transplanted directly from one organ to another during surgery when gloves and instruments serve as vehicles for the transportation of malignant cells. Another way in which malignant cells can "contaminate" normal tissues and organs is by entering a body cavity and coming in contact with a healthy organ. For example, malignant cells may break off from a diseased organ, enter the abdominal cavity, and attach themselves to an ovary or the **mesentery** (tissues that connect the internal organs to the abdominal cavity wall) (Fig. 8.3).

The **prognosis** (prediction of survival) for a patient with a malignancy depends on how much the malignant cells have attacked body tissues. Cancer that remains confined to the original site *(in situ)* and has not yet released its cells, even though the growth may have invaded underlying tissues, is much more easily removed or cured at this stage.

A *regional* malignancy is one in which cells from the original malignancy have spread to the tissues around the tumor, such as nearby lymph nodes. However, if the regional cancer is not treated or is inadequately treated, malignant cells may continue to grow and multiply, eventually breaking away and spreading or metastasizing throughout the body. This creates an *advanced cancer* that is often fatal.

Not all malignant cells metastasize, but most do. Patients with cancer often die from metastatic disease as cancer invades major organs and disrupts normal cellular processes.

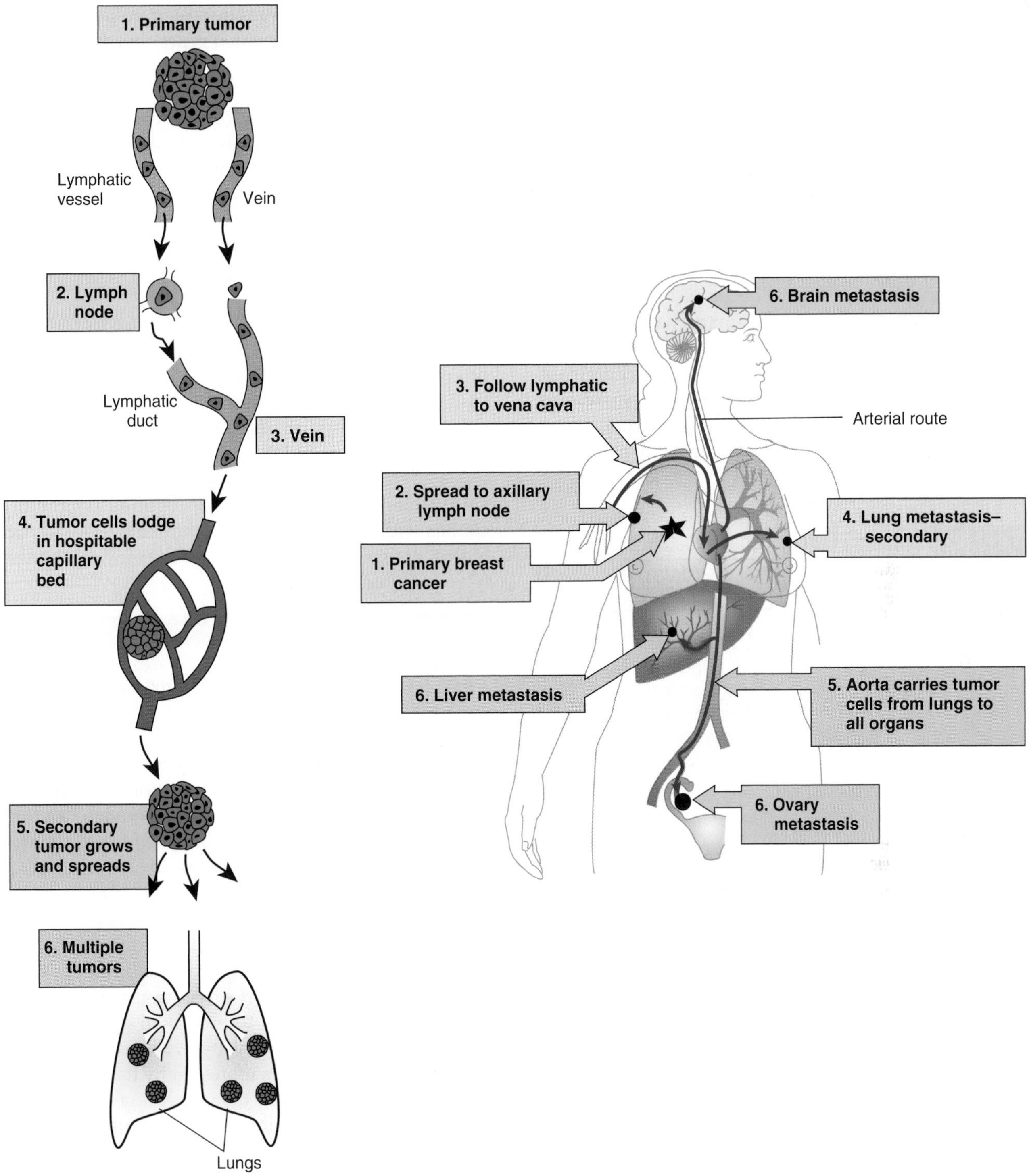

Fig. 8.3 Metastatic breast cancer. (From Hubert RJ, VanMeter KC: *Gould's pathophysiology for the health professions*, ed 6, St. Louis, 2018, Elsevier.)

> **? Think Critically**
>
> What are the characteristics of malignant cells that differ from those of normal cells?

GENETIC FACTORS

All cancer results from defects in the DNA of genes. These defects may be inherited or are caused by **mutation** (a permanent change in the DNA sequence of a gene) during a person's lifetime from exposures to chemicals or radiation. Often genetic mutations arise spontaneously for reasons that are unknown. Cancer-causing genes are known as oncogenes. An **oncogene** is a normal gene involved in cell growth and reproduction that becomes mutated and predisposes the cell to becoming cancerous. The defective gene tells the new cells to multiply at a higher rate. Normal cells go through a rapid cell death (apoptosis) when the cells are damaged. Activated oncogenes cause the cell to survive and expand instead of dying. This results in a tumor, or mass.

Tumor suppressor genes are healthy, normal genes that slow cell division, make cell repairs, and tell cells when to die.

CARCINOGENS

Each person's body has a different ability to withstand the effects of cancer-causing substances (**carcinogens**), to mount a healthy immune response, and to repair damaged DNA.

In the external environment, many harmful agents exist that are known or suspected to be carcinogenic. **Among these harmful agents are certain chemicals, sources of radiation, viruses, and other infectious agents** (Table 8.2). There are also some internal factors that affect an individual's ability to cope with malignant cells. The individual's immune system response, certain hormones and several inherited genes, and some medical conditions are thought to play a role in the development and progression of cancer.

Although cancer can strike at any age, older adults are more likely to develop cancer. **Immunocompetence**, or the capability of one's immune system to deal with foreign cells—bacterial, viral, or malignant—decreases with aging and is an important factor in the development of cancers. As a result, age is the single biggest risk factor for developing cancer.

Table 8.2 Common Carcinogenic Substances

SUBSTANCE	TYPE OF CANCER
Asbestos	Lung, peritoneal, pericardial
Benzene	Acute myelocytic leukemia
Tobacco	Lung, mouth, pharynx, larynx, esophagus, pancreas, bladder, kidney, colon, liver
Alcoholic beverages	Mouth, pharynx, larynx, esophagus, liver
Radon	Lung
Ionizing radiation	Leukemia, tumors of most organs
Sunlight (ultraviolet rays)	Skin
Diethylstilbestrol (prenatally)	Vaginal
Estrogens, synthetic	Endometrial
Androgens, synthetic	Liver
Vinyl chloride	Liver
Aromatic amines	Bladder
Arsenic (inorganic)	Lung, skin
Chromium	Lung
Nickel dust	Lung, nasal sinuses
Chronic hepatitis B or C infection	Liver
Human T-cell lymphotropic virus type 1 (HTLV-1)	Adult T-cell leukemia and lymphoma
Human papillomavirus (HPV)	Cervix, vagina, vulva, penis, anus, mouth, throat
Phenacetin	Renal pelvis, bladder
Alkylating agents (used for chemotherapy)	Acute myelocytic leukemia
Cyclosporine (used to prevent transplant rejection)	Non-Hodgkin lymphoma

CHEMICAL CARCINOGENS

More than 200 years ago (in 1775), Sir Percival Pott linked the occurrence of cancer to a substance in the environment when he observed that cancer of the scrotum was common among the chimney sweeps of London. He attributed this high incidence of cancer to repeated accumulations of soot on the skin of these young men, whose occupation required continuous contact with the coal soot in the chimneys they cleaned. Since that time, almost 500 different chemical carcinogens have been identified.

Think Critically

Identify carcinogens that you may be exposed to in your home or workplace. What can you do to reduce your exposure and decrease the risk of cancer?

Many of the cancer-producing substances in the environment are related to occupations that involve repeated exposure to these substances through handling or inhalation. **Petrofluorocarbons (polychlorinated biphenyls, or PCBs) and some pesticides (e.g., DDT) are known carcinogens.** Exposure to chemicals can decrease immunocompetence. For example, cancer of the skin often is related to the handling of pitch, asphalt, crude paraffin, and petroleum products. **Cigarette smoking is a known direct cause of cancer of the lung and is believed to be linked to esophageal, pancreatic, bladder, kidney, liver, and colon cancers.** Cigarette smoking is even more deadly than previously understood. In early 2014 the surgeon general's office released a report implicating tobacco use in several other diseases, including diabetes, colon cancer, and liver cancer (U.S. Department of Health and Human Services, 2014). Chewing tobacco has been directly related to cancer of the tongue and structures of the mouth and throat. Substances linked to the development of lung cancer are asbestos, radon, and chemical wastes from industry.

There is evidence that benzene, an ingredient in older unleaded gasoline, can cause certain types of leukemia. These are just a few of the chemical agents that can contribute to the development of cancer in humans.

Suppressing the immune system's normal response can result in the ability of cancer cells to evade the immune system's surveillance and in cancer. For example, immunosuppressive drugs used to suppress organ transplant rejection are a cause of non-Hodgkin lymphoma. Some hormones have also been linked to the growth and progression of cancer. Synthetic estrogens are linked to a higher incidence of breast and endometrial cancer. Ironically, some cancer drugs can harm the immune system and can predispose the patient to a secondary type of cancer.

EXOGENOUS HORMONES

The use of exogenous (external) hormones for the treatment of the symptoms of menopause, such as night sweats and hot flashes, has been linked to breast cancer. In women who are perimenopausal or postmenopausal, if hormones are used, a combination of progesterone and estrogen is recommended. However, long-term hormone replacement therapy is associated with an increased risk for breast cancer after 5 years of treatment. Each woman should discuss her personal risk for breast cancer with her health care provider before beginning hormone replacement therapy.

Health Promotion

Effects of Smoking

Encourage individuals who use tobacco to quit. Ninety percent of lung cancers in men and 79% in women are related to smoking. Use of tobacco in conjunction with the intake of alcohol is related to several other types of cancer.

CANCER PROMOTION

Some substances are thought to be involved in the promotion of cancer. **Promoters** are substances that are not carcinogenic by themselves but when combined with a known carcinogen, can lead to cancer development at a faster rate. Alcohol is such a substance. Cancer occurs at a faster rate in those who are heavy consumers of alcohol and who use nicotine than in those who use nicotine but do not drink alcohol. In this manner, alcohol is considered a promoter that is also a co-carcinogen. It is estimated that 90% of all head and neck cancers are related to a combination of tobacco and alcohol use.

PHYSICAL CARCINOGENS

Radiation

Radiation may originate from x-ray machines and radioactive elements or from the ultraviolet rays of the sun. These rays are capable of penetrating certain body tissues and causing the development of malignant cells in the affected area. The relationship of intense and prolonged exposure to radiation and the development of cancer was first discovered when a high incidence of leukemia occurred among people who pioneered studies of x-rays or who worked with radium or uranium. Survivors of the atomic blasts at Hiroshima and Nagasaki at the end of World War II had an unusually high incidence of leukemia.

There is continued concern about the danger that excessive radiation in the environment presents, especially the long-term effects that are not immediately apparent but may eventually prove to be related to malignancy. In addition to leukemia, cancers of the skin, bone marrow, breast, lung, and thyroid are believed to be closely linked to exposure to radiation.

The ultraviolet rays of the sun can produce skin cancer. The most common types of skin cancer (basal and squamous cell cancers) are found in areas of the body exposed to the sun and are related to the amount of lifetime sun exposure. The susceptibility of the individual also is a factor for developing skin cancer. People with fair complexions have less protective pigment and therefore are more likely to develop skin cancer from ultraviolet radiation than are people with darker skin. Severe sunburns before age 18 can lead to a more serious type of skin cancer called *malignant melanoma* in later life. Susceptibility to the development of malignant melanoma may be found to run in certain families.

Radon Gas

Radon gas is a colorless and odorless gas found with the decay of radioactive materials in rocks and soil. Radon gas can enter homes and businesses through cracks in the floors, walls, or foundations. When inhaled, these radioactive particles can damage cells that line the lung. Populations that live in areas that have more radon emission from the soil have a higher incidence of lung malignancy than do those that live in areas that are low in radon.

Viruses and Other Infectious Agents

In recent years research has established a causal link between viruses, bacteria, parasites, and malignancy. **Viruses are capable of introducing new genetic material into a normal cell and transforming it into a malignant one.** Furthermore, cell reproduction can be altered when viruses interact with carcinogens. Viruses have their own oncogenes, which when activated can reproduce and transform into malignant cells. In fact, at least 10 cancers have been identified as being driven by a virus. These viruses are known as *oncoviruses* because of their ability to cause cancer. After the **transformation** (change into something else) of a normal cell into a precancerous state, the malignant cell requires many conditions favorable to its multiplication and growth into a cancerous tumor.

Viruses such as the human immunodeficiency virus (HIV) can damage the immune system and indirectly cause cancer by allowing oncogenes to be expressed, leading to malignant transformation. Some cancers—such as Kaposi sarcoma—are seen only in HIV-infected or severely immunocompromised patients (see Chapter 11). HIV-infected people have a 10 times higher risk for developing non-Hodgkin lymphoma than uninfected people. The hepatitis B virus is carcinogenic for liver cancer. The Epstein-Barr virus is associated with the development of Burkitt lymphoma and cancer of the stomach. Cases of adult T-cell leukemia and lymphoma are caused by HTLV-1. Several types of the human papillomavirus (HPV) cause cervical carcinoma; cancers of the vagina, penis, and anus; and cancers of the head and neck.

Other infectious agents are also associated with cancer development. Cancer of the stomach is associated with the gram-negative bacterium known as *Helicobacter pylori,* which causes infection of the epithelial cells of the stomach. People infected with *H. pylori* have a 10% to 20% chance of developing a gastric (stomach) ulcer and a 1% to 2% chance of developing gastric cancer. The flatworm parasite *Schistosoma haematobium* can be found mostly in sub-Saharan Africa and the Middle East and is the most common parasitic infection in humans. The parasite enters the bladder, causing chronic infection and inflammation leading to bladder cancer. Early and complete treatment for infection can decrease inflammation and prevent some cancers caused by these infectious agents.

GENETIC PREDISPOSITION

Most cancers are caused by genes that are damaged (mutated) throughout the lifetime and not inherited. Genetic markers have been identified for colon cancer, prostate cancer, pancreatic cancer, and leukemia. However, only 5% to 10% of cancers are related to a directly inherited gene. Some people are more susceptible to these mutations.

Research has shown that some people have a genetic predisposition to various types of cancer. For example, breast cancer is more likely to occur in women who have a close female relative who developed breast cancer before age 50. When the breast cancer tumor suppressor genes *BRCA1* and *BRCA2* are inherited, this increases a woman's risk for breast cancer, but other factors may also determine whether a woman will actually develop breast cancer. These genes do not directly cause cancer, but those who have the genes are at a much higher risk for cancer. Because of this uncertainty, several assessment tools have been developed to estimate a woman's risk for breast cancer. These tools, which include the Gail model, the Claus model, and at least five other tools, ask women to supply information about well-known predictors for breast cancer (family history, personal history) and then provide an estimate of their risk. There are tools for other kinds of cancer as well. Hereditary nonpolyposis colorectal cancer (HNPCC), or Lynch syndrome, is an inherited genetic condition that greatly increases the risk for specific cancers, especially colon and endometrial cancers. The inherited mutation impairs DNA repair. People with this inherited mutation have an 80% chance of developing colon cancer, and women with this mutation have an 80% chance of developing endometrial cancer at a relatively young age.

Cultural Considerations

Race Factors

Some populations are at a higher risk for certain types of cancer. For example, of the four types of melanoma, African Americans are most susceptible to the acral lentiginous type, whereas whites are least susceptible to it. Lentigo maligna melanoma is found most often in Hawaii.

With the completion of the Human Genome Project, scientists continue to work to identify the genes that are related to specific cancers (Faherty, 2018). Current research is focused on finding genetic markers—or oncogenes—for other forms of cancer. Such markers, or the proteins they produce, could identify high-risk individuals who then might undergo more vigorous, regular diagnostic testing to detect any malignancy in the very earliest stages.

CONTRIBUTING FACTORS

INTRINSIC FACTORS

Age, sex, and race are considered "predisposing factors" for certain types of cancers. Predisposition simply means that, statistically, certain types of cancer strike particular age, sex, or racial groups more frequently than others. The risk for all cancers increases with age. Immune system functioning declines with age and may allow mutated cells to escape repair and become malignant. Approximately 76% of cancers occur in people ages 55 years and older.

Although some differences in cancer can be related to hormonal differences between males and females, it is thought that most differences in cancer incidence between the sexes result from health behaviors rather than real gender differences. Cancer of the esophagus is more common in men than in women, but this is more likely due to gastroesophageal reflux, triggered by behaviors such as smoking, alcohol, and late-night eating.

In terms of race, prostate cancer is far more common in black males than in white males. Breast cancer is more prevalent in white women than in Asian women.

DIETARY FACTORS

Obesity is strongly associated with the development of several cancers, including cancers of the pancreas, breast, esophagus, kidney, and endometrium. **At present, 15% to 20% of all cancer deaths in the United States are associated with obesity. Obesity is also associated with a 30% increase in breast cancer risk.** Being obese increases circulating blood glucose, insulin, cellular growth factors, and estrogens that can activate oncogenes and metabolic pathways that cause precancerous cells to grow and reproduce. There is evidence to suggest that diets high in fats, red meats, and processed meats and low in fruits and vegetables are related to the development of cancer, specifically breast, colorectal, and pancreatic cancers. Drinking alcoholic beverages is associated with developing head and neck cancer and cancers of the esophagus, breast, and liver. A diet high in fat has been linked to the risk of cancer recurrence, whereas a diet high in fruit intake is associated with fewer cancer relapses.

DISEASE FACTORS: DIABETES MELLITUS

There are now studies linking type 2 diabetes to the development of several cancers, including breast, prostate, pancreatic, esophageal, and colon cancers. Common cancer-promoting factors include obesity, insulin resistance, and inflammation in patients with type 2 diabetes.

CLASSIFICATION OF TUMORS

Tumors are often classified according to the organs or tissues from which they originated. More accurate naming can be achieved by adding modifying prefixes. For example, *osteosarcomas* arise from bone *(osteo),* and *adenocarcinomas* arise from glandular *(adeno)* structures.

Malignant growths are divided into four main types. A **sarcoma** arises from mesenchymal tissues (bone, muscles, and other connective tissues). A **carcinoma** originates in epithelial tissues (lining of organs, skin). These kinds of cancers make up most solid tumor cancers of the liver, kidney, breast, uterus, lungs, and tongue. Basal cell carcinoma is the most common cancer. It involves the deepest part of the outer layer of the skin. Another type of carcinoma is carcinoma in situ (in site). For example, ductal carcinoma in situ is a cancer in the milk ducts of the breast that has not spread to surrounding tissue. **Leukemia** and **lymphoma** are cancers of the blood-forming system. Malignancy of the pigment cells of the skin is called **melanoma**.

CANCER STAGING

One system that identifies cancers by how much the cancer or malignancy has spread is the **TNM staging** system. The three basic parts of the system are *T* for primary tumor, *N* for regional nodes, and *M* for metastasis. The number written beside each letter indicates how much the malignancy has spread and attacked other tissues. For example, T1, N0, M0 means that the tumor is small and localized (no involvement of regional lymph nodes and no metastasis). A label of T1, N2, M1 indicates a small (T1) tumor with moderate regional involvement (N2) that has metastasized to one distant site or organ (M1).

MEASURES TO PREVENT CANCER

Nurses play a critical role in the education of patients and families about sound ways to prevent cancer. **Each patient encounter is a time you can use to teach patients the following cancer prevention measures.**

NUTRITION AND EXERCISE FOR CANCER PREVENTION

Encourage maintenance of normal weight. Being overweight or obese is a risk factor in many cancers.

Encourage a healthy diet. Limit the intake of red meats and processed meats such as hot dogs, bacon, sausage, lunch meats like bologna, and processed chicken nuggets. Limit the intake of foods high in sugars, such as sodas, candy, and desserts. Limit foods high in saturated fats, such as cheese, butter, whole milk, and dairy products. Encourage the intake of whole grains, vegetables, and fruits. Eat at least 2½ cups of vegetables and fruits each day. Avoid drinking excessive amounts of alcohol, and limit salted, grilled, and smoked foods.

Encourage exercise. The ACS has the following physical activity recommendations for the prevention of cancer:

- **Adults:** Get at least 150 minutes of moderate-intensity activity or 75 minutes of vigorous-intensity activity each week. This can be spread throughout the week.
- **Children and teens:** Get at least 1 hour of moderate- or vigorous-intensity activity each day, with vigorous activity on at least 3 days each week.
- Limit sedentary behavior such as sitting or watching TV.

? Think Critically

You are caring for a patient who has a history of type 2 diabetes and who has just been diagnosed with cancer. What types and amounts of whole grains, fruits, and vegetables would you advise the patient to eat?

Nutrition Considerations

Minimizing the Risk for Cancer

- Eat a diet of brightly colored, varied fruits and vegetables, and balance daily caloric intake with exercise to maintain a healthy weight.
- Limit intake of red meats and processed meats. Eat fatty fish twice a week to increase intake of omega-3 fatty acids. Limit intake of saturated and trans fats. Substitute olive oil for cooking and salad dressings where possible.
- Eat five or more servings of a variety of vegetables and fruits each day. Include cruciferous vegetables (broccoli, cauliflower, cabbage) and those containing betacarotene (spinach, Swiss chard, turnip greens, beet greens, tomatoes, carrots, yellow squash, sweet potatoes).
- Choose whole-grain foods over processed (refined) grains; include beans, whole-grain cereals, flaxseed, whole-grain breads, and pastas to increase fiber intake daily. Avoid white potatoes, rice, and white bread. Substitute sweet potatoes, brown rice, and whole-grain bread.
- Keep alcohol consumption moderate: no more than two drinks or two glasses of wine or beer per day for men, and no more than one drink per day for women. No alcohol is best.
- Avoid smoked, salt-cured, nitrite-cured, and grilled or charred (blackened) foods.

Think Critically

Identify three specific changes you could make in your personal diet and exercise program that might decrease your risk for cancer. How would you change your diet and exercise plan?

ENVIRONMENT

Because groundwater is often contaminated with chemicals from fertilizers, pesticides, and industrial wastes, it is wise to know the chemical makeup of the local water supply. If the geographic area is highly contaminated, filtered or bottled water might help prevent further damage to immunocompetence and thereby decrease the incidence of cancer.

Patient Teaching

Avoiding and Limiting Exposure to Carcinogens

- Know which substances used in the household, yard, recreation, and workplace are carcinogenic.
- Decrease exposure to carcinogens by using protective clothing, gloves, and masks, as appropriate, when spraying pesticides or using chemicals.
- Keep areas well ventilated when using chemical cleaners indoors.
- Wash hands and any exposed skin thoroughly after using any compounds containing carcinogenic chemicals.
- Use a broad-spectrum sunscreen (protects against UVA and UVB rays) that has a sun protection factor (SPF) of 30 or higher and is also water resistant.
- Wear protective clothing and sunglasses when outdoors and avoid sunburns, tanning salons, and sunlamps to greatly decrease the incidence of skin cancer.
- Teach patients to *slip, slap, slop, strap—slip* on protective clothing, *slap* on a hat, *slop* on some sunscreen, and *strap* on sunglasses. Australians have the highest rate of skin cancer in the world and developed this useful saying as a reminder of how to reduce risk.
- Avoid swimming and playing water sports in contaminated waters. Avoid eating fish from waters that have chemical contamination.
- Wash or rinse fruits and vegetables before eating or cooking to decrease exposure to agricultural pesticides.

IDENTIFYING HIGH-RISK PEOPLE

Studies of the family and medical history and the lifestyle of individuals who have developed cancer have shown that some people are more likely to develop certain kinds of cancer. Table 8.3 shows information on high-risk groups published by the ACS to develop an awareness of the need for examinations to detect cancer early in those who are susceptible to developing a malignancy.

DETECTION OF CANCER

Cancer can strike any organ of the body, alter the function of critical organs such as the liver or kidneys, and result in numerous symptoms as it progresses. The purpose of screening for cancer in large segments of a population is to identify as many people with cancer in the early stages as possible. The signs and symptoms listed in the Health Promotion box are warnings for the person to seek medical advice to test for cancer.

Health Promotion

Warning Signs of Cancer

- Unusual bleeding or discharge
- A sore that does not heal
- A change in bowel or bladder habits
- A lump in the breast or other part of the body
- A nagging, persistent cough
- An obvious change in a mole
- Difficulty in swallowing

Older Adult Care Points

Older adults have a higher risk for developing cancer; their immune system is not as efficient as that of a younger person. Many cancer screening programs are suggested to begin at age 40 or 50.

At physical examination, certain tests are conducted to determine whether a malignancy is present. Recommendations made by the ACS for routine checkups and early detection of cancer are shown in Table 8.4.

One widely used technique to detect cancer is to examine cells under a microscope to determine whether they are malignant or premalignant. This technique is called **cytology**, and the most widely used cytology test is the Papanicolaou (Pap) smear to detect cervical cancer. A cytologic examination can be performed by obtaining a sample of secretions containing cells that have been released from adjacent tissue. The technique involves either scraping or brushing a sample of cells from the area or collecting body secretions that contain cells, such as cervical discharges, sputum, gastric washings, pleural fluid, or urinary washings. A specially trained technologist or pathologist examines the cells microscopically. If "suspicious" cells are found, the patient is referred to a health care professional for more extensive diagnostic tests. Another screening technique, used for colorectal cancer, is the simple test for **occult blood** (hidden blood) in the stool. This can be obtained through a fecal occult blood test (FOBT) or a newer test called the fecal immunochemical test (FIT). The person simply collects one or more stool specimens (depending on the test being used), applies a thin smear on the container provided, and returns the specimens to the health center, clinic, or clinical laboratory. **Occult blood**

Table 8.3 Major Risk Factors for Cancer

TYPE OF CANCER	RISK FACTORS	SIGNS
Lung	• Heavy smoker age >50 yr • Smoked a pack a day for 20 yr • Started smoking at age 15 yr or earlier • Exposure to environmental smoke • Exposure to asbestos, arsenic, certain chemicals in the workplace • Radiation or radon exposure • History of tuberculosis	Persistent cough, recurring pneumonia or bronchitis, blood in the sputum, chest pain
Breast	• History of breast cancer • History of some forms of breast biopsy • Close relatives with history of breast cancer • Early menarche; late menopause • Never had children; first child after age 30 yr • Lengthy exposure to cyclic estrogen • Higher educational and socioeconomic status • Consumption of alcohol	Lump in breast, nipple discharge, thickening, dimpling, nipple retraction, pain or tenderness of the nipple
Colon and rectum	• History of rectal polyps • Rectal polyps run in family • History of inflammatory bowel disease	Blood in stool, alteration in bowel pattern (e.g., constipation alternating with diarrhea)
Uterine and cervical	• Frequent sex in early teens or with many partners • History of HPV • Low socioeconomic status • Poor care during or after pregnancy • Smoking or history of smoking • Exposure to DES in utero	Unusual bleeding or discharge
Uterine and endometrial	• Estrogen therapy • Tamoxifen therapy • Late menopause (after age 55 yr) • History of infertility or failure to ovulate • Diabetes, high blood pressure, gallbladder disease, obesity • Pelvic irradiation	Unusual bleeding or discharge
Skin	• Excessive exposure to sun or tanning booth • Fair complexion • Work with coal tar, pitch, or creosote	Change in the size, color, or appearance of a mole or spot on the skin; scaliness, oozing, bleeding, or change in appearance of a bump or nodule; spread of pigmentation beyond the border; change in sensation of any skin lesion
Oral	• Heavy smoker and drinker • Use of smokeless tobacco • Poor oral hygiene • HPV	White patch in the mouth or on the tongue; nodules
Ovary	• History of ovarian cancer among close relatives • History of breast cancer • History of never having children	None until well advanced
Prostate	• Age >65 yr • Black ancestry • History of family incidence of prostate cancer	Difficulty urinating, hesitancy; blood in the urine; need to urinate frequently; pain in lower back, pelvis, or upper thighs
Stomach	• History of stomach cancer among close relatives • Diet heavy in smoked, pickled, or salted foods • Some link with blood group A	Nonspecific; indigestion, feeling of fullness or pressure; pain and weight loss are late signs
Pancreas	• Smoking or other recreational drugs	No signs
Bladder	• Smoking	Painless blood in the urine; need for frequent urination
Leukemia	• Down syndrome • Exposure to excessive radiation • Exposure to benzene (unleaded gas) • HTLV-1 infection • Philadelphia chromosome	Frequent infections, easy bruising, fatigue, weight loss, nosebleeds, paleness

DES, Diethylstilbestrol; *HPV,* human papillomavirus; *HTLV-1,* human T-cell lymphotropic virus type 1.

Table 8.4 Screening Guidelines for the Early Detection of Cancer in People With No Symptoms and Average Risk

CANCER SITE	POPULATION	TEST OR PROCEDURE	FREQUENCY
Breast[a]	Women, age >20 yr	Breast self-awareness	All women should be familiar with their own breasts and how they normally look and feel. Women should be encouraged to contact their health care providers about any changes.
		Mammography	Begin mammography at age 40, if desired. • Ages 45–54: annual • Ages 55 and older: biannual or annual, if desired • Continue mammography if life expectancy >10 yr
Cervix[b]	Women, ages 21–65 yr	Pap smear Human papillomavirus (HPV) DNA test	• Cervical cancer screening should begin at age 21. • Women ages 21–29 should be screened every 3 yr with conventional or liquid-based Pap smears. • Women ages 30–64 should be screened every 5 yr with both the HPV test and the Pap smear (preferred) or every 3 yr with the Pap smear alone (acceptable). • Women age >65 who have had normal results for the last 10 yr should discontinue testing and never restart. • Women who have had a total hysterectomy should stop cervical cancer screening. • Women vaccinated against HPV should follow the same cervical screening guidelines for all ages.
Colorectal[c]	Men and women, age >50 yr	Fecal occult blood test (FOBT) with at least 50% test sensitivity for cancer	Annual, starting at age 50. Testing at home with adherence to manufacturer's recommendation for collection techniques and number of samples is recommended. FOBT with the single stool sample collected on the clinician's fingertip during a digital rectal examination is not recommended. Guaiac-based toilet bowl FOBTs also are not recommended.[d]
		Fecal immunochemical test (FIT) with at least 50% test sensitivity for cancer or stool DNA test	Annual, starting at age 50 using the multiple stool take-home test.[d]
		Flexible sigmoidoscopy (FSIG)	Every 5 yr, starting at age 50. FSIG can be performed alone, or consideration can be given to combining FSIG performed every 5 yr with a highly sensitive FOBT or FIT performed annually.[d]
		Double-contrast barium enema (DCBE)	Every 5 yr, starting at age 50.[d]
		Colonoscopy	Every 10 yr, starting at age 50.[d]
		Computed tomography (CT) colonography	Every 5 yr, starting at age 50.[d]
Endometrial[c]	Women, at menopause	At menopause, women at average risk should be informed about risks and symptoms of endometrial cancer and strongly encouraged to report any unexpected bleeding or spotting to their health care provider.	For some women, history may dictate annual endometrial biopsy.

Table 8.4 **Screening Guidelines for the Early Detection of Cancer in People With No Symptoms and Average Risk—cont'd**

CANCER SITE	POPULATION	TEST OR PROCEDURE	FREQUENCY
Lung[e]	Current or former smokers ages 55–74 in good health with at least a 30 pack-yr history, are still smoking or have quit within the past 15 yr	Low-dose helical CT (LDCT)	Clinicians with access to high-volume, high-quality lung cancer screening and treatment centers should initiate a discussion about lung cancer screening with apparently healthy patients ages 55–74 who have at least a 30 pack-yr smoking history and who currently smoke or have quit within the past 15 yr. A process of informed and shared decision making with a clinician related to the potential benefits, limitations, and harms associated with screening for lung cancer with LDCT should occur before any decision is made to initiate lung cancer screening. Smoking cessation counseling remains a high priority for clinical attention in discussions with current smokers, who should be informed of their continuing risk of lung cancer. Screening should not be viewed as an alternative to smoking cessation.
Prostate[a]	Men, age >50 yr (African American, age >45 yr) Should make an informed decision with a health care provider whether to be tested	Prostate-specific antigen (PSA) test, with or without digital rectal examination (DRE)	Men who have at least a 10-yr life expectancy should have an opportunity to make an informed decision with their health care provider about whether to be screened for prostate cancer, after receiving information about the potential benefits, risks, and uncertainties associated with prostate cancer screening. Prostate cancer screening should not occur without an informed decision-making process. Research has not shown the benefits to outweigh the harm.
Cancer-related checkup	Men and women, age >20	During a periodic health examination, the cancer-related checkup may include examination for cancers of the thyroid, testicles, ovaries, lymph nodes, oral cavity, and skin, as well as health counseling about tobacco, sun exposure, diet and nutrition, risk factors, sexual practices, and environmental and occupational exposures.	

[a]From National Comprehensive Cancer Network (NCCN): *NCCN guidelines for detection, prevention, & risk reduction* (website): www.nccn.org/professionals/physician_gls/f_guidelines.asp#detection
[b]From American Society for Colposcopy and Cervical Pathology (ASCCP): *Screening guidelines* (website): www.asccp.org/Guidelines/Screening-Guidelines
[c]From American Cancer Society (ACS): *American Cancer Society guidelines for the early detection of cancer 2018* (website): www.cancer.org/healthy/findcancerearly/cancerscreeningguidelines/american-cancer-society-guidelines-for-the-early-detection-of-cancer
[d]Postitive tests should be followed by colonoscopy.
[e]From National Cancer Institute (NCI): *Lung cancer—non-small cell: screening* (website): www.cancer.net/cancer-types/lung-cancer-non-small-cell/screening

in the stool is not always an indication of cancer of the bowel or rectum. Other conditions, such as colitis, also can produce this symptom.

Other procedures used to identify lesions that are possibly malignant include radiologic studies (x-rays, mammography), endoscopy, sonography, magnetic resonance imaging (MRI), computed tomography (CT scan), clinical laboratory testing of enzymes and other substances in the blood, and studies specific to the system in which the cancer is suspected. Research continues to identify proteins produced by mutated DNA that might be used to diagnose various types of cancer. Tests for viruses are now being done to identify increased risk for some cancers. For example, a test for the presence of high-risk types of HPV is available to identify women at risk for cervical cancer.

DIAGNOSTIC TESTS

Biopsy

Biopsy of a tumor and examination of the cells obtained are required to firmly establish a diagnosis of malignancy in most neoplasms. Malignancies involving blood cells, such as in leukemia, are diagnosed by examining these cells through a bone marrow biopsy. A **biopsy** is the removal of living cells for the purpose of examining them under a microscope. The cells may be removed by surgical *excision* (cutting out) of a small part of a tumor, by the *aspiration* (suction) of cells through a needle introduced into the growth, or by brush biopsy. If the tumor is small, the entire growth may be removed. A pathologist uses a microscope to examine the specimen obtained.

If the sample is taken in the operating room, and the surgeon is waiting for the results to determine the extent of surgery needed to remove all malignant cells, the tissues may be frozen for quick examination. This technique is called *preparing a frozen section.*

Procedures such as fine-needle aspiration (FNA) and *percutaneous* (through the skin) large-core breast biopsy are used for diagnosing breast cancer without the disfigurement of traditional surgical breast biopsy. Breast biopsy is combined with imaging techniques such as ultrasound to verify correct placement of the biopsy needle. Then FNA is combined with computer analysis of the samples obtained.

Radiologic Studies

X-ray films may be the first step in examining the body for cancer. X-rays can be helpful in visualizing bone and hollow organ tumors. **Mammography** is a radiologic examination of the breast that is useful in diagnosing malignant growths or suspicious lesions that cannot be felt on examination. Newly developed three-dimensional (3D) mammograms (also called *tomosynthesis mammography*) are now commonly available. Recently, newer techniques have made it possible to create 3D images using the same radiation as the two-dimensional (2D) images. This makes tomosynthesis mammography superior to 2D mammography because it (1) better detects small invasive carcinomas and (2) reduces the rate of patient recalls (Hooly, Durand, & Philpotts, 2017). In some cases, mammography is combined with an ultrasound scan that uses sound waves to determine if a lump that can be felt is liquid filled (a cyst) or a solid mass that is more like a tumor.

The respiratory, digestive, and urinary tracts can be visualized on a radiograph if a **radiopaque** (not penetrated by x-rays) substance is used. The substance passes through the hollow organ and, because it is radiopaque, the inner structure of the organ is clearly demonstrated on the radiograph.

Another radiologic technique involves the use of a radioactive substance (*radionuclide* or *isotope*) that is given to the patient before the x-ray filming. The isotope is a "tumor-seeking" chemical that searches for a tumor and may concentrate around it. A special scanning apparatus records information about the concentration of the isotope in the area being examined. If the substance is concentrated in a tumor, the growth shows up as a "hot spot" on the screen of the scanning apparatus. If a tumor does not accept the isotope, the normal tissue around the tumor concentrates the isotope, and the tumor shows up as a "cold spot." This technique is commonly used in the investigation of thyroid tumors.

A commonly used radiologic scanning technique is *computed tomography* (CT). This method is noninvasive and involves relatively small amounts of radiation exposure for the patient.

In CT, the x-ray source moves past the patient in one direction while the film moves in another direction. In this way, 3D cross-sectional images, or "slices," of tissue can be obtained. Tumors, as well as other abnormal structures within the body tissues, can be seen in this way. *Positron emission tomography* (PET scan) is a nuclear imaging technique that produces 3D images of tracer within the body. In modern PET-CT scanners, 3D imaging is often accomplished with the aid of a CT scan performed on the patient during the same session in the same machine.

Another imaging technique is called *magnetic resonance imaging* (MRI). As in CT, MRI produces views of "slices" of tissue. MRI is very accurate in allowing the radiologist to see tumors and abnormalities that other techniques miss. It is currently used as a breast screening tool—in addition to mammography—only for patients at high risk for breast cancer (because of the need for increased screening and expense) based on family history. MRI can also be used in real time to monitor cancer treatments. Although the technique does not use ionizing radiation for imaging, the powerful magnetic field generated creates different safety concerns. Patients with pacemakers or certain metal fragments, clips, or shrapnel in the body cannot use MRI because the powerful magnets used in this technique can bend and twist metal and damage the body.

Endoscopy

An endoscope is an instrument used for direct visualization of internal body parts. It is designed so that it can be inserted and passed along the interior of hollow organs and cavities.

Types of endoscopes include the colonoscope for the colon, the bronchoscope for the trachea and bronchi, the laparoscope for the contents of the abdominal or pelvic cavity, and the cystoscope for inside the bladder. During an endoscopy, not only can the tumor or suspicious area be seen, but a sample of cells can be taken to be examined more precisely under a microscope (biopsy).

LABORATORY TESTS

No single blood test can establish a definite diagnosis of cancer, but certain tests are used to obtain specific

Box 8.1 Prostate-Specific Antigen (PSA) Test

- The patient should have no sexual activity for 24 to 48 hours before the test.
- Do not perform the test until after a urinary tract infection is cleared.
- Do not perform the test after recent urinary tract surgery.
- Collect a blood sample before digital examination.
- Prostatic acid phosphatase is collected to confirm an elevated PSA.
- The phosphatase level gives information about the extent of disease.
- Alkaline phosphatase is often elevated with bone cancer and liver metastasis.

information. A complete blood cell count that shows an extremely high white blood cell (WBC) count and the presence of blast cells is helpful in diagnosing leukemia. The presence of a high level of prostate-specific antigen (PSA) may indicate prostate cancer. Current recommendations include offering a baseline PSA test for men older than 50 years, to be repeated at various intervals depending on the patient's risk factors. Guidelines for performing a PSA test are provided in Box 8.1.

Specialized tests for **tumor markers** have been developed. These tests detect biochemical substances synthesized and released into the bloodstream by tumor cells. **Tumor markers are used not to confirm cancer but mainly to determine the response to therapy or to detect a relapse.** CA-125 is used to detect the presence of ovarian cancer or its recurrence after therapy. Carcinoembryonic antigen (CEA) and CA 19-9 are tests used to detect the recurrence of gastrointestinal, pancreatic, and liver cancer after initial treatment, and CA 27-29 is used most commonly to follow the progress of breast cancer treatment and later to check for recurrence.

NURSING MANAGEMENT

ASSESSMENT (DATA COLLECTION)

The first step is to find out whether the patient knows of the cancer diagnosis. You will then need to assess what the patient and family know about the illness and treatment plan. Some patients may suspect they have cancer but do not want to discuss it. One of your responsibilities is to assess how the disease is affecting the patient's body, quality of life, employment, and activities of daily living to plan comprehensive care.

A thorough assessment of the patient's symptoms and a good general physical assessment of the specific area of the body affected by cancer can provide a baseline for evaluation of changes in physical function caused by the cancer. A psychosocial assessment of the patient and family or significant others provides data that indicate psychosocial needs. You can then report these findings to the registered nurse (RN), who will refer the patient to resources for support and care.

Box 8.2 Common Nursing Problems for Patients With Cancer

- Altered nutrition due to increased metabolic demand from disease, nausea, vomiting, diarrhea, or mucositis
- Potential for infection due to bone marrow depression
- Pain, acute or chronic, due to effects of the tumor on body structures or due to cancer therapy
- Altered skin integrity due to surgical or radiation therapy
- Altered body image due to weight loss or hair loss
- Potential for injury to patient, staff, and visitors due to exposure to a radioactive implant
- Altered physical mobility due to restricted activity secondary to a radioactive implant
- Diarrhea and dehydration due to effects of cancer treatment
- Constipation due to effects of chemotherapy
- Altered urinary elimination due to radiation therapy or secondary to effects of chemotherapy
- Fatigue
- Insufficient knowledge of drugs and their potential side effects
- Altered self-care ability due to weakness and fatigue
- Fear of dying
- Limited coping due to the significance of cancer
- Altered family coping due to anxiety over the patient's prognosis

Finally, you and the RN should determine how to assist the patient to make the most of the personal resources and abilities that the patient currently possesses. This could mean helping with adjustment to the emotional effects of only recently receiving the diagnosis of cancer, or it could require helping the patient to deal with the pain and discomfort of advanced malignancy and to prepare for a peaceful death.

NURSING DIAGNOSIS/PROBLEM

Patients with cancer can have uncomfortable symptoms such as pain and develop complex organ system problems, depending on the stage of the disease. A large number of nursing problems or nursing diagnoses may be appropriate. Specific problems are chosen for the body systems and functions in which the disease or tumor is causing disruption of homeostasis. Often the patient and family require teaching about the cancer disease process and treatment. Common general patient problems associated with a diagnosis of cancer can be found in Box 8.2. Working with the RN, you can assist in providing the information that helps in choosing the right nursing diagnoses that fit the patient's problems.

PLANNING

Specific expected outcomes are written for each nursing problem or diagnosis chosen, as appropriate for the patient (Nursing Care Plan 8.1). Planning is a collaborative process that includes the patient, the family, the oncologist, the nurse practitioner or physician assistant,

Nursing Care Plan 8.1 Care of the Patient With Cancer

SCENARIO

Mr. Pole is receiving chemotherapy for leukemia. This is his third round of weekly intravenous treatments. His platelet count is down to 185,000; he has had difficulty eating as a result of mucositis and anorexia. He states that he is mildly nauseated most of the time. He is 15 lb underweight.

PROBLEM STATEMENT

Risk for infection related to bone marrow suppression.

SUPPORTING ASSESSMENT DATA

Objective: Receiving chemotherapy drugs that suppress bone marrow.

Goals/Expected Outcomes	Nursing Interventions	Selected Rationale	Evaluation
Patient will remain free of infection.	Monitor WBCs and absolute neutrophil count (ANC).	Neutropenia is a sign of immunosuppression. More susceptible to infection when WBCs <3000 and granulocyte count is <2000.	WBCs 3200; ANC 1.5.
	Assess for signs of infection every shift.	Elevated temperature may indicate infection.	Temp 98.8° F (37.1° C); no signs of infection.
	Teach good hygiene, mouth care, hand hygiene before meals and after using bathroom.	Hand hygiene prevents spread of infection.	Patient washing hands appropriately and using good hygiene.
	Use protective isolation techniques if needed.	If neutrophil count <500, protective isolation is necessary.	Isolation not yet initiated.
	Encourage good nutrition and hydration.	Good nutrition and hydration minimize irritation.	Taking sufficient food and fluid; continue plan.
	Give Neupogen as ordered.	Neupogen raises the WBC and neutrophil count.	Neupogen 300 mcg subcutaneously given 1 time/day.

PROBLEM STATEMENT

Risk for injury related to impaired blood clotting ability.

SUPPORTING ASSESSMENT DATA

Objective: Receiving chemotherapy (chemotherapy treatment lowers platelets and extends bleeding time).

Goals/Expected Outcomes	Nursing Interventions	Selected Rationale	Evaluation
Patient will remain free from hemorrhage.	Monitor blood count; assess for bleeding of gums or bruising and bleeding into joints every shift.	Blood count plays an important role in blood clotting and bleeding.	WBCs 3200; platelet count 180,000.
	Observe for signs of bleeding: hematuria, melena, etc.		No signs of bleeding.
	Refrain from needle sticks as much as possible.		
	Give stool softener as ordered to prevent straining at stool and bleeding. Prevent rectal bleeding.	Hard stools can initiate bleeding in the rectum.	Stool soft; continue plan. Stool softener administered.
	Do not take temperature rectally.		Oral temp: 98.8° F (37.1° C).
	Brush teeth with very soft brush or tooth sponge. Do not floss.	Prevent bleeding gums.	Appropriate dental hygiene.

PROBLEM STATEMENT

Risk for weight loss and loss of lean body mass due to nausea, vomiting, and mucositis.

SUPPORTING ASSESSMENT DATA

Subjective: "I feel nauseated."

Objective: Chemotherapy administration.

Nursing Care Plan 8.1 Care of the Patient With Cancer—cont'd

Goals/Expected Outcomes	Nursing Interventions	Selected Rationale	Evaluation
Patient will verbalize relief from nausea.	Keep room odor free; give mouth care before meals.	Odors may aggravate nausea.	
Patient will be able to eat with minimal discomfort.	Give ordered antiemetic before and during chemotherapy.	Antiemetics help prevent chemotherapy-induced nausea and vomiting (N&V).	Antiemetic 45 min before meals.
Patient will maintain present weight.	Assess mouth and mucous membranes every shift.	Sore mouth may reduce food intake.	Mucous membranes reddened, but intact.
	Give meticulous mouth care q2h.		Mouth care: 7, 9, 11, 1, and 3 o'clock.
	Use distraction, meditation, relaxation techniques.	N&V may be reduced with behavioral interventions.	Has not vomited this shift.
	Give small, frequent meals.	Experts recommend these dietary interventions.	Enriched shake taken between meals.
	Encourage added calories in meals and food supplements between meals.		

PROBLEM STATEMENT

Change in body image due to disease and treatment effects.

SUPPORTING ASSESSMENT DATA

Subjective: "I look awful; I don't want any visitors to see me."
Objective: Loss of considerable amount of hair from head.

Goals/Expected Outcomes	Nursing Interventions	Selected Rationale	Evaluation
Patient will adjust to new body image within 3 wk as evidenced by verbalization.	Encourage him to maintain sense of humor.	Humor is a positive coping strategy.	
	Use caps, head bandanna, and eyebrow pencil as needed.	Hair covering may reduce negative body image.	Checking on purchase of wig; family is bringing head scarves.
	Assure him that hair will eventually grow back.		
	Encourage verbalization of feelings; focus on strengths.	Verbalization is a positive coping technique.	Talking more about feelings regarding weight loss and appearance.
	Establish and maintain trusting relationship.		
	Assess spiritual needs; help patient achieve spiritual consolation.		Continue plan.
	Encourage him to obtain clothing that fits.		

PROBLEM STATEMENT

Psychological distress related to cancer diagnosis and fear of death.

SUPPORTING ASSESSMENT DATA

Subjective: "Do you really think the treatment will cure my cancer? I'm afraid that I'll go through all this and it will just come back in a few months."

Goals/Expected Outcomes	Nursing Interventions	Selected Rationale	Evaluation
Patient will verbalize fears and develop coping mechanisms to decrease fear.	Encourage verbalization and identification of specific fears.	Verbalizing fears makes them easier to face.	Is verbalizing fears; encouraged to do same with family.
	Help him to explore ways to cope with fears.	Knowing what to expect helps people plan.	Used to meditate; encouraged to do so.

Continued

Nursing Care Plan 8.1 Care of the Patient With Cancer—cont'd

Goals/Expected Outcomes	Nursing Interventions	Selected Rationale	Evaluation
	Assess spiritual needs; contact minister or other as patient desires.	Patients have their own beliefs about death.	Began teaching imagery techniques.
	Offer support by active listening, offering hope in some form, and being there for patient.	Active listening provides comfort and strength.	Continue plan.
	Encourage expression of fears to significant others.	When significant others are aware of the patient's fears, they have a better understanding of behavior.	

CRITICAL THINKING QUESTIONS

1. What is a nursing problem that may apply to a patient who is receiving chemotherapy?
2. Why should you be concerned about infection in a patient who is receiving chemotherapy?

the nursing team, the social worker, the oncology pharmacist, and other specialists on the health care team. At times, a home care nurse or an infusion therapy nurse is involved in care and should be included in the planning process. The health care team works directly with the patient and family, and typically an oncology case manager coordinates the plan of care for the patient.

◆ IMPLEMENTATION

See Nursing Care Plan 8.1 and sections later in this chapter for specific interventions.

◆ EVALUATION

Evaluation is based on determining whether the expected outcomes specified for the patient have been met. Assessment for signs of disease or treatment complications, side effects of therapy, nutritional status, and pain and emotional distress is conducted at each visit. The nursing care plan must be changed when the interventions initially chosen are not effective in meeting the desired outcomes. Collaboration with the patient and the other members of the health care team is important to the success of changes to the care plan.

COMMON THERAPIES, PROBLEMS, AND NURSING CARE

There are three traditional modes of therapy for malignancies: surgery, radiation, and chemotherapy. Hormone manipulation, immunotherapy with biologic response modifiers, and bone marrow or stem cell transplantation are treatments combined with traditional therapies as appropriate.

Each mode of treatment may be used individually or in combination with one or more of the other methods available. For example, chemotherapy may be used as treatment after surgical removal of a tumor. This is considered adjuvant chemotherapy, since it follows the initial treatment of surgery. The methods of treatment are chosen after consideration of the scientific information to support the treatment, the patient's goals, the patient's past medical history and physical condition, and the expected side effects of the treatments planned.

SURGERY

Surgery may be performed for a variety of reasons:

- To obtain a biopsy specimen
- As prophylaxis (preventive treatment), such as in the removal of the ovaries of a woman whose mother had ovarian cancer
- To determine the effectiveness of therapy by looking to see whether the initial tumor is reduced in size
- For palliation (offering relief), as in **debulking** (removing as much as possible) a tumor to prevent pressure on adjacent structures or obstruction of vessels or the gastrointestinal (GI) tract
- As an attempt at cure

Reconstructive surgery also is associated with cancer treatment. A woman who has had a breast removed by mastectomy may have the breast *reconstructed* using tissue from the patient's abdomen, back, or buttocks to form the reconstructed breast that is completed with a saline-filled breast implant. Other extremely mutilating forms of cancer surgery require reconstructive procedures after the initial procedure. Flap grafts in a patient who underwent radical neck surgery for cancer of the throat is an example.

Surgical removal of a malignant growth is the oldest method of treatment. It works very well for tumors that are easily accessible. Adjacent tissues that may contain malignant cells also are excised. Regional lymph nodes often harbor malignant cells, which can then travel to distant parts of the body and establish a new cancer site if not removed. Newer surgical procedures and techniques have significantly reduced the need for extensive surgical removal of adjacent tissues and structures. Radical mastectomy, for example, involved removal of the entire breast along with underlying pectoral muscle tissues and lymph nodes under the arm on the affected side. This procedure has been replaced almost completely by a modified radical mastectomy, or lumpectomy and sentinel node biopsy, combined with radiation and/or chemotherapy, which is far less traumatic and mutilating. If there is no evidence of metastasis, some patients are good candidates for simple removal of the tumor (*lumpectomy*). Rarely can surgery alone cure or control cancer, which is considered a systemic disease except for basal cell skin cancers. The use of radiation and/or chemotherapy during, after, and sometimes before surgery has decreased the need for extensive removal of adjacent tissues and is associated with decreased recurrence.

RADIATION THERAPY

Radiation therapy (RT) uses high-energy radiation from gamma rays or ionizing radiation beams. As part of cancer treatment, RT is used to control or kill malignant cells, to prevent tumor recurrence, or to relieve symptoms of pain or discomfort. Radiation therapy can also be given by implanting a radioactive element or substance in the patient, such as radioactive seeds implanted in the prostate to treat prostate cancer. Radiation therapy has been used before, during, and after chemotherapy in susceptible cancers. The effects of radiation are seen only in tissues within the radiation field or path; thus this type of therapy is a *local* treatment that targets cancer cells, but normal cells within the radiation field are also affected. Radiation therapy has both short- and long-term effects, depending on the area radiated. For example, a short-term effect is redness or peeling of the skin, whereas a long-term effect can be pulmonary fibrosis from radiation of the chest.

Ionizing radiation can have both an immediate and a delayed effect on malignant cells. Ionizing radiation can damage the cell membrane immediately, causing *lysis* (bursting) or decomposition of the cell, or it can cause a break in both strands of the DNA in the cell's nucleus. **When a cell is damaged in this way, it will not die until it attempts to divide and replicate itself. The rate at which a particular kind of cell undergoes mitosis determines how quickly the effects of radiation will occur.** This explains the delayed effects and side effects of radiation that appear after treatment ends. Normal cells have a greater ability to repair the DNA damage than do malignant cells. Some tissues are more sensitive to radiation than others, and this is taken into account when the physicist-provider calculates the dose of radiation needed to eradicate the tumor. The other factors considered are the sensitivity of the tumor to radiation, its location, and its size. Once calculated, the dose of ionizing radiation is *fractionalized,* meaning it is divided over many days to weeks, to deliver the optimal dosage with the least amount of effects to normal tissues. The *rad,* or *radiation absorbed dose,* is the unit used for measuring dosages of radiation.

External beam radiation (teletherapy) and brachytherapy are the two types of radiation delivery used to treat cancer. Teletherapy is *external*—the source of radiation is delivered to the outside body of the patient. Brachytherapy is *internal*—a sealed radiation source is placed inside or next to the area requiring treatment, so the source of radiation is a radioactive element or substance that has been implanted or injected into the body to provide low doses in focused areas.

Because of improvements in tumor localization, beam direction, megavoltage machines, planning and prescribing the field to be irradiated, and determining the precise dosage needed, radiation therapy is far more beneficial and less harmful than it was when it was first pioneered. With the *linear accelerator* and its partner, the *cyclotron,* the damage to normal tissue can be minimized by keeping the dosage or degree of penetration accurate and by aiming the rays from several different angles. The latter technique increases the concentration of the rays in the area of the tumor with a minimum of damage to overlying tissues. Cobalt-60 machines deliver gamma rays, and these machines are now much more efficient and precise than they were in the early years of radiation therapy.

External Radiation Therapy

The linear accelerator used for external radiation therapy produces extremely high-energy x-ray and electron beam irradiation that bombards the malignant cells and destroys them. Because malignant cells divide at an abnormally high rate, they are more susceptible to destruction than normal cells.

Modern radiation therapy has considerably reduced side effects. The use of *stereotactic* (exact positioning in space) surgery is effective for small brain tumors (Fig. 8.4). Many cancer research institutions have lead-lined surgical suites where intraoperative radiation therapy may be delivered directly to the affected area after tumor removal and before the incision is closed. Depending on the dosage (rads) given, the patient may not need to receive further radiation. This method has proven beneficial for cancers of the head and neck, abdomen, pelvis, and extremities and for patients with operable pancreatic cancer.

Nursing care of patients undergoing external beam radiation therapy. Nursing care goals related to cancer radiation therapy include (1) helping the patient and family cope with the diagnosis of cancer and understand the radiation therapy treatment and (2) teaching the patient and family how to recognize and manage the expected side effects of radiation. The patient who is receiving external beam radiation therapy has a planning visit before any treatments begin. The physicist plans the treatment dose and area. The patient is "marked" with very small (1 mm) semipermanent

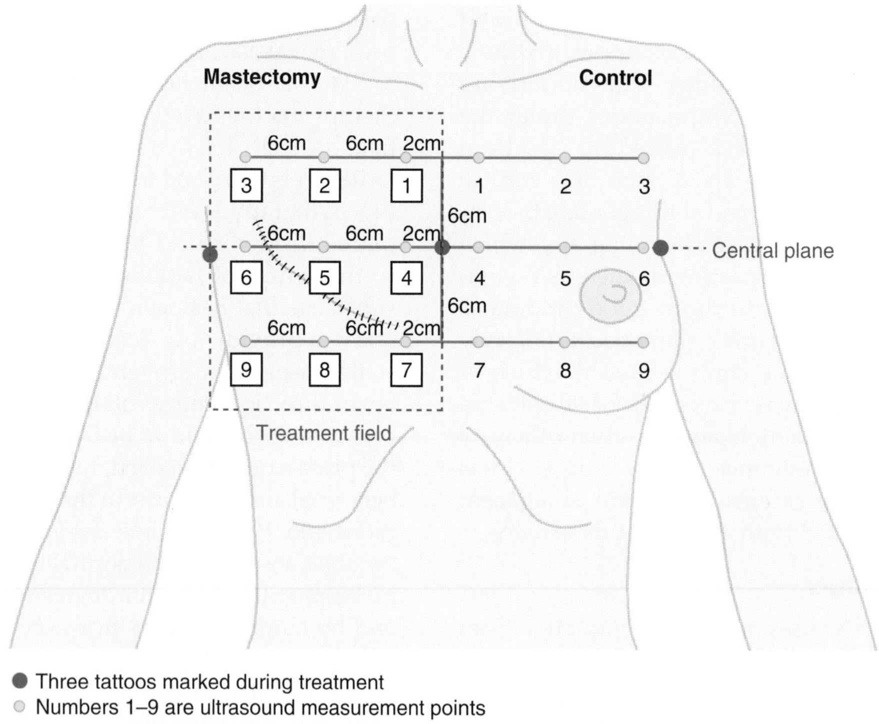

A

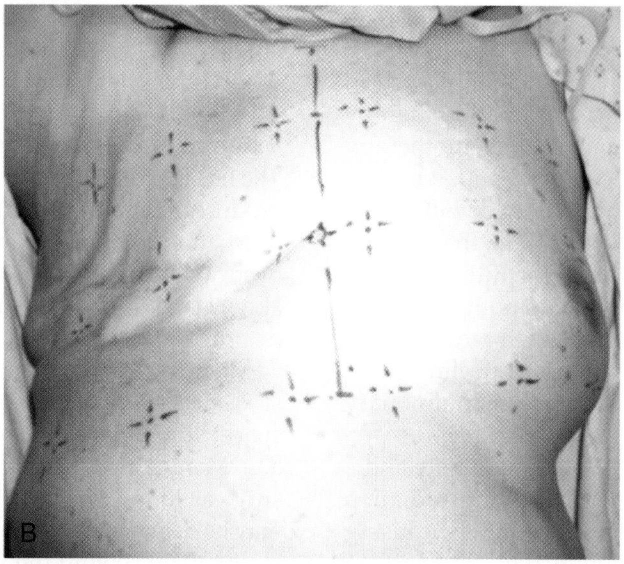

B

Fig. 8.4 **A,** Representation of points on the chest wall and contralateral nonirradiated breast. **B,** Points marked on the chest wall and contralateral nonirradiated breast prior to ultrasound (From Wong S, Kaur A, Back M, et al.: An ultrasonographic evaluation of skin thickness in breast cancer patients after postmastectomy radiation therapy, *Radiat Oncol* 6:9, 2011.)

tattoos to mark the corners and center of the area being treated.

Helping patients cope with external radiation therapy. A lack of knowledge about the side effects of radiation and how to cope with them can greatly add to the anxiety and stress that the patient feels. It is not unusual for a layperson to have some misconceptions about how radiation works, whether a patient can present a hazard to others while undergoing treatment, when the patient will begin to experience its effects, and how long it will be before the patient begins to recover from them.

Before the first treatment, the patient is told what therapeutic effects are anticipated, what it is like to have a treatment, and what to expect during the course of therapy. Because the patient will probably be treated on an outpatient basis, encourage the patient to keep their scheduled appointments but notify the clinic if cancellation is necessary. Someone should accompany the patient for initial treatments for emotional support. It is essential that time be set aside for you to establish a trusting relationship with the patient, to prompt and answer any questions about therapy, and to provide an avenue for communication throughout the course of treatment. Assure the patient that the source of radiation is in the linear accelerator machine only. It is not possible to "contaminate" others when receiving this type of radiation therapy.

Clinical trials may be available for the treatment of specific cancers, and enrollment may be available for certain patients who meet clinical trial criteria. The oncologist or radiation oncologist would provide this information to the patient and family. A comprehensive list of current clinical trials is available on the National Cancer Institute (NCI) website at http://www.cancer.gov/clinicaltrials.

Side Effects of Radiation Therapy

The most common side effect of radiation therapy is changes to the skin, known as *radiation dermatitis.* These changes can range from redness to rash and peeling of the skin. Changes to the skin can be temporary or permanent. Radiation to the scalp can result in permanent hair loss. Another common side effect of radiation is fatigue, thought to occur due to the lysis of tumor cells or the increased energy needed for repair of normal cells in the radiation path. Some degree of bone marrow suppression occurs with radiation, resulting in reduced immunity.

Patient Teaching

Skin Care During Radiation Treatment

- Shower or wash the radiated area once a day using warm water and mild soap; use a hand rather than a washcloth to wash the affected area. Dry with a soft, clean towel; pat, do not rub the skin. Do not remove the temporary ink (tattoo) markings from the skin during radiation treatment.
- Limit cold and sun exposure; when outdoors use a sunscreen with an SPF of at least 30 in the areas of the skin *not* being radiated. Radiation therapy makes the patient more susceptible to sunburn. Do not apply sunscreen to the affected skin.
- Do not use lotion, salve, or alcohol on the affected area unless prescribed by the radiologist.
- Do not remove any of the markings for radiation treatment. These will wear off over time.
- Wear loose, 100% cotton clothing over the irradiated area.
- Do not shave the area or use an electric razor without the radiologist's permission.

Skin care during radiation therapy. With the advanced methods and computerized delivery of radiation, there is much less trauma to the skin from radiation therapy than in previous years. In preparation for radiation therapy, the health care provider will outline the area to be exposed to radiation by marking it with indelible ink. The exposed area will need special care. Most clinics and hospitals have written procedures and precautions that are used to prevent unnecessary trauma to the exposed areas of skin.

Although skin damage is less now, the degree of reaction of the skin to radiation is individual and should be assessed daily, either by the patient or by a knowledgeable person. The oncology nurse working in the radiation department will assess the patient's skin on each visit, document expected findings, and report any severe skin problems to the health care provider.

Think Critically

Prepare a teaching plan for the care of the skin in a patient having external beam radiation to the chest.

Teaching the patient and family how to recognize and manage the expected side effects of radiation therapy and to understand when to call the health care provider is particularly important. The patient will feel less anxious when they know what to expect and how to perform self-care at home. It is essential to provide both verbal and written instructions to the patient and family. The verbal teaching allows the patient and family to ask questions for clarification. Written information should be simple to understand and provide a reference for when the patient is at home. Patients should be taught to bring a small notebook to write down instructions (if needed), to keep a list of questions they may have before the next visit, and to note any points on which they feel they need more information.

Internal Radiation Therapy

Radiation from *radioactive elements* has the same ionizing effect as that from linear accelerators; the only difference is the source of radiation. Internal radiation therapy, called **brachytherapy**, involves introducing a radioactive element (isotope) into the body and may be administered in different ways: (1) it can be placed in a *sealed* container and inserted in a body cavity at the tumor site or placed directly inside the tumor or (2) it may be administered in an *unsealed* form and taken orally or injected by syringe. The isotopes are unsealed sources of radiation. If radioactivity is a hazard, it is a problem only for the duration of the half-life of the isotope. The substance is eliminated through body secretions such as urine, feces, sweat, sputum, and vomit. Examples of unsealed sources are iodine-131, which is in a solution and is swallowed by the patient, and phosphorus-32 and gold-198, which are administered by injection. Because the thyroid gland readily takes up iodine, thyroid malignancies are often treated with iodine-131 delivered to the site of the tumor via the bloodstream.

To be effective, the radiation source must come into direct contact with the tumor tissue for a specified time. Most implants emit a lower level of radiation while in constant contact with the tumor cells. **Because the radiation source is within the patient, radiation is emitted for a period and can be a hazard to others. Nurses caring for patients who are receiving internal radiation must take extra precautions** (Box 8.3). During

Box 8.3 Precautionary Measures When a Patient Is Receiving Internal Radiation Therapy From a Sealed Source

- Place the patient in a private room.
- Place a sign on the patient's door indicating that they are receiving internal radiation therapy.
- Observe principles of time and distance. Limit time spent in the room. Work as quickly and as efficiently as possible. Avoid standing near the part of the patient's body where the radioactive element is located; stand at the shoulders or the feet depending on where the implant is located.
- Check all linens, bedpans, and emesis basins routinely to see if the sealed source has been accidentally lost from the tissue.
- If a sealed source is dislodged but has not fallen out of the patient's body, notify the x-ray department at once. If the source has fallen out, **do not pick it up with your bare hands.** Use forceps and place it in a lead container.
- Most patients are placed on bed rest and instructed to remain in certain positions so that emanations from the element will reach the correct area.
- Visitors should spend limited time in the room.
- No children or pregnant women should visit.

Box 8.4 Precautions When Caring for the Patient Receiving Internal Radiation From an Unsealed Source

- Observe the principles of time, distance, and shielding for radiation protection.
- Wear gloves when handling bedpans, bed linens, and the patient's clothing.
- Dispose of urine, feces, and vomitus according to policy.
- Handle dressings with forceps and dispose of them according to policy.
- Follow hospital procedure for disposal of patient's bed linens and clothing.

hospitalization for high-dose implanted radiation, children and pregnant women are not allowed to visit. Once the source of radiation is completely eliminated from the body, the patient and body waste are no longer considered radioactive.

As soon as an element becomes radioactive, it begins to lose its characteristic of radioactivity. The rate at which it becomes less radioactive is called its *half-life,* which is the amount of time it takes for half of its radioactivity to dissipate. The half-life of radium is about 1600 years, whereas the half-life of iodine is only about 8 days. Cesium-137 is a radioactive element with a half-life of 30.17 years and is frequently used to treat malignancies of the prostate, vagina, and uterine cervix. **It is important that nurses caring for a patient who is receiving sealed or unsealed sources of radiation know the element used, its half-life, and the ways in which it might be eliminated from the body in order to keep themselves and the patient safe. Nurses caring for these patients are specially trained for this task and follow hospital policy** (Box 8.4).

Some sources of radiation are small and emit very low doses of the radiation over time, until the radioactivity is completely lost. For example, brachytherapy for prostate cancer can be given in the form of tiny "seeds" placed within the prostate and left there.

Principles of Radiation Protection

In general, the amount of radiation you might receive while caring for a patient being treated with internal radioactive elements depends on three factors: (1) the distance between you and the patient, (2) the amount of time spent in actual proximity to the patient, and (3) the degree of shielding of the body that is provided.

Distance is an important factor in reducing exposure to radiation. Doubling one's distance from a radioactive element reduces the exposure to one fourth, and tripling the distance reduces it to one ninth (Fig. 8.5). Time spent near the source of radiation can be controlled when nursing care is planned to minimize time spent with the patient without sacrificing the quality of care given. The total time spent with a radioactive patient should be less than 30 minutes per shift.

Shielding from radiation exposure must take into account the type of rays being emitted. The denser the shielding material, the less the possibility of penetration by the rays, and the better the protection. A lead shield that is 1-cm thick offers the same amount of protection as 5 cm of concrete or 30 cm of wood. Lead aprons give protection from diagnostic x-rays but do not provide adequate shielding from the *gamma rays* emitted by radium, cesium-137, and cobalt-60. Anyone in proximity to—or in contact with—a source of radiation should wear a radiation dosimeter badge (Fig. 8.6). This badge measures the radiation dose that the individual has received through exposure to the source.

Hospitals where sealed sources of radiation are implanted into the body tissues to treat malignancies usually have written policies and procedures to guide personnel who are responsible for patient care. After the health care provider removes the source, the patient is no longer in need of special precautionary care. Special observations are necessary, however, in the event that a systemic reaction develops. Table 8.5 lists the most common side effects of radiation therapy. For appropriate nursing care of problems related to radiation therapy, see the Common Problems Related to Cancer or Cancer Treatment section later in the chapter.

CHEMOTHERAPY

Chemotherapy treatment protocols have been established for most types of cancer. Protocols are based on scientific evidence of their effectiveness in treating the type of cancer a patient has. A protocol will specify which drug or drugs to give for specific cancers, in what order to

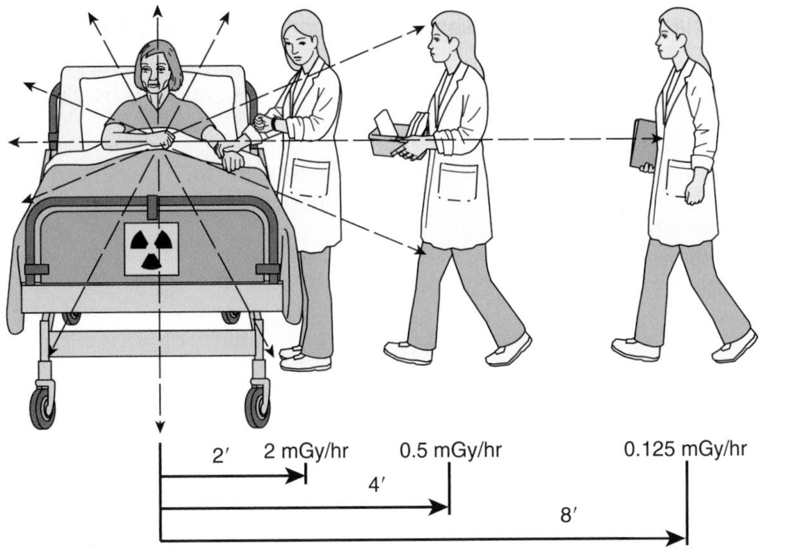

Fig. 8.5 Time, distance, and shielding in radiation exposure. The nurse nearest the source of radioactivity (the patient) is more exposed; at 2 feet, exposure is more than 15 times that of exposure at 8 feet. *mGy,* Milligray.

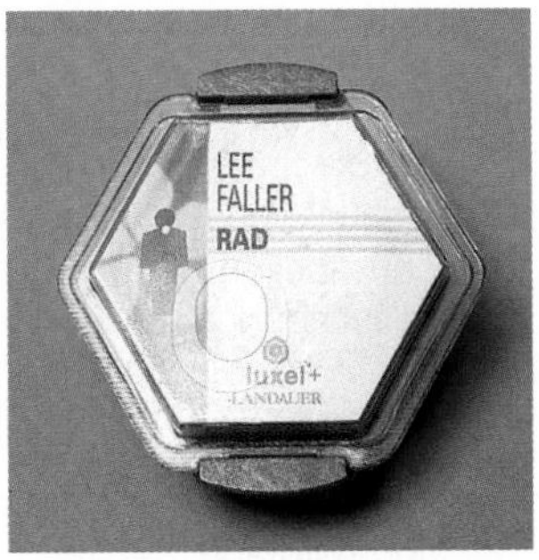

Fig. 8.6 Radiation dosimeter badge worn by personnel who might be exposed to radiation.

give them, and the time between each treatment. Which treatment is chosen depends on the type of cancer, if it has spread (metastasized), and the health of the patient. Chemotherapy may be given before surgery to shrink a tumor (neoadjuvant chemotherapy) or after surgery (adjuvant chemotherapy). Chemotherapy can also be given with other treatments such as immunotherapy.

Chemotherapy drugs are referred to as *antineoplastic* agents (Table 8.6). **The overall goal of antineoplastic drugs is to decrease the number of malignant cells in a generalized malignancy (such as leukemia), to reduce the size of a localized tumor, to relieve symptoms or prepare the patient for surgery, or to treat escaped cancer cells to prevent recurrence or metastasis.** Antineoplastic drugs are **cytotoxic** (poisonous to cells), and their damaging effects are not limited to only malignant cells. However, normal cells are better able to repair themselves more rapidly and effectively as compared to cancer cells.

Chemotherapy Administration

Drug combinations, known as *combination chemotherapy,* are used to treat certain types of cancers because different

Table 8.5 Common Side Effects of Radiation Therapy

TYPE AND AREA	EFFECT
External Radiation	
Head and neck	• Irritation of oral mucous membranes with oral pain and risk of infection • Loss of taste • Irritation of the pharynx and esophagus with nausea and indigestion • Increased intracranial pressure
Chest	• Inflammation of lung tissue with increased susceptibility to infection
Abdomen	• Nausea, vomiting, diarrhea, anorexia
Pelvis	• Diarrhea • Cystitis • Sexual dysfunction • Urethral and rectal stenosis
General side effects	• Skin: change in texture and/or color; moist desquamation (rare); alopecia • Blood: bone marrow depression with leukopenia, anemia, and thrombocytopenia • Depressed immune function • Fatigue
Internal Radiation	
General side effects	• Elevated temperature • Cervical implant: urinary frequency, diarrhea, nausea, vomiting, anorexia • Head and neck implant: mucositis, oral pain and risk of infection, anorexia

Table 8.6 Common Antineoplastic Drug Classes, Actions, and Major Side Effects

CLASSIFICATION AND EXAMPLES	ACTION	MAJOR SIDE EFFECTS[a]
Alkylating Agents		
Cyclophosphamide, doxorubicin, mechlorethamine, ifosfamide, melphalan, chlorambucil, busulfan, streptozocin, carmustin, lomustine, dacarbazine, temozolomide, thiotepa, altretamine, platinum (cisplatin, carboplatin, oxaliplatin)	Attach "alkyl groups" or organic side chains to the proteins in the cell, poisoning it; inhibit cell division	Bone marrow depression, nephrotoxicity with some Nausea, vomiting, diarrhea, dermatitis; hyperpigmentation Platinum: hearing loss
Antimetabolites		
Methotrexate, 6-mercaptopurine, 6-thioguanine, 5-fluorouracil, capecitabine, gemcitabine, cytarabine, fludarabine, pemetrexed	Interfere with a specific cell phase, thereby preventing replication Some inhibit enzymes that make essential cellular constituents; others attach to DNA, interfering with replication	Bone marrow depression, stomatitis, intestinal ulceration, nausea, vomiting, diarrhea
Antitumor Antibiotics		
Bleomycin, dactinomycin, doxorubicin, epirubicin, idarubicin, daunorubicin, plicamycin, mitomycin-C, mitoxantrone	Injure cells by direct interaction with DNA, causing distortion Interfere with DNA or RNA synthesis	Bone marrow depression, some cause cardiotoxicity; stomatitis, alopecia Bleomycin: pneumonitis and pulmonary fibrosis
Mitotic Inhibitors		
Vincristine, vinblastine, vinorelbine, etoposide	Interfere with mitosis Act during M phase of cell cycle to prevent cell division	Vincristine: peripheral neuropathy, constipation Vinblastine: bone marrow depression
Miscellaneous Agents		
Altretamine, asparaginase, etoposide, hydroxyurea, procarbazine, mitotane, teniposide, paclitaxel, imatinib mesylate, epirubicin, docetaxel, cladribine, rituximab, interleukin-2, interferon-alfa	Work in a variety of ways; consult information for each drug	Bone marrow depression is the major side effect of all except asparaginase and mitotane Asparaginase: pancreatic dysfunction Mitotane: central nervous system depression Paclitaxel: peripheral neuropathy
Hormone-Related Agents		
Anti-estrogens (fulvestrant, tamoxifen, toremifene), aromatase inhibitors (anastrozole, exemestane, letrozole), progestins (megestrol acetate), estrogens, anti-androgens	Lower circulating hormone levels to prevent hormone-related tumors	Hot flushes; deep venous thrombosis; cancer

[a]Each drug has specific side effects. Consult information on each individual drug before administration.

drugs are effective at different times in the growth and replication cycle of the tumor cell. This method offers the best chance of killing the most malignant cells. Chemotherapy is the preferred treatment for various kinds of leukemias, lymphomas, multiple myeloma, and many other solid tumors that have the ability to metastasize.

Techniques of administration of antineoplastic agents include intravenous, intra-arterial, intraperitoneal, intraventricular, and *intrathecal* (within a space of the spine). Cancers of the liver, ovary, and brain have sometimes shown better remission with intraventricular or intraperitoneal infusion treatment. An advance in chemotherapy has been the use of lower doses of multiple drugs to treat various types of malignancies. Chemotherapy drug dosages are based on *body surface area,* which considers both height and weight of the patient. Because side effects are lessened when lower doses of a drug are used, several drugs can be used in combination to hit all phases of the cell cycle, destroying more malignant cells. Chemotherapy drugs are classified as *hazardous drugs* and need careful handling in accordance with standards set by the Oncology Nursing Society and the institution's policies and procedures. **Chemotherapy is to be administered only by RNs who have completed an approved chemotherapy program**

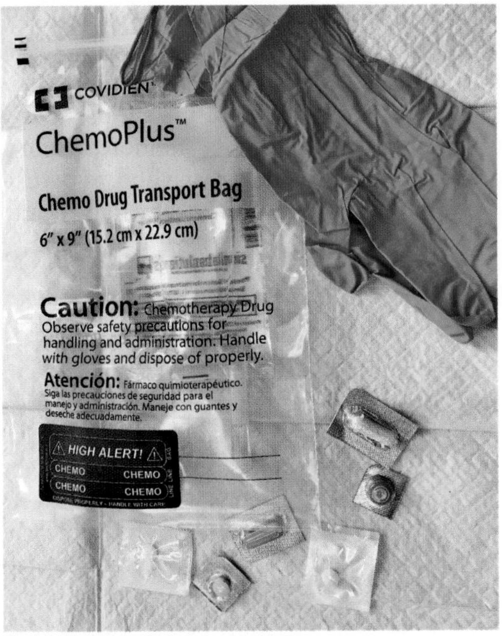

Fig. 8.7 Chemotherapy agents require special handling for the safety of the nurse administering the medication.

and have demonstrated competence in administering these agents. The licensed practical/vocational nurse (LPN/LVN) does not administer chemotherapy in the scope of their practice. ***However, responsibility for monitoring the patient during chemotherapy administration rests with all nurses providing patient care.***

IV administration of chemotherapy is the most common route, and an implanted injection port may be used as a long-term access to administer chemotherapy drugs that will be given over several weeks or months (Fig. 8.7). Nurses caring for IV sites where chemotherapy is given must wear special personal protective equipment (PPE) to prevent absorption of the drug on the skin or accidental splashing into the eyes and to handle patient urine or feces within 48 hours of chemotherapy administration. **Remember, most of these drugs are *teratogenic* (can cause birth defects), so handling of chemotherapy drugs should be avoided during pregnancy.**

Many antineoplastic drugs are **vesicants** (chemicals that cause tissue damage on direct contact) that can cause severe local injury if they leak into (infiltrate) the surrounding tissues from the vein into which they are administered. This is why the IV site is monitored closely throughout the entire infusion in accordance with the institution's policy. If **extravasation** (escape from the vein into the tissue) occurs, the infusion is stopped immediately. The type of treatment required depends on the drug and the amount that is extravasated. **Should extravasation occur, inform the RN, who will then follow the agency's policy and procedure, and also inform the health care provider and pharmacy.** Warm or cold compresses may be applied to the area, or antidotes may be injected into the affected area.

Table 8.7 Assessment for Toxic Effects of Chemotherapy[a]

SIDE EFFECT	INTERVENTION
Bone marrow suppression	Monitor red and white blood cell count and differential count for numbers of neutrophils and granulocytes; check platelet count.
Cardiotoxicity	Monitor for signs of congestive heart failure, such as pulmonary crackles, shortness of breath, tachycardia, weight gain, and peripheral edema. Monitor ECG.
Neurotoxicity	Monitor for weakness, paresthesias, sensory loss (particularly in feet), and decreased reflexes. Constipation and urinary hesitancy are other signs.
Pulmonary toxicity	Evidenced by pulmonary infiltrates and pulmonary fibrosis on x-ray. Monitor respiratory status closely; auscultate for decreased breath sounds and for crackles.
Hepatotoxicity	Monitor liver function tests: AST, ALT, bilirubin.
Nephrotoxicity	Monitor kidney function tests: creatinine and blood urea nitrogen. Monitor urine output.
Ototoxicity	Monitor for tinnitus or hearing loss.

[a]Many antineoplastic drugs are toxic to various organs of the body. Whenever a specific drug has one of these toxicities, include the specific assessment parameters for that toxicity in your regular assessment.
ALT, Alanine aminotransferase; *AST*, aspartate aminotransferase; *ECG*, electrocardiogram.

Oral Chemotherapy

Currently, a few chemotherapy drugs are available in an oral form to be taken by mouth. Oral anticancer drugs are just as toxic to the patient and to you or the person handling the drug as IV chemotherapy drugs. Since these drugs are given at home, the patient and family must be taught proper protection, correct administration, adherence, and how to manage drug side effects. Oral chemotherapy drugs should not be crushed, split, or chewed. These drugs are considered a biohazard and must be disposed of according to recommendations by the pharmacist.

Nursing Care of Patients Receiving Chemotherapy

Nursing care of the patient receiving chemotherapy requires special knowledge and skills. An oncology RN is a specialist who is able to give comprehensive nursing care because of professional education, training, or national certification in the specialty.

Antineoplastic drugs have toxic effects that must be assessed and monitored. Table 8.7 presents the assessments necessary to detect various types of organ toxicity. If a drug toxic to the reproductive system is chosen for a patient who desires children in the future, the patient will need to make a decision about banking sperm or eggs before beginning chemotherapy.

There are general principles that can be helpful to you if you are part of the team caring for a patient receiving chemotherapy for cancer or a patient who is experiencing some of the toxic side effects of antineoplastic drugs.

Side Effects of Chemotherapy

Not all antineoplastic drugs produce every toxic side effect, and the oncologist plans therapy so that destruction of malignant cells is maximized and toxicity is minimized. **The toxicity associated with chemotherapy is most evident in the cells of the body that have a short life span and therefore must continuously reproduce to provide the body with the normal cells it needs. These types of cells include the blood cells, hair follicles, and epithelial cells of the mucous membranes lining the digestive tract.** Patients can experience severe anemia, reduced immunity due to decreased WBCs, thrombocytopenia (decreased platelets) that affects blood clotting, alopecia (hair loss), mucositis (sores in the mouth), nausea and vomiting, or constipation or diarrhea.

Although the causes of the problems are different, assessment of the patient and symptomatic relief measures are the same. See Nursing Care Plan 8.1 for nursing interventions for selected problems that may be experienced by a patient receiving chemotherapy for cancer.

HORMONE THERAPY

Hormones are secreted by the endocrine glands, circulate in the body, and have effects on certain tissues. **Certain hormones can cause hormone-sensitive tumors to grow more rapidly, so decreasing the level of the hormone can slow tumor growth or prevent recurrence.** Hormone therapy, also known as *hormonal* or *endocrine therapy*, is used alone or as an adjunct to other types of cancer therapy. Many of these agents are used to block receptors and by this action work to prevent cancer cells from receiving normal hormonal growth stimulation.

Tamoxifen, a selective estrogen receptor modulator, is an example of an oral drug that produces metabolites that bind to the estrogen receptor on tumor cells, preventing tumor growth in women with breast cancer. Aromatase inhibitors are considered hormone inhibitors. Drugs such as letrozole (Femara) inhibit the production of estrogen, so the blood level of estrogen is decreased, slowing tumor growth in women with postmenopausal breast cancer. Tamoxifen has been shown to be chemopreventive for women with a high risk of breast cancer, and both drugs improve survival after breast cancer (National Cancer Institute, 2017). Side effects of hormone therapy depend on the type of hormone targeted. Women receiving estrogens or progestins may have irregular menses, fluid retention, and breast tenderness. All patients who take estrogen or progestins are at increased risk for venous thromboembolism (VTE). Androgens and the antiestrogen receptor drugs cause masculinizing effects in women. Chest and facial hair may develop, menstrual periods stop, and breast tissue shrinks. Patients may have some fluid retention. For men and women receiving androgens, acne and hypercalcemia are common, and liver dysfunction may occur with prolonged therapy.

IMMUNOTHERAPY: BIOLOGIC RESPONSE MODIFIERS

Biologic response modifiers (BRMs) are agents that manipulate the immune system in the hope of controlling or curing a malignancy with little or no toxic effect on normal cells. These agents either stimulate or suppress immune activity. The BRMs include interferons, interleukins, colony-stimulating factor (CSF), monoclonal antibodies, vaccines, gene therapy, and nonspecific immunomodulating agents. They essentially make the immune system function better. BRMs stimulate the immune system to recognize cancer cells and to institute action to destroy them. Some BRMs, such as CSF, work by enhancing a quicker recovery of the bone marrow after radiation or chemotherapy. CSF stimulates bone marrow to function more quickly. Neumega (interleukin-2) is a drug that stimulates thrombocyte (platelet) production. This drug is used to decrease the bleeding tendencies induced by chemotherapy and could help create new chemotherapy protocols that are more effective against cancer cells.

Two types of BRMs that are used to fight cancer are interleukins and interferons. **Interleukins help the immune system cells recognize and destroy abnormal cells. Interferons slow cell division in cancer cells, stimulate natural killer cells, delay the appearance of oncogenes, and assist cancerous cells to revert to more normal cells.** Both interleukins and interferons are manufactured using *recombinant* (artificial DNA sequence) DNA technology. Interleukin-2 is used for patients with melanoma, renal cell carcinoma, and lymphoma. Interferons are used effectively against leukemia, melanoma, multiple myeloma, carcinoid tumors, and renal carcinoma. Both interleukins and interferons are very expensive to manufacture. Patients receiving interleukins have generalized and often severe inflammatory reactions such as fluid shifts and capillary leak syndrome, which result in edema that affects the heart and lungs. Patients receiving high-dose BRM therapy may need to be in an intensive care unit (ICU) or on a monitored unit. These inflammatory effects occur during the days of active drug infusion and resolve after therapy completion. Neurologic symptoms associated with BRMs can be concerning and include severe depression, confusion, fatigue, somnolence, irritation or agitation, hallucinations, anxiety, and sleep problems. Early identification of these symptoms is an important nursing care activity. Other issues include fever, chills, rigors, and flu-like symptoms.

MONOCLONAL ANTIBODIES

Monoclonal antibodies (MoAbs) are manufactured using genetic engineering to make antibodies against certain cancer cells. MoAbs work by binding to antigens on the cell surface of the tumor, preventing the cancer cell from growing and dividing. Rituximab (Rituxan) and trastuzumab (Herceptin) are examples of commonly used MoAbs. Rituximab is used in the treatment of non-Hodgkin lymphoma, and trastuzumab is used for the treatment of breast cancer in patients who produce an excess amount of a protein called HER2/neu. Allergic reactions may occur in patients receiving monoclonal antibodies because of the incorporation of some nonhuman proteins. However, recently these antibodies have been "humanized," reducing the risk for allergic reactions. Nursing assessment is key for early recognition of a potentially life-threatening allergic reaction.

TARGETED THERAPIES

Targeted therapies are a newer form of cancer treatment that block the growth and spread of cancer by interfering with the specific cellular growth pathways or molecules involved in the growth and reproduction of cancer cells. The pathway or signal for cell division and growth is more active in cancer cells. Targeting these signal pathways blocks the activation of oncogenes and other factors in cancer cells, to slow or stop cell division. For example, one of these growth pathways in cancer is through the enzyme *tyrosine kinase* (TK). In the presence of TK, oncogenes are activated and cancer cell growth and reproduction are stimulated. When drugs such as tyrosine kinase inhibitors (TKIs) are given, the signal for turning on cell division (oncogenes) is blocked. An example of a TKI is imatinib mesylate (Gleevec). This drug binds to the enzyme TK and prevents its activation. The drug is useful in most types of chronic myeloid leukemia (CML).

Side effects common to most TKIs include nausea, vomiting, fluid retention, electrolyte imbalances, and bone marrow suppression (neutropenia, anemia, and thrombocytopenia).

BONE MARROW AND STEM CELL TRANSPLANTATION

Bone marrow transplantation (BMT) is mainly used to correct the severe bone marrow damage caused by chemotherapy or radiation. Sometimes whole-body irradiation is used to treat a hematopoietic cancer such as leukemia or Hodgkin disease. Irradiation of this sort totally incapacitates the body's bone marrow, and the patient would die if blood cells could not again be manufactured. Stem cells may be transplanted to overcome the devastating effects of chemotherapy or total body irradiation before BMT. BMT and stem cell treatment are discussed in Chapter 16.

COMMON PROBLEMS RELATED TO CANCER OR CANCER TREATMENT

The problems that can be experienced by cancer patients are complex and depend on both the location and the type of cancer and the therapy used to treat it. A discussion of the most common problems and the related nursing care is presented here.

ANOREXIA AND WEIGHT LOSS

Many cancer patients experience an alteration in taste that can be due to cancer progression (advanced cancer) or cancer treatment (chemotherapy, radiation to the oral cavity). Patients may complain of a metallic taste in the mouth. Commonly the first thing noticed is that red meat does not taste good. The taste of sweets also is altered. Anorexia (loss of appetite) often is associated with changes in taste and with mucositis (sores in the mouth) that can cause the patient great difficulty in eating and drinking. The loss of appetite can quickly lead to deficiencies of protein and calories. **A patient with anorexia can experience a significant weight loss (2 or more pounds per week) and may suffer from severe malnutrition.**

Patients with cancer should be taught to increase their protein intake to equal 1.5 g/kg (of weight) per day. The patient should be encouraged to eat small, frequent meals and add calorie-dense snacks. You should also refer the patient to a dietitian for counseling. Oral supplements should be used only if the patient has difficulty swallowing. It is important to note that older people with cancer are more likely to suffer malnutrition, with 90% experiencing weight loss during chemotherapy. Pharmacologic options for the treatment of anorexia or weight loss in cancer patients are limited and must be carefully selected to avoid unwanted side effects.

MUCOSITIS AND STOMATITIS

Patients undergoing chemotherapy may experience *mucositis,* or sores, in the mouth that can extend through the entire GI tract. *Stomatitis* is an inflammatory reaction in the mouth. Both mucositis and stomatitis can result in pain and interfere with eating and swallowing. For patients receiving chemotherapy, oral cryotherapy (using ice water or ice chips) can be used for the prevention of mucositis. Typically the RN giving the chemotherapy will instruct patients to suck on ice chips or to hold ice-cold water in their mouths before, during, and after the chemotherapy infusion. It is believed that the cold temperature decreases exposure of the oral mucous membranes to the mucositis-causing agents.

You should perform an assessment of the mouth and report any abnormal findings to the RN. The patient should be taught the importance of strict oral hygiene, including frequent tooth brushing with a soft brush or tooth sponges (toothettes), and to use gentle strokes. Tooth brushing should be followed by thorough mouth rinsing with plain water or saline. Rinsing the mouth is encouraged after meals and at bedtime. Teach patients to avoid mouthwashes that contain alcohol, as they dry and irritate the oral mucosa. Toothbrushes can be cleaned weekly in a home dishwasher or by rinsing them with a solution of liquid bleach or hydrogen peroxide and then rinsing with hot water.

Relief of the mouth pain of mucositis or stomatitis is provided by special topical compounds (such as Xylocaine Viscous) that are "swished and spit." Such compounds contain a topical anesthetic and an anti-inflammatory agent. **The patient is instructed *not* to swallow this solution.** The patient should avoid spicy foods, alcohol, and tobacco while undergoing treatment.

Radiation to the head or neck will produce some inflammatory changes in the mouth and often also in the pharynx and esophagus. Measures to combat this expected reaction include frequent oral intake of liquids that are not chemically irritating, the use of artificial saliva, and frequent and consistent mouth care.

Patients are encouraged to drink water as often as possible to help alleviate the discomfort of dryness of the mouth and tongue. However, drinking water will not completely resolve the problem. Artificial saliva combats mouth dryness in a different way and helps keep the mucous membranes soft and moist. It also helps to buffer the acidity in the mouth and thus to reduce irritation of the oral mucosa. Artificial saliva is available as a spray (Salivart) and a gel (Biotène OralBalance) and can be used by the patient as often as desired. It can be found at a local pharmacy or obtained from most online drugstores.

CHEMOTHERAPY-INDUCED NAUSEA AND VOMITING

Many cancer drugs are *emetogenic,* meaning they induce vomiting. Nausea often persists, even when vomiting is controlled. Chemotherapy-induced nausea and vomiting (CINV) may persist for 1 to 2 days after chemotherapy is given. A few drugs may trigger CINV almost as soon as the drug is started. Other drugs, such as cisplatin (Platinol), induce delayed nausea and vomiting that can continue for as long as 5 to 7 days after receiving it. CINV often can be well controlled with appropriate antiemetic therapy, especially with serotonin (5-HT3) receptor antagonists. Often steroids, such as dexamethasone, are added to enhance the effect of prescribed antiemetic drugs. Antiemetics are given *before* the nausea and vomiting begin. The nursing priority is to ensure adequate control of CINV. Teach patients to continue antiemetic drugs even when CINV appears controlled. **When the patient stops taking the drugs, teach them to start retaking the drugs at the first sign of nausea to prevent it from becoming uncontrollable.**

DIARRHEA

Many chemotherapy drugs and newer targeted therapies cause diarrhea because they affect the cells of the intestinal mucosa, causing inflammation. Radiation to the GI tract or pelvis can also result in diarrhea. Loperamide is recommended for uncomplicated mild to moderate diarrhea, and octreotide is recommended for severe diarrhea. Teach the patient to avoid high-fiber foods that encourage rapid evacuation from the bowel and to add low-fiber foods such as bananas and cheese to the diet. Cleansing the rectal area and applying petroleum jelly, A&D ointment, or Desitin cream helps decrease discomfort and protects the skin from breakdown. You must monitor the patient for signs of dehydration (loss of skin turgor, dry mucous membranes, and poor urine output) and electrolyte imbalance.

CONSTIPATION

Certain antineoplastic drugs, such as vincristine, vinblastine, and paclitaxel, cause constipation. Increasing fluids (as allowed), adding fiber to the diet, administering stool softeners and fiber laxatives, exercise, and monitoring vigilantly for the beginning signs of constipation are the usual measures taken. Suppositories or enemas may be necessary.

CHEMOTHERAPY-INDUCED PERIPHERAL NEUROPATHY

Chemotherapy-induced peripheral neuropathy (CIPN) is the loss of sensation (touch) or motor function of peripheral nerves from certain chemotherapy agents. The degree of CIPN is related to the dosage of the nerve-damaging drugs; higher doses lead to greater neuropathy. The results of CIPN on function are widespread, with the most common problems including loss of sensation in the hands and feet, impaired gait and balance, orthostatic hypotension, erectile dysfunction, neuropathic pain, loss of taste discrimination, and severe constipation. CIPN is a long-term consequence and may be permanent in some adults. No known evidence-based interventions are available to prevent CIPN; however, some patients have reduced pain and improved function and quality of life when taking duloxetine.

The priority for nursing care of patients experiencing CIPN is teaching them to prevent injury. Falls are more likely because of changes in gait and balance and decreased sensation in the feet. The loss of hand sensation may make some activities that require very fine motor skills (writing, buttoning clothing) difficult. Chemotherapy drugs such as the taxanes and platinum-based agents cause CIPN.

BONE MARROW SUPPRESSION

One of the most significant and potentially life-threatening side effects of chemotherapy is suppression of the bone marrow. Chemotherapy kills circulating blood cells and decreases the ability of the bone marrow to replace WBCs, red blood cells (RBCs), and platelets. It is the reduced WBCs, especially neutrophils, that greatly increases the patient's risk for infection and sepsis. Most of the infections arise from the overgrowth of the patient's own normal organisms. Decreased platelets increase the risk for bleeding, and a decline in RBCs can result in anemia. The risk for bone marrow suppression is related to the dose of chemotherapy received. Suppression of the bone marrow is typically temporary, occurring 7 to 10 days after the chemotherapy is given. Bone marrow suppression is the main reason why the dose of chemotherapy may be reduced or the treatment delayed until the marrow recovers.

The WBC count is closely monitored; a count of less than 3000/mm^3 indicates neutropenia. Filgrastim or sargramostim is given to raise the neutrophil and WBC counts. Often administration of these injectable agents begins before the WBC count drops too low. Thorough, frequent handwashing by the health care team, patient, and family helps reduce the danger of infection. You should maintain strict asepsis in all aspects of patient care. If the neutrophil count is below 500 mm^3, follow the policy and procedures for protective isolation to prevent infection. Teach the patient to report signs and symptoms of infection, such as fever, sore throat, burning on urination, or cough. If infection is suspected, specimens of blood, urine, and sputum may be collected for culture and sensitivity testing to identify the organism and the antibiotics or antifungal agents that can treat it.

The decreased RBC count and anemia resulting from chemotherapy place an increased workload on the heart and lungs as these organs attempt to oxygenate the body adequately. The most common symptom from anemia is fatigue. In the recent past, treatment with erythropoietin-stimulating agents (ESAs) such as epoetin alfa or darbepoetin alfa was done routinely to increase RBCs and decrease anemia. However, concerns about increased blood clots, strokes, heart attack, and even death need to be balanced against the potential benefits.

Patients with thrombocytopenia (low platelet count) can take measures to help lower the risk of bleeding. When the platelet count reaches a low of 50,000/mm^3, any small injury can lead to an episode of prolonged bleeding. At 20,000/mm^3, spontaneous bleeding that is difficult to control may occur. An infusion of platelets may be given to patients whose platelet count falls to 20,000/mm^3. Oprelvekin (Neumega) may be given to increase the production of platelets. The drug may cause fluid retention and increase the risk for heart failure and pulmonary edema. Other side effects include conjunctival bleeding, hypotension, and tachycardia. Teach patients to weigh themselves daily and keep a record. Remind them to immediately report sudden weight gain or dyspnea to the health care provider.

The patient must be handled gently. Using a lift sheet helps in turning and repositioning the patient. During severe thrombocytopenia, needle sticks for injections, laboratory specimens, and intravenous line starts are kept to a minimum. When a blood sample or IV access is needed, the smallest gauge needle possible for the task should be used. Once a needle is removed, apply pressure to the site for 5 to 10 minutes or until all bleeding stops. All urine and stool should be tested for the presence of blood. Ask the patient if they have abdominal pain. Abdominal girth is measured daily to check for internal bleeding. Assess the skin for the presence of petechiae (small spots on the skin from bleeding) or ecchymosis (bruising) and for any signs of abnormal bleeding.

Patient Teaching

Cancer Treatment and Infection Prevention

- Wash your hands well with an antimicrobial soap or alcohol-based hand rub frequently, especially:
  - Before eating
  - After using the toilet
  - After blowing your nose
  - After handling items many people have handled, such as railings, money, shopping carts, library books, newspapers, and pieces of mail
  - After touching a pet
  - After spending time in public
- Do not share personal care items (razor, toothbrush, toothpaste, washcloth, towels, deodorant, hand lotion, lipstick, etc.).
- Clean toothbrushes by running them through the dishwasher or soaking them in a bleach or hydrogen peroxide solution.
- Stay away from people with respiratory or other infections.
- Bathe daily if possible; use an antimicrobial soap.
- Examine the mouth daily for sores or white patches; perform mouth care frequently.
- Examine the skin, especially the feet, daily for signs of broken areas.
- Wash dishes, utensils, and items used in cooking in hot, sudsy water or run them through a dishwasher. Do not reuse drinking cups or glasses without washing them.
- Do not eat raw, uncooked foods. Eat only canned or cooked foods.
- If the WBC count is extremely low, maintain a low-bacteria diet by avoiding salads, raw fruits and vegetables, or undercooked meat.
- Do not handle garden flowers, plants, or earth.
- Do not clean out cat litter boxes or bird cages.
- Monitor temperature daily. No rectal suppositories or enemas are given, and rectal temperatures are contraindicated.
- Be careful not to nick or scratch the skin.
- Report the following signs of infection to your health care provider immediately:
  - Temperature over 100° F (38° C)
  - Sore throat
  - Persistent cough
  - Colored or foul-smelling drainage from wound or nose
  - Presence of a boil or abscess
  - Cloudy, foul-smelling urine or burning on urination

Patient Teaching

Prevention of Bleeding in the Patient With Thrombocytopenia

- Use a soft toothbrush and brush lightly; do not floss.
- Use only an electric razor or depilatory for shaving.
- Prevent constipation by increasing fluid and roughage in the diet; take a stool softener if needed.
- Avoid nonprescription drugs that inhibit platelet function such as aspirin, ibuprofen (Motrin, Advil), Alka-Seltzer, and cold medicines that contain these agents.
- Take measures to avoid injury; avoid contact sports or any activity where falling is a risk.
- If a bump or injury occurs, apply ice to the area for 1 hour.
- Avoid tight, constricting clothing or shoes.
- Do not wear jewelry with sharp edges.
- Use ample lubrication for intercourse; avoid anal intercourse.
- Blow your nose gently without occluding either nostril.

Think Critically

You came to work this morning with a slightly scratchy throat and a drippy nose. The charge nurse has assigned you to a cancer patient who has bone marrow suppression. What would you do in this situation?

CANCER-RELATED FATIGUE

Cancer-related fatigue (CRF) is a distressing and persistent feeling of tiredness or exhaustion from cancer or cancer treatment. It is estimated that 25% to 99% of patients with cancer have fatigue. This type of fatigue can last long after treatment for cancer has been completed. The cause of CRF is not completely known but may be related to biological processes from both cancer and treatment and can be complicated by reduced activity, sleep problems, and depression.

The Oncology Nursing Society proposed increased physical activity or exercise as a first-line treatment for CRF. There is not enough evidence to support the use of medications for the treatment of CRF. Nonpharmacologic recommendations for the treatment of CRF include increasing physical activity, minimizing bed rest and prolonged naps, maintaining a good balance between energy and activity, minimizing emotional distress, maintaining activities of daily living, and prioritizing activities.

Recommendations for increasing physical activity that are effective during and after treatment include yoga, resistance exercises, and walking. Using relaxation techniques *during* cancer treatment appears to be helpful in reducing CRF, but it is less effective once treatment is completed.

In addition, maintaining good nutritional status with high protein intake will help keep up energy levels. Supplemental feedings between meals often are necessary to ensure adequate calorie intake. Fluids should be increased to 2 to 3 L/day on day 3 of chemotherapy, unless contraindicated, to help flush the waste materials from the body.

ALOPECIA

Chemotherapy-induced alopecia (hair loss) is a common and distressing effect of many types of chemotherapy drugs. Alopecia resulting from chemotherapy is mostly temporary. Occasionally some chemotherapy agents, such as taxotere, have been reported to cause permanent hair loss in some women. Radiation therapy to the head almost always results in permanent hair loss. Scalp cooling during chemotherapy using approved caps can help prevent hair loss. Scalp cooling is thought to work by constricting blood vessels and therefore reducing blood flow to hair follicles. Although there have been concerns about ice caps protecting cancer cells in the scalp, two recent studies did not support this concern.

Hair regrowth begins about 1 month after chemotherapy ends. The patient should be informed that the new hair may differ in color or texture from the original hair. For women with long hair, cutting the hair short before chemotherapy reduces the distress of seeing large chunks of hair falling out. Before hair loss occurs, the patient also should be counseled to choose a wig or head cover to wear until the hair regrows. Hair loss usually begins by the second chemotherapy treatment. Some offices of the ACS have wigs donated by former patients that are available for loan. Whatever your patient decides, support their decision.

PAIN

Cancer pain can come from disease as it advances and invades other organs, bones, or soft tissue. Pain from cancer or its treatment is very common. It is estimated that as many as 75% of patients with cancer report pain as a frequent symptom following cancer treatment. Cancer pain is also treated differently from nonmalignant pain in that opioids are frequently used as a first-line therapy. Cancer pain also occurs with other symptoms and may be made worse by other symptoms such as sleeplessness, depression, or anxiety, significantly reducing the patient's quality of life. Despite evidence-based guidelines for the treatment of cancer pain, it may be undertreated. Chapter 7 discusses all modalities to control patients' pain. Recently, the opioid crisis in the United States has brought attention to the use of these medications in the control of cancer pain. Currently there is little evidence to help nurses understand the risk factors and extent of opioid abuse in the cancer patient population. A number of screening tools can be used to determine whether a patient is at risk for opioid misuse before the medication is prescribed and throughout treatment. Patients should be taught to lock up or store opioids out of sight to prevent friends or relatives from taking them to sell or use themselves.

Complementary and alternative therapies, such as acupuncture, can supplement medications for cancer pain but have limited effectiveness when used alone. Table 8.8 lists current oral and intravenous medications shown to be effective against cancer pain. Adjunctive

Table 8.8 **Drugs Commonly Used to Treat Cancer Pain**

DRUG	BRAND NAME	DURATION (h)	DOSAGE (mg)	SIDE EFFECTS
Common Oral Pain Relievers: Mild to Moderate Intensity				
Acetaminophen	Tylenol	3–4	650	Hepatic
Aspirin	Many brands	3–5	550	GI
Codeine	Many brands	3–5	32	CNS, GI
Hydrocodone combination	Vicodin	3–4	5	CNS, GI
Ibuprofen	Motrin, Advil	3–5	400	GI
Ketoprofen	Orudis	5–7	50	GI
Naproxen	Naprosyn	2–8	250	GI
Piroxicam	Feldene	24	20	GI
Propoxyphene	Darvon	4–6	65	CNS
DRUG	**BRAND NAME**	**DURATION (h)**	**PARENTERAL DOSE (mg)**	**ORAL DOSE (mg)**
Common Opioid Pain Relievers: Moderate to Severe Intensity				
Hydrocodone combination	Vicodin	3–4	5	CNS, GI
Oxycodone	Roxicodone	3–6	5	CNS, GI
Morphine	Generic	4–5	2.5–10	10–30
Controlled-release morphine	MS Contin	6–12	–	15
Hydromorphone	Dilaudid	3–4	1–4	2–8
Fentanyl	Duragesic	1–2	0.1	0.025
Oxycodone	Roxicodone	4–6	–	5–15
Controlled-release oxycodone	OxyContin	12	–	10
Codeine sulfate	Generic	4–6	–	15–60

CNS, Central nervous system; *GI*, gastrointestinal.

medications used alongside analgesics to help control cancer pain may include steroids, antidepressants, and antiseizure drugs. Pain should be reassessed 15 to 30 minutes after parenteral drug administration and 1 hour after oral drugs are given. Medication doses should be scheduled regularly and around the clock to maintain a therapeutic drug level to prevent pain recurrence. Since opioids are used frequently, a bowel program must be started using stool softeners and laxatives to prevent severe constipation, an adverse effect of opioids.

For adequate control, pain must be (1) assessed and documented regularly; (2) discussed openly with the patient and family; (3) addressed with options that are appropriate for the patient's diagnosis, physical condition, and goals; and (4) treated with the appropriate medication or combination of medications in a timely fashion. **The main factor for controlling cancer pain is to continue to seek a combination of different treatments until the pain is under control.**

Think Critically

A patient with advanced cancer tells you that the long-acting opioid currently being taken for pain control is not effective. How would you assess the patient's level of pain? What can you suggest to the health care provider to enhance the patient's pain relief?

FEAR AND INEFFECTIVE COPING

A cancer diagnosis brings with it feelings of fear and anxiety in a time of great stress and uncertainty. Patients lack knowledge about the disease and treatment options. Generally, at diagnosis patients fear death, and after treatment the fear is about recurrence of the disease. **Understanding the disease, treatment options, and what will be experienced during each type of treatment will greatly help to decrease the fear experienced by patients and families.** Knowing what to expect helps patients and families feel less fearful about the experience of surgery, chemotherapy, and the loss of control over their lives. Patients may also fear financial consequences of the disease and treatment, the inability to work or care for families, or changes in body image or sexuality. An assessment of the patient's and family's usual coping techniques is important in formulating the overall plan of care.

You must consider psychosocial and spiritual care when working with a patient with cancer because the disease will affect every aspect of their life in some way. Care of the cancer patient is a collaborative process that involves many members of the health care team. Refer the patient and family to the resources available to them, such as the social worker or psychologist, to help them through this time. Local chapters of the ACS have a wide variety of services available to patients and health care providers. Encourage the patient and the patient's partner to discuss concerns related to sexuality that may come from cancers of the breast, prostate, or reproductive organs. Intimacy is to be encouraged. Unless the patient is recovering from surgery, has pathologic fractures, or is severely immunosuppressed, sexual intercourse should not be prohibited. If sexual function has been altered by surgery or treatment, help the patient find other means of sexual expression and gratification.

Referral to a social worker may be needed to coordinate resources for treatment and care assistance.

ONCOLOGIC EMERGENCIES

An oncologic emergency is a cancer-related disorder that requires emergency medical or surgical treatment. Oncologic emergencies are classified as being metabolic, hematologic, or structural. There are six major oncologic emergencies:

1. *Tumor lysis syndrome:* A complication of cancer treatment that occurs when large amounts of tumor cells are destroyed (lysed) and tumor cell contents are released into the bloodstream. It is characterized by high potassium, phosphate, and uric acid levels and low blood calcium levels. An elevated potassium level may cause renal failure, cardiac dysrhythmias, or asystole. Treatment includes intravenous fluids and allopurinol.
2. *Hypercalcemia of malignancy:* An increased serum level of calcium may be caused by the release of calcium because of bone deterioration or the secretion of parathyroid hormone by a tumor. Patients with advanced disease of the breast or ovary or with lymphomas are most often affected. Very elevated calcium levels (above 11 mg/dL) result in severe mood changes, decreased cognitive function, headaches, seizures, decreased renal function, and GI symptoms (nausea, vomiting, anorexia, constipation). Patients are managed with vigorous intravenous hydration, calcitonin, bisphosphonates, prednisone, and even hemodialysis.
3. *Disseminated intravascular coagulation (DIC):* DIC is caused by abnormal activation of clot formation, resulting in widespread blood clotting (consumptive coagulopathy) and organ damage, followed by bleeding due to depletion of platelets and blood coagulation factors. This results in excessive bleeding. DIC is most often found in patients with acute leukemia due to the release of coagulation factors, fibrin, and cytokines. Patients may receive platelet transfusions, chemotherapy, and other blood products.
4. *Neutropenia:* Patients with cancers that involve the immune system, such as acute leukemia, or those receiving chemotherapy that suppresses the immune system are at risk for febrile neutropenia. Neutropenia is defined as an absolute neutrophil count of less than 500/mm^3. These infections are life-threatening, and patients are hospitalized for intravenous antibiotics and antifungals.
5. *Spinal cord compression (SCC):* Compression of the spinal cord results from a rapidly growing metastatic tumor that causes bone collapse and impingement of the spinal cord. Patients can have symptoms that range from severe back pain to leg weakness and/or loss of bowel or bladder function. SCC can result from aggressive myeloma, lymphomas, and solid tumors that metastasize to the bone. Treatments include surgery, high-dose steroids, and local radiation.
6. *Superior vena cava (SVC) syndrome:* This can be caused by compression from an expanding tumor (usually a lung cancer) near or around the SVC. Symptoms include edema of the face and arms, shortness of breath, cough, difficulty swallowing, and a high-pitched wheeze. Treatment includes intravenous steroids, diuretics, oxygen, and treatment of the underlying cancer.

When these emergencies occur, immediate action must be taken to prevent severe injury or death.

CARING FOR THE DYING CANCER PATIENT

PSYCHOLOGICAL PROCESS OF DEATH

Although an increasing number of cancer patients are surviving their disease through control or cure, cancer is still the second leading cause of death in the United States. It is estimated that 606,880 Americans will die of cancer in 2019 (Seigel, Miller, & Jemal, 2019). That amounts to 1600 patients who die of cancer every day. Nurses working with cancer patients need to understand the process of death and dying as well as grief. As a nurse, you will need to apply knowledge about these processes compassionately when caring for cancer patients and their families.

Grieving

Elisabeth Kübler-Ross introduced the world to the stages of grief and dying when her landmark book, *On Death and Dying,* was published in 1969. Kübler-Ross suggested that people go through five predictable stages as they learn to adapt to the processes of loss or impending death. Not everyone goes through all stages, nor do people go through the stages in any set order. These stages may apply to the grieving process when a body function or part is lost (such as a lost breast from cancer), a loved one dies, or one's own death is approaching (Box 8.5).

Box 8.5 Kübler-Ross's Stages of Dying

Denial (This can't happen to me!)
Anger (Why *me?*)
Bargaining (Yes me, *but* ...)
Depression (It *is* me, I give up ...)
Acceptance (I'm ready ...)

Box 8.6 Common Fears of Dying Patients

Almost all dying patients face varying levels of fear, which may include fear of:
- The unknown
- Abandonment and loneliness
- Loss of relationships
- Loss of experiences in the future
- Dependency and loss of independence
- Pain

Fear

The patient feels and expresses many powerful emotions as they approach the end of life. Almost all dying patients and families face varying levels of fear (Box 8.6). One of the most helpful things you can do is "be there" for the patient, encouraging them to share their feelings and expressing caring. A nurse who is compassionate and soothing provides comfort and strength for the patient. In the same way, when a patient displays behavior that is upsetting to the family, you can explain the behaviors to the family as normal for those going through the stages of grief and dying. These are times that both the patient and the family are in great need, and nursing support can be profoundly comforting.

When nurses care for dying patients regularly, they cannot help but reflect on their own mortality. It is important to review one's beliefs about death and dying and reaffirm those beliefs. In this way, it is possible to support patients who may have their own beliefs about the mysteries of death. When dealing with end-of-life situations, it is natural for patients to become reflective and consider their beliefs regarding life and death. Very often spiritual matters are considered whether these are connected to an organized religion or not. Table 8.9 provides some common spiritual beliefs and practices. Keep in mind that individuals do not always adhere to the stated beliefs of a religious organization. Find out from your patient what they feel is important. Research supports that many patients find comfort and strength in their spiritual beliefs when facing terminal illness. Nurses need to support this area that is meaningful to patients.

Take a periodic inventory of your ability to provide care without "burnout." If you come to the point where you can provide care only in a detached and distant manner, you can no longer be supportive, compassionate, and understanding. When this happens, it is time to take a break or to move on and let others provide care for the dying patient.

PALLIATIVE CARE

Palliative care is delivered by a multidisciplinary team of health care providers who work with patients with serious, life-threatening illnesses. The goal of palliative care is to provide relief of symptoms, with the goal of improving quality of life. Palliative care can be provided at home or in hospitals, clinics, or skilled care facilities. For example, a patient may receive palliative radiation to reduce the size of a tumor pressing on a body part, causing pain. The palliative care team also works with families, providing emotional and practical support.

Patients who have a shortened life expectancy of 6 months or less should be referred to hospice care. Like palliative care, hospice care can be delivered in different settings. Hospice care implies that treatment of the illness has stopped, and the focus is on comfort care, symptom relief, and emotional and spiritual care until the end of life.

Whether assisting the patient in the hospital or at home, certain comfort measures are required. Palliative care requires a specialized body of knowledge and skill that can be difficult to obtain and maintain if you are not routinely applying the skills. Clinical issues in both settings involve the following.

Anticipatory Guidance

You can prepare the family and patient by helping them anticipate the death to come: giving them guidance about physical changes, symptoms, complications that may arise, and decisions about possible hospice care. There are two stages of dying. In the *preactive phase,* patients know they are dying and exhibit this knowledge by withdrawing from social activities and attempting to put their affairs in order. This may take weeks or months. Patients often report seeing loved ones who have already died. They become restless, have slow wound healing, and begin to have dependent edema (swelling in extremities or even the entire body). When patients enter the *active phase* of dying (the final 2 to 3 days), they exhibit specific signs in breathing patterns and other body functions that indicate that death is imminent. The following are some active dying symptoms and associated nursing activities.

Terminal Hydration

A dying patient naturally and gradually reduces fluid intake. Dehydration can also increase as a result of the disease process. Also, a dry mouth and a feeling of thirst may be induced by the drugs being administered. You should be ready to educate the family about this process during the dying phase. Forcing the patient to eat or drink is discouraged. Many times, the course is for the patient to choose what to take and also to be allowed to refuse further nourishment. This is called *patient-endorsed intake.*

End-Stage Symptom Management

Many expected symptoms are related to metabolic changes at the end of life. The last few days of patient life have been studied extensively. Recognize these latter symptoms and either alleviate them or help explain them to the patient and family. Because comfort is the goal of palliative care, administering oral or sublingual medications is the preferred choice. As death draws

Table 8.9 Spiritual Beliefs and Practices Regarding Death

BELIEFS ABOUT TREATMENT	END-OF-LIFE RITUALS	AFTERLIFE BELIEFS
Christianity		
Roman Catholic		
No general guidelines. Individuals decide for themselves.	Sacrament of the sick, Holy Communion and anointing may be offered to the dying person.	Belief in life after death in the spiritual sense.
Protestant		
No general guidelines. Individuals decide for themselves.	No special rituals. Minister may perform extreme unction.	Belief in life after death in the spiritual sense.
Judaism		
The practice of medicine is a partnership with God. Relief of suffering is encouraged.	The dying person should never be left alone. It is against Jewish law to move or touch the actively dying person.	Orthodox and Conservative movements believe in life after death.
Buddhism		
Drugs that reduce consciousness may be distressing because the state of mind at death is very important.	Ideally the body should not be moved before the priest or monk arrives to recite prayers.	The death rituals are aimed at promoting human rebirth in the next life and preventing rebirth in lower forms.
Hinduism		
Alleviation of pain is not opposed. Pain control that does not affect mental clarity is preferred.	The Hindu dies at home if possible. Do not wash the body, as this is part of the funeral rites, and do not remove threads or jewelry that have been applied by the priest.	Belief in reincarnation and transmigration.
Islam		
Pain is a way to pay for sins, so some may not accept pain medication.	Family members or an imam (clergy) whisper in the ear the articles of faith, so that these are the last words the patient hears. The body should not be touched by non-Muslims after death.	Every soul will be judged after death based on the amount of good or evil that has been performed. According to this performance, individuals will be either rewarded or punished.
Nonreligious (Secular/Agnostic/Atheist)		
No general guidelines. Individuals decide for themselves.	No particular rites. Consult with the patient and family.	Death is the end. There is no further being. Agnostics believe that there is no way to know for certain what is beyond death.
Sikhism		
Everything that happens is the will of God. Treatment may or may not be accepted.	Hair and beard are left uncut; do not remove religious symbols. The family may wish to wash and lay out the body themselves.	Reincarnation is a cycle of rebirth. Salvation is liberation from this cycle. Salvation is achieved through disciplined meditation and spiritual union with God.

near, it may be possible to administer transdermal (fentanyl patches) and/or rectal pain medications as needed. Pain control at the end of life is an important goal, so nurses work with the health care provider to give the medications as ordered and notify the provider if the pain is not adequately controlled.

Dyspnea. When patients are near death and able to respond, they sometimes may feel as if they cannot get enough air. It is difficult to determine what causes this feeling, but several measures can be taken. Place the patient in Fowler position, adjust air temperature for the patient's comfort, and give medications such as bronchodilators as ordered. Oxygen via nasal cannula may be helpful as well. Morphine (sublingual or oral) is often given to ease breathing. It is important to remember that this feeling can be very frightening for both the patient and family members, and treatment to lessen discomfort is important. Noisy breathing can be heard at the end of life when patients can no longer clear their throats of normal secretions. Family members are often alarmed by this. Again, morphine can ease this symptom, and scopolamine or atropine, drugs that are known to reduce secretions, may be used to quiet the patient and quiet the breathing.

Delirium. Dying patients may experience hallucinations and/or altered mental status. Make sure the patient is in a comfortable position and that pain is controlled. Explain delirium with the patient's family and encourage the family to talk to the patient in quiet tones while remaining calm.

GET Ready for the Nclex® Examination!

Key Points

- Cancer cells begin growing as a result of a mutation in the DNA of genes in normal cells.
- Malignant cells can spread to other areas of the body.
- Tumors are classified according to the organs or tissues in which they first develop.
- Harmful agents that are potentially carcinogenic exist in the environment.
- Some people may have a genetic predisposition to some types of cancer.
- Age, sex, and race are considered predisposing factors for certain types of cancers.
- Changing certain lifestyle characteristics, such as quitting smoking, maintaining normal weight, reducing alcohol use, avoiding and limiting exposure to carcinogens, and eating a diet rich in fruits and vegetables, can lower the risk of cancer.
- Biopsy, cytology, radiologic studies, and laboratory tests are common methods used to diagnose and check the spread of cancer.
- Tumor markers detect biochemical substances synthesized and released into the bloodstream by tumor cells and are used mainly to determine response to a cancer therapy.
- Treatment modes of therapy for malignancies may include surgery, radiation, chemotherapy, hormone therapy, immunotherapy, and gene therapy.
- Nurses must protect themselves from overexposure to radiation.
- Antineoplastic chemotherapy drugs are effective at different times in the growth and replication phases of the tumor cell cycle.
- Many antineoplastic drugs can cause tissue damage on direct contact, so you must take care to protect patients from extravasation and administer the drugs into veins that have good blood flow. Chemotherapy is administered only by certified registered nurses.
- Biologic response modifiers manipulate the immune system to stimulate or suppress activity. These drugs assist the body in destroying cancer cells with minimal effect on normal tissue.
- Nausea, vomiting, diarrhea, constipation, pain, and fatigue are common complaints of cancer patients and require vigilant care.
- Cancer treatment may suppress the patient's bone marrow, and the patient may develop neutropenia, requiring that therapy be ceased for a period.
- Opioids plus a combination of interventions or different treatments are given to relieve cancer-related pain.
- Many cancer patients and their families go through the five stages of grief that are recognized in patients experiencing loss.
- Palliative care involves providing comfort for the dying patient and maintaining a high quality of life throughout the death process. Hospice care is indicated when cancer treatment stops and life expectancy is less than 6 months.

Additional Learning Resources

SG Go to your Study Guide for additional learning activities to help you master this chapter content.

Go to your Evolve website (http://evolve.elsevier.com/deWit/medsurg) for the following FREE learning resources:
- Animations, audio, and video
- Answers and rationales for questions and activities
- Glossary with pronunciations in English and Spanish
- Interactive Review Questions and more!

Review Questions for the NCLEX® Examination

1. What term would indicate to you that a substance in the environment can cause cancer to develop?
   1. Biologic
   2. Carcinogenic
   3. Emetogenic
   4. Immunotherapeutic

   NCLEX Client Need: Physiological Integrity: Reduction of Risk Potential
2. A 40-year-old woman is scheduled for external radiation therapy for breast cancer. What patient teaching instructions would be appropriate for this patient? *(Select all that apply.)*
   1. "Keep away from other family members until your radiation is completed."
   2. "Be sure you go to all scheduled radiation therapy appointments."
   3. "Protect your skin by applying lotion to the radiated area daily."
   4. "Keep out of the sun during radiation therapy."
   5. "Always wear snug-fitting clothing."

   NCLEX Client Need: Physiological Integrity: Reduction of Risk Potential
3. You are teaching a patient with neutropenia from cancer treatment about precautions to take during this time. Which of the following should be included in your teaching plan? *(Select all that apply.)*
   1. "Wash your hands frequently."
   2. "Eat only raw fruits and vegetables during this time."
   3. "Neutropenia is associated with abnormal bleeding."
   4. "You may experience a sore throat and fever; this is a normal response."

   NCLEX Client Need: Safe and Effective Care Environment: Safety and Infection Control
4. A patient receiving a chemotherapy agent that is a vesicant should be monitored for which adverse effect?
   1. Infiltration of the intravenous fluid containing the chemotherapy agent into the surrounding skin
   2. Orthostatic hypotension due to fluid expansion in the vascular system
   3. Dehydration due to the emetogenic effect of the drug
   4. The presence of blood in the urine or stool

   NCLEX Client Need: Physiological Integrity: Pharmacological Therapies

5. Which side effect of chemotherapy puts the patient at high risk for bleeding?
   1. Thrombocytopenia
   2. Elevated potassium
   3. Neutropenia
   4. Anemia

   NCLEX Client Need: Physiological Integrity: Pharmacological Therapies
6. A patient with cancer who is receiving chemotherapy asks you why her hair would fall out because of this treatment. What is your best response?
   1. "The cells of your hair fall out to show that the chemotherapy is working."
   2. "Chemotherapy can cause hair loss if you are lacking protein in your diet."
   3. "Chemotherapy affects all fast-growing cells, including normal cells."
   4. "You must have a low white blood cell count."

   NCLEX Client Need: Physiological Integrity: Pharmacological Therapies
7. A terminally ill female patient becomes increasingly confused and is having some hallucinations. Which nursing intervention(s) would be appropriate? *(Select all that apply.)*
   1. Discuss the patient's behaviors with the family.
   2. Encourage the family to talk to the patient in quiet tones.
   3. Apply physical restraints.
   4. Promote a calm environment.
   5. Force oral fluids.

   NCLEX Client Need: Physiological Integrity: Basic Care and Comfort
8. The family members attending to the needs of a dying patient express distress regarding the patient's noisy breathing. What would be your best action?
   1. Hold all pain medications.
   2. Administer atropine as ordered.
   3. Place the patient in supine position.
   4. Arrange for hospitalization of the patient.

   NCLEX Client Need: Physiological Integrity: Pharmacological Therapies
9. Which statement should be included in the teaching plan for a patient with thrombocytopenia?
   1. "Take your temperature every 4 hours."
   2. "Eat a diet that contains cooked foods only."
   3. "Use a soft-bristled toothbrush and do not floss."
   4. "Rinse your mouth with antiseptic mouthwash twice daily."

   NCLEX Client Need: Physiological Integrity: Reduction of Risk Potential
10. Which side effects can you expect to see in a patient receiving a biologic response modifier for cancer treatment?
    1. Severe alopecia
    2. Constipation and decreased appetite
    3. Cough and shortness of breath
    4. Fever, chills, and flu-like symptoms

    NCLEX Client Need: Physiological Integrity: Pharmacological Therapies

Critical Thinking Questions

Scenario A

A patient scheduled for chemotherapy today is experiencing a sore throat and slight fever but is afraid to inform the oncologist, fearing that treatment will be discontinued or delayed.

1. What would you tell the patient?
2. What teaching would you reinforce?

Scenario B

Ms. Allen went to her health care provider for a regular checkup and was told that she had malignant cells in the cervical secretions obtained from her Pap smear. She had a biopsy of the cervix, and this also contained malignant cells. She was admitted to the hospital, Cesium-137 was implanted in the cervix, and Ms. Allen was kept in bed in a private room during the treatment.

1. If you were assigned to give morning care to this patient, what special precautions would you take to protect yourself from excessive radiation?
2. What are some signs and symptoms you would watch for to determine whether Ms. Allen is having either a local or a systemic reaction to radiation?

Scenario C

A 19-year-old female college student is receiving chemotherapy for Hodgkin disease.

1. What short-term and long-term problems would you expect this patient to have?
2. To what health care professionals should you refer this patient?

Chronic Illness and Rehabilitation

9

http://evolve.elsevier.com/deWit/medsurg

Objectives

Theory

1. Demonstrate understanding of relevant nursing issues for patients with chronic illness and disability.
2. Recognize that *long-term care* is an umbrella term that describes a range of services and may provide varying levels of care.
3. Examine and identify patients at risk for problems associated with decreased physical mobility.
4. Describe the effect of decreased physical mobility on each of the major systems of the body and identify how they are interrelated.
5. Explain the general goals for a resident in a long-term care facility and how to meet those goals.
6. Describe the types of rehabilitation programs often associated with long-term care facilities and their scope of patient care.
7. Apply the goals of rehabilitation to patients with varying levels of disability.
8. Identify the members of the rehabilitation team and the collaborative care process and state the role of each.
9. Compare the role of licensed practical/vocational nurses (LPN/LVNs) in long-term care facilities with their role in acute care settings.

Clinical Practice

10. Choose nursing interventions to assist a patient with a chronic illness who is homebound.
11. Discuss with the charge nurse the measures that are used for safety and fall prevention in a long-term care facility.
12. Observe a rehabilitation team conference to see how a collaborative care plan is created or updated.
13. Based on assessment data, identify areas of psychosocial need for a home care patient and their caregivers.

Key Terms

chronic illness (KRŎN-ĭk ĬL-nĕs, p. 184)
disability (dĭs-ă-BĬL-ĕ-tē, p. 184)
hemiparesis (hĕm-ē-pă-RĒ-sĭs, p. 194)
impairment (ĭm-PĂR-mĕnt, p. 184)
long-term care (lŏng tĕrm kār, p. 189)
orthostatic hypotension (ōr-thō-STĀT-ĭk hī-pō-TĔN-shŭn, p. 189)
rehabilitation (rē-hă-bĭl-ĭ-TĀ-shŭn, p. 194)

Concepts Covered in This Chapter

- Functional Ability
- Self-Management
- Nutrition
- Elimination
- Mobility
- Safety
- Palliative Care
- Care Coordination

According to the Centers for Disease Control and Prevention (CDC, 2018), nearly half of all adults are diagnosed with one or more chronic health conditions, many of which can cause short-term or long-term disability. Cancer, stroke, diabetes, arthritis, and heart failure are just a few of the illnesses you will see in your clinical practice. Another major health condition, Alzheimer disease, affects about 10% of all adults over 65 years of age. In fact, Alzheimer disease is the only illness in the top 10 causes of death in the United States that cannot be prevented, slowed, or cured (Alzheimer's Association, 2017).

Patients with chronic illnesses and disabilities are cared for in a wide variety of practice settings. As a licensed practical/vocational nurse (LPN/LVN), you may have the opportunity to care for patients in long-term care facilities, rehabilitation facilities, outpatient clinics, primary care settings, and even at home. When you are working with patients who have a chronic illness or who are disabled, you will need to provide care and comfort, promote self-care for independent living, and foster patient well-being.

CHRONIC ILLNESS

The terms *chronic disease* and *chronic illness* are often used interchangeably by health care practitioners, yet they are quite different (Larsen, 2018). By chronic, we usually mean lasting longer than 3 months (National Center for Health Statistics, 2018). Chronic disease typically refers to the pathophysiologic process that leads to the medical diagnosis. Diabetes, hypertension, heart disease, cancer, neurologic disorders (such as multiple sclerosis and stroke), asthma, and musculoskeletal deformities (such as those from arthritis and osteoporosis) are common chronic diseases. Patients often have more than one chronic disease. The term **chronic illness**, on the other hand, is broad and refers to the lived experience of the patient with the chronic disease and their family (Larsen, 2018). Their experience is influenced by their perceptions of the illness, age, gender, culture, and socioeconomic status.

Terminology often associated with patients experiencing chronic illness include *disability, impairment,* and *handicapped*. According to the American Psychological Association (APA, 2018), a **disability** is linked to a person who has a condition or quality that is present when common activities such as walking, talking, reading, or learning are restricted. Some disabilities such as blindness or hearing loss are apparent to others, whereas others such as chronic depression are not. The term **impairment** refers to the dysfunction of a specific organ or body system.

In the past, the term *handicapped* was used to describe patients with chronic illness. This term is no longer acceptable as a description of an individual (APA, 2018), but it can be used to describe an obstacle imposed on an individual by some limit in the environment. For example, older buildings that do not have ramps handicap people who need wheelchairs. The environment is the problem, not the individual.

When chronic illness causes the loss of function, usual roles may be changed. The person may no longer be able to be the primary income provider or hold the positions in the workforce or community that formerly were held. Changes in the person's role affect the family as well. Daily patterns are altered to accommodate treatments and therapy and to cope with the problems of the disability. Sorrow is felt for all that has been lost. Spiritual distress may be experienced as the person is faced with the limitations of the illness or disability that has occurred. Holistic care that addresses spiritual and psychosocial needs as well as physical needs is essential.

Patients with a chronic illness and their families may feel powerless, especially during the phases of diagnosis and early treatment. Support for the patient's usual coping techniques—and teaching new ways to cope—help the patient effectively deal with the illness and the changes in life patterns it brings. Be instrumental in instilling hope for a good quality of life and in fostering resilience despite the illness (Edward, 2013).

PREVENTING THE HAZARDS OF DECREASED MOBILITY

Patients experience decreases in mobility to varying degrees and for different amounts of time. A multiple-trauma patient may be on bed rest for several weeks. A patient with advanced multiple sclerosis may be able to move around only with a wheelchair. A patient who experiences great difficulty breathing from advanced lung disease or heart disease may have very little energy and thus may not move around much. Patients with a spinal cord injury or brain damage from a stroke have body parts that are significantly decreased or even immobile. Patients who have pain or who have arthritic joints that cause pain with movement also tend to be less mobile. Patients who have any disorder requiring bed rest are at risk. All of these patients are subject to the problems of decreased mobility.

Evaluate each patient situation and determine whether the patient is at risk for problems related to decreased mobility. **Even if the patient is going to be immobile for only a few days, measures should be taken to prevent secondary problems.** Patients with disorders causing decreased mobility should be assessed for the degree of risk for the various associated problems, and interventions to prevent them should be initiated (Box 9.1). **Early effects of decreased mobility include a decrease in muscle strength, generalized weakness, easy fatigue, joint stiffness, decreased coordination, abdominal distention, and various metabolic changes detectable by laboratory testing.** Table 9.1 presents the more severe problems with measures for prevention when lack of activity occurs for more than a few days.

The prevention of problems related to decreased mobility begins the moment a patient first becomes ill or injured. Preventive actions must continue as long as the patient needs health care. The systems of the body work together as a whole, and lack of activity affects

Box 9.1 Disorders That May Cause Decreased Mobility

- Stroke
- Spinal cord injury
- Lower extremity amputation
- Head injury
- Multiple trauma
- Fractures of the knee, leg, ankle, hip, pelvis, or spine
- Neuromuscular disorders: multiple sclerosis, muscular dystrophy, amyotrophic lateral sclerosis, poliomyelitis, cerebral palsy, myasthenia gravis, etc.
- Congenital deformities
- Burns
- Advanced metastatic cancer
- Advanced stages of chronic disorders such as Parkinson disease, Alzheimer disease, or Huntington chorea
- Severe rheumatoid arthritis, osteoarthritis, and other forms of arthritis

Table 9.1 Prevention of the Common Hazards of Decreased Mobility

COMPLICATION	PREVENTION
Musculoskeletal	
Contractures	Range-of-motion exercises; maintain good body alignment; request physical therapy as needed
Foot drop	Foot support while in bed, range-of-motion exercises, encourage foot and ankle exercises as recommended by physical therapy and other members of the interdisciplinary team; use of foot splint
Osteoporosis	Range-of-motion exercises, ambulation if possible (walking); weight-bearing exercises; dietary consultation to ensure adequate calcium and vitamin D intake
Susceptibility to fractures	Weight-bearing exercises; maintain adequate nutritional status; assess fall risk and implement measures to prevent falls
Muscular atrophy	Passive or active range-of-motion exercises; reinforce exercises as prescribed by interdisciplinary team
Gastrointestinal	
Constipation	Increased activity level; increased fluid and fiber intake; administer stool softeners, laxatives as prescribed
Cardiovascular	
Increased venous stasis	Increased physical activity, compression hose as prescribed; range-of-motion exercises, sequential compression devices as prescribed
Thrombus formation	Increased physical activity, compression hose as prescribed; administer antiplatelet or anticoagulant drugs as prescribed
Embolism	Avoidance of leg massage; low-molecular-weight heparin injections as ordered
Neurologic	
Disorientation	Sleep-wake schedule in accord with light-dark pattern; reorientation (to person, place, and time); control of sensory stimulation; avoidance of sudden position changes; provide eyeglasses and/or hearing aids for patients as required
Renal/Urinary	
Urinary retention	Maintain fluid intake to avoid dehydration; high calcium and vitamin D intake may increase risk of kidney stones; monitor voiding patterns
Infection	Use evidence-based techniques to prevent catheter-associated urinary tract infections; use intermittent catheterization instead of indwelling if possible
Respiratory	
Pneumonia	Frequent repositioning in wheelchair or bed, incentive spirometry, respiratory exercises; notify health care provider if changes in respiratory status

more than one system. The effects vary depending on the general health of the individual, their age, the degree of decreased mobility, and the length of time of inactivity or bed rest. Lack of mobility may begin a cycle that leads to an ever-increasing loss of independence for the patient. As the patient becomes less able to move, they are less able to care for themselves and more dependent on quality care from others. Without care from others, they are at risk for adverse effects from decreased mobility. As the nurse, you can reduce that risk by helping the patient maintain functioning of each body system to the highest degree possible (Nursing Care Plan 9.1).

Older Adult Care Points

Although many older adults are active in their daily lives, some older adults may not be able to engage in regular physical activity. When mobility is decreased, muscle strength and flexibility is diminished due to disuse. It is much more difficult for these patients to regain mobility.

Assess the patient daily, looking closely at each body system in which a problem related to decreased mobility might occur. It is important to recognize signs and symptoms of each type of problem and understand how to intervene to decrease or prevent it. The assessment details and nursing care for each problem are discussed in the relevant chapters of this text.

CHRONIC ILLNESS AND REHABILITATION CARE

Rehabilitation care may be required for patients who are experiencing debilitation from a chronic illness or who have experienced complications from an acute illness or a traumatic accident. Some patients are transferred to a transitional unit or long-term care facility for a period of weeks for recovery after the most acute phase of illness or injury has passed. Many older adults who have several chronic problems and deficits in self-care enter long-term care facilities for the remainder of their lives. Other patients may enter a rehabilitation

Nursing Care Plan 9.1 Care of a Resident With Decreased Mobility

SCENARIO

Carl Sanders is an 83-year-old man with weakness and debilitation and has several chronic diseases. He has been transferred to a long-term care facility after a hospitalization for pneumonia.

PROBLEM STATEMENT/NURSING DIAGNOSIS

Altered physical mobility related to weakness, debility, illness, and age.

SUPPORTING ASSESSMENT DATA

Objective: Needs assistance to turn, reposition in the bed, and walk.

Goals/Expected Outcomes	Nursing Interventions	Selected Rationale	Evaluation
Resident will maintain present joint mobility.	Perform range-of-motion (ROM) on joints tid.	Regular ROM reduces risk of contracture, reduced joint mobility.	Active ROM done twice this shift.
Resident will perform active ROM of arms by discharge.	Assist to turn and reposition q2h.	Regular repositioning reduces risk of pressure injury.	Repositioned q2h.
	Place in high Fowler position for meals; assist to chair for lunch.	Reduces risk for aspiration when swallowing.	Up in chair for meals. Breath sounds clear on right side; slightly diminished in left base.

PROBLEM STATEMENT/NURSING DIAGNOSIS

Altered skin integrity related to decreased mobility and pressure over left trochanter.

SUPPORTING ASSESSMENT DATA

Subjective: "I can't move very much."

Objective: Too weak to reposition self; stage I pressure injury over left trochanter.

Goals/Expected Outcomes	Nursing Interventions	Selected Rationale	Evaluation
Resident will have no evidence of more pressure damage to skin.	Turn at least q2h and more frequently if possible.	Relieves pressure on dependent areas.	Position adjusted q1h.
	Use supports for positioning and cushioning for relief of pressure.	Prevents pressure injury and keeps body in good anatomic alignment.	On pressure-relief mattress; pressure-relief cushion in chair.
Stage I pressure injury will heal within 3 wk.	Keep reddened area clean and moist, with colloidal dressing in place; inspect every shift.	Cleanliness prevents infection. Clear film dressing seals in moisture while allowing inspection.	Clear dressing in place; reddening decreasing.
	Inspect all pressure points at least q4h.	Identifies skin problems.	Pressure points inspected q4h. No new reddened areas.
	Use turning sheet to turn resident.	Helps prevent shearing injuries from sliding resident on sheet.	Turning sheet used for turning.

PROBLEM STATEMENT/NURSING DIAGNOSIS

Constipation related to decreased mobility, lack of dietary fiber, decreased fluid intake.

SUPPORTING ASSESSMENT DATA

Subjective: "I feel constipated."

Objective: Only small amount of hard, dry stool passed once in last 4 days.

Goals/Expected Outcomes	Nursing Interventions	Selected Rationale	Evaluation
Resident will have normal bowel pattern by discharge.	Monitor frequency, amount, and consistency of stool with each bowel movement (BM).	Assessment can alert staff to need for stool softener or dietary consult.	No BM but is passing gas.
	Assist to bedside commode after breakfast every day. Provide privacy.	Sitting on commode and privacy promote ease of BM.	Small amount of stool, patient states stools were "hard" today. Notified provider to prescribe stool softener.
	Give stool softener daily as ordered.	Keeps stool soft.	Received stool softener.

Nursing Care Plan 9.1 Care of a Resident With Decreased Mobility—cont'd

Goals/Expected Outcomes	Nursing Interventions	Selected Rationale	Evaluation
	Increase fluids to 8 oz/h while awake.	Keeps stool soft.	Took in at least 6 oz of fluid each hour; continue plan.
	Increase fiber in diet.	Adds bulk, helping to prevent constipation.	Ate a bran muffin at breakfast. Dietary consult ordered.

PROBLEM STATEMENT/NURSING DIAGNOSIS

Potential for injury related to possible falls.

SUPPORTING ASSESSMENT DATA

Objective: Unsteady gait, two attempts to get out of bed without assistance. Occasional confusion during the night.

Goals/Expected Outcomes	Nursing Interventions	Selected Rationale	Evaluation
Resident will not sustain fall in facility.	Place call light and personal items within reach. Answer call light promptly.	Easy access to call light and rapid response from staff decrease risk of getting out of bed without assistance	Call bell and personal items on bed and bedside table within reach.
	Place an alarm device on the bed.	Alerts staff to attempt to get out of bed without assistance.	Bed alarm in place and functioning.
	Frequently reinforce instructions not to get up without assistance.		Reinforced not to get up without assistance q2h.
	Assist to bedside commode and back to bed.	Prevents falling.	Assisted to bedside commode after enema.
	Keep low light on in room at night to decrease confusion.	Light helps maintain orientation to room.	Placed instruction on Computer Care Plan.
	Check on resident frequently; anticipate needs.	Anticipating needs helps keep resident from arising without assistance.	Checked on resident every hour during this shift.

PROBLEM STATEMENT/NURSING DIAGNOSIS

Altered activity tolerance related to weakness and impaired mobility.

SUPPORTING ASSESSMENT DATA

Subjective: "I've really been sick; I'm so weak."

Objective: Unable to stand alone or transfer to chair; becomes short of breath with minimal exertion.

Goals/Expected Outcomes	Nursing Interventions	Selected Rationale	Evaluation
Resident will perform breathing exercises q2h while awake.	Assist to sitting position for deep-breathing exercises, use of spirometer, and coughing q2h.	Position can increase the chest excursion and allow for deeper breath.	Assisted to sit up and perform deep breathing and coughing. Used spirometer q2h.
Lung fields will remain clear.	Encourage adequate fluid intake.	Dehydration can increase tenacity of sputum.	Taking more fluid per hour (6 oz).
	Encourage to take deeper breaths during each commercial break when watching TV.	Aerates lower alveoli.	Encouraged to remember to take deep breaths during commercials on TV.
	Auscultate lungs each shift.	Detects changes in lungs.	Lungs clear on right side; slightly diminished sounds at left base.
	Turn q2h.	Helps prevent hypostatic pneumonia.	Turned q2h while in bed.
Resident will return to ambulation and other activities of daily living (ADLs) when possible.	Assist to sit in chair.	Ambulation increases respiratory activity.	Short stays in chair, increasing as tolerated.

PROBLEM STATEMENT/NURSING DIAGNOSIS

Risk for ineffective peripheral tissue perfusion related to venous stasis.

Continued

Nursing Care Plan 9.1 Care of a Resident With Decreased Mobility—cont'd

SUPPORTING ASSESSMENT DATA

Subjective: "I've been mostly in bed for over a week."

Objective: Has been inactive and in bed most of the time for the past 10 days. History of previous thrombophlebitis in right leg.

Goals/Expected Outcomes	Nursing Interventions	Selected Rationale	Evaluation
Resident will not have evidence of thrombophlebitis or deep venous thrombosis.	Encourage active ROM of legs, feet, and ankles q2h while awake.	Muscle movement compresses blood vessels, propelling blood to the heart.	Performing active ROM of legs, feet, and ankles after breathing exercises q2h.
	Keep TED hose smoothly in place except for 30 min while bathing.	Elastic hose places pressure on vessels, encouraging venous return to the heart.	TED hose reapplied after bath.
	Encourage adequate fluid intake.	Fluid prevents dehydration.	Offered fluid each time care provided.
	Visually inspect legs for reddening or swelling.	Reddening, swelling, or pain may indicate a thrombus or thrombophlebitis.	No reddening or swelling of legs and ankles.

PROBLEM STATEMENT/NURSING DIAGNOSIS

Risk for infection of the urinary tract related to decreased mobility, decreased fluid intake over past 4 days.

SUPPORTING ASSESSMENT DATA

Subjective: "I've had several bladder infections in the past."

Objective: Has been immobile for 10 days; urine is concentrated and slightly cloudy.

Goals/Expected Outcomes	Nursing Interventions	Selected Rationale	Evaluation
Resident will not develop a urinary tract infection.	Increase fluid intake to at least 3000 mL/day.	Promotes adequate hydration, maintains dilute urine.	Is increasing fluid intake this shift.
	Encourage fluid intake hourly until 2 h before bedtime.		Offering fluids each time care is given (q1–2h).
	Assess for bladder distention q4h.	Helps determine whether bladder is being emptied sufficiently.	No bladder distention; voiding sufficient quantities.
	Observe characteristics of urine for signs of infection.	Cloudy, foul-smelling urine may indicate infection.	Urine is yellow, clear, and without foul odor.
	Measure intake and output.	Helps evaluate fluid intake.	Intake 1800 mL this shift. Output 1465 mL this shift.

PROBLEM STATEMENT/NURSING DIAGNOSIS

Risk for social isolation related to lack of social interaction.

SUPPORTING ASSESSMENT DATA

Subjective: "I'm really sick of being in bed."

Objective: Confined to bed most of time without visitors; roommate is aphasic and cannot communicate verbally.

Goals/Expected Outcomes	Nursing Interventions	Selected Rationale	Evaluation
Resident will maintain social contact.	Bring phone to resident and assist to call family members and friends.	Phone calls maintain contact with family and friends.	Phoned wife this morning. Says will call friend later this evening.
	Ask volunteers to play cards with him.	Playing cards with another provides social interaction.	Requested volunteer to play cards for late afternoon.
	Visit his room frequently.	Stopping in room provides social contact.	In room q1h.
	Set up a schedule with family members for visits.	Spread out visits to help dispel loneliness.	Wife is trying to set up visiting schedule.

CRITICAL THINKING QUESTIONS

1. What other psychosocial problems might this resident have?
2. Once he is stronger and able to walk with assistance, what measures could you take to help prevent him from falling?
3. What types of activities will help him restore his muscle strength?

Older Adult Care Points

Older adults are at greatly increased risk for problems of decreased mobility because of the changes in the various body systems that normally occur with aging. Monitor closely for pressure sores as well as hypostatic pneumonia, constipation, urinary problems, and inadequate nutritional intake resulting from lack of appetite. Attention to range-of-motion exercises is very important and often neglected.

facility for an extended time to recover from major illness or trauma. Some patients are discharged home to continue with rehabilitation services in the home or as an outpatient.

Long-Term Care

Nurses have a significant role in **long-term care**. Many long-term care facilities have a registered nurse (RN; often with advanced education) as the director of nurses. RN supervisors typically manage the care for the entire facility on a 24-hour basis and delegate tasks to LPN/LVNs. An LPN/LVN often is the charge nurse, and certified nursing assistants (CNAs), patient care assistants, or restorative aides provide much of the basic direct care to the residents. An occupational therapist, physical therapist, speech pathologist, respiratory therapist, activity therapist, or other professional provides services as needed. A physician or advanced practice nurse supervises each resident's care program. Although the RN ultimately is responsible for the nursing care plan of each resident, the LPN/LVN charge nurse makes significant contributions to patient care. LPN/LVNs often admit the resident and may initiate the care under the direction of the RN.

Collaboration with the RN is essential to ensure that the plan is appropriate and complete. As an LPN/LVN, you may carry out certain treatments, provide wound care, assist with gathering assessment data from the residents, organize the shift's workload, administer medications, document assessment findings and care given, and delegate care tasks to patient care assistants.

Appropriate delegation is vital to your role as an LPN/LVN. You may assign specific tasks to the patient care assistants. For example, you may assign the patient care assistants to help residents with toileting, bathing, feeding, ambulation, or range-of-motion (ROM) exercises. Many are trained to transfer residents from bed to chair. A good understanding of how the patient care is delivered is important as you delegate these tasks.

Patient care assistants are often are the main direct caregivers in the long-term care facility. It will be important for you to establish rapport and show respect by appreciating their contributions and listening to their concerns, as they are vital to the overall welfare of the patient.

When planning care for residents in a long-term care facility, the LPN/LVN must keep in mind that the overall goals of care for the facility are to provide a safe environment, assist the resident to maintain or attain as much function as possible, promote individual independence, and **allow the resident to maintain or achieve as much autonomy as possible.**

Assignment Considerations

Appropriate Assignments

When assigning tasks to unlicensed assistants (unlicensed assistive personnel [UAP], patient care assistants, or restorative aides), you must know that they have shown competence at performing the task. Competencies of assistive personnel should be documented in their personnel files. Evaluation of task competence must be done at least annually. Give specific directions about what you want the person to do, how it is to be done, and what needs to be reported to you. You are responsible for the care of any resident or patient assigned to you. Do not assign unlicensed assistants to perform tasks for any patient or resident who is unstable.

Safety. Providing a safe environment for a group of residents, some of whom may be cognitively impaired, while allowing autonomy and independence is a great challenge. Two of the greatest safety concerns are to keep confused residents within the boundaries of the facility and to prevent falls. Those with physical disabilities need extra measures to ensure safety. Those with chronic physical conditions are more likely to experience mental illness. National Patient Safety Goals (The Joint Commission [TJC], 2019) have been developed specifically for long-term care and rehabilitation facilities (Box 9.2).

Fall prevention. The first step in the prevention of falls is to recognize which residents are at greatest risk (Box 9.3). All residents are assessed for the risk of a fall on admission and whenever their condition changes (Box 9.4). The next step to preventing a fall is to recognize hazards in the environment that could precipitate a fall (Box 9.5).

Restorative programs focus on muscle strengthening and balance. Residents who are at risk for **orthostatic hypotension** (blood pressure that falls with position change from supine to sitting or standing) are taught ways to decrease the risk of falling. Be alert to the fact that a resident who was previously ambulating safely may be weakened if they have been recently sick with fever, urinary tract infection, flu, a cold, vomiting, or diarrhea. A resident who is receiving diuretic therapy must be assessed frequently for fluid and electrolyte imbalance that could cause weakness, dizziness, or confusion. Residents on diuretic therapy must receive prompt assistance for toileting when assistance is requested. A resident who needs opioid therapy for pain or sedatives to sleep must be safeguarded. Instruct the resident to ring for assistance should the need to arise from the bed or chair occur. The bed should be kept in the low position.

Box 9.2 The Joint Commission's National Patient Safety Goals

The 2019 National Patient Safety Goals that specifically pertain to nursing care centers include the following:

- **Improve the accuracy of patient and resident identification.** Use at least two ways to identify residents when providing care, treatment, or services. For example, use the resident's name and date of birth. This is done to make sure that each resident gets the correct medicine and treatment. Blood samples or other specimens should be labeled in the presence of the patient or resident. The patient's room number or physical location is not used as an identifier.
- **Improve the safety of using medications.** Reduce the risk of harm to patients associated with anticoagulant therapy. Use unit-dose products for injectable medications. Follow agency protocols for initiation and maintenance of anticoagulant therapy. Assess the patient's drug and dietary history, as many foods and medications can interact with anticoagulants. Provide education about anticoagulant therapy to patients/residents and families about the importance of monitoring, drug-food interactions, compliance, and potential for adverse reactions. Maintain accurate patient and resident records of medication information.
- **Reduce the risk of health care–associated infections.** Use the hand cleaning guidelines from the Centers for Disease Control and Prevention or the World Health Organization. Use proven guidelines to prevent infection of the blood from central lines. Educate the patient and residents who are infected with drug-resistant organisms about infection prevention. Educate patients, residents, and their families about prevention of catheter-associated urinary tract infections and symptoms of urinary tract infection. Use written guidelines to safely insert and maintain urinary catheters.
- **Reduce the risk of patient and resident harm resulting from falls.** Assess patient or resident risk for falls and implement interventions to reduce falls based on their risk. Educate the patient and resident and, as needed, family on fall prevention strategies.
- **Prevent health care–associated pressure injury (decubitus ulcers).** Perform a skin assessment at admission and identify patients or residents at risk for pressure inujry. Participate in agency pressure injury prevention activities regularly.

! Safety Alert

Medication Assessment

Assess all medications a resident is taking to determine the risk of medication-induced postural hypotension or dizziness. This can contribute to falls. Don't forget to include over-the-counter and herbal medications as well as prescription medications.

Box 9.3 Problems and Disorders That Increase the Risk of Falls

- Musculoskeletal disorders that impair normal ambulation or balance
- Neurologic problems, such as peripheral neuropathy, that affect the feet
- Balance or gait problems resulting from stroke or inner ear problems
- Postural hypotension or dizziness caused by medications
- Impaired vision
- Impaired hearing
- Extreme weakness
- Oxygen deficit that may cause dizziness and loss of balance
- A history of previous falls

Box 9.4 Fall Risk Assessment

Place a check mark in front of the items that apply to the patient.

GENERAL INFORMATION

__ Age over 70 years
__ History of falls[a]
__ Confusion at times
__ Confused most of the time[a]
__ Impaired memory or judgment
__ Unable to follow directions[a]
__ Needs assistance with elimination
__ Visual impairment
__ Feels physically weak[a]

MEDICATIONS

__ Central nervous system suppressants (opioid, sedative, tranquilizer, hypnotic, antidepressant, psychotropic, anticonvulsant)
__ Medication that causes orthostatic hypotension (antihypertensive, diuretic)[a]
__ Medication that may cause diarrhea (cathartic)
__ Medication that may alter blood glucose levels (insulin, hypoglycemics)

GAIT AND BALANCE

__ Poor balance when standing[a]
__ Balance problems when walking[a]
__ Swaying, lurching, or slapping gait[a]
__ Unstable when making turns[a]
__ Needs assistive device (walker, cane, holds on to furniture)[a]

From Williams P: *deWit's fundamental concepts and skills for nursing*, ed 5, St. Louis, 2018, Elsevier.

[a]A check mark on any footnoted item indicates a risk for falls. A combination of four or more of the unfootnoted items indicates a risk for falls.

? Think Critically

Describe how you would determine a new resident's risk for falls. Can you identify points that should be included in the assessment of a high risk for a fall?

Box 9.5 Interventions to Help Prevent Falls

- Keep pathways free of objects.
- Remove loose rugs or secure with a nonslip pad.
- Place shoes and slippers underneath the bed or chair rather than in the pathway.
- Provide lighting without glare or deep shadows.
- Provide adequate lighting at night for the pathway from the bed to the bathroom.
- Wipe up spilled liquids immediately.
- Keep wheels on all equipment locked when stationary.
- Place belongings within easy reach to prevent leaning from the bed or chair.
- Check to see that the call bell is within reach before leaving the room.
- Promptly answer the call light to prevent the resident from arising without assistance.
- Encourage the use of supportive, sturdy footwear with nonslip soles for ambulation.
- Floor covering should not be slippery or highly patterned and should be easily navigated when ambulating in common footwear or with assistive devices.
- Encourage residents to crouch down rather than bend over to pick up something and to sit to dry the feet and pull on underwear and pants.
- Place grab bars by the toilet, in the bath or shower, along each set of stairs, and in the hallways.
- Provide chairs that are the proper height and depth to prevent "falling" into the chair or leaning far forward to arise from the chair.

Use of security devices and alternative measures. When a resident frequently forgets instructions to call for assistance, repeatedly attempts to get up and falls, or interferes with medical treatment by pulling out ordered tubes or scratching at wounds, the use of security devices may be necessary. However, these devices should be used only when all else has failed. Prior to initiating restraints, it is important that you work with the team to determine if there are any underlying causes of agitation or confusion that can be treated (Hartford Institute for Geriatric Nursing, n.d.).

Research has provided strong evidence that restraints increase rather than decrease the risk for injury (Walker et al., 2018). Chemical restraints are tranquilizers or sedatives that calm a resident and alter behavior. Physical and chemical restraint use is restricted by law and is applied only as a last resort for safety when a resident is exhibiting a threat to self or others.

The purpose of such statutes is to ensure that restraints are used to protect residents, not to hinder their movements for the staff's convenience. Alternative measures are always tried first (Box 9.6). When a security device is used, the least restrictive device is chosen. A variety of techniques help provide a restraint-free yet safe environment. **All security devices must be used only as a last resort and must be ordered by a health care provider.** If a qualified licensed nurse determines

Box 9.6 Measures Helpful to Prevent the Need for Security Devices

- Review medications to see if any are contributing to restlessness or confusion.
- Alert all team members of at-risk residents.
- Facilitate regular bowel and bladder function.
- Maintain regular sleep-wake practices and enhance bedtime activities to include restful music, warm milk or herbal tea, noise reduction activities, and avoiding TV watching immediately before bedtime.
- Enhance orientation by using calendars and clocks and making the identification of caregivers easily visible to the patient or resident.
- Communicate clearly with the patient or resident.
- Place a restless or high-risk resident in a room or location close to the nurses' station where they can be checked frequently and any attempts to get up will be more likely observed.
- Make sure that patients or residents are provided with their usual eyeglasses or hearing aids to enhance communication and orientation.
- Use validation to reaffirm the feelings and concerns of a resident with dementia.
- Provide a variety of activities that keep the resident engaged during the day.
- Provide familiar and cherished items that the resident can handle.
- Ask a family member to stay with the resident.
- Use a bed or chair alarm to alert nursing staff that the resident is attempting to get out of the bed or chair unassisted.
- Remain with unsteady, agitated, or confused residents when they are up and about.
- Leave another person in charge of your residents when leaving the unit for a meal break or other reason; specifically mention which residents need to be visually checked frequently.
- Provide social and diversional activities to a resident confined to a wheelchair or bed so that boredom does not cause the person to try to get up and seek activity.
- Maintain bed position at a level as low as possible.

Legal and Ethical Considerations

Considering Restraints

Patient deaths have occurred from improperly applied restraints. Laws require that they be used only after all other measures—such as sitters, family at the bedside, alarms, or distractions—have been tried and these other measures have failed. Documentation must be thorough, indicating specific alternative measures that have been tried and have failed. Document the time the restraint is applied, the condition of the patient at that time, interim assessments, the time the restraint is removed, and the condition of the patient at the time when the restraint is removed.

Box 9.7 Principles Related to the Use of Security and Safety Devices

- The use of safety or security devices must help the resident or be needed for the continuation of medical therapy.
- All devices that limit movement or immobilize must be ordered by a health care provider.
- Use the least amount of immobilization needed for the situation. For example, use mitts rather than wrist restraints if the resident cannot otherwise be prevented from pulling out tubes or lines.
- Apply the device snugly but not so tightly as to interfere with blood circulation or nerve function.
- If a security device is applied, check on the resident at least every 30 minutes or per agency policy. Assess for breathing, circulation, and possible nerve or skin impairment.
- An immobilization device must be removed and the resident's position changed at least every 2 hours. Active or passive exercises are performed for immobilized joints and muscles.
- Reassess the need for the security measure every 4 to 8 hours.
- Meet needs for food, fluids, and toileting and assess these needs every 2 hours.
- Assess pain and comfort level and provide interventions as necessary.
- Document alternative measures taken and their success or failure. Document all pertinent data related to assessments when security devices are in place, when they were applied, and when they were removed.
- The provider should be notified as soon as the security device is deemed no longer necessary.

the need for a chemical or physical security device in an emergency, the need is specifically documented when the security device is applied. A provider's order for the security device must be written within 24 to 48 hours. Box 9.7 presents the principles related to the use of security and safety devices.

A resident who is immobilized with a security device must be checked visually at least every 30 minutes to ensure that the resident's body is in good alignment and that there are no problems. These checks must be documented. Whenever you are in the patient's room, check skin color for circulation in the affected body parts. Residents must be turned or repositioned every 2 hours. Thorough assessment of skin and circulation is done at that time. The restraint should be removed immediately after the risk has been reduced.

Managing confusion and disorientation. For residents with mild confusion and disorientation, various techniques and measures are used to help maintain orientation or reduce agitation that can occur with confusion. Always make sure the resident has access to their eyeglasses and/or hearing aids to reduce sensory deficits. Adequate rest, sleep, fluids, elimination, pain control, and comfort measures are all recommended by the Hartford Institute for Geriatric Nursing. The environment can be structured so that the resident has visual reminders of the year, day, and time of day. Environmental aids such as a readable, up-to-date calendar; a clock; and the daily newspaper or local television or radio news will help. Remember, the priority is to maintain a safe environment

Consistency in mealtimes, scheduled activities, treatments, and daily personal care routine also can be helpful. Do not overwhelm the resident with options, but allow them to choose preferences during these activities (family members can be very helpful here). A time schedule for activities and events within the facility should be posted in large type where the resident can refer to it frequently. Decorations for the next upcoming holiday give clues as to the current season. Try to assign caregivers who are familiar to the resident, avoid placing the resident in unfamiliar situations, and be sensitive to the number of visitors the resident can tolerate without stress (this may be just one or two people at a time).

A positive and helpful approach is to respond continuously to the resident's confusion with honest and real information. Remember to assess the possibility of a physical cause for the confusion, such as urinary tract infection, constipation, dehydration, reduced oxygenation, or suboptimal pain control, when there is a change in the resident's usual ability to interact.

Late afternoon or evening confusion (often described as **sundown syndrome**, "sundowning," or "late-day confusion") can occur in some older adult residents. Residents most at risk are those with cognitive impairment and those who may have decreased ability to compensate for fatigue or stresses after a long day. Other factors that contribute to sundown syndrome include those that can disrupt the resident's normal routine, such as room changes, changes in roommate, changes in routine, decreased engagement in social activities, and social isolation. Interventions that have been effective in reducing sundown syndrome include activities such as group singing in late afternoon hours (Fig. 9.1), increasing the amount of daytime lighting between 7 A.M. and 9 P.M., and specialized training of nursing assistants (Scales, 2015; Yevchak, Steis, & Evans, 2012).

Other strategies may include keeping the call bell within reach and visiting the resident frequently to calm and reassure them. Moving the resident closer to the nurses' station, use of therapeutic touch, and other signs of caring may help minimize confusion. A bed alarm that alerts staff when the resident attempts to get out of bed is helpful. Door alarms that announce when the resident has left their room or designated area may be used in place of security devices and may prevent patients from wandering in unsafe areas. Keeping the resident active during the day and encouraging physical

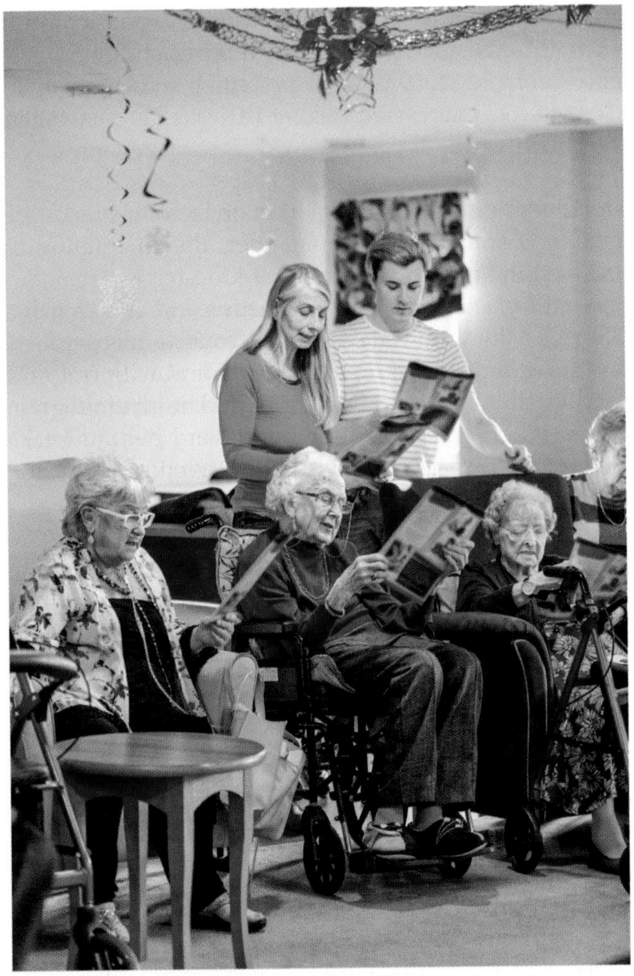

Fig. 9.1 Group singing intervention with residents in long-term care. (Copyright © SolStock/iStock.)

exercise helps promote sleep at night. **Listening to the resident to try to determine any possible cause of unrest or fear can often help solve the problem.**

Promoting independence. The move to a long-term care facility is a major upheaval, particularly when it is for the remainder of the person's lifetime. Specific goals should be set with the resident to encourage independence in activities of daily living (ADLs) and in recreational activity. Perhaps a resident can pursue a former hobby, such as knitting or playing the piano, if such activities are available. Adaptive devices and a consultation with the dietitian may provide all the assistance that is necessary for self-feeding once again. Other adaptive devices can make daily living considerably easier (Table 9.2). To promote a resident's independence, staff members should refrain from doing tasks that the resident is capable of doing themselves. For the resident who has had a stroke or suffers from debilitating arthritis or another musculoskeletal problem, use of adaptive devices can assist in the promotion of independence, provide some autonomy, and help maintain function (Fig. 9.2).

Table 9.2 Uses of Common Assistive-Adaptive Devices

DEVICE	USE
Buttonhook	Threaded through the buttonhole to enable patients with weak finger mobility to button shirts. Alternative uses include serving as a pencil holder.
Extended shoe horn	Assists in putting on shoes for patients with decreased mobility. Alternative uses include turning light switches off or on while the patient is in a wheelchair.
Plate guard and spork (spoon and fork in one utensil)	Applied to a plate to assist patients with weak hand and arm mobility to feed themselves. Spork allows one utensil for two purposes.
Gel pad	Placed under a plate or a glass to prevent dishes from slipping and moving. Alternative uses include placement under bathing and grooming items to prevent their movement.
Foam buildups	Applied to eating utensils to assist patients with weak hands to grasp and help feed themselves. Alternative uses include the application to pens and pencils to assist with writing or over a buttonhook to assist with grasping the device.
Hook and loop fastener (Velcro) straps	Applied to utensils, a buttonhook, or a pencil to slip over the hand and provide a method of stabilizing the device when the patient's hand grasp is weak.
Long-handled reacher	Assists in obtaining items located on high shelves or at ground level for patients who are not able to change positions easily.
Elastic shoelaces or Velcro shoe closure	Prevents the need for tying shoes.

Adapted from Ignatavicius DD, Workman ML, Rebar CR, et al.: *Medical-surgical nursing: critical thinking for collaborative care,* ed 9, St. Louis, 2018, Elsevier.

Maintaining function. Once a functional assessment has been completed, specific goals should be written to maintain the highest level of function possible for the resident. If the resident is ambulatory, exercise should be planned and encouraged on a daily basis. If the resident is not ambulatory, ROM exercises should be performed several times a day. Measures to promote

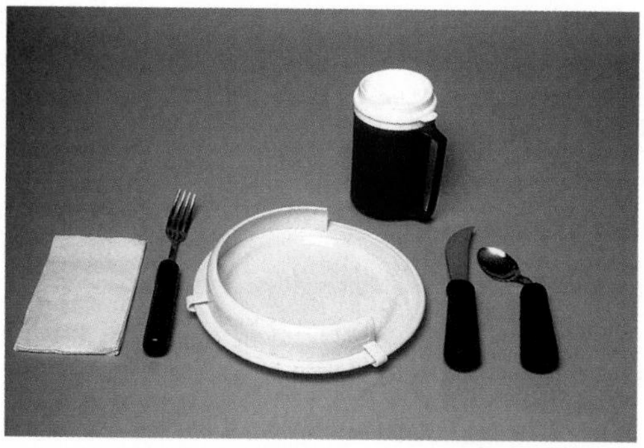

Fig. 9.2 Adaptive devices to promote independence in eating.

Clinical Cues

When residents understand that they have control of what happens, they maintain good adaptive skills. They are resilient and have the power to adjust and reduce stress. This helps resist adverse effects of chronic disease. **Activity theory** states that people will be happiest in direct proportion to how much activity they are able to maintain as they grow older. **Continuity theory** proposes that participation in activities and relationships that have been maintained over a long period contributes to a sense of well-being and allows a sense of integrity and continuity with the past. Finding out what activities have significant meaning for the resident, and seeing how those might be continued by making adaptations so that enjoying the activities is possible, can greatly enhance the quality of the resident's life and reduce the negative effects of chronic conditions.

Think Critically

Identify three ways to foster independence in a new right-handed resident who is still quite weak, has suffered a stroke, and has right-sided **hemiparesis** (weakness).

continued bowel and bladder continence are essential. Assessing patterns of elimination and providing assistance for toileting as needed is a basic part of promoting continued function and protecting the resident's dignity. If the resident has been temporarily incontinent because of illness or surgery, a bowel or bladder retraining program is appropriate. Chapters 28 and 33 discuss such programs.

Mental stimulation is essential to maintaining a high level of cognitive functioning. Although resident preference and values should be considered in group television viewing areas, the staff should consider working with the residents to plan segments of time to turn on informational programs that are interesting. Scientific shows, travel shows, public television specials, and similar programs can stimulate thinking and encourage the sharing of thoughts on a variety of subjects. Assisting residents to work crossword puzzles is another way to help them keep an active mind. When a resident cannot write or read because of poor vision, group work on a puzzle is an option. Card games promote mental stimulation as well as social interaction. Group activities such as bingo, group singing, holiday celebrations, and entertainment acts provide socialization and stimulation. Continuing interest in lifelong activities is a factor in successful aging for many.

Documentation. Documentation in a long-term care facility is somewhat different from documentation in the hospital or in home care. For long-term care documentation, an admission assessment and an extensive 38-page Minimum Data Set (MDS) form that is required by the federal government are filled out. Bowel and bladder training assessment forms and training program forms, weekly pressure ulcer reports, and 24-hour intake and output records are some of the other documentation forms used in the long-term care facility.

REHABILITATION

Rehabilitation is the process whereby a disabled person is helped to achieve optimal function. A primary goal of rehabilitation is to minimize the deficit from the condition and maximize the abilities that are intact. It involves measures to achieve the highest possible levels of physical, emotional, psychological, and social function and well-being. Rehabilitation is concerned with achieving a better quality of life. Most patients who require rehabilitation services are disabled as a result of a chronic illness. Others have become disabled from trauma incurred during an accident.

The need for rehabilitation services will continue to grow. Recent data suggest that more than 5 million people are living with some type of paralysis (Armour, Courtney-Long, Fox, Fredine, & Cahill, 2016). Most are younger than 65 years, female, and white. Nearly half are no longer able to work. Stroke is the most common cause of paralysis, and spinal cord injury, multiple sclerosis, and cerebral palsy round out the top four. Patients with moderate to severe traumatic brain injury may face disability for decades after the event (Andelic et al., 2018).

Several of the objectives for *Healthy People 2030* are rehabilitation oriented. These include objectives directed toward improving access to programs, increasing access to social and emotional support services, and improving access to interventions in the home and community-based settings. In addition, the World Health Organization (2013) supports the need for improving rehabilitation services for adults and children as well as the need for health care personnel to support and protect the rights and dignity of all persons with any kind of disability.

REHABILITATION PROGRAMS

Rehabilitation services are offered in freestanding rehabilitation hospitals, in general hospitals, and in skilled nursing homes where the patients stay for a few weeks.

Patients who have had a hip replacement often are placed in a skilled nursing facility for rehabilitation before returning home. Many communities have a hospital with an outpatient rehabilitation program for patients with cardiac and respiratory problems. Rehabilitation services may be scarce in rural areas, and patients who have suffered neurologic injury or loss of musculoskeletal function as a result of amputation, trauma, or disease often have to go to a rehabilitation center far from home. Programs within large cities are often available for vision or hearing rehabilitation. Community centers often have rehabilitation programs with water exercise for patients with severe arthritis. Most burn centers have comprehensive rehabilitation programs available for burn patients. Rehabilitation programs have a philosophy that is based on three beliefs:

1. Each person is unique, whole within themself, and interdependent with their own environment.
2. Independence can be achieved within the limits of disability when the person is a full participant in managing their own life.
3. The goal is to enable patients to mobilize their own resources, choose goals, and attain those goals through their own efforts.

Rehabilitation involves a team effort directed at holistic care and involves a variety of disciplines.

Older Adult Care Points

An older adult patient who has suffered a major loss of body function may not be initially receptive to rehabilitation efforts. It takes a skillful nurse to help motivate the patient to want to improve their functional ability. Sometimes introducing the patient to someone close to their own age who has been through a similar illness and has managed to regain some functions is the best "medicine." Gentle encouragement with praise for small efforts and accomplishments is better than trying to force the patient to perform exercises or practice tasks.

A pulmonary (respiratory) rehabilitation (PR) program teaches the patient self-care techniques that will help them attain a better quality of life. There are generally three components to a PR program:

1. Breathing exercises
2. Paced walking exercise
3. Correct use of inhaled medications

These components are usually mixed with medical therapy and may also include nutritional counseling, energy conserving techniques, and psychological counseling or group support. Patients are enrolled in the program for a number of weeks and interact with other patients who have the same problems. A nurse or respiratory therapist teaches the various breathing techniques, paced walking, and use of inhalers. The nurse conducts motivational group activities to increase the desire to participate in an exercise program and to display the benefits of following the program. Teaching how to avoid respiratory infections is reinforced. The nurse or respiratory therapist is available to encourage the patient and, while they exercise, to evaluate the patient's progress in using the techniques taught. Vital signs are monitored periodically to determine the effect of exercise on cardiac and respiratory function. Some rehabilitation centers provide respiratory services that wean the patient from the ventilator and then work with them to improve respiratory function and functional capacity for ADLs.

Cardiac rehabilitation programs are usually outpatient based and consist of several components:

- Monitored exercise to increase strength and endurance and build collateral circulation to the heart
- Diet counseling and education to lower cholesterol, triglycerides, and body fat
- Medication counseling regarding the purpose, administration, and side effects of the prescribed medications
- Vital sign monitoring to determine the effect of exercise on the cardiovascular system
- Group sessions on stress reduction techniques
- Support group sessions for those experiencing depression or anxiety after surgery or a myocardial infarction

Such cardiac rehabilitation programs usually have a physician, nurses, physical therapist, dietitian, and psychologist or social worker on staff.

Rehabilitation after knee surgery and other musculoskeletal injuries is often performed on an outpatient basis. Either the physical therapist goes to the home or the patient travels to the physical therapy facility. Supervised exercise is performed to increase ROM, decrease pain, strengthen muscles, promote ambulation, and improve balance.

Patients with neurologic damage from a spinal cord or head injury may need to spend several months in a rehabilitation facility. Because of insurance limitations, inpatient treatment is not always possible. Rehabilitation efforts then need to be continued at home.

THE REHABILITATION TEAM

Nurses who work with rehabilitation patients must be flexible and creative. Providing patient-centered care is essential. This means that the patient is not only a focus of the rehabilitation team but also a member of the team. Your function is to assist the patient to achieve an optimal state of wellness as **defined by the patient.** It is very important that nurses be nonjudgmental and not impose their own values and attitudes on their patients.

The rehabilitation nurse must be able to work collaboratively with other health team members. Besides the health care provider, occupational, physical, speech, cognitive, and recreational therapists; vocational counselors; and social workers are part of the team. You assist in ensuring that the patient correctly performs exercises and activities as instructed by each therapist and reinforce their teaching. A collaborative or interdisciplinary care

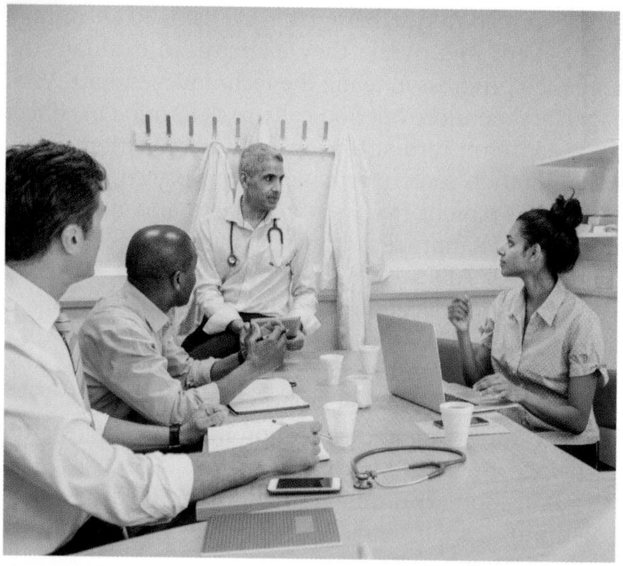

Fig. 9.3 The rehabilitation team conferring about the patient's care. (Copyright © SolStock/iStock.)

plan is followed so that each member of the team is aware of what treatment and education the patient is receiving. Both short- and long-term goals are set. This provides for continuity of interdisciplinary care, recognizing the critical importance of each discipline in promoting positive outcomes for the patient. Team conferences are scheduled regularly for members to collaborate on the patient's care and evaluate rehabilitation progress (Fig. 9.3).

The patient and family both undergo considerable stress during the rehabilitation period. Caregivers should assist the patient and family in developing positive coping techniques. A good sense of humor; gentle, firm people skills; patience; and the ability to provide solid encouragement are good tools for working with rehabilitation patients.

The philosophy of rehabilitation nursing is based on the recognition of the patient's need for independence. Learn to judge when the patient should be allowed to struggle to do something on their own, and learn to recognize when the patient's frustration is reaching a level at which assistance is needed.

Roles of the LPN/LVN in Rehabilitation

Often two levels of LPN/LVNs are employed in rehabilitation facilities, depending on the individual state practice act and facility protocols. One level is the LPN/LVN I, and the other level is the LPN/LVN II with intravenous (IV) therapy and Functional Independence Measure (FIM) certification. The LPN/LVN I does all nursing activities except for assessments and IV infusion therapy. The LPN/LVN II performs the same functions as the LPN/LVN I plus the tasks involved with IV infusions. At least 1 year of medical-surgical experience is required for employment as a nurse in a rehabilitation facility. The LPN/LVN initiates and participates in updating the team plan of care in collaboration with the RN to meet the patient's needs. The LPN/LVN assists with patient and family education by supporting the outlined teaching plan and reinforcing teaching. Any barriers to patient or caregiver readiness to learn are reported by the LPN/LVN to the supervisor. Recommendations are made by the nurses to team members on how to facilitate patient and caregiver learning. Learning outcomes are evaluated and documented. The LPN/LVN is an active participant and facilitator of both structured and nonstructured learning experiences. Leadership functions of the LPN/LVN are to supervise the patient care assistants, the CNAs, and the nursing rehabilitation technicians. The LPN/LVN acts as a preceptor for unlicensed personnel as needed and appropriate. As a member of the team, the LPN/LVN carries out all normal patient care nursing duties and provides input and feedback to the team. When assigned to do so, the LPN/LVN carries out quality improvement activities.

❖ NURSING MANAGEMENT

◆ ASSESSMENT (DATA COLLECTION)

After obtaining a thorough history, a physical and psychosocial assessment is performed for each patient to establish a baseline; to determine physical limitations, ability to perform ADLs, and amount of assistance needed; and to identify present psychosocial difficulties.

A skin risk assessment and fall risk assessment are performed (see Chapter 42 for the pressure ulcer risk assessment tool). Patients covered by Medicare will have data filled in on the section of the MDS pertinent to rehabilitation. The patient's home environment is examined before discharge to determine whether physical features of the home, such as stairs, narrow doorways, or access to bathroom facilities, will present a problem. Questions about the neighborhood, such as the location of shopping centers and types of transportation available, are asked. Inquiries about who does the grocery shopping, cooking, errands, and housework for the patient are made.

The patient's usual daily schedule and habits of everyday living are examined, including sleeping, waking, eating, elimination patterns, hygiene, grooming, sexual activity, working, and leisure activities. A *functional assessment* of how the patient's disability has affected their former usual patterns (Box 9.8) focuses on the patient's present ability to perform ADLs, such as toileting, bathing, dressing, grooming, and ambulating, as well as their ability to use the telephone, shop, prepare food, and perform housekeeping chores. Various assessment tools are used to determine the patient's ability to function. A common tool, the Katz Index of Independence in Activities of Daily Living (see Evolve website), helps evaluate how much assistance the patient needs for various activities.

The Baird Body Image Assessment Tool is often used to perform a psychosocial assessment, which includes evaluating self-esteem and body image. Use of defense

Focused Assessment

For the Rehabilitation Patient

After reviewing the patient's history, the following data are collected by asking pertinent questions regarding the function of each body system.

CARDIOVASCULAR
- Fatigue/weakness
- Chest pain
- Irregular heart rate or palpitations
- Dizziness
- Edema

RESPIRATORY
- Pain with breathing
- Shortness of breath
- Using accessory muscles to breath
- Cough (productive or nonproductive)

GASTROINTESTINAL/NUTRITION
- Difficulty swallowing
- Anorexia, nausea, vomiting
- Eating pattern; amount of oral intake
- Weight loss or gain
- Bowel status; change in stool
- Serum albumin levels

URINARY
- Voiding pattern
- Fluid intake
- Urinary retention
- Self-catheterization status
- Urinalysis and/or culture

NEUROLOGIC
- Motor function
- Sensation
- Cognitive abilities
- Assistive devices

MUSCULOSKELETAL
- Muscle strength
- Range of motion
- Fall risk assessment
- Assistive devices
- Safety measures

INTEGUMENTARY
- Skin condition
- Risk of skin breakdown
- Presence of lesions
- Measures to decrease risk of breakdown

DEGREE OF INDEPENDENCE
- Functional Independence Measure (FIM) scores per certified personnel assessment
- Ability for ADLs (Katz Index of Independence in Activities of Daily Living)

PSYCHOSOCIAL
- Alteration in roles
- Financial concerns
- Support system
- Self-concept
- Coping mechanisms
- Sexual concerns
- Employment/educational concerns
- Family strain
- Home environment alterations needed

MEDICATIONS
- Scheduled medications
- PRN (as needed) medications
- Over-the-counter medications
- Herbal medications
- Vitamins/dietary supplements

SAFETY
- All equipment in use checked for safety
- Risk assessments for falls and skin
- Prostheses applied correctly
- Adaptive equipment obtained

Box 9.8 Functional Independence Measure Scoring Categories

- Self-care
- Sphincter control
- Transfers
- Locomotion
- Communication
- Social cognition

A score of 0 or 1 is given in each category. Totaled scores indicate independent (6-7), modified dependence (3-5), or complete dependence (1-2).

mechanisms, level of anxiety, and usual coping techniques are explored. To ascertain the patient's response to loss, ask the patient to describe feelings related to the loss of a body part or body function. The patient's support systems and the family's coping abilities also are determined. As rehabilitation progresses, perform a vocational assessment so that the vocational counselor can assist the patient in finding appropriate training, education, or employment after discharge from the rehabilitation program.

Patients with life-changing illness or injury, those who have suffered major loss of body function or former roles, and those who have lost most of their independence and social contacts may suffer from anger and depression. Assessing mental outlook is an ongoing nursing function. Should several signs of severe depression become evident, consult with the health care provider. The patient must be kept safe. Determining suicide potential in the depressed patient is important. Chapter 47 discusses assessment and intervention for depression and suicidal thought.

Sexual concerns should be addressed during the rehabilitation period. Patients may feel more comfortable revealing these concerns to you as a member of the health care team that provides direct care. Never hesitate to report these concerns to the health care team and/or refer the patient to the RN, social services, a psychologist, or a sex therapist as your facility recommends. If you are not comfortable or knowledgeable in this role, never hesitate to contact another member of the health care team.

Think Critically

Explain the difference between a physical assessment and a functional assessment.

◆ NURSING DIAGNOSIS

Problem statements appropriate for the patient undergoing rehabilitation are listed in Box 9.9. Determining the nursing diagnosis is typically the responsibility of the RN, but as a member of the health care team the LPN/LVN can contribute to the plan of care on an ongoing basis.

◆ PLANNING

An interdisciplinary plan of care is devised for each rehabilitation patient. Periodic care conferences are essential for the members of the health care team to evaluate the progress of the patient, to share perceptions and ideas, and to revise the plan of care if it is not helping the patient meet established expected outcomes. Depending on the situation, the frequency of care conferences may vary. In some settings, these conferences may occur several times a week; others may occur once every 1 or 2 weeks or even once a month. Whatever the frequency, remember that you are an important part of the health care team by virtue of your frequent and direct patient contact. During the conference, both long-term and short-term goals will be determined. Expected outcomes are written for each problem.

Box 9.9 Problem Statements Common for Patients in Rehabilitation

- Altered physical mobility due to neuromuscular impairment, sensory-perceptual impairment, and/or pain
- Altered self-care ability (specify) due to perceptual or cognitive impairment and/or neuromuscular impairment
- Potential for altered skin integrity due to alteration in sensation, mobility, or nutritional status
- Potential for injury due to musculoskeletal weakness or perceptual or cognitive impairment
- Altered urinary elimination due to neurologic dysfunction or trauma or disease affecting spinal nerves
- Constipation due to neurologic impairment or decreased mobility
- Altered coping ability due to added stressors or situational crisis
- Altered family coping due to situational crisis and/or added stressors
- Altered home maintenance ability due to neuromuscular impairment or perceptual or cognitive impairment
- Insufficient knowledge for self-care and techniques for rehabilitation
- Altered body image due to loss of normal function or traumatic injury and/or scarring
- Altered sexual function due to neuromuscular impairment, pain, or impaired mobility

◆ IMPLEMENTATION AND EVALUATION

Interventions are carried out in a manner that encourages patients to do as much for themselves as possible. Positive feedback is given for even small accomplishments or attempts at self-care. Pace activities to help build endurance but reduce risk of excessive fatigue. Patients receiving rehabilitation interventions may be working with physical and occupational therapists, speech therapists, and recreational therapists. The health care team members will assist in timing activities for best patient outcomes (see the Rehabilitation Team Assessment Form on the Evolve website). Focus of care may include ADLs and instrumental activities of daily living (IADLs; Fig. 9.4). Speech therapists, activity therapists, and others will be involved in the implementation of the care plan.

Discharge planning is implemented from the time the patient enters rehabilitation. The family and patient will need resources within the community. Evaluation is performed by gathering data that show whether the goals and expected outcomes have been met.

HOME CARE

Most care in the community setting is given by home health and/or hospice agencies. Home health care is the preferred and most cost-effective method of health care delivery. Recent innovations in medical equipment

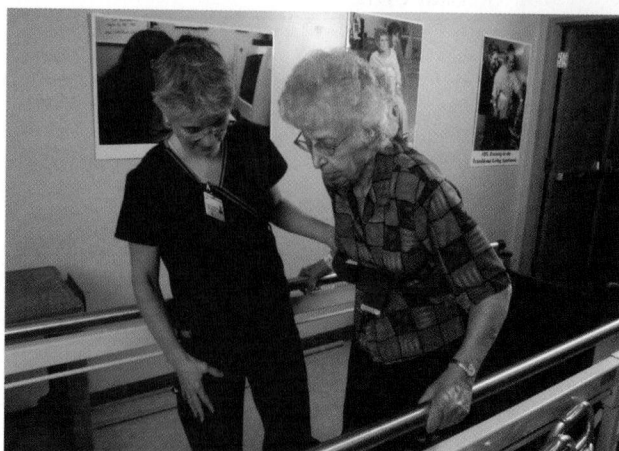

Fig. 9.4 Physical therapist working with a patient on ambulation and muscle strengthening.

have allowed more complex, high-technology care to be given at home. For the patient there are many benefits, both physically and psychologically. **The goal of home care is to keep the patient as well and independent as possible and enable them to live at home.** The LPN/LVN must have 1 year of experience working in an acute care facility before working in home care in most states.

For home care, the RN acts as case manager and coordinates the care of all of the health care providers involved in the patient's care. The RN is responsible for the plan of care and for seeing that care is delivered in an uninterrupted manner. This nurse must act as a liaison with the other care providers to ensure that all efforts effectively complement one another. The LPN/LVN may perform treatments, perform appropriate delegated duties of the RN, or provide care in the home on a daily shift basis.

Home care nursing can prevent a patient's expensive readmission to a hospital or entry into a long-term care facility. Home health care is family centered, and the family members are also responsible for the ongoing care of the patient. Home visits are made to intervene and see that the patient is provided comfort, to see that complications are prevented and health is improved, and to assist with rehabilitation (Fig. 9.5). Because home health care is family centered, **your philosophy must have a different focus. In the home care setting, the patient and family are in charge. You are a guest in the home and act as a consultant, coordinator of care, provider of skilled care, teacher, and advocate.**

In home care, the patient and family are seeking your services and must be treated as valued customers. You must learn to be nonjudgmental of the patient, the family, and the living arrangements. Together, you, the patient, and the family set goals for care and then establish the boundaries of your role. Should the living situation not be ideal, furnishings and equipment lacking, or the home dirty, establish trust with the patient and family before trying to accomplish major changes. Be sensitive to the patient's and family's cultural values, financial resources, and specific ways of doing things and try not to impose your own views. Work together with the patient and family to improve home safety, and share knowledge of available resources. **A home care nurse must be very flexible and creative in teaching patients and families ways to accomplish care of the patient while abiding by the principles of asepsis and safety.**

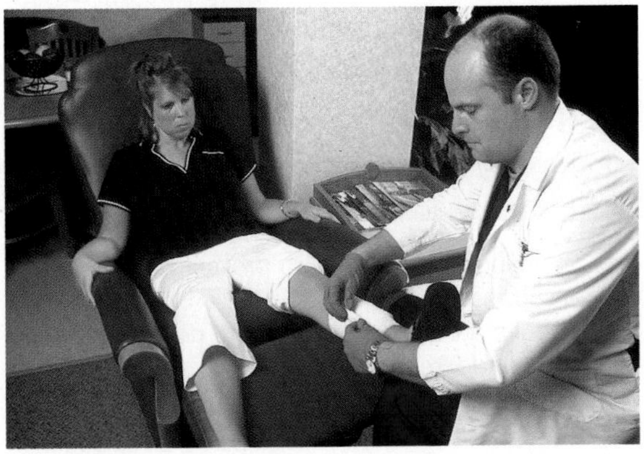

Fig. 9.5 Home health nurse changing a dressing.

Hospice care may be delivered in the home, long-term care facility, or hospital. Although the philosophy of hospice care was originally brought to the United States to support the death and dying of cancer patients, in the 1990s nurses and other health care providers realized the need for improvement in end-of-life care for all patients. Hospice and palliative care is now available to children and adults with chronic illnesses with a focus on supportive care at the end of life. This has made substantial improvements in the dying experiences for patients and their caregivers. For more information, see Chapter 8.

? Think Critically

Mrs. C. is diagnosed with advanced heart failure and wants to stay at home for as long as possible. On your first visit, Mrs. C. apologizes for not being able to wash the dishes or keep the house as clean as she would like. You also notice that she has several throw rugs in her home. What measures can you take to support her independence while reducing risk of falls or of infection?

A large percentage of the home care nurse's time with the patient is spent evaluating physical and psychosocial status, signs of complications, side effects of medications, and effects of therapy. Both the safety of the home and the quality of nutritional and basic care are evaluated. You are able to gather considerable useful data for the health care provider. Much time is spent consulting with providers by phone, providing updates on the patient's condition, seeking new orders, and collaborating about care needs. Each visit includes a physical assessment of the identified problems and of nutritional, home safety, elimination, skin, and psychosocial status. All findings are documented, as are data indicating that home health nursing care is still needed. Between visits, you may contact the patient or family to check on various aspects of care or to see whether there are any concerns. The patient and family may contact the agency or you at any time, and such phone calls are encouraged.

Other functions of the home health nurse include performing wound care and dressing changes, organizing medications for scheduled administration, monitoring blood sugar levels, drawing blood samples for laboratory testing, giving injections or teaching injection technique, monitoring pain control, and monitoring enteral feedings. Teaching self-care and rehabilitation techniques and monitoring progress and compliance with treatment are primary nursing functions that help control health care costs and keep the patient from needing hospitalization. The home care nurse needs to be a strong advocate for the patient's needs and treatment.

The home care nurse provides considerable psychosocial care for the patient and family. Sometimes, you are the only visitor the patient has. In this instance you become a sort of friend, providing social interaction as well as needed health care. You must become knowledgeable about negotiating the complex medical care system and obtaining supplies, medications, or services when the patient does not have money for them. A full knowledge of the community resources available to the patient is essential. Most home health agencies have lists of resources available. A medical social worker who has a liaison with the agency also can be of help. The hospital nurse stays out of financial concerns (except for referrals to the social worker) but must try to help the patient find remedies to financial problems so that stress will be reduced and energies can be directed at healing and techniques of self-care.

? Think Critically

What strategies would you use to obtain a shower chair for a patient who cannot afford to buy or rent one?

THE LPN/LVN IN HOME CARE

LPN/LVNs working in home care typically are under the supervision of an RN case manager. The LPN/LVN may be providing "private-duty" services for an unconscious patient who needs skilled care such as tracheal suctioning or tube feedings, performing home visits to change dressings or monitor blood sugar levels, or possibly acting as an in-agency supervisor by coordinating home health aide visits and supervising their work. The role of the LPN/LVN in home care is growing. The family provides assistance with personal care, and a home health aide may visit a few times a week to bathe the patient and shampoo hair. Homemaking is provided by family members or by a homemaker aide. "Sitters" may be hired to attend to the patient's needs at night if the family is not able to provide this service.

Nursing care plans are formulated, considering 24-hour needs, in collaboration with the patient, the family or relatives, and all other health care providers. Case conferences are conducted regularly, even if the case manager does them on the telephone with the others involved in the patient's care. Medicare requires a case conference every 60 days when more than one discipline is involved in the patient's care.

THE FAMILY CAREGIVER

When a patient has considerable disability and cannot function independently, a family member often becomes the main caregiver. Depending on the degree of dependence of the patient, the caregiver may have an overwhelming task in caring for the patient, maintaining the house, obtaining food and supplies, cooking, and coordinating therapy or health care provider appointments. The caregiver's usual life is disrupted, and social contacts are limited because of time constraints and fatigue. You must assess the caregiver's stress levels regularly.

Focused Assessment

Assessing Caregiver Stress

- What help do you have in caring for your spouse or relative?
- Are there more family members who might help?
- What are your cultural values related to caregiving?
- Have your sleep habits changed related to caregiving?
- Do you feel strained with all your family and caregiving responsibilities?
- Have you been feeling edgy or irritable lately?
- Are you feeling overwhelmed?
- Do you feel you cannot leave your relative alone?
- Have you been having crying spells?
- Are you having difficulty making decisions?
- Do you find you have trouble keeping your mind on what you are doing?
- Are you having frequent headaches, backaches, or muscle or stomach pain?
- Are you aware of the local support groups available for caregivers?
- Do you have any sources of support such as churches, clubs, or other groups?

Some home care agencies have an assessment tool for this purpose. When caregiver stress is high, calling the agency social worker for a consultation can provide either more help for the caregiver or a respite program that might provide the caregiver with a few days of needed rest and relaxation. A respite program provides room, meals, and care for a patient while the caregiver is relieved of all responsibility.

Get Ready for the NCLEX® Examination!

Key Points

- Chronic illness interferes with normal function for about 43 million people in the United States.
- Hazards of decreased mobility are numerous and can occur within just a few days for immobile patients.
- It is a nursing responsibility to prevent hazards of decreased mobility.
- Older adults are especially prone to developing problems of decreased mobility.
- LPN/LVNs often work as charge nurses in long-term care facilities under the direction of an RN director of nursing.

- The LPN/LVN often supervises the nursing assistants in long-term care facilities.
- Safety of residents is a primary goal in long-term care facilities.
- Much attention is directed to preventing resident falls.
- Security devices are used only to protect the resident or others and only as a last resort.
- Frequent assessment is essential when a security device is applied to a resident.
- Techniques to minimize confusion and disorientation are used consistently.
- Keeping the resident active during the day helps decrease nocturnal confusion.
- A goal of long-term care is to promote as much independence as possible for the resident.
- Long-term care facilities must help residents maintain or regain function.
- Rehabilitation helps a disabled person achieve optimal function.
- There are rehabilitation programs for patients with respiratory, heart, and musculoskeletal problems.
- Rehabilitation is a team effort of the patient and many health professionals.
- You assist with determining rehabilitation needs.
- Rehabilitation is carried out with a collaborative plan of care.
- Home care agencies provide continuing care in the community.
- LPN/LVNs are supervised by the health care provider or an RN in the home care environment.
- In the home care setting, the patient and family are in charge; you are a guest in the home.
- Home care nurses must be flexible and creative to accomplish needed care of the patient in the home.

Additional Learning Resources

SG Go to your Study Guide for additional learning activities to help you master this chapter content.

Go to your Evolve website (http://evolve.elsevier.com/deWit/medsurg) for the following FREE learning resources:
- Animations, audio, and video
- Answers and rationales for questions and activities
- Glossary with pronunciations in English and Spanish
- Interactive Review Questions and more!

Review Questions for the NCLEX® Examination

1. An 85-year-old diabetic man recovering from hip surgery has begun ambulating with a walker. Although he likes his independence, you are concerned that he may fall since he is early in his rehabilitation. You instruct him to please call for assistance when he gets out of bed. What can you do to help decrease his fall risk? *(Select all that apply.)*
   1. Make sure he knows how to use the call system and that the call bell is within reach.
   2. Place a bed alarm on the bed.
   3. Instruct him that he can only walk during the day and must use a bedpan at night.
   4. Place him in restraints when you are not available.

   NCLEX Client Need: Safe and Effective Care Environment: Safety and Infection Control

2. A 33-year-old man is admitted to the rehabilitation unit after a spinal cord injury from a motorcycle accident. What interventions can you perform to optimize the man's independence and self-esteem? *(Select all that apply.)*
   1. Assist him in identifying strategies he has used to problem solve in the past.
   2. Choose his meals for him.
   3. Refer him to a support group.
   4. Help him bathe and dress.

   NCLEX Client Need: Health Promotion and Maintenance

3. You give discharge instructions to an 80-year-old Asian woman who had open heart surgery. After detailing the importance of increasing activity, the patient smiles and nods her head. What is your next best action?
   1. Discharge the patient.
   2. Ask the patient to teach-back the instructions.
   3. Teach the patient's family about the plan of care.
   4. Repeat the instructions to the patient.

   NCLEX Client Need: Psychosocial Integrity: Reduction of Risk Potential

4. You admit a 70-year-old woman who has diminished hearing and bilateral cataracts. She is taking antihypertensive medications. A priority nursing problem would be:
   1. *Potential for injury.*
   2. *Altered communication ability.*
   3. *Insufficient knowledge.*
   4. *Altered activity tolerance.*

   NCLEX Client Need: Safe and Effective Care Environment: Safety and Infection Control

5. You provide discharge instructions on home safety to a 78-year-old woman. Which patient statement indicates a need for further teaching?
   1. "Scatter rugs would be useful in decreasing glare from shiny floors."
   2. "My favorite slippers can be stored underneath my bed."
   3. "I need to have a handyman install grab bars in the bathroom."
   4. "I need to be really careful when picking up something."

   NCLEX Client Need: Safe and Effective Care Environment: Safety and Infection Control
6. A 78-year-old woman is admitted with sudden onset of confusion and disorientation during the early evenings. Her family indicates that she is generally alert and oriented during the day. You would likely recommend:
   1. keeping lighting without glare or shadows on during the evening.
   2. promoting activity and physical exercise during the day.
   3. encouraging napping during the day.
   4. medicating with sleeping pills.

   NCLEX Client Need: Health Promotion and Maintenance
7. After failure of less restrictive measures, you decide to apply physical restraints to a confused older adult man. Which measure(s) must you include to ensure safe use of physical restraints? *(Select all that apply.)*
   1. Promptly attend to the toileting needs of the patient.
   2. Reevaluate use of the restraints every shift.
   3. Ensure adequate nutrition and hydration.
   4. Administer scheduled doses of sedative-hypnotics.
   5. Provide frequent range-of-motion exercises.

   NCLEX Client Need: Safe and Effective Care Environment: Safety and Infection Control
8. During a home visit, you find scatter rugs all over the house, the kitchen sink full of dirty dishes, a strong odor from the toilet, and several outdated food items in the pantry and refrigerator. The 76-year-old patient is coherent with occasional forgetfulness, disheveled with stained clothing, and generally ungroomed. A possible nursing problem would be:
   1. *Moral ambiguity*.
   2. *Powerlessness*.
   3. *Altered self-care ability*.
   4. *Altered nutrition*.

   NCLEX Client Need: Safe and Effective Care Environment: Safety and Infection Control
9. You suspect early complications of decreased mobility in a 45-year-old patient admitted to the unit after surgery for multiple stab wounds to the chest. What sign would you most likely find? *(Select all that apply.)*
   1. Increased muscle strength
   2. Generalized weakness
   3. Decreased breath sounds
   4. Limited range of motion
   5. Pain with repositioning

   NCLEX Client Need: Physiological Integrity: Reduction of Risk Potential
10. You reinforce the use of an incentive spirometer to a patient with a blunt chest injury. Understanding of nursing instructions is clear when the patient:
    1. exhales forcefully.
    2. takes rapid, shallow breaths.
    3. seals the mouthpiece during inhalation.
    4. tilts the incentive spirometer.

    NCLEX Client Need: Health Promotion and Maintenance

Critical Thinking Activities

Scenario A

Mr. Porter has been discharged home with continued care from nurses at a local home health agency after suffering a stroke that has left him with left-sided hemiplegia and dysphagia. His wife is concerned that she will not be able to provide care for him due to mild arthritis in her hands. You are assigned to provide daily in-home care for the next 2 weeks while the patient is receiving tube feedings.

1. What would be your priority assessments?
2. What information would you provide for the case manager and the physical therapist?
3. What would you teach Mr. Porter's wife about taking care of the equipment for his tube feeding?

Scenario B

Mrs. Robbins is a new resident in the long-term care facility where you work. She is alert and oriented. She needs assistance with bathing, dressing, and toileting because of arthritis and weakness and fatigue from heart failure. She can use a walker to ambulate short distances but does not like to do so.

1. What strategies would you use to promote greater independence for Mrs. Robbins?
2. What activities would you recommend to promote socialization for Mrs. Robbins?

The Immune and Lymphatic Systems

10

http://evolve.elsevier.com/deWit/medsurg

Objectives

Theory

1. Describe the body's innate (natural) immune response.
2. Compare and contrast the characteristics of innate and acquired immunity.
3. Describe the role of the lymphatic system in the immune response.
4. Identify the various ways in which immunity to disease occurs.
5. Analyze the factors that interfere with normal immune response.
6. Explain the role of immunizations in relation to immunity.
7. Compare and contrast the responsibilities of different members of the health care team in preventing infection in immunocompromised patients.

Clinical Practice

8. Identify assessments that indicate immune system function.
9. Describe precautions to be taken for patients with an impaired immune system.
10. Evaluate your patient's risk for infection during a clinical experience.

Key Terms

acquired immunity (ă-KWĪRD ĭ-MŪ-nĭ-tē, p. 210)
antibodies (ĂN-tī-bŏ-dēz, p. 204)
antigen-antibody response (ĂN-tĭ-jĕn ĂN-tī-bŏ-dē rē-SPŎNS, p. 209)
antigens (ĂN-tĭ-jĕnz, p. 207)
antitoxin (ĂN-tĭ-tŏk-sĭn, p. 209)
autoimmune disease (ăw-tō-ĭ-MŪN dĭ-ZĒZ, p. 208)
autoimmunity (ăw-tō-ĭ-MŪN-ĭ-tē, p. 210)
cell-mediated immunity (SĔL MĒ-dē-ā-tĕd ĭ-MŪ-nĭ-tē, p. 210)
complement system of proteins (PRŌ-tēnz, p. 210)
cytokines (SĪ-tō-kĭnz, p. 208)
homeostasis (hō-mē-ō-STĀ-sĭs, p. 205)
humoral immunity (HŪ-mŏr-ăl ĭ-MŪ-nĭ-tē, p. 208)
hyperpyrexia (hī-pĕr-pī-RĔX-ē-ă, p. 220)
iatrogenic (ī-ăt-rō-JĔN-ĭk, p. 211)
immune deficiency (ĭ-MŪN dĭ-FĬSH-ĭn-sē, p. 208)
immunization (ĭm-ū-nĭ-ZĀ-shŭn, p. 212)
immunoglobulins (ĭm-ū-nō-GLŎB-ū-lĭnz, p. 209)
innate immunity (ĭ-NĀT ĭ-MŪ-nĭ-tē, p. 210)
lysis (LĪ-sĭs, p. 209)
mediate (MĒ-dē-āt, p. 208)
neutropenia (nū-trō-PĒ-nē-ă, p. 220)
passive immunity (PĂ-sĭv ĭ-MŪ-nĭ-tē, p. 211)
stromal cells (STRŌ-măl SĔLZ, p. 208)
toxin (TŎK-sĭn, p. 209)

Concepts Covered in This Chapter

- Immunity
- Inflammation
- Infection
- Nutrition
- Health Promotion

ANATOMY AND PHYSIOLOGY OF THE IMMUNE AND LYMPHATIC SYSTEMS

ORGANS AND STRUCTURES

- Bone marrow produces a type of stem cell that is able to produce all types of blood cells (white blood cells [WBCs], red blood cells [RBCs], and platelets), which then *differentiate* (acquire individual characteristics) into the cells of the hematologic and immune systems (Fig. 10.1). B lymphocytes are produced and mature in the bone marrow and play a significant role in the humoral immune response.
- The thymus gland, located behind the sternum (breastbone), is where T lymphocytes mature and are released into the bloodstream.
- Lymph nodes and vessels circulate fluid called *lymph.* It contains nutrients such as proteins, glucose, monocytes, and lymphocytes. Lymph nodes (F 10.2) are also where most lymphocytes are i exposed to foreign antigens such as bac and viruses.

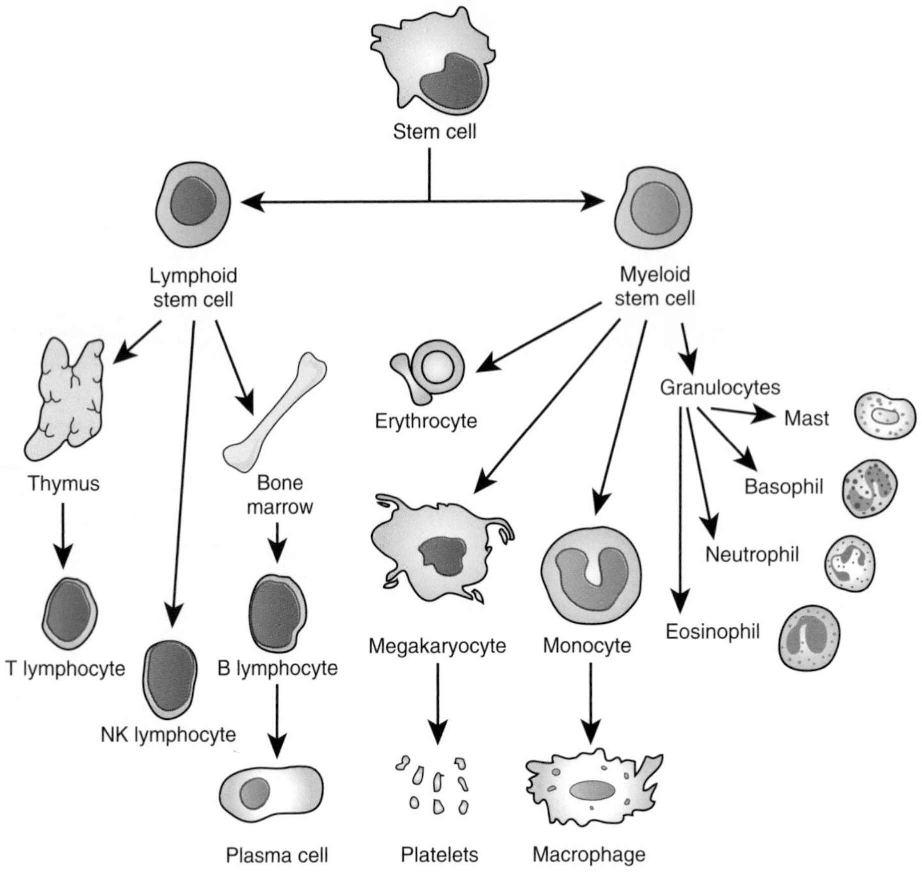

Fig. 10.1 Maturation of blood cells. *NK*, Natural killer.

- The lymph vessels are located near the blood vessels and capillaries. The lymph system removes what is left over after the plasma has delivered nutrients to the cells.
- The lymph fluid drains into large veins, blending with the plasma circulating in the bloodstream.
- Tonsils and adenoids are lymph tissues that guard the airway from inhaled microbes.
- The spleen filters blood, which allows lymphocytes to come into contact with any circulating organism, thus activating the appropriate lymphocyte response. It also filters out damaged or old RBCs, recycling the hemoglobin in the production of bilirubin.
- Peyer patches are lymphoid tissue typically found in the ileum portion of the small bowel. These patches help defend against ingested pathogens.

FUNCTIONS OF THE IMMUNE AND LYMPHATIC SYSTEMS

- The immune and lymphatic systems work together to guard the body against pathogens and to eliminate them if they manage to pass through external barriers.
- The neutrophils and macrophages of the hematologic system assist the immune system by phagocytosis when an antigen is encountered.
- Chemical mediators, plasma cells, and B and T lymphocytes play active roles in the immune response (Table 10.1).
- Both humoral and cellular immunity are carried out by the lymphocytic cells, a specialized type of WBC that originates in the bone marrow.
- T lymphocytes, which provide cell-mediated immunity, pass through the thymus and migrate to the lymph tissues throughout the body.
- B lymphocytes migrate to lymphoid tissue, where they wait in readiness to form either sensitized lymphocytes or **antibodies** (immunoglobulins that identify and neutralize foreign objects).
- The lymph system, in addition to facilitating the work of lymphocytes, also drains tissue fluid and puts it back into the circulation.
- Innate (natural) immunity is nonspecific immunity that is in humans when they are born and makes them not susceptible to diseases of other species.
- Immunity can be acquired actively or passively.

AGE IN RELATION TO THE IMMUNE AND LYMPHATIC SYSTEMS

- Neonates are susceptible to infection because they have an immature immune system.
- The thymus gland is largest during childhood and adolescence. After adolescence it begins to shrink in size, and its production of T lymphocytes decreases.
- Aging causes skin to become thin, less elastic, and more prone to injury. The skin is the first barrier encountered by pathogens.

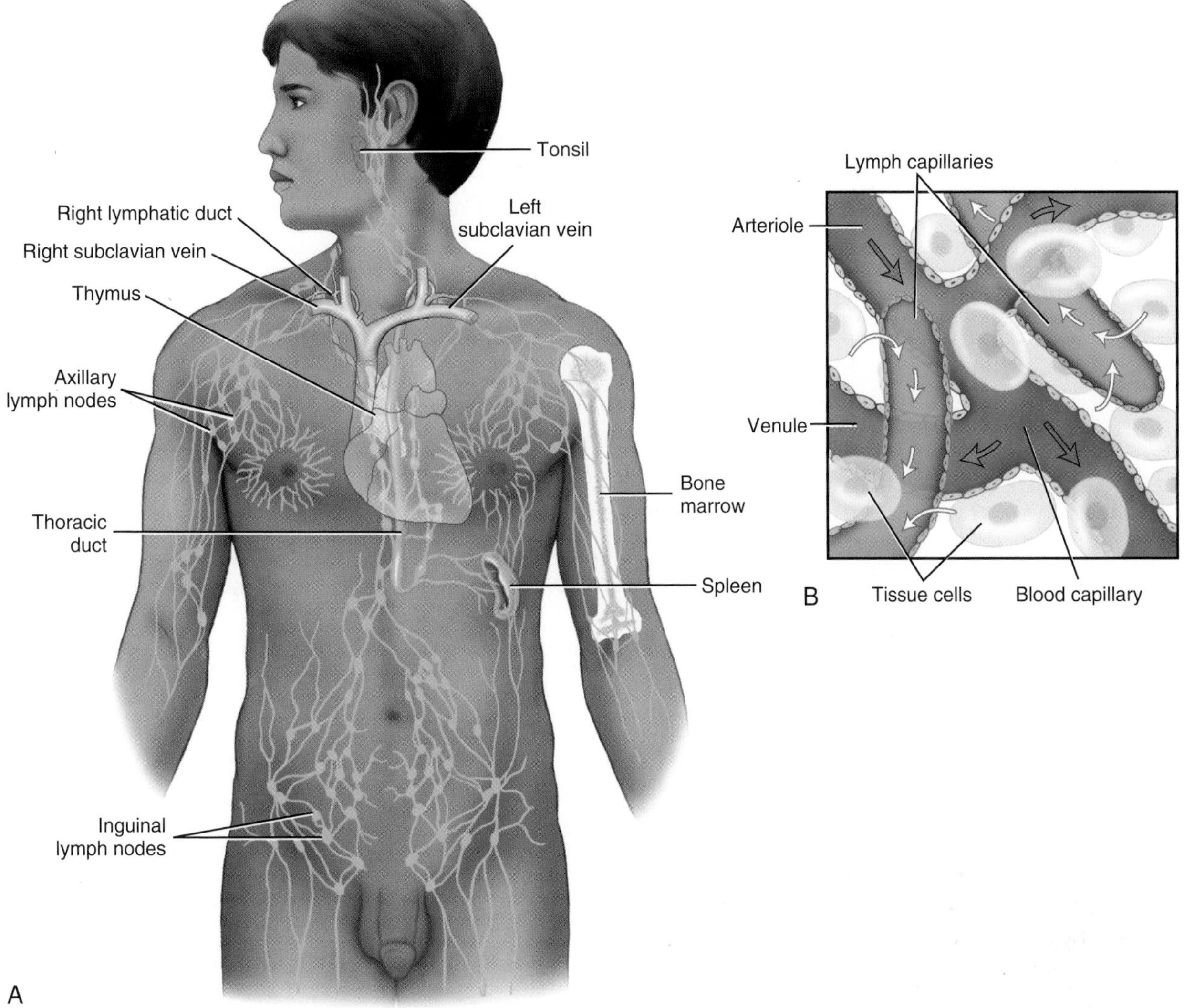

Fig. 10.2 **A,** Organs of the immune system and **(B)** structures of the lymph system. (From VanMeter KC, Hubert RJ: *Microbiology for the healthcare professional,* ed 2, St. Louis, 2016, Elsevier.)

- Decreased ciliary action in the respiratory system and gastrointestinal tract results in decreased removal of potentially harmful organisms.
- The presence of chronic diseases can decrease the immune response.

Additional information on the immune system is found in Chapter 6.

PROTECTIVE MECHANISMS OF THE IMMUNE AND LYMPHATIC SYSTEMS

The immune and lymphatic systems work together to defend against threats from multiple sources inside and outside the body. Some portion of the lymphatic system is found in every part of the body, including the central nervous system. Louveau and colleagues (2015) published their findings of the lymph system within the central nervous system, which until then had been thought not to exist. The sensory nervous system interacts with the lymphatic system by helping to alert the body to outside physical threats by relaying chemical signals back to the brain. Internally, the blood and lymphatic systems are constantly protecting against microscopic threats to **homeostasis** (tendency to maintain internal stability and balance). The hematologic system interacts in the production of specialized WBCs that help fight infection and rid the body of foreign invaders. The primary job of the immune system is to protect the body from agents that can cause disease.

The human body has multiple protective mechanisms. The first line of defense begins with the skin, tears, earwax, mucous membranes, and urinary tract. They all provide external barriers to prevent foreign substances and microorganisms from entering the body. Innate immunity is present in the body even before exposure to any unknown antigen occurs. This means that the body can recognize certain microorganisms as harmful, even without prior encounters, and immediately lodge a defense. The tissue damage created by the invading microorganisms releases certain chemicals within the

Table 10.1 Major Components of the Immune System and Their Functions

COMPONENT	FUNCTION
Antigen	Foreign substance or component of cell that stimulates an immune response
Antibody	Specific protein produced in a humoral response to bind with an antigen
Autoantibody	Antibodies against a self antigen; attacks body's own tissues
Bone marrow	Source of stem cells, leukocytes, and maturation of B lymphocytes
Thymus	Gland located in the mediastinum, large in children, decreasing size in adults; site of maturation and proliferation of lymphocytes
Lymphatic tissue	Contains many lymphocytes; filters body fluids, removes foreign matter, part of immune response
Cells	
Neutrophils	White blood cells: for phagocytosis; nonspecific defense; active in inflammatory process
Basophils	White blood cells: bind immunoglobulin E; release histamine in anaphylaxis
Eosinophils	White blood cells: participate in allergic responses
Monocytes	White blood cells: migrate from the blood into tissues to become macrophages
Macrophages	Phagocytosis; process and present antigens to lymphocytes for the immune response
Mast cells	Release chemical mediators such as histamine in connective tissue
B lymphocytes	Humoral immunity–activating cell becomes an antibody-producing plasma cell or a B memory cell
Plasma cells	Develop from B lymphocytes and secrete specific antibodies
T lymphocytes	White blood cells: cell-mediated immunity
Cytotoxic or killer T cells	Destroy antigens, cancer cells, virus-infected cells
Memory T cells	Remember antigens and quickly stimulate immune response on re-exposure
Helper T cells	Activate B and T cells; control or limit specific immune response
Natural killer (NK) lymphocytes	Destroy foreign cells, virus-infected cells
Chemical Mediators	
Complement	Group of inactive proteins in the circulation that when activated stimulate the release of other chemical mediators, promoting inflammation, chemotaxis, and phagocytosis
Histamine	Released from mast cells and basophils, particularly in allergic reactions; causes vasodilation and increased vascular permeability or edema, contraction of bronchiolar smooth muscle, and pruritus
Kinins (e.g., bradykinin)	Cause vasodilation, increased permeability (edema), and pain
Prostaglandins	Group of lipids with varying effects; some cause inflammation, vasodilation, increased permeability, and pain
Leukotrienes	Group of lipids, derived from mast cells and basophils, that cause contraction of bronchiolar smooth muscle and have a role in development of inflammation
Cytokines (messengers)	Includes lymphokines, monokines, interferons, and interleukins; produced by macrophages and activated lymphocytes; stimulate activation and proliferation of B and T cells (communication between cells); involved in inflammation, fever, and leukocytosis
Tumor necrosis factor (TNF)	A cytokine active in the inflammatory and immune response; stimulates fever and T cells
Chemotactic factors	Attract phagocytes to area of inflammation

From Hubert RJ, VanMeter KC: *Gould's pathophysiology for the health professions,* ed 6, Philadelphia, 2018, Elsevier.

body. These chemical triggers, such as histamine, lead to the activation of the inflammatory response, which then causes the blood and lymphatic systems to deliver certain types of WBCs, lymphocytes, proteins, and other nutrients to the affected area.

INFLAMMATORY RESPONSE

Trauma, pathogenic microorganisms, chemicals, or heat may cause injury to tissues inside and outside the body. The first step in the body's defense mechanisms against this invasion is inflammation or the inflammatory response (see Chapter 6). If the injury is close to the external surface of the body, there will likely be obvious redness and swelling, and the area may also be warm and tender to the touch. The delivery of select cells, proteins, and chemicals to the affected area increases blood flow to the site by dilating blood and lymphatic vessels upstream of the injury, resulting in warmth and redness. The same substances also affect downstream vessels, causing vasoconstriction and swelling. If the effects of swelling are not quickly controlled, the edema can compress nerve endings surrounding the area of injury, leading to a pain reaction.

The inflammatory response alone may be adequate in killing the invading organism by creating a hostile environment (see Chapter 6, Fig. 6.2). Protective proteins that are activated in the inflammatory response include the complement system of proteins. Several of these protein enzymes, when sequentially activated, form a membrane attack complex (MAC) that embeds itself in the cell membrane of the attacking microbe. This activation occurs when complement-binding sites are exposed on antibodies after they attach to antigens. This binding causes a break in the cell wall that allows ions, such as salt, to enter the cell. The salt is followed by water, which causes swelling and bursting of the microbe.

The same WBCs, lymphocytes, proteins, and chemicals respond to internal tissue injury. The results are not as readily visible but are detectable if appropriate assessments are conducted. The mechanisms of the inflammatory response combine with the immune response to eliminate foreign invaders (Fig. 10.3).

IMMUNE RESPONSE

The immune response is a remarkable series of complex chemical and mechanical activities that take place in the body. These activities involve (1) constant surveillance to detect the entry of foreign agents (**antigens**) as soon as they gain access to the body's cells, (2) immediate recognition of the agents as "nonself" (i.e., foreign or alien), and (3) the ability to distinguish one kind of foreign agent from another and to remember that particular agent if it appears in the body again at a later time. The lymphatic system, thymus, spleen, lymph nodes, bone marrow, and Peyer patches in the small intestine play a major role in the immune response (see Fig. 10.2). As previously mentioned, many different cells, proteins, and chemicals assist in the body's defense against invading agents.

The immune response is usually triggered by the body's identification of something as foreign, or nonself. This recognition is essential for the body to respond to

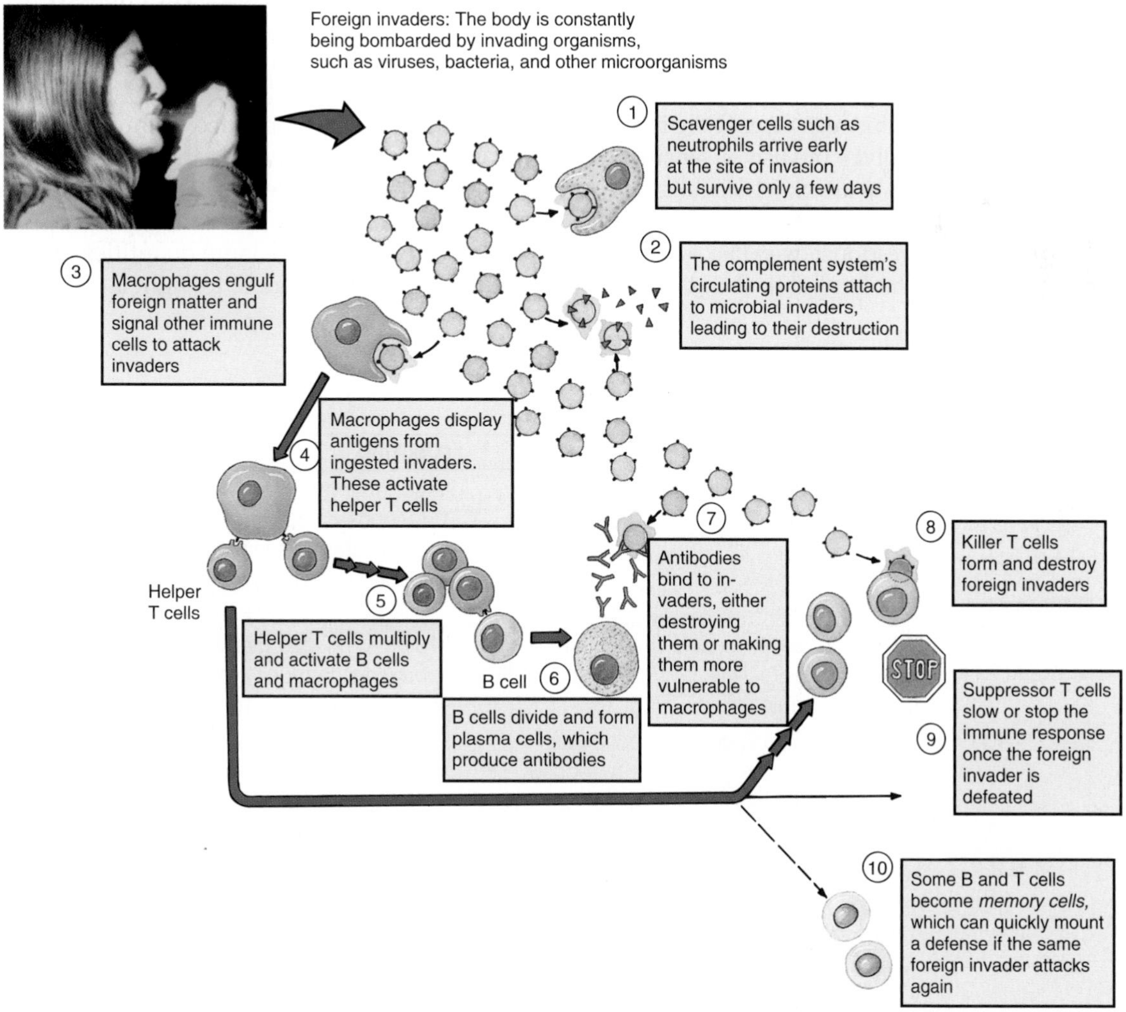

Fig. 10.3 Action of the immune response against foreign invaders. (From Huether SE, McCance KL: *Understanding pathophysiology*, ed 6, St. Louis, 2017, Elsevier.)

a foreign threat in an appropriate manner and to not react to tissues or cells that are typically recognized as "self." When an inappropriate response happens, one of two types of disorders occurs. If there is a lack of appropriate response, an **immune deficiency** is present. The second type of disorder occurs when the body produces an immune response to a self cell or tissue, causing an **autoimmune disease**. It is important to understand that although injury can activate a response by the immune system, massive trauma or chronic illness can also inhibit the ability of this vitally important system to respond effectively.

Types of Immunity

Once a foreign substance (antigen) has been detected and identified, the body responds in two general ways. **It immediately produces a protein (called an *antibody*) that is specifically designed to attack the *antigen*.** Examples of antigens include bacteria, viruses, fungi, and other infectious microorganisms, as well as the toxins they produce as they invade the body. Nonliving matter such as pollen, dust, and chemicals can also be antigens. For some people, certain foods are perceived by the body as antigens and result in an allergic reaction when those foods are eaten. Allergies to medications work by the same mechanism.

The immediate response is called a *humoral response*. *Humoral* refers to any fluid or semifluid. Lymphatic B cells are key to this response. There is also a delayed response that involves the use of sensitized lymphocytes (T lymphocytes) to attack whole cells, such as those of bacteria, viruses, and malignant (cancer) cells. This second kind of response is called a *cellular* or *cell-mediated* response. The lymphatic T and B cells interact with each other in complex ways. Both T cells and B cells are necessary for a normal immune response to occur. Acquired and inherited disorders can inhibit T- and B-cell activity.

The cells that **mediate** (bring about a reaction) the response are the T lymphocytes (produced in the bone marrow and matured in the thymus, therefore called "T").

Primary humoral response. Lymphocytic B cells are involved in humoral immunity and the production of antibodies. They arise from stem cells in the bone marrow and undergo a maturation process that involves bone marrow **stromal cells** (cells that contribute to the development of multiple tissues and blood cells) and their **cytokines** (messenger hormones). When mature, the B cells migrate to the lymph nodes. When stimulated by an antigen, a B cell becomes a plasma cell that secretes antibody molecules (also called *immune globulins*) into the bloodstream. The immune globulins secreted by the B cells are specific to the antigen they encounter. There are five classes of immune globulins (immunoglobulins; Ig): IgA, IgD, IgE, IgG, and IgM. Each immune globulin is able to attach to the kind of antigen for which it is made (Table 10.2). The antibody's ability to form a bond with its antigen is important to the destruction of the antigen, but it can sometimes result in damage to the body's own cells.

This is antibody-mediated immunity, or **humoral immunity** (Fig. 10.4). Some of the antigen-stimulated B cells become memory cells. This mechanism is the basis for acquired immunity. The memory cells reactivate the plasma cells to produce large quantities of the specific type of antibody needed to fight a particular type

Table 10.2 Immunoglobulins and Their Functions

CLASS	PERCENT OF TOTAL[a]	LOCATION	FUNCTION
IgG	75–85	Blood plasma	Major antibody in primary and secondary immune responses; activates complement system; inactivates antigen; neutralizes toxins; crosses placenta to provide immunity for newborn; responsible for Rh reactions
IgA	5–15	Tears, saliva, mucus, breast milk, gastrointestinal, pulmonary, prostatic, and vaginal fluids	Protects mucous membranes on body surfaces; provides immunity for newborn; prevents antigens on food from being absorbed
IgM	5–10	Attached to B cells; released into plasma during immune response	First Ig to respond to microbial invasion; activates complement systems; causes antigens to clump together; responsible for transfusion reactions in the ABO blood typing system
IgD	0.2	Attached to B cells	Receptor sites for antigens on B cells; binding with antigen results in B-cell activation
IgE	0.5	Produced by plasma cells in mucous membranes and tonsils	Binds to mast cells and basophils, causing release of histamine; responsible for allergic reactions; helps fight off parasitic invasion

From Applegate E: *The anatomy and physiology learning system*, ed 4, Philadelphia, 2011, Saunders.
[a]Immunoglobulins.

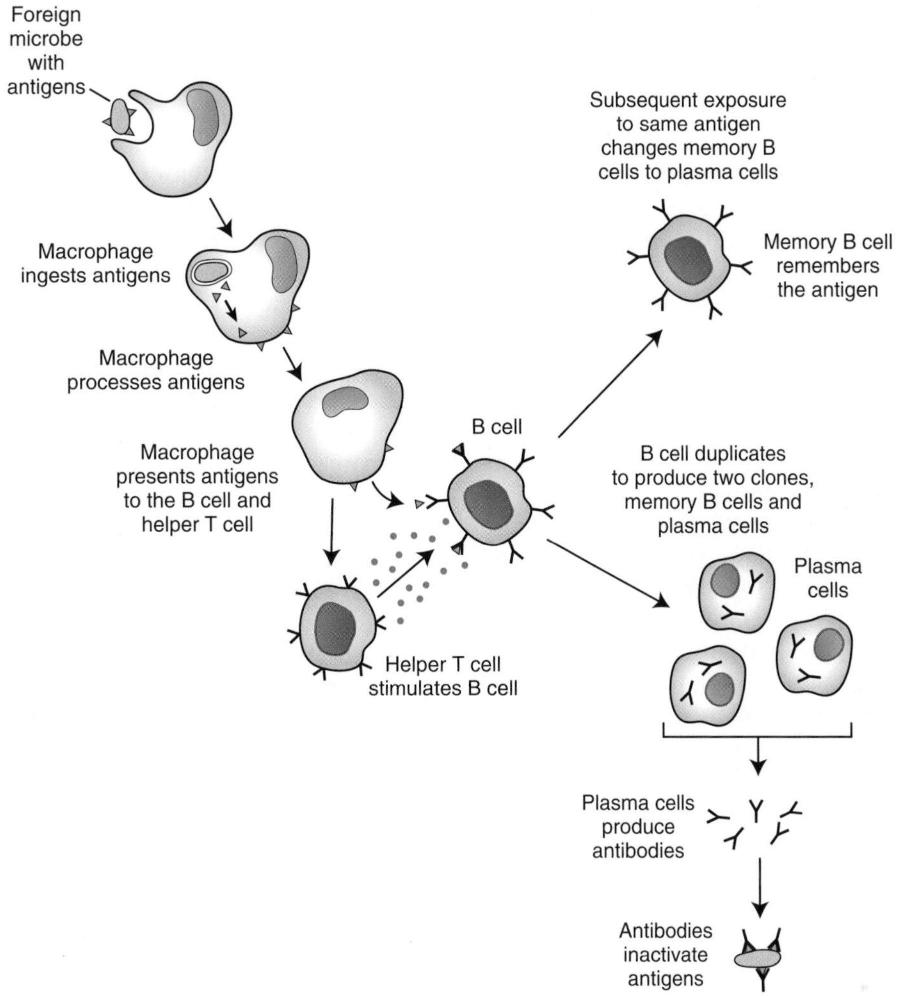

Fig. 10.4 Humoral (antibody-mediated) immunity.

of antigen when the same antigen enters the body a second time. It is an immediate and potent response, and antibodies continue to be produced for many months.

These antibodies are called **immunoglobulins**. Antibodies are found in the serum portion of blood and in other body fluids and tissues, including tears, saliva, breast milk, spinal fluid, interstitial fluid, lymph nodes, the spleen, and urine. An antibody can either destroy or inactivate its particular antigen by (1) mechanically harming it, (2) activating a complement system, or (3) causing the release of chemicals that affect the environment of the antigen.

Through a process called **lysis**, the antibody prepares the antigen for ingestion by damaging the outer membrane of the antigen's cell. The damaged cell then ruptures, making its contents accessible for digestion by phagocytes.

If the antigen is a **toxin** (poison) produced by a bacterial or viral cell, the antibody produced to fight it is called an **antitoxin**. This antitoxin can neutralize the poisonous chemical of the antigen by covering the antigenic agent. An antitoxin is therefore a specific type of antibody that acts through the process of *neutralization*.

To summarize this process, when a bacterium or other antigen enters the body, it may encounter a B lymphocyte that is specific for that bacterium or antigen. The B lymphocyte becomes a plasma cell that secretes IgM (antibody), which attacks the bacterium or antigen. After the particular bacterium or antigen is encountered for the first time, it takes 4 to 8 days for the B lymphocyte to produce immune globulins that can attack. If the same bacterium or antigen enters the body again several months or even years later, the immune globulin response by the memory cells is much quicker and the invading cells are attacked much sooner, typically 1 to 2 days after a reexposure. The major function of the humoral **antigen-antibody response** is to provide protection against acute, rapidly developing bacterial and viral diseases. The antigen-antibody response is also involved in allergic and transfusion reactions.

Secondary cellular response. **The second type of immunologic response of the body involves various interactions with antigens by T lymphocytes.** Unlike the humoral response, which takes place in the plasma, the cellular response involves whole cells called *sensitized* *lymphocytes* and occurs out in the tissues. They are said to be *sensitized* because they have been made sensitive to a specific antigen after their first contact with it. Subsequent exposure to the antigen to which they are sensitive triggers a host of chemical and mechanical activities, all designed to either destroy or inactivate the offending antigen.

Those lymphocytes destined to provide cellular immunity pass through the thymus and migrate to the lymph tissues throughout the body. These are called the *T lymphocytes* (the "T" is for *thymus*), and they are further divided into helper T cells, memory T cells, suppressor T cells, and sensitized T cells (killer cells). T cells provide defense against viral infections. Viruses are difficult to destroy because they inject themselves into host cells and reproduce themselves. T cells respond to foreign or abnormal molecules on the surface of cells. Host cells containing virus have small fragments of the virus slightly protruding from the cell membrane. T cells identify the virus fragment as foreign and kill the host cell. T cells and macrophages produce a variety of substances called *lymphokines* that help destroy antigens. Killer T cells attach themselves to cells bearing antigens and secrete toxic substances that kill the antigen-bearing cells. This cell-to-cell contact response is called **cell-mediated immunity** or cellular immunity (Fig. 10.5).

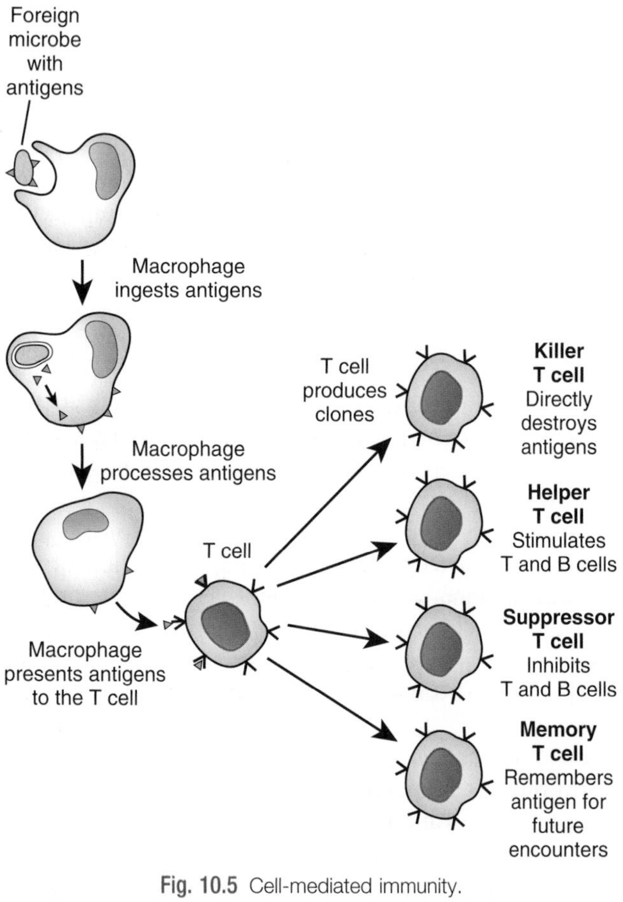

Fig. 10.5 Cell-mediated immunity.

The T lymphocytes mediate (indirectly accomplish) the cellular response. When an antigen is complex (e.g., a bacterium or another type of living cell), T lymphocytes that are specifically reactive with the particular antigen mediate the cellular response in several ways. These specific T lymphocytes enter the circulating fluids of the body from the lymphoid tissues, migrate widely, and react anywhere in the body where they encounter the particular antigen. Destruction of the antigen may occur by release of chemicals into the membrane of the target cell, by secretion of lymphokines such as interleukin-2 or T-cell growth factor, or by other processes. This direct contact by the T lymphocytes with an antigen is called *killer activity*, and such lymphocytes are named *killer T cells*. Cellular immune response is often called *delayed hypersensitivity*. The larger the amount of antigen present, the greater the response of sensitized T lymphocytes.

The **complement system of proteins** is a series of proteins produced in the liver that work with antibodies to destroy antigens. Similar to the inflammatory response, the complement system directly kills microbes by attaching to the cell wall and allowing salt and water into the cell, causing it to burst. The proteins of this system "complement," or assist, the immune system.

The T lymphocytes perform immune surveillance for the body by detecting cells that enter the host and have foreign antigens on their surface. T lymphocytes are also defensive cells that patrol the blood and tissues. Sensitized T lymphocytes are the cause of allergic reactions. T cells are responsible for the inflammatory response present in people with a variety of autoimmune diseases. **Autoimmunity** means that there is a defective cellular immune response, and antibodies are produced against normal parts of a person's body. These T lymphocytes, along with migrating macrophages, are responsible for rejecting transplanted organs as well. This is why transplanted tissue must have surface antigens that are very similar to those of the host (transplant recipient) tissue to be accepted by the host body.

Immunity Against Disease

There are two major types of immunity to specific disease: innate (natural) immunity and acquired (adaptive) immunity. **Innate immunity** is present at birth. **Acquired immunity** occurs through active production of antibodies when the body is invaded by pathogens or through an immunization that causes antibodies to a specific pathogen to form.

Innate (natural) immunity. Unique innate, or inborn, features of human cells make a person naturally immune to certain diseases. Humans are immune to some diseases simply by being human and are not susceptible to the same diseases as animals of other species. Some immunity is related to race, gender, or an inherited genetic makeup. Genetic factors present at birth may *predispose* individuals to immune disorders (Fig. 10.6).

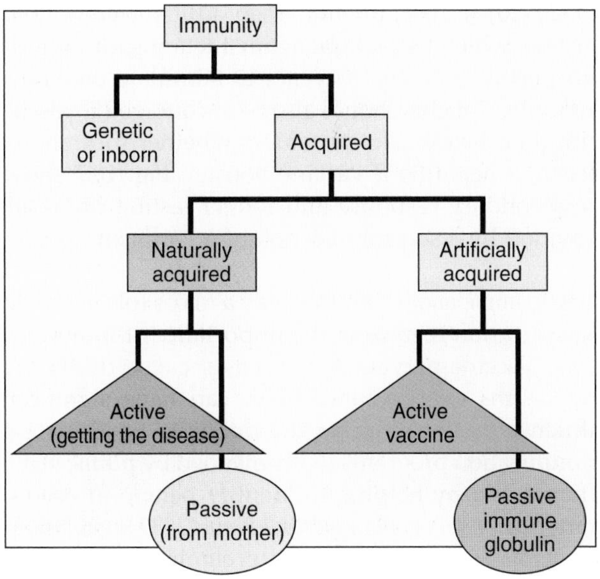

Fig. 10.6 Types of immunity. (From Herlihy B: *The human body in health and illness,* ed 6, Philadelphia, 2018, Elsevier.)

Acquired immunity. In acquired immunity, a person can either actively produce their own antibodies or passively receive antibodies produced by another person or animal (**passive immunity**). *Passive natural immunity* is the type that is transmitted from mother to baby. The mother passes antibodies to the fetus in utero or after birth through breast milk. When the fetus is in utero, it passively receives some natural immunity when antibodies from the mother's bloodstream pass through the placenta and mix with the blood of the fetus. Those maternal antibodies are then present in the infant's blood at birth. More immunity can be passed to the infant through breast milk. Breastfeeding is the best way to protect the newborn from infectious disease. Depressed immune function in the mother can limit the benefits typically received from breast milk to her baby.

Administration of human immune globulin to boost the immune system is an example of *passive artificial immunity.* Human immune globulin, formerly called gamma globulin, contains antibodies against not just one but many infectious diseases. It is developed from donated blood plasma and purified to prevent the spread of additional disease. This type of immune globulin is used when an individual has a humoral immunodeficiency; their body does not produce enough antibodies; or there is autoimmune destruction of platelets, RBCs, or nervous system tissues.

The blood serum from a horse that has been prepared with an injection of venom antigen contains ready-made antibodies and antitoxins against that antigen, producing snake antivenin. The same procedure is used to produce antivenin for black widow spider bites. Tetanus vaccines are made from inactivated tetanus toxin. Substances that provide passive immunity should be given as early as possible in the disease because they only protect against further tissue damage. It is important to note that immune globulins, regardless of the source, cannot reverse damage already done.

Passive immunity is usually time limited because the antibodies provided last only for a specific period.

> **? Think Critically**
>
> What type of immunity is provided by a "flu shot"?

Active naturally acquired immunity occurs when a person contracts and survives a disease. Once survival from a disease has occurred, the person is considered immune and will not contract that particular disease again (e.g., measles or chickenpox).

Active artificially acquired immunity occurs by vaccination or immunization. To provide active immunity to diseases by artificial means, the actual pathogenic microorganisms are grown and cultured in the laboratory. They are divided into single doses under rigid controls and made into vaccines. These specially treated microorganisms are weakened (attenuated) or killed so that they will stimulate the production of antibodies but will not cause the disease itself. Vaccines from cowpox, tetanus, polio, influenza, measles, mumps, chickenpox, and hepatitis A and B viruses are examples of immunizing agents used to produce an active immunity in humans.

This method of stimulating the production of immunizing substances in the body is successful in situations in which there is time to wait for the person to build up their own defenses. This immunity does not last indefinitely. The body must be reminded of the need to produce more antibodies. To achieve this, a booster dose of an immunizing agent is given to boost the memory of the specific B cells and cause them to actively produce more antibodies. This is one reason why a booster for tetanus is recommended every 10 years. Influenza vaccinations are given annually because the flu strains vary from year to year.

IMMUNE AND LYMPHATIC SYSTEM DISORDERS

With all the complexity of the human immune response, multiple natural areas of dysfunction occur. One of the more commonly encountered reasons for alteration in immune function not caused by pathogenic factors is **iatrogenic**—a condition caused by medical treatment. Current therapies for asthma, inflammatory disorders, autoimmune disorders, and organ transplantation are all aimed at suppressing or attenuating the body's natural immune response. Although this effect is helpful in addressing the primary disorder, it also makes the patient more vulnerable to infection or other autoimmune diseases. Many over-the-counter medications have antiinflammatory effects and are used to decrease pain caused by inflammation. The inflammation is the initiation of the immune process. Suppression of this response can hinder the body's ability to fight infection or disease.

Older Adult Care Points

Older patients are at risk for problems with immunity because of decreased immune function. They also are more likely to have chronic illness and decreased nutritional intake. For those in long-term care or assisted living facilities, living in close proximity to others makes transmission of communicable diseases easier if the appropriate Standard Precautions are not taken (see Chapter 6 and Appendix B).

Consumption of alcohol can alter the body's ability to launch an immune response. There are both long- and short-term effects of alcohol on the immune system. Two drinks can impair the ability of the B lymphocytes to produce antibodies and can affect T-cell activity. Long-term alcohol use leads to alteration in liver function and impaired nutrition, also altering immune function. Many other drugs, including cocaine, marijuana, and methamphetamines, also compromise the immune system.

Autoimmune disorders are caused by a malfunction of the body's immune system. When the body does not recognize tissues as self, defense mechanisms are launched against the body's own tissues. The trigger for this attack is largely unknown; however, some of these disorders are believed to be initiated by a systemic infectious process or by inherited factors that are still not fully understood.

Health Promotion

Maintaining a Healthy Immune System

A healthy immune system is a function of a healthy body. Eating right and getting enough rest and exercise are all important in maintaining resistance to infection and disease. Frequently skipping meals, eating unhealthy meals, sleeping too little, or not exercising weakens the immune system and makes people more susceptible to pathogens.

Clinical Cues

Treat any patient with chronic substance abuse as immunocompromised until proven otherwise.

PREVENTION OF IMMUNE AND LYMPHATIC SYSTEM PROBLEMS

Immunization

Before **immunization** and inoculation became commonplace, the only way an individual could acquire immunity was to contract a disease and survive. Today, immunity from immunizations is usually achieved by administering the vaccine in divided doses over weeks or months. This sets in motion the more powerful, longer lasting secondary immune responses. For example, infants are given immunizations at intervals during infancy and then periodically throughout early adolescence. The Centers for Disease Control and Prevention (CDC, 2018) recommends that adults receive *Tdap* vaccine, which helps fight against tetanus, diphtheria, and pertussis, every 10 years to stimulate continued immunity. Patients should also be encouraged to discuss with their health care providers whether they should receive a hepatitis B vaccine booster. Fig. 10.7 shows the secondary response and longer lasting immunity provided by a second injection of an antigen.

Nursing implications. Nurses play a major role in providing education regarding the importance of immunizations. Vaccine-preventable diseases cause disabilities and deaths every year. Nurses can have significant influence by encouraging the public to participate in immunization programs recommended by public health officials and by helping to identify people in need of immunization. A goal of *Healthy People 2030 Immunization and Infectious Diseases* is to reduce, eliminate, or maintain cases of vaccine-preventable diseases.

An important aspect of health teaching is to improve the general public's awareness of the importance of immunization as a means of preventing certain diseases and their consequences. Despite the availability of vaccines against poliomyelitis, measles, rubella, mumps, and other potentially dangerous diseases, there still are many children who have not been adequately immunized. This is particularly true in areas where people do not have easy access to the health care system. Nurses have a responsibility to inform the public about the purpose and importance of immunization in terms the layperson can understand.

Legal and Ethical Considerations

Immunizations

Immunizations are a proven way to decrease illness for individuals and the spread of diseases in communities. Some religious and cultural practices forbid immunizations. How can the needs of society be balanced with the rights of individuals?

Parents should be told why immunization is important for their children and be warned of the dangers faced by children who are not adequately immunized. This information must be presented in such a way that the parents do not feel threatened or badgered. Older adults and others who are particularly susceptible to influenza and pneumococcal pneumonia should also be immunized according to the recommendations of public health officials. Health care workers should be immunized annually for influenza so that they do not transmit the disease to susceptible patient populations. The CDC (2018) has recommended immunization schedules for people of all ages, including those who have never been vaccinated. The most current recommendations are available at http://www.cdc.gov/vaccines/schedules/index.html. Immunosuppressed individuals and others with allergies to vaccine components may not be able to be vaccinated. However, if those who can be

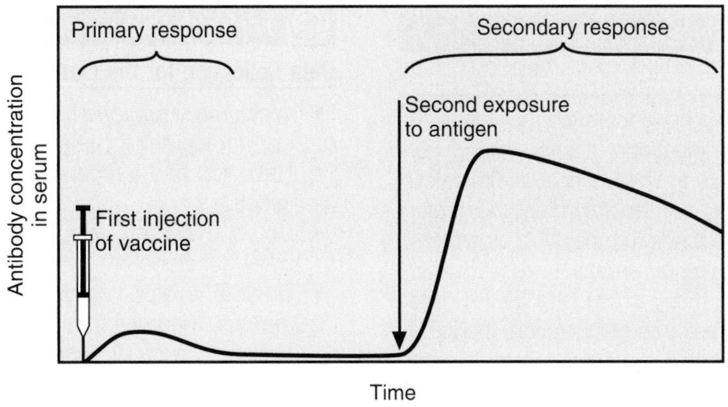

Fig. 10.7 Comparison of primary and secondary immune responses. (From Applegate E: *The anatomy and physiology learning system*, ed 4, Philadelphia, 2011, Saunders.)

immunized receive vaccinations, the spread of disease is limited, which indirectly protects the unvaccinated. This process is known as "herd immunity."

The Joint Commission (TJC) and the Centers for Medicare & Medicaid Services (CMS) have collaborated on standards that require all inpatients to be offered flu and pneumonia vaccinations as appropriate prior to discharge.

Circumstances that require modifying or postponing immunization include fevers, immune deficiency disease, immunosuppressive therapy, and administration of human immune globulin or plasma. Some immunizations, such as live attenuated influenza vaccine (which contains weakened live flu virus), are also contraindicated immediately before and during pregnancy and when a person is taking certain drugs, such as chemotherapy; however, the inactivated (killed virus) influenza vaccine is rarely contraindicated. Information inserts accompanying these vaccines identify the restrictions prohibiting the administration of an immunizing agent. The vaccine for tuberculosis (TB), bacillus Calmette-Guérin (BCG), is not routinely used in the United States because of the low incidence of TB. However, BCG is given in countries where TB is more prevalent, and individuals who have received the vaccine may have a positive TB skin test for a number of years.

Whenever an immunizing agent is to be administered, precautions must be taken to ensure, as much as possible, that the patient is not hypersensitive to the components of the agent. Religious orientation is also important to consider because some vaccine products are made using human blood products or pork or bovine material and are strictly forbidden by certain religious tenets. Common substances used in the manufacturing of vaccines include chicken embryos, horse or bovine extract, and preservative agents (CDC, 2018). These substances can produce a serious allergic reaction in people who are hypersensitive to them. Immunizing agents that are most often associated with anaphylaxis, a potentially fatal reaction, include tetanus antitoxin, botulism antitoxin, diphtheria antitoxin, rabies antitoxin, and antilymphocyte globulin. Federal law requires that a Vaccine Information Statement prepared by the CDC is provided to anyone receiving certain vaccinations (CDC, 2018).

It is imperative that a history of allergies in the patient and family be obtained before administering an immunizing agent. It also should be determined whether the patient has an immune deficiency disorder of any kind that would prevent a normal immune response to the immunizing agent. If a patient does have a history of allergies or an immune deficiency, the health care provider should be made aware of this fact before the immunizing agent is given. If the patient has had an allergic reaction to the specific agent the patient is supposed to receive, the vaccine must not be given.

There are serums that require a skin sensitivity test before they may be administered to a patient. Skin testing for sensitivity should not be confused with skin testing for diagnostic purposes. Testing for sensitivity is performed to determine whether a minute amount of the immunizing agent will produce a local reaction. If it does, the chances are the patient will have a severe reaction if the agent is given systemically. Botulism antitoxin is an example of a treatment for which a "scratch test" is mandated before its administration.

Despite these precautions, it is possible that a patient will suffer from hypersensitivity to an immunizing agent. To avoid serious problems, always be prepared to act quickly and effectively in such an emergency. In all patient care areas where immunizing agents are administered, emergency equipment should be readily available. As an extra precaution to ensure prompt treatment of a hypersensitivity reaction, it is advisable for people receiving immunizing agents to remain in the clinic or office for 15 to 20 minutes after an injection is given. This practice is in accordance with the National Patient Safety Goal of recognizing and quickly responding to changes in a patient's condition.

In addition to enhancing the immune system by administering immunizations, instruct the patient about other measures for maintaining a healthy immune system. Keeping the body healthy is the best way to preserve immune function. Not smoking, staying physically active, getting adequate rest, and eating a balanced diet are all measures that should be encouraged.

Complementary and Alternative Therapies

Garlic Assists Immune Action

Garlic has been used for centuries to increase resistance to the common cold and other infections. It has a variety of actions, including antilipidemic, antitriglyceride, antiplatelet, antioxidant, cancer preventive, and antimicrobial. It inhibits the growth of both gram-positive and gram-negative organisms and is effective against certain fungi, viruses, and helminths. Because garlic interacts with many drugs, the health care provider should be consulted before administration. It should not be used by pregnant women because it may induce labor. Patients taking anticoagulants need to know that it may extend their action.

NURSING MANAGEMENT

ASSESSMENT (DATA COLLECTION)

If the immune system is functioning normally but not activated, there will be an absence of physical signs and symptoms of an immune response or infection. When the system is activated and doing its job or is unable to mount an active defense, detectable physical signs and symptoms may become evident.

Because the function of the immune system is to guard the body against microbial invasion, it is important to assess for signs and symptoms of infection. These include fever, redness, swelling, and exudate from open skin areas. Patients who have a known infection but do not exhibit obvious signs and symptoms of infection should be evaluated for an immune deficiency. Another indicator of a depressed or inadequate immune response is recurrent infections or infections of common organisms to which individuals with normal immune systems are not susceptible. A thorough history should be gathered.

Previously diagnosed diseases that affect the immune system, immunizations, medications (including herbal supplements), allergies, and nutritional status are important areas to explore. The patient should also be questioned about any recent surgeries, blood transfusions, and diagnoses of chronic illnesses. Habits and lifestyle questions are also important to include in the data collection. Because diseases that affect the immune system can be transmitted through the exchange of blood and body fluids, asking about the use of illicit drugs and sexual history are very important. Information regarding smoking history and exposure to environmental and industrial radiation or pollutants should also be obtained.

Physical Assessment

The skin is a major defense against access to the body by microorganisms. It is important to do a thorough assessment of the skin to identify any potential entryways for organisms. Remember to assess those areas where catheters, tubes, and other medical devices may penetrate the skin barrier. The skin may show an excessive immune reaction, such as an allergic response resulting in hives, rash, or other skin eruptions.

Focused Assessment

Data Collection for the Lymphatic and Immune Systems

- What immunizations have you had? When were you last immunized for tetanus, diphtheria, and influenza?
- Have you had a recent infection or a recurrence of infection?
- Do you have any allergies to medications, food, or other substances?
- Do you have any chronic illnesses such as diabetes mellitus, rheumatoid arthritis, inflammatory bowel disease, Crohn disease, lung disease, renal disease, or human immunodeficiency virus (HIV) or acquired immunodeficiency syndrome (AIDS)?
- Have you ever had cancer? Radiation therapy? Chemotherapy?
- Have you recently had surgery or a blood transfusion?
- Do you get sick frequently?
- Have you recently traveled out of the country?
- What do you usually eat in a day?
- Has your weight changed lately?
- Do you smoke, drink, or use illicit drugs?
- Have you been exposed to industrial or agricultural chemicals?
- Have you been exposed to industrial radiation?
- Are you on any medications?
- Do you take any supplements or herbal preparations?
- Do you see a health care provider regularly?
- Are you under excessive stress at home or in your job?
- Are you sexually active? Do you use protection such as condoms? Are you monogamous?

Clinical Cues

Latex allergy can be another cause of redness at tube sites if the tube or the occlusive dressing contains latex.

When the immune response is activated, lymph nodes may become swollen and tender and can be evaluated by palpation. Nodes in the neck, axillae, and groin areas are those most commonly examined because they are closer to the skin surface. Data obtained from a head-to-toe physical assessment provide important information regarding immune and lymphatic system function.

Focused Assessment

Physical Assessment of the Lymphatic and Immune Systems

- Take vital signs, noting if there is an increase in temperature or pulse rate.
- Measure height and weight.
- Inspect the skin for color, turgor, texture, and presence of lesions.
- Assess extremities for edema.
- Inspect ears, eyes, nose, and throat for drainage, redness, or exudate.
- Palpate lymph nodes in the neck to identify enlargement or tenderness.
- Auscultate lung fields and assess work of breathing.
- Analyze laboratory results such as complete blood cell count (CBC), C-reactive protein, and antibody screening tests.

Diagnostic Tests, Procedures, and Nursing Implications

Skin testing. *Skin testing* is one of the most commonly used techniques to measure immunity and to identify people who may have a dormant infectious disease. These tests include the *Schick test* to determine susceptibility to diphtheria and the *TST* (Mantoux test) to identify those who might need treatment for TB. The Mantoux test and other tests for TB are discussed in Chapter 14.

Several types of skin testing may also be performed to identify allergens that are causing allergic symptoms in an individual. A scratch test (also called a prick or puncture test) involves dropping extracts of allergens into scratches made on the skin. Intradermal injection of allergens is used to detect allergies to insect venom or penicillin. Patches containing allergens that might cause contact dermatitis are placed in direct contact with the skin. Inflammation and itching identify those allergens that provoke the immune system.

Laboratory tests. Laboratory tests on blood and serum also give important information regarding the status of the immune system. A CBC gives information regarding the number of circulating WBCs. The differential indicates what percentage of the total WBC count is accounted for by the different cell types. An increased WBC count indicates that the immune system has been activated (Table 10.3). If a specific disease or condition is suspected, blood testing can determine whether antibodies to that disease or condition are present. A chemistry panel will be done to rule out other causes of any signs and symptoms. C-reactive protein will be measured to identify inflammation. Serum immunoglobulins will be measured to detect any deficiencies.

Imaging studies. The immune system is a multifaceted structure that does not lend itself to standard imaging techniques because its function takes place at the cellular level. Most imaging is done for research purposes.

Computed tomography (CT), magnetic resonance imaging (MRI), and positron emission tomography (PET) can all be used to evaluate the thymus gland and other tissue structures of the immune system. PET scanning can be helpful since the technique highlights active metabolic areas when tagged with the appropriate radioactive molecule. Newer technologies are allowing for microscopic real-time imaging of cells and tissues in a living person.

◆ NURSING DIAGNOSIS

Problems of the immune and lymphatic systems involve other body systems and may cause psychosocial problems as well. Problems are identified from the assessment and data collection. Table 10.4 lists the most common problems.

◆ PLANNING

Planning is based on the problems identified for the individual patient (see Table 10.4). General nursing goals include the following:

- Protect from infection
- Improve health status
- Maintain a high degree of wellness to promote optimal immune function

◆ IMPLEMENTATION

Nursing interventions include all methods to prevent the spread of infection. Meticulous adherence to Standard Precautions, including appropriate hand hygiene, is essential. Additional protection from infection may include implementation of protective isolation. Promotion of balanced, adequate nutrition is essential in maintaining or regaining optimal immune function.

Assignment Considerations

Instructing CNAs and UAP

When assigning patients or tasks to certified nursing assistants (CNAs) or unlicensed assistive personnel (UAP), remember to share that a patient is immunocompromised (very susceptible to infection) and that it is important to be extra diligent about complying with hand hygiene.

Psychosocial care to decrease fear, help deal with lifestyle or role changes, and reduce stress is important in caring for the whole person. Patient teaching regarding the disorder, treatment, signs of complications, and self-care is an effective way to reduce stress and fear. Nursing care for specific disorders of the immune and lymphatic systems is presented in Chapter 11.

◆ EVALUATION

Determining whether expected outcomes are being met includes assessing for signs and symptoms of immune function. This includes gathering physical data as well as monitoring laboratory and diagnostic study results for improvement. Temperature and other vital signs are also good indicators of immune function. General well-being and side effects of medications should also be monitored in evaluating the effectiveness of nursing and medical interventions.

COMMON PROBLEMS RELATED TO THE IMMUNE AND LYMPHATIC SYSTEMS

FEVER

A rise in body temperature typically signals a normal immune system response to infection. The rise in temperature is only one component for fighting off the invaders by promoting a hostile environment. There is a significant amount of evidence-based research that shows how fever is helpful to the immune system. However, there is continued controversy about when

Text continued on p. 220

Table 10.3 Diagnostic Tests for Disorders of the Immune and Lymphatic Systems[a]

TEST AND NORMAL RANGE	PURPOSE	DESCRIPTION	NURSING IMPLICATIONS
Complete Blood Cell Count (CBC)			
	Determines whether abnormalities are present in the numbers of blood cells or types of blood cells; assesses the amount of hemoglobin present Useful to diagnose anemia	Fill a lavender-top tube containing EDTA with a venous sample of blood. Use a site where there is little chance of dilution from intravenous solution. Mix the blood and the EDTA by gently rotating the tube.	Warn the patient that a "stick" is about to occur but that the pain will be short lived. Apply pressure directly to the puncture site after withdrawing the needle; at the antecubital space, do *not* have the patient flex the arm because this tends to cause a hematoma.
Erythrocytes Hemoglobin: females, 12.0–16.0 g/dL; males, 14.0–18.0 g/dL Red blood cell count: females, 4.2–5.4 million/mm^3; males, 4.7–6.1 million/mm^3 Hematocrit: females, 37%–47%; males, 42%–52%			
Leukocytes White blood cell (WBC) count: 5000–10,000/mm^3			
Differential Count			
Granulocytes Band neutrophils: 3%–5% of WBCs Segmented neutrophils: 54%–62% of WBCs Eosinophils: 1%–3% of WBCs Basophils: 0%–1% of WBCs			
Agranulocytes Lymphocytes: 28%–33% of WBCs Monocytes: 3%–7% of WBCs Thrombocytes (platelets): 150,000–400,000/mm^3 of blood Mean corpuscular hemoglobin (Hgb) (MCH): 27–31 pg/cell Mean corpuscular Hgb concentration (MCHC): 32–36 mg/dL Mean corpuscular volume (MCV): 80–96 μm^3			
Intranodal Lymphangiogram			
Normal-size vessels and nodes without filling defects	Detects abnormalities in the lymphatic system, such as leaks or obstruction	Ultrasound guidance is used to place a needle into a lymph duct. Ethiodized oil is injected as the contrast medium. The lymph vessels are then visualized by x-ray.	Repeat films may be taken in 24 h. Obtain written consent. Assess for allergy to iodine or shellfish. Explain procedure. Assess for signs of infection and oil embolism q4h for 24 h.
Contrast Enhanced Magnetic Resonance Lymphangiography			
Can map the central lymphatic system showing normal structures	Detects abnormalities in the lymphatic system	Ultrasound guidance is used to place a needle into a lymph duct. Gadolinium-based contrast is used. The lymph vessels are then visualized with MRI.	Gadolinium is eliminated by the kidneys, use is contraindicated for those with reduced renal function. The agent may be retained in tissues and cause health issues for some patients. Adequate information should be provided to the patient before the exam.
Spleen Ultrasound			
Proper size, shape, and position	Detects structural abnormalities of the spleen	An ultrasound probe is moved over the abdomen in the area of the spleen with the patient supine on the examining table.	Explain that the test typically takes about 30 min.

Table 10.3 Diagnostic Tests for Disorders of the Immune and Lymphatic Systems—cont'd

TEST AND NORMAL RANGE	PURPOSE	DESCRIPTION	NURSING IMPLICATIONS
Single-Photon Emission Computed Tomography (SPECT)			
Looks at the distribution of radiopharmaceuticals throughout the spleen	Detects anatomic changes in the spleen; identifies spleen rupture or hematoma Usually done in conjunction with a liver scan	A radioactive nuclide colloid is injected intravenously. Imaging is done 15 min after injection and takes up to 1½ h. The gamma camera rotates around the body. Schedule scan before tests using barium.	Explain that a substance will be injected and scanning will begin after about 15 min. Radiation exposure is minimal. The test takes about 60 min. Evaluate the ability of the patient to lay flat and still for over an hour and hold their breath when instructed. Sedation may be needed.
Immunoglobulins (Ig), Serum (Adults)			
IgG: 700–1600 mg/dL IgA: 70–400 mg/dL IgM: 40–230 mg/dL IgD: 0–10 mg/dL IgE: <214 international units/mL	Detects and monitors quantities of antibodies circulating in the blood Useful for monitoring hypersensitivity diseases, immune deficiencies, autoimmune diseases, and chronic infections	Serum is placed on a slide containing agar gel, and an electrical current is passed through the gel. The immune globulins are separated out and electrophoresed according to the quantity and difference in electrical charge.	No fasting or special preparation is required. Requires drawing 7–10 mL of blood. Values vary significantly with age. Make sure to use the correct age range and local lab reference values for interpreting the test.
Complement Assays			
Total serum complement (CH_{50}): 30–75 units/mL C3 (mature T cells): 75–175 mg/dL C4 (helper T cells): 22–45 units/mL	Monitors immune disorders, genetic complement deficiencies, and treatment response	In the presence of antibody/antigen complexes, the complement system is overly activated, and the complement components are "consumed" or used up.	No fasting or special preparation is required. Requires drawing 7–10 mL of blood.
C-reactive protein (CRP) <1.0 mg/dL	Detects the presence of an inflammatory process	CRP is initiated by antigen-immune complexes, bacteria, fungi, and trauma. It interacts with the complement system.	Explain that fasting may be required for 4–12 h. Water is permitted. Requires drawing a blood sample. Cigarette smoking can increase levels. Alcohol consumption can decrease levels. Estrogens and progesterones may cause increased levels. Statins, fibrins, and niacin may cause decreased levels.
Lymph Node Biopsy			
Negative for abnormal cells or infectious agents	Detects changes in tissue; identifies autoimmune disease or detects the spread of malignancy	Tissue is obtained by needle aspiration, excision, or needle punch using aseptic technique.	Fasting may be required. Sedation and/or local anesthesia will be administered. Biopsied material is placed in formaldehyde. Label and transport to the laboratory immediately. A dry, sterile dressing is applied to the biopsy site. Instruct the patient to watch for signs of infection: increasing pain, redness, swelling, purulent drainage, or fever >101° F (38.3° C).

Continued

Table 10.3 Diagnostic Tests for Disorders of the Immune and Lymphatic Systems—cont'd

TEST AND NORMAL RANGE	PURPOSE	DESCRIPTION	NURSING IMPLICATIONS
Culture			
	Determines organism responsible for infection	A sample of exudate, fluid, or tissue is taken from the suspected infected area.	The procedures for collecting bacterial, viral, and fungal samples are different. Consult agency protocol. Gather the correct culture tubes and culture media. Label all containers before collecting the specimen(s). Transport the specimen(s) to the laboratory immediately.

[a]Diagnostic tests for human immunodeficiency virus (HIV) are presented in Chapter 11. Bone marrow aspiration is covered in Chapter 16.
EDTA, Ethylenediaminetetraacetic acid; MRI, magnetic resonance imaging.

Table 10.4 Common Problem Statements and Interventions for Patients With Alteration in Immune and Lymphatic Function

PROBLEM STATEMENT	GOALS/EXPECTED OUTCOMES	NURSING INTERVENTIONS
Excessive Immune Response		
Altered breathing pattern due to excessive immune response	Patient will maintain a patent airway and adequate oxygenation.	Maintain patent airway. Assess respiratory function q2–4h. Provide supplemental oxygen as needed and ordered.
Altered thermoregulation due to inflammatory response	Patient will maintain core temperature within normal range.	Monitor temperature. Administer antipyretics as indicated. Initiate cooling measures if indicated. Monitor intake and output. Encourage fluid intake.
Potential for altered skin integrity due to allergens	Patient's skin will be intact and without redness or rash or hives.	Assess for rash or hives. Administer topical and systemic medications as ordered. Keep skin clean and dry; use lotions for lubrication. Refrain from bathing in hot water. Suggest use of ice to decrease itching. Keep nails short to reduce risk of injury from scratching. Provide distraction activities to shift focus from itching.
Anxiety due to threatened health status	Patient will assist with relieving symptoms through various techniques. Patient's anxiety will decrease by discharge.	Assess level of anxiety. If patient is having respiratory difficulty, stay with the patient. Explain to the patient what is being done to help them and what they can do to lessen the symptoms. Teach relaxation exercises.
Deficient Immune Response		
Potential for infection due to decreased resistance	Patient will remain free of infection or, if infection occurs, it will be promptly identified and treated.	Maintain infection control standards to prevent health care–associated infections. Assess for signs and symptoms of infection. Aggressively treat infection if it occurs. Instruct patient in techniques to prevent acquisition of infection.
Potential for social isolation	Patient will participate in social activities within ability.	Encourage interaction using technology to maintain relationships and prevent infections. Provide positive reinforcement when the patient participates socially. Provide education regarding modes of transmission so that social interactions can be safely undertaken.

Table 10.4 **Common Problem Statements and Interventions for Patients With Alteration in Immune and Lymphatic Function—cont'd**

PROBLEM STATEMENT	GOALS/EXPECTED OUTCOMES	NURSING INTERVENTIONS
Potential for altered thermoregulation due to illness	Maintain body temperature within normal range.	Monitor core body temperature. Maintain a comfortable ambient temperature. Restore/maintain temperature within patient's normal range.
Altered nutrition due to loss of appetite	Maintain stable weight.	Assess presence and degree of nausea or loss of appetite. Assist patient to make a dietary plan including favorite foods. Consult with dietitian and health care team. Offer frequent small meals. Promote an odor-free, relaxing atmosphere for meals.
Insufficient knowledge regarding disease process and prevention of infection transmission	Patient and family will verbalize understanding of disease process, treatment, and necessary precautions.	Assess readiness to learn. Provide information in multiple formats: verbal, visual media, written. Teach necessary precautions to prevent infection. Provide positive reinforcement. Use team and group teaching as appropriate. Provide access to other information sources. Refer to community agencies and support groups.
Lymph System Disorders		
Acute pain due to disease process	Patient's pain will be reduced and kept within range acceptable to patient.	Teach patient use of pain scale for reporting of pain. Accept patient's report of pain. Monitor vital signs. Provide comfort measures. Instruct and encourage relaxation, imagery, and diversional activities. Administer analgesics as needed to maintain acceptable comfort level. Encourage adequate rest periods. Work with patient and family to identify effective strategies for pain management.
Altered nutrition due to disease process	Patient will maintain present or ideal body weight.	Determine ability to chew and swallow. Identify patient food preferences. Offer frequent small meals. Weigh daily. Promote relaxing meal environment. Provide oral care before and after meals.
Loss of power due to disease process	Patient will become actively involved in care and will make choices related to care.	Assess patient's knowledge and perception of condition. Identify patient support systems. Listen to patient's expressions of feelings. Show concern for patient as an individual. Treat patient's decisions with respect. Encourage realistic goal setting. Provide opportunities for the patient to control as many events as restrictions allow.
Altered body image due to lymphedema	Patient will verbalize understanding of body changes.	Teach patient and family about pathophysiology of lymphedema. Institute measures to reduce lymphedema: elevation of extremity and use of pressure sleeve as ordered. Teach measures to prevent lymphedema recurrence. Support patient decision making. Refer to appropriate support groups.

to treat an elevation in body temperature. *Hyperthermia* or fever related to infections can cause discomfort, and excessive fever can lead to complications such as seizures. Decreasing body temperature by physical or pharmaceutical means promotes comfort for the individual but may decrease the effectiveness of the body's efforts to eliminate pathogenic microorganisms. Excessive fever (**hyperpyrexia**) is usually treated with antipyretics and cooling measures.

Nursing Management

Cooling measures can be as simple as removing excess coverings or as complex as using mechanical cooling blankets and cooled intravenous fluids. Usual nursing measures for decreasing body temperature include sponging with tepid water. Cold water is contraindicated because rapid cooling can induce shivering, which can drive the temperature back up.

The ideal treatment for fever is to address the cause. Appropriate antibiotic therapy can reduce fever by fighting the infection, if it is bacterial in origin. Allergic inflammatory responses can be treated with corticosteroids. Antiinflammatory medications such as aspirin, ibuprofen, or naproxen may also be administered to lower the temperature. A temperature above 100.4° F (38° C) is common in the first few postoperative days after a major surgery. The surgical trauma activates the inflammatory system; as the inflammation resolves, the fever resolves without treatment.

NUTRITION

Anorexia (decreased desire for food) often accompanies fever, infection, and use of some antimicrobial agents. Adequate amounts of fluid, calories, vitamins, and protein are essential in rebuilding tissues affected by infection and maintaining the immune system. Increased body temperature causes an increased metabolic rate. This increase in cellular metabolism uses more oxygen and water than under normal circumstances. Respiratory and heart rates increase with the core body temperature; therefore if a high temperature is not lowered and fluids replenished, the body ceases to function at an optimum level, which could lead to hypotension and shock.

Nursing Management

Offering favorite fluids and foods in small portions can sometimes tempt the appetite. When febrile, individuals often prefer cold or frozen items. Easily digested food items, such as soup, ices, pops, and clear (nonpulp) juices, are usually more tempting.

IMMUNOSUPPRESSION

Patients can be immunosuppressed either from the disease process or from medical treatment. This makes the person highly susceptible to common microorganisms. Patients who must take daily corticosteroids for any reason, such as those with chronic asthma, post–organ transplantation patients, or patients who are receiving chemotherapy, are immunosuppressed. Individuals with diabetes mellitus and chronic renal failure also have a depressed immune system.

Nursing Management

Hospital settings are known for having a high concentration of pathogens simply because of the variety of patient illnesses. In the hospital environment, **it is critical that all standard infection prevention and control protocols be implemented and followed by everyone without fail.** Patients with **neutropenia** (less than normal amount of WBCs) may need additional precautions. *Protective isolation precautions* refer to procedures that may be implemented to protect immunosuppressed patients from exposure to infectious microorganisms (see Chapter 6). In some cases, the precautions may also include restrictions on fresh fruits, vegetables, flowers, and visitors who may have an infectious disorder. Regardless of what is implemented, the principle is the same—preventing the transmission of potentially infective microorganisms to any patients, regardless of their immune status. These measures may include specially constructed rooms with positive airflow, monitoring of water purity, and monitoring of air vents for the presence of pathogenic microorganisms. The degree to which these measures are implemented is determined by the degree of immunosuppression. Any patient who is ill and hospitalized has an immune system under stress. Health care staff meticulously adhering to Standard Precautions and, if needed, Transmission-Based Precautions will help protect patients. Chapter 8 presents more on the care of neutropenic patients.

? Think Critically

What devices, tools, equipment, or other objects are routinely carried from patient to patient without disinfection? Where do they fit in the chain of infection? What can you do about reducing transmission of microorganisms?

Get Ready for the NCLEX® Examination!

Key Points

- The immune and lymphatic systems protect the body against microscopic threats to homeostasis.
- The inflammatory response is the first step in the immune response.
- Antibodies are proteins that fight antigens.
- B and T lymphocytes are major forces in fighting infection.
- The body produces a humoral (immediate) and cellular (delayed) response to antigens.
- Chronic consumption of alcohol can alter the body's ability to launch an immune response.
- Active artificially acquired immunity occurs by vaccination or immunization.
- Immunizations introduce pathogens to the body in a controlled way, allowing the body to produce antibodies to prevent future illness.
- You play a major role in providing patient education regarding the importance of immunizations to public health.
- Decreased immune response puts the patient at risk for infection.
- Measures such as hand hygiene and strict adherence to Standard Precautions should always be implemented, regardless of immune status, to prevent health care–associated infections.
- Good nutrition and healthy lifestyle choices are important for a healthy immune system.
- Immunosuppression can be caused by treatment for conditions such as asthma, autoimmune disorders, and cancer.

Additional Learning Resources

SG Go to your Study Guide for additional learning activities to help you master this chapter content.

Go to your Evolve website (http://evolve.elsevier.com/deWit/medsurg) for the following FREE learning resources:
- Animations, audio, and video
- Answers and rationales for questions and activities
- Glossary with pronunciations in English and Spanish
- Interactive Review Questions and more!

Review Questions for the NCLEX® Examination

1. You are teaching a patient ways to maintain a healthy immune system. Which of the following should be included? (*Choose all that apply.*)
   1. Eat plenty of fruit, vegetables, and protein.
   2. Take all medications as prescribed.
   3. Get adequate amounts of sleep at night.
   4. Stay hydrated by drinking at least 1 L of water per day.
   5. Stay physically active and exercise as tolerated.

   NCLEX Client Need: Health Promotion and Maintenance

2. The student demonstrates understanding of passive natural immunity when they make which statement?
   1. "Breastfeeding is the best way to enhance the infant's immunity."
   2. "Timely vaccination could easily provide protection from hepatitis."
   3. "The skin provides passive natural immunity for warding off diseases."
   4. "Administration of human immune globulins boosts the immunity."

   NCLEX Client Need: Physiological Integrity: Physiological Adaptation

3. The first protective line of defense the body has against pathogens is:
   1. the inflammatory response.
   2. killer T cells.
   3. gastrointestinal tract flora.
   4. the skin.

   NCLEX Client Need: Physiological Integrity: Physiological Adaptation

4. During a health promotion outreach for older adults, you discuss the physiologic changes in aging that increase susceptibility to infection. Which statement is true?
   1. "With advanced age, the skin becomes tough and leathery."
   2. "Decreased cilia in the lungs provide a more hospitable environment to harmful organisms."
   3. "Decreased normal flora in the intestines cause the harboring of pathogens."
   4. "Repeated infections build up immune responses."

   NCLEX Client Need: Physiological Integrity: Physiological Adaptation

5. A patient is newly diagnosed with an autoimmune thyroid disease. When you discuss the patient's questions and concerns, the patient asks, "What did the health care provider mean by autoimmune disease?" What is the most appropriate response?
   1. "The body's immune defenses fail to respond to the pathogenic agents."
   2. "Immune defenses are attacking the normal body cells."
   3. "There is a break in the body's defenses."
   4. "The provider was able to identify the underlying cause of the disorder."

   NCLEX Client Need: Psychosocial Integrity

6. You are assessing the condition of a sacral pressure ulcer on an immobilized patient. Which sign or symptom indicates the presence of infection?
   1. Warm to touch
   2. Pink wound surface
   3. Wound culture less than 10,000 colonies
   4. Purulent drainage

   NCLEX Client Need: Physiological Integrity: Physiological Adaptation

7. While caring for an immunocompromised patient, which action by a nursing assistant indicates a need for instruction and supervision by a licensed nurse?
   1. Reporting changes in the physical characteristics of the urine
   2. Allowing all family members in the patient's room at all times
   3. Meticulous hand hygiene before entering the patient's room
   4. Turning the patient while bathing them

   NCLEX Client Need: Safe and Effective Care Environment: Coordinated Care
8. During the data collection process, a patient indicates, "I take garlic pills to reduce my risk for cancer." What is an appropriate nursing response?
   1. "How much and how often do you take your garlic pills?"
   2. "Have you been screened for cancer?"
   3. "What other herbal medications are you taking?"
   4. "You sound worried. Could you talk more about it?"

   NCLEX Client Need: Health Promotion and Maintenance
9. Your patient receives a flu shot and a pneumonia vaccine prior to discharge. What type of immunity do these provide?
   1. Naturally acquired active immunity
   2. Artificially acquired active immunity
   3. Passive natural immunity
   4. Passive artificial immunity

   NCLEX Client Need: Physiological Integrity: Reduction of Risk Potential
10. Before receiving antivenin, a patient asks, "Why am I getting antivenin?" Which statement demonstrates that you have knowledge of the medication?
    1. "The antivenin provides a lifelong protection from any snake bite."
    2. "The antivenin must be given as early as possible to afford immediate reversal of the subsequent effects of the venom."
    3. "The antivenin reverses the effects of the poisonous snake bite."
    4. "The antivenin cannot be given to patients who are allergic to eggs."

    NCLEX Client Need: Physiological Integrity: Pharmacological Therapies

Critical Thinking Questions

Scenario A

Mr. Green, an 80-year-old farmer, is admitted with pneumonia. His vital signs are: temperature 103° F (39.4° C) (oral), blood pressure 136/78 mm Hg, heart rate 100 bpm, respirations 28 breaths/min, O_2 saturation 92% on room air, and no complaint of pain.

1. What assessment data indicate that the immune system is active?
2. Describe how the body is reacting to the lung infection. Which type of immunity will help fight the infection?
3. List appropriate nursing interventions for Mr. Green.

Scenario B

Mrs. Hope brings her newborn into the pediatrician's office. She is seeking information.

1. Mrs. Hope asks when she should bring her baby in for immunizations. What will you tell her?
2. Explain how immunizations help protect the body.
3. Discuss what information should be given so that Mrs. Hope could identify if her baby has had a reaction to an immunization.

Care of Patients With Immune and Lymphatic Disorders

11

http://evolve.elsevier.com/deWit/medsurg

Objectives

Theory

1. Discuss the key differences between primary and acquired immune deficiency disorders.
2. Summarize the ideal actions of therapeutic immunosuppressive drugs.
3. Discuss treatments for individuals who are HIV positive and how pre-exposure prophylaxis reduces the risk of contracting HIV.
4. Compare diagnostic tests for HIV and those used to monitor the immune status of individuals who are HIV positive.
5. Explain opportunistic infections (viral, bacterial, fungal, parasitic) that occur in patients who are HIV positive.
6. Identify four common disorders or diseases that are caused by autoimmune dysfunction.
7. Compare and contrast the two types of lymphoma, including how they are diagnosed.
8. Explain why the process of diagnosis and treatment for fibromyalgia would be difficult or frustrating for the patient.
9. Construct how an allergic reaction occurs during an excessive immune response.
10. Relate the nurse's role in helping a patient to control allergies.

Clinical Practice

11. During a clinical rotation, review the facility's policy for exposure to blood or body fluids from a patient.
12. List nursing measures for the prevention of infection for an immunocompromised patient.
13. Perform data collection on a patient in whom an immune-suppressant disorder is suspected.
14. Review a nursing care plan for a patient who has low immunity.
15. Write nursing interventions for a patient with fibromyalgia.
16. List the usual measures for treating an anaphylactic reaction and locate the necessary emergency equipment on your clinical unit.

Key Terms

acquired immunodeficiency syndrome (AIDS) (ă-KWĪRD ĭm-ū-nō-dĕ-FĬSH-ĕn-sē SĬN-drōm, p. 224)
allergy (ĂL-ĕr-jē, p. 247)
allodynia (ăL-ō-DĬN-ē-ă, p. 247)
anaphylaxis (ă-nă-fă-LĂK-sĭs, p. 247)
angioedema (ăn-jē-ōh-ĕ-DĒ-mă, p. 254)
atopy (ĂT-ōh-pē, p. 248)
disseminated (dĭ-SĔM-ĭ-nāt-ĕd, p. 245)
erythema (ĔR-ĭ-thē-mă, p. 239)
histamine (HĬSS-tă-mĭn, p. 248)
human immunodeficiency virus (HIV) (HŪ-măn ĭm-ū-nō-dĕ-FĬSH-ĕn-sē VĪ-rŭs, p. 224)
hyperalgesia (hī-pĕr-ăl-JĒ-zhă, p. 247)
hypersensitivity reactions (hī-pĕr-sĕn-sĭ-TĬV-ĭ-tē rē-ĂK-shŭnz, p. 247)
iatrogenic (ī-ăt-rō-JĔN-ĭk, p. 224)
immunocompetence (ĭm-yū-nō-KŎM-pĕ-tĕns, p. 223)
immunosuppression (ĭm-yū-nō-sū-PRĔSH-ŭn, p. 224)
lymphadenopathy (lĭm-făd'ĕ-NŎP-ă-thē, p. 244)
opportunistic infections (OIs) (ŏp-pŏr-tū-NĬS-tĭk ĭn-FĔK-shŭnz, p. 228)
patch test (pătch tĕst, p. 249)
primary immune deficiency disorders (PIDDs) (PRĪ-mār-ē ĭ-MYŪN dĕ-FĬSH-ĕn-sē dĭs-ŌR-dĕr, p. 224)
protease inhibitors (PIs) (prō-tē-ās ĭn-hĭb-ĭ-tŏrz, p. 232)
relapse (RĒ-lăps, p. 245)
remissions (rē-MĬ-shŭnz, p. 247)
replicate (RĔP-lĭ-kāt, p. 228)
retrovirus (rĕ-trō-VĪ-rŭs, p. 228)
reverse transcriptase (rē-VĔRS trănz-SCRĬP-tās, p. 228)
scratch test (skrătch tĕst, p. 249)
sentinel infections (SĔN-tĭ-nĕl ĭn-FĔK-shŭnz, p. 230)
suppression (sū-PRĔ-shŭn, p. 228)
syndrome (SĬN-drōm, p. 255)
systemic (sĭs-TĔM-ĭk, p. 224)
urticaria (ŭr-tĭ-KĀ-rē-ăh, p. 254)

Concepts Covered in This Chapter

- Immunity
- Inflammation
- Infection
- Patient Education
- Health Promotion
- Safety
- Care Coordination

IMMUNE FUNCTION AND DYSFUNCTION

An immune system that functions properly creates **immunocompetence**. When a threat to the body occurs, a competent immune system stimulates certain physiologic responses (i.e., the vascular system, initiation of chemical responses, and the release of white blood cells [WBCs]) to protect the body against invasion from microorganisms or toxins. Abnormal responses of the immune system are typically the result of an infection, medical therapy, or exposure to select toxins. These abnormal responses are divided into two basic categories: immune deficiency conditions and autoimmune disorders. Autoimmune disorders can be organ specific or **systemic** (generalized to the whole body).

In *immune deficiency conditions,* there is insufficient production of antibodies, immune cells, or both; the disorders may be congenital or acquired. A deficiency in the immune system leaves the body unable to resist foreign microbes or toxins. Common viral infections, such as influenza or infectious mononucleosis, can cause a short-term weakened immune response. Prolonged stress, lack of sleep, and inadequate nutrition and exercise can also depress the immune system.

Autoimmune disorders involve the overreaction or hypersensitivity to antigens from the external environment that causes the immune system to be unable to tell the difference between "self" (the body's own cells) and "nonself" (foreign cells). Autoimmunity can be organ specific, such as with type 1 diabetes mellitus in which the body attacks the pancreatic cells that produce insulin, or systemic, such as with systemic lupus erythematosus (SLE) in which antibodies that assault healthy cells throughout the body are produced.

IMMUNE DEFICIENCY CONDITIONS

There are two forms of immune deficiency: primary and acquired. In **primary immune deficiency disorders (PIDDs),** the cause is an inherited genetic mutation, and some PIDDs are detected during infancy or early childhood. Approximately 500,000 Americans have some form of PIDD, and approximately 15% of those are severely affected. Patients with this type of disorder experience repeated infections that clearly increase their risk of morbidity and mortality as well as the cost of health care. Refer to Box 11.1 for a modified list of PIDDs.

Acquired immune deficiency disorder can result from medications such as immunosuppressants that are used to prevent tissue or organ transplant rejection or chemotherapeutic agents to treat cancer that temporarily reduce the ability of the bone marrow to produce WBCs. **Acquired immunodeficiency syndrome (AIDS)** is perhaps the most commonly known disorder that is caused by the **human immunodeficiency virus (HIV).** This virus affects the body's ability to fight off an array of infections and diseases if recommended treatments are not followed.

Box 11.1 Primary Immune Deficiency Disorders

Autoimmune lymphoproliferative syndrome (ALPS)
Chronic granulomatous disease (CGD)
Common variable immunodeficiency (CVID)
Severe combined immunodeficiency (SCID)

Adapted from National Institute of Allergy and Infectious Diseases: Types of primary immune deficiency diseases (website): www.niaid.nih.gov/diseases-conditions/types-pidds.

THERAPEUTIC IMMUNOSUPPRESSION

A variety of disorders or conditions can be treated or controlled by medications or therapies such as corticosteroids, organ transplantation, chemotherapy, or radiation. However, some of these treatments can lead to chronic medical conditions or **iatrogenic** (a side effect of medical treatment) complications such as diabetes mellitus, osteoporosis, chronic infections, and significant weight gain. Drug-induced **immunosuppression,** often referred to as *therapeutically induced immunosuppression,* requires a delicate balance between the control of the body's immune response and the side effects. The ideal balance of therapeutic immunosuppressive drugs would inhibit the normal immune system response; defend against invasion from assorted pathogenic agents; and control the occurrence of the usual side effects, such as stomach ulcers and tremors (Box 11.2).

An example of iatrogenic immune suppression occurs with an organ transplant recipient. The patient must take multiple medications, such as mycophenolate mofetil (CellCept) and cyclosporine (Sandimmune), for the rest of their life (Table 11.1). Lifelong immunosuppressive therapy does not eliminate the danger of organ rejection or other health complications, and the drugs must be adjusted according to the systemic and immune responses of each patient and to prevent toxicity. This treatment regimen must be strictly followed, or the risk of organ rejection is increased from activation of the patient's own immune system to destroy the "foreign" organ.

There is significant evidence that use of antirejection medications increases the survival rate of patients with certain organ transplants. These immunosuppressive agents are also helpful in the management of autoimmune disorders such as multiple myeloma,

Box 11.2 Ideal Actions of Immunosuppressive Drug Therapy

- Offer a wide margin of safety between therapeutic and toxic dosing
- Produce selective effects on lymphoid cells without harming the rest of the body
- Suppress only the specific immune processes on the cells involved in causing the disease
- Require drug administration for a limited amount of time so the body's immune response becomes familiar with the foreign antigen and sees it as a part of the self
- Be effective against the immune processes of the body once the new immune response has been developed

Table 11.1 Types of Antirejection Medications

NAME	ACTION
Antithymocyte globulin	Immunosuppressive agent that selectively destroys T lymphocytes.
Basiliximab	Binds and blocks T cells from replicating and from activating B cells, thereby decreasing the production of antibodies that can lead to rejection.
Daclizumab	Inhibits the function of interleukin-2 (IL-2) receptors on the T cells, which prevents the cells from activating and stimulating the formation of antibodies.
Lymphocyte immune globulin	Reduces the number of circulating thymus-dependent lymphocytes in the blood.
Methylprednisolone	A corticosteroid with antiinflammatory properties.
Muromonab-CD3	Blocks the function of CD3 molecules in the membrane of human T cells.
Rapamycin	An antimicrobial that demonstrates antifungal, antiinflammatory, antitumor, and immunosuppressive properties and that inhibits IL-2 so the T and B cells are not activated.

Box 11.3 Examples of Diagnostic Tests to Detect an Autoimmune Disorder

- Complete blood cell count with differential
- Red blood cell count
- Creatinine level
- Antinuclear antibody (ANA)
- Bone marrow studies
- Serum protein
- Protein electrophoresis
- Immunoelectrophoresis
- T-cell and B-cell assays
- Enzyme-linked immunosorbent assays (ELISAs)

non-Hodgkin lymphoma, rheumatoid arthritis, and certain neoplastic growths.

DIAGNOSTIC TESTS AND TREATMENT OF IMMUNE DEFICIENCIES

In the early stages of an immune deficiency disorder, definitive diagnosis may be difficult. The health care provider must look at the complete health history, current complaints or symptoms, and physical examination findings so that the appropriate diagnostic studies can be performed (Box 11.3).

Some patients' immune systems have virtually no ability to respond to antigens because they are unable to produce lymphocytes that are sensitized or to synthesize antibodies, whereas others have a temporary minor defect in the humoral or cell-mediated immune response. In some types of immune deficiency, passive immunity can be accomplished by transfusing specifically sensitized lymphocytes to help the patient resist infection. Immune globulin (Ig) is a blood product that is given for the treatment of primary immunodeficiency diseases and certain other diseases in which antibody levels are low or dysfunctional. Immune globulin is also used to remove harmful antibodies and to block damage from immune cells. Administration of Ig may be given on a regular basis to provide passive immunity for those who are unable to produce their own antibodies. When impaired function of the bone marrow is involved, such as in leukemia, the patient may receive a bone marrow transplant to provide the stem cells that will eventually become immune bodies. To help prevent or combat infection in immunosuppressed patients, granulocyte colony-stimulating factor (filgrastim [Neupogen]) can be used to promote the growth of neutrophils, especially in patients with significant immunodeficiency.

As soon as an infection is evident, antimicrobial agents are usually given. However, these drugs can also be immunosuppressive and can lead to the development of multidrug-resistant organisms (MDROs), leaving the patient more vulnerable to infection and other complications. (Refer to Chapter 6 for more on MDROs.)

Treatment in an immunocompromised patient is aimed at controlling the disease or eliminating the condition that led to an inadequately functioning immune system. For some immune disorders, treatment consists of minimizing the effects of the illness in the immunosuppressed patient to optimize quality of life.

Older Adult Care Points

After age 70 years there is a definite decline in the function of the immune system. Many of the blood-forming tissues in the bone marrow are replaced with fat (lipids). B-cell numbers usually remain the same, but T-cell circulation is diminished.

NURSING MANAGEMENT

ASSESSMENT (DATA COLLECTION)

When an immune deficiency is suspected, information is obtained about the current physical status of the patient, such as general state of health, recent infections, how frequently they occur, and what symptoms were present. It is important to determine whether occupational or environmental exposure to assorted agents has occurred. Nutritional status should be assessed by measuring height and weight and inspecting the skin, hair, and overall appearance. If a significant decrease in weight is noted (usually greater than 10%), ask if it was intentional. If not, ask when the loss first started.

It is also essential to assess for risk behaviors such as intravenous (IV) drug use, multiple sexual partners, exposure to HIV, immunosuppressive drug therapy, alcohol consumption, and family history of genetic immune disorders.

Physical assessment should include palpation of the superficial lymph nodes in the neck, axilla, and groin to detect any abnormalities, as well as assessing the body systems involved in the patient's chief complaints. For example, if the patient tells you that they feel a bulge around their stomach, you would palpate both upper quadrants of the abdomen.

Body temperature should be closely monitored for significant changes, **although immune-deficient patients may not have a temperature elevation even in the presence of infection.** The body may not be able to recognize that an infection is beginning until much later in the process because of the body's impaired immune response. Therefore you must assess the whole patient because important signs or symptoms of potential complications can be easily missed if assessment is not performed correctly.

◆ NURSING DIAGNOSIS AND PLANNING

Problem statements for patients with immune deficiency should always include one regarding the potential for infection, which is a major problem. Psychosocial problems often accompany physical problems. Problem statements are based on the data gathered. The primary nursing goals when caring for a patient who has an immune deficiency are to (1) protect the patient from infection, (2) improve the health status, and (3) promote as high a degree of wellness as possible. Expected outcomes based on the patient problems might include the following:

- Patient will remain free from infection.
- White blood cell counts are within normal limits.

Planning care for the patient with an immune deficiency focuses on preventing exposure to pathogens. A patient whose immune deficiency is severe will likely need to be placed in protective isolation precautions. (See Chapter 16 for additional information on neutropenia.) Working with patients in this type of isolation requires more time because of the need for donning and removing personal protective equipment (PPE) before entering and on leaving the patient's room (see Chapter 6). Integrating care of this patient along with the rest of the patient assignments for the shift needs to be carefully planned. It is also important to teach patients with immune compromise the actions that should be taken once they are discharged from the hospital to prevent the onset of infection.

◆ IMPLEMENTATION

Proteins are needed to synthesize antibodies. If a patient has a condition or is on medications that suppress appetite or cause nausea, nutritional intake can be inadequate. Nutritional supplements may be added, and multiple small meals of high-protein foods chosen by the patient may need to be scheduled throughout the day. However, if the patient is on corticosteroid therapy, controlling overeating may be a challenge, and the patient must be carefully monitored for weight gain. Providing low-calorie snacks such as cooked vegetables and fruits instead of high-calorie chips, cookies, and sodas is helpful.

Patient Teaching

The Patient With Compromised Immunity

- Perform hand hygiene frequently and particularly before eating, after toileting, after petting an animal, after touching or shaking hands, and when returning home from shopping or errands.
- Maintain good personal hygiene by keeping the perineal area clean and dry.
- Obtain adequate rest daily to allow the body to function as well as possible.
- Use hand sanitizer after touching surfaces in public.
- Assess for signs of infection daily and report such signs immediately to the doctor.
- Take all prescribed medications per instructions.
- Refrain from mingling in crowds, especially during flu season. Wear a mask when in public.
- Avoid others who are displaying signs and symptoms of an infection.
- Avoid travel to areas with poor sanitation or inadequate health care facilities.
- Cook foods well and avoid eating raw, unwashed foods.
- Wash dishes in the dishwasher or with hot, soapy water.
- Clean thoroughly after use any cutting surfaces, knives, and food preparation areas that have come in contact with raw poultry, meat, and seafood.
- Do not dig in the soil or work with houseplants or manage cat litter.
- Use stress reduction techniques on a regular basis.

Think Critically

How would you explain to a patient why good-quality protein in the diet is important when an immune deficiency is present?

Safety Alert

Preventing Infection Among Immune-Deficient Patients

Protective isolation precautions are indicated when providing care to immune-deficient patients (see Chapter 6). It is well known that while providing nursing care, scrupulous hand hygiene is the standard of care for all patients, but for an immunocompromised patient this basic measure could mean the difference between life and death. Disinfect any object, such as your stethoscope, that may serve as a source of infection. Observe strict surgical aseptic technique when performing invasive nursing care procedures such as catheterization, dressing changes, and IV infusions.

Excessive stress can further depress immune function. Many factors related to family, employment, finances, or transportation can significantly increase the stress level for the patient or loved ones. As illness progresses, many patients may have difficulties at school or work. Collaboration with a social worker is often indicated. Referrals to community resources can greatly assist the patient and family in dealing with the added stress. You can be instrumental in teaching the patient stress-reduction strategies, such as light exercise, meditation, relaxation techniques, and guided imagery (see Chapter 7).

Providing instruction regarding the immune disorder, any therapies recommended for the patient, and follow-up care is an essential nursing intervention. Teach the patient and family to assess for signs of infection and to report them immediately. If traveling, the patient may need to use additional safeguards to ensure that they remain healthy.

◆ EVALUATION

Ensure that strict hand hygiene is being performed and adhere to Transmission-Based Precautions and protective isolation precautions. Check laboratory test results to assess whether immune function is improving. B-cell and T-cell assays are particularly important to monitor. Evaluate the patient for adequate recovery from any infection that might have been present, as well as for general well-being, appetite, weight changes, and side effects of medications or other therapies.

HUMAN IMMUNODEFICIENCY VIRUS AND ACQUIRED IMMUNODEFICIENCY SYNDROME

HIV/AIDS is one of the most commonly known immune deficiency disorders. When first identified in 1981, HIV/AIDS was a fatal disease, and the only treatments available were comfort measures and hospice care. Today there is still no cure, but there are now more than 40 medications approved by the U.S. Food and Drug Administration (FDA) to treat HIV/AIDS. If patients who are HIV positive are compliant with their HIV treatment, including routine testing to monitor overall health status and manage the effects of this chronic disease, the disease can be controlled and a good quality of life can be maintained (Fig. 11.1).

There are two forms of HIV infection. HIV-1 is the most common form in the United States, Europe, and Asia. Worldwide, 95% of cases are HIV-1. HIV-2 is widespread in West Africa. Research shows that HIV-2 spreads at a lower rate, has a lower plasma viral load, and takes longer to incubate, and individuals with this

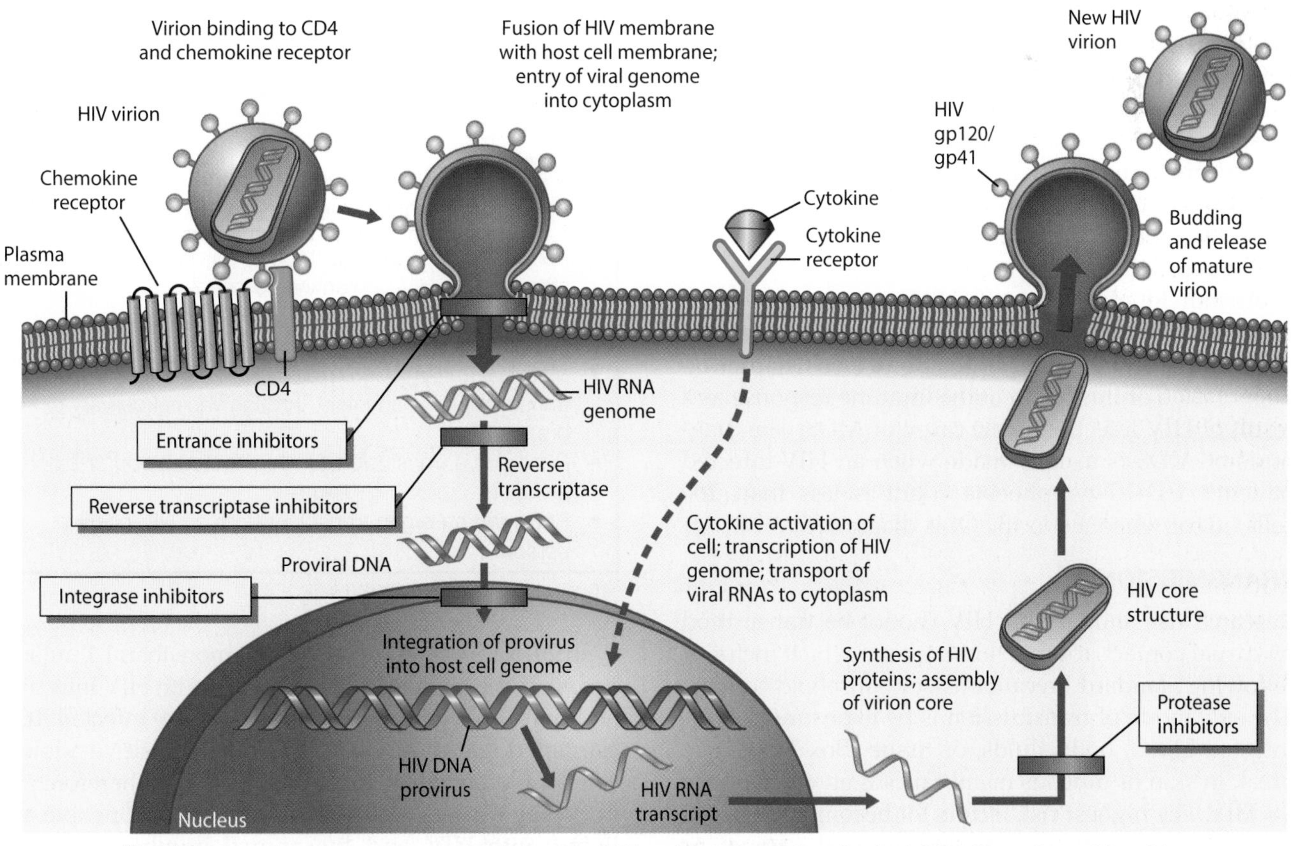

Fig. 11.1 Life cycle of human immunodeficiency virus *(HIV)* and the effects of medications. *DNA,* Deoxyribonucleic acid; *RNA,* ribonucleic acid. (From McCance KL, Huether SE: *Pathophysiology,* ed 8, St. Louis, 2018, Elsevier. Modified from Kumar V, et al.: *Robbins and Cotran pathologic basis of disease,* ed 9, Philadelphia, 2015, Elsevier.)

strain have less risk of developing AIDS (Avert, 2018). Laboratory criteria can recognize recent (occurring 10 to 33 days after exposure) or long-standing HIV infection (Centers for Disease Control and Prevention [CDC], 2018).

Clinical Cues

A person with AIDS also has HIV; however, a person with HIV does not necessarily have AIDS.

PATHOPHYSIOLOGY

HIV-1 and HIV-2 are retroviruses that have only ribonucleic acid (RNA) as their genetic material. A **retrovirus** differs from other viruses because of an enzyme called **reverse transcriptase**, which helps the virus **replicate** (reproduce) and place its genetic material in the deoxyribonucleic acid (DNA) of the host cell. The resulting new DNA continues the process of replication and produces as many as 2 billion viral particles a day that are released from the host cell into the circulatory system, infecting other cells in the body.

In a healthy immune system, the T cells that have the protein CD4 on their surface are known as *CD4 positive (CD4+)* and as *T helper cells.* Normally CD4+ T cells activate B cells, natural killer cells, and phagocytes. These cells participate in both cellular and humoral immunity. HIV primarily attaches to the CD4 cell wall receptors found on lymphocytes and some monocytes. The virus must go through several stages (Table 11.2) before it can effectively infect a host cell. Once infected with HIV, the host cell and the ability of the cell-mediated immune response is seriously impaired. Once the infection occurs in the CD4 lymphocytes and produces HIV, the CD4 cell itself dies. Overall, detection in the infected person's blood takes around 10 days for HIV-RNA and 25 days for HIV antibodies.

An individual infected with HIV becomes more prone to **opportunistic infections (OIs)**, including those derived from normal flora found in the body (see Chapter 6). **Suppression** or inhibition of the immune response as a result of HIV infection is the cause of AIDS. The diagnosis of AIDS is usually made when an HIV-infected patient's CD4 T-lymphocyte count is less than 200 cells/µL or when a specific OI is diagnosed.

TRANSMISSION

Research has shown that HIV cannot be transmitted by casual contact, routine nursing care (which includes following Standard Precautions), or household contact. The *only* mode of transmission is by exposure to HIV-infected blood, body fluids, or tissue (Box 11.4). Any break in skin or mucous membranes is an entry portal for HIV. The highest risk factors for becoming infected with HIV are having unprotected sex (oral, vaginal, or anal), sharing needles and syringes with an HIV-infected person, and maternal-fetal exposure.

Table 11.2 Life Cycle of Human Immunodeficiency Virus

STAGE	ACTION
Viral attachment	Virus binds to envelope protein of T cells or CD4 molecules, causing virus to fuse to host cell. HIV-1 injects proteins into the target T-cell cytoplasm.
Uncoating	Protective coating surrounding cell is dissolved, and genetic material is used to reproduce the virus.
Reverse transcription	Single-stranded RNA is transcribed into double-stranded DNA with the help of the enzyme reverse transcriptase. This phase is very error-prone and can lead to mutations.
Integration	The new DNA inserts into the cell nucleus.
Viral latency	Virus must wait for more protein building blocks to be formed by the cells to complete the reproductive process.
Final assembly	Viral protein production is activated, and T cells are modified by HIV-1 protease.
Budding	With its genetic material tucked away and a new outer coat made from the host CD4 cell's membrane, the newly formed HIV pinches off and enters into circulation, ready to start the whole process again.

Box 11.4 Additional Modes of Human Immunodeficiency Virus Exposure

- Percutaneous exposure through an open-bore needle stick with an HIV-contaminated needle
- Not using a latex condom or dental dam during sexual intercourse or activity
- Maternal transmission, referred to as vertical transmission, to an infant through vaginal delivery or breast milk
- Receiving a transfusion of HIV-infected blood or blood products
- Receiving an organ transplant from an HIV-positive person

In 2018 a CDC report stated that more than 1.1 million people in the United States are living with HIV infection and that 1 in 7 are unaware that they are infected. It is estimated that more than 50% of HIV-positive adolescents are unaware of their diagnosis and therefore are not being treated. An increasing number of people are living with HIV, and the annual number of newly diagnosed cases has been decreasing. In a CDC report that looked at data for 2015, the largest proportion of new cases (68%) was found in men who have sex with men (known as *MSM*). The second-highest rate (23%) of new HIV-positive cases was found in the heterosexual population, especially among those involved in high-risk behaviors (CDC, 2018). The increased numbers of heterosexual cases may be from bisexual MSM engaging in unprotected sex with female partners. Participating in unprotected (no form of barrier precaution such as a condom) anal intercourse with an HIV-positive partner increases the risk of exposure because of the microscopic tears that occur in the lining of the anus (a lining that is thinner than the vaginal walls) during sex.

EXPOSURE PROPHYLAXIS

Pre-Exposure

In 2012 the FDA approved the use of Truvada (tenofovir disoproxil fumarate [TDF] 300 mg and emtricitabine [FTC] 200 mg) in combination with safer sex practices for pre-exposure prophylaxis (PrEP). Daily oral PrEP has been shown to be safe and effective in reducing the risk of acquisition for HIV-1. Reducing the possibility of HIV infection, with its resulting morbidity, mortality, and cost to individuals and society, is the primary goal of PrEP. Therefore PrEP is recommended for at-risk individuals such as sexually active adult MSM, a non–HIV-infected sexual partner, and illicit drug injection users (IDUs). Before starting PrEP, acute and chronic HIV infection must be excluded by symptom history and HIV testing (Box 11.5). HIV status should be assessed every 3 months while taking PrEP to determine the feasibility of continuing this form of preventive therapy.

Box 11.5 Tests for Human Immunodeficiency Virus

- Rapid HIV antibody test
  - Can use blood, saliva, or urine
  - Results available within 10 to 20 minutes
  - If positive, HIV-1/HIV-2 antibody differentiation immunoassay is done from a blood sample
  - If the test is indeterminate, HIV-1 nucleic acid test (NAT) is performed
  - Blood sample
  - Polymerase chain reaction (PCR)
  - Can detect HIV in blood within 2 to 3 weeks of infection
  - Also used to determine viral load
  - Used to confirm whether an infant born to an HIV-positive mother is also positive for HIV
  - Sensitivity: 100%
- Immunofluorescent antibody assay (IFA)
  - Normal value: Negative
  - Sensitivity: 99.8%
- CD4 cell count[a]
  - Normal value: 500 to 1500 cells/μL
  - Values below 350 cells/μL prompt treatment
  - Values below 200 cells/μL, if accompanied by opportunistic infection, confirm diagnosis of AIDS

[a]Not an HIV test; used to monitor immune system function.

Patients should be taught that a prescription of oral PrEP is to be taken daily and not just coitally timed or taken intermittently.

Postexposure

Research has also found that postexposure prophylaxis (PEP) is more likely to be effective when the exposure is a single episode, such as unprotected sex (not using a latex condom) with an HIV-positive partner, and the PEP is initiated less than 72 hours after exposure. PEP is not appropriate for cases of multiple unprotected sexual exposures or frequent IDUs.

Health Promotion

People who take antiretroviral medications and have unprotected sex or who share needles and syringes with IDUs increase the risk of spreading the drug-resistant strains of HIV. Different factors can increase or decrease transmission risk. Three different studies have recently shown that taking antiretroviral therapy (i.e., medicines for HIV infection) prevented the sexual transmission of the infection to another person (HIV.gov, 2018). Taking the medications correctly is a key component in reducing the viral load.

Safer Sexual Practices

Barrier protection must be practiced with every sexual encounter to prevent transmission of HIV or other infectious diseases. Latex condoms are more impermeable than other types of condoms. Polyurethane and deproteinized latex condoms are available for those allergic to latex and provide protection from disease transmission. Condoms should not be stored in wallets, glove compartments, or hot or sunny areas because the temperature will degrade the integrity of the condom material. Lambskin condoms help prevent pregnancy but may allow the virus to seep through; therefore they do not prevent transmission of HIV. Spermicides may help in preventing pregnancy, but they may cause tissue irritation and thereby increase the risk of injury to the mucous membranes. **The only guaranteed way to prevent sexual transmission of HIV is through abstinence.**

Another unsafe practice is orogenital (fellatio or cunnilingus) or oroanal (rimming) stimulation without a barrier (dental dam). Direct contact with any body fluids, such as semen or vaginal secretions and blood, must be avoided when the partner has HIV. There is no reason for HIV-infected individuals to completely discontinue sexual activity. Touch and various forms of intimacy are important parts of any relationship. However, there is a need to reduce the risk of transmitting the virus to others and to prevent exposure to other sexually transmitted infections because additional infection is more difficult to treat when the immune system is compromised by HIV. It is important to note that if two people with HIV have sex with each other, condoms should still be used because one partner may have a drug-resistant strain of HIV and can transmit that resistance to his or her partner, thereby increasing the risk of failed drug therapy for the partner's HIV infection. Adequate treatment of HIV that results in suppression of the virus has been shown to be an effective strategy in prevention of sexually transmitted HIV.

Blood Products

Since 1985, all blood, blood products, and prospective organ donors have been screened for bloodborne pathogens such as hepatitis and HIV. According to the American Red Cross (2018), the current risk of contracting HIV from receiving a blood transfusion, blood products, or a donated organ or tissue is extremely small, about 1 in 2 million.

Vaccine Development

HIV mutates rapidly, and countless mutations have been found, making it difficult to develop an effective vaccine against HIV (CDC, 2018). Mutations are found in newly infected as well as chronically infected individuals. Clinical trials are currently in progress and show promise for a vaccine made up of multiple strains of HIV, according to a July 2018 report published in *The Lancet* (Barouch et al., 2018).

PREVENTION THROUGH EDUCATION

Providing basic, understandable information helps dispel the myths and fears associated with HIV/AIDS, and assessing for high-risk behaviors helps develop and implement individualized education. A nurse can contribute to the prevention of HIV/AIDS by obtaining accurate facts and by educating others—patients, colleagues, and the community—about individual roles in helping to prevent the spread of HIV as stated in the *Healthy People 2030* objectives (https://www.healthypeople.gov).

Cultural Considerations

Human Immunodeficiency Virus and Minorities in the United States

HIV reporting in the United States indicates that more than 74% of new HIV infections occur among minorities, specifically African Americans and Hispanics (CDC, 2018). Several factors may contribute to the increased incidence of HIV/AIDS among minority groups:

- Lack of culturally sensitive and high-quality information about HIV risk and prevention
- Socioeconomic status and limited access to health care
- Health beliefs concerning sexual practices, roles of women, the value of children, and HIV treatment
- The cost of antiretroviral therapy (ART)

Data from Centers for Disease Control and Prevention: HIV/AIDs: basic statistics (website): www.cdc.gov/hiv/basics/statistics.html.

SIGNS AND SYMPTOMS

A person's preexisting health status influences the length of time needed for the humoral (antibody-mediated) and cellular (cell-mediated) immune responses to lodge a defense against HIV. HIV has variable clinical presentations and latent periods without obvious symptoms. Often the initial signs and symptoms of infection are similar to flu: fever, fatigue, diarrhea, and loss of appetite. These symptoms may be ignored until the immune system begins to fail, as evidenced by the appearance of symptoms related to OIs considered **sentinel infections** (infections that indicate immunosuppression, leading to a diagnosis of HIV), such as oral thrush, recurrent infections, skin disorders, night sweats, swollen lymph glands, and significant unintended weight loss. It is typically at this point that the person seeks health care.

DIAGNOSIS

Testing is available through a health care provider, local public health clinic, community agency, or home test kit (see Box 11.5). Multiple FDA-approved home testing kits are available in the United States. These kits allow a person to anonymously perform the test and obtain the results in their own home. Follow-up with a health care provider is strongly recommended *regardless* of the test result.

Initial testing is done by an antigen-antibody immunoassay that detects HIV-1 and HIV-2 antibodies. If the test is positive, further testing is done to identify which HIV infection is present. If an exposure is suspected or reported and the antigen-antibody test is negative, an HIV-1 nucleic acid (NAT) test is performed (CDC, 2018).

It is estimated that 15% of HIV-infected patients are unaware of their infection and thus may be unintentionally infecting others (HIV.gov, 2017). This is why the CDC recommends that any sexually active person between ages 13 and 64 years be offered HIV testing at the time of a complete physical examination. The CDC recommends that separate written consent for HIV testing not be required, but the patient may decline the test when the health care provider is explaining what testing will be performed. Also not recommended is a requirement for counseling. Each state sets its own guidelines for providers. Currently all but two states have laws that reflect the CDC recommendations. The results of HIV antibody tests are confidential patient information and are protected by the Health Insurance Portability and Accountability Act (HIPAA). If the patient elects to "opt out" of HIV testing, a note about the declination should be documented in the clinical record.

MANAGEMENT OF HUMAN IMMUNODEFICIENCY VIRUS INFECTION

When an individual is confirmed to have HIV, a comprehensive history and physical examination for health status should be conducted, including additional baseline laboratory and diagnostic studies (Table 11.3). A CD4 lymphocyte count should be performed. If the count is less than 350 cells/mm^3, it is recommended that the patient initiate antiretroviral therapy (ART) and prophylaxis for OIs.

Table 11.3 Additional Laboratory and Diagnostic Studies for Patients Newly Diagnosed With Human Immunodeficiency Virus[a]

LABORATORY/DIAGNOSTIC STUDY	PURPOSE
HIV antigen-antibody immunoassay	Confirms diagnosis of HIV
CD4 count (reported as cells/μL)	Identifies what stage of HIV infection patient may be in; determines when to start ART and prophylactic therapy for OIs; should be obtained every few months to assess immune and/or therapeutic response and evaluate need for starting ART
Quantitative plasma HIV-RNA level, also known as HIV nucleic acid amplification test (NAT) (viral load, reported as copies/mL)	Estimates level of HIV replication; helps determine need for starting or effect of ART and whether it needs adjustment
Drug resistance test (genotype: mutations; phenotype: viral replication)	Determines which ART will be most effective; prevents further development of drug-resistant strains of HIV; should be done as early as possible
Complete blood cell count (CBC)	Assesses for anemia, leukopenia, and thrombocytopenia; certain ARTs may be less effective if any of these are present
Comprehensive chemistry panel (includes electrolytes, BUN/creatinine, liver enzymes, cholesterol, triglycerides, glucose)	Determines baseline kidney and liver function, as well as lipid profile; results can be used to determine potential for complications with proposed ART
Sexually transmitted infections	Establishes whether treatment is needed
Toxoplasma gondii IgG	Detects prior exposure; if positive in the newly diagnosed, patient is at increased risk of developing CNS difficulties when CD level is <100 μL
Hepatitis A, B, C	Determines prior exposure to hepatitis; also indicates need for vaccination against hepatitis A and B

Adapted from U.S. Department of Health and Human Services/Health Resources & Services Administration: HIV/AIDS Bureau: *Guide for HIV/AIDS clinical care*, 2014, with 2018 update.

[a]Additional testing may also include tuberculosis, PAP, and pregnancy tests for women; prostate-specific antigen level and prostate examination for men; cytomegalovirus antibody screening; varicella IgG test; and eye examination along with routine health maintenance examinations based on the age of the patient.

ART, Antiretroviral therapy; *BUN,* blood urea nitrogen; *CNS,* central nervous system; *IgG,* immunoglobulin G; *OIs,* opportunistic infections.

Choice of optimal therapy is based on clinical data and individual factors, such as past health status, medication history, quality-of-life issues, and patient expectations of therapy. The World Health Organization (WHO) has established standard criteria for staging HIV infection.

The most effective current treatment is ART, a combination of available drugs recommended for HIV. This therapy is also effective against other conditions common to HIV/AIDS. OIs are treated with drugs specific to their cause, and sometimes antimicrobials are given to prevent infection. Table 11.4 presents the current classes of antiretroviral medications with select nursing implications and side effects. Regardless of the medications prescribed, it must be stressed that the more compliant the patient is with the proposed treatment regimen, the less likely they are to experience OIs.

? Think Critically

How would you go about helping a patient who has HIV find a way to afford the medications needed to control the disease?

COMPLICATIONS

Opportunistic Infections

OIs are diseases caused by microorganisms commonly present in the environment or the body that cause disease only when there is a weakening or suppression of the immune system. They are caused by many types of organisms: virus, bacteria, fungi, parasites, and even protozoa. OIs are often the hallmark of a transition from HIV infection to AIDS (Table 11.5). Each OI is treated with specific medication. Effective ART prevents HIV from depleting the immune system, allowing the body to fight off infection, resulting in fewer OIs.

HIV Stages

Acute HIV infection develops within 2 to 4 weeks and may produce flu-like symptoms in some people. During this first stage, the HIV level in the blood is very high and can be transmitted to others. Antibody testing remains negative for approximately a month and a half. Chronic HIV infection is the second stage, also called asymptomatic HIV infection because most people do not have HIV-related symptoms. Even though they are asymptomatic, they are still able to spread the virus. Without treatment, chronic HIV usually advances to AIDS. For some people the time frame for onset of AIDS is weeks to months; for others it may take 10 years or longer. The third stage of HIV infection is AIDS, considered the terminal stage of the disease. The virus severely damages the immune system, and OIs and

Table 11.4 Antiretroviral Drugs Commonly Used to Treat HIV/AIDS

CLASSIFICATION	ACTION	NURSING IMPLICATIONS AND SIDE EFFECTS[a]
Nucleoside reverse transcriptase inhibitors (NRTIs)	Block conversion from RNA to DNA, thus preventing HIV genetic material from entering host cells	Monitor hepatic and renal function, complete blood cell count. Assess for signs of abdominal pain; nausea; vomiting; dizziness; neuropathy; difficulty in vision, hearing, touch, and balance. If sore throat, fatigue, shortness of breath, or flu-like symptoms occur, drug class may need to be modified or discontinued completely.
Nonnucleoside reverse transcriptase inhibitors (NNRTIs)	Act by binding to and disabling reverse transcriptase, a protein needed for replication of HIV	Monitor renal and hepatic function and, if on anticoagulants, coagulation levels. Monitor for headaches, dysphoria, dizziness, insomnia, and nightmares. Diarrhea occurs in some patients. Contraindicated in pregnancy.
Protease inhibitors (PIs)	Prevent the virus from using the enzyme protease to make copies of itself	Monitor serum lipid levels, glucose, bilirubin levels. Cause a higher incidence of nephrolithiasis. Most must be given with food, and adequate hydration is required.
Fusion inhibitors	Block HIV from entering the CD4 cells of immune system	Must rotate injection sites because of local irritation. Associated with a higher risk of pneumonia.
Entry inhibitors (CCR5 antagonists)	Block proteins on CD4 cells preventing entry of the HIV virus	Associated with a higher incidence of hepatotoxicity, severe rash, and systemic allergic reaction.
Integrase inhibitor	Block the integrase enzyme needed for HIV to make copies of itself	Monitor hepatic function. Can cause life-threatening and fatal skin reactions.
Postattachment inhibitors	Block the CD4 receptors, preventing HIV from entering the immune cells	May cause immune reconstitution inflammatory syndrome (IRIS), resulting in an increased response to a previously hidden infection.
Combination HIV medications	Contain two or more medications from two or more drug classifications	Current recommendations for treatment.
Pharmacokinetic enhancers	Increase the effectiveness of HIV medications	

Adapted from U.S. Department of Health and Human Services: AIDS info: *HIV treatment,* 2018. For the most current recommendations, visit the AIDS Education Training Center (AETC) website at https://aidsetc.org/resource-type/guidelines.

[a]Refer to current drug reference materials for drugs prescribed and review side effects and patient teaching recommendations.

cancers occur frequently. Without treatment, life expectancy is about 3 years.

Neoplasms

Kaposi sarcoma. Kaposi sarcoma (KS) is one of the most common causes of malignancy in HIV-positive people. KS is caused by the human herpesvirus type 8. KS does not usually cause death. KS appears as discolored areas on the skin but can also form inside the mouth, lungs, and intestines (Fig. 11.2). The skin discoloration may range from pink to red or purple. The lesions tend to darken over time. In people with olive or black skin, the lesions may appear dark brown or black. The discoloration is caused by the formation of many tiny blood vessels and cancer cells under the skin.

ART has been shown to halt or even eliminate the progression of skin lesions in some individuals and has decreased the incidence of KS. If KS has spread into internal organs and ART treatment is insufficient, chemotherapy or immunotherapy is used.

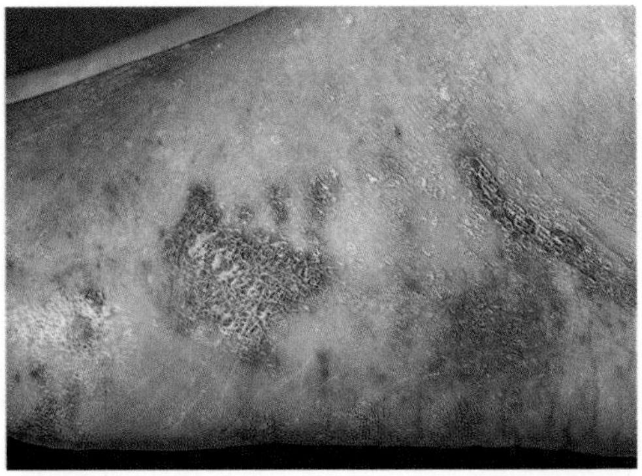

Fig. 11.2 Kaposi sarcoma. (From Van Meter KC, Hubert RJ: *Gould's pathophysiology for health professions,* ed 5, Philadelphia, 2015, Elsevier.)

Lymphomas. Lymphomas are tumors of the tissues and cells of the lymphatic system. Non-Hodgkin lymphoma (NHL) is the most common lymphoma in people with HIV/AIDS. Most cases of NHL in these patients are aggressive forms that include large B-cell lymphoma,

Table 11.5 Opportunistic Infections That Occur With Human Immunodeficiency Virus Infection

ORGANISM OR DISEASE	MANIFESTATIONS
Herpes simplex types 1 and 2	Type 1: vesicles and ulcerations on lips, oral membranes, and eye and possible meningitis; type 2: genital and/or perianal vesicles and ulcerations
Varicella zoster (chickenpox virus)	Vesicles along dermatomes (nerve tracts); "shingles" with itching and burning pain, low-grade fever
Cytomegalovirus	Retinitis; esophagitis; stomatitis; gastritis with diarrhea, cramps, anorexia, and weight loss
Hepatitis B and C	Often no symptoms; jaundice, dark urine, abdominal pain, loss of appetite, nausea, vomiting, joint pain
Mycobacterium tuberculosis	Respiratory and CNS, bone, skin, GI tract, liver, and spleen; productive cough, fever, night sweats, weight loss
Mycobacterium avium complex (MAC)	Respiratory and GI tract, other systems may be affected; nonproductive cough, fever, malaise, fatigue
Cryptococcosis	Fungal meningitis, fever, headache, seizures, motor dysfunction, altered mental status
Histoplasmosis	Fever, pneumonia, lymphadenopathy, weight loss, CNS symptoms
Coccidiomycosis (Valley fever)	Pulmonary infection, fever, purulent sputum, rash
Candidiasis	Thrush; esophagitis; vaginitis; yellow patches in mouth, GI tract, and vagina
Pneumocystis jirovecii (formerly *Pneumocystis carinii*, PCP)	Nonproductive cough, shortness of breath, fever, malaise, night sweats, fatigue, weight loss
Toxoplasmosis	Flu-like symptoms, inflammatory response
Cryptosporidiosis	Gastroenteritis, dehydration, malnutrition, debilitation

CNS, Central nervous system; *GI,* gastrointestinal.

primary CNS lymphoma, or Burkitt lymphoma. ART has improved outcomes by helping patients better tolerate treatments such as chemotherapy and immunotherapy.

Neurologic Complications

Cognitive disorders occur when HIV infection enters the central nervous system (CNS). Various names have been given to the alterations in the CNS produced by HIV. *HIV encephalopathy, AIDS dementia,* and *AIDS dementia complex* are all terms used to describe the changes in cognitive function, characterized by dementia, that occur in HIV/AIDS. The neurologic signs and symptoms displayed usually arise from the progression of the virus, but they also could be a result of OIs, tumors, or drug-related complications. The symptoms have a very subtle beginning and are difficult to differentiate from depression, Parkinson disease, and Alzheimer disease.

Treatment with ART appears to be the most effective intervention by targeting the primary cause of the problem. Nursing interventions focus on preventing the individual from doing harm to self or to others and ensuring that daily needs are being met.

❖ NURSING MANAGEMENT

◆ ASSESSMENT (DATA COLLECTION)

The assessment should include a review of signs and symptoms; functional level (ability to perform activities of daily living [ADLs]); safety; self-care abilities; support systems; financial status; risk behaviors; living environment; and understanding of disease process, transmission, and therapeutic regimen. The assessment of the functional level is an ongoing assessment using a tool such as the Karnofsky Performance Status Scale.

History and Physical Assessment

The history should include a general assessment of the patient's past and present status. Previous history of HIV testing, such as blood donations or military service, might be important for determining the timing of HIV infection. Current prescription medications and treatments should be documented, and documentation should include whether the patient is on any experimental, herbal, immune complex–boosting agents, or other complementary and alternative therapies. If the patient has been HIV positive for some time, it is important to obtain a history of OIs. Ask if there is any history of respiratory illnesses that increase risk for current problems, such as bacterial or opportunistic pneumonia, chronic obstructive pulmonary disease, or asthma. Assess for smoking history. Determine whether the patient has been tested for *Mycobacterium tuberculosis* (MTb)—if so, when, and what were the results? The neurologic history should include questions about pain or numbness in the extremities and changes in mental status (because HIV/AIDS can cause serious neurologic changes as the disease progresses). A sexual history is needed to ascertain risk behaviors such as multiple sexual partners, possible exposure to other sexually transmitted infections, and a history of substance use to determine the risk of transmission. Discussing notification of sexual or needle-sharing partners is essential.

A complete head-to-toe physical assessment should be performed.

Focused Assessment

Data Collection for the Patient With Human Immunodeficiency Virus

First gather a general health history, then:

- Obtain height and weight; note any loss from usual weight.
- Obtain vital signs. Assess for hypotension, orthostatic hypotension, and fever.
- Determine level of consciousness, orientation to time and place, cognition, and concentration ability.
- Assess for visual changes.
- Assess mouth condition and presence of any lesions.
- Determine whether there has been a change in eating pattern.
- Evaluate ability to swallow.
- Determine presence of nausea, vomiting, or diarrhea. If diarrhea is present, note the volume, quantity, and duration.
- Check lymph nodes for any swelling or hardness.
- Assess for dehydration and electrolyte imbalances.
- Auscultate the heart.
- Assess quality of respirations; auscultate breath sounds.
- Determine character of the cough and sputum, if cough is present.
- Assess condition of skin and mucous membranes.
- Assess for peripheral and periorbital edema and lymphedema.
- Identify any psychosocial issues that may complicate or enhance care.

When there is considerable weight loss, referral to a nutritionist or dietitian and providing written materials, such as how to plan a nutritious balanced diet using the U.S. Department of Agriculture's Choose My Plate (available at http://www.choosemyplate.gov/), can also be helpful. Changes in nutritional status could be caused by nausea, vomiting, or diarrhea related to the ART regimen.

Psychosocial History

The psychosocial assessment should include a history of interpersonal relationships, educational level, and career information. It is important to determine whether the patient has told their family of their HIV status. Examples of questions to ask include: Have you experienced multiple losses, such as your job, house, or partner? What is your living situation? Do you live with someone who is helpful? Referrals (such as community-based HIV/AIDS organizations) are needed if the patient does not have a support network.

Think Critically

A diagnosis of HIV affects a person's self-concept. How could you help a patient voice their feelings about the diagnosis and find an effective means to cope with the disease?

Table 11.6 identifies common patient nursing problems, expected outcomes, and interventions that may be associated with systemic, psychosocial, or specific body system responses to HIV/AIDS.

◆ PLANNING

A patient who is HIV positive can have significant issues related to finance, employment, housing, mental health, substance abuse, or other medical problems. HIV care is usually performed in an outpatient clinical setting, and the health care team may include the patient, nurses, health care providers, dietitian, pharmacist, case manager, and primary caregiver at home. Information related to the patient's social and economic status is critical for the team to develop and implement a successful treatment plan. The patient's ability to participate in the delivery of the plan of care must be periodically reassessed. If the patient is able to have a role in decisions and adjustments to the treatment plan, it increases the likelihood of compliance. The major nursing goals are listed in Box 11.6.

Instruct the patient on how to take the medication and which medications should be taken with or without food. By consistently taking antimicrobials and antiretroviral medications as ordered, less resistance to the drugs occurs, and the effectiveness of the drugs is thus prolonged.

Encourage social interaction and independence in activities as tolerated. Support groups can boost feelings of self-esteem and self-worth. Social interaction may reduce situational depression and can empower the patient. Promoting a positive attitude may reduce feelings of powerlessness. Referral to community-based HIV/AIDS organizations is appropriate, with the patient's consent.

◆ IMPLEMENTATION

In accordance with the CDC, Standard Precautions must be used consistently when caring for all patients (see Chapter 6 and Appendix B). Hand hygiene is critical

Box 11.6 Major Nursing Goals for Adults With Human Immunodeficiency Virus/Acquired Immunodeficiency Syndrome

- Prevent secondary bacterial, viral, and fungal infections.
- Prevent wasting resulting from malnutrition.
- Maintain or improve the present level of immune function.
- Maintain adequate social functioning.
- Maintain or improve current mental status.

Table 11.6 Problem Statements and Interventions for a Patient With Immune Deficiency or Autoimmune Disorder

PROBLEM STATEMENT	EXPECTED OUTCOMES	NURSING INTERVENTIONS
Potential for infection due to depressed immune function	Patient will exhibit no signs of infection; normal temperature.	Monitor body temperature daily. Monitor for outward signs of infections and for symptoms of opportunistic infection. Assess for signs of dehydration and altered mental status.
Altered gas exchange due to excessive lung secretions and shallow breathing	Patient's oxygenation will improve to within baseline levels within 3 wk of beginning treatment.	Encourage deep breathing and coughing as indicated. Conserve strength and oxygen by assisting with activities of daily living. Position patient to allow for maximum chest expansion. Monitor breathing patterns and breath sounds q4h. Provide supplemental oxygen as ordered. Monitor blood gases as ordered. Suction airway PRN.
Altered skin integrity due to multiple areas of skin abrasion and dehydration	No further areas of skin breakdown will occur. Areas of abrasion will heal within 2 wk.	Assess skin status q4h; assess for areas of excoriation, lesions, rashes, and discoloration. Report changes from baseline findings. Change linens as needed if diaphoresis or incontinence is present to keep skin clean and dry. Use elbow and heel protectors and special mattress if patient is bedridden. Encourage adequate fluid intake per physical status. Monitor intake and output. Assess for signs of dehydration or fluid overload/edema q4h.
Altered nutrition due to eating and swallowing difficulties	Patient will not experience further weight loss.	Assess patient's ability to take in food, chew, and swallow. Monitor weight twice a week. Record input and output. Administer antiemetics as ordered. Assess the availability of food within living situation. Assess ability of caregiver to meet patient's nutritional needs. Administer dietary supplements if required.
Pain due to pressure on nerves and discomfort from peripheral neuropathy	Pain will be controlled within tolerable levels within 4 days.	Assess pain level and patient's methods to relieve it. Relieve causes of pain by correcting underlying condition if possible. Administer pain medications as ordered; assess amount of relief provided by medication; if relief is not adequate, consult with provider for more effective protocol for pain relief; explore use of NSAIDs and antidepressant medications for pain relief in conjunction with other analgesics. Implement adjunctive therapies to assist with pain relief: massage, cold or hot applications, repositioning, distraction, meditation, imagery. Teach relaxation techniques.
Altered activity tolerance	Level of activity intolerance will improve within 1 mo.	Encourage periods of rest alternated with periods of activity; plan activities according to usual stamina levels; change schedule of activities as degree of fatigue indicates need; assist with activities of daily living as needed to conserve energy.
Limited coping ability due to diagnosis of life-threatening illness, fatigue, and anxiety	Patient will exhibit usual effective coping techniques to meet challenges of the illness.	Establish rapport with the patient, partner, and family. Assess past methods of effective coping. Assess patient's strengths. Schedule activities that may cause stress when the patient is most rested or has support person available. Review effective methods for problem solving.
Inability for self-care due to fatigue, deterioration of physical condition, mental changes, and neurologic impairment	Patient will accomplish as many activities of daily living as possible without undue fatigue. Patient will accept assistance with activities of daily living within 2 wk.	Assess ability to perform own activities of daily living. Provide assistance for activities the patient is unable to perform. Refer to occupational and physical therapy for assistive devices and home equipment needed. Instruct significant other and family members how to assist with activities of daily living.

NSAIDs, Nonsteroidal antiinflammatory drugs; *PRN,* as needed.

for health care providers, the patient, and the family to prevent secondary infections. Role modeling and teaching about the importance of hand hygiene happens during routine care. You must also teach about decreasing infection risk in the home setting.

◆ EVALUATION

A patient's expectations may not be the same as those of the health care team or the primary caregivers, so when outcomes are evaluated, variations in expectations should be addressed by all those involved. Monitoring laboratory tests to determine immune status, viral load, blood cell status, and effects of medications is a large part of the evaluation process.

HUMAN IMMUNODEFICIENCY VIRUS RISK IN PATIENTS OLDER THAN 50 YEARS

The life expectancy in the United States has increased to greater than 78.8 years (CDC, National Center for Health Statistics, 2017). People ages 50 years and older constitute about 45% of Americans diagnosed with HIV. The media tend to report more on younger populations with HIV/AIDS, including MSM, transgender individuals, the homeless, and IV drug users. Many older adults are single because of divorce or death of a spouse or partner. A persistent myth is that older adults are no longer interested in sex. Because pregnancy is not a consideration, condoms are typically not used as they should be. Also, erectile dysfunction medications allow sexual activity for longer periods in many men.

Many older adults are not aware of the risks, but old age is no barrier to becoming infected with HIV. The primary modes of transmission in adults older than 50 years are through heterosexual contact and sharing of contaminated needles among IV drug users. An older adult may ignore symptoms because of a belief that they are a normal part of aging. By the time an older at-risk adult is diagnosed, the survival rate is markedly less than that of a younger person. This is probably because of comorbidities (simultaneous presence of two chronic diseases or conditions in a patient) common to the older population. Skin and mucous membranes are more fragile in the older adult, possibly making transmission easier. Menopausal women are more vulnerable to HIV infection from sexual transmission because decreased estrogen levels cause thinning and decreased lubrication in the vagina. In the older population, the virus is also spread more easily because of the thinning and microscopic tearing of the anal mucosa. Educate this age group about the need for HIV testing in *both* partners before entering into a new sexual relationship and provide recommendations about using barrier techniques.

COMMUNITY EDUCATION AND CARE

All nurses should be alert to the possibility of transmission of HIV and the methods of prevention and should share this information with at-risk populations. Patients and their partners, families, and friends should all be included in the educational opportunities.

HUMAN IMMUNODEFICIENCY VIRUS CONFIDENTIALITY AND DISCLOSURE ISSUES

When a patient signs a form to release medical information, the form must also state whether the patient wants their HIV/AIDS diagnosis and treatment information released. If protected health information (PHI) is released without following HIPAA guidelines, a lawsuit and even loss of the nursing license may be the penalty for a nurse who is indiscreet and discloses PHI without specific patient authorization. For the patient, the consequences may be the loss of a job, housing, or insurance benefits and possible discrimination and rejection by families and friends.

Legal and Ethical Considerations

Confidentiality and Human Immunodeficiency Virus/Acquired Immunodeficiency Syndrome

The diagnosis of HIV/AIDS is a medical diagnosis and can be discussed among health care personnel like any other medical diagnosis for the purpose of rendering care to the patient and does not require a patient's consent. The right to disclose HIV status is regulated by the state in which you are working, but all states do require the reporting of new HIV/AIDS cases for public health statistical tracking. It is important for every licensed nurse to be aware of the state regulations and institutional policies. It is always preferable for the patient to disclose diagnostic information and HIV status to the family. If the patient has given permission (preferably in writing), the family can be informed about the health status and what progress or lack of progress is occurring.

Legal and Ethical Considerations

When a Nurse Has Human Immunodeficiency Virus

If a health care worker is HIV positive, there is a risk of transmitting the virus to others. What are the ethical, moral, and legal responsibilities to patients in such a situation?

BLOODBORNE PATHOGEN EXPOSURE AND HEALTH CARE WORKERS

The CDC and the Occupational Safety and Health Administration (OSHA), along with other health care agencies, have developed evidence-based guidelines to prevent exposure to blood, body fluids, and other potentially infectious material (OPIM) (see Chapter 6, Box 6.3). If the health care worker correctly follows these guidelines, the risk of being exposed is markedly reduced.

AUTOIMMUNE AND AUTOINFLAMMATORY DISORDERS

Autoimmune and autoinflammatory disorders are caused by the immune system reacting against the body's

Safety Alert

Possible Exposure to Human Immunodeficiency Virus

After an unintended exposure to the blood or body fluids of a person either who is HIV positive or whose HIV status is unknown, the need for PEP must be assessed within 2 hours. Exposure can be from a large-bore needle stick, significant mucosal contact with body fluids, or contact with body fluids via a break in the skin. The facility's Infection Preventionist or employee health office should be notified of the exposure. Two- or three-drug therapy, depending on the degree of determined risk, may be initiated as soon as possible after the exposure event. The drugs used are from different drug classes. The medications may need to be taken until HIV status from the source patient has been determined; if the patient is known to be HIV positive, the drugs should be taken for 4 to 6 weeks. If PEP is indicated, you may be unable to work for the first few weeks while taking the medications because of the significant side effects (i.e., headaches, nausea, vomiting, and diarrhea).

own cells. The three categories of disorders are classified according to how extensively the disorder affects body tissues: (1) *local,* which affects only a single organ or tissue; (2) *systemic,* which affect many organs or tissues; and (3) *mixed localized and systemic,* which can cause problems both in a localized area and systemically. The signs and symptoms produced by autoimmune and autoinflammatory disorders are similar; the main difference is the underlying cause of the problem. Autoinflammatory disorders are caused by a malfunction in the innate immune system, and autoimmune disorders are caused by problems in the adaptive immune system.

In *autoinflammatory diseases,* the innate or natural immune system reacts without a reason and without control. This inflammatory process produces fever and many times is a result of a genetic mutation. Autoinflammatory diseases are rare and include such conditions as familial Mediterranean fever.

In *autoimmune diseases,* the adaptive or acquired immune system is responsible for identifying and eliminating foreign threats. In autoimmune disease, the body does not identify its own tissues as "self" but as a foreign threat, so that the immune system is activated and destroys the cells identified as a threat. Some autoimmune diseases are hereditary; others are triggered by environmental factors or other illnesses. Box 11.7 lists the most common autoimmune conditions. Autoimmune conditions are fairly common, and significant research has been conducted to identify best treatment options.

SIGNS AND SYMPTOMS

Table 11.7 gives a partial list of diseases, with signs and symptoms, possibly caused by autoimmune or autoinflammatory mechanisms. Not all experts agree, but at

Table 11.7 Autoimmune Disorders and the Body Systems Affected

DISORDER	AREA AFFECTED	SIGNS AND SYMPTOMS
Systemic Autoimmune Disease		
Autoimmune hemolytic anemia	Red blood cells	Anemia, splenomegaly, hyperbilirubinemia, fatigue
Bullous pemphigoid	Skin, more typically on arms, legs, and trunk	Large fluid-filled vesicles on a swollen erythematous base
Goodpasture syndrome	Lungs and kidneys	Shortness of breath, hemoptysis, fatigue, edema, pruritus
Polymyalgia rheumatica	Large muscle groups, primarily neck, shoulders, upper arms, thighs, and hips	Moderate to severe aching and stiffness, fatigue, unintentional weight loss, anemia Can literally appear overnight; usually goes away on its own. Up to 15% develop temporal arteritis during or after symptoms appear.
Rheumatoid arthritis	Heart, lungs, joints, nerves, and skin	Variety of symptoms depending on what is most affected: fever, fatigue, joint pain and stiffness, deformity of the joints, shortness of breath, chest pain, edema, loss of sensation, rashes
Systemic lupus erythematosus (lupus)	Brain, heart, lungs, kidneys, joints, blood cells, and skin	Fatigue, weakness and lightheadedness, shortness of breath, chest pain, pruritus, rash, butterfly rash on the face in some cases
Temporal arteritis/giant cell arteritis	Arteries of the head and neck	Can affect all vessels within the body Symptoms vary depending on location Can have headache, loss of vision, chest pain, dyspnea, kidney failure, abdominal pain, weight loss, skin rash
Wegener granulomatosis (a form of vasculitis)	Nasal sinuses, lungs, and kidneys	Causes end organ damage and can be life threatening if not treated Rhinitis is generally first sign in most patients

Continued

Table 11.7 Autoimmune Disorders and the Body Systems Affected—cont'd

DISORDER	AREA AFFECTED	SIGNS AND SYMPTOMS
Local Autoimmune Diseases		
Addison disease	Adrenal glands	Slow progression. Affects the adrenal cortex, causing a deficiency in glucocorticoid hormones. Fatigue, dizziness, muscle weakness, diarrhea, diaphoresis, orthostatic hypotension, hyperpigmentation of the skin
Celiac disease	Gastrointestinal tract	Intolerance of gluten products; impaired nutrient absorption; abdominal pain; chronic diarrhea; vomiting; weight loss; pale, foul-smelling, or fatty stools
Crohn disease	Ileum and beginning of large colon	Persistent diarrhea, rectal bleeding, fever, loss of appetite, bloody stools
Grave disease (hyperthyroidism)	Thyroid gland	Tachycardia, tremors, nervousness, weight loss, intolerance to heat
Guillain-Barré syndrome	Peripheral nervous system	Ascending paralysis, starting in legs, then arms, then face Deep tendon reflexes disappear Some patients require mechanical ventilation until recovery occurs
Hashimoto thyroiditis (hypothyroidism)	Thyroid gland	Weight gain, coarse skin, drowsiness, intolerance to cold
Multiple sclerosis	Brain and spinal cord	Abnormal sensations, weakness, vertigo, vision problems, muscle spasms
Myasthenia gravis	Connection between nerves and muscles (neuromuscular junction)	Muscles weaken and tire easily, especially the eyes
Pernicious anemia (vitamin B_{12} deficiency)	Cells in stomach and intestines that absorb vitamin B_{12}	Anemia results in inadequate production of mature blood cells and maintenance of nerve cells and leads to fatigue and weakness; nerves can be damaged with resulting loss of sensation
Primary biliary sclerosis, primary sclerosing cholangitis, autoimmune hepatitis	Liver	Occurs more commonly in women Chronic cholestasis, which leads to destruction of the smaller bile ducts Fatigue, pruritus, hepatomegaly, jaundice, hyperpigmentation
Raynaud disease (isolated), also called primary Raynaud phenomenon	Fingers, toes, nose, ears	Can be triggered by changes in temperature or strong emotions. Has an unknown cause.
Raynaud phenomenon or secondary Raynaud phenomenon (accompanied by or caused by other autoimmune disorders [scleroderma, lupus]). Other possible causes include the categories of medications, occupational or hematologic.		Numbness and tingling in digits, which then become pale and turn blue because of lack of oxygen; as digits warm up, they turn red because of influx of blood Restricts blood flow of the microvascular system, can cause pitting ulcerations In some cases, gangrene requiring amputation
Type 1 diabetes mellitus	Islet (beta) cells of pancreas (insulin production)	Excessive thirst, appetite, and urination (initial symptoms) Can lead to significant multisystem disease (blindness, kidney failure, impaired circulation, amputations, especially of lower extremities)

Table 11.7 Autoimmune Disorders and the Body Systems Affected—cont'd

DISORDER	AREA AFFECTED	SIGNS AND SYMPTOMS
Mixed Localized and Systemic Autoimmune Disorders		
Scleroderma	Localized: skin Systemic: heart, lungs, kidneys, and intestines	Skin and connective tissue tightens and hardens Skin will have patches that are thick, white, or pale in the center surrounded by a purple border Heart may develop dysrhythmias; congestive heart failure and pericarditis can also occur Lungs become scarred (pulmonary fibrosis); pulmonary hypertension may develop Kidneys will release more protein into the urine; can trigger hypertension
Sjögren syndrome	Salivary glands, lacrimal glands, joints Can also affect lungs, lymphatic system, kidneys, and muscles	Dry eyes and mouth, gum disease, dental caries

Data from American Autoimmune Related Diseases Association (AARDA), 2018; Ignatavicius DD, Workman ML, Rebar CR, et al.: *Medical-surgical nursing: patient-centered collaborative care,* ed 9, St. Louis, 2018, Elsevier.

Box 11.7 Most Commonly Occurring Autoimmune Diseases

- Rheumatoid arthritis
- Systemic lupus erythematosus
- Celiac sprue disease
- Pernicious anemia
- Multiple sclerosis
- Scleroderma
- Psoriasis
- Inflammatory bowel disease
- Hashimoto disease
- Grave disease
- Sjögren syndrome
- Type 1 diabetes

this time more than 100 diseases are thought to be triggered by an alteration in immune function. Some of the diseases have other causes in addition to immune system dysfunction. General signs and symptoms usually include fever, fatigue, abdominal pain or digestive issues, swollen glands, joint pain, and swelling.

DIAGNOSIS

Diagnosing autoimmune and autoinflammatory disorders can be difficult. A detailed health history and complete physical examination must be conducted. Symptoms may be vague and intermittent and may occur over a period of years. The most commonly occurring conditions consistent with the presenting symptoms are ruled out first. It is usually after other diseases are ruled out that more in-depth genetics and other testing is done. This can be frustrating for patients who "just have not felt well for some time" and are looking for an explanation or diagnosis.

Blood tests, such as a complete blood cell count with differential, will typically be performed (see Box 11.3). Some immune disorders are associated with a specific antibody that can be detected in the blood. Other laboratory tests evaluating inflammation, such as an erythrocyte sedimentation rate (ESR) and C-reactive protein (CRP) levels, are not specific to immune disorders but may help confirm the diagnosis when used with other information. For disorders that are organ specific, a biopsy of the affected tissue may be used to confirm or exclude the diagnosis. For autoinflammatory disorders, genetic testing may be performed.

TREATMENT AND NURSING MANAGEMENT

Treatment falls into two categories: (1) replacement or support of lost or ineffective body function and (2) therapies targeted to halt the destructive process. The goal of physical, occupational, speech, or even psychological therapeutic interventions is to help the patient learn how to effectively deal with the disorder and be able to function at the highest achievable level for as long as possible. In medication therapy for autoimmune disorders, the chemical treatment is aimed at altering cell function to prevent further harmful effects, not kill the cells. However, some medications can minimize side effects, whereas others can cause additional medical complications. Other autoimmune disorders are discussed in relevant chapters (multiple sclerosis, Chapter 24; rheumatoid arthritis, Chapter 32; and psoriasis, Chapter 43).

SYSTEMIC LUPUS ERYTHEMATOSUS

Systemic lupus erythematosus (SLE), also known as lupus, is an autoimmune disease. The term *erythematosus* refers to the **erythema** (patchy congestion of capillaries of the skin with blood) that often accompanies the disease. As with most autoimmune disorders, the cause is largely unknown. Genetics, hormones, immunologic

Assignment Considerations

Protecting the Patient

Any health care team member that has a potentially infectious condition, such as a cold or the flu, should not be assigned to care for patients with alterations in immune function. If symptoms develop in the middle of the shift, the staff member should wear a mask and use meticulous hand hygiene until the assignments are reorganized.

response, and environmental influences may play a role in the development of this disease; however, no specific link has been established. In SLE, the body begins to produce abnormal antibodies that attack the target tissues or cells instead of foreign agents such as bacteria, fungi, and viruses. This assault can go on for years before onset of symptoms becomes evident and health care is sought.

SLE has a discoid form (skin is affected but internal organs are not), a systemic form (involves internal organs and is the most common type), and a drug-induced form (tends to be milder and less damaging to the body). Although SLE is incurable, symptoms can be treated.

Individuals of all ages have been diagnosed with SLE, but the typical age of onset appears to occur after puberty and peaks between 15 and 40 years of age. It occurs more often in women than men (a ratio of 11:1). The overall rate is 5 new cases per 100,000 individuals in the United States (CDC, 2018). Of note, African Americans and Hispanic women of childbearing age in the United States are affected more often than other ethnicities.

Etiology and Pathophysiology

SLE occurs from an abnormal reaction of the body's immune system, especially against proteins found in the nucleus of body cells. Inflammation of the muscles, blood vessel abnormalities, and immune complex deposition in tissues occur throughout the body. SLE usually waxes and wanes throughout the course of the disease. Some individuals have a very mild form of the disorder and have infrequent flare-ups with minimal symptoms. Others have severe, debilitating symptoms that, if left untreated, can lead to death.

Prolonged exposure to sunlight can initiate a flare-up of SLE, so use of sunblock and covering the skin are important. A variety of drugs, such as oral contraceptives (especially in women who test positive for the presence of antiphospholipid antibodies), sulfa-based antimicrobials, and penicillin, exacerbate lupus. In addition, hydralazine, procainamide, and minocycline are known to produce a lupus-like syndrome.

Signs and Symptoms

Signs and symptoms tend to come and go and include painful or swollen joints and muscle pain, extreme fatigue, unexplained fever, red rash usually on the face (malar rash or butterfly rash; Fig. 11.3), unusual loss of hair, sensitivity to the sun, weakness and profound fatigue, mouth ulcers, poor appetite, weight loss, abnormal menses, edema, and swollen glands. All body systems can be affected (Fig. 11.4). Weakness is a hallmark of the SLE disease process. It is not unusual to see skeletal abnormalities such as asymmetric arthritis, especially in the fingers, hands, wrists, and knees. Azotemia, hematuria, proteinuria, and pyuria indicate renal involvement, such as nephrotic syndrome or acute or chronic renal failure (see Chapter 34). Neurologic symptoms may include headaches, seizures, psychosis, and other cognitive disorders. Pleurisy may develop in the lining of the lungs and can lead to chest pain, shortness of breath, and pulmonary hypertension. Heart failure, pericarditis, and coronary disease may also be symptomatic of SLE (see Chapters 19 and 20).

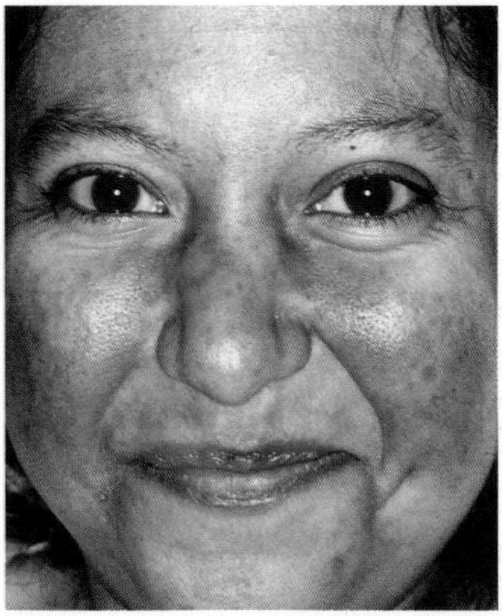

Fig. 11.3 The characteristic "butterfly" rash of systemic lupus erythematosus. (From Ignatavicius DD, Workman ML, Rebar CR, et al.: *Medical-surgical nursing: patient-centered collaborative care*, ed 9, St. Louis, 2018, Elsevier.)

Diagnosis

Currently no single test can confirm a diagnosis of SLE. A complete medical history is necessary to guide the diagnostic studies. To confirm SLE, a patient must have at least 4 of the 11 clinical presentations or laboratory test results performed for SLE. Typically the patient shows evidence of a multiorgan disorder. Initially serum blood studies, along with a urinalysis and tests for renal and liver function, are performed. Multiple antibody levels are obtained, and kidney and skin biopsies are performed.

A syphilis test measures antiphospholipid antibodies in the blood, which are known to be present in lupus, so a false-positive syphilis test is another indicator of SLE. Tests for signs of inflammation include obtaining ESR and CRP levels. Current research is focusing on identifying biomarkers that would indicate the presence of SLE.

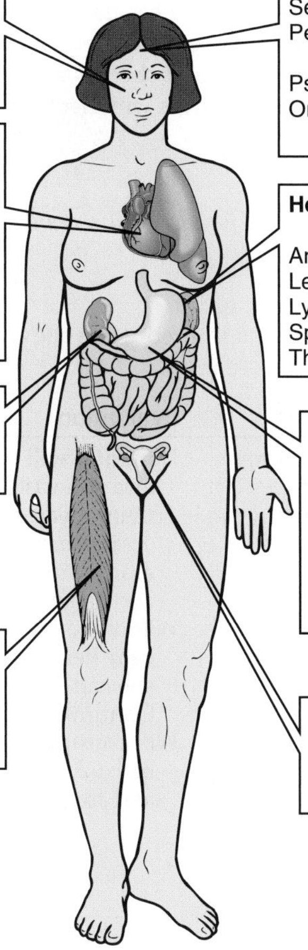

Fig. 11.4 Multisystem involvement in systemic lupus erythematosus. (From Lewis SL, Dirksen SR, Heitkemper MM, et al.: *Medical-surgical nursing: assessment and management of clinical problems,* ed 10, St. Louis, 2017, Elsevier.)

Treatment

There is no cure for SLE. Current treatments are targeted toward symptom control or management to prevent exacerbations, treat flare-ups when they occur, and minimize organ damage and long-term complications. Hydroxychloroquine, an antimalarial drug, aids in long-term control of SLE. Glucocorticoids, such as prednisone, are taken to reduce symptoms experienced during major flare-ups. Nonsteroidal antiinflammatory drugs (NSAIDs) are used to reduce inflammation and control pain. Dehydroepiandrosterone (DHEA), a mild male hormone, is given to treat hair loss, joint pain, fatigue, and memory issues. Immunosuppressant agents are given to suppress the immune system, thereby reducing the risk of a systemic attack. Immunosuppressive agents, such as azathioprine (Imuran), are used to interfere with immune function by damaging autoantibody-producing cells. Belimumab (Benlysta), an IV medication that targets B-lymphocyte stimulator (BLyS) protein, may reduce the number of abnormal B cells, which are believed to be a contributing factor in lupus. Rest, balanced diet, and exercise are also primary treatments for patients with SLE. Women with lupus are at higher risk for pregnancy complications, and those with antiphospholipid antibodies have an increased risk of miscarriage and preeclampsia. Oral contraceptives are not contraindicated in woman with mild lupus or who have a low risk of clotting.

Complementary and Alternative Therapies

Use of Alternative Therapies by Patients With an Immune System Disorder

Relaxation, meditation, reiki, and imagery can help decrease stress. Acupressure and acupuncture may help control pain. There is controversy regarding using herbal and other substances to boost the immune system because some can interfere with prescription medication. The health care provider should be consulted before starting use of complementary and alternative therapies.

Nursing Management

Assessment of the patient's ability to participate in ADLs is important. Joint pain is common, thus management of pain and assisting with mobility are priorities. Ongoing assessment of body systems is important to determine whether the disease process is affecting additional systems. Nursing Care Plan 11.1 presents interventions for the more common problems experienced by most patients with SLE.

Educate the patient about the disease and how to prevent possible complications. For example, any flu-like illness lasting for more than a few days should be reported to the health care provider. Review appropriate skin care, including the correct method of applying and reapplying sunblock with a sun protection factor (SPF) of 30 or higher. Infections can also exacerbate symptoms, so the patient should avoid being around anyone who is showing signs or symptoms of a communicable disease.

Patient Teaching

Skin Protection for Patients With Systemic Lupus Erythematosus

- Avoid direct sunlight and any other type of ultraviolet lighting, including tanning beds.
- Use an SPF 30 or higher sunblock when outdoors.
- Wear long pants, a long-sleeved shirt, and a wide-brimmed hat when in the sun.
- Cleanse the skin only with a mild soap that has a glycerin base.
- Dry the skin thoroughly by patting rather than rubbing it.
- Apply nonperfumed lotion liberally to dry skin areas at least twice a day.
- Avoid using alcohol-based skin care products, face powder, or other astringent agents.
- Use cosmetics that contain moisturizers.
- Inspect the skin daily for rashes and open areas.

Adapted from Ignatavicius DD, Workman ML, Rebar CR, et al.: *Medical-surgical nursing: patient-centered collaborative care,* ed 9, St. Louis, 2018, Elsevier.

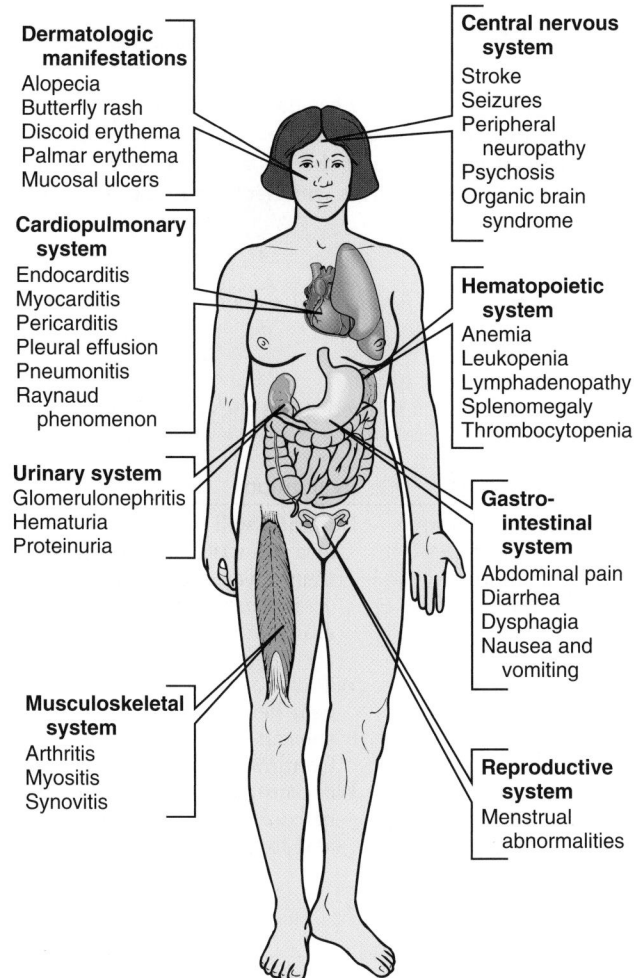

Nursing Care Plan 11.1 Care of a Patient With Low Immune Response

SCENARIO

Julie Hansen, age 37, has just been diagnosed with systemic lupus erythematosus (SLE). She has flat erythema in a butterfly pattern over the face, is complaining of joint pain in her knees and elbows, and has experienced constant fatigue and weakness for the past 6 months. Her erythrocyte sedimentation rate (ESR) is elevated, and she has a positive antinuclear antibody (ANA) test. Other tests helped confirm the health care provider's diagnosis. She lives with her husband, 12-year-old son, and 14-year-old daughter.

PROBLEM STATEMENT/NURSING DIAGNOSIS

Altered activity tolerance related to inflammatory nature of the disease as evidenced by need for increased rest and sleep and inability to keep up with household chores along with work.

SUPPORTING ASSESSMENT DATA

Subjective: States she cannot keep the laundry done or the house clean because she is so tired when she comes home from work; has been using more and more "fast food" for family dinners.

Goals/Expected Outcomes	Nursing Interventions	Selected Rationale	Evaluation
Patient will manage household along with work with help within 6 wk.	Explore chores that other family members may be able to take over.	Husband and children could help with cleaning, laundry, errands, and meal preparation.	Daughter will wash clothes and son will fold and put them away. Husband will do errands. All members will assist with meal preparation and cleanup.
	Assist to work out a schedule for rest periods at lunchtime, after work, and on the weekends.	Resting for 30 min at lunchtime eases fatigue.	Will try to find a place at or near her workplace where she can rest at lunchtime. Continue plan.
	Assist to plan meals for the week and to cook large quantities on the weekend that can be divided into individual meals and frozen for family dinners.	It is less fatiguing to cook large quantities of entrees once a week and to freeze portions than to prepare a dinner every day.	Will consider what meals might be cooked on the weekends and frozen. Continue plan.

PROBLEM STATEMENT/NURSING DIAGNOSIS

Chronic pain related to inflammation from disease process.

SUPPORTING ASSESSMENT DATA

Subjective: "My knees and elbows ache whenever I have walked for more than a block or used my arms to lift things frequently during the day."

Objective: Tenderness around elbow and knee joints.

Goals/Expected Outcomes	Nursing Interventions	Selected Rationale	Evaluation
Patient will experience fewer days of pain with regular use of antiinflammatory medication.	Instruct to take 400 mg of ibuprofen tid on a regular basis.	Keeping a steady blood level of the drug will help decrease and prevent inflammation.	States will begin taking the prescribed regimen of ibuprofen. Continue plan.
	Advise to let family lift heavy items and do chores requiring repetitive elbow motion or squatting.	Refraining from lifting, repetitive joint motion, and squatting helps prevent joint strain and added inflammation.	States will let family bring in groceries and put them away. Will remind family to pick up around the house every other day. Will refrain from gardening while bending down on her knees. Continue plan.

PROBLEM STATEMENT/NURSING DIAGNOSIS

Potential for altered skin integrity related to "butterfly" rash and sun sensitivity from disease process.

SUPPORTING ASSESSMENT DATA

Subjective: States sunburns very easily.

Objective: Inflamed rash in butterfly pattern over large part of face.

Nursing Care Plan 11.1 Care of a Patient With Low Immune Response—cont'd

Goals/Expected Outcomes	Nursing Interventions	Selected Rationale	Evaluation
Patient's skin will remain intact.	Instruct in proper skin care with mild soap and alcohol- and astringent-free products.	Avoiding harsh skin care products will help prevent excoriation and breaks in the skin.	States will check her skin care products for alcohol and astringents.
	Instruct to moisturize the skin twice daily.	Moisturizing products will help keep skin supple and prevent breaks.	Will begin moisturizing a second time a day before bedtime. Continue plan.
	Instruct to inspect the skin closely for any breaks or new lesions.	Finding breaks in the skin promptly and caring for them properly will help prevent infection.	Will begin to inspect skin after shower daily. Continue plan.
	Instruct to cover skin when out in the sun and to avoid ultraviolet rays as much as possible.	Protecting the skin from sunlight will help prevent flare-ups of the disease and will protect the skin from further damage.	Will wear suggested clothing of long sleeves, long pants, and a wide-brimmed hat when out in the sun.
	Instruct to use a sunblock product with an SPF of 30 or more when outdoors.	Sunblock helps prevent the damage that can occur from ultraviolet rays.	States will use sunblock daily on exposed parts of skin.
	Instruct to stop going to the tanning salon.	Ultraviolet light damages the skin and can cause a flare-up or progression of SLE symptoms.	States that she hates to give it up but will refrain from going to tanning salon.

CRITICAL THINKING QUESTIONS

1. What types of entrees could be prepared in advance in large quantities and then frozen in family-size portions?
2. What might you suggest as ways to rest at lunchtime when the patient is at work?

SPF, Sun protection factor.

DISORDERS OF THE LYMPHATIC SYSTEM

LYMPHOMA

Lymphoma is a form of lymphatic cancer that starts in the lymphocytes. These cells become malignant and multiply, crowding out the normal cells, which leads to the creation of solid tumors in the lymph nodes. The two main types of lymphoma are Hodgkin lymphoma (HL) and NHL. The primary differences between the two are the types of lymphocytes involved in the disease. If, under microscopic examination of tissue, Reed-Sternberg (R-S) cells are present, the patient has HL. If R-S cells are not present, the patient has NHL, which is further identified as B-cell and T-cell lymphoma and has around 30 subtypes. There are two main types of HL: classical HL and lymphocyte-predominant HL.

Classification and staging of these two diseases is complicated. It relies heavily on microscopic examination of tissues and diagnostic studies, including serum blood testing and select types of scans to determine the type and true extent of the disease. Many of the NHL subtypes look similar, but they are quite different and respond to different therapies with varying degrees of success.

Hodgkin Lymphoma

Etiology. HL, also known as *Hodgkin disease,* is one of the more curable forms of cancer when diagnosed and treated early. It accounts for less than 1% of all cancers. HL primarily affects young adults, but it can occur in those older than 55 years of age. Incidence rates are higher in whites than in African Americans. Treatment advances have improved survival rates, which are currently 86% at 5 years (American Cancer Society, 2018).

The cause of HL is not known, but there are possible genetic and environmental components that, in combination, can initiate the onset of this disease. Studies have shown that there is a 10 times higher risk of developing the disease in same-sex siblings of patients with HL. An association has been found among patients with HL who had few or no siblings, lived in a single-family home, were early in the family's birth order, and had few playmates. This form of life environment tends to decrease exposure to infectious agents at an early age, so the immune system is not exposed to as many microorganisms, and therefore fewer antibodies are produced. Other possible triggers are viral infections, such as Epstein-Barr and HIV. Previous exposure to various chemical agents has also been implicated.

Pathophysiology. The B cells in the immune system begin to develop atypical cells. The abnormal R-S cells have two unique features: (1) they rapidly replicate more defective B cells and (2) they do not die off as normal cells do. These R-S cells replace normal cells in the nodes and lymph tissue. The disease spreads from one area to another via the lymphatic system and can invade other body systems. As it progresses, the ability of the body to fight off infection can become severely impaired.

Signs and symptoms. More than 80% of cases present with **lymphadenopathy** (enlarged lymph nodes) above the diaphragm. The enlarged, painless lymph nodes can be felt easily in the neck, mediastinum, and axilla and less easily in the abdomen and inguinal (groin) area. The patient may also complain of abdominal fullness, fatigue, profuse night sweats, unintentional weight loss, and pruritus. High suspicion for HL exists when the patient has complaints of swollen lymph glands lasting for several weeks and no recent history of any type of infection. The patient will likely require a series of diagnostic studies. If there is a mediastinal mass of involved lymph tissue, the patient may have a nonproductive cough because of the narrowed airways from the swollen lymph glands. Many other organs can become affected, as shown in Fig. 11.5.

Diagnosis, treatment, and nursing management. A definitive diagnosis for HL is confirmed by the presence of R-S cells in the tissues obtained by biopsy of the lymph nodes. Radiographs, computed tomography (CT) scans, positron emission tomography (PET) scans, and bone marrow biopsy can also be used to help determine the extent or stage of the disease.

Treatment depends on the stage of the disease and whether involvement is above or below the diaphragm or both. Once the stage is known, the absence or the presence of one or more of the following symptoms is noted: unintentional weight loss of more than 10% of body weight over the previous 6 months; an unexplained fever greater than 100° F (38.5° C) for 3 days or longer; and profuse night sweats not related to weather conditions. In patients with four or more involved nodal areas who are older than 50 years and who have an ESR greater than 30, the outlook is less favorable.

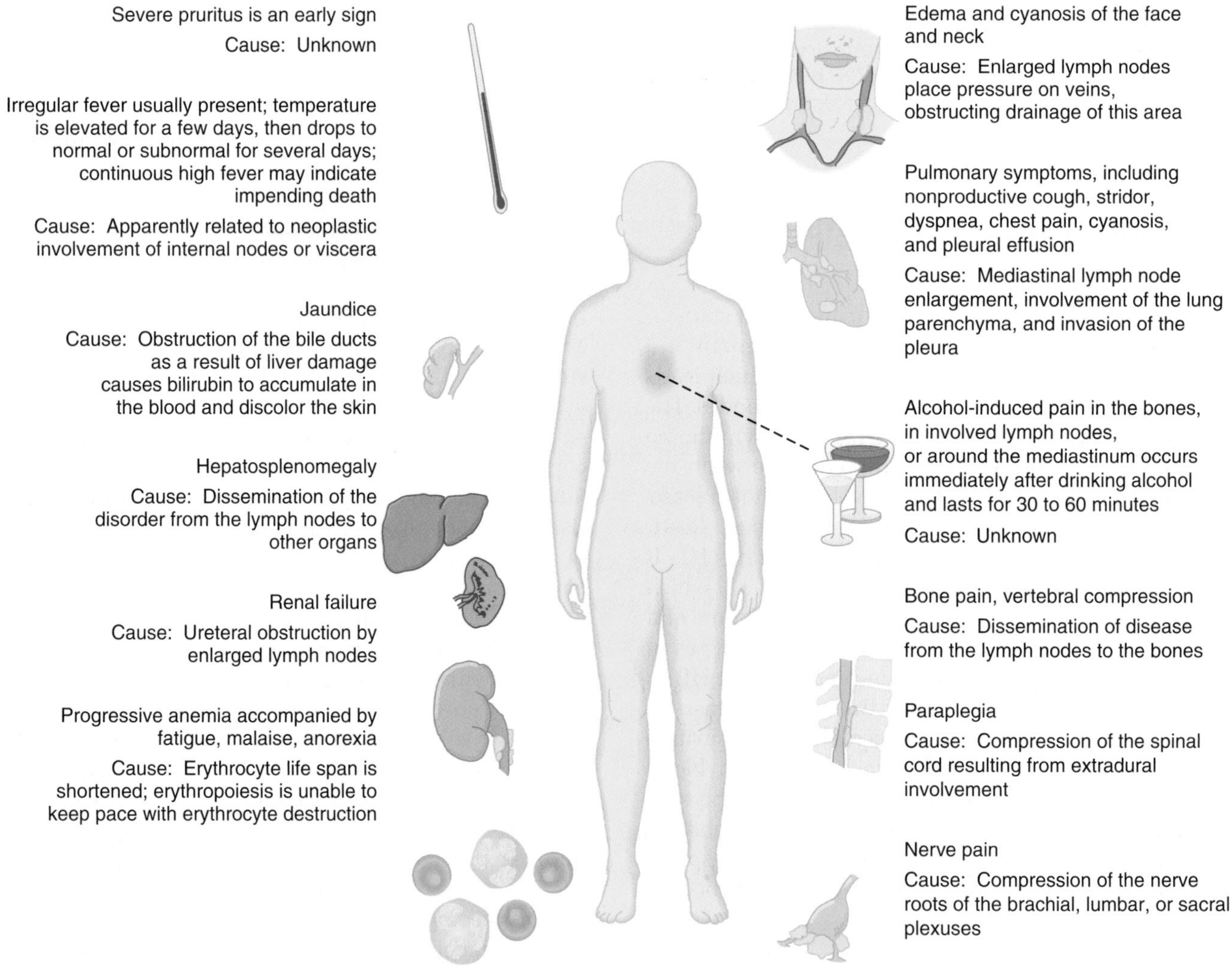

Severe pruritus is an early sign
Cause: Unknown
Irregular fever usually present; temperature is elevated for a few days, then drops to normal or subnormal for several days; continuous high fever may indicate impending death
Cause: Apparently related to neoplastic involvement of internal nodes or viscera
Jaundice
Cause: Obstruction of the bile ducts as a result of liver damage causes bilirubin to accumulate in the blood and discolor the skin
Hepatosplenomegaly
Cause: Dissemination of the disorder from the lymph nodes to other organs
Renal failure
Cause: Ureteral obstruction by enlarged lymph nodes
Progressive anemia accompanied by fatigue, malaise, anorexia
Cause: Erythrocyte life span is shortened; erythropoiesis is unable to keep pace with erythrocyte destruction
Edema and cyanosis of the face and neck
Cause: Enlarged lymph nodes place pressure on veins, obstructing drainage of this area
Pulmonary symptoms, including nonproductive cough, stridor, dyspnea, chest pain, cyanosis, and pleural effusion
Cause: Mediastinal lymph node enlargement, involvement of the lung parenchyma, and invasion of the pleura
Alcohol-induced pain in the bones, in involved lymph nodes, or around the mediastinum occurs immediately after drinking alcohol and lasts for 30 to 60 minutes
Cause: Unknown
Bone pain, vertebral compression
Cause: Dissemination of disease from the lymph nodes to the bones
Paraplegia
Cause: Compression of the spinal cord resulting from extradural involvement
Nerve pain
Cause: Compression of the nerve roots of the brachial, lumbar, or sacral plexuses

Fig. 11.5 Clinical manifestations and pathophysiologic basis of Hodgkin lymphoma. (From Black JM, Hawks JH: *Medical-surgical nursing: clinical management for positive outcomes*, ed 8, Philadelphia, 2009, Saunders.)

Chemotherapy can be given in all stages of the disease. Once it is completed, a more precise form of radiation therapy called *involved-node radiotherapy (INRT)* may be considered. Typically, INRT is delivered only to the affected areas of the body, so less damage occurs to the surrounding tissue. For stages I and II, administration of doxorubicin (Adriamycin), bleomycin, vinblastine, and dacarbazine (ABVD therapy), followed by INRT, has proven to be the most successful treatment. Stages III and IV disease show better improvement with mechlorethamine, vincristine (Oncovin), procarbazine, and prednisone (MOPP therapy) in combination with ABVD therapy. The number of cycles of chemotherapy depends on the stage of the disease, the response of the patient to the therapies, and whether a **relapse** (reappearance of abnormal cells) occurs. Patients may experience many complications from HL and the treatments. Examples of some of the adverse effects include permanent sterility, temporary hair loss, subclinical hypothyroidism, and an increased risk of developing cancer in other organs years after completing radiation therapy.

Nursing care should focus on symptoms the patient is currently experiencing and the side effects of the prescribed therapies. Prevention of health care–associated infections is essential. The problem statements/nursing diagnoses, expected outcomes, and interventions for patients with HL are the same as those for patients with leukemia (see Chapter 16).

Non-Hodgkin Lymphoma

Etiology and pathophysiology. Non-Hodgkin lymphoma (NHL) accounts for 4% of all cancers in the United States and is the seventh most common cancer in men and women (Cancer.net, 2018). The overall incidence is higher in men than in women. The National Cancer Institute estimated that in 2018, 74,680 new cases of NHL would be diagnosed and at least 19,910 people would die of NHL (American Cancer Society, 2018). Part of the increase has been linked to the increased number of patients with HIV and hepatitis C and those who have contracted an Epstein-Barr virus infection. The median age of diagnosis of NHL is 50 years of age. The overall rise in incidence is believed to be related to the continued advances in the successful diagnosis and treatment of a variety of diseases.

NHL is similar to HL, but NHL is less predictable and tends to spread to other body sites much more rapidly. There is also an abnormal proliferation of defective B cells or T cells in NHL. Only biopsy of pathologic lymph nodes and tumor tissue can provide a definitive diagnosis of NHL. There are several types of NHL. One type is an indolent, slow-growing form in which symptoms are usually not present until the advanced stages of the disease. Bone marrow involvement and intra-abdominal adenopathy may occur with this form of NHL, and it has a better prognosis if treatment is given in stage I or II of the disease. Usually radiation therapy is used because most indolent forms of NHL are nodular in shape.

The other forms of NHL are more aggressive; if treated with intensive chemotherapy, there is a survival/cure rate of 70% at 5 years and 60% at 10 years (American Cancer Society, 2016). The symptoms manifest early in the aggressive forms, and with vigorous therapy, there is a potential for cure. The rate of cure is reduced if NHL is diagnosed in a late phase. Five risk factors—**disseminated** (widely spread) tumors, elevated levels of lactate dehydrogenase, poor functional ability of the patient, age older than 60 years, and disease spread beyond lymph nodes—are used to predict the outcome of patients with the more aggressive forms of B-cell lymphoma, which is the most common type. Having none or one of the risk factors suggests a good outcome, but having four or five indicates a poor prognosis. When relapses occur, they typically do so within the first 2 years after treatment.

Signs and symptoms. NHL tends to have more widespread involvement of lymphoid tissue than is found in HL. Unlike HL, NHL typically shows up in one node, then one or more nodes are skipped, and then another node is affected (referred to as *noncontiguous*). NHL usually manifests as a unilateral, painless enlargement of a lymph node that may progress to generalized, painless lymphadenopathy. NHL tumors can occur in the brain, respiratory system, spleen, gastrointestinal (GI) tract, bone, or other parts of the body. As the disease progresses, the patient notices more symptoms, probably because of the increasing size of the affected lymph nodes. Symptoms related to other organs are site specific and can include complaints of high fevers, chills, drenching night sweats, unexplained weight loss, cough, dyspnea, chest pain, nausea, vomiting, a sense of fullness in the abdomen, and constipation. Hepatomegaly or splenomegaly occurs in about one third of patients. The nodes closer to the skin tend to be more easily palpated, are very pruritic, and may be either red or purple. Laboratory tests may show elevated liver enzymes. Physical examination may reveal a change in level of consciousness related to an elevation in intracranial pressure, especially in patients with aggressive NHL.

Diagnosis and treatment. The effectiveness of treatment depends on the stage of the tumor at the time of diagnosis and the type of lymphoma (indolent or aggressive). Staging considers the number and location of affected lymph nodes, whether the nodes are on one or both sides of the diaphragm, and whether the disease has spread to other tissues. To aid in staging, CT, magnetic resonance imaging (MRI), PET, or ultrasound can be used to determine the extent of tissue involvement and to assess therapeutic response after therapy has been completed. Biopsy of various body tissues may also be performed in one of three ways to determine the type of NHL: (1) excisional biopsy, in which an entire node is removed; (2) incisional biopsy, in which only a piece of the node is removed; or (3) fine-needle aspiration (FNA), in which a needle is used to aspirate tissue from the mass of cells. Bone marrow biopsy is usually performed after the diagnosis has been confirmed or is done to determine whether the disease has reached the bone marrow.

Treatment can be with chemotherapy or irradiation, depending on the stage of disease. Stage I or II or low-grade NHL may be cured with radiation therapy alone. Various combinations of drugs are used for other stages of the disease, depending on the type and aggressiveness. Cyclophosphamide (Cytoxan), hydroxydaunomycin (doxorubicin), vincristine (Oncovin), and prednisone (CHOP therapy) is standard treatment and has proven particularly effective for many stages when used with rituximab (Rituxan), a monoclonal antibody. Several other chemotherapy combinations are also often used, with rituximab as a maintenance therapy. Bone marrow transplantation, autologous stem cell transplantation, and immunotherapy with monoclonal antibodies are possible treatment options. A number of drugs provide radiolabeled monoclonal antibody agents. Once infused, these antibodies recognize and react to kill specific tumor cells. Other experimental therapies are under study.

Surgery may be attempted if the tumor is localized or as palliative care. Vaccines for this disease are currently in clinical trials.

Nursing management. Nursing care is directed toward supporting the patient through the diagnostic process and observing for and treating the side effects of radiation and chemotherapy. If bone marrow or stem cell transplants are performed, nursing care and patient education must focus on prevention of infection and other complications. Chapter 8 provides information on specific nursing problems/diagnoses and interventions for patients with cancer. Common problems for a patient with NHL include the following:

- Potential for infection due to neutropenia
- Risk for hemorrhage from thrombocytopenia
- Fatigue
- Nutritional deficit with weight loss

Expected outcomes might include the following:

- Patient will not experience infection.
- Patient will not experience hemorrhage.
- Fatigue will lessen after 6 weeks of treatment.
- Patient will gain 1 lb per week until desired weight is reached.

Nursing interventions are similar to those for the problems of leukemia (see Chapter 16).

LYMPHEDEMA

The lymphatic system drains water, proteins, lipids, and waste from the interstitial spaces throughout the entire body and returns them to the lymph nodes, where waste materials and foreign cells, such as bacteria, are filtered out. Once "clean," the lymph fluid returns to the lymphatic vessels, and the whole process is repeated. When the lymph system is unable to circulate normally, large amounts of fluid accumulate (**lymphedema**), causing swelling. If not controlled, this swelling can lead to further damage to surrounding nerves, blood vessels, and tissues.

There are two types of lymphedema: inherited and acquired. The inherited form (primary) is a congenital condition in which there is deficient growth of the lymphatic system, especially in a lower extremity. This condition chiefly affects women and most often becomes apparent during the middle teens to early twenties.

The acquired form (secondary) typically results from an obstruction caused by trauma to the lymph vessels and nodes, such as occurs during mastectomy when lymph nodes are removed, after radiation therapy, or after a liposuction procedure where some of the lymph nodes may have been damaged. Other causes of obstruction include extensive soft-tissue injury and scar formation and, in tropical countries, parasites that enter lymph channels and block them (e.g., elephantiasis). Patients may have a variety of symptoms, including restricted range of motion; heavy feeling; aching discomfort; recurrent infections; and thick, hard skin. An MRI or CT of the affected body part may help identify some other form of pathology. Lymphoscintigraphy is used to evaluate the integrity of the lymphatic system, determine whether there are any blockages, and evaluate patency and flow. Regardless of the cause, treatment goals are to minimize the effect of the disease process on the individual.

Lymphedema of an extremity often can be treated conservatively through light aerobic exercise and by using simple nursing measures. For example, the patient can be taught to wrap the extremity with an elastic bandage, beginning at the most distal portion and working up the extremity. This compression bandage may help minimize the degree of lymphedema. On the legs, compression stockings may be used. Pneumatic pumps and manual lymphatic drainage physically move the fluid from the affected location to an area where lymph drainage is still functional. Elevation of the affected extremity is also recommended. Meticulous skin care is needed to prevent cellulitis. Surgical intervention is palliative at best and is therefore controversial as a treatment option. There is no cure for this condition. Measures to manage lymphedema are lifelong. Prevention and treatment of lymphedema of the arm and hand after mastectomy are discussed in Chapter 39.

FIBROMYALGIA

In the 1970s, fibromyalgia was identified as a condition of chronic systemic pain and multiple symptoms that could not be explained as caused by any specific source or disease. The condition is still not fully understood. It is considered a problem with pain regulation and classified as a disorder of central sensitization (see Chapter 7). This disorder affects 10 million people in

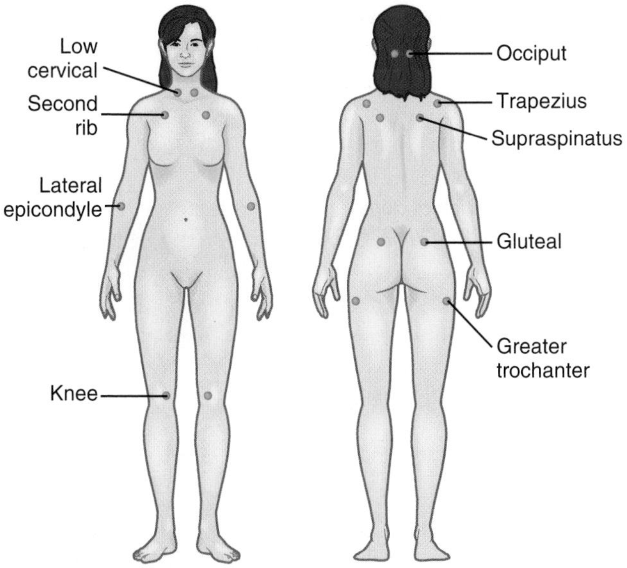

Fig. 11.6 Tender points in fibromyalgia. (From Lewis SL, Dirksen SR, Heitkemper MM, et al.: *Medical-surgical nursing: assessment and management of clinical problems*, ed 10, St. Louis, 2017, Elsevier.)

the United States. Of the 10 million people affected, 75% to 90% are women between 20 and 50 years of age. The change in pain perception can trigger fibromyalgia and its related symptoms. The most common feature of this disorder is musculoskeletal pain. It is typically described as diffuse or multifocal pain, with flare-ups and **remissions** (disease is under control), along with migration from one area of the body to another. Fibromyalgia interferes with a person's ability to perform ADLs and can cause significant fatigue and pain. Other disorders may occur in patients with fibromyalgia and may have similar symptoms or exacerbate symptoms. Chronic fatigue syndrome, irritable bowel syndrome, sleep disorders, and inflammatory rheumatic disease have all been associated with fibromyalgia.

Patients typically have either **hyperalgesia** (heightened response to painful stimuli) or **allodynia** (pain response to nonpainful stimuli). This disorder may also be caused by a deficiency in the neurotransmitters dependent on serotonin and norepinephrine within the CNS. The criteria, originally established in 1990 then updated in 2011 and most recently modified in 2016, include whether symptoms have been present for at least 3 months, pain in four of five regions, specific scoring on the widespread pain index and symptom severity scale, and that the diagnosis is valid even if other diagnoses are present (Fig. 11.6). Other symptom diagnostic criteria are sleep problems, poor cognition, fatigue, headaches, depression, and abdominal pain (Goldenberg, 2017).

There is no specific diagnostic test that can confirm the diagnosis of fibromyalgia, so treatment focuses more on symptom relief. Currently there are three medications approved by the FDA that help with pain management: the antiseizure medication pregabalin (Lyrica) and the antidepressants duloxetine (Cymbalta) and milnacipran (Savella). Low-dose antidepressants that can also be used include tricyclics, selective serotonin reuptake inhibitors (SSRIs), and benzodiazepines. NSAIDs and long-term use of narcotic pain relievers are not as effective in treating the pain experienced in this disorder because of the abnormal reactions of pain receptors. Additional treatment is based on the symptomatology and could include light exercise, massage therapy, guided imagery, dietary changes, and referral to a mental health provider. Nursing responsibilities include taking a detailed history of symptoms and measures the patient has tried to relieve the pain. Interventions should focus on helping the patient to manage fatigue, pain, activity intolerance, sleep disruption, and stress. The family should be included in the education process.

DISORDERS OF INAPPROPRIATE IMMUNE RESPONSE

ALLERGY AND HYPERSENSITIVITY

An **allergy** is an abnormal response to certain substances; it is considered a systemic immune disorder rather than a local one, and the reaction can be seen or expressed in one or more body systems. **Hypersensitivity reactions**, better known as allergic reactions, are the body's excessive response to a normally harmless substance. The severity of the condition can range from a mild rash to **anaphylaxis** (an extreme allergic reaction that is life-threatening).

Etiology and Pathophysiology

Exposure to microbes and illnesses can build up the immune system, and sanitizing the environment does not allow for these opportunities. The difficulty is to not overprotect from microorganisms while preventing serious illness. "Changes in lifestyle and environmental exposure, rapid urbanisation, altered diet and antibiotic use have had profound effects on the human microbiome, leading to failure of immunotolerance and increased risk of allergic disease" (Bloomfield et al., 2016, pg 213). Complex hereditary, environmental, and site-specific factors contribute to allergic reactions. In autoimmune disorders the immune system responds to the body's tissues and cells as though they are a threat; in allergic reactions, the body reacts to harmless environmental proteins or medications in similar ways.

Hypersensitivity reactions are divided into four types. Type I is an *immediate hypersensitivity* reaction that involves immunoglobulin E (IgE), mast cells, and eosinophils (e.g., anaphylaxis). Type II is an *antibody-mediated reaction* involving immunoglobulin G or M (IgG or IgM) attaching to cell surface antigens (e.g., drug-induced hemolytic anemia). Type III is an *immune complex–mediated reaction* involving bound antigen-antibody complexes being deposited in tissues, causing inflammation and tissue destruction (e.g. nephritis, allergic alveolitis). Type IV is a *T cell–mediated* or *delayed hypersensitivity reaction* involving cell-mediated immune reaction rather than antibodies (e.g., poison ivy dermatitis). As with all types of normal and abnormal immune responses, a reaction will not occur until an individual's body cells have been sensitized to the specific substance that triggers the response. This means that on first contact with the antigen (allergen), the body's immune system is triggered to produce IgE antibodies to recognize the specific antigen. On the second and subsequent contacts with the allergen, the antibodies specific to the allergen are rapidly produced and released into the circulating blood or in the lymphoid tissues, in larger and larger quantities. Because the number of antibodies is increased, they can be quickly transported to the location of the allergen, causing a more rapid and sometimes virulent allergic reaction. This type of reaction is typically seen within 15 to 30 minutes from exposure to the antigen and results from the increased production of mast cells and basophils from IgE antibodies. During this reaction, **histamine** is released from a mast cell mediator. When histamine is released because of an immune response, it triggers increased mucus secretions, vascular permeability, and vasodilation, which leads to tissue edema. Dilated blood vessels transport the IgE antibodies, histamine, and other chemicals to the site of exposure to the allergen (Fig. 11.7).

If the mast cells are IgE dependent, they typically produce only a localized allergic response. Examples of this are allergic conjunctivitis or allergy-induced asthma. A person who has **atopy** (a response that affects various parts of the body without being in direct contact with the allergen), such as is seen in eczema, tends to be hypersensitive to a variety of allergens.

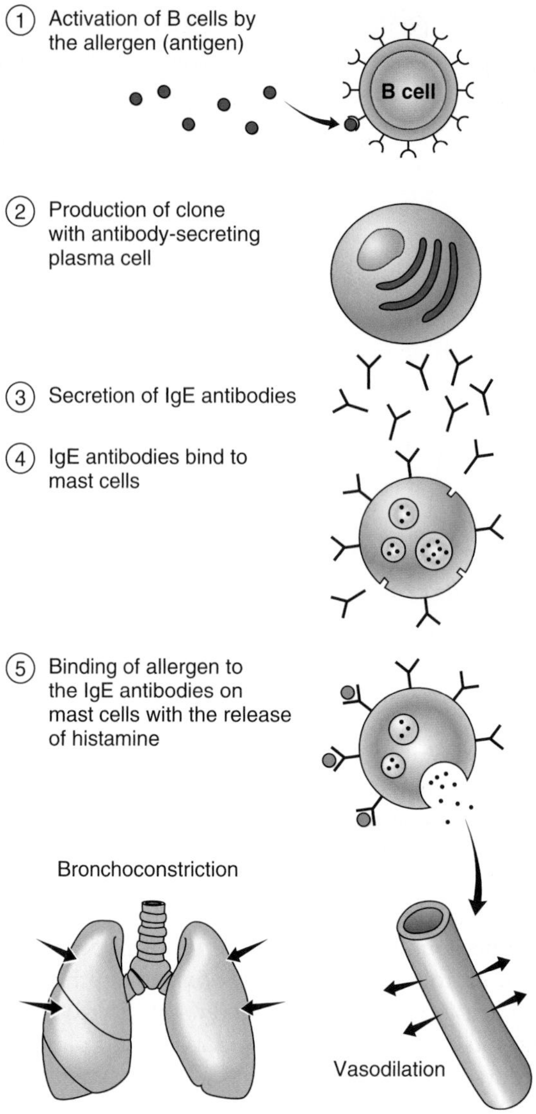

Fig. 11.7 Immediate-reaction allergy. *IgE,* Immunoglobulin E.

Signs and Symptoms

The body system most affected by the offending agent may present more specific symptoms. For example, when the nose and eyes are exposed to a contact allergen, symptoms of itchy, red, watery eyes; soft palate pruritus; clear rhinorrhea; and sneezing are common. Should the allergen be inhaled, the release of histamine can cause the contraction of smooth muscle tissues in the bronchioles of the lungs. These internal changes also produce an allergic response, notably erythema, edema, increased exudate, and breathing difficulties such as dyspnea and wheezing. Table 11.8 presents the four broad types of allergens.

Diagnosis

Identification of allergens. Identification of allergens can be a tedious process. Many times, more than one substance produces the symptoms of an allergy. Reactions to certain food products, animals, insect stings, drugs, and other substances that are out of the norm are noticeable because of the relationship between cause and effect. Ask about exposure to substances that appear to have or are known to cause an adverse response. Help the patient recognize that vague symptoms, such as consistently becoming "stuffed up" only at night when in bed, could be an allergic reaction, perhaps to their pillow.

Diagnostic tests. Two primary methods are used to test for allergies. One is performing a radioallergosorbent test, known as *RAST.* This test uses blood serum from the patient to determine whether the IgE to the suspected allergen is present. The major advantages to this type of allergy testing are that antihistamine medications can continue, it is safer for patients with serious heart and lung problems, there is no chance of an anaphylactic reaction, it is more useful to identify a true food allergy, and it can be used when severe skin conditions prevent skin testing. The disadvantages to the RAST are that it is more expensive than skin testing; it can take several days to weeks before results are known; and it is less specific, meaning that this test tends to produce more false-positive and false-negative results to allergens.

Table 11.8 Four Broad Categories of Allergens[a]

CATEGORY	METHOD OF EXPOSURE	TRIGGERS	EFFECTS
Contactants	Direct contact with mucosa, skin, or tissue	Dust, wool fabrics, detergents, soaps, lotions, cosmetics, plants such as poison ivy, dyes, metals in jewelry, and latex	Irritation to the conjunctiva of the eyes, urticaria, rashes, hives, dermatitis, and eczema
Ingestants	Swallowed	Food: citrus fruits, tomatoes, strawberries, cow's milk, wheat, eggs, dairy products, seafood, chocolate, nuts, monosodium glutamate (MSG), other preservatives, and artificial food coloring	Abdominal pain, flatulence, nausea, vomiting, and diarrhea
		Drugs: aspirin, barbiturates, anticonvulsants, and antimicrobials; any drug may cause an allergic reaction	Can also cause atopic dermatitis, rash, and dyspnea
Inhalants	Entry through nose or mouth	Dust mites, molds, pollen, fragrances, animal dander, insect feces, and some chemicals	Edema of nasal mucosa, allergic rhinitis or sinusitis, rhinorrhea, sneezing, laryngeal edema, coughing, dyspnea, bronchoconstriction, and wheezing
Injectables	Via needle (i.e., hypodermic, intramuscular, intravenous), animal or snake bites, and insect stings	Medications, vaccines, animal saliva, and snake or insect venoms	Swelling and pain at injection site, bruising, discoloration, and necrotic skin

[a]Any allergen can cause severe allergic reactions, including anaphylaxis and death, if not recognized and treated immediately.

The skin **scratch test** has been the most reliable method of allergy testing for more than 100 years. The skin is pricked by a needle, and a drop of the suspected allergen is applied to the area. A needle is then used to slightly scratch the skin just below the epidermis. The **patch test** is similar to the scratch test except that the allergen is placed on the surface of the skin and covered with an airtight dressing (patch). For both tests, a negative reaction occurs when there is no erythema, swelling, or complaint of itching. A positive reaction to either test is indicated by the appearance of a small (usually dime-size) wheal at the site of contact with the allergen and possibly by complaints of itching by the patient.

Drug allergy. A patient may have a confirmed allergy to a medication that is required and for which there are no alternatives. Before administration, a test dose of the drug may be given. For IV medications, a very small dose is given and then, at 10-minute increments, increasing amounts of the drug are infused until the full dose ordered by the health care provider is administered. Steroids, antihistamines, or other immune response–regulating medications may be given prior to the medication. Stay with the patient and closely monitor for signs and symptoms of a reaction during this process. Resuscitation drugs and emergency equipment must be immediately available. This process is repeated with each subsequent administration of the medication, and detailed documentation is required. If it is known in advance that the drug will be needed, the patient can be desensitized to the drug before its use.

Safety Alert

The Patient With Allergies

The medical record should be checked and the patient questioned about allergies before (1) giving medications or immunizations, (2) beginning radiographic studies using contrast media, and (3) minor or major surgery.

Food allergy. Even though other diagnostic methods are available to test for food allergies, a less expensive approach known as the *elimination diet* should be tried first. Teach the patient to read product labels to identify offending substances used in the preparation or preservation of the food item. Tell the patient to eliminate one food at a time and to keep a detailed diary, recording everything ingested each day, including the additives and preservatives in each food product. The patient should start with a food that is believed to be the cause of adverse reactions (e.g., itching, bloating). If symptoms persist for a week to 10 days after eliminating one food product (e.g., milk and dairy products), the patient can resume intake of that food and choose another one for elimination. This process continues until the offending food source is identified.

Latex allergy. Assess each patient for latex allergies because their presence may change the method of care delivery. Most patient care items, including gloves, Foley catheters, surgical drains, bandages, and condoms, are now latex free.

Safety Alert

Personal Protective Equipment

OSHA requires that employers furnish personal protective equipment for their employees at no cost to the employee, and nonlatex items should be made available for those with an allergy to latex. Severe latex allergies have caused some health care workers to change their work environment to one with little or no latex exposure.

Treatment

Drug therapy. Drugs that help alleviate systemic reactions to allergens include epinephrine, antihistamines, bronchodilators, corticotropin (adrenocorticotropic hormone), and cortisone (see Chapters 13 and 14 for specific drug information).

Antihistamines (histamine-blocking agents) help control the symptoms of hay fever and hives by preventing the release of histamine during an allergic reaction (Table 11.9). The histamine-blocking action relieves itching, decreases swelling of mucous membranes and production of secretions, and reduces other symptoms of an allergic reaction. Diphenhydramine (Benadryl) is commonly used orally and topically to counteract many allergic symptoms.

Table 11.9 Drugs Commonly Used to Treat Allergy

CLASSIFICATION	ACTION	SIDE EFFECTS	NURSING IMPLICATIONS
Antihistamines			
First-generation agents: tend to be short acting; impair concentration and can cause drowsiness			
Clemastine (Tavist Allergy)	Relieves acute symptoms of allergic response (itching, sneezing, excessive secretions, mild congestion)	Sleepiness, fatigue, dizziness, headache, dry mouth, urinary retention.	Teach patient to take with full glass of water; report palpitations, change in heart rate, change in bowel or bladder habits.
Diphenhydramine (Benadryl)	Competitively blocks the effects of histamine at peripheral H_1 receptor sites; has anticholinergic (atropine-like) and sedative effects	Patients vary in their sensitivity to these side effects.	Instruct patient not to use alcohol with antihistamines because of additive depressant effect. Is OTC in oral form. IV administration may be given in clinic or hospital setting.
Tripelennamine (PBZ)	Competes with histamine receptor sites	May cause palpitations, tachycardia, urinary retention or frequency.	Must take with food whole; do not crush.
Brompheniramine maleate (Dimetane)	Antagonist of histamine H_1 receptors	Severe constipation, urinary retention, dry mouth, blurred vision, tachycardia.	Do not use if patient is diagnosed with glaucoma.
Chlorpheniramine (Chlor-Trimeton)	Antagonist of histamine H_1 receptors; serotonin-norepinephrine reuptake inhibitor	Dizziness, blurred vision, euphoria, anxiety, increased appetite.	Do not use in patients with asthma or sleep apnea.
Promethazine (Phenergan)	Antihistamine and neuroleptic	Strong sedative effect, long-term use can lead to tardive dyskinesia.	Given preoperatively to some patients.
Second-generation agents: less likely to cause drowsiness			
Loratadine (Claritin)	H_1-receptor agonist with minimal sedative side effects; blocks H_1 receptors and blocks effects of histamines (vasodilation, increased capillary permeability)	Second-generation agents have limited affinity for brain H_1 receptors.	Teach patient to expect few if any side effects. Long-acting medication. Use with caution in patients with kidney or liver dysfunction.

Table 11.9 Drugs Commonly Used to Treat Allergy—cont'd

CLASSIFICATION	ACTION	SIDE EFFECTS	NURSING IMPLICATIONS
Cetirizine (Zyrtec)	Histamine H_1-receptor antagonist in the GI and respiratory tracts and the blood vessels	Causes minimal sedation; may cause headache.	Use with caution in patients with hepatic and renal disease.
Fexofenadine (Allegra)	Histamine receptor antagonist	Can cause menstrual cramping, diarrhea, nausea, and stomachache.	Rapid onset of action, no drug tolerance with prolonged use. Do not take with fruit juice.
Desloratadine (Clarinex)	Long-acting H_1-receptor antagonist	Can cause headache, diarrhea, or fever.	General interactions: do not take with alcohol or any form of tranquilizer or sedative.
Decongestants			
Oral			
Pseudoephedrine (Sudafed)	Stimulates adrenergic receptors on blood vessels, promotes vasoconstriction, and reduces nasal edema and rhinorrhea	CNS stimulation, causing insomnia, excitation, headache, irritability, increased blood and ocular pressure, dysuria, palpitations, tachycardia.	Advise patient of adverse reactions. Most states regulate the amount of pseudoephedrine that can be obtained per month. Is kept behind the counter and ID must be shown for purchase.
Phenylephrine (Suphedrin PE, Sudafed PE)	Same as above	Same as above.	Advise that some preparations are contraindicated for patients with cardiovascular disease, hypertension, diabetes, glaucoma, prostate hypertrophy, or hepatic and renal disease.
Topical (Nasal Spray)			Teach patient that these drugs should not be used for >3 days or >3–4 times/day; longer use increases risk of rhinitis medicamentosa.
Oxymetazoline (Dristan)	Blocks action of histamine	Headache, bitter taste, somnolence, nasal irritation.	Teach patient that it can cause irregular heart rate, insomnia, high BP. Stop medication and contact health care provider.
Phenylephrine (Neo-Synephrine)	Stimulates adrenergic receptors on blood vessels, promotes vasoconstriction, and reduces nasal edema and rhinorrhea	CNS stimulation, causing insomnia, excitation, headache, irritability, increased blood and ocular pressure, dysuria, palpitations, tachycardia.	Advise patient of adverse reactions.
Azelastine (Astelin [nasal spray]; Optivar [eye drops])	Histamine antagonist, mast cell stabilizer	Bitter taste, headache, nasal burning.	Advise patient not to drink alcohol or take other CNS depressants.

Continued

Table 11.9 Drugs Commonly Used to Treat Allergy—cont'd

CLASSIFICATION	ACTION	SIDE EFFECTS	NURSING IMPLICATIONS
Mast Cell Stabilizers			
Cromolyn (Gastrocrom, Opticrom)	Mast cell stabilizer, no bronchodilator activity	Anaphylactic reactions have occurred.	Dosage should be reduced if the patient has hepatic or renal impairment.
Nedocromil (Tilade, Alocril)	Mast cell stabilizer, no bronchodilator activity	Used for maintenance treatment of asthma and not for acute attacks.	Inhalation doses are given for asthma, and an ophthalmic solution is used for allergic conjunctivitis.
Corticosteroids			
Prednisone (Deltasone)	Glucocorticoid. In acute allergic reactions, is given to block the immune response. May be used for chronic management.	Immunosuppression. GI bleeding, osteoporosis. Can elevate BP, retain salt and water, increase elimination of potassium.	GI prophylaxis is needed. Monitor fluid and electrolyte status. Do not discontinue abruptly. Adherence to Standard Precautions and infection control principles.
Dexamethasone (Decadron)	Synthetic adrenocortical steroid, modifies the body's immune response	Immunosuppression. Elevation of BP, retention of salt and water, increased elimination of potassium are less likely to occur with the synthetic medication but may occur at higher doses.	Adherence to Standard Precautions and infection control principles. Do not discontinue abruptly.

BP, Blood pressure; *CNS,* central nervous system; *GI,* gastrointestinal; *IV,* intravenous; *OTC,* over the counter.

Antihistamines can cause drowsiness and impaired coordination, so there are restrictions on driving automobiles and operating machinery at the beginning of therapy. Other common side effects include dry mouth, urinary retention, weakness, and blurred vision. Antihistamines and decongestants can aggravate hypertension, narrow-angle glaucoma, and benign prostatic hyperplasia (enlarged prostate) and should be used with caution. Older adult men taking antihistamines may experience hesitancy while voiding, urinary retention, and difficulty with ejaculation; the offending drug should be discontinued if the problem cannot be resolved.

Antiinflammatory drugs such as corticotropin and cortisone are administered to reduce the inflammatory response that occurs in an allergic reaction. If the respiratory tract is involved, bronchodilators can be given to help relieve dyspnea and wheezing. Tranquilizers and sedatives may be ordered to promote the rest needed for successful recovery from a severe reaction and aid in relieving the stress that may have occurred. Local reactions involving widespread and deep skin lesions are treated with salves such as calamine lotion, wet compresses, and soothing baths. The patient must also be protected from a secondary bacterial infection.

Desensitization. When exposure to allergens cannot be avoided or if the symptoms cannot be managed successfully, desensitization (immunotherapy) may be suggested. The purpose is to decrease sensitivity to allergens. Regular injections of extremely small quantities of selected antigens are given daily, weekly, or monthly. The amount given is gradually increased until there is noticeable clinical improvement, and then a maintenance dosage is given. The program may last for years, but improvement should be noted about 6 to 24 weeks after it begins.

NURSING MANAGEMENT

ASSESSMENT (DATA COLLECTION)

Identifying or isolating the allergens that are causing the patient's symptoms requires time and diligence.

Households have common allergens such as pet dander, dust, dust mites, cosmetics, cleaning agents, and dyes in fabrics and materials used in home furnishings. Overstuffed furniture, heavy draperies, and thick carpets contribute by holding particulate matter. Removal of carpeting, routine cleaning as well as daily dusting and vacuuming, and elimination of dust-harboring furnishings can help remove some allergens. Compliance with daily dusting and vacuuming is more likely if the individual's allergy is severe, prompting every effort to control it. Electrostatic filters and top-quality vacuum cleaners with high-efficiency particulate air (HEPA) filters are essential for those with severe inhalant allergies. It may be necessary to part with a cherished family

Focused Assessment

Indicators of Allergic Response

GENERAL
- History of food intolerances; colic; abdominal cramping; bloating; or pain, vomiting, and diarrhea in the absence of general illness
- History of unusual reaction to any drug, food, insect sting, odor, or fumes
- History of recurrent respiratory problems or seasonal flare-ups of any symptoms
- History of fatigue, wheezing, or shortness of breath on exertion
- Exposure to new personal hygiene products or cleaning products

SKIN
- Itching, burning, dryness, scaling, irritations, inflammations, hives, rash (note symmetry and location), scratches, or urticaria

EYES
- Burning, itching, tearing, history of sties
- Redness, discoloration below eyes (allergic shiners), conjunctivitis, rubbing, or excessive blinking

NOSE
- History of nose twitching, stuffiness, recurring nosebleeds, sudden episodes of sneezing or snorting
- Allergic salute (pushing nose upward and backward with heel of hand), nasal polyps, nasal voice

MOUTH AND THROAT
- Open-mouth breathing, continual throat clearing, mouth wrinkling with facial grimaces, redness of throat, swollen lips or tongue, itchy palate

EARS
- History of hearing loss, drainage from ears

NECK
- Palpable, enlarged lymph nodes

Besides a food diary, the patient may need to keep track of any chemicals that are used (e.g., cosmetics, soaps, deodorants, household cleaners, garden products) for a few weeks. Recalling a family history of allergies and types of symptoms family members displayed may also prove helpful. Repeated assessments may need to be planned over a period of weeks or months if the patient is reactive to a variety of allergens.

Health Promotion

Nursing Goals for Patients With Hypersensitivity Reactions

- Assist in the diagnosis of hypersensitivity.
- Help the patient identify the substance or substances that trigger an allergic response.
- Assist the patient in devising ways to avoid or at least limit exposure to these allergens.
- Relieve the symptoms of an allergy.
- Decrease the exaggerated response to the allergens.
- Provide health teaching.

pet or to overcome the habit of smoking and ask others not to smoke. Purchase of HEPA filters for the heating and air conditioning unit may also be helpful. Molds grow in moist environments, so basements, building foundations, showers, and bathing areas are typically prone to mold growth. Routine cleaning and adequate ventilation can help reduce or eliminate mold growth in most homes. Houseplants should be removed if there is an allergy to mold. Dehumidifiers can reduce moisture in basements. Successful compliance with recommendations should reduce the frequency, severity, and symptoms of the allergic reaction.

Patients with allergy-induced skin conditions should be taught that a warm environment and sweating increase the sensation of itching. Advise the patient to keep cool without chilling and not to take excessively hot showers or baths. Over-the-counter topical lotions, as well as prescription medications and salves, can help relieve itching.

Avoiding exposure to allergens requires knowledge of the nature of the allergen, method of transmission, source or reservoir, and portal of entry. Alteration in habits and location may also help eliminate exposure. Successful management of hypersensitivity depends in large measure on the ability of the patient to understand the allergy and to follow the prescribed treatment regimen.

Think Critically

What actions would you suggest for removing allergens from the home environment to someone allergic to mold, animals, dust mites, and smoke?

ANAPHYLACTIC REACTION AND ANAPHYLACTIC SHOCK

Etiology and Pathophysiology

Anaphylaxis is a serious, life-threatening, whole-body allergic reaction. The cardiovascular system, respiratory system, GI system, and skin all contain copious amounts of mast cells. **Any agent that causes a severe hypersensitivity reaction can cause anaphylaxis.** Substances commonly known to cause hypersensitivity and possible anaphylaxis are listed in Box 11.8. For anaphylaxis to occur, the allergen usually needs to be delivered systemically before the sensitized mast cells are triggered to react. An example of this is the parenteral delivery of an antimicrobial agent such as penicillin. When the reaction occurs, the affected cells swell and rupture, with the subsequent release of histamine. Histamine causes dilation of small blood vessels, a pooling of blood, and release of fluid into tissues. This may lead to circulatory collapse and profound shock (Fig. 11.8). A less severe reaction usually occurs if the allergen is delivered by direct contact, inhalation, or ingestion.

Non–IgE-dependent allergens. IgE-mediated immune responses typically require repeated exposures for a

Box 11.8 Substances Known to Cause Hypersensitivity and Possible Anaphylaxis

DRUGS
- Aspirin
- Cephalosporins
- Chemotherapy agents
- Insulins
- Local anesthetics
- Nonsteroidal antiinflammatory drugs (NSAIDs)
- Penicillins
- Sulfonamides
- Tetracyclines

DIAGNOSTIC AND TREATMENT AGENTS
- Allergenic extracts for desensitization
- Blood products
- Iodine-containing contrast media used for radiographs

ANTITOXIN SERA
- Botulinum antitoxin
- Diphtheria antitoxin
- Poisonous spider antitoxin
- Snake venom antitoxin
- Tetanus antitoxin

FOODS
- Chocolate
- Milk
- Eggs
- Shellfish
- Fish
- Strawberries
- Wheat
- Nuts (especially peanuts)

INSECT STINGS
- Ants (particularly fire ants)
- Bees, hornets, wasps, yellow jackets

reaction to occur. In the non-IgE allergen response, a single encounter can lead to anaphylaxis or even death if not recognized immediately. Examples include iodine-based contrast agents for select radiologic studies and certain narcotics such as morphine and antibiotics such as vancomycin, especially if they are administered too rapidly.

Nurses must be alert for previous allergic reactions and identify patients who are likely to experience a serious reaction. Before administering any medication or drug, verify the patient's known allergies. Patients and families should be actively involved in knowing and reporting allergies. The National Patient Safety Goals view this as a safety measure. **Check all the areas in the medical record where allergies are usually documented.** For example, the home page of the patient's electronic health record may have an allergy alert on it; the medical history obtained by the health care provider should contain information related to allergies; and the medication administration record (MAR), the multidisciplinary care plan, and the nurse's admission history may also contain allergy information.

Clinical Cues

Allergies to seafood indicate intolerance to iodine. This means there is potential for an allergic reaction to iodine-based contrast agents used in radiologic imaging studies. Be certain that the shellfish or iodine allergy is noted on the home page of the medical record, on the MAR, and in other locations where allergies are likely to be noted.

Signs and Symptoms

An anaphylactic reaction requires immediate action. The appearance of hives (**urticaria**) or swelling beneath the skin (**angioedema**) may signal the onset of an anaphylactic episode. Hives or sudden outbreaks of **wheals** (small areas of swelling) on the skin that itch and burn may appear without subsequent anaphylaxis.

Tachycardia, decreased pulses, and a rapid drop in blood pressure signal circulatory collapse, which can occur very rapidly. The patient will also exhibit increasing dyspnea because of the narrowing of the air passages (bronchoconstriction), accumulation of mucus, and wheezing. If an airway is not maintained, convulsions may occur because of oxygen deprivation. Treatment must be started immediately to avoid hypoxic brain injury or death within a matter of minutes.

Emergency supplies should be readily available whenever vaccines, serum for passive immunization, and highly allergenic drugs are administered. Anaphylaxis may be prevented if complete information is obtained before administration. Premedication with steroids and/or antihistamines can be administered if a substance that the patient has shown sensitivity to in the past needs to be given.

Clinical Cues

Many patients report allergies to medications that are actually manifestations of side effects, intolerance, or nonallergic adverse reactions. Nausea, constipation, diarrhea, coughing, or drowsiness may be side effects of medications, but reactions to drugs that do not involve the immune system are considered nonallergic adverse reactions. Careful questioning of the patient can help distinguish what kind of reaction the patient has experienced in the past.

Diagnosis

There is no test to confirm the diagnosis of anaphylaxis; rather, it is the presenting symptoms, including sudden onset involving one or more body systems, producing one or more symptoms such as itching, hives, stridor, wheezing, or shock, that confirm the clinical diagnosis of anaphylaxis. Once the patient's condition has been stabilized, laboratory and other diagnostic tests may be performed to rule out other possible causes for the symptoms.

Treatment and Nursing Management

Treatment of anaphylaxis includes the following:

- Establishing a patent airway and administering oxygen to relieve the symptoms of dyspnea and hypoxia

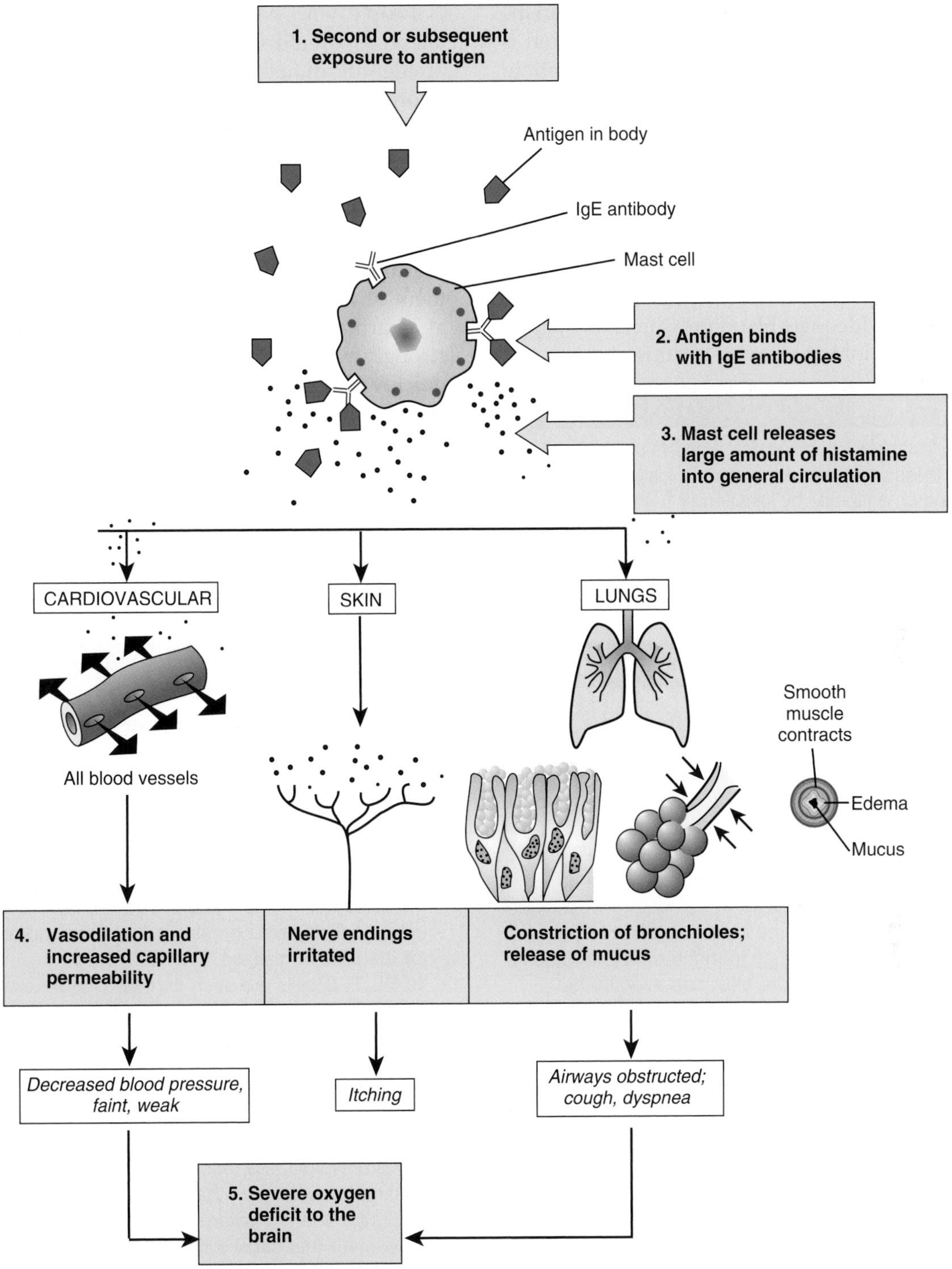

Fig. 11.8 The effects of anaphylaxis. (From Van Meter KC, Hubert RJ: *Gould's pathophysiology for health professions*, ed 6, St. Louis, 2018, Elsevier.)

- Administering IV epinephrine to counteract the effect of histamine: relax the bronchioles, increase the cardiac output, and elevate the blood pressure
- Administering antihistamine (e.g., diphenhydramine hydrochloride [Benadryl]) to stop the effects of the histamine released by the body cells
- Instituting measures to prevent or control shock
- Providing psychological support during the course of the **syndrome** (a group of symptoms that characterize a disorder or condition) and its treatment

When there is difficulty with breathing because of swelling in the airway, provide high-flow oxygen. Although the patient is still able to move air in and out, giving inhaled medications to relax the airways helps maintain air exchange. If these measures are not effective, an emergency intubation, tracheotomy, or cricothyrotomy may be necessary.

Epinephrine is given to counter the allergic reaction. It can be given IV, intramuscularly (IM), subcutaneously, or through an established endotracheal tube. IM injection is the preferred route of administration in the initial phases of the reaction. If IV administration is required, it should be given as a drip. **If the patient is taking beta blockers, these drugs will hinder the effectiveness of the epinephrine.** Diphenhydramine is also used to alleviate the symptoms of the allergic reaction. Corticosteroids may also be given to control the inflammatory response and reduce symptoms.

During the crisis, vital signs and respiratory effort must be monitored continuously. Adequate pharmacologic support and IV fluids are important to maintain perfusion and an adequate blood pressure. See Chapter 45 for additional information on treating shock.

? Think Critically

What is the first thing you would do if a patient starts complaining of shortness of breath and wheezing just after you have administered an antibiotic by injection or IV infusion?

People who have extreme sensitivities to certain allergens should carry a medical alert card or wear an identification bracelet or necklace that contains the information. Several companies offer "medical jewelry" that can relay pertinent information. It also is advisable for individuals who are highly allergic to stings from bees, wasps, or other insects or who are severely allergic to nuts or some other food to carry an EpiPen or a small kit containing epinephrine, syringe, needle, tourniquet, and diphenhydramine hydrochloride with them at all times. These pens and kits are available at pharmacies but require a prescription. They are strongly recommended by allergists because of how quickly an insect sting or inadvertent ingestion of a food can produce a fatal reaction in someone who is highly sensitive. It is also advised that the patient inform coworkers or family members where the kit can be found should it be needed.

Get Ready for the NCLEX® Examination!

Key Points

- In immune deficiency disorders there is an insufficient production of antibodies, immune cells, or both, and the disorders may be congenital or acquired.
- Immunosuppression may be used therapeutically for a variety of conditions, such as tissue transplants, rheumatoid arthritis, and NHL.
- Body temperature should be closely monitored for significant changes, although immune-deficient patients may not have a temperature elevation even in the presence of infection.
- HIV disease in the United States is now a chronic, controllable disease.
- HIV testing should be offered at the time of a complete physical examination to all sexually active patients.
- A barrier, such as a latex condom, should be used during insertive or receptive sexual intercourse to decrease the risk of acquiring HIV.
- Performing genotyping and phenotyping in a person newly diagnosed with HIV helps determine whether the person has any drug-resistant strains of HIV and guides therapy.
- The diagnosis of AIDS is made when the CD4 count is less than 200 cells/μL or by the presence of specific OIs.
- OIs secondary to AIDS cause increased morbidity and mortality.
- If a health care worker is exposed to the blood or body fluids of a patient with HIV, the occupational health department or the Infection Preventionist should be notified to assist with treatment and follow-up.
- ART is effective in controlling the HIV viral load and is also used to treat other conditions.
- Autoimmune disorders are believed to be caused by the immune system reacting to the body's own cells and are typically treated by suppressing the immune system.
- In SLE, the body produces abnormal antibodies that attack the target tissues or cells. Inflammation of muscles, blood vessel abnormalities, and immune complex deposition in tissue occur.
- Lymphoma starts in the lymph tissue when malignant lymphocytes multiply and crowd out normal cells; treatment depends on staging and the aggressiveness of the type of disease.
- In HL, R-S cells are seen on microscopic examination of tissue.
- In NHL, R-S cells are not present. NHL is further identified as B-cell or T-cell lymphoma.
- Nursing care for lymphomas focuses on preventing infection, managing the symptoms, and reducing the side effects of the therapies.
- In fibromyalgia, the most common feature is musculoskeletal pain that is diffuse and multifocal with flare-ups and remissions.
- Any agent that causes a severe hypersensitivity reaction can cause anaphylaxis.
- Nursing responsibilities in caring for patients with allergic conditions include assisting in the diagnosis of hypersensitivity, helping to identify substances that trigger an allergic response, assisting the patient to avoid or limit exposure to allergens, and relieving symptoms.
- Emergency equipment and medications must be available for an anaphylactic reaction, which is a life-threatening condition.

Additional Learning Resources

SG Go to your Study Guide for additional learning activities to help you master this chapter content.

Go to your Evolve website (http://evolve.elsevier.com/deWit/medsurg) for the following FREE learning resources:

- Animations, audio, and video
- Answers and rationales for questions and activities
- Glossary with pronunciations in English and Spanish
- Interactive Review Questions and more!

Review Questions for the NCLEX® Examination

1. You explain the health care provider's order to draw blood for HIV genotyping. The patient asks, "How does that help in my treatment?" What is the best explanation for the test?
   1. Confirms the presence of a viral autoimmune disease
   2. Informs how much of the virus has been replicated
   3. Determines the presence of any mutations in the virus
   4. Reveals the viral load or count of the virus

   NCLEX Client Need: Health Promotion and Maintenance
2. A patient known to be positive for HIV is admitted with oral thrush, recurrent vaginal yeast infections, and skin infections. What do these signs indicate?
   1. Opportunistic infection
   2. Antimicrobial resistance
   3. Resistant strain of HIV
   4. Sentinel infection

   NCLEX Client Need: Physiological Integrity: Physiological Adaptation
3. Which statement(s) is (are) true regarding HIV transmission? *(Select all that apply.)*
   1. Breast milk can harbor the virus.
   2. Proper use of PPE reduces the risk of disease transmission.
   3. Needle exchange programs facilitate the spread of the virus.
   4. Being assessed 2 hours after a bloodborne pathogen exposure decreases the risk of conversion.
   5. Monogamous relationships provide the best defense from the virus.

   NCLEX Client Need: Physiological Integrity: Physiological Adaptation
4. In determining the optimal therapy for a patient infected with HIV, what would you consider in developing a nursing care plan? *(Place in order of priority.)*
   1. Clinical data
   2. Compliance with therapy
   3. Medication tolerance
   4. Support system
   5. Patient expectations

   NCLEX Client Need: Health Promotion and Maintenance
5. A nurse is reviewing medication orders for a female patient with SLE who is positive for the presence of antiphospholipid antibodies. You would seek clarification from the health care provider about which type of medication?
   1. Oral contraceptives
   2. Hydroxychloroquine (antimalarial)
   3. Glucocorticoid medication
   4. NSAID

   NCLEX Client Need: Physiological Integrity: Pharmacological Therapy
6. A patient has the medical diagnosis of fibromyalgia. Which nursing problem is the highest priority on this patient's care plan?
   1. Airway congestion
   2. Inability to comply with treatment regimen
   3. Chronic pain
   4. Potential for fluid imbalance

   NCLEX Client Need: Safe and Effective Care Environment: Coordinated Care
7. You admit an older adult man with NHL. On initial assessment, you note that the patient is slightly confused, is irritable, is emaciated, has poor dentition, and is homeless. What is the priority nursing problem?
   1. Potential for infection
   2. Lack of coping ability
   3. Alteration in body image
   4. Inadequate knowledge of disease process

   NCLEX Client Need: Safe and Effective Care Environment: Safety and Infection Control
8. A systemic autoimmune disease affects more than one type of body tissue or organ. Which would be considered systemic autoimmune disease(s)? *(Select all that apply.)*
   1. Hodgkin lymphoma
   2. Rheumatoid arthritis
   3. Systemic lupus erythematosus
   4. Goodpasture syndrome
   5. Primary lymphedema

   NCLEX Client Need: Physiological Integrity: Physiological Adaptation
9. What are the advantages of performing a RAST? *(Select all that apply.)*
   1. The patient does not have to refrain from taking antihistamine medications.
   2. It is safer for patients with serious heart and lung problems.
   3. There is no chance of experiencing an anaphylactic reaction because it is performed on the blood.
   4. It can be used on patients whose skin condition is too severe to perform skin testing.
   5. The results can be obtained within several hours.
   6. It has greater specificity for allergens than other tests.

   NCLEX Client Need: Physiological Integrity: Reduction of Risk Potential

10. A patient with an immune deficiency disorder is very susceptible to infection. Which intervention(s) would be used in the care of this patient? *(Select all that apply.)*
    1. All health care workers should perform scrupulous hand hygiene.
    2. The patient should be instructed on how to wear PPE.
    3. The patient is placed in contact isolation as soon as possible.
    4. Caregivers with any type of infection should not be assigned to the patient.
    5. A high-protein diet with nutritional supplements is encouraged.

    NCLEX Client Need: Safe and Effective Care Environment: Safety and Infection Control

Critical Thinking Questions

Scenario A

A nursing assistant was instructed to clean up equipment that was used in a bedside procedure. She accidentally sustains a needle stick while putting a used syringe into an overly filled sharps container in the room of an HIV-positive patient. The nursing assistant is crying hysterically and unable to act on her own behalf.

1. What should you do first?
2. Outline the steps of treatment and reporting for this type of incident.
3. What factors may have contributed to the accident?

Scenario B

Marilyn Jost, age 15, is highly allergic to penicillin and bee stings. The last time she experienced a reaction to a bee sting on her leg, the entire limb became swollen. Marilyn is active in the teen church group and frequently goes on camping trips. Her health care provider has suggested that she wear an identification bracelet stating her allergies and that she carry an emergency kit when she is on a camping trip. Her mother sees no need for these precautions because Marilyn is a perfectly healthy girl. Marilyn says she would not know what to do with the kit if she did get stung by a bee or wasp.

1. How would you explain to Marilyn and her mother the need for the identification bracelet and the kit?
2. How would you go about teaching Marilyn to use the emergency kit?

The Respiratory System

12

http://evolve.elsevier.com/deWit/medsurg

Objectives

Theory

1. Describe the structure and function of the respiratory system.
2. Analyze three causative factors related to disorders of the respiratory system.
3. Summarize nursing responsibilities for patients undergoing diagnostic tests and procedures for disorders of the respiratory system.
4. Provide instructions to patients on measures to prevent long-term problems of the respiratory system.

Clinical Practice

5. Employ proper techniques for assessing the respiratory system.
6. Verify that problem statements or nursing diagnoses chosen for patients with problems of the respiratory system are appropriate.
7. Propose interventions for a patient who has a problem with oxygenation.
8. Teach a patient about smoking cessation.

Key Terms

adventitious (ăd-vĕn-TĬ-shŭs, p. 273)
antitussive (ăn-tĭ-TŬS-ĭv, p. 275)
aphonia (ă-FŌ-nē-ă, p. 271)
apnea (ĂP-nē-ă, p. 266)
bradypnea (brăd-ĕp-NĒ-ă, p. 271)
compliance (kŏm-PLĪ-ăns, p. 266)
crackles (KRĂK-ŭlz, p. 273)
cyanosis (sī-ă-NŌ-sĭs, p. 271)
dyspnea (DĬSP-nē-ă, p. 270)
expectorate (ĕk-SPĔK-tō-rāt, p. 259)
hypercapnia (hī-pĕr-KĂP-nē-ă, p. 266)
hypocapnia (hī-pō-KĂP-nē-ă, p. 277)
hypoxemia (hĭ-pŏk-SĒ-mē-ă, p. 266)
hypoxia (hī-PŎK-sē-ă, p. 274)
kyphosis (kĭ-FŌ-sĭs, p. 266)
orthopnea (ŏr-thŏp-NĒ-ă, p. 272)
perfusion (pĕr-FŪ-zhŭn, p. 267)
sputum (SPŪ-tŭm, p. 271)
stridor (STRĪ-dŏr, p. 274)
tachypnea (tăk-ĭp-NĒ-ă, p. 271)
ventilation (vĕn-tĭ-LĀ-shŭn, p. 266)
wheezes (WĒZ-ĕz, p. 273)

Concepts Covered in This Chapter

- Gas Exchange
- Perfusion
- Fatigue
- Patient Education

OVERVIEW OF ANATOMY AND PHYSIOLOGY OF THE RESPIRATORY SYSTEM

FUNCTIONS OF THE STRUCTURES OF THE UPPER RESPIRATORY SYSTEM

- Air passes through the nose, mouth, pharynx, larynx, and trachea and then into the lungs (Fig. 12.1).
- The nasal cavity is lined with mucous membrane that warms and moistens the air as it passes through.
- The mucous membrane secretes mucus, which traps dust particles and bacteria.
- The **cilia** (small, hairlike projections) propel the mucus toward the larynx, so that the person can swallow or **expectorate** it (cough up and spit out).
- The paranasal sinuses (maxillary, frontal, sphenoid, and ethmoid) are air-filled cavities lined with mucous membrane and situated among the facial bones around the nasal cavity (Fig. 12.2).
- The sinuses reduce the weight of the skull, produce mucus, and influence voice quality.
- The pharynx, consisting of the nasopharynx, oropharynx, and laryngopharynx, is about 5 inches long and extends from the back of the mouth to the esophagus.
- The pharynx is a passageway for moving air to the lungs and food to the esophagus.

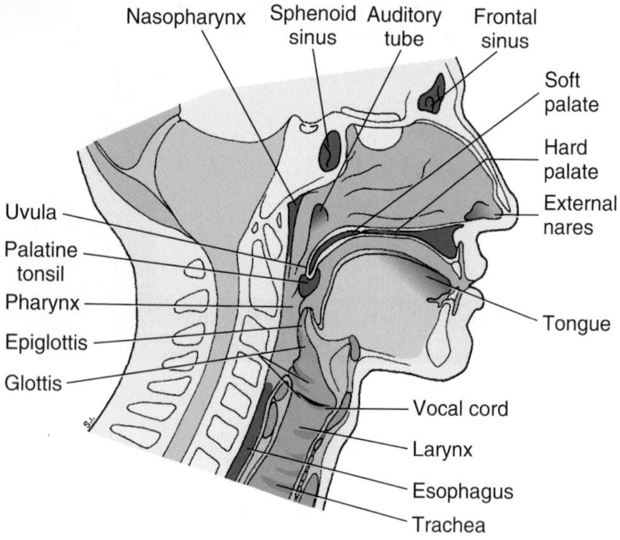

Fig. 12.1 Structures of the upper respiratory tract.

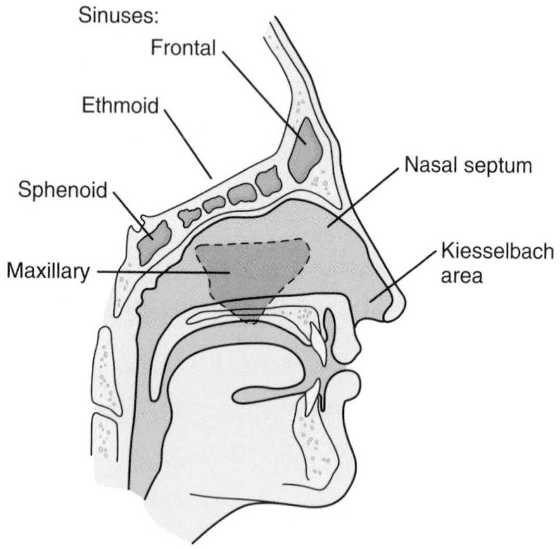

Fig. 12.2 The paranasal sinuses.

- The tonsils, which are part of the lymphatic system, are located in the oropharynx; the adenoids (also part of the lymphatic system) are located in the nasopharynx. If they become inflamed and enlarged, they may interfere with breathing. The epiglottis forms a hinged "door" at the entrance to the larynx.
- The larynx sits between the pharynx and the trachea. The vocal cords are located in the larynx.
- The trachea is made up of cartilage, smooth muscle, and connective tissue; is lined with mucous membrane; and extends from the larynx to the bronchi. It is the "windpipe" and carries air to the lungs.

Epiglottis Protection of the Airway

- When swallowing begins, the epiglottis closes over the larynx, preventing aspiration of food and secretions into the lungs. Food is then directed into the esophagus.
- When the swallowing reflex is weak or absent, aspiration is a risk.

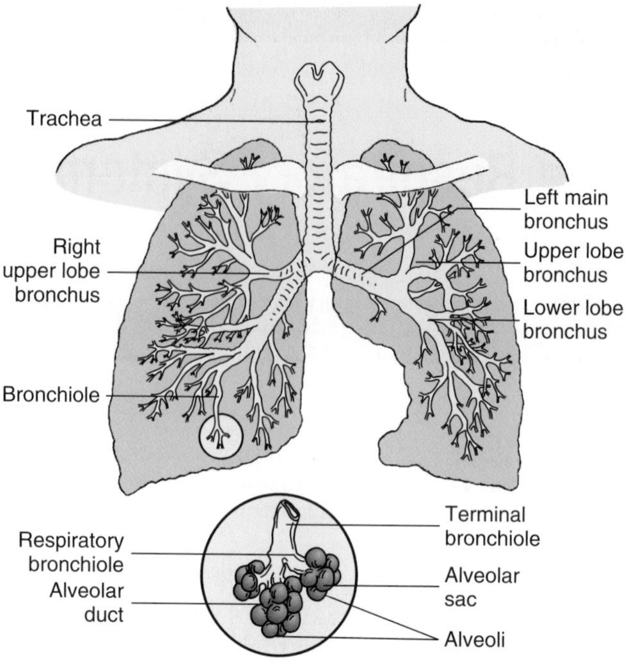

Fig. 12.3 Structures of the lower respiratory tract and alveoli.

Production of Speech in the Larynx

- The glottis is the space between the folds of the vocal cords, which are made up of mucous membrane attached to the front and back of the larynx.
- When air from the lungs exits through the larynx, it causes rapid opening and closing of the glottis. Movements of the mouth, lips, jaws, and tongue convert the sounds made by the rush of air through the glottis into speech sounds.

FUNCTIONS OF THE STRUCTURES OF THE LOWER RESPIRATORY SYSTEM

- On inhalation, after passing through the nose, pharynx, larynx, and trachea of the upper respiratory system, air enters the left and right bronchi, which branch off the trachea.
- The bronchi carry air into the lungs; the right lung has three lobes, and the left lung has two lobes.

Oxygen Delivery to the Alveolar Membrane for Diffusion Into the Blood

- The main bronchi divide into smaller and smaller bronchi and then divide into bronchioles that deliver the air to the alveoli (Fig. 12.3). The right bronchus has less of an angle than the left bronchus; inhaled foreign objects tend to go into the right bronchus.

Protection of the Lungs

- The **pleura** is a serous membrane of two layers. One layer, the visceral pleura, covers each lung, and the parietal pleura lines the inner wall of the chest cavity. These two layers make up the pleural sac, which encloses each lung and the chest wall and is an airtight compartment. **If the pleural sac is punctured, air will rush into the pleural cavity and collapse the lung.**

- The pleural cavity is a potential space between the pleural layers where there is normally only a small amount of fluid.
- This small amount of fluid between the two layers of pleura lubricates the pleural cavity and prevents friction between the pleural layers with inhalation and exhalation.
- The mucous membrane lining the many small branches of the bronchial tree contains tiny hairlike projections (cilia) that trap and propel small inhaled foreign particles toward the entrance of the respiratory tract; the cough reflex works to expel the secretions and particles.
- If the particles advance to the lungs, the alveoli contain macrophages that quickly destroy inhaled bacteria and other foreign particles.

CONTROL OF RESPIRATION

- The central nervous system controls both involuntary and voluntary respiration via the pons and the medulla. The vagus nerve supplies the pharynx, larynx, respiratory airways, and lungs.
- The brainstem chemoreceptors are sensitive to changes in carbon dioxide (CO_2) and hydrogen ions in the cerebrospinal fluid; the chemoreceptors in the aorta and the carotid arteries are sensitive to oxygen levels in the blood.
- The signals of changing levels of hydrogen ions (measured by pH), CO_2, and oxygen (O_2) trigger the respiratory center to send signals through the spinal cord and spinal nerves to the peripheral nervous system and to the phrenic and intercostal nerves that control the diaphragm and respiratory muscles.
- When CO_2 levels in the cerebrospinal fluid become higher than normal or the pH drops, the central receptors in the brainstem signal the nerves to initiate faster respiration to "blow off" the excess CO_2. Carbon dioxide levels give the primary signals for respiration.
- When arterial blood O_2 levels fall below normal, the respiratory centers in the aorta and carotid arteries signal the nerves to cause the lungs to inflate more fully, making the person breathe more deeply and at a faster rate.
- **When CO_2 levels are constantly high (as occurs with chronic lung disease such as emphysema), the body becomes accustomed to high CO_2 levels, and the respiratory drive is triggered by the receptors for low arterial O_2 instead of high levels of CO_2. Current research shows that CO_2 levels may rise if oxygen is administered, but this is *not* due to blunting of the hypoxic drive but to other vascular, ventilation, and perfusion changes. Oxygen must be given and titrated to maintain a pulse oximetry reading of 88% to 92%** (ABG normal values are listed in Table 12.1 under Arterial Blood Gas (ABG) Analysis.)

EFFECT OF THE BONES OF THE THORAX AND THE RESPIRATORY MUSCLES ON THE RESPIRATORY PROCESS

- Inspiration (inhalation) and expiration (exhalation) occur by movement of the diaphragm and the

Text continued on p. 266

Table 12.1 Diagnostic Tests for Respiratory Problems[a]

TEST/PURPOSE	DESCRIPTION	NURSING IMPLICATIONS
Pulse Oximetry (Spo_2)		
To noninvasively monitor arterial oxygen saturation (Sao_2)	Device attaches to earlobe, pinna of ear, or fingertip. Alternative placement with appropriate sensor: toe, forehead, bridge of nose.	Keep sensor intact on patient. Monitor and record Spo_2 readings.
To allow comparison of oxygenated hemoglobin to total hemoglobin	Sensor detects blood cells in capillaries using an infrared light source.	Report readings persistently below 95% to health care provider. Obstructions to blood flow, such as inflated BP cuff, peripheral artery disease, hypotension, or hypothermia, can cause false readings. Metallic nail polish and harsh ambient light also interfere with readings. Performed by the nurse at the bedside in home or clinic setting.
CO_2 Monitoring (Called Capnography When Equipment Displays a Waveform)		
To monitor adequacy of ventilation	Device can be part of an oxygen delivery system measuring end-tidal CO_2 ($ETCO_2$) or a skin sensor measuring transcutaneous CO_2 ($PtcCO_2$).	Make sure sensor is positioned properly to obtain readings. Explain the reason for the monitoring to the patient. Done at bedside by the nurse.
Sublingual CO_2 Level		
To detect early perfusion problems	Probe of handheld device is placed under the tongue.	Reading takes 60–90 s. Explain the procedure to the patient.

Continued

Table 12.1 Diagnostic Tests for Respiratory Problems—cont'd

TEST/PURPOSE	DESCRIPTION	NURSING IMPLICATIONS
Arterial Blood Gas (ABG) Analysis		
To determine whether there is adequate exchange of CO_2 and oxygen across alveolar membrane; to determine acid-base balance within the body; to determine hypoxemia	Useful for patients with respiratory disorders, problems of circulation and of blood distribution, body fluid imbalances, and acid-base imbalances.	Explain procedure to patient; arterial puncture is briefly painful. Apply firm pressure for 5–10 min after specimen is drawn. Compare laboratory results to normal values: pH: 7.35–7.45. Usually obtained by respiratory therapy or nursing personnel. In some states, phlebotomists need additional training to obtain arterial specimens.
	Arterial blood sample is drawn and tested for pH, PaO_2, $PaCO_2$, and HCO_3^-.	PaO_2: 80–100 mm Hg $PaCO_2$: 35–45 mm Hg HCO_3^-: 22–26 mm Hg
D-Dimer (Fibrin Split Products, Fibrin Degradation Products)		
To assess thrombin and plasmin activity	Blood test that provides assay of fibrin degradation.	No fasting is required.
Useful for assisting in the diagnosis of pulmonary embolism and disseminated intravascular coagulation (DIC)		Collect a venous blood sample in a light blue–top tube.
CBC		
To identify adequacy of hemoglobin to carry oxygen and to determine whether an infection is present	Provides information on red blood cells and the body's immune response.	Collect a venous blood sample in a lavender-top tube. Performed by the nurse or phlebotomist at the bedside in home or clinic setting.
Sputum Analysis		
To examine sputum from lower respiratory tract for bacteria, bacilli, or malignant cells; to determine color, consistency, and sensitivity of bacteria to specific antibiotics	Sputum specimen is examined and cultured for bacteria; acid-fast stain and Gram stain are done for tuberculosis bacillus; cytologic studies may be done to search for malignant cells. If bacteria are present, sensitivity studies to antibiotics are performed. Nucleic acid amplification can detect *Mycobacterium tuberculosis* earlier than culture and should be interpreted in correlation with acid-fast results.	Explain that specimen is desired from lower areas of lungs; may require respiratory therapy to obtain proper specimen or coaching in proper coughing technique. Best specimen is obtained in morning before eating or mouth care. Provide mouth care after obtaining specimen. Specimen is expectorated into sterile container.
Pulmonary Function Tests (PFTs)		
To determine integrity of mechanical function and gas exchange function of the lungs: volume of air lung can hold; rate of flow of air in and out of the lung; and elasticity, or compliance, of lung Bedside testing of pulmonary function	Patient breathes in as much air as possible and then breathes out as much air as possible into a spirometer, indicating the forced vital capacity (FVC); forced expiratory volume in 1 s (FEV_1) is measured. Other measurements include total lung capacity (TLC), vital capacity (VC), tidal volume (TV), functional residual capacity (FRC), and residual volume (RV). Slow vital capacity (SVC), forced vital capacity (FVC), peak expiratory flow rate (PEFR, PF), and maximum inspiratory pressure (MIP) *or* negative inspiratory force (NIF) are components of a bedside PFT.	Should not be done within 1–2 h of eating. No smoking for 4–6 h before test. Patient is not to take any drugs causing sedation. Patient may be instructed to stop bronchodilator and corticosteroid medications before the procedure. Explain procedure to patient. *Post test:* Monitor vital signs and allow patient to rest because test can be fatiguing. Some of the readings can be obtained at the bedside for an inpatient. Most full studies are done in a pulmonary function laboratory as an outpatient procedure. Spirometry measurements can be done at the bedside of a patient able to follow instructions.

Table 12.1 Diagnostic Tests for Respiratory Problems—cont'd

TEST/PURPOSE	DESCRIPTION	NURSING IMPLICATIONS
Chest Radiograph (X-Ray)		
To determine pathologic conditions in the lungs, such as pneumonia, lung abscess, tuberculosis, atelectasis, pneumothorax, and tumor; also gives indication of heart size and any abnormalities of bony structures	Front, back, and lateral views may be taken; fluoroscopy may be used to visualize lung and diaphragm movement.	For outpatient procedures, tell patient to remove clothes down to the waist and put on gown provided so that it ties in back. Will be asked to take a deep breath and hold it while the radiograph is taken. Portable x-rays can be taken when the patient is unable to stand or be transported to the stationary x-ray equipment.
Chest Computed Tomography (CT)		
To visualize the organs and tissues of the chest, looking for injury, abnormalities, or disease such as tumors and blood clots	A series of images are taken by x-ray and analyzed by the computer, producing longitudinal and cross-sectional views. High-resolution CT, which shows more detail, may be used. Helical CT can produce 3D images.	Patient must be able to lie flat and still for several minutes. Must be done in the imaging department. Provide information about the test.
	Contrast agent may be used.	Check for sensitivity to iodine, shellfish, or the specific contrast medium. Check renal function with creatinine level.
CT Fluoroscopy		
Used to assist with timing of helical scanning and for interventional procedures	Continuous imaging is done to guide therapy.	Same as for CT scan.
CT Angiography		
Used to assess blood flow through the lungs	Contrast is injected venously, and blood flow deficits are identified.	Same as for CT scan with contrast.
Positron Emission Tomography (PET) Scan		
A nuclear medicine procedure that evaluates the metabolism of tissues; used to identify cancerous growths and to follow the treatment	Glucose molecules are combined with a radioactive tracer. Rapidly dividing cells take up the glucose for fuel; the tracer allows for imaging of the tissue. Tracers may be attached to other molecules depending on what imaging is desired.	PET scans can be combined with CT. Notify the provider if the patient is allergic to iodine, aspartame, or saccharin. No caffeine, alcohol, or tobacco within 24 hours of the procedure.
Magnetic Resonance Imaging (MRI)		
Used primarily to assess abnormal masses, chest wall, heart, and blood vessels	Does not use radiation to obtain images. Uses a very strong magnetic field, electric field gradients, and radio waves to generate an image. The primary effect is on hydrogen ions. Most of the hydrogen ions in the body are in H_2O. MRI is a better imaging technique for soft tissues (organs) since they are made up mostly of water.	MRI is contraindicated for patients with metal implants due to the strong magnetic field. Check with the implanting physician or the patient literature regarding safety for MRI. Pacemakers and other implanted devices can be MRI compatible.
Ultrasound		
To identify fluid in the pleural space or for needle guidance when performing a thoracentesis	Ultrasound technology is used for imaging the chest cavity.	No special prep. Can be done at bedside.

Continued

Table 12.1 Diagnostic Tests for Respiratory Problems—cont'd

TEST/PURPOSE	DESCRIPTION	NURSING IMPLICATIONS
Lung Ventilation and Perfusion Scan (V-Q Scan)		
Nuclear medicine procedure to assess lung ventilation and lung perfusion; to locate pulmonary embolism and diagnose tumor, emphysema, bronchiectasis, or fibrosis; CT angiography has replaced the V-Q scan for diagnosing pulmonary embolus	*Perfusion scan:* An IV injection of radionuclide-tagged, macroaggregated albumin is given; decreased blood flow to any part of the lung is shown by decreased radioactivity in that area. *Ventilation scan:* Radioactive gas is inhaled and, when scanned, presents a pattern of ventilation in the lungs.	Assess for allergies. Ask patient to remove all metal jewelry from around the neck. Assure patient that amount of radioactivity used is very small and is not harmful. An IV access will be inserted. Patient will be asked to hold breath for a short period for the ventilation scan.
Pulmonary Angiography		
To visualize pulmonary vasculature; to locate abnormalities	Radiopaque contrast agent is injected via a venous catheter into the right side of the heart or the pulmonary artery. Radiographs are taken; fluoroscopy is used.	Check consent form. Assess for allergy to dye. Explain that patient may feel warm flush as contrast is injected. The test will be done in a special procedure room in the imaging department by a physician. *Post test:* Monitor vital signs and check dressing for signs of bleeding. The femoral vein is used for access, so bleeding is not as common as with arterial access. If procedural sedation was used, monitor patient per policy.
Bronchoscopy		
To inspect bronchi; to remove foreign objects or mucous plugs; to biopsy lesions	Preoperative sedation may be given. Throat is sprayed with local anesthetic and/or the patient is asked to gargle with topical anesthetic agents. With neck hyperextended, a flexible fiberoptic bronchoscope is guided into bronchi; biopsies are taken if needed, bronchial washings may be done, and debris is suctioned. Oxygen is administered; a patent IV line is necessary in case emergency drugs are needed and for administration of procedural sedation.	Keep patient NPO for 6 h before test. IV access is initiated. Check consent form; administer preoperative sedative. Give mouth care just before test. *Post test:* For 2–4 h, monitor vital signs, pulse oximetry readings, and level of consciousness. Observe for bleeding, dyspnea, wheezing, discomfort, and swelling of face and neck; sputum may be slightly blood-tinged at first. Position patient on side until gag reflex has returned. Check for return of gag reflex by having patient take small sips of water. When gag reflex has returned, the patient may eat. The procedure must be performed in a negative airflow room with HEPA filtration. All personnel in the room must use personal protective equipment appropriate to airborne precautions. Procedural sedation should be administered only by a nurse credentialed to do so. The procedure is performed by a physician usually with assistance from respiratory therapy.
Laryngoscopy		
Direct: To detect or remove lesions, polyps, or foreign bodies in the larynx or to obtain biopsy specimens or tissue for culture	*Direct:* A fiberoptic laryngoscope is used; sedation and local or general anesthetic are administered. Performed by a physician in a surgical facility.	*Direct:* Patient should be NPO for several hours before procedure. Administer preprocedure medications; ensure that respiratory status will be monitored closely. Advise that the room will be darkened. An ice collar may be applied post procedure. A mild sore throat and hoarseness may occur.

Table 12.1 Diagnostic Tests for Respiratory Problems—cont'd

TEST/PURPOSE	DESCRIPTION	NURSING IMPLICATIONS
Indirect: To assess function of the vocal cords or to obtain tissue for biopsy	*Indirect:* A laryngeal mirror, head mirror, and light source are used. Inspection is performed at rest and during phonation. Performed by a physician. Can be done in an office or clinic setting.	*Indirect:* Patient will be upright for procedure. *Post procedure:* Keep patient NPO until gag reflex has returned. Encourage fluid intake.
Mediastinoscopy		
To inspect the mediastinum and biopsy mediastinal lymph nodes To gain information from biopsies about lung metastasis, sarcoidosis, and granulomatous infections	Mediastinoscope is inserted via a small incision made at the suprasternal notch by a physician in an operating room.	Informed consent is required. Preoperative and postoperative care are the same as for other surgeries. The patient remains NPO after midnight the night before a morning procedure. Administer preoperative sedation before the procedure. *Post procedure:* Observe for crepitus around insertion site indicating air from pneumothorax. Observe for distended veins and pulsus paradoxus because a hematoma may be preventing cardiac filling (cardiac tamponade).
Thoracentesis		
To remove pleural fluid, instill medication, or obtain fluid for diagnostic studies	With local anesthetic and ultrasound guidance, a large-bore needle is inserted through the chest wall into the pleural space, and fluid is withdrawn with a syringe or into vacuum bottles by a physician at the patient's bedside. Aseptic technique must be used. Specimens are obtained for culture, microscopic examination, and stains. Medication may be instilled.	Requires signed consent. Explain procedure to patient. Take baseline vital signs. Position patient sitting, facing side of bed, and leaning over the overbed table with arms crossed on it; pillows or the back of a chair can also be used. Monitor respirations and skin color during procedure. Assist patient to remain still. Chest radiograph may be ordered after procedure. Monitor vital signs q15min for 1 h or until stable, then routinely. Auscultate breath sounds frequently. Rapid breathing, cyanosis, hemoptysis, changes in breath sounds, and tachycardia should be reported immediately. Chart amount and appearance of fluid and condition of patient. Send specimens to the laboratory as ordered.

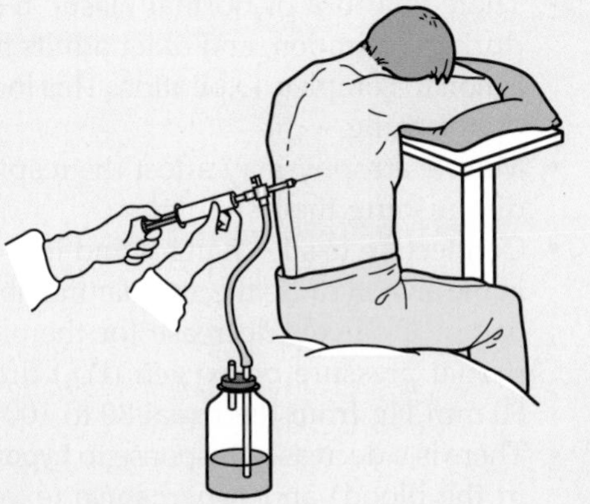

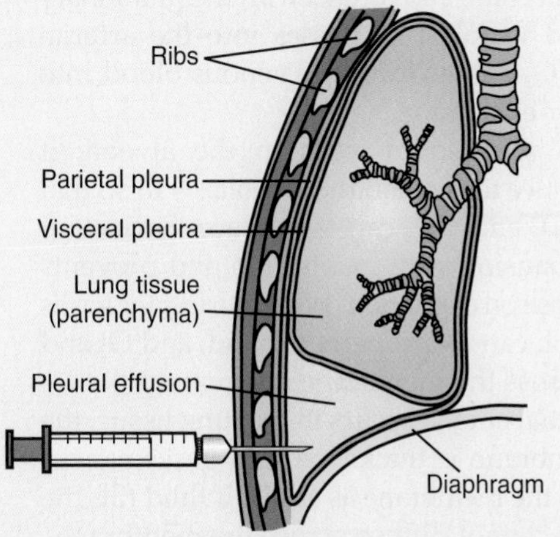

[a]For tuberculosis test, refer to Chapter 14.

3D, Three-dimensional; *BP,* blood pressure; *CBC,* complete blood cell count; CO_2, carbon dioxide; H_2O, water; HCO_3^-, bicarbonate ion; *HEPA,* high-efficiency particulate arresting; *IV,* intravenous; *NPO,* nothing by mouth; $PaCO_2$, partial pressure of arterial carbon dioxide; PaO_2, partial pressure of arterial oxygen.

intercostal muscles in the chest wall. During normal breathing, about 500 mL of air moves in and out of the lungs with each breath. The diaphragm is the primary respiratory muscle.

- When the diaphragm contracts, it moves downward; the other chest muscles contract, pulling the rib cage up and out, expanding the lungs and creating an area of negative pressure. Air from the atmosphere, which has a positive pressure, flows into the lungs.
- When the muscles relax, the rib cage moves back to its normal position, and the lungs return to a resting position, causing air to be passively pushed out in exhalation.
- **If damage to the spinal cord occurs above the level where the phrenic nerve branches off to control the diaphragm (C4), voluntary respiration ceases.**
- If the muscles of the diaphragm and chest (intercostals) are paralyzed, **apnea** (absence of breathing) occurs.
- The thoracic cage—composed of the thoracic vertebrae, the sternum, and the ribs—forms a stable unit that allows the respiratory muscles to function correctly. If any bones of the thorax or chest wall are injured or fractured, breathing can be affected. **Compliance** describes the elasticity of the lungs or how easily the lungs inflate; when compliance is decreased, the lungs are more difficult to inflate. Chronic obstructive pulmonary disease (COPD) and aging alter compliance because of damage in the alveoli.
- **Weakness of the respiratory muscles, such as occurs with neuromuscular diseases, also causes decreased respiratory ability.**
- **Kyphosis** (inward curvature and collapse) of the spine constricts the thoracic cavity and restricts the capacity of the lungs to expand fully.

FACTORS THAT AFFECT THE EXCHANGE OF OXYGEN AND CARBON DIOXIDE

- Alveoli are tiny air sacs covered with a permeable membrane that come into contact with the pulmonary arterioles and venules; O_2 passes into the arterial blood, and CO_2 passes from the venous blood into the alveoli for exhalation.
- Surfactant is secreted by cells in the alveoli; it decreases surface tension on the alveolar wall so that diffusion of O_2 and CO_2 can take place. Surfactant facilitates expansion with inspiration and prevents alveolar collapse on expiration. When surfactant levels are low, alveoli cannot properly expand, and O_2 and CO_2 cannot cross the membrane adequately.
- When interstitial edema occurs in the lung tissue, the alveolar membrane is thickened and gases cannot diffuse across the membrane as easily. If fluid fills the alveoli, gases cannot diffuse across the membrane.
- Edema in the lungs occurs with infectious processes such as pneumonia and in disorders such as congestive heart failure.
- The major portion of the O_2 (about 97%) attaches to the heme portion of the hemoglobin molecule carried by the **erythrocytes** (red blood cells) and forms **oxyhemoglobin**. The plasma also transports a portion of each gas; about 3% of O_2 is dissolved in the plasma.
- CO_2, a cellular waste product, combines with water, forming carbonic acid (H_2CO_3); **dissociation** (uncombining) occurs, forming hydrogen ions and bicarbonate ions. About 77% of CO_2 is transported in the blood plasma in the form of bicarbonate ions. The remaining 23% of CO_2 combines with hemoglobin and is carried to the lungs. In the lung, the process reverses and the bicarbonate ions combine with hydrogen ions to form carbonic acid, which then dissociates into water and CO_2. The CO_2 diffuses across the alveolar membrane and is exhaled. The ability of the lungs to acquire oxygen is measured clinically by pulse oximetry (Spo_2). The ability of the lungs and chest to move air in and out of the body is called **ventilation** and is clinically measured by end-tidal CO_2 ($ETCO_2$ or capnography).

EFFECTS OF AGING ON THE RESPIRATORY SYSTEM

- The decrease in the immune system's efficiency makes older adults more susceptible to upper respiratory infections.
- Aging results in a decreased cough reflex and an increased potential for aspiration.
- Osteoporosis may cause kyphosis, which impinges on lung expansion.
- Adults age 70 years and older have some degree of change in connective tissue that causes decreased elasticity and affects lung function and ventilation.
- Total body water decreases to 50% after age 70 years; thus mucous and respiratory membranes are not as moist, and mucus becomes much thicker.
- There is some impairment of the ciliary action, which makes it more difficult for older adults to remove mucus, and retained mucus provides a breeding ground for bacterial infection.
- There is a loss of normal elastic recoil of the lung during expiration, and older adults must use muscle action to complete expiration. This increases the work of breathing.
- Muscle atrophy may affect the respiratory muscles, diminishing their strength.
- Connective tissue changes and loss of elastic tissue in the alveoli cause the alveolar membranes to become baggy. O_2 levels decrease for the older adult, with partial pressure of oxygen (Po_2) dropping to 75 to 80 mm Hg from the usual 80 to 100 mm Hg.
- There is a decreased response to **hypoxemia** (O_2 deficit in the blood) and **hypercapnia** (excessive amounts of CO_2 in the blood).

CAUSES OF RESPIRATORY DISORDERS

Trauma or disease can affect structures of the respiratory system, nerves controlling respiration, or diffusion of

Box 12.1 Terms Commonly Used in Respiratory Care

- *Diffusion:* The movement of oxygen and carbon dioxide across the alveolar-capillary membrane. It takes place between the gas in the alveolar spaces and the blood in the pulmonary capillaries.
- *Elastance:* The extent to which the lungs are able to return to their original position after being stretched or distended.
- *Hypoxemia:* Deficient oxygenation of the blood. Clinically measured by Spo_2.
- *Hypoxia:* A broad term referring to diminished availability of oxygen to the body tissues.
- *Lung compliance:* The ability of the lungs to distend in response to changes in volume and pressure of inhaled air. Lung compliance first increases and then decreases with age as the lungs become stiffer and the chest wall more rigid.
- *Perfusion:* The delivery of fluid through the blood vessels to body tissues.
- *Pulmonary hygiene:* Methods used to clear secretions from the airways.
- *Resistance:* The force working against the passage of air. The major determinant is the radius of the airway.
- *Respiratory failure:* An abnormality of gas exchange with either an excess of carbon dioxide or a deficit of oxygen, or both.
- *Shunting:* Intrapulmonary shunting is the diverting of blood so that it does not take part in the gas exchange at the alveolar sites. When intrapulmonary shunting occurs, blood enters the left side of the heart without being oxygenated. It is therefore a possible cause of hypoxemia.
- *Surfactant:* A complex lipoprotein produced by cells lining the alveoli, which lowers surface tension within the alveoli. It prevents collapse of the lung by stabilizing the alveoli and decreasing capillary pressures.
- *Ventilation:* The movement of air from the external environment to the gas exchange units of the lung and back to the environment. It can be spontaneous or done by a mechanical ventilator. Clinically measured by CO_2.

O_2 or CO_2 across the alveolar membranes. **Perfusion** (blood flow into cellular tissue) is essential to provide oxygen to the cells of the body. Blood must flow past the alveolar membrane for *diffusion* (Box 12.1) of O_2 and CO_2 to take place. Cardiac disease, emboli, and other disorders of the heart and pulmonary blood vessels may cause problems in the respiratory system.

The respiratory system is particularly susceptible to harmful substances in the environment. Inhalation of bacteria and other organisms can quickly produce an infection in either the upper or the lower respiratory tract. Tobacco smoke, allergens, poisonous gases, and other toxic substances cause irritation and inflammation of the air passages and can lead to chronic inflammation, obstructive diseases, and tumors. There may be a familial tendency related to sensitivity to these toxins, which may result in asthma and other lung problems.

Box 12.2 Factors That Increase Risk for Respiratory Infection

- Age older than 65 years
- Cigarette smoking
- Residing in an extended care facility
- Chronic respiratory disorders (includes asthma)
- Congenital or chronic cardiovascular disorders
- Chronic renal disease
- Diabetes mellitus or a chronic metabolic disorder
- Compromised immune response

There are two major types of ventilatory diseases: *restrictive* and *obstructive*. **Restrictive diseases are characterized by decreased lung capacity or compliance.** The expansion of the lung and chest wall is limited either by abnormalities in the bony structures **or by inability of the lung tissue to expand.** Arthritis increases stiffness of the chest wall and results in a decreased ability of the chest cavity to expand and contract. Scoliosis and kyphosis decrease the size of the chest cavity. **Pneumothorax** (collapsed lung) diminishes lung surface; neuromuscular disorders weaken the strength of the muscles of respiration (e.g., myasthenia gravis), and disorders of the lung (e.g., pneumonia, atelectasis, and fibrosis) increase stiffness and decrease lung volume.

Obstructive pulmonary diseases are characterized by problems moving air into and out of the lungs. Narrowing of the openings in the tracheobronchial tree increases resistance to the flow of air, making it difficult for O_2 to enter and contributing to air trapping; therefore exhalation is also difficult. Asthma, emphysema, and chronic bronchitis are examples of obstructive lung diseases. Tumors in the lung can also obstruct airflow to the alveoli.

RESPIRATORY DISORDERS

PREVENTION

The best ways to prevent infection and inflammation of the respiratory system are to practice hand hygiene frequently; stay out of crowds, especially during cold and flu season; refrain from smoking; avoid known allergens as much as possible; maintain adequate nutrition; and obtain sufficient rest to help keep the immune system healthy. Nurses should identify persons who have a high risk for infection (Box 12.2) and refer them for appropriate vaccinations or teaching.

Allergy to airborne substances causes the mucous membranes of the nose and sinuses to become irritated and inflamed. When these membranes are inflamed, bacteria and viruses can more easily invade the cells and cause infection. By controlling inhaled allergens, the incidence of upper respiratory infection (URI) can be decreased.

Older Adult Care Points

Older adults do not acquire upper respiratory infections more frequently than other age groups, but due to a decreased immune system response and chronic illness they more frequently have complications.

Elimination of widespread respiratory diseases such as the common cold and influenza is not possible; therefore nurses must practice good hand hygiene and use Standard Precautions and airborne or droplet precautions when working with patients with respiratory infections as per the Centers for Disease Control and Prevention (CDC) guidelines. For certain groups such as older adults and the chronically ill, immunization against influenza and pneumonia is an effective means of reducing the incidence of respiratory disease. Health care providers, nurses, and others involved in providing health care should also be immunized. Among the more serious reactions to influenza vaccine are allergic reactions, fever, malaise, or muscle soreness. Current research indicates that in rare occasions influenza vaccinations may increase the risk for Guillain-Barré syndrome (CDC, 2017). This immune-mediated disorder occurs in about 1 in 100,000 individuals. The incidence of Guillain-Barré syndrome has been noted to be higher in the patient population that had influenza than in the group that just received the vaccine, so vaccination is recommended. The vaccine is prepared from chicken embryos, therefore screening patients for egg allergy is important; nonegg formulations are available. One of the most important preventive measures of lung tissue injury is avoiding prolonged and repeated inhalation of irritating substances. Such substances include tobacco smoke (first or second hand), industrial gases, coal dust, particulates from agricultural activities, soot and other carbons, and air polluted by automobile exhaust. *Healthy People 2030* goals include addressing outdoor air quality as well as reducing "illness, disability and death related to tobacco use and secondhand smoke exposure." Smoking cessation efforts are supported by increasing insurance coverage for evidence-based interventions, increasing smoke-free environments, and strengthening tobacco laws. The Joint Commission has developed Core Measures for the assessment and treatment of tobacco use. Nurses participate by identifying patients at risk for tobacco-related disease and encouraging cessation programs.

Think Critically

Identify three changes in lifestyle that might prevent you or a family member from developing a chronic or serious respiratory disorder.

DIAGNOSTIC TESTS AND PROCEDURES

Table 12.1 presents the most common diagnostic tests performed for problems of the respiratory system. A complete blood cell count with hemoglobin and hematocrit

Health Promotion

Smoking and Tobacco Cessation

The Agency for Healthcare Research and Quality (AHRQ, 2018) provides a guide for clinicians that states the following: There are "five **A**s" for helping your patients to quit smoking: **Ask** about tobacco use. **Advise** about the health benefits of quitting. **Assess** readiness to quit. **Assist** in creating a cessation plan. **Arrange** follow-up. For those patients who are resistant to the five **A**s model, an alternative model is the "Five Rights." Help the patient identify the personal **Relevance, Risks, Rewards,** and **Roadblocks,** and **Repeat** these at every visit. Other toolkits and strategies are available on the AHRQ website.

determinations is done to detect any deficiency in the oxygen-carrying capacity of the blood. An elevated white blood cell count may indicate the presence of infection. Anterior-posterior and lateral chest radiographs are usually ordered when the patient has a lower respiratory tract problem that does not resolve quickly.

Diagnostic Visual Examination of the Nose, Mouth, and Throat

The interior of the nose, mouth, and pharynx and the tonsils can be inspected using a tongue blade and a good source of light. The nose is inspected for redness, swelling, discharge, and lumps. Using a nasal speculum, the head is tilted upward, and the inside of the nares is inspected for pallor, redness, swelling, and polyps and for mucus color, consistency, odor, and amount. The hard and soft palates are inspected, and the mobility of the soft palate is evaluated by asking the patient to say "ah." The pharynx can be brought into view by asking the patient to say "ee." Presence of inflammation, lesions, plaques, or exudates is noted. The paranasal sinuses are assessed by observing for purulent discharge in the nares and by palpating over the sinus areas for tenderness. Sometimes sinus radiographs are ordered. Magnetic resonance imaging may be ordered to locate tumors and pathologic abnormalities of the esophagus and larynx.

Throat Culture

The most common reason for culturing pharyngeal secretions is to establish a definitive diagnosis of infection with *Streptococcus pyogenes* (strep throat). Rheumatic heart disease and glomerulonephritis can result if strep throat is not properly identified and treated. A "rapid strep test" is commonly performed in the health care provider's office or ambulatory clinic. A throat culture also is sometimes taken to establish a diagnosis of pneumonia, tonsillitis, meningitis, or whooping cough. These diseases can be particularly harmful to older adults, the debilitated, or very young patients.

Tuberculosis Tests

Sputum testing for acid-fast bacilli is ordered when tuberculosis (TB) is suspected. Sputum specimens should be collected just after the patient awakens in the morning. Ideally a total of three specimens on 3 consecutive days should be collected. Suctioning may be required to obtain the specimen. Airborne isolation precautions should be used until TB has been ruled out. Some strains of TB are resistant to conventional drug therapies. A test for TB drug susceptibility called *microscopic observation drug susceptibility (MODS)* assay can produce results more rapidly and for less cost than standard cultures (Sertel Şelale & Uzun, 2018). Current technology allows for molecular detection of drug resistance (MDDR), which examines TB DNA sequencing. In 2018 whole genome sequencing (WGS) began, allowing for identification of new strains of TB (CDC, 2017). A blood test has replaced the tuberculin skin test used for TB screening in many settings. The test identifies T-cell response to the TB antigens. Like the skin test, this test only identifies the activation of the body's immune response to the TB organism and does not distinguish between active and latent disease (CDC, 2017).

Lung Function Tests

Pulmonary function tests (PFTs) are useful in screening gross abnormalities in the respiratory system. Complete testing includes measurement of various volumes, flows, resistance, muscle strength, and arterial blood gases. This testing is usually done as an outpatient. There are multiple ways to obtain the various reading; some are directly measured, and some are calculated (Table 12.2). Bedside spirometry testing is also done with portable equipment and at minimum includes *forced vital capacity (FVC)* and *forced expiratory volume in 1 second* (FEV_1).

The results of pulmonary function tests are listed in Table 12.2. Fig. 12.4 shows the various subdivisions of total lung capacity.

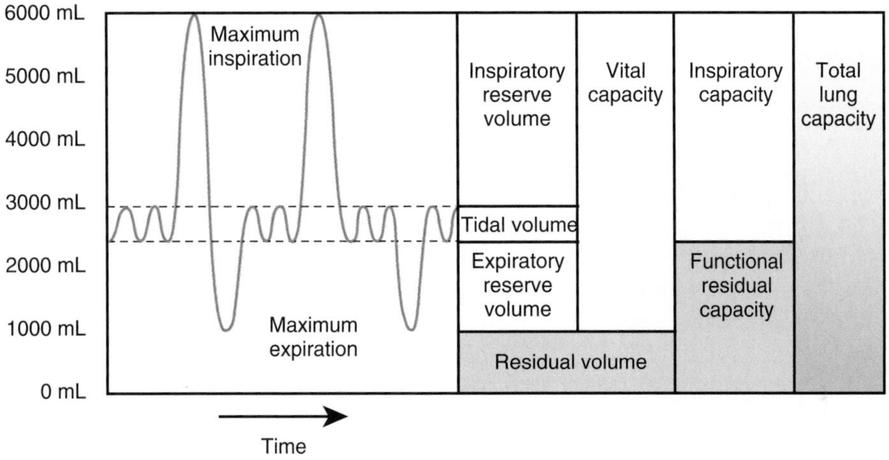

Fig. 12.4 Comparison of respiratory volumes and capacities as measured by spirometry. (Volumes can vary by age, gender, height, or weight.)

Table 12.2 Clinical Application of Pulmonary Function Testing

TERMINOLOGY	DEFINITION	CLINICAL IMPLICATIONS
Forced vital capacity (FVC)	Maximum amount of air forcefully inspired or exhaled	Affected by diseases that restrict airflow. Is used to identify reversible airway obstruction.
Forced expiratory volume in 1 s (FEV_1) (In complete testing, FEV is measured at 0.5, 1, 3, and 6 s.)	Volume forcefully expired in the first second after a full inspiration	Gives an estimate of how quickly the lungs empty. Helpful pre and post administration of bronchodilators to evaluate effect.
FEV_1/FVC	Calculation from FVC and FEV_1	Gives an indication of any airflow limitations.
Vital capacity (VC)	Volume of gas measured from a slow, complete expiration without force after a maximal inspiration	Decreases may be associated with respiratory muscle weakness or restrictive lung and chest wall diseases.
Total lung capacity (TLC)	The volume of gas the lung can hold at the end of a maximal inspiration	Obstructive lung diseases show a normal or increased TLC; restrictive diseases show a decrease in TLC.
Tidal volume (TV)	The volume of gas either inspired or exhaled during each normal breath	Decreased in restrictive and neuromuscular diseases.

Continued

Table 12.2 Clinical Application of Pulmonary Function Testing—cont'd

TERMINOLOGY	DEFINITION	CLINICAL IMPLICATIONS
Functional residual capacity (FRC)	The volume of gas remaining in the lungs after a quiet breath	Volume is usually reduced in obese individuals.
Residual volume (RV)	The volume of gas remaining in the lungs after a maximal expiration	Increased in COPD.
Inspiratory reserve volume (IRV)	Maximum amount of additional air that can be inspired at the end of a normal inspiration	Increases with exercise.
Expiratory reserve volume (ERV)	The maximum amount of additional air that can be exhaled at the end of normal expiration	ERV/VC ratio is calculated. High ratios suggest stiff lungs, and low ratios could mean increased resistance such as in asthma.
Maximum inspiratory pressure (MIP), also called negative inspiratory force (NIF)	Pressure generated by inhaling as strongly as possible against a completely occluded mouthpiece	Diminished in diseases affecting respiratory muscles.
Peak expiratory flow rate (PEFR)	Flow rate of exhalation is measured during forceful expiration starting with full lung inflation	Useful in monitoring status of patients with COPD and asthma.

COPD, Chronic obstructive pulmonary disease.

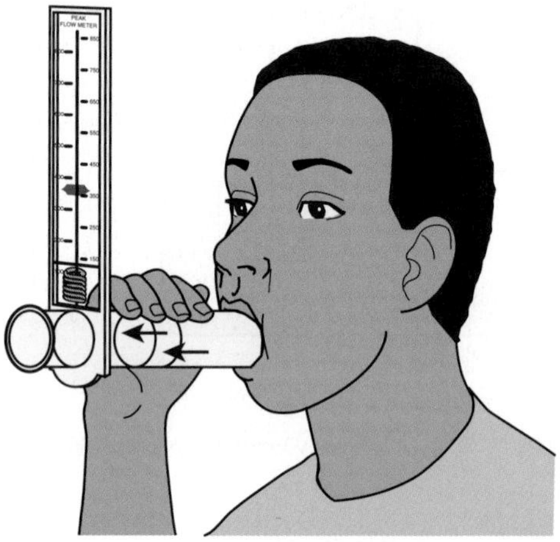

Fig. 12.5 Use of a peak flowmeter to measure peak expiratory flow volume.

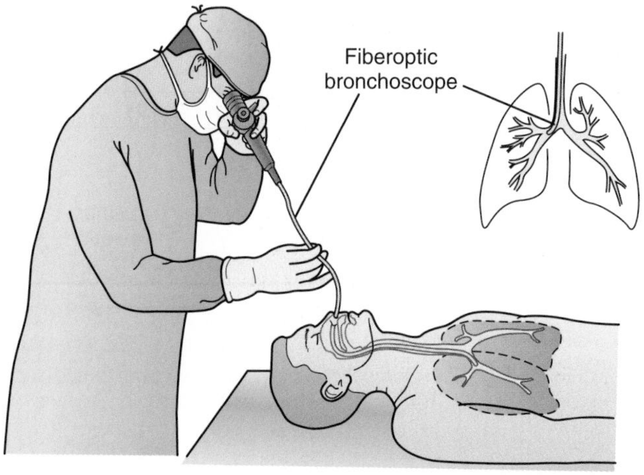

Fig. 12.6 Fiberoptic bronchoscopy.

Peak Flowmeter

Patients with asthma or COPD are often asked to check their peak expiratory flow with the use of a peak flowmeter (Fig. 12.5). Normal peak flow values for adults are based on age, gender, height, and underlying lung disorder. Normal values range from 300 to 700 L/min but are assessed by comparison against a patient's baseline values. While standing or sitting upright, the patient exhales into the mouthpiece; a small arrow points to the maximum expiratory flow volume. The peak flowmeter is useful for knowing when additional medications are needed to prevent acute exacerbation of disease.

Lung Biopsy

When tumor is suspected, a lung biopsy may be obtained by bronchoscopy (Fig. 12.6) or using a thoracoscopic approach or open thoracotomy. Postprocedure care includes observing sputum for blood and monitoring vital signs closely. Nothing is given by mouth until the gag reflex returns. A surgical biopsy will require the usual postoperative care, including monitoring for bleeding, shortness of breath, and infection.

❖ NURSING MANAGEMENT

◆ ASSESSMENT (DATA COLLECTION)

History Taking

Observe respiratory function while you are talking with the patient and ask about frequency of URIs, known inhalant allergies, and sinus problems. If the patient is in obvious respiratory distress or complains of **dyspnea** (difficult breathing), ask only a few questions about the present illness and chief complaint. Later, during a formal admission interview and informal discussions with the patient and family, obtain more information to plan individualized nursing care.

Chest pain can occur with frequent coughing, pleurisy, or trauma to the lungs; however, whenever there is a complaint of chest pain, seek additional information and always consider cardiac problems. Patients with sinus problems may complain of headache, malaise, a bad taste in the mouth, nasal congestion or obstruction, purulent drainage from the nose, and painful upper teeth. Those with pharyngitis often report a sore or "scratchy" throat, malaise, headache, and sometimes a cough. Dysphagia also might be a problem for patients with pharyngitis because swallowing involves pushing the food back against the inflamed oropharynx. **Hoarseness and loss of the voice (aphonia) are common symptoms of laryngitis.** Hoarseness or a sore throat that lasts longer than 2 weeks should be noted because this may assist in the early detection of throat malignancy.

Focused Assessment

Data Collection for the Respiratory System

HISTORY TAKING

- Chief complaint and precipitating factors
- New onset of dyspnea or orthopnea
- Cough frequency with or without sputum production
- Measures used for symptom relief
- Medications, over-the-counter medicines, supplement use
- Personal smoking history, family smoking history
- History of respiratory disorders, such as asthma
- History of allergy or hay fever
- History of conditions such as sinusitis or bronchitis
- History of night sweats or tuberculosis
- History of other lung diseases, injuries, or surgeries
- History of alcohol consumption
- Occupational and environmental respiratory hazards
- Influenza and pneumonia immunization

PHYSICAL ASSESSMENT

- Skin color, peripheral and central
- Rate, depth, rhythm, and character of respiration; pulse oximetry readings; CO_2 readings
- Restlessness or agitation
- Posture: need to be upright or to lean forward
- Nose: deviation, flaring of nostrils, discharge, patency of nares
- Trachea position, palpation of neck lymph nodes
- Sinus pain on palpation
- Shape of chest and symmetry of chest expansion
- Use of accessory muscles for respirations: intercostal or supraclavicular retractions
- Shape of fingers, angle of nail bed
- Cough: frequency, characteristics
- Sputum: amount, character, color, presence of blood
- Listen for abnormal breath sounds or absence of breath sounds in a systematic pattern
- Any wheezes, fine or coarse crackles, or "rubs"?
- Do abnormal sounds clear up when patient coughs?

Older Adult Care Points

When assessing an older adult patient, it is important to obtain a thorough smoking history and a history of alcohol intake throughout adulthood. **Approximately 90% of throat cancer occurs in people who both smoke and immoderately drink alcohol,** and it is four times more common among men (American Cancer Society, 2017).

Physical Assessment

If the patient is not experiencing respiratory distress, start the assessment at the head and end with lung auscultation. There may be facial puffiness over inflamed sinuses. Palpation of the neck may reveal enlarged lymph nodes. Observe skin color; **cyanosis** (bluish discoloration) of the skin is not a reliable indicator of hypoxemia. **Cyanosis occurs late in the process of oxygen depletion** and could indicate problems of circulation or hemoglobin deficiency. However, the presence of cyanosis is always a concern and prompts further assessment.

Note the posture of the patient, the amount of effort exerted to breathe, the way abdominal muscles and other accessory muscles of respiration are used, the number of words that can be said between breaths, and the rate and character of respirations. Is respiration rapid (**tachypnea**) or slow (**bradypnea**)? Is chest expansion equal when a breath is taken? Are there retractions? Is kyphosis or scoliosis present? Does the patient display or report coughing? A *productive* cough is moist and deep, often accompanied by rhonchi or wheezing, and ends in production of sputum. A *nonproductive* cough is dry and harsh, and no sputum is produced. **Sputum** refers to material brought up from the bronchial tree. It is not mucus from the sinuses, nasal secretions, or saliva. Table 12.3 describes various characteristics and implications of sputum specimens.

A patient with COPD may lean forward in a sitting position and use the abdominal muscles to force air out of the lungs. Other indications of difficulty breathing are elevating the shoulders and ribs, tensing the neck and shoulder muscles, and flaring the nostrils. A retraction of the spaces below and around the sternum also might be observed in a patient in respiratory distress. Obstructive disorders can cause enlargement of the front-to-back (anterior-posterior) measurement of the chest wall, giving a barrel-like appearance to the chest (Fig. 12.7) because of the presence of trapped air in the lungs and inadequate recoil. Over time there is a gradual elevation of the resting level of the diaphragm, which produces an increase in the size of the chest wall. Exhaling through pursed lips is a clue to obstructive disorders. By exerting back pressure into the lungs, the alveoli stay open longer, allowing for trapped air to escape. Clubbing of the fingers (Fig. 12.8) may be seen in patients with lung tissue or heart disease, gastrointestinal disorders, or genetic causes. The cause of clubbing has not been identified (Schwartz, 2017). Note the number of pillows the patient uses to prop themself up in bed or if the head of the bed needs to be raised to facilitate breathing. This position indicates **orthopnea**.

Clinical Cues

Restlessness, agitation, or mental confusion or an increase in heart rate are early indicators of inadequate oxygenation of the blood. Make sure you have a baseline assessment of mental status and vital signs to be able to identify early changes.

Table 12.3 Characteristics of Sputum and Possible Causes[a]

CHARACTERISTIC	POSSIBLE CAUSE
Thick, tenacious, and "ropey"; difficult to cough up	Chronic bronchitis, emphysema
Scant, sticky, rust colored	Pneumococcal pneumonia
Frothy, pinkish or blood tinged	Pulmonary edema
Yellow, yellow-green, or grayish yellow, with foul odor or taste	Pulmonary infection
Blood tinged, bloody, or blood streaked	Tuberculosis, ulcerated pulmonary vessel, or bronchogenic carcinoma
Large amounts	Pneumonia or bronchitis
Scanty	Asthma
Very thick and viscous	Inadequate hydration
Large amounts, foamy, purulent, foul odor	Bronchiectasis

[a]Normal sputum is white and slightly viscous and has no odor or taste.

To auscultate the lungs, first eliminate room noise and instruct the patient to sit up, if possible, so that the bed or back of the chair is not interfering with chest expansion. Ask the patient to remain quiet and to breathe slowly and deeply through the mouth. Listen to one full

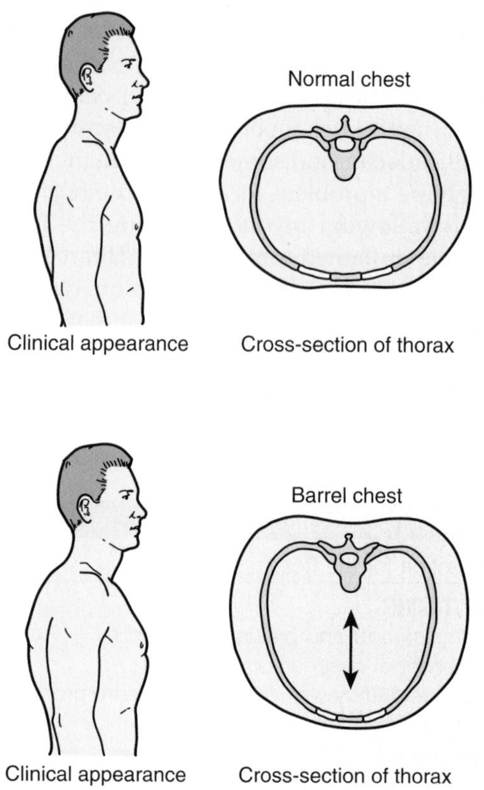

Fig. 12.7 Barrel chest typical of a patient with chronic obstructive pulmonary disease.

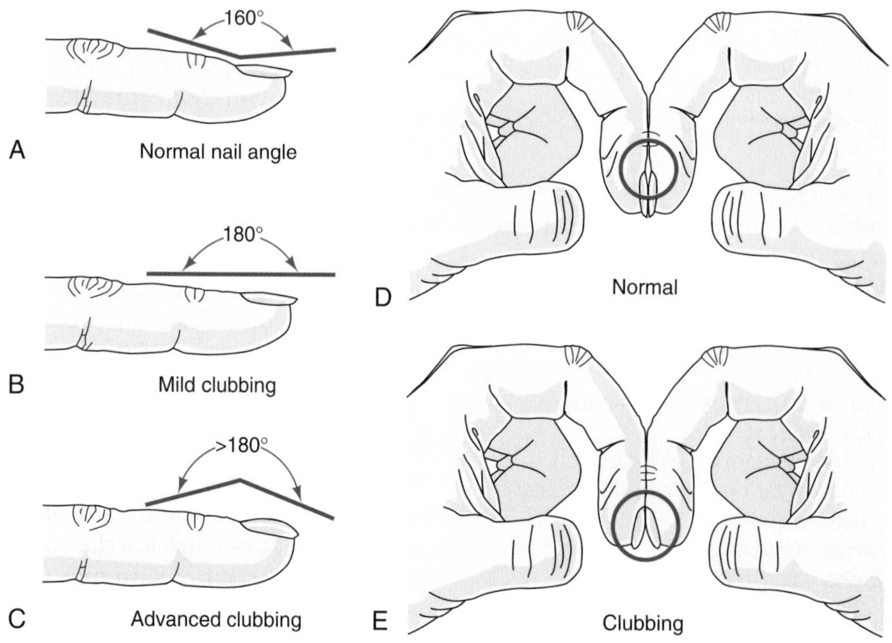

Fig. 12.8 Clubbing of fingers. **A,** Normal fingernail angle is 160 degrees. **B,** Early mild clubbing appears as a flattened angle between nail and skin (180 degrees). **C,** Advanced clubbing shows a rounded (clubbed) fingertip and nail. **D and E,** To assess clubbing by Schamroth's diagnostic method, place the nails of the second digits together. Obliteration of the normal diamond-shaped space between the nails is an abnormal finding, signifying clubbing. (From Copstead LC, Banasik JL: *Pathophysiology*, ed 5, Philadelphia, 2012, Elsevier.)

breath in each location (Fig. 12.9). Place the stethoscope diaphragm against the skin with moderate pressure. Move from one side of the midline of the chest to the other side; compare the sounds. Begin above the clavicles and progress downward in the intercostal spaces to above the sixth rib. On the back, start above the scapula and progress downward along the sides of the spine, and then toward the lateral areas above the tenth thoracic vertebra. Laterally, listen in the midaxillary line in three descending locations to just above the diaphragm. If the patient is short of breath, begin posteriorly at the bases of the lungs and work upward because the patient may not be able to cooperate for the full sequence. Table 12.4 presents sounds normally heard in various locations. Audio clips of normal and abnormal breath sounds are located on the Evolve website.

Clinical Cues

Clean your stethoscope with alcohol or a disinfectant wipe between patients to decrease health care–associated infections. Do not loop the stethoscope around your neck; place it in a pocket after cleaning.

Listen for abnormal or **adventitious** sounds. **Wheezes** are a whistling, musical, high-pitched sound produced by air being forced through a narrowed airway. They are common in patients with asthma. Another type of coarse or sonorous wheezing sound (also known as *rhonchi*) is coarse, low-pitched, rattling sounds caused by secretions in the larger air passages. **Crackles** are produced by air passing through moisture in the smaller airways. *Fine crackles* are high in pitch and can be heard in patients who have atelectasis, fibrosis, pneumonia, or early congestive heart failure. *Coarse crackles* are louder and low in pitch and are heard in patients with bronchitis, pulmonary edema, and resolving pneumonia. **Fine crackles sound similar to the sound produced by rubbing hairs between the fingers close to the ear.**

Clinical Cues

If crackles are heard, have the patient take a deep breath and cough. Listen again. If the crackles are no longer present, atelectasis has been cleared.

Another abnormal sound is that of a **pleural friction rub**, which is a grating or scratchy sound similar to creaking shoe leather or an opening squeaky door; it occurs when irritated visceral and parietal pleura rub against each other. This also produces pain. The sound (and pain) will stop if the patient is asked to hold the breath.

Table 12.4 Normal Lung Sounds

TYPE OF SOUND	LOCATION WHERE NORMALLY HEARD[a]	DESCRIPTION OF SOUND
Vesicular breath sounds	Over lung tissue to level of sixth intercostal space	Low to medium pitch with a soft whooshing quality; inspiration is two to three times the length of expiration
Bronchovesicular breath sounds	Over the mainstem bronchi, below the level of the clavicles, beside the sternum; posteriorly: between the scapulae	Moderate to high pitch with a hollow, muffled quality; equal time of inspiration and expiration
Bronchial breath sounds	Over the trachea above the sternal notch (these sounds are abnormal elsewhere and often indicate atelectasis)	High pitch with a loud, harsh, tubular quality; inspiration half as long as expiration

[a]See Fig. 12.9.

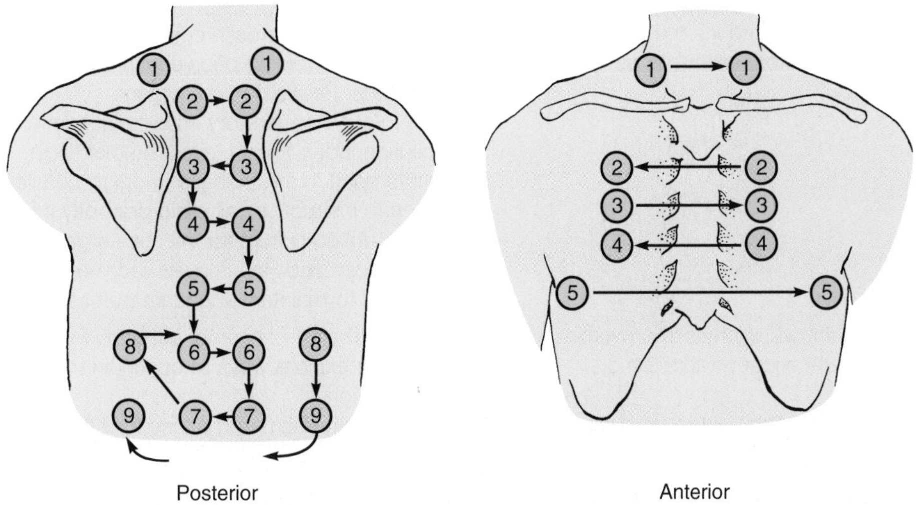

Fig. 12.9 Sites for auscultation of the lungs.

Stridor ("croaking" sounds) can be heard (without using a stethoscope) when there is partial obstruction of the upper air passages. These sounds are typically heard in children with croup but can also occur in adults with upper airway obstruction. The inflammation that is producing the obstruction often also affects the larynx, producing hoarseness. It is important to distinguish between airway swelling and foreign body obstruction as a cause of stridor. Presence of stridor requires prompt assessment and intervention.

? Think Critically

How does shortness of breath affect a person's ability to speak?

◆ NURSING DIAGNOSIS

A variety of patient problems and nursing diagnoses arise when breathing is altered or impaired. Lack of oxygen intake or distribution may cause fatigue and decreased ability to engage in activity. Alteration in roles, coping ability, and body image may cause psychosocial issues. Pain from coughing or surgery on the respiratory system requires nursing interventions. Specific nursing diagnoses are chosen depending on the patient's actual problems. Table 12.5 provides common problem statements for patients with respiratory problems. Other problems may be included in the care plan as they relate to secondary problems.

◆ PLANNING

A patient who has chronic **hypoxia** (oxygen deficiency) moves more slowly, takes more time to answer questions, and has less energy. For patients with a respiratory disorder resulting in hypoxia, consider comfort measures, time needed for eating or feeding, time for patient education, and psychosocial needs. Working with patients who have dyspnea requires planning extra time to accomplish treatments and care.

Table 12.5 Common Problem Statements, Expected Outcomes, and Interventions for Patients With Respiratory Disorders

PROBLEM STATEMENT	GOALS/EXPECTED OUTCOMES	NURSING INTERVENTIONS
Altered gas exchange due to decreased airflow and respiratory muscle fatigue	Patient will use modified breathing techniques to facilitate improved gas exchange.	Instruct in techniques of pursed-lip breathing, diaphragmatic breathing, deep breathing, and effective coughing; teach relaxation techniques. Review medication dosages and schedule and proper technique for use of measured-dose inhaler with patient; assess effectiveness and compliance. Encourage use of incentive spirometer. Monitor pulse oximetry and CO_2 levels before, during, and after exertion. Begin stepped exercise program to improve plan for pacing activities of daily living.
Altered airway clearance due to viscous sputum	Patient will maintain a clear airway. Fluid intake will increase to 3000 mL/day. Patient will demonstrate proper use of nebulizer.	Explain effect of inadequate fluid intake on liquidity of mucus; assess what fluids patient likes; advise to drink 8 oz of fluid every hour while awake; suggest use of room humidifier at home; review technique for using nebulizer and mucolytic agents. Obtain peak flow readings before and after nebulizer treatment.
Potential for respiratory infection due to compromised respiratory system and decreased resistance	Patient will reduce the number of respiratory infections per year.	Review ways to decrease contact with respiratory infectious organisms: avoiding people with colds, flu, and other infections; frequent hand hygiene. Teach to avoid respiratory irritants; stay in house when air pollution index is high; avoid smoke, dust, and cold air. Observe sputum for changes in color, consistency, odor, and amount; instruct to call clinic promptly if signs of infection occur; obtain culture for infective organism if indicated. Give influenza and Pneumovax vaccines. Encourage to maintain adequate nutrition.
Potential for decreased self-esteem due to inability to do ordinary activities	Patient will express improvement in self-concept within 3 mo. Patient will be able to resume desired activities within 3 mo.	Allow to verbalize concerns; assist to focus on possible activities; explore ways of continuing favorite activities using modifications. Give encouragement and praise for efforts in stepped exercise program.

Table 12.5 Common Problem Statements, Expected Outcomes, and Interventions for Patients With Respiratory Disorders—cont'd

PROBLEM STATEMENT	GOALS/EXPECTED OUTCOMES	NURSING INTERVENTIONS
Altered activity level due to dyspnea	Patient will be able to perform bathing and dressing without dyspnea within 3 mo. Patient will participate in and comply with stepped exercise program. Patient will display increased ability to tolerate activity by walking short distance without breathlessness.	Encourage use of pursed-lip and diaphragmatic breathing. Begin stepped exercise program as soon as acute respiratory infection has resolved. Alternate activity with rest periods, beginning with small increments of activity. Use oxygen as prescribed during acute episodes of dyspnea.
Anxiousness due to hypoxia and dyspnea	Patient will verbalize that anxiety has lessened within 1 wk.	Allow to verbalize concerns within ability to speak without becoming dyspneic. Encourage use of pursed-lip and diaphragmatic breathing to decrease dyspnea. Teach best positions to decrease dyspnea. Teach relaxation techniques; encourage practice. Interact with calm, reassuring manner. Refer to community support groups.
Potential for health problems due to continued smoking	Within 1 wk patient will look at alternative ways to quit smoking. Patient will begin a smoking cessation program within 3 wk.	Explain the harmful effects of continued smoking. Motivate patient to quit smoking by emphasizing benefits of increased stamina and decreased dyspnea. Introduce to various methods and programs for quitting smoking. Get referral from health care provider for interventions requiring prescriptions. Introduce to people with equivalent lung disease who have quit smoking. Praise any effort at decreasing or quitting smoking.

The nursing goals for patients with a respiratory disorder are to:

- Promote oxygenation
- Prevent infection
- Prevent further lung damage
- Promote rehabilitation

Specific expected outcomes are individualized for each patient (see the Nursing Care Plans in Chapters 13 and 14).

◆ IMPLEMENTATION

Examples of interventions and teaching for patients with respiratory disorders are presented in Table 12.5. Interventions are discussed later in this chapter and in Chapters 13 and 14.

◆ EVALUATION

Effectiveness of interventions for and treatment of patients with respiratory disorders is based on improved breathing pattern, pulse oximeter readings, arterial blood gas values, and lung sounds. Decreases in coughing, sputum production, wheezing, and signs of infection are other parameters that indicate improvements. Patient reports of lessened dyspnea, as well as of more energy and ability to perform more self-care and other activities, indicate that interventions are effective. Reassessment is an ongoing nursing activity for patients with respiratory problems.

COMMON RESPIRATORY PATIENT CARE PROBLEMS

AIRWAY MAINTENANCE

A cough is usually a reflex triggered by a foreign substance or some other irritant in the respiratory tract. Coughing can be beneficial and should be encouraged if it is effective in clearing the air passages and removing accumulations of stagnant mucus. Explain that deep-breathing and coughing maneuvers help remove sputum and decrease the likelihood of complications, such as pneumonia. (See Chapter 4 for deep-breathing and coughing maneuvers and the Evolve website for Teaching Guidelines.)

If coughing is excessive, the patient will tire and the respiratory tissues and thoracic structures can be traumatized, so **antitussive** agents may be used to inhibit the cough reflex in the cough center in the brain. Many sedative cough mixtures contain codeine or other drugs that decrease the desire to cough. The liquefying agents and diluents thin secretions and help the patient expectorate (cough up secretions). Adequate hydration is the most effective method to liquefy secretions so they can be expectorated. Cough syrups are given to soothe the nerve endings in the upper respiratory mucosa. These medications are given in small doses to coat and protect the throat. **Water should not be taken immediately after a cough syrup, because it rinses off the topical application of the medication.**

In bacterial infections and chronic respiratory diseases, the sputum often is foul smelling, leaving a bad taste in the mouth and offensive breath odor. Mouth care is especially needed before meals, when the taste or odor of the sputum may adversely affect appetite. **Frequent mouth care also helps remove pathogenic microorganisms from the oral cavity and thereby diminishes the possibility that they will be aspirated deep into the air passages.**

Mechanical suctioning is indicated when the patient cannot clear the airway of excessive amounts of secretions. Removing secretions from the nose, mouth, and throat is a relatively safe and simple procedure. However, deep tracheal suctioning—whether through the nose, mouth, or endotracheal tube—should only be performed using strict aseptic technique and by someone experienced in the correct procedure.

The need for suctioning is based on patient assessment. Some patients may require suctioning only once or twice daily to remove deeply situated pools and plugs of mucus that cannot be coughed up. Others require suctioning every 10 to 15 minutes to clear their air passages. Remember, the purpose of suctioning is to facilitate breathing and to allow for an adequate exchange of CO_2 and O_2 in the lungs. Even though the procedure may be necessary, suctioning removes oxygen and is uncomfortable for the patient.

ALTERED BREATHING PATTERNS

Dyspnea or Breathlessness

Administer O_2 as prescribed. Use a calm manner and assure the patient that everything possible is being done to bring relief of dyspnea. Coach the patient to perform pursed-lip and diaphragmatic breathing (see Chapter 14).

The high Fowler position is best for patients with dyspnea. Proper positioning and support allow the respiratory muscles to function at maximum efficiency. For severe dyspnea, the orthopneic position is most effective. *Orthopnea* means that the patient has trouble breathing when supine. The patient should sit upright, lean over the overbed table (which is padded with pillows), and elevate and round the shoulders to allow maximum expansion of the lungs (Fig. 12.10).

Pressure from organs, fluid, or tissue below or near the lungs and diaphragm can impair breathing. A full stomach can contribute to dyspnea by limiting the amount of space available for expansion of the lungs. Abdominal distention resulting from edema or collection of flatus and fecal material can also make breathing more difficult. Obesity is a risk factor for dyspnea.

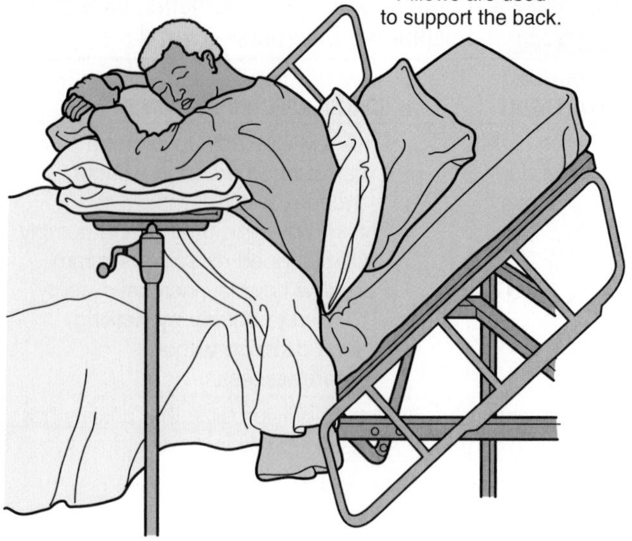
Pillows are used
to support the back.
Other pillows are placed on an overbed table to support the
weight of the arms, shoulders, and head.

Fig. 12.10 Orthopneic position.

Dyspnea may or may not be a result of *hypoxemia* (low blood oxygen levels). *Hypoxia* (low levels of tissue oxygen) results from not enough oxygen being delivered in the bloodstream to the tissues. For oxygen to reach the tissues, the patient must be breathing adequately, have a patent airway, have lung tissue able to exchange gases, and have adequate hemoglobin to carry the oxygen and adequate blood flow to deliver the oxygen. Alteration in any of these can affect delivery of oxygen to tissues.

The tissues most sensitive to changes in oxygen levels include the brain and heart; therefore clinical signs and symptoms of hypoxia show up first in these organs. Alterations in brain function include restlessness, anxiety, and confusion. Subtle changes in cognitive ability may not be noticed initially. If hypoxia is not identified and corrected, vital signs will be affected. The heart rate will increase in an attempt to increase oxygen delivery. Blood oxygenation is monitored by pulse oximetry (Spo_2), which reflects the arterial oxygen saturation (Sao_2). An Spo_2 greater than 95% is considered normal, and an Spo_2 of 92% or less (at sea level) suggests hypoxemia.

Hypercapnia

Hyperventilation, hypoventilation, and the effect of these abnormal breathing patterns on the acid-base balance of body fluids are discussed in Chapter 3. Ventilation is the movement of air in and out of the lungs. The body's ventilation ability is measured by CO_2 levels. Levels of exhaled CO_2 can be monitored by devices inline to oxygen delivery systems (Fig. 12.11). Blood CO_2 levels can be monitored by equipment similar to that used to assess pulse oximetry. CO_2 levels obtained from these devices are similar to arterial blood gas Pco_2 levels. Capnography is the measurement and display of CO_2 levels. Hypercapnia (also called *hypercarbia*) is the retention of excessive amounts of CO_2. It is the result

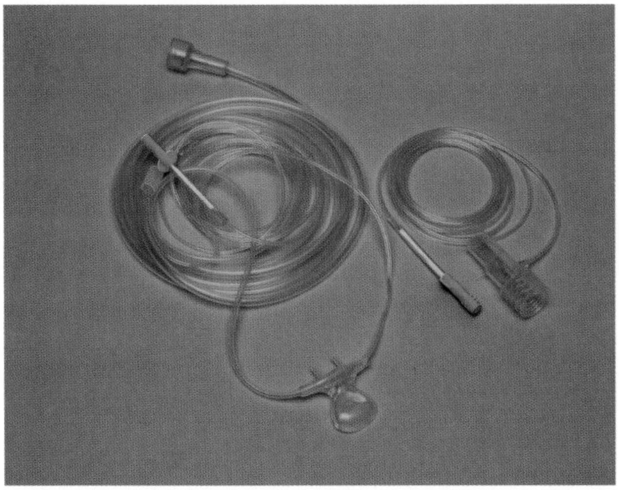

Fig. 12.11 Nasal cannula with end-tidal carbon dioxide ($ETCO_2$) detection device.

of hypoventilation, during which the usual amount of CO_2 is not eliminated by exhalation.

Hypocapnia

Hypocapnia, which is a deficit of CO_2, occurs as a result of hyperventilation and can result in respiratory alkalosis. Conditions associated with hypocapnia include (1) those in which there is an increased metabolic rate, such as thyrotoxicosis, persistent fever, and acute anxiety; (2) salicylate overdose; and (3) improper use of mechanical ventilation.

Clinical signs of respiratory alkalosis include hyperactive neuromuscular reflexes, tetany, carpopedal spasms, vertigo, blurred vision, and diaphoresis. Blood gas analysis will show a low partial pressure of arterial carbon dioxide ($Paco_2$) and a high pH (alkalinity). CO_2 monitoring devices will show low levels of CO_2. Since 2012 the AHRQ has recommended use of transcutaneous O_2 ($PtcO_2$) and transcutaneous CO_2 ($PtcCO_2$) monitoring for patients requiring close observation of oxygenation and ventilation status. Most facilities require this monitoring for patients who are receiving patient-controlled analgesia (PCA), and The Joint Commission mandates monitoring during procedural sedation.

Respiratory Failure

Carbon dioxide is a respiratory stimulant; hence **the body responds to excessive levels of CO_2 by increasing the rate and depth of respirations.** However, if the respiratory centers in the brain are exposed to higher than normal levels of CO_2 over a long time, they cease to react and do not adjust respirations in response to mildly elevated CO_2 levels. Without intervention the accumulation of CO_2 can cause a decreased level of consciousness up to and including coma.

Respiratory failure is defined by arterial blood gases: arterial oxygen (PaO_2) is below 50 mm Hg and the partial pressure of carbon dioxide (PCO_2) is equal to or greater than 50 mm Hg. Cardiac arrest can result from respiratory failure because of hypoxia and acid-base changes.

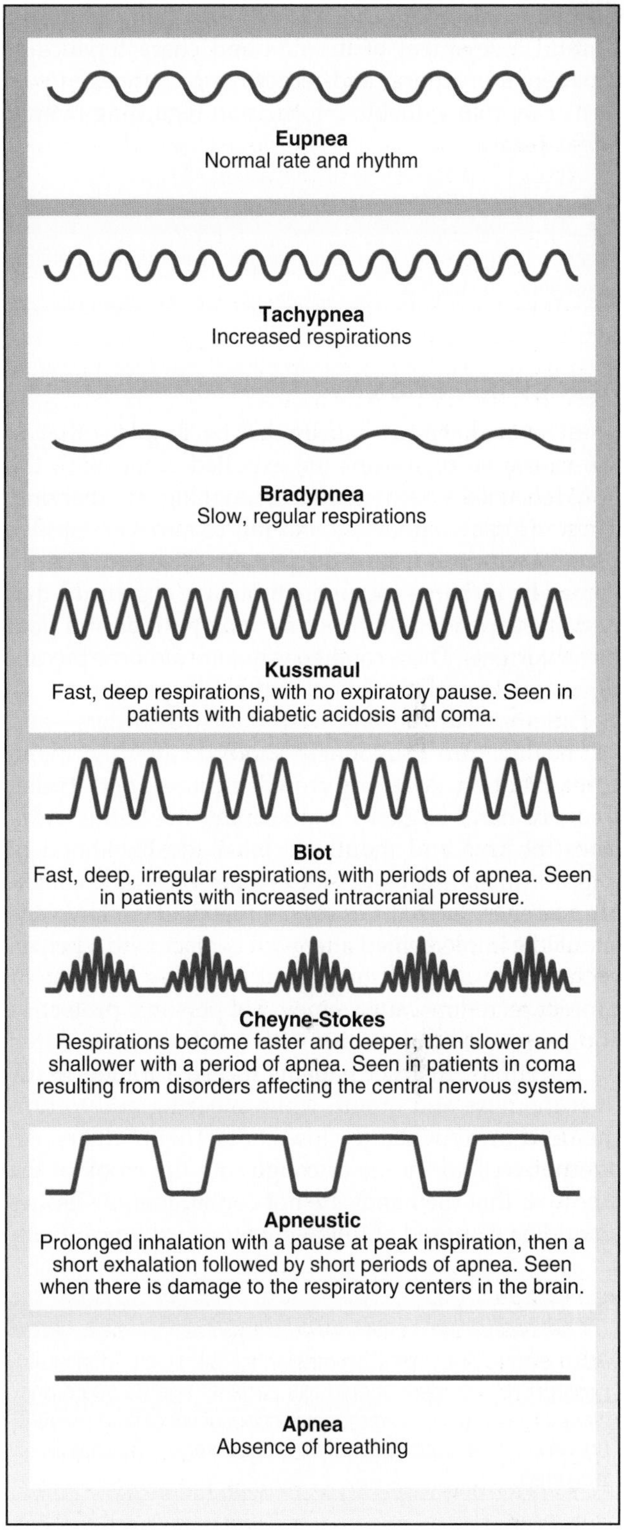

Fig. 12.12 Respiratory patterns. (From Williams P: deWit's fundamental concepts and skills for nursing, ed 5, St. Louis, 2018, Elsevier.)

Other Ineffective Breathing Patterns

Additional respiratory patterns are shown in Fig. 12.12. Diseases, trauma, changes in neurologic function, and metabolic disorders can all alter breathing patterns. Careful assessment of the rate and characteristics of a patient's breathing and recognizing changes in patterns can give valuable information regarding overall clinical status.

? Think Critically

Name four nursing interventions that will help a patient experiencing dyspnea.

RISK OF INFECTION

Many acute URIs are transmitted by droplets; that is, the causative organisms are expelled along with the liquid secretions released during coughing and sneezing. These droplets are heavy and fall to surfaces rapidly, usually within 3 feet of the patient. Diseases that are spread by airborne contamination have organisms that remain suspended in the air for long periods and float on air currents. These conditions require airborne precautions and special masks for health care personnel.

Patients with chronic respiratory disorders—and all health care personnel—should carefully avoid contamination. Avoiding crowded places, performing frequent hand hygiene, and keeping the hands away from the face and mouth decrease the likelihood of infection. Standing to the side of a person who is coughing and sneezing reduces contamination. Hand hygiene should be implemented after each contact with a person with a respiratory disorder that produces airborne or droplet secretions, after removal of personal protective equipment, or after contact with articles contaminated by secretions. Instruct patients to use a folded tissue over the nose and mouth while sneezing and to turn the head away when in close contact with others. An alternative is to sneeze or cough into the crook of the elbow so that the hands are not contaminated. Tissues should be disposed of following Standard Precautions.

Older Adult Care Points

According to The Joint Commission's (2018) Core Measures, health care providers should ask patients age 65 years and older if they have received pneumococcal vaccine to prevent pneumococcal bacteremia and encourage vaccination if indicated.

ALTERATIONS IN NUTRITION AND HYDRATION

Anorexia and inadequate nutrition are common in patients with respiratory disorders, particularly when the disorders are chronic. The patient may have an impaired sense of taste or smell, or sputum can leave a bad taste in the mouth or cause nausea. The patient may fear that chewing and swallowing will bring on an attack of coughing or may be so tired that eating or preparing food is too exhausting.

Keep the patient's environment clean, uncluttered, and orderly. Dispose of used tissues promptly. Frequent oral hygiene and mouth care before meals can help diminish mouth odor and nausea and improve taste. Smaller, more frequent feedings of nutritious liquids and foods are preferable to three large, heavy meals.

Because there is increased energy expenditure when breathing is difficult, many patients have difficulty maintaining weight, even when they take in normal amounts of calories. Supplements such as Pulmocare have an increased fat content and provide more calories in smaller quantities and decrease the dietary production of CO_2. **When a patient is receiving mechanical ventilation, caloric needs rise.** Sometimes total parenteral nutrition or lipid infusions are necessary to prevent malnutrition for patients on ventilators.

A fluid deficit is likely in patients with respiratory disorders because there is an increased loss of fluid in respiratory secretions. The patient usually breathes through the mouth and exhales large amounts of moisture from the body. Unless contraindicated, an intake of at least 3000 mL of liquid should occur each day. This intake may include low-sodium bouillon, fruit juices, and other liquids in addition to water.

Humidifying the air breathed by the patient is an effective way to minimize dehydration and moisturize the air passages. Humidification is especially important for patients whose secretions are thick and tenacious and difficult to cough up. Humidification of inhaled air is discussed in Chapter 14.

FATIGUE

Hypoxia produces a loss of energy because it causes a disturbance in cellular metabolism. Patients with respiratory disorders often have hypoxia and use their energy to struggle for breath and cough up secretions.

Patients with respiratory disorders, whether acute or chronic, have some degree of intolerance to physical activity and therefore need periods of rest throughout the day. Treatments and medications should be scheduled so that the patient can rest without interruption. To conserve energy, the patient should intermittently take short naps. Deep-breathing exercises and coughing techniques should be planned whenever the patient is able to do them with or without some assistance. These activities should be followed by good mouth care and a short period of uninterrupted rest. The goal of nursing care should be to achieve a satisfactory balance of rest and activity.

Get Ready for the NCLEX® Examination!

Key Points

- Inhalation of infectious organisms and chemical irritants causes respiratory problems.
- Cardiac disease can interfere with blood supply to the lungs and distribution of gases.
- There are two major types of ventilatory diseases: restrictive (decreased lung volume) and obstructive (narrowed air passages).
- Restrictive conditions, such as scoliosis and kyphosis, decrease lung capacity.
- Obstructive disorders cause problems moving air in and out of the lungs. Asthma, emphysema, and chronic bronchitis are obstructive disorders.
- Prevention of respiratory problems includes good health practices: rest, nutrition, personal hygiene, and avoiding known allergens. At-risk persons should be immunized against influenza and pneumonia.
- The incidence of respiratory ailments decreases for people who stop smoking.
- Effectiveness of interventions and treatment is identified by improvements in breathing pattern, $PtcO_2$ and SpO_2 readings, arterial blood gas values, and lung sounds. Decreased cough, sputum production, wheezing, and dyspnea are other parameters.
- Positioning in high Fowler position or sitting with shoulders hunched and arms resting on the knees with legs apart eases breathing.
- Signs of respiratory acidosis are excessive PCO_2 and rapid respirations.
- Signs of respiratory alkalosis are tetany, carpopedal spasms, vertigo, blurred vision, diaphoresis, and low PCO_2 and high pH.
- Respiratory failure is defined as PaO_2 below 50 mm Hg and PCO_2 equal to or greater than 50 mm Hg.
- Abnormal respiratory patterns include Biot respirations, Cheyne-Stokes respirations, Kussmaul respirations, and apneustic respirations.
- Respiratory infections are transmitted by airborne or droplet secretions.
- Anorexia and inadequate nutrition are common with chronic respiratory disease.
- Patients should drink at least 3000 mL of liquid per day to help thin secretions. Humidification of air can help prevent drying of mucous membranes.

Additional Learning Resources

SG Go to your Study Guide for additional learning activities to help you master this chapter content.

Go to your Evolve website (http://evolve.elsevier.com/deWit/medsurg) for the following FREE learning resources:

- Animations, audio, and video
- Answers and rationales for questions and activities
- Glossary with pronunciations in English and Spanish
- Interactive Review Questions and more!

Review Questions for the NCLEX® Examination

1. A 59-year-old male patient with hypertension and COPD states that he is having trouble breathing. He appears to be in distress and has labored breathing. Put in order of priority the nursing actions to be taken.
   1. Take vital signs, including pulse oximetry reading.
   2. Report condition to health care provider.
   3. Raise the head of the bed.
   4. Auscultate lung sounds.

   NCLEX Client Need: Physiological Integrity: Reduction of Risk Potential
2. You are caring for several patients who are scheduled for diagnostic testing for respiratory disorders. The patient who needs postprocedural care that includes frequent vital signs is the patient who had:
   1. capnography.
   2. a D-dimer test.
   3. a ventilation and perfusion scan.
   4. bronchoscopy.

   NCLEX Client Need: Physiological Integrity: Physiological Adaptation
3. You are caring for a patient who is short of breath. The degree of shortness of breath can be assessed by which of the following?
   1. Ability to speak
   2. Breath sounds
   3. Capnography
   4. Nail bed color

   NCLEX Client Need: Physiological Integrity: Reduction of Risk Potential
4. You are caring for a patient who has asthma. Which lung sound would you expect to hear when auscultating this patient's lung fields?
   1. Fine crackles
   2. Stridor
   3. Pleural friction rub
   4. Wheezes

   NCLEX Client Need: Physiological Integrity: Physiological Adaptation
5. You should observe for and report which abnormal breathing pattern that is most likely to occur in patients with increased intracranial pressure?
   1. Cheyne-Stokes respirations
   2. Kussmaul respirations
   3. Biot respirations
   4. Apneustic respirations

   NCLEX Client Need: Physiological Integrity: Reduction of Risk Potential
6. You attend to the nutritional needs of a patient with chronic respiratory disease by providing oral care. What is the best rationale for this nursing action?
   1. Low energy states diminish appetite.
   2. Respiratory secretions leave a bad taste.
   3. Chewing is believed to induce coughing spells.
   4. Nasal congestion reduces the flavor of food.

   NCLEX Client Need: Physiological Integrity: Basic Care and Comfort

7. You are caring for a patient who has had a thoracentesis with the removal of 800 cc of fluid. What finding would you expect in the physical assessment of the patient post procedure?
   1. Slow heart rate
   2. Clear lung sounds
   3. Increased blood pressure
   4. Improved ventilation

   NCLEX Client Need: Physiological Integrity: Reduction of Risk Potential
8. While obtaining sputum for culture and sensitivity, you note that the specimen is thick, tenacious, and "ropey." This finding is most likely to be present in which disorder?
   1. Pneumococcal pneumonia
   2. Pulmonary edema
   3. Chronic bronchitis
   4. Tuberculosis

   NCLEX Client Need: Physiological Integrity: Physiological Adaptation
9. On initial assessment of a patient diagnosed with an acute exacerbation of COPD, you are likely to find which sign(s) and symptom(s)? *(Select all that apply.)*
   1. Tensing of the shoulder muscles
   2. Inability to tolerate sitting up
   3. Flaring of the nostrils
   4. Ability to complete sentences with no effort
   5. Sternal retraction

   NCLEX Client Need: Physiological Integrity: Physiological Adaptation
10. A 72-year-old patient has just returned to the nursing unit after a lung biopsy. You watch closely for signs of which condition?
    1. Hypotension
    2. Hypercapnia
    3. Hyperventilation
    4. Hypovolemia

    NCLEX Client Need: Physiological Integrity: Reduction of Risk Potential
11. An 80-year-old male patient with COPD states that he is short of breath. You observe orthopnea, increased work of breathing, respiratory rate of 40, and a pulse oximetry reading of 69%. What should be done next for this patient?
    1. Obtain an arterial blood gas
    2. Place the head of the bed at a 60-degree angle
    3. Auscultate lung sounds
    4. Place on high-flow oxygen

    NCLEX Client Need: Physiological Integrity: Reduction of Risk Potential
12. A 40-year-old mother of two teenagers has a history of asthma and COPD. She is currently hospitalized with pneumonia. She is anxious and worried about her family. What interventions are appropriate to implement? *(Select all that apply.)*
    1. Administer antianxiety medication
    2. Have the social worker see her
    3. Ask the patient about her concerns
    4. Arrange a family conference
    5. Notify the health care provider

    NCLEX Client Need: Psychosocial Integrity

Critical Thinking Questions

Scenario A

Mr. Keelog is an older adult man who may have cancer of the larynx. He will undergo diagnostic procedures to confirm this diagnosis. You observe that he is not currently having respiratory distress and can answer your questions. He appears willing and able to listen to information.

1. What questions should you ask to identify if Mr. Keelog has risk factors for cancer of the larynx?
2. Identify at least four questions you would ask Mr. Keelog about his present status.
3. Describe the teaching plan that would be used for a patient undergoing a direct laryngoscopy.
4. What other diagnostic tests would have been done on this patient?
5. How can this type of cancer potentially be prevented?

Scenario B

Ms. Tiber has had frequent bouts of bronchitis. Her health care provider tells her that this disorder has caused some COPD.

1. What measures would you teach her to make breathing easier?
2. Why is it important to be cautious in giving oxygen to a patient with COPD? What might happen?

Scenario C

Mrs. Clampett is an older adult woman who comes to the clinic for an annual flu vaccination. She would like a "good physical check of my lungs" and information about how to prevent respiratory disorders.

1. What questions should you ask in obtaining a history about potential respiratory problems?
2. Describe how you would auscultate her lungs.
3. If you heard an abnormal lung sound such as "fine crackles," what would you do?

Care of Patients With Disorders of the Upper Respiratory System

13

http://evolve.elsevier.com/deWit/medsurg

Objectives

Theory

1. Recognize symptoms of disorders of the sinuses, pharynx, and larynx.
2. Describe the postoperative care for a patient undergoing a tracheostomy.
3. Prioritize emergency measures for a patient with an airway obstruction.
4. Present a nursing care plan for a patient who had a laryngectomy.
5. Analyze safety factors to be considered when caring for a patient with a tracheostomy.

Clinical Practice

6. Institute measures to stop epistaxis.
7. Provide tracheostomy care.
8. Devise interventions for the psychosocial care of a patient who has undergone a laryngectomy.
9. Visit a patient who has a permanent tracheostomy and ask them to share some of their successful coping strategies.

Key Terms

crepitation (KRĔP-ĭ-tā-shŭn, p. 288)
endotracheal intubation (ĔN-dō-TRĀ-kē-ăl ĭn-tyū-bā-shŭn, p. 289)
epistaxis (ĕp-ĭ-STĂK-sĭs, p. 284)
follicular pharyngitis (fōl-ĭk-yĕ-lĕr fĕr-ĭn-jī-tĭs, p. 285)
laryngectomy (lăr-ĭn-JĔK-tō-mē, p. 288)
laryngitis (lăr-ĭn-JĪ-tĭs, p. 285)
laryngoscope (lăr-ĭn-JĔ-skōp, p. 289)
lozenges (LŎZ-ĕn-jĕz, p. 285)
obturator (ŎB-tŭ-ră-tŏr, p. 290)
pharyngitis (fĕr-ĭn-jī-tĭs, p. 285)
rhinitis (rī-NĪ-tĭs, p. 281)
rhinoplasty (RĪ-nō-plăs-tē, p. 288)
stoma (STŌ-mă, p. 289)
tracheostomy (trā-kē-ŎS-tō-mē, p. 288)

Concepts Covered in This Chapter

- Gas Exchange
- Inflammation
- Infection
- Communication
- Safety

DISORDERS OF THE NOSE AND SINUSES

The upper respiratory tract includes the nose and sinuses, mouth, pharynx, and larynx above the vocal cords. The larynx below the vocal cords and the trachea are considered lower airway structures but are frequently involved in upper airway conditions. Upper respiratory infections (URIs) include viral and bacterial infections resulting in cold, flu, pharyngitis, rhinosinusitis, epiglottitis, laryngotracheitis, and pertussis. Trauma and allergies also cause nose and sinus disorders.

UPPER RESPIRATORY INFECTIONS AND RHINITIS

The common cold—acute viral **rhinitis**—is an inflammation of the nose and upper respiratory tract. Other names for a cold include nasopharyngitis, rhinopharyngitis, acute coryza, and head cold. It is the most prevalent infectious disease among people of all ages. Many different strains of viruses can produce the symptoms of a common cold, which makes total immunity unlikely and developing a vaccination problematic. Avoiding exposure to those who have a cold and maintaining a state of good health are the only ways one can avoid "catching" a cold.

Etiology and Pathophysiology

Viruses are spread by airborne droplet sprays from infected people during breathing, speaking, coughing, and sneezing or by direct hand contact with a contaminated object and then contact between that hand and mucous membranes. Viruses can live on surfaces for prolonged periods. A chill, fatigue, physical or emotional stress, a compromised immune status, or inflammation caused by allergic rhinitis make one more susceptible to contracting an upper respiratory virus.

Allergic rhinitis may have many of the symptoms of a cold, except there is no fever. It is caused by reaction of the nasal mucosa to an allergen, such as pollen or dust.

Signs, Symptoms, and Diagnosis

The common cold usually starts with a mild sore throat or a hot, dry, prickly sensation in the nose and back of the throat. Within hours after the onset of a cold, the nose becomes congested with increased secretions; the eyes begin to water; and sneezing, malaise, and an irritating, nonproductive cough appear. The invading organism causes inflammation and swelling of the mucosa. Muscle aches and headache may occur. There usually is no elevation of temperature; if a fever does develop, it is low grade (<101° F [<38.3° C]), as is typical with viral infections. In most instances, a cold will last 7 to 11 days, but it may take up to 14 days before all symptoms are gone.

Safety Alert

Use of Zinc

The use of zinc to decrease the recovery time from a cold is recommended by many health care providers. The Centers for Disease Control and Prevention (CDC) has issued a warning regarding the use of intranasal zinc. Using these preparations may result in anosmia (loss of the sense of smell) (CDC, 2017).

Treatment and Nursing Management

There is no cure for the common cold. It is important to distinguish a cold from other URIs that may be bacterial and need antibiotic therapy or are conditions that in some patients can lead to more severe illness.

The treatment of allergic rhinitis is symptomatic. Antihistamines, steroids, and sprays that stabilize the mucous cell membranes are often prescribed (Table 13.1). The patient is taught to avoid the offending allergens as much as possible. This may include filters for room air. If the disorder is severe, an allergy evaluation is indicated so that a desensitization program can be started.

Complementary and Alternative Therapies

Alternative Treatment for an Upper Respiratory Infection

Echinacea; goldenseal; or a combination of herbs, minerals, vitamins, and amino acids such as those contained in over-the-counter products can be taken at the first sign of a cold or before going into crowded areas during cold season. These substances are believed to boost the body's immune response.

A major goal in the care of a common cold is prevention of a secondary bacterial infection. Individuals with a cold should avoid contact with others to avoid contracting a bacterial infection or giving their viral infection to someone else. A person with a cold is contagious for about 3 days after symptoms first appear.

Colds are spread by droplet infection, and most people realize that coughing and sneezing will spread viruses. Coughing and sneezing into tissues does limit the viruses' travel by air, but the viruses are also very likely to be on the person's hands, where they can be transferred to anything touched. Hand hygiene is

Table 13.1 Drugs Commonly Used to Treat Allergic Rhinitis and Sinusitis

CLASSIFICATION	ACTION	NURSING IMPLICATIONS	PATIENT TEACHING
Antihistamines			
First-Generation Antihistamines			
Diphenhydramine (Benadryl) Clemastine (Tavist) Brompheniramine (Dimetane) Chlorpheniramine (Chlor-Trimeton)	Relieve sneezing, excessive secretions, itching, and nasal congestion Block histamine binding by binding with H_1 receptor sites	Tend to cause sedation and slow reaction time May cause stimulation in some people May cause GI side effects: anorexia, constipation or diarrhea, or epigastric distress May cause urinary retention or frequency	Warn patient not to operate machinery and that driving may be dangerous because of sedation; this usually passes after the first 2 wk of treatment. Ask patient to report changes in heart rate, palpitations, or urinary retention or frequency. Warn that alcohol will have additive depressant effect.
Second-Generation Antihistamines			
Loratadine (Claritin) Fexofenadine (Allegra) Cetirizine (Zyrtec) Desloratadine (Clarinex) Levocetirizine (Xyzal)	Relieve sneezing, excessive secretions, itching, and nasal congestion. Are less likely to cross the blood-brain barrier, producing less drowsiness than first-generation antihistamines	Have limited attachment to H_1 receptors in the brain Do not cause sedation, and have less effect on reflexes Do not affect bladder function	Instruct not to take with alcohol or other CNS-active drugs. Warn not to take with any monoamine oxidase inhibitor. These drugs are more expensive than first-generation drugs.

Table 13.1 Drugs Commonly Used to Treat Allergic Rhinitis and Sinusitis—cont'd

CLASSIFICATION	ACTION	NURSING IMPLICATIONS	PATIENT TEACHING
Corticosteroid Sprays			
Beclomethasone (Beconase) Budesonide (Rhinocort) Flunisolide (Nasalide) Fluticasone (Flonase) Triamcinolone (Nasacort) Ciclesonide (Omnaris) Mometasone (Nasonex)	Inhibit inflammatory response Have low systemic absorption with normal doses	Use can result in nosebleeds. Directing the nozzle away from the septum may help prevent nosebleeds. If saline irrigation is used as an adjunctive treatment, it should be performed prior to the nasal spray.	Teach to use on a daily basis rather than PRN. Instruct to discontinue if infection occurs. May initially cause some burning in nostrils.
Mast Cell Stabilizer			
Cromolyn sodium spray (Nasalcrom)	Stabilizes mast cells, preventing inflammatory reaction	Minimal side effects	Instruct to begin 2 wk before pollen season starts and use throughout pollen season to prevent allergy symptoms. May be used prophylactically for isolated allergy (i.e., cat). Instruct to use 10–15 min before exposure.
Decongestants			
Oral Pseudoephedrine (Sudafed) *Spray* Oxymetazoline (Dristan) Phenylephrine (Neo-Synephrine) Saline nasal spray or rinse[a]	Promote vasoconstriction by stimulating adrenergic receptors on blood vessels Reduce nasal edema and rhinorrhea	May cause insomnia, headache, irritability, dysuria, palpitations, or tachycardia Can cause rebound nasal congestion	Some products are contraindicated for patients with hypertension, cardiac disease, glaucoma, diabetes, prostatic hypertrophy, or liver or renal disease. Teach to use only three or four times a day for no more than 3 days.
Other Categories			
Intranasal Antihistamines Azelastine (Astelin) Olopatadine intranasal (Patanase)	Topical H_1 receptor antagonists Inhibit the release of histamine May help relieve nasal congestion	May be absorbed systemically in some patients, producing sedation	Instruct not to use if patient has glaucoma or prostatic hypertrophy.
Intranasal Anticholinergic Agents Ipratropium (Atrovent)	Inhibits vagally mediated reflexes Chemically related to atropine Reduces nasal secretions	Works best if used regularly at evenly spaced intervals	Teach that it may cause dry or bloody nose, throat irritation, or bad taste in mouth.

[a]Saline nasal sprays and rinses wash away pollen and dust, thin secretions, and soothe the nasal mucosa.
CNS, Central nervous system; *GI*, gastrointestinal; *H_1*, histamine-1; *PRN*, as needed.

important in the prevention of spreading infection to others, and patients should also be taught not to share personal-use items, such as drinking glasses.

The patient should stay indoors, preferably in bed or resting, during the first few days of the illness. Fluid intake should be increased. Fruit juices are recommended, especially citrus juices, because of their vitamin C content. Mild nonprescription analgesics can help relieve the muscle aches and headache of a cold.

Decongestant nose drops or sprays containing vasoconstrictors such as oxymetazoline (for the relief of nasal congestion) can have a rebound effect, leaving the nose "stuffier" if used for more than 3 days. Frequent use of saline nasal spray decreases congestion without

Older Adult Care Points

Older adults should be encouraged to stay away from people who have a cold or URI because older adults have decreased immune function and if a cold develops, a secondary infection is more likely. Older patients should continue the extra fluids and rest until symptoms are resolved.

Safety Alert

Caution With Aspirin

The U.S. Surgeon General, the Food and Drug Administration, the CDC, the American Academy of Pediatrics, the National Reye's Syndrome Foundation, and the World Health Organization recommend that aspirin and combination products containing aspirin not be given to children under 19 years of age during episodes of fever-causing or viral illnesses. Adults taking anticoagulants or nonsteroidal antiinflammatory drugs should take aspirin only under the direction of their health care provider because aspirin will further prolong the clotting time.

side effects. Antibiotics are not given because a cold is a viral infection.

A bacterial infection, which requires medical treatment, is likely present when a "cold" persists for more than 7 to 10 days without improvement or if the patient begins to feel worse, has a temperature of 101° F (38.3° C), and develops chest pains or coughs up purulent sputum.

Think Critically

What are the various ways you can prevent contracting a cold?

SINUSITIS

Sinusitis is an inflammation of the mucosal lining of the sinuses and can be caused by infection or by allergies (allergic rhinitis). *Rhinosinusitis* is the preferred term because the nasal mucosa is almost always inflamed along with the sinuses. Viral infections are the most common cause of rhinosinusitis. Sinusitis often occurs after colds or other respiratory infections and during periods of uncontrolled allergic rhinitis. The nasal passages can be blocked by a deviated septum, which may occur congenitally; by injury to the nose; or by nasal polyps. Polyps occur from repeated inflammation of the nasal mucosa and are tissue growths that obstruct airflow. People with a deviated nasal septum or allergy problems tend to have recurrent sinusitis.

As exudate accumulates in the sinuses, pressure builds up, causing pain. Symptoms include tenderness over the sinuses, purulent drainage from the nose, nasal obstruction, and sometimes a nonproductive cough. The upper teeth may become painful.

Treatment of sinusitis includes relieving pain, promoting sinus drainage, controlling bacterial infection, reducing inflammation, and preventing recurrence. Hot, moist packs over the sinus area can be helpful. Inhaling moist steam keeps mucous membranes moist, and equipment for sinus irrigation to help promote drainage is available at drugstores. Medications are prescribed to promote decongestion or vasoconstriction and to reduce swelling, to promote drainage, and to relieve pain. The infection may be treated with an antibiotic or antiinfective agent, often for at least 10 days. Rest, reduced stress, a balanced diet, and control of allergies can help prevent recurrence. Fluid intake should be increased. There is no scientific evidence for the common belief that dairy products increase the thickness of secretions or produce mucus. In studies, individuals who believe that mucus production increases with dairy products reported increased mucus.

Think Critically

How would you know if you or a patient has a sinus infection rather than just a common cold?

Acute or chronic sinus infection can cause a variety of complications, including septicemia, meningitis, and brain abscess. When sinus infection is chronic, surgery to clean out the sinuses may be necessary. A deviated septum can be surgically repaired, and polyps can be removed endoscopically if medical treatment is unsuccessful.

Complementary and Alternative Therapies

Treatment of Allergic Rhinitis and Sinusitis

Allergens in contact with mucous membranes prompt the inflammatory response. Eliminating the allergens can minimize the inflammation symptoms. Use of a neti pot or other device to irrigate the sinuses will rinse out the allergens. A nasal filter device can be used to prevent the allergens from getting into the nasal passages.

EPISTAXIS

Epistaxis (nosebleed) is a common occurrence and usually results from crusting, cracking, or irritation of the mucous membrane covering the front (anterior) of the nasal septum. Anterior bleeds are the most common (90% to 95%). Blood loss is usually minimal, but about 6% of nosebleeds require medical attention. Decreased humidity, excessive nose blowing, allergy with inflammation, and nose picking may cause nosebleeds. Overuse of nasal spray, street drug use (particularly "snorting"), and tumors are other causes. Any condition or medication that prolongs bleeding time or lowers the platelet count may predispose an individual to nosebleeds. Nosebleeds can also result from trauma, hypertension, and blood disorders such as leukemia. They are common in boys during pubescence.

Bleeding from the nose is the only sign of epistaxis. When epistaxis occurs, the patient should sit forward and apply direct pressure by pinching the nose just below the bone, close to the face, for 10 to 15 minutes. This position prevents blood from running down the back of the throat. Cold compresses or ice may be applied to the nose to constrict the blood vessels. If there is still bleeding at the end of a 10- to 15-minute period, repeat the process (Fig. 13.1). If bleeding continues, the patient should go to the emergency department, where a provider will cauterize the bleeding vessels, solidly pack the nose, or insert a small balloon device to stop the bleeding (Fig. 13.2). Once bleeding stops, the patient should rest quietly for a few hours and be instructed to avoid bending over and not to blow the nose, pick at it, or rub it for 24 hours after the nosebleed has stopped.

Clinical Cues

If a patient is having an active nosebleed, instruct them to spit the blood into a basin or tissue rather than swallowing it. Accumulation of blood in the stomach will eventually cause nausea and vomiting, and the patient's cooperation will help you assess the amount of bleeding and may help prevent aspiration of the blood.

Patients on anticoagulants and antiplatelet medications are at increased risk of nasal bleeding when nasal cannula oxygen is administered for prolonged periods, causing drying of the mucosa.

PHARYNGITIS

Etiology and Pathophysiology

Pharyngitis (inflammation of the pharynx), usually called a *sore throat,* may be caused by a virus, bacteria, or fungus. Most cases are viral. Acute **follicular pharyngitis** ("strep throat") is caused by beta-hemolytic streptococcal infection. Fungal pharyngitis occurs with long-term use of antibiotics or inhaled corticosteroids and in patients with immunosuppression, such as occurs with HIV/AIDS or during cancer treatment. **Laryngitis** (inflammation of the larynx with diminished voice or hoarseness) may occur if the infection progresses into the larynx. If the inflammation extends to the epiglottis, epiglottitis occurs; this is more common in children. Epiglottitis can cause an acute airway obstruction and should be monitored closely.

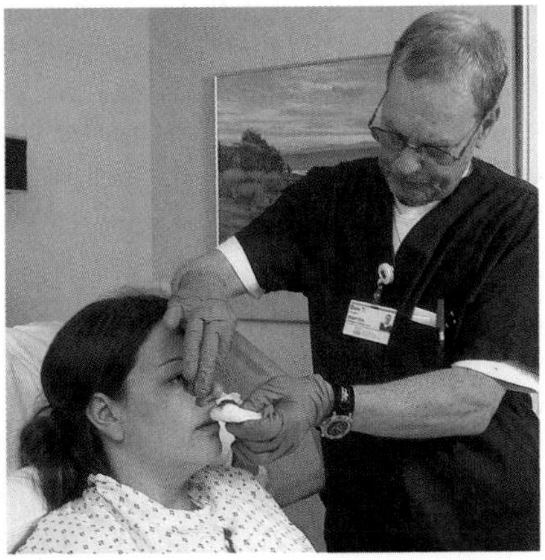

Fig. 13.1 Stopping a nosebleed by applying pressure to the nose.

Signs, Symptoms, and Diagnosis

The symptoms of pharyngitis include a dry, "scratchy" feeling in the back of the throat; mild fever; headache; and malaise. The throat, tonsils, palate, and uvula may be involved and will be reddened. If swelling of these structures is present, dysphagia may occur. Discomfort when swallowing one's own saliva is common but does not usually inhibit the ability to take adequate fluids and nourishment. With laryngitis, the voice may become hoarse or absent. The usual course for uncomplicated pharyngitis or laryngitis is 3 to 10 days. The diagnosis of pharyngitis is confirmed by clinical signs and symptoms. A throat culture is often performed to confirm or rule out streptococcal infection.

Treatment and Nursing Management

Uncomplicated viral pharyngitis usually responds to conservative measures, such as rest, warm saline gargles (½ to 1 tsp of table salt added to a glass of warm water), throat **lozenges** (small medicinal tablets that dissolve in the mouth), antiseptic sprays, plenty of fluids, and a mild analgesic for aches and pains.

Bacterial pharyngitis requires antibiotic therapy, particularly if the infecting organism is *Streptococcus.* Chronic pharyngitis may require diagnostic procedures to determine the underlying cause and therapeutic measures such as humidification and filtering of

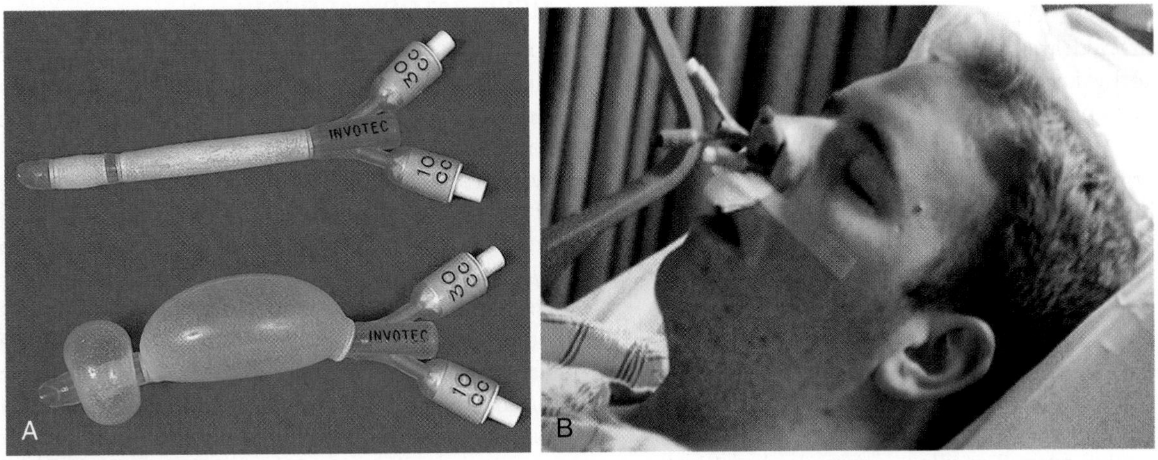

Fig. 13.2 A nasal balloon device **(A)** is being used to control bleeding from epistaxis **(B).** (Courtesy Invotec Corp., Jacksonville, Fla.)

environmental air. Fungal pharyngitis is treated with an antifungal agent but may be difficult to control in immunocompromised individuals.

TONSILLITIS

Etiology and Pathophysiology

An infection with inflammation of the tonsils is usually caused by viruses such as those causing the common cold. Group A streptococcus is the most common organism causing bacterial infections. Symptoms are somewhat similar to those of pharyngitis. Acute tonsillitis may occur repeatedly, especially in those who have a low resistance to infection.

Tonsillitis caused by the Epstein-Barr virus is called glandular fever or infectious mononucleosis.

Signs, Symptoms, and Diagnosis

Acute tonsillitis occurs more commonly in young children. Symptoms include high fever, sore throat, general malaise, pain referred to the ears, and chills. Inspection of the throat reveals redness and swelling of the tonsils and surrounding tissues with patches of yellow exudate. The white blood cell count becomes elevated.

Chronic tonsillitis usually produces an enlargement of tonsillar and adenoidal tissues. Chronic infection produces less dramatic symptoms than acute tonsillitis, but discomfort still occurs. A person with chronic tonsillitis and enlarged adenoids has frequent colds and appears to be in poor health.

Diagnosis is by physical examination and history. If a streptococcal infection is suspected, a throat culture or a "rapid strep test" may be performed.

Treatment

A throat culture is performed before treatment to check for the presence of *Streptococcus,* which can cause rheumatic fever or glomerulonephritis if not treated promptly. Acute tonsillitis is treated with warm saline throat gargles and the administration of specific antibiotics (usually penicillin) to destroy the pathogen. Nursing measures include bed rest, fever management, and a liquid diet to minimize trauma to the tissues and maintain hydration.

Surgery is used to treat tonsillitis when it is recurrent or when enlargement of the tonsils and adenoids obstructs airways. Surgery is considered if the patient has more than six episodes of streptococcal tonsillitis per year (Shah, 2018).

> **? Think Critically**
>
> What would be appropriate foods to offer a patient with pharyngitis or tonsillitis?

Nursing Management

Preoperative care. Tonsillectomy and adenoidectomy are generally done on an outpatient, same-day surgery basis. Preliminary laboratory testing and patient education begin before the patient is admitted. Physical preparation of the patient involves administering preoperative medications as ordered, restricting the use of aspirin or other nonsteroidal antiinflammatory medications, and restricting the patient's diet for 6 to 8 hours before surgery. An elevation of temperature or any signs of URI should be reported because surgery is usually postponed if these signs are present.

Postoperative care. Although patients usually recover rapidly from tonsillectomy and adenoidectomy and rarely suffer any complications, be vigilant for signs of hemorrhage. **Vital signs are checked frequently, and the patient is observed for frequent swallowing or clearing of the throat, which may indicate bleeding. Restlessness can be another clue to excessive bleeding.** Sneezing, coughing, and vomiting can cause bleeding. An ice collar or ice pack may be placed around the neck to reduce swelling and pain. A side-lying position when drowsy or semi-Fowler position when fully awake will help maintain a patent airway. The postoperative diet usually consists of cold or warm liquids, progressing to semisolid foods, for the first 24 hours. Avoiding red foods can help in distinguishing between ingested food and blood. Citrus fruits, hot fluids, and rough foods should be avoided until the throat has completely healed. Straws are not used because sucking may cause bleeding. Note that stools may be black due to the swallowing of blood. Written instructions for routine care, pain management, and emergency circumstances are reviewed with the caregiver and patient.

> **? Think Critically**
>
> What sign would alert you to the probability that a tonsillectomy patient is experiencing bleeding and that the blood is running down the throat where you cannot see it?

OBSTRUCTION AND TRAUMA

AIRWAY OBSTRUCTION AND RESPIRATORY ARREST

Laryngeal edema caused by the inflammation of an infection or an allergic reaction, a crush injury of the larynx, or a foreign object or food that goes down the airway rather than the esophagus may obstruct the airway. If a person seems to be choking, encourage forceful coughing if possible. If the person cannot breathe or speak, they may make the universal signal for choking, signaling for help by grasping at the throat with the hands (Fig. 13.3). If breathing is obstructed, abdominal thrusts should be performed (American Heart Association, 2015). The arms are wrapped around the victim from behind. One hand makes a fist with the thumb inward, then the fist is positioned just above the umbilicus. The other hand wraps around the fist. Upward thrusts are delivered into the abdomen to try to dislodge anything stuck in the

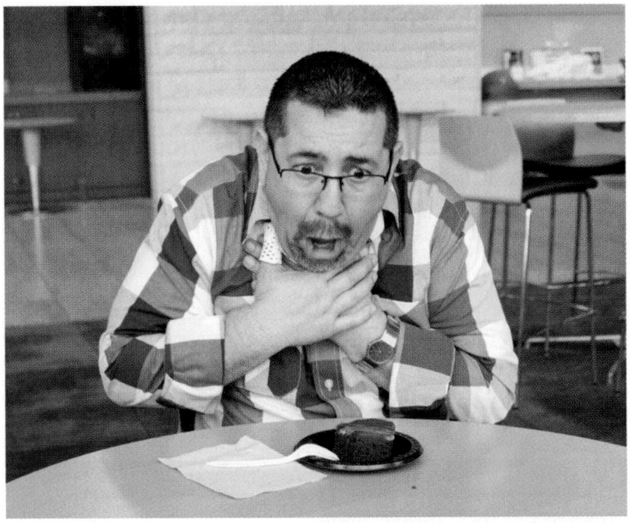

Fig. 13.3 The hands grasping the throat is the universal signal for choking.

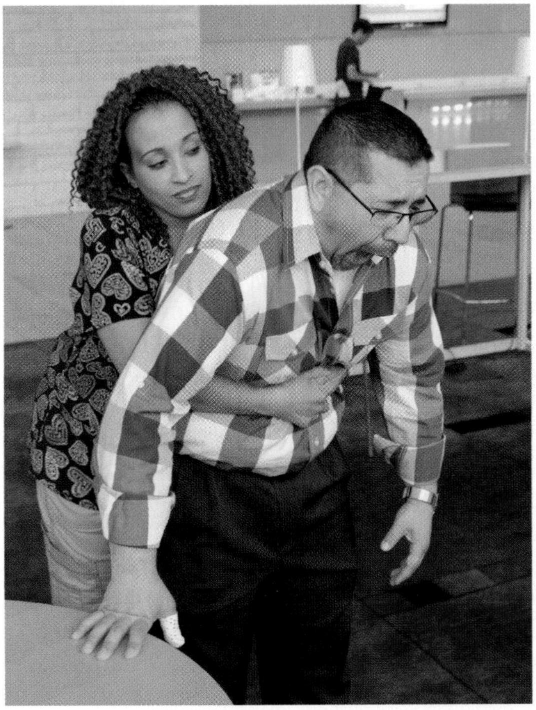

Fig. 13.4 Abdominal thrust.

airway (Fig. 13.4) (see Chapter 44). **In an unconscious adult or child older than 1 year, the most common cause of airway obstruction is the tongue.** An artificial airway may be orally or nasally inserted; it helps to keep the tongue in place (Fig. 13.5).

If the airway is obstructed for an extended period, the hypoxia may cause the heart to stop. If the obstruction is cleared but the patient has no pulse, cardiopulmonary resuscitation must be started (see Chapter 45).

OBSTRUCTIVE SLEEP APNEA

Obstructive sleep apnea (OSA) is a condition in which, during sleep, the person is making breathing effort but there is no or extremely limited airflow. Muscle relaxation at the back of the throat is the most common cause, allowing the tongue to fall back and block the airway. Snoring is common with this condition, and sleeping partners are usually the first to notice the problem. Daytime symptoms include fatigue, morning headaches, and difficulty concentrating. Physical examination of patients with OSA typically reveals obesity, enlarged neck circumference, and hypertension. A sleep study should be performed to determine the severity of the condition. Those with mild apnea may be treated with conservative measures such as weight loss, avoiding alcohol for 4 to 6 hours before bed, and sleep position modification. The first-line therapy for sleep apnea is nasal continuous positive airway pressure (CPAP) applied with nasal prongs. If that is unsuccessful, bilevel positive airway pressure (BiPAP) may be tried with a face mask or nasal mask (see Chapter 14, Fig. 14.10). Oral appliances may be used to maintain an airway. If noninvasive therapies fail, the patient can be offered surgical interventions, including implantable devices that stimulate the nerves leading to muscles controlling the palate and tongue or surgical alteration of the upper airway. Untreated sleep apnea can contribute to myocardial infarction or stroke. Since 2012, clinical guidelines require capnography (carbon dioxide [CO_2] monitoring)

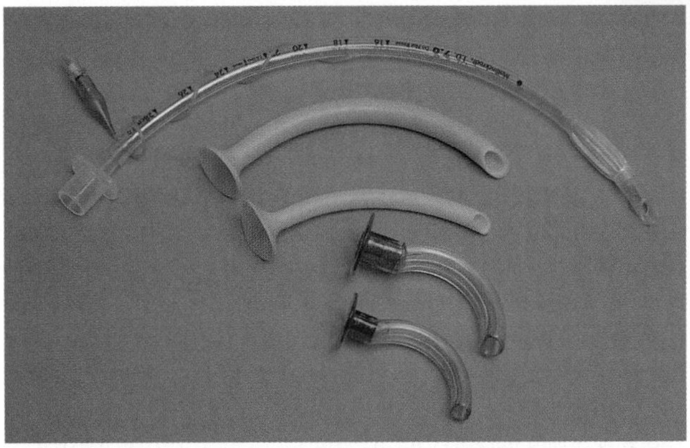

Fig. 13.5 Types of airways inserted during a respiratory emergency (endotracheal *[top]*, nasopharyngeal *[middle]*, and oropharyngeal *[bottom]*). (From Williams P: *deWit's fundamental concepts and skills for nursing*, ed 5, St. Louis, 2018, Elsevier.)

Clinical Cues

You can insert nasal or oropharyngeal airways. If indicated, an endotracheal tube would be inserted by a health care provider, respiratory therapist, or nurse anesthetist. Your role in this emergency procedure is to obtain the emergency airway equipment, including a laryngoscope, a 5- to 10-mL syringe, a manual resuscitation bag (Ambu bag), suction equipment, lubricant, a stylet, an endotracheal tube, and a securing device. You may also be required to oxygenate the patient using the resuscitation bag, administer medications for rapid sequence intubation, or assist in making the equipment available to the clinician performing the intubation.

for postoperative patients with OSA in addition to routine pulse oximetry monitoring after any surgical procedure (The Joint Commission, 2018).

NASAL FRACTURE

Nasal fracture often results from sports injuries, motor vehicle accidents, or physical assault and is the most common type of facial fracture. If the cartilage or bone is not displaced, complications are unlikely and no treatment is needed. Displacement of the cartilage or bone can interfere with airflow, cause deformity of the nose, and become a potential spot for infection.

Diagnosis is by visual inspection for deformity, a change in nasal breathing, and presence of **crepitation** (grating sound or a feeling of rough surfaces rubbing together) on palpation. It is important to determine whether other facial bones are also fractured. Imaging studies should be ordered if additional fractures are suspected. If the patient is seen within the first 24 hours after injury, a closed reduction is most often performed using local or general anesthetic. Treatment includes pain relief and the use of ice or cold compresses to reduce swelling.

If the fracture is severe, **rhinoplasty** (surgical reconstruction of the nose) may be performed to improve airflow and cosmetic appearance. Nasal packing, internal and/or external splints, or sutures may be used to stabilize the septum postoperatively. The patient will be given specific instructions depending on the procedure performed. Drainage from the nose is expected, and a drip pad of folded gauze is secured as a "mustache" dressing beneath the nose.

The patient is observed for frequent swallowing postoperatively, which could indicate posterior nasal bleeding. Vital signs are monitored closely, and the amount of drainage on the dressing is observed. The patient should be encouraged to rest in a semi-Fowler position. Cool compresses are used to decrease nose and facial swelling. Forceful coughing and straining at stool (Valsalva maneuver) should be avoided. Saline spray is used intranasally to help remove dried blood and clots. Over-the-counter analgesics are usually adequate for pain control. After recovery from anesthesia, the patient is typically discharged to recuperate at home. It may take 6 to 12 months before the end result of the surgery is evident.

CANCER OF THE LARYNX

Etiology and Pathophysiology

It was predicted that there would be 13,150 new cases of cancer of the larynx in 2018 (American Cancer Society [ACS], 2017). A clear association has been made between cigarette or cigar smoking, excessive use of alcohol, and the development of laryngeal cancer. Lack of fruits and vegetables in the diet, gastroesophageal reflux disease, immunosuppression, and infection with human papillomavirus or *Helicobacter pylori* have all been linked to increased incidence of cancer of the larynx. Exposure over long periods to environmental pollutants, such as asbestos, paint fumes, or wood or coal dust, has been shown to be associated with increased risk (ACS, 2017). The most common malignant tumor of the larynx is squamous cell carcinoma. It grows from the mucous membrane lining the respiratory tract. Metastasis may occur to the lung.

Signs, Symptoms, and Diagnosis

The larynx (sometimes called the *voice box*) is directly involved with the production of vocal sounds. A tumor of the larynx will quickly produce persistent hoarseness that does not respond to the usual methods of treatment.

Health Promotion

Signs of Possible Throat Cancer

Tell patients to seek medical attention if the following signs of cancer of the larynx or throat occur:

- Hoarseness that lasts more than 3 weeks
- Sore throat that lasts more than 2 weeks
- Consistent pain in or around the ear when swallowing
- Difficulty swallowing
- Dry, persistent cough for no known reason
- Blood in phlegm or saliva that lasts more than a few days
- Lumps or knots on the neck indicating enlarged cervical lymph nodes

After the cancer has spread beyond the vocal cords (and is much more difficult to treat), the symptoms may include difficulty in swallowing or breathing, halitosis, blood-tinged sputum, fatigue and weakness, a sensation of having a lump in the throat, cough, enlarged lymph nodes in the neck, pain in the region of the Adam's apple, or an airway obstruction.

Diagnosis is established by visualizing the larynx with a laryngoscope, by a computed tomography scan (may be combined with a positron emission tomography [PET] scan) of the larynx and throat, by magnetic resonance imaging, and by microscopic examination of a sample of tissues taken from the site.

Treatment

Once the type of cancer is determined, it is staged for appropriate treatment. Outpatient treatment is common. Radiation alone is 85% effective in treating early cancer of the larynx. Radiation may be combined with endoscopic laser cordectomy for certain types of lesions. Brachytherapy (also called internal radiotherapy) along with external beam radiation (or external radiotherapy) is used for certain types of lesions. When possible for organ preservation, the surgeon may perform a partial **laryngectomy**, in which the thyroid cartilage is split and only the tumor and involved portion of the larynx and vocal cords are removed. A partial laryngectomy does not permanently eliminate voice sounds. A **tracheostomy** (surgical opening into the trachea) may be performed to facilitate breathing temporarily, but the **stoma** (opening) is eventually closed, and the patient may resume talking after the affected area is completely healed.

Chemotherapy may be the initial treatment in some cases of laryngeal cancer. Combinations of chemotherapy and radiation may also be used first. These treatments are used to shrink the malignancy so that it can be removed surgically. The goal is to preserve as much function as possible.

A total laryngectomy is performed if the tumor has progressed to surrounding tissues, radiation therapy has failed, or better survival can be obtained by the more aggressive surgery. The surgeon excises the entire larynx and may remove all or part of the following structures: epiglottis, thyroid cartilage, hyoid bone, cricoid cartilage, and two or more rings of the trachea (Fig. 13.6). Near-total laryngectomy preserves voice production and swallowing and is used when possible.

If the tumor has extended to the lymph nodes, neck dissection is performed on the side of the lesion. In a radical neck surgery, all the muscle, lymph nodes, and soft tissue from the lower edge of the mandible to the clavicle and from the top of the trapezius muscle to the midline are removed. A modified radical neck dissection is more commonly performed and excises only the lymph tissue and surrounding structures directly affected by the cancer. A permanent tracheostomy is performed at the same time. A laryngectomy tube, which is shorter and wider than a tracheostomy tube, is put into place before discharge. After the stoma is completely healed and matured, about 6 weeks after surgery, the tube can be taken out as long as there is no compromise of the airway.

Extensive surgeries will often include placement of a feeding tube for nutrition until the surgical site is sufficiently healed to allow for swallowing. For patients with tracheal or laryngeal procedures, a swallow evaluation should be performed before food or fluids are resumed.

When the patient is discharged from the hospital, a visiting nurse, clinic nurse, or occupational therapist will work with the patient on eating skills if indicated. Some patients will have to rely on a feeding tube if they cannot master the swallowing procedure without aspiration. The indwelling tube may then be replaced with a gastrostomy tube.

? Think Critically

How can you help decrease the incidence of cancer of the larynx?

Endotracheal intubation and tracheostomy. **Endotracheal intubation** means that an endotracheal tube is inserted into the trachea through the nose or the mouth with the use of a **laryngoscope**. In some settings video laryngoscopes may be used for better accuracy in placement. An endotracheal tube is placed for airway protection against aspiration, when there is upper airway obstruction, and when mechanical ventilation is necessary.

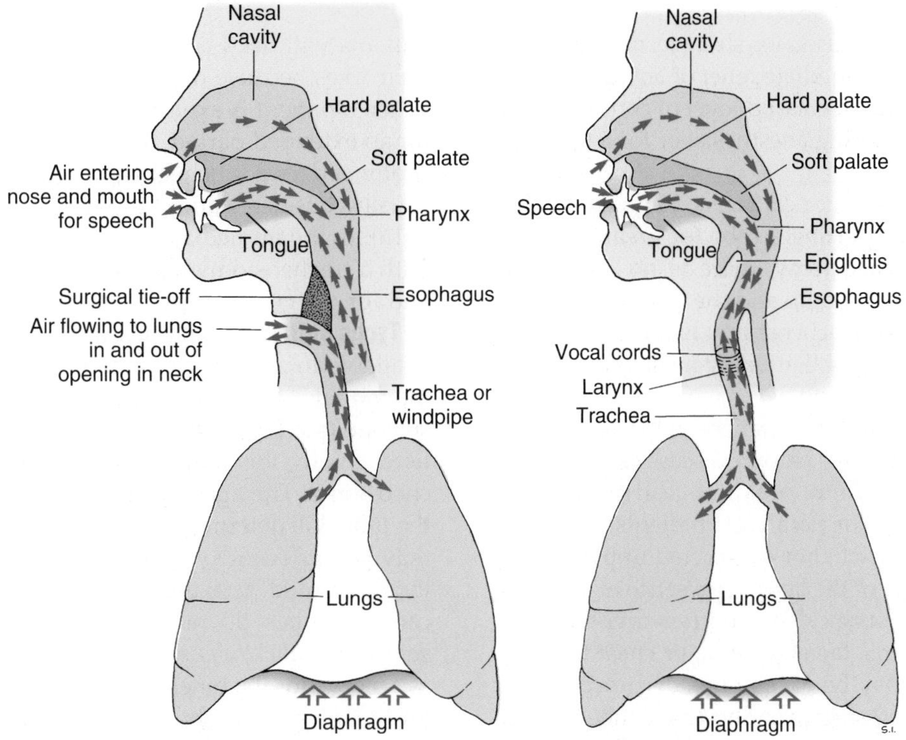

Fig. 13.6 Airflow after laryngectomy *(left)* and in a normal respiratory tract *(right)*.

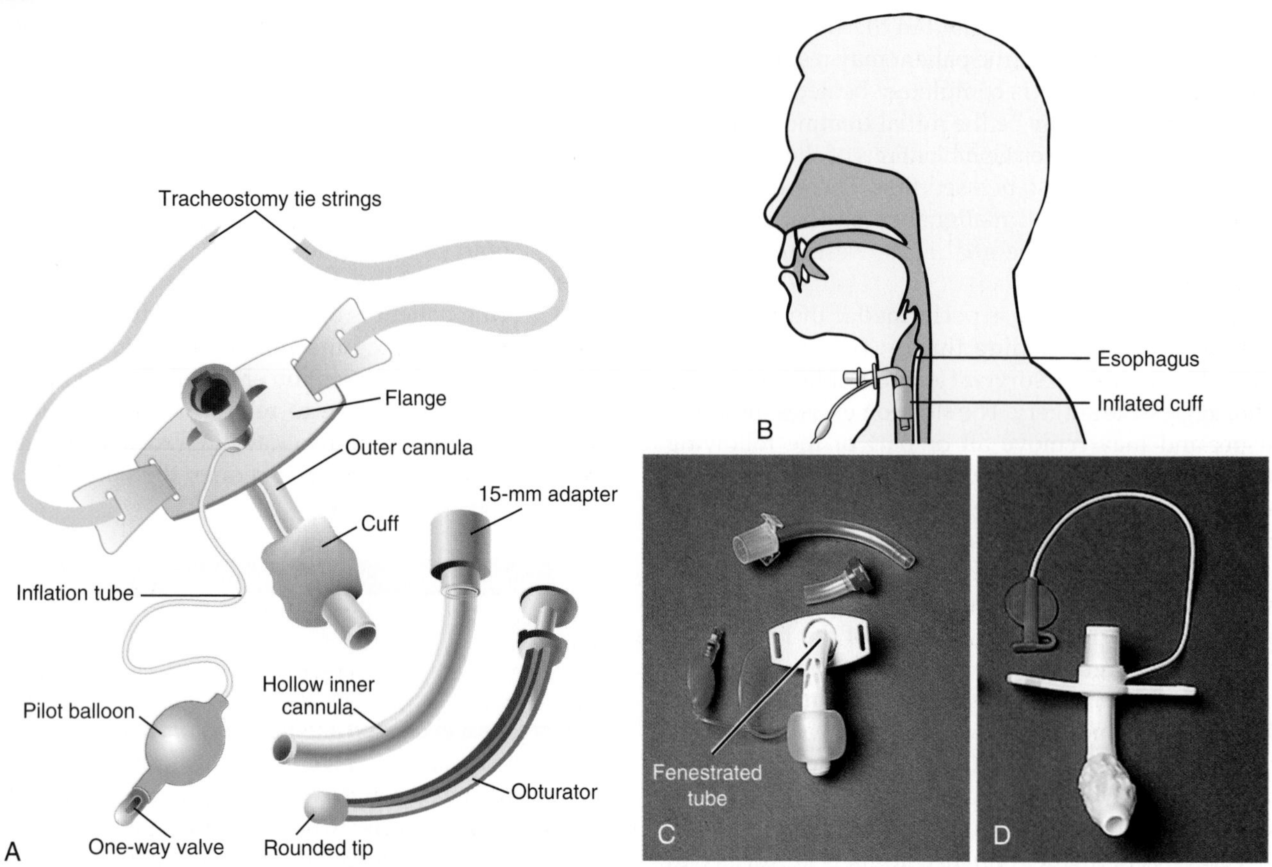

Fig. 13.7 Types of Tracheostomy Tubes. A, Parts of a tracheostomy tube. **B,** Tracheostomy tube inserted in airway, shown with cuff inflated. **C,** Fenestrated tracheostomy tube with cuff, inner cannula, decannulation plug, and pilot balloon. **D,** Tracheostomy tube with foam cuff and obturator. Cuff is deflated on tracheostomy tube. (From Lewis S, Bucher L, Heitkemper MM, et al.: *Medical-surgical nursing: assessment and management of clinical problems,* ed 10, St. Louis, 2017, Elsevier.)

Endotracheal tubes are used for short-term respiratory support, such as for immediate relief of airway obstruction; for patients with decreased level of consciousness because of trauma; during anesthesia; or for a few days postoperatively.

A tracheostomy is a surgical incision into the trachea for the purpose of inserting a tube for breathing. In a patient with a tracheostomy, there is no connection between the nose and mouth and the lower respiratory system (Fig. 13.7, *B*). Tracheostomy is done:

- To assist or control ventilation by mechanical means over a prolonged period
- To facilitate suctioning of secretions in the air passages when the patient with a chronic disease cannot cough
- To prevent aspiration of oral and gastric secretions (as in unconscious or paralyzed patients)
- To bypass a constricted or obstructed upper airway (e.g., from edema of the larynx, presence of a foreign body or tumor, surgical procedures involving the neck, severe burns, facial trauma, or chest trauma)

Tracheostomy may be an emergency procedure or elective surgery. If passing an endotracheal tube through the mouth is impossible or extremely difficult, a tracheostomy may be done to provide an airway. Some patients will need a tracheostomy tube for the rest of their lives because of anatomic changes in the throat. When a patient is expected to need an artificial airway for an extended period, tracheostomy is preferred over prolonged endotracheal intubation. Tracheostomy is usually considered after 1 to 3 weeks of intubation (Hyzy, 2016). In the immediate postoperative period, patients with a tracheostomy may need mechanical ventilation and/or oxygen therapy (see Chapter 14).

Types of tracheostomy tubes. Tracheostomy tubes are available in a variety of materials and styles. Most of the models are made of polyvinyl chloride (plastic) or silicone (see Fig. 13.7). Tubes made of metal alloys are used chiefly for patients who need a permanent tracheostomy. The age of the patient and the purpose of the tube will determine what features are selected. They may be cuffed or uncuffed and may have a reusable inner cannula or a disposable inner cannula. Single-cannula tubes do not have an inner cannula. In a *double-cannula tracheostomy tube,* the outer cannula acts as a sleeve for the inner cannula, which can be removed for cleaning. The **obturator** (insertion guide) is used during insertion as a guide (the tip, shaped like an olive, extends beyond the end of the tube) to protect against scraping the sides of the trachea with the sharp edge of the tube (see Fig. 13.7, *A*).

Fenestrated tubes have a small opening in the outer cannula that allows some air to escape through the larynx (see Fig. 13.7, *C*). This helps prepare the patient for the time when the tracheostomy tube will be removed and breathing occurs normally again. If the fenestrated tube is cuffed and the cuff is not inflated, the airflow allows for speech. A one-way tracheostomy valve box can be fitted into the tube opening. It allows air to be inhaled through the tracheostomy opening, but the valve closes when the patient exhales. This diverts the exhaled air through the larynx and enables the patient to speak.

A *cuffed tracheostomy tube* has a small balloon encircling its tracheal end. When the balloon is inflated, it fills the space between the outside of the tracheostomy tube and the trachea, thereby providing a seal and preventing the escape of air around the tube. When positive pressure mechanical ventilation is administered, the air passes through the tracheostomy tube *only*, thus providing sufficient pressure to inflate the lungs. The cuffed tracheostomy tube may offer some protection against aspiration of mucus and fluids; however, the use of the cuffed tube does not replace careful nursing observation or interventions to prevent aspiration.

Foam-cuffed tracheostomy tubes have the cuff filled with a sponge-like material that is fully expanded at rest. To insert the tube, air must be withdrawn from the cuff so that the foam compresses, allowing for placement (see Fig. 13.7, *D*). When in place, the cuff inflation line is left open to air, which allows for compression and expansion of the cuff with tracheal movement. Because of this, minimal pressure is exerted on the tracheal wall, decreasing the risk of tissue damage or necrosis.

Nursing Management

A patient with a new tracheostomy requires very specialized nursing care, especially if mechanical ventilation through the tube is required. **Immediate postoperative care focuses on maintaining a patent airway and observing for hemorrhage.** During the first 24 hours, the patient is monitored continuously for signs of respiratory distress. If the patient is unable to cough to remove mucus and drainage, tracheal suctioning is necessary. If the lumen is not kept open, the patient will suffocate. Suctioning is done with strict sterile technique to prevent infection. See Nursing Care Plan 13.1. Adequate humidification of the inhaled air prevents drying of mucous membranes, and hydration of the patient helps to thin secretions.

The lungs should be auscultated (1) before suctioning to assess the need and (2) afterward to verify that the procedure successfully cleared the airways. Head-to-toe assessment is performed as for any surgical patient (see Chapter 5).

When the patient has a tracheostomy tube with a cuff, the cuff must be inflated just enough to seal the trachea without causing extreme pressure against the tracheal wall; otherwise depression of the surface blood vessels in the tracheal wall will cause necrosis. Cuff pressure is checked with a manometer each shift and each time the degree of cuff inflation is changed.

> **Clinical Cues**
>
> When you are suctioning a patient with a tracheostomy or endotracheal tube and using a sterile suction kit, ask an assistant to accompany you to deliver oxygen before and during the procedure (as needed). Oxygenation of the patient will prevent desaturation, and the assistance of a helper allows you to maintain sterile technique. Patients on mechanical ventilation can be preoxygenated with the ventilator and may have an inline suction device attached to the airway.

> **Assignment Considerations**
>
> **Reporting on a Patient With a Tracheostomy**
>
> Instruct the unlicensed assistive personnel (UAP) to immediately report coughing episodes or coarse gurgling sounds produced by a patient with a tracheostomy. Explain that you must be notified so that you can perform an immediate assessment and possible suctioning to alleviate an airway obstruction.

Preventing infection is another nursing responsibility. The incision is an open wound with minimal dressings and is an ideal entryway for infectious organisms. Tracheostomy care is a sterile procedure until the stoma is well healed. **When changing the ties or Velcro tube holder of the tracheostomy tube, the tube should be manually held in place; otherwise the tube may be dislodged by coughing.** (Coughing frequently occurs when the tube is moved or manipulated.)

If the patient will go home with a tracheostomy, techniques for suctioning and providing the necessary tracheostomy care are taught to both the patient and a family member or caregiver.

> **Patient Teaching**
>
> **Home Care of a Tracheostomy**
>
> The patient and family should be taught the following points:
>
> - Clean the stoma with normal saline and cotton-tipped sterile applicators, removing all secretions, on a daily basis and as needed.
> - Replace the commercially split gauze pad around the tube as frequently as needed when it becomes soiled. (Do not cut regular gauze pads, because the loose threads can be aspirated.)
> - It is best to have two people help change the ties or tube holder because movement of the tube can easily cause the patient to cough and expel the tube from the stoma.
> - Prepare the new ties before loosening the old ones. If a device with self-sticking ties is used, attach the new holder before removing the soiled holder.
> - Hold the tube securely in place with thumb and forefinger while the ties are loose.
> - Stand to the side of the stoma when providing care because if the patient coughs, mucus may be expelled.

Nursing Care Plan 13.1 Care of a Patient With a Laryngectomy

SCENARIO

Mr. Collins had a supraglottic laryngectomy 5 days ago. He is having difficulty adjusting to his tracheostomy and frequently chokes when trying to eat or swallow secretions. He indicates, with pencil and paper, that he does not feel he can learn to speak again and is very anxious about choking; he is withdrawn.

PROBLEM STATEMENT/NURSING DIAGNOSIS

Alteration in airway clearance related to secretions resulting from surgery and tracheostomy.

SUPPORTING ASSESSMENT DATA

Objective: Unable to cough out secretions; becomes hypoxic when secretions build up, decreasing airflow.

Goals/Expected Outcomes	Nursing Interventions	Selected Rationale	Evaluation
Airway will remain patent	Assess respiratory effort and rate; auscultate upper airways to determine needs for suctioning on a frequent basis. Observe ostomy site for secretions.	If rate or respiratory effort increases, the airway may be obstructed. Coarse sounds heard in the upper airways or secretions at ostomy site indicate need for suctioning.	Respiratory rate varies; 18/min if patient is relaxed. Rate of 28–30/min when anxious or trying to cough out mucus. (Suctioning improves respiratory rate when mucus is cleared.)
	Suction as needed.	Suctioning secretions clears airway.	Suctioning is effective.
Patient will learn to suction own tracheostomy effectively by discharge.	Encourage patient to assist with procedure (e.g., have patient hold water for moistening catheter).	Having patient assist with small steps helps him develop confidence for home care.	Patient is making attempts to learn suctioning technique.
	Teach to attach catheter to suction tubing; teach to suction self using mirror.	Knowledge and practice are essential for self-care.	Beginning to attempt to cough out secretions and suction.
	Praise for all attempts.	Praise reinforces patient's efforts and learning.	Positive reinforcement given for any attempt.
	Point out advantages of not being dependent on others for care of airway.	Provides incentive to learn self-care.	States he wants to be independent.
Patient will learn to clear tracheostomy by coughing effectively.	Medicate for discomfort and encourage patient to cough to remove secretions without suctioning.	Lessened discomfort makes it possible to cough effectively.	Analgesia provided as ordered.
	Assist to an upright position of at least 45 degrees.	Sitting upright allows for full expansion of chest cavity.	Able to place self in an upright position and reposition self as needed.
	Remind to hold tissues in front of tube rather than the mouth.	Secretions will be coughed out of the tube.	Holding tissues in front of tube when coughing.
	Instruct to breathe deeply for several seconds and to forcefully cough two or three times using the abdominal muscles.	Use of abdominal muscles increases the force and depth of the cough.	Able to perform deep coughing with support and coaching.

PROBLEM STATEMENT/NURSING DIAGNOSIS

Altered skin integrity related to surgical incisions.

SUPPORTING ASSESSMENT DATA

Objective: Supraglottic laryngectomy and tracheostomy.

Goals/Expected Outcomes	Nursing Interventions	Selected Rationale	Evaluation
No infection at incision sites as evidenced by absence of redness, swelling, or purulent discharge.	Clean around tracheostomy stoma with normal saline; q4–8h change gauze pad PRN (as needed).	Cleans away bacteria and helps prevent infection.	No evidence of infection. Slight redness around tracheostomy stoma.
Skin integrity will be intact within 6 wk.	Change tracheostomy ties or holder at least q24h and as needed.		Skin is intact; no redness or signs of irritation.
	Observe for signs of infection.	Early recognition ensures prompt treatment.	No signs of infection. Continue plan.

Nursing Care Plan 13.1 Care of a Patient With a Laryngectomy—cont'd

PROBLEM STATEMENT/NURSING DIAGNOSIS

Altered verbal communication ability related to loss of larynx.

SUPPORTING ASSESSMENT DATA

Subjective: No verbal communication.

Objective: Laryngectomy and tracheostomy.

Goals/Expected Outcomes	Nursing Interventions	Selected Rationale	Evaluation
Effective communication will be established	Assist patient to use dry erase board or paper and pencil for communication; show patience.	Provides for some means of communication.	Using communication tools.
Patient will show interest in learning new style of speech within 6 wk.	Reinforce teaching from the speech therapist and encourage efforts.	It is important to recognize and celebrate progress.	Practicing exercises taught by speech therapist
	Obtain order for visit from rehabilitated patient who has mastered some form of speech.	Seeing an example reinforces the possibility of regaining a form of speech.	Visit scheduled.
	Encourage affiliation with community support group.	Support from people with a similar problem helps decrease feelings of isolation and helplessness.	Advised about support group. Continue plan.

PROBLEM STATEMENT/NURSING DIAGNOSIS

Potential risk for aspiration related to choking when trying to swallow.

SUPPORTING ASSESSMENT DATA

Subjective: Writes that he does not feel he will be able to swallow or eat by mouth again.

Objective: Chokes when he tries to swallow saliva; tends to aspirate.

Goals/Expected Outcomes	Nursing Interventions	Selected Rationale	Evaluation
Patient will not experience injury from aspiration of food or fluids.	Place in an upright position before eating or medication administration and maintain for at least 1 h.	Gravity facilitates the downward movement of the food bolus.	Able to place self in an upright position; acknowledges need to remain upright for 1 h after eating.
	Teach to hold his breath and perform the Valsalva maneuver while swallowing.	Valsalva maneuver closes the glottis over the tracheal opening in the throat, preventing food from entering the trachea.	Practicing but having trouble coordinating the breathing and Valsalva maneuver and swallowing.
Patient will learn to swallow without aspirating within 6 wk.	Teach to keep neck relaxed forward, take small bite of food, keep chin toward chest, swallow, then forcibly exhale.	Exhaling forcibly after swallowing will expel particles that accidentally end up in the trachea.	Is still choking when he tries to swallow. Revise plan: Obtain consultation with speech therapist for swallowing exercises.

CRITICAL THINKING QUESTIONS

1. What psychosocial problems might Mr. Collins experience?
2. How can you motivate Mr. Collins to participate in suctioning his tracheostomy?

Psychological support of the tracheostomy patient and family is essential. The patient must learn to breathe in a totally different way and cannot speak or call out for help. A Passy-Muir speaking tracheostomy valve (Fig. 13.8) may be used by some patients. Verbal reassurance will show awareness of apprehension and readiness to help. Explanations about what is being done and why it is being done are given each time tracheostomy care is provided. Teaching begins as soon as the patient is alert after the tracheostomy tube is placed. The patient may experience grief over losing their natural voice and the change in eating. The patient will need help in facing a future in which they will not be able to speak normally. A radical neck dissection may create body image disturbance because the procedure can be somewhat disfiguring. Initially, depression is common.

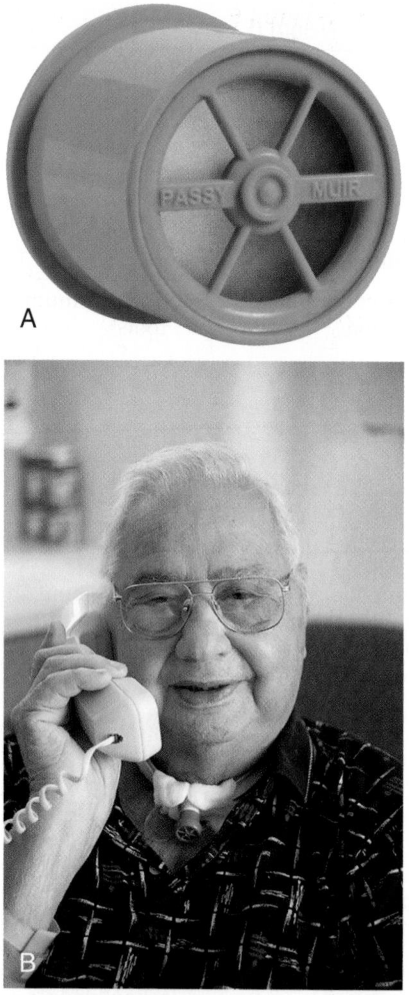

Fig. 13.8 **A,** Passy-Muir speaking tracheostomy valve. **B,** Patient using a Passy-Muir valve. (Courtesy Passey-Muir, Inc., Irvine, Calif.)

Contact with others who have had the surgery may help the patient focus on the benefits of lifesaving surgery.

The laryngectomy patient needs to be provided with a means of communication, such as a pad and pencil, a dry erase board, a picture board device, or electronic devices with appropriate software.

Once the tracheal stoma is healed, protection of the tracheal opening from dust and lint can be accomplished through the use of a simple gauze covering or high-necked clothing. The patient also should be told to avoid swimming and to use care when taking a shower or tub bath so that water is not aspirated through the opening. To protect the patient from inhalation of extremely cold air (the patient no longer breathes through the nose and mouth, which normally warm the inspired air), they may wear a small scarf over the opening during the winter. A stoma cover may be used to retain moisture.

Rehabilitation. Proper rehabilitation is important in the acceptance of surgery and its consequences. The speech therapist helps the patient master a new form of speech.

Nutrition Considerations

Assisting the Patient With Swallowing After a Partial Laryngectomy

- Explain that swallowing food without choking is possible.
- Arrange a visit from a partial laryngectomy patient who has mastered the technique.
- Begin practice with soft or semisolid foods.
- Supervise initial practice and explain that someone needs to be with the patient when they eat until swallowing without choking is mastered.
- Teach to swallow by asking the patient to:
  - Take a deep breath and bear down to close the vocal cords.
  - Place a small bite of food in the mouth.
  - Tip the chin toward the chest and swallow.
  - Emit a cough to rid the throat of any food particles.
  - Swallow again.
  - Cough again.
  - Begin breathing normally again.
- Offer encouragement for each effort.

Many people can learn esophageal speech; first they master the art of swallowing air and then moving it forcibly back up through the esophagus; then they learn to coordinate lip and tongue movements with the sound produced by the air passing over vibrating folds of the esophagus. The sounds may be somewhat hoarse but are more natural than those produced by an artificial larynx. For patients who cannot master esophageal speech, a tracheoesophageal prosthesis can be implanted. A fistula is made between the esophagus and trachea; a silicone prosthesis is inserted after the fistula heals. The patient covers the opening of the prosthesis with a finger or closes a special valve that diverts air from the lungs up through the trachea into the esophagus and out of the mouth. Lip and tongue movements form speech as the air is expelled.

An electronic artificial larynx is a battery-powered device that is applied externally to the skin of the esophagus to simulate speech. The sounds are not voicelike but are understandable and make it possible for the patient to communicate (Fig. 13.9).

Another option is an electronic speech aid that has a small tube device that can be inserted into the mouth. The patient can push a button device implanted in the throat that allows diaphragmatic speech.

Throughout the United States, groups have been organized for laryngectomy patients who wish to get together for social and rehabilitation purposes.

Think Critically

Identify all of the health care professionals who would be involved in the collaborative care of a patient undergoing a total laryngectomy and radical neck dissection.

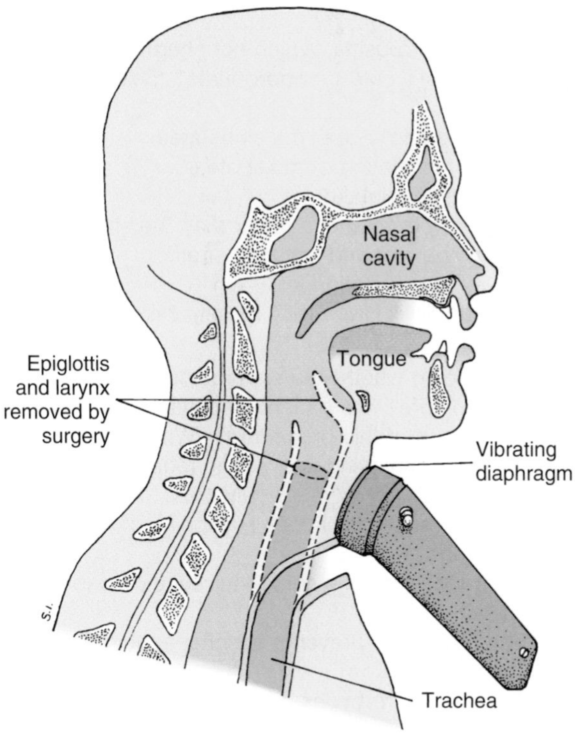

Fig. 13.9 External electronic larynx. The vibrating cap of the electronic larynx is held against the throat with sufficient pressure to maintain firm contact. Sound vibrations are transmitted into the lower portion of the pharynx and transformed into speech by the normal movements of the tongue, lips, and teeth.

COMMUNITY CARE

One of the primary aspects of community care for nurses is to promote immunization for influenza and pneumonia. Remind the public that frequent hand hygiene and covering the mouth when coughing or sneezing are simple measures that prevent the spread of URIs.

HOME CARE

Home care nurses follow up with patients who have had surgery or need further teaching or assessment. **Reminding patients to take all prescribed antibiotics as directed is very important in preventing the development of disease-resistant strains of bacteria** (CDC, 2017). The home care nurse will also help patients with throat cancer or surgeries to address nutritional concerns, provide wound care, supervise self-care techniques for care of a tracheostomy, and provide psychosocial support.

Tracheostomy care in the home setting differs from hospital procedures. In the home, suction catheters may be used longer and can be disinfected for reuse. Once the stoma is healed, the patient learns to adapt supplies to their needs. You can help identify community resources that can help meet the needs of the patient.

EXTENDED CARE

Extended care facility nurses must be vigilant for signs of URI among residents to prevent the spread of infection. If you have a contagious URI, do not expose your older adult patients. Stay at home or diligently wear a mask and perform hand hygiene. Adequate protein stores and hydration will promote immunity for your patients. Timely immunization against influenza and pneumonia is a top priority. Assist residents with hand hygiene and remind everyone to cover sneezes and coughs to decrease the spread of URIs within the facility.

Get Ready for the NCLEX® Examination!

Key Points

- If a cold persists or high fever develops, the patient should obtain medical attention.
- Rhinitis may be allergic in origin. If it interferes with lifestyle or productivity, desensitization is an option.
- Sinusitis symptoms include headache, fever, tenderness over the sinuses, purulent drainage from the nose, painful upper teeth, and malaise. A nonproductive cough may be present.
- Epistaxis is caused by many factors, such as irritation from nose blowing, hypertension, trauma, blood dyscrasias, decreased humidity, and nose picking. Apply direct pressure to the nose for 10 to 15 minutes to stop bleeding; cold compresses or ice is helpful.
- Pharyngitis is inflammation of the pharynx, or sore throat, that is viral, bacterial, or fungal in origin. Treatment for viral pharyngitis is rest, warm saline gargles, throat lozenges, and a mild analgesic. A throat culture and antibiotics are common for bacterial pharyngitis.
- Treatment and nursing interventions for tonsillitis consist of warm saline gargles, throat lozenges, rest, and antibiotics.
- When a tonsillectomy is performed, check vital signs frequently; keep the patient on their side or abdomen for as long as there is drainage from the throat; and limit diet to soft, nonirritating foods until the throat is no longer sensitive. Observe for frequent swallowing, which may indicate blood running down the throat.
- Rhinoplasty is performed for severe nasal fracture; the postoperative priority is to monitor for and control bleeding.
- Risk factors for cancer of the larynx include smoking, immoderate alcohol use, chronic laryngitis, and abuse of vocal cords. Persistent hoarseness is a first sign of cancer of the larynx; later signs are pain in the throat, coughing, dysphagia, a lump in the throat, or pain in the region of the Adam's apple. Surgical treatment for laryngeal tumor is laser treatment, partial or total laryngectomy, and possible radical neck dissection.

- Endotracheal intubation or tracheostomy provides an artificial airway. Major concerns of an artificial airway are maintaining an open airway and preventing infection.
- Promote immunization for influenza and pneumonia. Teach prevention of infection by hygiene measures—proper hand hygiene and covering the mouth when coughing or sneezing.

Additional Learning Resources

SG Go to your Study Guide for additional learning activities to help you master this chapter content.

Go to your Evolve website (http://evolve.elsevier.com/deWit/medsurg) for the following FREE learning resources:

- Animations, audio, and video
- Answers and rationales for questions and activities
- Glossary with pronunciations in English and Spanish
- Interactive Review Questions and more!

Review Questions for the NCLEX® Examination

1. On initial assessment, a patient who just had a tonsillectomy and an adenoidectomy is restless and swallows frequently. What is the most likely explanation?
   1. Excessive thirst
   2. Swelling in the neck
   3. Bleeding
   4. Sore throat

   NCLEX Client Need: Physiological Integrity: Reduction of Risk Potential
2. A 45-year-old man who is eating steak suddenly rises from his seat. His hands are grasping his throat. What actions should be performed? Identify the correct sequence.
   1. Position your open hand just above the umbilicus.
   2. Wrap your arms around the man from behind.
   3. Deliver upward squeeze thrusts.
   4. Ask the man if he is choking.

   NCLEX Client Need: Physiological Integrity: Physiological Adaptation
3. When caring for a patient who had a rhinoplasty, you should perform which intervention(s) in the immediate postoperative period? *(Select all that apply.)*
   1. Observe for frequent swallowing.
   2. Monitor amount of drainage on dressing.
   3. Position patient flat on the back.
   4. Apply warm compresses.
   5. Provide humidified oxygen.

   NCLEX Client Need: Physiological Integrity: Reduction of Risk Potential
4. The spouse of a patient with a tracheostomy asks, "What is the purpose of the cuff on the tracheostomy tube?" What is the best response?
   1. "It holds the tube in place."
   2. "It allows the ventilator to deliver a full breath of air."
   3. "It prevents the development of pneumonia."
   4. "It reduces the risk for tracheal wall necrosis."

   NCLEX Client Need: Physiological Integrity: Physiological Adaptation
5. A patient has sinusitis. Which nonpharmacologic intervention(s) would be appropriate? *(Select all that apply.)*
   1. Apply ice packs over the sinus area.
   2. Suggest inhalation of moist steam.
   3. Increase fluid intake.
   4. Position with the head lower than the shoulders.
   5. Encourage rest and reduced stress.
   6. Use a sinus irrigation kit.

   NCLEX Client Need: Physiological Integrity: Basic Care and Comfort
6. While deciding whether to sign the surgical consent for tracheostomy, the patient's spouse asks, "What is the purpose of this procedure?" Which response(s) demonstrate(s) nursing knowledge regarding the procedure? *(Select all that apply.)*
   1. "The procedure facilitates suctioning of respiratory secretions."
   2. "The procedure prevents recurrence of respiratory arrest."
   3. "The procedure prevents hospital-acquired pneumonia."
   4. "The procedure bypasses an obstructed upper airway."
   5. "The procedure is a temporary airway for face and neck injuries."

   NCLEX Client Need: Physiological Integrity: Physiological Adaptation
7. A 55-year-old man with a new tracheostomy is unable to cough. Breath sounds are diminished. Pulse oximetry is 88% on 100% humidified air. What is the priority nursing action?
   1. Provide positive pressure ventilation.
   2. Suction respiratory secretions.
   3. Administer pain medications.
   4. Humidify inhaled air.

   NCLEX Client Need: Physiological Integrity: Physiological Adaptation
8. A patient is newly diagnosed with a squamous cell carcinoma of the larynx. What is an early sign and symptom for this diagnosis?
   1. Crepitation
   2. Hoarseness
   3. Frothy sputum
   4. Drooling

   NCLEX Client Need: Health Promotion and Maintenance
9. A student is caring for a patient diagnosed with OSA. The patient is not convinced that the CPAP machine is worth the effort. What is the most important reason for the patient to receive treatment?
   1. Use of the CPAP machine will decrease the risk of pneumonia.
   2. Use of the CPAP machine will improve energy levels.
   3. Untreated OSA can lead to heart attack and stroke.
   4. Untreated OSA can lead to upper airway cancers.

   NCLEX Client Need: Health Promotion and Maintenance

10. A nurse is caring for a patient who is postoperative for tonsillectomy. Within the first 24 hours, which food item would be the most appropriate to offer the patient?
    1. Orange juice
    2. Warm tea
    3. Snack crackers
    4. Popsicles

    NCLEX Client Need: Basic Care and Comfort

Critical Thinking Questions

Scenario A

Mr. Kim has undergone diagnostic procedures to confirm suspected cancer of the larynx. He has been admitted to the hospital for a laryngectomy.

1. What is the primary postoperative issue related to Mr. Kim's nutritional status?
2. Identify interventions and teaching points that will allow Mr. Kim to eat and swallow safely.
3. Devise a postoperative nursing care plan for Mr. Kim, including interventions for psychosocial problems.
4. What resources in the community could be suggested to help Mr. Kim adjust to his laryngectomy?

Scenario B

Mr. George has undergone a total laryngectomy and radical neck dissection.

1. What structures would have been removed during this surgery, and how would Mr. George's life be affected?
2. How often should Mr. George's tracheostomy be suctioned?
3. How might you facilitate communication with Mr. George during the postoperative period?

Scenario C

You are not scheduled to work today or tomorrow, and you are glad because you don't feel very well and suspect that you might have a cold.

1. What are the signs and symptoms of the common cold?
2. What measures will you take to prevent the spread of the virus to your family?
3. Describe the interventions you will use to manage your own symptoms at home.

14 Care of Patients With Disorders of the Lower Respiratory System

http://evolve.elsevier.com/deWit/medsurg

Objectives

Theory

1. Discuss appropriate nursing care for patients with bronchitis, influenza, pneumonia, empyema, and pleurisy.
2. Choose nursing interventions appropriate for the care of patients with the problem statements Alteration in airway clearance, Altered breathing pattern, Altered gas exchange, and Fatigue due to hypoxia.
3. Explain ways a nurse can contribute to prevention and prompt treatment of tuberculosis.
4. Summarize the pathophysiologic changes that occur during an asthma attack.
5. Evaluate problems that occur with aging that may cause a restrictive pulmonary disorder.
6. Describe the specifics of nursing care for a patient who has had thoracic surgery and has chest tubes in place.

Clinical Practice

7. Complete a nursing care plan, including home care, for a patient with chronic obstructive pulmonary disease.
8. Review nursing interventions for a patient with a tracheostomy who is receiving oxygen therapy.
9. Teach a patient how to use a peak flowmeter.
10. Observe a respiratory therapist (RT) who is responsible for a patient on a mechanical ventilator and identify how RTs and nurses work together to deliver safe care.

Key Terms

aerosols (ĂR-ō-sŏlz, p. 326)
asthma (ĂZ-mă, p. 309)
atelectasis (ă-tē-LĔK-tă-sĭs, p. 302)
bronchiectasis (brŏng-kē-ĔK-tă-sĭs, p. 307)
bronchodilators (brŏng-kō-DĪ-lā-tĕrz, p. 323)
cor pulmonale (kŏr pŭl-mō-NĂ-lē, p. 315)
crepitus (KRĔP-ĕ-tŭs, p. 321)
emphysema (ĕm-fĭ-SĒ-mă, p. 309)
health care–associated pneumonia (HCAP) (hĕlth kār ĕ-SŌ-shē-ā-tĕd nū-MŌ-nē-ă, p. 301)
hemoptysis (hē-MŎP-tĭ-sĭs, p. 303)
hemothorax (hē-mō-THŌ-răks, p. 318)
hospital-acquired pneumonia (HAP) (HŎS-pĭ-tăl ă-KWĪRD nū-MŌ-nē-ă, p. 301)
intrathoracic (ĭn-tră-thōr-RĂ-sĭk, p. 320)
latent TB infection (LTBI) (LĀ-tĕnt, p. 302)
leukotriene (lĕw-kō-trī-ēn, p. 326)
nebulizer (NĔ-bū-lī-zĕr, p. 326)
pleurisy (PLŪR-ă-sē, p. 306)
pneumonectomy (nū-mō-NĔK-tō-mē, p. 317)
pneumonia (nū-MŌ-nyă, p. 299)
pneumothorax (nū-mō-THŌ-răks, p. 318)
polycythemia (pŏl-ē-sī-THĒ-mē-ă, p. 309)
sarcoidosis (săr-koy-DŌ-sĭs, p. 306)
subcutaneous emphysema (sŭb-kū-TĀ-nē-ĕs ĕm-fĭ-SĒ-mă, p. 321)
thoracentesis (thŏ-ră-sĕn-TĒ-sĭs, p. 307)
thoracotomy (thō-ră-KŎT-ō-mē, p. 320)
thrombolytic (thrŏm-bō-LĬT-ĭk, p. 317)
tuberculosis (TB) (tū-BĔR-kū-LŌ-sĭs, p. 302)
ventilator-associated pneumonia (VAP) (VĔN-tĭ-lā'tŏr ĕ-SŌ-shē-ā-tĕd nū-MŌ-nē-ă, p. 301)

Concepts Covered in This Chapter

- Self-Management
- Acid-Base Balance
- Cellular Regulation
- Perfusion
- Gas Exchange
- Inflammation
- Infection
- Mobility
- Fatigue
- Anxiety
- Patient Education
- Collaboration
- Caregiving

RESPIRATORY INFECTIOUS DISEASES

ACUTE BRONCHITIS

Acute bronchitis is often an extension of an upper respiratory infection involving the trachea *(tracheobronchitis)* and is usually viral in origin. Other causes of acute bronchitis include inhalation of physical or chemical agents such as dust, automobile exhaust, industrial fumes, and tobacco smoke.

Early symptoms of acute bronchitis are similar to those of the common cold. Cough producing some sputum is the most common symptom. Sore throat, runny or stuffy nose, headache, muscle aches, and fatigue are also typical. The health care provider relies on history and signs and symptoms for diagnosis.

Symptomatic treatment includes humidification using either warm or cool moist air. Cough suppressants or bronchodilators are used to reduce coughing and soothe the irritated tracheal and bronchial mucosa. Nutrition and fluid balance should be maintained. Rest is recommended to prevent progression from an acute condition to a chronic one. Antibiotics are used if a sputum culture identifies specific bacterial organisms.

INFLUENZA

Etiology

Influenza is an acute, highly infectious disease of the upper and lower respiratory tracts that occurs in isolated cases or in epidemics. Every year there are between 9 and 36 million cases (not all cases are confirmed by testing) resulting in between 140,000 and 710,000 hospitalizations and between 12,000 and 56,000 deaths (Centers for Disease Control and Prevention [CDC], 2018). There are four major types of influenza viruses (A, B, C, and D) and numerous subtypes. Types A and B are responsible for the seasonal disease epidemics each year. Type C causes a mild respiratory illness and does not cause epidemics, and Type D affects cattle. Seasonal flu is spread by direct and indirect contact with infected people by coughing and sneezing and by virus transferred from contaminated hands to objects. It is extremely virulent and usually affects young adults first and then spreads to the very young and very old in the community.

Pathophysiology

The influenza viruses affect the respiratory mucosa, causing inflammation and destruction of tissue, which sheds the virus into the secretions. The inflammation may involve the lungs, pharynx, sinuses, and eustachian tubes. The damaged tissue provides an environment for the growth of bacteria that cause secondary infection.

Signs and Symptoms

The first symptoms of influenza appear suddenly 2 to 3 days after exposure and include headache, fever (often 101° to 103° F [38° to 40° C]), chills, and muscle aches. Sore throat, hacking cough, runny nose, nasal congestion, sensitivity to light, nausea, vomiting, and diarrhea can also occur. Virus is usually shed for 1 to 2 days before the onset of symptoms.

Diagnosis

Chest radiographs and auscultation are usually normal. The white blood cell count is normal or slightly below normal. Diagnosis is usually based on clinical findings. To confirm the diagnosis, viral culture, serology, rapid molecular assays, or rapid influenza diagnostic tests (RIDTs) that are antigen detection assays may be used. Immunofluorescence assays are another type of RIDT. The CDC (2018) recommends testing only when the results will alter treatment decisions.

Treatment and Nursing Management

Antibiotics are given only if there is evidence of bacterial infection secondary to the viral infection. Antibiotics are not effective against viral illness and are contraindicated. Antiviral medications may be used in specific patient populations. If a person is known to be at high risk for influenza and has been exposed to type A influenza, the health care provider may choose to provide prophylaxis with an antiviral agent such as amantadine (Symmetrel), rimantadine (Flumadine), zanamivir (Relenza), or oseltamivir (Tamiflu). These drugs must be started within 48 hours of the start of symptoms.

Uncomplicated influenza usually is managed more effectively by nursing interventions than by drugs or other forms of medical treatment. Nursing interventions for patients with flu symptoms might include:

- Increase oral fluid intake to at least 3000 mL per 24 hours, unless contraindicated.
- Encourage patient to take analgesics when discomfort first appears.
- Offer saline gargles for a sore throat.
- Administer suppressant cough medicine at bedtime and during the night as prescribed.
- Perform mouth care at least every 4 hours, before each meal, and more frequently if the patient reports a bad taste in the mouth or has halitosis from sputum.
- Cater to the patient's food and drink preferences within the limits of dietary restrictions.
- Give antipyretics and use cooling measures to reduce high fever.
- Humidify inhaled air.
- Splint chest and abdomen with a pillow during coughing attacks.
- Apply emollient to the lips and nares as needed.
- Clear the nostrils as much as possible to prevent mouth breathing.
- Provide for periods of uninterrupted rest.
- Protect from and monitor for secondary infections such as pneumonia, otitis media, and sinusitis because the weakened immune system causes greater susceptibility.
- Teach frequent hand hygiene after coughing or handling used tissues.

PNEUMONIA

Etiology and Pathophysiology

Pneumonia is an extensive inflammation of the lung with either consolidation of the lung tissue as it fills with exudate or interstitial inflammation and edema. It can affect one (most common) or both lungs. Lobar pneumonia is a serious condition affecting an entire lobe of the lung and is usually caused by *Streptococcus*

Health Promotion

Protection from Influenza

The 2017 Advisory Committee on Immunization Practices recommended annual influenza vaccination for the following groups (Grohskopf et al., 2017)):

- People at high risk for influenza-related complications and severe disease, including:
  - Children ages 6 to 59 months
  - Pregnant women
  - People older than 50 years
  - People of any age with certain chronic medical conditions
- People who live with or care for persons at high risk, including:
  - Household contacts who have frequent contact with people at high risk and who can transmit influenza to those individuals
  - Health care workers

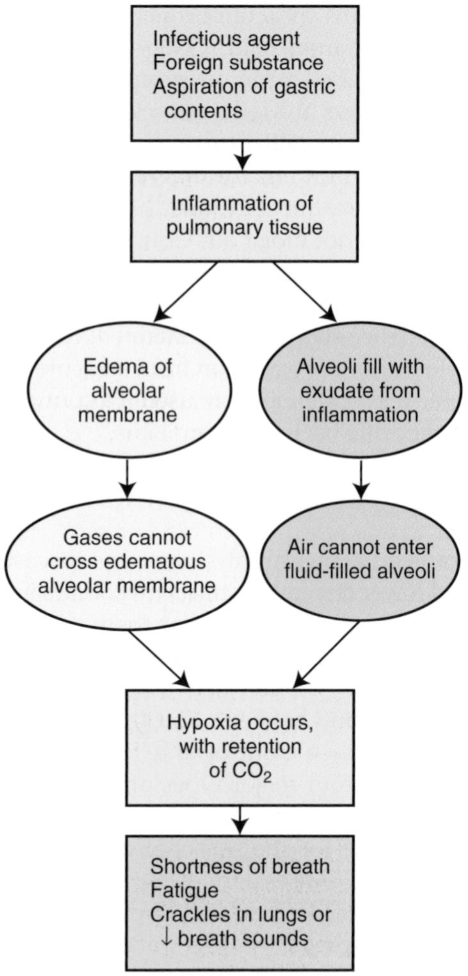

Concept Map 14.1 Pathophysiology of pneumonia. CO_2, Carbon dioxide.

pneumoniae. In 2015, 57,062 people died of pneumonia in the United States; it is the eighth leading cause (combined with influenza) of death in the United States (National Vital Statistics Reports, 2017). Bacteria or viruses may cause pneumonia; bacterial pneumonia is more common and is associated with greater symptoms and risks. Pneumonia is classified as community acquired or hospital acquired. Viral pneumonia does not produce exudate; it causes interstitial inflammation and tends to be less severe than bacterial pneumonia. Any respiratory infection in an already debilitated patient can have severe consequences. In otherwise healthy individuals, viral pneumonia is usually a mild, self-limiting illness. *S. pneumoniae* (pneumococcus) is the most common cause of bacterial pneumonia. Pathogenic microorganisms are always present in the upper respiratory tract; pneumonia can occur when resistance is lowered by some other factor, such as chronic disease, alcoholism, debilitation, physical inactivity, or extremes in age (very young or very old). In many instances pneumonia occurs after an influenza infection. Concept Map 14.1 presents the pathophysiology of pneumonia.

Pneumonia also can result from inhalation of irritating gases *(chemical pneumonia)* or accidental aspiration of foods or liquids that cause a pneumonitis progressing to pneumonia *(aspiration pneumonia). Hypostatic pneumonia* results from lying in bed for extended periods because of the lack of physical exercise and inadequate aeration of the lungs. Fungi also may cause opportunistic pneumonia in immunocompromised patients. Fungi found in the environment in defined geographic regions or fungi normally found in the body can both cause pneumonia in patients with congenital or acquired immunocompromise.

Prevention

People who are older than 65 years and those with chronic respiratory disease should receive the pneumococcal pneumonia vaccine. A second dose may be needed 5 years after the first dose for immunocompromised patients or those older than 65 years.

A variety of nursing interventions can help prevent pneumonia, including:

- Strengthening the patient's natural defenses and avoiding infection.
- Ensuring frequent turning, coughing, and deep breathing for postoperative patients or those who are otherwise unable to ventilate their lungs adequately.
- Watching for vomiting and initiating a side-lying position for patients with decreased consciousness, such as patients recovering from anesthesia.
- Maintaining elevation of the head of the bed at 30 to 45 degrees for patients at risk for aspiration with meals or who are receiving tube feedings (unless contraindicated).
- Avoiding thin liquids for patients who are at risk for aspiration.
- Faithfully following principles of cleanliness and asepsis when caring for debilitated patients and those most susceptible to infection.
- Encouraging the pneumonia vaccine for those most at risk for developing the disease.
- Encouraging immunization against influenza.

Patients are at risk for **health care–associated pneumonia (HCAP)** (formerly known as *nosocomial pneumonia*). These at-risk circumstances include **hospital-acquired pneumonia (HAP)**, in which symptoms occur more than 48 hours after admission, or **ventilator-associated pneumonia (VAP)**, in which pneumonia occurs 48 to 72 hours after endotracheal intubation. HCAP is also associated with nursing home or long-term care; intravenous (IV) therapy, chemotherapy, immunosuppressive treatment, and wound care; severe chronic obstructive pulmonary disease (COPD); and child care facilities, hospitals, and dialysis centers (CDC, 2018). HAP is a major problem that lengthens hospital stays and increases the cost of health care. VAP is the most common health care–associated infection (HAI); however, vigilant and aggressive nursing and respiratory care can greatly decrease the incidence.

People who are on gastrointestinal acid–suppressive therapy should be educated that this may make them more susceptible to community-acquired pneumonia. The research shows that long-term use increases the risk of pneumonia, particularly in the older adult population (Zirk-Sadowski et al., 2018). Normal gastric acid helps prevent pathogens from colonizing the upper gastrointestinal tract, where they can then be introduced into the respiratory tract.

Signs, Symptoms, and Diagnosis

In typical infectious pneumonia, there is usually a high fever accompanied by chills, a cough that produces rusty or blood-flecked sputum, sweating, chest pain that is made worse by respiratory movements, and a general feeling of malaise and aching muscles. Diagnosis is confirmed by chest radiograph, which reveals densities in the affected lung.

In atypical pneumonia (also called walking pneumonia), body temperature can be normal or subnormal; breath sounds can be normal with perhaps only occasional crackles and wheezes; and there may be no pleural involvement and therefore no pain, dry cough, or feeling of extreme fatigue. Chest radiography reveals diffuse, patchy areas of density. Symptoms tend to be more systemic than pulmonary. Headache, abdominal pain, diarrhea, and myalgias are common.

Treatment

Typical pneumonia is treated with IV or oral antibiotic agents, such as erythromycin, macrolides (clarithromycin [Biaxin]), cephalosporins, aminoglycosides, or fluoroquinolones such as ciprofloxacin (Cipro).

Safety Alert

Fluoroquinolones

In July 2018 the U.S. Food and Drug Administration (FDA, 2018) strengthened the warning about the potential hypoglycemia and mental health side effects of fluoroquinolones. Hypoglycemia can lead to coma. The mental health side effects include disturbances in attention, disorientation, agitation, nervousness, memory impairment, and delirium.

Atypical pneumonia caused by *Mycoplasma* species usually is treated with erythromycin, clarithromycin, or azithromycin. Viral, atypical pneumonia requires no antiinfective therapy, but antiviral medication may be administered. *Pneumocystis jirovecii* (formerly *Pneumocystis carinii* and still referred to as PCP) infection associated with acquired immunodeficiency syndrome (AIDS) is treated with trimethoprim-sulfamethoxazole (Bactrim) given IV or orally depending on the severity of the infection. According to practice guidelines, the first antibiotic dose should be administered within 4 hours of presentation whenever the admission diagnosis is community-acquired pneumonia. The timeliness of this therapy is related to decreased mortality rates. Supplemental oxygen (O_2) is provided as needed. Some patients require mechanical ventilation.

Complementary and Alternative Therapies

Treatment for Pneumonia

Barberry root bark is used against bacteria, fungi, and viruses as well as other organisms and is an alternative treatment for pneumonia. It has antimicrobial action against both gram-positive and gram-negative bacteria. It should not be used during pregnancy because it can cause spontaneous abortion.

Think Critically

Identify five signs or symptoms found on assessment that might correlate with a diagnosis of pneumonia.

Nursing Management

The nursing care plan for a patient with pneumonia should include interventions to:

- Promote oxygenation
- Control elevated temperature
- Maintain nutritional and fluid intake
- Provide adequate rest
- Monitor vital signs and respiratory status
- Relieve pain and discomfort
- Provide good oral hygiene
- Prevent irritation of the lungs by smoke and other irritants
- Avoid secondary bacterial infections

Clinical Cues

The first signs of decreasing oxygenation may be restlessness or confusion. The patient may want to sit upright to allow for better chest excursion. Respiratory rate will increase, and later there will be flaring of the nares, then retraction of intercostal muscles if the condition worsens. Cyanosis is a very late sign.

The patient should breathe deeply and cough 5 to 10 times each hour while awake to prevent atelectasis, which can lead to pneumonia. It is important to assess for signs of increasing impairment of gas exchange. Unless contraindicated, fluid intake should be increased to 2500 to 3000 mL/day. Because abdominal distention, nausea, and vomiting also may accompany pneumonia, nursing interventions to deal with these problems may be indicated. Other problems include altered states of consciousness (delirium and confusion) or the development of such complications as empyema and congestive heart failure. For young adults, convalescence with rest should extend for at least a week after acute symptoms subside. Older adults require several weeks before usual activities can be resumed without experiencing fatigue.

ATELECTASIS

Atelectasis is an incomplete expansion, or collapse, of alveoli. It may occur from compression of the lungs from a lesion in the thorax, a decrease in surfactant, or bronchial obstruction that prevents air from reaching the alveoli. Postoperatively it results from retained secretions that accumulated during anesthesia, positioning on the operating room table for an extended period without movement, and hypoventilation related to surgical pain. It usually is a reversible condition. Breath sounds are diminished when the airways are collapsed, and oxygen saturation (SaO_2) will decrease. Treatment consists of expelling secretions by coughing. Deep breathing and use of the incentive spirometer help keep the alveoli open and functional.

Clinical Cues

If your postoperative patient has crackles in the bases of the lungs, have them take several deep breaths and cough. Listen again; if the crackles are gone, atelectasis has just been cleared.

Older Adult Care Points

Older adults are at higher risk for influenza and pneumonia because of a less efficient immune system, decreased action of cilia, and decreased elasticity and tone of respiratory muscles.

- Confusion or altered mental status often is the most obvious sign of atypical pneumonia in older adults.
- It may take 6 to 12 weeks after a bout of pneumonia for an older adult patient to be able to resume normal activities without experiencing acute fatigue.
- Older adult patients may never quite regain the former level of wellness after a serious episode of pneumonia.
- Teach older adults to seek medical attention quickly if symptoms of pneumonia occur.

FUNGAL INFECTIONS

The most common fungal lung infections are coccidioidomycosis, aspergillus, and histoplasmosis. Coccidioidomycosis occurs primarily in the western United States, and exposure occurs by inhaling dust during desert recreational activities or when working in occupations that require digging in the earth. Living in an agricultural community where plowing stirs up dust also contributes to exposure. Typically there are no symptoms or mild respiratory symptoms, but 40% will have cough, fever, pleuritic chest pain, myalgias, and arthralgias. Sometimes a flat red rash with dark red papules occurs. Aspergillus is also transmitted by inhalation of spores that are commonly found in the environment in mold. A wide range of diseases is possible from an allergic response to an invasive form causing sepsis. Symptoms include cough, wheezing, fever, and dyspnea. Histoplasmosis occurs in central and eastern portions of North America. The fungus lives in moist soil such as that in which mushrooms grow, on the floors of chicken houses and bat caves, and in bird droppings. Clinical signs are fever, fatigue, cough, dyspnea, and weight loss over 1 to 2 months.

Other fungal respiratory infections, such as blastomycosis, cryptococcosis, and candidiasis, are seen mostly in immunocompromised people or those with cystic fibrosis. PCP is found only in immunocompromised patients and is highly lethal (see Chapter 11). Although classified as a fungal infection, PCP does not respond to antifungal treatment, and trimethoprim-sulfamethoxazole (Bactrim) is the preferred therapy. Fungal infections are diagnosed by history, signs and symptoms, and positive skin test reaction to the fungus or serology testing.

TUBERCULOSIS

Etiology

Pulmonary **tuberculosis (TB)** is an infectious disease characterized by lesions within the lung tissue. The lesions may degenerate and become necrotic, or they may heal by fibrosis and calcification. The causative organism is the true tubercle bacillus *Mycobacterium tuberculosis.* **Latent TB infection (LTBI)** refers to an infection with *Mycobacterium tuberculosis* but no current active disease. LTBI may develop into active TB if the immune system is weakened by a serious illness such as human immunodeficiency virus (HIV) or when the system is less efficient, as with advanced age.

Tuberculosis is spread through airborne particles that carry the TB bacilli and are inhaled by a susceptible individual. The droplets can remain suspended in the air for several hours. Infection most often occurs after prolonged exposure, but not everyone contracts the disease, even after close and extensive contact with infected persons.

Cultural Considerations

Ethnic Occurrence of Tuberculosis

American Indians, Alaska Natives, Asian/Pacific Islanders, black non-Hispanics, and Hispanics have a high incidence of TB. The disease is most prevalent in people older than 65 years within these groups. For the first few years of residence in the United States, new immigrants from areas where TB is prevalent have incidence rates similar to those in their former country.

Tuberculosis is a major health problem throughout the world and the third leading cause of death for an infectious agent worldwide (Baylor, 2018; World Health Organization [WHO], 2018). The incidence of TB in the United States has been declining steadily since 1992. In 2017 TB cases in the United States occurred among foreign-born persons at 15 times the rate for U.S.-born persons. The majority of new cases (>80%) result from activation of LTBI (CDC, 2018).

Pathophysiology

Mycobacterium is an acid-fast, aerobic, slow-growing bacillus. When the organism enters the lungs, a local inflammatory reaction occurs, usually in the upper lobe. It takes 2 to 12 weeks for organisms to replicate in sufficient numbers to prompt enough of an immune response to be detected by a TB skin test. If an exposure is suspected, a second skin test will be performed 8 to 10 weeks later. Bacilli migrate to the lymph nodes and activate a cell-mediated hypersensitivity response. This triggers granuloma formation with influx of macrophages and lymphocytes at the site of inflammation. The bacillus is walled off, forming a *tubercle.* Caseous necrosis (a core of cheeselike material) develops in the center of the tubercle. In a healthy person the initial lesions may heal and become latent before any signs or symptoms of the disease occur. Over time the tubercles eventually calcify. Bacilli may remain viable in a dormant state inside the tubercle for many years. In the unhealthy individual, the bacilli spread to other parts of the lung and to other organs.

Signs and Symptoms

The onset of TB is gradual; a patient may have an active, progressive lesion before symptoms appear. Typical symptoms are cough, low-grade fever in the afternoon, anorexia, loss of weight, fatigue, night sweats, and sometimes **hemoptysis** (blood in sputum). Tight or dull chest pain and mucopurulent sputum may occur as the disease progresses. Persons with LTBI are asymptomatic and have a negative chest radiograph.

Older Adult Care Points

The older adult population may not experience the expected signs and symptoms of TB because the immune response is not as strong. In many instances active TB infections present as chronic pneumonitis.

Diagnosis

Early detection of TB is of great importance because:

- The anti-TB drugs are more effective in the early stages of the disease.
- The period of disability is much shorter.
- The complications are fewer.
- The spread to others can be prevented.

Tuberculin skin testing. Food handlers, those working with children, and health care workers must be tested periodically. Others who are symptomatic or have been exposed to someone with TB should be tested. Skin testing for TB is done by the Mantoux test. In this test, 0.1 mL of purified protein derivative (PPD) tuberculin is injected intradermally. The test is called the *tuberculin skin test (TST)* (formerly known as *PPD test*). The test is positive when the swelling at the site of injection is more than 5 mm in diameter 48 to 72 hours after injection in people who have a history of contact with infectious TB or in immunocompromised patients. Induration of more than 10 mm in diameter is positive in recent immigrants from countries where TB is prevalent, in medically underserved groups, and in the homeless (Fig. 14.1). For those persons at low risk, induration of more than 15 mm is considered positive. Skin testing is contraindicated only for those who have had a severe reaction. Vaccination with bacillus Calmette–Guérin (BCG) is not a contraindication but must be considered when interpreting the results (CDC, 2018).

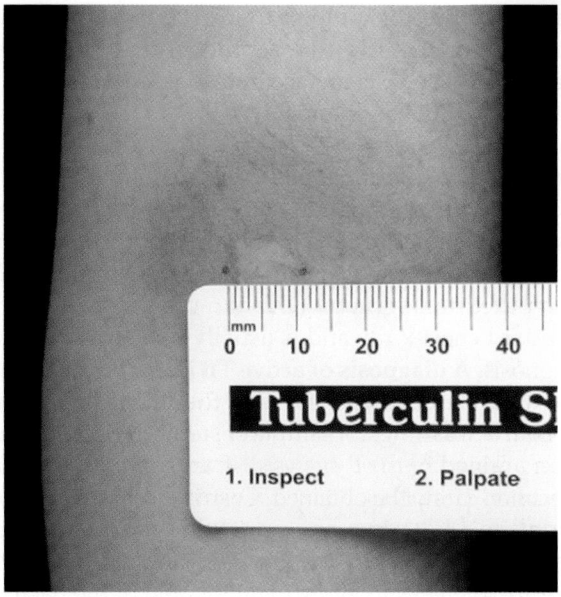

Fig. 14.1 Positive tuberculin skin test. Raised area (induration) is measured, not the entire reddened area. (Courtesy Centers of Disease Control and Prevention: Tuberculosis tuberculin skin testing, 2016, https://www.cdc.gov/tb/education/ssmodules/pdfs/2017SelfStudy_Module3.pdf.)

A positive TST indicates that the person has been infected with the tubercle bacillus; however, it does not indicate whether the disease is active or inactive, only that the body tissues are sensitive to tuberculin. A positive reaction indicates a need for further evaluation. Once positive, subsequent TSTs will always be positive.

Blood testing. Two blood tests are approved by the FDA: the QuantiFERON-TB Gold (QFT-GIT) and T-SPOT.TB test (T-Spot). The tests are interferon gamma release assays (IGRAs) that measure the patient's immune system reaction to TB. They do not distinguish between active and latent TB. They are less likely to produce false-positive readings and require only one visit to the clinic or office for a blood draw, rather than the two required for the TST (the second visit is for reading the result). The tests are accurate even for people who have had BCG vaccination.

Radiographic examinations and sputum cultures. A radiographic examination of the chest may or may not reveal tubercular lesions in the lung, but calcified and healed lesions usually can be seen on radiographs. Computed tomography (CT) is more sensitive than a standard chest x-ray and is usually not necessary for a diagnosis. **A diagnosis of active TB is established when the tubercle bacillus has been found in the sputum or gastric washings.** A sample of stomach contents may be examined *(gastric analysis)* if an adequate sputum specimen cannot be obtained. Gastric washings are done rarely in adults but are more common in children. Sputum cultures are slow growing, and culture results take 1 to 3 weeks to allow identification of the bacillus. The culture report also indicates to which medications the organism is sensitive.

Treatment

Uncomplicated pulmonary TB is managed in the outpatient setting. Only those who are extremely debilitated or suffering from another chronic illness are hospitalized. Treatment of active TB consists of taking at least four drugs for an extended period (Table 14.1). The drugs are given in varying combinations and on varying numbers of days per week. The treatment protocols outline the initial 2-month phase followed by several options for the continuation phase of either 4 or 7 months. Noncompliance is an issue because of side effects, the requirement to avoid alcohol, and the long duration of therapy. Drug combinations that make compliance easier for patients are available: Rifamate, which contains rifampin (RIF) and isoniazid (INH), and Rifater, which contains RIF, INH, and pyrazinamide (PZA). Effective cure can be obtained within 6 to 9 months for most patients with pulmonary TB. A two-drug regimen of INH and rifapentine (RPT) on a once-weekly dosing schedule for 12 weeks is used for LTBI.

Complementary and Alternative Therapies

Vitamins Aid in Treatment of Tuberculosis

Multiple studies have shown that vitamin D is effective in preventing the conversion of LTBI into active TB and has shortened the recovery time for active TB. Vitamin C is showing promise in helping TB medications be more effective (American Society for Microbiology, 2018).

A new drug, pretomanid, seems to be extremely effective in quickly killing TB and is in phase III clinical trials (Drugbank, 2018). A shorter treatment time could improve compliance with medication therapy. There is an increase in the incidence of multidrug-resistant TB, and patients with these infections do not fare well. For this reason, directly observed therapy (DOT) is recommended for patients who are known to be at risk for noncompliance with therapy. DOT involves visual observation of the ingestion of each required dose of medication for the entire course of treatment. Electronic directly observed therapy (eDOT) is being used to help meet the needs of patients and lessen the demand on resources. A public health nurse administers the medication at a clinic site. Follow-up visits are necessary for 12 months after completion of therapy to monitor for the presence of resistant strains.

Legal and Ethical Considerations

Noncompliance With Medication

When someone is found to have TB and the person is noncompliant with the treatment, is it legal or ethical to compel the person to come for treatment? What will happen if the person is allowed to remain in the community without treatment?

Nursing Management

A complete history and assessment of TB risk factors are needed. A focused assessment of the respiratory system is performed (see Focused Assessment in Chapter 12).

Nursing objectives are to control the spread of the infectious agent, promote immunity, and strengthen potential recovery in a patient with an infectious disease. Problem statements or nursing diagnoses for the patient with TB may include:

- Altered breathing pattern due to decreased lung capacity.
- Absence of compliance due to lack of knowledge of disease process and long-term requirements for treatment.
- Altered activity tolerance due to fatigue, febrile status, and poor nutritional status.
- Altered nutrition due to anorexia, fatigue, and productive cough.

Control of infection. Airborne infection isolation in addition to Standard Precautions (see Appendix B) are recommended for hospitalized patients who have active TB and are just beginning drug therapy. The patient is placed in a negative-pressure isolation room with an anteroom. A high-efficiency particulate air (HEPA) respirator mask that tightly fits the face or a powered air purifying respirator (PAPR) is required for all personnel when caring for the patient. The home care patient does not need airborne infection isolation because family members have already been exposed by the time of diagnosis. Patients and families should be educated about the importance of medication compliance and the basic principles of infection control: covering the mouth when coughing or sneezing, disposing of tissues in plastic bags, practicing good hand hygiene, and wearing a mask when in contact with crowds until medication effectively suppresses the infection. Sputum examinations are required monthly during treatment.

Table 14.1 **Drugs Commonly Used in the Treatment of Tuberculosis**

DAILY DOSAGE	OTHER DOSING SCHEDULES	MOST COMMON SIDE EFFECTS	TEST FOR SIDE EFFECTS	REMARKS
Primary Drugs				
Isoniazid (INH) 5 mg/kg up to 300 mg/24 h PO or IM (can be given IV)	15 mg/kg PO weekly, or IM 2 or 3 times a week Usual dose 900 mg total	Peripheral neuritis, hypersensitivity, jaundice	AST/ALT monthly Drug levels: 3–5 mg/L at 2 h	Bactericidal agent. Pyridoxine as prophylaxis for neuritis; 25–50 mg/24 h as treatment.
Ethambutol (EMB) (Myambutol) 15–25 mg/kg PO up to 1600 mg/24 h	35–50 mg/kg PO twice a week up to 4000 mg or 20–35 mg/kg	Optic neuritis (reversible with discontinuation of drug; very rare at 15 mg/kg), skin rash	Baseline and monthly red-green color discrimination and visual acuity Drug levels: 2–6 mg/L at 2 h	Use with caution with renal disease or when eye testing is not feasible.
Rifampin (RIF) (Rifadin) 10 mg/kg up to 600 mg/day PO or IV	10 mg/kg PO or IV 2 or 3 times a week up to 600 mg/day	Rash, hepatitis, febrile reaction, purpura (rare)	AST/ALT monthly in patients with preexisting liver disease Drug levels: 8–24 mg/L at 2 h	Bactericidal agent. Orange secretion color. Affects action of other drugs.
Pyrazinamide (PZA) 15–30 mg/kg up to 2 g/day PO	50 mg/kg PO twice weekly up to 2 g/dose	Hyperuricemia, hepatotoxicity	Uric acid, AST/ALT	Under study as first-line drug in short-course regimens.
Rifabutin (RBT) 5 mg/kg (300 mg) PO	5 mg/kg (300 mg) PO 2 or 3 times a week	Causes discoloration of urine Neutropenia, leukopenia	CBC	May be used as a substitute for RIF.
Rifapentine (RPT) 600 mg PO once a week for 4 mo during continuation phase	600 mg twice a week during intensive phase	Hypertension, headache, dizziness	Hepatic enzymes, bilirubin, CBC	May be used once a week in combination with INH in select patients in the continuation phase of treatment.
Secondary Drugs				
Streptomycin (SM) Capreomycin (Capastat) Cycloserine (Seromycin) Ethionamide[a] (Trecator) Kanamycin[a] (Kantrex) Levofloxacin[a] Moxifloxacin[a] Amikacin[a]				These drugs are reserved for special situations such as drug intolerance or resistance.

Adapted from Lewis SL, Bucher L, Heitkemper MM, et al.: *Medical-surgical nursing: assessment and management of clinical problems,* ed 10, St. Louis, 2017, Elsevier.
[a]Not approved by the U.S. Food and Drug Administration for use in the treatment of tuberculosis.
ALT, Alanine aminotransferase; *AST,* aspartate aminotransferase; *CBC,* complete blood cell count; *IM,* intramuscularly; *IV,* intravenously; *PO,* orally.

When sputum cultures are negative and the clinician evaluates the effectiveness of the treatment, the patient is considered no longer infectious and may resume work and other usual social activities.

Close contacts are monitored with skin or blood testing. If the TST or IGRA result is positive, the contact is treated with INH, RPT, or RIF depending on whether the type of TB is known to be drug resistant. HIV-positive, pregnant, or breastfeeding individuals as well as infants and children have specific recommended drug combinations and doses. The CDC website has the most current treatment recommendations.

Promotion of immunity. Improving living conditions and carrying out sound health practices are essential to maintaining a natural resistance to TB. The populations most at risk for contracting TB are those with an insufficient immune system. That is why the very young and the very old as well as those with immunosuppression from disease or disease treatment are at increased risk.

Several vaccinations are in clinical trials in the hopes of boosting immunity to the TB organism. Good ventilation and healthful living can prevent the spread of TB.

Support. When a person first learns that they have tuberculosis, they will need support in sorting out their feelings and overcoming any fears and misinformation they might have.

It is also important that the patient name all close contacts, so that they can be notified and appropriately tested and treated. Giving the names of contacts may be very difficult for the patient because of the social stigma that is still attached to TB in certain cultural groups.

EXTRAPULMONARY TUBERCULOSIS

It is possible for the tubercle bacillus to attack and damage parts of the body other than the lungs. This is called *extrapulmonary* or *miliary tuberculosis.* The areas most commonly affected are the lymph nodes, bones, meninges, digestive system, urinary system, and reproductive system. Presenting signs and symptoms are dependent on the body system affected. Tuberculosis of the spine, called *Pott disease,* can cause *kyphosis,* or "hunchback," but the condition is rare in the United States.

OCCUPATIONAL LUNG DISORDERS

Coal dust; dust from hemp, flax, and cotton processing; and exposure to silica in the air can cause work-related lung disorders. Asbestos exposure may cause mesothelioma, a rare cancer of the chest lining (American Lung Association, 2018). Asbestos exposure also causes scarring of lung tissue. The other exposures cause obstruction of small airways or scarring and loss of elasticity and compliance. Occupational history is part of the respiratory assessment.

RESTRICTIVE PULMONARY DISORDERS

Restrictive pulmonary disorders are caused by decreased elasticity or compliance of the lungs or decreased ability of the chest wall to expand. Disorders of the central nervous system or of the neuromuscular system can cause a restrictive lung disorder. Myasthenia gravis and arthritis are examples of extrapulmonary causes. *Kyphosis* of the spine or severe *scoliosis* may hamper lung expansion, but the lung tissue remains normal. Obesity is becoming a major cause of restrictive lung disease.

INTERSTITIAL PULMONARY DISEASE

Sarcoidosis

Sarcoidosis is a multisystem inflammatory disease characterized by granulomas primarily in the lungs and intrathoracic lymph nodes. This disease causes fibrotic changes in the lung tissue and other tissues over time. A cellular immune response seems to be responsible, but the exact cause is unknown. Sarcoidosis is 10 times more common in African Americans than in whites, and most cases occur between ages 20 and 40 years. The fibrotic changes cause a reduction in functional lung tissue. Most patients (>75%) recover with treatment only for symptoms. Patients with extrapulmonary or persistent pulmonary disease are treated with corticosteroids.

Pulmonary Fibrosis

Pulmonary fibrosis occurs from environmental pollutants, some medications, and interstitial lung diseases that scar the lungs. Occupational inhalation of lung irritants, smoking, and radiation treatments to the chest are risk factors. Signs and symptoms are exertional dyspnea, nonproductive cough, and inspiratory crackles and sometimes clubbed fingers. Diagnosis is by high-resolution CT scanning and pulmonary function testing. There is a 20% to 25% survival rate at 10 years after diagnosis. Treatment is with pirfenidone or nintedanib antifibrotic medications and for more advanced cases with sildenafil to treat pulmonary hypertension. Lung transplantation is an option for some patients.

PLEURITIS

Pleuritis, also called pleurisy—an inflammation of the pleura—is most commonly caused by infection but can also be caused by medications, lupus, and rheumatoid arthritis. Pleuritic pain is sharp and abrupt in onset and is most evident on inspiration. This causes shallow breathing. A pleural friction rub may be heard. Treatment is aimed at the underlying cause and at providing pain relief. Lying on the affected side or splinting the affected side during coughing may provide some relief. An intercostal nerve block may be performed for severe pleuritic pain.

PLEURAL EFFUSION

Pleural effusion is a collection of fluid in the pleural space. Pleural fluid accumulation is characterized as transudative or exudative. Transudate is a thin fluid containing no protein that passes from cells into interstitial spaces or through a membrane. A transudate occurs in noninflammatory conditions that cause changes in chest pressures such as congestive heart failure, chronic liver failure, or renal disease. Exudate is thicker and contains cells, proteins, and other substances. Exudative pleural effusion is usually from pleural and lung inflammation but can be caused by any organ system through a variety of mechanisms.

When pleuritis is accompanied by effusion of serous fluid, the health care provider may perform a **thoracentesis** (removal of fluid from the pleural cavity) for diagnostic tests or symptom relief. It is not uncommon for as much as 500 mL to be removed during a thoracentesis (see Chapter 12, Table 12.1).

EMPYEMA

Empyema occurs when the fluid within the pleural cavity becomes infected and the exudate becomes thick and purulent. Most empyemas are secondary to pneumonia, but 20% are secondary to complications of thoracic surgery, chest tube insertion, or thoracentesis. Treatment includes drainage of the fluid by one or more chest tubes attached to a closed drainage system and antibiotics. A specimen of the fluid is sent for a culture and sensitivity, which determines the choice of antibiotic therapy. If the source of the empyema is from pneumonia, the organism causing the pneumonia is usually also responsible for the empyema.

OBSTRUCTIVE PULMONARY DISORDERS

Obstructive pulmonary disorders are characterized by problems with moving air out of the lungs, contributing to air trapping, thus making exhalation difficult. Asthma, emphysema, bronchiectasis, cystic fibrosis, and chronic bronchitis are examples of diseases that cause chronic airflow limitation (CAL).

Obstructive disorders can be caused by cigarette smoking (tobacco and other forms) and any other inhalation of irritants, chemicals or particles from air pollution, agricultural chemicals, volcanic eruptions, fumes, and organic or inorganic dusts. Another factor is genetic. **Alpha-1 antitrypsin (AAT)** is a serum protein that inhibits the activity of the enzyme **elastase**, which tends to break down lung tissue. In the absence of AAT, lung tissue is more easily destroyed by the enzyme. Patients with a deficiency of AAT may develop severe lung disease at an early age. Cystic fibrosis is also genetically acquired.

BRONCHIECTASIS

Bronchiectasis is a chronic respiratory disorder in which the bronchi walls are thickened. It occurs as a result of frequent respiratory infections or inflammation. Frequent aspiration of food particles can also cause the condition. In the United States, about one third of all bronchiectasis is caused by cystic fibrosis.

CYSTIC FIBROSIS

Cystic fibrosis (CF) is a genetic disease (more common among whites) in which there is excessive mucus production because of exocrine gland dysfunction. The lungs, intestines, sinuses, reproductive tract, sweat glands, and pancreas are all affected. It is diagnosed by history, physical examination, and genetic testing or a positive sweat test.

Lung damage occurs in CF because of excessive secretion of abnormally thick mucus, impairment of ciliary action in the lungs, airway obstruction, and repeated infections, which cause scarring. It was once a pediatric disease because children with CF died before reaching adulthood. Individuals with CF now live into their 40s and beyond with aggressive respiratory treatment and antibiotics. Current research has identified that the gene that causes CF can be damaged in more than one way. Ivacaftor is a new treatment that is effective in supplying the chemicals missing as a result of gene malfunction. The FDA approved ivacaftor in 2017 for use in people ages 2 years and older who have at least 1 of 23 mutations of the gene causing CF (Cystic Fibrosis Foundation, 2017). These medications treat the problem rather than the symptoms, and the progress made so far is encouraging and has improved life for many patients. Treatment of symptoms includes bronchodilators, expectorants, oral pancreatic enzymes, double doses of fat-soluble vitamins, and mucolytics. A high-protein, high-calorie, moderate-fat diet is prescribed. Dornase alfa (Pulmozyme) reduces the frequency of respiratory infections and improves pulmonary function for patients with CF by decreasing the viscosity of sputum. DNase, a recombinant deoxyribonucleic acid (DNA) medication, is also used to reduce the thickness of the sputum. Breathing exercises and chest physiotherapy are used daily. A handheld device called a flutter valve, which looks like a fat pipe, is used to loosen secretions. By exhaling actively into the pipe, the device causes vibrations of the airway walls, loosening secretions so that they can be coughed up. Lung transplantation is a possible lifesaving measure. The Cystic Fibrosis Foundation is hopeful that the new drug therapies will eliminate the need for lung transplantations in patients with CF.

CHRONIC OBSTRUCTIVE PULMONARY DISEASE

The WHO uses the term *COPD* to describe a condition that includes the related diseases *emphysema* (Fig. 14.2) and *chronic bronchitis.* **Also related is chronic obstructive asthma** (Fig. 14.3). Approximately 12 million people in the United States have COPD, and 12 million have impaired lung function with probable underlying COPD. Annually, 120,000 deaths occur as a result of COPD (National Institutes of Health, 2018).

Etiology and Diagnosis of Chronic Obstructive Pulmonary Disease

Smoking and AAT deficiency are causes of emphysema and chronic bronchitis. Passive smoke, biomass fuel use, and occupational exposure are other risk factors. Tobacco smoke exposure accounts for as much as 90% of COPD risk, including smoking and secondhand smoke. AAT deficiency is the cause of less than 1% of cases.

Firefighters, welders, farmers, and others who have repeated exposure to dust and particulate matter are in the high-risk group. Diagnosis is by history, physical assessment, and spirometry readings before and after bronchodilator treatment. A chest radiograph is not useful in diagnosing COPD, but it can help rule out other causes of the symptoms.

Treatment of Chronic Obstructive Pulmonary Disease

COPD is a chronic disorder treated with bronchodilators and antiinflammatory agents to maintain a stable condition. Risk for exacerbation is categorized for appropriate treatment. Reduced exposure to lung irritants such as open cooking fires, smoking, and air pollution also helps prevent further deterioration. Smoking cessation is very important. Influenza and pneumococcal vaccines help prevent infections that cause COPD exacerbations. Pulmonary rehabilitation programs are also recommended, and supplemental O_2 is given for hypoxemia. Respiratory rehabilitation programs can help increase exercise tolerance and improve quality of life.

O_2 should be titrated to maintain an oxygen saturation of 88% to 92%. COPD patients have adjusted to chronic hypoxia and to high carbon dioxide (CO_2) levels. Closely monitor the pulse oximetry readings and titrate the O_2 as needed.

Nutrition is very important for patients with COPD because the extra work of breathing uses more calories and anorexia may be present. Extra protein is required to repair damaged tissues. It is beneficial to maintain as normal a weight as possible for height and age.

For COPD exacerbations, IV steroids, noninvasive ventilation, and additional bronchodilators are given.

For severe emphysema, surgical interventions have been shown to be helpful in selected patients. Lung volume reduction surgery (LVRS) removes portions of damaged lung tissue. This allows for greater expansion of the residual tissue. This intervention has had more success for patients with upper-lobe emphysema. Lung transplantation may be considered for patients who meet selection criteria.

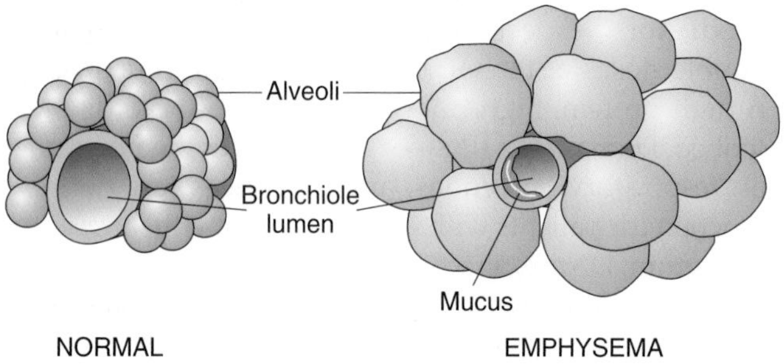

Fig. 14.2 Alveoli in emphysema. (From Banasik JL: *Pathophysiology*, ed 6, St. Louis, 2019, Elsevier.)

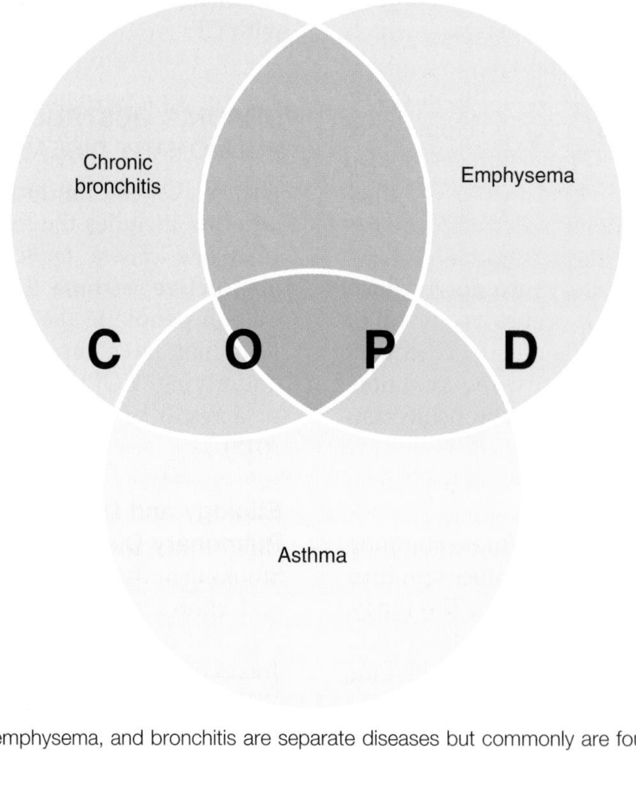

Fig. 14.3 Asthma, emphysema, and bronchitis are separate diseases but commonly are found in combination.

Nutrition Considerations

Nutritional Suggestions for Patients With Chronic Obstructive Pulmonary Disease

The following tips may help patients with COPD:

- Drink six to eight glasses of noncaffeinated fluids per day to keep mucus thin and easier to cough up. Check with your health care provider if you are on fluid restrictions.
- Rest before eating.
- Avoid overeating and avoid foods that cause gas or bloating because a distended stomach may make breathing more difficult.
- Eat four to six small meals a day rather than three regular meals, to decrease stomach fullness and reduce fatigue.
- Eat a well-balanced diet with adequate protein.
- Avoid lying down for an hour after eating.
- If you become short of breath while eating or right after meals:
  - Take small bites and chew food slowly.
  - Choose foods that are easy to chew.
  - Use your oxygen cannula while you eat.
- Take in sufficient calcium via dairy products, vegetables, and supplements—steroid medications put you at risk for osteoporosis.
- Cook when feeling most energetic; make extra portions and freeze them for easy, quick, reheatable dinners.

Think Critically

List five nursing interventions that might help your patient with COPD prevent episodes of dyspnea.

EMPHYSEMA

Pathophysiology

In **emphysema**, there is destruction of alveolar and alveolar-capillary walls producing emphysematous blebs. This leads to large, permanently inflated alveolar air spaces. Air that is inhaled becomes trapped, and it becomes harder to exhale air than to inhale it (see Fig. 14.2). As emphysema progresses, lung elasticity decreases. The blebs decrease the surface area for gas exchange.

Signs and Symptoms

Dyspnea is an early symptom of emphysema. Coughing with small amounts of mucoid sputum is present and more common in the morning. As the disease progresses, dyspnea worsens and eventually interferes with activities of daily living. The diaphragm becomes permanently flattened by overdistention of the lungs, the muscles of the rib cage become rigid, and the ribs flare outward. The patient develops a "barrel chest" (see Chapter 12, Fig. 12.7).

To compensate for the loss of normal muscular action, the patient begins to use the neck and shoulder muscles. The shoulders are held high in an attempt to enlarge the space for lung expansion. The patient may look anxious or tense. The skin has a pink tone in whites even though hypoxia may be present. Early in the disease process CO_2 is usually not retained, and therefore an acid-base imbalance is unlikely. As the disease progresses, both hypercapnia and hypoxemia as well as chronic respiratory acidosis are usually present. Treatment includes inhaled bronchodilators and steroids. Oxygen is given for hypoxia.

CHRONIC BRONCHITIS

Pathophysiology

In chronic bronchitis there is excess secretion of thick, tenacious mucus that decreases ciliary function, interferes with airflow, and causes inflammatory damage to the bronchial mucosa. Airways become edematous and narrowed, and air trapping occurs. Initially the larger airways are affected, and then the smaller airways also become obstructed. Inflammation of the bronchi is considered chronic when a recurrent cough is present for at least 3 months of each year for at least 2 years. Respiratory infections occur frequently because the thick mucus provides a growth medium for bacteria.

Signs and Symptoms

Symptoms can range from a mildly irritating "cigarette" cough in the morning with production of small amounts of sputum to a severe, disabling condition. The latter extreme is characterized by increased resistance to airflow, hypoxia, and development of hypercapnia (excess CO_2).

Pulmonary function testing reveals an increased residual volume caused by the premature closure of the narrowed airways during exhalation. The patient has a marked increase in partial pressure of arterial carbon dioxide ($Paco_2$) levels and a marked decrease in partial pressure of arterial oxygen (Pao_2) levels. **The retention of CO_2 and deficiency of O_2 give the skin and/or mucous membranes a reddish-blue color.** The reddish color is also related to an increase in the red blood cell count (**polycythemia**) that is an attempt by the body to compensate for chronic hypoxia. Hemoglobin and hematocrit levels are elevated for patients with chronic bronchitis. Table 14.2 presents a comparison of emphysema, chronic bronchitis, and asthma.

ASTHMA

Etiology

Factors implicated in the occurrence of asthma include allergens, viruses and other infectious agents, occupational and environmental toxins, exercise, perfumes, genetics, obesity, and emotional stress. *Healthy People 2030* objectives include reducing deaths, hospitalizations, emergency department visits, and activity limitations related to asthma.

Pathophysiology

Asthma is a chronic lung disease characterized by reversible airway obstruction, airway edema or swelling from

Table 14.2 Comparison of Pulmonary Emphysema, Chronic Bronchitis, and Asthma

CLINICAL FEATURES/ CHARACTERISTICS	EMPHYSEMA	CHRONIC BRONCHITIS	ASTHMA
Age of onset (years)	40–50	30–40	95% <5
Pathophysiology	Destruction of alveolar walls Loss of elasticity, impaired expiration, hyperinflation	Increased mucus secretion, inflammation and infection, obstruction of airways	Inflammation, bronchoconstriction, increased mucus, obstruction in the small airways. Repeat attacks lead to damage.
Health history	Generally healthy	Frequent URI, acute episodes	Hypersensitivity reaction type I
Smoking	Usually	Usually	
Clinical Features			
Barrel chest	Yes	May be present	May be present
Weight loss	May be severe in late disease	Uncommon	Uncommon
Shortness of breath	Absent early; pronounced late in disease	Early symptom; especially with activity	Primary symptom; worse with activity
Decreased breath sounds	Yes	Variable	Ominous sign
Wheezing	Usually absent	Variable	Present
Sputum	Absent or develops late in disease	Early sign; frequent infections with purulent sputum	Thick, tenacious
Cyanosis	Usually absent; appears late in disease with low PaO_2	Yes; worsens as disease progresses	Some
Cor pulmonale	Occasional	Common	Rare
Polycythemia	May appear in advanced disease	Commonly present	Rare
Blood gases	Normal until late in disease	May display hypercapnia Hypoxemia common	May display hypercapnia May display hypoxemia

PaO_2, Partial pressure of arterial oxygen; *URI*, upper respiratory infection.

inflammation, and increased airway hypersensitivity to a variety of stimuli. With asthma, a precipitating factor creates inflammation of the airways, which causes bronchospasm and edema. Cough usually indicates obstruction of the larger airways. Dyspnea, another common symptom, is indicative of inflammation of the airways, mucosal edema, and excessive secretion of mucus, which cause a plugging of the small airways. With bronchoconstriction, there is further obstruction and narrowing of the airways, limiting airflow (Fig. 14.4 and Concept Map 14.2).

Signs, Symptoms, and Diagnosis

Diagnosis is by history, physical examination, pulmonary function testing, and chest radiograph. The symptoms may be continuous or episodic. Findings include wheezing, cough that is worse at night, difficulty breathing, and chest tightness.

Unrelieved asthma attacks become *status asthmaticus* and are very serious. **Respiratory distress without wheeze is an ominous sign for the asthma patient;**

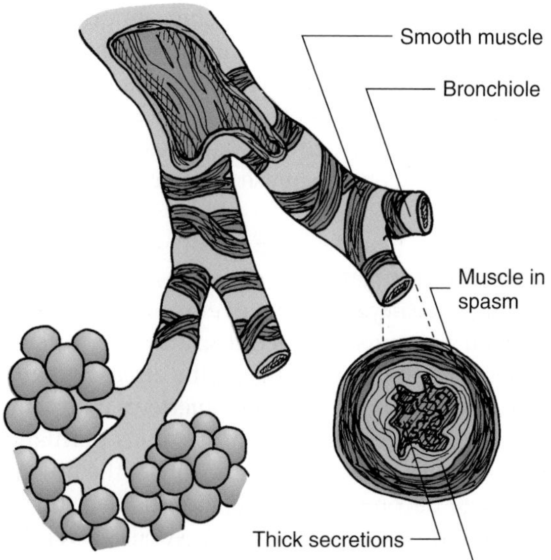

Fig. 14.4 Asthma.

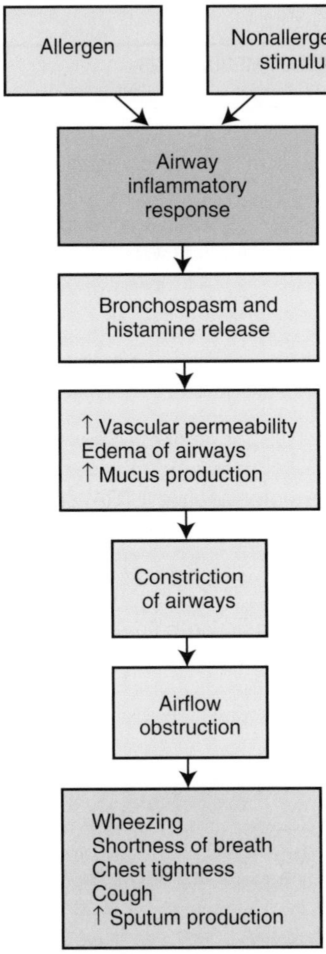

Concept Map 14.2 Pathophysiology of asthma.

this suggests further constriction with very little air movement. Patients and nurses must know that a severe, acute asthma attack can cause death from hypoxia.

Clinical Cues

If your patient takes an angiotensin-converting enzyme (ACE) inhibitor, teach them to report a cough (which can be caused by this medication). Excessive coughing can trigger or worsen an asthma attack.

Treatment

Asthma is classified based on the degree and frequency of symptoms and treated by a step system. See Table 14.3 for an example of treatment for adults. Symptom control is managed by increasing or decreasing the treatment step as needed. The goals of medical treatment are to manage the underlying symptoms and include:

- Minimizing irritation of the air passages and relieving obstruction by secretions, edema, or bronchospasm
- Preventing or controlling infection and allergy
- Increasing the patient's tolerance for activity
- Determining the best drug combinations in the smallest dosages that will control symptoms

Bronchodilators in the form of beta-adrenergic agonists and inhaled glucocorticoids are mainstays of therapy. Theophyllines or anticholinergic agents such as ipratropium bromide (Atrovent), mucolytics, and antibiotics may also be prescribed (Table 14.4). Oxygen is prescribed for moderate and severe hypoxemia. For acute episodes of hypoxemia, O_2 is given to raise the Spo_2 to 92% or greater. Systemic glucocorticoids are given for acute episodes.

Clinical Cues

A metered-dose inhaler (MDI) is incorrectly used much of the time. The inhaler should be held 1 to 2 inches in front of the mouth. A slow, deep breath is started through the mouth, then the activator is depressed as the deep breath is completed, inhaling the medication and room air. Dry powder inhalers require a seal around the mouthpiece. There is no propellant in the device, and the deep, fast inhalation is what delivers the medication to the lungs. No room air should enter around the mouthpiece.

Asthma patients are taught to use a peak flowmeter to determine the drug dosage needed to control the asthma, to predict the effectiveness of therapy, and to detect airflow obstruction buildup before it becomes serious and requires hospitalization (see Chapter 12, Fig. 12.5). Peak flow monitoring is based on the greatest airflow velocity that can be produced during a forced expiration that starts from fully inflated lungs.

Patient Teaching

Using a Peak Flowmeter

Peak flow should be monitored daily. Readings are recorded and compared with the baseline of the patient's personal best peak flow. If a reading is 60% below the patient's best, treatment should be adjusted. When the reading is in the "green zone," airflow is normal; in the "yellow zone," the usual airflow has decreased and routine medications should be increased; and in the "red zone," rescue medications are needed and the health care provider should be notified. To properly use a peak flowmeter, instruct the patient to:

- Set the pointer to zero.
- While standing, take a deep breath.
- Put the mouthpiece in the mouth and clamp the lips firmly around it for a tight seal.
- Blow into the meter as hard and as fast as possible.
- Record the value and reset the pointer.
- Rest for a couple of breaths.
- Repeat the procedure for a total of three readings.
- Record the highest reading on the peak flow sheet.

Clinical Cues

When a patient has respiratory distress in an emergency situation, apply high-flow O_2 and monitor the saturation level with a pulse oximeter. **Observe and monitor continuously.** Immediately alert the registered nurse (RN) and the health care provider. If there is a history of COPD, the O_2 rate should be changed after the respiratory crisis has resolved to achieve the ordered Spo_2 levels.

Table 14.3 Asthma Severity and Step Treatment

CLINICAL MANIFESTATIONS	TREATMENT RECOMMENDATIONS
Intermittent	
Well controlled with step 1. Symptoms or episodes occur less than once a week. Episodes or exacerbations are short, lasting only a few hours. Symptoms are present at night no more frequently than twice per month. FEV_1 is normal between episodes. During episodes or exacerbations, FEV_1 is at least 80% of normal. FEV_1/FVC is normal.	**Step 1** As-needed low dose inhaled corticosteroids (ICS)-formoterol Low dose ICS taken whenever inhaled short acting beta agonist (SABA) is taken
Mild	
Symptoms or episodes occur more than twice a week but not daily. Symptoms are present at night three or four times per month. During episodes or exacerbations, FEV_1 is at least 80% of normal. FEV_1/FVC is normal.	**Step 2** Daily low dose ICS, or as needed low dose ICS-formoterol Leukotriene receptor-agonist (LTRA) or low dose ICS taken whenever SABA taken
Moderate	
Symptoms occur daily and cause limitation to activity. Symptoms or episodes occur more than once a week. Symptoms are present at night at least once per week. During episodes or exacerbations, FEV_1 is only 60%–80% of normal. FEV_1/FVC is reduced 5%.	**Step 3** Low dose ICS-long acting beta agonist (LABA) Medium dose ICS, or low dose ICS + LTRA
Severe	
Episodes or exacerbations are frequent and severely limit physical activity. Symptoms are frequently present at night. During episodes or exacerbations, FEV_1 is less than 60% of normal. FEV_1/FVC is reduced more than 5%. PEF variability is greater than 30%.	**Step 4** Medium dose ICS-LABA High dose ICS, add-on tiotropium or add-on LTRA **Step 5** High dose ICS-LABA Refer for phenotypic assessment ± add-on therapy, e.g. tiotropium, anti-IgE, anti-IL5/5R, anti-IL4R Add low dose oral corticosteroids (OCS), but consider side effects

Adapted from Global Initiative for Asthma: Global strategy for asthma management and prevention, 2019 (website): www.ginasthma.org.
FEV_1, Forced expiratory volume in 1 second; *FVC,* forced vital capacity; *PEF,* peak expiratory flow.

Table 14.4 Commonly Prescribed Drugs for Chronic Obstructive Pulmonary Disease and Asthma[a]

CLASSIFICATION	ACTION	NURSING IMPLICATIONS	PATIENT TEACHING
Bronchodilators			
Short-Acting Beta-Adrenergic Agonists (SABA)			
Albuterol (Proventil, Ventolin) Pirbuterol (Maxair) Levalbuterol (Xopenex)	Stimulates beta-adrenergic receptors, producing bronchodilation Increases ciliary action and mucus clearance Selectively stimulates beta-adrenergic receptors, producing bronchodilation	All may be administered by MDI. Some can be administered orally or by nebulizer. Monitor tachycardia, BP changes, nervousness, palpitations, muscle tremors, and dry mouth. May cause nausea, headache, insomnia, and hypokalemia. Acts in 5–10 min and lasts for 3–4 h.	Should not be used in patients with cardiac disorders or angina. Increase fluid intake; watch for signs of potassium deficit. Wait 5 min before using a glucocorticoid inhaler (antiinflammatory). Teach to use MDI correctly.

Table 14.4 Commonly Prescribed Drugs for Chronic Obstructive Pulmonary Disease and Asthma—cont'd

CLASSIFICATION	ACTION	NURSING IMPLICATIONS	PATIENT TEACHING
Anticholinergics			
Ipratropium (Atrovent)	Causes bronchodilation by blocking action of acetylcholine	Do not mix with cromolyn sodium. Use cautiously in those with narrow-angle glaucoma, prostatic hypertrophy, or bladder neck obstruction.	Do not take more than two puffs at a time. Avoid excessive use of caffeine.
Ipratropium and albuterol (Combivent)	Causes bronchodilation by stimulating beta-adrenergic receptors and blocking action of acetylcholine		
Tiotropium bromide (Spiriva)	Causes bronchodilation by inhibiting receptors on the smooth muscle		
Long-Acting Beta-Adrenergic Agonists (LABA)			
Salmeterol (Serevent) Formoterol (Foradil) Olodaterol (Striverdi Respimat)	Relaxes bronchial smooth muscle, producing bronchodilation	Monitor for tachycardia, muscle tremors, hypokalemia. Salmeterol should be combined with fluticasone (Advair). Formoterol should be combined with budesonide.	Not to be used for acute symptoms or exacerbations.
Methylxanthine Derivative			
Aminophylline (Theo-Dur, Slo-Bid, Uniphyl, Aerolate, Uni-Dur)	Relaxes bronchial smooth muscle, improves diaphragm contractility, increases ciliary action and mucus clearance, stimulates respiration and pulmonary vasodilation, improves exercise tolerance	Administered orally or IV. CNS effects cause nervousness, irritability, headache, and insomnia. Causes tachycardia, BP changes, dysrhythmias, muscle twitching, flushing, anorexia, nausea and vomiting, epigastric pain, and diarrhea. Several drugs may increase theophylline levels. Monitor theophylline levels.	Length of drug action is decreased by smoking. Take with food to decrease GI effects. Lie down if dizziness occurs. Take medication regularly and only as prescribed. Teach to take pulse. Instruct not to use OTC medications without checking with health care provider. Wear an ID bracelet stating asthmatic status. Check interactions with herbal products.
Antiinflammatory Agents/Inhaled Corticosteroids (ICS)[b]			
Beclomethasone (Vanceril, Beclovent) Triamcinolone (Azmacort) Flunisolide (AeroBid) Fluticasone (Flovent) Budesonide (Pulmicort) Ciclesonide (Alvesco) Mometasone (Asmanex)	Provides antiinflammatory and immunosuppressive effect, decreasing edema in airways Decreases mucus secretion	All can be administered by MDI. Work synergistically with beta-adrenergic agonists. May affect potassium and glucose levels. Monitor weight. May mask infection. Monitor for edema. May have transient unpleasant taste.	Rinse mouth after each use of inhaler to prevent oral fungal infection. Do not discontinue use abruptly. Wash inhaler with warm water and dry after each use.
Cromolyn (Intal) Nedocromil (Tilade)	Stabilizes cell membranes possibly by inhibiting release of histamine and SRS-A by acting on mast cells	Cromolyn nebulizer may be preferred for some patients if MDI is inadequate.	Therapeutic response may occur within 2 wk, but doctor may suggest a 4- to 6-wk trial. Some patients may experience a bad taste with nedocromil.

Continued

Table 14.4 **Commonly Prescribed Drugs for Chronic Obstructive Pulmonary Disease and Asthma—cont'd**

CLASSIFICATION	ACTION	NURSING IMPLICATIONS	PATIENT TEACHING
Combination Agents			
Leukotriene Receptor Antagonists (LTRA)			
Zafirlukast (Accolate) Montelukast (Singulair)	Blocks action of leukotrienes in the lung once they are formed Provides both bronchodilation and antiinflammatory effects	Administered orally. May cause headache, dizziness, nausea, vomiting, diarrhea, fatigue, or abdominal pain. Not to be used for acute asthma episodes.	Should take drug 1 h before or 2 h after meals daily. Increase fluid intake. Do not stop taking other asthma medications.
Leukotriene Inhibitor			
Zileuton (Zyflo)	Inhibits the synthesis of leukotrienes, providing bronchodilation and antiinflammatory effect	Administered orally. Monitor liver enzymes. May cause dizziness, insomnia, dyspepsia, and abdominal pain. May interfere with warfarin (Coumadin) therapy and theophylline. Is not used to treat acute asthma attacks.	Check all medications and OTC drugs for ephedrine, which will increase stimulation. Teach to avoid alcohol. Notify health care provider of nausea, vomiting, anxiety, or insomnia. Continue to take even if symptom-free.
Immunomodulators			
Omalizumab (Xolair) Subcutaneous injection	Decreases mast cell mediator release from allergen exposure	Currently FDA is reviewing the possible association between omalizumab and an increased risk of heart attack, abnormal heart rhythm, heart failure, and stroke.	Subcutaneous dose is administered every 2–4 wk.
Phosphodiesterase 4 Inhibitors			
Roflumilast	Reduces the release of inflammatory mediators, countering tissue damage	Not a bronchodilator; is not used for acute bronchospasm. Increased risk of adverse psychiatric effects.	Can be taken with or without food. Risk of weight loss. Consult with provider before using OTC medications.
Cilomilast	Reduces the release of inflammatory mediators Reduces mucus hypersecretion and airway remodeling	Not a bronchodilator; is not used for acute bronchospasm.	Nausea is the principal side effect.
Mucolytic			
Acetylcysteine (Mucomyst)	Breaks down mucoproteins by enzyme action Decreases viscosity and aids in mobilization of secretions	Administered by nebulizer. Nausea and vomiting may occur. May cause bronchospasm or hemoptysis. Usually combined with bronchodilator. Monitor respirations.	Warn that secretions may become profuse. Teach that unpleasant odor will decrease with use. Discoloration of solution after bottle is opened does not impair its effectiveness.

[a]Many other drugs are also prescribed for asthma.
[b]Systemic corticosteroids (hydrocortisone, methylprednisolone, or prednisone) may be administered orally or intravenously when severe or refractory asthma attacks occur.
BP, Blood pressure; *CNS,* central nervous system; *FDA,* U.S. Food and Drug Administration; *GI,* gastrointestinal; *IV,* intravenously; *MDI,* metered-dose inhaler; *OTC,* over the counter; *SRS-A,* slow-reacting substance of anaphylaxis.

COMPLICATIONS OF CHRONIC OBSTRUCTIVE PULMONARY DISEASE

Pulmonary Hypertension

Pulmonary hypertension (PH) is high blood pressure in the blood vessels of the lungs. Lung pressures are measured during right heart catheterization using a pulmonary artery catheter.

The WHO has five classifications based on the cause of the PH. Type 1 involves increased pressure in the pulmonary arterial system from drugs and toxins, connective tissue disease, heredity, HIV, or other causes. Type 2 develops from left heart disease. Type 3 is due to lung diseases (COPD) and/or hypoxemia. Development of chronic pulmonary blood clots is the cause of type 4. Type 5 captures all other causes, including the unknown. Medications to reduce pressure in the lung vasculature are given, and underlying causes are treated. Patients with type I PH have the poorest prognosis; survival rate at 5 years from diagnosis is 57% (Rubin & Hopkins, 2018).

Cor pulmonale. **Cor pulmonale** is enlargement of the right side of the heart as a complication of PH caused by constriction of the pulmonary vessels in response to hypoxia. To overcome the increased pressure in the lungs, the right side of the heart must pump more forcefully, causing enlargement. Constant hypoxia stimulates erythropoiesis, with resulting polycythemia and increased viscosity of blood. Eventually right-sided heart failure causes systemic venous congestion, which manifests as distended neck veins, right upper quadrant tenderness from an engorged liver, peripheral edema, weight gain, gastrointestinal distress, and ascites. Treatment is continuous low-flow O_2 and medications to treat both the heart failure and the fluid volume overload.

Gastroesophageal reflux disease. Gastroesophageal reflux disease (GERD) is twice as likely to occur in patients with COPD. It can worsen the symptoms of COPD; the reflux of acid in the esophagus stimulates bronchoconstriction, and microaspiration may contribute to lung tissue damage (Houghton et al., 2016).

Nursing Management and Rehabilitation

Rehabilitation and education of the patient and family are the chief long-term goals of nursing intervention. With proper home care, patients with chronic lung disease can live longer and have a higher quality of life, reduce the number of hospitalizations and health care provider visits, and have fewer psychosocial problems related to inactivity and a feeling of hopelessness. This means working with the patient, identifying specific difficulties they are experiencing, assessing current ability to cope with those difficulties, and devising plans to accomplish specific goals for improvement. To prevent frequent hospitalizations for acute flare-ups of the disease, the patient should be taught how to avoid bronchial irritation and infection and identify such complications as right-sided heart failure (cor pulmonale) or pneumonia.

It is very important for the family to be educated on the need for appropriate exercise and activity and on the patient's natural desire for independence. Families may be overprotective because the episodes of dyspnea are very distressing.

Patient Teaching

Instructions for Patients With Chronic Respiratory Disease

- See the nutrition suggestions for patients with COPD.
- Normal sputum is white and slightly viscous and has no odor or taste. Changes in sputum should be reported to your health care provider.
- When you exert yourself, as in lifting something or getting up from a chair, exhale slowly through pursed lips. You should do the same when you are walking for exercise. It is natural to hold your breath during exertion, so you may need practice exhaling on exertion.
- Practice your breathing exercises every day without fail.
- Try to avoid crowds during the cold and flu seasons.
- Do not take over-the-counter drugs unless directed by your health care provider. They can interact with your prescribed drugs. Antihistamines can dry out the mucus even more and make it more difficult for you to clear your air passages.
- Do not smoke or inhale the tobacco smoke of others.

Smoking cessation. All patients should be encouraged to quit smoking; however, smoking cessation is critically important for those with asthma or COPD because quitting in the early stages of COPD can slow the progression of the disease. After quitting smoking, pulmonary function gradually improves, and after 10 to 20 years the chance of lung cancer is again equal to that of a nonsmoker. Smoking cessation information must be offered to all inpatients as part of The Joint Commission's Core Measures. Hospitals are required to track efforts and report them as part of the accreditation process. In addition to community resources such as support groups and information sessions, nicotine patches, nicotine gum, nicotine nasal spray, and nicotine inhalers can help wean patients off the addictive nicotine. Prescription medications such as bupropion (Wellbutrin), an antidepressant that helps alleviate some nicotine withdrawal symptoms, and varenicline (Chantix), which prevents withdrawal symptoms, are currently being used and might be most effective in combination use.

Work with the patient to develop a plan that seems possible to achieve. Decreasing stress levels and improving coping techniques aid success for patients who are trying to quit smoking. Help patients review what has helped or hindered their past attempts to quit. Identify social settings that contribute to smoking and explore substitute activities. Encourage patients to share their decision to quit with friends and family and ask friends and family not to undermine the attempt to quit. Set a definite stop-smoking date and include specific ways to reach the goal. Exercise is a good distracter for the urge to use tobacco. A support group can be very helpful. Encouragement and praise for progress in quitting smoking are essential components of the treatment program. The American Lung Association has both literature and community programs available to assist patients.

Psychosocial care. The patient often needs help with adjustment to alterations in roles and lifestyle. They may have problems with self-esteem, body image, and sexuality that stem from their chronic disease. A trusting relationship between nurse and patient facilitates discussion of personal concerns and provides a means to explore possible solutions or adaptations for problems in these areas. Referral to community support groups also can be beneficial because the patient then has an opportunity to see and hear how others in their situation have learned to cope and adapt.

Patient and family teaching. The teaching plan for a patient with a restrictive airway disease is extensive and includes:

- Management of medications and side effects
- Use of respiratory therapy measures and care of equipment
- Management of dyspnea
- Control of the immediate environment and avoidance of allergens
- Maintenance of nutrition
- Balancing exercise and adequate rest
- Awareness of signs of complications
- Need for close medical supervision

Education of the patient and family can be overwhelming; allow enough time for them to gain confidence in one aspect of care before introducing more information. An action plan for patient education and self-management can be helpful. See www.nhlbi.nih.gov, www.lung.org, www.cic.gov, or other online sources for an asthma action plan.

Most patients with chronic respiratory disease have difficulty getting sufficient rest and sleep because of dyspnea, anxiety, and decreased mobility. Sedatives and tranquilizers are contraindicated because they tend to depress respiration. Tension and anxiety often can be relieved if the patient is taught some relaxation techniques, but it takes a bit of practice to use them whenever relaxation is needed (see Chapter 7). Simply telling a patient to relax or to stop worrying is not helpful; they are using almost every muscle in their body to struggle for breath or are extremely tense in anticipation of breathlessness. Some patients become very agitated and talkative. You should display a calm attitude, stay with the patient, and encourage them to breathe, not talk.

LUNG CANCER

Etiology

Lung cancer is the leading cause of cancer deaths worldwide. In the United States in 2018 there were about 234,030 new cases of lung cancer and 154,050 deaths (American Cancer Society, 2018). Lung cancer typically occurs in people 40 years of age or older. **Cigarette smoking is the primary cause (90%).** A person living with a smoker has twice the risk of lung cancer as someone not regularly exposed to smoke. Other risk factors are increasing air pollution, asbestos exposure, lung diseases such as TB and COPD, and radon exposure. About 15% of men and 22% of women diagnosed with lung cancer survive more than 5 years. The percentage is low because often lung cancer is not detected until it is at an advanced stage.

Pathophysiology

Non–small cell lung cancer (NSCLC) includes adenocarcinoma, squamous cell carcinoma, and large cell carcinoma and accounts for about 85% of all lung cancers. Small cell lung cancer (SCLC) makes up the other 15%. Small cell or "oat" cell tumors grow rapidly and are often located near a major bronchus in the central part of the lung. Non–small cell tumors are usually found in the lung periphery and have undifferentiated cells that have slow growth and tend to metastasize.

Chronic irritation of the epithelial tissue in the lung causes changes in cell structure. This makes the tissue more vulnerable to the carcinogens and irritants inhaled when smoking or breathing air with particulate matter. Dysplasia develops, and the tumor grows. Common sites of metastases for cancer of the lung are the brain, bone, and liver.

Signs and Symptoms

At first there are few symptoms, usually only a cough and some wheezing. As the tumor grows larger, the patient may have some pain or discomfort in the chest, exertional dyspnea, and expectoration of blood-streaked sputum. More specific symptoms depend on the location and size of the malignant tumor and the areas to which it has metastasized. If, for example, the malignancy has involved the esophagus, there will be ulceration, bleeding, and dysphagia. Tumors pressing against the trachea can produce hoarseness and paralysis of the vocal cords. Fatigue, anorexia, and weight loss are common because lung cancer is usually advanced when discovered.

Diagnosis

Multiple tests are used to diagnose and stage lung cancer. These include chest radiograph; sputum cytology; low-dose CT; positron emission tomography (PET); cytology of specimens obtained by mediastinoscopy, bronchoscopy with endobronchial ultrasound, electromagnetic navigation, or thoracentesis; fine-needle biopsy of the tumor; and video-assisted thoracoscopic surgery (VATS).

Treatment

Treatment is based on the type of cancer—small cell or non–small cell—and its stage. It may be possible to remove the affected area of the lung by surgery if the malignancy is in its earliest stages and is localized. Surgical procedures include wedge resection, in which a small area of the lung is removed; segmental resection, which includes removal of lung tissue and surrounding blood vessels and bronchioles; lobectomy, with removal of an entire lobe of the lung; and **pneumonectomy**, in which an entire lung is removed. Lobectomy is the most common procedure used for SCLC. Radiation may be used before and after surgery; however, some types of lung cancers are radiation resistant. Small cell tumors respond dramatically to chemotherapy and radiation, but if the disease is extensive, the malignancy tends to recur because of metastasis that occurred before diagnosis.

NSCLC is very aggressive and difficult to treat; unless caught in the very early stages, the prognosis for this cancer is not good. The treatment for stage I and II lesions is surgical resection. For higher stages, combinations of one or two chemotherapy drugs, biotherapy agents, and radiotherapy are used, depending on the stage of the cancer and the symptoms of the patient. Current research is focusing on the genetic characteristics of individual tumors and tailoring chemotherapy to target the specific tumor. Identification of the mutations in genes has produced medications that take advantage of the weakness in the gene. Some of the medications help destroy the cancerous tissue, and others slow the progression.

Nursing Management

Care of a patient undergoing thoracotomy for cancer of the lung is discussed later in the chapter. See Chapter 8 for nursing care of patients with cancer. You must educate the patient about tests and treatments; this may help to reduce the patient's and the family's anxiety.

PULMONARY VASCULAR DISORDERS

PULMONARY EMBOLISM

Etiology and Pathophysiology

Pulmonary embolism (PE) occurs when a pulmonary vessel is plugged with a mass or clot. Emboli can occur in solid, liquid, or gas forms and can occur from fracture of a long bone (fat embolus), from amniotic fluid during childbirth, from air introduced through a central line, or from clots formed elsewhere in the body (such as from a deep venous thrombosis or thrombi that form in the heart when the patient has dysrhythmias). Regardless of the origin of the embolus, there is interference with blood flow in the lung distal to the point where the embolus lodges. The obstruction causes shunting, and blood is blocked from flowing past the alveoli, which prohibits receiving O_2 or giving up CO_2. The consequences of PE can be minor or life threatening.

Older adults are especially prone to developing deep venous thrombosis (DVT) when they are immobilized from surgery or for a major illness. Long airplane flights and sitting for long periods with the legs crossed are other potential causes of DVT. All hospitalized patients are screened for their DVT risk and appropriately anticoagulated and/or managed with sequential compression stockings as part of The Joint Commission's Core Measures. Most pulmonary emboli are a result of thrombus formation that then becomes mobile and travels to the lungs.

Signs and Symptoms

Symptoms depend on the size and location of the clot in the lung and whether it is one clot or multiple small clots. The general symptoms are respiratory distress with dyspnea, chest pain, cough, hemoptysis, and anxiety. Hypotension, tachycardia, or confusion may occur. A sudden onset of dyspnea and a drop in SpO_2 in a patient at risk of thrombus formation is very suggestive of PE.

Diagnosis

Diagnosis is made by ruling out other problems, such as heart failure, and by tests to support a diagnosis of PE. A clinical pretest probability score should first be determined, based on presence of symptoms and risk factors. Plasma D-dimer testing is recommended when a PE is initially suspected (see Chapter 12, Table 12.1). Computed tomographic pulmonary angiography (CTPA) is ordered (unless contraindicated, in which case a ventilation/perfusion scan is performed; Ouellette, 2018). The CTPA will help with the diagnosis of PE or identify another cause for the symptoms. Other tests include a chest radiograph, an echocardiogram, arterial blood gases (ABGs), and an electrocardiogram (ECG). These tests look for other causes of symptoms and do not diagnose a PE.

Treatment

Oxygen therapy is initiated to decrease hypoxia. Treatment depends on the size and location of the embolus and the stability of the patient. Intravenous heparin is usually begun in patients who might require invasive tests or treatments or when long-term therapies have not been decided. Stable patients are started on injectable low-molecular-weight heparin and may be transitioned to oral anticoagulants for the recommended 3 months of treatment. **Thrombolytic** (dissolves thrombi) therapy using alteplase or reteplase is reserved for large emboli that cause hemodynamic instability. Pulmonary embolectomy may be beneficial to patients with severe right ventricular dysfunction and cardiogenic shock. An inferior vena cava (IVC) filter may be placed to prevent future clots from traveling to the lungs from the lower extremities. Recent reports of complications related to the filters have made placement of the device controversial (Aggarwal et al., 2017).

Nursing Management

Initial care for a patient who might be experiencing a PE is to remain calm, stay with the patient, raise the head of the bed to a high Fowler position, begin O_2 therapy to maintain O_2 saturation above 92%, assess vital signs, notify the health care provider of the patient's symptoms, start a peripheral IV, and administer IV or subcutaneous heparin when it is ordered. Prepare the patient for the diagnostic tests and for probable treatment. Prevention is the best intervention, and DVT prophylaxis is implemented for all inpatients. Early identification and notification of the provider of any change in condition indicating possible PE is an important nursing responsibility. The patient is kept on bed rest in the semi-Fowler position initially, but turning, deep breathing, and coughing are important to prevent atelectasis.

PULMONARY HYPERTENSION

Pulmonary hypertension (PH) was discussed earlier as a complication of COPD. It is also caused by the four other mechanisms listed earlier. Type 1 is pulmonary arterial hypertension (PAH); all others are labeled PH. The classic symptoms are dyspnea and fatigue. Other symptoms are chest pain with exertion, dizziness, and syncope.

There is no cure for PH, but treatment can improve or relieve symptoms and increase the quality and length of life. Treatment of an underlying cause can help improve symptoms. Drug therapies are concentrated on lowering pulmonary pressures by vasodilating the vessels. Calcium channel blockers and the prostacyclin epoprostenol (Flolan) promote pulmonary vasodilation. Calcium channel blockers are administered orally, but epoprostenol must be administered continuously through a permanent central catheter and a portable infusion pump. Other medications include oral phosphodiesterase type 5 inhibitors, endothelin-receptor antagonists, and soluble guanylate stimulators. Anticoagulants, diuretics, digoxin, and supplemental O_2 may be used according to guidelines. Lung transplantation is reserved for patients with PH who do not respond to epoprostenol and who progress to severe right-sided heart failure.

LUNG TRANSPLANTATION

Lung transplantation is a viable option for a variety of end-stage lung diseases. Options include single lung, bilateral lung, and heart-lung transplantation. Patients must undergo extensive evaluation and psychological counseling and meet stringent criteria. There must be no history of malignancy within 2 years, no active TB, no substance addiction (e.g., alcohol, tobacco) for 6 months, and no renal or liver impairment. The average wait for a patient scoring in the 50th percentile for transplant viability is 6 to 7 months. The most common cause of death after lung transplantation is infection, which often occurs within 4 to 6 weeks of surgery. Immunosuppressive therapy is lifelong to prevent organ rejection. After transplantation and stabilization, patients enter a rehabilitation program to improve physical endurance.

CHEST INJURIES

The major complications of chest trauma involve either the lungs and air passages or the heart and major blood vessels, and the patient can deteriorate rapidly. Major concerns in the care of patients with chest injuries are:

- Maintenance of an airway
- Ensuring adequate ventilation
- Treatment of circulatory problems to ensure circulation of oxygenated blood

(See Chapter 45 for additional information about chest trauma.)

PNEUMOTHORAX AND HEMOTHORAX

Pneumothorax and **hemothorax** often occur as a result of a blunt (nonpenetrating) or penetrating injury to the chest wall. These conditions can cause partial or total collapse of one or both lungs. The space within the pleural membranes is an airtight compartment with *negative pressure*. This negative pressure allows for the tidal movement of air in and out of the lungs. However, if there is a break in the airtight compartment—either along the surface of the lung or from outside the pleural sac—air rushes in and collapses the lung. **Pneumothorax is a threat in chest injury and usually present in the period after thoracic surgery.** The condition also can occur spontaneously when there is a rupture of the alveoli. This is called *spontaneous pneumothorax*. Tall, thin people and smokers are more prone to spontaneous pneumothorax. Cases have occurred after scuba diving, flying, or mountain climbing.

A pneumothorax may require nothing more than rest and the administration of O_2 to relieve discomfort. If the amount of air in the pleural space is minimal, a large-bore needle may be used to aspirate it or a one-way chest valve device may be placed. For greater amounts of air or fluid, a thoracostomy tube (chest tube) may be inserted and connected to water-seal drainage to remove the air and allow re-expansion of the lung (Fig. 14.5).

Hemothorax is the presence of blood within the pleural cavity caused by laceration of the lung, heart, or blood vessels within the thorax. The accumulation of blood in the pleural cavity can cause partial or total collapse of the lung. There also is the possibility of mediastinal shift in hemothorax and the likelihood of impaired venous return to the heart. The blood is removed with a thoracostomy tube and chest drainage.

For a patient with pneumothorax, hemothorax, or a combination of the two—hemopneumothorax (Fig. 14.6)—assess for a history of acute or chronic respiratory disease, accidental injury to the chest, or chest surgery. The patient may complain of sudden chest pain or a feeling of tightness in the chest. There is an increase in both pulse rate and rate of respirations, a drop in blood pressure, and the absence of normal chest movements and absent or diminished breath sounds on the affected side.

? Think Critically

You come upon an automobile accident and stop to assist. You have your stethoscope in your car. Name three assessment criteria that would lead you to believe that the driver of the vehicle has suffered a pneumothorax.

LUNG DISORDERS

PULMONARY EDEMA

Pulmonary edema is an abnormal collection of fluid in the interstitial spaces of the lung and inside the alveoli.

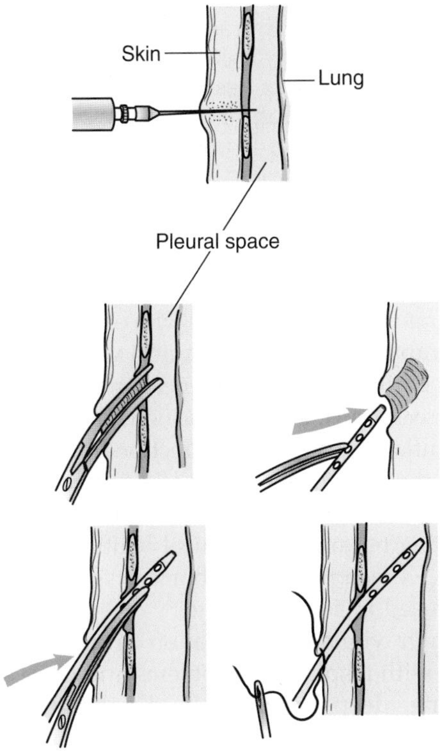

Fig. 14.5 Insertion of a thoracostomy tube (chest tube).

Acute pulmonary edema is a medical emergency. Pulmonary edema is classified as cardiogenic or noncardiogenic depending on the cause. Left ventricular heart failure is a common cause. See Chapter 19 for assessment and treatment of heart failure. Noncardiogenic causes include neurogenic pulmonary edema drowning, acute glomerulonephritis, inhalation injury, allergic reaction, and acute respiratory distress syndrome (ARDS).

Nursing care involves placing the patient in high Fowler position. Oxygen is started immediately, and continuous positive airway pressure (CPAP) or intubation may be necessary. Furosemide is given for fluid diuresis, and morphine reduces anxiety and the workload on the heart. Drugs for the underlying heart disorder or other condition also are administered. You must closely monitor intake and output and perform continuous respiratory and cardiac assessment to evaluate the effectiveness of treatment.

ACUTE RESPIRATORY DISTRESS SYNDROME

Etiology and Pathophysiology

Acute respiratory distress syndrome (ARDS) is a form of acute lung injury (ALI) that results from pulmonary changes that occur with sepsis, major trauma, major surgery, or any critical illness. When the alveolar capillary membrane is injured, it becomes more permeable to intravascular fluid. Alveoli fill with fluid, and O_2 and CO_2 cannot cross the membrane into and out of the capillaries. Pulmonary edema and lung stiffness occur, resulting in severe hypoxemia. ARDS is particularly dangerous when a patient has multisystem disorders; the mortality rate in these patients is 25% to 40%. Improvements in treating the underlying cause as well as interventions for ARDS have improved survival rates.

Signs, Symptoms, and Diagnosis

Dyspnea, tachypnea, tachycardia, and hypoxemia occur. Auscultation may reveal fine, scattered crackles. There is increasing hypoxemia and respiratory alkalosis from the tachypnea. As ARDS progresses, symptoms worsen

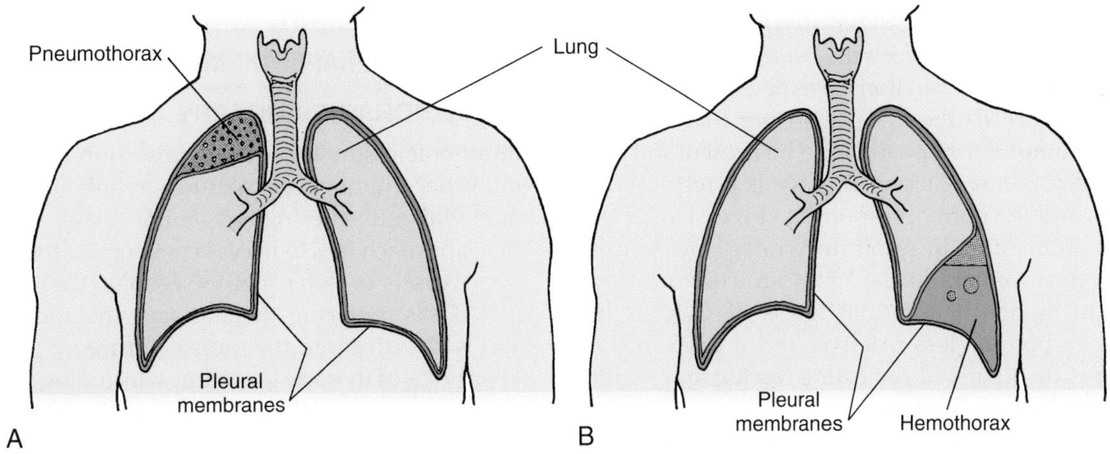

Fig. 14.6 A, Pneumothorax. **B,** Hemothorax.

because of increased fluid accumulation and decreased lung compliance. The onset may be as soon as 12 to 48 hours after the initiating event.

Diagnosis is by physical presentation, history of a disorder or event known to cause ARDS, ABG determination, and chest radiograph. The chest radiograph will show bilateral infiltrates, sometimes called *whiteout,* in the absence of heart failure. The sudden onset and hypoxemia despite supplemental O_2 complete the diagnosis. The Pao_2 is divided by the fraction of inspired oxygen (Fio_2); if the result is 200 or less, the diagnosis is ARDS. Results of less than 300 constitute a diagnosis of ALI.

Treatment and Nursing Management

Treatment for ARDS is ventilatory support with low tidal volumes to prevent additional pressure-related lung injury, positive end-expiratory pressure (PEEP) or CPAP, treatment of the underlying disorder, careful fluid and electrolyte management, and total care for basic needs. Drug therapies have not been shown to be an effective intervention for ARDS. Because infection and sepsis are often the cause of ARDS, early administration of appropriate antibiotics is essential to halt the infectious process.

Nutritional support is essential in prevention of complications and modulation of the stress response. Enteral nutrition is the preferred route of administration. Prone positioning has been shown to improve oxygenation but not overall survival. Patients with ARDS will be on mechanical ventilation in an intensive care setting.

RESPIRATORY FAILURE

Respiratory failure is the result of insufficient O_2 or excessive CO_2. The disorder can occur acutely or as a chronic condition.

Hypoxemic respiratory failure (type I) occurs when Pao_2 is lower than 60 mm Hg and a normal or low Pco_2 is present. This is a result of insufficient oxygen passing from the alveoli to the capillaries. For example, in pneumonia or with a massive pulmonary embolism, fluid fills the alveoli and interferes with gas exchange at the alveoli-capillary interface.

Hypercapnia (also called *hypercarbia*) is the result of hypoventilation, during which the usual amount of CO_2 is not eliminated by exhalation. In hypercapnic respiratory failure (type II) the Pco_2 is greater than 50 mm Hg. It is common for hypoxemia to be present in type II respiratory failure. Carbon dioxide is a respiratory stimulant, and the normal response to excessive levels of CO_2 is an increase in respiratory rate. However, if the respiratory centers in the brain are continuously exposed to higher-than-normal levels of CO_2, as in COPD, they become less reactive, and a drop in the respiratory rate occurs. Chronic lung disease may result in a chronic state of respiratory failure. Many patients live in a constant hypoxic state and are always short of breath. Abruptness of onset and severity of symptoms identify the acuteness of the condition. Signs and symptoms of respiratory failure include restlessness, agitation, or confusion. An increase in respiratory rate, pulse, and blood pressure signals a physiologic attempt to compensate for inadequate oxygenation. The patient may sit upright and bend forward and be unable to speak without pausing for breath. Diaphoresis and retraction of accessory respiratory muscles occur as the work of breathing increases. Cyanosis is a late sign of hypoxemia. The outcome can be cardiac arrest from respiratory acidosis.

> **! Safety Alert**
>
> **Recognition of and Response to Changes in Patient Condition**
>
> An essential National Patient Safety Goal is to improve the recognition of and response to changes in patient condition. Particularly for patients who are at risk for retaining CO_2, do not assume that lethargy and drowsiness are secondary to the patient's having had a "restless, sleepless night." Assess breathing patterns and respiratory rate and carefully compare the current mental status to baseline. Check pulse oximetry and transcutaneous CO_2 ($PtcCO_2$) readings. Notify the health care provider if you suspect respiratory failure and obtain an order for ABGs.

Respiratory failure is treated with oxygen and respiratory therapy, including mechanical ventilation, noninvasive ventilatory support, measures to reduce and remove secretions, drugs to reduce bronchospasm and airway inflammation, and correction of acidosis. Treatment of the underlying cause is also necessary. Acute respiratory failure will be managed in an intensive care unit setting because mechanical ventilation is usually required. Extracorporeal membrane oxygenation (ECMO) may be used in some patients.

Through vigilant observation and assessment of patients with respiratory problems and close attention to turning, deep breathing, and coughing, you can often prevent respiratory failure. Nursing measures are incorporated to relieve anxiety and agitation. Monitoring fluid balance is particularly important when there is concurrent heart or multiorgan failure.

COMMON THERAPEUTIC MEASURES

INTRATHORACIC SURGERY

Intrathoracic surgery, such as resection of lung tissue and other pulmonary structures, requires opening the chest wall and entering the pleural cavity. An intrathoracic approach is also necessary to repair the heart and great vessels or defects of the esophagus.

VATS is replacing the standard **thoracotomy** (incision with entry into the thorax) for many procedures. About 70% of thoracic procedures, including pulmonary resections, biopsy or resection of mediastinal tumors or masses, and drainage of pleural effusions, can be performed in this manner. As with laparoscopic procedures performed in the abdominal cavity, several incisions are made to introduce the scope, camera, and necessary instruments. At any time, a VATS procedure can be converted to an open thoracotomy if needed.

Preoperative Care

Assessment of the patient's respiratory status before thoracic surgery depends on whether the surgery is elective or emergent. If there is time, a health history as well as subjective and objective assessment data should be obtained before the surgery (see Chapter 12).

Preoperatively, efforts are made to improve the respiratory status of the patient as much as possible. Special exercises may be prescribed to strengthen the chest, shoulder, and accessory muscles of respiration and to remove accumulated secretions from the air passages.

When standard thoracotomy is to be performed, arm and leg exercises are taught preoperatively to prevent thrombophlebitis and problems with movement. Movement of the arm may be very painful because of positioning during surgery or the surgical involvement of muscles that control the arm. "Frozen" (immobile) shoulder can occur if the arm is not exercised. With VATS, this complication is less likely to occur.

Preoperative patient education focuses on teaching information to improve lung ventilation and to prepare for postoperative equipment such as chest tubes, suctioning, mechanical ventilation, and use of an incentive spirometer.

Postoperative Care

During the immediate postoperative period, nursing assessment and intervention focus on routine positioning, turning, coughing, and deep breathing; procedure-specific observations; and attention to chest tubes and the closed drainage system. A patient who has had thoracic surgery should be ambulatory as soon as possible. An advantage of VATS is that the patient is out of bed and into a chair within 4 to 6 hours of surgery; pain is less. The standard thoracotomy patient has a 4- to 6-week recovery, whereas the VATS patient resumes activities of daily living in 3 to 4 days and can return to work within 1 week. To promote early mobility, pain management is essential. Surgical pain causes the patient to take shallow breaths and limit movement that causes pain. Adequate pain management will facilitate deep breathing and mobility, both of which are essential in preventing complications.

Special observations include watching for signs of pneumothorax, hemothorax, or both; observing for symptoms of respiratory distress; and auscultation and palpation of the upper chest and neck for swelling caused by **subcutaneous emphysema** (an accumulation of air or gas under the skin, which feels like bubble wrap on palpation). Subcutaneous emphysema is also called **crepitus** and can occur when air leaks into the tissues around chest tubes. It could be a sign of malfunctioning of the drainage system and should be reported. Inspecting the drainage system for air leakage is essential. Assessing for signs of infection, both respiratory and incisional, is also a nursing responsibility.

Gastric distention and paralytic ileus are possible complications of standard thoracic surgery. **Distention of the stomach and intestines is particularly hazardous for the patient who has had a thoracotomy because distention can cause these organs to push up on the diaphragm and impair ventilation, which is already compromised by the surgery.**

Positioning for comfort, optimal ventilation, and adequate drainage of the operative site is important during post-thoracotomy care. In most cases the patient is allowed to lie on the back and operative side. Many surgeons do not permit lying on the unaffected side because this position diminishes the expansion of the good lung. When the patient has a tube inserted for drainage from the operative site, lying on the operative side facilitates the flow of drainage. Care must be taken when positioning the patient to prevent kinking of the chest tubes.

An understanding of the surgical procedure performed and a careful adherence to mobility orders are essential for safe movement of thoracotomy patients. A pneumonectomy patient has had an entire lung removed. Over time the body will accommodate for the space previously occupied by the lung; however, in the immediate postoperative period certain positions may put tension on the bronchial stump. Surgeon preference will dictate acceptable patient positioning for any thoracic surgery.

Care of patients with chest tubes and closed drainage. Regular and frequent monitoring of patients with chest tubes, with an understanding of why the tube has been placed, will help with early identification of problems requiring intervention. It will also allow for assessment of effectiveness of the therapy (Fig. 14.7). There are three major areas of assessment:

1. The respiratory status of the patient
2. The site at which the tube is inserted into the chest and the length of the tube (for kinks or clots)
3. The amount and character of the drainage in the collection chamber

The patient is assessed for ease of breathing, pain or discomfort, level of consciousness and orientation, and anxiety and restlessness. The rate and character of respirations are noted, as are breath sounds. The entry site is assessed for unusual drainage, infection, integrity of sutures, and the presence of subcutaneous emphysema. The chest tube will be attached to a drainage system. Commercial disposable plastic water-seal drainage systems are the most common. The drainage system should (1) provide for drainage of air and blood from within the pleural cavity and (2) allow for gradual re-expansion of the lung by isolating the intrathoracic pressure from atmospheric pressure. Fig. 14.8 shows a disposable system. Note that the water in the left-hand chamber serves as a suction control chamber. When the unit is attached to wall suction, there will be bubbling in the compartment. The level of fluid determines the amount of suction applied to the chest. Increasing the wall suction will increase the bubbling but does not change the degree of suction. Slow, gentle suction is adequate. The middle chamber is the water-seal chamber that prevents air from entering the chest cavity. Tidaling (movement with breathing) should occur in this chamber. If air is being removed from the chest, bubbles might be observed in this chamber. The collection chamber—located on the far right of the device—is calibrated for accurate measurement of drainage from the chest. When caring for a patient with a closed drainage system, the following precautions should be kept in mind:

- Remember that the pleural cavity is an airtight compartment. The apparatus and all connections must remain airtight at all times; all connections should be taped.
- Do not allow the tubing to become kinked or obstructed by the weight of the patient.
- Never pin the tubing to the bedclothes.
- Do not empty chest tube drainage containers. The system must remain closed. Replace the unit when the drainage chamber is full.
- The system operates by gravity and must remain below the patient's chest level at all times.
- The amount of drainage expected will vary according to why the tube was inserted. Find out from the surgeon how much drainage is expected and when to call.
- If the chest tube becomes unattached, do not clamp the tube; place the end of the tubing in a container of sterile water. This creates a "water seal" and can prevent tension pneumothorax. Temporary clamping may be performed by the surgeon to assess lung function or occasionally by the RN to check for the source of air leaks.
- Persistent bubbling in the water-seal chamber indicates an air leak. Fluid in the chamber *should* fluctuate with inhalation and exhalation. Occasional bubbles may appear with breathing, sneezing, or coughing. If a pneumothorax is present, bubbling will occur with inspiration, as air is forced out of the area of the pneumothorax.

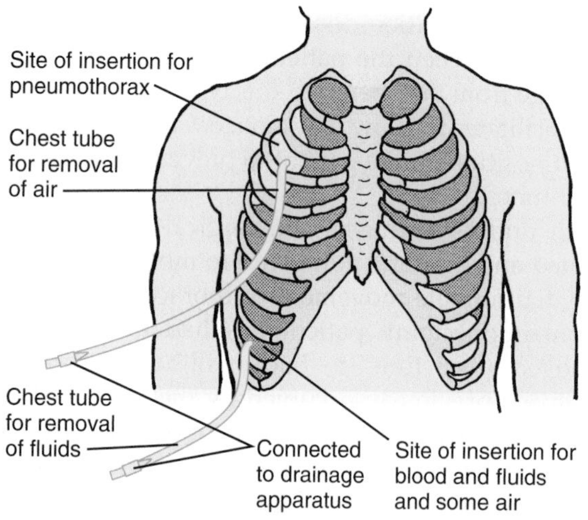

Fig. 14.7 Location of sites for insertion of chest tubes for drainage of air and fluids.

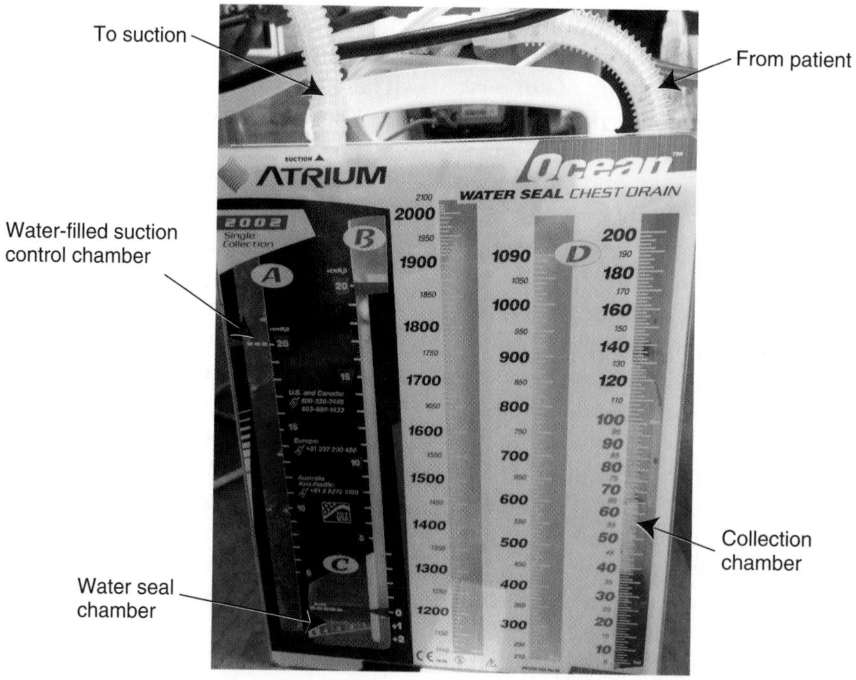

Fig. 14.8 Disposable water-seal drainage system; note the three chambers.

- A "puffed-up" appearance of the patient's chest or neck could be subcutaneous emphysema.
- Dressings may be reinforced but are not changed except by order of the surgeon. Dressings must be occlusive and not allow air in around the chest tube.

Other devices such as a flutter valve, or Heimlich valve, may be substituted for chest drainage systems. This valve permits the flow of air and fluid from the pleural space into a collection area but prevents the return flow of air or fluid; the Heimlich valve is inserted between the chest tube and the drainage collection apparatus or may be used without a collection device if only air is being evacuated.

Ambulatory patients may be using a small, portable chest drainage system that has only one chamber with a dry seal and does not contain water. The system is used for certain patients who have less than 500 mL of drainage daily. The collection chamber must be emptied when full. Several other devices are available for chest drainage for home care patients. Each comes with specific care directions.

A dry-suction system is sometimes used in place of water-seal suction. It provides more consistent flow because the suction adjusts automatically to changes in the patient's pleural pressure or to fluctuations in wall suction pressure. The regulator within the unit is preset to –20 cm H_2O but can be changed to range from –10 to –40 cm H_2O.

Specialized chest drainage systems are used to collect the patient's blood from the chest after surgery so that it can be reinfused in an autologous transfusion.

The patient should be medicated 30 to 60 minutes before the removal of a chest tube. When the surgeon removes the chest tubes, the incision is covered with a dressing containing sterile petroleum jelly to close off the opening so that air does not enter the pleural space. This type of dressing is also applied if a chest tube is accidentally pulled out. Auscultate the lungs after chest tube removal to verify that a pneumothorax has not occurred. Eventually the incision will seal itself. A sample plan with interventions for a patient having thoracic surgery is shown in Nursing Care Plan 14.1.

? Think Critically

Your patient is 1 day postoperative from an open thoracotomy. What would you do if the fluid in the drainage chamber of the closed drainage system had not increased over the past 4 hours?

? Think Critically

Your patient is 1 day postoperative from a standard thoracotomy. While assessing the patient, you notice that the water in the closed drainage system's water-seal chamber is not fluctuating with the patient's breathing. What would you do?

MEDICATION ADMINISTRATION

Bronchodilators are drugs that directly act on and relax the smooth muscle of the bronchi and thereby relieve bronchospasms. Box 14.1 lists general nursing implications for these drugs. Liquefying agents help thin the bronchial secretions, making them less tenacious. Antiinfective agents used for respiratory infections include the tetracyclines, penicillins, cephalosporins, macrolides (azithromycin), and fluoroquinolones (ciprofloxacin [Cipro]).

Box 14.1 General Nursing Actions for the Administration of Chronic Obstructive Pulmonary Disease and Asthma Medications

When giving any medication, you should:

- Follow the standard procedures for checking identification of the patient, using the "Six Rights," verifying allergies, and monitoring for side effects and drug interactions.
- Verify that the medication is appropriate for the patient considering the current clinical condition.

When giving inhaled corticosteroids (ICS):

- Know how to use the delivery device so you can teach the patient the correct technique. Many are dry powder and have different ways of providing the dose.
- Have the patient rinse their mouth well and spit out the rinse water. ICS cause tissue irritation and may even result in oral thrush if the mouth is not rinsed thoroughly.

When giving bronchodilators:

- Auscultate the lungs to ascertain the types of lung sounds present and take vital signs.
- Use these drugs cautiously in patients with cardiac disease because they affect heart action.
- Follow correct procedure for inhaling the drug: shake the inhaler gently before using, clear the nose and throat, take a deep breath, relax, and completely exhale before inhaling drug.
- When the patient is taking theophylline, check drug serum levels; the therapeutic range is 5 to 15 mcg/mL. If the level is above 20 mcg/mL, withhold the drug and notify the health care provider.

Regarding possible side effects or adverse effects of the medications, you should:

- Warn the patient about the possibility of paradoxical bronchospasm and advise them to consult the provider if this happens before administering another dose of bronchodilator.
- Tell the patient to chew sugarless gum or suck on hard candy to relieve a dry mouth.
- Monitor the patient for specific side effects of each drug; general side effects of bronchodilators are dry mouth, insomnia, nervousness, dizziness, palpitations, gastrointestinal upset, and changes in blood pressure.

For all respiratory medications, you should:

- Monitor the patient for effectiveness of the drug by performing a respiratory assessment.

Nursing Care Plan 14.1 Care of a Patient With Lung Cancer

SCENARIO

A 62-year-old female smoker with a diagnosis of early lung cancer is scheduled for a right thoracotomy with lobectomy. She has no other medical problems except mild arthritis, for which she occasionally takes aspirin.

PREOPERATIVE PROBLEM STATEMENT/NURSING DIAGNOSIS

Insufficient knowledge related to postoperative care for thoracotomy.

SUPPORTING ASSESSMENT DATA

Subjective: "I've never had surgery before."

Goals/Expected Outcomes	Nursing Interventions	Selected Rationale	Evaluation
Patient will verbalize understanding of postoperative routine of frequent monitoring of vital signs, chest tube care, and respiratory treatments.	Explain purpose and show tubes, drainage apparatus, and oxygen equipment. Explain need for early ambulation. Describe methods of pain control.	Being familiar with equipment and what to expect after surgery decreases fear of the unknown.	Verbalizes understanding of what equipment is for. Says will try to ambulate this afternoon. States understanding of PCA pump for pain control. Outcomes met.
Patient will demonstrate use of spirometer and coughing and deep-breathing exercises.	Teach deep breathing, coughing, use of incentive spirometer. Obtain return demonstration.	Learning the techniques before surgery facilitates postoperative performance.	Uses spirometer correctly and can demonstrate coughing and deep breathing.
Patient will be mobile and active after the surgery to prevent postoperative complications.	Teach leg exercises; flex and extend ankles and knees, circular rotation of ankles, and gluteal tightening. Ambulate to determine preoperative abilities.	Teaching before surgery empowers patient and provides time to practice techniques and ask questions. Ambulating before surgery gives baseline information.	Is practicing leg exercises enthusiastically. "Hope I can keep this up after surgery." Ambulates independently with steady gait. Easily walks full length of preop teaching unit without distress.

POSTOPERATIVE PROBLEM STATEMENT/NURSING DIAGNOSIS

Risk for altered gas exchange related to surgical removal of portion of lung and possible complications.

SUPPORTING ASSESSMENT DATA

Objective: Thoracotomy and lobectomy.

Goals/Expected Outcomes	Nursing Interventions	Selected Rationale	Evaluation
Patient will display normal respiratory rate and normal oxygenation before discharge.	Position on back or operative side; turn, cough, deep-breathe, and use incentive spirometer q2h; splint incision with small pillow to minimize pain.	Position allows good lung to fully expand. Incentive spirometer use opens alveoli, promoting better gas exchange and preventing atelectasis.	Assisted to turn q2h; using spirometer and coughing q2h. Splints incision when coughing.
	Administer oxygen as ordered.	Oxygen saturation should be maintained at ordered parameter.	Receiving oxygen at 3 L via nasal cannula.
	Monitor vital signs and respiratory effort and auscultate lung fields q4h; pulse oximetry readings q1h, monitor blood gas levels.	Respiratory rate, lung sounds, blood gas levels, and pulse oximetry readings provide data regarding respiratory status and can indicate decline or improvement.	BP 134/82, P 85, RR 28/min. Left lung with normal breath sounds; right lung with diminished sounds in bases and absent over middle lobe area. Sao_2 95% average.
	Encourage use of PCA to promote better cooperation with respiratory therapy, coughing, and deep breathing, but avoid oversedation and respiratory depression.	If pain is minimized, patient is able to more fully expand the lungs and to perform coughing and deep-breathing exercises.	Using PCA appropriately; pain at 4 on a scale of 1–10.

Nursing Care Plan 14.1 Care of a Patient With Lung Cancer—cont'd

Goals/Expected Outcomes	Nursing Interventions	Selected Rationale	Evaluation
	Maintain intact, functioning closed water-seal drainage system.	Intact system prevents air from entering pleural space and collapsing lung.	Chest drainage system intact with 150 mL drainage.
	Observe for signs of subcutaneous emphysema.		No subcutaneous emphysema; no signs of respiratory distress (i.e., labored, uneven respirations; no subjective SOB).
	Monitor abdomen for signs of distention or ileus.	Distention can cause pressure on diaphragm and decrease lung expansion.	Abdomen soft and nondistended.

POSTOPERATIVE PROBLEM STATEMENT/NURSING DIAGNOSIS

Potential for infection related to surgical incision and chest tubes.

SUPPORTING ASSESSMENT DATA

Objective: Thoracotomy and lobectomy; chest tube in place.

Goals/Expected Outcomes	Nursing Interventions	Selected Rationale	Evaluation
No signs of infection as evidenced by clean incision, temperature in normal range, normal WBC count, and clear breath sounds during hospitalization.	Use aseptic technique for dressing changes and care of chest tube.	Prevents introduction of pathogenic organisms.	Very small amount of pink-tinged drainage on old dressing. Dressing changed, as ordered, with aseptic technique. Incision intact.
	Assess temperature trends q24h; monitor WBC count.	Provides data that might indicate beginning of infection.	Temp 99.4° F (37.4° C) CBC results pending.
	Observe wound for signs of infection.	Early detection and reporting results in early intervention.	No redness, swelling, or pain to surrounding tissues. Dressing dry and intact.
	Protect from people with infections.	Helps prevent exposure to respiratory infection.	Note placed on door advising visitors, who may have infection, to check with nurses before entering.
	Maintain adequate nutrition and fluid intake.	Adequate fluid and nutrition are required for healing.	Taking clear liquids. IV line patent at 125 mL/h.
	Auscultate lungs each shift and as needed for changes in respiratory status.	Auscultating at the beginning of the shift establishes baseline for comparison.	Breath sounds clear but diminished in bases and absent over right middle lobe.
	Administer antibiotics as ordered.	Antibiotics may be ordered prophylactically because of weakened immune system.	Antibiotics are en route from the pharmacy, will be administered as soon as available.

PROBLEM STATEMENT/NURSING DIAGNOSIS

Anxiety related to diagnosis of cancer of the lung, treatment, and prognosis.

SUPPORTING ASSESSMENT DATA

Subjective: "I'm scared. I don't want to die of cancer. Will I have to have chemotherapy? Will there be a lot of pain?"

Objective: Anxious look on face.

Goals/Expected Outcomes	Nursing Interventions	Selected Rationale	Evaluation
Patient will be less anxious about treatment and disease process by discharge.	Establish trusting relationship; use active listening.	A trusting relationship promotes sharing of feelings and fears.	Using active listening, but patient is not verbalizing details.
	Encourage verbalization of fears and concerns; answer questions honestly.		

Continued

Nursing Care Plan 14.1 Care of a Patient With Lung Cancer—cont'd

Goals/Expected Outcomes	Nursing Interventions	Selected Rationale	Evaluation
	Engender hope; discuss what patient can do to optimize chances of survival: quit smoking, exercise program, diet, relaxation techniques, stress reduction.	Hope allows patient to focus on the future. Active participation in her own survival is empowering and increases feelings of control over the disease.	Reminded that many people have lived for many years after having lung cancer. Discussed aids for quitting smoking. Not willing to try relaxation exercise yet.
	Advise that oncologist will discuss modes of treatment when pathology report is completed. Type of tumor, growth, and aggressiveness dictate treatment.	Giving correct information and explaining why more information is not immediately available helps decrease anxiety.	Advised that oncologist would be in tomorrow morning to talk about options. States that she would like to have her family present for that discussion.
	Assure that pain control is possible.	Fear of pain and uncertainty about ability to withstand pain is a major source of anxiety.	Visibly relieved when reassured about pain management. Continue plan.

CRITICAL THINKING QUESTIONS

1. Why should this patient not be positioned on the nonoperative side after surgery?
2. What would you do if you noticed that the suction control chamber on the disposable water-seal chest drainage system was not bubbling?

BP, Blood pressure; *CBC*, complete blood cell count; *IV*, intravenous; *P*, pulse; *PCA*, patient-controlled analgesia; *RR*, respiratory rate; SaO_2, oxygen saturation; *SOB*, shortness of breath; *WBC*, white blood cell.

Corticosteroids are a major part of inhalation therapy for patients with COPD. Inhaled steroids at doses used routinely for COPD and asthma are not significantly absorbed systemically and do not produce the same side effects as oral steroids. Acute respiratory problems are sometimes treated with systemic corticosteroids, either oral or IV. When corticosteroids are prescribed, the patient must be aware that steroids may blunt the inflammatory response normally seen in early infection. Long-term steroids should not be abruptly discontinued; these drugs must be slowly tapered over several days. Oral steroids contribute to potassium loss, and replacement may be necessary. Blood glucose is closely monitored for elevation. Gastrointestinal prophylaxis is recommended to counter gastric irritation.

Antihistamines are used to treat respiratory symptoms of an allergic disorder. They reduce the secretions and swelling of the nasal and bronchial mucosa. Decongestants are prescribed for symptoms of the common cold and sinusitis. **Leukotriene** inhibitors and **immunomodulators** help control asthma symptoms by blocking the activity of substances that mediate inflammation.

Aerosols are fine suspensions of very small particles of a liquid or solid that dispense as a gas. Several delivery systems provide aerosolized medications. MDIs are used to deliver a variety of drugs to respiratory patients. The patient should be taught to use an MDI properly. MDIs deliver liquid medication, and dry powder inhalers (DPIs) deliver the dose in powder form. Bronchodilators, liquefying agents, and some antiinfective agents may be administered directly onto the mucous membranes of the respiratory tract by a **nebulizer** (device producing a fine spray) and mechanical ventilator.

A nebulizer can provide aerosolized medications via mouthpiece, face mask, face tent, or tracheostomy collar. Nebulizers are available for use at home. In the hospital, the nebulizer is attached to oxygen so that hypoxemia can be treated as medication is being administered. Nebulizer treatments are usually 20 to 30 minutes long and are given two, three, or four times a day.

The patient is taught to breathe through the mouth during the treatment. They should sit in a comfortable chair. Halfway through the treatment and after the treatment, deep breathing and coughing are performed to raise loose mucus.

HUMIDIFICATION

Without adequate water and humidity, mucous secretions become extremely thick and tenacious, and the mucous membranes become dry, crusted, irritated, and more susceptible to invasion by pathogenic microorganisms. For O_2 delivery of 4 L/min or less, humidification is not necessary. Room air is not artificially humidified. At low flow rates, the largest volume of inhaled gas is room air, and the normal physiologic mechanisms function to humidify the inhaled O_2 and room air. With tracheostomies and high-flow O_2 delivery, humidification is needed. Highest humidification is achieved with warmed fluids, although room temperature fluid can be used.

PULMONARY HYGIENE

Patients with chronic pulmonary disease can benefit from a program of pulmonary hygiene that is designed to remove secretions and to enable more efficient exchange of O_2 and CO_2. Pulmonary hygiene programs include administering prescribed drugs; humidifying inhaled air; medication therapy via nebulizer, DPI, or MDI; chest physiotherapy; and breathing exercises. Several devices are available to help clear mucus and open airways, and these devices can be used at home.

Chest physiotherapy includes postural drainage (when possible) and percussion and vibration. *Postural drainage* involves positioning the patient so that the forces of gravity can help remove secretions deep in the bronchi and lungs (Fig. 14.9). Tapping, clapping, and vibrating techniques are used primarily for cystic fibrosis for the purpose of dislodging mucus plugs so that they can be coughed up more easily. The health care provider or physical therapist will give specific directions, and therapy must be provided by someone who has been instructed in the proper technique. Family

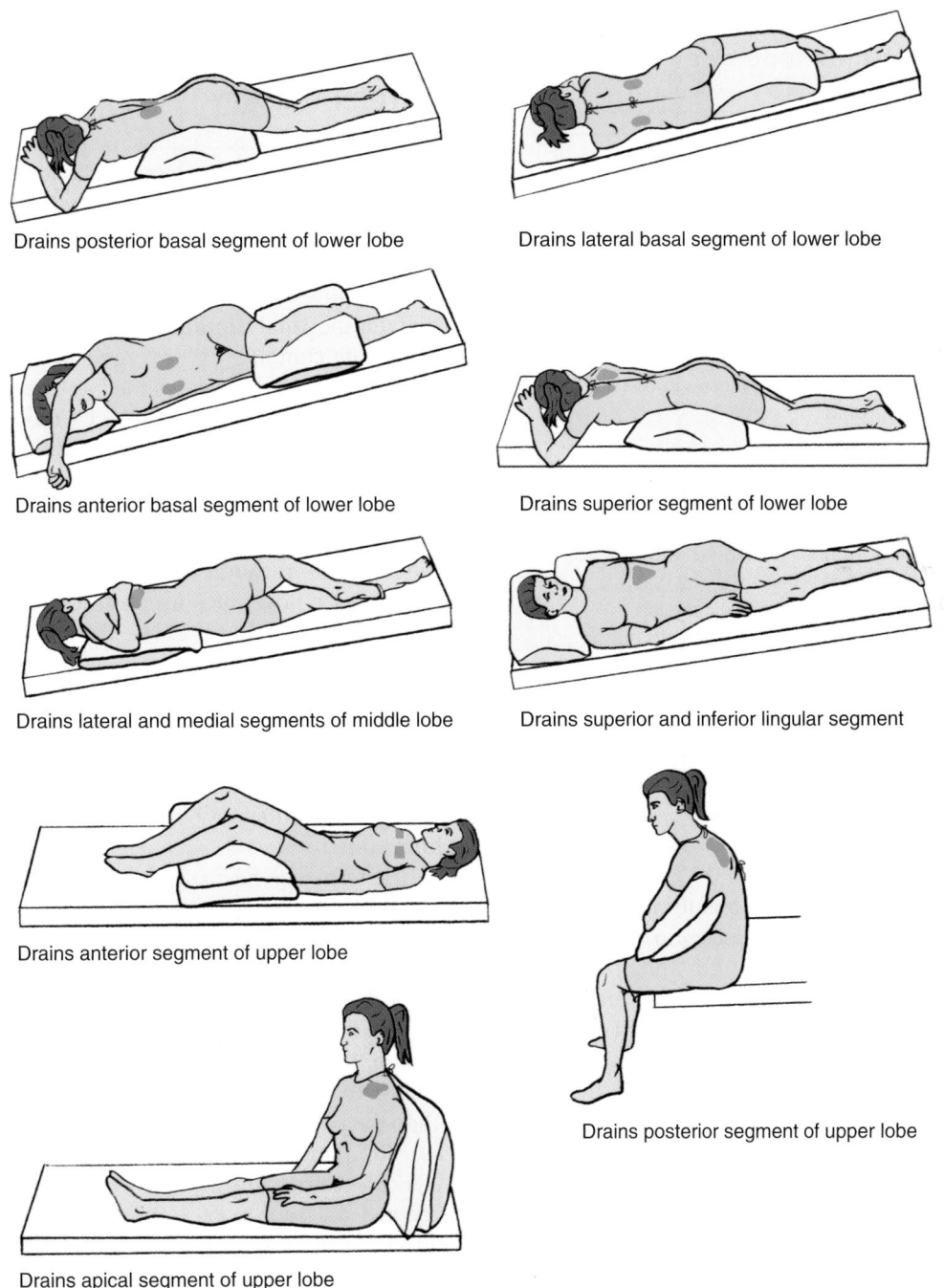

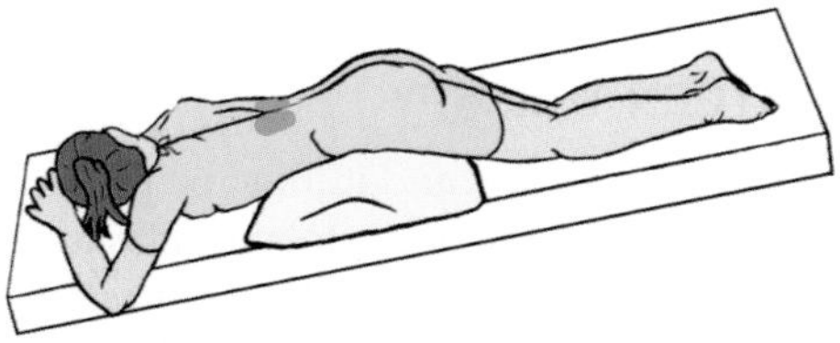

Drains posterior basal segment of lower lobe

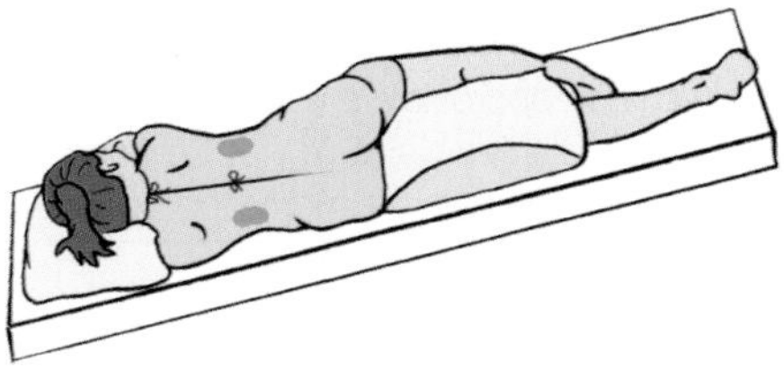

Drains lateral basal segment of lower lobe

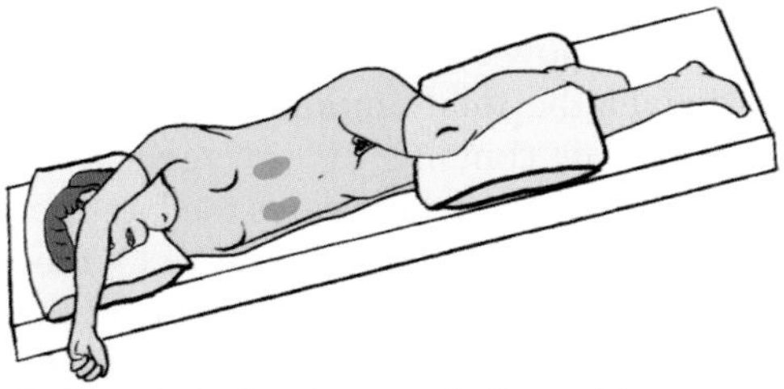

Drains anterior basal segment of lower lobe

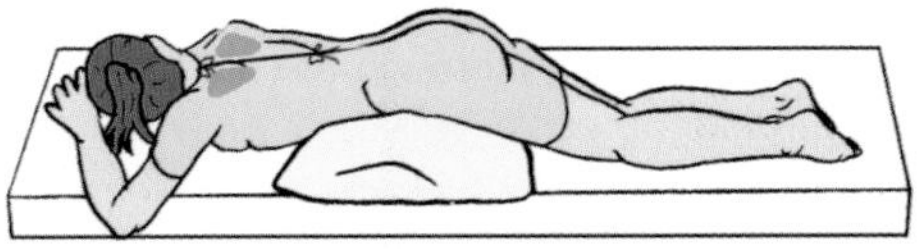

Drains superior segment of lower lobe

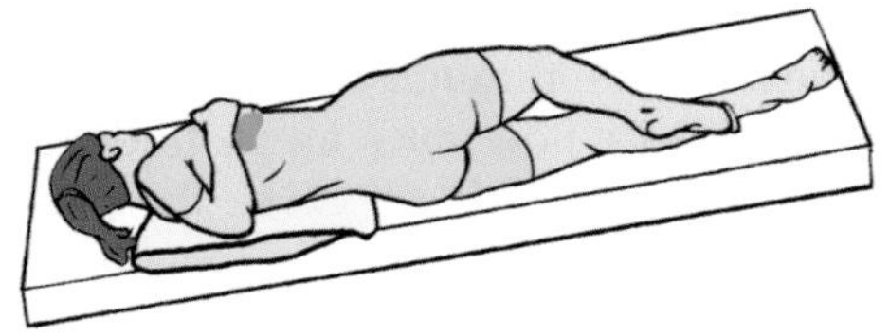

Drains lateral and medial segments of middle lobe

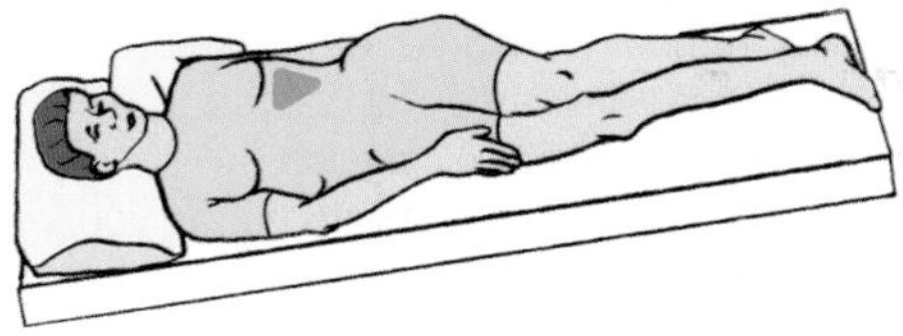

Drains superior and inferior lingular segment

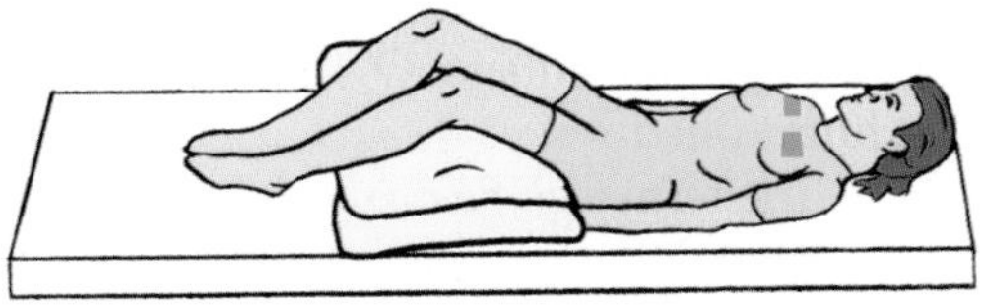

Drains anterior segment of upper lobe

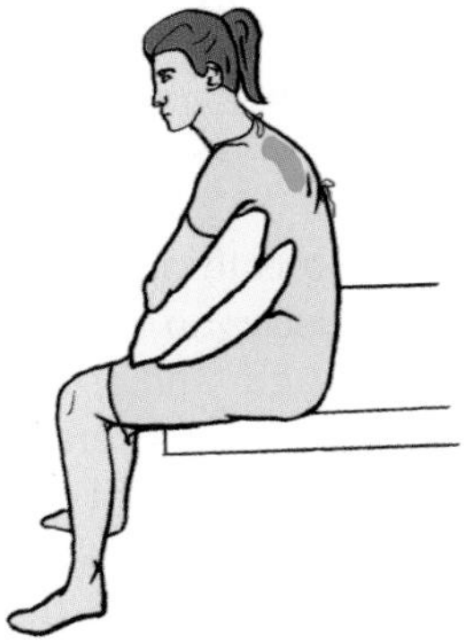

Drains posterior segment of upper lobe

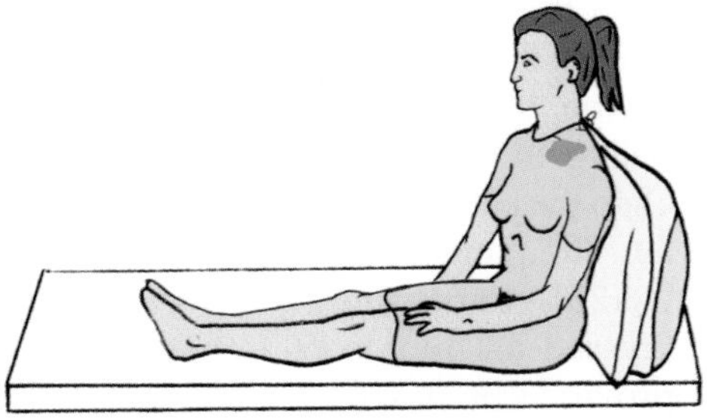

Drains apical segment of upper lobe

Fig. 14.9 Positions for postural drainage. (From Williams P: *deWit's fundamental concepts and skills for nursing,* ed 5, St. Louis, 2018, Elsevier.)

members can be taught the procedures, if needed, for home care.

Because there is likely to be some gagging during coughing episodes that take place during postural drainage, it is best to carry out the procedure before meals, when the stomach is relatively empty and vomiting is less likely. If the patient is to have postural drainage only once a day, drainage should be done in the morning to remove secretions that have accumulated during the night. After postural drainage is completed, good mouth care—including brushing the teeth and using a refreshing mouthwash—should be performed.

Older Adult Care Points

Older adult patients with osteoporosis are at risk for fractures of the vertebrae and ribs. Clapping should not be used on these patients; vibrating techniques are more appropriate.

Patient Teaching

Pursed-Lip Breathing

- Sit up tall and move the back away from the chair; place the feet about shoulder-width apart. Lean forward slightly with hands or elbows on the knees.
- Close the mouth and breathe in through the nose.
- Purse the lips as though to gently whistle or blow out a candle; keep the lips and cheeks relaxed.
- Blow through relaxed pursed lips, exhale slowly, and do *not* force the air out of the lungs (this can bring about the collapse of the airway structures).
- Breathe out slowly without puffing out the cheeks; control the flow of exhaled air as if you wanted to cause a candle to flicker but not extinguish.
- Take twice as much time to let the breath out as you did to take it in.
- Tense the abdominal muscles to force as much air from the lungs as possible.
- Use pursed-lip breathing during any physical activity.
- Refrain from holding your breath when lifting objects or performing other physical activities.

The purpose of performing breathing exercises is to strengthen the abdominal muscles so that they can push upward against the diaphragm and assist in the expiration of air from the lungs. These exercises also help overcome rigidity of the thorax so that the lungs can inflate and deflate more easily. Patients who follow the exercises prescribed for them often find that they can lead more active and useful lives than formerly possible because their exertional dyspnea is less severe (Berry, 2017). The muscles of their body are stronger; thus there is less risk for complications that accompany immobility. The exercises also help patients cough up secretions that would otherwise remain in the lower bronchi and serve as a growth medium for bacteria or a cause of atelectasis.

Patient Teaching

Abdominal (Belly) or Diaphragmatic Breathing

- Initially practice lying down.
- Lie on the back with the knees bent. Take a deep breath through the nose with the abdomen relaxed and, with the palm of one hand, feel the abdomen rise. Exhale slowly to a count of four.
- Exhale slowly through pursed lips, tightening the abdominal muscles that push the diaphragm up, forcing more air out of the lungs.
- Once comfortable with the abdominal breathing technique, use it when standing or sitting. This type of controlled breathing will provide more endurance during physical activity.

OXYGEN THERAPY

Oxygen is a drug, and it must be prescribed and administered in specific doses to avoid O_2 toxicity. The dosage of O_2 is stated in terms of *concentration* and *rate of flow.* Methods of administration are divided into high-flow and low-flow systems (Fig. 14.10 and Table 14.5).

Low-flow systems supplement O_2 needs but do not deliver the total amount of O_2 needed by the body. Room air contains 21% oxygen. Every liter of 100% oxygen delivered increases the FiO_2 (fraction of inspired oxygen) by 3%. The amount of O_2 the patient receives depends on rate and depth of breathing. Nasal cannula provides low flow and should not exceed 5 L/min flow. Higher flow rates cause drying and cracking of nasal mucosa. If a mask system is used, it is important that the flow rate through the mask is a minimum of 6 L/min. Lesser flow rates are not adequate to wash out exhaled CO_2 and will cause the patient to rebreathe exhaled CO_2.

High-flow oxygen delivery systems provide O_2 levels high enough to completely supply the needs of the patient. They do not rely on the patient's breathing to provide the set amount of O_2. For prolonged periods of high-percentage O_2 delivery, the gas should be humidified.

The term *high-flow oxygen* is used to signify a specific oxygen delivery system that is different from standard systems. Normally O_2 is delivered through a cannula, mask, or tent that is supplied to the device directly from the O_2 source at a specific liter flow. High-flow oxygen therapy provides humidified O_2 from the source to the high-flow machine. Compressed air is also delivered to the machine. The machine then sends the O_2 to the patient at high flow rates using the compressed air. The patient receives the prescribed percentage of O_2 (21%–100%) and the flow rate ordered for the compressed air (up to 60 L/min). This therapy can be provided by nasal prongs or mask. By delivering the O_2 under pressure, better gas exchange occurs.

Short-term O_2 therapy, which is the administration of O_2 to treat hypoxemia, is given to achieve an SpO_2

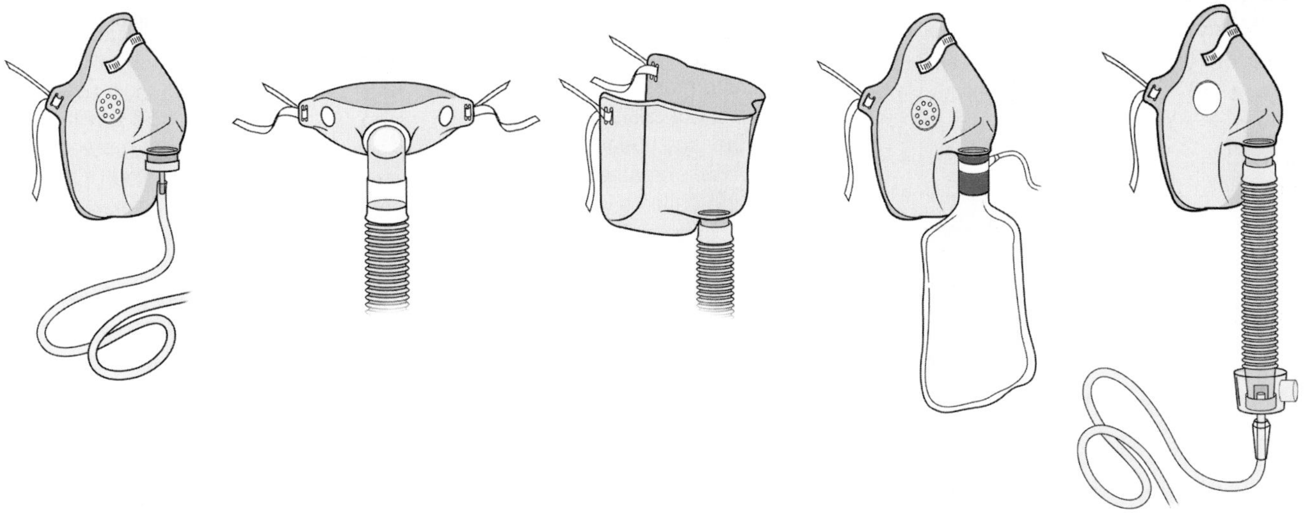

Fig. 14.10 Various oxygen delivery devices. (From Williams P: *deWit's fundamental concepts and skills for nursing,* ed 5, St. Louis, 2018, Elsevier.)

Table 14.5 Advantages and Disadvantages of Common Oxygen Delivery Devices

METHOD	O_2 DELIVERY	ADVANTAGES	DISADVANTAGES	NURSING IMPLICATIONS
Nasal cannula (nasal prongs)	Low concentrations; dependent on rate and depth of breathing *Flows:* 1 L = 24% O_2 2 L = 28% O_2 3 L = 32% O_2 4 L = 36% O_2 5 L = 40% O_2 6 L = 44% O_2	Patient can move about, eat, and talk while receiving O_2. Most COPD patients can tolerate 2 L/min flow.	Restless patients can easily dislodge the prongs. Risk of skin irritation at nares, ears, and cheeks. If drying of mucosa occurs, warm humidified O_2 should be supplied.	The curve of the prongs should be facing down toward mouth when inserted in nose; check frequently because patients tend to replace the prongs incorrectly. Make sure prongs are patent.
Simple face mask	Low to medium concentrations; 35%–50% can be achieved with flow rate of 6–12 L/min.	Delivers 40%–60% O_2 quickly for short-term therapy.	Requires a tight seal to deliver higher concentrations of O_2; some patients feel claustrophobic. Device must be removed for patient to eat, drink, or take medications. Muffles voice when talking. Requires at least 5-L flow to prevent accumulation of CO_2 in mask.	Wash and dry under mask and wipe out mask q1–2h. Mask must fit snugly. May need to pad straps at ears to prevent skin irritation and possibly necrosis.
Partial nonrebreather mask	Higher concentrations; 80%–90% at flow rates of 10–20 L/min.	Mask is lightweight; reservoir contains 100% O_2 for breathing. One tab on the mask prevents limitation on the amount of exhaled CO_2 that is "rebreathed" by the patient.	Risk of tissue pressure injury with long-term use. Cannot be used with high humidity.	Flow of O_2 should be high enough that the bag does not deflate during inspiration. Check skin under straps frequently.

Continued

Table 14.5 **Advantages and Disadvantages of Common Oxygen Delivery Devices—cont'd**

METHOD	O_2 DELIVERY	ADVANTAGES	DISADVANTAGES	NURSING IMPLICATIONS
Face tent	Delivers up to 60% oxygen.	Better tolerated than a face mask because it is not sealed on the face. Good for mouth breathers and patients with blocked nasal passages.	Cannot deliver high levels of O_2.	Needs to be well fitted. Flow needs to be >5 L/min to prevent rebreathing of exhaled CO_2.
Venturi mask	Delivers consistent FiO_2 regardless of breathing pattern. Concentration and liter flow marked on mask apparatus; available for 24%, 28%, 35%, 40%, and 60% O_2.	Good for delivering low, constant O_2 concentrations to patient with COPD.	Discomfort and risk of skin irritation. Must be removed for eating, drinking, and taking oral medications. Talking is muffled.	Air ports must not be occluded. Check skin contact areas frequently.
Transtracheal catheter	Delivers O_2 efficiently.	Flow requirement is reduced 60%–80%, increasing time O_2 is available from portable source. Catheter is less visible. Less nasal irritation occurs.	Catheter replacement is an invasive procedure. Not appropriate for someone with excessive mucus production.	Patient and family teaching about catheter replacement.
Tracheostomy collar	Delivers O_2 and humidification via tracheostomy; must be connected to a nebulizer with FiO_2 set at 24%–100%.	Adds humidity to help prevent drying of the tracheal mucosa. Loses some O_2 flow because collar is not tight fitting and sits loosely over the tracheostomy.	Must drain condensation in tubing often. Risk of respiratory infection.	Drain condensation from tubing into receptacle, being careful not to allow fluid to go into tracheostomy. Remove and clean collar device and check skin under straps at least q4h.
T-bar (Briggs adapter)	Delivers O_2 and humidification to tracheostomy or endotracheal tube; must be connected to a humidifier FiO_2 set at 24%–100%.	Attaches directly to the tracheostomy. Adds humidity to prevent drying of the tracheal mucosa.	Must drain condensation in tubing often. Risk of respiratory infection.	Drain condensation from tubing into receptacle; be careful not to get fluid into tracheostomy. Remove and clean T-bar device q4h.

COPD, Chronic obstructive pulmonary disease; *FiO_2*, fraction of inspired oxygen.

between 94% and 98%. In patients at risk for worsening of hypercapnia (COPD), the target SpO_2 is between 88% and 92% (Cousin, Wark, & McDonald, 2016). You or the respiratory therapist titrates the O_2 delivery to achieve the intended outcome.

Outward signs of hypoxia vary among patients, but dyspnea, restlessness, and confusion are the most common signs. Blood gas analysis is the most reliable indicator. For bedside assessment, pulse oximetry is quick and noninvasive and gives a snapshot of oxygen saturation.

Long-term O_2 therapy for patients with asthma or COPD is used to:

- Relieve hypoxemia
- Reverse tissue hypoxia and its signs and symptoms
- Allow the patient to function better mentally and physically, thereby increasing self-reliance

Oxygen orders for long-term management are prescribed in liters per minute or a specific FiO_2.

Nursing Management

Check the O_2 delivery system at the beginning of the shift and then periodically to verify that the flow is set according to the health care provider's order or that the target SpO_2 is being maintained. Check the tubing to see that it is not kinked and that it is connected to the O_2 source. Make sure that the patient is wearing the delivery device. Oxygen is not explosive; however, oxygen does support combustion, which means that a spark or flame can cause a major fire. **Smoking is not allowed when O_2 is used. The tubing should be kept off the floor, and the connections should be handled aseptically to prevent contamination of the system. Most health care facilities are smoke-free institutions, but patients and families need to be taught safety principles if O_2 is to be used at home. Open flames for cooking are also a risk.**

When oxygen therapy is discontinued, it is usually done gradually. The patient is "weaned" from dependence on oxygen by gradually reducing the dosage, until room air is tolerated.

? Think Critically

Describe the assessment points you would cover at the beginning of the shift for a patient who is receiving oxygen therapy. Consider both the patient and the oxygen setup system.

MECHANICAL VENTILATION

Mechanical ventilation is needed when the patient cannot maintain adequate ventilation because of respiratory, neurologic, or neuromuscular problems or trauma. In the acute care setting the most commonly used method is positive-pressure ventilation.

The pressure delivered is greater than that within the airway and alveoli; therefore gas flows into the lungs, either assisting or controlling inhalation. When the pressure is released, exhalation is passive without effort by the machine or the patient. Ventilators are classified by how the inspiratory cycle is terminated. An endotracheal tube or tracheostomy tube must be in place for use of most mechanical ventilators (see Chapter 13).

Pressure-cycled ventilators deliver air into the lungs up to a preset pressure. The Babybird and the Siemens Servo are examples of this type. These are mainly used for infants and children.

Volume-cycled ventilators deliver a preset volume of gas with preset pressure limits. Adequate tidal volumes will be delivered even when airway resistance is great (e.g., in patients suffering from severe obstructive lung disease). If the ventilator meets too much pressure, an alarm sounds to indicate that the correct tidal volume is not being delivered. This is commonly caused by excessive secretions in the lungs, and suctioning is needed.

High-frequency jet ventilation provides good ventilation with the use of relatively small tidal volumes at *very* high respiratory rates. The oxygenation and ventilation are accomplished by gas diffusion and convection rather than by a high flow of gas. Because the intrathoracic pressures needed for this type of ventilation are much lower, there are fewer complications (e.g., barotrauma, hypotension, and pneumothorax) than with other types of ventilation.

Modes of Ventilation

In *controlled-mode ventilation,* the machine is set to deliver a fixed number of breaths per minute, at a set volume. The machine does not allow for spontaneous respirations. Controlled-mode ventilation is used during periods of central nervous system depression, such as during anesthesia, sedation, and drug overdose.

Assist-mode ventilation decreases the work of breathing for the patient. When the patient takes a breath, the machine delivers a set tidal volume. Assist-mode ventilation is combined with the control function to provide an assist-control mode. If the patient's respiratory rate falls, the machine will deliver a set number of breaths per minute; if the patient initiates a breath, the machine finishes it at the set tidal volume. The patient can breathe above the rate set on the ventilator. *Intermittent mandatory ventilation (IMV)* and *synchronized intermittent mandatory ventilation (SIMV)* are the most common modes of ventilation found in critical care settings. These allow the patient to breathe spontaneously and yet provide a preset number of ventilator breaths at a preset tidal volume, to ensure adequate ventilation without respiratory muscle fatigue. SIMV is triggered by the patient's inspiratory effort to initiate the machine breath. During mechanical ventilation, it is possible for a patient's respiratory muscles to weaken from lack of use. One of the advantages of SIMV mode is that the patient's respiratory muscles are at work during spontaneous breathing, keeping the muscles toned, which makes it easier to wean the patient from the ventilator.

In PEEP, the pressure in the airways never falls below a certain level (usually between 5 and 15 cm H_2O). This holds the smaller air passages open, thus limiting atelectasis. It also expands alveoli so that there is more time for gas to diffuse across the membrane and correct hypoxemia. PEEP is used for ARDS and respiratory failure. PEEP increases intrathoracic pressures, which can diminish venous return to the heart, thereby decreasing cardiac output and blood pressure.

Pressure support ventilation. In pressure support ventilation (PSV), the patient breathes spontaneously, but PSV decreases the work of drawing gases through the ventilator tubing, thus decreasing patient fatigue. PSV is used as an adjunct to standard ventilator modes. PSV has proven very beneficial during weaning from IMV.

Continuous positive airway pressure. CPAP and bilevel positive airway pressure (BiPAP) can be used for patients who are breathing spontaneously but are showing signs of hypoxemia. It is used for infants with mild respiratory distress syndrome (RDS) and for adults in the early stages of respiratory failure. The therapy can be delivered via the ventilator in an intubated patient, usually for weaning purposes. CPAP and BiPAP not delivered through an artificial airway are considered *noninvasive positive pressure ventilation (NPPV).*

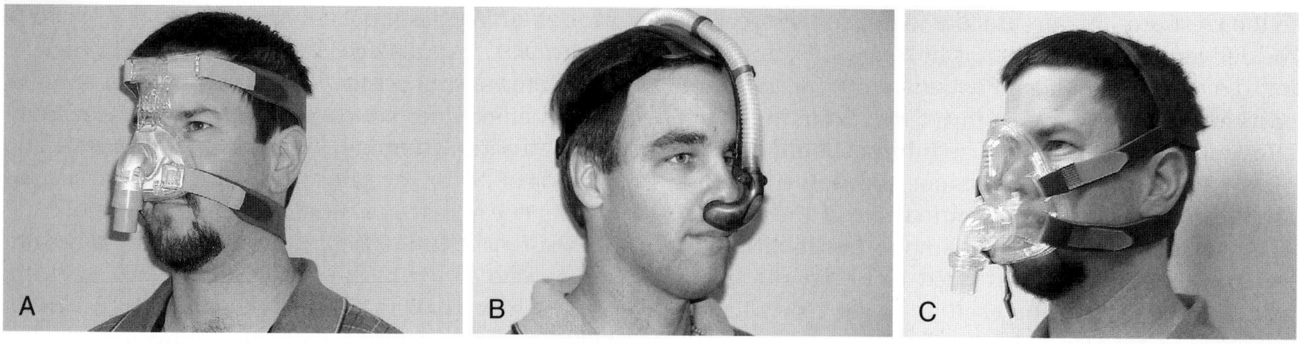

Fig. 14.11 Management of sleep apnea often involves sleeping with noninvasive positive pressure ventilation (NPPV) delivered through **(A)** a nasal mask, **(B)** nasal prongs, or **(C)** a face mask. The pressure supplied by air coming from the compressor opens the oropharynx and nasopharynx. (From Cairo JM: *Mosby's respiratory care equipment*, ed 10, St. Louis, 2018, Elsevier.)

Noninvasive positive pressure ventilation. NPPV is used in the hospital and in the home to provide ventilation assistance for patients who need help with oxygenation or air movement. NPPV may be used to improve oxygenation and ventilation so that endotracheal intubation is not needed. It is only used in spontaneously breathing patients who can maintain their own airway. Carefully monitor CO_2 levels, oxygen saturation, hemodynamic stability, level of consciousness, ability to clear secretions, and ability to tolerate the mask or prongs. If treatment outcomes are not met, intubation with mechanical ventilation may be necessary. In the home setting, NPPV is used in the form of CPAP or BiPAP primarily for sleep apnea. The delivery devices use room air and not O_2 for gas delivery. The primary function is to keep positive pressure in the airway to prevent it from closing during sleep. Delivery of supplemental O_2 is not a goal of the therapy (Fig. 14.11).

Nursing Management

Care for a patient who is receiving mechanical ventilation requires extensive training and supervised practice. The patient will require protection from infection, continuous monitoring of vital signs, observation for hypoventilation and hyperventilation, measurement of intake and output, and prevention of disabilities from inactivity. Mechanical ventilation may be a short-term therapy or a chronic support for those who cannot breathe on their own. When caring for a patient on mechanical ventilation, you should:

- Check the health care provider's order each shift and then check the ventilator for the proper settings: mode, FiO_2 (the oxygen concentration that is delivered), respiratory rate, tidal volume, peak inspiratory pressure, and if PEEP or CPAP is ordered.
- Check alarms to see that they are turned on. Alarms should not be turned off when disconnecting the patient to suction because the alarms may not be reactivated.
- Keep tubing clear of pooled water; empty the water into an appropriate receptacle as needed.
- Check for tension or stretching of the ventilator tubing every time a patient is repositioned.

The patient is observed for signs of complications, such as gastric distention, pneumothorax, and impaired cardiac output from decreased venous return, and the need for increasingly higher pressures to deliver the set tidal volume, which can indicate stiffening of the lungs (decreased compliance). Prevention of ventilator-associated pneumonia includes multiple nursing interventions. Auscultate the lung fields to be certain that both lungs are being ventilated. Monitor ABG levels to determine the effectiveness of ventilation treatment.

! Safety Alert

Preventing Ventilator-Acquired Pneumonia

Use of a "ventilator bundle" helps prevent ventilator-acquired pneumonia. The Agency for Healthcare Research and Quality recommends (1) regular oral care with chlorhexidine, (2) continuous removal of subglottic secretions, (3) change of ventilator circuit only if visibly soiled or malfunctioning, (4) selective oral or digestive decontamination, and (5) prophylactic probiotics (Timsit et al., 2017).

For ventilation to be effective, the lungs must be kept clear of secretions. Many patients can cough up secretions and do not need to be suctioned; others may need frequent suctioning. Endotracheal and tracheal suctioning must be done with strict aseptic technique because of the high risk of respiratory infection. In intubated patients an inline suction catheter is used for secretion removal.

An intubated patient on a ventilator cannot talk, so alternative means of communication such as a dry erase board, VitalVoice communication device, electronic device, or paper and pencil are offered. In the acute phase of mechanical ventilation, patients may be sedated. Nurses and other staff need to communicate with the patient, assuming that they can hear what is being said, and explain all procedures and activities.

Additional calorie intake is needed just to maintain weight when a ventilator is used. Continuous enteral feeding is the method most often used to prevent malnutrition in these patients. You should monitor nutritional parameters.

If a ventilator alarm sounds and the problem cannot be located quickly, the patient should be disconnected from the machine and ventilated with a manual resuscitator bag and oxygen until the problem is solved.

? Think Critically

You have just assisted another nurse in turning a patient who is being mechanically ventilated. The patient has been positioned on the left side, and the ventilator is on the right side of the bed. What would you check before you leave the bedside?

COMMUNITY CARE

Home care nurses may be the first to notice that a patient needs home oxygen therapy; also, chronic respiratory patients must be monitored for early signs of complications, such as heart failure. Most patients diagnosed with sleep apnea are using BiPAP or CPAP machines in the home, and home health nurses monitor and teach about use of the machine. Outpatient clinic nurses may be the first to notice that respiratory patients are having an increased number of sick days and an increased severity with each episode. Careful history and screening should be conducted to determine whether there is an occupational exposure to an irritant or if the patient is developing hypersensitivity. You can advocate for spirometry because it is a good test for detecting nonmalignant occupational lung diseases. Community nurses participate in infection control by identifying and referring potential and active cases of tuberculosis within the community.

Working with patients to promote compliance with their exercise and medication regimen is a primary function of the nurse in the community. Teaching use of the peak airflow meter and the MDI can save health care dollars by decreasing serious episodes of acute respiratory dysfunction. *Rehabilitation* (see Chapter 9) of chronic respiratory patients is directed at:

- Improving breathing
- Improving activity tolerance
- Decreasing infection
- Preventing acute episodes

Get Ready for the NCLEX® Examination!

Key Points

- Symptoms of influenza are headache, fever, chills, and muscle aches, followed by hacking cough, runny nose and nasal congestion, and sensitivity to light.
- Hospital-acquired pneumonia can often be prevented by use of aseptic technique and good respiratory care. Older adults are at special risk for pneumonia.
- Symptoms of bacterial pneumonia are high fever, chills, cough with rusty sputum, chest pain, diaphoresis, malaise, and aching muscles. There will be diminished or abnormal breath sounds.
- Fluids (unless contraindicated) should be increased for patients with respiratory infections.
- Treatment of tuberculosis requires multiple medications for a period of 6 to 9 months (see Table 14.1).
- Restrictive lung disorders include pleurisy, pleural effusion, pulmonary fibrosis, kyphosis, severe scoliosis, and arthritis of the chest wall.
- Chronic obstructive lung disorders include emphysema, chronic bronchitis, and asthma. Smoking cessation is one of the most important measures in the treatment of obstructive lung disease.
- Emphysema causes destruction of the terminal respiratory units and narrowed, stiff airways with loss of lung elasticity; it causes air trapping and CO_2 retention.
- Chronic bronchitis causes inflammation, excess secretion of mucus, chronic cough, increasing resistance to airflow, and hypoxia. In asthma, bronchospasm and excessive secretion of mucus with bronchoconstriction cause decreased airflow and hypoxia. A severe asthma attack can kill, if not relieved.
- Patients with COPD are taught diaphragmatic breathing and pursed-lip breathing techniques to assist aeration of the lungs.
- The primary cause of lung cancer is cigarette smoking. Symptoms of lung cancer include cough, wheezing, chest discomfort, exertional dyspnea, and expectoration of blood-streaked sputum. Treatment includes surgery, radiation, chemotherapy, and biotherapy agents.
- Signs and symptoms of pulmonary embolus are dyspnea, chest pain, cough, hemoptysis, and anxiety. Anticoagulant therapy is used for prevention or treatment of pulmonary embolus.
- Pneumothorax and hemothorax decrease lung capacity; treatment includes chest tubes and a closed drainage system.
- Pulmonary edema is a medical emergency. Symptoms include severe dyspnea; orthopnea; noisy respirations; pink frothy sputum; pale, cold, clammy skin; anxiety; restlessness; and possibly confusion.
- ARDS is life threatening and is treated with ventilatory support with PEEP.
- Respiratory failure occurs as type I hypoxemic failure and type II hypercapnic failure.
- Frequent respiratory assessment is essential for a patient with chest tubes. Nursing care includes positioning on the back or on the operative side or according to health care provider orders, checking tubing for kinks, and reporting abnormal chest drainage.
- O_2 is a medication used to treat hypoxemia and can be toxic. High concentrations of O_2 are used for patients

with COPD for short periods, titrating to desired SpO_2, because it can cause further CO_2 retention.

- Mechanical ventilation may be necessary after chest surgery and for respiratory failure, ARDS, flail chest (see Chapter 45), and neuromuscular disorders that interfere with the respiratory muscles. Nursing care includes carefully checking ventilator settings each shift, ensuring that alarms are on, auscultating the lungs to be sure that both lungs are being ventilated, suctioning as needed, administering nutritional therapy, and observing for complications.

Additional Learning Resources

SG Go to your Study Guide for additional learning activities to help you master this chapter content.

Go to your Evolve website (http://evolve.elsevier.com/deWit/medsurg) for the following FREE learning resources:

- Animations, audio, and video
- Answers and rationales for questions and activities
- Glossary with pronunciations in English and Spanish
- Interactive Review Questions and more!

Review Questions for the NCLEX® Examination

1. You are caring for a patient with signs and symptoms of influenza. What home care for this respiratory condition would be appropriate?
   1. Schedule adequate periods of exercise and activity.
   2. Provide warming measures.
   3. Restrict fluid intake.
   4. Consider analgesics and antipyretics.

   NCLEX Client Need: Physiological Integrity: Pharmacological Therapies

2. A 58-year-old man is admitted with bacterial pneumonia. He has high fever accompanied by chills, a cough productive of rust-colored sputum, and a general feeling of malaise. The medical diagnosis is confirmed by:
   1. blood cultures.
   2. chest radiographs.
   3. white blood cell count.
   4. bronchoscopy.

   NCLEX Client Need: Physiological Integrity: Reduction of Risk Potential

3. Which patient is at greatest risk for developing a pulmonary embolism? The patient who:
   1. has a central line that was started 2 days ago.
   2. is 3 months pregnant with her first child.
   3. has been immobile for 1 week and is mildly dehydrated.
   4. is ambulating 2 days after abdominal surgery.

   NCLEX Client Need: Physiological Integrity: Reduction of Risk Potential

4. A frail 40-year-old woman is admitted with complaints of fever, fatigue, coughing, difficulty breathing, and weight loss. Place the following nursing interventions in priority order.
   1. Auscultate lung sounds.
   2. Assess work of breathing and oxygen saturation.
   3. Review the health care provider's orders and implement.
   4. Weigh the patient.

   NCLEX Client Need: Physiological Integrity: Reduction of Risk Potential

5. A person having a tuberculosis (TB) blood test would need further teaching about the test if they stated which of the following?
   1. "I will only have to make one trip to have the test done."
   2. "This test is okay even though I have had a BCG vaccination."
   3. "This test evaluates my body's response to TB."
   4. "This test will determine if I have active or inactive TB."

   NCLEX Client Need: Health Promotion and Maintenance

6. A nursing student is reviewing signs and symptoms with a group of people who are at risk for lung cancer. You would intervene if the student says which of the following?
   1. "Weight loss and fatigue are the first symptoms to manifest."
   2. "An occasional cough or wheezing is typically the first sign."
   3. "Hoarseness could occur if a tumor presses against the vocal cords."
   4. "Deep bone pain could occur because the cancer may spread to the bones."

   NCLEX Client Need: Health Promotion and Maintenance

7. Which action is appropriate in the care of a patient who is on mechanical ventilation?
   1. Instruct the respiratory therapist to check the ventilator settings and alarms.
   2. Auscultate the lungs bilaterally to ensure that both lungs are being ventilated.
   3. Disconnect the alarms before suctioning or before turning the patient.
   4. Perform endotracheal suctioning every 15 minutes, using sterile technique.

   NCLEX Client Need: Physiological Integrity: Reduction of Risk Potential

8. A 55-year-old man was admitted for complaints of a recurring, irritating "smoker's" cough with small amounts of sputum and was diagnosed with chronic bronchitis. What is the most likely clinical finding?
   1. Weight loss
   2. Decreased white blood cells
   3. Dry mucous membranes
   4. Elevated hemoglobin and hematocrit

   NCLEX Client Need: Physiological Integrity: Reduction of Risk Potential

9. A patient is immobilized and has been lying in bed for an extended period. What nursing intervention(s) should be done to prevent hypostatic pneumonia? *(Select all that apply.)*
   1. Avoid immunizations because of weakened state.
   2. Assist the patient to turn at least every 2 hours.
   3. Instruct the patient to cough and deep-breathe.
   4. Allow nothing by mouth to prevent aspiration.
   5. Practice scrupulous hand hygiene.

   NCLEX Client Need: Physiological Integrity: Reduction of Risk Potential

10. You admit a patient who was diagnosed with active pulmonary tuberculosis. What nursing intervention(s) would help control the spread of the disease? *(Select all that apply.)*
    1. Implementing airborne isolation
    2. Prohibiting visitors
    3. Wearing a HEPA respirator mask when providing direct patient care
    4. Explaining the importance of covering the mouth when smiling
    5. Practicing good hand hygiene

    NCLEX Client Need: Safe and Effective Care Environment: Safety and Infection Control

Critical Thinking Questions

Scenario A

You are assigned to take care of Janet Blair, a 26-year-old married mother of two small children who has pneumococcal pneumonia. She is receiving oxygen by nasal cannula at 3 L/min and has "activity as tolerated" ordered. IV antibiotics are being administered, and she is receiving nebulization treatments from respiratory therapy. She is very weak, has a temperature of 104.6° F (40.3° C), and sometimes experiences delirium.

1. What would be an appropriate plan of care for Janet?
2. How would you evaluate the effectiveness of the nursing interventions listed on the plan of care?
3. What psychosocial problems might Janet have? How would you help her with these?

Scenario B

Mrs. Wester is 62 years old. She has had emphysema for several years but has not sought help in coping with the problems associated with the chronic lung disease. While in the hospital with an acute respiratory infection, she becomes very depressed and says she will never be able to take care of herself again because of her breathlessness. She has not been taught any techniques for pulmonary hygiene. She is not willing to give up smoking.

1. What do you think might be the attitude of some health care professionals regarding Mrs. Wester's problems? What is your personal response to Mrs. Wester's situation?
2. Devise a teaching plan to help her with her problem of fatigue and breathlessness.
3. List interventions that would be appropriate in helping with her nutritional and hydration needs.

Scenario C

Mr. Cohen is admitted to the hospital for a lobectomy. His diagnosis is early lung cancer. He is 56 years old and has worked in a cotton mill since he was 16. He is slightly underweight but is physically strong and has an optimistic outlook about his surgery and chances for recovery.

1. What special preoperative instruction would you expect Mr. Cohen to need?
2. What nursing interventions would you expect to be on his postoperative nursing care plan?
3. How would you help Mr. Cohen deal with the diagnosis of cancer, treatment, and prognosis?

Scenario D

Mr. Azale has recently been diagnosed with asthma. He is coming to the clinic for ongoing management of the condition. He wants to understand the disease and be an active participant in his own health care.

1. Prepare a teaching plan to help him understand his condition and self-care.
2. Describe what you would tell Mr. Azale about the possibility of having a severe acute asthma attack.

15 The Hematologic System

http://evolve.elsevier.com/deWit/medsurg

Objectives

Theory

1. Summarize the structures and functions of the hematologic system.
2. Differentiate between the various types of blood cells and their functions.
3. Distinguish factors that may alter the function of the hematologic system.
4. Explain ways in which the nurse might help prevent blood disorders.
5. Relate at least five different kinds of information that can be obtained from a complete blood cell count (CBC).
6. Illustrate ways to accomplish hemostasis.
7. Apply the nursing process to patients with hematologic system disorders.

Clinical Practice

8. Explain the procedure and care for a patient receiving bone marrow aspiration.
9. Perform a focused assessment on a patient with a problem of the hematologic system.
10. Plan appropriate nursing interventions for patients with hematologic system disorders.

Key Terms

agranulocytosis (ăh-grăn-ū-lō-sī-TŌ-sĭs, p. 340)
aplastic anemia (ā-plăs-tĭk ă-NĒ-mē-ă, p. 340)
dyscrasias (dĭs-KRĀ-zhē-ăz, p. 340)
erythropoiesis (ĕ-rĭth-rō-pō-Ē-sĭs, p. 337)
hemarthrosis (hē-măr-THRŌ-sĭs, p. 346)
hematocrit (hē-MĂT-ŏ-krĭt, p. 342)
hemolysis (hē-MŎL-ĭ-sĭs, p. 340)
iatrogenic (Ī-ă-trō-JĔN-ĭk, p. 340)
jaundice (JĂWN-dĭs, p. 344)
leukopenia (lū-kō-PĒ-nē-ă, p. 340)
melena (MĔL-ĕh-nă, p. 346)
petechiae (pĕ-TĒ-kē-ă, p. 344)
phagocytosis (făg-ō-sī-TŌ-sĭs, p. 337)
polycythemia (pŏl-ē-sī-THĒ-mē-ă, p. 344)
thrombocytopenia (thrŏm-bō-sĭt-ō-PĒ-nē-ă, p. 340)

Concepts Covered in This Chapter

- Fluid and Electrolytes
- Perfusion
- Clotting
- Inflammation
- Tissue Integrity

OVERVIEW OF ANATOMY AND PHYSIOLOGY OF THE HEMATOLOGIC SYSTEM

FUNCTIONS OF BLOOD

- Transportation of water, oxygen, nutrients, hormones, enzymes, and medications to the cells
- Transportation of carbon dioxide (CO_2) and other waste products away from the cells
- Regulation of fluid volume and electrolyte distribution
- Regulation of pH and acid-base balance with its buffering ability
- Regulation of body temperature
- Providing clotting factors for hemostasis

COMPONENTS OF BLOOD

- Blood is composed of formed elements and plasma (Fig. 15.1).
- The formed elements are erythrocytes, neutrophils, lymphocytes, monocytes, eosinophils, basophils, and platelets.
- Plasma contains proteins, water, salts, dissolved gases (such as CO_2), bicarbonate (HCO_3^-), hormones, glucose, and wastes.
- The plasma proteins are albumin, globulins, and fibrinogen.

FUNCTIONS OF THE PLASMA PROTEINS

- Albumin raises osmotic pressure at the capillary membrane, preventing fluid from leaking into the tissue spaces. (Osmotic pressure is discussed in Chapter 3.)
- The alpha and beta globulins work as carriers for drugs and lipids by combining with them and

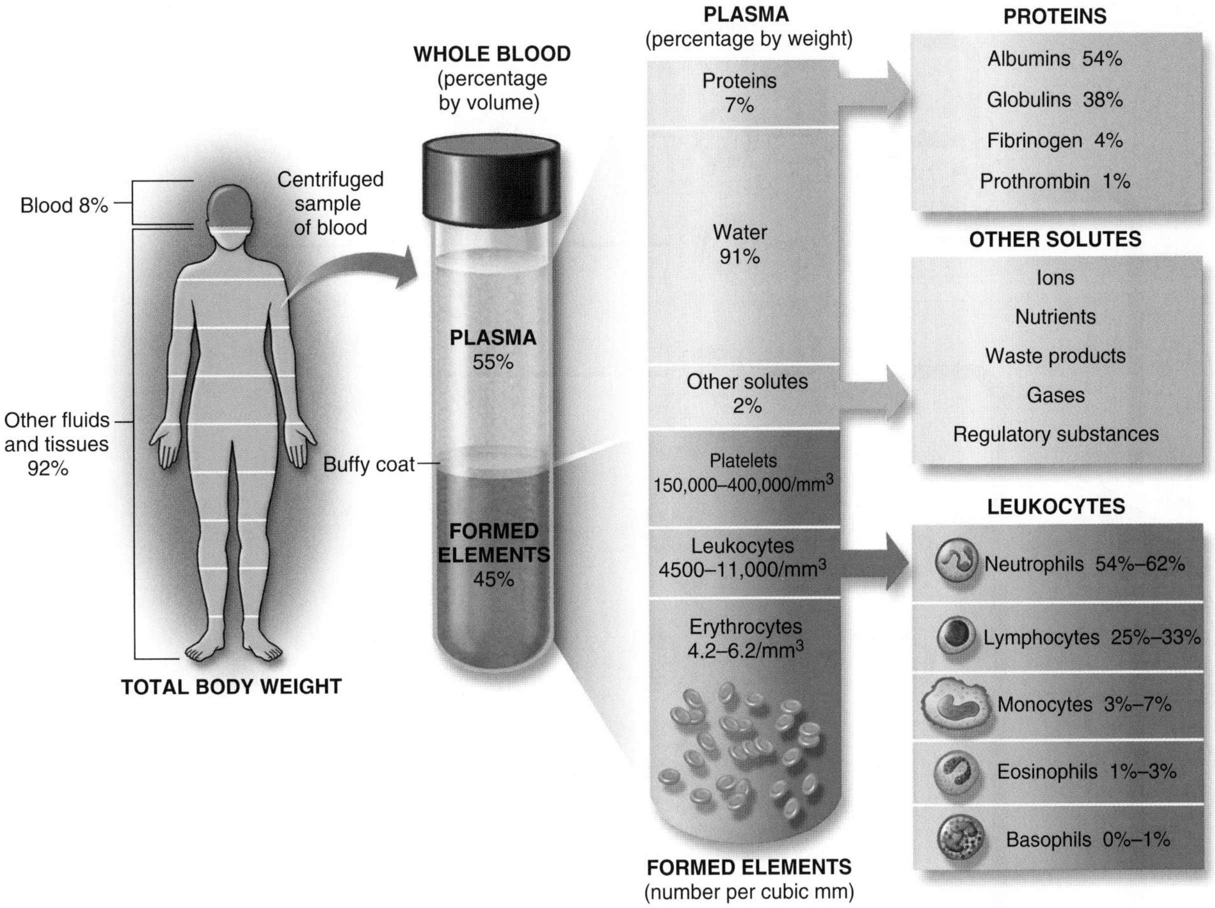

Fig. 15.1 Components of blood. (From Patton KT, Thibodeau GA: *The human body in health and disease*, ed 7, St. Louis, 2018, Elsevier.)

transporting them throughout the body; gamma globulins act as antibodies.
- Fibrinogen is essential to the formation of blood clots.

PRODUCTION OF BLOOD CELLS

- Blood cells develop from stem cells located in the bone marrow through **erythropoiesis** (Fig. 15.2).
- The kidney makes most of the body's erythropoietin, which then prompts erythrocyte production by the bone marrow.
- Erythropoiesis requires iron; vitamins B_{12}, C, and E; folic acid; and amino acids—most of which are obtained from proteins.

FUNCTIONS OF THE RED BLOOD CELLS

- Red blood cells (RBCs, or erythrocytes, the most numerous of the blood cells) contain hemoglobin, which carries oxygen to the cells and a portion of CO_2 away from the cells.
- Each person has a hereditary blood type based on the antigens on the RBCs. This can be A, B, AB, or O.
- The normal laboratory range of RBCs for adults is 4.2 to 6.2 million/mm^3 and varies by gender.
- The normal laboratory range for hemoglobin in adults is 12 to 18 g/dL and varies by gender.
- Decreased numbers of RBCs or decreased hemoglobin results in a reduction in the amount of oxygen that can be carried to the cells of the body.
- RBCs live for approximately 120 days.
- The spleen and the liver remove old, damaged RBCs.

FUNCTIONS OF THE WHITE BLOOD CELLS

- White blood cells (WBCs, or leukocytes) provide the first line of defense against microbial agents.
- The normal adult laboratory range for total leukocytes (WBCs) is 4500 to 11,000/mm^3; they have a life span of about 13 to 20 days.
- Leukocytes migrate from the bone marrow cells into the tissues and are carried by the bloodstream to locations where they are needed.
- Leukocytes are divided into granulocytes (meaning "with granules") and agranulocytes (meaning "without granules") in the cell nucleus (see Fig. 15.2).
- Granulocytes are divided into neutrophils, eosinophils, and basophils and are produced in the red bone marrow.
- Neutrophils make up 54% to 62% of the WBC count and work by engulfing and destroying bacteria through the process of **phagocytosis**, which means "to consume or swallow up other cells or particles."

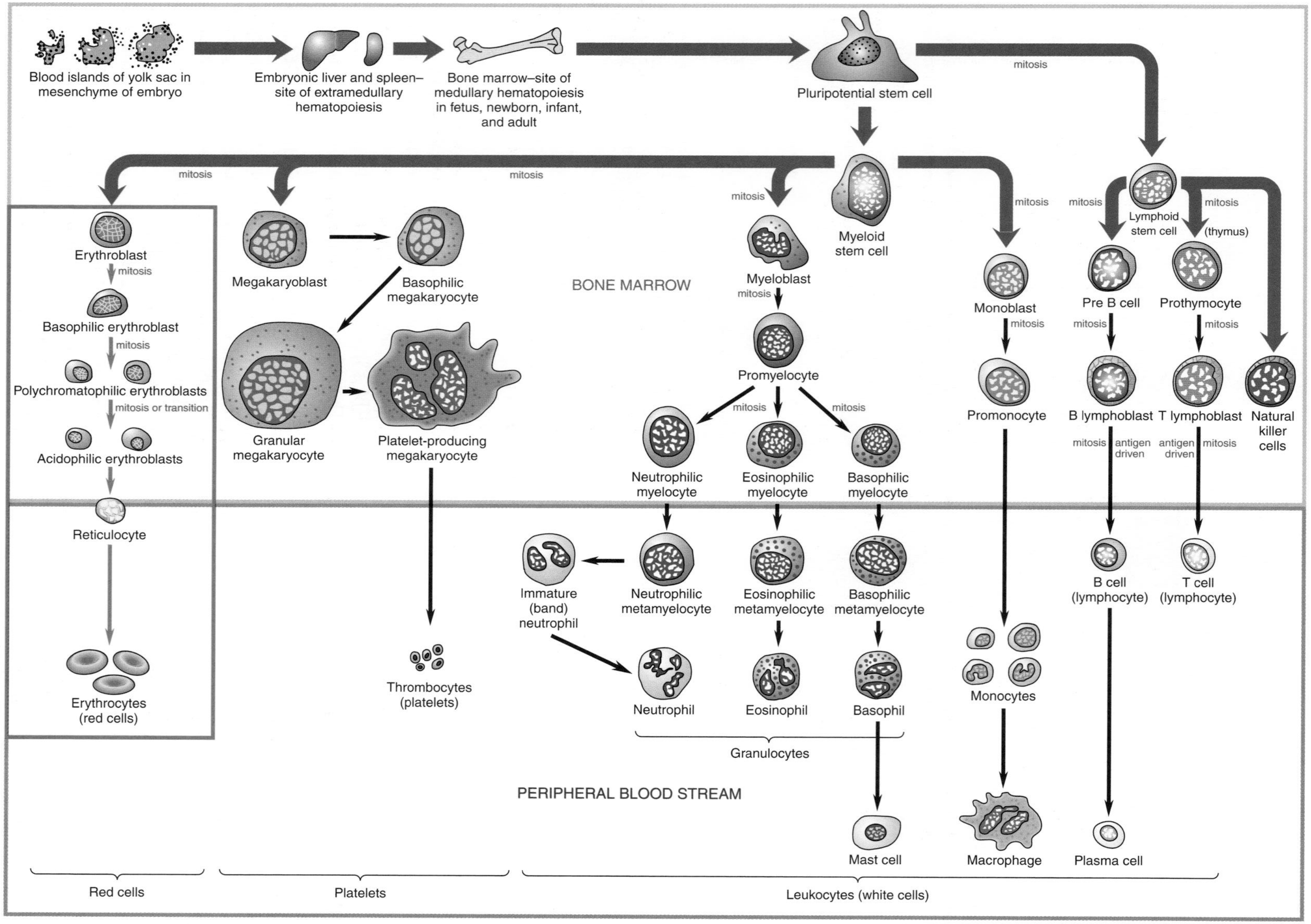

Fig. 15.2 Maturation of human blood cells. (From Banask JL, Copstead LC: *Pathophysiology*, ed 6, St. Louis, 2019, Elsevier.)

- An infection in the body stimulates increased production of neutrophils, resulting in a higher-than-normal WBC count, or leukocytosis.
- Eosinophils, which make up 1% to 3% of the total WBCs, help detoxify foreign proteins; eosinophils increase in number during allergic reactions and in response to parasitic infections.
- Basophils, which compose up to 1% of the total WBC count, release histamine in response to allergens and help prevent clotting in the small blood vessels.
- Agranulocytes consist of lymphocytes and monocytes. They are produced in the red bone marrow and in lymphatic tissue.
- Lymphocytes, which account for 25% to 33% of WBCs, are produced in the red bone marrow and the lymphatic tissue. Lymphocytes occur as B cells and T cells. B lymphocytes change into plasma cells that produce immunoglobulins responsible for the humoral immune response.
- Some T cells are killer cells that fight antigens and provide cell-mediated immune response (see Chapter 10).
- Monocytes compose 3% to 7% of the WBCs and become macrophages (large mononuclear monocytes) that migrate into the tissues, where they become phagocytes, fighting infection and ridding the body of foreign substances. They engulf bacteria and foreign substances and eliminate them from the body.
- A differential blood cell count gives information about the numbers of different types of leukocytes present in the blood and about the type of inflammatory process that is occurring.

PLATELETS AND THEIR FUNCTION

- Platelets, also called *thrombocytes,* are fragments of megakaryocytes that are produced by the bone marrow.
- Platelets provide the first line of protection, after vasospasm (contraction of a vessel), to prevent bleeding by promoting clotting when the wall of a blood vessel has been damaged.
- Platelets are involved in maintaining hemostasis through a complex process that balances the production of the clotting and dissolving factors.
- Fibrin strands derived from the plasma protein fibrinogen attach to aggregated platelets to help form a clot.
- Platelets are small, formed elements of the blood active in the clotting process. Platelets tend to adhere to damaged or uneven surfaces and to clump together.
- The normal laboratory platelet count range for adults is 150,000 to 400,000/mm^3; the life span of a platelet is about 10 days.
- Although the body can withstand a substantial drop in the number of platelets, when the platelet count is low, there is risk of spontaneous bleeding into the skin, kidney, brain, and other internal organs.

INTERACTION OF THE LYMPHATIC SYSTEM WITH THE VASCULAR SYSTEM

The lymphatic system consists of lymph nodes, lymph channels, the spleen, and the thymus gland (see Chapter 10). The spleen, located in the upper left abdominal cavity below the diaphragm and behind the stomach, filters the blood, removing pathogens, old blood cells, and debris, and produces lymphocytes (see Fig. 10.2). It is a reservoir for extra blood; in response to hemorrhage, it contracts, and by contraction the spleen releases some of its stored blood into the cardiovascular system. If the spleen is removed, its functions are taken over by other lymph tissue and by the liver.

Lymph vessels collect fluid and protein from the interstitial spaces and return them to the bloodstream. Lymph nodes (bundles of lymphatic tissue) filter out leukocytes and cell debris from inflammations and infections before the lymph is returned to the bloodstream.

CHANGES OF THE HEMATOLOGIC SYSTEM THAT OCCUR WITH AGING

Plasma volume decreases after age 60 years; older individuals have less blood volume. This means less blood reserve in case of blood loss. In addition, bone marrow activity decreases by about 50% as years advance; the marrow becomes infiltrated with fat and fibrotic tissue. Reduced bone marrow inhibits full production of blood cells, so the immune response is decreased, making the older person more susceptible to infection. There is less antibody response to foreign proteins, a decreased secretion of intrinsic factor from the stomach, and decreased absorption of vitamin B_{12}, which may lead to megaloblastic (pernicious) anemia from vitamin B_{12} deficiency. Anemia is not a normal sign of aging, and its presence should prompt a thorough investigation as to the cause.

In older adults, new cells are produced at a slower rate, and correction of anemia becomes a longer process. Antibody response to vaccines is also decreased. There is now a super-strength flu vaccination for patients age 65 years and older that is intended to compensate for this decreased response.

When blood loss occurs, an older adult patient is at greater risk for hypovolemia and shock. Blood is more prone to coagulate because platelets tend to aggregate more with advancing age, and there are alterations in clotting activity. The increased incidence of thrombosis in coronary and cerebral arteries may be related to changes in clotting activity. Daily low-dose aspirin sometimes is prescribed to counteract this phenomenon.

Pigment loss and yellowish cast to the skin are common changes associated with aging; these routine skin changes make pallor and jaundice more difficult to discern in older adults.

CAUSES OF HEMATOLOGIC DISORDERS

Hematology is the study of blood, blood components, and blood-forming tissues. The lymphatic system, which drains the fluid from the spaces around each cell and channels it into the circulatory system, is discussed in Chapter 10. Anemias, blood loss and hemorrhage, and hemolysis are all types of hematologic disorders you may encounter during patient care. Several disorders that interfere with normal function of the blood are inherited. Hemophilia, sickle cell disease, and thalassemia types of anemias are examples. Accidental tearing or cutting of the vessels of the cardiovascular system and surgery cause bleeding and loss of blood. Blunt trauma to the spleen, such as might occur in an automobile accident, may cause tearing and massive internal hemorrhage. Chemicals and transfusions of the wrong blood type can cause **hemolysis** (destruction of RBCs).

Cultural Considerations

Genetic Hematologic Tendencies

- African Americans have the highest incidence of sickle cell disease.
- Megaloblastic anemia is more prevalent among those of Scandinavian descent and among African Americans.
- People of Middle Eastern origin may have a genetic predisposition to thalassemia.
- Whites have a higher incidence of leukemia, followed by Hispanics.

Some blood disorders are **iatrogenic**; that is, they are brought on by medical treatment. For example, blood **dyscrasias** (imbalance in numbers of types of cells) or other pathologic conditions of the blood can be induced through at least four kinds of actions:

- Bone marrow suppression, which interferes with the production of blood cells
- Interference with normal cell function
- Destruction of the blood cells by cytotoxic drugs
- Destruction of cells by a transfusion reaction of mismatched blood

Some antineoplastic drugs, for instance, act to depress the bone marrow, which inevitably causes a reduced supply of blood cells. Other drugs, such as phenytoin (Dilantin), primidone (Mysoline), and oral contraceptives, can produce anemia by interfering with the absorption and use of folic acid, a substance needed to produce RBCs. Diuretics such as furosemide (Lasix) and hydrochlorothiazide (HydroDIURIL) sometimes cause **leukopenia** (decreased numbers of WBCs), **aplastic anemia** (deficient cell production resulting from a bone marrow disorder), and abnormally low counts of platelets and granulocytes. Procainamide hydrochloride (Pronestyl) and quinidine, which are used to correct dysrhythmias of the heart, also can cause **thrombocytopenia** (too few platelets), **agranulocytosis** (decrease in granulocyte production), and aplastic anemia. Most drugs are powerful chemicals that are capable of producing undesirable side effects, even though the drugs can be of great value.

Box 15.1 Factors That May Alter Function of the Hematologic System

GENETIC DISORDERS
- Hemophilia
- Sickle cell disease
- Agranulocytosis

HEMORRHAGE (ANEMIA)
- Surgical blood loss
- Blood loss from childbirth or spontaneous abortion
- Traumatic blood loss
- Gastrointestinal (GI) bleed

ANEMIA
- Iron deficiency
- Folic acid deficiency
- Megaloblastic anemia
- Chronic slow blood loss
- Aplastic anemia

HEMOLYSIS
- Blood transfusion reaction
- Genetic types of anemia

BONE MARROW SUPPRESSION
- Antineoplastic agents used in treatment of cancer
- Radiation treatment used for cancer
- Excessive exposure to ionizing radiation
- Exposure to toxic chemicals that damage bone marrow
- Drugs that suppress the bone marrow

BONE MARROW PROLIFERATION OR ABNORMALITY
- Leukemia

Clinical Cues

If a patient is showing signs of a blood disorder, review the medications that are being taken and note their side effects.

Nutritional deficiencies, such as low protein or lack of vitamin C, can interfere with erythropoiesis and normally functioning blood cells. Abnormal RBCs are more prone to rapid destruction, which can result in anemia. Bone marrow damage from toxic substances may also interfere with the production of blood cells. Malignant conditions such as leukemia cause growth of abnormal blood cells and interfere with the production of normal cells. Box 15.1 presents factors that alter hematologic system function.

PREVENTION OF HEMATOLOGIC DISORDERS

When considerable blood is lost through hemorrhage, the patient becomes anemic. Sometimes excessive blood loss can occur during menstruation. Prevent hemorrhage

Nutrition Considerations

Nutrients Needed for Building Red Blood Cells (Erythropoiesis)

NUTRIENT	ROLE IN ERYTHROPOIESIS	FOOD SOURCES
Cobalamin (vitamin B_{12})	RBC maturation	Red meats, especially liver
Folic acid	RBC maturation	Green leafy vegetables, liver, meat, fish, legumes, whole grains
Iron	Hemoglobin synthesis	Liver and muscle meats, eggs, dried fruits, legumes, dark green leafy vegetables, whole-grain and enriched bread and cereals, potatoes
Vitamin B_6	Hemoglobin synthesis	Meats (especially pork and liver), wheat germ, legumes, potatoes, cornmeal, bananas
Amino acids	Synthesis of nucleoprotein	Eggs, meat, milk and milk products (cheese, ice cream), poultry, fish, legumes, nuts
Vitamin C	Conversion of folic acid to its active forms; aids in iron absorption	Citrus fruits, green leafy vegetables, strawberries, cantaloupe

RBC, Red blood cell.

after surgery or childbirth by vigilantly assessing the amount of blood loss and by instituting measures to stop the loss if it is excessive.

Clinical Cues

The average amount of blood loss from menstruation is less than 80 mL per cycle. Estimating blood loss from menstruation or childbirth is difficult. The recommendation from the Association of Women's Health, Obstetric and Neonatal Nurses (AWHONN) is to weigh pads, dressings, and any item with blood. One gram of weight equals one milliliter of blood (AWHONN, 2015).

Nurses can help prevent anemia by promoting proper nutrition and by educating the public about the possibility of nutritional anemia. Nutritional anemia is a particular concern for individuals who subsist mostly on "fast food" or who for various reasons are not able to consume a healthful diet.

Older Adult Care Points

An older adult, especially one who lives alone, is at high risk of poor nutrition. Problems with arthritis, vision, and chronic diseases make it more difficult for older adults to shop for food and to prepare food. As a result, an older adult may substitute cookies, toast, or cereal for a well-balanced meal. It is important to obtain a food intake history.

Monitoring patients for drug side effects and alerting the health care provider should blood-related side effects occur can prevent a serious blood disorder from developing. Carefully monitoring blood transfusions and promptly reporting any untoward reaction may decrease the incidence of hemolysis from a reaction.

DIAGNOSTIC TESTS AND PROCEDURES

Most testing for hematologic disorders is done on the blood itself with a sample obtained from simple venipuncture. Explain the venipuncture procedure and the purpose of the test to the patient. Many patients have a great fear of needles. Others are concerned about having what seems like a lot of blood withdrawn. A few words of assurance and explanation can do much to relieve anxiety about a needle stick and to promote cooperation. Use Standard Precautions (see Appendix B) and aseptic technique for the venipuncture and the correct tubes for each sample.

Health Promotion

Preventing Blood Disorders

- Caution the public about the dangers of exposure to ionizing radiation and harmful chemicals to help decrease the incidence of blood disorders related to harmful substances.
- Suggest genetic counseling (for the possibility of transmitting a genetic blood disorder to offspring) to those adults who have such a genetic disorder.
- Inform patients about medications they are taking that can cause blood disorders; remind patients to be alert for signs of excessive bruising or easy bleeding. Suggest that CBCs be checked periodically, for monitoring purposes.

Think Critically

The CBC of your patient shows the following values:
- RBCs: 4.8 million/mm^3
- WBCs: 6.7 million/mm^3
- Hemoglobin: 10.2 g/dL
- Platelets: 250,000/mm^3

What abnormalities, if any, do these results indicate?

Leukocyte counts provide information about infection and possible immune disorders (see Chapter 10). Data about the number of platelets are valuable in diagnosing a variety of diseases affecting—or affected by—the clotting of blood. There are at least 12 different types of hemoglobin in human blood. The types are designated by letters—for example, hemoglobin A is normal adult hemoglobin, hemoglobin F is normal fetal hemoglobin, and hemoglobin S is found in sickle cell disease. A **hematocrit** is a test that measures the volume of blood cells in relation to the volume of plasma. When there has been a loss of body fluids but no loss of cells (as in dehydration), the cell volume is high in proportion to the amount of liquid (plasma) in the bloodstream (i.e., the hematocrit rises). When either hemorrhage or anemia has depleted the supply of cells, the blood cell volume is low. Table 15.1 presents the most common diagnostic tests and related nursing care for the hematologic and lymphatic systems.

Clinical Cues

- Increased numbers of eosinophils often indicate allergy.
- A viral infection prompts the production of additional lymphocytes.
- Bacterial infection stimulates the production of neutrophils, and segmented neutrophils (segs) increase.
- Ongoing bacterial infections cause immature neutrophils to appear in the blood as *bands* (immature forms of segmented granulocytes). This is referred to as a "shift to the left."
- A "shift to the right" occurs when there are more mature neutrophils than usual; this occurs with anemia from vitamin B_{12} or folic acid deficiency.

Table 15.1 Diagnostic Tests for Disorders of the Hematologic System

TEST AND NORMAL RANGE	PURPOSE	DESCRIPTION	NURSING IMPLICATIONS
Complete blood cell count (CBC)	Determine whether abnormalities are present in the numbers of blood cells or types of blood cells; assess the amount of hemoglobin present. Useful to diagnose anemia. Elevated WBC count may indicate infection.	Fill a lavender-top tube containing EDTA with a venous sample of blood. Use a site where there is little chance of dilution from intravenous solution. Mix the blood and the EDTA by gently rotating the tube.	Warn the patient that a "stick" is about to occur but that the pain will be short-lived. Apply pressure directly to the puncture site after withdrawing the needle; at the antecubital space, do *not* have the patient flex the arm because this tends to cause a hematoma.
Erythrocytes			
Hemoglobin: females: 12.0–16.7 g/dL; males: 13.0–18.0 g/dL			
RBC count: females: 4.2–5.4 million/mm^3; males: 4.7–6.1 million/mm^3			
Hematocrit: females: 37%–47%; males: 42%–52%			
Leukocytes			
WBC count: 5000–10,000/mm^3			
Differential Count			
Granulocytes Band neutrophils: 3%–5% of WBCs Segmented neutrophils: 54%–62% of WBCs Eosinophils: 1%–3% of WBCs Basophils: 0%–1% of WBCs			
Agranulocytes Lymphocytes: 28%–33% of WBCs Monocytes: 3%–7% of WBCs			
Thrombocytes (platelets): 150,000–400,000/mm^3 of blood			
Mean corpuscular hemoglobin (Hb) (MCH): 27–31 pg/cell			
Mean corpuscular Hb concentration (MCHC): 32–36 g/dL			
Mean corpuscular volume (MCV): 80–95 μm^3			
Erythrocyte Sedimentation Rate (ESR)			
Males: 0–22 mm/h Females: 0–29 mm/h	To detect inflammation and infection.	Fill a blue-top tube with venous blood. The laboratory determines the rate at which the RBCs settle.	Explain that this test helps diagnose an inflammatory process but is nonspecific.
Hemoglobin Electrophoresis			
Hemoglobin A_{1c}: 3%–5% Hemoglobin A_2: 2%–3.5% Hemoglobin F: 0%–2.1%	Useful in diagnosing various types of anemia. Useful for diagnosis and monitoring of diabetes mellitus.	Performed on venous sample using lavender-top tube with EDTA.	Same as for CBC.

Table 15.1 Diagnostic Tests for Disorders of the Hematologic System—cont'd

TEST AND NORMAL RANGE	PURPOSE	DESCRIPTION	NURSING IMPLICATIONS
Blood Typing			
ABO Rh testing	Used to determine blood type. Useful for detecting unexpected antibodies.	Performed on venous sample using red-top tube. Some specific types of ABO/Rh tests use lavender-top tube with EDTA.	Same as for CBC.
Tests for Anemia			
Ferritin, serum: 40–200 ng/mL Total iron-binding capacity: 300–360 mcg/dL Saturation 20%–50%	Detect reason for anemia.	Obtain a venous blood sample of 5–7 mL in a red-top tube.	Same as for CBC.
Reticulocyte count 0.5%–2%, or 30,000–130,000 per microliter.	Helps distinguish between different types of anemia. Monitors bone marrow function.	Same as for CBC.	Same as for CBC.
Coagulation Tests			
Activated partial thromboplastin time (APTT): 20–25 s	Determine abnormalities of clotting time.	Performed on a venous blood sample; use a blue-top tube.	Same as for CBC; pressure may need to be applied longer than usual if the patient has an abnormal clotting time or is on heparin or warfarin therapy.
Prothrombin time (PT): 12–14 s is usually reported as INR—some labs do not report the PT. International normalized ratio (INR) Normal: 1–2 Prevention and treatment of VTE, PE, VHD: 2–3	Standardized blood clotting test for tests run at different laboratories.		
D-Dimer			
Negative: <0.5 mcg/mL	Provides assay of fibrin degradation to assess thrombin and plasmin activity. Useful for diagnosing PE and disseminated intravascular coagulation (DIC).	Collect blood sample in a blue-top tube.	No fasting is required.
Sickle Cell Testing			
Hemoglobin S	Tests for the presence of hemoglobin S.	Performed on a venous blood sample; use a lavender-top tube.	Patient may be anxious about the result; be sensitive to patient emotions. Positive result indicates need for genetic counseling.
Monoclonal (M) Protein Testing			
Presence of monoclonal protein (Bence-Jones proteins) in the urine is abnormal. Serum protein electrophoresis	Assists in the diagnosis of multiple myeloma.	Obtain a 10-mL fresh morning specimen of urine in a clean container. Must be refrigerated or tested immediately. In a 3.5 mL gold-top tube collect a minimum of 1 mL of blood.	Explain the procedure to the patient.

Continued

Table 15.1 Diagnostic Tests for Disorders of the Hematologic System—cont'd

TEST AND NORMAL RANGE	PURPOSE	DESCRIPTION	NURSING IMPLICATIONS
Blood Tests for Leukemia (in Addition to CBC and Bone Marrow Aspiration and Biopsy)			
Immunophenotyping	To identify what type of leukemia is present.	Bone marrow or blood cells are checked for surface antigens to determine if they are lymphocytes or myeloid cells.	Blood test. Patient may need additional information when the results are known.
FISH (fluorescence in situ hybridization)	Identifies biomarkers in hematologic neoplasms.	Looks at genes or chromosomes in cells and tissues.	Testing can be done on bone marrow cells or blood cells.
Flow cytometry	Assesses immune cell function.	Measures the number of cells in a sample, the number of live cells and characteristics of the cells, presence of tumor markers.	Can test blood cells, bone marrow cells, or tissue samples.
IgVH gene mutation test		Checks for *IgVH* gene mutation.	Patients with an *IgVH* mutation have a better prognosis.
Bone Marrow Aspiration and Biopsy			
Normal cell counts	Help diagnose blood disorders. Assist in identifying certain anemias, leukemia, and thrombocytopenia.	Cells are withdrawn by needle from the sternum or iliac crest. Leukocytes, platelets, and erythrocytes are examined in the various stages of development to determine abnormalities.	Explain that the aspiration is done at the bedside. Seek an order for prebiopsy medication to decrease the discomfort. Explain that there is a feeling of pressure when the needle is inserted and sharp, brief pain when the marrow is aspirated. The area of aspiration is surgically prepped. The patient must hold perfectly still. Pressure is applied to the site afterward to prevent hematoma formation. Posttest, observe for swelling and tenderness, indicating continued bleeding or infection.

Note: Normal values differ among laboratories.
EDTA, Ethylenediaminetetraacetic acid, an agent used to reduce blood clotting; *PE,* pulmonary embolism; *RBC,* red blood cell; *VHD,* valvular heart disease; *VTE,* venous thromboembolism; *WBC,* white blood cell.

NURSING MANAGEMENT

ASSESSMENT (DATA COLLECTION)

History

Assess patients for signs and symptoms that indicate abnormalities in the blood. Abnormal symptoms result from too little circulating blood or too little hemoglobin, too few platelets, deficiency of normal neutrophils or lymphocytes, and too many abnormal blood cells. **When there is insufficient hemoglobin to carry oxygen to the cells, signs of oxygen deficit occur.** Perform a focused assessment to obtain an appropriate history. Inquire about renal disease, which may be a cause of anemia.

Physical Assessment

Skin. Although pallor may be a sign of anemia, it is not the most reliable sign. Many other factors can affect a person's complexion and skin color, including thickness of the skin, amount of skin pigment, and number and distribution of blood vessels near the surface of the skin. Pale mucous membranes or pale conjunctiva of the eye are better indicators of anemia. A very ruddy complexion with a red, florid appearance is typical of an excessive number of RBCs (**polycythemia**).

Jaundice, or a yellowing discoloration of the skin and sclera of the eyes, can occur as a result of excessive destruction of RBCs (hemolysis). When RBCs are ruptured, bilirubin is released. The pigment eventually finds its way into the bloodstream, where it causes jaundice. If hemolysis is occurring, the urine will often contain bilirubin, giving urine a brown tea color.

Bruises; purplish patches; and small, red, pinpoint lesions (**petechiae** [Fig. 15.3]) are typical of thrombocytopenic purpura, a hemorrhagic disease sometimes

Focused Assessment

Data Collection for the Hematologic System

HISTORY TAKING

Ask the patient the following questions:

- Do you or does anyone in your family have a genetic blood disorder (hemophilia, thalassemia, sickle cell trait or disease, aplastic anemia, agranulocytosis, or thrombocytopenic purpura)?
- What is your occupation?
- Have you ever been told you had anemia?
- Do you become easily fatigued?
- Do you have frequent sore throats or other infections?
- Do you frequently feel as though you have a fever?
- Do you ever have night sweats?
- Are your joints painful? Do they swell?
- Do you bruise easily or develop pinpoint blood spots?
- Do you suffer from itching?
- Do you have any swollen lymph nodes in the groin or armpits?
- Do you ever have tingling or numbness in the extremities?
- Do you have frequent headaches? Palpitations?
- Have you become more irritable than usual?
- Do you get dizzy frequently? Do you suffer fainting spells?
- Do you get short of breath when you walk a short distance or when you climb stairs?
- Do your gums bleed when you brush your teeth? Does your tongue get sore? Do you have frequent mouth sores?
- Do you have any difficulty eating?
- How much alcohol do you drink in a day?
- Do colds or infections seem to last a long time for you?
- Do you often feel fatigued even when not doing much?
- Have you been exposed to chemicals, such as pesticides, cleaning agents, or industrial chemicals of any kind?
- Have you ever noticed that you have black, tarry-looking stool? Smoky or brown urine?
- Do you have stomach pain or indigestion or have you ever had an ulcer?
- Are your menstrual periods unusually heavy?
- What do you usually eat for each meal?
- Are you often cold when others are not?
- Are there cultural factors you would like considered?
- What are your expectations of treatment?

PHYSICAL ASSESSMENT

Head and Neck

- Color of conjunctiva and sclera of eye
- Condition of gums, oral mucous membranes, and tongue
- Presence of enlarged cervical lymph nodes

Skin

- Color (pale) (check conjunctivae, palms of hands, and roof of the mouth in people with dark skin)
- Condition of fingernails (brittle, spoon-shaped)
- Presence of ecchymoses or petechiae
- Jaundice
- Nasal or gingival bleeding
- Hair (dry, brittle, thinning)

Chest and Abdomen

- Presence of swollen lymph nodes in armpits or groin
- Rapid respirations; shortness of breath on exertion
- Rapid pulse rate at rest
- Widened pulse pressure (greater distance between systolic and diastolic pressure)
- Epigastric tenderness
- Abdominal distention

Extremities

- Presence of swollen or painful joints
- Quality of pulses, skin color

Urine and Stool

- Signs of blood

Clinical Cues

When assessing skin color and hue, use natural light whenever possible because fluorescent lighting can alter the perception of color. Also, be aware of clothing, bed linens, or other colors that might alter the results of skin assessment.

Older Adult Care Points

- Older adults bruise more easily because of thinner skin and greater fragility of blood vessel walls.
- Antiplatelet medications, omega-3 fatty acids, vitamin E, ginkgo biloba, and some prescription drugs also may make older adults more prone to bruising.
- Bruising is not necessarily an unusual sign in this age group. However, frequent large bruises and bruising with no known cause should be investigated.

associated with a decrease in the number of circulating platelets. For dark-skinned people, check the palms of the hands and soles of the feet for petechiae. Bleeding under the skin and formation of bruises in response to the slightest trauma are common in anemias, leukemias, and diseases affecting the bone marrow and spleen. These appear as darker areas on brown-skinned people.

Cyanosis, or a bluish tint to the skin, can indicate hypoxia resulting from inadequate numbers of circulating erythrocytes. The gums or the roof of the mouth are the best places to check for a bluish color in dark-skinned people. Cyanosis is a late sign of hypoxemia, whereas increase in respiratory rate is an earlier sign.

Mucous membranes. Nutritional deficiencies contributing to anemia and resultant hypoxia may cause sore and painful gums and tongue. The patient may have difficulty chewing and eating. The tongue may be smooth and beefy red. Bleeding of the gums may occur with tooth brushing when the platelet count is low.

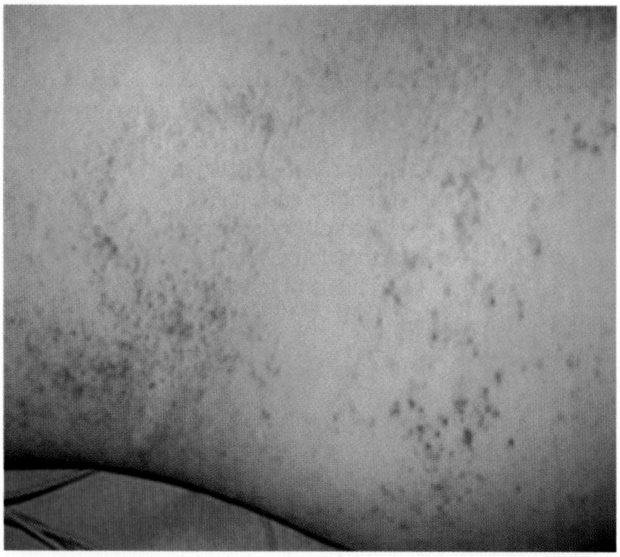

Fig. 15.3 Petechial rash located on the abdomen. (Courtesy National Library of Medicine, Lister Hill National Center for Biomedical Communications. Retrieved from https://openi.nlm.nih.gov/detailedresult.php?img=PMC3366531_tropmed-86-911-g001&query=petechiae+of+skin&it=xg&req=4&npos=12.)

Abdomen. Stomach pain or nausea can be caused by bleeding ulcers (a common cause of chronic blood loss). Black, tarry stools or coffee-ground emesis indicates gastrointestinal (GI) bleeding. Hiatal hernia also can cause iron deficiency anemia.

> **Assignment Considerations**
>
> **Observing for Blood**
>
> If a nursing assistant will be assisting the patient with toileting, remind the assistant to check the stool for signs of **melena** (dark stool containing blood pigments) and the urine for a smoky color (indicating blood).

Swollen and painful joints. Bleeding into the joints (**hemarthrosis**) is not uncommon in certain kinds of anemia or in hemophilia. This might be evidenced by swelling and slight redness in the area of the joints, or the patient may move more slowly and with obvious discomfort.

Lymph tissue involvement. Enlarged lymph nodes occur in a number of blood disorders, as well as in infections and immune disorders. The nodes most often inspected and palpated are those under the arm, in the neck, and in the inguinal (groin) region. Lymph node enlargement is often found while bathing a patient or helping with activities of daily living (ADLs).

Enlargement of the spleen, which also accompanies polycythemia and several other blood disorders, might be described by the patient as a feeling of fullness on the left side of the upper abdomen. Palpate the abdomen gently in a patient with a suspected blood disorder. Do not palpate deeply if there is tenderness in the area of the spleen because this could cause rupture of the spleen.

> **Assignment Considerations**
>
> **Changes to Report**
>
> When assigning tasks to a certified nursing assistant (CNA) or unlicensed assistive personnel (UAP), ask the person to report any swellings they notice when assisting the patient with bathing. State that the patient may bruise easily and ask for a report of any new bruised areas or patient complaints of bleeding of gums or elsewhere.

Mental state. Dizziness and altered mental function are often found in patients with blood disorders. Irritability, dizziness, difficulty concentrating, and headache may be caused by a decreased supply of oxygen to the brain. Depression often accompanies the chronic lack of energy, difficulty in eating and enjoying food, and the many other problems from which patients with blood disorders often suffer.

> **Older Adult Care Points**
>
> An older adult who has developed megaloblastic anemia may present with confusion and a loss of mental faculties. This state initially may be believed to be Alzheimer disease or dementia. A blood count is important to establish the correct diagnosis.

Activity intolerance. Physical activity increases the demand for oxygen, but if there are not enough circulating RBCs to carry the necessary oxygen, the patient becomes physically weak and unable to engage in physical activity without severe fatigue and shortness of breath. Note whether the patient is able to do things independently or needs help to complete specific ADLs.

> **Think Critically**
>
> Name four signs or symptoms you might encounter when taking a patient's history that could indicate your patient is anemic.

◆ NURSING DIAGNOSIS

Problem statements or nursing diagnoses for hematologic and lymphatic disorders are based on the problems the disorders cause for the patient. Problem statements or nursing diagnoses commonly associated with hematologic disorders are listed in Table 15.2. They must be individualized for each patient.

◆ PLANNING

Plan nursing care to provide rest periods for the patient. For patients with anemia, plan dietary teaching or consultation with the dietitian. **Patients with a blood abnormality are at higher risk for infection, so it is**

Table 15.2 **Common Problem Statements/Nursing Diagnoses, Expected Outcomes, and Interventions for Patients With Blood Disorders**

PROBLEM STATEMENT/ NURSING DIAGNOSIS	GOALS/EXPECTED OUTCOMES	NURSING INTERVENTIONS
Altered nutrition related to iron deficiency blood loss or vitamin B_{12} deficiency	Protein levels will be within normal limits within 6 wk. Hemoglobin levels will be within normal range within 3 mo. CBC will show increasing RBCs and Hb within 3 wk. The patient will administer own vitamin B_{12} injections on a regular schedule or take the ordered oral dose.	Teach the patient about foods that meet required needs. Obtain dietary consultation as needed. Administer iron preparation; if liquid, give through straw. Give iron with juice or food containing vitamin C. Warn that stool may be greenish-black. Monitor CBC count for evidence of increase in RBCs and Hb. Administer vitamin B_{12} as ordered; advise that lifetime therapy is needed.
Altered tissue integrity related to inflammation of mucous membranes	Patient will perform mouth care diligently on schedule. Patient will display normal-appearing mucous membranes.	Give gentle mouth care before meals and q2h. Provide bland, easily chewed foods.
Altered activity tolerance related to decreased RBCs or Hb	Patient will use oxygen as ordered. Patient will alternate activities with rest. Patient will seek assistance with ambulation when dizzy.	Administer oxygen by nasal cannula at 3–6 L/min as ordered for patient with sickle cell crisis. Space activities, allowing rest periods for patient with fatigue. Assist with ADLs to prevent fatigue. If dizzy, caution to change position slowly; call for assistance with ambulation.
Pain related to ischemia and swollen joints	Patient will verbalize that pain is controlled by analgesics. Patient will verbalize that pain has decreased within 48 h.	Elevate swollen joints and apply hot or cold packs. Teach to avoid strenuous exercise. Position for comfort. Administer analgesics as ordered PRN.
Potential for injury due to low platelet count	Patient will have no new hematoma formation or other evidence of bleeding.	Assess for signs of internal bleeding (bruises, blood in urine or stool); measure abdominal girth daily. Minimize trauma; handle gently. Apply ice packs and gentle pressure if hematoma seems to be forming. Monitor administration of platelets PRN. Use small-gauge needle for injections; rotate sites. Avoid injections if possible. Apply pressure to puncture site or any invasive procedure for 10 min. No rectal meds. Use toothettes/no toothbrush.
Potential for infection due to decreased leukocytes	Patient will have no evidence of infection.	Observe for early signs of infection and report. Take temperature q4h. Use strict aseptic technique for wound care and invasive procedures. Use protective isolation as needed. Teach patient good personal hygiene. Avoid sick people, crowds. Maintain integrity of skin and mucosa. Administer antiinfective drugs precisely as ordered.
Insufficient knowledge due to substances that damage bone marrow	Patient will verbalize knowledge of drugs and chemicals that are harmful to the bone marrow within 1 wk.	Assess for exposure to substances that could have damaged the bone marrow. Teach about drugs and chemicals that are harmful to bone marrow and how to prevent damage. Seek feedback to validate understanding of content taught.

Continued

Table 15.2 Common Problem Statements/Nursing Diagnoses, Expected Outcomes, and Interventions for Patients With Blood Disorders—cont'd

PROBLEM STATEMENT/ NURSING DIAGNOSIS	GOALS/EXPECTED OUTCOMES	NURSING INTERVENTIONS
Anxiety due to unknown outcome of diagnostic tests and knowledge of disease, treatment, and prognosis	Patient will verbalize purpose and expected experience for each diagnostic test ordered. Patient will verbalize fears regarding disease, treatment, and prognosis.	Provide teaching regarding each diagnostic test. Encourage verbalization of fears. Offer emotional support to patient and family. Refer to support groups.
Decreased self-esteem due to inability to perform usual activities	Patient will define ways to cope with physical limitations. Patient will verbalize strengths. Patient will discuss possibility of seeking counseling.	Assist to cope with limitations of the illness. Help plan ways to maintain appropriate activity. Help to focus on the things that still can be done. Obtain counseling referral if psychological disturbance indicates need.
Altered family functioning due to expenses of treatment and possible death of patient	Patient and family will seek assistance from community resources as needed. Patient and family will verbalize understanding of disease, treatment modalities, and their implications.	Refer leukemia patient and family to community resources, such as the American Cancer Society, for assistance. Assist family and patient to understand the disease, treatment modalities, and their implications. Encourage attendance for all family members in a support group. Obtain referral to social worker for further assistance. Encourage open communication within family.

ADLs, Activities of daily living; *CBC,* complete blood cell count; *Hb,* hemoglobin; *PRN,* as needed; *RBCs,* red blood cells.

extremely important to use aseptic technique. Patients with a blood abnormality should not be exposed to people who are ill with contagious diseases, such as colds or influenza. Nursing goals include the following:

- Prevent infection.
- Conserve the patient's energy and prevent undue fatigue.
- Correct nutritional deficiencies.
- Provide treatment to halt or slow the disease process.
- Control pain or discomfort.
- Identify and promptly report complications.

Specific expected outcomes are written for individualized problem statements or nursing diagnoses.

◆ IMPLEMENTATION

Handle patients with blood dyscrasias gently to prevent bruising and hematomas. Take care to apply pressure for 5 to 10 minutes after injections or venipuncture. Good skin care is essential because the skin acts as a protective barrier against infection. Teach about nutrition and medication administration, prevention of infection, and measures to prevent bleeding. Pain control is important for patients with sickle cell anemia in crisis, patients with hemophilia with hemarthrosis, and patients with advanced leukemia.

Think Critically

When caring for a patient who has been in an automobile accident and has sustained trauma to the trunk of the body, what laboratory values should you check daily?

See Table 15.2 for specific interventions for patients experiencing blood disorders. Other interventions are included in the discussion of the various disorders in Chapter 16.

◆ EVALUATION

The evaluation process provides data to determine whether the specific outcome criteria are being met for each patient. Monitor laboratory values for blood counts and determine whether counts are improving to determine whether treatment and nursing actions are meeting the patient's needs. Assess for side effects and evaluate how the patient is tolerating the medication or other treatment for the underlying disorder.

Clinical Cues

When a patient with leukemia is undergoing chemotherapy, evaluate the blood count results to confirm that safe levels of leukocytes and platelets are present before administering another dose of a drug that inhibits their production.

COMMON PROBLEMS RELATED TO DISORDERS OF THE HEMATOLOGIC SYSTEM

EXCESSIVE BLEEDING

When injury has occurred or spontaneous bleeding happens, you should immediately apply pressure to stop the bleeding (Fig. 15.4). Severe bleeding can lead to irreversible hypovolemic shock and circulatory collapse

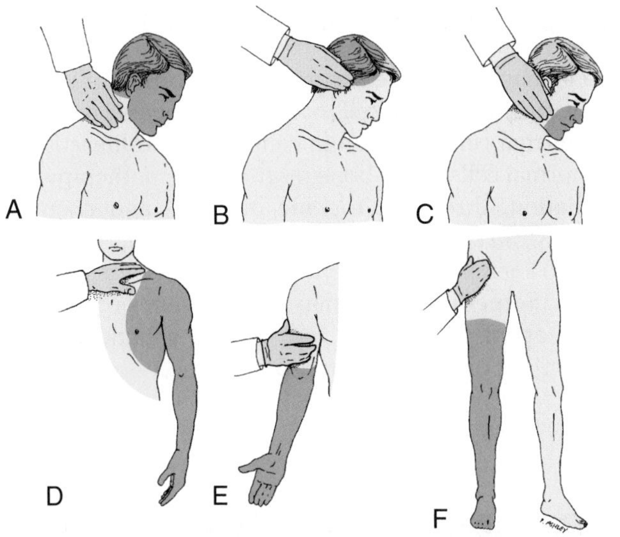

Fig. 15.4 Locations of commonly used digital pressure points to stop hemorrhage. The screened areas are those within which hemorrhage may be controlled by pressure on a specific artery. **A,** Carotid artery. **B,** Temporal artery. **C,** External maxillary artery. **D,** Subclavian artery. **E,** Brachial artery. **F,** Femoral artery.

Box 15.2 Techniques to Control Bleeding[a]

- Position the body part that is bleeding over a firm surface and immobilize the part.
- Place a sterile dressing or clean cloth over the wound.
- With gloved hand, place the flat palm of the hand or several fingers to apply direct pressure on the wound continuously for 5 minutes.
- Check whether bleeding has stopped after 5 minutes; if bleeding is still occurring, apply pressure continuously for another 10 minutes.
- When bleeding has stopped, gently remove hand pressure and apply a pressure dressing over the cloth or dressing by folding another dressing or piece of cloth several times and tying it firmly over the wound.
- Check circulation distal to the wound to be certain that the pressure dressing is not so tight that circulation below the wound is cut off.
- Reinforce the dressing as needed by applying yet another layer of dressing as blood soaks through; do not remove previously applied dressings.
- If direct pressure will not stop the bleeding and bleeding is considerable, apply pressure over the artery leading to the wound. **(Cut off arterial flow only as a last resort.)**
- Check for adequate pressure over the artery by determining a lack of pulse distal to the wound and patient report of a sensation of tingling and numbness in the wound area.

[a]Severe bleeding can lead to irreversible hypovolemic shock from loss of intravascular fluid and to circulatory collapse.

from loss of intravascular fluid. Blood loss from an artery is bright red and will gush forth in spurts at regular intervals as the heart contracts. Blood from a severed or punctured vein leaks slowly and steadily and is dark red. Box 15.2 presents methods of controlling bleeding. If bleeding occurs in a patient who does not have sufficient clotting factors, a transfusion of that factor, platelets, or fresh frozen plasma will be ordered. See Chapter 16 for information on transfusions. If blood loss is internal and pressure cannot be applied, surgical intervention will be needed to control the bleeding. Early recognition and reporting of the patient's change in condition is essential in providing prompt lifesaving care.

EXCESSIVE CLOTTING

Patients with certain disorders, such as polycythemia vera, and patients with high platelet counts are at risk for increased clotting. Watch for symptoms of phlebitis (see Box 15.1). Monitor circulation by checking peripheral pulses and skin color regularly.

Clinical Cues

Blood loss in the GI tract from an ulcer, tumor, or hiatal hernia can be in small amounts or in an amount large enough to make stool appear black (melena). Loss of 50 to 75 mL of blood from the upper GI tract is required before melena will appear.

FATIGUE

Help decrease fatigue by spacing activities throughout the day, with frequent rest periods. Assure the patient that stamina will improve as RBC count and hemoglobin rise. Work with the patient and family to decrease chores and expectations while fatigue is being experienced. Fatigue is common with anemia, and it affects all aspects of the patient's life.

ANOREXIA

Serve small, frequent meals high in protein, vitamin C, and iron, unless contraindicated. Provide mouth care before each meal. Offer foods that are appealing to the patient. Keep the eating environment pleasant and free of odors. Ask family to sit with the patient, to offer socialization and encouragement during meals.

PAIN

If the patient is experiencing pain, all comfort measures should be used. Assess pain level at least every 4 hours and medicate as ordered. Teach relaxation and imagery and assist the patient to perform these techniques (see Chapter 7). For joint pain, positioning and use of cold or heat may be effective. Pain may escalate quickly for a patient with sickle cell anemia who is in crisis, so assess pain level at least every 2 hours.

INFECTION

When a patient is moderately to severely anemic, the oxygen-carrying capacity of the blood is considerably decreased. Less than optimal tissue perfusion and tissue hypoxia make it easier for pathogens to invade and cause infection. When WBCs are decreased or abnormal, there are fewer cells to fight infection. Patients with abnormalities of the blood need to be taught how to protect themselves from infection. Good hand hygiene is essential. Staying away from crowds and individuals with infections is necessary. Getting enough sleep and eating a well-balanced diet help keep the immune system as healthy as possible under the circumstances. Prophylactic antibiotics may be given in certain situations. Precautions for patients who are prone to infection because of neutropenia are discussed in Chapters 8 and 10.

If the patient develops an infection, close monitoring of therapy and symptoms is needed. Rest, plenty of fluids, and sufficient protein and vitamin C are required to help the patient heal.

BONE MARROW FAILURE

Bone marrow failure occurs from abnormal cells overcrowding the normal cells or from inadequate production of normal cells. Leukemia causes overproliferation of abnormal cells in the bone marrow. Chemotherapy and radiation, thrombocytopenic purpura, and chemical toxicity can be factors in bone marrow failure. Predisposition to anemia, thrombocytopenia, and decreased WBCs occur. Sometimes bone marrow recovery occurs if the toxic agent is avoided, but usually a bone marrow transplant or stem cell transplant is necessary.

Get Ready for the NCLEX® Examination!

Key Points

- When the number of RBCs or hemoglobin is decreased, the amount of oxygen that reaches the cells is reduced.
- Leukocytes are the first line of defense against microbial agents.
- Neutrophils perform phagocytosis.
- Lymphocytes such as B cells and T cells destroy foreign proteins.
- Platelets are the first line of cell protection to prevent bleeding when trauma has occurred.
- When the platelet count is low, spontaneous bleeding may occur.
- Bone marrow activity decreases by 50% in older adults.
- Blood in older adults coagulates more easily because of platelet *aggregation* (sticking together).
- Hemophilia, sickle cell disease, and certain types of anemias that cause blood disorders are inherited.
- Blood dyscrasias may be caused by drugs, radiation, or toxic substances (see Box 15.1).
- Nutritional deficiencies can cause anemia.
- A CBC with a differential count (count of the different types of WBCs) can help diagnose many blood disorders (see Table 15.1).
- Bone marrow aspiration is used to diagnose a variety of blood disorders.
- A history is gathered and a focused physical assessment is performed for patients with a suspected blood disorder.
- There are common problem statements or nursing diagnoses appropriate for patients with a blood disorder (see Table 15.2).
- Preventing infection, conserving energy, controlling pain, and correcting the underlying cause are the goals of care for patients with a blood disorder.
- Patients with blood disorders must be handled gently.
- Checking serial CBCs is part of the evaluation process.
- Methods to stop bleeding should be taught to patients and families.
- Self-care measures are taught to each patient to prevent infection.

Additional Learning Resources

SG Go to your Study Guide for additional learning activities to help you master this chapter content.

Go to your Evolve website (http://evolve.elsevier.com/deWit/medsurg) for the following FREE learning resources:

- Animations, audio, and video
- Answers and rationales for questions and activities
- Glossary with pronunciations in English and Spanish
- Interactive Review Questions and more!

Review Questions for the NCLEX® Examination

1. For a patient with the clinical finding of leukocytosis, you should:
   1. initiate protective isolation precautions.
   2. inspect for signs of active bleeding.
   3. anticipate a possible health care provider order for antibiotic coverage.
   4. schedule periods of rest and activity.

   NCLEX Client Need: Physiological Integrity: Pharmacological Therapies

2. For an older adult patient admitted for recent falls, which clinical finding(s) relative to the hematologic system would be associated with the aging process? *(Select all that apply.)*
   1. Decreased hematocrit and red blood cells
   2. Decreased antibody buildup from flu immunization
   3. Prolonged prothrombin time and sedimentation rate
   4. Increased neutrophils to fight infection
   5. Increased coagulability, which predisposes to clots

   NCLEX Client Need: Safe and Effective Care Environment: Safety and Infection Control

3. A patient works in a chemical plant. When answering an assessment question, they tell you that they wear protective clothing, mask, and equipment when handling any chemicals and they avoid coming into contact with radiation. These precautions will:
1. make the work environment safe.
2. decrease the risk for blood disorders.
3. decrease the risk for idiopathic thrombocytopenia purpura.
4. protect against megaloblastic anemia.

NCLEX Client Need: Health Promotion and Maintenance

4. A patient is told that their hematocrit is very low. What symptom would you expect the patient to experience?
1. Increased energy because of the increased percentage of red blood cells
2. Fatigue related to reduced oxygen transport
3. Reduced mobility caused by decreased lubrication of the joints
4. Increased thirst from salt retention

NCLEX Client Need: Physiological Integrity: Physiological Adaptation

5. A patient displays purple spots and patches characteristic of thrombocytopenia purpura. This assessment finding is found in which of the following?
1. Vitamin B_{12} deficiency
2. Platelet deficiency
3. Iron deficiency anemia
4. Bruising of the skin

NCLEX Client Need: Physiological Integrity: Physiological Adaptation

6. A nurse formulates the following expected outcome for a patient admitted with hemarthrosis: "The patient will have no new hematomas or other evidence of bleeding." The most appropriate nursing intervention would be to:
1. suggest the patient use a soft toothbrush.
2. handle the patient very gently, protecting joints.
3. keep the skin well lubricated.
4. place the patient on a mechanical soft diet.

NCLEX Client Need: Health Promotion and Maintenance

7. A nurse taking care of an older adult woman with megaloblastic anemia demonstrates understanding of the functional implications by:
1. promoting adequate rest.
2. actively listening to the patient's concerns.
3. monitoring for bleeding.
4. administering antibiotics.

NCLEX Client Need: Physiological Integrity: Reduction of Risk Potential

8. After removing a peripheral vascular access device, you note bleeding at the site. Put the following nursing actions in order of priority:
1. Check blood pressure.
2. Check for other areas of bleeding.
3. Apply direct pressure.
4. Elevate the extremity.

NCLEX Client Need: Safe and Effective Care Environment: Coordinated care

9. A nurse initiates neutropenic precautions for a patient who has undergone chemotherapy. Which nursing action(s) would be considered appropriate? *(Select all that apply.)*
1. Use clean technique for wound care and invasive procedures.
2. Use transmission-based isolation precautions as needed.
3. Allow all visitors as desired.
4. Maintain integrity of skin and mucosa.
5. Provide analgesics as needed.

NCLEX Client Need: Safe and Effective Care Environment: Safety and Infection Control

10. An 80-year-old patient with megaloblastic anemia is admitted after a fall that resulted in a fractured hip. In preparing for surgical repair of the hip, a CBC is done. Which of the following results is most concerning?
1. Hgb 6.0 g/dL
2. Hct 17%
3. RBCs 2.2 million/mm^3
4. WBCs 2000/mm^3

NCLEX Client Need: Physiological Integrity: Reduction of Risk Potential

Critical Thinking Questions

Scenario A

You come upon an automobile accident and stop to help.
1. The first victim has a gash in the thigh, and blood is spurting at regular intervals from the wound. What method would you use to stop the bleeding?
2. The second victim has a bleeding wound on the forehead. What method would you use to stop the bleeding?

Scenario B

Mr. Jones has a disorder that has caused leukopenia. He lives alone. To prepare him for discharge home, you need to provide teaching.
1. What would you teach him about preventing infection?
2. What would you suggest regarding visitors who wish to see him?
3. What would you tell him about performing necessary errands?

Scenario C

Your 38-year-old male patient has a history of seizures and takes phenytoin. He has developed mild hypertension and takes hydrochlorothiazide to control his blood pressure.
1. What would you teach him about measures to prevent blood disorders?
2. What would you recommend to him for monitoring possible problems?

16 Care of Patients With Hematologic Disorders

http://evolve.elsevier.com/deWit/medsurg

Objectives

Theory

1. Examine the causes of the various types of anemias.
2. Develop a plan of care for a patient with an anemia.
3. Explain the pathophysiology and care of sickle cell disease.
4. Compare cell abnormalities of polycythemia vera with those of leukemia.
5. Formulate a teaching plan for a patient with leukemia.
6. Interpret laboratory values for patients experiencing coagulation disorders.
7. Summarize the problems and treatments that a patient with hemophilia faces.

Clinical Practice

8. Considering the goals of care, write expected outcomes for each of the appropriate problem statements for a patient with a blood disorder.
9. Prepare to provide preprocedure and postprocedure care for the patient undergoing a bone marrow aspiration.
10. Perform an assessment on a patient with a suspected hematologic disorder.
11. Assist with the development of a plan of care for an adult with leukemia.
12. Assess for signs and symptoms of disseminated intravascular coagulation.

Key Terms

allogeneic (ĂL-ō-JĔN-ĭk, p. 373)
anemia (ă-NĒ-mē-ă, p. 352)
autologous (ăw-TŎL-ŏ-gŭs, p. 369)
disseminated intravascular coagulation (DIC) (dĭ-SĔM-ĭ-nāt-ĕd ĭn-tră-VĂS-cū-lăr kō-ăg-ū-LĀ-shŭn, p. 369)
ecchymoses (ĕk-ĭ-MŌ-sēz, p. 366)
erythropoiesis (ĭ-rĭth-rō-pōĭ-Ē-sĭs, p. 353)
hemarthrosis (hē-măr-THRŌ-sĭs, p. 368)
hemolysis (hē-MŎL-ĭ-sĭs, p. 353)
hypovolemia (hī-pō-vō-LĒ-mē-ă, p. 352)
leukapheresis (lū-kă-fĕ-RĒ-sĭs, p. 363)
purpura (PŬR-pū-ră, p. 366)
splenomegaly (splē-nō-MĔG-ă-lē, p. 360)
stomatitis (stō-mă-TĪ-tĭs, p. 365)
thrombocytopenia (thrŏm-bō-sīt-ō-PĒ-nē-ă, p. 366)

Concepts Covered in This Chapter

- Fluid and Electrolytes
- Cellular Regulation
- Perfusion
- Gas Exchange
- Clotting
- Inflammation
- Tissue Integrity
- Pain

DISORDERS OF THE HEMATOLOGIC SYSTEM

ANEMIA

In the human body, healthy red blood cells (RBCs) carry oxygen to tissues. A balance is maintained between the production of new RBCs and the disposal of old, "worn-out" RBCs. Anemia occurs when something interferes with this balance or interferes with the maturation of cells. **Anemia** is a state in which there are insufficient numbers of functioning RBCs, or a lack of hemoglobin (Hb), to meet the demands of the tissues for oxygen. Anemia is not a disease; it is a symptom of a disease or pathologic process. It can be chronic or acute.

Etiology

There are three major classifications of anemia, according to cause:

- Anemia resulting from blood loss
- Anemia resulting from a failure in blood cell production
- Anemia associated with a destruction of RBCs

Rapid, severe bleeding leads to anemia from blood loss, **hypovolemia** (decreased volume of circulating blood), and potentially shock. A blood loss that leads to anemia may result from severe trauma to the blood vessels and massive hemorrhage, or the blood loss may be more gradual, as from a small, bleeding peptic ulcer that causes a chronic blood loss (Table 16.1).

Anemia caused by a failure in cell production is the result of either a deficiency of certain substances necessary for the formation of RBCs or abnormal functioning of bone marrow. Examples of this type of anemia are:

- Nutritional anemia, in which there is an inadequate intake of foods containing proteins, folic acid, and iron

Table 16.1 Clinical Manifestations of Acute Blood Loss

VOLUME LOST	CLINICAL MANIFESTATIONS
10%	None
20%	At rest, no signs or symptoms; slight postural hypotension when standing; tachycardia with exercise
30%	Blood pressure and pulse normal when supine; postural hypotension and tachycardia with exercise
40%	Below-normal blood pressure, central venous pressure, and cardiac output at rest; rapid, thready pulse and cold, clammy skin
50%	Shock and potential death

Adapted from Lewis SL, Bucher L, Heitkemper MM, et al.: *Medical-surgical nursing: assessment and management of clinical problems,* ed 10, St. Louis, 2017, Elsevier.

- Anemia resulting from bone marrow suppression caused by toxic substances
- Megaloblastic (pernicious) anemia, in which there is faulty absorption of specific nutrients, such as vitamin B_{12}
- End-stage renal disease (ESRD), in which erythropoietin is not produced by the kidney so RBC production is not stimulated.

Anemia caused by destruction of RBCs may be inherited or acquired. Hemolytic anemias, in which RBCs are destroyed prematurely in the body, have many causes. Hemolytic anemia can be a result of genetic defects that affect cell structure, causing the cells to disintegrate quickly. Some of the hemolytic anemias, such as *thalassemia* and *sickle cell disease,* are inherited, whereas others are acquired when erythrocytes are exposed to poisonous agents, such as chemicals or certain bacterial toxins.

Immune reactions can cause blood cell **hemolysis** (destruction of RBCs). The presence of toxins in the blood, infections such as malaria, transfusion reactions, and changes in blood chemistry may cause RBC hemolysis. Blood incompatibility in the newborn *(erythroblastosis fetalis)* is another cause.

Pathophysiology

Iron deficiency anemia occurs when total body iron is insufficient and **erythropoiesis** (the production of RBCs, as from the bone marrow) is diminished. The lack of iron impedes the formation of Hb (Concept Map 16.1). In *megaloblastic anemia,* an autoimmune disease, the intrinsic factor is missing from the gastric juices, and vitamin B_{12} is not absorbed without it. Vitamin B_{12} acts as a coenzyme in conjunction with folate metabolism and is important in the use of iron and protein for the manufacture of RBCs. The result of the missing intrinsic factor is that the RBC production is decreased, and those RBCs that are produced are abnormal in their structure and function

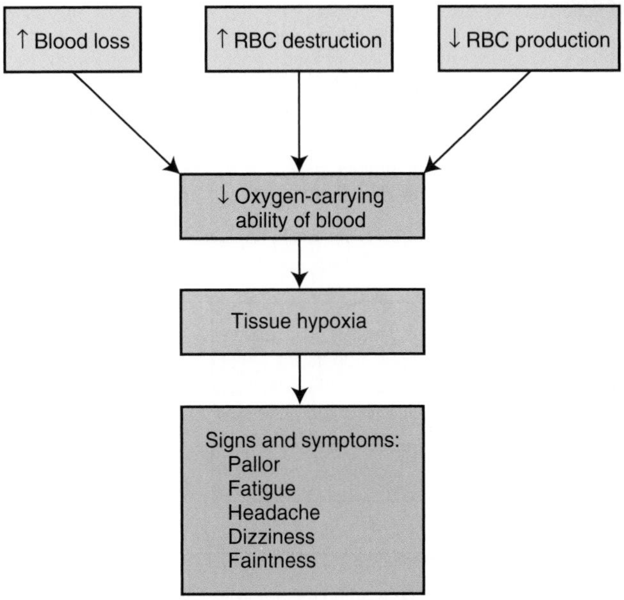

Concept Map 16.1 Pathophysiology of anemia. *RBC,* Red blood cells.

(Concept Map 16.2). To treat this condition, vitamin B_{12} will be given and any folic acid deficiency corrected.

Hemolytic anemias associated with excessive destruction of RBCs are quite rare. When RBCs are not normal, they break up easily or are destroyed by the body more quickly than are normal RBCs. This RBC destruction causes the anemia.

Anemia occurs during ESRD when there is a deficiency of production of *erythropoietin,* a substance necessary to stimulate the creation of RBCs in the bone marrow. This problem is usually corrected by the administration of erythropoiesis-stimulating agents (ESAs), including epoetin alfa (Epogen, Procrit) and darbepoetin alfa (Aranesp) (U.S. Food and Drug Administration [FDA], 2017). These drugs are used to improve RBC production in patients receiving chemotherapy, undergoing major surgery, and with other conditions where transfusion might be necessary if the body cannot provide adequate RBCs. **Oxygen transport depends on the number and condition of the RBCs and the amount of Hb they contain.**

Clinical Cues

When a patient has had gastric bypass surgery or a gastrectomy, there is a risk of megaloblastic anemia from the resultant decrease of available intrinsic factor. Observe for signs of megaloblastic anemia in these patients.

Patients who take medications over a long period that suppress gastric acid secretion (histamine-2 inhibitors, proton pump inhibitors) must be watched for signs of megaloblastic anemia. Supplementation with vitamin B_{12} may help prevent this problem.

Signs and Symptoms

Signs and symptoms of anemias from causes other than rapid bleeding depend on whether the anemia is mild,

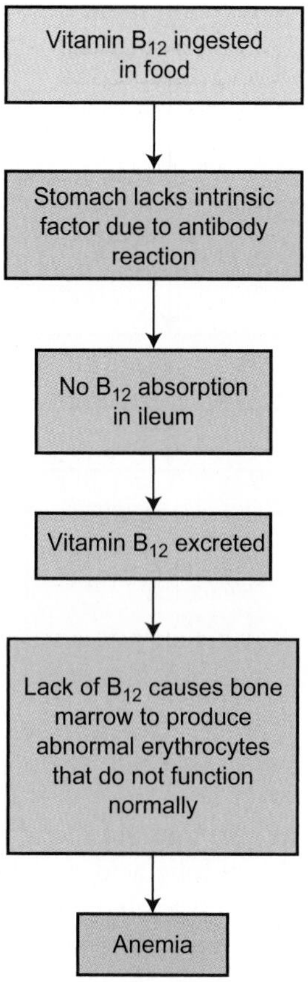

Concept Map 16.2 Pathophysiology of megaloblastic anemia.

Table 16.2 Signs and Symptoms of Severe Anemia

BODY SYSTEM	SIGNS AND SYMPTOMS
General	Sensitivity to cold, lethargy, weight loss
Eyes	Blurred vision, blue sclera, yellowing of or pale conjunctiva, retinal hemorrhage
Skin	Pallor of face and palms, pruritus, jaundice, pale nail beds, pale mucous membranes, stomatitis, brittle nails
Cardiovascular	Palpitations, tachycardia, angina, systolic murmur, widened pulse pressure, intermittent claudication, CHF, possible MI
Respiratory	Tachypnea, orthopnea, dyspnea at rest
Gastrointestinal	Anorexia, difficulty swallowing, glossitis, enlarged liver, enlarged spleen, smooth tongue
Musculoskeletal	Bone pain, leg cramps, weakness, cold extremities
Neurologic	Headache, dizziness, impaired thinking, irritability, depression, fatigue, insomnia

CHF, Congestive heart failure; *MI,* myocardial infarction.

moderate, or severe. Signs and symptoms of mild anemia (Hb 11 to 13 g/dL) are mild headache, palpitations, and dyspnea on exertion. Moderate anemia (Hb 8 to 10 g/dL) may include brittle nails, sore tongue, pallor, chronic fatigue, headache, and dizziness or faintness. Table 16.2 presents the many signs and symptoms of severe anemia (Hb <8 g/dL). Tachypnea and tachycardia may develop with severe anemia because of the decreased ability of the blood to transport sufficient oxygen to the tissues.

Diagnosis

The microscopic appearance of the RBCs in a film of blood that has been spread over a slide (a peripheral smear) gives information about abnormalities in size, shape, and color of erythrocytes circulating in the patient's bloodstream. The complete blood cell count (CBC) and differential cell count results are used to diagnose the presence of anemia. Measuring the quantity of Hb determines whether the cells have sufficient amounts of Hb to carry adequate oxygen to the body. An Hb less than 12 g/dL in women and less than 13 g/dL in men is the definition of anemia.

The prefix *normo-* refers to "normal"; the suffix *-cyte* refers to "cells"; the suffix *-chrom* refers to "color"; and the suffix *-ic* means "having the quality of" or "characterized by." Thus a normocytic, normochromic anemia is characterized by cells that are normal in size and color but that have a deficiency in the number of RBCs and a low hematocrit. **This type of anemia usually occurs as a result of sudden blood loss.**

A hypochromic, microcytic anemia is characterized by decreased levels of Hb (not enough color) and small (micro) cells. **This type of anemia is typical of an iron deficiency anemia.**

Treatment

Correcting the underlying problem and then building up replacement blood cells treats anemia from chronic, slow blood loss. Anemia caused by inadequate iron, folic acid, or protein intake is managed with oral iron supplements, vitamins, and diet adjustment. If the anemia is serious, blood transfusions may be given or intravenous (IV) iron preparations may be administered.

Megaloblastic anemia is treated by regular administration of vitamin B_{12}, by injection, orally, sublingually, or intranasally. Because the deficiency of intrinsic factor prevents adequate absorption of this vitamin from food, it also inhibits gastric absorption of the medication, so the sublingual route results in more drug being absorbed. There must be sufficient folic acid in the diet or by supplement. Table 16.3 presents the medications most commonly prescribed for hematologic disorders.

For *hemolytic anemia,* the underlying cause is found and corrected (if possible), and then the blood volume is rebuilt with added iron and appropriate diet or administration of an ESA. If the anemia is severe, blood transfusion may be indicated.

Nutrition Considerations

Common Foods High in Iron and Folic Acid

FOODS HIGH IN IRON

- Beef liver
- Blackstrap molasses
- Chicken liver
- Cooked oatmeal
- Cooked prunes
- Cooked shrimp
- Dried apricots
- Egg yolks
- Kidney beans
- Lean beef
- Lima beans
- Whole grains
- Prune juice
- Raisins
- Spinach and green leafy vegetables
- Turkey

Adding raw spinach to dinner salads and snacking on raisins or dried apricots can quickly improve iron intake. Iron-enriched cereals and breads also can be added to the diet.

FOODS HIGH IN FOLIC ACID

- Asparagus
- Beef
- Fish
- Cabbage
- Brussels sprouts
- Broccoli
- Legumes (kidney beans, etc.)
- Liver
- Eggs
- Whole grains

Note: Many of the foods high in iron also are high in folic acid.

Think Critically

Your patient, who has suffered a blood loss and is now anemic, complains that they are short of breath. Explain how blood loss might affect respiration.

Focused Assessment

Data Collection When Anemia Is Suspected

HEALTH HISTORY

Ask the patient the following questions:

- Have you had any recent blood loss or trauma?
- Do you have chronic liver, endocrine, gastrointestinal, or renal disease?
- What medications, vitamins, supplements, or herbal products do you take?
- What surgeries have you had and when?
- Have you ever had radiation treatments or chemotherapy?
- Is there a history of genetic blood disorders in your family?
- Has your appetite or weight changed?
- Have you noticed any changes in your urine or stool?
- Are you experiencing shortness of breath, weakness, or fatigue?
- Have you noticed any heart palpitations?
- Do you get frequent headaches?
- Have you noticed any changes in vision or dizziness?
- Do you have pain or itching anywhere?
- Do you become cold when others are not?

PHYSICAL ASSESSMENT

Check for the following:

- *Skin:* Pale skin and mucous membranes; pale conjunctiva, yellowing of sclera; cracks in lips; brittle, spoon-shaped fingernails (Fig. 16.1); jaundice; petechiae; ecchymoses; dry, brittle, thinning hair
- *Respiratory:* Tachypnea, orthopnea, dyspnea on exertion or at rest
- *Cardiac:* Tachycardia, systolic murmur, angina, ankle edema
- *Gastrointestinal:* Sore mouth, stomatitis, beefy red tongue, abdominal distention, enlarged liver or spleen
- *Neurologic:* Headache, dizziness, confusion, irritability, ataxia (unsteady gait), paresthesia

PERTINENT LABORATORY VALUES

- CBC, serum iron, ferritin, folate, cobalamin (vitamin B_{12}), stool for guaiac, urinalysis, serum erythropoietin

NURSING MANAGEMENT

ASSESSMENT (DATA COLLECTION)

Whenever a patient complains of fatigue, headaches, or shortness of breath, anemia should always be considered. A CBC and data regarding physical signs and symptoms are collected.

NURSING DIAGNOSIS

Problem statements or nursing diagnoses are based on the clinical findings. Common problem statements include:

- Altered activity tolerance due to weakness and fatigue
- Altered gas exchange due to decreased hemoglobin
- Altered nutrition due to poor diet and anorexia
- Insufficient knowledge regarding nutrition and medication regimen

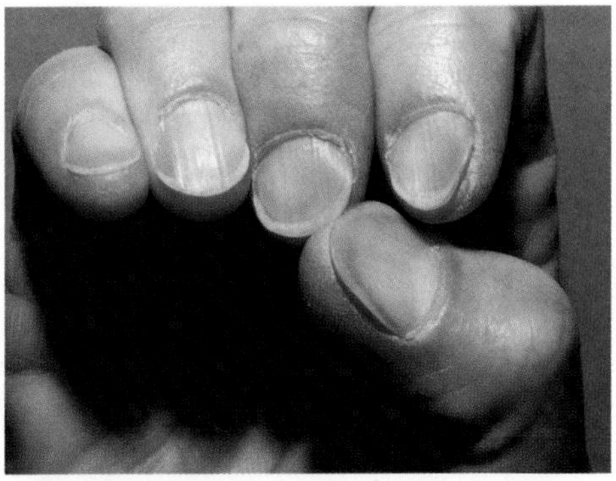

Fig. 16.1 Thin, concave (spoon-shaped) nails with raised edges may be seen on people with iron deficiency anemia.

Table 16.3 Drugs Commonly Used to Treat Disorders of the Hematologic System[a]

CLASSIFICATION	ACTION	NURSING IMPLICATIONS	PATIENT TEACHING
Mineral			
Ferrous sulfate (Feosol, Fer-In-Sol) Ferrous gluconate (Fergon) Ferrous fumarate (Feostat, Ircon) Ferric citrate Iron sucrose IV (Venofer) Sodium ferric gluconate IV, ferumoxytol IV, ferric carboxymaltose IV	Increases elemental iron as a component in the formation of hemoglobin. Used to treat iron deficiency anemia.	May cause GI upset: nausea, diarrhea, or constipation; monitor for constipation. Tell patient that oral form will turn stool black. Do not give with milk, which reduces absorption. Dilute elixir in juice and give through a straw to prevent staining of the teeth. Do not crush enteric-coated or sustained-release tablets or capsules. Patients with asthma or more than one drug allergy are premedicated with methylprednisolone prior to IV infusion. Give slowly at first to determine patient's reaction.	Take oral form with orange juice or other vitamin C–rich food. Avoid taking iron with milk products. Keep out of reach of children because it is toxic. Have Hb checked according to health care provider's schedule to check response to medication. Eat foods high in iron. Increase fluids and roughage if constipation occurs.
Vitamins			
Folic acid (Folvite)	Promotes normal erythropoiesis; used in certain types of anemia.	May interfere with anticonvulsant blood levels. Chloramphenicol interferes with absorption. Increase foods high in folic acid.	Have blood count monitored according to provider's schedule to determine effectiveness of therapy.
Vitamin B_{12} cyanocobalamin (Rubramin, Anacobin); methylcobalamin; hydroxobalamin	Acts as coenzyme for cell replication and hematopoiesis. Used in megaloblastic anemia, other GI disorders that decrease vitamin B_{12} absorption, and cases of dietary deficiency.	Give subcutaneously or IM daily for 5–10 days and then once monthly for maintenance. Can cause anaphylactic reaction when given IV. Deficiency more common in strict vegetarians.	Teach importance of maintaining monthly injections for life to prevent further episodes of megaloblastic anemia. Encourage increased intake of vitamin B_{12} in diet if deficiency is diet related.
Antimetabolite			
Hydroxyurea (Hydrea)	Inhibits DNA synthesis. Used to reduce episodes of sickling in sickle cell anemia. Used to eradicate abnormal cells in leukemia, myeloma, polycythemia vera, and some solid tumors.	Discontinue if WBC count is $<2500/mm^3$ or platelet count is $>100,000/mm^3$. Capsule granules may be mixed with water if taken immediately. May cause GI problems: stomach upset, stomatitis, vomiting, diarrhea.	Use cautiously in presence of renal dysfunction. Radiation therapy increases toxicity. Monitor intake and output. Monitor for infection. Monitor blood counts for neutropenia, thrombocytopenia, and bone marrow suppression. Use caution to avoid exposure to infection and to report signs or symptoms of infection promptly. Increase fluid intake to maintain adequate hydration. Give mouth care q4h to prevent stomatitis. Report bleeding to the provider.

Table 16.3 **Drugs Commonly Used to Treat Disorders of the Hematologic System—cont'd**

CLASSIFICATION	ACTION	NURSING IMPLICATIONS	PATIENT TEACHING
Biologic Response Modifiers			
Epoetin alfa; erythropoietin (Epogen, Procrit)	A natural hormone produced by recombinant DNA techniques that controls rate of RBC production. Stimulates the bone marrow, functioning as a growth factor. Used to combat reduced production of erythropoietin in end-stage renal disease, increase RBC production in anemias, boost RBCs postoperatively instead of blood transfusion.	Also used for patients with anemia secondary to chemotherapy and in patients with rheumatoid arthritis who experience anemia from therapy. May be used to increase RBCs in anticipation of autologous blood transfusion before surgery.	May cause seizures. Monitor blood count closely; dosage may need to be reduced if hematocrit rises too rapidly. Monitor blood pressure closely; may cause rise. May cause pain in limbs and pelvis. Explain the purpose of the injections. Remind that the drug must be refrigerated; discard after 6 h at room temperature.
Filgrastim (Neupogen)	Stimulates production, maturation, and activation of neutrophils.	CBC with differential before beginning therapy and twice weekly thereafter. Monitor BP; may cause transient increase.	Teach to inform provider if fever, chills, severe bone pain, chest pain, or palpitations occur.
Pegfilgrastim (Neulasta)	Regulates production of neutrophils within bone marrow. Increases phagocytic activity.	CBC and differential before therapy and routinely thereafter. Monitor for allergic reaction (i.e., peripheral edema). Assess muscle strength. Observe mouth for stomatitis, mucositis.	Inform of possible side effects and how to watch for allergic reaction. Remind that regular blood counts are important.

[a]Chemotherapy drugs are discussed in Chapter 8.
BP, Blood pressure; *CBC*, complete blood cell count; *DNA*, deoxyribonucleic acid; *GI*, gastrointestinal; *Hb*, hemoglobin; *IM*, intramuscularly; *IV*, intravenously; *RBC*, red blood cell; *WBC*, white blood cell.

◆ PLANNING

Expected outcomes are written for the specific individual problem statements chosen to resolve the patient's problems. For the problem statements listed, outcomes might include:

- Within 1 month patient will be able to perform hygiene, dressing, and grooming activities without needing to rest between activities.
- Within 2 months patient will be able to carry out usual daily activities without shortness of breath or fatigue.
- Patient will eat three nutritious meals per day, containing sufficient iron, folic acid, vitamin C, and protein daily.
- Patient will verbalize understanding of dietary and medication regimen within 1 week.

◆ IMPLEMENTATION

Intervention is based on an understanding of the kind of anemia affecting the patient. Anemia from blood loss presents problems quite different from those related to chronic—and possibly incurable—aplastic or hemolytic anemia. For patients with anemia that interferes with clotting and that tends to cause bleeding episodes, nursing actions are directed toward preventing the episodes. For any patient with anemia severe enough to cause fatigue, assist with activities of daily living and provide planned rest periods.

Nursing functions include administering blood, iron, vitamin B_{12}, and folic acid and monitoring for desired effects. Patients are educated about needed dietary adjustments. Patients should be taught that iron is absorbed more readily if vitamin C is simultaneously present in the gastrointestinal (GI) system. Taking iron medication with orange juice provides the necessary vitamin C.

Analgesia for headache or joint pain is given as ordered, and the patient is monitored for adverse side effects. More problem statements commonly associated with hematologic problems, including anemia, and lists of appropriate interventions are included in Chapter 15, Table 15.2.

Older Adult Care Points

- Iron supplements should be taken 1 hour before or 2 hours after a meal, as long as they do not cause GI distress.
- Many older adults have chronic conditions that require daily medication. Antacids and many other drugs interfere with iron absorption.
- Check all drugs a patient is receiving to determine whether drug interactions might interfere with iron absorption.

◆ EVALUATION

Evaluation data are gathered to determine whether expected outcomes are being met. Laboratory values are particularly important when evaluating the care of a patient with anemia. However, equally important are data showing that the problems caused by the anemia are resolving.

APLASTIC ANEMIA

Aplastic anemia (a rare disorder) may develop after a viral infection, as a reaction to a drug, or because of an inherited tendency. The disease is characterized by bone marrow depression and is believed to probably be an immune-mediated disease. RBC, white blood cell (WBC), and platelet levels are decreased. The toxic effects of certain substances can be responsible for aplastic anemia. Some of these agents include benzene; insecticides; drugs such as chloramphenicol (Chloromycetin), phenylbutazone (Butazolidin), and sulfonamides; some anticonvulsants; gold compounds used to treat rheumatoid arthritis; and alkylating agents or antimetabolites used in chemotherapy. Many other drugs can cause aplastic anemia, but this adverse effect is rare. Radiation exposure is another factor in the development of the disorder.

Safety Alert

Monitor Drug Side Effects

It is your responsibility to monitor blood studies carefully for all patients who are receiving any drug that is potentially damaging to the bone marrow.

Think Critically

What chemical products in your home or garage can cause bone marrow depression?

Impairment or failure of bone marrow function leading to the loss of stem cells is the cause of aplastic anemia (Concept Map 16.3). With aplastic anemia, the bone marrow has decreased cells and increased fatty tissue. In addition to the signs and symptoms of iron deficiency anemia, ecchymosis, petechiae, and hemorrhage related to low platelet count also occur. Infection is common and may not cause an inflammatory response because of the very low leukocyte count. There is often frequent bleeding in the mouth.

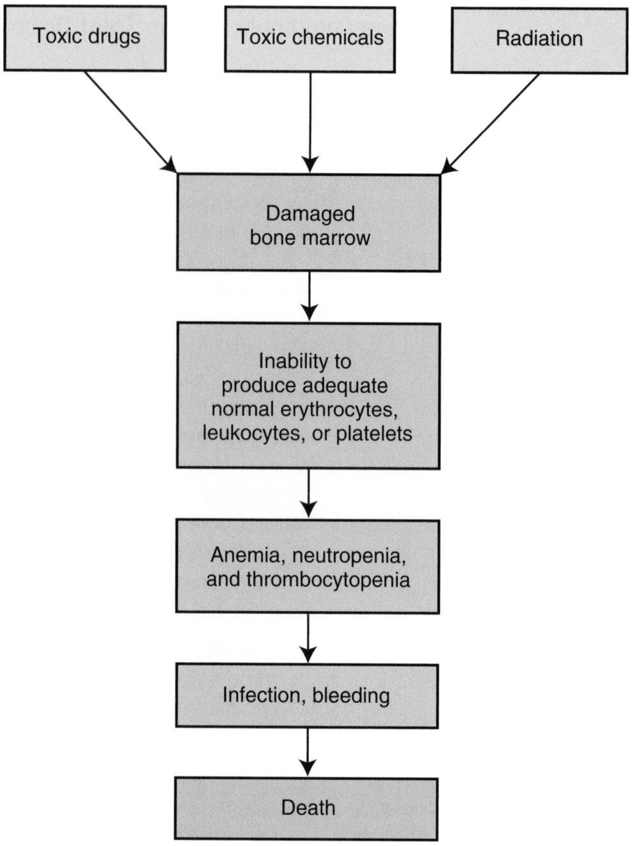

Concept Map 16.3 Pathophysiology of aplastic anemia.

Diagnosis is by blood count with differential, bone marrow biopsy, and ruling out other disorders. **Aplastic anemia causes an emergency situation.** Treatment must eliminate any identifiable underlying cause. Packed RBCs and platelets are administered. Antibiotics are given for identified infection; oxygen is sometimes administered to patients with low erythrocyte counts. Hematopoietic cell transplantation (HCT) (or bone marrow transplantation) is the treatment of choice for patients younger than 50 years. Immunosuppressive therapy plus eltrombopag, a hematopoietic agent and colony-stimulating factor, may be used if HCT is not available or appropriate.

Prevention of hemorrhage and infection is a top priority (see the Evolve website for patient teaching guidelines). Psychological support of the patient and family is important when they are faced with this life-threatening condition. Safety measures are priorities. Actions for problems of weakness and fatigue are the same as those presented for anemia earlier in the chapter. Other common nursing interventions are included in Chapter 15, Table 15.2. See Chapter 8 for precautions and actions for patients with disseminated intravascular coagulopathy and neutropenia and for safety measures when thrombocytopenia is present.

SICKLE CELL DISEASE

Etiology

Sickle cell disease is a genetic disorder in which the gene is inherited from both parents (homozygous gene)

Clinical Cues

Cells for use in HCT can be obtained from peripheral blood, umbilical cord blood, or bone marrow. Up to now, most stem cells were obtained from bone marrow and the term *bone marrow transplant* was commonly used. HCT covers all sources of cells, not just bone marrow.

Health Promotion

Dangers of Toxic Agents

All nurses should promote public education about the dangers of toxic agents. It is vitally important that people read and follow the label instructions on all cleaning agents, insecticides, and chemical compounds.

(Table 16.4). Sickle cell disease is characterized by gene mutations that cause production of abnormal hemoglobin S rather than hemoglobin A. Sickle cell disease is found in 8% to 10% of African Americans but also affects Hispanics, South Asians, Caucasians from southern Europe, and people from Middle Eastern countries.

Sickle cell trait is heterozygous, meaning that the person has an inherited gene for the trait from one parent only. People with the heterozygous trait for sickle cell are carriers; they can transmit the gene to their children even when they themselves do not show signs of the disease. Therefore genetic counseling and adequate screening for early detection of the disease are considered extremely important to control sickle cell anemia.

Pathophysiology

The defective hemoglobin S (HbS) polymerizes (chemical change forming a compound) when hypoxia is present, causing them to assume a sickle shape, blocking blood vessels, breaking apart, and forming thrombi that cause organ damage. Sickle cells are destroyed by the body very quickly, causing anemia. HbS has a life span of 10 days compared to 120 days for normal hemoglobin.

In the United States many patients with sickle cell anemia live into their mid-40s. The most common cause of death is acute organ failure from impaired circulation.

Signs and Symptoms

Sickle cell disease indicates the presence of HbS; as long as the cells are not causing blockages in circulation, there are no symptoms. When cells clump, blood flow is impaired and the signs and symptoms are those that indicate lack of oxygen and blood flow, such as pallor, lethargy, and pain. Periodic episodes of pain are called *sickle cell crisis* and indicate lack of blood flow in small vessels. The problems from interrupted normal blood flow affect many organs (Fig. 16.2). Painful swelling of the hands and feet related to bone infarction from the sickled cells (hand-foot syndrome) may occur. After sickle cell crisis, signs typical of anemia occur because the abnormally shaped cells are very fragile, break easily, and are destroyed. The RBC and hemoglobin counts can drop very quickly during a crisis.

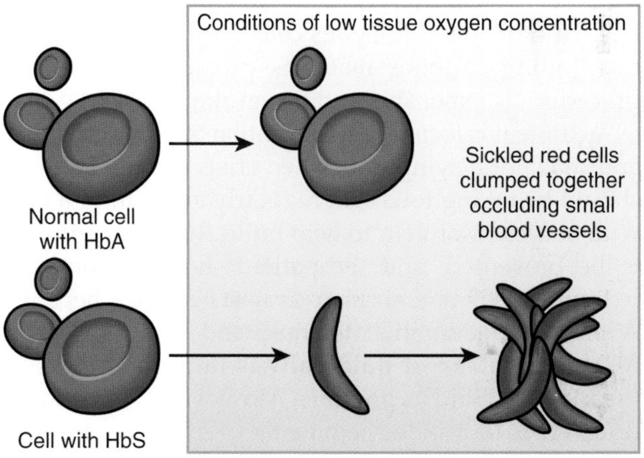

Fig. 16.2 Sickling of red blood cells occurs when tissue oxygen is low. (From Ignatavicius DD, Workman ML, Rebar CR, et al.: *Medical-surgical nursing: patient-centered collaborative care,* ed 9, Philadelphia, 2018, Elsevier.)

Table 16.4 Comparison of Four Types of Anemia

CHARACTERISTIC RBC	ETIOLOGY	ADDITIONAL EFFECTS
Iron Deficiency Anemia		
Microcytic, hypochromic Decreased hemoglobin production	Decreased dietary intake, malabsorption, blood loss	Only effects of anemia
Megaloblastic Anemia		
Megaloblasts, immature nucleated cells	Deficit of intrinsic factor due to immune reaction	Neurologic damage Achlorhydria
Aplastic Anemia		
Often normal cells Pancytopenia	Bone marrow damage or failure	Excessive bleeding and multiple infections
Sickle Cell Anemia		
RBC elongates and hardens in "sickle" shape when O_2 levels are low—short life span	Recessive inheritance	Painful crises with multiple infarctions Hyperbilirubinemia

From Hubert RJ, VanMeter KC: *Gould's pathophysiology for the health professions,* ed 6, St. Louis, 2018, Elsevier.
O_2, Oxygen; *RBC,* red blood cell.

Diagnosis

Most cases are diagnosed in infancy with blood testing of newborns. Whether newborn, child, or adult, high-performance liquid chromatography (HPLC) is the test of choice for diagnosis. The testing identifies the presence and amounts of abnormal hemoglobin. Another test called *thin-layer isoelectric focusing* uses the electrical properties of cells to identify variations. During crisis, there will be elevations of serum bilirubin because of the hemolysis of the abnormal RBCs. Skeletal x-rays reveal bone and joint abnormalities.

Treatment

Sickle cell disease is a chronic condition that is not reversible at this time. In 2017, the *New England Journal of Medicine* published an article in which a teenager in France was treated with an autologous hematopoietic stem cell transplantation (HSCT) where the cells were genetically modified to deliver an antisickling variant of hemoglobin. There were no symptoms of sickle cell disease 2 years after the procedure (Ribeil et al., 2017). Multiple clinical trials continue for similar treatments. HSCT not using autologous cells has been successful, but finding a donor match is problematic and the procedure is expensive and has multiple risks.

Treatment is focused on prevention of sickle cell crisis and managing symptoms when crisis occurs. Patients should be taking folic acid regularly and eating a diet with sufficient protein to help build RBCs. Infection is to be prevented, and the patient should receive all recommended immunizations against influenza, hepatitis A and B, pneumonia, tetanus, and other diseases. **Adequate intake of fluid daily is important to keep the blood as fluid as possible.** Alcohol and recreational drugs are to be avoided because they can cause complications. Quick attention for illness should be sought.

The drug hydroxyurea (Hydrea) has been found to reduce the frequency of sickling episodes. Patients taking this drug have shown a decrease in the number of hospitalizations, painful episodes, acute chest syndrome, and mortality (Rodgers & George, 2018). An alternative medication for those who cannot tolerate hydroxyurea is pharmaceutical grade L-glutamine. It can also be used in addition to hydroxyurea (Nihara et al., 2018). If a crisis occurs, the patient may be treated at home with bed rest, adequate fluid intake, and analgesics. Pain control is important during a crisis. Narcotic analgesia with morphine is administered on a continuous basis, usually by patient-controlled analgesia (PCA) pump. If the patient's hemoglobin drops considerably or their condition suddenly deteriorates, they are hospitalized, given oxygen and IV fluids, and transfused with packed RBCs. An attempt is made to mobilize the sickled cells and to prevent damage to major organs. Infection is treated with appropriate antibiotics.

There are many complications of sickle cell disease, including cholecystitis, stroke, pulmonary embolus, congestive heart failure, and damage to all major organs (Fig. 16.3). One of the most common problems is leg ulcers from impaired circulation to the legs and feet. Protecting the feet and lower legs from injury is important because small wounds tend to develop into difficult-to-heal ulcers.

Nursing Management

Nursing care is aimed at relieving the symptoms from complications of the disease and minimizing organ damage. Patients are taught to avoid high altitudes, vigorous exercise, and iced liquids. Patients are to maintain adequate fluid intake, refrain from smoking, and obtain treatment for infections promptly. Adequate rest is important because patients with sickle cell anemia experience fatigue. **Assessment for adequate pain relief is a top priority** (Field, Vichinsky, & DeBaun, 2018). Intake and output will be monitored to prevent overloading the patient with fluid. Oxygen therapy is instituted if the patient is hypoxic (oxygen therapy helps prevent further cellular damage).

POLYCYTHEMIA VERA

Polycythemia vera is a neoplastic disorder resulting in overproduction of RBCs. WBC numbers sometimes also increase but not to the degree that they do in leukemia. The major cause of polycythemia vera is a mutation in the *JAK2* gene, which is a protein switch that tells the cells to grow. What prompts the gene mutation is not known, but the condition is not hereditary. The blood becomes thick from the increased numbers of cells, blood vessels become distended, and blood flow is sluggish. Because of the sluggish flow, there is a tendency to develop blood clots. Blood pressure is elevated and the heart hypertrophies. Bleeding is common in areas of distended blood vessels. Signs and symptoms of polycythemia vera include a reddish face with deep red–purplish lips, fatigue, weakness, dizziness, headache, enlarged spleen (**splenomegaly**), and congested liver. Minor injury may result in excessive bleeding.

Diagnosis includes a genetic test for the JAK2V617F mutation. This mutation is positive in 95% of cases of polycythemia vera.

Treatment is aimed at reducing the number of blood cells and preventing complications. Phlebotomy, antineoplastic agents, and radiation therapy are all used. In phlebotomy, a blood vessel is pierced, and blood is drawn off. As much as 500 mL of blood at a time may be withdrawn every 2 to 3 months. Ruxolitinib is a *JAK1/2* inhibitor that has been approved for use in patients who cannot take hydroxyurea or in whom it has not worked. **Increased fluid intake is essential to decrease blood viscosity, and aspirin is used to decrease platelet clumping and clot formation.**

A secondary polycythemia may develop in response to prolonged hypoxia and increased erythropoietin secretion. Secondary polycythemia does not have the same effects as primary polycythemia. In addition, 20% of patients develop acute myelogenous leukemia (AML).

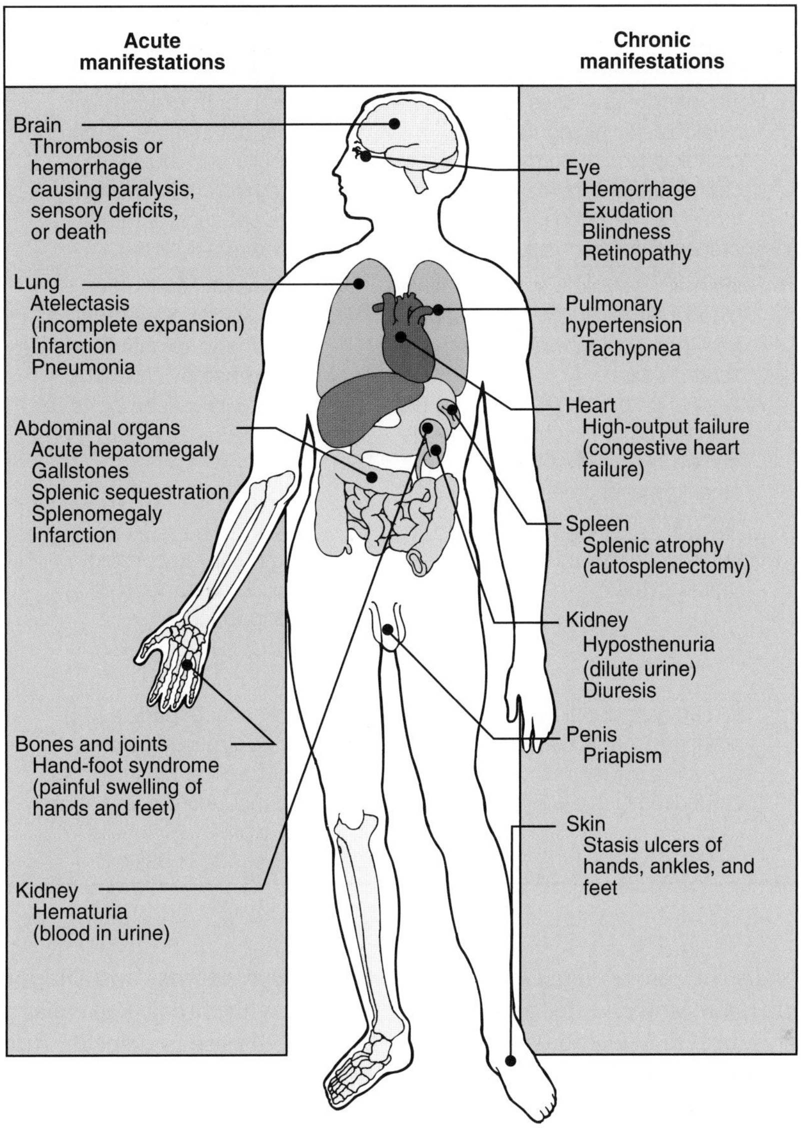

Fig. 16.3 Clinical manifestations and complications of sickle cell disease. (From McCance KL, Huether SE: *Pathophysiology*, ed 8, St. Louis, 2019, Elsevier.)

LEUKEMIA

The word *leukemia,* translated literally, means "white blood." Since the disease is a cancer of the bone marrow, which produces WBCs, it is aptly named. There are various types of leukemia, some more likely in children and some found primarily in adults. Specific leukemia type, age, and physical condition determine the best treatment options (Table 16.5).

Etiology

Leukemia is a cancer and, as with other types of cancers, the exact cause is not known. There are factors considered to be closely linked with the development of leukemia. **Exposure to ionizing radiation in relatively large doses is one such factor. Another is exposure to certain chemicals, such as benzene, that are toxic to bone marrow.** Benzene is an ingredient in lead-free gasoline, and the incidence of leukemia has risen since lead-free gasoline has been in use. The amount of exposure to benzene and other chemicals that cause bone marrow suppression is unknown, and this amount possibly varies among individuals. **It is prudent to be careful about breathing gasoline fumes and using household chemicals and pesticides.** The third factor is the retrovirus known as *human T-lymphotropic virus 1 (HTLV-1),* which causes human T-cell leukemia. People with an abnormal number of chromosomes and chromosomal translocations are at a greater risk for developing acute lymphocytic leukemia. About 90% of patients with chronic myelogenous leukemia have the Philadelphia chromosome.

Malignant production of WBCs is the actual cause of the disease. DNA becomes damaged, and abnormal cell production results.

Pathophysiology

An acute leukemia is one in which there is a large number of immature cells, called *blasts.* These cells do not mature and stay in the bone marrow, impairing the

Table 16.5 Types of Leukemia

TYPE	PATHOPHYSIOLOGY	DEMOGRAPHICS	STAGING
Acute myelogenous (AML)	Bone marrow produces abnormal myeloblasts leading to granulocytes. Abnormal red blood cells and platelets may also be formed by the bone marrow. There are 8 different subsets of AML.	Occurs in both children and adults but is more common in adults and affects men more often than women. Five-year survival rate is approximately 26%.	Based on microscopic examination of the myeloblasts and number of myeloblasts.
Chronic myelogenous (CML)	Bone marrow makes too many white blood cells (WBCs). Can change from slowly progressing to an acute form. Abnormal chromosome (Philadelphia chromosome; Ph chromosome) is formed by the breaking apart of other chromosomes and recombines into the cancer gene.	Affects mostly adults. For those whose gene mutation responds to targeted cancer therapy (imatinib), 5-year survival can be up to 90%.	Based on the WBC count at the time of diagnosis and number of myeloblasts.
Acute lymphocytic (ALL) (also called acute lymphoblastic leukemia)	Bone marrow makes too many lymphocytes.	Occurs mostly in children. Most common form of childhood leukemia. Survival rate is >85%.	Based on microscopic examination of the lymphocytes. WBC count may also be used.
Chronic lymphocytic (CLL)	Too many abnormal lymphocytes are produced in the bone marrow, crowding out normal cells. Hairy cell leukemia is a rare subtype of CLL.	Primarily affects people >55 years. Rare in children. Most common type of adult leukemia. Affects men more than women. Five-year survival rate is 82%.	Based on the WBC count at the time of diagnosis.

production of healthy cells. In chronic leukemia, the abnormal cells build up at a slower rate, allowing production of some normal cells. Leukemias are also classified by the origin of the abnormal cells. Myeloid leukemia arises from the bone marrow, whereas lymphoid leukemia has its origin in the lymphatic system. There are four main types of leukemia: acute myelogenous leukemia (AML), chronic myelogenous leukemia (CML), acute lymphocytic leukemia (ALL), and chronic lymphocytic leukemia (CLL).

Each year about 60,300 people will develop leukemia, and 24,370 people in the United States will die of it (Leukemia & Lymphoma Society, 2018). In acute leukemia there is a sudden, rapid growth of immature blast or stem cells, rapid progression of the disease, and a short survival if the disease is not treated.

Chronic forms of leukemia have a more gradual onset, a slower disease progression, and a relatively longer survival time. CLL is common in men older than 50 years and accounts for one third of the new cases of leukemia annually. CML is most common in young and middle-age adults. CML can progress to the acute form, with a poorer prognosis.

Leukemia has three major effects:

1. Increased numbers of abnormal, immature leukocytes
2. Accumulations of these cells within the bone marrow
3. Eventual infiltration of the malignant cells throughout lymph nodes, spleen, and other organs of the body

Signs, Symptoms, and Diagnosis

Patients with chronic leukemias are often asymptomatic, and the disease is detected during a regular physical examination and routine CBC. Other signs and symptoms of leukemias include fever, headaches, bone pain, pallor, weakness, fatigue, malaise, frequent or persistent infections (sore throat, flu, etc.), swollen lymph nodes, enlarged spleen, bone pain, weight loss, and easy bleeding or thrombosis. Diagnosis is made by using the history, physical examination, CBC with differential, and bone marrow studies to rule out other disorders.

Safety Alert

Chemotherapy

Although it is not within the scope of practice of licensed practical/vocational nurses (LPN/LVNs) in most states to administer IV chemotherapy, oral chemotherapy agents are frequently given. Many of the IV and oral chemotherapy drugs require special handling for the safety of the nurse. Know the safety protocols for any medications requiring special precautions.

Treatment

Treatment is aimed at:

- Slowing down the growth of the malignant blood cells
- Maintaining a normal level of RBCs, hemoglobin, and platelets

- Managing the symptoms and meeting the special needs of each patient
- Exploring possible "curative" therapies such as HCT

Acute leukemia treatment consists primarily of chemotherapy with a combination of antineoplastic agents targeted at different phases of the cell cycle. The drug therapy is divided into three phases: induction, consolidation, and maintenance. *Remission induction therapy* is initiated at the time of diagnosis and consists of an intensive combination chemotherapy aimed at achieving a complete remission of symptoms. *Consolidation therapy* is another course of the same agents, or others, at a different dosage level, and the goal is to achieve cure. *Maintenance therapy* is usually oral chemotherapy at lesser doses taken for 2 to 5 years to maintain remission.

Older Adult Care Points

Patients older than 65 years require reduced dosages of chemotherapeutic drugs (to prevent toxicity) because they have decreased kidney and liver function and the drugs are not metabolized as quickly in older adults as they are in younger persons.

Radiation therapy is sometimes used as a supplement to increase the success of treatment and to decrease discomfort from enlarged organs (spleen, liver). Cure is sometimes possible, as has been evidenced in children with ALL. Results in adults have not been as good. HCT is a possibility for patients who have had an initial remission with chemotherapy. Currently monoclonal antibody treatment combined with HCT is showing promising results in selected patients. Chimeric antigen receptor (CAR) T-cell therapy involves taking the patient's T cells, modifying them in the laboratory so that the cells recognize cancer cells, and reinfusing the T cells so that they kill the cancer. Chronic lymphocytic leukemia—the most common leukemia seen in older adults—is not treated until the patient experiences symptoms. At that time a combination of chemotherapy agents is used. **Leukapheresis** (separation of WBCs) may be done to reduce the massive number of circulating leukocytes that clog organs and cause damage. Blood is drawn, the unwanted WBCs are separated out, and the remainder is returned to the patient.

Chronic myelogenous leukemia is treated with chemotherapy. Once the initial therapy controls the disease, HCT is recommended. The treatment protocols rely extensively on tyrosine kinase inhibitors (TKIs).

Transfusions of blood components are prescribed for leukemia patients to maintain a near-normal blood picture. Platelet transfusion during or after chemotherapy often is necessary. Antibiotics may be given prophylactically during chemotherapy and are started immediately on signs of infection because the body's defense mechanisms are seriously compromised. Box 16.1 lists the treatments used for the various types of leukemia.

Box 16.1 Treatment for Specific Types of Leukemia

ACUTE LYMPHOCYTIC LEUKEMIA (ALL)

- Induction: vincristine, prednisone, cyclophosphamide, doxorubicin, and L-asparaginase
- Consolidation: including cytarabine and methotrexate
- Maintenance: 6-mercaptopurine, methotrexate, steroids, and vincristine. Methotrexate is given intrathecally throughout.
- Philadelphia chromosome–positive patients receive tyrosine kinase inhibitors (TKIs)
- Blinatumomab (monoclonal antibody)
- Tisagenlecleucel (chimeric antigen receptor [CAR] T-cell therapy)

CHRONIC LYMPHOCYTIC LEUKEMIA (CLL)

- Not treated until symptoms appear: weight loss >10% over 6 months, night sweats >1 month, extreme fatigue, fever related to leukemia for longer than 2 weeks
- Chemotherapy agents: fludarabine, ibrutinib, cyclophosphamide, rituximab, pentostatin, mitoxantrone, vincristine, doxorubicin, prednisone
- Monoclonal antibodies are used for specific types of CLL.
- Venetoclax, a Bcl-2 inhibitor, is newly approved. Bcl-2 helps keep cancer cells alive; through its inhibition, cancer cells die.

ACUTE MYELOGENOUS LEUKEMIA (AML)

- All-trans retinoic acid (ATRA) is started when APL (a subtype of AML) is suspected and combined with anthracycline-based chemotherapy after diagnosis.
- Induction: anthracycline, cytarabine
- Remission therapy: cytarabine and HCT
- Ivosidenib, a targeted agent for adults with relapsed or refractory AML
- Gemtuzumab ozogamicin (monoclonal antibody)

CHRONIC MYELOGENOUS LEUKEMIA (CML)

- Initial therapy: TKIs. There are multiple TKI medications, and the specific drug and dose recommended depends on age, blood counts, spleen size, and other criteria.
- Accelerate phase: TKIs, omacetaxine
- Blast phase: HCT, TKIs

Nursing Management

A thorough health assessment is performed, and specific problems are identified. Problem statements for a patient with leukemia include those appropriate for anemia, leukopenia, and thrombocytopenia. Patient problems to be addressed are:

- Potential for infection
- Abnormal bleeding
- Anemia
- Nutritional alteration with severe anorexia and weight loss
- Psychosocial problems related to the effects of the disease as well as the prescribed treatment
- Alteration in comfort

Collaboration with the dietitian and the pharmacist is a key point in nursing care of a patient with leukemia.

Nursing Care Plan 16.1 presents care for common problems of patients with leukemia.

Infections from bacteria, viruses, and fungi are the most common cause of death in people with leukemia. Infection is a threat either because of abnormal function of bone marrow that is characteristic of the disease or because of suppression of bone marrow function as a result of therapy. Nursing measures to prevent infection are essential, as is vigilant assessment for early signs (see Chapter 8 for information about risk for infection from the effects of chemotherapy or radiation).

Abnormal bleeding as a result of a very low platelet count is the second most common and dangerous complication of leukemia. Observation of the patient, awareness of the patient's current platelet count, and prevention of trauma to body tissues and blood vessels as a result of low platelets are primary concerns in nursing management.

Safety Alert

Prevent Bleeding

For a patient with a low platelet count, whenever venipuncture is performed, an injection is administered, or an IV catheter or needle is discontinued, pressure over the site must be maintained for at least 10 minutes to prevent continuous oozing.

Older Adult Care Points

- Older adult patients already have decreased immune system function. When leukemia develops, or is treated, these patients are at very high risk for infection.
- Older adult patients cannot tolerate hemorrhage, and so hemorrhage must be carefully guarded against.
- Other conditions may affect appetite. Emphasis on an appropriate diet, supplements, good nutritional status, and excellent mouth care can make a marked difference in the quality of life of an older adult with leukemia.

Nursing Care Plan 16.1 Care of the Patient With Leukemia

SCENARIO

James Cathcart, a 42-year-old man, has acute myelogenous leukemia (AML). He is undergoing outpatient chemotherapy and is being followed at home by a home care agency nurse.

PROBLEM STATEMENT/NURSING DIAGNOSIS

Potential for infection related to low WBCs.

SUPPORTING ASSESSMENT DATA

Objective: WBCs 2000/mm^3.

Goals/Expected Outcomes	Nursing Interventions	Selected Rationale	Evaluation
Patient will remain free of infection.	Monitor temperature daily. Report elevation >100.4° F (>38° C) that lasts for more than 4 h.	Temperature elevation may indicate beginning infection.	Temp remains at 99.2° F (37.3° C).
	Teach patient and family to perform hand hygiene frequently.	Hand hygiene helps prevent infection.	Hand hygiene used consistently.
	Use meticulous hand hygiene when caring for patient.	Helps prevent transmission of microorganisms.	
	Have patient deep-breathe q2h while awake.	Respiratory exercises help prevent respiratory infection from pooled secretions.	Using incentive spirometer regularly.
	Administer transfusion of granulocytes as needed.	Granulocyte transfusion provides WBCs to help fight infection.	Transfusion not ordered yet.
	Caution to eat only cooked fruits and vegetables.	Raw foods often carry bacteria that could cause infection.	States understands need to eat only cooked foods.

PROBLEM STATEMENT/NURSING DIAGNOSIS

Fatigue related to chemotherapy side effects.

SUPPORTING ASSESSMENT DATA

Subjective: States has no energy; frequently falls asleep.

Objective: RBCs 3.2 million/mm^3, Hct 33 mL/dL.

Goals/Expected Outcomes	Nursing Interventions	Selected Rationale	Evaluation
Patient will be able to bathe and dress self without assistance.	Provide bathing assistance daily as needed, encouraging self-care.	Conserves patient's energy.	Bathing assistance given daily, now able to dress self.
	Encourage resting between care activities.	Prevents undue fatigue.	Is resting between activities.
	Encourage to perform activities of daily living (ADLs) in small segments.	Preserves energy.	Is combing hair and brushing teeth.

Nursing Care Plan 16.1 Care of the Patient With Leukemia—cont'd

PROBLEM STATEMENT/NURSING DIAGNOSIS

Altered family functioning related to loss of patient's income.

SUPPORTING ASSESSMENT DATA

Subjective: Patient too weak to work; wife seeking full-time employment.

Goals/Expected Outcomes	Nursing Interventions	Selected Rationale	Evaluation
Patient's wife will cope effectively as primary wage earner.	Assist wife with defining alternatives for employment.	Helps focus direction for employment.	Wife is considering possible alternatives.
	Arrange consultation with social worker to coordinate patient's care when wife returns to work.	Social worker can arrange in-home assistance.	Social services appointment made.
	Suggest community resources that might help wife find employment.		Wife given list of community resources for employment.

PROBLEM STATEMENT/NURSING DIAGNOSIS

Potential for bleeding related to decreased platelets.

SUPPORTING ASSESSMENT DATA

Objective: Platelets 106,000/mm^3.

Goals/Expected Outcomes	Nursing Interventions	Selected Rationale	Evaluation
Patient will not experience episodes of bleeding.	Monitor CBC and platelet counts.	Will detect further decrease in platelets.	CBC remaining stable, but platelets down to 104,000/mm^3.
	Instruct to report oozing of blood from the gums.	Alerts to potential for impending bleeding episode.	No oozing of blood.
	Instruct to observe stool and urine for signs of bleeding.		
	Administer stool softener to prevent constipation.	Soft stool will not injure rectal mucosa, causing bleeding.	Stool soft without signs of blood.
	Instruct to use soft toothbrush or toothettes to clean teeth.	Helps prevent small breaks in mucosa or skin that might cause bleeding.	Using soft toothbrush and electric razor.
	Instruct to use an electric razor to shave.		
	Assess home for safety concerns.	Loose rugs are a fall risk; furniture placement may promote bumps, leading to bruises.	Safety assessment of home completed, recommendations made.

CRITICAL THINKING QUESTIONS

1. What measures are necessary for a patient who is immunosuppressed from chemotherapy and is susceptible to infections?
2. How could you help boost Mr. Cathcart's self-esteem now that he must give up his role as the family wage earner?

Anemia and its associated problems of fatigue, hypoxia, GI upsets, and cardiovascular complications affect patients with leukemia. The anemia can result from the disease itself, from excessive bleeding, or from the therapy administered. Nursing measures previously described for a patient with anemia are appropriate to the care of a patient with leukemia. Colony-stimulating factor drugs sometimes are used to counteract the anemia and neutropenia caused by treatment for leukemia. However, these drugs may stimulate the growth of abnormal cells, making the patient's condition worse, and so they are used with caution.

Nutritional problems arise from a number of conditions. **Extreme weight loss and cachexia are nearly always seen in patients with advanced cancer.** Failure to eat sufficient amounts of nutritious foods is not the only reason this is so. As explained in Chapter 8, metabolic changes that occur with the proliferation of malignant cells in the body also are responsible for weight loss and emaciation. If nursing measures to alleviate or minimize **stomatitis** (inflammation of the mouth), nausea, and vomiting are not effective, parenteral nutrition may be indicated. Enteral and parenteral nutrition should be thoroughly discussed by the health care team, patient, and family before implementation near end of life. If the nutritional deficit is secondary to HCT therapy, nutritional supplementation or replacement can be beneficial (Kim et al., 2018).

Tumor lysis syndrome results from rapid cell destruction during chemotherapy. Killing the leukemia cells releases intracellular contents into the circulation, causing a rapid change in blood chemistry. The syndrome consists of hyperuricemia, hyperkalemia, hyperphosphatemia, hypocalcemia, and acute kidney injury. Monitoring laboratory values, assessing renal function, and reporting significant changes to the health care provider are extremely important. The emotional effect of a diagnosis of cancer and the psychosocial needs of the cancer patient and the family are discussed in Chapter 8.

> **? Think Critically**
>
> Why is it common for a patient with leukemia to have frequent infections? What causes this problem? When caring for a leukemia patient, what parameters would you need to assess to detect early signs of infection?

COAGULATION DISORDERS

THROMBOCYTOPENIA

Thrombocytopenia occurs when the platelet count drops to less than 150,000/mm^3 and can be a life-threatening condition. Causes include bone marrow depression from chemotherapy or radiation, autoimmune diseases, bacterial and viral infections, disseminated intravascular coagulation (DIC), and overfunction of the spleen. Certain drugs, such as nonsteroidal antiinflammatory drugs (NSAIDs) and thiazides, also can result in platelet deficiency. Increased use of heparin preparations for deep vein thrombosis prophylaxis has led to more instances of heparin-induced thrombocytopenia. Heparin triggers antibodies that prompt platelet activation, resulting in formation of clots and depletion of platelets. While platelet counts are low, the primary problem is clotting.

Immune thrombocytopenic purpura (ITP) is the most commonly acquired thrombocytopenia. It is an autoimmune disease in which there is abnormal destruction of circulating platelets. In ITP the platelets are covered with antibodies. In the spleen, these platelets are recognized as foreign and are destroyed by macrophages. This disorder commonly occurs in women between 20 and 40 years of age. The chronic form of ITP has a gradual onset, with transient remissions.

Many patients with thrombocytopenia are asymptomatic. Signs and symptoms of thrombocytopenia include **purpura** (purple spots and patches and small areas of multiple petechiae in the skin and mucous membranes) or large bruised areas caused by hemorrhage that are called **ecchymoses** (Fig. 16.4). Bleeding can occur in any part of the body. Hemorrhage is the major danger.

Some patients recover spontaneously. Otherwise, corticosteroids are administered to reduce the rate of platelet destruction and IV immunoglobulin or, for select patients, IV Rho immunoglobulin. Splenectomy usually results in lifelong remission in acute conditions. In chronic cases the outcome is less predictable. Platelet transfusions are used only for significant clinical bleeding. Fostamatinib was recently approved by the FDA. It is a spleen tyrosine kinase (SYK) inhibitor and is used to block the destruction of the platelets by the spleen.

Nursing care is focused on prevention of bleeding by careful handling of the patient, close observation for signs of spontaneous bleeding, and quick intervention. Invasive procedures are used only when essential. Patients are taught to avoid activities that might induce bleeding (see Chapter 8).

MULTIPLE MYELOMA

Multiple myeloma is a disease in which neoplastic plasma cells infiltrate the bone marrow and destroy bone. In 2018 30,770 new cases were expected in the United States. Men are affected twice as often as women, and the disease occurs in African Americans twice as often as in whites. The disease usually occurs after age 40 years, with the average age at diagnosis being 65 years.

Etiology and Pathophysiology

The cause of multiple myeloma is unknown. Risk factors include a family tendency toward the disease; ionizing radiation; and exposure to herbicides, insecticides, and chemicals (particularly benzene). Genetic factors and viral infections may play a role.

In multiple myeloma, abnormal plasma cells multiply out of control in the bone marrow. These abnormal cells produce excessive amounts of abnormal immune globulin and cytokines. The accumulation of the abnormal cells (tumors) in the bone marrow disrupts normal RBC, leukocyte, and platelet production. The disruption of normal cell production leads to anemia, impaired immune response with susceptibility to infection, and bleeding tendencies. The tumors disrupt normal bone marrow function and weaken the bone, predisposing the patient to frequent fractures.

Signs, Symptoms, and Diagnosis

The onset of multiple myeloma is gradual, and symptoms appear when the skeletal system is heavily involved. The patient may experience backache, bone pain that is worse with movement, or pathologic fractures and severe pain. Multiple myeloma is diagnosed by a combination of x-ray studies, bone marrow biopsy, and blood and urine tests. The appearance of light chains from the abnormal immune globulins in the urine, or Bence-Jones proteins, is a diagnostic sign. Because the bone destruction during multiple myeloma releases calcium, a hypercalcemia that may lead to kidney stone formation and renal impairment occurs. The CBC will show anemia, leukopenia, and thrombocytopenia. Bone marrow studies show large numbers of immature plasma cells.

Treatment

Chemotherapy and HCT are used to combat the disease. Pain control is a primary concern. Hypercalcemia and osteoporosis often develop, and patients must be monitored and treated for these complications. Measures must be taken to prevent pathologic fractures.

Chemotherapy regimens are individualized to the patient based on the results of testing. Bortezomib (Velcade), lenalidomide (Revlimid), and dexamethasone

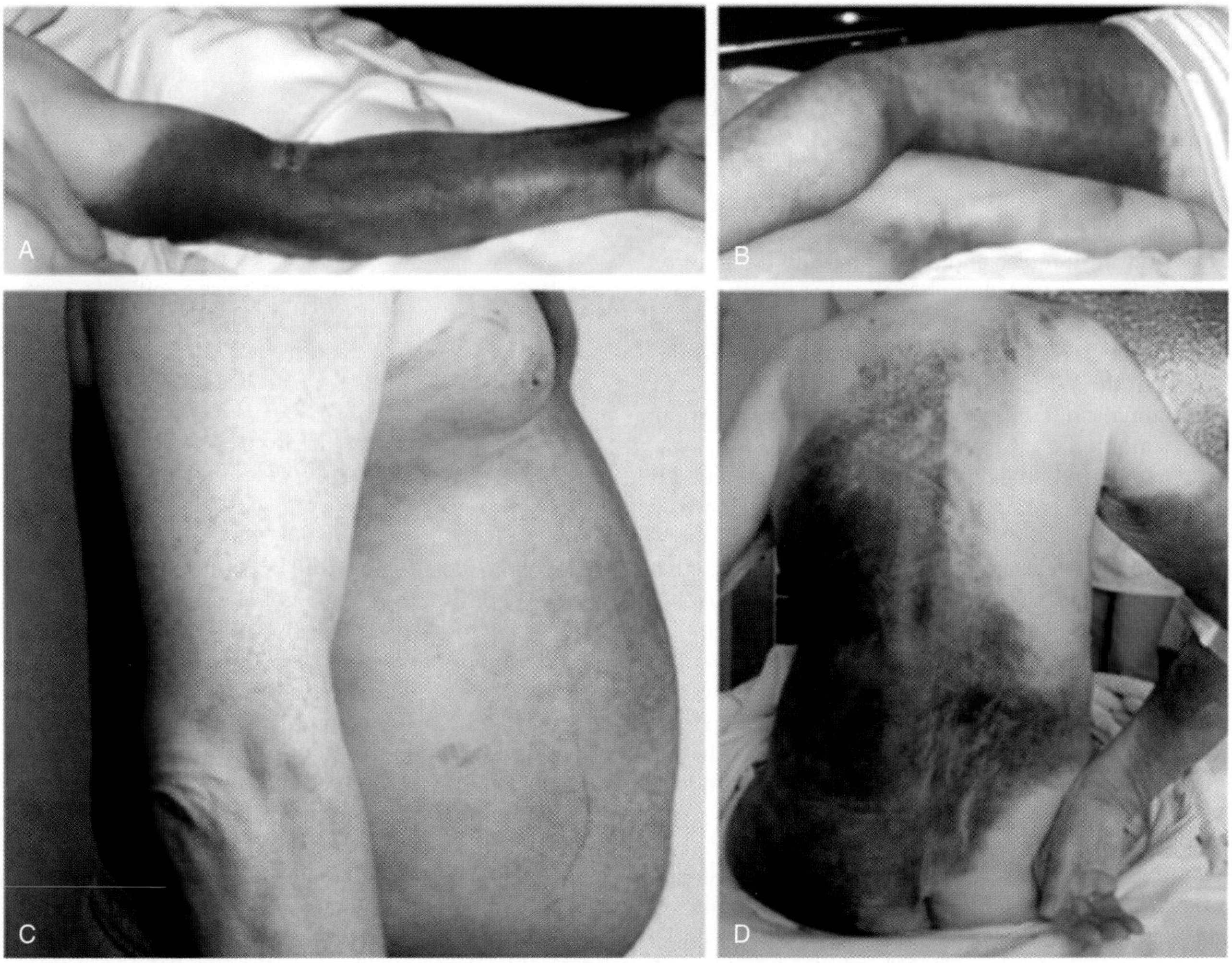

Fig. 16.4 Extensive subcutaneous ecchymoses of the **(A and B)** limbs, **(C)** abdomen, and **(D)** thorax in a patient with acquired hemophilia A. (Courtesy National Library of Medicine, Lister Hill National Center for Biomedical Communications. Retrieved from https://openi.nlm.nih.gov/detailedresult.php?img=PMC2896368_1756-0500-3-161-1&query=ecchymosis+spontaneous&it=xg&req=4&npos=29)

constitute first-line therapy. Adjunctive therapy includes radiation to target areas of pain, erythropoietin, plasmapheresis, and surgical intervention. Bisphosphonates such as etidronate (Didronel), pamidronate (Aredia), or zoledronic acid (Zometa) inhibit bone breakdown and thereby decrease skeletal pain and hypercalcemia.

Nursing Management

Supportive care for the many complications of the disease and treatment is provided. Encouraging adequate hydration with an intake of 3 to 5 L of fluid a day to minimize problems from hypercalcemia is a priority. Pain assessment and management are crucial to the quality of life for the patient. Acetaminophen and NSAIDs are used along with narcotic analgesics. Care is taken when moving the patient because of the potential for fractures.

Psychosocial care is essential because the disease has remissions and exacerbations and is eventually fatal. The nursing care for a patient with a neoplastic disorder is discussed in Chapter 8. The patient and family must be taught about the signs and symptoms of hypercalcemia and instructed to report these signs and symptoms immediately to the health care provider. Measures to prevent falls must be instituted, both in the hospital and in the home. Mental status is monitored closely, and measures to protect the patient are instituted if confusion arises.

> **Assignment Considerations**
>
> **Assisting Patients With Blood Disorders**
>
> When enlisting the aid of a nursing assistant to help with positioning, moving, or toileting the patient, remind the assistant that the patient is very prone to bruising, bleeding, or fractures (as the case may be). Do not assign ambulation of a patient with multiple myeloma to assistive personnel because any slight bump or twist of the body may cause a fracture.

GENETIC BLEEDING DISORDERS

Etiology

Hemophilia is an inherited X-linked disorder in which there is a deficiency of specific clotting factors. Classic hemophilia, or *hemophilia A* with a factor VIII deficiency, affects 20.6 in 5000 males in the United States. *Hemophilia B,* or Christmas disease, causes a deficiency of factor IX. Christmas disease affects 1 in 30,000 male births. Because of the deficiency in the clotting system, both types of hemophilia are characterized by delayed blood coagulation that produces a prolonged period of bleeding after injury or surgery. These types of hemophilia almost always occur in males and are genetically transmitted through the mother. Although the mother does not have the disease herself, she and all her female descendants can transmit classic hemophilia to their offspring. Female carriers of the X-linked recessive condition are usually asymptomatic but under certain conditions may exhibit mild hemophilia.

Acquired hemophilia can affect both men and women, but the disease is rare. Hemophilia can develop as a result of formation of antibody to the clotting factors in blood transfusions, in patients with collagen vascular disease, or after a drug reaction. Idiopathic occurrence may be seen in people older than 50 years of age.

VonWillebrand disease (VWD) is a genetic disorder in which the VonWillebrand clotting factor is absent or defective. This protein binds factor VIII, helping to form clots. In its absence or dysfunction, platelets do not clump correctly. It affects men and women equally.

Pathophysiology

In all types of hemophilia and VWD, there is a decrease in the amount of activity of one of the 11 different clotting factors normally present in blood and essential to the formation of clots. The blood of a patient with hemophilia A forms a clot immediately after injury by platelet aggregation (clumping), but the clot breaks down and does not effectively stop bleeding because of lack of fibrin. In VWD there is a decrease in the activity of factor VIII, which prohibits the initial platelet plug. In hemophilia B, factor IX does not play its normal role in continuing activation of other factors to form a stable clot.

There are varying degrees of severity in the types of hemophilia, depending on the amount of the factor present and the role of the factor in clot formation. For patients with mild cases (those who have 25% to 50% of the deficient factor present in the serum), symptoms may not appear at all until a severe injury or surgery is followed by prolonged bleeding and the hemophilia is thus discovered. In very severe cases (those in which less than 1% of the factor is present), the affected individuals may bleed spontaneously without injury, and severe hemorrhage can develop very quickly whenever an injury does occur.

Signs and Symptoms

The most obvious symptom of hemophilia and VWD is bleeding. The hallmark of hemophilia is bleeding into joints, causing loss of mobility and unequal extremity lengths. Bleeding also occurs internally, with leakage of blood into the intestinal wall or peritoneal cavity and into the deeper tissues of the body. **Hemarthrosis**—bleeding into the joints—produces swelling, pain, warmth, and limitation of movement similar to that experienced by patients with rheumatoid arthritis (Fig. 16.5). Hemarthrosis is the primary problem for most patients with hemophilia. If the bleeding occurs in the intracranial spaces and thereby increases intracranial pressure, the patient may experience convulsions and brain damage that can be fatal. Other serious complications from internal bleeding in a person with hemophilia include obstruction of the airway as a result of hemorrhage into the neck or pharynx and intestinal obstruction resulting from bleeding into the intestinal wall or peritoneum. Bleeding in VWD presents as a history of "bleeding problems" such as frequent nosebleeds, easy bruising, and longer than normal bleeding after injuries or minor surgical procedures.

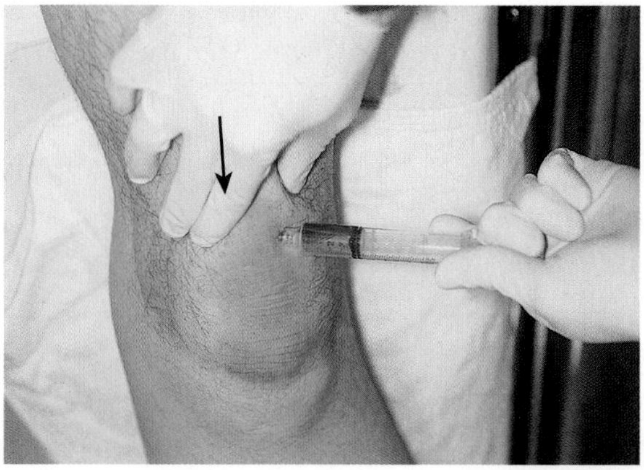

Fig. 16.5 Aspiration of the knee to relieve the hemarthrosis common in hemophilia. (From Roberts JR, Hedges JS: *Clinical procedures in emergency medicine,* ed 5, Philadelphia, 2009, Saunders.)

Diagnosis and Treatment

Diagnosis is by history, physical examination, CBC, coagulation profile, and tests for the various clotting factors in the blood. In the more common types of hemophilia, transfusion of the missing blood factors prevents bleeding. Recombinant forms of factor VIII and factor IX are available and administered IV at various dosages and intervals based on clinical data.

For mild hemophilia A and for some subtypes of VWD, desmopressin acetate (DDAVP), which is a synthetic form of vasopressin, may be given to stimulate an increase in factor VIII and von Willebrand factor. Tranexamic acid (Cyklokapron) and aminocaproic acid (Amicar) are sometimes administered to inhibit fibrinolysis by increasing clot stability. Monoclonal antibodies such as emicizumab or rituximab are used to alter or restore the function of clotting factors.

Analgesic drugs and corticosteroids may be used to treat the joint inflammation and pain caused by hemarthrosis and by the common resultant arthritis. Safe analgesics include acetaminophen, oxycodone, codeine, and tramadol. Prophylactic factor treatment may be administered before dental procedures or in advance of other invasive diagnostic tests and unavoidable surgery.

Safety Alert

Avoid Taking Aspirin

Aspirin must never be taken by patients with hemophilia because aspirin increases the bleeding problems due to its antiplatelet properties. Patients must read the labels on every over-the-counter preparation to be certain that drug products do not contain aspirin or acetylsalicylic acid.

Many patients with hemophilia have been receiving blood products for a number of years. Prior to 1992, screening tools for human immunodeficiency virus (HIV) were not available for donated blood products. Unfortunately, many older patients have been infected with HIV or hepatitis C virus from contaminated plasma concentrates. Better screening and processing have resulted in no new infections with hepatitis or HIV associated with blood products used by hemophilia patients since 1998 (Centers for Disease Control and Prevention [CDC], 2017).

Nursing Management

In addition to administering the necessary clotting factors, interventions include elevating the injured body part, applying cold packs, controlling pain, observing for further bleeding, and providing psychological support for the patient and family. You should also encourage genetic counseling for family members, if this counseling has not occurred previously.

DISSEMINATED INTRAVASCULAR COAGULATION

Disseminated intravascular coagulation (DIC) is a complicated disorder that usually occurs in conjunction with tissue destruction. It is not a disease but a complication of a significant clinical condition. It accompanies serious problems, such as severe trauma, gram-negative sepsis, shock, respiratory distress syndrome, malignancy, transfusion reaction, amniotic embolus, and abruptio placentae (separation of the placenta from the uterine wall).

Damaged tissue liberates tissue thromboplastin, creating a state of excessive clotting in the microcirculation throughout the body. When excessive clotting depletes the body's clotting factors, bleeding follows, which may lead to hypotension or shock. DIC can present as a life-threatening emergency or can be a chronic subclinical process.

The first signs of DIC are usually continued bleeding from an injection or IV site, extensive bruising in areas of injury, ecchymoses where there has been no trauma, and petechiae. There may be oral, vaginal, or rectal bleeding. Laboratory studies will reveal a decreased hemoglobin and low platelet count. The international normalized ratio (INR) (prothrombin) and activated partial thromboplastin times will be increased. The fibrinogen level is reduced, and the fibrin degradation products level is increased. The D-dimer result is elevated.

Treatment consists of correcting the underlying problem (e.g., trauma, infection). Vascular volume is maintained with fluid replacement and vasopressor medications. Mechanical ventilation may be needed for support of oxygenation and ventilation. Packed RBCs are given to support circulation and perfusion. Fresh frozen plasma may be given to replace clotting factors if significant bleeding is present, and platelets may be transfused if platelet levels are below 10,000 μL (Leung, 2018).

As a nursing priority, be alert to the possibility of the development of DIC whenever a patient has a condition that predisposes to it. Early detection of external bleeding and monitoring sensorium and vital signs for indications of internal bleeding are both extremely important.

Chronic DIC is more likely to present with thromboembolic complications because clotting factors are not used up quickly and replacement products are manufactured by the body, keeping pace with those consumed by clots. Many patients with malignancies have no symptoms but laboratory tests show evidence of coagulation and clot breakdown. These patients have a subclinical DIC. Some types of leukemia also cause chronic DIC. If clinical symptoms are present, they are represented by the organs or organ systems affected by the clotting.

THERAPIES FREQUENTLY USED IN THE MANAGEMENT OF HEMATOLOGIC DISORDERS

TRANSFUSIONS

A blood transfusion involves the administration of a blood component. To minimize the risks of circulatory overload, infection, transfusion reaction, and other problems related to the administration, blood usually is transfused only when there has been a large blood loss, when the patient has a deficiency of a blood component, or when there must be a total blood exchange in a newborn. Table 16.6 shows some commonly used blood products, the usual amount given per transfusion, and reasons why each is used.

Autologous (originating in one's self) blood transfusion is commonly used when the patient's own blood can be collected and reinfused. Blood is collected either during or after surgery (such as from chest drainage), or blood is donated by the patient during the weeks before surgery for later use. Laboratory procedures that separate the various components by centrifuge or other means allow for the administration of only the particular element of blood needed by a particular patient.

Several artificial substitutes for human blood are being tested, but none of them can provide all of the functions of human blood. So far the FDA has only approved substances being used in clinical trials.

Table 16.6 Blood Products and Their Use

COMPONENT	VOLUME	INFUSION TIME	INDICATIONS
Packed red blood cells (PRBCs)	200–250 mL	1–4 hr	Anemia; hemoglobin <6 g/dL, depending on symptoms
Washed red blood cells (WBC-poor PRBCs)	200 mL	1–4 hr	History of allergic transfusion reactions Bone marrow transplantation patients
Platelets			
Pooled	About 300 mL	15–30 min	Thrombocytopenia, platelet count <20,000/mm^3 Patients who are actively bleeding with a platelet count <50,000/mm^3
Single donor	200 mL	30 min	History of febrile or allergic reactions
Fresh frozen plasma	200 mL	15–30 min	Deficiency in plasma coagulation factors Prothrombin or partial thromboplastin time 1.5 times normal
Cryoprecipitate	10–20 mL/unit	15–30 min	Hemophilia A or von Willebrand disease Fibrinogen levels <100 mg/dL
White blood cells (WBCs)	400 mL	1 hr	Sepsis; neutropenic infection not responding to antibiotic therapy

Adapted from Ignatavicius DD, Workman ML, Rebar CR, et al.: *Medical-surgical nursing: critical thinking for collaborative care,* ed 9, St. Louis, 2017, Elsevier.

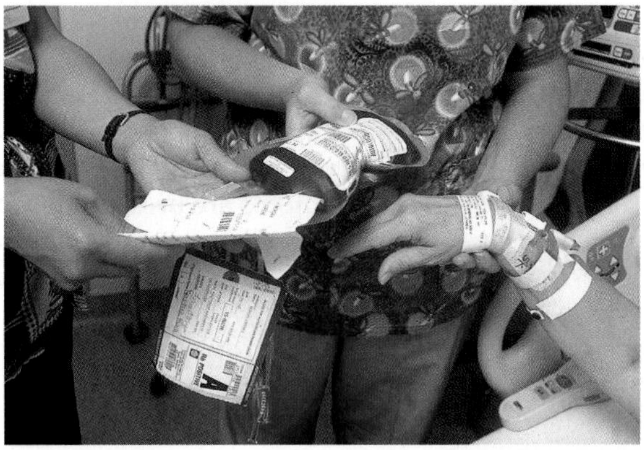

Fig. 16.6 Two nurses must check the label on the blood product bag, the blood administration form of the blood bank, and the patient's armband and blood bracelet.

Special precautions are always taken when any blood component is given. Blood banks have written procedures and policies for withdrawing and dispensing blood for transfusion.

Legal and Ethical Considerations

Consent for Blood Administration

The patient must have signed a consent form to receive a blood transfusion. If the patient is unable to sign and the condition is life-threatening and no family member is reachable, the health care provider may make the decision to transfuse the patient.

Blood products are always checked by two nurses before administration (Fig. 16.6). Check facility policy and state law for procedures. Some facilities require that two registered nurses (RNs) check the blood, and some allow a LPN/LVN with appropriate training to be one of the two licensed nurses.

Legal and Ethical Considerations

Check the LPN/LVN Role

Some states have expanded their LPN/LVN practice act to include the administration of blood products. Check your state's nurse practice act to see if that procedure is within legal practice in your state.

All blood bank and agency policies must be strictly followed to decrease the possibility of an adverse reaction or the administration of wrong blood to the wrong patient.

Nursing Management

Determine whether the patient has an IV site already established and note what size catheter is in place. If rapid infusion is needed, give blood through at least an 18-gauge catheter. Slower infusions can be given through 20-14 gauge devices. Ensure patency of the infusion site before obtaining blood products from the blood bank. The only solution that should be used is 0.9% saline. No other fluids or medications should be given with the blood or blood components unless they are FDA approved. The administration set is primed and set up prior to obtaining the blood.

Older Adult Care Points

- Vessels in older adults are fragile. A 22-gauge cannula may be used for transfusion to older adults.
- Blood products should be transfused more slowly, to allow an older adult's body time to adjust to the added fluid.
- Careful assessment for fluid overload during and after the transfusion is essential. Signs of fluid overload are rapid, bounding pulse; hypertension; dyspnea; and visibly swollen veins.

After obtaining the blood from the blood bank, it must be infused within 4 hours. If the blood is not going to be infused, it can be returned to the blood bank if it has been out of the refrigerator for no more than 30 minutes. Blood infusion sets can be used for 4 hours or for two units of blood. If a second unit of blood can be infused in the 4-hour window, the same administration set can be used. All blood must be filtered. Filters may be built into the administration set or added to the tubing (Gorski et al., 2016). Blood products are typically between 200 and 300 mL. It is important to assess the patient and how well they may tolerate the colloid fluid volume in the time frame required. If a unit of blood is to be given slower than over 4 hours, request that the blood bank divide the unit.

Safety Alert

Blood Product Safety

Blood bags should never be heated in a microwave oven or placed in hot water. No other solution or drug is ever administered through the same line or to the same site through which blood is infusing because destruction of the cells might occur or a precipitate that could cause emboli might be formed.

Think Critically

If there has been carelessness in the proper identification method used to ensure that the right blood is given to the right patient and the patient has a reaction, could you be sued for negligence?

Transfusion Reaction

The word *reaction* means sensitivity to the blood itself or sensitivity to the preservatives or other substances that have been added to a solution. Reactions to RBCs are the result of incompatibility between blood types. Antigens on the surfaces of RBCs can bring about a reaction when exposed to blood that is not the same type and is incompatible. The antigen-antibody reaction causes the cells to clump together and obstruct the flow of blood through the capillaries. A major blood reaction usually results from giving the wrong blood to the patient. A mild reaction is usually caused by antibodies in the donor blood and not the RBCs themselves.

Safety Alert

Signs and Symptoms of a Transfusion Reaction

The symptoms of a transfusion reaction may be so mild that they go unnoticed or so severe that death is the outcome (Table 16.7). In milder cases, the patient may develop a rash, hives, itching, or facial flushing. In more severe reactions, the patient may experience a variety of problems, including shock.

Diphenhydramine hydrochloride (Benadryl) may be ordered IV if itching or hives occur. In severe anaphylactic reactions the treatment is the same as for anaphylaxis caused by any extreme hypersensitivity. Other signs of reaction include the patient's temperature rising 2 degrees above the starting temperature. In any significant reaction, the infusion is stopped, the IV kept patent, and the health care provider notified. Follow the policies of the facility if a reaction occurs. As long as there are no signs of adverse reaction, the patient is assessed and vital signs are taken every 30 to 60 minutes until the transfusion is completed, depending on agency policy.

Think Critically

Your patient is receiving a unit of packed RBCs. When you assess them after the first hour of the transfusion, the pulse rate has increased from 78 to 84, they are slightly restless, and they are complaining of discomfort in the back. The temperature has risen from 98.4° F to 99° F. They have no skin rash and deny nausea. What would you do?

LEUKAPHERESIS

Leukapheresis is a procedure performed to clear excessive WBCs from the blood. Leukapheresis may be performed directly on the patient, or the procedure may be performed on separated blood products. When performed directly, the patient is connected to a blood separator machine. Blood is drained a bit at a time from the patient, the WBCs are washed out of the blood, and the RBCs and plasma are returned to the patient. This treatment is used to lower the WBC count in patients with CML and is sometimes used to treat certain immune disorders, such as myasthenia gravis.

BIOLOGIC RESPONSE MODIFIERS: COLONY-STIMULATING FACTOR THERAPY

Research with DNA-recombinant techniques has developed drugs that stimulate the bone marrow to produce erythrocytes or neutrophils. Erythropoietin (Epogen) is given parenterally to patients who have decreased erythropoietin resulting from end-stage renal disease or who have suppressed bone marrow from the toxicity of chemotherapy given for malignancy, rheumatoid arthritis, or HIV.

Granulocyte colony-stimulating factor (G-CSF; Neupogen, Neulasta) is given parenterally to combat neutropenia. It is used for patients with bone marrow suppression from chemotherapy, particularly for those with non–blood-related malignancies. Granulocyte-macrophage colony-stimulating factor (GM-CSF; Leukine) accelerates the recovery of bone marrow after autologous HCT in patients with ALL, Hodgkin disease, or non-Hodgkin lymphoma who have undergone total destruction of the bone marrow during therapy.

HEMATOPOIETIC CELL TRANSPLANTATION (HCT)

HCT is aimed at providing healthy blood cell–producing capability when the patient's own bone marrow is faulty or has been destroyed by chemotherapy or irradiation

Table 16.7 Acute Transfusion Reactions

TYPE	CAUSE	CLINICAL MANIFESTATIONS AND MANAGEMENT	PREVENTION
Acute hemolytic reaction	Infusion of ABO-incompatible blood or components containing ≥10 mL RBCs. Antibodies in the recipient's plasma attach to antigens on transfused RBCs, causing RBC destruction.	Chills, fever, low back pain, flushing, tachycardia, tachypnea, hypotension, dark urine, shock, death. Stop transfusion. Treat shock if present. Maintain BP with IV colloid solutions. Treat other symptoms as needed for comfort while maintaining BP. Monitor hourly urine output. Dialysis may be required if renal failure occurs. Notify health care provider and implement protocol for laboratory follow-up.	Meticulously verify and document patient identification from sample collection to component infusion. Most ABO compatibility reactions are a result of the wrong blood to the wrong patient.
Allergic reactions	Antibody-mediated response to donor plasma proteins.	Itching, urticaria. Antihistamines are given and the transfusion continued.	If a previous allergic reaction has occurred, premedication with an antihistamine may be given.
Nonhemolytic febrile reactions	Sensitization to donor WBCs, platelets, or plasma proteins. Sensitivity to foreign plasma proteins.	Chills, hypertension, tachycardia, dyspnea. Stop the transfusion. Antipyretics for fever. Additional medications usually not indicated.	In patients with repeated reactions, premedication with antipyretics may be helpful and/or use of leukoreduced blood products.
Circulatory overload	Fluid administered faster than the circulation can accommodate.	Dyspnea, hypertension, pulmonary congestion, headache, tachycardia, distended neck veins. Place patient upright with feet in dependent position. Administer prescribed diuretics, oxygen, and morphine.	Adjust transfusion volume and flow rate based on patient size and clinical status. Have blood bank divide unit into smaller aliquots for better spacing of fluid input. Giving a diuretic before, during, or after blood products can be helpful. A usual transfusion rate is 2–2.5 mL/kg/h.
Bacterial contamination	Transfusion of bacterially infected blood components. Contamination can occur from the donor, through the collection and testing process up to transfusion to the patient, including not using aseptic technique for administration.	Onset of chills and fever, nausea, vomiting, tachycardia, dyspnea, hypotension, or shock. Treat BP with fluids and vasopressors if necessary. Antibiotics should be started as soon as possible. Oxygen as needed to support respirations.	Collect, process, store, and transfuse blood products according to blood banking standards and infuse within 4 h of removal from the blood bank.
Transfusion-related acute lung injury (TRALI)	WBC activation occurs affecting pulmonary capillaries resulting in leakage. Pulmonary edema occurs without circulatory overload.	Rapid onset of dyspnea and tachypnea. May have fever, cyanosis, and hypotension. Fluids, vasopressors, and corticosteroids are given. Diuretics have no role.	There are no prevention strategies, but early recognition and treatment may prevent fatalities.

Adapted from Lewis SL, Bucher L, Heitkemper MM, et al.: *Medical-surgical nursing: assessment and management of clinical problems,* ed 10, St. Louis, 2017, Elsevier; Sandler SG: *Transfusion reactions,* 2017, Medscape. Retrieved from https://emedicine.medscape.com/article/206885-overview.
BP, Blood pressure; *IV,* intravenous; *RBC,* red blood cell; *WBC,* white blood cell.

during attempts to rid the body of leukemic or other cancer cells. The cells used for transplantation can be **allogeneic** (from another person) or *autologous* (from the patient).

Peripheral stem cells, stem cells from umbilical cord blood, or from bone marrow are used for transplantation. If the transplant is to be autologous, cells are taken from the patient during a period of remission of disease—either by bone marrow aspiration or by pheresis (for peripheral stem cells). Allogeneic bone marrow is harvested from a human leukocyte antigen (HLA)–matched person. The HLA match is determined by tissue typing. Finding a good HLA match is difficult; there is only a 25% chance of matching with the patient's own sibling.

Cultural Considerations

Bone Marrow Donations

Most people willing to donate bone marrow are white. There is a 75% chance of an HLA match for a white patient and donor marrow. Far fewer African Americans have signed up at the bone marrow registry, and the chance for an HLA match for an African American patient is about 25%. Efforts are being made to encourage African Americans to become bone marrow donors.

Bone marrow harvest is done in the operating room, where multiple aspirations from the iliac crests are performed. The marrow is filtered and may be purged to rid autologous marrow of cancer cells or to rid the allogeneic marrow of T cells. Nursing care after harvest consists of monitoring the dressings for bleeding and medicating the donor for pain in the hip area. Nonaspirin analgesics often are sufficient to control pain.

The patient undergoes a conditioning regimen to rid the body of malignancy or to obliterate the diseased bone marrow. This usually takes 5 to 10 days. The process involves intensive high-dose chemotherapy and often includes total body irradiation. The patient experiences all the side effects of these treatments: bone marrow suppression, diarrhea, stomatitis, severe nausea, and vomiting. The patient is at extreme risk for infection. Meticulous supportive and preventive nursing care is essential during and after this phase.

At least 2 days after the end of chemotherapy, the stem cell infusion takes place, through a central line, over approximately 30 minutes. If the stem cells are from an allogeneic donor, the infusion takes place right after procurement. The process of engraftment begins as the cells find their way to the marrow-forming locations in the patient's bones and establish themselves there. Engraftment takes 2 to 5 weeks and is considered successful when the patient's erythrocyte, leukocyte, and platelet counts begin to rise. Until engraftment is complete, the patient is at dire risk of infection and hemorrhage. Other complications include failure of engraftment and graft-versus-host disease, in which the cells see the patient's tissues as foreign and mount an immune attack.

OXYGEN THERAPY

Low concentrations of oxygen may be administered to relieve severe dyspnea and hypoxia during the acute phase of a blood disorder. Target SpO_2 should be no more than 98% to 99%. The treatment is mostly symptomatic, but it does offer some relief if there is sufficient hemoglobin to carry the oxygen to the tissues. With sufficient oxygen saturating the hemoglobin tissue, ischemia may be prevented. The care of a patient receiving oxygen therapy and the need for careful monitoring of blood gases are discussed in Chapter 14.

IRON THERAPY

Iron is one of the principal elements in the production and maturation of RBCs. When the body lacks iron, the amount of hemoglobin is decreased in the RBCs, making them very small and pale in color. In simple iron deficiency anemia, the condition is relieved by administering iron salts. The iron preparations most often used are ferrous sulfate and ferrous gluconate. Ferric citrate (Auryxia) is also available since FDA approval in 2017.

Although iron salts are absorbed better from an empty stomach, they are irritating to the GI tract. There will be fewer gastric upsets if this medication is given in divided doses and immediately after meals. The patient should be warned that taking iron salts by mouth produces greenish-black stools and that there is no cause for alarm if this change in the color of stools occurs. Because iron salts may form deposits on the teeth and gums, causing a discoloration, the liquid forms of this medication should be given through a straw. After administration of each liquid dose, the teeth should be thoroughly cleansed and the mouth well rinsed. Research has shown that dosing iron three times per day may not be the best schedule. The morning dose of iron increases the blood level of iron, which stimulates hepcidin (a hormone from the liver that regulates iron levels in the blood) and prevents further absorption of doses of iron taken later in the day (Harper, 2018). Current practice guidelines recommend dosing on every other day (Schrier, 2018a).

Some patients suffer such severe gastric disturbances from the oral intake of iron salts that the medication must be given by another route. Patients who are anemic because of gastric or intestinal bleeding cannot take iron by mouth because the irritation aggravates their condition. Ferric carboxymaltose injection (Injectafer) and ferumoxytol injection (Feraheme) are approved for IV administration. They are newer preparations and do not have the same risk for severe side effects like older medications. The medications have been shown to be effective and well tolerated by patients. Intramuscular (IM) administration of iron is not recommended.

Vitamin C usually is given with iron because it enhances iron's absorption. If a pharmaceutical preparation of vitamin C is not prescribed, the patient can take the iron salts with orange juice or another juice that is a good source of vitamin C.

Think Critically

What would you teach a home care patient who is complaining that the iron medication is causing a mild nausea, stomach discomfort, and constipation?

VITAMIN B_{12} THERAPY

Vitamin B_{12} has two main functions in the body. First, vitamin B_{12} is needed for RBCs to develop into mature, normally functioning cells; second, vitamin B_{12} is necessary for nerve cells to function normally. Another B-group vitamin, folic acid, also is needed for RBC maturation, but it has no effect on the nervous system. Vitamin B_{12} is used to treat megaloblastic anemia.

Injections of vitamin B_{12} are given daily for the first few weeks and later may be spaced a week apart. As the patient improves, vitamin B_{12} injections may be necessary only once a month, but injections must continue for the duration of life for patients with megaloblastic anemia. Cyanocobalamin can be given orally, intranasally, or by IM or deep subcutaneous injection; methylcobalamin can be given orally, sublingually, IM or IV; and hydroxcobalamin is given by IM injection or IV infusion. Vitamin B_{12} can be administered so that it best fits the needs of the patient.

In addition to taking supplemental iron and vitamins, patients with nutritional anemia should eat nutritionally balanced, high-protein meals.

Nutrition Considerations

Hints for Adding Protein to the Diet

- Mix dry skim milk into the milk called for in recipes.
- Provide between-meal shakes made with commercial protein powder available at the grocery or health food store.
- Add dry skim milk to hot or cold cereal, scrambled eggs, soups, gravies, meat loaf or meatballs, casseroles, and desserts.
- Add diced or ground meat to soups and casseroles.
- Drink commercial canned high-protein drinks (available from pharmacies) between meals or use instant breakfast drink mix.
- Add cream cheese or peanut butter to breakfast breads.
- Eat peanut butter on crackers, apples, celery, or toast for snacks.
- Eat desserts made with eggs.
- Eat commercial high-protein bars for snacks, available at grocery, health food, or sporting goods stores.

SPLENECTOMY

Indications for surgical removal of the spleen include:

- Severe trauma to and rupture of the spleen
- Splenomegaly causing destruction of blood cells
- Blood disorders caused by the spleen

If the spleen is removed, the other organs of the monocyte-macrophage system take over many of its functions. Individuals who no longer have a functioning spleen are at very high risk for developing life-threatening infections, especially those caused by pneumococci. It is recommended that these persons receive the Pneumovax vaccine. They are advised to consult a health care provider and take preventive antibiotics as prescribed when they experience even a seemingly trivial respiratory infection.

A patient with a ruptured or torn spleen is in immediate danger of hemorrhage and shock. Whenever an accidental blow, stab wound, or gunshot wound occurs in the vicinity of the spleen, the patient must be watched closely for signs of internal bleeding, such as an expanding abdomen and increased pain. After surgery, the patient is observed for early signs of infection, abdominal distention, and other more general complications of abdominal surgery.

COMMUNITY CARE

Patients with blood disorders are treated in many different places in the community. Patients undergoing chemotherapy may attend an outpatient clinic to receive the doses of the drugs they need. Support groups for patients with the various disorders may meet in hospitals, clinics, churches, schools, or other community locations. Patients with sickle cell disease or hemophilia may attend ambulatory clinics.

Patients with blood disorders are commonly treated as home care patients. An older adult patient with megaloblastic anemia who is homebound may need a nurse to give vitamin B_{12} injections and draw laboratory specimens for periodic blood counts. Patients with leukemia are commonly followed at home during chemotherapy and recovery periods. Patients with sickle cell problems are more likely to be treated in the home setting after the initial crisis period is over. In some instances blood products are administered at home. Some types of chemotherapy agents are given in the home setting, and the patient must be monitored for all of the adverse effects that such therapy can cause.

Home care nurses must do considerable patient and family teaching about prevention of infection, prevention of and treatment for bleeding episodes, appropriate nutrition, and regulation of medication. The home care nurse manager will coordinate care for patients with their health care provider, pharmacist, home infusion company, home health aide, and family.

Get Ready for the NCLEX® Examination!

Key Points

- Anemia results in insufficient oxygen being carried to cells for the body's needs.
- Anemias result from blood loss, failure in blood cell production, or excessive destruction of RBCs.
- Hypovolemia from blood loss may result in shock.
- Blood cell production requires protein, folic acid, and iron.
- Megaloblastic anemia results from lack of intrinsic factor and faulty absorption of vitamin B_{12}.
- There are a variety of causes of hemolytic anemia, some of which are genetic.
- A CBC and differential (peripheral smear) are used to diagnose blood disorders.
- Sickle cell disease is a genetic inherited disorder in which the affected gene is transmitted from both the father and the mother.
- The main method of sickle cell crisis prevention is hydration and hydroxyurea therapy; the primary treatment is rehydration and pain control.
- Abnormal hemoglobin causes RBCs to sickle when oxygen tension in the blood is lowered.
- There are many signs and symptoms and problems for those with sickle cell disease (see Fig. 16.3).
- Nursing care for sickle cell disease and crisis is aimed at relieving the symptoms of complications and minimizing organ damage.
- Treatment of anemia is aimed at curing the underlying disorder and providing nutrients or supplements needed for building RBCs.
- Aplastic anemia can be life-threatening and may require HCT.
- Polycythemia vera causes blood to become too thick and predisposes to blood clots.
- Thrombocytopenia affects the platelets and causes bleeding that can be life-threatening.
- Nursing care for thrombocytopenia focuses on preventing bleeding.
- There are four major types of leukemia: chronic lymphocytic, chronic myelogenous, acute lymphocytic/lymphoblastic, and acute myelogenous.
- Agents that are toxic to the bone marrow are a key factor in the development of leukemia.
- Leukemia is acute or chronic, according to the phase of cell development present and the symptoms.
- A patient with leukemia may be asymptomatic or may have fever, malaise, and frequent infections.
- Treatment for leukemia is aimed at slowing or eliminating the growth of malignant blood cells and maintaining normal levels of RBCs, hemoglobin, and platelets.
- Hematopoietic cell transplantation is an option for certain types of leukemia.
- Infection and hemorrhage are two major complications of leukemia.
- Hemophilia is mostly an inherited disorder affecting the blood's ability to clot.
- Bleeding into the joints is the major problem of hemophilia.
- Blood factor replacement is the treatment for hemophilia.
- DIC occurs in conjunction with many disorders.
- There is clotting in the microcirculation and bleeding in acute DIC.
- Blood transfusions must be administered very carefully because reactions can be serious or fatal.
- Patient consent is needed before blood component transfusion.
- There are many signs and symptoms of a blood transfusion reaction (see Table 16.7).
- If there is any sign of a serious transfusion reaction, the transfusion is stopped immediately.
- Iron, vitamin C, folic acid, and vitamin B_{12} supplementation are used to treat anemias.

Additional Learning Resources

SG Go to your Study Guide for additional learning activities to help you master this chapter content.

Go to your Evolve website (http://evolve.elsevier.com/deWit/medsurg) for the following FREE learning resources:
- Animations, audio, and video
- Answers and rationales for questions and activities
- Glossary with pronunciations in English and Spanish
- Interactive Review Questions and more!

Review Questions for the NCLEX® Examination

1. While reviewing the laboratory results for a patient who had gastric bypass surgery last year, you note that the amount of red blood cells has decreased remarkably. You suspect that the anemia is related to:
   1. vitamin B_{12} deficiency.
   2. chronic renal failure.
   3. iron deficiency.
   4. bone marrow suppression.

   NCLEX Client Need: Physiological Integrity: Reduction of Risk Potential
2. An emergency department patient has a gunshot wound to the abdomen. If you find a profusely bleeding abdominal wound, you should anticipate which signs and symptoms of profuse blood loss? *(Select all that apply.)*
   1. Increased blood pressure
   2. Rapid, weak pulse
   3. Cold, clammy skin
   4. Urine output greater than 50 mL/h
   5. Decreased blood pressure

   NCLEX Client Need: Physiological Integrity: Reduction of Risk Potential

3. The patient is prescribed Feosol oral medication for a mild anemia. Which patient statement indicates a need for further teaching about this medication?
   1. "The medication is absorbed best on an empty stomach."
   2. "The medication is more effective if I drink orange juice as well."
   3. "I should take the medication with milk."
   4. "I should increase fluids and fiber to prevent constipation."

   NCLEX Client Need: Health Promotion and Maintenance
4. You are assessing a new admission with AML. You have asked the patient about symptoms and they reply, among other things, that they are very tired. You understand that this symptom is caused by:
   1. excessive amounts of lymphocytes, causing perfusion problems to the brain and muscles.
   2. excessive WBC production, which increases cellular activity, using energy resources.
   3. excessive production of abnormal cells, including RBCs, decreasing the amount of functional hemoglobin.
   4. excessive metabolic rate due to leukemia, increasing cellular production, and requiring increased nutrients that are lacking.

   NCLEX Client Need: Physiological Integrity: Physiological Adaptation
5. A nurse is caring for a patient who had multiple traumatic injuries. You note blood in the urine and the feces. Suspecting DIC, you expect which laboratory result?
   1. Increased hematocrit
   2. Elevated platelet count
   3. Increased activated partial thromboplastin time
   4. Decreased D-dimer

   NCLEX Client Need: Physiological Integrity: Reduction of Risk Potential
6. Your patient has been diagnosed with multiple myeloma. What are some considerations while planning nursing care for this patient? *(Select all that apply.)*
   1. Be very gentle while moving the patient.
   2. Encourage frequent mobility activities.
   3. Delegate the care to a nursing assistant.
   4. Know that psychosocial care is essential.
   5. Place the patient in protective isolation.
   6. Medicate as ordered for bone pain.

   NCLEX Client Need: Safe and Effective Care Environment: Safety and Infection Control
7. A patient with sickle cell crisis may display which signs and symptoms on assessment?
   1. Ruddy complexion and elevated RBCs
   2. Joint pain and low platelet count
   3. Leukocytosis and frequent sore throat
   4. Ischemia pain and poor circulation

   NCLEX Client Need: Physiological Integrity: Physiological Adaptation
8. Which measure(s) should a patient with leukopenia institute to prevent infection? *(Select all that apply.)*
   1. Avoid eating salads, raw fruits, and raw vegetables.
   2. Stay within the home.
   3. Wash hands after handling the mail.
   4. Do not get close to pets.
   5. Increase activity as tolerated.
   6. Do not reuse dishes or eating utensils without washing them first.

   NCLEX Client Need: Safe and Effective Care Environment: Safety and Infection Control
9. After the first few minutes of transfusing packed RBCs, the patient has a temperature of 101.5° F (38.6° C), heart rate of 120 beats/min, and blood pressure of 90/50 mm Hg with complaints of back pain. The priority nursing action would be:
   1. flush the line with normal saline.
   2. stop the transfusion.
   3. notify the health care provider.
   4. administer diphenhydramine (Benadryl).

   NCLEX Client Need: Physiological Integrity: Reduction of Risk Potential
10. A patient with cancer who has undergone HCT, chemotherapy, and total body irradiation is under close observation. You would continue protective isolation until the patient begins to show signs of improvement when engraftment takes place. Engraftment would be expected in what time frame?
    1. 2 to 3 days
    2. 2 to 5 weeks
    3. 1 to 2 months
    4. 1 year or longer

    NCLEX Client Need: Safe and Effective Care Environment: Safety and Infection Control

Critical Thinking Questions

Scenario A

Mrs. Hutton is a young mother who has three small children. She is admitted to the hospital with a severe anemia. Her hemoglobin is 7.5 g/dL, and her red blood cell count also is very low. Mrs. Hutton confides in you that she has never eaten as she should, especially when she was a teenager. With the added strain of having children to care for at home, she does not take the time to cook the meals she knows they should have because she is so tired all the time. Her husband makes a good salary, but Mrs. Hutton is under the impression that an adequate diet would cost more than they can afford at present.

1. How can you teach the patient the value of nutritious food and help her with shopping practices that would provide her family with food items that are not expensive?
2. Which foods that are high in iron would you suggest she include in her diet?
3. What practical suggestions could you make to help Mrs. Hutton cope with fatigue?

Scenario B

Mr. Tate is a 24-year-old who has acute lymphocytic leukemia. He is receiving chemotherapy with cyclophosphamide, vincristine, prednisone, and doxorubicin. He is experiencing many of the problems associated with a blood disorder, as well as the problems caused by the side effects of the potent drugs he is receiving.

1. Describe the physiologic problems Mr. Tate is likely to experience as a result of the disease and the therapy.
2. Identify psychosocial concerns that Mr. Tate might have.

Scenario C

Mr. Harris, a 72-year-old white man, has just been diagnosed with chronic myeloid leukemia (CML). He has started chemotherapy with hydroxyurea and imatinib.

1. What do you need to teach Mr. Harris about the drugs he is taking? Will he be on other drugs to control the side effects of this chemotherapy?
2. His wife asks whether he would be eligible for bone marrow transplantation. How should you answer?

Scenario D

Mrs. Solter, age 82, is to receive a transfusion of packed RBCs because she is very anemic and not responding to oral medication. You are assigned to assist with the transfusion and to monitor the patient.

1. What are the priorities of care for this patient at this time?
2. Mrs. Solter asks what this transfusion will do for her. How would you respond?
3. What is the proper sequence of actions you would take if Mrs. Solter experienced a transfusion reaction while the blood product is infusing?

17 The Cardiovascular System

http://evolve.elsevier.com/deWit/medsurg

Objectives

Theory

1. Discuss the normal anatomy and physiology of the cardiovascular system.
2. Examine the risk factors and incidence of cardiovascular disease.
3. Explain ways to modify risk factors for the development of cardiovascular disease.
4. Choose ways in which nurses can contribute to the prevention of cardiovascular disease.
5. Compare the diagnostic tests, specific techniques, and procedures for assessing the cardiovascular system.
6. Present three likely problem statements for patients who have common problems of cardiovascular disease and list the expected outcomes and appropriate nursing interventions for each.

Clinical Practice

7. Teach patients about the more common diagnostic tests and procedures to diagnose and evaluate cardiovascular diseases.
8. Assist patients to form plans to modify cardiovascular disease risk factors.
9. Assess for cardiovascular abnormalities in assigned patients.

Key Terms

arteriosclerosis (ăr-tē-rē-ō-sklĕ-RŌ-sĭs, p. 383)
atherosclerosis (ăth-ĕr-ō-sklĕ-RŌ-sĭs, p. 381)
bruit (brū-Ē, p. 396)
cardiac output (KAR-dē-ăk ŎWT-pŭt, p. 379)
coarctation (kō-ărk-TĀ-shŭn, p. 383)
dysrhythmia (dĭs-RĬTH-mē-ă, p. 382)
ejection fraction (ē-JĔK-shŭn FRĂK-shŭn, p. 379)
endocarditis (ĔN-dō-kăhr-DĪ-tĭs, p. 383)
hypertension (hī-pĕr-TĔN-shŭn, p. 383)
infarct (ĬN-farkt, p. 383)
intermittent claudication (ĭn-tĕr-MĬT-ĕnt klăw-dĭ-KĀ-shŭn, p. 393)
ischemia (ĭs-KĒ-mē-ă, p. 383)
palpitations (păl-pĭ-TĀ-shŭnz, p. 403)
pericarditis (pĕr-ē-kăhr-DĪ-tĭs, p. 383)
rubor (RŪ-bŏr, p. 397)
stroke volume (strōk VŎL-yŭm, p. 379)
syncope (SĬN-kō-pē, p. 397)

Concepts Covered in This Chapter

- Self-Management
- Fluid and Electrolytes
- Nutrition
- Perfusion
- Inflammation
- Tissue Integrity
- Fatigue
- Stress

OVERVIEW OF ANATOMY AND PHYSIOLOGY OF THE CARDIOVASCULAR SYSTEM

THE STRUCTURES OF THE HEART AND THEIR FUNCTIONS

- The heart wall consists of three layers. The epicardium is the outer layer of tissue; the myocardium is the middle layer of muscle fibers that contract to pump blood; and the endocardium is the lining of the inner surface of the heart chambers.
- A membranous sac, the pericardium, surrounds the heart.
- The pericardium is a double-layered sac. The double layer helps provide a barrier to infection, prevents displacement of the heart, and contains pain and other receptors that elicit reflex changes in heart rate and blood pressure.
- The pericardial space contains a thin layer of fluid (30 to 50 mL).
- The four chambers of the heart make up two coordinated pumps: the right-side pump is a low-pressure system; the left-side pump is a high-pressure system.
- The right atrium and right ventricle receive deoxygenated blood from the vascular system and pump it through the lungs.

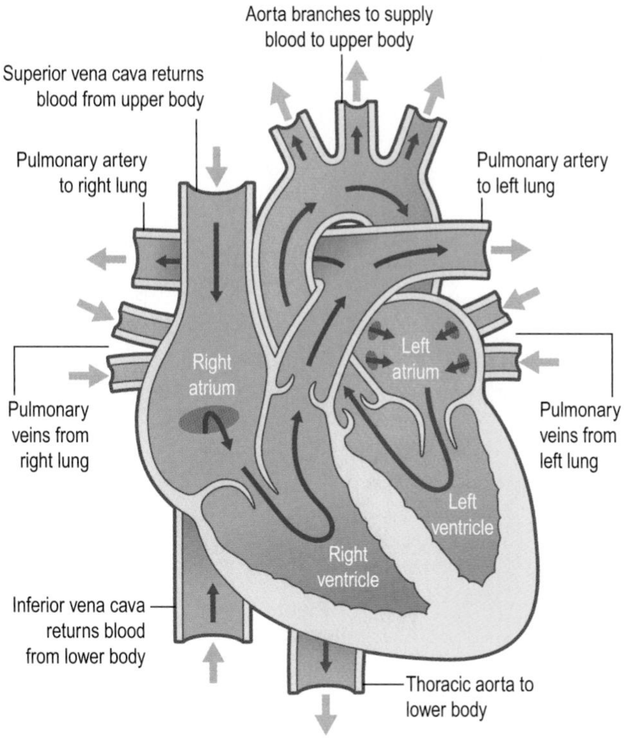

Fig. 17.1 Direction of blood flow through the heart. (From Waugh A, Grant A: *Ross and Wilson anatomy and physiology in health and illness*, ed 13, St. Louis, 2018, Elsevier.)

- The left atrium and left ventricle receive oxygenated blood from the lungs and pump it through the systemic circulation (Fig. 17.1).
- A septum separates the right and left sides of the heart.
- The cardiac valves direct the flow of blood through the heart chambers.
- Blood enters the right atrium via the superior and inferior vena cava and goes to the right ventricle through the tricuspid valve.
- Blood leaves the right ventricle through the pulmonic (or pulmonary) valve and goes into the pulmonary artery to circulate in the lungs, exchanging carbon dioxide for oxygen. The pulmonary artery carries blood away from the heart, so it meets the definition of *artery*, but it carries deoxygenated blood. The left atrium receives oxygenated blood from the pulmonary veins, and the mitral valve controls the flow from the atrium into the left ventricle. Pulmonary *veins* carry blood toward the heart but come from the lungs with oxygenated blood.
- The left ventricle ejects the blood through the aortic valve into the aorta and the systemic circulation.
- The coronary arteries branch from the aorta and supply the cardiac muscle with blood during diastole (Fig. 17.2). Blood flow in the coronaries is restricted during systole because of muscle contraction.
- The left coronary artery divides into the anterior descending and the circumflex arteries, providing blood for the left atrium and the left ventricle.
- The right coronary artery supplies the right atrium, right ventricle, and part of the posterior wall of the left ventricle, as well as the atrioventricular node of the cardiac conduction system (see Fig. 17.2).
- The heart is located within the mediastinum and is tilted forward and to the left side of the chest.
- The point of maximal impulse (PMI) can normally be felt between the fifth and sixth ribs on a line dividing the left clavicle in half. Listen to the apical heart rate at this location.

CONTRACTION OF THE HEART TO PUMP BLOOD

- The heart's pumping action is sparked by specialized pacemaker cells and conduction fibers that initiate spontaneous electrical activity, causing muscle contractions that result in a heartbeat.
- The conduction pathways are located in the myocardium and transmit the electrical impulse throughout the heart.
- The sinoatrial (SA) node is located in the right atrium and is called the "pacemaker" of the heart because it normally initiates the electrical impulses.
- The atrioventricular (AV) node (or junction) is located in the lower part of the right atrium. It relays the impulse from the SA node to the bundle of His and throughout the ventricles via the Purkinje fibers (Fig. 17.3).
- The heart rate and rhythm are influenced by the autonomic nervous system; factors affecting the autonomic nervous system can speed up or slow down the heart rate.

THE CARDIAC CYCLE

- The cardiac cycle consists of contraction of the muscle (systole) and relaxation of the muscle (diastole).
- The heart pumps out about 5 L of blood every minute.
- The amount of cardiac output depends on the heart rate, the amount of blood returning to the heart (venous return or preload), the strength of contraction, and the resistance to the ejection of the blood (afterload).
- **Stroke volume** equals the amount of blood ejected by a ventricle during one contraction.
- **Cardiac output** equals stroke volume multiplied by the heart rate.

THE EJECTION FRACTION

- The **ejection fraction** is the percentage of blood that is ejected from the left ventricle during systole.
- A normal ejection fraction is 50% to 70%.
- As ejection fraction decreases with heart failure, tissue perfusion diminishes.
- A decreased ejection fraction causes backup of blood into the pulmonary vessels.
- Too much blood and the increased pressure in the pulmonary vessels can cause pulmonary edema.

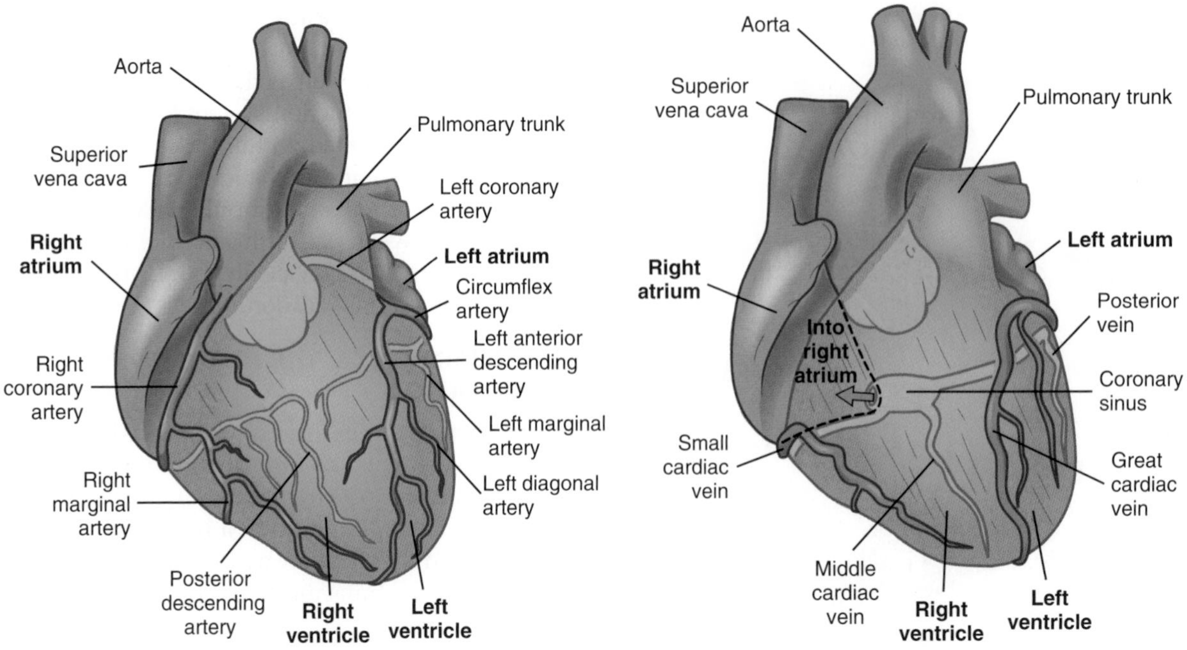

Fig. 17.2 A view of the coronary arterial system. *Left,* Arteries. *Right,* Veins. (From Lewis SL, Bucher L, Heitkemper MM, et al.: *Medical-surgical nursing: assessment and management of clinical problems,* ed 10, St. Louis, 2017, Elsevier.)

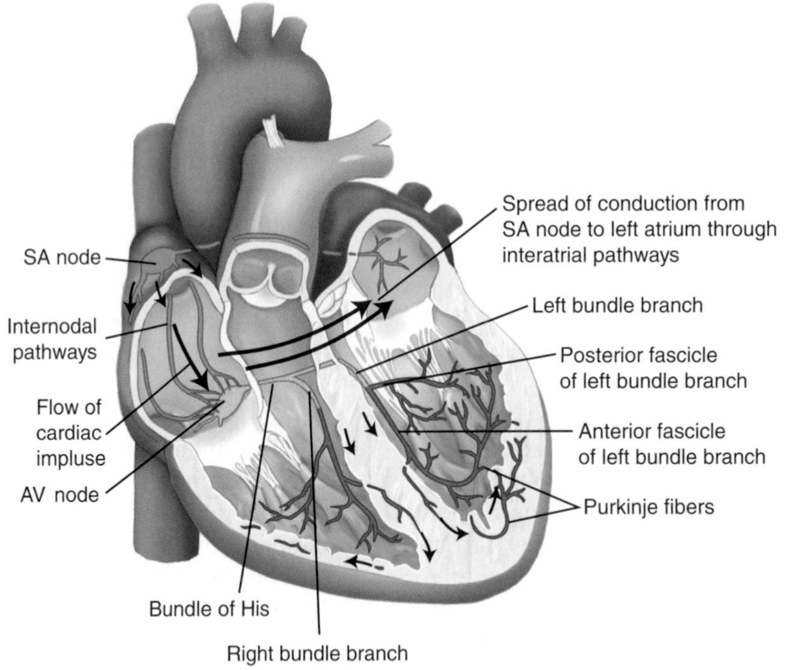

Fig. 17.3 The cardiac conduction system. *AV,* Atrioventricular; *SA,* sinoatrial. (From Lewis SL, Bucher L, Heitkemper MM, et al.: *Medical-surgical nursing: assessment and management of clinical problems,* ed 10, St. Louis, 2017, Elsevier.)

BLOOD FLOW THROUGHOUT THE BODY

- Three types of blood vessels make up the vascular system: arteries, veins, and capillaries. These vessels conduct the blood from the body tissues to the heart-lung circulation and from the heart back to the tissues.
- Arteries carry oxygenated blood away from the heart (Fig. 17.4). Veins carry oxygen-depleted blood back to the heart for reoxygenation by the lungs (Fig. 17.5).
- Small veins, *venules,* and small arteries, *arterioles,* are connected by the capillaries. It is in the capillaries that the oxygen is transported to cells and waste products are removed from them.
- The aorta is the largest artery in the body, and it receives blood from the left ventricle.
- The inferior and superior vena cava are the largest veins in the body and empty blood into the right atrium of the heart.

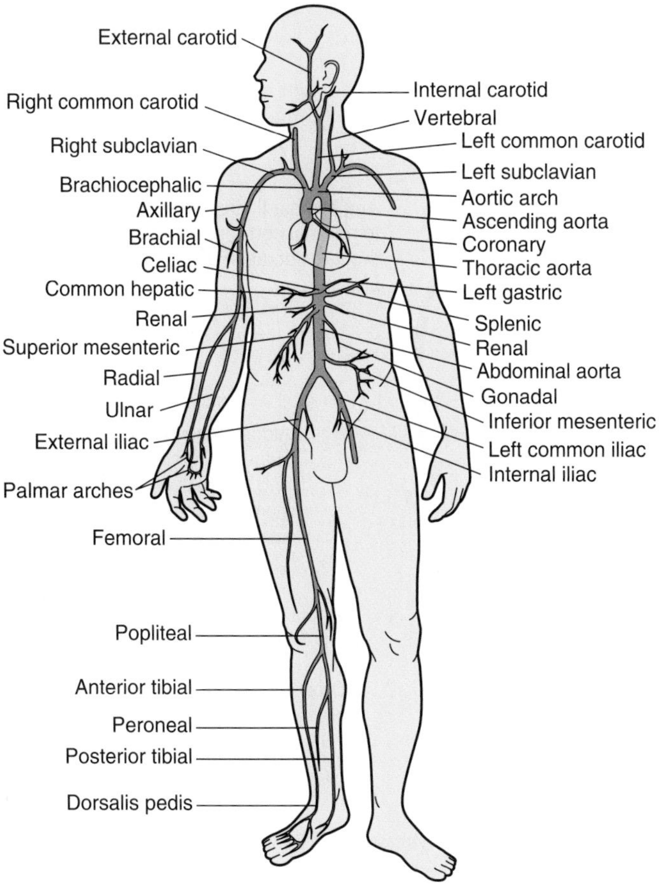

Fig. 17.4 Major arteries in the body.

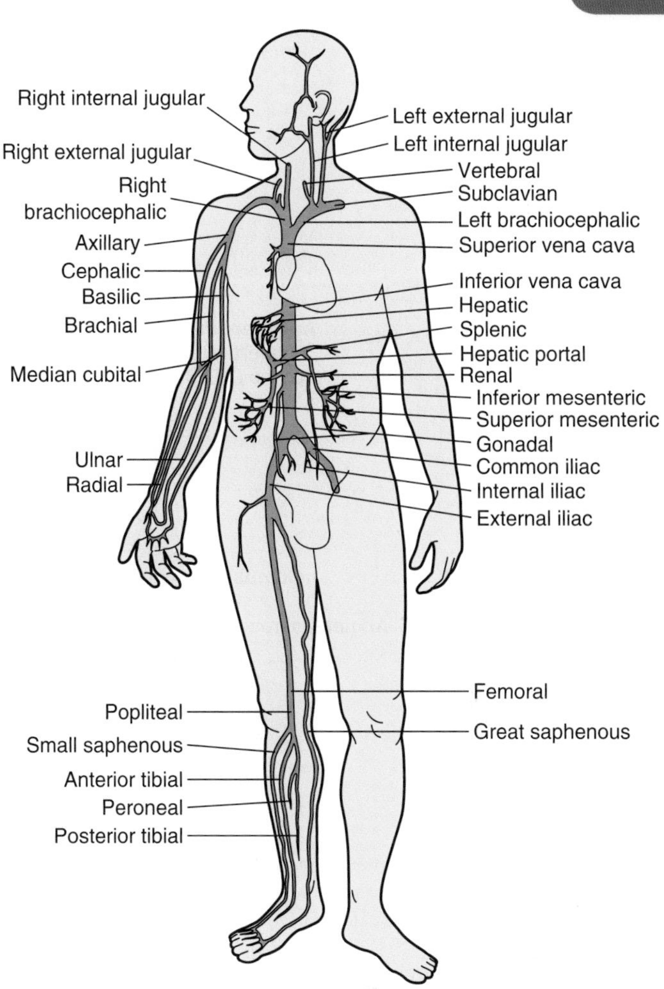

Fig. 17.5 Major veins in the body.

- Arteries are elastic and accommodate changes in blood flow by constricting or dilating.
- Three layers of tissue make up the artery wall. The outer layer *(tunica adventitia)* is connective tissue, the middle layer *(tunica media)* is smooth muscle, and the inner layer *(tunica intima)* consists of endothelial cells.
- Veins have the same three layers but with less smooth muscle and connective tissue. The veins are thinner and less rigid and thus can hold more blood.
- The heart pumps blood through the arterial system with each contraction. Skeletal muscle contraction, respiratory movements that change pressures in the chest, and constriction of the veins propel blood back to the heart.
- Sets of valves in the medium and large veins open and close, keeping blood flowing toward the heart against gravity.
- For blood to circulate, the arteries must be unobstructed, and they must be able to dilate and constrict as necessary to regulate the blood flow. Veins also must be patent, their valves must function normally, and surrounding muscles must contract so that venous blood is continually being moved in the direction of the heart.

BLOOD PRESSURE

- Arterial blood pressure is the force that the blood exerts against the walls of the aorta and its branches.
- The blood pressure is greatest during ventricular contraction, or *systole,* when blood is ejected into the aorta.
- Diastolic pressure is the pressure when the ventricles are in the relaxation phase, or *diastole,* just before the next contraction of the ventricles.
- The difference between the systolic blood pressure and the diastolic blood pressure is called the *pulse pressure.*
- If the diameter of blood vessels becomes smaller because of atherosclerosis, blood pressure is increased with the effort of forcing the blood through the smaller opening. **Atherosclerosis** is the condition in which fibrous plaque with fatty deposits forms in the interior layers of the arteries, causing narrowing.
- If there is an increase in the volume of fluid in the blood vessels, the pressure within the vessels increases, and the heart must work harder to pump the increased volume of fluid through the vessels.
- If blood volume decreases, the kidneys secrete the enzyme renin in the blood (Fig. 17.6).
- Renin acts on certain blood proteins to produce angiotensin I.
- Angiotensin I is converted to angiotensin II by angiotensin-converting enzyme from the lungs.

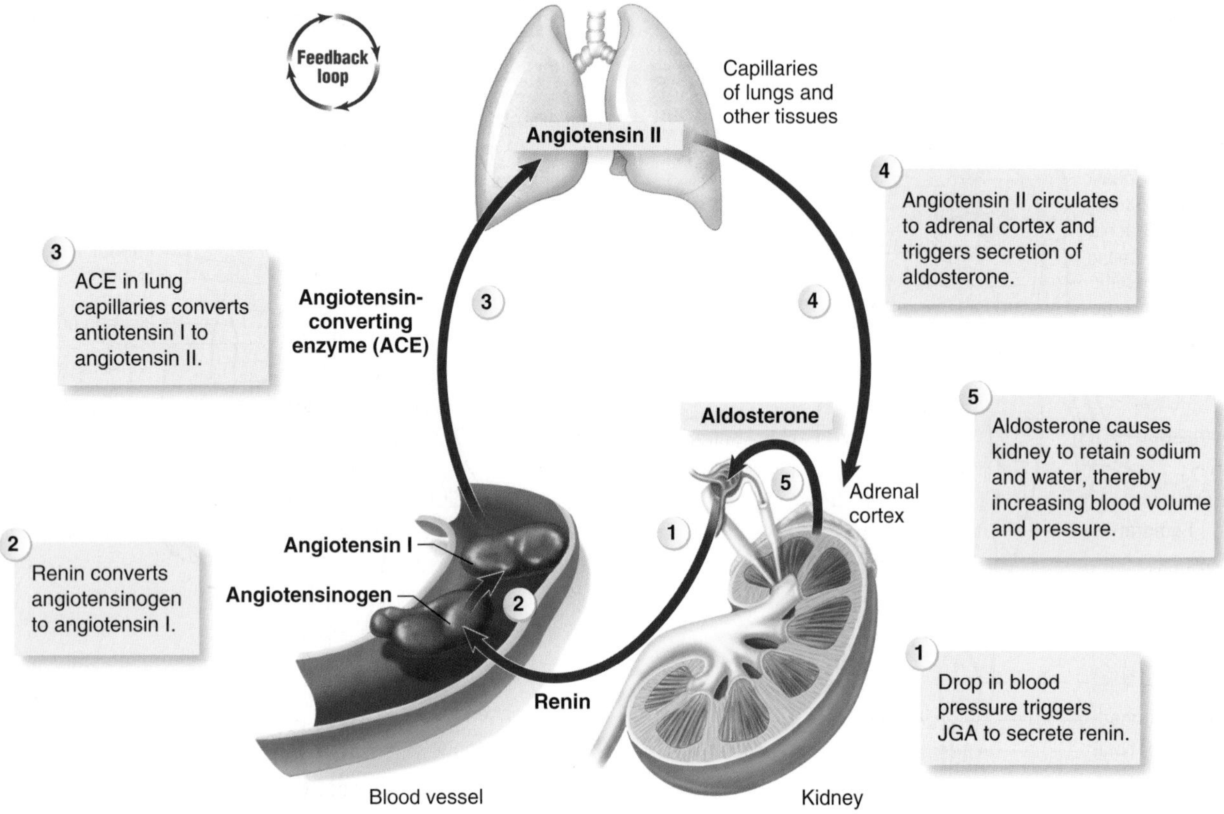
Feedback loop
Capillaries of lungs and other tissues
Angiotensin II
4
Angiotensin II circulates to adrenal cortex and triggers secretion of aldosterone.
3
ACE in lung capillaries converts antiotensin I to angiotensin II.
Angiotensin-converting enzyme (ACE)
3
4
Aldosterone
5
Aldosterone causes kidney to retain sodium and water, thereby increasing blood volume and pressure.
5
Adrenal cortex
1
2
Renin converts angiotensinogen to angiotensin I.
Angiotensin I
Angiotensinogen
2
1
Drop in blood pressure triggers JGA to secrete renin.
Renin
Blood vessel
Kidney

Fig. 17.6 The renin-angiotensin-aldosterone system. (From Patton KT: *Anatomy and physiology*, ed 10, St. Louis, 2019, Elsevier.)

- Angiotensin II acts directly on the blood vessels, causing them to constrict, increasing resistance to blood flow in the peripheral vessels. Angiotensin II also stimulates the adrenal gland to release aldosterone, causing sodium and water retention by the renal tubules. The retained sodium and water increase the blood volume, causing blood pressure elevation and improved cardiac output.
- Blood flow is affected by the amount of resistance in the vessels and by the viscosity of the blood.
- Vascular resistance is controlled by the nervous system, hormones, blood pH, and ions that regulate the diameter of the vessels.
- **When the vessel diameter increases, resistance falls and blood pressure decreases. When vessel diameter decreases, resistance rises and blood pressure increases.**
- The sympathetic nervous system plays a major role in regulating vessel diameter because it prompts the release of the hormones norepinephrine and epinephrine that cause vasoconstriction.
- Blood viscosity is affected by the hydration status of the body. When dehydration occurs, blood viscosity increases; thicker blood causes an increase in blood pressure due to increased resistance.

CARDIOVASCULAR SYSTEM CHANGES RELATED TO AGING

- The aging heart becomes stiffer and contractile ability decreases, resulting in decreased stroke volume.
- The coronary arteries become tortuous and dilated and have areas of calcification.
- The cardiac valves become thickened, particularly the mitral and aortic valves, which are subject to higher pressures. A systolic murmur is common in those older than age 80 years.
- The SA node loses about 40% of its pacemaker cells over time, predisposing to cardiac **dysrhythmia** (abnormal rhythm) or SA node failure.
- The aorta becomes stiffer, contributing to an increase in systolic blood pressure because the left ventricle must pump against greater resistance.
- The arterial walls thicken and lose elasticity, making them less able to adjust to changes in volume and to comply with sympathetic stimulation.
- Varicose veins develop as veins lose their elasticity, valve function decreases, and the leg muscles weaken and atrophy from decreased exercise.
- Platelet aggregation and increased coagulation potential lead to a greater incidence of thrombus formation, deep vein thrombosis, and thrombophlebitis.
- Chronic health problems and failing eyesight often lead to decreased activity, predisposing to vascular problems.

CARDIOVASCULAR DISEASE

Cardiovascular disease (CVD) affects 1 in 3 people in the United States, and more than 800,000 people die in the United States as a result of cardiovascular problems each year (Benjamin et al., 2018). Cardiovascular disease is responsible for the largest portion of Medicare funds spent each year. Together with the heart, the vascular system provides the body with nutrients and oxygen needed for life. The vascular system also transports metabolic wastes that are excreted by the lungs and the kidneys. When a disorder of the cardiovascular system occurs, homeostasis is upset. Many of the disorders that afflict the cardiovascular system can be prevented or controlled.

WOMEN AND HEART DISEASE

Heart disease incidence in women is almost equal to that in men. More women than men die each year of heart disease. The risk factors are similar to those for men: high cholesterol, high blood pressure, and obesity. Other factors play a bigger role for women, such as diabetes, metabolic syndrome, smoking, and mental stress.

Health Promotion

Preventing Cardiovascular Disease in Women

- Participate in regular physical activity—at least 40 minutes three or four times a week.*
- Maintain cholesterol levels as indicated by risk stratification.
- Refrain from smoking.*
- Do not consume more than one alcoholic drink per day.
- Obtain and maintain a healthy weight to reduce the chance of type 2 diabetes.* Type 2 diabetes increases the risk of cardiovascular disease.
- Maintain a body mass index (BMI) below 25.
- Discontinue use of estrogen contraception or supplementation as soon as possible.
- Reduce the amount of trans fat in the diet.
- If diabetes is present, keep fasting blood sugar below 100 mg/dL.
- If hypertension is present, take medication regularly to keep blood pressure below 130/80 mm Hg (below 115/75 mm Hg is optimal).
- Incorporate stress reduction techniques into the daily lifestyle because increased stress is a risk factor for cardiovascular disease.*

*These factors play an even larger role in prevention of heart disease in women than in men.

Think Critically

Think of and explain two physiologic reasons why older adults are more at risk for hypertension.

CAUSES OF CARDIOVASCULAR DISORDERS

Causes of cardiovascular disorders can be congenital or acquired. Narrowing of the aorta (**coarctation**), holes in the septum, or abnormal formation of a cardiac valve can occur congenitally. Acquired defects include narrowing or hardening of the blood vessels from **arteriosclerosis** (thickening and loss of elasticity) or atherosclerosis (buildup of plaque) and aneurysms of the large vessels. Inflammation of the valve structure may cause narrowing (stenosis) or incomplete closure (insufficiency) of the heart valves. Alteration of the myocardial muscle tissue by extra growth with thickening (hypertrophy) or fibrosis may occur as a result of systemic **hypertension** (persistently elevated blood pressure), pulmonary hypertension, or valve problems. Lack of adequate blood supply (**ischemia**) or **infarct** (area of tissue that has died from lack of blood supply) may occur from coronary artery disease. Deterioration of the pacemaker cells and conduction fibers related to hypertrophy or inflammation of tissues may cause conduction disorders affecting heart rhythm.

Heart failure is a complication of many cardiovascular diseases, as discussed in Chapters 18-20. When the heart is not able to pump enough blood to meet the body's needs for oxygen and nutrients, *heart failure* is diagnosed. Damage to the muscle, changes in vascular tone, and various other disease processes can cause or contribute to heart failure.

Disturbances in any part of the heart's conduction system can result in an increase in heart rate (tachycardia), a slowing of the heart rate (bradycardia), and disturbances in the rhythm of the heartbeat (dysrhythmias).

Infection and inflammation also can take their toll on the structure and function of the heart. **Endocarditis**, inflammation within the lining and valves of the heart, and **pericarditis**, inflammation of the sac surrounding the heart, can occur as primary diseases, but they are more often secondary to infection and inflammation elsewhere in the body. An example is rheumatic heart disease, which occurs after a streptococcal infection and damages heart valves.

Substances in the blood, such as excess carbon dioxide and certain drugs, can affect the rate and rhythm of the heart through their effect on the autonomic nervous system. The heart also responds to physiologic changes that indicate a need for more or less oxygen.

The arterial walls can be injured by several factors. Hypertension causes a mechanical injury by applying increased pressure continuously on the arterial walls. For each increment of 20/10 mm Hg above a pressure of 115/75, the risk of CVD doubles (World Health Organization [WHO], 2018). Elevated levels of total cholesterol and decreased levels of high-density lipoprotein cholesterol (HDL-c) lead to increased fatty deposits in the arterial walls, causing a narrowing of the vessels. Chemical toxins such as nicotine from tobacco and the toxins caused by renal failure cause injury to the arterial walls. Substance abuse with alcohol, stimulants, and recreational drugs is damaging to the cardiovascular system (see Chapter 48).

Physiologic disorders such as diabetes mellitus and metabolic syndrome directly cause physical changes in the vessel walls, leading to more rapid arteriosclerosis, an increased rate of atherosclerosis, and an earlier onset of hypertension.

Obesity, a sedentary lifestyle, and stress are all directly related to the increased incidence of atherosclerosis and hypertension. Smoking, and the changes it causes in the vessel walls, is directly related to arteriosclerosis of the peripheral vessels and decreased circulation in the lower extremities. Long-term hypertension causes arteriosclerosis and is a direct factor in the development of aortic aneurysm in many patients. Hypertension in some cases cannot be prevented, but it can be managed with diligent therapy and cooperation of the patient.

PREVENTION OF CARDIOVASCULAR DISEASE

Cardiovascular disease as the underlying cause of death accounts for about 1 in 3 deaths in the United States, totaling 836,546 deaths annually (Benjamin et al., 2018). Heart disease remains the major cause of death in the United States. Cardiovascular diseases also account for a large percentage of the chronic illnesses that disable, to some degree, a large portion of the U.S. population.

There are many kinds and degrees of heart disease. Advances in medical science have made it possible either to cure or to successfully manage a large number of cardiovascular problems. This management has allowed longer life for many people by prevention of heart failure, strokes, and myocardial infarctions in the older population. There has been a decline in deaths from heart disease since the mid-1980s because of improved emergency treatment of persons experiencing a coronary occlusion ("heart attack"), improved education of the public regarding ways to prevent cardiovascular disease, and teaching about the warning signs of a heart attack. Every nurse has a responsibility to assist with public education about heart disease.

Health Promotion

Know the Warning Signs of a Heart Attack

- **Chest discomfort:** A feeling of tightness, pressure, or a crushing or squeezing pain lasting more than a few minutes or returning after easing. In women, discomfort that radiates to the back or abdomen.
- **Pain or discomfort in other areas of the upper body:** Arms, shoulder, back, neck, jaw, or the top of the stomach. Women often have jaw or back pain.
- **Shortness of breath:** May occur with or without chest discomfort.
- **Breaking out in a cold sweat,** nausea, or lightheadedness with or without chest discomfort.
- **Feeling of impending doom** that does not go away. Or unusual fatigue in women.
- **Chest pain** unrelieved by prescribed doses of nitroglycerin.

Call 911 or emergency number immediately—get help! Take an aspirin.

Nonmodifiable risk factors are those that cannot be prevented by an individual. However, control of diseases such as hypertension and diabetes mellitus and the reduction of high cholesterol are possible. Because hypertension and diabetes are factors in the development of atherosclerosis, controlling them can help prevent the early onset of heart disease. If a person with diabetes can keep the hemoglobin A_{1c} below 6%, the risk of atherosclerosis is decreased (McCulloch, 2018). Management of hypertension is one of the major factors in heart disease prevention.

Table 17.1 presents the risk factors for cardiovascular disease. Metabolic syndrome is a strong indicator of cardiovascular risk and is diagnosed when three or more of the components in Box 17.1 are present (Wang, 2017). More than 50 million Americans meet the criteria. Modifiable risk factors are the major focus for education to prevent heart disease. Cigarette smoking–related health problems are heavy contributors to heart disease, and smoking is a key factor in sudden cardiac death. Other chemicals, whether legal or illegal, can contribute to cardiovascular disease or cause stroke, hypertension, or sudden cardiac death. Cocaine causes vasoconstriction and is believed to speed up the atherosclerosis process. Also, cocaine has been known to cause sudden cardiac death or stroke in susceptible individuals. Research is finding that the ingestion of both alcohol and cocaine greatly increases the chance of cardiac death. Methamphetamine increases heart rate, causes vasoconstriction that can lead to hypertension, and speeds up electrical conduction, potentially causing dysrhythmias and myocardial infarction (MI) (National Institute on Drug Abuse, 2017).

Clinical Cues

To stop smoking, many patients are using e-cigarettes. Have the patient verify with their health care provider if that is a good strategy based on the patient's health history. Studies are reporting mixed results as to the health benefit of electronic versus traditional cigarettes.

Think Critically

Identify two risk factors you can modify to decrease your risk of heart disease.

Although systolic blood pressure rises as a natural process of aging because arteries become less elastic, systolic hypertension should be treated in older adult patients. The guidelines for management of hypertension recommend implementing antihypertensive medications for individuals 60 years or older who have a systolic blood pressure at or above 130 mm Hg or a diastolic blood pressure above 80 mm Hg (Whelton et al., 2018).

Hypertension in older adults is associated with an even higher risk of heart disease, stroke, and death from coronary thrombosis. Hypertension has been associated with more rapid memory loss and loss of cognitive function in some research studies.

Table 17.1 Risk Factors for Cardiovascular Disease

UNMODIFIABLE RISK FACTORS	SIGNIFICANCE
Heredity	Children of parents with cardiovascular disease are more likely to develop the same problem. Researchers have identified 67 different DNA sites that increase risk. The more sites inherited, the higher the risk (Harvard Medical School, 2017).
Race	African Americans experience high blood pressure two to three times more frequently than whites. Consequently the risk of heart disease in this group is higher.
Sex	Males experience more heart attacks than females earlier in life. After age 65 years, the death rate from heart disease increases in women.
Age	Four out of five people who die of a heart attack are age 65 years or older. Increasing age increases risk.
MODIFIABLE RISK FACTORS	**MEANS OF MODIFICATION**
Obesity	Keep weight within normal limits through diet and exercise. Reduce abdominal obesity.
High cholesterol	Implement a low-fat diet and exercise; take medication as prescribed. Target levels of cholesterol are individually set.
Hypertension	Keep blood pressure less than 120/80 mm Hg.
Diabetes	Maintain good glycemic control by keeping blood glucose within normal limits (<100 mg/dL).
Tobacco/ nicotine use	Quit smoking. Do not use smokeless tobacco or e-cigarettes; nicotine by any route affects blood vessels.
Sedentary lifestyle	Maintain an exercise program of 30-min sessions three to five times a week. Any level of increased activity is helpful.
Excessive stress	Use stress reduction techniques regularly, such as exercise and relaxation techniques; reduce hostility; maintain a positive support system.
Excessive alcohol intake	Limit alcohol consumption to no more than recommended levels: men, 2 drinks/day; women, 1 drink/day.
Drug use	Do not use cocaine, methamphetamine, or other recreational drugs.

Nurses can play an important role in teaching others about hypertension, support patient efforts to prevent the disease and its long-term consequences, and contribute to reducing the incidence of the harmful effects of hypertension by participating in community screening programs and education. Nurses and other health care professionals have an obligation to serve as models for a healthy lifestyle.

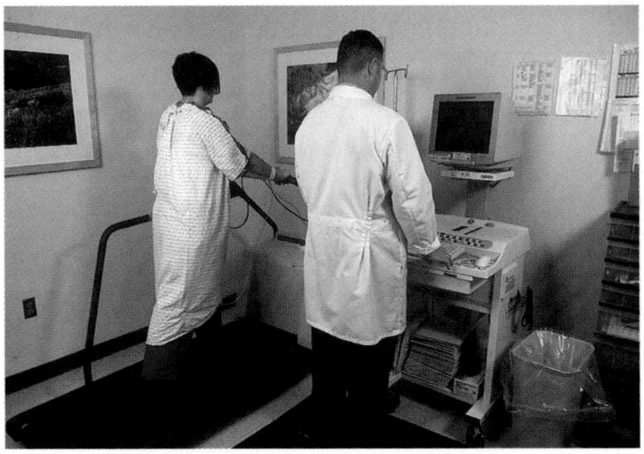

Fig. 17.7 Cardiac treadmill stress test.

Box 17.1 Metabolic Syndrome Components

- Elevated waist circumference indicating abdominal obesity: *men,* greater than 40 inches (102 cm); *women,* greater than 35 inches (88 cm)
- Elevated triglyceride level: greater than 150 mg/dL
- Reduced high-density lipoprotein cholesterol level: *men,* less than 40 mg/dL; *women,* less than 50 mg/dL
- Elevated blood pressure: at or above 130/85 mm Hg
- Elevated fasting blood glucose level indicating insulin resistance: 100 mg/dL or greater

DIAGNOSTIC TESTS AND PROCEDURES

In addition to a routine physical examination and medical history, the health care provider has access to a number of procedures and tests to help diagnose cardiovascular disease (Fig. 17.7). Noninvasive procedures usually are performed first and in general give less detailed information about cardiovascular structure and function. Specific cardiovascular diagnostic tests and their nursing implications are listed in Table 17.2.

Cardiac Monitoring

Continuous monitoring of cardiac rate and rhythm often is done by *telemetry.* Disposable electrodes and wire leads are applied to the patient and are connected to a battery-operated transmitter unit. The wave pattern signals are sent to a monitor in a central station, where they are continually observed. This allows patients to walk around the nursing unit while being monitored. The wave pattern signals may also be displayed on a bedside monitor when continuous observation of the electrocardiogram (ECG) is needed.

Cardiac monitors can detect specific dysrhythmias (abnormal variations of heart rhythm), automatically store the wave pattern, and alert you to the abnormality with an alarm. Cardiac monitoring is used for patients experiencing an acute cardiac disorder, after cardiac

Text continued on p. 392

Table 17.2 Common Diagnostic Tests for the Cardiovascular System

TEST	PURPOSE	PROCEDURE	NURSING IMPLICATIONS
Electrocardiography (12-lead electrocardiogram [ECG])	Records electrical impulses of the heart to determine rate, rhythm of heart, site of pacemaker, and presence of injury at rest	Small electrodes are placed on the chest and extremities to show conduction patterns in different directions of electrical flow. **Signal-averaged ECG** can be used for patients at high risk for serious ventricular arrhythmias. It takes longer than a standard ECG; monitoring takes approximately 10 min, and signals are averaged.	Inform patient that there is no discomfort with this test. Maintain electrical safety. Normal finding: normal ECG.
Holter monitor (ambulatory ECG) Multiple devices in addition to the Holter monitor are available. All record the ECG over hours or days during regular activities of daily living.	Correlates normal daily activity with electrical function of the heart to determine whether activity causes abnormalities	Patient wears a small ECG recorder for 6, 12, or 24 h while doing usual tasks. A diary is kept to show at what time the various activities were performed and any symptoms experienced. The record is analyzed to correlate any dysrhythmia with the activity at that time.	Remind patient that all activities must be recorded in the diary: brushing teeth, climbing stairs, sexual intercourse, bowel movements, sleeping, etc. Caution patient not to remove the electrodes and not to get the recorder or wires wet. Instruct patient to wear a loose shirt during test.
Loop recorder Implantable External	Continuously records ECG to determine if an arrhythmia is the cause of symptoms (e.g., syncope, palpitations, or dizziness)	A small device that records ECG activity for several months. The device can be implanted under the skin with local anesthesia or attached externally to the skin with long-term adhesive. The implanted device can be left in place for up to 3 yr.	The implanted device requires a small skin incision that will need assessment and care similar to that for any surgical incision.
Exercise ECG stress test (treadmill)	Records electrical activity of the heart during exercise Insufficient blood flow and oxygen can be identified by the abnormal waveforms they produce	Small electrodes are placed on the chest, and a tracing is made while the patient exercises on a treadmill, bicycle, or stairs. The degree of difficulty of the exercise is increased as the test continues to see how the heart reacts to increasing work demands. Vital signs are continuously recorded. May be combined with radionuclide imaging or echocardiograph. Health care provider is present.	Requires a signed consent form. Instruct patient to wear comfortable clothes and walking shoes. Light meal 2–3 h prior, then NPO. Regular medications are given. Chest is shaved as needed for electrode placement. Inform patient that the test will be stopped if chest pain, severe fatigue, or dyspnea develops.
Chemical stress test with dipyridamole, adenosine, regadenoson (may be used with nuclear imaging), or dobutamine	Used for those who cannot exercise for an ECG stress test	Continuous 12-lead ECG monitoring is performed, and the drug is administered. Blood pressure and pulse are taken and recorded q15min. The drug effect increases cardiac workload to identify whether cardiac ischemia results. The patient is NPO during the test.	Mild nausea or headache may occur. Explain that patient will lie on back for the test.

Table 17.2 Common Diagnostic Tests for the Cardiovascular System—cont'd

TEST	PURPOSE	PROCEDURE	NURSING IMPLICATIONS
Echocardiography	Useful in evaluating size, shape, and position of structures and movement within the heart Test of choice for valve problems Can evaluate blood flow through the heart and determine ejection fraction	An ultrasound probe that emits sonar waves is guided over the chest wall while the patient is supine or turned on the left side. Test takes 30–60 min. May be done in combination with the exercise (stress) test.	Inform patient that there is no discomfort, although conduction jelly may feel cool. Normal finding: no abnormalities of size or location of heart structures; normal wall movement.
Stress echocardiogram	Detects differences in left ventricular wall motion before and after exercise	Resting echocardiogram images are obtained. The patient exercises; within 1 min, postexercise images are obtained. May be done in conjunction with a chemical stress test.	Explain the procedure and the importance of returning to the examining table immediately after exercising. Instruct patient not to consume heavy meal beforehand and to abstain from using tobacco or caffeine for 6–8 h before test. Tell patient to wear walking shoes.
Venous ultrasound of the legs (lower extremity Doppler)	Assesses occlusion or thrombosis in a vein	A water-soluble gel is applied to bare skin in the area to be assessed. A Doppler transducer is passed over the area of the vessel. A grayscale image of the vessel is obtained with color depicting the blood flow velocity.	Instruct patient to abstain from smoking for 30 min before the test.
Impedance plethysmography	Estimates blood flow in a limb based on electrical resistance present before and after inflating a pneumatic cuff placed around the limb Detects deep vein thrombosis	Measurements of electrical resistance are taken before and after a pneumatic cuff placed around the limb is inflated. Electrodes are placed on opposite sides of the limb.	Instruct patient to wear loose clothing. Explain that some discomfort may occur during inflation of the cuff. The patient is placed on an examination table and positioned supine in a relaxed, comfortable position. The limb is properly positioned, and electrodes and the pneumatic cuff are applied.
Nuclear imaging (myocardial perfusion scan, myocardial perfusion imaging, thallium scan, sestamibi cardiac scan, and nuclear stress test)	Evaluates blood flow in various parts of the heart Determines areas of infarction	A radioactive tracer is injected IV; radioactive uptake is counted over the heart by a gamma scintillation camera. May be done in conjunction with an exercise ECG stress test and/or chemical stress test.	Explain that the radioactivity used is a very small amount and lasts only a few hours. Explain that a camera will be positioned over the heart. ECG electrodes are placed on the chest; scanning is done 10–15 min after injection; can be done as an outpatient procedure. May be done in two parts a few hours apart.

Continued

Table 17.2 Common Diagnostic Tests for the Cardiovascular System—cont'd

TEST	PURPOSE	PROCEDURE	NURSING IMPLICATIONS
Multiple-gated acquisition (MUGA) scan (radionuclide angiography)	Determines area and extent of myocardial infarction (MI) Assesses left ventricular function	^{99m}Tc is injected IV and is taken up by areas of infarction, producing hot spots when scanned. Multiple serial images are obtained. Best results occur when done 1–6 days after a suspected MI.	Inform patient that radioisotopes will be given IV and that it will be necessary to lie still while the machine scans the heart. The patient's glucose level must be between 60 and 140 mg/dL. If scan is combined with exercise, patient will need to be NPO and must abstain from using tobacco and caffeine for 24 h before the test.
Computed tomography (CT) scan **CT angiography**	Determines size and condition of aortic aneurysm Coronary vessels may be imaged	Noninvasive unless dye contrast is used. Patient is positioned on scanning table and moved under the scanner. Other medications may be given to slow down heart rate.	Instruct patient in necessity of holding still during scan.
Magnetic resonance imaging (MRI) **Magnetic resonance angiography (MRA)**	Evaluates cardiac tissue integrity, detects aneurysms, determines ejection fraction, and determines patency of proximal coronary arteries	Noninvasive magnetic resonance is used to depict tissue images. IV gadolinium is injected as a contrast medium for MRA.	Explain about the cylinder within which the patient will be positioned. Warn that there will be loud noises from the machine. Administer antianxiety medication if needed and ordered; provide ear protection.
Positron emission tomography	Evaluates myocardial perfusion	Baseline images are obtained, then a radioactive tracer is injected IV. Several scans will be done to provide different angles. Medications (same as used for chemical stress testing) may be given to increase heart rate. Additional images are obtained to see if there are areas of decreased blood flow with increased activity.	Inform patient that radioisotopes will be given IV and that it will be necessary to lie still while the machine scans the heart. The patient's glucose level must be between 60 and 140 mg/dL. If scan is combined with exercise, patient will need to be NPO and must abstain from using tobacco and caffeine for 24 h before the test.

Table 17.2 Common Diagnostic Tests for the Cardiovascular System—cont'd

TEST	PURPOSE	PROCEDURE	NURSING IMPLICATIONS
Transesophageal echocardiogram (TEE)	Provides images of the wall thickness, heart valve structure and function, atrial septum, and presence of clots, and can calculate ejection fraction	Pharynx is anesthetized with topical agent. With patient in left side-lying position, an endoscopic transducer is placed in the esophagus and positioned behind the heart. Recordings of the images are made. Test takes about 20 min.	Patient must be NPO for 4–6 h before test. Initiate IV access before test for sedation. Apply ECG leads for monitoring during test. Monitor pulse oximetry, end-tidal CO_2, and BP. Observe patient after test until sedation has worn off.
Angiogram (venogram)	Identifies thrombi within the venous system. Rarely used because noninvasive images provide adequate information.	A tourniquet may be placed on the extremity, and dye is injected into the affected extremity. Radiographs are taken at timed intervals. Also used to identify venous stenosis.	Requires a signed consent form. Assess for allergies to radiopaque contrast. Hydrate patient before the procedure. Tell patient it takes 30–90 min and that a warm flush may be felt when the dye is injected.
Arteriogram	Visualizes arterial anatomy and vascular disease in carotid, vertebral, aorta, renal, coronary, and peripheral arteries	A catheter is placed via the femoral artery into the desired artery. Radiopaque contrast is injected while x-ray (fluoroscopy) images are obtained. Digital subtraction techniques obliterate bony structures from the views. A balloon may be used during the procedure to open constricted areas. A stent may be placed in the vessel to keep it open.	Requires a signed consent form. Patient must be NPO for 2–8 h before test. Mark peripheral pulses before procedure. Check renal function and coagulation studies before test and alert provider of abnormal values. Mucomyst may be administered a day before and after the test to prevent dye-induced nephropathy. Warn patient that dye acts as a diuretic and may cause some bladder distention during the test. Metformin must be discontinued before and after the test for several days to prevent renal damage.

Continued

Table 17.2 Common Diagnostic Tests for the Cardiovascular System—cont'd

TEST	PURPOSE	PROCEDURE	NURSING IMPLICATIONS
Cardiac catheterization with coronary angiography; also called a *left heart catheterization (LHC)*	Assesses size and patency of coronary arteries and presence of collateral circulation Identifies pressure gradients for the aortic and mitral valves Assesses pumping action of the left side of the heart by measuring the ejection fraction of the left ventricle	Catheter is inserted into an artery. Femoral artery is commonly used but may use radial or axillary arteries. With local anesthetic and procedural sedation, using fluoroscopy, the catheter is threaded up the aorta to the coronary arteries, which come off the aorta just past the aortic valve. Contrast media is injected to visualize the size and shape of the coronary vessels. A separate catheter is used to pass through the aortic valve into the left ventricle. Contrast is injected into the chamber to visualize wall motion and calculate ejection fraction.	Requires a signed consent form. Patient must be NPO for 6–8 h before test. Assess patient for allergy to iodine, shellfish, or contrast dye. Have patient void before giving preoperative medication. Record baseline vital signs and mark location of pedal pulses. Inform patient that procedure involves being on a narrow table with a camera that rotates to different angles, patient will have an IV, and must lie still during test. Procedural sedation is used.
During the procedure *intravascular ultrasound (IVUS)* may be performed.	Assesses degree of narrowing of coronary vessels and the type of material causing the narrowing (e.g., calcium, clot, or plaque)	An ultrasound catheter may be advanced into the coronary artery to image the lumen of the vessel. This is accomplished through the existing vascular access and through the catheters already in place. It is done as an adjunct procedure to the LHC.	ECG leads, BP cuff, O_2 saturation monitor, CO_2 monitor will be in place during the test. Patient may be asked to cough or turn head during the procedure. Assess peripheral pulses with vital signs and question patient about numbness or tingling. Inspect insertion site for bleeding or signs of hematoma. If femoral insertion site was used, keep patient flat and leg extended for ordered time. If a closure device was used at the arterial puncture site, patient may be able to ambulate within 2 h. Encourage fluids unless contraindicated to flush contrast from body.

Table 17.2 Common Diagnostic Tests for the Cardiovascular System—cont'd

TEST	PURPOSE	PROCEDURE	NURSING IMPLICATIONS
Electrophysiology studies	Measure and record electrical activity from within the heart to determine the area of origin of the dysrhythmia and the effectiveness of the antidysrhythmic drug for the particular dysrhythmia	Three to six electrodes are placed in the heart through the venous system. Electrodes are attached to an oscilloscope that records the intracardiac and external ECG waveforms simultaneously. After baseline tracings are taken, the cardiologist tries to trigger the dysrhythmia that is to be studied by programmed electrical stimulation through the electrodes. Once the dysrhythmia is triggered, an antidysrhythmic drug is administered to determine its effectiveness in stopping the abnormal rhythm. Studies may take 1.5–4 h; serial studies may be done on different days.	Provide psychological support for the patient, who is commonly fearful of having dysrhythmias induced. Antidysrhythmic drugs may be stopped 24 h or more before the test to eliminate them from the patient's system. Assure the patient of constant monitoring and that emergency equipment and staff will be on hand. Keep patient NPO after midnight. Patent IV line is required. Electrodes are placed using fluoroscopy. Patient will be supine on an x-ray table. The femoral vein is most commonly used; the groin is shaved, and local anesthesia is used. Post-test care: much the same as for cardiac catheterization.
Hemodynamic monitoring via pulmonary artery (PA) (Swan-Ganz) catheter Placement of a PA catheter for diagnostic purposes is called a *right heart catheterization.*	Determines pressure, flow, and oxygenation within the right side of the heart and pulmonary vessels	A special catheter, infusion system, transducer, and a monitor are prepared, and the catheter is placed by the provider, usually under fluoroscopic guidance.	The system must be calibrated to perform properly. Readings are taken in the right atrium, right ventricle, and pulmonary artery, including pulmonary wedge pressures. Cardiac output may also be measured. Other data can then be calculated.
Laboratory Tests[a]			
B-type natriuretic peptide (BNP)	Determines degree of HF	Obtain 5–7 mL of venous blood; use an EDTA lavender-top tube.	No fasting is required.
C-reactive protein (CRP)	Level increased with inflammation	Obtain one tube of venous blood; use red-top tube.	Some laboratories require fasting; water is permitted. Low risk: <1 mg/dL High risk: >3 mg/dL
Serum lipids	Elevation of cholesterol is a risk factor for atherosclerotic heart disease.	Use red-top serum separator tube (SST). Upon collection, the tube is inverted 6–12 times to accelerate the clotting process and separate the serum from the clot.	Patient is NPO except for noncaloric liquids for 12 h. Normal ranges: Cholesterol: 150–200 mg/dL HDL: 30–80 mg/dL LDL: 60–180 mg/dL (with two or more risk factors, <73 mg/dL) Triglycerides: 40–150 mg/dL

Continued

Table 17.2 Common Diagnostic Tests for the Cardiovascular System—cont'd

TEST	PURPOSE	PROCEDURE	NURSING IMPLICATIONS
Myoglobin	Is released by all damaged muscles, including the heart	Obtain 5 mL blood; use a red-top tube. Apply pressure to venipuncture site.	No fasting is required. An elevated level can help confirm an MI. A nonelevated level rules out an MI. Normal value: <90 mcg/L
Troponin I (Tn I) Troponin T (Tn T)	Proteins specific to heart muscle are released into the circulation with heart muscle damage	Troponin I and T require different tubes for collection. Serial samples are usually drawn.	Levels may elevate within 4–6 h after MI, peak within 10–24 h, and return to normal within 10 days. Normal values: Tn I: <0.3 mcg/L Tn T: <0.1 mcg/L
Creatinine phosphokinase (CPK)	CPK is an enzyme found mainly in the heart, brain, and skeletal muscle	Serial samples are drawn over a 2-day period.	Elevated within 4–8 h after heart attack (may also rise with injury to other muscles). Peaks within 12–24 h; returns to normal levels within 3–4 days. Normal ranges: Men: 55–170 international units/L Women: 30–135 international units/L
CK-MB (creatinine kinase)	Isoenzyme of CPK that is primarily found in the heart	Serial samples may be evaluated.	Elevates within 2–6 h after an MI, peaks within 12–24 h, and returns to normal within 3 days. CK-MB is specific to myocardial injury. Normal value: <3 ng/mL
Homocysteine	An amino acid (a building block of protein) usually present in the blood as a result of eating meat	Obtain blood sample; use a blue- or purple-top tube.	10- to 12-h fast is required. Normal ranges: Men: 5.2–12.9 μmol/L Women: 3.7–10.4 μmol/L Elevated level is considered an independent risk factor for ischemic heart disease. There are no current guidelines that recommend use of the test, and most insurance will not cover the significant cost.
Myeloperoxidase (MPO)	Found in heme and is an antimicrobial enzyme biomarker for predicting risk for cardiovascular disease	Obtain 0.5-mL blood; use a yellow-top tube.	No fasting required. Normal value: <6 units/mL Detects or assists in ruling out microangiitis of the arteries.

[a]Electrolyte values are listed in Chapter 3, Table 3.3.
[99m]Tc, Technetium-99m; *BP*, blood pressure; *CO_2*, carbon dioxide; *EDTA*, ethylenediaminetetraacetic acid; *HDL*, high-density lipoprotein; *HF*, heart failure; *IV*, intravenously; *LDL*, low-density lipoprotein; *NPO*, nothing by mouth; *O_2*, oxygen.

surgery, after pacemaker insertion, and for patients with a potential for developing dysrhythmias. Fig. 17.8 shows proper placement for telemetry leads.

Specific Tests for Vascular Disorders

Diagnosing a vascular problem begins with a history and physical examination that includes a variety of tests for risk factors for vascular disorders. A complete blood cell count (CBC); urinalysis; blood lipid and cholesterol assessment (including high-density lipoprotein [HDL] and low-density lipoprotein [LDL]); or sequential multiple analyzer (SMA, also called a *metabolic panel*) panel that screens liver and kidney function, electrolytes, and blood glucose are ordered. If blood pressure is elevated, tests of thyroid, adrenal glands, kidneys, and renal arteries are done to rule out the possibility of another disease that might cause secondary hypertension. Hyperthyroidism, Cushing syndrome, pheochromocytoma, nephrosclerosis, and renal arterial stenosis all elevate blood pressure.

Doppler flow studies are performed to detect a venous thrombus when one is suspected and to assess the patency of the carotid arteries. Angiography may be performed to determine areas of narrowing in arteries or to detect a blockage. Computed tomography (CT) angiography may be used to detect emboli in the lungs or blockages in coronary arteries. An echocardiogram may be performed to assess wall motion of the heart, valve function, and ejection fraction.

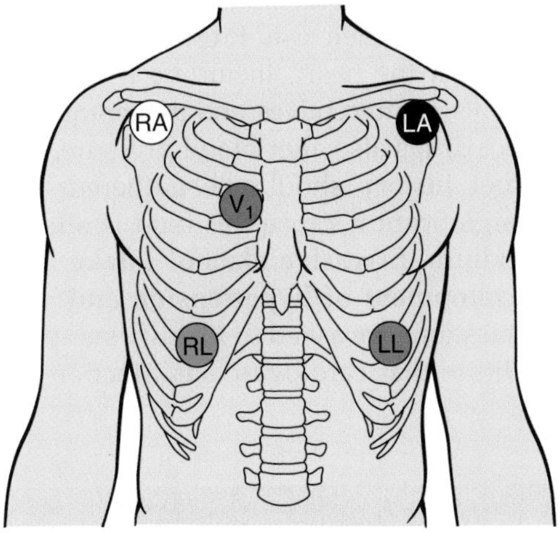

Fig. 17.8 Placement of the most commonly used telemetry leads. *LA*, Left arm; *LL*, left leg; *RA*, right arm; *RL*, right leg; *V_1*, chest lead corresponding to the V_1 on a 12-lead electrocardiogram.

The ankle-brachial index (ABI) is an inexpensive, noninvasive bedside screening test to evaluate arterial status in the lower extremities (Fig. 17.9). A regular blood pressure cuff is placed above the malleolus. Another blood pressure cuff is positioned over the brachial artery. A Doppler probe is used to check the systolic end point at the dorsalis pedis and the posterior tibial sites. The brachial blood pressure is measured. The ABI is calculated by dividing the systolic ankle pressure by the systolic brachial pressure. An ABI of 1 or more is considered normal. An abnormal ABI indicates arterial disease and can confirm a vascular cause for ischemic pain in the legs at rest and **intermittent claudication** (cramping pain in the muscles brought on by exercise and relieved by rest). This pain is most common in the calves of the legs, but it also can affect the muscles of the thighs and buttocks. Chronic occlusive arterial disease commonly causes pain described as burning and tingling, with numbness of the toes. It is most noticeable at night when the patient is in bed.

See Table 17.2 for diagnostic tests used to detect other problems in the vascular system. Serum cholesterol and lipids are also discussed in Chapter 18.

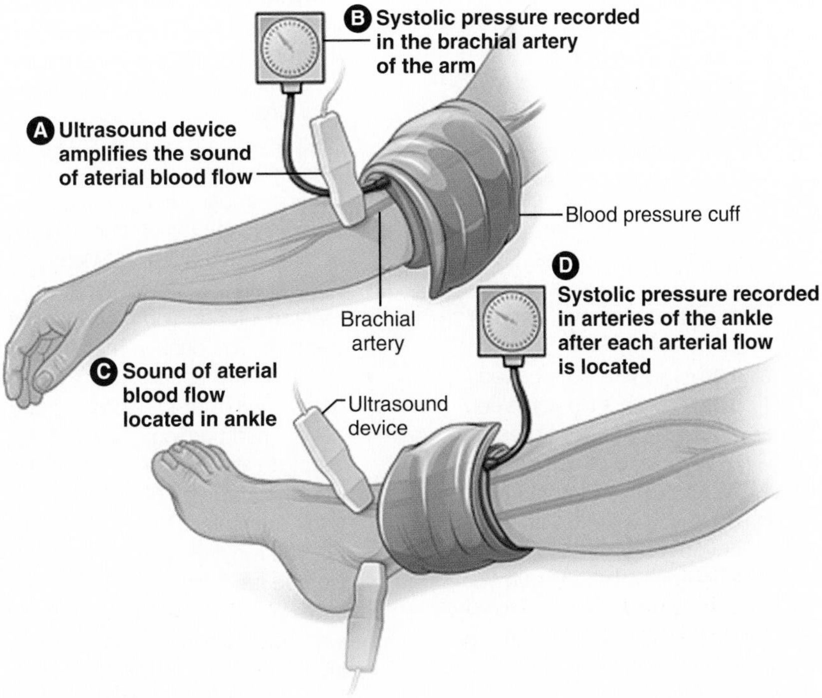

Fig. 17.9 Ankle-brachial index. (From National Heart, Lung, and Blood Institute; National Institutes of Health; U.S. Department of Health and Human Services.)

Think Critically

Identify four teaching points to be covered for the patient who will undergo an arteriogram.

NURSING MANAGEMENT

ASSESSMENT (DATA COLLECTION)

History Taking

It is important to determine whether the patient has risk factors for cardiovascular disease. Much of this information is obtained by the health care provider or nurse practitioner during history taking and by the admitting nurse during a complete nursing assessment. Some additional information, however, will be gathered in less formal interactions when the patient becomes more relaxed and comfortable with the nurses providing care.

Information concerning the patient's actual eating habits, such as snacking on "junk" food or daily consumption of several drinks containing caffeine, is more likely to be obtained during nursing care activities than during the initial assessment. Data concerning stressors in the patient's life and their response to them are more easily assessed while interacting over time.

An understanding of the patient's perception of their condition and overall health is necessary to plan appropriate teaching. The effectiveness of your communication with the patient will determine the quality of subjective data obtained. Many over-the-counter (OTC) drugs can cause vasoconstriction and elevate blood pressure. Cold remedies, decongestants, and diet pills are particularly noted for having this effect. Patients sometimes do not consider OTC items as medications and do not report their use. Prescription medications also may affect the heart, including bronchodilators, anticoagulants, contraceptives, and psychotropic medications. Street drugs also alter blood pressure. A careful, specific diet history should be gathered. Fast-food intake is significant because this food is often high in fat and sodium. **Excessive alcohol intake is a factor in the development of hypertension and cardiomyopathy.** Questions are asked to identify symptoms that might indicate that cardiovascular function has been impaired.

Focused Assessment

Data Collection for the Cardiovascular System

HISTORY TAKING

Ask the following questions:

- Do you ever have any chest discomfort or pain? What does it feel like? What, if anything, seems to bring it on? What makes it worse? How long does it last? Is it worse when you breathe in deeply? What gives relief? Does the pain radiate (spread) to other parts of the body—for example, down the arm or up into the neck or jaw, or to the upper abdomen? Is it localized, or does it cover a large area? On a scale of 1 to 10, with 10 being the worst and 0 being none, how do you rate your pain? Do you have numbness, tingling, nausea, sweating, shortness of breath, anxiety, or dizziness when you have chest pain?
- Have you or any member of your family ever been told that you have diabetes mellitus; cardiovascular, thyroid, or renal disease; arteriosclerosis; hyperlipidemia; atherosclerosis; peripheral vascular disease; a blood disorder; gout; kidney disease; or an immune disorder such as lupus erythematosus?
- Do you become easily fatigued? Dizzy or lightheaded?
- Do you become short of breath? When? Do you sleep on more than one pillow? Is your shortness of breath worse after physical activity? What kind of activity? When walking up steps? Does it occur when you are at rest? Does resting relieve it? Do you wake up at night short of breath or feeling like you are suffocating? Does sitting up on the side of the bed or getting up give you relief?
- Do you have a cough? What kind? Dry and hacking, or wet and productive? What does the sputum look like? Is there ever any blood in your sputum?
- Do you notice your heart beating very fast or pounding in your chest (palpitations)? Does it skip a beat?
- Have you ever fainted or felt like you were going to faint?
- Do you get up in the night to urinate? How many times do you get up each night?
- Have you noticed any sudden weight gain or swelling in the feet and legs?
- Do you experience pain in your legs when walking?
- Are your feet always cold?
- Have you ever had a bad injury to either leg?
- Have you ever had a deep vein thrombosis (DVT) or thrombophlebitis?
- What medications do you take that are prescribed by your health care provider? What over-the-counter medications do you take? Do you take herbals? Do you use recreational drugs?
- Do you smoke? Have you ever smoked? How much and for how long? Do you use nicotine in any form—smokeless tobacco, e-cigarettes, patches?
- Do you drink alcohol? What do you usually drink? How many drinks do you have? About how many times a week do you drink something alcoholic?
- What do you usually eat? Can you tell me what you generally eat for breakfast, lunch, and dinner? Do you have a midmorning, midafternoon, or evening snack? What do you eat for a snack? Do you eat fast food often? What type of fast food? What do you usually drink at meals? Do you drink liquids between meals?
- Do you regularly add salt to your food?
- Do you have leg pain at night?
- Have you ever had a sore on your foot or lower leg that was slow to heal?
- How would you rate your stress levels? What do you do to cope with or reduce stress?

Think Critically

How would you phrase questions about alcohol intake or drug use so that the patient will answer honestly?

Physical Assessment

Significant findings include abnormal or extra heart sounds, crackles in the lungs, or pink frothy sputum indicating pulmonary edema.

Cultural Considerations

Diet and Culture

Food is at the center of most family and social activities. Society and family culture determine eating habits. In some cultures and ethnic groups, food is part of religious observances. When teaching a heart-healthy diet, be aware that you are not just asking someone to change food consumption, but also affecting family traditions and valued rituals.

Chest pain, if present, should be further assessed using the "PQRST" memory device (Table 17.3). Other significant findings might be a bluish cast to skin; pallor or diaphoresis (sweating); clubbing of the fingers; or pitting edema of the feet, ankles, or sacral area (see Chapter 3, Fig. 3.5). There may be distended jugular veins, an abnormal rate or volume of pulses, or a pulse deficit. A pulse deficit is the difference between the apical and radial pulse rate when they are counted at the same time.

An apical pulse rate should be taken for all patients on admission. Privacy should be provided before baring the chest, and the room should be warm. Heart sounds are auscultated at least every 8 hours on all patients who have a known dysrhythmia or a potential for dysrhythmia, a valve problem, or heart failure (Fig. 17.10).

Table 17.3 "PQRST" For Pain Assessment[a]

FACTOR	QUESTIONS TO ASK
Precipitating events	What events or factors precipitated or caused the pain or discomfort?
Quality of pain or discomfort	What does the pain or discomfort feel like? Is it aching, dull, sharp, tight, heavy pressure, etc.?
Radiation of pain	Where is the pain located? Does it radiate to the back, arms, jaw, teeth, shoulder, or elbow?
Severity of pain	On a scale of 0–10, with 10 being the most severe, how do you rate the pain?
Timing	When did the pain or discomfort begin? Has it changed since it started? Has this type of pain occurred before?

[a]This memory device is used to assist in obtaining information from any patient experiencing chest pain or discomfort.

Focused Assessment

Physical Examination of the Cardiovascular System

When assessing the cardiovascular system, check for:

- Skin color, temperature, and texture
- Facial expression: signs of pain or anxiety
- Vital signs
- Heart sounds: S_1, S_2, abnormal sounds, murmurs
- Apical pulse rate and rhythm; presence of pulse deficit
- Quality of peripheral pulses; compare them bilaterally
- Breath sounds: presence of crackles in lung bases
- Shape of fingers: presence of clubbing (see Chapter 12, Fig. 12.8)
- Appearance of neck veins: presence of venous jugular distention
- Abdomen: presence of distention; abdominal pulsation
- Ankles and feet: presence of edema and degree
- General body appearance: presence of edema
- Weight: gain of 2 lb or more over a few days
- Varicosities in lower extremities

Clinical Cues

Chest pain should be considered cardiac in origin until another cause can be ruled out. Many things can cause chest pain, but it is important to always think "cardiac first."

The diaphragm of the stethoscope is placed over the bare skin at the mitral area to listen to the apical pulse. S_1 (lub) and S_2 (dub) should be distinguished. S_1 occurs with the closing of the AV valves during systole. S_2 is the closure of the pulmonic and semilunar (aortic) valves during diastole. Extra sounds or gallops may occur as S_3 sounds. Splitting of the S_2 sound may be normal in children and young adults but may be abnormal in adults. S_4 is usually heard just before S_1 and can indicate various heart diseases.

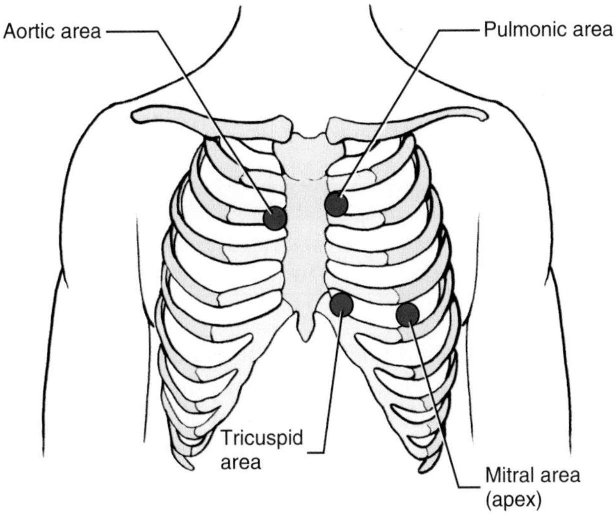

Fig. 17.10 Sites for auscultation of heart sounds. S_1 is loudest at mitral and tricuspid areas. S_2 is loudest at aortic and pulmonic areas. Listen in the mitral area for S_3 and S_4 sounds. (From Williams P: *deWit's fundamental concepts and skills for nursing,* ed 5, St. Louis, 2018, Elsevier.)

Box 17.2 Scale for Grading Pulse Quality

0	Absent
+1	Weak, thready
+2	Light volume
+3	Normal volume
+4	Full, bounding

The bell of the stethoscope is used to listen for heart murmurs. **It must be placed lightly on the skin for the sounds to be heard.** Murmurs usually have a "swooshing" sound from turbulent blood flow. Murmurs are commonly the result of damaged valves, causing abnormal blood flow in the heart. Because heart sounds typically are very soft, ask the patient to refrain from talking and turn off the television or other sources of extra sound while listening. (Just remember to turn it back on.) Having the patient roll to the left side or lean forward may make the sounds louder and clearer.

Older Adult Care Points

The thickening of valve leaflets with age may cause a systolic murmur common in persons older than age 80 years.

Pulses. Check the arterial pulses and determine the pulse rate, rhythm, and character (force) of the pulse (Box 17.2). When performing a cardiovascular assessment, the radial pulse should be assessed and compared with the apical pulse. The apical pulse should be counted for a full minute. The carotid, femoral, popliteal, and pedal pulses should also be palpated and compared bilaterally, noting quality and character (Fig. 17.11). The quality of pulses is graded as to their intensity. The character of the pulse is its regularity (see Box 17.2).

If pulsations are weak or undetectable, use a Doppler device to check them. A Doppler measures the velocity of blood flow through a vessel with ultrasound waves. It can sense weak pulsations even in severely narrowed arteries. Dopplers may have a stethoscope or handheld probe attachment (Fig. 17.12).

Think Critically

Recall the correct way to locate a dorsalis pedis and a posterior tibial pulse. Demonstrate the technique to a classmate.

Examine the abdomen with the patient lying supine to observe for a visual abdominal pulsation from the aorta. This indicates the presence of an aneurysm. If a pulsation is seen, DO NOT palpate the abdomen.

Bruits. A whooshing or purring sound (a **bruit**) is made either when blood passes through a turbulent area of an artery possibly caused by a partial obstruction or when the blood is flowing rapidly. To detect bruits, listen with the bell of the stethoscope applied lightly over the skin of the carotid arteries, abdominal aorta, and femoral arteries.

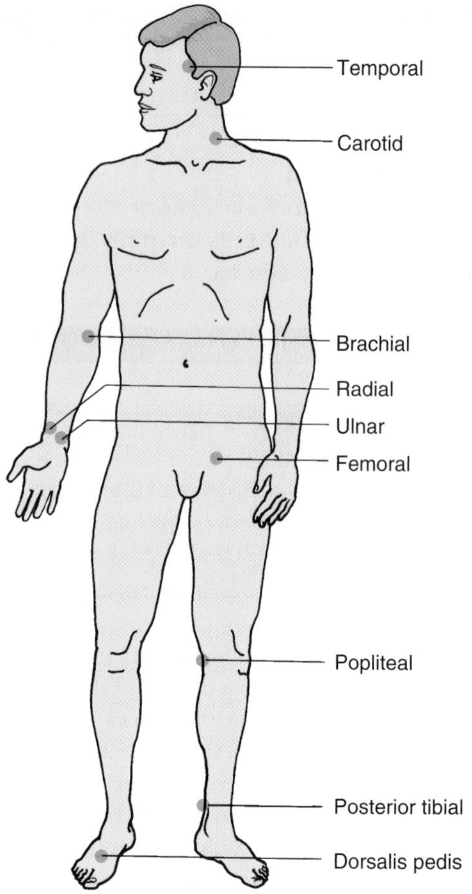

Fig. 17.11 Palpation sites for arterial pulse.

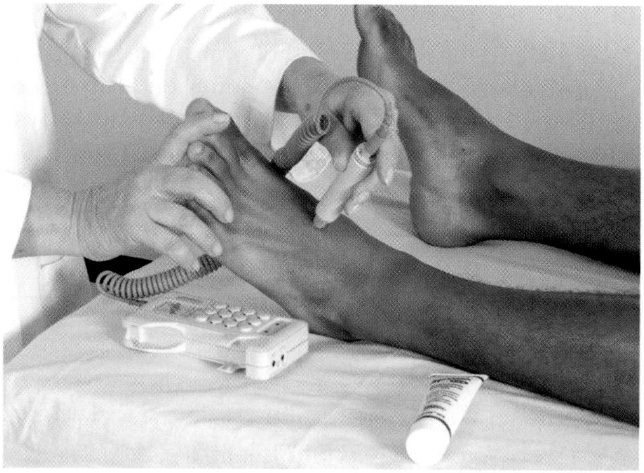

Fig. 17.12 The Doppler stethoscope is used to detect a faint pulse. (From Jarvis C: *Physical examination and health assessment*, ed 7, St. Louis, 2016, Elsevier.)

Blood pressure. For more accurate readings, be certain the patient has not had a cigarette or any caffeine for the past 30 minutes. Blood pressure should be carefully measured with the correct cuff size. The cuff should fit the upper arm with the lower edge 2.5 cm (1 inch) above the antecubital space. If the cuff is too narrow, the pressure will be falsely elevated. Cuffs are available in child, normal adult, and large adult sizes. The inflatable portion of the cuff must be centered over the brachial artery, and its length should cover at least 80% of the extremity's circumference when positioned correctly. The pressure should be taken lying supine, sitting, and standing for a thorough assessment. Standing blood pressure measurements also are important when a patient is started on a new medication, particularly an angiotensin-converting enzyme (ACE) inhibitor. Blood pressure should be measured on both arms. The arm on which the cuff is placed should be supported at heart level, and the feet should be supported or be on the floor. The patient should be resting quietly for 5 minutes before the measurement is taken. The equipment used should be calibrated, and the valve should open and close smoothly. The cuff should be deflated slowly and smoothly to obtain a correct diastolic reading. Automatic blood pressure machines must regularly be calibrated and checked for accuracy.

Orthostatic or postural hypotension occurs when the blood pressure drops when a person stands. Orthostatic or postural hypotension is a common cause of **syncope** (fainting) in older patients. A decrease of 20 mm Hg systolic pressure or a drop of 10 mm Hg diastolic pressure within 3 minutes of standing is orthostatic hypotension.

Older Adult Care Points

The blood pressure of older adult patients is usually lower right after a meal. For accurate readings, assess blood pressure between meals.

Skin. Tissues in light-skinned people who are receiving an adequate supply of oxygenated blood appear pink and rosy, whereas tissues deprived of normal amounts of arterial blood appear pale and mottled. In dark-skinned people, the mucous membranes will be rosy and pink if oxygenation is adequate. However, the environment must be taken into account. Pale and mottled skin also can indicate that the patient is cold. Reddish-blue color can indicate venous insufficiency.

One way to assess arterial blood flow more accurately is by having the patient elevate their feet and legs above the level of the heart for 1 to 3 minutes until pallor occurs. Have the patient lower the legs to a dangling position while sitting. Compare both feet, noting the time necessary for pinkness to return (usually about 10 seconds). Note the time it takes for the veins of the feet and ankles to fill (usually about 15 seconds). For those with dark skin, inspect the soles of the feet for color change and use a light shining at an angle to visualize vein filling.

Return of color to the lowered feet is delayed in arterial insufficiency. If there is severe peripheral arterial disease, the dangling feet soon take on a dusky red color (**rubor**). The skin may be shiny and taut.

A cold environment and immobility will cause the extremities to feel cold to the touch. However, when a patient experiences persistent coldness of an extremity in a warm environment, peripheral arterial disease should be suspected. When observing a patient for signs of arterial disease, note differences in skin temperature in various areas of the same limb, as well as differences between limbs.

Skin that is chronically malnourished because of decreased blood supply has a characteristic appearance: the skin appears smooth, shiny, and thin, and there is little or no hair on its surface. The nails are thick and yellow.

Edema is either present, absent, pitting, or nonpitting. Pitting means that a fingertip pressed into the area for 5 seconds leaves an indentation. Pitting is graded on a scale from 1+ to 4+ depending on how deep the skin can be depressed and how long the indentation remains. Review Chapter 3 for assessment and staging of edema.

The capillary refill test has traditionally been used to check peripheral circulation. A fingernail or a toenail is squeezed over the bed of the nail to cause blanching; the pressure is removed and an observation is made of how quickly the color returns. Normally the color returns immediately; less than 2 seconds is considered normal. Although it is a good gross assessment of circulation to the extremity, this test may be unreliable because many factors can cause a decrease in time for color to return. This test is most useful for determining whether circulation is occluded by constriction or thrombosis above the area and has been shown to be a "red flag" warning in the assessment of children. A new device is available that squeezes the finger and uses optical sensors to identify color change, eliminating the subjectivity of human interpretation.

◆ NURSING DIAGNOSIS, PLANNING, IMPLEMENTATION

Table 17.4 presents general problem statements or nursing diagnoses, expected outcomes, and nursing interventions for patients experiencing cardiovascular problems. Problem statements or nursing diagnoses may be added to the care plan for problems secondary to treatments, such as drug side effects or complications from surgery or preexisting diseases of other body systems.

A goal of community nursing is the promotion of healthful living to prevent cardiovascular disease. A concerted effort is being made to decrease childhood obesity as a method of decreasing risk for cardiovascular disease in adulthood. Blood sugar management in patients with diabetes and blood pressure control in those with hypertension are important for preventing vascular complications.

When planning care for cardiovascular patients, it is important to schedule nursing activities to conserve the strength of the patient and prevent excessive fatigue. Patients undergoing telemetry monitoring should not

Table 17.4 Common Problem Statements, Expected Outcomes, and Interventions for Patients With Heart Disorders

PROBLEM STATEMENT/ NURSING DIAGNOSIS	GOALS/EXPECTED OUTCOMES	NURSING INTERVENTIONS
Cardiac Disorders		
Altered activity tolerance due to decreased perfusion	Patient will not experience undue fatigue performing activities with changes in vital signs.	Space activities of daily living and nursing procedures to prevent undue fatigue. Encourage use of oxygen as ordered. Implement actions to promote rest.
Potential for altered tissue perfusion due to dysrhythmia or complications of myocardial infarction (MI) or heart failure (HF)	Patient will not experience serious dysrhythmia and will have a stable ECG. Patient will not experience complications from MI or HF.	Monitor ECG or telemetry tracings, observing for changes and life-threatening dysrhythmias. Assess for complications: Monitor lungs for crackles. Check for jugular venous distention. Auscultate for changes in heart sounds, extra sounds, changes in rhythm. Assess respirations for increasing dyspnea. Assess for signs of inflammation or infection; check temperature trend, white blood cell (WBC) level. Assess for chest pain on exertion or at rest. Monitor for central and peripheral edema. Assess trends in daily weight. Assess trends in 24-h intake and output. Monitor vital signs.
Potential for altered cardiac output due to dysrhythmia or ineffective cardiac muscle action	Patient will demonstrate adequate cardiac output with normal pulses, vital signs, skin color, and urine output.	Assess apical pulse every shift. Administer antidysrhythmic and cardiotonic medications as ordered. Observe for side effects of medications. Assess for adequate perfusion: Check peripheral pulses. Assess color of extremities and around mouth. Assess mentation. Monitor urine output (related to perfusion of kidneys). Auscultate lungs for crackles every shift. Assess level of fatigue. Treat impaired oxygenation and fluid imbalance. Give stool softeners or laxatives, as ordered, to prevent straining at stool (Valsalva maneuver) and slowing of pulse or stopping of heart.
Altered gas exchange due to cardiac failure	Patient will not experience impaired oxygenation; SpO_2 within normal limits and PO_2 between 80 and 100.	Place in high Fowler position. Administer oxygen, as ordered. Feed frequent small meals to decrease oxygen demand. Administer diuretics as ordered. Monitor intake and output. Enforce fluid restrictions. Assist with activities of daily living (ADLs). Promote relief of anxiety. Give morphine, as ordered, to ease breathing and decrease anxiety. Monitor lung sounds, pulse oximetry, and blood gases. Assist to use incentive spirometer q2h as ordered.
Altered self-care ability due to fatigue, weakness, or dyspnea	Patient will increase performance of own ADLs of 1–3 metabolic equivalents (METs) within 1 wk.	Assist with all ADLs as needed. Plan nursing treatments to provide rest periods. Encourage to do small tasks of ADLs as condition improves. Assist to turn in bed q2h. Assess skin every shift and when turning. Provide mouth care before meals to stimulate appetite.

Table 17.4 **Common Problem Statements, Expected Outcomes, and Interventions for Patients With Heart Disorders—cont'd**

PROBLEM STATEMENT/ NURSING DIAGNOSIS	GOALS/EXPECTED OUTCOMES	NURSING INTERVENTIONS
Fear due to life-threatening illness	Patient will verbalize feelings and fears regarding life-threatening condition. Patient will identify own best coping mechanisms.	Perform a spiritual assessment. Determine usual coping style. Support in coping mechanisms. Obtain clergy if patient desires contact. Provide privacy for prayer and devotions. Assist to express fears to reduce anxiety. Keep informed of what is being done for treatment and what to expect. Inform of positive gains toward wellness. Allow state of denial in acute stage; denial may be protective. Provide time with loved ones. Provide therapeutic touch if patient is accepting. Assess cultural meanings of events to patient. Actively listen to the patient's fears and concerns. Offer realistic reassurance as appropriate.
Decreased ability for home maintenance due to fatigue, dyspnea, and activity intolerance	Appropriate home services will be in place before discharge.	Refer for social services consultation. Consider home health care services. Offer information on homemaker aide services. Consult with family regarding ongoing care of patient at home. Collaborate with patient regarding plans for home care.
Vascular Disorders		
Altered tissue perfusion due to vascular damage from elevated blood pressure	There will be no further tissue injury as evidenced by skin color, temperature, and integrity the same or improved in 2 wk. Patient's blood pressure will be within normal range within 3 mo.	Assess blood pressure; determine effectiveness of therapy. Administer medications to lower blood pressure. Discourage intake of caffeine and excess sodium. Discourage smoking. Teach to arise slowly and stabilize before walking to counteract postural hypotension effect from medication. Teach anxiety- and tension-reduction techniques to decrease blood pressure. Encourage regular rest, relaxation, and exercise program.
Potential for injury due to obstructed blood flow	Patient will not develop thrombosis or emboli. Thrombosis will resolve within 10–14 days.	Assess for signs and symptoms of deep vein thrombosis and impaired blood flow. Maintain activity restrictions as ordered. Elevate affected extremity as ordered. Increase fluid intake to 3000 mL/day unless contraindicated. Administer anticoagulants as ordered; monitor for side effects. Teach to prevent future episodes by encouraging not to sit with legs crossed, not to sit for long periods, and not to put pressure on the back of the knees. Apply elastic stockings or sequential pneumatic devices to promote venous return.
Potential for bleeding due to surgical revascularization	Patient will not develop bleeding or decreased perfusion.	Check incisions for bleeding q1–2h × 24 h, then q4h × 6, then every shift. Assess for internal hematoma by checking sensation below surgical area. Assess for adequate blood flow by checking pulses distal to incision on same schedule. Assess skin color and temperature above and below incision when checking for bleeding. Reinforce dressing as needed; change dressing per orders, using strict aseptic technique.

Continued

Table 17.4 Common Problem Statements, Expected Outcomes, and Interventions for Patients With Heart Disorders—cont'd

PROBLEM STATEMENT/ NURSING DIAGNOSIS	GOALS/EXPECTED OUTCOMES	NURSING INTERVENTIONS
Pain related to decreased blood flow and edema	Patient will verbalize adequate pain control attained from analgesics and comfort measures provided.	Assess type and location of pain experienced. Handle gently and avoid jarring the bed. Use a bed cradle or footboard to prevent pressure from bed linens. Administer analgesics and antiinflammatory agents as ordered. Apply heat as ordered; monitor closely to prevent burns. Teach relaxation techniques, imagery, or distraction to decrease pain. Elevate edematous extremity. Apply elastic stockings or sequential pneumatic devices to encourage venous return and decrease edema. Medicate for sleep as ordered if discomfort is interfering with rest.
Altered activity tolerance related to pain in legs when walking	Patient will develop own activity program within 3 wk. Patient will exercise regularly according to devised program.	Collaborate with physical therapist to encourage prescribed exercises. Assist to plan walking, swimming, or cycling program.
Altered body image related to: Diagnosis of chronic illness Edema and dilated veins in the legs Loss of limb by amputation Inability to maintain former lifestyle	Patient will verbalize feelings regarding diagnosis, body changes, and needed lifestyle changes. Patient will identify personal strengths and coping mechanisms within 3 wk. Patient will become as independent as possible in tasks of daily living within 2 mo.	Allow to express feelings about illness and disease process. Assist through the grief process. Assist to identify personal strengths. Reinforce coping mechanisms that have been helpful before. Be with patient for first dressing change. Clarify misconceptions about physical limitations after amputation. Involve patient in care of the wound after initial period of adjustment. Foster independence in tasks of daily living. Assist to explore lifestyle changes. Encourage significant others in their support of the patient. Teach ways to decrease risk of further amputation.
Altered tissue integrity related to: Ulcer from decreased circulation Surgical wound (Potential for infection may be used here also.)	Tissue will show signs of healing within 1 wk. Patient will not develop a wound infection.	Use strict aseptic technique for wound care. Treat and dress wound per health care provider's orders. Promote adequate nutrition to promote healing. Administer medication, as ordered, to prevent infection. Position affected limb as ordered. Maintain correct body alignment.
Potential for altered tissue integrity related to bed rest and impaired circulation	Patient will not develop impaired tissue integrity.	Inspect pressure points q2h. Turn at least q2h. Maintain smooth linens on bed; provide appropriate padding to prevent pressure areas. Keep skin clean and dry. Refrain from raising the knee section of the bed. Encourage foot and ankle exercises every hour while patient is awake. Prevent shearing when patient is moving in bed by using a lift sheet and two people to turn the patient. Use mechanical lifts when indicated and special beds for complicated skin lesions. If skin breakdown occurs, notify provider immediately and provide appropriate wound care.

Table 17.4 Common Problem Statements, Expected Outcomes, and Interventions for Patients With Heart Disorders—cont'd

PROBLEM STATEMENT/ NURSING DIAGNOSIS	GOALS/EXPECTED OUTCOMES	NURSING INTERVENTIONS
Insufficient knowledge due to inadequate information about disease process, medications, and self-care	Patient will verbalize knowledge of disease process and ways to prevent further damage. Patient will verbalize how to take medications and side effects to report. Patient will demonstrate self-care techniques.	Explain what is happening in the body to cause the decreased blood flow. Allow time for questions. Instruct in ways to decrease risk factors. Teach self-care methods, including exercises, skin care, foot care, dietary changes, and lifestyle changes. Teach about medications, including schedule of administration, action, side effects, and what to report to the provider. Encourage regular visits to the provider.
Inadequate health maintenance due to refusal to follow treatment regimen	Patient will verbalize barriers in complying with treatment regimen and lifestyle changes. Patient will discuss with health care team strategies to overcome barriers. Patient will demonstrate compliance with treatment regimen.	Reinstruct about disease process. Explore problems with treatment regimen. Allow patient to express feelings about lifestyle changes. Explore ability to obtain and afford medications. Explore any difficulty in swallowing medications. Explain progression of disease and consequences of poor control; discuss complications and effect on lifestyle. Seek support system for compliance with treatment program. Give praise for each attempt at compliance. Respect the patient's right to make decisions about compliance.
Potential for injury due to: Embolus or bleeding from anticoagulant medication Circulatory occlusion from embolus	Coagulation times will remain within safe therapeutic range. Patient will have no signs of bleeding. Patient will have no signs of embolus.	Encourage activity as ordered. Monitor laboratory values: international normalized ratio (INR) or activated partial thromboplastin time (APTT); notify provider when values are outside of accepted therapeutic limits. Assess urine and stool for signs of blood. Assess patient for excessive bruising, bleeding gums, nosebleeds, or bleeding at puncture sites. Check injectable anticoagulant dosages and IV admixtures with another nurse before administration to verify correct ordered dosage and rate of infusion. Assess for signs of embolus: chest pain, shortness of breath, change in level of consciousness, sudden headache, or other neurologic signs.

ECG, Electrocardiogram; *IV*, intravenous.

be disconnected from their monitor for any extended time. Check whether the patient may shower before disconnecting the telemetry device. **Reconnect the leads immediately afterward.**

Clinical Cues

Know what the patient's last blood pressure and pulse measurements were before going to the room with cardiovascular medications. Often you will need to take an apical pulse rate and blood pressure reading before administering certain medications. You need to know what those measurements were previously to properly evaluate the patient's status. Plan time to take these measurements and record them.

When a patient has a history of thrombosis, plan measures to prevent recurrence regardless of the patient problem that is currently the focus of treatment. If the patient has peripheral arterial disease, be alert to prescribed medications that may cause further vasoconstriction. Understanding the patient's overall condition allows for individualized care specific to the patient.

A large part of what you do for a patient with a cardiovascular disorder is to monitor the condition and determine whether treatment is effective. Considerable time is spent on teaching patients about the disease, self-care, and medications. It is very important to monitor side effects or adverse effects of medication and to teach the patient what effects to report.

Remember that any patient experiencing fatigue or weakness takes longer to accomplish the tasks of daily living. Space nursing actions appropriately. Watch the patient receiving cardiac drugs for postural hypotension;

have them sit on the edge of the bed for a couple of minutes before getting up and beginning to walk. This will help prevent falls. Use this as a teaching moment for medication side effects. The patient information given is that the medication may cause dizziness. If they were to become dizzy, it would most likely be upon standing. They should follow the same instructions at home when getting up from a lying or sitting position. Specific nursing interventions are discussed with the various disorders in the following chapters.

Collaboration

Cardiovascular patients often are being treated by the physical therapist, dietitian, and respiratory therapist, as well as by the primary health care provider, cardiovascular specialist, and nurse. It is important to consult with the other health professionals involved in the patient's care. Early collaboration with the discharge planner is important to provide continuity of care after discharge.

◆ EVALUATION

Evaluation involves both subjective and objective data. Use good communication skills to ask the right questions to gather the required information from the patient. Ask the patient to describe any "different" feelings they have experienced. Inquire about changes in appetite and bowel movements that could indicate possible medication side effects. Check laboratory values for therapeutic drug levels before giving doses of medication and note the latest blood levels of electrolytes. Assess for signs and symptoms of drug toxicity and for fluid or electrolyte imbalance. Ask yourself whether the patient is showing signs indicating that the medication you are giving is effective. The nursing care plan should be checked daily to evaluate whether each nursing action is effective. If an action is ineffective, it should be stopped and a new action should be devised to resolve the problem.

It is important to look at serial blood pressure readings to evaluate the effectiveness of treatment and of nursing interventions. Pressures that are consistently higher than normal between medication doses indicate a need to change either the dosage or the medication. Trends in assessments give more information than isolated information.

Carefully evaluating pulses and comparing them bilaterally are important parts of nursing care for patients with problems of the cardiovascular system. Writing a good description of the quality and character of the pulses monitored in your notes will give coworkers an accurate assessment baseline on which to evaluate changes.

It is important to determine whether skin color and temperature have changed since the last assessment. Accurately measure and document areas of discoloration in the medical record. Monitor ulcerated areas closely and measure and photograph per policy the areas to determine whether healing is occurring. Evaluate the color of the healing tissue and presence of exudate. If the wound is growing or not improving, the nursing actions or treatment must be changed.

Often you must rely on subjective data from the patient to evaluate whether treatment and nursing actions are effective. Increases in peripheral circulation may be evident only by a decrease in pain or an ability to walk farther without pain.

COMMON PROBLEMS OF PATIENTS WITH CARDIOVASCULAR DISORDERS

FATIGUE AND DYSPNEA

When the coronary arteries fail to supply adequate oxygen to the cells of the heart muscle, the heart is unable to perform as it should, especially when extra demands are placed on it. The result is a general hypoxia of the tissues throughout the body, which causes fatigue and dyspnea on exertion. In the early stages of heart disease, the patient may be only slightly aware of the inability to do as much physical work as they formerly could.

Activity may be restricted for MI and severe congestive heart failure (CHF). The patient may independently perform activities of daily living (ADLs), with the nurse monitoring for shortness of breath or return of admitting symptoms. The patient should be cautioned against any strenuous activity, and response to activity should be monitored via telemetry to watch for dysrhythmias or excessive heart rate changes. The amount of energy used in activity is expressed in *metabolic equivalents (METs)*. Chapter 20, Box 20.4, shows the metabolic equivalents for various activities. The MET level and exercise tolerance are assessed, and targets are set for the rehabilitation process.

Criteria used to determine whether a cardiac patient is tolerating an activity include the following:

- The heart rate does not rise more than 20 beats per minute over the baseline rate.
- Systolic blood pressure does not drop.
- There is no complaint of chest pain, dyspnea, or severe fatigue.
- There is no abnormal heart rate or rhythm.

The progress of activity often is jointly supervised by a physical therapist and a nurse. More information on cardiac rehabilitation is presented in Chapter 9.

EDEMA

Edema is an accumulation of fluid in the interstitial fluid compartment. It becomes a problem in heart disease when blood flow into or out of the heart is inhibited, causing a backup of body fluids in the vascular space, which in turn causes fluid to relocate to the tissues.

Continually assess the fluid balance of a patient with cardiac disease by looking for signs of abnormal collections of fluid in the body tissues. Daily weight change is considered the best indicator of fluid buildup. Check the feet and ankles of ambulatory patients for signs of dependent edema, and watch patients on bed rest for signs of swelling in the area of the sacrum, buttocks, and thighs. Observe for progressive signs of shortness of breath and auscultate lung fields each shift to detect crackles—a sign of beginning pulmonary congestion. Observe the jugular veins for prominence when the patient is in an upright position; prominent veins may indicate fluid overload and CHF.

> **Clinical Cues**
>
> A weight gain of 2 to 3 lb or more in 2 to 3 days or less indicates fluid retention.

Nursing responsibilities include recording the patient's weight daily before breakfast, supervising fluid restriction, accurately measuring intake and output, and assessing for signs of both fluid deficit and fluid overload. Older adult patients on fluid restriction and diuretics can easily become dehydrated.

Therapeutic measures to control edema include the administration of diuretics and restriction of sodium and, possibly, the restriction of fluid. You must observe for adverse effects of medication, such as electrolyte imbalance and postural hypotension. Potassium supplementation may be ordered for a patient who is experiencing hypokalemia or to prevent hypokalemia in patients taking non–potassium-sparing diuretics.

> **Safety Alert**
>
> **Signs of Hypokalemia**
>
> Be alert for the following signs of hypokalemia: fatigue, muscle weakness, muscle cramps, drowsiness, confusion, new onset of bradycardia, or postural hypotension. Hypokalemia may cause life-threatening dysrhythmias.

PAIN

Chest pain can be a symptom of a life-threatening heart event. Each episode of pain is carefully assessed by noting when it started; the location and radiation pattern; degree of pain on a scale; activity before onset; associated symptoms such as nausea, diaphoresis, or **palpitations**; and vital signs.

Anginal pain caused by narrowed coronary arteries can interfere with the patient's lifestyle as well as cause discomfort. As myocardial oxygen need increases with activity, adequate blood flow cannot be provided. Stable angina pain is treated with nitroglycerin, oral nitrates, oxygen, reassurance, and careful monitoring for relief. Nitrates and other medications that dilate coronary arteries to promote better blood flow and decrease ischemia are used to control or prevent anginal pain.

If pain is not relieved, emergency care should be implemented. The goals of treatment are to restore oxygen supply to the heart and relieve the symptoms. Morphine, nitroglycerine, and oxygen are given as well as low-dose aspirin—not to decrease pain but to decrease the stickiness of platelets to prevent further clot occlusion of coronary arteries (Zafari, 2018). For chronic chest pain not related to acute MI, oral pain medications may be used in addition to other interventions. The patient's pain may be increased because of nervousness and anxiety, and you can do much to help relieve pain by providing a restful environment, interacting therapeutically with "active listening," and balancing rest with prescribed physical activity.

> **Clinical Cues**
>
> If chest pain is not relieved after administering three nitroglycerin sublingual tablets (or spray) 5 minutes apart, notify the health care provider. Institute oxygen therapy according to agency protocol, monitor vital signs, and stay with the patient. The patient may be experiencing an MI. (Do check to make certain that the nitroglycerin causes tingling under the tongue. If not, the tablets may be too old and will not work. The tablets are very light sensitive.) Nitroglycerin can cause a significant decrease in blood pressure and mild to severe headache. Monitor for these side effects. At home, 911 should be called if the first nitroglycerin dose has not relieved the pain within 5 minutes, and an aspirin should be taken.

Sleep deprivation and fatigue can increase the pain. Turning, administration of medications, visiting, exercise, and procedures should be coordinated so that the patient is not disturbed more than necessary.

Determining those factors that seem to trigger an attack can identify stressors that the patient may be able to avoid. Relaxation and other noninvasive techniques to manage pain are discussed in Chapter 7.

ALTERED TISSUE PERFUSION

In peripheral vascular disease, blood flow may be sluggish or altered by constriction of the vessels. The smooth muscles of the arterial walls respond to temperature by constricting in the presence of cold and extreme heat and relaxing in the presence of warmth. Therefore the nursing care plan should include (1) providing a warm environment for the patient; (2) covering the hospitalized patient with warm blankets or dressing them in warm clothing; and (3) instructing the patient to avoid extremes of cold and heat.

The constricting effect of extreme heat rules out the use of local applications of heat therapy. In addition to the danger of burning the patient because of decreased sensitivity to extremes of temperature, local heat increases metabolic activity in the tissues to which it is applied and therefore further disrupts the balance of supply and demand for blood flow to all the tissues.

> **Think Critically**
>
> What would you recommend to an older adult home care patient to keep their lower extremities warm during the winter? The patient does not have the funds to keep the house heated above 68° F (20° C).

A second consideration is that of *pressure* against the walls of the blood vessels. Constricting clothing, elastic materials in underclothing, tight socks, and other form-fitting clothing is avoided. Frequent position changes are essential; position must be changed at least every 2 hours.

Patients with poor venous circulation can benefit from periodic elevation of the lower extremities above the level of the heart to facilitate venous return of blood to the heart. Well-distributed support of the vessels near the surface of the body will help improve venous return. To provide this kind of support, the health care provider may prescribe an elastic bandage or fitted elastic stockings. The stockings or elastic bandage should be applied early in the morning, before the legs are placed in a dependent position, because the blood vessels are less congested after a prolonged rest. Bandages and hose should be applied by beginning at the feet and working upward to avoid trapping blood in the lower leg. To stay in place, the stockings have a band at the top. The skin under this area should be assessed to make sure the stockings are not constricting blood flow. The patient should have two pairs of elastic hose and should wash the hose after each day's wearing. Elastic hose should be replaced every 6 months because they lose their elasticity. When stockings are removed, the heels should be checked for pressure areas. **Elastic stockings are not used for patients with arterial disorders.**

Exercise is especially beneficial to patients with decreased blood flow. Flexion of leg muscles helps "pump" venous blood back up to the heart against gravity. Walking is ideal exercise for ambulatory patients. Bedridden patients will need range-of-motion (ROM) exercises and the other kinds of muscular movements described in Chapter 31. Use of a treadmill for patients who cannot exercise by walking outside is very beneficial. A stationary bicycle is another alternative.

In addition to mechanical factors, certain chemical factors affect the constriction of blood vessels. Nicotine, which is inhaled with tobacco smoke, has the effect of producing spasmodic narrowing of the peripheral arteries. Patients with arterial insufficiency are encouraged to stop smoking. Used in conjunction with a community smoking cessation support program, the booklet *You Can Quit Smoking*, available from the Agency for Healthcare Research and Quality at https://www.uspreventiveservicestaskforce.org/Page/Document/UpdateSummaryFinal/tobacco-use-in-adults-and-pregnant-women-counseling-and-interventions1, can be very helpful.

Alcohol is a mild vasodilator when taken in moderate amounts. Unless the patient has moral or religious convictions against its use, the health care provider may approve a daily intake of a specific, small amount of wine or liquor. It is important to find out whether alcohol will interfere with the action of medications being taken or cause problems for other coexisting diseases.

Health Promotion

Drink in Moderation

Promote proper use of alcohol for those who consume alcoholic beverages. Moderate alcohol intake for a man is two drinks in any 1 day. For a woman, the appropriate amount is one drink per day. One drink is 1½ ounces of alcohol, 4 ounces of wine, or 12 ounces of beer.

Drugs that are helpful to relieve vasoconstriction and improve blood flow are prescribed. These drugs are of value only when the arteries are still capable of dilating. Severely sclerosed vessels respond very poorly to therapy of this kind.

IMPAIRED TISSUE INTEGRITY

Tissues that have a diminished blood supply are subject to severe and permanent damage from the slightest injury because the normal processes of healing and repair are impaired. Arterial and venous stasis often lead to chronic leg ulcers.

These ulcers are particularly distressing to patients because they heal very slowly and many never heal completely. Patients must be taught to avoid conditions that contribute to injury of the extremities and to report any injury, no matter how minor.

Prevention of leg ulcers includes (1) wearing elastic bandages or support hose; (2) proper positioning and exercise; (3) preventing injury to the feet and legs; and (4) avoiding extremes of heat and cold and other mechanical and chemical factors that contribute to obstruction of blood flow. Information on care of a patient with a venous stasis ulcer is provided in Chapter 18.

Get Ready for the NCLEX® Examination!

Key Points

- Cardiovascular disease is the leading cause of death in the United States.
- The heart and vessels become stiffer with age, and older adults have less cardiac reserve.
- Atherosclerosis and arteriosclerosis are major contributors to cardiovascular disease.
- Close to one third of the population in the United States has elevated blood pressure.
- Control of hypertension and obesity could lower the incidence of cardiovascular disease.
- Peripheral pulses should be compared bilaterally.
- Blood pressure should be taken—using correct technique—with the patient lying, sitting, and standing.

- Comprehensive nursing care plans should be holistic and may need to include problems secondary to the cardiovascular disease.
- Planning should include time management because many heart medications need to be given as close to the prescribed time as possible to maintain a steady blood level of the drug.
- Collaboration with other health care team members assists in providing consistent, thorough care for patients with cardiovascular disorders.
- Evaluation involves ECG monitoring, checking blood levels of electrolytes, obtaining laboratory values for cardiac drugs to determine adequate dosing or toxicity, and monitoring blood counts for adequate red blood cells and hemoglobin to carry sufficient oxygen to the tissues of the body.
- Fatigue and dyspnea occur when the heart cannot pump sufficiently to carry adequate oxygen and nutrients to the tissues.
- Activity during cardiac rehabilitation is measured in metabolic equivalents; activity is started slowly and may progress according to the body's response.
- Heat therapy is applied cautiously to the extremities of patients with peripheral vascular disease.
- When blood volume is more than the heart can handle, there are changes in concentration and pressure, causing edema.
- Daily weight change is the best indicator of fluid buildup.
- Watch patients who have fluid imbalances for accompanying electrolyte imbalances.
- Measures to reduce or prevent edema are often needed for patients with peripheral vascular disease.
- Nitroglycerin, morphine, aspirin, and oxygen are the drugs of choice for myocardial pain.
- Anginal pain is treated with nitroglycerin and other drugs to promote arterial vasodilation.
- Decreasing anxiety and promoting rest may decrease anginal pain.
- It is very important to encourage patients with cardiovascular disease to quit smoking because nicotine is a vasoconstrictor.
- Patients with peripheral vascular disease have difficulty healing lower leg and foot wounds.

Additional Learning Resources

SG Go to your Study Guide for additional learning activities to help you master this chapter content.

Go to your Evolve website (http://evolve.elsevier.com/deWit/medsurg) for the following FREE learning resources:

- Animations, audio, and video
- Answers and rationales for questions and activities
- Glossary with pronunciations in English and Spanish
- Interactive Review Questions and more!

Review Questions for the NCLEX® Examination

1. Which statement(s) regarding drug use and the risk of cardiac disease is (are) true? *(Select all that apply.)*
 1. The vasodilation effects of cocaine hasten atherosclerosis.
 2. Sudden cardiac death is associated with cocaine use.
 3. Methamphetamine dilates blood vessels.
 4. Cigarette smoking contributes heavily to heart disease.
 5. Methamphetamine can cause myocardial infarction.
 NCLEX Client Need: Health Promotion and Maintenance

2. The ankle-brachial index test is ordered for a patient experiencing signs of peripheral vascular disease. Which patient statement indicates that further teaching about the test needs to occur?
 1. "I'll be lying down for this examination."
 2. "The test is noninvasive."
 3. "My brachial and pedal pulses will be checked and compared."
 4. "My brachial and ankle blood pressure will be taken."
 NCLEX Client Need: Physiological Integrity: Reduction of Risk Potential

3. Morphine 6 mg is ordered for a man admitted with chest pain and a probable myocardial infarction. On hand is morphine 10 mg/mL. You should give ____ mL to the patient. *(Fill in the blank.)*
 NCLEX Client Need: Physiological Integrity: Pharmacological Therapies

4. During initial assessment of an older adult, you find that the skin appears smooth, shiny, and thinned with little or no hair on the surface. Which nursing diagnosis should be on the care plan?
 1. *Altered peripheral tissue perfusion.*
 2. *Potential for infection.*
 3. *Acute pain related to decreased perfusion.*
 4. *Fluid volume deficit.*
 NCLEX Client Need: Physiological Integrity: Physiological Adaptation

5. When providing care for a patient with cardiac disease, you understand that the patient is at risk for alteration in cardiac output. Which of the following has the most potential to affect cardiac output?
 1. Antihypertensive medications
 2. Dysrhythmias
 3. Chest pain
 4. Atherosclerosis
 NCLEX Client Need: Physiological Integrity: Reduction of Risk Potential

6. You weigh a patient with congestive heart failure and determine that there is a net weight gain of 3 lb within the last 24 hours. The patient states that they are short of breath. Place in priority order the nursing actions to take.
 1. Listen to lung sounds.
 2. Place nasal cannula O_2 starting at 2 L/min.
 3. Raise the head of the bed.
 4. Notify the health care provider.
 5. Take vital signs, including pulse oximetry.
 NCLEX Client Need: Physiological Integrity: Physiological Adaptation

7. You administer two consecutive sublingual nitroglycerin tablets to a patient complaining of moderate chest pain. If the patient's blood pressure is 148/88 mm Hg with continued chest pain, the next nursing action would be to:
   1. administer morphine sulfate.
   2. get an IV cannula inserted.
   3. give another sublingual nitroglycerin.
   4. provide emotional support.

   NCLEX Client Need: Physiological Integrity: Pharmacological Therapies
8. When interviewing a patient complaining of moderate chest pain, what question(s) should be asked? *(Select all that apply.)*
   1. Who witnessed the pain?
   2. What does the pain or discomfort feel like?
   3. What relaxation strategies were implemented?
   4. Where is the pain located?
   5. To where does the pain radiate?

   NCLEX Client Need: Physiological Integrity: Physiological Adaptation
9. A nurse assesses an 83-year-old patient and finds a diastolic murmur on auscultation of the heart. The priority action should be to:
   1. stop the examination and call the health care provider.
   2. document the finding in the chart.
   3. inquire if other members of the family have a murmur.
   4. realize that such a murmur is normal in this age group.

   NCLEX Client Need: Physiological Integrity: Physiological Adaptation
10. A patient is receiving a drug that may cause postural hypotension. For safety, you should instruct the patient to do what? *(Select all that apply.)*
    1. Increase fluid intake to prevent dehydration.
    2. Arise slowly from a lying to a sitting position.
    3. Sit on the side of the bed until not lightheaded before standing.
    4. Stand holding on to the bed rail to stabilize before walking.
    5. Always ask for assistance when up and moving around.

    NCLEX Client Need: Physiological Integrity: Pharmacological Therapies

Critical Thinking Questions

Scenario A

Debra Johnson, a 20-year-old African American college student on your campus, comes to the health center complaining of frequent headaches. The assessment data show that she is 5′4″ tall, weighs 170 lb (77 kg), temp 98.8° F (37° C), P 82, RR 14, and BP 154/90 mm Hg. She smokes about half a pack of cigarettes per day. She has a heavy academic schedule and rarely exercises. She eats a lot of "food on the run" at the local fast-food places. Her mother and uncle both have hypertension.

1. Which of her data are abnormal for her age?
2. What risk factors does she have for cardiovascular disease?
3. Which risk factors are modifiable?

Scenario B

Akio Sukura, a 64-year-old man, comes to the emergency department after experiencing chest pain and diaphoresis. His ECG is abnormal. He is scheduled for a cardiac catheterization.

1. Is a consent required for this procedure? If so, would he be able to sign it?
2. What questions would you need to ask him when preparing him for this diagnostic test?
3. What are the priorities of care related to this diagnostic test after the procedure is finished?

Scenario C

Jackson Smith, a construction worker, comes to the clinic. The health care provider suspects that he has peripheral vascular disease.

1. What are the risk factors for this type of cardiovascular disease?
2. What diagnostic tests might be ordered for him?
3. Why would it be important to assess for signs of diabetes mellitus as well?

Care of Patients With Hypertension and Peripheral Vascular Disease

18

http://evolve.elsevier.com/deWit/medsurg

Objectives

Theory

1. Explain the pathophysiology of hypertension.
2. Identify the complications that can occur as a consequence of hypertension.
3. Briefly describe the treatment program for the different stages of hypertension.
4. Contrast the pathophysiology of arteriosclerosis with that of atherosclerosis.
5. List four factors that contribute to peripheral vascular disease.
6. Explain the signs, symptoms, and treatment of aneurysm.
7. Prepare a teaching plan for a patient with Raynaud syndrome.
8. Discuss the etiology and care for thrombophlebitis and deep vein thrombosis.
9. Summarize how venous insufficiency may lead to a venous stasis ulcer.
10. Compare venous stasis ulcer with arterial leg ulcer.
11. List types of surgery performed for problems of the peripheral vascular system.

Clinical Practice

12. Develop and implement a teaching plan for a patient who has hypertension.
13. Choose the points to be included in the teaching plan for a patient who has experienced thrombophlebitis.
14. Institute a teaching plan for a patient undergoing anticoagulant therapy.
15. Differentiate between venous and arterial insufficiency during a physical assessment.
16. Prepare a nursing care plan for a patient with arterial insufficiency.
17. Identify three likely problem statements for patients who have vascular disease and list the expected outcomes and appropriate nursing interventions for each.

Key Terms

aneurysm (ĂN-yū-rĭzm, p. 420)
bruit (brū-Ē, p. 423)
cellulitis (sĕl-ū-LĪ-tĭs, p. 417)
embolus (ĔM-bō-lŭs, p. 416)
gangrene (găng-GRĒN, p. 423)
hypertension (hī-pĕr-TĔN-shŭn, p. 407)
intermittent claudication (ĭn-tĕr-MĬT-ĕnt klăw-dĭ-KĀ-shŭn, p. 416)
rubor (RŪ-bōr, p. 416)
scleropathy (sklĕr-ŎP-ă-thē, p. 430)
stent (stĕnt, p. 419)
thrombophlebitis (thrŏm-bō-flĕ-BĪ-tĭs, p. 416)
thrombus (THRŎM-bŭs, p. 419)
varicose veins (VĂR-ĭ-kōs VĀNZ, p. 429)

Concepts Covered in This Chapter

- Nutrition
- Perfusion
- Clotting
- Inflammation
- Tissue Integrity
- Pain
- Fatigue
- Health Promotion

HYPERTENSION

Hypertension is defined as persistently high blood pressure. This means a systolic pressure that is equal to or greater than 130 mm Hg and a diastolic pressure that is equal to or greater than 80 mm Hg when taken at least twice and averaged on two different occasions 2 weeks apart. The diastolic pressure is the focus of treatment. It reflects the amount of pressure being exerted against the vessel walls while the heart is in its phase of relaxation and there is no added pressure from blood being forced out of the left ventricle and into the arteries. Table 18.1 presents ranges for the classification of hypertension based on the 2017 guidelines developed by multiple professional organizations.

Hypertensive individuals usually die of long-term damage to the end organs or target organs—that is, from damage to the brain, heart, and kidneys. More than half of the deaths associated with persistent and unrelieved hypertension are caused by myocardial infarction (MI). Immediate causes of death related to high blood pressure include cerebral hemorrhage and heart failure.

Think Critically

What are two physiologic reasons why older adults are at greater risk for hypertension?

Table 18.1 Blood Pressure Classification

CLASSIFICATION	SYSTOLIC	DIASTOLIC	PATIENT ACTION
Normal	Less than 120	Less than 80	Monitor if risk factors are present.
Elevated blood pressure	120–129 and	Less than 80	Nonpharmacologic interventions: modify diet, increase exercise, lose weight, stop smoking.
High			
Stage 1	130–139 or	80–89	Nonpharmacologic interventions + antihypertensives and/or diuretics may be prescribed.
Stage 2	140 or higher or	90 or higher	Nonpharmacologic interventions + additional antihypertensive drug(s) may be prescribed.

From: ACC/AHA/AAPA/ABC/ACPM/AGS/APhA/ASH/ASPC/NMA/PCNA (2017) Guideline for the Prevention, Detection, Evaluation, and Management of High Blood Pressure in Adults. Paul K. Whelton, Robert M. Carey, Wilbert S. Aronow, et al. *Journal of the American College of Cardiology* 71(19):e127–e248, 2018; DOI: 10.1016/j.jacc.2017.11.006.

ETIOLOGY

Hypertension is classified as primary or secondary. The etiology of primary hypertension is believed to be related to genetic and environmental causes, whereas secondary hypertension is caused by multiple other conditions, including renal, vascular, and endocrine disorders (Alexander, 2018).

In 5% to 8% of patients, the hypertension is secondary to another disorder. Acute stress, excessive alcohol intake, sickle cell disease, arteriosclerosis, coarctation of the aorta, eclampsia of pregnancy, renal disorders, endocrine disorders, and neurologic disorders are examples of secondary causes. Amphetamine use, chronic nonsteroidal antiinflammatory drug (NSAID) use, and tyramine-containing foods such as beer and wine taken with monoamine oxidase inhibitors (MAOIs) contribute to secondary hypertension. Female hormone therapy and nicotine use appear to be contributing factors in some people. If the underlying disorder can be detected and treated successfully, the problem of secondary hypertension is eliminated or more easily controlled. If no underlying disease can be identified as elevating the patient's blood pressure, the patient is considered to have primary hypertension.

Table 18.2 presents the nonmodifiable and modifiable risk factors for hypertension. In many cases a loss of excess weight alone can return a slightly elevated blood pressure to normal. A moderate reduction of salt intake has been effective in lowering the blood pressure of some patients with mild or moderate hypertension. There is continuing research on the relation of race, gender, and ethnicity to the incidence and effects of hypertension.

Cultural Considerations

Hypertension and Racial Predisposition

In a recent study it was shown that American Indians, native Hawaiians, and Asians tend to have hypertension at almost the same rate as African Americans, who have long been known to have a higher incidence (Young et al., 2018).

The rising incidence of childhood obesity has resulted in an increase in the incidence of hypertension. Health promotion activities targeting nutrition and exercise habits of children are increasing.

PATHOPHYSIOLOGY

Blood pressure equals the amount of blood pumped out of the heart (cardiac output) multiplied by the systemic vascular resistance. If the diameter of blood vessels becomes smaller because of atherosclerosis or vasoconstriction, blood pressure increases with the effort to force the blood through the smaller opening. If there is an increase in the volume (amount) or viscosity (thickness or consistency) of fluid in the blood vessels, the pressure within the vessels increases and the heart must work harder to pump the fluid through the vessels. A pathologic response to stress can result in an elevation in blood pressure by stimulating the sympathetic nervous system, which releases epinephrine, causing peripheral vasoconstriction and increased heart rate. Insulin, glucose, and lipoprotein abnormalities related to metabolic syndrome are common in primary hypertension. In some instances of hypertension, an excess of renin is secreted by the kidneys. Renin acts on a substance called *angiotensinogen,* converting it to angiotensin I. Angiotensin I is converted to angiotensin II by angiotensin-converting enzyme (ACE). Angiotensin II acts directly on the blood vessels, causing them to constrict, and stimulates the adrenal gland to release aldosterone. Angiotensin thereby increases resistance to blood flow in the peripheral vessels and causes retention of sodium and water by the renal tubules through the influence of aldosterone (see Chapter 17, Fig. 17.6). The retained sodium and water increase the blood volume, causing increased cardiac output and elevation of blood pressure. Concept Map 18.1 shows the pathophysiology of hypertension.

Older Adult Care Points

The stiffening of arteries that occurs with arteriosclerosis is a natural part of aging. The baroreceptors that normally help adjust blood pressure become less sensitive with age. The lack of elasticity of the vessels and the decreased sensitivity of the baroreceptors cause older adults to be at risk for orthostatic (postural) hypotension when changing position. An elevation of systolic pressure above normal should still be treated in this age group.

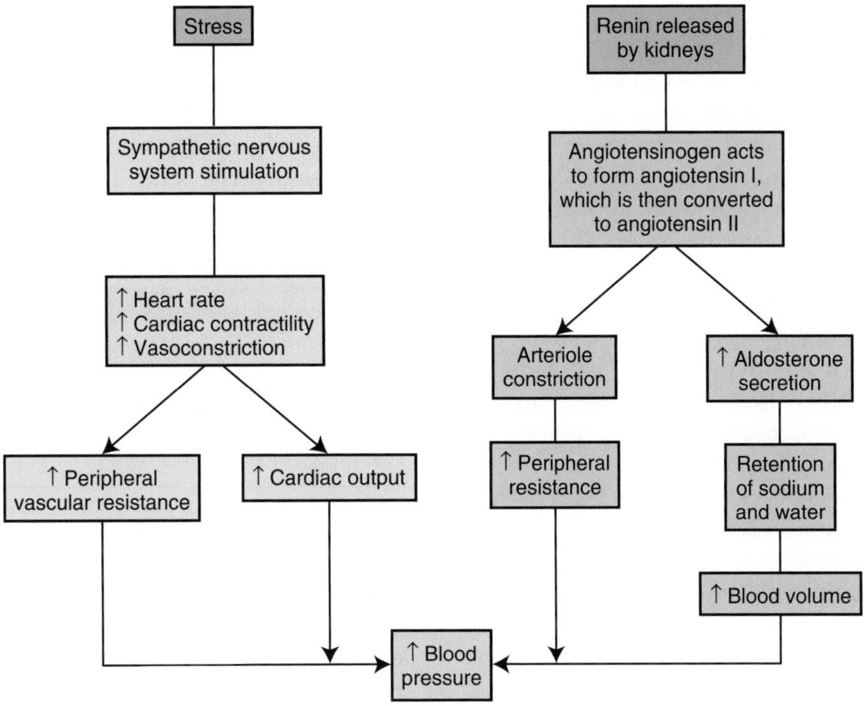

Concept Map 18.1 Pathophysiology of hypertension.

Table 18.2 Nonmodifiable and Modifiable Risk Factors for Primary Hypertension

Nonmodifiable Risk Factors	
Age	Systolic blood pressure (SBP) rises with age. After age 50 years, SBP >140 mm Hg is a cardiovascular risk factor.
Gender	Until age 55 years, hypertension is more prevalent in men; after age 55 years, it is more prevalent in women.
Ethnicity/race	Incidence is much higher in African Americans.
Family history	A close relative with hypertension increases a person's risk for developing it.
Modifiable Risk Factors	
Alcohol	Excessive alcohol intake is strongly associated with hypertension. Daily intake should be limited to 1 oz for those with hypertension.
Cigarette smoking, smokeless tobacco, e-cigarettes	Nicotine contributes to arteriosclerosis and thereby to hypertension. People with hypertension who smoke are at greater risk for cardiovascular disease.
Diabetes	Diabetes accelerates atherosclerosis and leads to damage of the large vessels. Hypertension is twice as prevalent in diabetics as in nondiabetics.
Obesity	Central body obesity in particular is associated with the development of hypertension. When combined with other factors in metabolic syndrome, the risk of hypertension is increased even more.
Stress	Stress increases peripheral vascular resistance and stimulates sympathetic nervous system activity. If stress responses become excessive, they can contribute to the development of hypertension.
Elevated serum lipids	Elevated cholesterol and triglycerides are risk factors for atherosclerosis. Atherosclerosis contributes to hypertension in many individuals.
Excess dietary sodium	High sodium intake contributes to hypertension in some patients.
Decreased kidney function	Hypertension is more prevalent with an estimated glomerular filtration rate (GFR) less than 60 mL/min.
Decreased physical activity	Decreased physical activity is a cardiovascular risk factor, increasing blood pressure (BP) and contributing to obesity.

SIGNS, SYMPTOMS, AND DIAGNOSIS

Hypertension has been called the "silent killer" because in early stages it does not usually cause discomfort or any other subjective signs and symptoms to indicate its presence. About one third of those who have hypertension are not aware of it. Signs may appear only in the later stages when damage has been done to the target organs—that is, the kidneys (renal ischemia and nephrosclerosis), brain (arteriosclerosis and microaneurysm), aorta (aortic aneurysm), eyes (retinal damage), and heart (left ventricular hypertrophy and reduced cardiac output). **Patients with symptoms may complain of headache, dizziness, blurred vision, blackouts, irritability, angina, dyspnea, or fatigue.**

Hypertensive patients develop coronary heart disease at a rate two to three times greater than that of persons with normal blood pressure. Examination of the blood vessels of the retina will reveal any damage to the retinal vessels. This retinal assessment gives an indication about how much damage the high blood pressure has done to vessels throughout the body. If retinal damage has occurred, it is an indication that the person's hypertension is moderate to severe.

Diagnosis is based on blood pressure readings on at least two occasions 2 weeks apart. An electrocardiogram (ECG), echocardiogram, and cardiac stress test may be ordered to determine whether any damage has been done to the heart muscle.

TREATMENT

The goals of treatment are (1) reduction of high blood pressure and (2) long-term control to decrease the risk of stroke, heart attack, loss of vision, and kidney disease. The target is to control blood pressure at or below 120/80 mm Hg. Treatment is individualized, using a stepped care approach. For elevated blood pressure, smoking cessation, weight reduction, sodium restriction, alcohol restriction, exercise, a low-fat diet, and stress control are instituted. Sodium should be kept to less than 2400 mg/day with the DASH (Dietary Approaches to Stop Hypertension) eating plan. Alcohol intake should not exceed one serving of liquor, wine, or beer per day for women or two servings per day for men. Aerobic exercise of 30 to 45 minutes on most days of the week is recommended. If blood pressure reaches Stage 1, a diuretic or antihypertensive drug is prescribed. In Stage 2, all of the above continue and other medications are added.

Patients with more severe hypertension often require more than two drugs to attain control. The dose of each drug is increased as needed to achieve the desired blood pressure level unless side effects occur. In the event of side effects, another drug is substituted. Newer blood pressure medications are very expensive, and cost is a concern for many patients. Some drug companies have programs to help patients who cannot afford their medications. If a potassium-wasting diuretic is prescribed, the patient is taught to increase dietary potassium intake. A potassium supplement is added to treatment, and electrolyte levels are monitored regularly.

Patients should monitor their blood pressure at home and keep records of the readings. Periodic visits to the health care provider's office for regular examinations are necessary. The better the blood pressure is controlled and kept within normal limits, the less damage there will be to the target organs.

Safety Alert

Licorice that is found in herbal teas as well as in black licorice candy, if consumed in large amounts, can increase blood pressure. If non–potassium-sparing diuretics are taken together with licorice, dangerously low potassium levels may result (Schonwald, 2017).

Antihypertensive Therapy

The drugs prescribed to reduce blood pressure work by decreasing blood volume, cardiac output, or peripheral resistance. Table 18.3 and Box 18.1 list examples of the drugs most commonly prescribed for hypertension and relevant nursing interventions. Medications used to treat hypertension reverse or block conditions causing elevated blood pressure. Diuretics address fluid volume. Most of the "blockers" or "inhibitors" (renin, ACE, calcium channel, angiotensin II receptor) stop the progression of a process that results in vasoconstriction (peripheral resistance), causing elevation in blood pressure.

The blood pressure of older adult patients who are taking antihypertensive medications should be measured when they are sitting and when standing. Many of these medications can cause orthostatic hypotension. Normally when standing, the blood vessels respond by vasoconstricting to maintain blood flow. Most antihypertensives block this effect. Measuring blood pressure with the patient standing will reveal whether the medication is reducing the blood pressure too much. Assess patients receiving antihypertensives for dizziness, confusion, syncope, restlessness, and drowsiness, which may indicate hypotension.

Patient Teaching

Safety Measures to Prevent Falls for Patients With Orthostatic Hypotension

Teach patients who experience the side effect of orthostatic hypotension from medication to:

- Rise slowly from a lying to a sitting position; do not hold the breath while arising. Sit for 1 minute before standing; stand slowly while holding on to a stable object. Stand for 1 minute before walking.
- While seated, flex and rotate the feet several times before attempting to stand; plant feet firmly on the floor before standing.
- When walking, do not turn the head or body abruptly.
- When feeling unsteady while standing, call for assistance before walking.
- Report lightheadedness or sudden dizziness.
- Use the bathroom before meals and try to avoid getting up for 30 to 60 minutes after meals.

Table 18.3 **Drug Classifications Used for Patients With Vascular Disorders**

TYPE OF DRUG	ACTION
Diuretics	
Thiazides and Related Drugs Hydrochlorothiazide (Esidrix, HydroDIURIL, Dyazide) Chlorthalidone (Thalitone) Metolazone (Zaroxolyn) Indapamide (Lozol)	These drugs increase the excretion of water, sodium, potassium, and chloride by blocking the reabsorption of sodium and chloride.
Loop Diuretics Bumetanide (Bumex) Furosemide (Lasix) Torsemide (Demadex)	These drugs work in the loop of Henle to block reabsorption of sodium and chloride. This prevents passive reabsorption of water and promotes its excretion. These drugs produce the greatest amount of diuresis.
Potassium-Sparing Diuretics Amiloride hydrochloride (Midamor) Spironolactone (Aldactone) Triamterene (Dyrenium)	These drugs block the action of aldosterone in the distal nephron. This prevents the promotion of sodium uptake in exchange for potassium secretion usually caused by aldosterone, and potassium is "spared" (not secreted) and sodium is excreted. These drugs cause very little diuresis.
Antihypertensives	
Adrenergic Inhibitors ***Beta Blockers*** Atenolol (Tenormin) Propranolol (Inderal) Metoprolol (Lopressor, Toprol XL) Timolol (Apo-Timol) Bisoprolol (Zebeta) Esmolol (Brevibloc) Nebivolol (Bystolic)	Blockade of the beta-1 receptors lowers cardiac output by decreasing heart rate and contractility. Action on the beta-1 receptors in the kidney decreases the release of renin, which is a factor in rising blood pressure. Beta-adrenergic receptors are blocked, which prevents epinephrine and norepinephrine from attaching to the receptor site, preventing the vasoconstriction they would produce.
Alpha Blockers Doxazosin (Cardura) Prazosin (Minipress) Terazosin (Hytrin)	These drugs block alpha-1 stimulation on arterioles and veins, preventing sympathetic vasoconstriction. This action results in vasodilation, reducing peripheral vascular resistance and venous return to the heart.
Alpha-Beta Blocker Labetalol (Normodyne, Trandate) Carvedilol (Coreg)	These drugs block both alpha-1 and beta-1 receptors, producing decreased heart rate, contractility, peripheral vascular resistance, and venous return.
Angiotensin-Converting Enzyme (ACE) Inhibitors Benazepril (Lotensin) Captopril (Capoten) Enalapril (Vasotec) Fosinopril (Monopril) Lisinopril (Prinivil) Quinapril (Accupril)	These agents lower blood pressure by inhibiting the conversion of angiotensin I into angiotensin II, thereby preventing vasoconstriction. They also restrict volume expansion mediated by aldosterone.
Angiotensin II Receptor Blockers Candesartan (Atacand) Eprosartan (Teveten) Irbesartan (Avapro) Losartan (Cozaar) Olmesartan (Benicar) Telmisartan (Micardis) Valsartan (Diovan)	These agents lower blood pressure by blocking the action of angiotensin II, thereby preventing vasoconstriction.
Calcium Channel Blockers Amlodipine besylate (Norvasc, Lotrel) Diltiazem (Cardizem) Nicardipine (Cardene) Nifedipine (Procardia) Verapamil (Calan, Isoptin)	These drugs reduce blood pressure by causing dilation of arterioles. Calcium channels are blocked, preventing the influx of calcium that promotes constriction.

Continued

Table 18.3 Drug Classifications Used for Patients With Vascular Disorders—cont'd

TYPE OF DRUG	ACTION
Central-Acting Agents	
Clonidine (Catapres) Guanabenz (Wytensin) Methyldopa (Aldomet)	These agents act within the brainstem to suppress sympathetic impulses to the heart and blood vessels. This action decreases the release of norepinephrine by sympathetic nerves, reducing activation of peripheral adrenergic receptors, and promotes vasodilation. These agents also decrease heart rate and cardiac output.
Peripherally Acting Adrenergic Blockers	
Guanethidine (Ismelin) Guanadrel (Hylorel)	These agents reduce blood pressure by blocking adrenergic receptors in the postganglionic sympathetic neurons and causing decreased sympathetic stimulation of the heart and blood vessels.
Direct-Acting Vasodilators	
Hydralazine (Apresoline) Minoxidil (Loniten)	These agents reduce blood pressure by promoting arteriole vasodilation.
Direct Renin Inhibitors	
Aliskiren (Tekturna)	This new class of drugs inhibits renin secretion from the kidney, reducing angiotensin I and angiotensin II, inhibiting vasoconstriction.

Box 18.1 General Nursing Interventions for the Administration of Diuretics and Antihypertensive Drugs

DIURETICS

- Follow all medication "Rights." Instruct the patient on the medication's action and side effects, assess for drug allergies, check for possible interactions, document after administration, and assess effectiveness.
- Check for sulfa allergy. Thiazide and thiazide-like diuretics are related to sulfonamides. Patients allergic to sulfas may have adverse reactions.
- Monitor intake and output to determine the amount of diuresis and the drug's effectiveness.
- Track the patient's weight daily to determine the drug's effectiveness; evaluate for decreased edema.
- Check all drugs the patient is receiving for drug interactions with the diuretic drug to prevent toxicity or lack of absorption. Several diuretics are ototoxic, and this adverse effect may be potentiated by other ototoxic drugs.
- If possible, administer the diuretic dose in the morning; if a second dose is required, give it mid-afternoon to avoid sleep interference from the need to urinate.
- Provide assistance with urination in a timely manner (answer call bell quickly).
- Assess for signs of dehydration and hypotension; take blood pressure on a set schedule. Older adults are prone to excessive diuresis and can quickly become dehydrated.
- Monitor diabetic patients for increased blood glucose levels when taking loop or thiazide diuretics because these drugs may cause hyperglycemia.

Regarding possible side effects or adverse effects of the drug, you should:

- Monitor potassium levels frequently if the patient is taking a potassium-wasting diuretic; assess for signs of hypokalemia: weakness, tremor, muscle cramps, change in mental status, cardiac dysrhythmia.
- If the patient also is taking digoxin, consult the health care provider before administering the dose if the potassium level is below 3.5 mEq/L or if the patient exhibits signs of hypokalemia because hypokalemia increases risk of fatal cardiac dysrhythmia in patients taking digoxin.
- If a patient is taking a potassium-sparing diuretic and potassium level is above 5.2 mEq/L, or if signs of hyperkalemia develop (abnormal cardiac rhythm), consult the provider before administering the dose.
- Monitor blood pressure. If blood pressure drops considerably, speak with the provider before giving another dose of the drug.
- Monitor the patient for signs of constipation, which is a possible side effect of diuresis.
- Monitor patients with a history of deep vein thrombosis (DVT) for recurrence because diuretics reduce circulating fluid volume.
- Monitor for and educate the patient on side effects or adverse effects of the particular drug taken. The most common general side effects are constipation, electrolyte disturbance, gastric upset, and hypotension. Adverse effects are dehydration, ototoxicity, hyperglycemia, and hyperuricemia.
- Monitor the patient for signs of allergic reaction, such as rash or itching.

Teach patients taking a diuretic to:

- Expect a frequent need to urinate and an increased volume of urine.
- Report any new heartbeat irregularity.
- Report any signs of ringing of the ears, roaring sounds, a feeling of fullness in the ears, or decreased hearing.
- Eat foods high in potassium, such as bananas, orange juice, cereals, meats, tomatoes, potatoes, and raisins, daily unless taking a potassium-sparing diuretic.
- If taking a potassium-sparing diuretic, restrict foods high in potassium.
- Take a potassium supplement regularly if one is prescribed.

Box 18.1 General Nursing Interventions for the Administration of Diuretics and Antihypertensive Drugs—cont'd

- Increase fiber in the diet if prone to constipation; consult provider if constipation occurs. Older adult patients who are inactive are more prone to constipation.
- Watch for signs of postural hypotension, such as dizziness or lightheadedness, when changing position. Encourage patients to arise slowly from a supine position and to sit for 1 minute before standing. (Older adults are particularly prone to this side effect.)
- Avoid the sun or take precautions; do not use a sunlamp when taking a loop or thiazide diuretic because the medication may cause photosensitivity.
- Watch for signs of gout (tenderness or swelling of joints) when taking a loop or thiazide diuretic and notify the provider if these occur. Loop diuretics may cause an increase in uric acid levels.
- When taking spironolactone, menstrual irregularities or impotence may occur; report these occurrences to the provider.

ANTIHYPERTENSIVE DRUGS

- Establish that the patient is not hypotensive before giving a dose of an antihypertensive drug. If the patient's blood pressure is below normal levels, consult the provider before giving the dose.
- Monitor the heart rate for bradycardia or tachycardia. Follow specific parameters for administration of the specific drug; some drugs may cause bradycardia, and others may cause tachycardia.
- Ask the provider for blood pressure parameters when giving antihypertensives for afterload reduction to a patient with a normal or slightly low blood pressure.
- Inquire about any dizziness. If dizziness has been occurring, measure blood pressure standing and sitting to determine whether the patient is experiencing orthostatic hypotension; several antihypertensives may cause orthostatic hypotension.
- Note contraindications and precautions for each specific drug the patient is taking. Angiotensin-converting enzyme (ACE) inhibitors are contraindicated during pregnancy.
- Check all drugs the patient is receiving for drug interactions to prevent toxicity or increased severity of side effects. Many antihypertensive drugs have a depressant effect on the heart.
- Monitor blood pressure readings to evaluate effectiveness of the drug.

Regarding possible side effects or adverse effects of the drug, you should:

- Monitor the patient for the side effects of each drug administered.
- Monitor serum glucose levels in patients with diabetes who are taking a beta blocker because the drug may mask hypoglycemia.
- Monitor lipid levels for changes in patients taking beta blockers because these drugs interfere with lipid metabolism.
- Observe for hypersensitivity reactions such as rash; ACE inhibitors may cause hypersensitivity.
- Monitor patients for signs of congestive heart failure, such as edema; beta blockers, calcium channel blockers, and other drugs that decrease cardiac output may precipitate heart failure in patients with borderline cardiac function.
- Check the skin of patients using a clonidine patch for signs of irritation, a potential side effect of the patch. Be certain the old patch is removed when applying a new one.
- Give the first dose of an ACE inhibitor at bedtime because it often causes hypotension.
- Monitor the potassium level of patients taking an ACE inhibitor. Because it suppresses the release of aldosterone, it increases potassium retention.
- Monitor liver function tests for patients taking centrally acting drugs, such as clonidine, because these drugs may cause liver damage in some patients.
- Monitor renal function tests in patients taking hydralazine because this drug may cause renal impairment.

Teach the patient taking an antihypertensive to:

- Monitor blood pressure regularly and record the readings.
- Alter lifestyle factors that contribute to hypertension, such as smoking, excess weight, excessive stress, excessive alcohol ingestion, high-salt diet, and lack of exercise.
- Rise slowly from a lying position and stabilize before standing for a couple of minutes.
- Report alteration in sexual response because some of the antihypertensive drugs may cause impotence.
- Report persistent side effects and any adverse effects of the drug.
- Monitor for weight gain from retention of sodium and water by weighing at least twice a week; report weight gain of more than 2-3 lb to the provider.
- Report signs of ankle edema because several of the antihypertensive drugs can precipitate congestive heart failure.
- Be aware that methyldopa may cause dark urine for the first few weeks of therapy.
- Avoid abruptly discontinuing centrally acting antihypertensives, such as clonidine, because rebound hypertension may occur.
- Check with the provider before taking over-the-counter drugs because many are contraindicated in hypertension.
- Comply with medication therapy even when blood pressure is normal because long-term compliance is the key to preventing the organ damage that hypertension can cause.
- Set own goals for lifestyle changes and medication therapy; a patient-directed program has a better chance of success.
- Notify the provider if a persistent dry cough develops after starting on an ACE inhibitor medication.

COMPLICATIONS

Hypertensive Crisis

Hypertensive emergency is a life-threatening situation in which the blood pressure rises higher than 180/120 mm Hg and there is indication of target organ damage. Symptoms may include severe headache, blurred vision, seizures, nausea, and change in level of consciousness. It may occur if a patient has stopped taking antihypertensive medication, or it may be secondary to another disease process such as renal stenosis. The patient is placed in the intensive care unit and treated with intravenous (IV) emergency drugs, such as IV sodium nitroprusside (Nipride), nicardipine (Cardene IV), nitroglycerin, or labetalol (Normodyne), to lower the blood pressure. A reduction in blood pressure to 160/100 mm Hg is desired over the first 2 hours. Blood pressure is monitored every 5 to 15 minutes. Medication is adjusted to reduce the pressure slowly to prevent renal, cerebral, or coronary ischemia. **Hypertensive urgency** occurs when the blood pressure rises to 180/110 mm Hg but there are no signs or symptoms of target organ damage. This is a more common occurrence. The patient is observed in the emergency department and treated with oral medication. The patient is directed to follow up with their primary care provider.

❖ NURSING MANAGEMENT

◆ ASSESSMENT (DATA COLLECTION)

The patient should be assessed for indications of modifiable and nonmodifiable risk factors for cardiovascular disease. Physical assessment of the cardiac system should be performed. Assessment of blood pressure and documentation of levels and potential influences on values is an important aspect of nursing care. The patient's blood pressure should be taken lying supine, sitting, and standing for a thorough assessment.

Older Adult Care Points

The blood pressure of older adult patients can be affected by other coexisting diseases. As people live longer, more chronic illnesses develop. Blood pressure management must take into consideration all medical conditions.

◆ NURSING DIAGNOSIS AND PLANNING

Common problem statements for a patient with hypertension include:

- Potential for organ injury due to complications of hypertension.
- Insufficient knowledge (disease process, medications) due to new diagnosis of hypertension.
- Altered nutrition due to obesity, high-fat diet, or high sodium intake.
- Anxiety due to potential complications of disease process.

Expected outcomes for a patient with hypertension may include:

- The patient will not experience retinopathy.
- The patient's blood pressure will return to normal limits.
- The patient will verbalize an understanding of teaching related to medications and the disease process.
- The patient will lose 10% of body weight in a designated period.
- The patient will be able to choose low-fat and low-sodium items from a variety of menus.

◆ IMPLEMENTATION

Nursing interventions consist of assisting the patient to make necessary lifestyle changes that will help control the blood pressure and slow further atherosclerosis. Diet changes are often the most difficult for the patient. It is best to work with the patient's current dietary likes and dislikes, modifying methods of food preparation to decrease sodium and fat content.

Sources of hidden sodium should be identified, and the patient should be taught how to read food labels. A dietitian referral or providing contact information to community groups that encourage healthful eating and promote exercise may be helpful.

Patients who need to increase potassium intake are taught to include citrus fruits and juices, bananas, dried beans, tomatoes, and potatoes in their diet. The person who does the shopping and food preparation must be included in the diet instruction process. **Weight loss is the most important lifestyle change for obese patients.** The goal is a weight that is within 15% of ideal body weight.

If caffeine restriction is recommended, teach the patient to gradually decrease their caffeine consumption so that they will not experience withdrawal symptoms, such as headache and nervousness. Remind the patient that many types of soft drinks, as well as coffee, tea, and chocolate, contain caffeine. Most of these beverages are available in decaffeinated formulas, which still contain some caffeine but much less than the regular formulas. Because it produces vasoconstriction, nicotine has a major effect on blood vessels and blood pressure. Stopping smoking or use of smokeless tobacco products can be a difficult task for many patients. Core Measures call for counseling and an information packet on smoking cessation to be given to the patient. An exercise program that fits the patient's personality, ability, and preference should be designed. Walking to work from a parking lot a few blocks away, climbing stairs instead of using elevators, and a daily walk in the neighborhood often are sufficient. Other patients might prefer to use a stationary bicycle or treadmill. The object is to work on something that the patient will continue to do for the rest of their life.

Weight loss will begin to occur if the patient is faithful to the prescribed diet and exercise program. As their weight decreases, remind the patient of the direct effect these efforts have had on the blood pressure. Even a

Nutrition Considerations

Decreasing Sodium in the Diet

Instruct a patient who must reduce sodium in the diet to:

- Avoid "convenience" foods: ready-mixed sauces, frozen dinners, cured or smoked meats (including lunch meats), canned soups, and prepared salad dressings, unless the label truly indicates low sodium content.
- Be aware that regular canned vegetables often contain a large amount of sodium; in some instances rinsing will greatly decrease the sodium content. Use fresh or frozen vegetables or those canned without sodium when possible.
- Check soft drink labels for sodium content; avoid those that contain more than 140 mg of sodium.
- Check cereal box labels for sodium content; switch to a lower sodium cereal, such as shredded wheat.
- Use one fourth to one half the amount of salt that a recipe calls for.
- Avoid adding salt to food after cooking.
- Make a salt substitute of ½ tsp garlic powder mixed with 1 tsp each of basil, black pepper, marjoram, onion powder, parsley, sage, savory, and thyme; or use a product such as Mrs. Dash or lemon pepper instead of salt. (Note that many "salt substitutes" use potassium chloride, which might be dangerous for some patients and helpful to others.)
- Fast-food and other restaurants are required to supply nutrition information, including sodium content. Make wise choices.
- Do not eat preserved or commercially prepared smoked meats, such as bacon, hot dogs, salami, pastrami, ham, smoked turkey, or sausage.
- Read all labels on food containers, looking for the words *salt* and *sodium* and the letters *NaCl.*
- Check condiments for amount of sodium. Catsup, soy sauce, steak sauce, and others are high in sodium.

Cultural Considerations

Cultural Diet Variations

Working with patients from diverse cultures who have very different diets can be a challenge. Encouraging fat and sodium restriction in a cultural diet requires working with the patient to discover food preferences and food preparation patterns inherent in the family.

moderate weight loss of 7 to 12 lb (3 to 5 kg) can reduce blood pressure. Positive reinforcement should be given for even small amounts of weight loss.

Stress reduction requires an evaluation of lifestyle. Meditation, yoga, leisure activities, or just saying no to extra obligations can all decrease stress. Help the patient determine where their stressors are and what can be done practically to manage them. Lifetime compliance with diet, exercise, stress reduction, and medication plans is difficult for most patients. Alternative therapy may help.

Complementary and Alternative Therapies

Grapeseed Extract for Hypertension

Grapeseed extract is an alternative medicine treatment for hypertension that also helps decrease cholesterol.

Many patients do not understand or accept that it is up to them to control their disease. They do well for several months or a few years, but then because they feel well (while their blood pressure has been controlled), they stop taking their medication and gradually return to previous lifestyle patterns. By teaching them what high blood pressure does to the blood vessels and to the heart, brain, eyes, and kidneys, you can do much to encourage patients to follow the treatment plan for life. Instruct patients on how to monitor their blood pressure at home to engage them in their care and track effectiveness of treatment. Each patient needs continuing encouragement for maintaining blood pressure control.

Patient Teaching

Complications of Uncontrolled Hypertension

The following information should be included in the teaching plan of a patient at risk for noncompliance with treatment of hypertension:

- Hypertension can cause damage to arteries, making them less elastic. This places an increased workload on the heart. This may cause MI, left ventricular hypertrophy, aortic aneurysm, and congestive heart failure.
- Small vessel damage to the brain disrupts circulation and may lead to dementia, transient ischemic attacks (TIAs), and ischemic stroke.
- Hypertension may cause an already weakened area in a blood vessel to rupture. This may cause an intracranial bleed known as a *hemorrhagic stroke.*
- Hypertension may cause damage to the small vessels of the kidney and may lead to kidney failure.
- Hypertension damages the arteries of the eye, causing the formation of clots or occurrence of hemorrhage that may lead to blurred vision or blindness.

There are many resources to help hypertensive patients manage their illness more effectively. The American Heart Association, Heart Center Online, the National Institutes of Health, and many others offer educational materials for patients with hypertension. *Healthy People 2030* goals and objectives have been written for hypertension.

Ensure that the patient understands the needed lifestyle changes and how to accomplish behavior modification. The patient may be referred to a local support group as a resource in the management of their health.

◆ EVALUATION

Consistent maintenance of blood pressure within prescribed limits is a primary indicator of effectiveness of disease management. Evaluate the patient's knowledge

Health Promotion

Assessment for and Management of Hypertension

Blood pressure should be assessed every time there is contact with a health care provider. All adults should have their blood pressure assessed at least once a year, even if it has always been within normal limits. A patient with hypertension requires intense teaching to assist in achieving health management goals. Blood pressure should be monitored regularly at home with an automatic blood pressure cuff that can be purchased at any pharmacy or most department stores. Some automated blood pressure cuffs have a feature that uploads the results to a smartphone via Bluetooth. This makes the information easily available for the provider at visits. For patients who enjoy technology solutions, this can be a motivator to track blood pressure.

of prescribed medications, including use, side effects, and administration. Knowledge of dietary management, exercise activities, stress management, and smoking cessation should be discussed at follow-up sessions. The patient's compliance with the management of hypertension is critical to preventing or minimizing complications of the disease process.

ARTERIOSCLEROSIS AND ATHEROSCLEROSIS

Arteriosclerosis (hardening of the arteries) is a general term for a variety of arterial changes. Arteriosclerosis occurs with aging as degenerative changes occur in the small arteries and arterioles. The disorder is characterized by thickening of the artery walls that progresses to hardening as calcium deposits form. Vessel elasticity is lost. The thickening and calcification reduce the diameter of the vessels and cause slowing of blood flow. This may lead to ischemia and necrosis in various tissues. *Atherosclerosis* is another form of artery narrowing. Lipids are deposited within the vessel walls and combine with cells, fibrin, and cell debris to form plaques. The plaque grows and extends into the lumen of the artery, where inflammation or erosion causes the plaque to be exposed to the blood. This triggers clotting and subsequent blocking of the vessel by a clot (see Chapter 20, Fig. 20.1).

Atheromatous plaque with thrombi forms primarily in the larger arteries (aorta, femoral), the carotid, and the coronary arteries. Diabetes mellitus, particularly when uncontrolled, speeds the development of arteriosclerosis and atherosclerosis. Hypertension is a major factor in arteriosclerosis. Any artery in the body can develop atherosclerosis. When vessels delivering blood to the extremities, heart, and brain narrow because of plaque formation, serious consequences can result.

PERIPHERAL VASCULAR DISEASE

Peripheral vascular disease (PVD) involves narrowing or obstruction of peripheral blood vessels and loss of function. These vessels may be in the arms, neck, abdomen, or lower extremities (Fig. 18.1). Peripheral blood vessels include all blood vessels, both veins and arteries, except those in the heart and brain.

Other causes of peripheral vascular problems include spasm of the smooth muscles in the arterial walls (e.g., Raynaud disease), structural defects in the arteries (aneurysms), trauma, or **embolus** (blood clot or debris that travels and lodges in a blood vessel) that causes occlusion. Peripheral venous problems are caused by defective valvular function and formation of **venous thrombosis** (blood clots), which may be accompanied by **thrombophlebitis** (inflammation of a vein).

Prevention of PVD is focused on decreasing atherosclerosis and arteriosclerosis, controlling diabetes mellitus, controlling hypertension, and preventing smoking. Smoking cessation is important because nicotine causes vasoconstriction, resulting in elevation of blood pressure and decreased blood flow through the vessels.

PERIPHERAL ARTERIAL DISEASE (ARTERIAL INSUFFICIENCY)

Etiology and Pathophysiology

The most common etiology of peripheral arterial disease (PAD) is atherosclerosis. The vessel walls become narrowed or the lumen obstructed, leading to loss of blood flow to the extremity. Restriction of arterial blood flow may cause arterial ulcers. Cessation of blood flow in the arteries leads to ischemia and tissue death (necrosis). PAD may be acute or chronic. Embolism is the most common cause of acute interruption of arterial blood flow. PAD may occur in any peripheral artery and frequently occurs in the carotid arteries.

Signs, Symptoms, and Diagnosis

Obtain a complete history and physical examination of the patient. Table 18.4 compares the signs and symptoms of arterial and venous disorders to help identify which part of the vascular system is affected. Signs and symptoms of PAD of the lower extremities include **intermittent claudication** (pain when walking that diminishes at rest), pain at rest, tightening pressure in calves or buttocks, and ischemic changes. Blood pressure in the extremity affected by PAD is lower. This is identified by obtaining an ankle-brachial index (ABI).

Patients with PAD have pallor in the affected extremity when the leg is elevated and **rubor** (dark redness) when the leg is dependent. The skin may appear tight and shiny. Hair is usually absent on the affected extremity, and the toenails are thickened. Pulses are diminished or absent. There also is a temperature change distal to the occlusion. Wounds on the lower leg are difficult to heal. The severity of these symptoms depends on the extent of the lesion, degree of occlusion, and amount of collateral circulation that has been established.

If severe ischemia occurs from occlusion of arterial blood flow, tissue distal to the occlusion blanches, becomes cold, hurts, and eventually becomes numb as

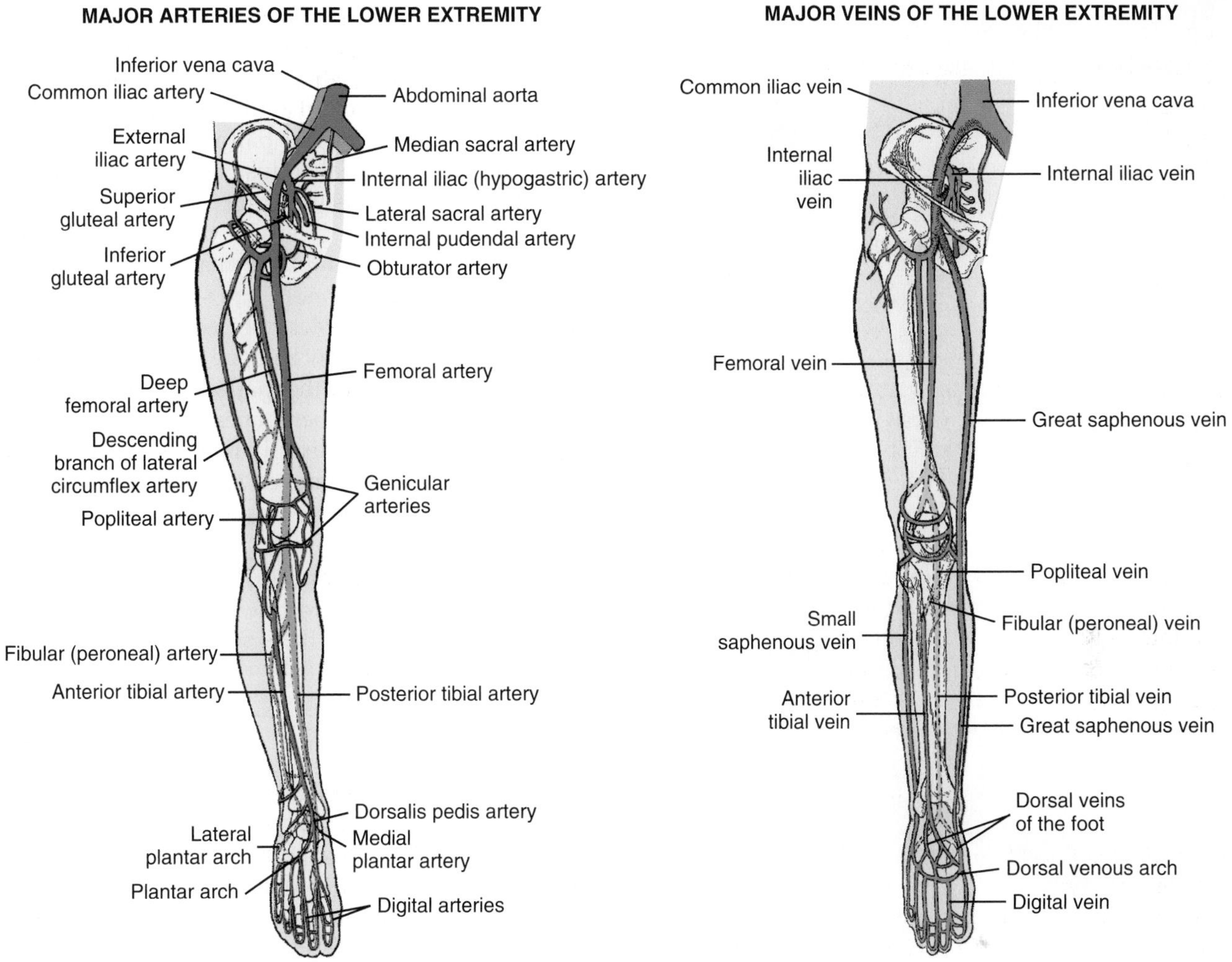

Fig. 18.1 The peripheral vascular system: veins and arteries of the lower extremities. (From Patton K: *Anatomy and physiology*, ed 10, St. Louis, 2019, Elsevier.)

Table 18.4 Differences in Signs and Symptoms of Arterial and Venous Disease

CHARACTERISTIC	ARTERIAL DISEASE	VENOUS DISEASE
Pulses	Diminished, weak, or absent	Strong and symmetric; may be difficult to palpate if edema is present
Skin	Pallor, dependent rubor; thin, dry, shiny, cool	Mottling with brown pigmentation at ankles, veins may be visible; legs or feet bluish when dependent; dermatitis; warm at ankle
Edema	Absent or mild	Present, particularly around ankle and in foot
Ulceration	On toes or at pressure points on feet	At bones of ankle
Necrosis and gangrene	Likely	Unlikely
Pain	Intermittent claudication when walking; sharp, stabbing, gnawing; lessens when at rest	Aching, cramping, particularly when dependent; may have nocturnal cramps
Nails	Thick, brittle (normal in older adults)	Normal
Hair	Hair loss distal to area of occlusion (hair loss normal in older adults)	Normal

necrosis occurs. Ischemic areas of the lower leg and foot may develop skin breakdown without injury. *Arterial ulcers* with a sharp edge and a pale base may form and are quite painful. These ulcers are very slow and difficult to heal (Fig. 18.2). This is particularly true for diabetic patients. The affected part may develop **cellulitis** and edema and become gangrenous, necessitating amputation (Figs. 18.3 and 18.4). The toes and foot are most often affected. Many times ulcerations can occur and progress in diabetic patients due to diabetic neuropathy

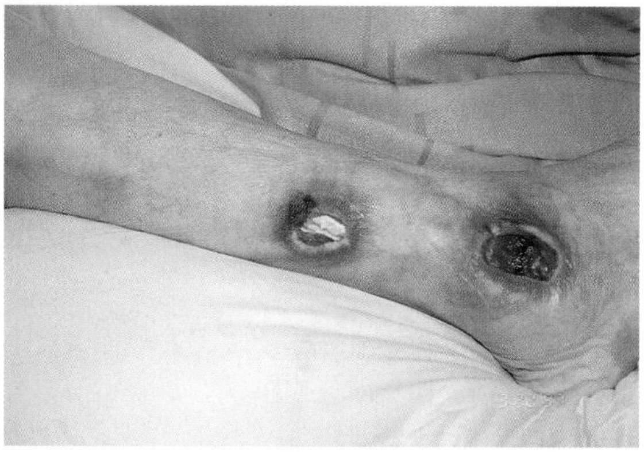

Fig. 18.2 Patient with peripheral arterial disease who has arterial ulcers of the lateral malleolus and distal and lateral portion of the leg. Note the round, smooth shape. (From Black JM, Hawks JH: *Medical-surgical nursing: clinical management for positive outcomes,* ed 8, Philadelphia, 2009, Saunders.)

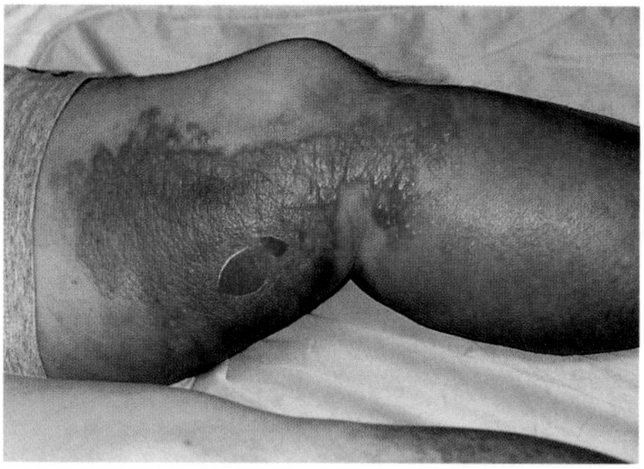

Fig. 18.3 Patient with cellulitis of the legs. (From *Mosby's dictionary of medicine, nursing, and health professions,* ed 10, St. Louis, 2017, Elsevier.)

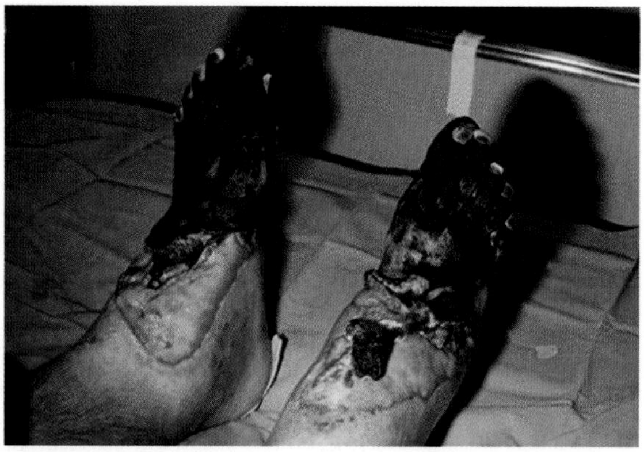

Fig. 18.4 Patient with gangrene of the toes. (Courtesy Cameron Bangs, MD.)

altering the usual pain that accompanies the condition and causes patients to seek early treatment.

An arterial thrombosis can occur as a vessel is narrowed by atherosclerosis. Atherosclerotic plaque ruptures, platelets aggregate at the roughened area, and a clot (thrombus) forms, which may occlude the vessel. If the clot breaks loose and travels, it becomes an arterial embolus and causes acute occlusion of an artery distal to the plaque. **Signs and symptoms of embolus or thrombus occlusion of an extremity artery are the five *P*s: pain, pulselessness, pallor, paresthesia, and paralysis.** Acute arterial occlusion may be treated with percutaneous intravascular procedures. The artery is accessed, and the clot can be removed by special catheters; balloon angioplasty may be performed to open the lumen of the vessel, and stents may be placed to keep the vessel open. Many procedures that previously required surgery can now be done in a procedure room with fluoroscopy and the patient given procedural sedation rather than general anesthesia. Thrombolytic therapy may be given directly into the clot within the artery if it cannot be removed successfully.

Older Adult Care Points

Hair loss is a natural occurrence with aging, as is thickening of fingernails and toenails. These signs alone are not reliable indicators of vascular problems in the extremities in older adults.

Diagnosis of PAD is made using the ABI (see Chapter 17, Fig. 17.9). The normal value is 1 (i.e., the systolic pressure is the same at the ankle and brachial artery sites). Radiographic and ultrasound procedures also may be performed.

Treatment

The best treatment for arterial occlusive disease is regular exercise. A regular walking program results in substantial improvement. Patients are instructed to walk until the claudication pain starts and then rest until the pain goes away. This cycle is repeated until patients are able to walk 45 to 60 minutes daily. Smoking cessation is also a key factor in improvement of peripheral arterial occlusive disease (Dominguez, 2018). Some dietary supplements have proven helpful in increasing circulation.

Complementary and Alternative Therapies

L-Carnitine

Several research studies have shown that L-carnitine, a natural substance found in muscle, heart, brain, and nerve cells, may be beneficial in improving the exercise capacity of individuals with PAD. L-Carnitine, especially in the form of propionylcarnitine, improves muscle recovery after exercise. L-Carnitine can be found in many foods, with higher concentrations in red meat and dairy products. It is supplied as a dietary supplement in 50- to 500-mg tablets. Recommended dosage for individuals with PAD is 600 to 1200 mg three times per day or 750 mg twice daily. Side effects are few; however, dosages in the upper range may cause diarrhea, hyperactivity, and insomnia.

Areas of ulceration are kept clean and free from pressure. Bed rest may be initially prescribed, but walking has been shown to help circulation. Dry eschar is left in place. Debridement is performed only by a qualified health professional. Moist interactive dressings are used on the clean and granulating ulcer to promote healing. The goal of treatment of PAD is directed toward increasing blood flow through the peripheral arteries and decreasing the risk of clot formation in the vessels. Antiplatelet agents and platelet inhibitors may be used alone or in combination with other drugs. Aspirin is the most commonly used antiplatelet agent. It prevents the aggregation of platelets in the arteries. Platelet inhibitors, such as clopidogrel (Plavix), may be prescribed. Patients experiencing intermittent claudication may achieve relief of symptoms when prescribed pentoxifylline (Trental) or cilostazol (Pletal). These drugs increase blood flow by inhibiting clot formation in the vessel. Patients experiencing acute ischemia may receive thrombolytic therapy. Alteplase (tPA, Activase) and tenecteplase (TNKase) are the drugs of choice for thrombolysis. Cholesterol-lowering drugs (e.g., atorvastatin [Lipitor], simvastatin [Zocor], ezetimibe [Zetia]) have been shown to be effective by decreasing low-density lipoprotein (LDL) and increasing high-density lipoprotein (HDL) levels, thus reducing plaque deposits in the arteries.

Clinical Cues

Medications to treat PAD or thrombosis may cause serious adverse reactions. The major adverse reaction is bleeding. Observe the patient for and immediately report evidence of excessive bruising or bleeding, prolonged clotting after a needle stick, hematuria, changes in vital signs, or changes in neurologic signs.

Percutaneous transluminal angioplasty (PTA) may be performed to open an artery to reduce claudication symptoms and improve extremity perfusion. A catheter is introduced into the artery, and when the proper spot is reached, a balloon is inflated multiple times to dilate the vessel, promoting better blood flow. A metal or mesh **stent** (tubular device to give support to a vessel interior) may be placed to prevent narrowing or closure of the artery (see Chapter 20, Fig. 20.5 for a similar stent illustration). If the plaque has a significant calcium component, it may be difficult to dilate the vessel. Atherectomy may be done by several techniques, removing plaque by laser, cutting, or abrading. By removing the plaque, the diameter of the vessel is enlarged, allowing for increased blood flow. Stenting is usually performed to maintain vessel patency. Interventional procedures can prevent the need for open surgical intervention.

Surgical or interventional treatment of PAD is a palliative measure only. It does not cure the disease or halt the atherosclerotic process. It can, however, relieve ischemic pain, help prevent amputation, and add years to a patient's life. The purpose of vascular surgery is to revascularize and nourish cells in the affected area in a patient where percutaneous intervention failed or is not adequate to treat the disorder.

An aortoiliac bypass or a femoropopliteal bypass is performed to correct arterial occlusion of the leg to prevent the need for amputation. A synthetic graft is placed to divert blood around the obstructed area. Fig. 18.5 shows a schematic of a femoropopliteal bypass graft surgery. Postoperative care is the same as for other operative procedures but includes careful assessment of pulses distal to the graft to detect **thrombus** (clot) formation. As with any vascular surgery, extra attention is paid to assessment for signs of bleeding. An aortoiliac bypass requires both an abdominal incision and a groin incision. Blood pressure management is extremely important to maintain blood flow in the graft. Hypotension will cause slowing of the blood flow and potential thrombosis formation, whereas hypertension puts significant stress on the graft sutures, risking bleeding. Because of the condition of the patient's cardiovascular system, the very patients who need the grafting are the poorest surgical candidates. Percutaneous interventions are used more frequently for this patient population. A hyperbaric oxygen chamber is sometimes used for patients with severely compromised circulation to a lower extremity to increase tissue oxygen and prevent amputation.

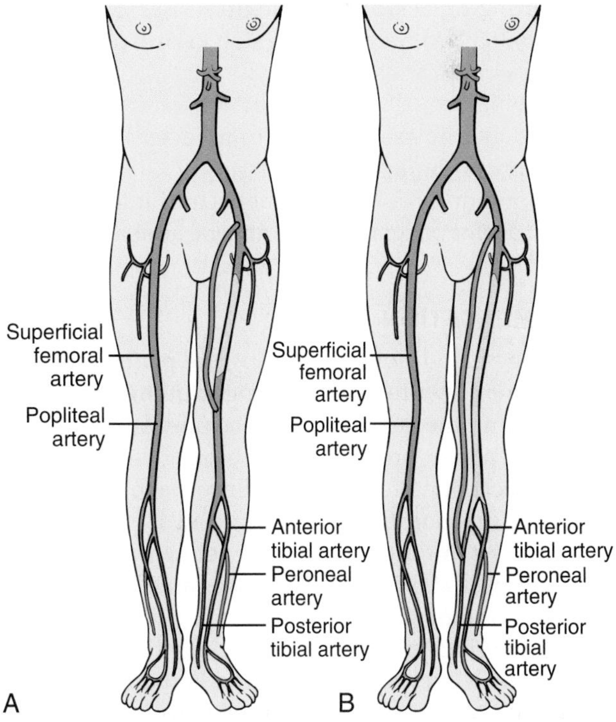

Fig. 18.5 Femoropopliteal bypass graft. **A,** Femoropopliteal bypass graft around an occluded superficial femoral artery. **B,** Femoropopliteal bypass graft around occluded superficial femoropopliteal and proximal tibial arteries. (From Monahan FD, Neighbors M, Sands JK, et al.: *Medical-surgical nursing: health and illness perspective,* ed 8, St. Louis, 2007, Mosby.)

NURSING MANAGEMENT

ASSESSMENT (DATA COLLECTION)

Perform a physical assessment of the patient's affected extremity at least every 4 hours or per facility protocol. Feet should be assessed for warmth, paresthesia, pain, and pulses. All findings must be documented, including any changes. If ulcers are present, assessment and documentation of skin integrity should be included. A major nursing role is early detection and prevention of complications.

NURSING DIAGNOSIS AND PLANNING

The major nursing care goals for patients with PAD are (1) maintaining arterial blood flow to the lower extremities; (2) protecting tissues from further injury from pressure and constriction of blood flow; and (3) preventing wound infection.

Problem statements for a patient with PAD may include:

- Altered peripheral tissue perfusion due to narrowed vessels.
- Altered skin integrity due to ulcers on lower extremities.
- Potential for injury due to loss of peripheral circulation.
- Acute pain due to ischemia to lower extremities.

Expected outcomes may include:

- The patient will not experience loss of skin integrity.
- Peripheral pulses will remain palpable or prompt reporting of lack of palpable pulses.
- The patient will report reduction in pain level in the lower extremities.

Rehabilitation of the patient requires instruction and guidance in special exercises to increase collateral circulation to the legs. See Chapter 17, Table 17.4 for other common problem statements and interventions appropriate for patients with peripheral arterial occlusive disease.

IMPLEMENTATION

Encourage blood flow by keeping the patient and the environment warm. Constricting clothing is to be avoided, and the bed should not be raised at the knees to prevent added pressure on the back of the knees and further occlusion of blood flow. Encourage the patient to change position frequently while awake. The lower extremities should be positioned below heart level to facilitate arterial blood flow. The legs are elevated only if edema is impeding circulation.

Encouraging exercise is especially beneficial to patients with decreased blood flow. Walking regularly every day is best for the ambulatory patient. Swimming also is good because it applies light pressure to the surface of the legs and requires muscle action that encourages venous return. Patients on bed rest should be encouraged to do foot and leg exercises at least once each hour.

> **? Think Critically**
>
> Rhonda, a 63-year-old executive, is experiencing worsening intermittent claudication. Describe how you would interact with her to develop an exercise program that could lessen her symptoms.

Patients should dress in warm, nonrestrictive clothing and should avoid becoming cold. Blankets may be added for additional warmth. The room temperature should be maintained at the patient's comfort level.

Tobacco use, especially smoking, contributes to PVD because of the vasoconstrictive effect of nicotine. Other chemicals in cigarettes directly damage blood vessels, accelerating the development of atherosclerosis. Staff are required to offer hospitalized patients smoking cessation information. Referral to a smoking cessation program, providing support group information, and teaching regarding the adverse effects of smoking all may have been attempted on previous occasions. Know that each encounter is an opportunity for the patient to be receptive to the information. Information concerning the effects of alcohol on vascular disorders, surgical interventions, patient teaching, and interventions to prevent leg ulcers can be reviewed in Chapter 17.

> **? Think Critically**
>
> Describe the specific actions you would take to help a patient recognize the need to establish a smoking cessation program.

EVALUATION

Evaluation of the effectiveness of the plan of care involves assessing changes in peripheral pulses and skin integrity. Improvement or extension of vascular ulcers should be documented in writing and photographed periodically (e.g., weekly). Note changes in color, sensation, and temperature of the lower extremities. The patient's perception of pain level should be documented using a scale of 0 to 10. Evaluate the patient's level of compliance with establishing an exercise routine. Include type, frequency, and tolerance of exercise activities. Evaluate the patient's ability to meet established goals and revise the plan as needed.

ANEURYSM

Etiology

Aneurysms—outpouchings of the wall of an artery resulting from a structural defect in the layers of the arterial wall—occur in a weakened area of a blood vessel. Aneurysms usually are the result of plaque formation, genetic predisposition, or hypertension. Aneurysms may also occur in areas weakened by trauma or surgical procedures. Aortic aneurysms can occur in the area below the diaphragm (abdominal aneurysm) or on the ascending aorta in the chest (thoracic aneurysm). An abdominal aortic aneurysm is usually located below the kidneys. Long-term hypertension and smoking are risk factors, particularly in men.

Congenital malformations, diabetes mellitus, and hyperlipidemia predispose to various types of aneurysm. However, atherosclerosis and hypertension are believed to be the major factors in their development. Atherosclerotic plaque weakens the vessel wall, and hypertension puts extra pressure on the weakened walls. Cerebral aneurysm is discussed in Chapter 23.

Pathophysiology

An aneurysm can occur along any artery. Blood flow may become stagnant along the wall of the aneurysm, and clots can form. The clots can cause occlusion by thrombosis; alternatively, a clot may break away from the thrombosis to become an embolus that travels and lodges elsewhere. Once an aneurysm develops, it continues to grow larger. Aneurysms may eventually rupture if not repaired.

Aortic dissection of the medial layer of the arterial wall can occur, causing bleeding between layers of the wall and increasing pressure on surrounding structures. As the dissection extends, blood flow through the arterial branches of the aorta becomes blocked. Blood flow slows to the organs those branches feed. Dissection occurs more frequently than aneurysm, particularly in men who are hypertensive. Although dissection and aneurysm are two different problems, they can occur together and have similar risk factors.

Signs, Symptoms, and Diagnosis

Aneurysms often cause no obvious symptoms. Patients with an abdominal aortic aneurysm (AAA) may report back pain or a feeling of pressure and may have a visible pulsation of the abdomen. An aortic aneurysm in the thoracic area may cause substernal or tracheal pressure and difficulty with breathing. Diagnosis of aneurysms is difficult because of lack of symptoms during formation. Physical examination and screening of patients with a family history may be the best means of early detection. The presence of an aneurysm can be verified by chest or abdominal radiograph, ultrasound, magnetic resonance imaging (MRI), or computed tomography (CT) scans. Men who have hypertension and a smoking history should undergo ultrasound screening for AAA. Often abdominal or thoracic aneurysms are discovered when the patient has a scan or x-ray for some other reason. AAA rupture is a medical emergency. About 65% of patients with a ruptured AAA die before reaching the hospital (Rahimi, 2017). Emergent surgery to stop the hemorrhage and repair the aneurysm is indicated for patients who present to the emergency department.

Aortic dissection usually causes abrupt, excruciating pain. The pain radiates to the back, chest, abdomen, or extremities. Peripheral pulses are diminished. The patient may be in hypotensive shock because of blood loss if rupture occurs. It can be rapidly fatal, with many patients dying before arrival at the emergency department.

Treatment

If an aortic aneurysm is detected early, it usually can be surgically repaired before it dissects or ruptures. The size and location of the aneurysm guide the need for surgical intervention. Thoracic and abdominal aneurysms do not warrant surgical intervention until the risk of rupture is higher than the risk of the surgery. The patient is evaluated every few months with ultrasound tracking of the size of the aneurysm. Surgery may be performed when AAAs are approximately 6 to 8 cm in diameter and thoracic aneurysms are 5.5 to 6.5 cm in diameter. Patients may be prescribed antihypertensive drugs, such as beta blockers, to reduce the pressure on the arterial walls. If symptoms occur, surgical intervention may be necessary to prevent rupture of the aneurysm.

Surgery for aortic aneurysm involves replacing the area of the vessel wall that is weakened with a graft (open abdomen or chest surgery) or inserting a stent graft into the vessel (percutaneous intravascular insertion). The open surgery requires access to the aorta, where the aneurysm is opened, graft material is placed, and then the vessel is closed around the graft material. Placing a stent graft is a minimally invasive procedure and is used for patients who are not good candidates for open surgical repair of the aneurysm. A wire mesh stent covered with fabric is percutaneously placed in the area of the aneurysm (Fig. 18.6). Small incisions in the groin are used to access the femoral artery. The stent grafts are positioned in the abdominal aorta and usually down the right and left femoral arteries. The graft provides support to the vessel wall and allows blood to flow through the stent, thus reducing pressure on the vessel wall. The aneurysm is then monitored frequently.

❖ NURSING MANAGEMENT

◆ ASSESSMENT (DATA COLLECTION)

Careful physical assessment is needed to detect the presence of an aneurysm. Immediately report findings of pulsations in the abdomen or other structures in which this is abnormal. Changes in peripheral pulses should be noted; clots from the aneurysm may embolize, affecting perfusion. Information concerning family history of aneurysm should be gathered during the patient history interview. Assessment of pain patterns—especially changes in intensity and location—is needed to identify progression of the patient's condition, which may be life-threatening.

◆ NURSING DIAGNOSIS AND PLANNING

The main goal for a patient with an aneurysm is the prevention of rupture. Rupture of an aneurysm is a medical emergency and causes rapid hypovolemic shock, which can lead to death. Advise the patient to report any change in symptoms, such as pain intensity, apprehension, lightheadedness, or any unusual sensation. Problem statements for a patient with an aneurysm may include:

- Potential for injury from possible rupture or dissection of aneurysm.

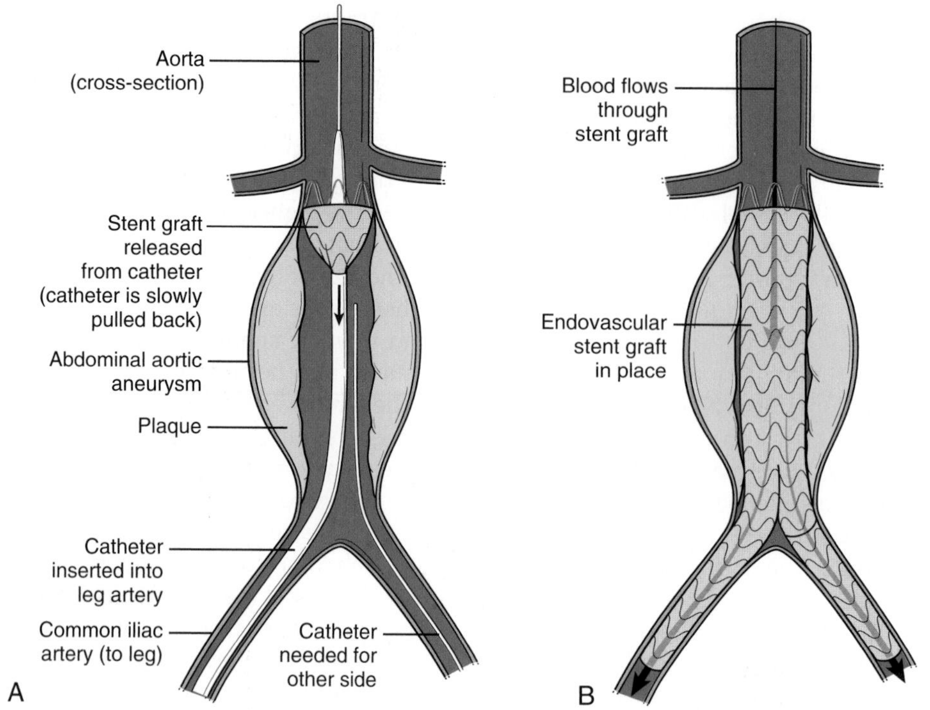

Fig. 18.6 The placement of a stent graft in an aortic aneurysm. **A,** A catheter is inserted into an artery in the groin (upper thigh). The catheter is threaded to the abdominal aorta, and the stent graft is released from the catheter. **B,** The stent graft allows blood to flow through the aneurysm. (Redrawn from National Heart, Lung, and Blood Institute, National Institutes of Health (NIH), Department of Health and Human Services [DHHS]: How is an aneurysm treated? 2011. Available at https://www.nhlbi.nih.gov/health/health-topics/topics/arm/treatment.)

- Acute pain due to pressure of aneurysm on body structures and nerves.
- Insufficient knowledge due to management of medical condition.

Other problems will depend on the location of the aneurysm and whether there is leaking. Expected outcomes might be:

- The patient will not experience rupture or dissection of the aneurysm.
- The patient will report absence of pain.
- The patient will verbalize understanding of management of medical condition.

◆ IMPLEMENTATION

Presurgical patient education is important. The patient must be taught signs and symptoms that should be reported to the health care provider immediately. Teaching concerning the medical and surgical treatment regimen should be included along with what to expect postoperatively.

> **? Think Critically**
>
> You detect a pulsation in a patient's abdomen during physical examination. The patient states that it has been present for several years and the health care provider is "watching it." List signs and symptoms that could indicate a need for surgical intervention.

The surgical procedure and nursing care depend on the location of the aneurysm and the procedure performed. If aortic aneurysm is treated by thoracotomy or abdominal surgery, the care is similar to that for other types of thoracic and abdominal surgery. The main difference is that you must also carefully assess pulses and function distal to the repair site. Renal function must be watched closely because blood flow to the kidneys is briefly cut off when the aorta is clamped for surgical repair of an abdominal aneurysm.

The patient may spend 24 to 48 hours in an intensive care unit postoperatively. Assist the patient to deep-breathe and use an incentive spirometer every 1 to 2 hours if not intubated. Coughing is not encouraged, but should it occur the incision should be splinted with a pillow or folded bath blanket. Paralytic ileus may occur for a few days after abdominal surgery, and a nasogastric tube may be in place. Auscultate the abdomen every shift for the return of bowel sounds. Adequate pain medication is needed.

A patient undergoing thoracic aortic aneurysm repair will have chest surgery that uses a cardiopulmonary bypass machine. The care is the same as for other chest surgery patients. Chest tubes will be in place. These patients are especially at risk for atelectasis and pneumonia. Pain management is necessary to promote adequate respiratory effort. Cardiac dysrhythmias may be a problem, depending on the location of the repair.

A patient having an endovascular repair may be placed on a telemetry or medical-surgical unit. Observation for bleeding from the procedure site is the priority assessment. Frequent checks of pulses distal to the endovascular stent graft and procedure sites are important to verify patency.

◆ EVALUATION

Objective data—including vital signs, neurologic status, distal pulses, and respiratory status—should be assessed. Subjective data—including pain level and loss of sensation—should also be determined. Evaluation of the patient's understanding of teaching related to the disease process, potential complications, follow-up appointments, medications, and recommended lifestyle changes should be assessed and appropriate revisions made to the nursing care plan.

CAROTID ARTERY DISEASE

When atherosclerosis has narrowed the carotid arteries leading to the brain, the signs and symptoms include carotid **bruit** (a purring sound heard with a stethoscope), confusion, transient vision loss, fainting, extremity weakness or paralysis, or other strokelike signs of decreased blood flow to the brain. The condition is treated by carotid endarterectomy or carotid artery angioplasty with stenting. The most benefit from surgery is attained if surgery is performed when the artery has more than 70% stenosis (occlusion) (Rodriguez, 2017). The goal of both procedures is to prevent the occurrence of stroke (see Chapter 23).

Specific postoperative care for endarterectomy includes assessing for signs of bleeding, for pressure from hematoma on the trachea (evidenced by increasing hoarseness), and for neurologic problems caused by thrombosis or embolus. Neurologic signs are monitored every 2 to 4 hours.

Clinical Cues

There is risk for cerebrovascular accident (stroke) after carotid endarterectomy. Assess the patient for signs of disorientation, hoarseness, impaired speech, impaired swallowing, hemiparesis, facial asymmetry, aphasia, and hypertension. These findings should be reported immediately to the surgeon. Because there may be swelling in the neck that may occlude the airway, observe for difficulty breathing.

If surgery is not indicated, the patient is taught to maintain adequate hydration and to comply with drug therapy for hypertension, diabetes, and hyperlipidema, if applicable. Teaching is provided regarding prescribed antiplatelet or anticoagulant drugs. Signs and symptoms of further problems are reviewed, and the patient is advised to call 911 for emergency assistance if sensory or motor deficits appear.

THROMBOANGIITIS OBLITERANS (BUERGER DISEASE)

Etiology and Pathophysiology

Thromboangiitis obliterans, or Buerger disease, is one of approximately 20 disorders that cause inflammation in blood vessels. The conditions may be primary disorders or caused by other diseases. Thromboangiitis obliterans is a primary condition not caused by atherosclerosis, but it involves inflammation and thickening of small and medium-size arteries. Occlusion of the vessels in the hands and feet is usually noted first. The disease occurs more often in men than women and is commonly found in people from the Middle East, the Far East, India, and Southeast Asia. There is increasing incidence of the disease in women older than age 50 years. Moderate to heavy cigarette smoking is directly linked to the progression of the disease. It may be classified as an allergic response in some people in whom the body reacts to properties in nicotine.

SIGNS, SYMPTOMS, DIAGNOSIS, AND TREATMENT

The signs and symptoms include numbness and tingling of the toes or fingers in cold weather, pain in the feet, and intermittent claudication that progressively becomes more severe. The pain is intense. Ulcerations and **gangrene** (death of tissue) may occur. Diagnosis is made through patient history, symptoms, and angiography. **Cessation of smoking is the single most important treatment factor.** Cigarette smoking must be stopped immediately. Those who do not stop smoking are at great risk for gangrene and amputation of fingers or toes. Exercise may be used to increase circulation in the legs and feet.

❖ NURSING MANAGEMENT

◆ ASSESSMENT (DATA COLLECTION), NURSING DIAGNOSIS, PLANNING, AND EVALUATION

The most important nursing role is patient teaching and reinforcement of the need for smoking cessation. Assessment of the extremities for skin impairment is essential. Pain management is needed due to the ischemic pain. Nursing care and teaching is the same as for PAD.

RAYNAUD DISEASE AND RAYNAUD PHENOMENON

Etiology and Pathophysiology

The etiology of Raynaud disease is unknown. Raynaud disease is characterized by spasm of the arteries of the upper and lower extremities. The body has an exaggerated response to cold and stress, resulting in bilateral vasospasm. The disease occurs most commonly in young women. It mostly affects the fingers and toes. Raynaud disease can be a primary disorder or may occur secondary to another disease such as lupus erythematosus, rheumatoid arthritis, or scleroderma. In the latter instance it is known as Raynaud phenomenon and often occurs on only one side of the body.

Blood vessels normally constrict in cold environments; however, with Raynaud disease, this process is excessive. The affected body part changes color. When the spasm stops, there typically is burning pain and throbbing. In about 10% of those affected, the disease progresses

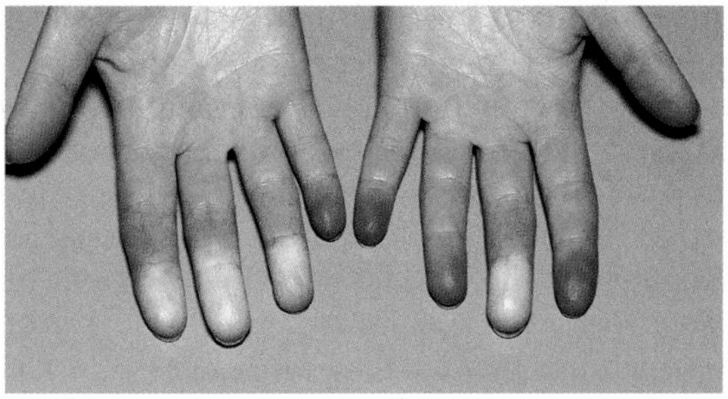

Fig. 18.7 Raynaud phenomenon. (From Hallett JW, et al.: *Comprehensive vascular and endovascular surgery*, ed 2, Philadelphia, 2009, Elsevier.)

to the point at which ischemia from arterial spasm is so severe that gangrene occurs and amputation is necessary.

Signs and Symptoms

Signs and symptoms of Raynaud disease include the following:

- Fingers and toes may display a series of color changes from white to blue to red; these changes are evident on the dorsal surface of the hands and feet (Fig. 18.7).
- The patient may experience numbness or a prickly sensation on warming and relief of stress.
- There may be decreased sensory perception.
- Edema may be present.
- Discomfort may occur in the extremity.

Diagnosis and Treatment

Diagnosis of Raynaud disease is usually made by evaluation of patient symptoms. The health care provider may order laboratory studies such as antinuclear antibody (ANA) test to determine the presence of autoimmune disorders. Medical therapy consists of stress control, avoidance of exposure to cold, and smoking cessation. Calcium channel blockers may be used to dilate capillaries in the hands and feet. The synthetic prostaglandin iloprost (Ventavis) dilates arterial beds throughout the body and extremities. Other drugs such as alpha blockers and vasodilators may be used to achieve vasodilation in the small blood vessels in the hands.

Nursing Management

The major nursing intervention for Raynaud disease is teaching the patient to protect extremities and prevent injury. The patient should be taught to dress warmly when in cold environments. Clothing should be layered and nonrestrictive. Hat, gloves, and warm socks should be worn. The patient should be taught to wear protective gloves when reaching into ovens and when handling extremely cold items. Teach the patient to avoid cold temperatures when possible, to manage stress, and to stop tobacco use. Caffeine intake should be limited.

Evaluate the progression of symptoms, including changes in skin color and sensation. Any changes in skin integrity should be noted. The patient's compliance with recommended lifestyle changes should be evaluated and the plan revised as needed to assist the patient to meet established goals.

> **Health Promotion**
>
> **Smoking Cessation**
>
> Encourage smokers with vascular disorders to seek smoking cessation programs in their communities. The American Lung Association's program "Freedom from Smoking" is offered free of charge online at the American Lung Association website. Group programs are offered in many communities, hospitals, American Lung Association affiliates, and community-based health programs. A variety of products are available to decrease and prevent nicotine cravings during the cessation process. Assessment of progress with smoking cessation should occur at each visit with a health care provider.

VENOUS DISORDERS

SUPERFICIAL THROMBOPHLEBITIS

The body is continuously forming small clots as needed and breaking them down when not needed. Alteration in this normal physiologic occurrence can be caused by several factors. Virchow's triad identifies conditions such as vessel trauma, venous stasis (or turbulence), and abnormal coagulability as factors that cause the small clots to grow into bigger clots. Superficial thrombophlebitis that occurs in a patient receiving IV therapy may be caused by chemical or mechanical irritation of the vessel. If not identified and treated, bacteremia may occur, resulting in *septic thrombophlebitis*. Decreasing hospital-acquired bloodstream infections is a National Patient Safety Goal, and strict asepsis when inserting or accessing IV sites can help meet this goal. Superficial thrombophlebitis can occur spontaneously or as a complication of medical or surgical interventions and usually occurs in the lower extremities. It is usually a self-limiting disease but as mentioned above can progress to a more serious condition.

Signs, Symptoms, and Diagnosis

Redness and tenderness along the course of the vein accompanied by swelling are the usual presenting symptoms. Laboratory testing for hypercoagulability and to check inflammation status is performed. White blood cell (WBC) count as part of the complete blood cell count (CBC) will help identify if an infection has occurred. An ultrasound demonstrating thickened, inflamed, and noncompressible veins confirms the diagnosis.

Treatment and Nursing Management

Treatment for thrombophlebitis depends on the severity of the condition. If the IV is implicated as a cause, the IV catheter site will be changed to a new location. For mild tender areas, treatment with analgesics such NSAIDs is usually adequate. Elastic support may also be used. More severe thrombophlebitis will be treated with elevation and heat. Treatment is primarily symptomatic. If there is concern about the thrombus enlarging or affecting the deep veins, fondaparinux or low-molecular-weight heparin injections will be implemented. If infection is present, antibiotics will be given.

DEEP VEIN THROMBOSIS

Deep vein thrombosis (DVT) occurs most commonly in the iliac and femoral veins, but upper extremity DVT accounts for 5% to 10% of all incidences. Because DVT can lead to embolization from the thrombus to the lungs, DVT prophylaxis is recommended for all hospitalized patients and is included in The Joint Commission's National Patient Safety Goals.

Signs, Symptoms, and Diagnosis.

Classic signs and symptoms include pain, swelling, and redness (Fig. 18.8). However, only about 50% of patients with DVT report pain, and many are asymptomatic. Edema may be unilateral or bilateral and can be mistaken for dependent edema. Upper extremity DVT is more likely to present with pain, swelling, and arm fatigue.

Etiology and Pathophysiology

People who are immobile for a long time are very susceptible to DVT. Prolonged surgeries, spinal cord damage and paralysis, and chronic heart failure all contribute to venous stasis. Immobility with the legs dependent in car or airplane travel for long periods also promotes venous stasis. Trauma or external pressure or internal pressure from hypertension may damage the endothelium. Inflammation of the vessel leads to aggregation of blood components at the site of the inflammation. A clot forms at the inflammation site, leading to obstruction of blood flow. If not treated, the clot may become an embolus that may travel from the legs to the lungs, resulting in pulmonary embolus.

Smoking, female hormone replacement, estrogen-based contraceptives, corticosteroids, and various blood disorders are contributing factors to blood hypercoagulability. Obesity and dehydration also contribute to increased coagulability.

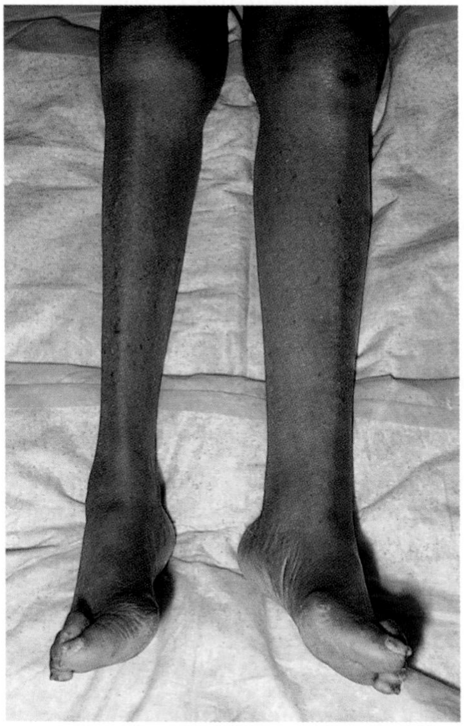

Fig. 18.8 Patient with deep vein thrombosis. (From Swartz MH: *Textbook of physical diagnosis: history and examination*, ed 7, Philadelphia, 2014, Elsevier.)

Older Adult Care Points

Older adult patients who have problems with mobility or stress incontinence tend to drink less fluid so that they do not have to visit the bathroom as often. This can lead to dehydration and more viscous blood, which in turn can predispose to thrombus formation in those susceptible to this disorder. Encourage adequate fluid intake to promote circulation and provide a means for convenient toileting for these patients. The occurrence of DVT or thrombophlebitis increases with advanced age.

Patients particularly at risk for DVT are those having orthopedic surgery; those who smoke; and those who have diabetes, lung disease, blood disorders, PVD, sepsis, or cancer. If DVT is not resolved, the interaction of the clot with the vessel wall results in destruction of venous valves and development of venous insufficiency. *Embolism* may develop when a portion of a DVT in a leg breaks loose and travels to the lungs. The embolus lodges in small vessels, especially those in the pulmonary system. Blood flow is interrupted, and loss of oxygenation to the lung may occur. The condition can be life-threatening (see Chapter 14). When a pulmonary embolus is suspected, place the patient in a high Fowler position, provide oxygen and reassurance, notify the health care provider, and stay with the patient. Medication for pain and anxiety may be ordered; tests to determine whether a pulmonary embolus has occurred will be ordered.

Patients are encouraged to stay off their feet and to elevate their legs. Support stockings are to be worn after the acute phase.

Think Critically

What teaching points would you include for a 52-year-old female hair stylist who is being discharged after hospitalization for thrombophlebitis of the right leg?

Clinical Cues

Whenever a patient has a known DVT, watch for signs of pulmonary embolus: dyspnea, hemoptysis, tachypnea, tachycardia, chest pain, decreased oxygen saturation, a feeling of impending doom, cyanosis, and possibly coughing and altered mental status. These signs indicate an emergency situation.

Treatment

Inpatient medical treatment for DVT usually consists of IV heparin. Low-molecular-weight heparin (LMWH), such as enoxaparin (Lovenox) by injection, may be used for inpatient management and is increasingly being used for outpatient treatment. Fondaparinux (Arixtra), a factor Xa inhibitor, may be used instead of enoxaparin. After initial IV or subcutaneous injection of anticoagulation treatment, oral anticoagulation is started with warfarin sodium (Coumadin), rivaroxaban (Xarelto), edoxaban (Lixiana), dabigatran (Pradaxa), betrixaban (Bevyxxa), or apixaban (Eliquis). Anticoagulation is continued for 3 to 12 months (Patel, 2017). Anticoagulants will not dissolve the clot but may prevent new ones. The body dissolves the clot on its own over time.

Thrombolytic therapy may be used to dissolve the thrombus if vessel obstruction is severe; the agents used are the same as those listed for arterial thrombolysis. There is a high risk of bleeding with these drugs, and a compelling reason must be present for their use because in time the body will dissolve the clot without intervention. Sequential compression devices (SCDs) may be prescribed, or compression stockings may be fitted for daily use. Stockings must fit properly and be kept smooth. The compression forces blood from the superficial veins into the deep veins, decreasing venous stasis. Compression stockings are removed only for bathing and are changed and laundered daily. They must be replaced after 6 months because the elastic quality decreases. Ambulation as soon as it is not prohibited by pain and swelling is recommended. There is no evidence that ambulation will dislodge a DVT and cause a pulmonary embolus, as has been believed for many years (Patel, 2017).

If a patient is considered at risk for further embolus formation from DVT and is not a candidate for anticoagulation, a *vena cava filter* will be inserted. The device is placed in the inferior vena cava (IVC) below the kidneys to prevent pulmonary emboli. With the use of a special catheter threaded into the vena cava, the device is positioned and deployed. The metal cage device catches the emboli, and the body slowly dissolves and disposes of them. IVC filters come in different shapes and configurations, but they all do the same thing.

Post-thrombotic syndrome (PTS) is a potential complication for 50% of patients with DVT. While the body is dissolving the clot, there is continued inflammation at the site. This causes permanent damage in the vessel (PTS) and may lead to venous insufficiency. The latest consensus is that compression stockings after DVT do not help prevent PTS. Current research is focusing on more aggressive DVT treatment to remove the clot so it does not remain in contact with the vessel wall. Thrombolytic therapy delivered directly into the clot, percutaneous thrombectomy, angioplasty, and stenting are all being examined with the goal of preventing PTS.

Heparin-induced thrombocytopenia (HIT) may occur when unfractionated or LMWH is used for several days to weeks. It is heralded by a sudden decrease in platelet count. If HIT occurs, heparin administration must be stopped.

NURSING MANAGEMENT

ASSESSMENT (DATA COLLECTION)

Assess patients at risk for DVT each shift for signs and symptoms. Assessment should include:

- Observation of the extremity for asymmetric size
- Areas of warmth and redness over a vein
- Calf pain and/or tenderness
- Pitting edema of the affected extremity
- Measurement of calf circumference
- Body temperature greater than 100.4° F (38° C)

Nursing management of a patient with thrombophlebitis from DVT includes assessment and documentation of the color, warmth, circumference, and pulses of the affected extremity. Explain the importance of adhering to the prescribed level of physical activity and explain the potential complications of noncompliance. Make certain that the patient receives medications as prescribed. Warm, moist compresses to the affected extremity may be ordered. Emphasize the importance of this treatment. Develop a discharge teaching plan related to the disease process, medications, activity level, home care, and follow-up. Components of teaching may include:

- Avoidance of sitting for long periods with the legs down
- Avoidance of standing in one place for long periods
- Management with NSAIDs
- Application of compression stockings
- Preventive measures

NURSING DIAGNOSIS, PLANNING, AND IMPLEMENTATION

Early ambulation postoperatively helps promote circulation and reduces the risk of clot formation. Encouraging patients on bed rest to change position and perform leg and ankle exercises each hour while awake can do much to decrease the incidence of DVT. Venous thrombosis occurs fairly commonly during long plane flights or car trips. Staying well hydrated, exercising the leg and calf muscles frequently during the trip, and walking every 1 to 2 hours help prevent clots from occurring. Wearing support hose while standing aids venous return and helps prevent thrombosis in those who have varicose veins (Lew, 2017).

Problem statements or nursing diagnoses, expected outcomes, and interventions are presented in Nursing Care Plan 18.1.

EVALUATION

Decrease in leg circumference and adequate blood flow to the extremity as evidenced by color, warmth, and lack of edema indicate that interventions for DVT are working. Evaluation of interventions for thrombophlebitis include checking for decreased redness and swelling.

Decreased redness, swelling, and pain indicate resolution of the thrombophlebitis. Evaluation of patient success in meeting goals would include compliance with medications and demonstrated evidence of understanding of discharge teaching. Often subjective data from the patient must be relied on to evaluate whether treatment and nursing actions are effective.

Nursing Care Plan 18.1 Care of a Patient With a Deep Vein Thrombosis

SCENARIO

Mrs. Hanson, age 72, fainted at the airport after returning from a cross-country plane trip of 6 hours. She was unconscious at the scene and woke up when medical personnel arrived. She had a heart rate of 20 when checked by the paramedics, and her heart rate returned to a normal range before she arrived at the hospital. She was admitted to a telemetry floor for observation.

She has now developed pain in her right calf, and her lower leg is swollen, with a hot, tender area in the midcalf region. She has been placed on a continuous heparin drip.

PROBLEM STATEMENT/NURSING DIAGNOSIS

Altered peripheral tissue perfusion due to presence of clot in vein and inflammation, decreasing venous circulation.

SUPPORTING ASSESSMENT DATA

Subjective: "My leg wasn't swollen like that earlier."

Objective: Reddened, warm, tender area on midcalf. Temperature 101.2° F (38.4° C). Leg circumference increased compared with left leg.

Goals/Expected Outcomes	Nursing Interventions	Selected Rationale	Evaluation
Circulation will be maintained in the right leg with decrease in swelling and no evidence of skin breakdown.	Encourage ambulation as tolerated; keep right lower leg elevated when in bed.	To prevent formation of further clot and help venous circulation.	Up to the bathroom several times during the day. Right leg elevated when in bed.
Thrombosis will begin to resolve by discharge as evidenced by normal temperature and no calf tenderness, redness, or swelling.	Early ambulation.	Maintains venous circulation.	Walking as much as tolerated.
	Warm packs to right leg; handle right leg gently.	Provides comfort, decreases edema.	Leg circumference decreased by 0.5 cm.
	Encourage increase in fluid intake.	Assists in reducing blood viscosity.	Intake 2000 mL this shift.
	Apply compression stockings smoothly, removing only for bathing.	Assists with venous return and prevents blood pooling.	Compression stockings in place.

PROBLEM STATEMENT/NURSING DIAGNOSIS

Pain secondary to inflammation and swelling.

SUPPORTING ASSESSMENT DATA

Subjective: "My leg really hurts." Complains of pain 8/10 in right calf.

Objective: Reddened, warm, tender area on midcalf.

Goals/Expected Outcomes	Nursing Interventions	Selected Rationale	Evaluation
Pain level will be maintained at or below 5 on a 10-point scale	Administer analgesia for aching and tenderness.	Helps relieve pain.	Analgesic administered × 2. States is more comfortable. Pain level 3.
	Warm, moist packs to right calf as needed.	Promotes comfort	Warm, moist pack kept in place for 2 h.
	Offer nonpharmacologic measures, repositioning, teach relaxation techniques, activities for diversion.	Promotes comfort without the use of medications.	Patient requested and was taught imagery techniques. States it helped to take her mind off the pain. Her family is bringing in a crossword puzzle book this evening.

PROBLEM STATEMENT/NURSING DIAGNOSIS

Potential for bleeding related to heparin drip and initiation of oral anticoagulants.

Continued

Nursing Care Plan 18.1 Care of a Patient With a Deep Vein Thrombosis—cont'd

SUPPORTING ASSESSMENT DATA

Objective: Heparin drip 50,000 units in 500 mL at 25 mL/h. Warfarin 2 mg orally to be started tonight.

Goals/Expected Outcomes	Nursing Interventions	Selected Rationale	Evaluation
Patient will have no bleeding from heparin as evidenced by no signs of bleeding externally and normal vital signs.	Maintain heparin drip on IV pump at ordered rate; assess IV site q1h for infiltration.	Prevent formation of additional thrombi.	Heparin drip continuous; IV site without redness or swelling.
Patient will verbalize measures to take to prevent injury while on anticoagulants.	Observe for bleeding of gums, excessive bruising, blood in urine or stool, nosebleeds, and abdominal pain with rigidity.	Heparin can cause bleeding.	Slight bleeding of gums. Bruising from previous needle sticks. No evidence of blood in urine or stool; bowel sounds present all four quadrants, abdomen soft.
	Monitor Hb and hematocrit to detect blood loss.	May indicate need to change infusion rate or administer protamine sulfate if excessive blood loss occurs.	No change in Hb and hematocrit.
	Monitor aPTT and advise health care provider immediately if values rise above 2½ times the control value or above therapeutic range.	Allows for adjustment of heparin dosage to keep it within therapeutic range.	aPTT two times control value.
	Hold pressure over any needle stick for 5 min.	Heparin extends bleeding time.	No excessive bleeding with laboratory draws.
	Instruct patient to move around carefully, trying not to hit head on anything or bump into things.	Injury could cause bruising and hematoma formation	Slight bruising noted on buttocks.
	Handle patient very gently.	Prevents bruising.	No new bruising.

PROBLEM STATEMENT/NURSING DIAGNOSIS

Potential for altered gas exchange secondary to pulmonary embolus.

SUPPORTING ASSESSMENT DATA

Objective: Presence of right calf DVT demonstrated on ultrasound.

Goals/Expected Outcomes	Nursing Interventions	Selected Rationale	Evaluation
Patient will have no alteration in gas exchange as evidenced by continuously maintaining Spo_2 greater than 96% on room air.	Maintain heparin drip at ordered rate.	Prevent formation of additional thrombi.	Heparin drip continuous.
Any change of Spo_2 below 3% of baseline or development of tachypnea will promptly be reported to the provider.	Spo_2 continuously monitored. Vital signs including respiratory rate assessed q4h.	Sudden drop in Spo_2 or increase in respiratory rate could indicate a pulmonary embolus.	Spo_2 98% on room air. Respiratory rate 16.
Patient will not experience embolus or other DVT during hospitalization.	Caution not to sit with legs crossed in the bed.	Crossing the legs decreases venous return and promotes blood pooling in the extremity. Sitting causes dependent pooling in legs.	States understands not to cross legs while lying in bed or sitting up.
	Caution to use support stockings correctly so they do not bunch up, causing a tourniquet effect.	Can decrease venous return and cause pooling in extremities.	States she understands that stockings should be smoothed out and not bunched up.

Nursing Care Plan 18.1 Care of a Patient With a Deep Vein Thrombosis—cont'd

PROBLEM STATEMENT/NURSING DIAGNOSIS

Insufficient knowledge due to new diagnosis and medication treatment plan.

SUPPORTING ASSESSMENT DATA

Objective: No previous DVT diagnosis and has never taken warfarin.

Goals/Expected Outcomes	Nursing Interventions	Selected Rationale	Evaluation
Patient will verbalize danger signs to report to provider, proper dosage of medications, and dietary considerations before discharge.	Teach the following: avoid foods high in vitamin K (give list).	Vitamin K counteracts the action of warfarin.	Patient identified foods high in vitamin K that are in her routine diet and states "I will be consistent in the amount of these foods in my diet."
	Avoid over-the-counter medications and drugs that might extend clotting time or interfere with action of warfarin (e.g., aspirin).	Some over-the-counter drugs have anticoagulant actions that may increase risk of complications of drug therapy.	States understands to check with provider before using over-the-counter medications.
Patient will verbalize understanding of need for regular medical follow-up and periodic laboratory tests of clotting times before discharge.	Instruct her to maintain close contact with provider to monitor clotting times.	Monitoring of INR important to evaluate effectiveness of warfarin therapy.	Verbalizes need to keep appointments for follow-up laboratory studies.
	Explain dosage schedule. Give written instruction sheet.	Provides reference for safe administration of drug.	Given written instructions to be followed when taking warfarin. Verbalized understanding.
Patient will completely stop smoking within 1 mo.	Give smoking cessation information. Get order for nicotine patch or other assist product. Refer to support group.	Cigarette smoking constricts vessels and contributes to blood coagulability.	Is willing to work with a smoking cessation counselor.
Patient will establish a walking program when acute stage has resolved.	Assist to establish walking schedule.	Walking promotes venous return by calf muscles compressing the veins.	Is thinking about a walking schedule.
	Caution not to sit with legs crossed or to sit for long periods without elevating legs.	Crossing the legs decreases venous return and promotes blood pooling in the extremity. Sitting causes dependent pooling in legs.	States understands not to sit with legs crossed or for long periods with legs dependent.
	Caution not to wear constricting clothing.	Tight clothing can decrease venous return and cause pooling in extremities.	States she understands not to wear tight clothing items.

CRITICAL THINKING QUESTIONS

1. List the signs and symptoms of pulmonary embolism.
2. What assessment data would you expect to find indicating that the treatment of a patient with deep vein thrombosis was successful?

aPTT, Activated partial thromboplastin time; *Hb*, *hemoglobin; IV*, intravenous.

VARICOSE VEINS

Varicose veins are enlarged and tortuous veins that are distorted in shape by accumulations of pooled blood. Veins that develop varicosities have incompetent valves that allow reflux of blood from the deep to the superficial veins. The increased blood flow and resultant pressure on the vein walls cause the vessels to dilate and become tortuous.

Varicosities usually occur in the saphenous veins and perforator veins in the ankle. Congenital or family disposition that leads to loss of vessel wall elasticity is a primary cause. Standing for long periods, obesity, and pregnancy are contributing factors. Trauma, DVT, and inflammation that results in vein valve damage are secondary causes. Individuals who must be on their feet a great deal are encouraged to wear support stockings to promote venous return.

Signs and symptoms of varicose veins include dilated, twisted-appearing, superficial vessels on the

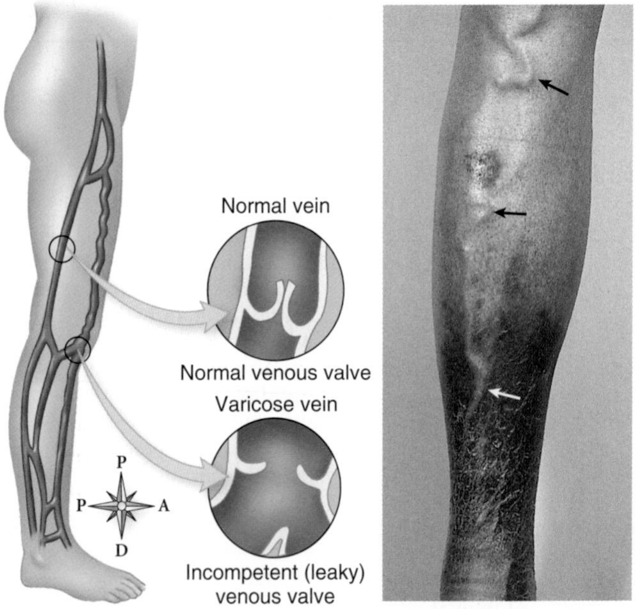

Fig. 18.9 Varicose veins. (From Patton KT, Thibodeau GA: *The human body in health and disease,* ed 7, St. Louis, 2018, Elsevier.)

Think Critically

Identify two lifestyle changes you could make that would decrease your risk of a vascular disorder later in life.

Older Adult Care Points

Varicose veins develop in older adults as the veins lose their elasticity and the leg muscles weaken and atrophy from decreased exercise.

legs. Swelling of the foot and ankle on the affected leg may occur by the end of the day, and swelling is often accompanied by aching. The patient may complain of pain, itching, or both along varicose veins (Fig. 18.9). The legs may feel full and heavy during walking or exercise. Diagnosis is made by thorough physical assessment and patient history.

Treatment

Treatment of varicose veins includes using elastic support hose, exercising the legs and feet periodically throughout the day, and elevating the legs whenever possible. Prolonged standing, sitting, or crossing the legs is to be avoided. Weight reduction is recommended for patients who are obese. Exercises such as walking or swimming are beneficial because the muscle contraction encourages venous return to the heart. Some herbs are helpful for varicose veins.

Knee-high elastic stockings or elastic wraps should be used to support venous circulation. See Chapter 17 for correct use and application of support garments.

Exercise is especially beneficial to patients with decreased blood flow. Walking is the ideal exercise for ambulatory patients. If a patient is unable to ambulate, promote venous return through range-of-motion (ROM) exercises and other kinds of muscular movements. Any activity that causes contraction of the leg muscles will help move venous blood from the legs to the heart.

Complementary and Alternative Therapies

Herbs for Varicose Veins

Several herbs have been found to be helpful for patients with varicose veins (but should not be used during pregnancy and lactation):

Bilberry: May cause constipation; affects blood glucose levels, may increase the action of anticoagulants; check drug and herbal interactions

Butcher's broom: Not to be used by patients with hypertension or prostatic hypertrophy

Gotu kola: Also helpful for hypertension

Horse chestnut: Check for interactions with other drugs the patient is taking; do not use with hypoglycemics, salicylates, or anticoagulants

Patients need to be aware of potential side effects of herbs as well as prescribed medications.

Clinical Cues

Follow directions carefully and measure the patient's calves and legs before choosing a pair of elastic stockings. Accurate fit is crucial to effective treatment. If standard sizes do not coincide with the measurements, custom stockings may need to be purchased.

Medications such as NSAIDs (e.g., aspirin, ibuprofen) may be used for aching. Surgical procedures may be used when medical treatment is ineffective. Small varicosities can be treated by **sceropathy**, which involves injecting an agent that will sclerose the vessel, causing it to dry up and wither. Endovenous occlusion using a laser is performed by placing a catheter within the vein under duplex ultrasound guidance; a laser heats the vessel, causing it to collapse and close off. It can be performed in an office setting or outpatient ambulatory surgery site. Compression stockings are worn for 1 to 2 weeks after the procedure. Patients ambulate immediately after the procedure for 30 to 60 minutes and 1 to 2 hours per day for 1 to 2 weeks. A similar procedure uses radiofrequency energy for closure of the vessel. Vein stripping may be performed for severe cases; a less invasive technique is called *PIN (perforate invaginate) stripping*. In this procedure only two small incisions are used, and the vein is removed much like pulling a sock off inside out. It can be done in an office setting but also may be performed in an operating room.

CHRONIC VENOUS INSUFFICIENCY

Etiology and Pathophysiology

Chronic venous insufficiency is common among older adults. Many cases are caused by congenital absence of the valves in the veins. It can also occur when the venous valves are damaged and can affect the superficial low-pressure vessels or the higher pressure deep venous system, such as occurs with severe cases of DVT. When valves are damaged or absent, there is retrograde venous blood flow, and blood pools in the legs. Swelling results, with increasing venous pressure and stasis of blood flow. The condition may lead to venous stasis ulcers.

Venous return occurs by the pumping action of the calf muscles against the venous walls. When valves are incompetent, venous return is compromised, and flow goes both ways in the vessel. The increased pressure leads to leakage of red blood cells into the tissues. The breakdown of the red blood cells releases hemosiderin, which causes a brownish skin color (Weiss, 2017). Fibrous tissue replaces subcutaneous tissue around the ankle. The skin becomes thick and hardened.

Signs, Symptoms, and Diagnosis

Signs and symptoms of chronic venous insufficiency include chronically swollen legs; thick, brownish skin around the ankles; and itchy, scaly skin (Fig. 18.10). Stasis dermatitis is common. Venous stasis ulcers often occur (Fig. 18.11). Infection and cellulitis occur if an ulcer is untreated. Diagnosis is made through physical assessment and patient history.

Treatment and Nursing Management

Treatment is the use of knee-high elastic support stockings and elevation of the legs for 8 of 24 hours each day. Teach the patient to avoid prolonged standing or sitting and to sleep with the foot of the bed elevated 6 inches. Legs should not be crossed when sitting, and tight, restrictive clothing should be avoided. Legs should be elevated above heart level whenever possible.

VENOUS STASIS ULCERS

Diabetic patients with venous insufficiency are at high risk for venous stasis ulcers because of compromised circulation in the extremities and a slow rate of healing. The ulcers may extend deeply into the tissue and are very slow and difficult to heal because of tissue congestion and edema that prevent nutrients from reaching the cells. The ulcer may begin as a small, tender, inflamed area and becomes very painful. With the slightest trauma, the skin breaks and the ulcer enlarges. It is imperative that patients with venous insufficiency be taught the extreme importance of good foot and leg care. Teach the patient about proper self-care and signs of beginning skin breakdown. The slightest injury to an ischemic area can take a very long time to heal and can easily become infected because the blood supply is inadequate to provide the usual leukocyte defenses. Any injury to an affected extremity, no matter how minor, should be reported to the health care provider immediately.

Treatment for an ulcer consists of leg elevation, a moist dressing, and compression. A culture is performed to determine whether infection is present. Saline or mild soap is used to clean around the ulcer. A lanolin-type lotion is used to keep skin moist and supple. The

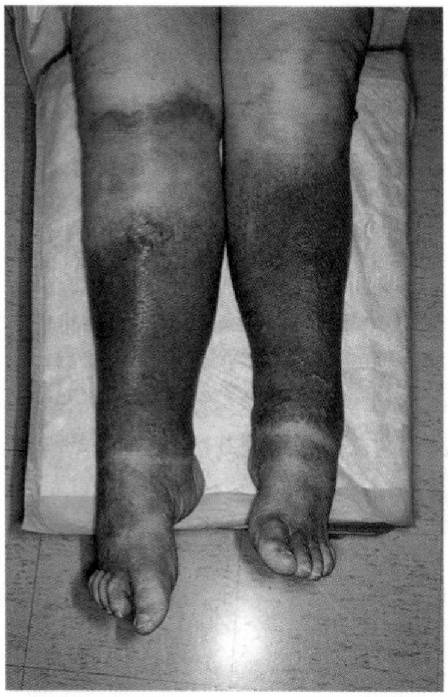

Fig. 18.10 Characteristic skin changes in a patient with venous insufficiency. (From Swartz M: *Textbook of physical diagnosis: history and examination*, ed 7, Philadelphia, 2014, Elsevier.)

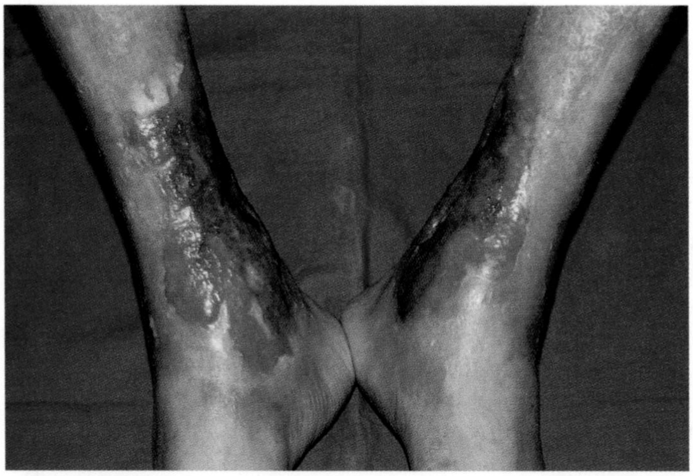

Fig. 18.11 Venous stasis ulcer. (From Swartz MH: *Textbook of physical diagnosis: history and examination*, ed 7, Philadelphia, 2014, Elsevier.)

dressing to be used depends on the condition of the ulcer and the amount of exudate produced. A vacuum-assisted drainage device may be needed for excessive drainage. The wound may need a graft to heal completely. Venous stasis ulcers can take weeks to months to heal. Compression dressings are not used if arterial insufficiency is also present. Compression therapy options include compression stockings, elastic tubular support bandages, intermittent compression devices, a paste bandage such as Unna boot, or placement of two to four layers of compression dressings to the affected area. Venous return is accomplished as the patient moves their leg and achieves pressure on the calf muscles. Compression dressings can be placed over wound dressings. The dressings help reduce ulcer pain, keep the wound moist, and assist debridement. The dressing is changed from every 2 to 3 days to every few weeks depending on the type of dressing applied.

For success, the underlying venous problem must be treated. A graft may be necessary to heal the ulcer. A split-thickness graft or bioengineered skin may be used. Advise the patient to avoid injury to the graft site. Patients are placed on bed rest for several days after grafting to protect the site. Give the patient considerable support because treatment is long, recurrent, and tedious. Patients with stasis ulcers commonly become depressed. Praise for compliance with instructions and for any small gains made toward healing can do much for a patient's morale.

NURSING MANAGEMENT

ASSESSMENT (DATA COLLECTION)

Subjective information is gathered during history taking. A nutritional assessment is essential. Objective assessment data should include status of the skin, noting color, warmth, and moisture. Stasis dermatitis may be present, and pruritus and edema are common. Document the location, size, and presence of exudate and its color and odor, and include a photograph. Obtain a patient statement of pain at the site on a scale of 0 to 10. Assess the patient's experience with pain, including intensity, when pain occurs, and how it is relieved. Assess arterial pulses and determine the pulse rate, rhythm, and character (force) of the pulse. For diagnostic tests, refer to Chapter 17, Table 17.2.

NURSING DIAGNOSIS AND PLANNING

Problem statements are chosen based on those assessment data that indicate problems for the patient. Common problem statements associated with vascular disorders are listed in Chapter 17, Table 17.4. Nursing diagnoses may be added to the care plan for problems secondary to treatments, such as drug therapy or surgery. Other problem statements sometimes used include:

- Insomnia related to pain in the legs while at rest.
- Decreased self-esteem related to inability to perform usual roles because of chronic leg ulcers.

Focused Assessment

Data Collection for Vascular Disorders

Gather data on the following while interviewing the patient.

HEALTH HISTORY
- Family history of hypertension, cardiovascular disease, stroke, hyperlipidemia, aortic aneurysm, diabetes mellitus, or PVD
- History of trauma to the lower extremities
- Personal history of any PVD
- All medications taken on a regular basis (prescribed and over-the-counter medications)
- History of tobacco use, especially smoking
- History of alcohol use
- Dietary practices, especially sodium and fat intake
- Current or history of central nervous system occurrences, such as dizziness, headaches, or loss of consciousness
- Occurrence of edema in the legs, feet, or ankles
- Occurrence of leg pain during walking (When? How is it relieved?)

PHYSICAL ASSESSMENT
- Color of skin of the neck
- Observe for jugular vein distention
- Auscultate carotid arteries for presence of bruit
- Auscultate heart sounds and note any abnormalities
- Assess for any visible abdominal pulsation over aorta
- Auscultate over aorta in abdomen for presence of bruit
- Assess peripheral pulses and compare bilaterally
- Assess blood pressure on both arms, sitting and standing
- Assess skin for temperature, color, appearance, lesions, dryness, presence or absence of hair on legs
- Note presence of varicosities
- Assess capillary refill

Appropriate exercise is important to treat vascular disease. Collaborate with the health care provider and physical therapist about activity, exercises, and the reinforcement of teaching. Work with the dietitian to promote the patient's adequate nutrient intake for healing. Specific expected outcomes must be written on an individual basis (see Chapter 17, Table 17.4).

IMPLEMENTATION

A major role of a nurse caring for a patient with venous insufficiency is to monitor the condition and determine whether treatment is effective. Chapter 17, Table 17.4 lists helpful interventions for the most common problem statements associated with problems of the vascular system. Nursing interventions for selected problems in a patient with a venous stasis ulcer are summarized in Chapter 17, Table 17.4.

EVALUATION

Evaluate the patient's response to treatment to determine effectiveness and potential development of complications. Carefully evaluating pulses and comparing them bilaterally are important parts of nursing care for patients with problems of the vascular system. Documenting a good description of the quality and character of the monitored pulses in the nursing notes will give coworkers an accurate assessment baseline on which to evaluate changes in the pulse (see Chapter 17, Box 17.2).

It is important to determine whether skin color and temperature have changed since the last assessment. Ulcerated areas are monitored closely, measured, documented in writing, and photographed to determine whether healing is occurring. The color of the healing tissue and presence of exudate also are evaluated. Documentation of the characteristics of any exudate should be included. If the wound is enlarging or not improving, the nursing actions or treatment must be changed.

Subjective data from the patient help evaluate whether treatment and nursing actions are effective. Increases in peripheral circulation may be evident only by a decrease in pain or an ability to walk farther without pain. The patient should be able to demonstrate understanding of the disease process, preventive measures, medications, signs and symptoms to report to the health care provider, and follow-up care.

COMMUNITY CARE

Many patients with vascular disease are treated in outpatient clinics and their homes. Patients who have venous stasis ulcers are often treated by a home health nurse. With early discharge after surgery, many patients receive postoperative care in the home. Patients with arterial bypass may be referred for rehabilitation exercise programs at a rehabilitation center. Your role in these settings is focused on ongoing assessment, coordination of care with other members of the health care team, monitoring progress and compliance with treatment, and patient education.

Include careful monitoring of the blood pressure for the presence of hypertension. Patients should be aware of expected blood pressure levels and critical levels to report to the health care provider. Evaluate the home care patient's understanding of medication, diet, and exercise to accomplish optimal management of hypertension.

Some patients may have the capability of monitoring their coagulation status through home monitoring devices. This is especially important for patients who are taking drugs such as warfarin. There are multiple devices on the market for home testing of international normalized ratio (INR). The patient then has more information to manage their coagulation status, and missed laboratory appointments are prevented. Be aware of patient use of these devices and ensure that the patient is using them correctly.

Get Ready for the NCLEX® Examination!

Key Points

- Hypertension is more prevalent and more severe in African Americans than in other minority groups and whites.
- Treatment of hypertension involves measures to assist the patient to maintain blood pressure at or below 120/80 mm Hg.
- Antihypertensive drugs work by decreasing blood volume, cardiac output, or peripheral resistance.
- Nursing care of patients with hypertension includes counseling and education about lifestyle changes, diet, weight control, stress relief, and exercise.
- Noncompliance with the medical regimen for hypertension can result in heart problems, dementia, blindness, stroke, and kidney failure.
- Obesity, stress, and sedentary lifestyle contribute to the incidence of atherosclerosis and hypertension.
- Atherosclerosis is the most common cause of PVD.
- Arterial wall injury may be caused by hypertension, deposit of fatty plaque, chemical toxins, or diabetes mellitus.
- Disorders of peripheral arteries lead to ischemia.
- Quitting smoking, maintaining a low-fat diet, controlling diabetes mellitus, and following an exercise program decrease the incidence of PAD.
- Signs and symptoms of PAD include intermittent claudication, pain at rest, and ischemic changes. The five *P*s are pain, pulselessness, pallor, paresthesias, and paralysis.
- The best treatment for arterial insufficiency is exercise—specifically, walking.
- Long-term hypertension and atherosclerosis are factors in the development of aneurysms.
- Aneurysms in the aorta may be repaired by surgical resection and graft or stent insertion.
- An aortic aneurysm rupture often causes death.
- The etiology of Raynaud disease is an exaggerated response to cold environment and stress.
- Carotid occlusion is signified by a carotid bruit, confusion, blackouts, extremity weakness or paralysis, temporary loss of vision, or other neurologic strokelike symptoms.
- Treatment for carotid stenosis includes carotid endarterectomy or stenting.
- Thrombophlebitis is the development of a clot and inflammation of a vein.
- DVT is a clot in a deep vein occluding blood flow.
- The effects of a thrombus depend on the location and size of the clot and the degree of obstruction to blood flow.
- The etiology of DVT includes immobility, trauma, surgery, cancer, dehydration, and abnormal clotting.
- Treatment of DVT may include IV heparin, subcutaneous agents, oral anticoagulants, and hydration.

- Medical management of DVT includes elevation of the extremity when seated, compression stockings, ambulation, warm moist packs, NSAIDs, and sometimes antibiotics.
- Varicose veins are enlarged, tortuous veins engorged with pooled blood.
- The symptoms of varicose veins include fatigue, a feeling of heaviness in the legs after prolonged standing or sitting, pain, and itching along the course of the blood vessel.
- Medical management of varicose veins involves compression stockings, treatment of obesity, and exercise.
- Surgical treatment of varicose veins may include scleropathy, vein stripping or PIN stripping, ligation, or endovenous laser treatment.
- Venous insufficiency occurs from damaged valves in veins and pooling of blood.
- Venous stasis ulcers are skin lesions, usually on the lower leg, from venous insufficiency.
- Treatment for venous stasis ulcers includes acute debridement, dressings, compression, and prevention of infection.

Additional Learning Resources

SG Go to your Study Guide for additional learning activities to help you master this chapter content.

Go to your Evolve website (http://evolve.elsevier.com/deWit/medsurg) for the following FREE learning resources:

- Animations, audio, and video
- Answers and rationales for questions and activities
- Glossary with pronunciations in English and Spanish
- Interactive Review Questions and more!

Review Questions for the NCLEX® Examination

1. A 40-year-old woman complains of leg swelling and a feeling of heaviness and fullness during walking. She describes itching on the lower leg and on inspection has a twisted-appearing swelling in her legs. The patient most likely will be treated for:
   1. venous stasis ulcers.
   2. deep vein thrombosis.
   3. arterial insufficiency.
   4. varicose veins.

   NCLEX Client Need: Physiological Integrity: Physiological Adaptation
2. A nurse reinforces discharge instructions to a patient who is diagnosed with chronic venous insufficiency. Which instruction(s) should be included? *(Select all that apply.)*
   1. "Take a low-dose aspirin every day."
   2. "Consider swimming for exercise."
   3. "Avoid wearing tight clothing."
   4. "Use elastic wraps at night."
   5. "Decrease fluid intake to help prevent edema."
   6. "Elevate the legs above the level of the heart as much as possible."

   NCLEX Client Need: Health Promotion and Maintenance
3. If a patient complains of intermittent claudication, you would expect which clinical finding?
   1. Strong, symmetric peripheral pulses
   2. Skin mottling
   3. Rubor when legs are dependent
   4. Continual pain

   NCLEX Client Need: Reduction of Risk Potential
4. A patient diagnosed with peripheral arterial disease complains of a sudden onset of pain in the right foot. Identify the nursing actions in priority order.
   1. Notify the health care provider.
   2. Note the color, temperature, and capillary refill of the foot.
   3. Check for pedal and posterior tibial pulses.
   4. Check vital signs.

   NCLEX Client Need: Physiological Integrity: Physiological Adaptation
5. A patient is started on antihypertensive medications. Which patient statement indicates effectiveness of teaching?
   1. "I will be able to perform sit-ups in the morning."
   2. "I need to take the medication when I feel dizzy."
   3. "The medication helps reduce the incidence of a blood clot."
   4. "Sudden changes in position may cause dizziness."

   NCLEX Client Need: Physiological Integrity: Pharmacological Therapies
6. You are receiving a patient who had angioplasty and stenting of the right femoral artery. Which nursing intervention would take priority in the immediate postoperative period?
   1. Assessing the right femoral artery pulse
   2. Monitoring for signs of fluid overload
   3. Determining range of motion
   4. Checking right pedal pulses

   NCLEX Client Need: Physiological Integrity: Reduction of Risk Potential
7. You are reinforcing the health care provider's instructions to an older adult woman who is newly diagnosed with hypertension. The patient does not speak the same language as you and is legally blind. What is the best nursing action?
   1. Use a certified translator to provide instructions.
   2. Speak slowly and use hand motions to describe information.
   3. Use a loud voice and speak directly into the patient's ear.
   4. Provide written instructions for the family.

   NCLEX Client Need: Health Promotion and Maintenance
8. A 54-year-old man complains of pain when walking and numbness of the lower extremities. On examination, you note that both extremities are pale and cool to touch. The highest priority nursing diagnosis would be:
   1. *Altered peripheral tissue perfusion.*
   2. *Altered activity tolerance.*
   3. *Altered fluid volume.*
   4. *Potential for injury.*

   NCLEX Client Need: Physiological Integrity: Reduction of Risk Potential

9. A patient with PAD is prescribed a daily dose of aspirin. You accurately explain the prescription by stating:
   1. "Aspirin controls the body temperature to reduce vasoconstriction."
   2. "Aspirin helps prevent formation of clots."
   3. "Aspirin protects the blood vessels from injury."
   4. "Aspirin reduces pain associated with inadequate tissue perfusion."

   NCLEX Client Need: Physiological Integrity: Pharmacological Therapies

10. You promote lifestyle modifications to a 39-year-old man who is diagnosed with prehypertension. Which lifestyle modification(s) should be recommended? *(Select all that apply.)*
    1. Smoking cessation
    2. Restrict sodium intake to 4000 mg/day
    3. Exercise 30 minutes per day on most days of the week
    4. Limit alcohol intake to two drinks per day
    5. Low-fat diet
    6. Stress reduction measures

    NCLEX Client Need: Physiological Integrity: Reduction of Risk Potential

Critical Thinking Questions

Scenario A

Mrs. Dunn is being discharged from the hospital after being treated for arterial insufficiency in both lower extremities. The health care provider requests that Mrs. Dunn receive instruction in the care of her feet and legs before discharge.

1. What findings do you expect on physical examination of Mrs. Dunn's legs?
2. What medication and treatment do you expect the provider to prescribe? Why are these prescribed?
3. List five priority teaching points for Mrs. Dunn.

Scenario B

Ms. Yao, age 27, developed a DVT in her left thigh after surgery to repair a fractured right femur. She is receiving IV heparin and will transition to warfarin starting tomorrow.

1. Describe the pathophysiology of DVT. How does Ms. Yao's diagnosis relate to development of DVT?
2. Identify essential information you need to safely administer the medications prescribed.
3. Develop a teaching plan for Ms. Yao.

Scenario C

Mr. Tompkins, age 66, who is hypertensive and only recently quit smoking, has been diagnosed with a 3-cm AAA.

1. What treatment would you expect for him?
2. What signs and symptoms of complications would you teach him?
3. What measures could he take to help prevent the aneurysm from growing and rupturing?

19 Care of Patients With Cardiac Disorders

http://evolve.elsevier.com/deWit/medsurg

Objectives

Theory

1. Contrast left-sided and right-sided heart failure.
2. Discuss treatment of systolic and diastolic heart failure.
3. Apply the nursing assessment specific to a patient who is admitted with heart failure.
4. Identify life-threatening heart rhythms from a selection of cardiac rhythm strips.
5. Examine usual treatment for atrial fibrillation, third-degree heart block, and ventricular tachycardia.
6. Explain nursing responsibilities in the administration of cardiac drugs.
7. Determine under what circumstances cardiac surgery is appropriate treatment.
8. Analyze the nurse's role in caring for patients with heart disorders in a long-term care facility or in their home.
9. Develop a teaching plan with dietary recommendations for heart disease.

Clinical Practice

10. Develop a plan of care for a patient who has heart failure.
11. Perform a basic physical assessment on a patient who has a mitral valve stenosis and dysrhythmia.
12. Use the nursing process to care for assigned patients who have cardiovascular disorders.
13. Safely administer medications for patients with cardiac disorders.
14. Provide support to patients undergoing diagnostic testing and treatment for cardiac disorders.
15. Develop a teaching plan for patients with a newly implanted pacemaker or implantable cardioverter-defibrillator (ICD).

Key Terms

ablation (ăb-LĀ-shŭn, p. 454)
arrhythmias (ă-RĬTH-mē-ăz, p. 445)
atrial fibrillation (Ā-trē-ăl fĭ-brĭ-LĀ-shŭn, p. 449)
cardiac tamponade (KĂR-dē-ăk tăm-pŏn-ĂD, p. 455)
cardiomyopathy (kăr-dē-ō-mī-ŎP-ă-thē, p. 456)
cardioversion (kăr-dē-ō-VĔR-zhŭn, p. 448)
dysrhythmias (dĭs-RĬTH-mē-ăz, p. 445)
effusion (ĕ-FŪ-zhŭn, p. 455)
ejection fraction (ē-JĔK-shŭn FRĂK-shŭn, p. 439)
endocarditis (ĔN-dō-kăhr-DĪ-tĭs, p. 454)
friction rub (FRĬK-shŭn, p. 455)
infarct (ĭn-făhrkt, p. 445)
palpitations (păl-pĭ-TĀ-shŭnz, p. 446)
pericardiocentesis (pĕr-ĭ-KĂR-dē-ō-sĕn-TĒ-sĭs, p. 455)
pericardiotomy (pĕr-ĭ-KĂR-dē-ŏt-ō-mē, p. 455)
pulsus paradoxus (PŬL-sŭs păr-ă-DŎK-sŭs, p. 455)

Concepts Covered in This Chapter

- Functional Ability
- Self-Management
- Fluid and Electrolytes
- Nutrition
- Perfusion
- Clotting
- Inflammation
- Infection

DISORDERS OF THE HEART

HEART FAILURE

More than 5 million Americans have heart failure (HF), and approximately 550,000 are newly diagnosed each year. The prevalence of HF is increasing, and it is a major chronic condition. Half of patients diagnosed with HF will die within 5 years. African Americans have a higher incidence of HF and have higher mortality rates than other populations. HF can occur at any time the heart muscle is prevented from fulfilling its function as a pump and circulator of blood. HF may be acute or chronic, mild or severe. The New York Heart Association scale identifies four stages of HF, classed according to exercise tolerance. The American Heart Association (AHA) has identified stages of HF from A to D. The "A" stage includes individuals who have no structural heart problems but are at high risk for HF (Table 19.1). Early recognition of risk factors and prevention of HF is being promoted (Yancy et al., 2017).

Etiology

The most common causes of HF are coronary artery disease and uncontrolled hypertension. Other factors that contribute to weakness of the heart muscle are toxins, infection, anemia, myocarditis, dilation from

Table 19.1 Classification and Staging of Heart Failure

New York Heart Association Function Classification	
CLASS	**ACTIVITY TOLERANCE**
I	Ordinary physical activity with no symptoms
II	Dyspnea with long-distance walking, climbing two flights of stairs, or strenuous activity
III	Dyspnea and fatigue with short-distance walking or climbing one flight of stairs
IV	Dyspnea at rest or with very little activity
Adapted from the New York Heart Association Heart Failure Symptom Classification System. Retrieved from https://www.chf-solutions.com/heart-failure-classifications/	
American Heart Association/American College of Cardiology Staging of Heart Failure	
STAGE	**DEFINITION**
A	At risk for heart failure but no heart damage
B	Structural heart disease present, no heart failure symptoms
C	Past or present heart failure symptoms
D	Advanced disease needing ongoing treatment

blood backup behind diseased valves, and damage from myocardial infarction (MI) (Concept Map 19.1). Toxins include cocaine, excessive alcohol, certain chemotherapy drugs, nonsteroidal antiinflammatory drugs (NSAIDs), and thiazolidinediones used for diabetes. Cardiac dysrhythmias also can contribute to HF. (Coronary artery disease [CAD] and MI are discussed in Chapter 20, with cardiac surgery.)

Older Adult Care Points

Heart failure is the most common reason for hospitalization among adults age 65 years or older. As life spans continue to extend, more and more older adults will develop HF related to hypertension and CAD.

Pathophysiology

The key words to understanding HF are *congestion* and *increased pressure*. Congestion develops because the heart is unable to move the amount of blood it receives efficiently through the system. This may occur because the heart muscle is too weak or because the blood vessels throughout the body are narrowed and constricted (because of atherosclerosis or arteriosclerosis). Therefore the vessels cannot accommodate a normal supply of blood, causing the heart muscle to become exhausted trying to overcome the resistance (pressure) in the vessels. Poorly functioning valves may cause the chambers to dilate from blood backup, further decreasing pumping ability. A myocardium damaged by infarct, infection, ischemia, or other factors is not an efficient pump and cannot manage the volume of blood in the circulation. Box 19.1 lists factors that precipitate HF.

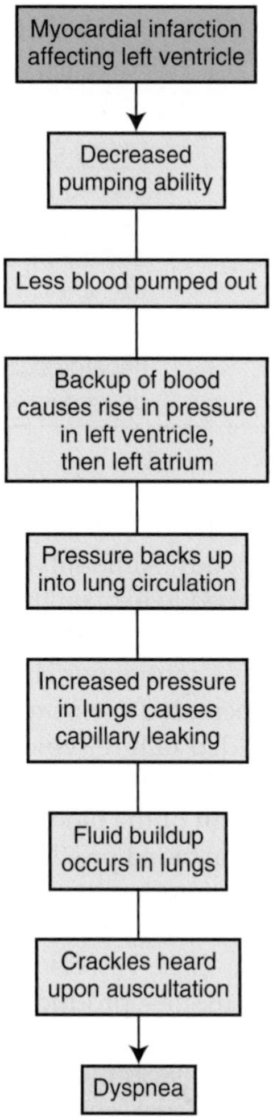

Concept Map 19.1 Pathophysiology of heart failure after a myocardial infarction.

Box 19.1 Factors That Can Precipitate Heart Failure

- Anemia
- Systemic infection (sepsis)
- Myocardial infarction or ischemia
- Pulmonary embolism
- Uncontrolled hypertension
- Thyroid disorders
- Dysrhythmias
- Pericarditis, myocarditis, or endocarditis
- Chronic pulmonary disease
- Physical, emotional, or environmental stress

Older Adult Care Points

Aging processes also contribute to arteriosclerosis and stiffening of the heart muscle. The combination of high blood pressure, diabetes, and age greatly contributes to the number of older patients who develop HF.

HF may be classified as right-sided HF or left-sided HF. The heart has two pumps: a right-sided and a left-sided pump. The right-sided pump receives blood from the body and pumps it to the lungs for oxygenation. The left-sided pump receives blood from the lungs and

Table 19.2 **Comparison of Left-Sided and Right-Sided Heart Failure**

	RIGHT-SIDED HEART FAILURE	LEFT-SIDED HEART FAILURE
Selected etiology	Pulmonary stenosis, pulmonary hypertension, severe emphysema, right ventricular MI	Hypertension, coronary artery disease, MI, mitral or aortic valvular disease
Pathophysiology	Increased pump pressure is needed to eject blood into pulmonary arteries. The myocardium of the right atrium and ventricle becomes thickened, and contraction strength weakens.	Weakness of the left ventricle results in reduced cardiac output with backup of blood into the atrium and the pulmonary system.
Signs and symptoms	Fatigue; edema in sacrum, legs, feet, ankles; hepatomegaly; abdominal distention as a result of ascites; weight gain; dyspnea	Fatigue; dyspnea; wheezing; orthopnea; sleep apnea; pulmonary edema (pink, frothy sputum); pallor; clammy skin

MI, Myocardial infarction.

pumps it out to the body. Although the terms *right-* and *left-sided failure* are used to explain the physiology, clinically it is rare to see pure right- or left-sided failure. The circulatory system is a continuous circle, and eventually all congestion or increased pressure affects both sides of the heart. Left-sided failure typically occurs first. If the muscle wall of the left ventricle cannot contract effectively, not enough of the blood is ejected from the ventricle; this residual blood prevents part of the blood from the lungs from entering the left side of the heart. This causes fluid to back up into the pulmonary vessels. The pressure within those vessels increases, and fluid leaks into the lung tissue—producing congestion and eventually pulmonary edema. If not corrected, left-sided failure, because of the backup of blood and increased pulmonary artery pressure, will soon lead to failure of the right side of the heart. Table 19.2 compares the signs and symptoms of left-sided and right-sided HF.

Primary right-sided HF is commonly caused by chronic pulmonary disease. The right ventricle does not usually have to generate a lot of pressure to pump blood to the lungs. Normal systolic pressure in the right ventricle is about 25 mm Hg. Chronic lung disease causes scarring, which makes it harder for the ventricle to eject blood into the pulmonary circulation. This increased resistance requires the right ventricle to squeeze harder, generating more pressure and causing inadequate ejection. This makes it difficult for entry of the venous blood returning to the heart. As pressure in the peripheral vessels increases, the fluid from the intravascular fluid compartment begins to leak into the interstitial compartment. This produces edema. When the right side of the heart fails, the edema is first evident in the lower extremities *(dependent edema)* (Fig. 19.1). Also, fluid accumulates in the liver and abdominal organs as the portal circulation becomes involved. Alteration of blood flow to the kidneys may lead to impaired renal function, preventing normal excretion of urine and causing more accumulation of body fluids. Inadequate circulation to and from the brain may cause mental confusion and irritability.

The systemic backup of blood that occurs in right-sided HF will eventually lead to left-sided HF because the heart will have to pump against increasing pressure in the aorta and systemic circulation. The circulatory system is exactly that: a system. Failure of one component affects the entire system.

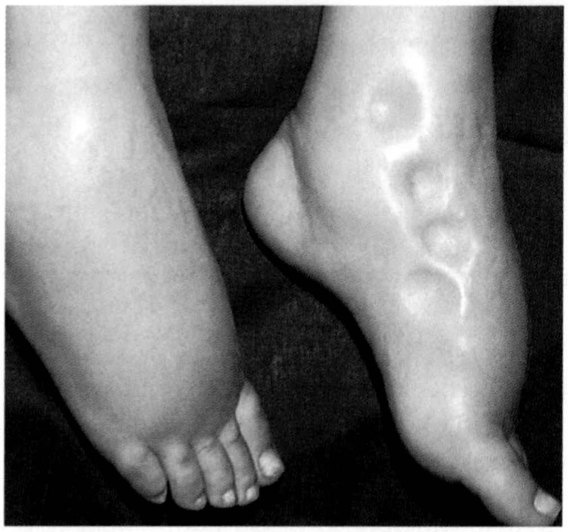

Fig. 19.1 Dependent, pitting edema. (From Bloom A, Watkins PH, Ireland J: *Color atlas of diabetes*, ed 2, St. Louis, 1992, Mosby.)

Think Critically

Describe the changes that occur with chronic hypertension that may cause HF.

Left-sided HF is subdivided into systolic and diastolic HF. In the cardiac cycle, diastole is the part of the cycle in which the heart is resting and filling with blood. During this time the valves between the atria and ventricles (tricuspid and mitral) are open. Most of the blood entering the ventricles does so passively by the pressure in the system during diastole. Right before the ventricles are ready to contract (systole), the atria contract and "top off the tank," contributing about 20% of the volume. Systole occurs, and the exit valves open in the ventricles (pulmonic and aortic), allowing ejection of blood into the circulation. Disorders leading to HF that cause problems with filling are called *diastolic failure*, and those that affect ejection of blood are called *systolic failure*.

Systolic failure. Systolic failure is caused by anything that interferes with ejection of blood from the ventricles. Muscle dysfunction, problems from MI, dilated cardiomyopathy, and aortic or pulmonic stenosis may lead to systolic failure. Inability of the heart to pump an adequate amount of blood to meet the needs of the body can lead to problems in other organs. **Ejection fraction** is the percentage of the filling volume pumped out with each ventricular contraction. In a normal heart, ejection fraction is 55% to 70%. This means that 30% to 45% of the blood is left in the ventricle, which allows the body to increase cardiac output when needed by increasing the force of contraction (through release of epinephrine, responsible for the fight-or-flight response) and ejecting more blood. An ejection fraction of 40% or less is a marker of systolic HF.

Diastolic failure. Diastolic failure occurs when conditions prevent the filling of the heart with blood. Tricuspid and mitral stenosis, cardiac tamponade, or constrictive cardiomyopathy can cause diastolic failure. Decreased filling results in decreased stroke volume and cardiac output. Ejection fraction is normal in primary diastolic failure. Medical literature refers to *diastolic failure* as HF with preserved ejection fraction (HF*p*EF). A hallmark of diastolic failure is neck vein (jugular) distention.

Evidence is emerging that HF with a reduced ejection fraction (HF*r*EF) and HF*p*EF are separate clinical conditions that require very different treatments. Ejection fraction can be determined with echocardiography or left heart catheterization and is a key feature in determining the correct treatment.

? Think Critically

Can you explain to a patient in simple terms what happens in the body when systolic HF occurs?

Signs, Symptoms, and Diagnosis

Initially, compensatory mechanisms prevent symptoms of HF. Heart rate rises to increase output, and the ventricles hypertrophy to pump out more blood with each contraction. In left-sided failure compensatory mechanisms eventually weaken the heart, and the blood backs up into the pulmonary vessels, pressure within those vessels increases, and fluid leaks into the lung tissue, producing congestion. Fatigue and shortness of breath (SOB) are first noticed with activity and when lying down. If failure progresses, pulmonary edema occurs. There is no single diagnostic test for HF, and diagnosis is made primarily on clinical signs and symptoms and careful history. Helpful diagnostic tests include chest x-ray, echocardiogram, electrocardiogram (ECG), magnetic resonance imaging (MRI), electrolytes, complete blood cell count (CBC), and brain natriuretic peptide (BNP). BNP measures the level of a protein released when myocardial cells are stretched. A level greater than 500 pg/mL is consistent with HF when other symptoms are present (see Table 19.2).

Advanced systolic HF signs are S_3 and S_4 heart sounds. Weight gain of 2 to 3 lb in 24 hours or 5 lb in 1 week occurs as fluid is retained. Dyspnea is present, and crackles or wheezes are heard in the lungs.

? Think Critically

You auscultate the lung sounds of a patient with HF. You hear crackles in the bases and up to mid-chest. What is the significance of this finding?

Treatment

There are multiple causes of HF, but the clinical signs and symptoms are the same. Identification and treatment of the underlying cause of HF should be initiated. Dysrhythmias are controlled. Surgical correction of valve or septal abnormalities may reverse HF. Medical treatment is largely symptomatic and depends on the type and degree of HF present. Drugs and other therapies are used to reduce or eliminate the symptoms and complications of HF, but they only control the condition; they do not cure it. AHA 2017 Heart Failure Guidelines outline strategies for early identification of patients at risk for HF and implementation of interventions to prevent the disease or decrease its effects. For patients experiencing HF, efforts are made to (1) reduce the demand for oxygen and the workload of the heart, (2) strengthen the heart's pumping action, (3) relieve venous congestion in the lungs, and (4) minimize sodium and water retention in the tissues. Some clinical trials have shown that early intervention with appropriate drug therapies can reverse some of the ventricular dysfunction found in HF (Borlaug & Colucci, 2018).

To accomplish the goals of medical intervention, the following may be prescribed:

- Angiotensin-converting enzyme (ACE) inhibitors and angiotensin-receptor blockers (ARBs) decrease the workload of the heart by causing vasodilation; as a result, blood pressure is reduced (Table 19.3). ACE inhibitors and ARBs also play a role in reducing fluid retention.
- Beta-adrenergic blockers (e.g., metoprolol [Toprol XL]) are used to slow the rate if tachycardia is causing the HF, thereby decreasing oxygen demand. Beta blockers are used cautiously, as they can also cause HF and are not recommended in HF*p*EF.
- Diuretics, especially loop diuretics, are prescribed to reduce fluid retention in the lungs and lower extremities. Watch for ototoxicity with these drugs. Thiazide diuretics such as hydrochlorothiazide (Hydrodiuril) may also be prescribed. Measures are taken to prevent electrolyte imbalances from the use of these drugs.
- Digitalis is occasionally used to increase the force of heart contraction (i.e., an inotropic agent) and slow the rate, thereby increasing cardiac output. The most commonly used drug in this category is digoxin

Table 19.3 **Drugs Used to Treat Heart Failure**[a]

CLASSIFICATION	EXAMPLES	USE
Diuretics		
Loop	Furosemide (Lasix), bumetanide (Bumex)	Remove excess fluid, waste potassium
Potassium sparing	Triamterene (Dyrenium), amiloride (Midamor)	Remove fluid but not potassium
Thiazide	Hydrochlorothiazide Metolazone (Zaroxolyn)	Remove fluid but waste potassium
Angiotensin-converting enzyme inhibitors	Enalapril (Vasotec), captopril (Capoten), lisinopril (Zestril)	Prevent vasoconstriction
Angiotensin-receptor blockers	Losartan (Cozaar), valsartan (Diovan), irbesartan (Avapro)	Produce vasodilation and salt and water excretion
Beta-adrenergic blockers	Atenolol (Tenormin), metoprolol (Lopressor), nadolol (Corgard)	Reduce blood pressure, slow heart rate
Calcium channel blockers	Amlodipine (Norvasc), diltiazem (Cardizem), nifedipine (Procardia), verapamil (Calan), nicardipine (Cardene)	Produce vasodilation and reduced heart rate
Vasodilators (nitrates)	Nitroglycerin (Nitrostat, Nitro-Bid), isosorbide (Isordil)	Dilate blood vessels; decrease preload and relieve shortness of breath; relieve myocardial ischemia
BNP analog	Nesiritide (Natrecor)	Alleviates dyspnea
Inotropics		
Beta-adrenergic agonists	Dobutamine (Dobutrex), dopamine (Intropin)	Increase cardiac contractility and cardiac output
Phosphodiesterase inhibitors	Milrinone (Primacor)	Reduces preload and afterload; causes vasodilation; increases cardiac contractility
Digitalis	Digoxin	Increases cardiac contractility
Hyperpolarization-activated cyclic nucleotide-gated (HCN) channel blocker	Ivabradine (Corlanor) (approved for use in the United States on April 15, 2015, in a very select group of patients)	Directly acts on the sinoatrial (SA) node to reduce heart rate, reduce myocardial workload, and prevent angina

See Chapter 18, Table 18.3 and Box 18.1, and Table 19.4 for further information and nursing implications for these drugs.
[a]The choice of drugs depends on the type of heart failure and whether the left ventricle function is normal.
BNP, Brain natriuretic peptide.

(Lanoxin). Several large doses of the drug are given initially, followed by a lower, regular-maintenance dosage. This drug is not recommended for older adult white women because it increases mortality rates in this group.

- Venous vasodilators such as isosorbide dinitrate (Isordil) and nitroglycerin (NTG), which relax and dilate blood vessels, allow the vessels to accommodate larger percentages of the total blood volume.
- Morphine is prescribed if pulmonary edema is present to relieve anxiety and make breathing easier.
- Benzodiazepines may be used for anxiety and reduction of emotional stress.
- Limited physical activity or bed rest in semi-Fowler or high Fowler position will decrease the workload of the heart and help breathing.
- Oxygen therapy will optimize the amount of oxygen available to be delivered to the tissues.
- Intravenous inotropes (dobutamine, norepinephrine, milrinone) may be used for acute systolic HF to improve cardiac contractility.

Other treatments may include:

- The pumping action of the atria and ventricles may be synchronized for more efficient pumping by use of a biventricular pacemaker. This procedure is called *cardiac resynchronization therapy (CRT);* pacing wires attached to a pulse generator are placed in the heart to send electrical impulses to the right and left ventricles so they contract at the same time. In a standard pacemaker, only the right ventricle is stimulated to cause ventricular contraction. CRT is the treatment of choice when drug therapy does not control HF.
- A left ventricular assist device (LVAD) may be used to help with the heart's pumping action. This device is implanted in the patient's abdomen or chest and attached to the heart. These devices have proven to be beneficial to adults diagnosed with severe HF. The device may be used while the patient is awaiting transplantation and, with continued research, may potentially eliminate the need for transplantation in some patients (Fig. 19.2).

Nutrition Considerations

Guidelines for a Heart-Healthy Diet

- Limit foods high in saturated fat, trans fat, and cholesterol. Limit meat intake to no more than 6 oz of cooked *lean* meat and skinless poultry (singly or in combination) per day. Fix main dishes with pasta, rice, beans, or vegetables mixed with small amounts of lean meat, poultry, or fish to create "low-meat" dishes. Restrict intake of organ meats, such as liver, brains, chitterlings, kidney, gizzards, and sweetbreads, because they are very high in cholesterol.
- Avoid trans fat as much as possible. Read product labels. Limit food high in saturated fat, including tropical oils and partially hydrogenated vegetable oils.
- Cook using little or no fat; broil, bake, roast, poach, stir-fry, microwave, or steam foods rather than frying them.
- Eliminate as much fat as possible by trimming meat and skinning poultry before cooking. After browning meats, drain off all fat. Chill soups, stews, and so on, and then skim off fat before reheating to serve.
- Use fats with no more than 2 g of saturated fat per tablespoon. Olive, canola, corn, or safflower oil and liquid and tub margarines are good choices.
- Eat fish at least twice a week. Fatty fish such as salmon, mackerel, and tuna are best.
- Eat five to seven servings of fruit and vegetables per day. Use fresh or frozen vegetables and fresh fruit or fruit canned in juice rather than high-fructose corn syrup.
- Increase intake of fiber and carbohydrates by eating six or more servings of whole-grain products, such as cereals and breads, per day. Check labels to see that the product really contains *whole* grains.
- Use skim or 1% fat milk and nonfat or low-fat yogurt, cheeses, and ice creams.
- Limit consumption of egg yolks to three or four per week, including those in baked or cooked items. Check store packages for listing of eggs or egg yolk as an ingredient.
- Eat less than 1500 mg of salt (sodium chloride) per day.
- Have no more than one alcoholic drink per day if you are a woman and no more than two per day if you are a man. Examples of one drink are 12 oz of beer, 4 oz of wine, or 1½ oz of 80-proof spirits.

Note: The heart-healthy diet is promoted by the American Heart Association.

- Temporary placement of a small catheter-based pump may help improve left ventricular function. The catheter is placed via standard femoral artery approach and is passed through the aortic valve into the left ventricle, where it remains. The catheter pulls blood from the ventricle and expels it in the aorta, offloading some of the work of the ventricle.
- Surgery to reduce the size of an enlarged heart (ventricular restoration surgery) may be effective for some patients. The less effective portions of the left ventricle are removed, and the remaining muscle is reattached and shaped to form a more efficient pump. Sometimes the heart enlarges again.
- Heart transplantation may be the only alternative for patients with advanced HF who do not respond to other medical or drug treatment. Heart transplantation is discussed in Chapter 20.

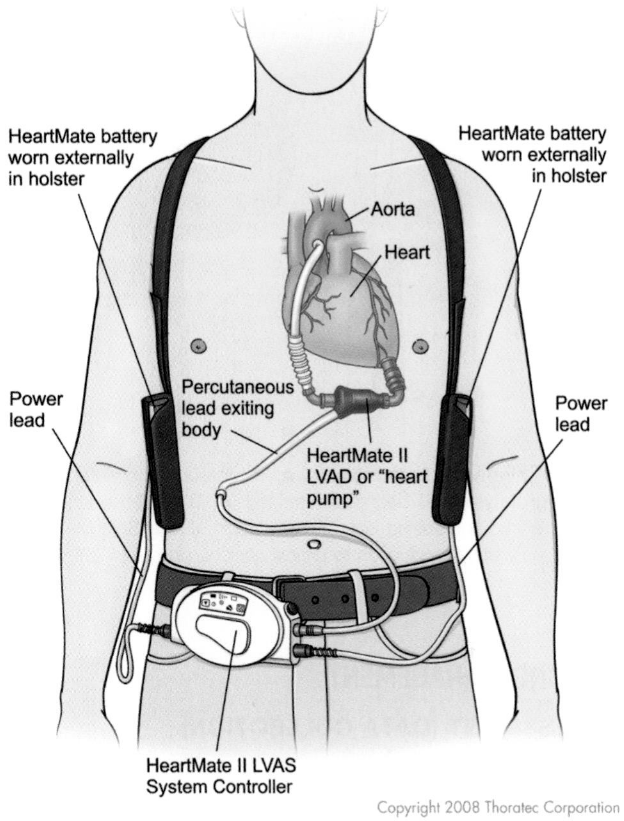

Fig. 19.2 HeartMate II left ventricular assist device (LVAD). (Reproduced with permission of Abbott, © 2019. All rights reserved. HeartMate and HeartMate II are trademarks of Abbott or its related companies.)

Short-term treatment for severe HF can be accomplished with an intra-aortic balloon pump (IABP). The IABP is positioned in the descending aorta and is designed to increase blood supply to the myocardium and decrease the workload. The balloon inflates during diastole, thus increasing perfusion to the coronary arteries. The balloon deflates during systole, making it easier for the left ventricle to eject blood (Fig. 19.3).

Acute pulmonary edema. Acute pulmonary edema (acute left ventricular failure) is a medical emergency that must be treated promptly. A patient with this condition has severe dyspnea; a cough productive of frothy, pink-tinged sputum; tachycardia; and moist, bubbling respirations with cyanosis. Nursing interventions for acute pulmonary edema include placing the patient in high Fowler position to relieve the dyspnea; administering oxygen, diuretics, morphine, and other prescribed drugs; limiting and monitoring activity; and assessing cardiopulmonary status.

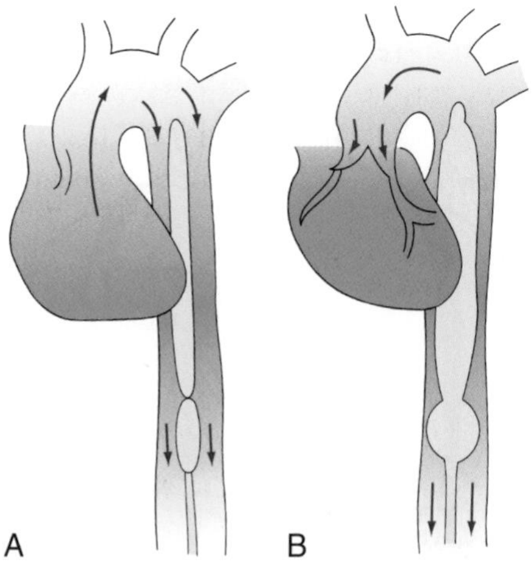

Fig. 19.3 Intra-aortic balloon pump. **A,** The balloon is deflated at the beginning of systole to decrease afterload. **B,** The balloon is inflated during diastole, increasing coronary perfusion. (From Sole ML, Klein DG, Moseley MJ: *Introduction to critical care nursing*, ed 7, St. Louis, 2017, Elsevier.)

NURSING MANAGEMENT

ASSESSMENT (DATA COLLECTION)

The effects of HF can range from very mild to extremely serious. A thorough nursing assessment can help identify specific patient care problems. Data guide the health care provider in the evaluation of the patient's response to medical treatment and the decision to continue or change prescribed drugs and other therapies. It is important to ask the patient if clothes, rings, or shoes fit tighter than previously, indicating edema. Is pedal edema worsening or improving? Obtain an accurate weight. What has the trend of weight been? Feelings of breathlessness or having to catch the breath in midsentence may indicate fluid in the lungs and left-sided HF. Are crackles present in the lungs? Inquire how much activity causes SOB. Does the patient have paroxysmal nocturnal dyspnea (PND) (wakes up at night with SOB) or onset of nocturia (being awakened by the need to urinate)? Ask about medication compliance and any problems or side effects noted. Assess the diet to determine usual sodium, fat, and calorie intake, and obtain a smoking history.

> **Clinical Cues**
>
> It is important for patients who have been diagnosed with HF that is well controlled *(compensated)* to weigh themselves daily at home and to record the weight. If the patient can see that fluid weight gain is occurring, they may be able to avert a trend back into *decompensated* HF by adjusting diuretic medication, decreasing sodium intake, treating infection, and decreasing activity and resting more.

Significant Findings Indicating That Heart Failure Is Occurring

Left-sided failure:

- Increasing fatigue.
- Dyspnea and a dry, hacking cough.
- Crackles heard on auscultation of the lungs.
- Pale, cool, and clammy skin, which are signs of poor peripheral circulation.
- Diminished peripheral pulses.
- Dizziness, confusion, restlessness, and difficulty concentrating and remembering because of diminished blood flow to the brain.
- Gradually increasing heart rate, even when the patient is at rest; increased heart rate occurs when the heart attempts to increase cardiac output.
- Extra heart sound (S_3, S_4).
- Decreased blood pressure as the ventricles fail.

Right-sided failure:

- Weight gain without a change in caloric intake.
- Dependent, pitting edema (assess feet and ankles in an ambulatory patient or one sitting up most of the time). Assess thighs and sacral region in a patient confined to bed. Patient may feel "bloated" and experience a loss of appetite and nausea because of diminished venous return from abdominal organs, liver enlargement resulting from increased pressure in the portal veins, edema in the intestine, and accumulations of fluid in the abdominal cavity.
- Jugular venous distention; visible jugular vein pulsation more than 4.5 cm above the clavicle when the patient is in a semi-Fowler position.
- Reduced urinary output, which reflects the kidney's response to poor perfusion by retaining sodium and water; need to urinate at night (nocturia).
- Blood pressure increased from fluid overload.
- Waking up at night after a few hours of sleep because of PND.

> **Clinical Cues**
>
> Nocturia and PND occur after a few hours of lying down because fluid that has been sequestered in the extremities has had a chance to return to the circulation. The increase in fluid volume overloads the heart, leading to the HF symptom of PND. The kidneys receive more blood flow and eliminate more fluid.

NURSING DIAGNOSIS AND PLANNING

The main problem statements or nursing diagnoses for patients with HF are listed in Nursing Care Plan 19.1 (see also Chapter 17, Table 17.4). Plan extra time when caring for patients with HF because fatigue, possible lack of mobility, and oxygen deficit cause these patients to move slowly and need more time to accomplish the activities of daily living

IMPLEMENTATION

HF is a chronic disease. Patients with mild HF may be cared for at home with intermittent hospitalization as needed. They require instruction in self-care. Instruction includes balancing rest with physical activity, limiting sodium intake, and following other dietary restrictions.

The entire family should be included in dietary teaching. Teach self-administration of medications and awareness of adverse side effects that must be reported. Review the dangers of drug-drug interaction when taking nonprescription drugs, particularly NSAIDs. Reconcile medications. Immunize the patient against seasonal flu and pneumonia. Modify lifestyle according to patient needs (diet, smoking, physical activity). Teach symptoms that should be reported to the health care provider if they become worse or appear for the first time. An objective of *Healthy People 2030* is to reduce hospitalizations of adults with HF as the principal diagnosis. Thorough patient teaching and nursing follow-up helps achieve this objective.

Nursing Care Plan 19.1 Care of a Patient With Heart Failure

SCENARIO

Miguel Garcia, age 60 years, is admitted to the nursing unit with exacerbation of left- and right-sided heart failure. Physical examination reveals 3+ pitting edema of the right lower extremity and 4+ pitting edema of the left lower extremity. He is in acute respiratory distress and is positioned in high Fowler position to facilitate breathing. He is receiving oxygen with a simple mask at 8 L/min. T 98° F (36.6° C), P 96, R 28, BP 160/90, Spo_2 90%, Wt. 255 (20-lb increase).

PROBLEM STATEMENT/NURSING DIAGNOSIS

Altered gas exchange due to fluid in lung tissue.

SUPPORTING ASSESSMENT DATA

Subjective: States has difficulty breathing while lying down.

Objective: Spo_2 90% on 8 L oxygen, elevated respiratory rate, sitting up to facilitate breathing.

Goals/Expected Outcomes	Nursing Interventions	Selected Rationale	Evaluation
Spo_2 95% on room air.	Assess vital signs and Spo_2 q2h. Report increase in respiratory rate or decrease in oxygen saturation.	Change in vital signs and oxygen saturation may indicate improvement or deterioration of condition.	Spo_2 remains within 93%–95%. The respiratory rate is 12–22/min. The heart rate remains between 60 and 100 bpm.
	Increase oxygen to maintain Spo_2 at level specified by health care provider.	Maintain oxygen saturation at levels that indicate effective gas exchange.	Spo_2 94%. O_2 at 5 L/min by nasal cannula
	Assess lung sounds at least q4h.	Changes in lung sounds indicate positive response to therapy or need to modify treatment plan.	Lung sounds clear on right, fine crackles on left.
	Maintain Fowler position as needed for comfort. Teach patient pursed-lip breathing.	Promotes optimum expansion of thoracic cavity to facilitate breathing and improve gas exchange.	Head of bed at 45 degrees.

PROBLEM STATEMENT/NURSING DIAGNOSIS

Altered activity tolerance due to fluid in lungs, fluid retention in lower extremities.

SUPPORTING ASSESSMENT DATA

Subjective: States feet have become more swollen over the past 3 days.

Objective: Pitting edema both lower extremities, dyspnea on exertion, crackles in bases bilaterally.

Goals/Expected Outcomes	Nursing Interventions	Selected Rationale	Evaluation
Patient will be able to complete activities of daily living and personal hygiene without fatigue.	Assess activity tolerance. Assist with personal hygiene initially. Monitor oxygen saturation. Provide frequent rest periods. Coordinate care with other health care providers to conserve energy.	Provides guidelines for planning care activities. Conserves patient energy. Scheduling activities to maximize energy use prevents overtiring. Prevents fatigue.	Able to complete partial bath. Becomes fatigued, requires assistance. Patient remains fatigued.

PROBLEM STATEMENT/NURSING DIAGNOSIS

Fluid volume overload due to heart failure as evidenced by pulmonary and venous congestion.

SUPPORTING ASSESSMENT DATA

Subjective: Patient reports nonproductive cough.

Objective: 3 to 4+ edema both lower extremities; crackles in lung bases on auscultation.

Continued

Nursing Care Plan 19.1 Care of a Patient With Heart Failure—cont'd

Goals/Expected Outcomes	Nursing Interventions	Selected Rationale	Evaluation
Lung fields will be clear, pitting edema in lower extremities 0–1+.	Assess lung sounds q4h.	Identifies changes in condition.	Fine crackles on auscultation. Less distress.
	Assess lower extremities each shift.	Identifies effectiveness of drug therapy.	2+ pitting edema bilaterally.
	Elevate legs	Helps move fluid from the tissues back into the circulation so it can be removed by the kidneys.	2+ pitting edema bilaterally—less than on admission.
	Administer diuretics as prescribed by the provider.	To reduce fluid retention through diuresis.	Urinary output 2500 mL q8h.
	Maintain accurate intake and output. Daily weights.	Identify positive or negative response to treatment.	Weight 245 lb.

CRITICAL THINKING QUESTIONS

1. List three additional problem statements that are appropriate for this patient.
2. List five items to be included in the discharge teaching plan for this patient.
3. What assessment data might indicate a worsening of this patient's condition?
4. What assessment data might indicate improvement of this patient's condition?

Patient Teaching

Instructions for Patients Taking Warfarin (Coumadin)

Teach the patient who has been prescribed warfarin to:

- Take the medication at the same time every day.
- Keep appointments for international normalized ratio (INR) blood tests or perform the test at home.
- Take a missed dose as soon as it is remembered on the day it is due. Do not double up on the dose the next day if the previous dose was forgotten.
- Check all medications, all over-the-counter preparations, and all herbs for possible interactions with warfarin.
- Wear a medical alert bracelet and carry a wallet ID card indicating warfarin use.
- Tell all medical personnel that warfarin is being taken.
- Eat foods containing vitamin K in consistent amounts weekly; asparagus, beans, broccoli, cabbage, spinach, cauliflower, brussels sprouts, kale, and mustard greens are high in vitamin K and should not be eaten in large quantities. Fish, rice, and yogurt also contain vitamin K.
- Avoid consuming more than one or two alcoholic drinks per day.
- Use an electric razor if prone to nicking the skin when shaving.
- Use a soft toothbrush.
- Blow the nose gently.
- Report unusual bleeding or bruising to the health care provider.
- Report signs of intestinal bleeding (blood in the stool) and blood in the urine.

It is of vital importance to monitor patients with HF for electrolyte imbalances, especially imbalance of sodium or potassium. **Electrolyte imbalances may cause serious cardiac dysrhythmias.**

Patients with chronic HF will need encouragement to follow the prescribed regimen. A chronic disease management program is advised based on multiple studies over the past decade indicating better outcomes (Centers for Disease Control and Prevention [CDC], 2018). If treatment does not stop the progress of the disease, the patient may be admitted to the hospital for reevaluation and a change in therapies. Sometimes the patient's heart continues to fail despite aggressive therapy, and pulmonary edema and liver and renal failure occur.

Older Adult Care Points

An older adult patient who is experiencing HF often is taking many medications. With decreased kidney function, it is especially important to look for drug interactions and to monitor for signs and symptoms of toxicity. Loop diuretics continue to work even after excess fluid is eliminated. Monitor older adult patients for signs of dehydration such as decreased urine output and confusion.

Think Critically

Why does weighing the patient daily help you evaluate the treatment for HF? How would you know that the treatment is not effective?

Assisting hospitalized patients with activities of daily living will decrease oxygen demand. Scheduling all activities to promote as much rest as possible is a high priority. Activity is alternated with rest throughout the day. Several pillows may be required to achieve a comfortable bed position. Monitoring intake and output is very important. Daily weight is recorded at the same time each day, preferably before breakfast. Careful attention to frequent repositioning and skin care is essential because edematous tissue breaks down easily. Particular attention should be given to the sacral area as a pressure point susceptible to skin breakdown for a patient on bed rest. Bed rest causes venous pooling, and deep vein thrombosus (DVT) prophylaxis should be implemented. Heparin or enoxaparin may be used unless the patient is already on antiplatelet or anticoagulant medication for another condition. Elastic stockings or sequential compression devices and leg exercises should be used. Careful ongoing physical assessment is essential. Nursing interventions for selected problems in a patient with HF are summarized in Nursing Care Plan 19.1. Instructional materials regarding smoking cessation are offered to *all* smokers on admission and discharge, and patients are counseled about the importance of quitting smoking (Centers for Medicare & Medicaid Services, 2018). *Tobacco treatment*, the term used by The Joint Commission, is a stand-alone core measure and is not specific to any one diagnosis because smoking cessation is key to controlling many diseases. Discharge instructions include (1) activity level, (2) diet, (3) discharge medication, (4) follow-up appointment, (5) weight monitoring, (6) what to do if symptoms worsen, and (7) when to notify the health care provider.

Patients with HF*r*EF (ejection fraction <40%) should receive a prescription for an ACE inhibitor, an ARB medication, or an angiotensin receptor–neprilysin inhibitor (ARNI). Providing education about warning signs of worsening condition (decompensation), exercise needs, diet compliance, and lifestyle changes greatly helps symptom control (Yancy et al., 2017).

◆ EVALUATION

Patients with HF require extensive treatment with medication and lifestyle changes. Evaluate objective and subjective data to determine whether expected outcomes are being met. Note subjective data related to activity tolerance, respiratory status, comfort, and understanding of teaching related to the disease process and self-management. Understanding of the medication regimen is key to the patient's progress. The cardiovascular system should be monitored for improvement of status. Observe the patient for improvement of symptoms, including edema, respiratory quality, and activity tolerance. Improvement is an indication of patient progress.

CARDIAC DYSRHYTHMIAS

A normal heart generates electrical impulses and sends them through an electrical conduction system signaling the atria and ventricles to contract. An abnormal heart rhythm occurs when the conduction system or heart muscle is not functioning normally. The goal for a beginning nurse is to be able to determine when the tracing is not a normal sinus rhythm.

Etiology

Alterations in the conduction of cardiac electrical impulses that create heart rate and rhythm may be the result of congenital abnormalities, electrolyte disturbances, too much caffeine, illegal drug use, stress, or medication side effects. Valvular disorders, damage to the heart from **infarct** (area of necrosis caused by ischemia), thyroid problems, infective endocarditis, and problems in the autonomic nervous system also cause rhythm disturbances. Abnormal rhythms are called **arrhythmias** or **dysrhythmias**.

Box 19.2 Evaluating an Electrocardiogram Rhythm Strip

- Obtain a 6-second strip (35 large graph squares).
- Find the QRS. If the rate is too slow or too fast, check the patient before proceeding. Calculate the rate. Count the number of QRS complexes in the 6-second strip and multiply by 10. Measure with calipers from R wave to R wave throughout the tracing to determine whether the rate is regular. Do all the QRS complexes look the same?
- Look directly in front of the QRS for the P wave. Is there a P wave in front of every QRS? Do the P waves all look alike? Measure the P-R interval. Is it normal (0.12 to 0.20 second or 3 to 5 little boxes)? Does it vary?
- Measure the QRS duration. Is it normal (0.04 to 0.12 second or 1 to 3 little boxes)?
- Are there any abnormal beats? Is the QRS wide or normal? Do the beats come in early?

Pathophysiology

The sinoatrial (SA) node generates electrical impulses 60 to 100 times per minute. Each impulse travels through the atria to the atrioventricular (AV) node (or junction), which delays the impulse slightly, then relays it via the bundle of His and the Purkinje fibers to the ventricles, causing them to contract (Fig. 19.4). Box 19.2 describes the procedure for evaluating an ECG strip. If the SA node fails to produce an electrical impulse, the AV node will initiate an impulse at 40 to 60 beats per minute (bpm). If neither the SA nor the AV node is functioning, the Purkinje fibers in the ventricles will initiate an impulse at a slower rate. When there is disruption of the normal electrical conduction in the heart, an abnormal heart rhythm occurs.

Signs and Symptoms

Normal pulse rate is 60 to 100 bpm. Fig. 19.5 shows the ECG pattern of normal sinus rhythm. A pulse below 60 bpm is labeled *bradycardia*. Bradycardia may or may not be a problem. Athletes often have a bradycardia without a pathologic condition because their hearts are so well conditioned that they are very efficient. Whether a bradycardia requires treatment depends on whether the patient has symptoms of decreased blood flow. Symptomatic bradycardia is treated with atropine or pacing. In an emergency, external pacing pads may be used until a different mode of pacing can be implemented.

If the heart rate rises above 100 bpm, the patient has a dysrhythmia known as *tachycardia*. Sinus tachycardia

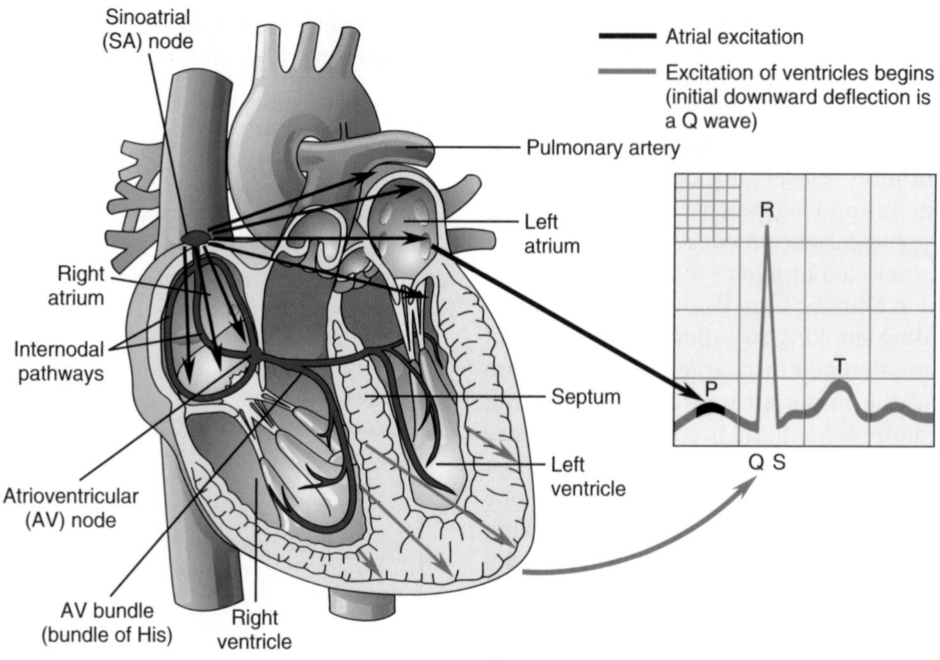

Fig. 19.4 Cardiac conduction system. (From Banasik JL, Copstead LC: *Pathophysiology*, ed 6, St. Louis, 2019, Elsevier.)

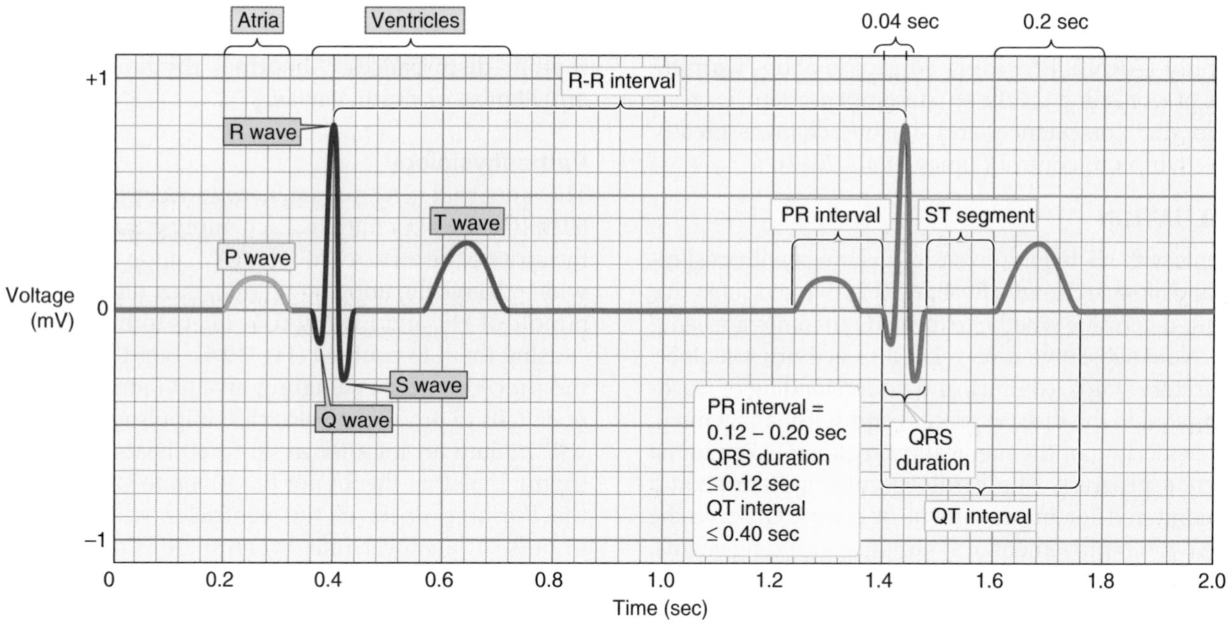

Fig. 19.5 Electrocardiogram tracing of normal sinus rhythm. (Modified from Boron WF, Boulpaep EL: *Medical physiology*, ed 3, Philadelphia, 2017, Elsevier.)

with a rate of 100 to 150 bpm is usually caused by pain, fever, stress, hypovolemia, or hypoxia. Increasing heart rate is the body's response to the need for increased blood flow. It is managed by treating the underlying condition.

When the heart beats too fast, the ventricles do not have adequate time to fill with blood and therefore cannot pump effectively. As a result, cardiac output falls. Heart rates over 150 bpm are considered "too fast" for most patients. Again, signs and symptoms of decreased blood flow determine how urgently treatment needs to be administered. When the heart is not stimulated to contract at the correct rate or in an effective manner, adequate blood is not pumped out to the body. Symptoms the patient may experience include dizziness, **palpitations** (abnormally rapid throbbing or fluttering of the heart), fatigue, chest pain, hypotension, and loss of consciousness; death may occur. The severity of the symptoms depends on whether the abnormal rhythm significantly decreases cardiac output and whether the dysrhythmia is persistent.

It is important to be able to recognize a normal heart rhythm so that abnormalities can be quickly identified (see Box 19.2). The most important component in delivering appropriate treatment is assessment of the patient. The overall health of the patient will determine whether a specific dysrhythmia requires immediate reporting or treatment. Some rhythms are more likely than others to cause decreased cardiac output. The heart rate is the single best indicator as to how the patient may be tolerating a heart rhythm. The ECG will give additional information about the specific source of the problem, but bedside assessment is key in delivering the correct therapy. The name of the rhythm indicates where the electrical impulse originated to cause the QRS. Sinus rhythms originate in the sinus node; for ventricular rhythms, an impulse starts in the ventricles. Rhythms can be too fast or too slow, or the patient can be pulseless.

Cardiac Dysrhythmias—Too Slow

As stated previously, a pulse rate below 60 bpm is a bradycardia. The only time a bradycardia is treated is if the patient has symptoms of decreased cardiac output. The heart fills during diastole, which is the flat line part of the ECG. The amount of blood in the ventricles pumped out multiplied by the number of times per minute the heart pumps is cardiac output. If the heart does not beat enough times per minute to generate enough blood flow, symptoms occur. Slow heart rates can be caused by hypoxia, electrolyte imbalances, infection, drugs, hypoglycemia, and other treatable conditions. There also may be disease of the conduction system causing the "pacemaker" of the heart—the SA node—to malfunction. *Sinus bradycardia* is the most common form of bradycardia. The rhythm looks like a normal sinus rhythm except for the rate.

Heart block. Bradycardias can also be produced by conduction problems such as heart blocks. Normally when the SA node fires, it sends the electrical signal through the atria and then to the ventricles through the AV node (also called the *AV junction*). In heart block the signal is stopped either temporarily or permanently at the AV junction. Heart block is either first, second, or third degree. The higher the degree, the more significant the block and the more likely it is to produce bradycardia.

In *first-degree heart block,* impulse conduction between the atrium and the ventricle is consistently lengthened beyond 0.2 seconds. First-degree block can be temporary or permanent. It often occurs after open heart surgery or an MI. Digoxin, calcium channel blockers, and beta blockers may cause this arrhythmia. It usually does not cause hemodynamically significant symptoms.

Second-degree heart block has two types. The first is *Mobitz I or Wenckebach,* which displays a normal R-R interval on the ECG and increasingly lengthened P-R intervals until a P wave appears without a QRS complex because the impulse was not conducted to the ventricles. This causes a "pause" in the rhythm. The cycle then begins again after the AV node has rested for that one beat. Parasympathetic tone or drug effect from digoxin, calcium channel blockers, beta blockers, or disorders such as electrolyte imbalance, Addison disease, and endocarditis is a possible cause. The arrhythmia is most often transient and rarely progresses to third-degree heart block; it is considered benign.

Type II second-degree heart block (Mobitz II) is a more severe heart block. The AV node blocks certain beats from traveling through to the ventricles. P waves are seen without a following QRS. There may be a single or multiple P waves without a QRS. The P-R interval is constant throughout. The rhythm can be regular or irregular. This rhythm is dangerous because it may progress to third-degree heart block and is most often caused by ischemia. This arrhythmia often occurs after open heart surgery. Bradycardia may be the result, and the patient may or may not be symptomatic depending on the ventricular rate. If the patient is symptomatic, a temporary transvenous pacemaker may be inserted, followed by a permanent pacemaker if needed.

In *complete heart block (third-degree heart block;* Fig. 19.6, *B*) the AV node does not conduct atrial impulses to the ventricles. The atria contract on their own, and an "escape" stimulus from the ventricle provides a slow ventricular rhythm. Cardiac output falls drastically. This dysrhythmia can be life threatening, but many times an adequate heart rate is present to allow time for interventions.

If a rhythm strip has more P waves than QRS complexes, the rhythm is Type I or Type II second-degree heart block or third-degree heart block. All bradycardia is treated the same, so initially, specific identification is not necessary to implement correct therapy.

> **Clinical Cues**
>
> Any time a person states that they have noticed an irregular or rapid heartbeat, ask how much caffeine is being consumed each day. If consumption is minimal, ask about medications being taken, such as decongestants. Ask about the person's stress level. The problem may disappear when the precipitating factor is removed.

Cardiac Dysrhythmias—Too Fast

Any fast heart rate has the potential to be clinically significant. It is during diastole that the heart fills with blood. When heart rate increases, the time spent in diastole significantly shortens, reducing the time for filling to occur.

Supraventricular tachycardia (SVT) (Fig. 19.6, *A*) is a rhythm that originates in or above the bundle of His ("above" the ventricles). SVTs include atrial flutter or fibrillation, atrial tachycardia, and junctional tachycardia. The heart rate will be greater than 150 bpm, and the QRS will be of normal duration. At this heart rate the origin of the impulse is almost impossible to identify, so the term *SVT* communicates that the rhythm is not

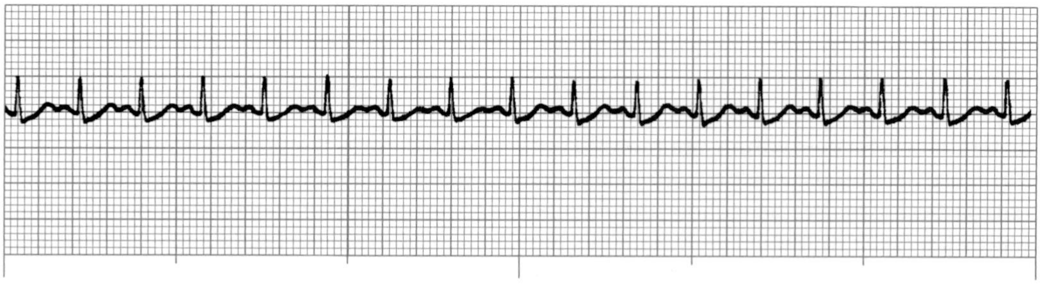

A

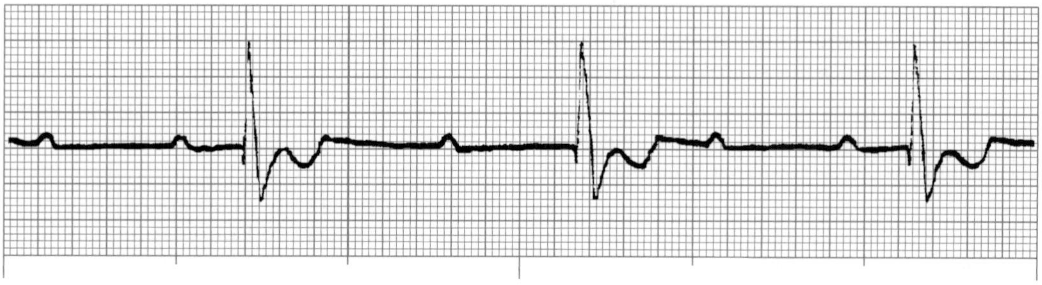

B

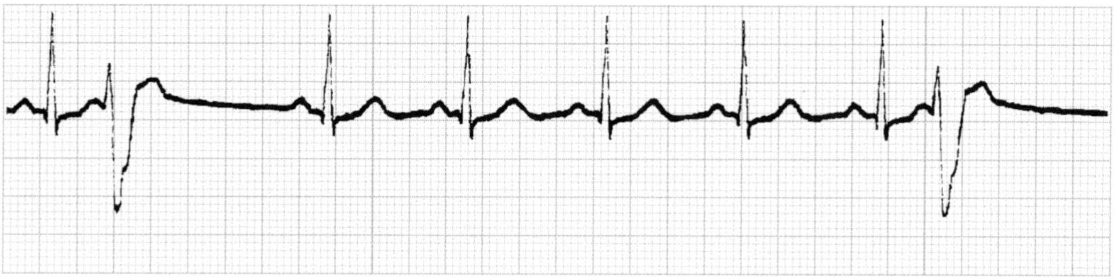

C

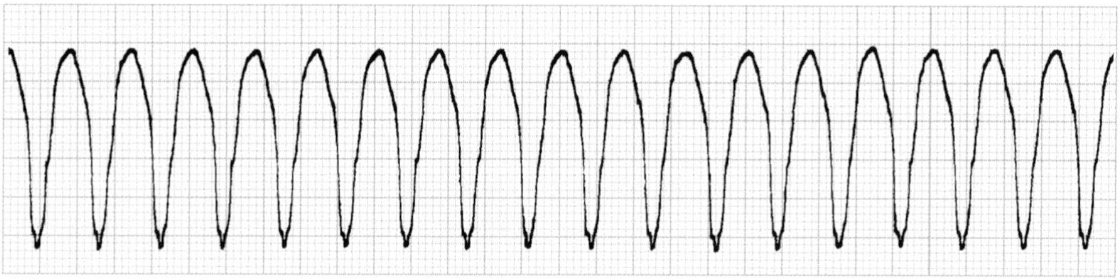

D

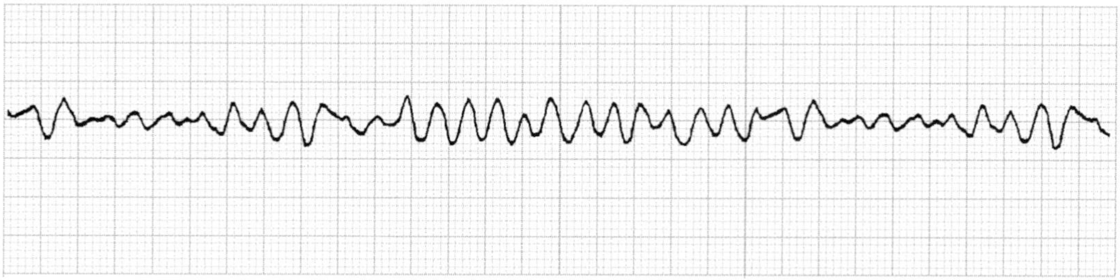

E

Fig. 19.6 Electrocardiogram patterns of abnormal and life-threatening dysrhythmias. **A,** Supraventricular tachycardia. **B,** Complete (third-degree) heart block. **C,** Sinus rhythm with premature ventricular contractions. **D,** Ventricular tachycardia. **E,** Ventricular fibrillation. (From Aehlert B: *EKGs made easy*, ed 6, St. Louis, 2018, Elsevier.)

ventricular tachycardia. If the patient is unstable, a synchronized **cardioversion** will be implemented. For stable patients, vagal maneuvers and drug therapies will be used.

Ventricular tachycardia. *Ventricular tachycardia (VT)* is a potentially life-threatening dysrhythmia that is generated from one or more focal points in the ventricle at a very fast rate (usually 120 to 200 bpm) (Fig. 19.6, *D*). The patient may be awake and alert without symptoms or just not feeling well. Or the patient may be pulseless. **The ECG tracing will not tell if the patient has a pulse; feel for the pulse.** VT occurs in bursts, short runs, or as a sustained rhythm. The length of time this rhythm continues and the underlying condition of the heart determine how well the body can tolerate it. The atria do not have a chance to contract and push blood into the ventricles. The ventricles contract too fast to allow for adequate filling with blood. Cardiac output falls drastically. VT can quickly deteriorate into ventricular fibrillation or cardiac standstill. Treatment depends on whether the dysrhythmia is sustained and how well the patient is tolerating the rhythm. If the patient is symptomatic with changes in blood pressure, pulse, and level of consciousness, the VT is unstable; synchronized cardioversion starting at 100 joules (biphasic) is the treatment. If the patient is not unstable, treatment with oxygen and amiodarone (Cordarone) is provided. VT is usually caused by cardiac ischemia or any condition or substance that causes myocardial irritability.

Atrial fibrillation. New-onset **atrial fibrillation** usually presents with a very rapid heart rate. Patients are admitted with "a fib with RVR"—atrial fibrillation with rapid ventricular response. In a normal heartbeat, the atria provide the "atrial kick," which is about 20% of the blood volume for the ventricles to pump out. When atrial fibrillation happens, the atrial kick is lost, and the fast heart rate decreases filling time. Some patients are lightheaded, have a decreased blood pressure, and are clammy. Atrial fibrillation may occur with HF, coronary artery disease, hyperthyroidism, or chronic obstructive pulmonary disease (COPD). Instead of atrial contraction there is quivering. P waves are not visible on the ECG tracing. There are only a lot of tiny, erratic bumps visible. Because the AV node cannot respond to the huge number of impulses, it conducts impulses to the ventricle in an erratic manner, resulting in irregular heart rhythm. The rhythm is **irregularly irregular.** Treatment is with loading doses of diltiazem or digoxin, amiodarone, or a beta blocker. If drug treatment is unsuccessful, synchronized cardioversion is performed to convert to a normal sinus rhythm.

Atrial fibrillation predisposes the patient to clot formation in the atria. The quivering rather than pumping of the atria allows blood to pool, leading to formation of clots. The atria both have an anatomic feature called an appendage. On the right the appendage is triangular shaped and can cause some blood pooling. The left atrial appendage is shaped more like a wind sock and has a significant potential for blood pooling during atrial fibrillation. Patients with chronic atrial fibrillation are usually placed on oral anticoagulant therapy. Teach the patient the importance of taking the medication as directed by the health care provider. Dislodged clots from the right atrium can cause pulmonary embolus, and clots from the left side can travel to the brain, resulting in stroke or possibly death. Several devices to block off the opening to the left atrial appendage are available and in use for patients in which anticoagulation is contraindicated or impractical. This prevents blood pooling and clot formation (Fig. 19.7). Multiple other techniques and devices are in clinical trials.

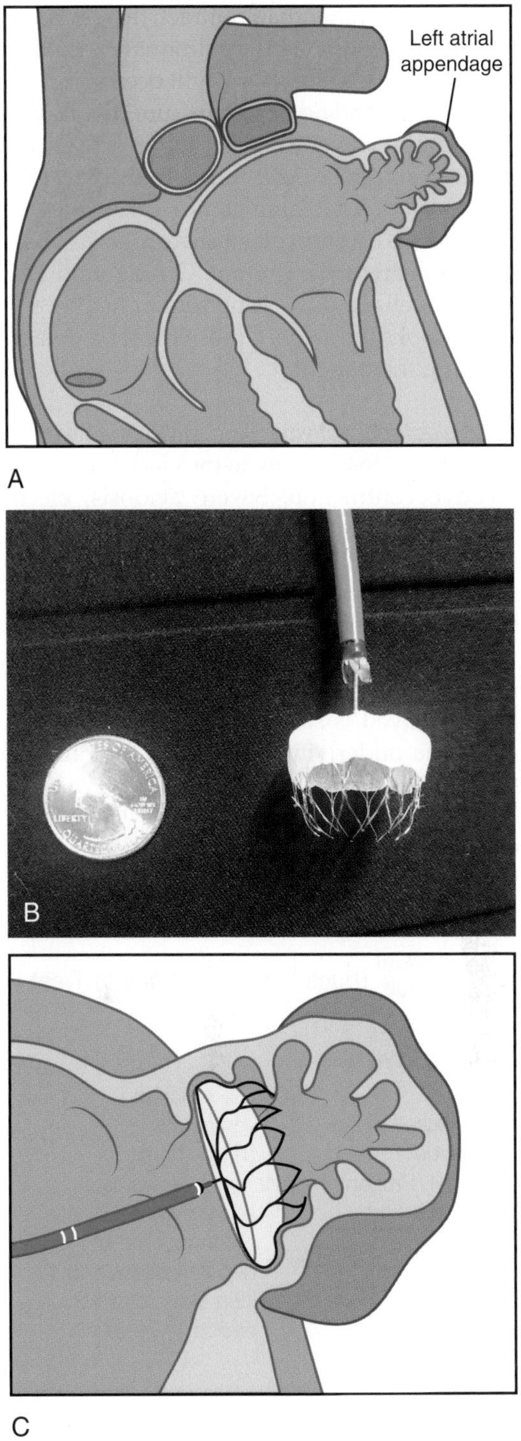

Fig. 19.7 **A,** Left atrial appendage. **B,** Left atrial appendage occlusion device. **C,** Watchman closure device placed.

Older Adult Care Points

With increased age the left ventricle and cardiac valves thicken and the amount of fibrous tissue and fat in the SA node increases, which decreases the number of pacemaker cells the SA node contains. These changes make individuals older than 75 years more prone to cardiac dysrhythmias. Failure of the SA node and the need for a pacemaker are common. Thyroid studies should be performed for patients older than 65 years who have atrial fibrillation because thyroid problems can be a cause. Hypothyroidism or hyperthyroidism may also aggravate HF.

Cardiac Dysrhythmias—Absent Pulse

Ventricular fibrillation. *Ventricular fibrillation (VF)* is a chaotic random firing of all the ventricular cells. The ventricles quiver rather than contract; there is no cardiac output, and without cardiopulmonary resuscitation (CPR) and defibrillation, death will occur (Fig. 19.6, *E*). There is no pulse and no blood pressure. The ECG shows coarse electrical waveforms varying in size and shape, and no intervals can be determined. Immediate intervention is required. The same clinical picture can occur with pulseless VT. Ventricular tachycardia was discussed earlier as a tachycardic rhythm. On the monitor there is no way to tell if a pulse is present or not because the waveform looks the same; a pulse must be determined by assessing the patient.

Pulseless electrical activity. Sometimes the heart muscle is not capable of responding to the electrical signal with an effective contraction. Severe acidosis, electrolyte imbalances, profound hypovolemia, and other disorders keep the myocardium from contracting because of the toxic environment. The signal is sent and a QRS appears on the ECG, but there is no pulse. The rhythm on the monitor can be anything that would normally be expected to have a pulse generated. The most common rhythm displayed is sinus tachycardia. CPR and correction of the underlying disorder is the only way to regain a pulse.

Premature beats (ectopic beats). An extra heartbeat that interrupts the regularity of the rhythm can be caused by an impulse coming from the atria, junction, or ventricles. Because they occur outside of the normal location, they are considered *ectopic*. They are usually beats that come in early and are labeled according to which part of the heart is responsible for the QRS.

Premature ventricular contractions. The *premature ventricular contraction (PVC)* appears on the ECG as an early beat without a P wave and with a wide QRS complex. A ventricular impulse causes a ventricular contraction; it is labeled *premature* because it comes in early (Fig. 19.6, *C*). A pause usually occurs after the premature beat. The patient perceives a PVC as a skipped beat because the PVC is not efficient at pumping blood and may not generate enough blood flow to be felt at a pulse point. An apical and radial pulse deficit may be detected. The ventricular irritability causing PVCs may be from caffeine, drugs, or increased emotional stress. Hypoxia, hypokalemia, and myocardial ischemia also may trigger PVCs. A few PVCs are not abnormal, but when there are more than six or seven in a minute, cardiac output may fall. If PVCs are persistent and symptomatic, antidysrhythmic drugs are used to control them (Table 19.4). Three or more PVCs in a row are considered ventricular tachycardia. PVCs may not all look alike. This indicates more than one area of irritability in the heart muscle. PVCs should be reported to the health care provider when they occur frequently or have

Table 19.4 Drugs Commonly Used to Treat Dysrhythmias

EXAMPLES	ACTION	NURSING IMPLICATIONS	PATIENT TEACHING
Class I Antidysrhythmics			
IA Quinidine sulfate Procainamide (Pronestyl, Procan) Disopyramide (Norpace) IB Lidocaine (Xylocaine) Phenytoin (Dilantin) Tocainamide (Tonocard) Mexiletine (Mexitil) Moricizine (Ethmozine) IC Flecainide (Tambocor) Propafenone (Rythmol)	*Uses:* Atrial and ventricular dysrhythmias *Actions:* Slows the sodium channel, prolongs time of depolarization, and increases refractory period	*Quinidine:* Monitor for cinchonism: tinnitus, headache, nausea, vertigo, and disturbed vision. Observe for changes in ECG pattern. If patient is taking digitalis, monitor for digitalis toxicity; quinidine can double digoxin levels. Cimetidine increases effects of quinidine. Quinidine may enhance action of anticoagulants. Monitor for diarrhea. Monitor drug level. *Procainamide:* Monitor for systemic lupus erythematosus–like syndrome: joint pain; hepatomegaly; unexplained fever; soreness of the mouth, throat, or gums. Discontinue medication if this occurs. Observe for side effects or adverse effects of particular drug administered. Monitor electrolyte levels; watch for postural hypotension, especially if patient is taking antihypertensives.	Instruct to report signs of adverse effects of the drug. Report noticeable changes in cardiac rhythm to the health care provider. Advise to take quinidine with meals to prevent GI upset. Advise to minimize citrus fruit intake; it changes the urine pH and decreases excretion of quinidine. Procainamide is absorbed best on an empty stomach; if GI upset occurs, instruct to take immediately after a meal.

Table 19.4 Drugs Commonly Used to Treat Dysrhythmias—cont'd

EXAMPLES	ACTION	NURSING IMPLICATIONS	PATIENT TEACHING
Class II Antidysrhythmics (Beta Blockers)			
Propranolol (Inderal) Atenolol (Tenormin) Carvedilol (Coreg) Esmolol (Brevibloc) Nadolol (Corgard) Sotalol (Betapace) Metoprolol (Lopressor, Toprol XL)	*Uses:* Atrial and ventricular dysrhythmias *Action:* Slow SA node impulses	Monitor for signs of CHF; monitor pulse and blood pressure, watching for bradycardia and hypotension. Monitor electrolytes. Carefully monitor blood sugar in diabetic patients.	Instruct not to discontinue the drug abruptly. Notify provider if skin rash, confusion, fever, sore throat, or unusual bleeding or bruising occur. Monitor weight and report gain of >2 lb/wk. Report edema or shortness of breath.
Class III Antidysrhythmics (Potassium Channel Blockers)			
Amiodarone (Cordarone) Dofetilide (Tikosyn) Ibutilide (Corvert) Sotalol (Betapace)	*Uses:* Supraventricular and ventricular dysrhythmias *Actions:* Increase the refractory period and action potential duration	Check for drug interactions and for side or adverse effects of specific drug administered. Monitor heart rhythm, blood pressure, and pulse. Monitor renal function.	Instruct to report adverse reactions to specific drug being taken. Advise of need for provider supervision. Report any new heart rhythm irregularities.
Class IV Antidysrhythmics (Calcium Channel Blockers)			
Verapamil (Calan, Isoptin, Verelan) Diltiazem (Cardizem)	*Use:* Paroxysmal supraventricular tachycardia (PSVT) *Action:* Converts PSVT to normal sinus rhythm by slowing conduction time through the nodes	Monitor heart rate and rhythm; watch for signs of CHF. Observe for hypotension and edema. Use very cautiously with beta blockers.	Instruct to report signs of edema, shortness of breath, or weight gain of >2 lb in 1 wk. Notify provider of new changes in heart rhythm.
Other Agents			
Atropine	Vagolytic action blocks vagal tone, allowing heart rate to increase.	Used to raise the heart rate, monitor rate and rhythm.	Explain goal of use.
Digoxin (Lanoxin)	Increases contractility while decreasing heart rate.	Monitor heart rate for expected decrease.	Teach signs and symptoms of toxicity: visual changes, anorexia, nausea, vomiting, diarrhea, headache, confusion, new dysrhythmia.
Adenosine (Adenocard)	Slows conduction through the AV node and blocks AV reentry pathways.	Monitor for expected decreased heart rate.	Monitor for dizziness, blurred vision, facial flushing, nausea, dyspnea, bronchospasm, new dysrhythmia, and chest pressure.
Magnesium sulfate	Slows SA node rate and prolongs conduction time. Promotes movement of calcium, potassium, and sodium in and out of cells and stabilizes excitable membranes.	Used to correct digitalis toxicity, to aid in correction of ventricular dysrhythmias, and with myocardial irritability.	Monitor for muscle weakness, flushing, confusion, nausea, cramps, diarrhea, and circulatory collapse.

AV, Atrioventricular; *CHF,* congestive heart failure; *ECG,* electrocardiogram; *GI,* gastrointestinal; *SA,* sinoatrial.

multiple shapes or when the patient has several in a row or shows signs of decreased cardiac output.

Premature atrial contractions. *Premature atrial contraction (PAC)* happens when an ectopic electrical focus fires before the next SA node impulse is due, thereby depolarizing the atria. An abnormally shaped P wave appears on the ECG before the QRS wave. The impulse is routed to the AV node and then to the ventricles, causing normal ventricular contraction. PACs are common and do not often produce symptoms. PACs result from sympathetic nervous system stimulation, such as occurs with anxiety, hypoxia, or ischemia.

Premature junctional contractions. Early junctional beats can also occur and are called *premature junctional contractions (PJCs).* They look much like PACs but usually do not have a P wave in front of the early beat. They do not cause hemodynamic compromise and are difficult to distinguish from PACs. A full discussion is not within the scope of this text.

Premature beats can occur in many different rhythms. Most of the premature beats are caused by irritability of the tissue. The more frequently the premature beats occur, the more concern you should show.

There are many types of cardiac dysrhythmias. Nurses assigned to a critical care or telemetry unit take a special course in dysrhythmia recognition to learn the patterns, significance, and treatment of each type. All nurses should be able to recognize life-threatening dysrhythmias.

Diagnosis and Treatment

Disorders of the cardiac conduction system are diagnosed by a 12-lead ECG, by continuous ECG monitoring, and by patient history (see Chapter 17, Table 17.2). Drug therapy is effective in correcting or controlling dysrhythmias in many cases. A variety of antiarrhythmic agents may be used alone or in combination to regulate the heartbeat (see Table 19.4). Oxygenation, acid-base status, and electrolyte balance are watched carefully and corrected as needed. Early recognition and correction of abnormalities decreases the occurrence of life-threatening dysrhythmias.

Synchronized cardioversion. Patients who experience tachycardia or rhythms that do not respond to drug therapy may be treated with *synchronized cardioversion.* A mild electrical shock is delivered to the heart at a specific time in the cardiac cycle to interrupt the abnormal rhythm and begin a new, normal rhythm of electrical impulse and contraction. The procedure is done emergently when the patient is unstable and requires immediate intervention. It also can be done electively as a scheduled procedure, primarily to convert atrial fibrillation to a normal rhythm. The patient is given a sedative before the procedure. Signed consent is required. The procedure may be performed in the cardiac catheterization laboratory or in the emergency department by the health care provider. Resuscitation equipment must be at hand. The patient must be monitored for response to treatment, including heart rate, rhythm, and blood pressure.

Cardiac pacemakers. Cardiac pacemakers may be used to manage chronic and life-threatening dysrhythmias and are used to support heart rate when bradycardia occurs. Advances in pacemaker technology have led to units that are programmable for single- and dual-chambered control. A pacemaker can be used to pace the atria and one or both ventricles. Some units can override a dysrhythmia and keep the heart at a more steady rhythm. There are rate-responsive pacemakers, in which the pacemaker automatically adjusts to the patient's level of activity. When the patient exercises, the heart rate increases (similar to the normal SA node response).

Pacing can be a temporary measure if the problem is an emergent, transient condition, such as drug toxicity. An external pacemaker often is used in the emergency department. Electricity is passed through the chest wall via external pads. It causes uncomfortable muscle contractions as current passes through the chest, so it is used only until another mode of pacing is available.

A temporary transvenous pacemaker is placed if a transient rhythm such as heart block develops after an MI or drug toxicity. Transvenous pacemakers are inserted by fluoroscopy with local anesthesia. The leads are attached to an external power source. Patient consent is required, and a sedative is given to the patient before the procedure. Epicardial pacemaker wires are often placed during cardiac surgery for quick use should the patient need pacing in the postoperative period. The wires are brought through the chest wall and are attached to an external power source. When the wires are no longer needed, the surgeon will remove them by pulling them out (the wires can easily be dislodged).

Clinical Cues

Patients are at risk for cardiac tamponade when the epicardial pacer wires are pulled. Monitor patients for signs and symptoms of bleeding into the pericardial sac, including sharp chest pain, dyspnea, hypotension, cyanosis, tachycardia, paradoxical pulse, and distended neck veins.

A permanent pacemaker is implanted for SA node dysfunction, heart block, or treatment of chronic HF. All pacemakers have the same function: to produce effective heartbeats. A permanent pacemaker is inserted in the operating room or cardiac catheterization laboratory to ensure an aseptic environment (Fig. 19.8). The pulse generator is placed in a skin pocket below the right or left clavicle.

Nursing Management

If inserting a pacemaker is not an emergency procedure, there will be opportunities to assess the patient's

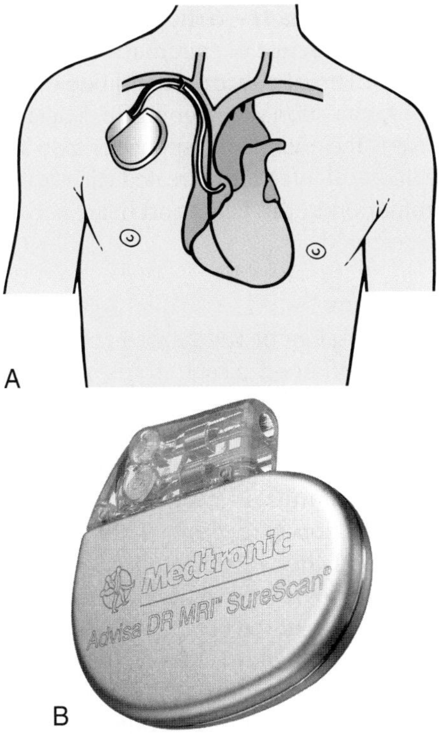

Fig. 19.8 Thoracic placement of permanent pacemaker and transvenous pacing wires. **A,** Placement of pacemaker and wires. **B,** Pacemaker. (**A,** From Lewis SL, Bucher L, Heitkemper MM, et al.: *Medical-surgical nursing: assessment and management of clinical problems,* ed 10, St. Louis, 2017, Elsevier. **B,** Reproduced with permission of Medtronic, Inc.)

knowledge of and understanding about having their heart rate regulated. Assess the patient's learning needs, seek to identify the source of any fear, and gauge the level of anxiety.

Think Critically

How would you approach discussion with an older adult patient who is fearful of getting a permanent pacemaker?

Both the American Heart Association and the manufacturers of pacemakers provide illustrated booklets to help patients learn more about their cardiac pacers. You can go over these booklets with the patient and perhaps show a demonstration model and explain how it works.

Older Adult Care Points

Older patients who have SA node disease and resulting cardiac dysrhythmias can achieve a far better quality of life with an implanted pacemaker. Many patients are fearful of the surgery required and can benefit from talking with another patient who has had a successful pacemaker implantation.

Postoperative nursing care for patients with a permanent pacemaker includes continuous monitoring of heart rate, rhythm, blood pressure, and temperature. Patients are also monitored for hematoma formation at the site of insertion. The battery in a pacemaker should last 6 to 9 years, depending on how frequently pacing is required.

Patient Teaching

Instructions for a Patient With a Permanent Pacemaker

A patient who has had a permanent pacemaker implanted should receive these instructions before discharge:

- Avoid lifting the arm away from the body on the pacemaker side until your health care provider says you may progress to normal activity. Lifting may dislodge the leads from their positions.
- Keep the incision dry for at least 4 days after the surgery.
- Check for redness, swelling, drainage, or fever and report such findings to your provider immediately.
- Refrain from activities that might cause a direct blow to the pacemaker.
- Use cellular or cordless phones on the ear opposite the pacemaker.
- Stay away from high-output electrical generators or large magnets such as a magnetic resonance imager. Such devices can interfere with pacemaker function.
- Monitor your pulse daily and report to the provider if it drops below the set rate.
- Carry a pacemaker information card with you at all times.
- Wear a medical alert bracelet or necklace at all times.
- Keep follow-up appointments with your provider to check the insertion site and to check pacemaker function.
- **Microwave ovens are safe to use, and airport security screening should not cause a problem with the function of the pacemaker. Travel is not restricted.**

The patient must understand the importance of periodic evaluations of their condition for the rest of their life. Some pacemakers have a telephone monitoring device that allows calling a monitoring station to have the pacemaker checked or a telemetry device that sends a report automatically every night. Instructions for the use of the pacemaker and monitoring device are included in the owner's manual.

Implantable cardioverter-defibrillators. Implantable cardioverter-defibrillators (ICDs) are used for patients who have an episode of a life-threatening dysrhythmia. They are also indicated in some patients with cardiomyopathy and decreased EF that are at increased risk of lethal dysrhythmias. The defibrillator is implanted in the same way as a pacemaker. The pulse generator is slightly larger than that for a regular pacemaker because it requires a high-capacity battery. ICDs monitor the heartbeat and provide an electrical shock similar to that delivered in cardiac defibrillation or cardioversion when a life-threatening rhythm is detected. Most ICDs can pace as well as defibrillate. The patient is warned to avoid exposure to strong magnetic fields such as microwave towers, transformers and electrical transmitters, electrical generators, handheld security devices at airports, and arc welding equipment. The patient should not lean over the alternator of a running car or boat motor. A magnetic field will temporarily inactivate the device. Moving away from the magnetic source will restore normal function.

Radiofrequency catheter ablation. When drugs will not control supraventricular or ventricular tachydysrhythmia, the irritable focus can sometimes be destroyed with radiofrequency catheter **ablation**. Electrophysiologic studies are completed in a specialized cardiac catheterization laboratory to pinpoint the irritable focus. A specially trained health care provider then uses radiofrequency waves to destroy the irritable focus via heat and subsequent scarring. The procedure may affect the normal conduction system, requiring the implantation of a permanent pacemaker.

INFLAMMATORY AND INFECTIOUS DISEASES OF THE HEART

The tissues of the heart are subject to the same inflammatory conditions that affect other parts of the body. The inflammation may be present in the inner lining (**endocarditis**), the heart muscle (myocarditis), or the sac surrounding the heart (pericarditis). Inflammation may be from an infectious source or from a noninfectious cause.

INFECTIVE ENDOCARDITIS

Etiology

Infective endocarditis (IE) is an infection of the endocardial surface of the heart. It may affect the heart valves, the walls, or a septal defect in the heart. IE was formerly called *bacterial endocarditis (BE),* or *subacute bacterial endocarditis (SBE),* but it can be caused by organisms other than bacteria.

Infective endocarditis may be caused by bacteria, viruses, or fungi. Ports of entry are the oral cavity, particularly with dental procedures; the skin, from surgery or invasive procedures; and infections in the body. Intravenous drug use with unclean needles is a major cause of endocarditis. Patients with irregularity or injury to the endocardium are at risk for organisms sticking to the surface and growing. Rheumatic fever causes injury to the heart valves. The heart valves are covered by the endocardium.

Older Adult Care Points

Systemic infections of the respiratory tract, urinary tract, gastrointestinal tract, or skin often are the causes of endocarditis in older adults. The immune system function decreases with age, making older adults more susceptible to IE. Diagnosis is difficult because symptoms are usually vague. The aortic valve is most often affected.

Although antibiotics—particularly penicillin—have decreased the incidence of rheumatic fever, the danger is still present. Throat culture should be performed any time there is a question whether group A beta-hemolytic *Streptococcus* is the organism responsible for a sore throat. If the streptococcal infection is treated early with antibiotics, inflammation in the heart and heart valve injury is usually prevented.

Pathophysiology

The inflamed tissues of the heart become rough and swollen. The inflamed tissue traps organisms. The bacterial growth on the valves are called *vegetations.* Vegetations decrease the effectiveness of the valve. Damage to the valve from bacteria may require valve replacement. The mitral valve is the most common location of infection (Fig. 19.9). Arterial emboli may occur if pieces of the vegetation break off and travel. As mentioned previously, where an embolus lodges depends on the side of the heart from which it emerges: Emboli from the right side of the heart become pulmonary emboli; those from the left side of the heart usually go to the brain but can travel to other organs.

Signs, Symptoms, Diagnosis, and Treatment

The signs and symptoms of IE vary considerably. The sedimentation rate or C-reactive protein (CRP) and leukocyte count are elevated, and signs of low-grade intermittent fever are evident. A blood culture will be positive. The spleen becomes enlarged. Splinter

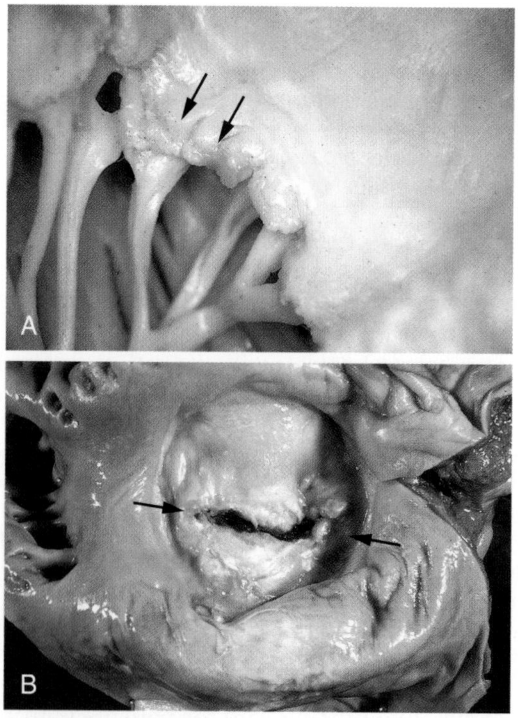

Fig. 19.9 A, Thickening and valve leaflet distortion from infection and inflammation of the endocardium. **B,** Mitral stenosis. (From Kumar V, Abbas A, Fausto N: *Robbins & Cotran's pathologic basis of disease,* ed 10, Philadelphia, 2018, Elsevier.)

hemorrhages (thin black lines) can occur under the nails, and there may be petechiae (pinpoint red spots) inside the mouth, in the conjunctivae, and above the clavicles. Echocardiography or transesophageal echocardiography (TEE) confirms the diagnosis. Fatigue, chills and sweats, malaise, anorexia, muscle aches, and headache may occur.

An existing cardiac murmur may worsen, or a new murmur may appear as a valve is damaged. Cardiac dysrhythmias may appear. There may be complaints of sharp, stabbing chest pain. Each instance of endocarditis further damages the heart valves. The scar tissue that occurs as the inflammation subsides may cause the valve to leak, resulting in regurgitation (lack of closure), or the valve leaflets may become thickened and calcified, causing narrowing or stenosis. The mitral and aortic valves are most commonly affected. When mitral or aortic stenosis or regurgitation causes symptoms sufficient to interfere with the patient's usual lifestyle, surgery becomes necessary. Stenosis and regurgitation of cardiac valves may eventually cause HF.

Older Adult Care Points

The valve leaflets thicken with age; this gives rise to the common systolic murmur heard in persons older than 80 years. This murmur does not indicate cardiac inflammation.

Treatment for IE is with antibiotics for 4 to 6 weeks for the underlying infection. NSAIDs are used to decrease inflammation. Pain medication is provided. Medications for dysrhythmia and HF are administered for those complications. Repair of congenital cardiac problems, such as atrial or ventricular septal defect, may be performed.

Safety Alert

Infective Endocarditis

Viridans streptococci, bacteria found in the mouth, are responsible for about 50% of cases of infective endocarditis. Regular dental care is very important. The health care provider should be advised of all cardiac history before any invasive procedure so that appropriate prophylactic treatment can be provided.

PERICARDITIS

Pericarditis is inflammation of the pericardium (the sac that encloses the heart). Pericarditis may be caused by cancer and its treatment, systemic connective tissue disease, infectious organisms, renal failure, trauma, or tissue damage from an MI. The serous fluids that typically are produced by inflammation may cause an **effusion** (accumulated fluid) in the pericardium. If the effusion becomes large, it presses on the ventricle, restricting filling, which can affect the cardiac output. Should the fluid become excessive, **cardiac tamponade** may occur as the fluid severely limits filling, resulting in little blood available to be pumped out of the heart (Fig. 19.10). If unresolved, the heart cannot supply the body with needed oxygen and nutrients, and death occurs.

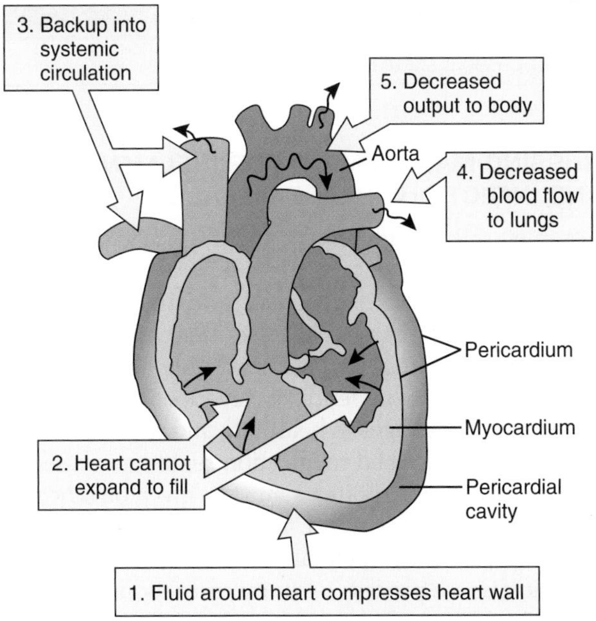

Fig. 19.10 Effects of pericardial effusion. (From Gould BE: *Pathophysiology for health professions*, ed 6, St. Louis, 2018, Elsevier.)

Symptoms of pericarditis include fever, tachycardia, chest pain eased by sitting up and leaning forward, dyspnea, and a pericardial **friction rub**. The rub is a high-pitched scratchy sound heard with the diaphragm of the stethoscope placed at the left sternal border at the third intercostal space. The ECG will show changes.

Dressler syndrome is pericarditis with effusion occurring from inflammation after an MI. It appears 1 to 12 weeks after infarct. When effusion is present, there may be malaise and fatigue related to decreased cardiac output and decreased perfusion of the tissues with oxygen. Assess for fever, muffled heart sounds, tachycardia, restlessness, anxiety and confusion, distended neck veins, and **pulsus paradoxus**—a drop in systolic blood pressure greater than 10 mm Hg on inspiration. This can be noted when measuring the blood pressure.

Diagnosis of pericarditis is made by history and physical examination and confirmed by ECG, echocardiogram, computed tomography (CT) scan or MRI, and laboratory studies of CRP, CBC, and erythrocyte sedimentation rate (ESR). **Pericardiocentesis** will be performed if effusion is interfering with cardiac output. The procedure may be done at the bedside or in a procedure room. The fluid extracted is analyzed to determine a cause of the inflammation. Restrictive pericarditis may be treated by **pericardiotomy** and creation of a window in the pericardium. Pain is controlled with medication.

Think Critically

Which patients should you watch for signs of pericarditis?

NURSING MANAGEMENT FOR INFLAMMATORY AND INFECTIOUS HEART DISEASE

Complete a thorough history and physical examination and document all data as a baseline assessment. Any abnormalities should be noted and included in the nursing care plan. Assess heart sounds carefully. Assess vital signs on a regular basis and note abnormalities. The patient may experience an elevation in temperature in addition to changes in heart rate and rhythm. Adherence to the prescribed medication regimen is essential to care. Ordered medications must be given on schedule. The teaching plan should include information about the drugs, as well as detailed information about the specific disease process. Activity restrictions are determined by patient tolerance. Make the patient as comfortable as possible and reinforce the rationale for the prescribed activity level. Oxygen administration may be required; discuss the importance of this treatment with the patient. Include evaluation of the patient's physical status, assessment of the patient's understanding of the home care requirements, and teaching related to medications and treatment in discharge planning. Home intravenous (IV) antibiotics may be required for weeks after discharge. Advise that prophylactic antibiotic therapy is necessary before dental procedures that involve gingival manipulation or bleeding. If the patient is at high risk for IE, prophylaxis may be needed before other invasive procedures.

Think Critically

Why is it important to assess a patient with IE for lung, brain, and abdominal organ abnormalities?

CARDIOMYOPATHY

Cardiomyopathy is a group of diseases that affect the structure or function of the heart. The risk of cardiomyopathy is increased in systemic hypertension, with chronic excessive alcohol intake, during pregnancy, and in those who have had a systemic infection. The heart enlarges and becomes an inefficient pump. There are three main types of cardiomyopathy: dilated, hypertrophic, and restrictive (Box 19.3).

The major problems exhibited by patients with cardiomyopathy are HF and dysrhythmias. Signs and symptoms of cardiomyopathy include dyspnea, activity intolerance, angina, dizziness, hypertension, and palpitations. Diagnosis is made through history and chest x-ray, cardiac catheterization, echocardiography, ECG, or MRI or CT scans. Medical treatment for cardiomyopathy includes drugs to increase contractility (such as digoxin), antihypertensive drugs, diuretics, antiarrhythmic drugs, and anticoagulants. Severe cardiomyopathy can be rapidly fatal. These patients are possible candidates for a heart transplant. Because of the possibility of cardiac arrest, families are taught CPR. In later stages, an LVAD may be used to rest the heart or as a bridge to heart transplantation. An LVAD can be external or can be implanted. The patient may have an ICD implanted.

Box 19.3 Three Main Types of Cardiomyopathy

DILATED

Characterized by extensive enlargement of the ventricles with impairment of contraction. Causes include chemotherapy, alcohol abuse, infection, inflammation, poor nutrition, and connective tissue disorders. Advances to heart failure.

HYPERTROPHIC

Increased growth of left ventricle muscle. May be hereditary as an autosomal dominant gene or be caused by hypertension or hypoparathyroidism. Sudden death may occur.

RESTRICTIVE

Stiffened ventricles prevent adequate relaxation after systole, affecting ventricular filling. Caused by systemic diseases such as amyloidosis or sarcoidosis. Progresses to right-sided heart failure. Is the least common of the three types of cardiomyopathy.

Heart transplantation is indicated when conventional treatments are no longer effective and the patient has a projected life span of 1 year or less. Transplants due to cardiomyopathy account for 99% of heart transplants. Any organ transplantation is coordinated through a regional office affiliated with The United Network of Organ Sharing (UNOS). UNOS is a private nonprofit organization contracted by the federal government to oversee the transplant system in the United States. It maintains wait lists and matches donors and recipients. Surgical procedures are done in approved regional medical centers. After surgery and recovery, patients return to their home communities. It is likely that the patient will be admitted to a facility in their community that is not a transplant center. You should understand that the patient will be taking multiple antirejection medications that will blunt the immune system, making them susceptible to infection. When the donor heart was transplanted, the normal nerve connections to the sympathetic and parasympathetic nervous systems were disrupted. The transplanted heart will not respond to medications targeted to these systems. If heart failure symptoms occur, they are most likely indicating rejection of the transplanted heart. Most rejection is identified by biopsy during routine checks prior to symptoms occurring. Heart transplantation is discussed further in Chapter 20.

CARDIAC VALVE DISORDERS

Mitral and aortic valve disorders are the most common cardiac valve disorders.Tricuspid and pulmonic valve

Clinical Cues

Takotsubo cardiomyopathy, also known as *broken heart syndrome* or *stress cardiomyopathy*, can occur abruptly in patients with no underlying cardiac disease. Signs and symptoms are similar to those for an acute MI, and it can be diagnosed only when a left heart catheterization is performed. No coronary blockages are found, the ejection fraction is reduced, and there is evidence of dysfunction of the left ventricle. The images obtained of the left ventricle show a shape similar to a Japanese ceramic octopus trap, a takotsubo. The dysfunction is believed to be caused by increases in circulating hormones such as adrenaline that are released with stress. Most patients recover without long-term consequences.

problems are rare. Tricuspid problems are usually from IV drug abuse or rheumatic fever. Pulmonic stenosis is congenital. In addition to congenital abnormalities, untreated hypertension, MI, and IE can cause cardiac valve disorders. The AHA published guidelines for valvular heart disease in 2014 with an update in 2017. Valve disorders are staged, and treatment recommendations are made according to the severity of the disease.

Mitral valve prolapse (MVP) occurs when the valve leaflets and tendonlike cords supporting the valve weaken and prolapse into the left atrium during systole. This is most often a benign condition. MVP is typically asymptomatic but can cause chest pain, palpitations, exercise intolerance, or fainting. A midsystolic click heard at the apex is characteristic of MVP.

MITRAL STENOSIS

Mitral stenosis is most commonly caused by rheumatic fever. This disorder is occurring less frequently as the incidence of rheumatic fever from Group A *Streptococcus* declines. Other causes are systemic lupus erythematosus, rheumatoid arthritis, and related conditions. Valve leaflet thickening and calcification cause stiffening. Left atrial pressure rises, and the left atrium dilates, causing backup pressure in the lungs. Pulmonary pressure increases, pulmonary congestion occurs, and over time the right ventricle hypertrophies.

The first symptom may be dyspnea on exertion. Paroxysmal nocturnal dyspnea (sudden dyspnea at night), palpitations of atrial fibrillation, and a dry cough may occur. If untreated, right-sided HF may eventually occur. Atrial fibrillation may be present. A diastolic murmur that is rumbling is heard on auscultation. Treatment is based on the stage of mitral stenosis identified by intracardiac pressures and clinical symptoms.

MITRAL REGURGITATION (INSUFFICIENCY)

Rheumatic heart disease is the main cause of mitral regurgitation. Papillary muscle rupture from ischemic heart disease, a congenital anomaly, and infective endocarditis are other causes. Fibrosis and calcification, other causes, or insufficiency prevent the valve from closing completely during systole. Backflow of blood into the left atrium occurs as the ventricle contracts. In diastole, the blood flows back into the left ventricle along with the normal blood flow. This increased volume must be ejected with the next contraction. The left ventricle and left atrium dilate and hypertrophy to accomplish the ejection. More women than men develop mitral regurgitation.

Symptoms take decades to emerge. Fatigue and weakness from reduced cardiac output are early signs. Dyspnea on exertion and orthopnea are later developments. There may be complaints of palpitations, anxiety, and atypical chest pain. Atrial fibrillation may occur. Right-sided HF causes jugular venous distention, hepatomegaly, and pitting edema. Auscultation at the apex reveals a high-pitched systolic murmur. A third heart sound occurs when regurgitation is severe.

AORTIC STENOSIS

Aortic stenosis is the most common valve disorder in the United States. Atherosclerosis with degenerative calcification of the valve is a common factor in older adults. Congenital valve malformations and rheumatic fever are causes in younger patients. The aortic valve opening narrows and obstructs left ventricular outflow during systole. The increased pressure required to eject the blood causes left ventricular hypertrophy. Eventually cardiac output is decreased to the point that the body's demands cannot be met during exertion. Systolic HF begins, and pulmonary congestion produces symptoms. When the pressure gradient across the valve is significantly increased and the ejection fraction decreases, aortic valve replacement is recommended (Nishimura et al., 2017).

Dyspnea, angina, and syncope on exertion are classic symptoms of aortic stenosis. Later, extreme fatigue, weakness, and peripheral cyanosis become apparent. A narrowed pulse pressure is found when blood pressure is measured. Auscultation reveals a systolic crescendo-decrescendo murmur.

Older Adult Care Points

Older adults with long-term hypertension are at risk for aortic stenosis because of increased atherosclerosis and stiffening of the aorta. Carefully assess the aortic valve sounds of older adult patients, especially if hypertension is not well controlled.

AORTIC REGURGITATION (INSUFFICIENCY)

Infective endocarditis, congenital abnormalities, long-term hypertension, and Marfan syndrome (a rare genetic connective tissue disease) are factors in aortic regurgitation. The valve leaflets do not close properly during diastole, allowing backflow of blood from the aorta into the left ventricle. The left ventricle dilates and hypertrophies from the greater blood volume.

Symptoms do not appear until left ventricular failure happens. Dyspnea on exertion, orthopnea, and paroxysmal nocturnal dyspnea begin. Nocturnal angina with diaphoresis and palpitations particularly when lying on the left side occur late in the disease. The pulse is bounding, and pulse pressure is widened with increased systolic pressure and decreased diastolic pressure. On auscultation there is a high-pitched, blowing diastolic decrescendo murmur.

TREATMENT OF VALVE DISORDERS

Treatment depends on the valve affected and the degree of impairment. Yearly monitoring and drug therapy for symptoms is standard when disease is not severe. Later, heart surgery for valve replacement may be needed. Newer techniques allow for an endovascular approach to some valve replacements or repair.

Medical Treatment

Diuretics, beta blockers, digoxin, and oxygen along with rest are used to improve symptoms of HF and dysrhythmias. Atrial fibrillation is corrected with drug therapy and/or cardioversion. If atrial fibrillation cannot be converted to a normal sinus rhythm, drugs such as diltiazem, metoprolol, or amiodarone will be administered to slow ventricular response rate. Patients with chronic atrial fibrillation are prescribed regular anticoagulant therapy. Medical treatment is not the treatment of choice. Interventional procedures are the only effective treatment for the problem.

Surgical Treatment

When valvular disease becomes severe, surgery is required to correct the problem. Reparative procedures are becoming more common. Balloon valvuloplasty is sometimes used to open stenosed valves. It is performed with a balloon-tipped catheter. The catheter is threaded via the femoral artery into the heart and to the diseased valve. The balloon is inflated to enlarge the opening, then is deflated and removed. However, it is questionable as to how long the valve will stay open. Often the stenosis recurs within 6 months.

Direct commissurotomy occurs during cardiopulmonary bypass with open heart surgery. Thrombi are removed from the atria, and the leaflets are incised, along with calcification debridement. This opens the valve orifice.

Mitral valve annuloplasty (reconstruction) is performed for acquired mitral regurgitation. The valve ring (annulus) that attaches to the leaflets and supports them is made smaller with sutures or tucks. Leaflets are repaired as well to provide good closure of the valve at systole.

Valve Replacement

Replacement may be performed as an open heart procedure with cardiopulmonary bypass or as minimally invasive surgery. Many mechanical (prosthetic) and biological (tissue) valves are available (Fig. 19.11). Mechanical valves require lifetime anticoagulation postoperatively because of the possibility of clot formation. Biological valves may be from a pig (porcine), from a cow (bovine), or from a human cadaver. Biological valves do not require postoperative anticoagulation therapy. Biological valves tend to wear out in about 15 years, requiring replacement. Mechanical valves are more durable. Bioprosthetic valves that use tissue for the leaflets and a manufactured supporting structure also can be used.

Transcatheter aortic valve replacement (TAVR) is an emerging technology that allows for replacement of the aortic valve via a percutaneous approach rather than a thoracotomy. A catheter is threaded from the groin (or other arterial access site) through the aorta to the aortic valve. A valvuloplasty is performed on the stenotic

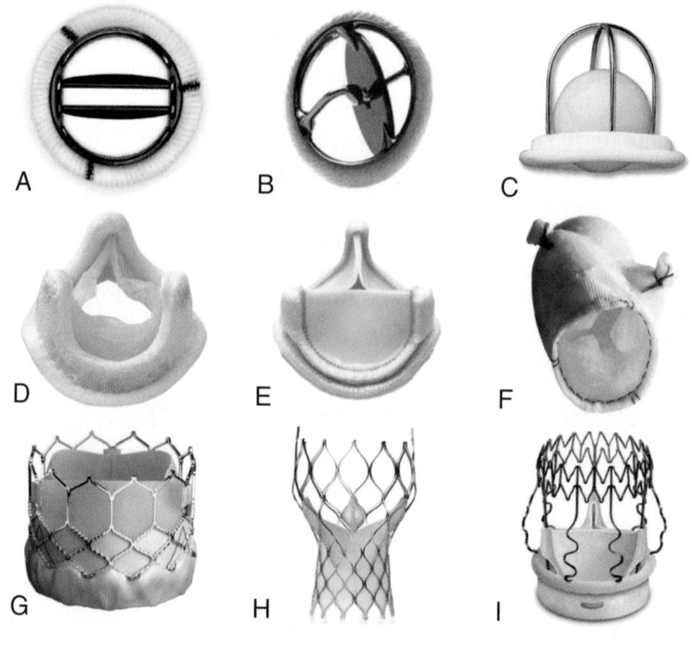

Fig. 19.11 Examples of mechanical and biological tissue valves for valve replacement. **A,** Bileaflet St. Jude mechanical valve. **B,** Monoleaflet Medtronic Hall mechanical valve. **C,** Caged-ball Starr-Edwards mechanical valve. **D,** Stented porcine Medtronic Mosaic bioprosthetic valve. **E,** Stented bovine pericardial Edwards Magna bioprosthetic valve. **F,** Stentless porcine Medtronic Freestyle bioprosthetic valve. **G,** Transcatheter balloon-expandable Edwards SAPIEN 3 bioprosthetic valve. **H,** Transcatheter self-expanding Medtronic CoreValve Evolut bioprosthetic valve. **I,** Sutureless Sorin Perceval bioprosthetic valve. (**A–E, G, H,** From Bonow RO, Mann DL, Zipes DP, et al.: *Braunwald's heart disease: a textbook of cardiovascular medicine*, ed 11, St. Louis, 2019, Elsevier. **F,** From Seeburger J, Weiss G, Borger MA, Mohr FW: Structural valve deterioration of a CoreValve prosthesis 9 months after implantation, *Eur Heart J* 34:1607, 2013. **I,** Courtesy LivaNova PLC/Sorin Group.)

valve. The replacement valve is then carefully positioned and deployed. The patient is sedated, and the procedure is performed in a hybrid operating room/catheterization laboratory suite.

Nursing Management for Cardiac Valve Disorders

The primary nursing goals for patients with cardiac valve disease are to maintain adequate cardiac output, to control dysrhythmias, and to prevent or control HF. Assessing the patient for signs of developing HF, teaching the patient about prescribed medications, and preparing the patient for surgical procedures should all be included in the nursing plan of care. See Chapter 17 for common problems and interventions for complications related to valve problems.

Valve surgery is most often an elective procedure. Preoperative and postoperative care is very similar to that of coronary artery bypass graft surgery (see Chapter 20). Patients taking anticoagulation drugs preoperatively must stop taking them about 72 hours before the procedure. Any needed dental work is obtained before the valve replacement to decrease the chance of infective endocarditis.

Patients with mitral stenosis may have pulmonary hypertension and stiff lungs. Postoperatively, respiratory status must be monitored very closely during weaning from the ventilator. Patients undergoing aortic valve replacement are at higher risk of postoperative hemorrhage. Be particularly alert for bleeding. Monitor cardiac output closely and watch for signs of HF. Fatigue is a common problem during convalescence. Rest and activity must be balanced carefully. For those with a mechanical valve, teach about the care needed when taking an anticoagulant.

COMMON THERAPIES AND THEIR NURSING IMPLICATIONS

The medical treatments most commonly used to manage heart disease include (1) oxygen therapy, (2) pharmacologic agents, (3) surgical and interventional procedures, and (4) dietary controls. Education and rehabilitation of the cardiac patient also must be included in the plan of care. Surgical treatment of cardiac conditions most often is used to correct structural defects of the heart and great vessels. Interventional procedures correct blockages, repair structures, or are for implantation of therapeutic devices.

OXYGEN THERAPY

Administering supplemental oxygen to relieve the dyspnea and hypoxemia of a cardiac patient is a routine therapeutic measure. Any patient experiencing chest pain is started on low-dose oxygen. Responsibilities regarding oxygen therapy for a cardiac patient are primarily concerned with observation to determine a patient's need for supplemental oxygen, maintenance of the ordered Spo_2, and the response to therapy once oxygen has been initiated. It is important to be alert for signs of changing oxygen needs, such as increased pulse rate and symptoms of cerebral anoxia, including irritability, confusion, and disorientation.

> **Clinical Cues**
>
> The patient's Po_2 should be maintained between 95% and 99%. If Po_2 falls lower than 93% consistently, notify the health care provider. Oxygen saturation by blood gas determination should be 94 to 100 mm Hg. Patients with a history of pulmonary disease such as emphysema may normally exhibit an oxygen saturation between 89% and 92%.

PHARMACOLOGIC AGENTS

Many types of drugs are used to treat heart disorders (see Tables 19.3 and 19.4). Digitalis in its various forms is used less frequently than in the past. However, it is a potent drug that can produce serious toxicity. **Classic symptoms of digitalis toxicity are yellow-green halos around lights, nausea, diarrhea, and confusion.** Digitalis can be very effective in treating certain kinds of cardiac disorders, but its therapeutic range is quite narrow. A therapeutic dose is only about one third less than the dose that will induce toxicity.

> **Clinical Cues**
>
> Some health care providers may not want a dose of digitalis held if the patient's pulse rate is below 60 bpm, as long as there are no signs of digitalis toxicity. If the pulse rate is less than 60, check the provider's order before administering the medication.

> **Think Critically**
>
> List four signs and symptoms that might indicate your patient is experiencing digitalis toxicity.

A wide array of medications is used to manage hypertension and related disorders. Most of the agents block some portion of the renin-angiotensin system, the effect being to prevent vasoconstriction. Diuretics are also indicated as a therapy for hypertension.

Antilipids are used to control the atherosclerotic process. Blood glucose management is necessary to prevent vascular damage. Nicotine patches are used to help patients with smoking cessation. They do deliver nicotine, so while the lung damage may be minimized, the effect of nicotine is still present.

Anticoagulants are prescribed to inhibit the formation of clots within blood vessels and the heart. Anticoagulants do not dissolve clots that have already formed, but they can prevent existing ones from growing larger and can interfere with the development of new clots. Long-term anticoagulant therapy is necessary for patients with chronic atrial fibrillation or mechanical valve replacement.

DIETARY CONTROL

The National Heart, Lung, and Blood Institute cites obesity as a risk factor for cardiac disorders. When obesity is present in conjunction with other factors, such as metabolic syndrome, hypertension, high cholesterol levels, diabetes mellitus, smoking, or family history of heart disease, the likelihood of cardiovascular problems is increased.

Many health professionals consider self-help groups to be most successful in assisting people to lose weight and then keep their weight within normal range once the excess is lost. These groups include Weight Watchers, TOPS (Take Off Pounds Sensibly), and Overeaters Anonymous. Studies have shown that the behavior modification techniques these groups use are very successful. To prevent heart disease and decrease the factors that predispose one to cardiovascular disease, the American Heart Association recommends several measures.

Health Promotion

Heart-Healthy Lifestyle Recommendations

- With daily activities plus exercise, use up as many calories as you consume. To calculate, multiply current weight by 15 if moderately active; if sedentary, multiply weight by 13.
- Follow a heart-healthy diet (see Nutrition Considerations: Guidelines for a Heart-Healthy Diet).
- Limit portion sizes to recommended amounts.
- Exercise with physical activity at least 30 minutes a day.
- Avoid inhaled smoke and smokeless tobacco products.

Increased fiber will lower cholesterol even without cutting down on dietary fat. Adults should consume about 35 g of fiber per day; the national average consumption is about 12 g. Increasing fiber in the diet also lowers the risk of cancer and helps with weight control by maintaining a feeling of fullness for longer.

Foods containing trans fat increase the cholesterol level, especially low-density lipoprotein. Patients should be taught to read food labels for the presence of trans fat. Many community hospitals sponsor weight management programs. Local chapters of the American Heart Association provide pamphlets and other sources of information about diet. AHA resources can also be found on the website at www.heart.org.

A high intake of sodium is believed to contribute to the development of high blood pressure. Limiting sodium intake is an important part of preventing and treating hypertension. Several cookbooks that make low-sodium, low-cholesterol meals easier to plan and prepare are sponsored by the AHA and organizations. The fact that the tendency to develop cardiovascular disease is familial gives the patient and the family good reason to develop good eating habits and to eat more heart-healthy foods.

Think Critically

How could you specifically change your eating habits in a way that would help you follow a more heart-healthy diet?

COMMUNITY CARE

Patients with infectious and inflammatory disease of the heart are sent home after a few days in the hospital. A home care nurse is usually assigned to supervise any ordered IV antibiotic infusion and to carefully assess the patient on a regular basis. The importance of taking prescribed NSAIDs for inflammation is discussed. A thorough heart and lung assessment is performed at every visit. You teach the patient or family how to infuse the antibiotics and how to care for the IV or peripherally inserted central catheter (PICC) line. The importance of tracking temperature daily is stressed. Signs and symptoms to report to the health care provider are reviewed, including new or increased chest pain, dysrhythmia, fatigue, shortness of breath, change in level of consciousness, sharp abdominal pain, or dependent edema. Assessment for signs and symptoms of adverse reactions is performed. Repeat blood cultures and CBCs are drawn at intervals to determine effectiveness of treatment.

Nurses in long-term care settings must be vigilant for beginning signs of HF because many older adult residents have had chronic hypertension, previous MIs, or previous episodes of HF. Whenever a resident has an infection, an increased demand is placed on the heart, and HF can develop quickly if the heart is already compromised. Episodes of vomiting or diarrhea or of dehydration cause electrolyte imbalances that can lead to dysrhythmias. Heart rates and rhythms should be monitored closely, and fluid and electrolyte replacement should begin early in the course of the illness.

Get Ready for the NCLEX® Examination!

Key Points

- HF is the inability of the heart to pump as it should, and pressure changes cause blood to back up into lungs and systemic circulation.
- Systolic HF is identified by an ejection fraction of 40% or less.
- Diastolic HF results when filling of the ventricles is impaired. A primary sign is jugular venous distention.
- Medical treatment of HF includes limited activity initially; oxygen therapy; medications such as ACE inhibitors or ARBs, digoxin, loop diuretics, and antihypertensive drugs; restricted sodium intake; and smoking cessation.

- Recording daily weight and keeping accurate intake and output records are essential.
- Assist the patient to maintain fluid restrictions as required.
- Disruption of normal SA node conduction leads to dysrhythmias; lack of normal regular myocardial contraction decreases cardiac output.
- Life-threatening dysrhythmias include ventricular tachycardia, ventricular fibrillation, pulseless electrical activity, and asystole.
- Dysrhythmias causing decreased cardiac output include severe bradycardia, atrial fibrillation, complete heart block, supraventricular tachycardia, and frequent PVCs.
- Dysrhythmias are diagnosed using 12-lead ECG, continuous ECG monitoring, patient history, and electrophysiologic testing.
- Failure of the heart's natural pacemaker may require an artificial pacemaker.
- Artificial pacing can be temporary or permanent, external, transvenous, or internal.
- ICDs may be used in patients with an episode of ventricular tachycardia or ventricular fibrillation or in those at risk for developing fatal arrhythmias.
- Inflammation of the heart may occur as endocarditis, myocarditis, or pericarditis.
- Medical treatment includes rest to reduce workload of the heart, antiinfective drugs to control infection, and surgery to replace or repair valves damaged by the inflammatory process.
- Severe cardiomyopathy is treated by heart transplant.
- Cardiac valve disorders are caused by congenital defect, rheumatic fever, endocarditis, or long-term hypertension.
- Valve disorders include stenosis and regurgitation (insufficiency).
- Valve disease, if left untreated, often progresses to HF.

Additional Learning Resources

SG Go to your Study Guide for additional learning activities to help you master this chapter content.

Go to your Evolve website (http://evolve.elsevier.com/deWit/medsurg) for the following FREE learning resources:

- Animations, audio, and video
- Answers and rationales for questions and activities
- Glossary with pronunciations in English and Spanish
- Interactive Review Questions and more!

Review Questions for the NCLEX® Examination

1. A nurse answers the call light of a patient admitted with HF. The patient states that they are short of breath and appears to be in distress. Identify the nursing actions in priority order.
   1. Apply supplemental oxygen.
   2. Raise the head of the bed.
   3. Notify the health care provider.
   4. Check vital signs.
   5. Listen to lung sounds.

   NCLEX Client Need: Physiological Integrity: Physiological Adaptation
2. A patient is admitted with a cardiac dysrhythmia. The morning laboratory values show potassium as 6.1 mg/dL. What action is most important to take first?
   1. Encourage intake of extra fluid.
   2. Notify the health care provider immediately.
   3. Check the breakfast tray for sodium-containing foods before serving.
   4. Check the patient's vital signs.

   NCLEX Client Need: Physiological Integrity: Physiological Adaptation
3. The delivery of a mild electrical shock at a specific time of the cardiac cycle to interrupt an abnormal rhythm and to possibly initiate a normal rhythm is which of the following?
   1. Synchronized cardioversion
   2. Defibrillation
   3. Pacemaker initiation
   4. Electrophysiology study

   NCLEX Client Need: Physiological Integrity: Reduction of Risk Potential
4. After pacemaker implantation, it is important to teach the patient to:
   1. stay away from microwave ovens.
   2. count their pulse regularly.
   3. refrain from swimming.
   4. use a safety razor to shave.

   NCLEX Client Need: Health Promotion and Maintenance
5. A 48-year-old patient is admitted for tachycardia, shortness of breath, and chest pain eased by sitting up and leaning forward. You auscultate a high-pitched scratchy sound at the left sternal border of the chest. The patient most likely has:
   1. heart failure.
   2. pericarditis.
   3. pneumonia.
   4. aortic stenosis.

   NCLEX Client Need: Physiological Integrity: Physiological Adaptation
6. Which assigned patient would take priority for immediate attention?
   1. A patient with infective endocarditis who has an antibiotic dose due
   2. A patient awaiting aortic stenosis surgery who is complaining of pain
   3. A patient with systolic HF whose weight is up 1.5 lb today
   4. A patient with dysrhythmia whose heart rate has dropped to 42 bpm and who is dizzy

   NCLEX Client Need: Safe and Effective Care Environment: Coordinated Care
7. A patient has HF and atherosclerosis. Which patient statement regarding healthy food choices demonstrates a need for further teaching?
   1. "I can have an egg two to three times per week."
   2. "I need to watch my red meat intake but can have all the cheese I want."
   3. "I should read labels to see how much sodium and fat a serving contains."
   4. "Canned goods are often high in sodium."

   NCLEX Client Need: Health Promotion and Maintenance

8. You explain the importance of reducing salt in the diet to a Hispanic man who was recently diagnosed with HF. The relatives are at the bedside with the patient. An appropriate nursing action would be to:
   1. involve the youngest male in the family to translate.
   2. ensure patient privacy by directing the relatives out of the patient's room.
   3. determine who does the cooking in the family.
   4. include all relatives in the diet teaching.

   NCLEX Client Need: Health Promotion and Maintenance
9. While discussing HF with a student, a nurse explains that the underlying weakness of the left ventricle results in reduced cardiac output and backup of fluid in the pulmonary system. The student nurse anticipates which sign or symptom?
   1. Edema in the sacrum, legs, feet, and ankles
   2. Hepatomegaly
   3. Crackles in the lungs
   4. Ascites

   NCLEX Client Need: Physiological Integrity: Physiological Adaptation
10. The patient asks you, "Why am I taking lisinopril (Zestril)?" An accurate response would be:
    1. "The medication increases the force of contraction of the heart."
    2. "The medication increases the heart rate."
    3. "The medication helps prevent vasoconstriction."
    4. "The medication causes excretion of extra fluid."

    NCLEX Client Need: Physiological Integrity: Pharmacological Therapies

Critical Thinking Questions

Scenario A

Mr. Jenkins, age 56 years, is admitted to the telemetry unit with a diagnosis of atrial fibrillation with RVR. Physical assessment reveals a restless, apprehensive man with an irregular heart rate of 155 bpm and dyspnea.

1. Describe the rhythm you expect to note on the telemetry monitor.
2. What treatment do you expect the health care provider to prescribe for Mr. Jenkins?
3. List five priority teaching points you should establish for Mr. Jenkins if he continues in atrial fibrillation.

Scenario B

Mr. Zulic, age 76 years, received a permanent pacemaker to correct complete heart block. He is 1 day postoperative and preparing for discharge home.

1. What are the indications for a pacemaker?
2. Describe the types of pacemakers and indications for their use.
3. Describe preoperative and postoperative nursing interventions when caring for a patient receiving a pacemaker.

Scenario C

Mr. Postma, age 72 years, is diagnosed with systolic heart failure. He has been experiencing fatigue and shortness of breath when walking the dog for 1 mile and has gained 5 lb over the past 2 weeks.

1. What stage of heart failure is Mr. Postma in? What symptoms does he have, supporting this stage?
2. What would you expect to be prescribed for him?
3. What topics should your teaching plan cover?

Care of Patients With Coronary Artery Disease and Cardiac Surgery

20

http://evolve.elsevier.com/deWit/medsurg

Objectives

Theory

1. Examine the risk factors for coronary artery disease.
2. Illustrate the pathophysiology of coronary artery disease.
3. Outline nursing interventions to care for a patient experiencing angina, including medication administration and patient teaching regarding diagnostic procedures.
4. Explain the pathophysiology of myocardial infarction.
5. Compare and contrast the symptoms of and care for stable angina with those of STEMI.
6. Develop a nursing care plan for a patient experiencing a myocardial infarction.
7. Relate the nursing care of a patient undergoing cardiac surgery.
8. Discuss five complications of cardiac surgery.

Clinical Practice

9. Develop a teaching plan for a patient with coronary artery disease.
10. Identify signs and symptoms that indicate a patient may be experiencing a myocardial infarct.
11. Administer medications to patients experiencing cardiac disorders.
12. Collaborate with other health care providers to care for patients after cardiac surgery.
13. Contribute to discharge planning for a patient after cardiac surgery.

Key Terms

angina pectoris (ăn-JĪ-nă PĔK-tŏr-ĭs, p. 464)
atherosclerosis (ăth-ĕr-ō-sklĕ-RŌ-sĭs, p. 463)
coronary artery bypass graft (CABG) (KŌR-ŏ-nār-ē AR-tĕr-ē BĪ-păs grăft, p. 476)
coronary insufficiency (KŎR-ō-nĕr-ē ĭn-să-FĬSH-ăn-sē, p. 464)
drug-eluting stent (drŭg e-LŪ-tĭng stĕnt, p. 477)
infarction (ĭn-FĂRK-shŭn, p. 471)
metabolic equivalent (MET) units (MĔT-ă-bŏl-ĭk ē-KWĬV-ă-lĕnt YŪ-nit, p. 476)
myocardial infarction (MI) (mī-ō-KĂR-dē-ăl ĭn-FĂRK-shŭn, p. 463)
necrosis (nē-KRŌ-sĭs, p. 464)

Concepts Covered in This Chapter

- Perfusion
- Clotting
- Inflammation
- Pain
- Anxiety
- Patient Education
- Health Promotion
- Collaboration

CORONARY ARTERY DISEASE

Coronary artery disease (CAD) is a progressive disease leading to narrowing or occlusion (blockage) of the coronary arteries. The coronary arteries are responsible for supplying oxygen and nutrition to the myocardium (see Chapter 17, Fig. 17.2). As the coronary vessel narrows, the patient may experience symptoms of ischemia, such as chest tightness and angina. When a sudden obstruction to blood flow through one or more major coronary arteries occurs and cuts off oxygen and nutrients to the cardiac cells, a **myocardial infarction (MI)** occurs. With rapid intervention, the amount of infarcted tissue can be limited.

ETIOLOGY

A major factor in the development of CAD is atherosclerosis, in which plaque containing cholesterol and lipids is laid down within the walls of the arteries as fatty streaks. Plaque can occur in the cerebral vessels, the aorta, and arteries other than the coronaries. Coronary arteries are smaller, and narrowing here produces symptoms sooner than in the larger vessels. **Atherosclerosis** is one form of arteriosclerosis. *Arteriosclerosis* is a general term for disorders that cause thickening and loss of elasticity of the arteries.

Factors such as age (older than 40 years), gender, and race contribute to the disease; however, these characteristics cannot be modified. Those who have had one or more immediate family members develop or die of CAD during middle age are considered at high risk for the disorder. Postmenopausal women and women who use oral contraceptives or hormone replacement therapy are at greater risk of CAD than are women outside these categories.

Cultural Considerations

Ethnicity and Coronary Artery Disease

The incidence of coronary artery disease is disproportionately higher in African Americans, especially African American males. Research continues to determine the etiology of this finding and the approaches to decrease the incidence. Ethnicity-based treatment of heart disease is also explored because research has demonstrated that some classifications of medications are more effective for persons of diverse ethnicity.

PATHOPHYSIOLOGY

The process of atherosclerosis begins during late childhood, when streaks or islands of fatty material are laid down on the inner walls of the arteries. Low-density lipoprotein (LDL) is the major contributing factor to the formation of this fatty material. Plaques accumulate, particularly where there has been irritation or inflammation of the blood vessel from smoking, hypertension, diabetes, or infection. Later, the plaques become fibrous as a result of inflammation and healing. The plaque area protrudes into the artery, decreasing the vessel's size (Fig. 20.1). Over time, the plaque begins to calcify, causing rigidity of the vessel wall. The further narrowing of the coronary arteries causes **coronary insufficiency** (decreased or insufficient blood flow). Obstruction occurs from this process and forms thrombosis. Arterial spasm may contribute to deficient blood flow and consequent heart muscle damage.

Older Adult Care Points

Compared with the coronary blood flow in a 25-year-old, coronary blood flow in a 60-year-old is decreased. Older adults have less cardiac reserve, meaning that any added oxygen demands may compromise the coronary circulation and the heart's ability to pump properly.

There is a proven link between hyperlipidemia or high levels of LDL and triglycerides and atherosclerosis. High levels of homocysteine and episodes of inflammation causing an elevated level of C-reactive protein (CRP) are also factors in the development of atherosclerosis.

As CAD progresses, the coronary vessels become narrower, decreasing blood supply to the myocardium. This can result in **angina pectoris** (chest pain), which is a problem with supply and demand. The narrowed vessels cannot provide enough oxygenated blood to meet the needs of the muscle. When plaque areas rupture, the rough edges cause platelet clumping and clotting (thrombosis). When the blockages occur in the very small arteries that branch out from the coronary arteries, it is called *microvascular disease (MVD)*; this is more common in women (American Heart Association [AHA], 2017). This lack of blood supply leads to ischemia and eventually **necrosis** (cell death) of the myocardium (MI). If significant loss of muscle tissue occurs, the heart muscle is unable to pump effectively, and cardiac output is reduced. Cardiac dysrhythmias and death may occur if medical intervention is not obtained.

Box 20.1 Signs and Symptoms of Coronary Artery Disease

- Chest discomfort, including feeling of tightness, aching, burning
- Chest pain (angina pectoris) radiating to the arm, jaw, or back
- Dyspnea (shortness of breath)
- Palpitations or tachycardia
- Nausea and vomiting
- Undue fatigue (particularly in women)
- Weakness and inability to complete usual activities without chest pain or dyspnea

SIGNS AND SYMPTOMS

Signs and symptoms of CAD are related to the lack of oxygen supply to the myocardium and the inability of the heart to pump blood effectively to oxygenate tissues and cells (Box 20.1). Angina pectoris, acute coronary syndrome (ACS), or sudden cardiac death may occur.

Classic signs of angina in men include chest discomfort that may be described as pressure, heaviness, or squeezing. The pain is located in the midchest area and may radiate to the neck, jaw, or arm. Women may state that they feel short of breath or nauseated or have vomiting or abdominal pain. The chest pain present may be described as a sharp pain (Fig. 20.2).

DIAGNOSIS

Diagnosis of CAD is accomplished through tests such as electrocardiogram (ECG), echocardiogram, cardiac stress test, cardiac angiography (cardiac catheterization), computed tomography (CT) angiogram, or magnetic resonance angiogram. Laboratory testing for risk factors includes lipid panel, blood glucose, and hemoglobin A_{1c} (HbA_{1c}).

TREATMENT

A low-fat diet, weight control, and exercise are prescribed to lower cholesterol and total lipids (Fleming et al., 2016). If elevated cholesterol and triglyceride levels cannot be lowered by a low-fat diet and exercise, lipid-lowering drugs are prescribed (Table 20.1). These medications are not effective alone and may not reduce cholesterol levels to the point of eliminating the risk for CAD. Several herbs and supplements have shown the ability to lower cholesterol. Advise patients to consult with their health care provider before taking over-the-counter medications or herbs.

NURSING MANAGEMENT

Patients should be encouraged to adopt a healthy lifestyle, including exercise and a diet low in saturated fat. Obtain a referral to a dietitian and assist the patient

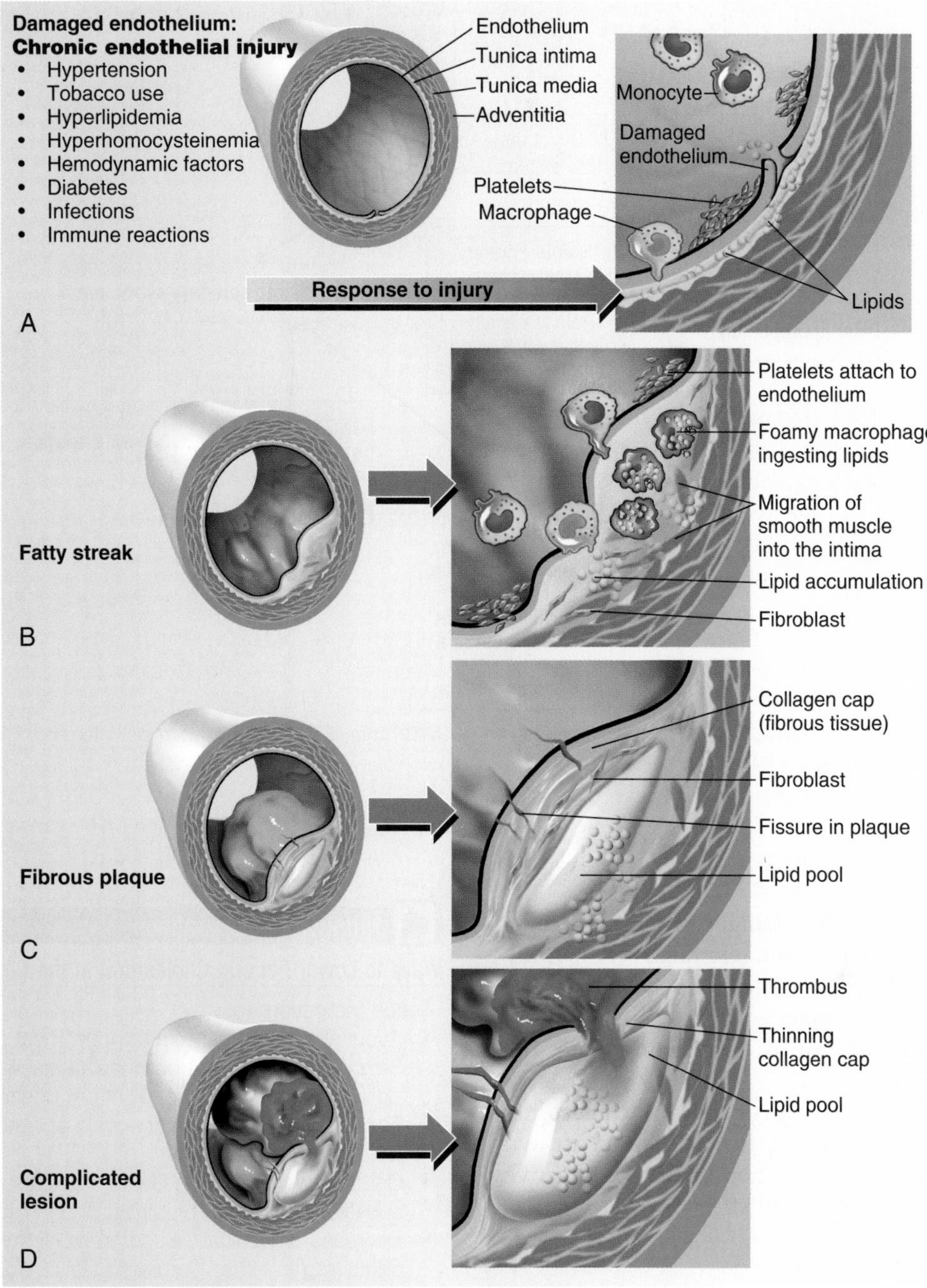

Fig. 20.1 Progression of atherosclerosis. **A,** Damaged endothelium. **B,** Fatty streak and lipid core formation. **C,** Fibrous plaque (raised plaques are visible: some are yellow; others are white). **D,** Complicated lesion (thrombus is red; collagen is blue). (From McCance KL, Huether SE, Brashers VL, Rote NS: *Pathophysiology: the biologic basis for disease in adults and children,* ed 8, St. Louis, 2019, Elsevier.)

Complementary and Alternative Therapies

Herbs and Supplements That Naturally Lower Cholesterol

The following have been found to lower cholesterol in patients with hyperlipidemia:

- Garlic
- Omega-3 fatty acids
- Red rice yeast
- Milk thistle
- Fiber
- Phytosterols
- Soy
- Coenzyme Q_{10}

Patients who choose to use these substances should check for interactions with other medications they are taking. Some of the substances only lower cholesterol and LDL; others raise high-density lipoprotein (HDL). Management of hypertension and blood glucose levels is also important because they contribute to CAD development.

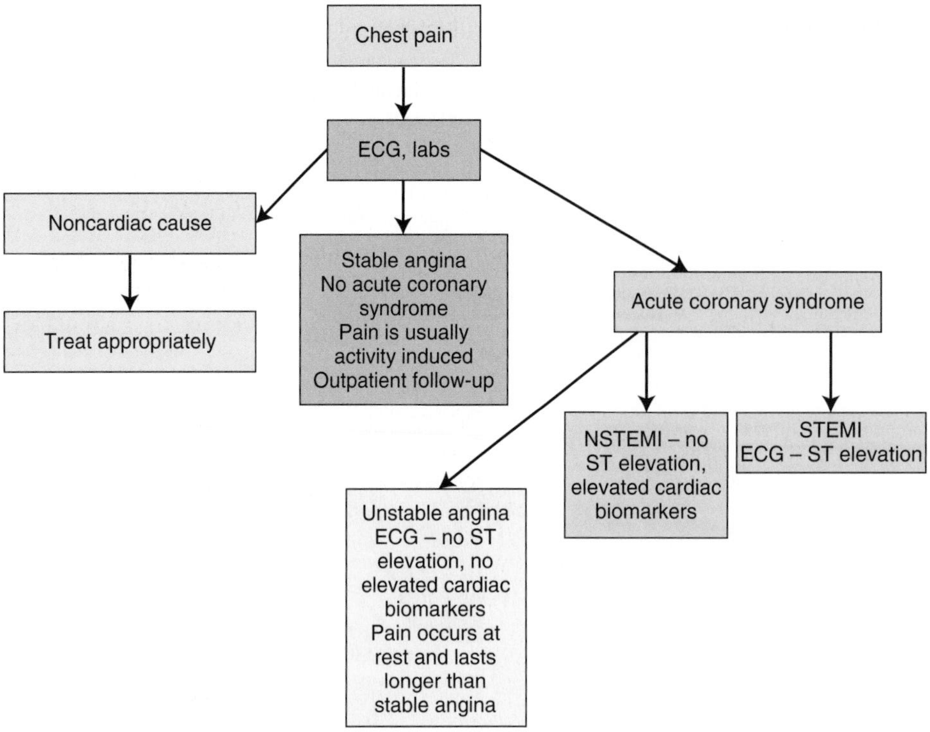

Fig. 20.2 Chest pain diagnosis. *ECG,* Electrocardiogram; *NSTEMI,* non–ST-elevation myocardial infarction; *STEMI,* ST-elevation myocardial infarction.

by reinforcing the need for changes in dietary habits. A cardiac rehabilitation program referral is very helpful. The program will help the patient choose an exercise regimen that they can manage over the long term. Emphasize the importance of maintaining a normal body weight.

If the patient is on a statin drug to lower cholesterol, remind them that they need to have blood drawn periodically to determine whether the drug is effective and to monitor for serious side effects.

ANGINA PECTORIS

Angina pectoris (chest pain) occurs when blood supply to the heart is decreased and need is increased. The ischemia (inadequate blood and oxygen supply) of the heart tissue causes pain. Angina may be caused by vessel narrowing due to atherosclerosis or arterial spasm (sudden constriction). Any activity that increases the heart's workload increases its need for oxygen. When the narrowed coronary arteries cannot deliver adequate amounts of blood to meet normal needs, the patient experiences an angina attack.

Signs, Symptoms, and Diagnosis

Anginal pain or discomfort may vary in individuals, but in most cases it is described as a dull pressure or ache under the sternum or pain that radiates to the neck or jaw. The pain may also radiate down one or both arms. Angina sensation is seldom sharp or stabbing. The feeling may be described as suffocating. The pain

Nutrition Considerations

Ways to Lower Fat and Cholesterol in the Diet

Teach the patient to:

- Avoid all fried foods; trim fat from meat and stick to 3-oz portions of meat per meal (a piece the size of a deck of cards). Remove skin from poultry.
- Eat fish with omega-3 fatty acids at least twice a week (salmon, mackerel, tuna).
- Use egg whites or Egg Beaters as cholesterol-free egg substitutes, both for breakfast and in recipes.
- Decrease or eliminate all commercial baked goods containing trans fat, saturated fat, or high levels of fat. Check the labels. Pies, doughnuts, croissants, and pastries are very high in fat.
- Use unsaturated fats for home baking and cooking. Avoid palm oil, coconut oil, lard, bacon fat, and hydrogenated vegetable shortening. Use olive oil whenever possible in salad dressings and for cooking. Do not use cube margarine that contains trans fats.
- Microwave bacon on paper towels to decrease the amount of fat; use turkey bacon rather than pork bacon.
- Check the amount of fat in cheeses and choose the lower-fat varieties. Eat only small amounts of cheese.
- Drink nonfat milk and use a nondairy, no-cholesterol creamer if you must have creamer in your coffee.
- Decrease the use of all dairy products and use only the low-fat or nonfat varieties.
- Eat more high-fiber whole grains, fruits, and vegetables.

Table 20.1 Drugs Commonly Used to Treat Hypercholesterolemia

DRUG	ACTION	COMMON SIDE EFFECTS	NURSING INTERVENTIONS
Bile Acid Sequestrants			
Cholestyramine (Questran, Locholest, Prevalite) Colestipol (Colestid) Colesevelam (Welchol)	Bind bile acid in the GI tract, resulting in decreased absorption of cholesterol	Abdominal pain, constipation, nausea. Because the medications decrease the reabsorption of bile acids, they can decrease the absorption of some medications.	Instruct patient to take before meals. Instruct to mix with 4–6 oz liquid. Advise drug may cause constipation and to increase fluid intake if not contraindicated. May need stool softeners. Counsel patient to continue low-fat diet and exercise. Take 4 h before or after other medications.
Fibric Acid Derivatives			
Gemfibrozil (Lopid) Clofibrate (Atromid) Fenofibrate (Tricor, Antara, Lipofen, Triglide, Trilipix) Lovaza	Reduce triglyceride production by the liver	Abdominal pain, diarrhea, epigastric pain. Can cause muscle toxicity if used with some statins. Interferes with metabolism of warfarin. Warfarin dose should be decreased.	Encourage to keep appointments for follow-up laboratory studies. Encourage to notify health care provider if symptoms of side effects occur.
HMG-CoA Reductase Inhibitors (Statins)			
Atorvastatin (Lipitor) Lovastatin (Mevacor) Fluvastatin (Lescol) Simvastatin (Zocor) Rosuvastatin (Crestor) Pitavastatin (Livalo) Pravastatin (Pravachol)	Inhibit the enzyme HMG-CoA reductase, which is responsible for synthesis of cholesterol	Abdominal pain, constipation, diarrhea, flatus, heartburn, rash	Teach to notify provider if severe muscle pain and weakness occur. Encourage to keep follow-up appointments and have periodic laboratory work performed. Pregnancy category X. Advise female patients to notify provider immediately if pregnancy is suspected. Notify provider of alcohol intake. May be at risk for liver disease. Do not drink grapefruit juice while on some statins.
Cholesterol Absorption Inhibitor			
Ezetimibe (Zetia)	Inhibit intestinal absorption of cholesterol	Possible headache and mild GI distress; infrequent	Can be used along with other antilipemics. Do not use for those with active liver disease. Take bile acid sequestrant 2 h before or 4 h after this drug. Obtain periodic lipid levels and liver function enzymes.
Niacin: Contains Nicotinic Acid			
Niacin (Nicobid, Nicotinex, Niacor, Slo-Niacin, Novo-Niacin)	Inhibit formation and secretion of VLDL and LDL	Flushing and itching of face and upper body, nausea and vomiting, indigestion, orthostatic hypotension	Monitor liver function when patient is taking high doses. Instruct to take aspirin or NSAID 30–60 min before dose to decrease flushing. Take niacin with food. Increase folic acid intake if homocysteine levels rise.
PCSK9 Inhibitors: Monoclonal Antibodies			
Alirocumab (Praluent) Evolocumab (Repatha)	Decreases the degradation of LDL receptors.	The medication is injected subcutaneously weekly or monthly based on the specific preparation. Injection site irritation, swelling, and itching may occur.	Drug companies are investigating oral compounds of these medications.

GI, Gastrointestinal; *HMG-CoA,* 3-hydroxy-3-methylglutaryl coenzyme A; *LDL,* low-density lipoprotein; *NSAID,* nonsteroidal antiinflammatory drug; *PCSK9,* proprotein convertase subtilisin/kexin type 9; *VLDL,* very low–density lipoprotein.

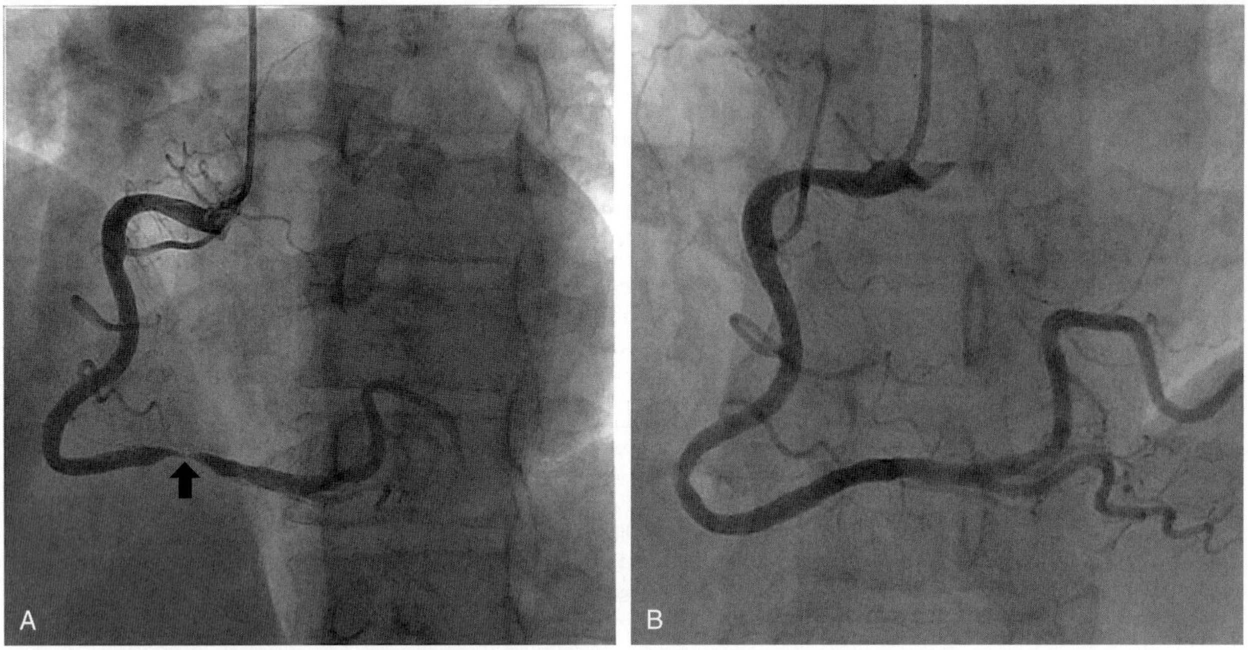

Fig. 20.3 **A,** Stenosis *(arrow)* of the right coronary artery. **B,** Right coronary artery with stent in place. (From Holte E, Vegsundvåg J, Wiseth R: Direct visualization of a significant stenosis of the right coronary artery by transthoracic echocardiography: a case report, *Cardiovasc Ultrasound* 5:33, 2007.)

Clinical Cues

- Because statins can injure muscle tissue and are toxic to the liver in some patients, blood should be drawn for levels of creatinine kinase (CK; an enzyme released from damaged muscle) and for liver enzymes. Elevated liver enzymes may indicate toxic damage to the liver.
- Patients should be told to report any unexplained muscle tenderness or pain persisting for more than a few days. When a statin drug is started, baseline blood values should be obtained before therapy. Laboratory tests for liver enzymes are recommended at the start of therapy and only when clinically indicated. Grapefruit juice should not be consumed when taking a statin drug. Grapefruit juice interferes with the metabolism of the drug, which can lead to increased serum levels and risk of toxicity (U.S. Food and Drug Administration [FDA], 2017).

can occur between the shoulder blades. In women, there may be no chest pain but just a tenderness to touch or a burning or tingling sensation. Patients may think they are experiencing indigestion or esophageal reflux. Shortness of breath without chest discomfort may also occur.

Stable coronary artery disease (SCAD) (formerly called stable angina) can be induced by stressors such as exercise or emotion. It can also occur spontaneously. Coronary artery disease is an ongoing process unless interrupted by change in lifestyle and medications. Although stages of the disease have had various labels, the symptoms exhibited are not a true reflection of the underlying pathology. Any patient exhibiting angina symptoms should be evaluated by a health care provider.

Medical diagnosis is established based on history, clinical signs and symptoms, and diagnostic testing. Response of the heart muscle to increased oxygen demands can be determined by exercise stress testing in a stable patient. If noninvasive testing is positive, cardiac catheterization with coronary angiography may be performed (Fig. 20.3). Echocardiography may be ordered to rule out a valve disorder or to evaluate left ventricular function. Laboratory levels of blood lipids will be tested, and cardiac enzymes may be ordered to rule out an MI. An electrocardiogram is a standard diagnostic procedure.

Treatment

The treatment of SCAD is mostly symptomatic, with emphasis on eliminating those factors that are known to precipitate an attack in the individual patient. With guidance and teaching, the patient may soon be able to correlate certain activities with an attack and thereby learn to avoid one whenever possible. Nitroglycerin, nitrates, calcium antagonists, and beta blockers are used in combination with drugs to lower cholesterol and prevent platelet aggregation. A low daily dose of aspirin (81 mg up to 325 mg) or other antiplatelet medication such as clopidogrel (Plavix) may be prescribed for the treatment of SCAD. Antiplatelet medications help prevent clotting and may prevent a thrombus that could cause an MI. Nitroglycerin administered sublingually is the most common drug for treatment of angina. An aerosol spray and a buccal form of the drug are also available.

Nursing Management

Collect data that assist in determining the type of angina the patient is experiencing. Patients with a history of angina may experience increased episodes when exposed to very cold environments. Externally cold temperatures result in vasoconstriction. The patient should be instructed to wear warm clothing when exposed to cold and may consider remaining indoors when the weather is extremely chilly. Nursing interventions for selected problems related to SCAD are summarized in Nursing Care Plan 20.1.

Nursing Care Plan 20.1 Care of the Patient With Angina

SCENARIO

Mrs. Ralston, age 63 years, came to the emergency department with shortness of breath and chest pain. She is admitted to the telemetry unit for unstable angina and evaluation of cardiac status. Cardiac enzymes are negative for myocardial infarction (MI). She has a history of chest pain and dyspnea precipitated by physical or emotional exertion. Her body mass index (BMI) is 30, and she has a history of smoking two packs of cigarettes per day for 40 years.

PROBLEM STATEMENT/NURSING DIAGNOSIS

Acute pain due to cardiac ischemia.

SUPPORTING ASSESSMENT DATA

Subjective: States she took five nitroglycerin tablets before admission with no relief of chest pain.

Objective: BP 100/70, HR 90, R 26. O_2 sat 92% on 5 L oxygen via nasal cannula.

Goals/Expected Outcomes	Nursing Interventions	Selected Rationale	Evaluation
Pain will be relieved within 15 min.	Assess level and duration of angina.	Determine severity of pain and need for additional intervention.	Pain relieved after two nitroglycerin tablets 5 min apart.
	Teach to notify nurse and lie down and rest when pain occurs.	Early intervention for pain relief and assessment of change in condition.	Nurse notified within 5 min of onset of pain.
	Assess vital signs during episodes of angina and medication administration.	Recognize side effects such as hypotension and patient's response to treatment.	Blood pressure maintained within 4 mm Hg of level at beginning of episode.
	Apply oxygen to maintain O_2 saturation greater than 95%.	Increases available oxygen to cardiac muscle.	Saturation 96% on 3 L nasal cannula oxygen.

PROBLEM STATEMENT/NURSING DIAGNOSIS

Anxiety related to diagnostic tests and recurrent chest pain.

SUPPORTING ASSESSMENT DATA

Subjective: Asks, "Are you sure I didn't have a heart attack this time?"

Objective: Scheduled for cardiac catheterization in the A.M.

Goals/Expected Outcomes	Nursing Interventions	Selected Rationale	Evaluation
Patient will verbalize that anxiety has decreased within 12 h.	Assess level of anxiety. Administer medication if appropriate.	Increased anxiety can precipitate episodes of angina.	States is less anxious.
	Allow patient opportunity to express concerns.	Active listening will help reduce patient's anxiety.	Patient verbalized fear of dying from heart attack or complications of procedures.
Patient will verbalize understanding of cardiac catheterization.	Provide information related to cardiac catheterization.	Adults desire straightforward information concerning their medical status.	Verbalized understanding of procedure. Some anxiety.
	Answer questions or refer to appropriate health care provider as needed.	Provides level of control for decision making.	Encouraged to write down a list of questions for the provider. Seemed more relaxed that she had a plan.

PROBLEM STATEMENT/NURSING DIAGNOSIS

Insufficient knowledge regarding effect of diet on medical condition or methods to improve cardiac health.

SUPPORTING ASSESSMENT DATA

Subjective: "I just can't exercise, and I don't understand how to choose and cook foods without salt or frying."

Objective: Wt. 195 lb, elevated cholesterol, resting HR 98.

Continued

Nursing Care Plan 20.1 Care of the Patient With Angina—cont'd

Goals/Expected Outcomes	Nursing Interventions	Selected Rationale	Evaluation
By discharge, patient will be able to verbalize how to choose foods that are low in fat and sodium.	Assess current knowledge of food content and reading food labels.	Provides starting point for teaching.	Patient able to choose low-fat and low-sodium foods from a menu list.
	Refer for outpatient dietitian consult.	Expert knowledge of dietitian needed to determine caloric needs and develop nutrition plan.	States has dietitian consultation appointment.
	Print out patient education materials on appropriate food choices.	Patient can read and have a knowledge base for meeting with dietitian.	States she is willing to learn and will look over the materials.
Patient will establish regular exercise program. Patient will learn a new method of stress reduction.	Determine whether patient is candidate for cardiac rehabilitation program. Make referral after collaboration with provider.	Provide structured, monitored exercise program that also includes dietary and emotional counseling.	States she will consider participation in a cardiac rehabilitation program if funds are available.
	Refer to social services for assistance with financial concerns.	Social workers can assist with financial resources.	Contacted social services for consultation.
	Collaborate with patient and provider about evaluation of emotional status that may interfere with ability to remain compliant.	Stress reduction will help her cardiac status as well as allow her to focus on maintaining her exercise program.	Patient states that she will use meditation to help calm herself down so she can participate fully in her treatment plan.

PROBLEM STATEMENT/NURSING DIAGNOSIS

Inadequate health maintenance due to continued cigarette smoking.

SUPPORTING ASSESSMENT DATA

Subjective: "I have tried to quit smoking, but it just doesn't work."

Goals/Expected Outcomes	Nursing Interventions	Selected Rationale	Evaluation
Patient will agree to enter a community smoking cessation program.	Assess willingness to reduce amount of or stop smoking.	Patient must be internally motivated for optimal success.	Patient states she has tried many times to stop smoking with limited success.
	Provide nicotine patch while in the hospital.	Hospitals are nonsmoking facilities. The patch will help reduce craving for nicotine.	Since she has not been able to smoke since admission, she states that she has a good start this time and maybe can be successful.
	Teach complications related to heart disease and smoking.	Provide understanding of roles of smoking and vasoconstriction that lead to episodes of angina.	States she understands need to quit smoking and the effect smoking has on her health.
	Refer to social services for community programs available; give a smoking cessation packet of information.	Social services personnel are aware of community resources that can benefit patient care.	Identified smoking cessation program within patient's neighborhood in nearby church. Patient states she will contact program before discharge.

CRITICAL THINKING QUESTIONS

1. What are five risk factors for coronary artery disease? What are the related complications?
2. Provide a teaching plan for a patient with angina. Include commonly used medications and side effects.
3. What is the most commonly used medication for angina or chest pain? How should it be administered?
4. What information about Mrs. Ralston's living situation would be helpful to know?

Clinical Cues

Sublingual nitroglycerin tablets should be kept in a cool, dark place and should be carried by the patient at all times. Patients should frequently check the expiration date on the bottle and replace the nitroglycerin tablets accordingly. If the mouth is dry, a sip of water should be taken before placing the tablet under the tongue. If possible, the patient should lie down when using nitroglycerin. After taking the first dose, if the pain has not subsided, emergency services should be contacted. In the hospital, a baseline blood pressure (BP) should be measured, a tablet given, and then the pressure should be checked again in 5 minutes. If the pain has not eased or the pressure has risen, another tablet is placed under the tongue. Check the BP again in 5 minutes. It will likely decrease. If the BP has not decreased significantly and if the pain is still present, administer a third sublingual tablet. Notify the health care provider immediately if the pain worsens or does not resolve after the three tablets. If oxygen is available, administer it according to hospital policy while waiting for communication from the provider.

ACUTE CORONARY SYNDROME AND MYOCARDIAL INFARCTION

If ischemia is prolonged and not quickly reversed, acute coronary syndrome (ACS) occurs. ACS includes unstable angina, non–ST-elevation myocardial infarction (NSTEMI), and ST-elevation myocardial infarction (STEMI). All patients with heart disease should be taught the signs of MI and be advised that the best survival rate is directly related to obtaining medical attention as quickly as possible. About 720,000 Americans experience an MI annually and 114,023 die from MI. The incidence of heart disease, including MI, continues to rise among women. Women are more likely to experience heart attacks after reaching menopause; however, poor dietary habits, sedentary lifestyle, and increased levels of stress contribute to the development of cardiovascular disease earlier in life for an increasing number of women.

Etiology and Pathophysiology

An MI is usually caused by thrombosis resulting from a ruptured atherosclerotic plaque. Sustained arterial spasm can also produce angina pain or even MI. Tissue ischemia occurs when oxygenated blood is not supplied to tissues (usually causing chest pain), and tissue death occurs when blood flow is stopped for a prolonged period.

An **infarction** is an area of necrosis in tissue caused by an obstruction to the flow of blood to that area for a prolonged period (Fig. 20.4). In an MI, there is an area of necrosis (cell death) in the heart muscle. That portion of the heart muscle cannot contract normally to help pump blood out of the heart. Dead tissue does not return to normal, and scar tissue forms and interferes with the normal functions of pumping and electrical conduction. The prognosis for patients who experience an acute MI depends on the location and the amount of heart tissue that is damaged. If a large area of the heart is affected, instant death may occur. Smaller ischemic areas may heal if treated promptly and effectively. As the coronary vessels narrow over time, small blood vessels are formed

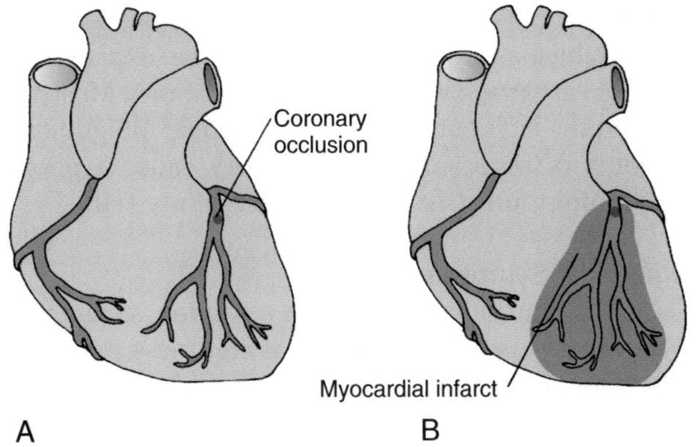

Fig. 20.4 **(A)** Occlusion of a major coronary artery leads to **(B)** area of infarct resulting from ischemia.

Patient Teaching

Guidelines for Patients With Angina

Patients who experience anginal attacks are taught to:

- Avoid eating heavy meals.
- Avoid physical activity for an hour after meals to prevent excessive oxygen demands.
- Take nitroglycerin before heavy physical activity that is known to cause an attack, such as intercourse or sports activities.
- Avoid exposure to cold; do not walk into a cold wind.
- Decrease controllable risk factors, such as lifestyle stress, obesity, hypertension, and improper diet.
- Adopt a graduated exercise program.
- Stop smoking.
- Learn meditation or other deep relaxation techniques.
- Take a sublingual nitroglycerin tablet and lie down at the beginning of an anginal attack. Make certain that the tablet produces a tingling sensation where it contacts the mucous membrane. If the pain does not ease or go away after the first dose, call 911. Nitroglycerin may be repeated twice more at 5-minute intervals for a total of three tablets if the pain persists.
- Check the pulse rate once daily if taking a calcium channel blocker or a beta-adrenergic blocker. These drugs should never be stopped abruptly; call the health care provider if the heart rate drops below 60 beats per minute.
- Rise slowly from a supine or sitting position because of potential postural hypotension.
- Cleanse area of previous application of nitroglycerin patch when applying a new dose.
- Keep appointments for regular checkups.
- Obtain sufficient rest daily.
- Avoid high environmental temperatures and high humidity; stay in air-conditioned areas when such conditions occur because they increase cardiac workload.
- Nitrates may initially cause a headache and hypotension.

that supply oxygen to the myocardium. A patient with a well-established collateral circulation may experience a milder heart attack with fewer complications. Most MIs occur in the left ventricle, the main "pump." Significant amounts of myocardial tissue injury cause a poorly functioning pump, leading to heart failure (HF).

Signs and Symptoms

Classically, during an MI there is a sudden, severe pain in the chest, usually described as tightness, pressure, squeezing, or crushing, that is not relieved by nitrates or rest. The patient also shows symptoms of dyspnea; nausea with or without vomiting; wheezing; and ashen, clammy, cool skin. Signs of shock with pallor, profuse sweating, and anxiety may occur. The heart rate may be very fast (tachycardia) or very slow (bradycardia), or the pulse may be irregular. In older adults, the attack may manifest as fatigue, syncope (temporary loss of consciousness), or weakness. Women often complain of recent episodes of extreme fatigue, with inability to complete daily activities without prolonged rest periods. These episodes may be accompanied by chest pressure, followed by eventual return to a full energy state. Feelings of "indigestion" are common. **Women tend to present with atypical symptoms such as sharp pain, fatigue, and weakness during an MI.** Denial is a significant factor in not seeking quick treatment and can lead to increased heart damage (Zafari, 2018).

Although these symptoms are usually present in an acute MI, they are not always severe, and in some cases patients have described their pain as mild. Sometimes the patient only experiences pain in the left arm, jaw, or back. Some people experience a "silent" MI, in which no symptoms are perceived. **It is paramount for the patient to seek quick medical attention when experiencing any new onset of chest pain.** The window of time to prevent significant myocardial damage is narrow (about 6 hours), and the sooner medical treatment is started for an MI, the greater the chance of saving myocardium and preserving life.

Older Adult Care Points

Older adult patients may never complain of chest pain when having an MI. Associated symptoms such as indigestion, nausea, dyspnea, and confusion are more common complaints.

Diagnosis

An ECG will be performed promptly when a patient is having symptoms that could indicate ACS. STEMI or NSTEMI will be ruled in or ruled out based on the ECG. Changes occur in the QRS complex, ST segment, and T wave when ischemia or damaged tissue occurs. A chest x-ray will rule out other possible causes of the symptoms, such as a thoracic aortic aneurysm. When there is necrotic tissue anywhere in the body, the white blood cell count increases and the sedimentation rate rises. Within 24 hours of an acute attack, the temperature of the patient with MI rises slightly, and mild leukocytosis appears.

In addition to the clinical manifestations, ECG changes, and other diagnostic tests, laboratory determinations of specific enzymes are used to establish a diagnosis of MI and evaluate the extent of damage done to the heart muscle (Table 20.2). Troponin levels are the preferred biomarker for diagnosis. Serum troponin T and troponin I are elevated within a few hours of MI. Troponin is found only in cardiac tissue. CK isoenzymes, lactic dehydrogenase (LDH), and LDH isoenzyme levels are observed over a 72-hour period. The CK is fractionalized into CK-MB, an enzyme that is found only in heart muscle. Other isoenzymes are CK-MM, found in skeletal muscle, and CK-BB, found in brain tissue. The level of CK-MB rises in 4 to 8 hours and begins to decline in 12 to 24 hours; LDH level increases 24 to 48 hours after an MI and stays high for up to 2 weeks. The most significant laboratory finding for diagnosis of MI is an elevated troponin level, especially if accompanied by an elevated CK-MB. Myoglobin levels rise with cardiac damage and do not diagnose MI but can rule out MI.

Table 20.2 Laboratory Tests Performed to Determine Myocardial Infarction

TEST	NORMAL VALUE	SIGNIFICANCE OF ABNORMAL VALUE
Troponin I (Tn I) Troponin T (Tn T)	<0.3 mcg/L <0.1 mcg/L	Specific to heart muscle damage. Levels may elevate within 4–6 h after MI, peak within 10–24 h, and return to normal levels within 10 days.
CPK (creatinine phosphokinase)	Men: 55–170 international units/L Women: 30–135 international units/L	Elevated within 4–8 h after heart attack (may also rise with injury to other muscles). Peaks within 12–24 h, returns to normal levels within 3–4 days.
CK-MB	<3 ng/mL	Elevates within 2–6 h after MI, peaks within 12–24 h, and returns to normal within 3 days. CK-MB is specific to myocardial injury.
Myoglobin	0–85 ng/mL	Detects muscle damage to myocardium. Presence of myoglobin is not diagnostic of MI, but absence of myoglobin rules out MI.

Other laboratory tests are listed in Chapter 17, Table 17.2.
CK, Creatinine kinase.

Cardiac catheterization with angiography may be performed soon after the patient is admitted to the emergency department if MI is the probable diagnosis. This provides immediate, definitive diagnosis and treatment for occluded vessels.

Safety Alert

Intravenous Contrast (Dye)

If the patient is diabetic and takes metformin, hold the drug before the contrast-dye procedure. If the procedure is done as an emergency, metformin should be held for 3 days afterward. Metformin and contrast have an adverse effect on kidney function. When any patient has received contrast for a diagnostic test, promote good hydration by either oral or intravenous (IV) fluids. Keeping the patient hydrated will increase the rate of urine flow, dilute the urine, and help prevent kidney damage as the contrast is excreted.

Magnetic resonance imaging (MRI), echocardiography, and a technetium-99m sestamibi scan may be performed to determine whether there is myocardial dysfunction.

Think Critically

How would you prepare the patient who has experienced a probable MI for the diagnostic tests they will most likely undergo? What teaching is required?

Treatment

Outside the hospital, a trained emergency medical team should be called immediately. The patient should chew and swallow an aspirin when the symptoms of MI occur. If the patient shows signs of cardiac or respiratory arrest, help should be called and cardiopulmonary resuscitation (CPR) should be started immediately. If an automated external defibrillator (AED) is available, bystanders or family should initiate its use. Many public areas, such as airports and shopping malls, have AEDs available, and these can be used by individuals trained in CPR. The AED will detect and treat possible shockable rhythms until emergency personnel are on the scene and take over care. It is recommended that a 12-lead ECG is done in the field and transmitted to the receiving hospital. This is not available in all areas but is becoming more common.

As soon as a patient with an acute MI is brought to the emergency department, measures are taken to relieve pain, decrease ischemia, and prevent further circulatory collapse and shock. The MONA (morphine, oxygen, nitrates, aspirin [if not already taken]) regimen is initiated. Oxygen via nasal cannula or mask is started, IV access is obtained for administration of fluids and emergency drugs, and the patient is placed on a cardiac monitor. The Joint Commission has Core Measures in place for patients admitted with an MI (Box 20.2).

Sublingual nitroglycerin is given unless contraindicated. Drugs administered IV to control pain in a patient with acute MI are morphine sulfate or hydromorphone hydrochloride (Dilaudid). Morphine is the drug of choice because of its vasodilation property. **Pain medication given IV has a shorter duration, and doses must be repeated more frequently to keep the patient comfortable.** A bolus of heparin will be given and a heparin drip started to prevent the clot from enlarging. A nitrate infusion also may be started. Antidysrhythmia drugs are given as indicated for abnormal ECG rhythms. Close assessment of respiration is essential because the drugs for pain can depress respiration at a time when the heart's oxygen demand is increased. Pulse oximetry is instituted quickly to measure oxygen saturation.

If STEMI is indicated on the ECG, measures are implemented to address the complete occlusion of a coronary artery. The patient may immediately undergo cardiac catheterization and balloon angioplasty with placement of stents to restore blood flow. In many communities, facilities with cardiac catheterization capabilities may be designated as STEMI-receiving hospitals. Protocols are in place to fast-track the diagnosis and mobilization of intervention teams to quickly treat a patient experiencing an MI. If cardiac catheterization is not available, thrombolytic therapy may be considered to dissolve the clot occluding the coronary artery.

Thrombolytic therapy is started preferably within 6 hours but can be given up to 12 hours after the onset of symptoms to prevent necrosis of the myocardium and is indicated when the ECG shows ST-segment elevation (Rivera-Bou, 2017). To meet the Core Measures, standard thrombolytics should be given within 30 minutes of arrival to the hospital. Agents used intravenously to dissolve the clot include alteplase (tPA, Activase), tenecteplase (TNKase), and reteplase (Retavase). These drugs are contraindicated in patients who have severe, uncontrolled hypertension or a history of a hemorrhagic stroke, gastrointestinal (GI) bleed, intracranial or intraspinal surgery within the past 2 months, a brain tumor, arteriovenous malformation, or aneurysm. After one of

Box 20.2 The Joint Commission Core Measures for Myocardial Infarction

- Aspirin administered upon arrival at the hospital
- Beta blocker started within 24 hours of arrival
- Thrombolytic agent administered within 30 minutes of hospital arrival or percutaneous coronary intervention (PCI) within 90 minutes of arrival
- Aspirin or other antiplatelet therapy at discharge
- Beta blocker therapy continued at discharge
- Angiotensin-converting enzyme (ACE) inhibitor or angiotensin receptor blocker (ARB) therapy at discharge for left ventricular ejection fraction less than 40%

Think Critically

A patient has chest pain. The health care provider orders laboratory studies. Which results may indicate MI versus an episode of angina?

these agents is infused, a heparin drip may be started to prevent reocclusion. When a patient is not a candidate for thrombolytic therapy, heparin and low-dose aspirin may be administered to prevent further thrombosis.

? Think Critically

How would you explain the thrombolytic therapy used when a patient has acute coronary occlusion?

Nursing Management

In the acute phase of MI, nursing care is directed toward the following:

- Preparing the patient for possible percutaneous coronary intervention (PCI) or thrombolytic therapy
- Relieving pain
- Administering ordered medical therapy and observing for side effects
- Monitoring for signs of complications of MI, such as dysrhythmia, HF, pulmonary edema, pericarditis, cardiogenic shock, or cardiac arrest (Table 20.3)
- Maintaining a patent IV access at all times

Table 20.3 Signs and Symptoms of Complications After Myocardial Infarction

COMPLICATION	SIGNS AND SYMPTOMS
Dysrhythmia	Irregular pulse; abnormal ECG pattern. Ventricular fibrillation is the most common complication after MI. Report more than six PVCs per minute, heart rate >120 or <40 bpm.
Heart failure (HF)	Dyspnea; pedal edema; sacral edema; crackles in lung bases; distended neck veins; enlarged, tender liver; weight gain of more than 2 lb in 24 h; pulmonary edema.
Cardiogenic shock	Significant drop in systolic blood pressure (>20 points); diaphoresis; rapid pulse; cold, clammy skin; gray skin; restlessness.
Papillary muscle dysfunction	Mitral valve regurgitation with systolic murmur; dyspnea, pulmonary edema, and decreased cardiac output.
Ventricular aneurysm	Outpouching of ventricular wall may cause HF, dysrhythmias, and angina. May cause formation of thrombi that lead to a stroke.
Pericarditis	Pericardial friction rub on auscultation; chest pain aggravated by movement and lessened by sitting up and leaning forward.
Dressler syndrome	Occurs 4–6 wk after MI. Chest pain, fever, friction rub, pleural effusion, and arthralgia.

bpm, Beats per minute; *ECG,* electrocardiogram; *MI,* myocardial infarction; *PVCs,* premature ventricular contractions.

In the recovery phase of MI, nursing care is directed toward the following:

- Decreasing anxiety and stress for the patient. Explain the function of all equipment and tests in simple terms. Explain the routine of frequent assessment and tests so that the patient will know what to expect. Decrease the family's anxiety by reinforcing what the health care provider has told them about the patient's condition and treatment.
- Monitoring physical status by performing a thorough cardiovascular assessment every 4 to 8 hours and monitoring vital signs every 2 to 4 hours.
- Recording daily weight and comparing with previous weight. Intake and output are accurately recorded and compared with previous amounts.
- Promoting rest.
- Monitoring tolerance of activities of daily living (ADLs) and ambulation.
- Assisting with rehabilitation activities.

Patients with damage to the myocardium are admitted to the critical care unit (CCU) or telemetry where they are initially kept on bed rest. Physical activity is gradually increased according to the patient's individual condition and response to activity. An IV line or a saline lock is maintained to provide a route for administration of emergency drugs to control BP and dysrhythmias.

Vital signs and Spo_2 are continuously monitored by electronic means and are assessed every 15 minutes to 2 hours. The temperature may be slightly elevated. Continuous ECG monitoring is essential to provide an accurate evaluation of the status of the heart. If death occurs, it is most likely within the first 24 hours of an MI and is caused by ventricular fibrillation.

A heart-healthy diet is ordered when the patient's vital signs have stabilized. A stool softener is given to decrease the risk of bradycardia, which can be caused by straining to have a bowel movement. Potassium and magnesium are monitored closely because imbalances can cause dysrhythmias. Medication to correct dysrhythmia is given as needed (see Table 19.4). A beta-adrenergic blocker, such as metoprolol (Toprol XL, Lopressor), may be ordered to decrease the heart's workload. An angiotensin-converting enzyme (ACE) inhibitor such as captopril (Capoten) may also be given. Oxygen via mask or nasal cannula is administered to maintain Spo_2 at 95% or greater. Various IV drugs may be used to regulate BP or to control dysrhythmias. While in the CCU, if hemodynamic instability is present, a pulmonary artery flow-directed catheter (Swan-Ganz type) may be inserted to monitor central venous pressure (CVP), pulmonary artery pressure (PAP), pulmonary capillary wedge pressure (PCWP), and cardiac output, which give a better picture of the injured heart's ability to pump. A temporary pacemaker may be inserted if the patient develops a persistent bradycardia causing symptoms of inadequate cardiac output. External pacing patches can be used for emergency pacing. A transvenous temporary pacing wire will be placed as soon as possible.

Rare but deadly complications of MI requiring surgical repair are ventral septal defect, a ventricular aneurysm, or papillary muscle rupture.

CARDIOGENIC SHOCK

If the left ventricle is badly damaged, cardiogenic shock may occur. Signs and symptoms are those that accompany decreased cardiac output, such as decreased BP, confusion, restlessness, diaphoresis, rapid and thready pulse, increased respiratory rate, cold and clammy skin, and diminishing urinary output to less than 20 mL/h. The patient is cared for in the CCU, where a variety of drugs aimed at improving cardiac output may be administered.

An intra-aortic balloon pump (IABP) may be used to ease the heart's workload while it begins to heal (see Chapter 19, Fig. 19.3). This device uses a balloon catheter positioned in the aorta that inflates during diastole and deflates during systole, effectively decreasing the workload of the heart and increasing blood flow through the coronary arteries. Only registered nurses who are certified in the care of patients on an IABP are assigned to care for these patients. See Chapter 45 for further information on shock.

Intermediate Care

When very frequent assessment and monitoring are no longer essential and the patient can participate in their personal hygiene activities without detrimental effects on the healing heart tissues, they are transferred out of the CCU into a telemetry, or "step-down," medical unit. For some patients, this move is frightening because they know they will no longer have a nurse giving them constant attention. Every effort is made to assure the patient that they are making progress toward recovery and no longer need intensive care. While the patient is on the telemetry unit, physical activities are gradually increased according to ability to tolerate exercise, as evidenced by stable heart rate, BP, and respiratory rate. There is close monitoring for symptoms of excessive strain on the heart, such as dysrhythmia or dyspnea, or for the development of complications. These measures may minimize damage from an MI, but the patient still has CAD, requires treatment, and must attend to lowering their risk factors.

If the patient received successful thrombolytic therapy or percutaneous coronary intervention (PCI), they may have averted significant myocardial damage and not require CCU care after the MI. Patients with a STEMI who arrive for treatment before significant left ventricular damage has occurred may be sent to telemetry after PCI and are hospitalized for only 24 to 48 hours. Intensive teaching needs to occur to help the patient access resources to enable the lifestyle changes needed to prevent another MI.

Rehabilitation

A variety of emotional and behavioral responses may occur after an MI (Box 20.3). The patient and family may need help and support as they work to make the necessary adjustments. Many hospitals offer an outpatient cardiac rehabilitation program to help the patient make lifestyle changes to reduce future risk of cardiac problems. The program provides counseling on dietary changes for a heart-healthy diet; stress reduction techniques; reduction of risk factors, such as avoiding tobacco use; controlling hypertension and diabetes; and a supervised exercise program with continuous ECG monitoring for 4 to 6 weeks. Such programs have been found to be effective in decreasing cardiac death and HF (Wenger, 2018). Progressive, supervised exercise is continued for an additional 8 to 12 weeks, and then a

Box 20.3 Emotional and Behavioral Responses to Acute Myocardial Infarction

DENIAL
- May have history of ignoring symptoms related to heart disease
- Minimizes severity of medical condition
- Ignores activity restrictions
- Avoids discussing MI or its significance

ANGER
- Is commonly expressed as "Why did this happen to me?"
- May be directed at family, staff, or medical regimen

ANXIETY AND FEAR
- Fears death and long-term disability
- Overtly manifests apprehension, restlessness, insomnia, tachycardia
- Less overtly manifests increased verbalization, projection of feelings to others, hypochondriasis
- Fears activity, recurrent heart attacks, and sudden death

DEPENDENCY
- Is totally reliant on staff
- Is unwilling to perform tasks or activities unless approved by health care provider
- Wants to be monitored by ECG at all times
- Is hesitant to leave CCU or hospital

DEPRESSION
- Experiences mourning period concerning loss of health, altered body function, and changes in lifestyle
- Realizes seriousness of situation
- Begins to worry about future implications of health problem
- Shows manifestations of withdrawal, crying, anorexia, apathy
- May have more evident depression after discharge

REALISTIC ACCEPTANCE
- Focuses on optimum rehabilitation
- Plans changes compatible with altered cardiac function

CCU, Critical care unit; *ECG,* electrocardiogram; *MI,* myocardial infarction.
From Lewis SL, Heitkemper MM, Bucher L, et al.: *Medical-surgical nursing: assessment and management of clinical problems,* ed 10, St. Louis, 2017, Elsevier.

maintenance program is devised that the patient can do independently. A support group consisting of other individuals who have the same condition or have had similar surgery often is available. Most insurance coverage will pay for the exercise program because it has been highly successful in helping people to develop and maintain a healthier lifestyle and to reduce risk factors.

One area of major concern is sexuality. The patient may be fearful of resuming intercourse, thinking that it may cause a heart attack. The partner often has these fears also. Both partners need reassurance that resumption of normal sexual activities will be possible. The patient may need to take a more passive role during intercourse, at least for a while, using alternate positions that cause less strain and less oxygen demand. The patient should be told that the workload of intercourse with a known partner is equal to climbing a flight of stairs. If a flight of stairs can be climbed without much change in heart rate, respirations, or blood pressure, intercourse should not cause harm. The health care provider should discuss this area with the patient and their partner, but if the provider does not, ensure that the proper information is given. Sexual dysfunction may be a side effect of some medications.

Patients should be taught to plan sexual activity for times when they are well rested and to avoid an environment that is too hot or too cold. It is best to space such activity at least 2 hours after eating a meal or drinking any alcohol. Nitroglycerin should be used prophylactically if intercourse causes angina symptoms. If angina does occur, the patient should cease activity, place a nitroglycerin tablet under their tongue, lie down, and rest.

Levels of physical activity are designated through **metabolic equivalent (MET) units**. One MET is the amount of oxygen needed by the body at rest. The patient's rehabilitation program slowly progresses stepwise to higher energy expenditures over a period of months (Box 20.4).

Rehabilitation involves three major aspects: (1) a program of increasing activity based on the patient's individual progress and needs; (2) instruction of the patient and family about the nature of the illness and the rationale for every aspect of its management; and (3) assistance to the patient and family as they work toward the goal of accepting the limitations imposed and the changes in lifestyle that may be required. The goal is to have the patient and family continue with heart-healthy living even after the formal program ends.

SURGICAL AND NONSURGICAL TREATMENT OPTIONS

PERCUTANEOUS CORONARY INTERVENTION

If only a few areas of stenosis are identified, a PCI may be performed. The patient may have a percutaneous transluminal coronary angioplasty (PTCA) rather than **coronary artery bypass graft (CABG)** to improve blood

Box 20.4 Energy Expenditure in Metabolic Equivalents

LOW-ENERGY ACTIVITIES (<3 METS OR <3 CAL/MIN)

Activities in Hospital

Resting supine
Eating
Washing hands, face

Activities Outside Hospital

Sweeping floor
Painting, seated
Driving a car
Sewing by machine

MODERATE-ENERGY ACTIVITIES (3–6 METS OR 3–5 CAL/MIN)

Activities in Hospital

Sitting on bedside commode
Showering
Using bedpan
Walking at 3 to 4 mph

Activities Outside Hospital

Bricklaying
Ironing, standing
Cycling at 5.5 mph on level ground
Golfing
Dancing

HIGH-ENERGY ACTIVITIES (6–8 METS OR 6–8 CAL/MIN)

Walking 5 mph
Performing carpentry
Ascending a flight of stairs
Mowing lawn using walking mower

VERY-HIGH-ENERGY ACTIVITIES (>9 METS OR >9 CAL/MIN)

Cross-country skiing
Running faster than 6 mph
Cycling faster than 13 mph
Shoveling heavy snow

cal, Calories; *METs,* metabolic equivalent units; *mph,* miles per hour.
From Lewis SL, Heitkemper MM, Bucher L, et al.: *Medical-surgical nursing: assessment and management of clinical problems,* ed 10, St. Louis, 2017, Elsevier.

Patient Teaching

Guidelines for Recovery From an MI

Teach the patient to:

- Recognize the signs of recurrent MI and seek immediate medical attention should they occur. These are chest pain, diaphoresis, nausea, and anxiety.
- Adopt a lifetime regular, graduated exercise program.
- Alter controllable risk factors: reach and maintain a normal weight; cease smoking; keep alcohol consumption at a moderate level (no more than 1.5 oz per day); keep cholesterol within normal limits; control hypertension; continue on a low-fat, low-sodium diet individualized to taste.
- Reduce stress and learn relaxation techniques.
- Take medications as ordered and monitor for side effects.

It is important to stress to the patient that they have control over their rehabilitation and prognosis. They alone have full control over lifestyle changes and the treatment program. When the patient feels that they, rather than the health care provider, is in control, they are much more likely to remain on the treatment program.

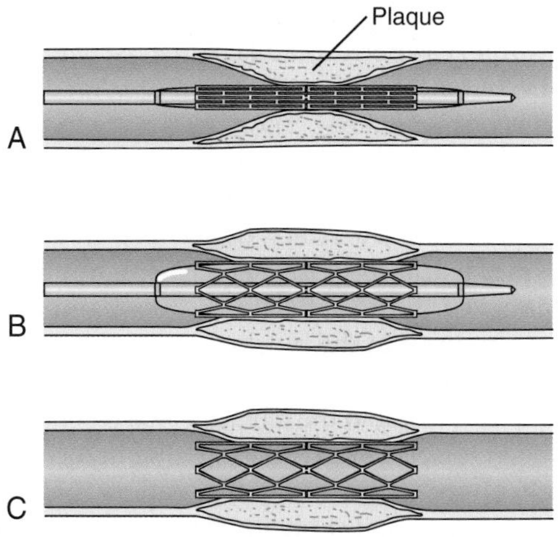

Fig. 20.5 Placement of coronary artery stent. **A,** The stent is positioned at the site of stenotic lesion. **B,** The balloon is inflated, expanding the stent. The balloon is then deflated and removed. **C,** The implanted stent is left in place. (From Lewis SL, Bucher L, Heitkemper MM, et al.: *Medical-surgical nursing: assessment and management of clinical problems,* ed 10, St. Louis, 2017, Elsevier.)

flow. PTCA is a nonsurgical interventional technique to open blocked coronary arteries. It is performed in the cardiac catheterization laboratory using fluoroscopy. A catheter with a balloon tip is threaded into the blocked artery, and when the narrowed area is reached, the balloon is inflated, pushing aside the plaque and widening the interior of the artery. To maintain patency of the vessel, a coronary stent is usually placed. A stent is made of stainless steel and acts as a brace for the artery wall. A bare metal or **drug-eluting stent** may be placed in the artery to help maintain patency of the vessel (Fig. 20.5). Several manufacturers provide drug-eluting stents. They all have a coating of a drug that is released slowly over several weeks after placement. The drug coatings are medications that are used in cancer treatment. The purpose is either to suppress cell growth so that the body does not occlude the vessel with new cells or to decrease inflammation with immunosuppressants to reduce swelling and promote healing. Research has shown that the drug-eluting stents may reduce the need to restent the vessels over time because of cellular hyperplasia as the body adjusts to the foreign body. During the procedure a glycoprotein (GP) IIb/IIIa inhibitor such as abciximab (ReoPro), tirofiban (Aggrastat), eptifibatide (Integrilin), or direct thrombin inhibitor bivalirudin (Angiomax) may be given as an IV infusion to reduce platelet aggregation. When a stent is placed, the patient must take antiplatelet agents, such as aspirin, and/or clopidogrel (Plavix) for up to 1 year after placement. A loading dose of antiplatelet medication is usually given before the patient leaves the cardiac catheterization laboratory; this reduces the need for infusions. Thoroughly assess the status of the patient after cardiac catheterization. The patient may be up and about within 2 to 4 hours when an arterial closure device is used to seal the procedure site. Distal pulses on the affected leg must be assessed frequently, and the groin area must be assessed for the presence of hemorrhage or a hematoma. If the radial artery approach was used, the patient will have a pressure device in place at the procedure site. The pressure will gradually be released until the device can be removed. The patient has no ambulation restrictions immediately post procedure except possibly needed help due to grogginess from procedural sedation. Renal function should be monitored because of potential adverse effects of contrast dyes used during the procedure.

CABG may be indicated if there is multivessel disease or a critical lesion that puts a large portion of myocardium at risk. Depending on the nature of the risk, patients may go emergently to the operating room (OR) from the cardiac catheterization laboratory or may be scheduled at a later time.

Other procedures to remedy clots and plaque are laser angioplasty, thrombectomy, and atherectomy. Laser angioplasty breaks up the clot. Rheolytic thrombectomy uses low-pressure, high-speed saline jets to break up the clot. Atherectomy devices either excise and retrieve plaque or destroy it. These procedures are sometimes used when a patient has reocclusion after CABG and PTCA. CABG surgery is covered in the section on cardiac surgery.

Studies are ongoing to determine whether a regimen consisting of a very low–fat diet, regular exercise, reduction of stress, and practice of relaxation techniques can reverse CAD without surgery. These methods have been effective in people who have the discipline needed to maintain the program.

Clinical Cues

Patients may have a genetic resistance to clopidogrel (Plavix). For clopidogrel to inhibit platelets it must be activated by a sequence mediated by the liver. P2Y12 platelet function testing can identify resistance.

TRANSMYOCARDIAL LASER REVASCULARIZATION

For patients who are critically ill and are not candidates for PTCA or CABG, transmyocardial laser revascularization (TMR) is an option. This procedure may be available to patients with severe chest pain that limits their ability to perform ADLs, who have a history of CABG, and who have no other treatment options. The procedure is done with general anesthesia without use of cardiopulmonary bypass (heart-lung machine), and the heart is approached through a small thoracotomy incision. A carbon dioxide or holmium:YAG laser is used to drill multiple tiny holes in the heart's left ventricle. These channels heal on the outside of the heart and over time heal on the inside. The mechanism that causes improvement in patient symptoms is not well understood. Postoperatively the patient will have a chest tube and be monitored in the CCU.

CARDIAC SURGERY

The term *open heart surgery* refers to the use of the heart-lung machine during the procedure. The machine functions as an artificial heart (pump) and lung (oxygenator). Because all this is done outside the patient's body, the procedure is called *extracorporeal circulation.* The surgeon inserts large tubes in the vena cava and reroutes the unoxygenated venous blood through the heart-lung machine. There, the blood is exposed to an atmosphere of oxygen in which an exchange of gases takes place (carbon dioxide is released, and oxygen is taken up), and the oxygenated blood is returned to the patient via the aorta. The blood may be cooled so that the patient's body temperature is lowered (hypothermia), thereby reducing the body's metabolic needs during surgery.

Open heart surgery technically means that the chest is opened, the heart is stopped, and blood is routed through a heart-lung machine. The term is used for any procedure during which these conditions take place. Some procedures are done with minimally invasive techniques not requiring a sternotomy. In others, the heart is not stopped, and "off-pump" (beating heart) surgery is performed. Congenital heart defects, valve replacements, bypass of clogged coronary arteries, and heart transplant are conditions requiring surgical repair.

Coronary Artery Bypass Graft Surgery

CABG surgery is performed (1) when ischemia cannot be controlled medically or (2) to prevent greater occlusion and consequent MI. The CABG surgery bypasses the artery that is blocked, replacing it with sections of a vein or artery taken from another part of the patient's body. The mammary artery or sections of saphenous vein or radial artery are grafted. The mammary artery is left attached to the subclavian artery, and the other end is sewn distal to the blockage in a coronary artery. Saphenous vein or radial artery grafts are sewn to the aorta and then distal to the blockage in a coronary artery. These new vessels supply blood to the myocardium. If an open approach is used, the patient will have a midsternal incision; if saphenous veins are used for the grafts, the patient will have leg incisions. A small dressing (Fig. 20.6, *B*) will be seen if an endoscopic approach was used. Fig. 20.7 shows CABG procedures using vein grafts or the internal mammary artery.

Older Adult Care Points

Older adult patients tolerate CABG surgery well, but the recovery period is longer because of the slower healing rate and decreased ability of the body to handle this degree of physical stress.

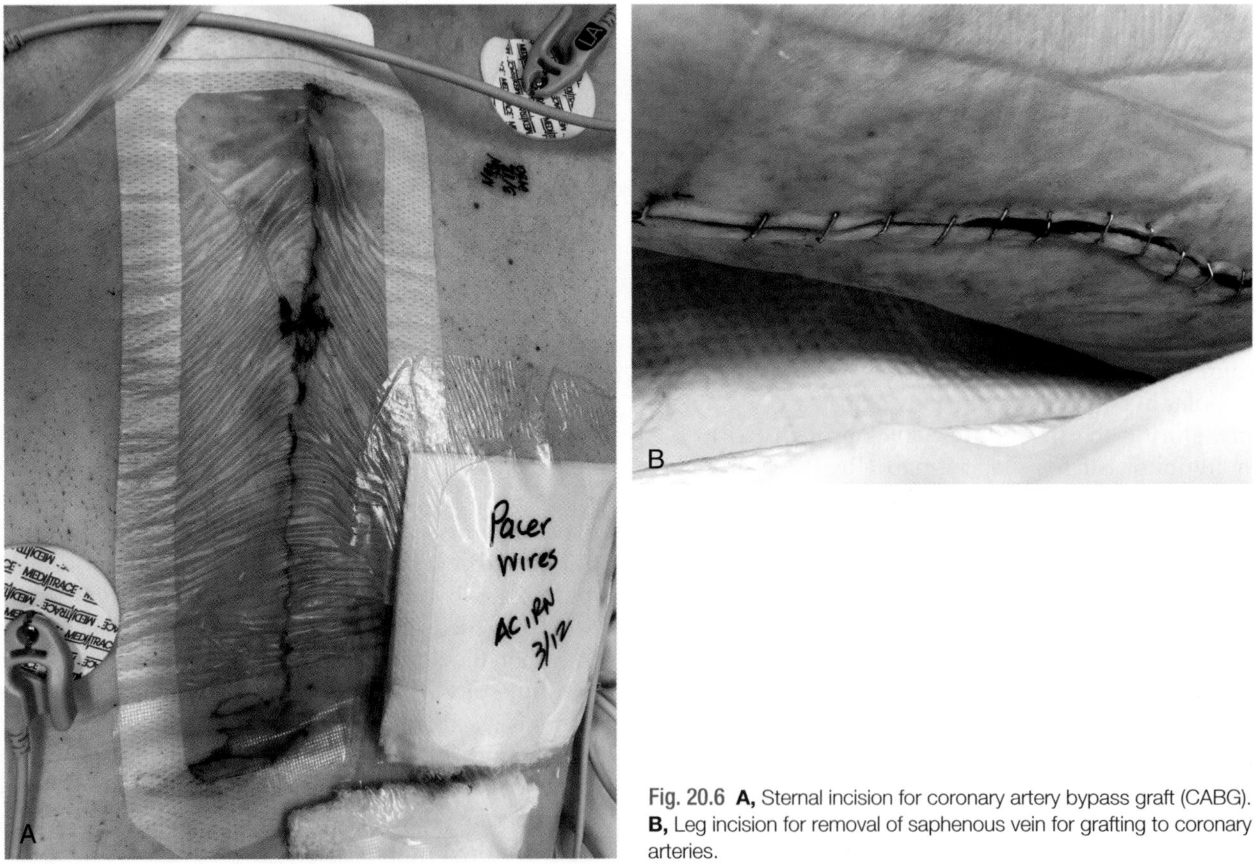

Fig. 20.6 **A,** Sternal incision for coronary artery bypass graft (CABG). **B,** Leg incision for removal of saphenous vein for grafting to coronary arteries.

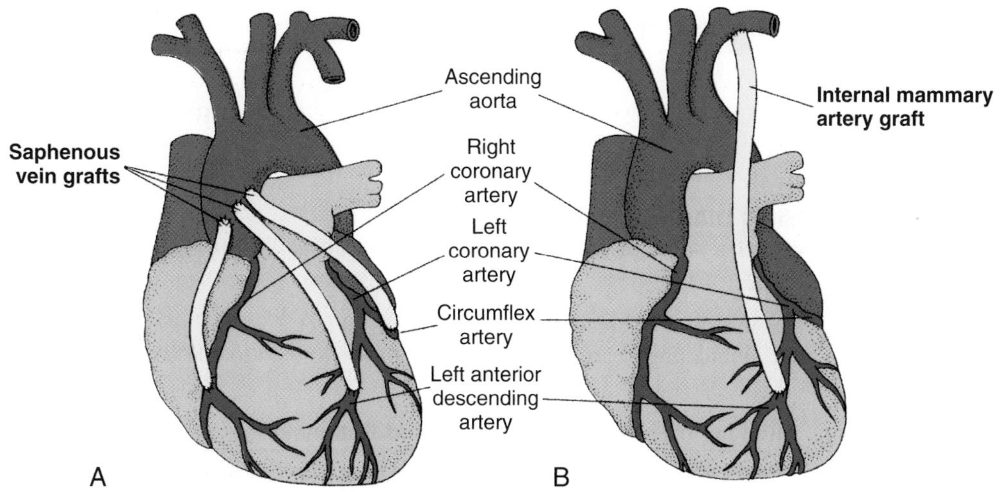

Fig. 20.7 Two methods of coronary artery bypass grafting. **A,** Saphenous vein grafts. **B,** Internal mammary artery graft.

An off-pump coronary artery bypass technique for CABG procedures—minimally invasive direct coronary artery bypass (MIDCAB)—does not require stopping the heart's activity and therefore does not require using the heart-lung machine. MIDCAB procedures are performed on only the vessels in the front of the heart because the access allows contact with only those arteries. Use of robotic assistance is becoming more common in all aspects of surgery. The advances in technology are being applied to coronary bypass and intracardiac procedures. Coronary bypass surgery does not cure the disease; it only relieves the symptoms and may prevent myocardial damage from total occlusion of a coronary artery. After the surgery, anginal chest pain disappears in about 65% of patients, and another 25% show improvement. Many of those patients who had a coronary artery bypass in the past 10 years are returning for a second operation because the grafted arteries or venous bypass grafts have become occluded. A greater emphasis is being placed on the need for adherence to lifestyle changes to prevent a second operation. Nursing Care Plan 20.2 summarizes care of a patient after cardiac surgery.

Heart Transplant

Heart transplants are performed for selected patients who have a history of hospitalizations for HF, need a left ventricular assist device (LVAD), need increasing types and doses of medications or documentation of decreased oxygen supplied to the body as measured by VO_2 (VO_2 is the amount of oxygen consumption by the tissues of the body), have good renal function, and are psychologically stable. There is some flexibility with the age requirements.

Candidates for heart transplant undergo psychological evaluation and a thorough physical assessment. Patients must also be evaluated for the ability to remain in compliance with health care instructions and for the ability to obtain and comply with antirejection medication protocols. Transplant patients must take immunosuppressants and other medications for the remainder of their lives. Very few donor hearts are available, and the waiting lists are long. Allocation of available organs is determined by evidence-based criteria with oversight of the United Network for Organ Sharing (UNOS). In addition to meeting transplant criteria, patients are limited by geography. A heart can be out of the donor body for only 4 to 6 hours if it is to be successfully transplanted into the recipient. Patients who receive a heart transplant face considerable financial cost, a life of taking immunosuppressive drugs that have many serious side effects (including risk for infection), and the constant threat of organ rejection. However, the benefits are considerable, with an average 1-year survival rate of about 85% to 90%, a 3-year survival rate of about 75%, and a 5-year survival rate of 60% (Eisen, 2018). A significant number of heart transplant patients survive beyond 10 years.

Transplant patients must adhere to strict dietary and exercise regimens to prevent the new heart from becoming affected with problems that led to the original HF. Heart transplants are performed in highly specialized medical centers. Patients who are too unstable for care in the home may remain in the hospital for an extended period until a heart is available. Other patients may be given a special pager for notification of an available heart. These patients must be available for immediate admission to the hospital. Patients awaiting a heart transplant are placed on a national waiting list. A heart may be available within 24 hours, or one may be months away. Unfortunately, some patients die before a suitable heart is available. There has been increasing success with use of LVADs and mechanical artificial hearts in providing needed perfusion for patients awaiting transplant surgery. For some patients who are not a candidate for transplant, smaller, fully implanted LVADs have been used as the intervention to support and improve perfusion (see Chapter 19, Fig. 19.2).

Nursing Care Plan 20.2 Care of a Patient After Cardiac Surgery

SCENARIO

Mr. Jacobi, age 57 years, was transferred to the telemetry unit after a coronary artery bypass graft (CABG) and is 2 days postoperative. Mr. Jacobi is married and has three teenage children. He plans to return to his job as a truck driver after surgical recovery.

PROBLEM STATEMENT/NURSING DIAGNOSIS

Altered activity tolerance due to preoperative deconditioning and postsurgical hemodynamic changes.

SUPPORTING ASSESSMENT DATA

Subjective: States, "I'm feeling weak and short of breath" after ambulating 30 feet.

Objective: RR 32, Spo_2 90% after ambulating short distance, Po_2 increases to 95% to 100% when returned to chair, RR decreased to 24.

Goals/Expected Outcomes	Nursing Intervention	Selected Rationale	Evaluation
Patient will be able to ambulate 50 feet in hallway without complaints of weakness and dyspnea.	Assess Spo_2 continuously and vital signs before and after ambulation.	Provides baseline values for evaluation.	Spo_2 96%, no complaints of weakness by third postoperative day.
	Provide safety during ambulation (e.g., follow with wheelchair, use gait belt, instruct to use handrails).	Prevent falls if hemodynamic changes occur.	Patient did not sustain fall.
	Provide rest periods every 15 feet.	Improves success of ambulation.	Patient able to ambulate 100 feet without rest period by third postoperative day.
	Gradually increase distance of ambulation as condition stabilizes.	Physical conditioning decreases the workload on heart and facilitates patient recovery.	Patient ambulated 100 feet three times per day without complaints of weakness and dyspnea by third postoperative day. Continue plan.

PROBLEM STATEMENT/NURSING DIAGNOSIS

Altered skin integrity due to thoracotomy and saphenous vein graft.

SUPPORTING ASSESSMENT DATA

Subjective: Patient asks about care of wounds to chest and left lower leg.

Objective: Incisions to midsternum and left lower leg. Both incisions intact, no areas of redness or wound dehiscence.

Goals/Expected Outcomes	Nursing Intervention	Selected Rationale	Evaluation
Surgical incisions will remain intact and free of signs of infection.	Assess and document status of incision at the beginning of each shift.	Determines changes in status of wound, such as development of redness, edema, opening of suture lines.	Midsternal incision intact, no signs of infection. Incision to left lower leg slightly edematous, ½-inch opening of wound on fourth postoperative day. Continue to monitor.
	Assess vital signs.	Elevated temperature and heart rate may indicate beginning of wound infection.	HR 72, T 100° F (37.8° C).
	Provide wound care as ordered.	Keeps incisions free of drainage, irritants, and pathogens.	Wounds are clean and dry with no signs of infection.
	Include wound management in discharge teaching plan.	Provides knowledge to prevent and recognize complications associated with wound healing.	Demonstrated appropriate wound care. Verbalized signs and symptoms of infection.

PROBLEM STATEMENT/NURSING DIAGNOSIS

Acute pain due to midsternal and leg surgical incisions.

Nursing Care Plan 20.2 Care of a Patient After Cardiac Surgery—cont'd

SUPPORTING ASSESSMENT DATA

Subjective: States, "It hurts too much to do these breathing exercises and walk."

Objective: Unable to reach incentive spirometer goals; SpO_2 94% or ambulation goals.

Goals/Expected Outcomes	Nursing Intervention	Selected Rationale	Evaluation
Patient will verbalize pain level of no more than 5 during use of incentive spirometer	Assess pain level before deep-breathing exercises and use of incentive spirometer. Provide pain medication as needed. Teach to splint incision during respiratory exercises.	Patient will be more likely to complete exercises if he is more comfortable.	Completes breathing exercises without pain medication by third postoperative day.
Patient will be able to ambulate maintaining a pain level of 6 or less.	Medicate prior to activity.	Activity will increase pain, so proactively medicating will allow achievement of pain goal.	Able to ambulate 100 feet with pain goal achieved.

PROBLEM STATEMENT/NURSING DIAGNOSIS

Insufficient knowledge related to postoperative care after discharge from hospital.

SUPPORTING ASSESSMENT DATA

Subjective: States, "I don't know how I can manage all this at home. When can I return to work?"

Objective: Patient anxious, irritable during discussion of discharge planning.

Goals/Expected Outcomes	Nursing Intervention	Selected Rationale	Evaluation
Patient and wife will demonstrate knowledge of home care instructions, including wound management, medications, exercise, diet, activities of daily living (ADLs), when to notify health care provider, and when to return to work.	Provide instructions concerning medications, wound care, ADLs.	Knowledge of expectations increases confidence and reduces anxiety.	Demonstrated understanding of instructions.
	Refer to dietitian or nutritionist for dietary requirements.	The dietitian can help the family understand the dietary requirements and how to adapt their traditional diet to comply.	States understands diet instructions and will attempt to follow them. Wife also states understanding.
	Collaborate with provider concerning additional instructions, such as return to work and cardiac rehabilitation recommendations.	Expert knowledge may be needed to provide appropriate information.	Patients states understanding of how to make an appointment with cardiac rehabilitation and when he may expect to return to work.
	Reinforce information as provided by provider.	Patients may not question a provider even if they do not understand all they were told. You are in the best position to reinforce the information given by the provider.	Verbalized disappointment that he will be unable to return to work for at least 8 wk. May require part-time work for longer period.
	Assess level of understanding of discharge instructions.	Baseline for developing discharge plan.	Verbalized understanding of discharge instructions.
	Provide opportunity to verbalize concerns.	Reduces patient anxiety.	Verbalized concerns openly, stated some anxiety relieved.

CRITICAL THINKING QUESTIONS

1. List five additional nursing problem statements that are appropriate for a patient after cardiac surgery.
2. List five additional priority assessments you should complete for this patient.

Nursing Care of Patients Having Cardiac Surgery

Preoperative care. Before cardiac surgery, the patient undergoes diagnostic tests and examinations, mostly on an outpatient basis. The teaching plan should include expectations during the preoperative and postoperative periods. There is considerable apprehension on the part of both the patient and the patient's family when faced with open heart surgery. If the surgery was emergent, teaching must be done post procedure.

The patient is given information about the procedure, explaining what to expect and what kind of equipment will be used. Admission occurs early the morning of surgery. Specific information regarding what medications to take and which ones to stop is included in the preoperative instructions. See Nursing Care Plan 20.2 for care of the patient after cardiac surgery.

Postoperative care. During the early postoperative period, the patient remains in a CCU, where specialized cardiac monitoring equipment is used and highly skilled personnel are in constant attendance. Cardiac rate and rhythm are monitored closely. For patients who had an open heart procedure, chest tubes for drainage and proper reexpansion of the lungs are in place for 24 hours. The patient often continues to receive mechanical ventilation for a few hours after surgery. Once consciousness has fully returned, weaning from the ventilator is begun if oxygenation is adequate and extubation occurs. Chest tubes are usually removed before the patient is moved out of the CCU. Temporary epicardial pacemaker leads may be in place and may or may not be connected to a pacemaker pulse generator. Usually a multilumen central line is in place for medication delivery and fluid maintenance, as well as an arterial line and pulmonary artery line for hemodynamic monitoring. If saphenous vein or radial artery grafts were used, there will be leg and arm incisions to care for along with the chest incision. Urine output is initially monitored hourly for 8 hours and thereafter every 2 hours to detect signs of decreased perfusion to the kidneys.

After the first 12 to 24 hours, the surgeon will assess the patient's condition and decide whether transfer to a step-down unit is appropriate. The patient will continue to need special nursing care and continuous ECG monitoring. Vital signs must be taken and recorded at frequent intervals; urinary output is monitored closely. Lung sounds and oxygenation are priority assessments. Daily weight is monitored to assess fluid balance.

Coronary artery bypass surgery can produce many special problems related to rehabilitation of the patient. Postoperative care is directed at preventing infection to the surgical sites, managing wounds, monitoring for complications, and promoting rehabilitation. The physiologic symptoms that can persist into the home recovery period include fatigue and weakness, incisional discomfort, edema in the donor leg, dysrhythmias, loss of appetite, and unusual physical sensations. Depression for weeks to months may occur after heart surgery. Patients should be alerted to this possibility and referred for assistance if this occurs. Women are more likely than men to experience depression after heart surgery, and their cases are more severe.

Most patients do not experience all these problems during the home recovery period after coronary artery bypass surgery, and some have relatively trouble-free recovery periods. It is important that bypass surgery patients and their families realize that bypass surgery is not a cure for CAD. Bypass surgery is simply one form of therapy for a chronic condition that will require continued management to slow the disease process and reduce the incidence of life-threatening events in the person's life.

With an uncomplicated recovery, the patient is usually discharged home within 3 to 7 days and referred to a cardiac rehabilitation outpatient program.

Cardiac transplant patients are at risk for organ rejection, infection, and development of CAD in the new heart. Heart biopsies are performed regularly. Posttransplant malignancy is a known risk factor and is believed to result from the prolonged immunosuppression. Skin cancer is the most common malignancy after organ transplant.

COMMUNITY CARE

With early discharge from the hospital after surgery, many patients have continuing care from home health nurses. Patients recovering from cardiac surgery, MI, atherosclerotic heart disease, angina, or valvular heart disease all may be referred to a cardiac rehabilitation program. The goal of such programs is to reduce risk of further heart problems or death.

Home care nurses care for many patients diagnosed with heart disease. The goals of home care are to monitor the patient's condition and to prevent complications, such as life-threatening dysrhythmias, MI, and congestive heart failure (CHF). Nurses supervise the medication regimen, monitor weight gain, draw blood for laboratory tests to determine drug levels and electrolyte status, and assess for beginning signs of complications. By detecting complications early, patients can be treated at home rather than at the hospital, thereby decreasing costs of care.

Many residents in long-term care facilities have cardiac disorders. Assessing changes in condition is a high priority. If changes can be identified quickly, the severity of a complication can be reduced in this population. It is important to know each resident's history.

Get Ready for the NCLEX® Examination!

Key Points

- High levels of cholesterol (LDL) contribute to development of atherosclerosis, a major factor in occlusion of coronary vessels.
- Ischemia occurs as blood supply is decreased to the myocardium.
- A cardinal sign of myocardial ischemia is angina pectoris (chest pain).
- SCAD may be treated medically or by PCI.
- *Acute coronary syndrome* is an umbrella term for a group of symptoms indicating severe myocardial ischemia or necrosis.

- Nitrates (nitroglycerin) are the most commonly used drugs to treat angina.
- Patients should be monitored for hypotension and development of a throbbing headache while taking nitroglycerin.
- When a coronary artery becomes completely obstructed, necrosis of myocardial tissue (MI) occurs.
- Necrotic myocardial tissue cannot perform its function of pumping.
- Diagnosis of MI is made by patient history, ECG, and serum cardiac enzyme levels.
- A patient is given an aspirin tablet if an MI is suspected. Aspirin helps prevent further clot formation.
- Emergency care for a patient suspected of experiencing an MI includes oxygen; IV access; cardiac monitoring; pain management, usually with IV morphine sulfate; ECG; and management of dysrhythmias. These activities are done promptly if STEMI is suspected.
- Medications prescribed after MI may include nitrates, antihypertensive drugs, anticoagulants, beta blockers, ACE inhibitors, and antidysrhythmic drugs.
- Cardiac catheterization is likely to be performed on a patient experiencing an MI.
- Nursing care after cardiac catheterization includes cardiac monitoring, maintaining the patient in a supine position with the legs straight for at least 2 hours, monitoring the femoral area for hematoma formation, assessing peripheral pulses frequently, and monitoring urinary output. Or monitoring the radial access area if the radial artery was used.
- Stents may be placed to maintain patency of coronary vessels in an attempt to prevent the need for CABG. Stents may be placed during PTCA.
- CABG may be needed when a patient's angina cannot be controlled by medical means or when there is myocardial damage caused by occlusion of one or more coronary vessels.
- A heart transplant may be needed for a patient with end-stage left ventricular heart failure.
- Patients receive physical and psychological assessment before acceptance into a cardiac transplant program. Family counseling is also advisable.
- Donor hearts are not readily available; therefore patients must be carefully screened to determine the most appropriate recipient.
- Patients who are candidates for cardiac transplant must be advised of potential complications, the need to follow through on dietary and exercise recommendations, and the need to continue medications, such as immunosuppressants, for the remainder of their lives.
- Nursing care of patients after heart transplant includes intense monitoring in the CCU; assessing for signs of complications; wound management; administration of emergency, antirejection, and appropriate cardiac drugs; pain management; assessment of respiratory function; and initial return to physical activity such as out of bed to chair.
- Discharge planning should prepare the patient for return home and the beginning of care in the community.
- Monitoring the patient's understanding of and compliance with prescribed medications is an important responsibility of the home health nurse.

Additional Learning Resources

SG Go to your Study Guide for additional learning activities to help you master this chapter content.

Go to your Evolve website (http://evolve.elsevier.com/deWit/medsurg) for the following FREE learning resources:
- Animations, audio, and video
- Answers and rationales for questions and activities
- Glossary with pronunciations in English and Spanish
- Interactive Review Questions and more!

Review Questions for the NCLEX® Examination

1. After reviewing risk factors for cardiac disease, a patient is prescribed atorvastatin (Lipitor) to reduce cholesterol levels. You must include which instruction(s)? *(Select all that apply.)*
   1. Report any muscle weakness.
   2. Avoid exposure to sunlight.
   3. Keep appointments for laboratory work.
   4. Drink grapefruit juice.
   5. Maintain a low-protein diet.
   NCLEX Client Need: Physiological Integrity: Pharmacological Therapy

2. A patient asks you, "What causes angina pectoris?" An accurate response would be:
   1. "It is caused by the decreased blood flow to the coronary arteries resulting from shunting of the blood."
   2. "It is caused by a decreased blood flow to the myocardium resulting from partial obstruction of the coronary arteries."
   3. "It is caused by poor oxygenation of the coronary arteries resulting from poor gas exchange across the alveolar basement membrane."
   4. "It is caused by the inflammation of the sternal cartilage."
   NCLEX Client Need: Physiological Integrity: Physiological Adaptation

3. A patient is diagnosed as having attacks of angina pectoris. As part of the discharge instructions, the patient is instructed on the appropriate storage and use of sublingual nitroglycerin. Which of the following patient statements indicates a need for further instructions?
   1. "The tablets should be kept in a cool, dark place."
   2. "I need to lie down after I take the medication."
   3. "I can take the tablet every 15 minutes for angina pains."
   4. "The expiration date on the bottle is important."
   NCLEX Client Need: Physiological Integrity: Pharmacological Therapy

4. A 44-year-old patient is admitted with sudden, severe chest tightness unrelieved by rest or nitroglycerin and profuse sweating. Which test would exhibit an elevated level only if the patient has had an MI?
   1. Serum troponin
   2. Blood urea nitrogen
   3. Myoglobin level
   4. Prothrombin time

   NCLEX Client Need: Physiological Integrity: Reduction of Risk Potential
5. Immediate therapeutic measures provided for a patient entering the hospital with an acute myocardial infarction include which measure(s)? *(Select all that apply.)*
   1. Morphine sulfate
   2. Oxygen therapy
   3. Furosemide
   4. Nitroglycerin
   5. Aspirin

   NCLEX Client Need: Physiological Integrity: Physiological Adaptation
6. Which food has been found to reduce cholesterol levels?
   1. Garlic
   2. Onion
   3. Ginger
   4. Nutmeg

   NCLEX Client Need: Physiological Integrity: Reduction of Risk Potential
7. The health care provider explains the treatment options to a Hispanic woman diagnosed with occlusion of multiple coronary vessels. Before signing an informed consent, the patient is most likely to defer her health care decisions to her:
   1. oldest adult son.
   2. oldest adult daughter.
   3. brother-in-law.
   4. husband.

   NCLEX Client Need: Psychosocial Integrity
8. A patient has experienced an MI and has ST-segment elevation on the ECG. The priority problem would be:
   1. altered gas exchange.
   2. limited coping ability.
   3. altered tissue perfusion.
   4. altered activity tolerance.

   NCLEX Client Need: Physiological Integrity: Reduction of Risk Potential
9. Postoperative nursing care of a patient who has undergone CABG includes which priority intervention(s)? *(Select all that apply.)*
   1. Assessing cardiac rate and rhythm
   2. Encouraging use of an incentive spirometer
   3. Monitoring liver enzymes
   4. Assessing bowel sounds
   5. Managing pain

   NCLEX Client Need: Physiological Integrity: Physiological Adaptation
10. After the change-of-shift report, which of the following assigned patients should you attend to first? The patient with:
    1. stable vital signs who returned 40 minutes ago after a PCTA.
    2. an MI complaining of a headache who was transferred from the CCU earlier.
    3. stable angina whose chest pain was relieved by two nitroglycerin tablets 2 hours ago.
    4. unstable angina who is having chest pain, shortness of breath, nausea, and anxiety.

    NCLEX Client Need: Physiological Integrity: Physiological Adaptation

Critical Thinking Questions

Scenario A

Ms. Trotter, a 62-year-old woman, comes to the clinic for her annual examination results. Her cholesterol level is 260 mg/dL, with HDL 30 mg/dL and LDL 220 mg/dL. She has a family history of atherosclerosis and heart disease. She asks about the danger of her high cholesterol level.

1. Describe to her how atherosclerosis can lead to heart problems.
2. Help her identify ways to decrease her cholesterol level and raise her HDL level.
3. Describe to her the symptoms of heart problems that she should report to her health care provider.
4. Have her identify the symptoms that might indicate a heart attack and what she should do if they occur.

Scenario B

Mrs. Yee, a 50-year-old woman, comes to the emergency department complaining of a burning, squeezing sensation in her chest and a feeling of nausea. She is diaphoretic and apprehensive.

1. Compare and contrast the symptoms of heart attack for men and women.
2. Describe the probable emergency treatment of Mrs. Yee in the emergency department.
3. What laboratory tests may be ordered to evaluate for possible MI? What is a significant ECG finding indicating MI?

Scenario C

Ms. O'Hare, a 45-year-old woman, is on the list for a heart transplant. She has an LVAD and is waiting at home.

1. What signs and symptoms would indicate that Ms. O'Hare is no longer stable enough to wait at home?
2. Describe the purpose of the LVAD.
3. Develop a discharge teaching plan for Ms. O'Hare after transplant.

The Neurologic System*

21

http://evolve.elsevier.com/deWit/medsurg

Objectives

Theory

1. Define the vocabulary particular to problems of the nervous system.
2. Examine the differences in the actions of the sympathetic and parasympathetic nervous systems.
3. Devise four specific ways in which a nurse can contribute to preventing neurologic disorders.
4. Provide rationale for the appropriate preparation and postprocedure care for patients undergoing lumbar puncture (spinal tap), electroencephalogram (EEG), and radiologic studies of the brain and cerebral vessels.
5. Demonstrate techniques used for assessment of the nervous system.
6. Compare and contrast the various signs and symptoms of the common problems experienced by patients with nervous system disorders.

Clinical Practice

7. Gather a pertinent history for a patient with a nervous system problem.
8. Demonstrate a "neuro" check.
9. Score the neurologic status of a patient with a nervous system disorder according to the Glasgow Coma Scale.

Key Terms

accommodation (ăk-kŏm-ē-DĀ-shŭn, p. 501)
afferent (ĂF-ĕr-ĕnt, p. 488)
aphasia (ă-FĀ-zhă, p. 510)
Babinski reflex (Bab-INS-key RĒ-flĕks, p. 496)
calculi (KĂL-kū-lī, p. 508)
caloric testing (kăl-Ō-rĭk, p. 503)
clonus (KLŌ-nŭs, p. 496)
delirium (dĕ-LĬR-ē-ŭm, p. 510)
dysphagia (dĭs-FĀ-jē-ă, p. 508)
efferent (ĔF-ĕr-ĕnt, p. 488)
extensor posturing (ĕks-TĔN-sōr pŏs-CHŪR-ĭng, p. 502)
flexor posturing (FLĔK-sōr pŏs-CHŪR-ĭng, p. 502)
hemiparesis (hĕm-ē-pă-RĒ-sĭs, p. 507)
hemiplegia (hĕm-ĭ-PLĒ-jă, p. 507)
nystagmus (nĭs-TĂG-mŭs, p. 496)
quadriplegia (kwŏd-rĭ-PLĒ-jă, p. 507)
synapse (SĬN-ăps, p. 487)
tetraplegia (TĔT-ră-PLĒ-jă, p. 507)

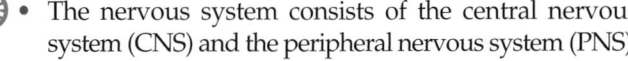

Concepts Covered in This Chapter

- Functional Ability
- Self-Management
- Intracranial Regulation
- Mobility
- Sensory Perception
- Cognition
- Clinical Judgment

ANATOMY AND PHYSIOLOGY OF THE NEUROLOGIC SYSTEM

ORGANIZATION OF THE NERVOUS SYSTEM

- The nervous system consists of the central nervous system (CNS) and the peripheral nervous system (PNS).

CNS

- The CNS is made up of the brain and spinal cord (Fig. 21.1).
- The brain is divided into the cerebrum, diencephalon, cerebellum, and brainstem, which each perform various functions (Fig. 21.2). Table 21.1 lists the functions of the various divisions of the brain.
- The brainstem consists of the midbrain, pons, and medulla.
- The spinal cord extends from the medulla to the level of the first lumbar vertebra.
- The spinal cord is a conduction pathway for impulses going to and from the brain and also serves as a reflex center for nerve impulse transmission. Sensory impulses travel to the brain on ascending conduction pathway tracts; motor impulses travel on descending tracts.
- Pyramidal tracts are conduction pathways that begin in the cerebral cortex and end in the spinal cord.

*Refer to an anatomy and physiology text for a thorough review of the complex nervous system.

Table 21.1 Functions of the Divisions of the Brain

DIVISION	FUNCTION
Cerebrum	Center of intellect and consciousness. Receives and interprets sensory information; controls voluntary movements and certain types of involuntary movements; responsible for thinking, learning, language capability, judgment, and personality; stores memories.
Cerebellum	Responsible for coordination of movement, posture, and muscle tone that are the mechanisms of balance.
Diencephalon (consists of two parts)	
Thalamus	Relay center between spinal cord and cerebrum.
Hypothalamus	Controls body temperature, appetite, and water balance; links nervous and endocrine systems.
Brainstem (consists of three parts)	
Midbrain	Mediates visual and auditory reflexes; controls cranial nerves III and IV and certain eye movements.
Pons	Links various parts of the brain; helps regulate respiration.
Medulla oblongata	Contains reticular formation that regulates heartbeat, respiration, and blood pressure; controls center for swallowing, coughing, sneezing, and vomiting; relays messages to other parts of the brain.

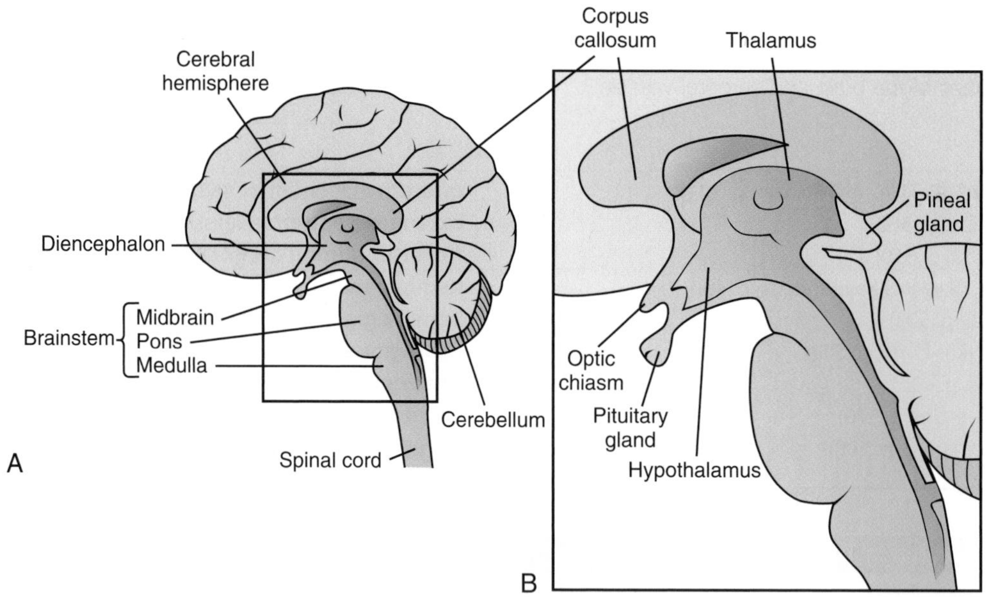

Fig. 21.1 **A,** Main divisions of the central nervous system. **B,** Diencephalon (thalamus and hypothalamus).

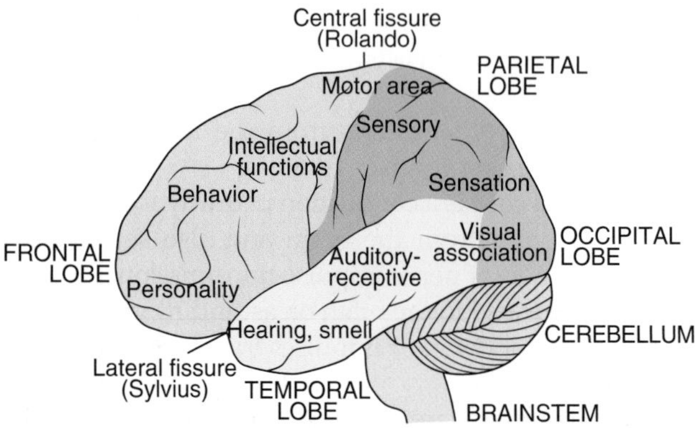

Fig. 21.2 Specialized functions of the lobes of the cerebrum.

These tracts control skeletal muscle movement. All other conduction pathways are extrapyramidal tracts, and they control muscle movements associated with posture and balance.

PNS

- The PNS is composed of the sensory organs—eyes, ears, taste buds, olfactory receptors, and touch receptors—12 pairs of cranial nerves, and 31 pairs of spinal nerves and ganglia that link the sensory organs, muscles, and other parts of the body to the brain and spinal cord. The distribution pathways of the spinal nerves are called *dermatomes* (Fig. 21.3).

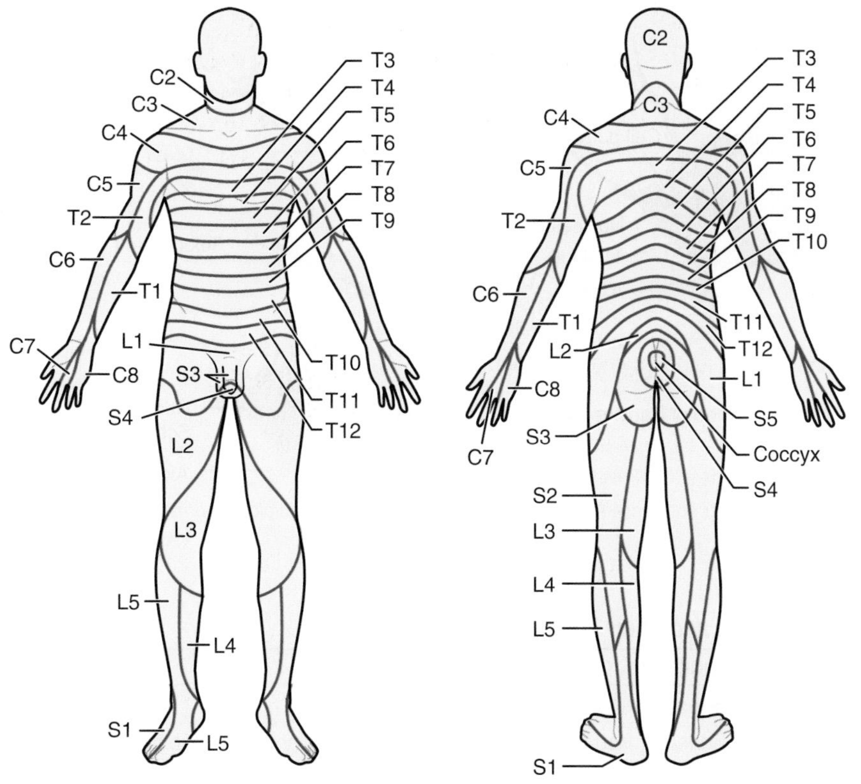

Fig. 21.3 Dermatomes (cutaneous innervation of spinal nerves). Stimulation of the skin in the depicted area for each nerve causes reflex activity. *C,* Cervical spinal nerves; *L,* lumbar spinal nerves; *S,* sacral spinal nerves; *T,* thoracic spinal nerves. (From Ignatavicius DD, Workman ML, Rebar CR, et al.: *Medical-surgical nursing: critical thinking for collaborative care,* ed 9, St. Louis, 2018, Elsevier.)

- Of the 12 pairs of cranial nerves, some are sensory nerves and others are motor nerves (Table 21.2).

NERVES AND THE CONDUCTION OF IMPULSES

- Neurons react to stimuli, conduct impulses, and influence other neurons.
- The axons of many neurons, bundled together and wrapped in connective tissue, make up a nerve (Fig. 21.4). Ganglia are collections of nerve cell bodies outside the CNS; within the CNS, they are referred to as a *nucleus*.
- When in a state of polarization, neurons have the capacity to become excited (stimulated). They also can conduct that stimulus along the nerve pathways.
- A stimulus is a physical, chemical, or electrical event that changes the cell membrane and initiates conduction of the stimulus as an electrical impulse along the nerve pathway.
- The stimulus travels from one neuron to another across a **synapse** (the space between two neurons).
- A neurotransmitter secreted by the neuron is necessary for transmission of an impulse across the synapse (Table 21.3). Acetylcholine, dopamine, and norepinephrine are the major neurotransmitters.
- Neurotransmitter substances are secreted at the synapse, and these diffuse across the synapse to stimulate the postsynaptic membrane on the next neuron. **When the neurotransmitter is absent or decreased at the synaptic junction, the stimulus cannot travel along the nerve pathways normally.**
- Impulses either travel in a reflex arc, going to the spinal cord and traveling back to an effector site, or travel along nerve pathways to the brain to be interpreted.
- After impulse interpretation, a message may be sent out from the brain through the spinal cord or cranial nerves (PNS) for appropriate action to be taken. In other words, a stimulus produces a response.
- Many axons are surrounded by a myelin sheath that is a white, fatty covering. The myelin sheath is an excellent electrical insulator, and it speeds the conduction of nerve impulses. **When myelin is destroyed, as in multiple sclerosis, impulse transmission is slowed or stopped.**

CONTROL OF THE BODY

- Body functions for homeostasis and those of voluntary mechanisms are controlled by the somatic nervous system (SNS) and the autonomic nervous system (ANS).
- The functions of the SNS result in moving skeletal muscles.
- SNS movement may be conscious and voluntary or reflex-type activity that does not involve a conscious decision.

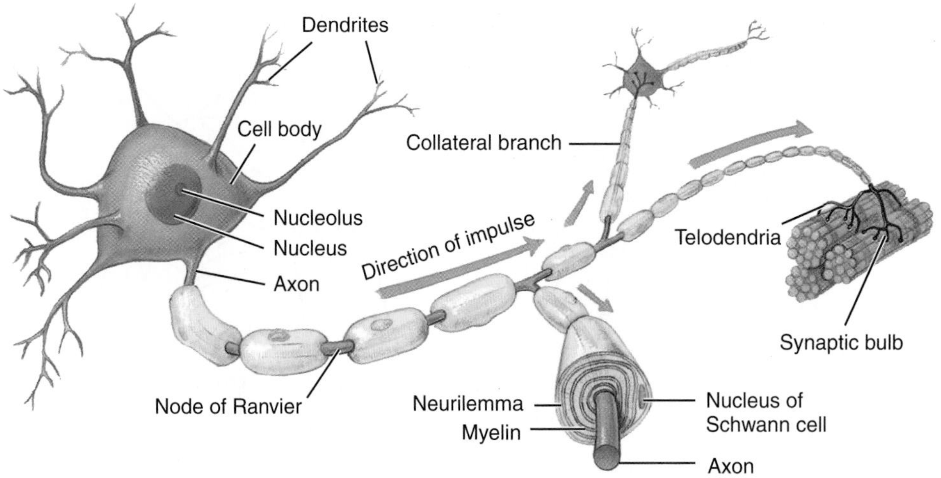

Fig. 21.4 Structure of a neuron. (From Applegate E: *The anatomy and physiology learning system,* ed 4, Philadelphia, 2011, Saunders.)

Table 21.2 The Cranial Nerves and Their Functions

TYPE	FUNCTION
Olfactory (CN I)	*Sensory:* smell
Optic (CN II)	*Sensory:* visual acuity, field of vision, pupillary response (afferent impulse)
Oculomotor (CN III)	*Motor:* eyelid elevation, extraocular eye movement, pupil size, convergence, pupillary constriction (efferent impulse)
Trochlear (CN IV)	*Motor:* extraocular eye movement (inferior and lateral)
Trigeminal (CN V)	*Sensory:* corneal reflex *Motor:* facial sensation; chewing, biting, lateral jaw movement
Abducens (CN VI)	*Motor:* extraocular eye movement (lateral)
Facial (CN VII)	*Sensory:* taste *Motor:* facial muscle movement, including muscles of expression; lacrimal gland and salivary gland control
Acoustic (CN VIII)	*Sensory:* hearing, sense of balance
Glossopharyngeal (CN IX)	*Sensory:* sensations of the throat, taste (posterior tongue) *Motor:* gagging and swallowing movements
Vagus (CN X)	*Sensory:* sensations of posterior tongue, throat, larynx; impulses from heart, lungs, bronchi, and gastrointestinal tract *Motor:* initiation of swallowing and phonation
Spinal accessory (CN XI)	*Motor:* shoulder movement and head rotation
Hypoglossal (CN XII)	*Motor:* tongue movement, articulation of speech

- The ANS is found in both the CNS and the PNS and affects cardiac or other smooth muscle tissue and prompts glands to produce secretions.
- The ANS helps maintain homeostasis by regulating organ systems.

INTERACTION OF THE PERIPHERAL NERVOUS SYSTEM AND THE CENTRAL NERVOUS SYSTEM

- The PNS is subdivided into an afferent division and an efferent division. The **afferent** division carries impulses to the CNS; the **efferent** division carries impulses away from the CNS.
- The reflex arc is a simple conduction pathway that uses a receptor (a sensory neuron centered in the spinal cord) and a motor neuron located in an effector (skeletal muscle). A stimulus travels from the sensory receptor through the spinal cord and back to the effector, causing action (Fig. 21.5).
- Reflex arcs are important to most functions of the body, including maintaining an upright position.
- The cranial and spinal nerves are part of the somatic subsystem and respond to changes in the outside world. Because these nerves initiate voluntary action, the somatic system often is called the *voluntary system.*
- The autonomic system of the PNS is active in maintaining internal body balance *(homeostasis)* and is automatic (involuntary) in its actions.

Table 21.3 Neurotransmitters That Affect Transmission of Nerve Impulses

NEUROTRANSMITTER	LOCATION	FUNCTION	COMMENTS
Acetylcholine	CNS and PNS	Generally excitatory but is inhibitory to some visceral effectors	Found in skeletal neuromuscular junctions and in many ANS synapses
Norepinephrine	CNS and PNS	May be excitatory or inhibitory depending on the receptors	Found in visceral and cardiac muscle neuromuscular junctions; cocaine and amphetamines exaggerate the effects
Epinephrine	CNS and PNS	May be excitatory or inhibitory depending on the receptors	Found in pathways concerned with behavior and mood
Dopamine	CNS and PNS	Generally excitatory	Found in pathways that regulate emotional responses; decreased levels in Parkinson disease
Serotonin	CNS	Generally inhibitory	Found in pathways that regulate temperature, sensory perception, mood, onset of sleep
Gamma-aminobutyric acid (GABA)	CNS	Generally inhibitory	Inhibits excessive discharge of neurons
Glutamic acid (glutamate)	CNS	Generally excitatory	Facilitates signals between nerve cells and plays a role in learning and memory
Endorphins and enkephalins	CNS	Generally inhibitory	Inhibit release of sensory pain neurotransmitters; opiates mimic the effects of these peptides

From Crossman AR, Neary D: *Neuroanatomy: an illustrated colour text*, ed 5, Edinburgh, 2015, Churchill Livingstone.
ANS, Autonomic nervous system; *CNS*, central nervous system; *PNS*, peripheral nervous system.

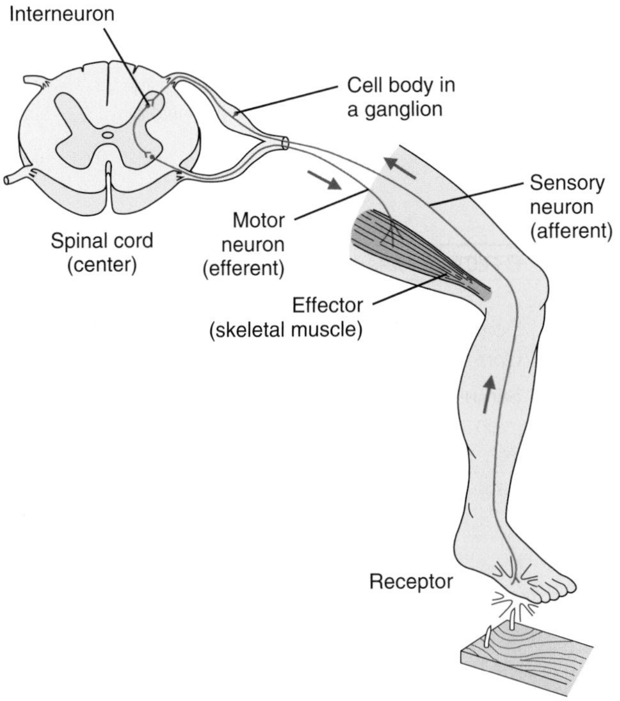

Fig. 21.5 Components of a generalized reflex arc.

- The autonomic system is divided into the sympathetic nerves, which mobilize energy to initiate changes aimed at maintaining or restoring homeostasis, and the parasympathetic nerves, which conserve and restore energy that has been used to maintain homeostasis.
- **Sympathetic and parasympathetic nerves have opposite effects on many organs** (Fig. 21.6 and Table 21.4).

PROTECTION OF THE CENTRAL NERVOUS SYSTEM

- The bones of the skull and the vertebral column form the outer layer of protection for the brain and the spinal cord.
- The meninges are protective membranes that cover the brain and are continuous with the membranes covering the spinal cord. The meninges consist of the pia mater, which covers the brain; the arachnoid, which encases the entire CNS; and the dura mater, which is a tough membrane protecting the brain and spinal cord.
- The subarachnoid space is located between the pia mater and the arachnoid membrane and is where the cerebrospinal fluid (CSF) circulates (Fig. 21.7).
- CSF serves to cushion and protect the brain and spinal cord. It is formed continuously as a filtrate from the blood in specialized capillary networks in the choroid plexus, located in the ventricles of the brain. It is reabsorbed by the arachnoid villi of the arachnoid membrane at the same rate at which it is formed. The volume of CSF normally stays constant (see Fig. 21.7).
- **Normal CSF pressure measured during lumbar puncture is 100 to 180 cm water pressure (cm H_2O) when side lying and 200 to 300 cm H_2O when sitting.** When there is an excess of fluid in the subarachnoid space, the CSF pressure rises above normal.

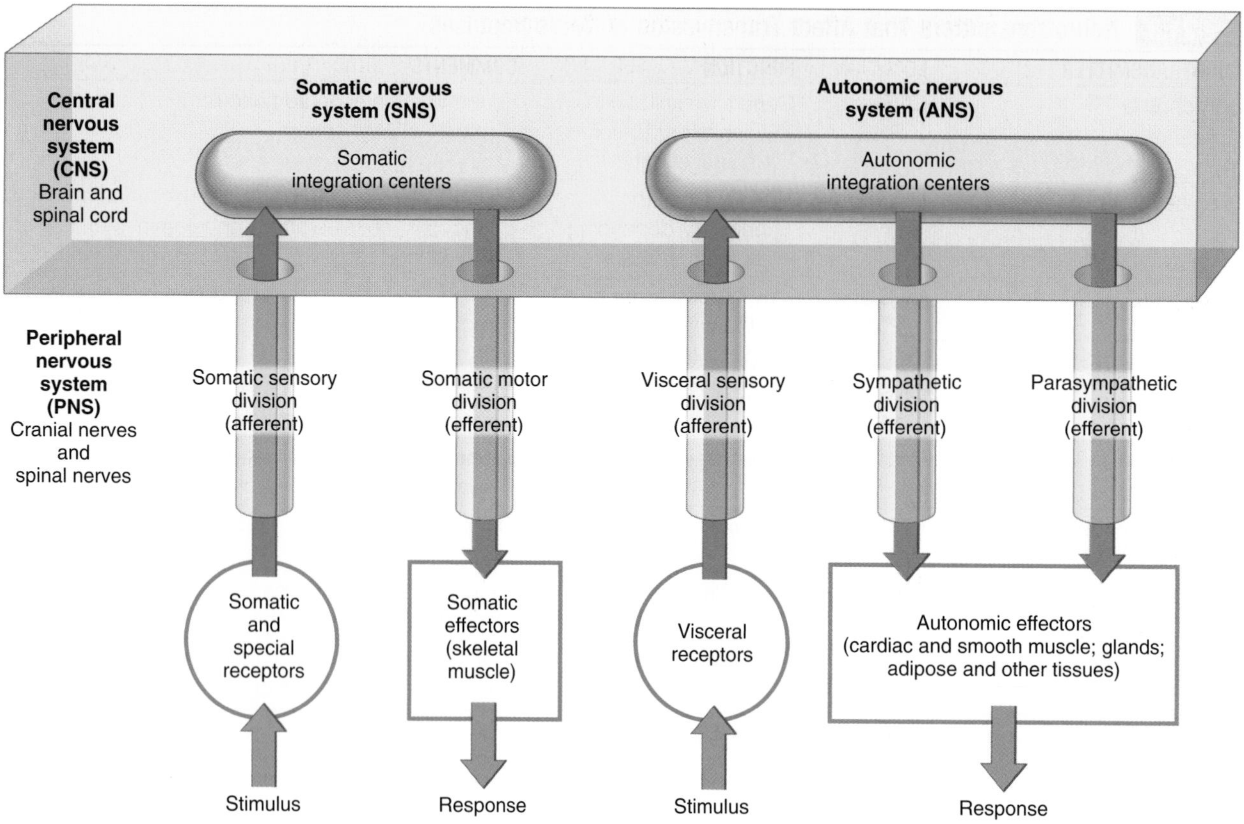

Fig. 21.6 Organizational plan of the nervous system. Diagram summarizes the scheme used by most neurobiologists in studying the nervous system. Both the somatic nervous system *(SNS)* and the autonomic nervous system *(ANS)* include components in the central nervous system *(CNS)* and peripheral nervous system *(PNS)*. Somatic sensory pathways conduct information toward integrators in the CNS, and somatic motor pathways conduct information toward somatic effectors. In the ANS, visceral sensory pathways conduct information toward CNS integrators, whereas the sympathetic and parasympathetic pathways conduct information toward autonomic effectors. (From Patton K: *Anatomy and physiology,* ed 10, St. Louis, 2019, Elsevier.)

Table 21.4 Autonomic Effects on Various Organs of the Body

ORGAN	EFFECT OF SYMPATHETIC STIMULATION	EFFECT OF PARASYMPATHETIC STIMULATION
Eye		
Pupil	Dilated	Constricted
Ciliary muscle	Slight relaxation (far vision)	Constricted (near vision)
Glands: nasal, lacrimal, parotid, submandibular, gastric, pancreatic	Vasoconstriction and slight secretion	Stimulation of copious secretion (containing many enzymes for enzyme-secreting glands)
Sweat glands	Copious sweating (cholinergic)	Sweating on palms of hands
Apocrine glands	Thick, odoriferous secretion	None
Blood vessels	Most often constricted	Most often little or no effect
Heart		
Muscle	Increased rate Increased force of contraction	Slowed rate Decreased force of contraction (especially of atria)
Coronary arteries	Dilated ($beta_2$); constricted (alpha)	Dilated
Lungs		
Bronchi	Dilated	Constricted
Blood vessels	Mildly constricted	Dilated
Gut		
Lumen	Decreased peristalsis and tone	Increased peristalsis and tone
Sphincter	Increased tone (most times)	Relaxed (most times)
Liver	Glucose released	Slight glucose synthesis
Gallbladder and bile ducts	Relaxed	Contracted

Table 21.4 Autonomic Effects on Various Organs of the Body—cont'd

ORGAN	EFFECT OF SYMPATHETIC STIMULATION	EFFECT OF PARASYMPATHETIC STIMULATION
Kidney	Decreased output and renin secretion	None
Bladder		
Detrusor	Relaxed (slight)	Contracted
Trigone	Contracted	Relaxed
Penis	Ejaculation	Erection
Systemic arterioles		
Abdominal viscera	Constricted	None
Muscle	Constricted (alpha-adrenergic) Dilated (beta-adrenergic) Dilated (cholinergic)	None
Skin	Constricted	None
Blood		None
Coagulation	Increased	None
Glucose	Increased	None
Lipids	Increased	None
Basal metabolism	Increased up to 100%	None
Adrenal medullary secretion	Increased	None
Mental activity	Increased	None
Piloerector muscles	Contracted	None
Skeletal muscle	Increased glycogenolysis Increased strength	None
Fat cells	Lipolysis	None

From Hall JE: *Guyton and Hall textbook of medical physiology*, ed 13, Philadelphia, 2016, Elsevier.

BLOOD FLOW TO THE CENTRAL NERVOUS SYSTEM

- The brain requires a constant flow of oxygen to function.
- Neurons are very sensitive to oxygen and die quickly when deprived of oxygen. **The brain's neurons cannot survive anoxia for more than 4 to 6 minutes.**
- Arterial blood flow is delivered via the right and left carotid arteries anteriorly and the right and left vertebral arteries posteriorly. The vessels all converge at the base of the brain into the circle of Willis (Fig. 21.8). This maintains blood flow even if one part has a narrowing or blockage.
- The venous blood exits the cerebral circulation via the jugular veins.
- The brain can autoregulate the flow of blood for a constant supply. Blood provided to the brain arrives in waves consistent with the pulsatile flow from each heartbeat. The vessels into the brain constrict or dilate as needed so that the brain receives a continuous supplied of oxygenated blood.

INTRACRANIAL PRESSURE (ICP)

- The pressure within the skull is normally 5 to 15 mm Hg.
- The volume of brain tissue, CSF, and cerebral blood flow determine the ICP.
- Disorders causing swelling of brain tissue, increased CSF, or increased blood flow (or decreased venous drainage) will all increase ICP.
- ICP greater than 20 mm Hg requires treatment.
- Prolonged elevation of ICP will compromise brain tissue and cause injury or death of neurons.

SPECIAL CHARACTERISTICS OF THE NERVOUS SYSTEM

- Although some cells in the PNS have an outer membrane called the *neurilemma* (or Schwann sheath) that may regenerate after damage, cells of the CNS do not have this capability. **Once destroyed, cells in the brain cannot be replaced,** but other brain cells may pick up their function.
- In the PNS, the Schwann cells can regenerate the myelin sheaths that wrap around the axons in the PNS.

AGING-RELATED CHANGES IN THE NERVOUS SYSTEM

- There is a loss of neurons with aging, and brain weight may drop considerably after age 70 years; there is no loss of intellectual function attributable to this loss of neurons.
- The number of functioning dendrites decreases with aging. This decrease causes slower impulse transmission and resultant slower reaction time in older adults.

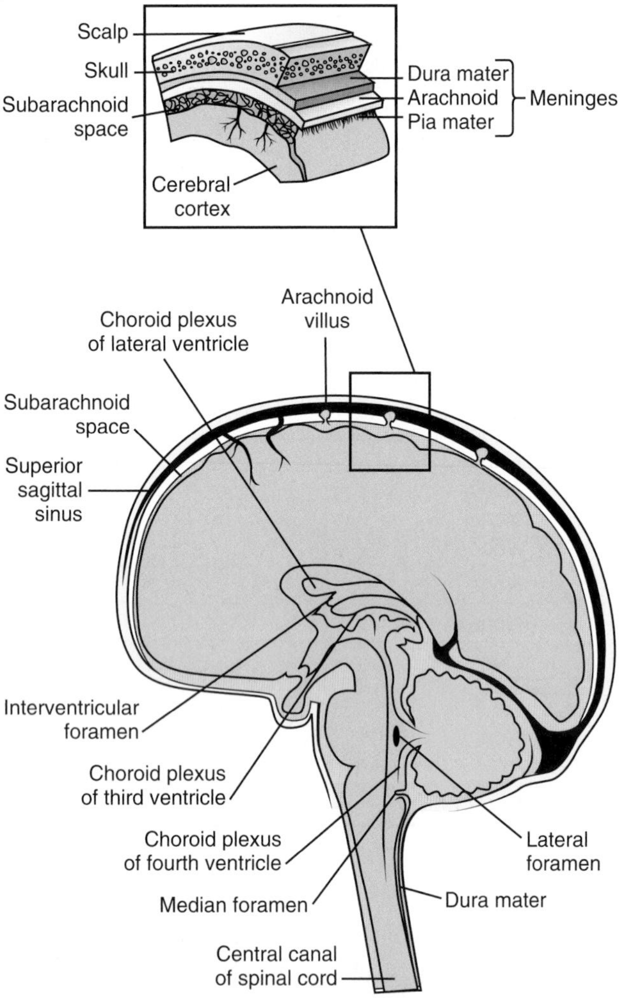

Fig. 21.7 Flow of the cerebrospinal fluid. *Inset,* Meninges covering the brain.

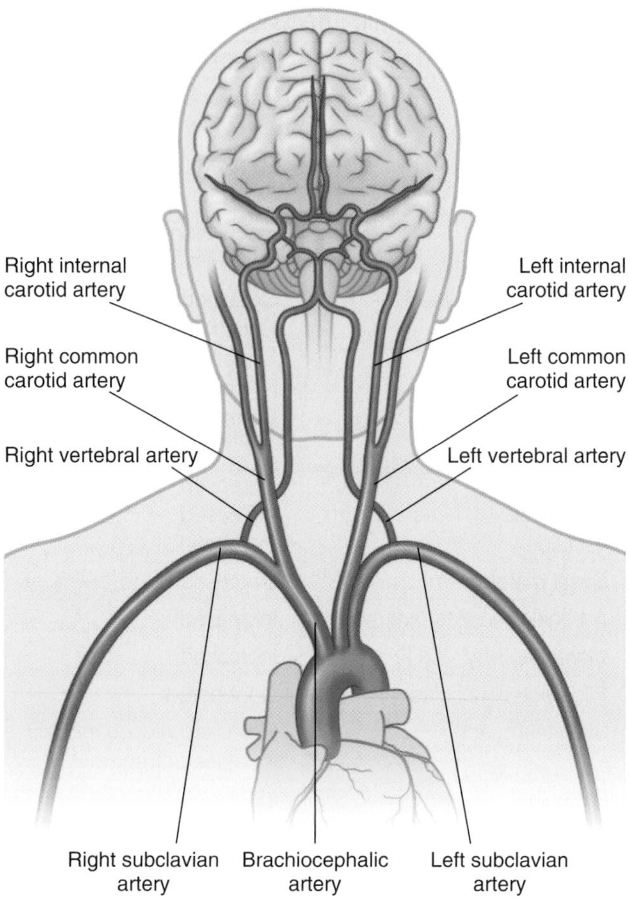

Fig. 21.8 Arteries forming the circulus arteriosus (circle of Willis). (From Grant A, Waugh A: *Ross and Wilson anatomy and physiology in health and illness,* ed 13, St. Louis, 2018, Elsevier.)

- Blood flow to the brain is decreased with advanced age; this makes older adults more susceptible to permanent damage if blood flow to the brain is further compromised.
- Loss of neurons and slower nerve conduction cause a decrease in efficiency of the ANS with advanced age.
- In late adulthood, changes can cause decreased sensation. Tremors may occur without rigidity, and tendon reflexes may be hypoactive.
- Body homeostasis is more difficult for older adults to maintain or regain. Exposure to prolonged cold or to excessive heat may cause death. Adaptation to physiologic stress takes much longer, and recovery often is incomplete.
- The aging process affects recent, short-term memory, but long-term, distant memory is often not affected. The ability to learn is not affected by aging, but the learning process is slower. It takes longer to process new information. Abstract reasoning ability slowly diminishes with advancing age, and perception may become impaired.
- Decreases in secretion of the neurotransmitters norepinephrine and dopamine occur with advanced age, and there is an increase in monoamine oxidase, which can affect cognitive function, gait, and balance.
- Pupils decrease in size with advanced age, and more light is needed for reading.

CAUSATIVE FACTORS INVOLVED IN NEUROLOGIC DISORDERS

Many factors can affect neurologic function, including genetic and acquired developmental disorders. Infections and inflammation, benign and malignant tumors, vascular or neuromuscular degeneration, and metabolic and endocrine disorders can all cause damage to or interfere with normal function of the nervous system. Chemical or physical trauma often causes permanent damage to the brain or spinal cord. Box 21.1 lists by category the most common neurologic disorders in adults.

PREVENTION OF NEUROLOGIC DISORDERS

The nervous system coordinates all sensory and motor activities by receiving, interpreting, and relaying

Box 21.1 Classification of Common Neurologic Disorders

GENETIC OR DEVELOPMENTAL DISORDERS
- Cerebral palsy
- Muscular dystrophy
- Huntington disease (chorea)

TRAUMA
- Head injury
- Penetrating brain injury
- Spinal cord injury
- Ruptured intervertebral disk

CEREBROVASCULAR
- Cerebrovascular accident
- Ruptured aneurysm
- Arteriovenous malformation
- Migraine, cluster headache

TUMOR
- Brain tumor
- Spinal cord tumor

INFECTION
- Meningitis
- Encephalitis
- Brain abscess
- Spinal abscess
- Poliomyelitis
- Guillain-Barré syndrome

NEUROMUSCULAR DISORDERS
- Multiple sclerosis
- Myasthenia gravis
- Amyotrophic lateral sclerosis

DEGENERATIVE DISORDERS
- Parkinson disease
- Alzheimer disease

CRANIAL NERVE DISORDERS
- Bell palsy
- Trigeminal neuralgia

messages that are vital to the proper performance of all the body's activities. Respiratory, circulatory, digestive, and endocrine functions all depend on an intact and normally functioning ANS.

Nurses can help prevent neurologic problems in many ways. The goals for *Healthy People 2030* encourage health protection through education about safety and responsible self-care.

EVALUATION OF NEUROLOGIC STATUS

The complete neurologic examination performed by the health care provider systematically measures the ability of the body to perform its myriad motor and sensory functions. Mental acuity, memory, and emotional stability also are assessed. A complete neurologic examination is a very long procedure and is usually not indicated for the hospitalized patient. Components of the complete assessment are routinely done on every patient, and more detailed evaluations are completed for patients with neurologic disorders. Assessment of cognitive function is part of every patient encounter. Cognitive changes may be the first sign of hypoxia, a drug reaction, or other conditions affecting the nervous system but not caused by a disease process of the system.

Health Promotion

Protecting the Nervous System

- Encourage people to wear helmets when biking, inline skating, skateboarding, or riding motorcycles and when involved in other sports activities that may lead to head injury.
- Remind people that wearing safety hats or helmets when in a workplace where head injury is a danger reduces the number of injuries.
- Review safety precautions when diving and swimming. To help prevent spinal cord injury, never dive into water of unknown depth.
- Encourage people to fasten their seat belts before putting the car into gear.
- Be certain that children are fastened into appropriate restraints.
- Wear mask, gloves, long pants, and long-sleeved shirt when spraying with insecticide; wash up immediately afterward and change clothes.
- Refrain from using recreational drugs because they can affect the cardiovascular system and can cause a stroke.

Teaching about the dangers of recreational drug use, such as the possibility of stroke from the use of "crack" cocaine or methamphetamine and the potential for accidents while under the influence of some drugs, is another area for public education. Informing the public about the damaging effect of too much alcohol on brain cells, as well as the increased incidence of alcohol-induced accidents, is yet another area for education.

Control of hypertension and cholesterol can reduce the number of strokes and the damage they cause. Teaching people to recognize the symptoms of stroke and to seek early treatment may prevent permanent disability.

NURSING MANAGEMENT

ASSESSMENT (DATA COLLECTION)

Neurologic nursing requires special training and experience in observation, clinical judgment, and specific skills to help patients cope with myriad problems. You not only must be aware of subtle changes in the patient's condition but also must recognize the significance of these changes and act promptly when medical attention is needed. Licensed practical/vocational nurses (LPN/LVNs) assist registered nurses (RNs) with the gathering of data for the neurologic assessment.

Patient History

Because neurologic disorders can be present in conjunction with or in addition to disorders of other body systems, include questions about neurologic status in

Assignment Considerations

Reporting Observations

If a patient with a neurologic problem that may affect the level of consciousness is assigned to a certified nursing assistant (CNA) for bathing and morning care, remember to remind the assistant to report to you any change in wakefulness, irritability, speech, eye appearance, gait, or balance. It is best not to assign a patient who has already shown some signs of deteriorating level of consciousness to a CNA.

the initial and ongoing assessments of all patients. For example, a surgical patient could have had a previous stroke or could have a history of seizures or an existing neuromuscular disease such as multiple sclerosis. Although these may not be the primary reason for admission to a hospital, they will certainly influence the course of the illness or injury for which admission occurred.

Focused Assessment

Data Collection for the Neurologic System

When gathering a history for a patient who may have a neurologic problem, ask the following questions:

- Do you or does any member of your family have any genetic disorder of the nervous system?
- Have you ever had a seizure or been told you have epilepsy?
- Have you ever had difficulty in speaking, concentrating, remembering, or expressing thoughts? Have you noticed any changes in these functions?
- Have you had any changes in muscle strength or coordination?
- Have you ever injured your head?
- Have you ever had a very high fever?
- Have you had any severe sinus, ear, tooth, or facial skin infection?
- Do you recall any episodes of tremors, muscle spasms, fainting, dizziness, ringing in the ears, or blurred vision?
- Have you had any "blackout" spells?
- Have you noticed any changes in taste or smell?
- Do you have any numbness or tingling in the extremities?

Physical Assessment

A basic nursing assessment of neurologic function is performed on all patients. Patients who are suspected of experiencing a neurologic problem will receive a more in-depth assessment. Basic neurologic assessment includes assessment of level of consciousness and mental acuity, muscle strength, and presence of any deficit (speech, swallowing, unilateral weakness). Depending on the patient's status, a mixture of the following assessments may be conducted.

Vital signs. Assessing and recording temperature, pulse, respirations, and blood pressure are essential. The patient's temperature is important and may be elevated for a number of reasons. Infection or damage to the temperature control mechanisms within the brain from increasing ICP may be present.

Changes in blood pressure, particularly a rise in systolic pressure and a widening pulse pressure, may indicate an increase in ICP. After prolonged ICP elevation the pulse may become slow and bounding, and breathing may become irregular and labored. Changes in breathing pattern often indicate a problem with neurologic control of respiration. Any identified change must be reported to the health care provider promptly.

Clinical Cues

When the systolic and diastolic pressure readings are farther apart, a widening pulse pressure has occurred. For example, if the blood pressure was 128/78 mm Hg earlier and is now 136/64 mm Hg, there is a widened pulse pressure. Notify the health care provider when the pulse pressure widens.

Current vital signs should be compared with those from the previous several days to determine any changes or trends. Look for changes in blood pressure, pulse rate and quality, and respiratory pattern and for rising temperature.

Mental function and level of consciousness. Patients experience varying levels of consciousness and ability to respond. It is necessary to determine where the patient is in relation to level of consciousness (LOC), the extremes being alert, wakefulness, and deep coma (no responsiveness at all).

When observing a patient to determine LOC, the best assessment is based on established criteria or standards that are understood by the observer as well as by others who will be reading the results of the observations. The Glasgow Coma Scale (GCS) is a tool that is universally used in one form or another for this purpose (Table 21.5). The patient's LOC is scored in three different categories. The first category is eye opening, the second is best motor response, and the third is best verbal response. A number is assigned for each category depending on what the assessment reveals. Assessment in the first and last categories determines whether the patient can respond to voice commands or to pain or does not respond at all. Verbal responses are evaluated according to whether the patient is oriented and "making sense," confused, making inappropriate remarks, incomprehensible, or silent. **The score in each area is added together, with the optimal score being 15, which indicates a fully alert patient. A score of 3 indicates a totally comatose patient.** A score of 8 or less indicates coma level. Some of the criteria for assessing LOC include: Does the patient awaken easily? Are they oriented to person (self as well as others), place, and time? Are they able to follow commands? Do they fail to respond to any stimulus, even physically painful ones? Are they restless? Combative? Do they respond to pain with abnormal posturing?

Table 21.5 Level of Consciousness Scales

Glasgow Coma Scale	SCORE[a]
Eye Opening	
Spontaneous	4
To sound	3
To pain	2
Never	1
Motor Response	
Obeys commands	6
Localizes pain	5
Normal flexion (withdrawal)	4
Abnormal flexion posturing	3
Extension posturing	2
None	1
Verbal Response	
Oriented	5
Confused conversation	4
Inappropriate words	3
Incomprehensible sounds	2
None	1
FOUR Score Scale	**SCORE[b]**
Eye Response	
Eyelids open or opened, tracking or blinking to command	4
Eyelids open but not tracking	3
Eyelids closed, but open to loud voice	2
Eyelids closed, but open to pain	1
Eyelids remain closed to pain	0
Motor Response	
Thumbs-up, fist or peace sign	4
Localizing to pain	3
Flexion response to pain	2
Extension response to pain	1
No response or generalized myoclonus status	0
Brain Stem Reflexes	
Pupil and corneal reflexes present	4
One pupil wide and fixed	3
Pupil or corneal reflexes absent	2
Pupil and corneal reflexes absent	1
Absent pupil, corneal and cough reflex	0
Respiration	
Not intubated, regular breathing pattern	4
Not intubated, Cheyne Stokes breathing pattern	3
Not intubated, irregular breathing	2
Breathes above ventilator rate	1
Breathes at ventilator rate or apnea	0

[a]A score of 8 or less indicates coma. The highest possible score is 15.
[b]A score of 4 or less indicates a poor prognosis. The highest possible score is 16.
From Wijdicks E, Bamlet W, Maramattom B, et al.: Validation of a new coma scale: the FOUR Score, *Ann Neurol* 58(4):585–593, 2005.

The FOUR (Full Outline of UnResponsiveness) score developed by Eelco Wijdicks, a neurologist at the Mayo Clinic, is becoming the preferred scale to assess comatose or intubated patients who cannot speak. A score of 0 to 4 is assigned in each of four categories: eye, motor, brainstem, and respiratory function. A score of 0 indicates no function, and a score of 4 indicates normal function (see Table 21.5) (Nair et al., 2017).

Coma scales were initially developed for prehospital use. The patient could be scored in the field and then in the emergency department to see if there was improvement or deterioration of their condition. The use of the scales has been generalized to the hospitalized patient and is part of a routine assessment for many facilities.

? Think Critically

If your patient's blood pressure was 138/84 mm Hg and is now 146/76 mm Hg, what is happening? Is the ICP probably increasing or decreasing?

For an alert patient, note changes in mental function by asking questions to determine orientation to person, place, and time: "What day is today? What month is it? Where are you now?" Memory lapses may be assessed by asking the patient what city they live in, what state they reside in, what the last major holiday was, and so on. Thinking can be evaluated by asking the patient to add three numbers together; to count by sixes; or to solve a simple puzzle, such as "If a man goes to the store and purchases four oranges at 40 cents each, two apples at 60 cents each, and two bananas for 46 cents, how much did he spend?" (Allow pencil and paper to be used.) If the patient can read English, hand them a card with a command written on it, such as "walk to the sink" or "turn on your right side" (assuming that they are physically capable of performing such a task).

Judgment can be grossly tested by assessing whether the patient has been making rational choices in their day-to-day life and by asking them what they would do in a particular situation. Additional information may be obtained by administering the Mini-Mental State Examination (MMSE). It contains many of the above questions and has a scoring scale to interpret the results.

Neurologic and neuromuscular status. While watching the patient perform morning activities of daily living (ADLs), basic assessment of cranial nerves and motor function can be performed. Assess the following: Does the face move symmetrically when the patient smiles? Is speech clear when they answer questions? Do they move left and right extremities without noticeable problems? Is there anything abnormal about the gait as they move across the room or down the hall? Do they have difficulty eating or swallowing? Observe the pupils of the eye for size and equality. Pupils should be equal size and should constrict and dilate readily when the environmental light changes (Fig. 21.9). Can

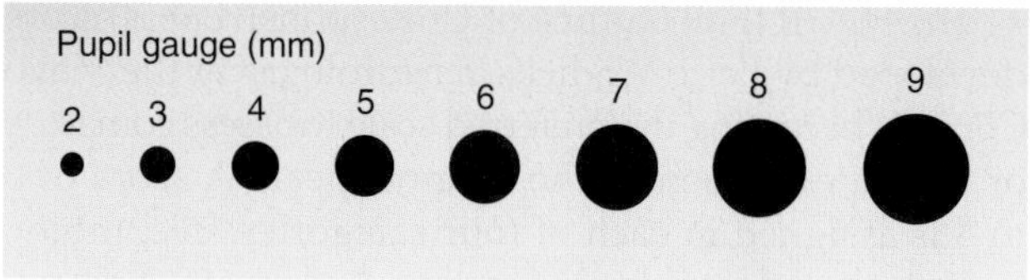

Fig. 21.9 Pupil gauge (mm). (From Williams P: *deWit's fundamental concepts and skills for nursing,* ed 5, St. Louis, 2018, Elsevier.)

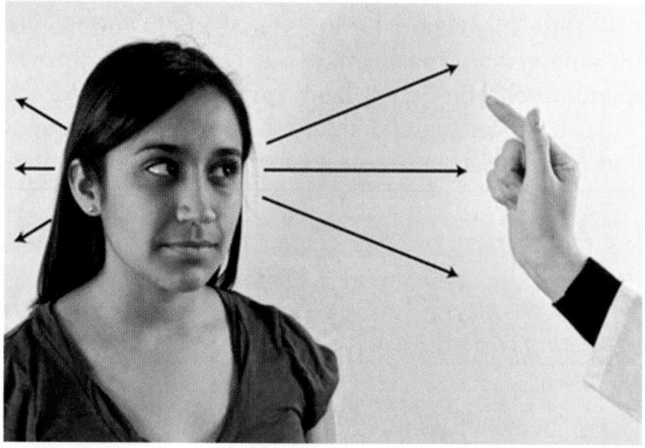

Fig. 21.10 Checking the cardinal positions of eye movement. (From Jarvis C: *Physical examination and health assessment,* ed 7, St. Louis, 2016, Elsevier.)

the patient hear you if you speak to them when their back is turned? Do they seem as alert as usual? Are they having any trouble with balance?

Evaluate the extraocular muscle movements. Ask the patient to follow your finger while you move it through the cardinal positions of gaze (Fig. 21.10). Note whether both eyes move together (conjugate) or one deviates. If there is deviation, it is important to note the direction of the deviation. Note any quick back-and-forth oscillation (**nystagmus**) of the eye at the end points of each direction. Nystagmus can indicate abnormality, such as multiple sclerosis, or can be a side effect of medication, such as phenytoin (Dilantin).

Neuromuscular assessment is concerned with the function of the motor pathways. Test each of the upper and lower extremities. Ask the patient to follow verbal commands such as "raise your left leg," "bend your right knee," "touch your left elbow with your right hand," and "touch your face with your left hand." Have them push against the palms of your hands first with one foot and then with the other to test the strength of the leg muscles. To test muscle strength, have the patient extend their arms in front of them, and press down on each arm one at a time while asking them to try to raise the arm. If the patient has an extremity that is not responding, another stimulus may be necessary to test it. Pronator drift is determined by having the patient hold their arms out in front of their body with palms up and eyes closed. If weakness is present, the weak limb will drift downward and the hand will turn inward (pronating). More sophisticated tests include electromyography (Table 21.6).

The portion of the neurologic examination assessing coordination and balance evaluates functions controlled by the higher centers of the brain, the cerebrum and cerebellum. The patient is asked to stand with their feet together and to close their eyes (Romberg test). If the sense of balance is normal, a steady posture will be maintained and there will not be swaying from side to side. Next ask the patient to walk across the room; as they do so, assess the gait. Then stand in front of the patient, hold up a finger, and ask the patient to touch your finger and then their own nose; move your finger to different locations in front of the patient. This tests both the ability to follow directions and coordination. This assessment can be done when getting the patient out of bed for other activities. If physical therapy is working with the patient, they may do a balance test. The test is not performed on bedbound or hemodynamically unstable patients.

A **reflex** is an action or movement that is built into the nervous system and does not need the intervention of conscious thought to take place. In other words, it is an automatic response. The knee jerk is an example of the simplest type of reflex. When the knee is tapped, the nerve that receives this stimulus sends an impulse to the spinal cord, where it is relayed to a motor nerve. This causes the quadriceps muscle at the front of the thigh to contract and to move the leg upward. This reflex, or simple reflex arc, involves only two nerves and one synapse. The leg begins to jerk up while the brain is just becoming aware of the tap on the knee (see Fig. 21.5).

The knee jerk, or patellar reflex, tests nerve pathways to and from the spinal cord at the level of the second through fourth lumbar nerves. In addition to testing the patellar reflex, a neurologic examination might include testing the biceps reflex (pathways for the fifth and sixth cervical nerves), triceps reflex (seventh and eighth cervical nerves), brachioradialis reflex (fifth and sixth cervical nerves), and Achilles tendon reflex (first and second sacral nerves). Reflexes are graded as follows: 0/5 = absent; 1/5 = weak response; 2/5 = normal; 3/5 = exaggerated response; and 4/5 = hyperreflexia with clonus. **Clonus** is a continued rhythmic contraction of the muscle while there is continuous application of the stimulus.

Another reflex action widely used as a diagnostic aid in CNS disorders is the plantar reflex known as the **Babinski reflex**, which is elicited by firmly stroking a blunt object such as a key along the sole of the foot. In a normal response to this stimulus, the toes will bend downward. In a *positive* Babinski reflex, the great toe bends backward (upward) and the smaller toes fan outward. A positive Babinski reflex in an adult who is not under the influence of chemical substances indicates an abnormality in the motor control pathways leading from the cerebral cortex (Fig. 21.11).

The 12 cranial nerves (CNs; designated as CN I through CN XII) control both sensory and motor

Table 21.6 **Diagnostic Tests for Neurologic Disorders**

PURPOSE	DESCRIPTION	NURSING IMPLICATIONS
Skull and Spine Radiographs		
To detect fractures, bone loss, and other bony abnormalities	Radiographs are taken of the desired area from various angles.	Explain that the test is noninvasive. Advise that the patient will have to move into various positions.
Lumbar Puncture (Spinal Tap) (see Fig. 21.13)		
To determine whether CSF pressure is elevated; to determine whether there is a blockage to the flow of CSF; to inject medications; to obtain fluid for chemical analysis and culture	Health care provider performs a sterile puncture into the arachnoid space, using local anesthetic, between L3 and L4 or L4 and L5; opening pressure is obtained; fluid is aspirated and placed in sterile test tubes labeled 1, 2, and 3. Fluid is analyzed for color, pH, cell count, protein, chloride, and glucose; a culture is usually done. Local anesthetic is used.	Procedure requires a signed consent form. Obtain sterile lumbar puncture tray, local anesthetic, sterile gloves, and tape. Assist patient into position with back bowed, head flexed on chest, and knees drawn up to the abdomen. Patient may be lying or sitting. Assist patient to maintain position and to hold still during procedure. Reassure patient and provide emotional support. Personnel must wear a mask during procedure. *Postprocedure:* Appropriately label tubes with patient data and transport them to the laboratory immediately. Keep patient flat in bed for 1 h or longer after procedure to reduce headache and encourage fluid intake unless contraindicated. Observe the site for signs of drainage and inflammation.
Electroencephalography (EEG)		
To detect abnormal brain wave patterns that are indicative of specific diseases, such as seizure disorder, brain tumor, CVA, head trauma, and infection; to determine cerebral death	May be performed while patient is asleep, drowsy, or undergoing stimulation such as hyperventilation or rhythmic bright light. Test may be done at the bedside or in the EEG laboratory. Tracing is taken with patient in reclining chair or lying down. Electrodes are applied to the scalp with an electrode paste. Test takes 45 min-2 h.	Explain purpose of test to the patient; the test is not painful, and it is similar to an ECG for the heart. It detects electrical activity in the brain. Hair should be clean and dry. No sleeping pills or sedatives the night before test; check with provider regarding other drugs to be held; restrict coffee, tea, caffeine, and alcohol for 24–48 h. If a sleep EEG is ordered, patient may need to be kept up most or all of the night before the test; do not keep NPO, as hypoglycemia can affect the test. *Postprocedure:* Wash hair to remove the electrode paste. *Nothing touches the patient during the procedure.*
Magnetoencephalography (MEG)		
Preoperative brain mapping or use in epilepsy surgery	A biomagnetometer machine detects the small magnetic fields generated by neurons.	The test is done in a magnetically shielded room to block out extraneous signals. It is often done in conjunction with MRI. *Postprocedure:* Care is the same as for EEG.
Electromyography (EMG)		
To measure electrical activity of skeletal muscle at rest and during voluntary activity to determine abnormalities in muscular contraction, nerve dysfunction, or dysfunction in the nerve to muscle communication; helpful in diagnosing neuromuscular, peripheral nerve, and muscular disorders	With the patient sitting in a chair or lying on a table, needle electrodes are inserted in selected muscles for certain conditions. Surface electrodes may be used for other conditions. Tracings of electrical activity are taken with the muscles at rest, then with various voluntary activities that produce muscle contraction. The test takes 1–2 h depending on how many muscles are tested.	Procedure requires a signed consent form. Explain the procedure to the patient; tell them that there is discomfort when the needle electrodes are placed but not the surface electrodes. Check with provider regarding medications to be withheld; muscle relaxants, cholinergics, and anticholinergics can influence test result. There is no food or fluid restriction. If serum enzymes are ordered, they should be drawn before the EMG.

Continued

Table 21.6 Diagnostic Tests for Neurologic Disorders—cont'd

PURPOSE	DESCRIPTION	NURSING IMPLICATIONS
Myelography		
To detect spinal lesions, intervertebral disk problems, tumors, or cysts	Contrast medium is injected into the spinal canal, and fluoroscopic examination and radiographs are made. The study is contraindicated if the patient has increased ICP. The patient is placed prone and strapped to the x-ray table for the spinal puncture; as the contrast medium is injected, the table is tilted. After the test, if oil-based medium was used, it is withdrawn. The patient is kept in bed with head of bed elevated 60 degrees or flat depending on the contrast medium used. Procedure takes 1 h. Rarely performed.	Procedure requires a signed consent form. Explain what to expect. Patient may feel a warm flush when contrast medium is injected. Bowel evacuation regimen may be ordered the night before. Keep NPO for 4–8 h before procedure. Check for medications to be withheld before and for 48 h after test. Assess for allergy to iodine or shellfish. Dress in myelogram pajamas; administer preoperative sedative or analgesic if ordered. *Postprocedure:* Monitor VS q30min × 2 h, then hourly × 4 h. Assess pulses and sensation in extremities; monitor urinary output; catheterize as ordered if patient cannot void in 8 h; encourage increased fluid intake. Observe for signs of meningitis.
Computed Axial Tomography (CAT or CT Scan); Xenon CT; Intrathecal Contrast-Enhanced CT		
To examine the brain from many different angles, obtaining a series of cross-sectional images that provide views from three dimensions To identify hematomas, tumors, cysts, hydrocephalus, cerebral atrophy, obstruction to CSF flow, and cerebral edema	May be done with or without contrast enhancement. Patient lies on a narrow table that moves so that the head is inside the circular opening of the machine. A security strap is used. CT scanner produces a narrow x-ray beam. Various clicking and whirring noises are heard as the machine rotates the scanner for different views. The test takes about 15 minutes. A lumbar puncture is needed for an intrathecal contrast-enhanced CT.	Procedure requires a signed consent form. Explain the procedure and what patient will see, hear, and feel. If contrast is used, the patient will feel a warm flush and have a metallic taste in the mouth as it is injected. Assess for allergy to iodine or shellfish. Remove all hairpins, jewelry, and metal from the head and neck. Patient may need to be sedated if they are prone to claustrophobia; the table can be uncomfortable for those with arthritis or back problems. They will be able to communicate with the technician. *Postprocedure:* Lumbar puncture postprocedure care if done.
Cerebral Angiography		
To visualize the structure of the cerebral arteries to determine the presence of stricture, tumor, aneurysm, thrombus, bleeding, or hematoma	Radiopaque contrast is injected through a catheter positioned in the common carotid artery, and a series of radiographs is taken. The femoral artery is usually used to enter the arterial system, and then catheters are positioned as needed depending on what is being imaged. Fluoroscopy is used during the procedure. Digital subtraction angiography (DSA) is done by using the computer to eliminate background images. Test takes 1–2 h. The test may also be performed with CT imaging rather than fluoroscopy–CT angiography.	Procedure requires a signed consent form. Assess for allergy to iodine and shellfish. Explain procedure; patient will be supine on x-ray table; local anesthetic will be used to introduce the catheter; an IV line will be started for administration of procedural sedation; patient will feel a flush as the dye is injected. Patient should be NPO 8–12 h before test; anticoagulants are discontinued beforehand. May be given preprocedure sedative, antihistamine, or steroid to decrease possibility of allergic reaction to dye. *Postprocedure:* Assess for bleeding at catheter site; assess distal pulses; perform neurologic checks; monitor VS q15min × 2 h, then hourly × 4 h or until stable.

Table 21.6 Diagnostic Tests for Neurologic Disorders—cont'd

PURPOSE	DESCRIPTION	NURSING IMPLICATIONS
Radionuclide Imaging (Brain Scan)		
To detect an intracranial mass: tumor, abscess, hematoma, or aneurysm	A radioisotope is administered IV. Abnormal tissue usually absorbs more of the isotope than normal tissue. After a 1- to 3-h waiting period for absorption, a scintillation scanner is used to image the brain. The test takes 30 min-1 h.	Explain the procedure; patient will sit or lie on a table; the scanner makes clicking noises; the amount of radioactivity is very low and is not dangerous to the patient or others. Patient will need to lie or sit still during the scanning. A drug may be given the night before to block uptake of the radioactive element by the thyroid and salivary glands. There is no food or fluid restriction; no special aftercare.
Magnetic Resonance Imaging (MRI)		
To visualize soft tissue without the use of ionizing radiation; provides excellent images of soft tissue, eliminating bone; can visualize lesions undetected by CT scan To detect white matter areas in nervous system that represent demyelination, as in multiple sclerosis	An electromagnet is used to detect radiofrequency pulses produced by alignment of hydrogen protons in the magnetic field. Computer produces tomographic images with high contrast of area studied. Cannot be used in the presence of metal. A contrast agent often is used for better visualization and definition of specific structures.	Inform patient that the test is painless; no dietary restrictions. Remove all metal objects before test. Screen the patient for hidden sources of metal, such as bullet fragments, iron filings, aneurysm clips. MRI is contraindicated for patients with pacemakers unless special precautions are taken. Patient must be still during test. Explain that the body part to be imaged is moved inside a large machine; some patients become claustrophobic. The machine generates a loud noise when scanning; headphones or ear protection is supplied. Patient will be able to communicate with the technician. Requires a signed consent for use of contrast media.
Magnetic Resonance Angiography (MRA)		
To evaluate intracranial and extracranial blood vessels and for diagnosing cerebrovascular disease; is rapidly replacing cerebral angiography	Similar to MRI. Uses differing signals of flowing blood to collect data. May be enhanced with use of contrast media.	Explain the need for lying completely still for 1 h. May require sedation. Screen patient for any metal on body before test. Requires a signed consent for use of contrast media.
Magnetic Resonance Spectroscopy (MRS)		
Measures biochemical changes in the brain. Can detect tissue changes in stroke, epilepsy, and tumors	Uses MRI to gather information about chemical composition of brain tissue using the magnetic properties of the chemicals.	Same as for MRI.
Positron Emission Tomography (PET)		
To assess for cell function, damage in brain tissue caused by Alzheimer disease, Parkinson disease, stroke, tumors, or a seizure focus	Radioactive material is given and provides differing color in areas of cellular activity on imaging.	Procedure requires a signed consent form. Explain that an IV will be inserted. Patient is to avoid sedatives or tranquilizers before test and to avoid intense physical activity for 24 h before test. Ask to empty bladder before scanning starts. Patient may be asked to perform various activities during the test.
Single-Photon Emission Computed Tomography (SPECT)		
To visualize glucose or oxygen metabolism in the brain and to visualize blood flow Assesses cell function like PET but does not give as high resolution images as PET	Radiolabeled compounds are injected, and their single-photon emissions are scanned. Images are made of the accumulated radiolabeled compounds.	Same as for PET.

Continued

Table 21.6 Diagnostic Tests for Neurologic Disorders—cont'd

PURPOSE	DESCRIPTION	NURSING IMPLICATIONS
Ultrasound Arteriography (Doppler Flow Studies)		
To study flow and determine areas of constriction or obstruction in cerebral arteries To detect arterial spasm	Noninvasive test. Doppler image scanning device is used with computer to visualize anatomy of major cerebral arteries.	Tell patient that the test is noninvasive and painless. A small Doppler wand is positioned over particular "window" areas on the skull (temples), and with the computer, sound waves are directed so as to produce an image of the interior arteries and their blood flow. No special preparation or aftercare.
Carotid Duplex Doppler Studies		
To determine whether blood flow in carotid arteries is decreased or blocked	Sound waves graph a picture of blood flow in the carotid arteries.	Explain that the test is noninvasive and painless. Patient will lie flat with head turned to one side and then the other as metal wand passes along the artery.
Evoked Potential Studies		
To measure response of the CNS to visual, auditory, or sensory stimulus and helpful in detecting tumor of CN VIII, blindness in infants, or brainstem lesions; also useful in diagnosing multiple sclerosis	May be done in conjunction with EEG. Electrodes are used to pick up and transmit impulses to a computer while a stimulus is delivered to the patient. Signals are displayed on a screen, and data are stored for later interpretation.	Explain the procedure to the patient. Visual-evoked potentials: stimulus may be a bright flashing light or checkerboard patterns. Somatosensory-evoked potentials require stimulation of a peripheral sensory nerve with a mild electric shock. Auditory brainstem-evoked potentials use various noises or tone bursts through earphones. Discomfort is minimal. Test takes 30–60 min.
Cerebrospinal Fluid Analysis and Culture		
To detect abnormalities that are indicative of specific neurologic problems and determine which organism is responsible for infection	CSF is obtained by lumbar puncture. It is analyzed for color, cell count, protein, chloride, and glucose. The fluid is cultured to detect the presence of organisms; CSF pressure also is measured. Normal CSF values for the adult are: Color: clear Cell count (WBCs): 0–8 mm^3 Protein: 14–45 mg/dL Chloride: 118–132 mEq/L Glucose: 40–80 mg/dL Pressure: 70–150 cm H_2O or <20 mm Hg	Follow lumbar puncture procedure. Label the test tubes as 1, 2, and 3 and be certain they are filled with at least 3 mL of CSF in this order. Do not refrigerate the tubes; transport to the laboratory immediately. Maintain Standard Precautions (see Appendix B).
PLAC (Lipoprotein-Associated Phospholipase A_2; Lp-PLA_2)		
To detect enzyme marker for increased ischemic stroke risk	This substance is thought to be partly responsible for atherosclerosis formation.	Explain that this is a simple blood test. Results take 7–10 days.

CN, Cranial nerve; *CNS*, central nervous system; *CSF*, cerebrospinal fluid; *CVA*, cerebrovascular accident; *ECG*, electrocardiogram; *ICP*, intracranial pressure; *IV*, intravenous; *MRI*, magnetic resonance imaging; *NPO*, nothing by mouth; *VS*, vital signs; *WBCs*, white blood cells.

activities within the head and neck (see Table 21.2). Table 21.7 explains how to perform a basic assessment of CN function.

Pupillary reactions. Changes in pupil size in response to a bright light are commonly used to determine whether the areas of the brainstem that help control consciousness are functioning normally. Cranial nerves II and III control pupil movement. When ICP rises

Clinical Cues

A mnemonic for remembering the CN names is as follows:

*"On Old Olympus's Towering Top A Finn Very Gladly Viewed A Hop" (**O**lfactory, **O**ptic, **O**culomotor, **T**rochlear, **T**rigeminal, **A**bducens, **F**acial, **V**estibulocochlear, **G**lossopharyngeal, **V**agus, **A**ccessory, **H**ypoglossal).*

Table 21.7 Quick Gross Assessment of Major Cranial Nerves

CRANIAL NERVE TESTED	QUICK METHOD OF TESTING[a]
Olfactory	Have patient smell a sample of ground coffee, perfume, and pickle juice.
Optic	Test visual acuity with a Snellen eye chart. Test visual fields by asking patient to hold the head still and identify items on various areas of a chart.
Oculomotor, trochlear, and abducens	Assess pupil size, direct and consensual constriction, and accommodation. Assess the cardinal fields/directions of gaze.
Trigeminal	Ask patient to clamp jaw shut, open the mouth against resistance, open the mouth widely, move the jaw from side to side, and make chewing motions. Test sensation by placing a warm and then a cold item on various portions of the face. Ask whether item is warm or cold.
Facial	Observe the face for symmetry; ask patient to smile, frown, raise the eyebrows, tightly close the eyes, whistle, show the teeth, and puff out the cheeks.
Vestibulocochlear (or acoustic)	Whisper from varying distances and locations behind the patient and ask patient what was said. Test equilibrium with Romberg test: ask patient to stand with feet only slightly apart and eyes closed. Observe for swaying of the body.
Glossopharyngeal and vagus	Ask patient to open mouth wide and say "Ah." Place tongue depressor on first third of tongue to flatten it and observe movement of the uvula and palate; they should rise symmetrically with the uvula at midline. Assess gag reflex by touching each side of the pharynx; there should be a brisk response. Have patient swallow a bit of water.
Spinal accessory	Ask patient to elevate the shoulders with and without resistance, turn the head to each side, resist attempts to pull the chin back toward the midline, and push the head forward against resistance.
Hypoglossal	Ask patient to open mouth wide, stick out tongue, and rapidly move it from side to side and in and out. Watch for deviation from midline. Apply pressure to cheek and ask patient to push tongue against hand to check for strength.

[a]These maneuvers do not check for every function of these cranial nerves but will provide data indicating whether a more thorough assessment is needed.

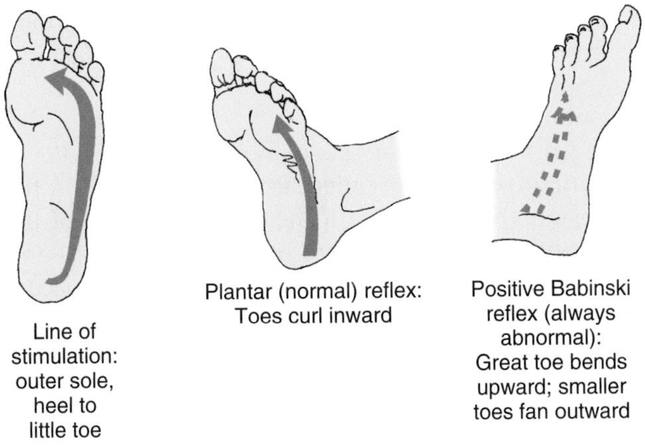
Line of stimulation: outer sole, heel to little toe
Plantar (normal) reflex: Toes curl inward
Positive Babinski reflex (always abnormal): Great toe bends upward; smaller toes fan outward

Fig. 21.11 Babinski reflex.

beyond a certain point, pressure on these nerves causes changes in the pupils. Although pupils of equal size are considered normal, some people have pupils that are unequal in size. The size of the pupils also may vary from person to person (see Fig. 21.9). It is best to measure pupil size rather than estimate it. The size of the pupils in relation to each other is more important that the actual millimeter size, which changes with ambient light

Examine the pupils in a room with low light, when the pupils would usually be dilated. Direct a bright light into each eye from the side while the other eye is covered. Observe whether the pupil into which the light shines constricts and whether it does so briskly or sluggishly *(direct reflex)*. Finally, shine the light into each eye while watching to see if the pupil constricts in the other eye *(consensual reflex)* (Table 21.8). **When pupils have been previously reactive, changes in pupil size or reactivity may signal an emergency, and the health care provider must be notified immediately.** To test for **accommodation** (eyes able to focus on both near and far objects), ask the patient to look at an object across the room away from the light source and then to look at your fingers held about 6 inches from the eyes. The lenses should change shape and the pupils constrict. Normal pupil responses often are charted as "PERRLA," meaning "pupils equal, round, and reactive to light with accommodation."

Pupils that remain dilated and fixed in the presence of a bright light indicate brain damage if there are no drugs in the system that affect the pupils. One pupil that remains fixed and dilated indicates increased ICP. If both pupils remain constricted, there probably is damage to the pons.

Table 21.8 Pupillary Abnormalities and Possible Causes

ASSESSMENT DATA	APPEARANCE	POSSIBLE CAUSES
Unilateral, fixed, dilated pupil. Unreactive to light. May be accompanied by ptosis and deviation to side and downward.	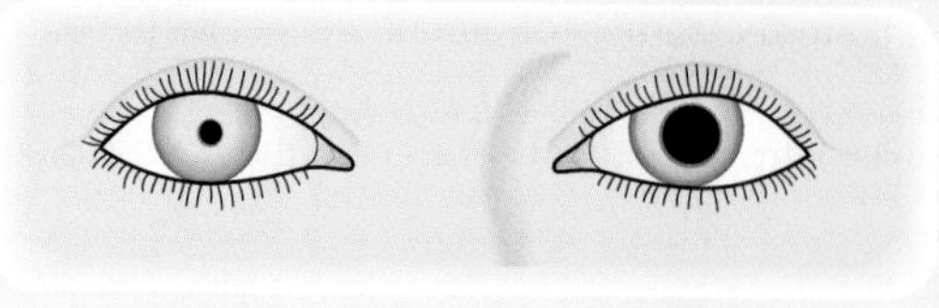	Damage to oculomotor nerve related to increased intraocular pressure, compression of oculomotor nerve, head trauma with epidural or subdural hematoma
Bilateral dilated and fixed pupils that do not react to light.	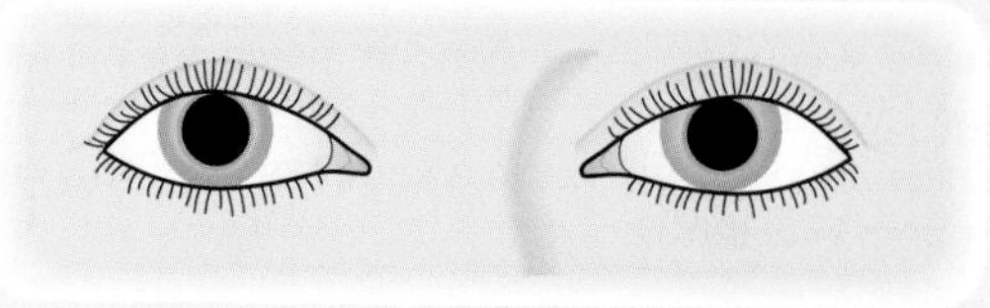	Hypoxia associated with cardiopulmonary arrest Pressure on midbrain Severe CNS disorder Anticholinergic drug overdose
Bilateral small, fixed pupils that do not react to light. Accompanied by motor deficits, drowsiness, confusion, headache, vomiting, incontinence when caused by damage to diencephalon.	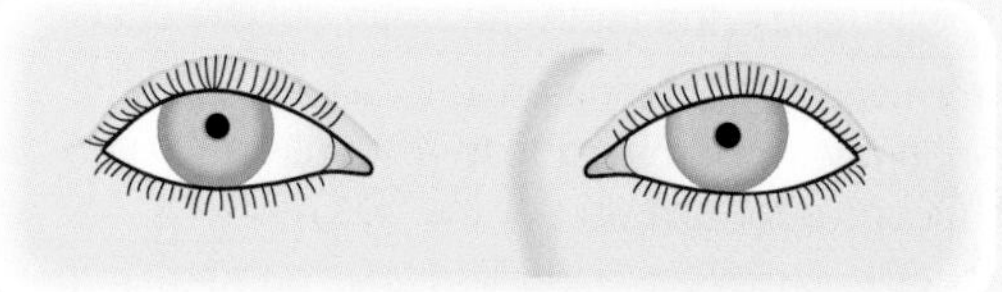	Side effect of opiates such as morphine Miotic eye drops Hemorrhage into the pons Damage to the diencephalon
Unequal pupil size; both pupils react to light unless there is underlying pathology.	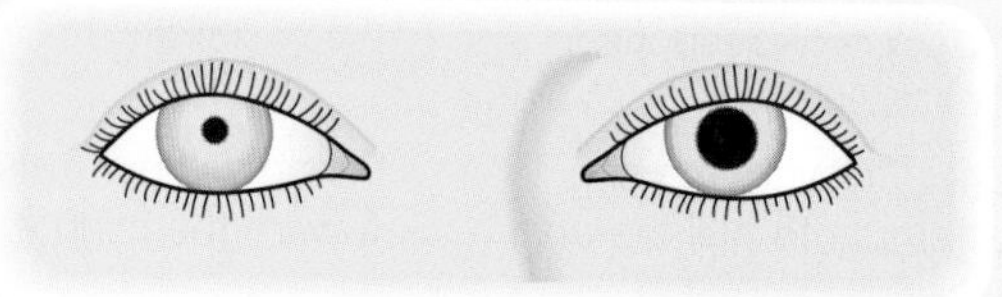	Ocular inflammation Congenital aberration Adhesion, as of iris to cornea or lens Disturbance of neural pathways

CNS, Central nervous system.

Although changes in the pupils, such as unequal constriction or decreased rate of constriction, indicate increased ICP, sometimes changes in pupils can be caused by medications. For example, atropine and scopolamine can produce dilated pupils, and opiates, miotics, and street drugs can cause constriction (see Table 21.8).

Decreased Level of Consciousness

If the patient does not respond to voice commands at all, and deafness is not an issue, test the degree of unconsciousness. First use a louder voice to try to arouse the patient; then, if they do not respond, gently shake them as you would to awaken a child. If that is not successful, painful stimuli may be applied. A central pain response may be elicited by firmly pinching the trapezius muscle at the angle of the shoulder and neck, slightly twisting and increasing pressure for 10 to 20 seconds. Applying pressure above the eye by placing a thumb under the orbital rim beneath the middle of the eyebrow and pushing upward is used if there is no response to the trapezius twist. One other alternative method is to apply pressure to the angle of the mandible with the thumb. Peripheral pain response is evaluated by using a pen or pencil and applying pressure to the nail bed near the cuticle. Historically a sternal rub has been used to evaluate a pain response. This is no longer recommended since damage to tissue and bruising occurs with the method.

The levels of response to pain are:

- Purposeful withdrawal from the stimulus or an attempt to push it away
- Nonpurposeful response, in which the patient may frown or move the arm or leg in a random fashion
- Posturing
- Failure to respond at all

Posturing that may be exhibited includes **flexor posturing** (previously called *decorticate*), which is the extension and stiffening of the legs, adduction of the arms with the forearms bent upward, and wrists and fingers flexed on the chest. This type of posture occurs with damage to the cortex. **Extensor posturing** (previously called *decerebrate*), in which the arms are stiffly extended and held close to the body, the wrists are flexed outward, and the legs are stiff with toes pointed downward (plantar flexion), may also occur. This response means that there is damage to the midbrain or brainstem, which indicates a very serious injury (Fig. 21.12). The response may be "lateralized," wherein only one side of the body shows typical flexor or extensor posturing. A patient may also display a flexor response on one side and an extensor response on the other. An important aspect of neurologic assessment is to look for changes in the patient from each day to the next. Bilateral flaccidity is usually present when there is no response at all.

For a comatose patient, tests are performed to determine brainstem function. After ruling out spinal

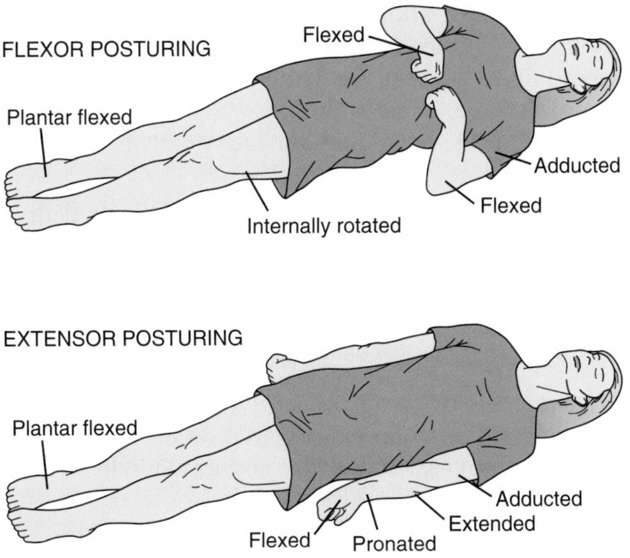

Fig. 21.12 Flexor and extensor posturing indicating brain injury.

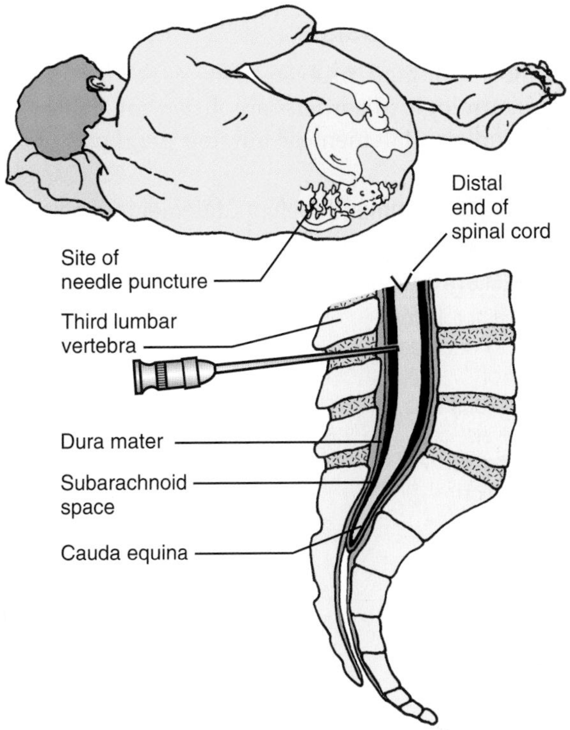

Fig. 21.13 Lumbar puncture technique.

cord injury, the oculocephalic ("doll's eye") and/or oculovestibular reflexes are assessed. For the doll's eye reflex, the examiner places a hand on each side of the patient's head, using the thumbs to gently hold open the eyelids. While watching the patient's eyes, the head is rotated briskly to one side, and eye movement is observed in relation to head movement. If the brainstem pathways are intact, the eyes appear to move in a direction opposite to that of the head movement; that is, if the head is rotated to the right, the eyes appear to move to the left. This finding is a "positive" doll's eye reflex and indicates an intact brainstem. If the eyes remain stationary and do not appear to move and passively follow the head motion, the result is a "negative" doll's eye reflex and is abnormal. After ensuring that the tympanic membrane is intact, the oculovestibular reflex is assessed by **caloric testing**. With the patient's head elevated at least 30 degrees, 20 to 200 mL of cold or ice water is instilled into the ear with a catheter-tipped syringe. While the external ear canal is irrigated, the patient's eye movements are observed. Normally the eyes will show nystagmus, darting away from the irrigated ear. Absence of eye movement may indicate a brainstem lesion. Caloric testing may induce immediate vomiting in patients with a normal response.

The "neuro" check. Monitoring the neurologic status of a patient with a known neurologic disorder includes a "neuro" check on a set schedule. It is performed to determine whether increased ICP is present or ICP is rising. For example, monitoring is necessary after a traumatic head injury, after ingestion of an overdose of a drug or other chemical, when a stroke has occurred or is suspected, or for any other condition in which the patient has lost or may lose consciousness. A neurologic assessment flow sheet is used to chart assessment data so that the trend in function of each area can be quickly identified (see the Evolve website for a neurologic assessment flow sheet). Four areas are monitored: vital signs, LOC, pupil reaction, and motor function. Neuro checks may be ordered as frequently as every 15 minutes or at intervals from 2 to 8 hours.

Assignment Considerations

The Neuro Check

Although the measuring of vital signs can be assigned to assistive personnel, the gathering of data for the neuro check should not be delegated. It is important to compare current data with previous data and to carefully assess neuromuscular and pupillary response.

Think Critically

You arrive at the home of an older adult woman who has severe heart disease and atherosclerosis and is very weak. Her spouse says she is confused and lethargic and that she would not eat breakfast. He is worried. As her nurse, what specific assessments would you perform to determine whether she has suffered a cerebrovascular accident (CVA)?

Diagnostic tests. The diagnostic tests most commonly used to evaluate the neurologic system are presented in Table 21.6. Basic physiologic testing is also performed to rule out disease in some other system that might be affecting the nervous system. A nerve or muscle biopsy may be performed to determine pathologic changes in these tissues. Fig. 21.13 shows the technique used for lumbar puncture.

◆ NURSING DIAGNOSIS

The most common problem statements for patients with neurologic disorders are listed in Table 21.9. Each problem statement or nursing diagnosis chosen for the patient should be individualized to fit the situation. Problems included in a care plan vary according to whether the patient is in the acute stage, recovery stage, or rehabilitative stage of the disorder. General expected outcomes for each problem statement

Table 21.9 Common Problem Statements, Goals/Expected Outcomes, and Nursing Interventions for Patients With Neurologic Disorders

PROBLEM STATEMENT	GOALS/EXPECTED OUTCOMES	NURSING INTERVENTIONS
Potential for injury due to decreased level of consciousness, paralysis, or decreased sensation	Patient will have no evidence of injury or trauma.	Side rails up at all times when patient is unattended. Bed in low position when patient is unattended. Pad side rails if seizure activity or restlessness indicates need. Provide eye care for unconscious patient and if corneal (blink) reflex is absent; lubrication and eye patch or shield as needed. Position carefully, protecting extremities from contact with side rails. Maintain correct body alignment. Administer anticonvulsants as ordered to prevent seizure activity. Protect from thermal injury. Use hand mitts to prevent injury from dislodging tubes.
Altered breathing pattern to neurologic disruption of respiration	Maintain a patent airway. Maintain an SpO_2 of 95%–99%. Patient will have no evidence of pulmonary infection.	Assess respiratory status q2–8h depending on patient condition. Position to maximize open airway and to promote chest expansion. Insert oropharyngeal airway as ordered. Suction secretions PRN as ordered. For controlled ventilatory support: auscultate to verify that both lungs are inflating. Check ventilator settings with those ordered. Promptly respond to all alarms. Remove excess water gathering in ventilator tubing PRN. Suction patient using sterile technique as ordered PRN. Monitor blood gas values for changes. Provide frequent mouth care (i.e., q2–4h) and other ventilator-associated pneumonia prevention strategies. Monitor hydration status.
Altered physical mobility due to CNS deficit, weakness, paralysis, or fatigue	Patient will maintain mobility of all joints. Patient will have no evidence of contractures. Patient will regain optimal physical mobility that is neurologically possible.	Perform passive ROM or supervise active ROM qid. Position flaccid extremities in anatomically correct positions during rest. Teach ROM exercises to patient and family. Teach transfer techniques to hemiplegic patient and family. Collaborate with physical therapist to maximize activity.
Altered skin integrity due to impaired mobility, decreased sensory awareness, or decreased sensation	Patient's skin will remain intact.	Inspect pressure points for redness, warmth, tenderness, or edema each time patient is turned. Thoroughly inspect skin every shift. Position and pad joints to prevent pressure ulcers. Formulate regular turning and repositioning schedule and stick to it. Use special mattress or special bed to enhance skin protection. Teach patients in wheelchairs to shift weight q15min. Teach patient and family to inspect pressure areas and skin for beginning signs of breakdown.
Altered self-care ability due to neurologic impairment: paresis, paralysis, decreased LOC, or confusion	Patient will meet self-care needs of hygiene, toileting, feeding, and grooming. Patient will resume self-care at level physiologically and neurologically possible.	Assist with hygiene, toileting, feeding, and grooming as needed. Assist patient to set small, attainable goals for self-care. Explain and demonstrate specific ADLs in small, one-task segments. Obtain and demonstrate adaptive devices to assist with ADLs. Offer patience, support, and encouragement for each attempt at self-care. Maintain chart of self-care improvement to track achievement so that patient can see progress.

Table 21.9 Common Problem Statements, Goals/Expected Outcomes, and Nursing Interventions for Patients With Neurologic Disorders—cont'd

PROBLEM STATEMENT	GOALS/EXPECTED OUTCOMES	NURSING INTERVENTIONS
Altered nutrition due to inability to swallow or danger of aspiration	Patient's nutritional status will remain adequate as evidenced by normal weight and adequate levels of serum protein.	Institute tube feeding as needed. Check tube placement before initiating each feeding. Check residual before each intermittent feeding or q4h for continuous feedings; if greater than 150 mL or more than half of previous feeding, replace and delay next feeding for 1–2 h (or per facility protocol). Position patient with head of bed up at least 30 degrees when feeding and for 30–60 min after feeding. Monitor for adverse side effects such as diarrhea. Flush tube with 30–60 mL water after each feeding. Instill ordered amount of water between feedings to maintain hydration. Monitor glucose levels after initiation of feedings until blood glucose is stable. Check weight at least twice a week. Monitor intake and output. *For patient with dysphagia who can take oral feedings:* Serve semisoft foods. Provide six small meals per day; provide nonstressful atmosphere with few distractions for mealtime. Teach to sit upright with head slightly forward and neck flexed; encourage to place food on strongest side of mouth and tongue; encourage to take small bites at a time. Remain with patient to decrease fear of choking; keep suction at hand and turned on during meal. Ensure privacy for meal to decrease embarrassment about drooling, dropping food, or choking. (See Chapter 28.)
Altered elimination, diarrhea, or bowel incontinence due to decreased level of consciousness, neurogenic impairment, or side effects of medications	Patient will have normal bowel movements as evidenced by soft, formed stool. Patient will attain bowel continence.	Monitor bowel movements and evaluate regularity based on nutritional intake. Administer stool softeners, rectal suppositories, or enemas as ordered for constipation. Check for and remove fecal impaction if it occurs, guarding against spinal dysreflexia in the paralyzed patient. Institute bowel training program if needed (see Bowel Training Program). If diarrhea occurs, determine cause and alleviate if possible. Administer antidiarrheal if ordered. Keep rectal area clean and dry; protect rectal mucosa. Monitor hydration status; evaluate intake and output.
Altered neurologic function due to disease or injury	Patient will respond to family interaction as evidenced by movement, hand squeezing, eye opening, or speech. Patient will return to alert state as evidenced by proper orientation to person, time, and place.	Speak of current events or daily happenings while providing care. Encourage family members and friends to speak to patient of day's occurrences or fun times in past. Play music on the radio that is to the patient's taste. Play movies or shows on topics of interest to the patient. Ask questions and patiently listen for a response. Have the family record sounds from the patient's home and work environment.
Social isolation due to immobility and intellectual limits imposed by neurologic impairment	Patient will have social interaction with visiting friends. Patient will maintain relationships with family members and loved ones. Patient will make new friends among support group members.	Encourage friends and family to visit. Instruct friends and family on how to interact with the patient. Encourage patient to discuss their feelings regarding social contact. Encourage participation in an appropriate support group. Encourage development of a social network. Encourage participation in church, civic, volunteer, and social groups in community. Provide referrals to community job-retraining resources if patient is unable to resume former employment or lifestyle.

Continued

Table 21.9 Common Problem Statements, Goals/Expected Outcomes, and Nursing Interventions for Patients With Neurologic Disorders—cont'd

PROBLEM STATEMENT	GOALS/EXPECTED OUTCOMES	NURSING INTERVENTIONS
Altered family coping due to role changes, uncertainty of the future, and financial constraints	Each family member will demonstrate appropriate coping methods.	Assess strengths of each family member; look for signs of stress. Refer to appropriate counseling services as needed.
	Each family member will regain an optimistic outlook.	Provide opportunity for verbalization of fears and concerns and feelings about patient's changed condition.
	Each family member will accept the patient in their changed state.	Refer to social worker and community resources for support services.
	Each family member will use referrals to support groups and community resources.	Arrange for psychological counseling or family therapy as needed. Encourage contact with appropriate support group. Initiate interaction and honest communication between patient and family members when patient and each member is ready. Teach problem-solving methods if coping skills are weak.

ADLs, Activities of daily living; *CNS,* central nervous system; *LOC,* level of consciousness; *PRN,* as needed; *qid,* four times a day; *ROM,* range of motion; *Spo_2,* peripheral oxygen saturation.

are presented in Table 21.9 along with appropriate interventions.

◆ PLANNING

Overall goals for patients with neurologic disorders depend on whether there is a physiologic possibility that full function may be regained. When permanent neurologic deficit occurs, as may occur with some spinal cord injuries, the ultimate goal is for the patient to function at the highest physiologic level. This requires adjusting to limitations imposed by the neurologic deficit so that the patient may live life in a meaningful way. A goal for all patients with neurologic disorders is to prevent injury, whether from complications of immobility, accidents related to lack of sensation, aspiration from difficulty in swallowing, or any of the other problems that the neurologic deficit may cause.

Caring for patients with neurologic deficits can be very time consuming and requires considerable patience and understanding. If the patient has any weakness, paralysis, or decreased sensation in the extremities or is confused, disoriented, aphasic, or otherwise incapacitated, providing care will take more time than usual. Extended time must be included in the daily work plan. When a patient is comatose or paralyzed, it is best to team up with another helper to provide care and to turn or reposition the patient. By working together, care is smoother and less taxing. If the patient is to be cared for at home upon discharge, make sure that the case manager and social worker are fully aware of the functional status so that adequate resources are available to the family members caring for the patient. Respite care may be available and is very helpful in allowing caregivers to take a break from the physical and psychological stress of caregiving.

◆ IMPLEMENTATION

Interventions for each problem statement concerning neurologic disorder problems are listed in Table 21.9. Patients should be given information about the disorder and taught about diagnostic tests and self-care. Positive coping skills should be reinforced and ongoing support offered. Interventions are discussed in the following section on common care problems and with the specific neurologic disorders in Chapters 22, 23, and 24.

◆ EVALUATION

Evaluation of interventions is performed to determine whether goals are being met. Are the interventions chosen helping to meet the specific expected outcomes written? If not, the plan needs to be changed. Progress in the patient experiencing a neurologic deficit is often slow. It may take a considerable time for improvement to be noted. Long-term goals of a realistic nature are appropriate. Keep in mind that certain types of neurologic deficits, such as those caused by spinal cord severance, may not improve. Goals are based on preventing complications rather than improving function.

COMMON NEUROLOGIC PATIENT CARE PROBLEMS

Neurologic disorders and illnesses cause many of the same problems. Whether the patient has encephalitis, has a head injury, is recovering from cranial surgery, has suffered a stroke, or has multiple sclerosis or Parkinson disease, they may need nursing intervention in one or more of the following areas.

ALTERED BREATHING PATTERN

Weakness of the diaphragm or respiratory muscles or interruption of normal brain function may occur with a variety of neurologic disorders. Monitor the adequacy of respiratory effort and promote a patent airway and chest expansion. Elevating the head of the bed 30 degrees allows the diaphragm to drop more easily and promotes chest expansion. When consciousness is depressed, the tongue may be flaccid and fall back, blocking the airway. Positioning the patient on the side allows the tongue to fall to the side and opens the airway. Insertion of an oropharyngeal or nasopharyngeal airway may be indicated. Make sure that positioning of the patient for improved breathing is not contraindicated by a neurologic injury.

Assisting the patient with deep breathing and the use of an incentive spirometer can help prevent atelectasis and improve ventilation. Respiratory assessment is performed every shift and includes auscultating the lungs for signs of atelectasis or retained secretions and judging the quality of respiratory effort. If respiratory efforts are considerably impaired, the patient may need intubation and mechanical ventilation. Interventions for patients undergoing mechanical ventilation are presented in Chapter 14.

ALTERED MOBILITY

You, the physical therapist, and the patient work together to help the patient cope with muscle weakness or paralysis. Activities such as proper positioning and range-of-motion (ROM) exercises are started immediately to preserve proper alignment of joints and limbs and prevent contractures and muscle atrophy. Assistive devices, such as splints and slings, may be used. Patients with **hemiplegia** (paralysis and loss of sensation in an extremity) are taught to become aware of arm or leg placement when turning or transferring to a chair to prevent injury to the affected extremity.

For example, a patient with left hemiplegia from a CVA may neglect their paralyzed side. They must therefore be taught to attend to the affected side of their body by scanning it frequently. To prevent discomfort in the shoulder and arm on the affected side and to prevent dislocation of the shoulder, take care not to pull on the affected arm or shoulder during transfers or ambulation. Support the affected arm with pillows or an armrest to keep it from dangling when the patient is seated. Use a sling for comfort and to promote better balance when ambulating and transferring the patient.

Patients with hemiplegia are taught, step by step, the safest way to transfer from the bed to a wheelchair and back and how to use assistance from others. They are also taught how to care for and protect their skin in areas of decreased sensation.

Patients with **hemiparesis** (one-sided weakness) are taught how to strengthen their muscles and use assistive devices, such as walkers, crutches, or canes, to walk. They are taught the best ways to get out of bed and into and out of a chair. Patients with **tetraplegia** (four limbs paralyzed) are helped to learn to cope with this drastic life-changing alteration and how their energies might be directed toward different but attainable goals. (An older term for tetraplegia is **quadriplegia**.)

All patients with a recent impairment of mobility need help with the grieving process, support in establishing healthy and effective coping patterns, and assistance with depression.

Attention to pain relief and muscle spasm is necessary for these patients to achieve the highest level of rehabilitation possible. Paralyzed extremities are susceptible to edema; to decrease this problem, extremities should be elevated when the patient is at rest. The patient needs to be turned frequently to prevent complications from pressure and sluggish circulation.

Older adult patients may suffer joint stiffness from arthritis. Assess joints for tenderness and pain before performing ROM exercises and be gentle and considerate when turning and repositioning them.

SKIN INTEGRITY

Take measures to promote skin integrity. Place the patient on a special bed, mattress, or protective mattress cover or pad; inspect pressure points frequently; and keep the skin clean and dry. Chapter 9 discusses the effects of immobility on each body system, along with the nursing activities necessary to prevent disabilities resulting from inactivity. The principles and practices presented in that chapter are relevant to the nursing care of a patient with a neurologic disorder that produces some type of paresis or paralysis and of a patient who is unconscious.

Denervated skin is more susceptible to skin breakdown than tissues with an intact nerve supply, so extra effort must be made to maintain skin integrity.

ALTERED SELF-CARE ABILITY

Neuromuscular impairment may interfere with the patient's ability to perform hygiene activities and other ADLs. They may need assistance with bathing, grooming, oral hygiene, dressing, eating, and toileting. Work with the patient as their condition dictates, assisting with techniques to perform self-care despite disability when possible, offering encouragement, and praising any effort at accomplishing a self-care task.

Inability to carry out the most basic of self-care activities can erode a person's sense of independence and self-esteem. The ability to feed, clothe, and take care of toileting is an important part of independence. Regaining some level of self-care in these areas is of particular concern to the adult who, because of neurologic dysfunction, may have to relearn ways to perform the simplest of daily activities.

If the patient is unconscious, the mouth must be kept clean to avoid infection of the parotid gland. The lips are cleansed and lubricated at frequent intervals, because mouth breathing makes them excessively dry. Moistening of the mouth may be accomplished by wet foam sponges. To fully cleanse the mouth, teeth, gums, and tongue should be brushed a minimum of twice per day. This cleansing may be done by turning the patient to the side; turning on the oral suction device;

and brushing the teeth, gums, and tongue with fluoride toothpaste and a soft bristled brush. Using an irrigation syringe filled with water in one hand and the oral suction device in the other allows rinsing of the mouth while preventing aspiration of the liquid. It is easiest for two caregivers to work together to rinse and suction the mouth. Each time the mouth is cleansed, the patient should be positioned on the opposite side to ensure thorough cleansing of each side of the mouth. Oral suction should be available and turned on any time mouth care is given to a patient who has a weakened gag reflex, cannot swallow normally, or has weakness of the facial muscles. Studies show that tooth and tongue brushing decreases iatrogenic infection significantly.

When the patient cannot shut their eyes, you or a caregiver must provide care to prevent keratitis or corneal ulceration. The eyelids are cleansed with warm, sterile water or normal saline every few hours to remove discharge and debris. Artificial tears or a lubricant is instilled as prescribed to prevent dryness. If the corneal reflex is absent, an eye shield or patch is placed over the eye. The eyelid is closed before a patch is applied. The eyes are examined each day for signs of inflammation.

The ability of relatives to learn how to care for the patient, and their willingness to do so, are important parts of assessing and planning for rehabilitation. Goals for rehabilitation must be realistic and mutually agreed on by the patient, the family, and the health care team.

Assistive devices help patients with neurologic deficits to feed and dress themselves. Occupational therapists can help the patient relearn how to perform elementary tasks necessary for daily living. Patients are retaught how to feed themselves; how to get in and out of a bed or a chair; how to select and put on clothes and fasten them; and how to bathe, brush teeth, and comb hair.

Provide assistance when the patient cannot do a task completely and—most of all—provide encouragement and praise for efforts made. **When pursuing self-help rehabilitation, remember that the patient tires easily; tasks must be spaced apart so that energy is available to achieve them.** Pushing the patient to try another task when they are too tired only sets them up for failure and frustration.

DYSPHAGIA

Every patient who has suffered a neurologic insult (damage) from head injury, stroke, or intracranial surgery should have the swallowing reflex assessed. A bedside nursing swallow screening should be performed to determine if it is safe to give oral medications prior to the speech therapist doing a formal examination. With the patient sitting upright in bed, give them a spoonful of water. Observe for the ability to swallow without choking, if the voice sounds gurgly or wet, or if water dribbles out of the corner of the mouth. If the spoonful of water is tolerated, have the patient drink 60 cc of water. Do not use a straw. If the patient tolerates the 60 cc of water without exhibiting swallowing difficulty, the bedside screening is passed. Check periodically that the patient automatically swallows saliva before offering water. Patients who have paresis from a stroke or who suffer from myasthenia gravis or other neurologic disorders often have difficulty swallowing (**dysphagia**). Those patients who have difficulty eating are at risk for nutritional disorders and aspiration pneumonia. Patients with dysphagia should be sitting upright or in a high Fowler position to eat. Depending on the mechanism of the dysphagia, various head positions may be used to facilitate passage of food without aspiration. For some patients, a more recumbent position might be used. It is recommended to not lay flat for 30 minutes after eating. A nonstressful meal environment without distractions is best because stress makes dysphagia worse.

When the patient cannot swallow without choking or aspirating, tube feeding is necessary. When the patient is receiving nutrients by tube, the caloric intake should be assessed frequently. Tube-fed patients are weighed daily on initiation of the feeding and then twice a week after they have stabilized. Intake and output are recorded and evaluated. Interventions for the patient receiving tube feedings are outlined in Chapter 28.

BOWEL AND BLADDER FUNCTION

Many patients with CNS disorders experience temporary or permanent urinary or fecal incontinence. Some patients experience constipation or urinary retention. Bowel and bladder function need to be regulated so that incontinence does not lead to skin breakdown. Constipation or urinary retention can lead to organ dysfunction if not promptly corrected.

Bladder Training Program

Bladder training is a program designed to help a patient with some degree of loss of normal bladder function and a resulting disturbance of voiding and bladder control. Loss of control can occur in a variety of neurologic disorders, including stroke, spinal cord injury, and tumors and lesions of the spinal cord.

The purposes of a bladder reconditioning program are to prevent urinary complications such as infection and **calculi** (stones) and to allow the patient freedom from fear of embarrassment and loss of self-esteem. Calculi are less likely to develop when there is a high fluid intake and frequent, complete emptying of the bladder. Skin integrity is more likely to be maintained if not in frequent contact with urine.

Bladder function is assessed to determine the optimal neural and muscular control that can be realistically expected in view of the physiologic cause of loss of control. In developing a bladder reconditioning program, the patient's mental and emotional ability to cooperate and take an active part in carrying out the program is evaluated.

Spinal cord injuries and lesions produce what is known as a *cord bladder* or *neurogenic bladder*. Patients with disorders of this type are not aware of the need to void and must be trained in techniques to initiate voiding and emptying the bladder.

A bladder training program usually begins with a 2-hour schedule for toileting. The patient should attempt to drink 2000 to 3000 mL of fluid between waking up and 6 P.M. Coffee, tea, alcoholic beverages, and soda with caffeine should be avoided after dinner because they have a diuretic effect. The patient is toileted before retiring for the night. The maintenance of an accurate training record is essential. A trial of 6 weeks is necessary before determining whether the training is successful. Various drugs that affect the voiding process, such as oxybutynin chloride (Ditropan), flavoxate hydrochloride (Urispas), tolterodine (Detrol), darifenacin (Enablex), fesoterodine (Toviaz), trospium (Sanctura), mirabegron (Myrbetriq), or solifenacin (VESIcare), may be helpful for certain types of patients. Assess whether the medication is beneficial.

Patients who have nerve damage and paralysis are trained in specific techniques to empty the bladder. The Credé maneuver, in which the open hand is pressed over the bladder area and directed toward the suprapubic area, can facilitate emptying a flaccid bladder. This maneuver is effective in patients with a spinal injury at L2 or below. It is controversial, and studies are in process to determine whether it is universally safe and which patients would best benefit. Self-catheterization is taught to patients with paraplegia so that they are not dependent on an indwelling catheter or on other people for their urinary elimination (Abrams & Wakasa, 2018; see also Chapter 34).

Some patients are candidates for the implantation of an artificial sphincter to control bladder release of urine. More and more types of successful devices are developed each year, but these are primarily for patients who have no neurologic control over the bladder.

Every patient undertaking a bladder retraining program needs a great deal of understanding and encouragement and a positive attitude to be successful. Praise for each small achievement should be given. Intermittent incontinence should be expected and not looked on as "failures." Achieving total continence takes considerable time and effort but is possible for many patients.

Bowel Training Program

Bowel training is used to correct incontinence or prevent constipation and impaction in patients with neurologic disorders or injuries. The bowel training program begins with an assessment of the specific patterns of elimination. It also helps to know the patient's former bowel pattern before illness or injury. Did they regularly rely on the use of enemas or laxatives? Have they been prone to constipation? Next, establish whether the patient is aware of the urge to defecate or has any warning of evacuation.

Bowel training for either constipation or incontinence should incorporate an exercise program that is within the patient's ability, a high-fiber diet, and adequate liquid intake during the day. An accurate recording of bowel movements correlated with times of oral intake over a 2- to 3-day period will help establish the most opportune times to try to stimulate evacuation and thus establish a habit. If incontinence occurs at specific times after eating, toileting 30 minutes sooner and using a rectal suppository or a gloved finger to stimulate the urge to defecate may alter the pattern. Gradually the use of the suppository is discontinued.

For patients who are prone to constipation and incontinence, increasing liquid intake and administering a stool softener can be effective. If this does not work, a planned regimen of suppository or enema use may be necessary to assist with evacuation at a desired time, thus preventing incontinence.

All patients need to be comfortable when attempting to evacuate the bowel. A raised, padded toilet seat, handrails, and perhaps a footstool can provide enough comfort to allow the patient to relax so that evacuation can occur naturally. Privacy is essential. Remember to provide privacy for bedridden patients. Most of all, a positive attitude is needed by staff members. Many times, if the health care team and the patient are optimistic and patient, success can be achieved.

PAIN

Many patients with neurologic disorders experience pain. The pain often is chronic in nature. Work with the patient to identify the characteristics of the pain, its location and spread, its intensity, and how it is affecting the patient's life. Determination as to whether the pain is nociceptive, neuropathic, or "other" will help guide treatment. Review Chapter 7 for more specific information.

A trusting relationship between you and the patient is necessary for teaching to be assimilated. Teaching the patient about pain and its relief; the adverse effect of stress, anxiety, and unpleasant stimuli; and the benefits of distraction from the pain become part of the plan. Pain may cause difficulty in sleeping. Pharmacologic agents specific to the type of pain and nonpharmacological methods for pain control are used.

? Think Critically

How would you determine whether a patient who has a decreased level of consciousness is experiencing pain?

Depression often occurs with chronic pain and lack of sleep. The combination of an antidepressant and pain medication often is more effective for chronic pain control than either type of drug used alone.

CONFUSION

Patients with brain tumors, head injuries, and strokes, as well as degenerative diseases, may experience confusion and deficits in memory, intellectual ability, or judgment. Confusion may be acute and short term, or it may be a permanent state. Confusion also may be mild or severe and may be accompanied by anxiety, agitation, and refusal to cooperate. The person is in a state of disorientation, and until the symptoms subside, they cannot behave rationally. They must be supported and protected, or they may injure themselves. In states of severe (acute) confusion (**delirium**), the patient may experience hallucinations, delusions, and severe agitation. This is usually an acute, short-term state caused by fever or metabolic imbalance. Patients who experience confusion after a head injury often become combative as their ICP rises. It is not advisable to restrain these patients; be very careful to stay out of range of flailing arms. Delirium and dementia are more fully described in Chapter 46.

Be alert to signs of confusion in any patient with a CNS problem. Subjective and objective assessment data include the following:

- Loss of orientation to person, place, or time
- Inability to cooperate fully with simple tasks and requests, such as eating and bathing
- Inappropriate statements or inappropriate answers to questions
- Restlessness and agitation
- Hostility and anxiety
- Hallucinations or delusions
- Other signs of inability to maintain control over thought processes and behavior

A patient who is confused needs above all else a stable and calm environment. Their thought processes are, in a sense, "fractured" and somewhat beyond their control. Stimuli entering the brain are frightening and threatening, and they simply cannot make sense of most of what is going on around them. A calm, consistent, and orderly approach combined with a set daily routine is most helpful.

Attention to the safety of the patient is a priority. Family members must be taught measures to protect a patient who wanders, is disoriented, or lacks judgment.

Confused patients need a dependable, consistent schedule. If agitation or confusion causes undesirable behavior, the use of distraction can be beneficial. Handing the patient an item, leading them from the area, or decreasing environmental stimuli (turning off the television or radio) can calm the patient.

Patients with memory loss who can still read benefit from written instructions and from a posting of the day's schedule of activities. Measures to protect patients and deal with confusion are presented in Chapter 46.

Older Adult Care Points

Older adults typically have several chronic illnesses requiring medications. Polypharmacy is an increasing issue that needs to be evaluated to determine if confusion is related to a pathophysiologic process or a drug effect.

APHASIA

Aphasia is a defect in the ability to express oneself in speech or writing, or an inability to comprehend spoken or written language. Aphasia is caused by disease or injury of the brain centers controlling language comprehension and expression, located in the Wernicke area of the left cerebral hemisphere.

Aphasia may be *receptive, expressive,* or *global.* A person with receptive aphasia has difficulty interpreting communications in either spoken or written form. With expressive aphasia, the person has difficulty expressing themselves in speech or writing. Global aphasia occurs when the person has a combination of receptive and expressive aphasia. Aphasias vary in degree and in type of deficit. For example, a person may be able to write a message but not form the words to say it.

A comprehensive assessment of a patient who has aphasia usually is a team effort carried out under the leadership of a specially trained speech therapist. Nurses and others responsible for the care of the aphasic patient can assist by noting specific abilities or inabilities of the patient to communicate with them.

Focused Assessment

Determining the Type of Aphasia Problem

Questions to ask when evaluating the type and degree of aphasia that a patient is experiencing include the following:

- Can the patient understand yes or no questions? Are their responses of "yes" and "no" reliable (i.e., does that seem to be what they mean)?
- Can they point to or look toward objects you have named that are in their line of vision?
- Can they name the objects?
- Are they able to follow simple directions (e.g., "Turn your head.")?
- Can they repeat simple words? Complex words?
- Can they repeat sentences?
- Can they follow simple written requests?
- Can they write answers to questions?

A patient who suddenly has a problem speaking or understanding words or signs is likely to feel isolated and extremely frustrated unless an effort is made to establish some means of communicating with them as quickly as possible. Once the patient's specific problem is identified, which could be relatively simple or extremely complex, measures are taken to help the patient communicate as fully as their condition will allow.

Goals for the care of aphasic patients are focused on stimulating communication without undue frustration. Categories of treatment include those that are to improve language function and those that are to facilitate communication by whatever means is effective. Reaching these goals may take weeks or months, but there are helpful principles and techniques that can be used by all members of the health team and by family members and friends.

Perhaps the most important rule is to avoid talking to an aphasic person as if they are mentally incompetent. The inability to communicate does not mean a lack of intelligence. The patient should be spoken *to*, not spoken *about* as if they cannot hear and understand what others are saying in their presence.

Speak slowly and distinctly in a normal voice while facing the patient. Use body language and sign language to communicate if it seems to help the patient. Your facial expressions, posture, and gestures can often say more than the words you are saying.

Give aphasic patients time to respond to questions. Do not ask more than one question at a time. It takes longer for an aphasic person to process what is being said. If you need to repeat a statement or question, use *exactly* the same words. The patient may have comprehended only half of the sentence the first time. Only one person should speak at a time. Be certain to establish eye contact with the patient before speaking. Keep the environment orderly, relaxed, and relatively free from distractions that make it difficult to concentrate on communicating.

The speech therapist will plan the patient's speech therapy program and will share with you the details of how best to work with each patient. Some general guidelines include the following:

- Give praise for attempts at communication and for each correctly expressed word or sentence.
- Do not correct the patient's pronunciation, as they are liable to become too frustrated and give up speaking.
- Be very patient.

Problems with aphasia sometimes resolve spontaneously in 3 or 4 months after a CVA. Total speech rehabilitation can take many months and may never reach the pre-aphasia level. If aphasia is permanent, work with the patient in the use of picture boards, word boards, writing tablets, or electronic communication devices to allow them to communicate needs and thoughts to the best of their ability.

? Think Critically

Identify three specific techniques you might use to assist a patient with aphasia to communicate their needs.

New technology is changing our lives daily. Laptops and tablets have programs that can assist aphasic patients through various techniques, such as giving phonemic cues. Often if a patient is just given the first sound of a word, they can say the complete word.

Writing treatments are used as therapy. Techniques using current technology such as touch screens, adaptive keyboards, and texting are in routine use.

All of these techniques are helpful in improving communication. Whatever techniques are chosen, they should not be used in a condescending manner; an adult patient should always be treated respectfully.

The plan of care for an aphasic patient should not neglect the physical condition of the mouth and tongue. Good oral hygiene is needed to keep the oral mucosa clean and moist and in optimal condition so that it is easier for the patient to form words. Coexisting conditions require treatment and interventions to put the patient in the best possible condition to improve communication and overall health.

ALTERED SEXUAL FUNCTION

Sexual dysfunction from a lesion in neural pathways should be dealt with by allowing expression of the patient's concerns, beliefs, and feelings. Sexual counseling by someone skilled in working with patients with neurologic deficits should be initiated. As technology has advanced, a better understanding of neural pathways is emerging regarding arousal and orgasm in the patient with an injured spinal cord. This knowledge is providing information for the exploration of treatments and interventions to help the patient with sexual expression. Alternative techniques for meeting sexual needs should be explored. Many patients can lead a sexually satisfying life with teaching and treatment.

PSYCHOSOCIAL CONCERNS

The multiple stresses, alteration in roles, and changes in body image and self-esteem that result from a chronic neurologic disorder can be overwhelming. The patient will need time and assistance in adapting to an altered body image. Be accepting of the patient's expression of anxiety, anger, denial, regression, and depression. Work to support the patient emotionally, attempting to establish realistic hope for quality of life. Exploring the patient's previous methods of coping with adversity, as well as their support systems, talents, and desires, provides clues for how best to help. Jointly establishing small, accomplishable goals can do much to rebuild self-esteem.

Collaboration with the social worker concerning referral to support groups and interaction with others with similar disabilities who are coping well can prove most beneficial. The social worker can also assist with referral to community agencies that offer support services, financial assistance, and job retraining, if pertinent. The patient needs a way to be a productive member of society and to contribute to the welfare of their family. The county or state office of vocational rehabilitation may also help with funding.

Reentry into the community and a normal social life are other areas for intervention. Often the patient has been out of touch with their normal social circles for many months during the illness and recovery process. Strategies should be discussed before discharge regarding how social contact is to be reinstated.

ALTERED FAMILY FUNCTIONING

A chronic neurologic disorder that disrupts normal function for the patient also disrupts normal roles within the family. Family lifestyle is altered, and changes in roles may lead to family conflict. Family members often feel powerless, ambivalent toward the patient, angry, and guilty for having angry feelings. Family members need to be included when educating the patient about their disorder, the possibility of remissions and exacerbations, and the self-care measures necessary. Everyone needs time to adjust to the situation. Referrals to counseling and support groups can be very helpful.

Get Ready for the NCLEX® Examination!

Key Points

- Nerve pathways travel through the spinal cord receiving messages from the peripheral nervous system, transmitting them to the brain for processing and then back to the peripheral muscles.
- Reflexes do not travel to the brain for processing but travel as sensory input to the spinal cord and motor movement results.
- Neurons are the functional unit of the nervous system. Glial cells are support structures.
- Messages are sent via electrical stimulation of cells and neurotransmitters located in the synapses.
- When deprived of oxygen, neurons die quickly.
- Cerebral blood flow is autoregulated by the brain.
- Prolonged elevation of ICP damages neurons.
- Many changes occur with aging, and after age 70 years the brain atrophies somewhat.
- Reflexes diminish or are lost as age advances.
- Preventing accidents and head injuries by teaching safety practices reduces the number of neurologic injuries.
- Discouraging recreational drug use helps prevent neurologic damage.
- Teaching patients how to reduce risk factors for stroke can prevent the devastation that a stroke can inflict.
- Vital signs, mental function, neuromuscular status, papillary reactions, and level of consciousness are parts of the physical assessment and are always performed as part of the "neuro" check.
- A thorough history is gathered, focusing on areas of neurologic function (see Focused Assessment: Data Collection for the Neurologic System).
- Nursing care is individualized, with problem statements or nursing diagnoses, outcome objectives, and interventions chosen to alleviate the various problems (see Table 21.9).
- Every effort is made to maintain effective breathing for neurologic patients.
- Many neurologic patients experience impaired mobility, and nurses attempt to prevent the associated potential problems.
- Assisting with ADLs when patients have self-care deficits is a major part of nursing care for patients with neurologic disorders.
- Specific techniques are needed for patients with dysphagia to prevent aspiration.
- Many patients with bowel or bladder incontinence can regain continence through bowel and bladder retraining programs.
- Pain control can be a difficult issue because most pain medications dull the sensorium and will interfere with accurate neurologic assessment and signs of decreasing level of consciousness.
- Many patients with neurologic disorders become confused, and there are special techniques nurses use to assist these patients.
- Learning to work with an aphasic patient is essential to providing appropriate care.
- When appropriate, neurologic patients should be referred for sexual counseling.
- When a family member has a neurologic deficit, it affects the whole family and can disrupt normal family functioning; families need help to learn to cope.

Additional Learning Resources

SG Go to your Study Guide for additional learning activities to help you master this chapter content.

Go to your Evolve website (http://evolve.elsevier.com/deWit/medsurg) for the following FREE learning resources:
- Animations, audio, and video
- Answers and rationales for questions and activities
- Concept Map Creator
- Glossary with pronunciations in English and Spanish
- Interactive Review Questions and Exercises and more!

Review Questions for the NCLEX® Examination

1. You demonstrate understanding of the physiologic changes in the nervous system associated with aging by:
   1. providing extra time for the patient to process and answer questions.
   2. teaching the patient how to perform activities of daily living.
   3. finishing the patient's sentences when they are responding to questions.
   4. communicating slowly and loudly with low-pitched tones.

   NCLEX Client Need: Health Promotion and Maintenance
2. A nurse scrapes an object along the sole of a patient's foot and notes that the great toe bends upward and the smaller toes fan outward. The clinical finding is suggestive of:
   1. sensory abnormality of the cortex.
   2. motor abnormality of the cortex.
   3. cerebellar tissue destruction.
   4. a normal finding.

   NCLEX Client Need: Physiological Integrity: Physiological Adaptation

3. You assess consensual reflex of the eyes. To do this, you:
   1. shine a light in one eye and observe for any change in the other eye's pupil.
   2. have the patient look at an object in the distance and then at your fingers 6 inches from the eyes, observing for pupil constriction.
   3. have the patient look as far in one direction as possible to determine whether the eyes go back and forth rapidly.
   4. hold a tissue to the corner of the eye to see whether the patient blinks.

   NCLEX Client Need: Physiological Integrity: Reduction of Risk Potential
4. Which nursing intervention(s) would be appropriate when providing care for a patient with right hemiplegia from a stroke? *(Select all that apply.)*
   1. Reminding the patient to pay attention to the left side
   2. Protecting the right extremities during transfers
   3. Supporting the unaffected arm with pillows
   4. Using a sling on the affected arm to promote better balance
   5. Initiating ROM exercises

   NCLEX Client Need: Physiological Integrity: Basic Care and Comfort
5. While reviewing a patient's chart you note that the patient has a condition known as *expressive aphasia.* What responses might you expect from the patient upon showing the patient a key and asking, "What is this?"
   1. The patient responds, "Argh ooh."
   2. The patient looks away and gazes out the window.
   3. The patient responds, "It is a key, and it is used to eat my food."
   4. The patient does not respond.

   NCLEX Client Need: Physiological Integrity: Physiological Adaptation
6. You are conducting a "neuro" check on a patient who is admitted with a stroke. Which assessments will be done? *(Select all that apply.)*
   1. Direct light reflex
   2. Balance and coordination
   3. Plantar reflex
   4. Vital signs
   5. Muscle strength
   6. Alertness and orientation

   NCLEX Client Need: Physiological Integrity: Reduction of Risk Potential
7. You are providing discharge instructions to an older adult male who experienced a stroke. You notice that the patient seems indifferent to teaching. You must consider:
   1. talking to the spouse or daughter.
   2. involving the entire family in the care of the patient.
   3. sending the patient to a long-term care facility.
   4. stopping and trying again later.

   NCLEX Client Need: Psychosocial Integrity
8. When giving instructions to a patient with some dysphagia, further teaching is needed if the patient states:
   1. "I must sit upright when I eat."
   2. "I can watch my crime show on TV while I eat."
   3. "I should stay upright after eating for at least 30 minutes."
   4. "I should be calm and unhurried when eating."

   NCLEX Client Need: Physiological Integrity: Reduction of Risk Potential
9. With an open hand, you press over the flaccid bladder of a patient. When questioned regarding this nursing action, an appropriate response would be:
   1. "The technique increases the muscle tone of the bladder."
   2. "The maneuver facilitates removal of urinary sediments."
   3. "The technique assists with complete bladder emptying."
   4. "The technique reduces the incidence of bladder irritation."

   NCLEX Client Need: Physiological Integrity: Basic Care and Comfort
10. You use the Glasgow Coma Scale to evaluate the neurologic responses of a patient. The patient opens their eyes to pain, makes incomprehensible verbal sounds, and extends their extremities with pain. The score would suggest:
    1. locked-in syndrome.
    2. brain death.
    3. coma.
    4. lethargy.

    NCLEX Client Need: Physiological Integrity: Reduction of Risk Potential

Critical Thinking Questions

Scenario A

Mr. Lawson is to have several diagnostic tests to determine the cause of his neurologic symptoms, which include headache, visual disturbance, muscular weakness, and personality change.

1. How would you explain an electroencephalogram to Mr. Lawson? A computed tomography scan? Magnetic resonance imaging?
2. If you are to assess Mr. Lawson's "neuro signs" and he is using eyedrops for glaucoma that constrict the pupils, how would you evaluate his pupillary responses?

Scenario B

Mr. Horton has experienced a CVA and has incontinence of urine.

1. How would you institute a bladder training program for him?
2. What would you do to protect his skin, and his dignity, during the bladder training?
3. If bladder training cannot be accomplished, what is the best way to handle his urinary elimination?

22 Care of Patients With Head and Spinal Cord Injuries

http://evolve.elsevier.com/deWit/medsurg

Objectives

Theory

1. Describe the types of injuries that result from head trauma.
2. Compare and contrast the signs and symptoms of subdural hematoma and epidural hematoma.
3. Explain why an epidural hematoma causes an emergency situation.
4. Determine appropriate nursing assessments for the patient with a subarachnoid hemorrhage or an intracerebral bleed.
5. Illustrate the pathophysiology of increasing intracranial pressure in a patient who has experienced brain injury.
6. Review the reasons why an older adult is more at risk for an intracranial bleed from a head injury.
7. Explain the possible ramifications of spinal cord injury.
8. Plan appropriate nursing interventions necessary to provide comprehensive care for a patient who has suffered a C5 spinal cord injury.
9. Analyze and review the symptoms of low back pain and correlate them with their causes.

Clinical Practice

10. Teach a family member how to properly assess and care for a patient who has suffered a concussion.
11. Perform a neurologic check on a patient who has suffered head trauma.
12. Participate in a collaborative care planning conference for a patient who has sustained a spinal cord injury.
13. Prepare a plan for teaching self-care measures to a patient who suffers from low back pain.

Key Terms

concussion (kŏn-KŬ-shŭn, p. 514)
contralateral (kŏn-tră-LĂT-ĕr- ăl, p. 517)
contusion (kŏn-TŪ-zhŭn, p. 516)
coup-contrecoup injury (kū KŎN-trĕ-kū IN-jŭ-rē, p. 514)
epidural hematoma (Ĕ-pĭ-DŪ-rŭl hē-mă-TŌ-mă, p. 516)
hydrocephalus (hī-drō-SĔF-ă-lăs, p. 523)
intracerebral hematoma (ĭn-trăh-sĕ-RĒ-brăl hē-mă-TŌ-mă, p. 516)
ipsilateral (ĭp-sĭ-LĂT-ĕr-ăl, p. 517)
nuchal rigidity (NŪ-kăl rĭ-JĬ-dĭ-tē, p. 516)
papilledema (păp-ĭl-ĕ-DĒ-mă, p. 521)
quadriplegia (kwŏd-rĭ-PLĒ-jă, p. 524)
subarachnoid hemorrhage (sŭb-ŭ-RĂK-noid HĔM-rĭj, p. 516)
subdural hematoma (sŭb-DŬ-rŭl hē-mă-TŌ-mă, p. 516)
subluxation (sŭb-lŭk-SĀ-shŭn, p. 524)

Concepts Covered in This Chapter

- Functional Ability
- Family Dynamics
- Self-Management
- Intracranial Regulation
- Inflammation
- Cognition
- Sexuality
- Mobility
- Coping

TRAUMATIC BRAIN (HEAD) INJURIES

Traumatic brain injuries (TBIs) account for 2.5 million emergency department (ED) visits and 56,000 deaths annually in the United States. The direct medical costs and indirect costs (lost productivity) for TBIs total approximately $76.5 billion (Rajajee, 2018).

ETIOLOGY

The most common modes of injury identified by ED visits were falls, being struck by an object, and motor vehicle crashes. A **coup-contrecoup injury**, or an *acceleration-deceleration injury,* occurs when the head is moving rapidly and hits a stationary object, such as a windshield. The contents within the cranium hit the inside of the skull *(coup)* and then bounce back and hit the bony area opposite the site of impact, causing a second injury *(contrecoup;* Fig. 22.1). Males have a higher occurrence of TBI than females. Risk factors for head injury include lower socioeconomic status, alcohol and drug use, and underlying psychiatric and cognitive disorders.

CONCUSSION

The mildest form of TBI is **concussion**, which is defined by the Quality Standards Subcommittee of the American Academy of Neurology as a "trauma-induced alteration in mental status that may or may not involve loss of consciousness" (Evans & Whitlow, 2018). The clinical symptoms observed in a concussion are thought to

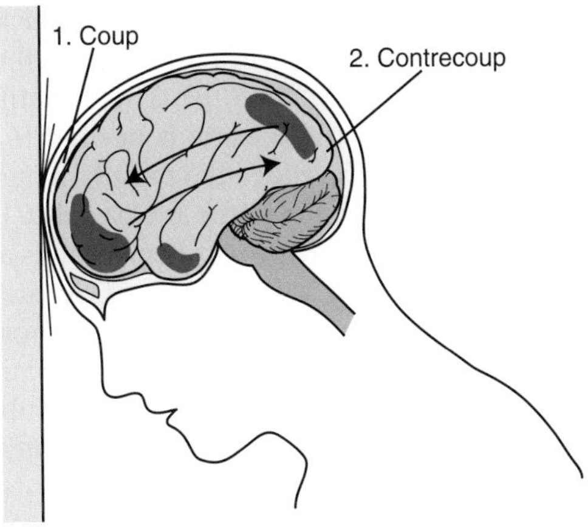

Fig. 22.1 Coup-contrecoup (acceleration-deceleration) injury.

reflect a disturbance in function rather than a structural injury. Microscopic injury to the axons and glial structures may occur and are not visible on imaging studies.

SIGNS, SYMPTOMS, AND DIAGNOSIS

The signs and symptoms of concussion include headache or "pressure" in the head; balance problems or dizziness; nausea or vomiting; confusion or memory problems; feeling sluggish, hazy, foggy, groggy, or just "not right." Multiple scoring systems are used, including the Glasgow Coma Scale, Full Outline of UnResponsiveness (FOUR) Score, and Standardized Assessment of Concussion (SAC), which was developed for use with athletes.

TREATMENT

If a brain injury that can be seen on imaging studies has occurred, the injury is managed according to its type. Most concussions are diagnosed at a health care facility based on clinical signs and symptoms, and then the patient is sent home with discharge instructions that are intended to promote recovery and identify complications. The main treatment is rest and sleep to allow the brain to heal. The patient is instructed to gradually resume normal activities, not doing too much too fast. Return to work or recreational activities should be cleared by the health care provider. Sustaining another concussion within 10 days puts the patient at risk for long-term problems. Most providers will not allow resumption of activities that could produce concussion for 1 to 2 weeks after symptoms have subsided. Patients are instructed to contact their provider if they do not feel back to normal within 1 week, as further testing may be needed.

SKULL FRACTURE

Trauma to the head may result in fracture of the skull. Fractures are categorized by location, appearance, degree of compression, and whether they provide direct access to sinuses, the oropharynx, the ear, or the skull through a skin wound. A fracture is considered an open fracture when it allows the brain and meninges to be exposed to locations that contain microbes. Open fractures require immediate intervention. Any skull fracture is of concern because the force required to break the skull is also transmitted to the underlying brain tissue, causing injury.

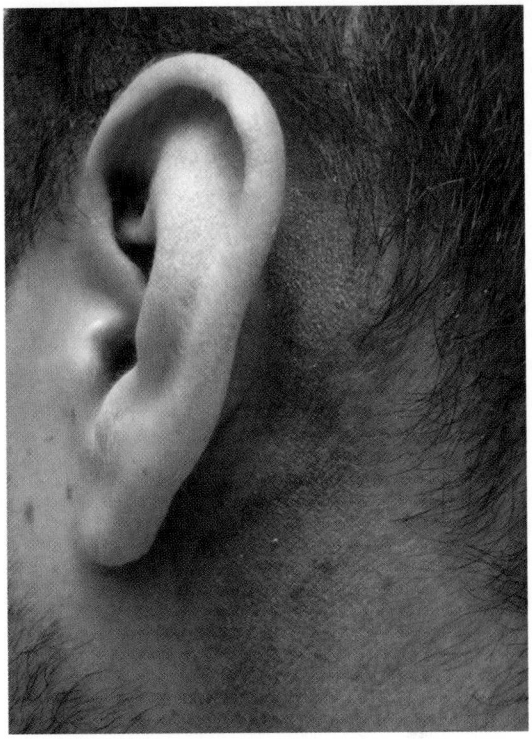

Fig. 22.2 Battle sign. (From Parillo JE, Dellinger RP: *Critical care medicine: principles of diagnosis and management in the adult*, ed 5, Philadelphia, 2019, Elsevier.)

Linear fractures are "cracks" with no bone displacement and are sometimes called "hairline" fractures. If the fracture crosses a vascular channel, a blood vessel may be damaged, resulting in bleeding. Fractures that do not cause bone displacement are left to heal without treatment other than what might be needed for injury to the brain. When a depressed skull fracture occurs, there is usually bruising, contusion, or laceration of the underlying brain tissue by the bone, with the inflammatory changes that occur with any wound. Surgical intervention is required to remove bone fragments and prevent further brain injury.

Basilar skull fractures are usually linear and occur in the bones that cradle the brain, which is the base of the skull. Because of its location, fractures of this bone cannot be seen on standard imaging. The fracture may be diagnosed by the clinical signs of a cerebrospinal fluid (CSF) leak or bleeding into other structures. Otorrhea (fluid from the ears) or rhinorrhea (fluid from the nose) may be observed within hours to days after injury. The fluid may be bloody or clear. Ecchymosis around the eyes (raccoon eyes) and ecchymosis behind the ear (Battle sign) (Fig. 22.2) are both indicators of basilar skull fracture.

Older Adult Care Points

The brain atrophies with age and does not take up as much space in the cranial vault. This allows for more movement and more potential for torn vessels and contusions on the brain when an accident occurs that involves a head injury.

BLEEDING

Contusion, hematoma, or hemorrhage may occur with any TBI. Many TBIs result from falls in the older adult, and many of these older adults are on antiplatelet or anticoagulant medications for other conditions. This increases the bleeding risk.

In a **contusion**, the brain tissue is bruised, blood from broken vessels accumulates, and edema develops. This could lead to the development of increased intracranial pressure (ICP).

Subdural hematoma is a common result of head injury. When a blow is delivered to the head, it may rupture the blood vessels that lie between the arachnoid membrane and the tough, fibrous dura mater. As the blood leaks under the dura mater (subdural), the hematoma becomes larger, pressing against the brain tissue (Fig. 22.3, *A*). Subdural hematomas tend to result from venous bleeding and may take time to bleed enough to cause changes in ICP.

Older Adult Care Points

Because the brain of an older adult tends to move more in the cranial vault when head trauma occurs, small vessels may be torn, putting these patients more at risk for a slow-developing subdural hematoma. Use of antiplatelet and anticoagulant medications increases this risk. When such an injury occurs, the person should be watched for several months for signs of personality change, decreasing level of consciousness (LOC), increased irritability, and other signs of increased ICP.

An **epidural hematoma** occurs more rarely, but when it does, there is rapid leakage of blood from the middle meningeal artery (or rarely from some other vessel) into the space between the dura and the skull, which quickly elevates ICP (Fig. 22.3, *B*). This constitutes a medical emergency. A craniotomy is needed to repair the damaged vessel and relieve the rapidly rising pressure before death occurs from the increased ICP.

A **subarachnoid hemorrhage** can also occur as a result of TBI. The subarachnoid space is where CSF circulates, so bleeding into this area circulates the blood throughout the spinal dural sac and predisposes the patient to developing hydrocephalus. Bleeding into the subarachnoid space may be evidenced by **nuchal rigidity** (neck pain with flexion).

An **intracerebral hematoma** may occur within the brain from a blow to the head (Fig. 22.3, *C*). This bleeding occurs into the brain tissue and not within the meningeal layers. Because of its location within brain tissue, surgical removal is usually not possible.

SIGNS AND SYMPTOMS

The severity of brain damage from a head injury is best judged by the symptoms presented by the patient, a neurologic assessment, the history of the type of injury received, and whether and for how long the victim lost consciousness. The outward symptoms of scalp injury are usually obvious; these include bruising, swelling, lacerations, and bleeding. The actual damage to the underlying brain tissue is not as easy to identify and needs to be assessed carefully.

Clinical Cues

Historically, it was thought that testing rhinorrhea fluid for dextrose would determine if the fluid was CSF or normal nasal discharge. It was found that this method was not reliable. Visual inspection is still in use. Collect about a quarter-teaspoon of the fluid on a white gauze pad. Within a few minutes the serous fluid will wick away from the blood cells, leaving a pink spot surrounded by a yellow ring (halo). The halo sign is indicative of CSF (Fig. 22.4).

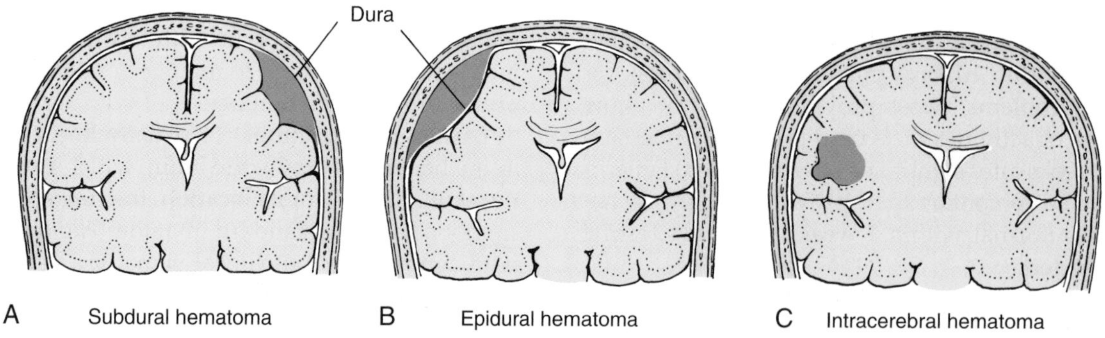

Fig. 22.3 **A,** Subdural hematoma. As a result of trauma to the head, small ruptured blood vessels leak blood into the space under the dura mater (slower than an epidural bleed). **B,** Epidural hematoma, the result of a head injury that tears a large meningeal artery, has caused a rapid bleed with a large amount of blood above the dura mater. If not relieved, subdural and epidural hematomas can be fatal. **C,** Intracerebral hematoma. Small vessels within the brain have torn and bled. (From Black JM, Hawks JH: *Medical-surgical nursing: clinical management for positive outcomes*, ed 8, Philadelphia, 2009, Saunders.)

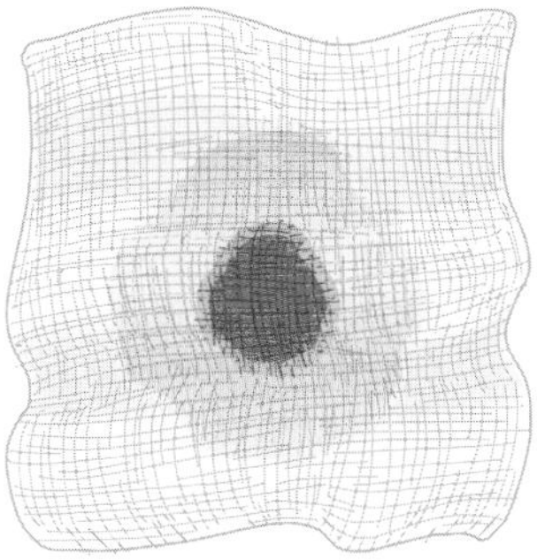

Fig. 22.4 Assessing for the halo sign on fluid from the nose or ear after a head injury. The blood will draw together in the middle of the gauze pad, leaving a yellow ring (halo) around the blood, indicating the presence of cerebrospinal fluid.

Box 22.1 Decreasing Levels of Consciousness (LOCs)

- *Alert:* Responds appropriately to questions and commands with little stimulation. Attends to surroundings.
- *Confused:* Somewhat disoriented to surroundings, time, or people. Judgment may be impaired. Needs to be cued to respond to commands.
- *Lethargic:* Drowsy but easily aroused; needs gentle touch or verbal stimulation to attend to commands.
- *Obtunded:* More difficult to arouse and responds slowly to stimulation. Needs repeated stimulation to maintain attention and to respond to the environment.
- *Stuporous:* Responds to vigorous stimulation only slightly; may only moan or mutter in response.
- *Comatose:* No observable response to stimulation.

A concussion causes a disruption of the normal function of the central nervous system (CNS) and may result in amnesia regarding the event and headache. A contusion can cause an alteration in LOC and may cause seizures. Box 22.1 shows the downward progression of decreased LOC.

A subdural hematoma may be acute, subacute, or chronic, building up over time. An acute intracerebral bleed causing hematoma formation is accompanied by unconsciousness, hemiplegia on the **contralateral** (opposite) side, and a dilated pupil on the **ipsilateral** (same) side. However, the symptoms indicating a slow buildup of pressure within the skull are more subtle and less easily detected.

Signs of epidural hematoma may include unconsciousness at the time of the injury, a brief lucid interval followed by decreasing LOC, headache, nausea and vomiting, and dilation of the ipsilateral pupil. The patient is observed for signs of increased ICP as well as other focal changes (see Increased Intracranial Pressure later in this chapter).

Subarachnoid hemorrhage classically presents with a severe headache, often described as the "worst headache of my life." This is accompanied by nausea and vomiting, nuchal rigidity, and back pain. Photophobia and visual changes are also common.

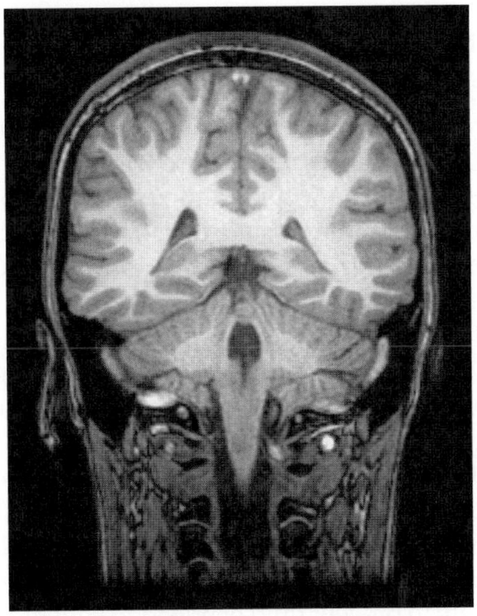

Fig. 22.5 Magnetic resonance imaging midline sagittal view of the brain. (From Leonard PC: *Building a medical vocabulary with Spanish translations*, ed 10, St. Louis, 2018, Elsevier.)

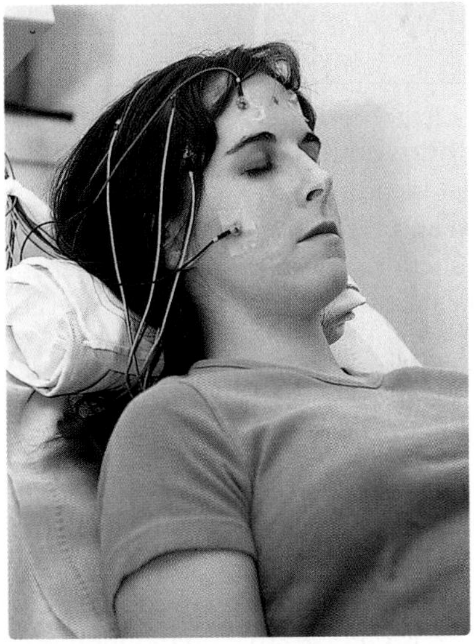

Fig. 22.6 Electroencephalogram (EEG). (From Fuller G, Manford M: *Neurology*, ed 3, London, 2011, Churchill Livingstone.)

DIAGNOSIS

The diagnostic tests and examinations commonly used to determine the extent of head injury include a radiograph of the skull, a computed tomography (CT) scan, magnetic resonance imaging (MRI) with or without contrast, positron emission tomography, evoked potentials, and electroencephalography (Fig. 22.5 and 22.6; see Chapter 21, Table 21.6).

Think Critically

Why should every patient who has sustained a head injury be monitored closely for 24 to 48 hours?

TREATMENT

Initially, patients with a head injury usually are treated conservatively. If the injury causes an increase in ICP or involves a compound fracture of the skull, surgical debridement of the wound and removal of splintered bone from the brain tissues or elevation of the skull fragment is performed. All measures to keep ICP from rising are instituted for serious head injuries.

A patent airway must be secured and the head raised 20 to 30 degrees, with the body in correct alignment. Elevation helps reduce ICP by promoting venous drainage from the head. Keeping the neck in a neutral position allows for unimpeded venous drainage. Neurologic signs are monitored closely. An intravenous (IV) line is inserted for access for diuretic drugs, if needed, and for administration of fluid. Intravenous fluids are infused very slowly to prevent fluid overload that would increase ICP. Diuretics are used to decrease vascular volume and keep ICP as low as possible.

> **? Think Critically**
>
> Why would you check for a patent airway before performing a neurologic assessment on a patient with a head injury?

Surgical Intervention

Intracranial bleeding is treated surgically as indicated by location and type. The hematoma or blood is evacuated by suction or surgical instruments. Epidural hematoma necessitates immediate, emergency craniotomy to prevent death from increased ICP. The craniotomy procedure is described in Chapter 23 along with surgeries of the brain.

Preoperative period. A patient with a brain bleed is quickly prepared for surgery. If indicated, the operative site is shaved after the patient is under anesthesia. For planned surgery, a shampoo may be ordered the evening before surgery. Preoperative preparation is the same as for other surgeries. Any scalp lesions or other unusual conditions that are noted at this time should be reported.

Postoperative period. During the immediate postoperative period, the patient who underwent a craniotomy is in the intensive care unit for continuous monitoring. Essentially, care will be the same as that for any patient in danger of increasing ICP. Additional postoperative care of a patient who has undergone intracranial surgery includes the following:

- Positioning the patient according to written orders from the attending surgeon. **Make no exceptions.** Positioning is important to prevent added increases in ICP.
- Keeping the neck in midline, usually maintaining head of the bed (HOB) at 30 degrees, and preventing excessive hip flexion to promote venous drainage from the head and keep the ICP from rising (Rajajee, 2018).
- Treating increased body temperature to prevent secondary injury.
- Preventing constipation. Straining a stool increases ICP.
- Providing adequate pain control.
- Administering anticonvulsant medications, corticosteroids, and prophylactic antibiotics as ordered.
- Reporting promptly any changes in the neurologic status of the patient.

NURSING MANAGEMENT

If it has been determined that there is indeed leakage of spinal fluid through the nose, ear, or an open head wound, special precautions must be taken to prevent infection, and the health care provider must be notified. The special precautions include the following:

- Keep the patient on bed rest with the head of the bed elevated 20 to 30 degrees.
- Cover a draining ear with a sterile gauze pad, changing the pad periodically to look for drainage. Apply a moustache dressing for nasal drainage.
- Instruct the patient *not* to blow the nose or pick at it; blowing may increase ICP, and picking may allow entry of microorganisms.
- Coughing and sneezing can increase drainage or enlarge the opening. Medicate as needed.
- Do not plug the nose or ear if there is drainage of CSF because blockage may increase ICP.
- If drainage persists, surgical intervention may be needed.
- Manage bowel activity to prevent straining at stool.

Continued neurologic assessments are an integral part of care. Specific problem statements are listed in Nursing Care Plan 22.1. Specific instruction is required for the observation of a patient treated in an ED for head injury and released to go home. The long-term outcome for patients who have suffered a severe head injury is unpredictable. Recovery is a long process, and improvement may occur over many months to years in some patients. Disabilities may be lifelong.

INCREASED INTRACRANIAL PRESSURE

ETIOLOGY AND PATHOPHYSIOLOGY

Because the skull is a closed bony structure in adults, it is unable to expand. **Any lesion or fluid accumulation that begins to take up space within the cranial cavity causes an increase in the pressure within the cavity.** The Monro-Kellie doctrine indicates that 80% of the cranial vault is taken up by brain tissue, 10% by CSF, and 10% by cerebral blood flow. If any one of these three elements increase, pressure rises. The body shunts some CSF to the spinal dural sac, and some blood flow can be reduced. Medications can be given to reduce brain edema, shrinking cells. Although these measures can help, they do not prevent increased ICP. Therefore any swelling of the brain tissue from injury or surgery; leakage of blood from ruptured cerebral vessels;

Nursing Care Plan 22.1 Care of a Patient With a Head Injury and Increased Intracranial Pressure

SCENARIO

Ryan, an 18-year-old male who suffered a head injury in an automobile accident, is groggy but arousable.

PROBLEM STATEMENT/NURSING DIAGNOSIS

Potential for altered cerebral perfusion related to increased ICP from head injury.

SUPPORTING ASSESSMENT DATA

Subjective: Hit right side of head on dashboard.
Objective: Nondepressed linear skull fracture, alteration in LOC, confused as to where he is, what day it is; somewhat combative.

Goals/Expected Outcomes	Nursing Interventions	Selected Rationale	Evaluation
Patient will not display further increase in ICP.	Monitor neurologic status hourly using the appropriate scale per facility policy, Glasgow Coma Scale (GCS), or FOUR score scale; notify health care provider of any pupil changes or signs of increasing ICP, such as widening pulse pressure, change in respiratory pattern, slowing of pulse, increase in temperature, or decrease in LOC.	GCS provides good estimate of neurologic status.	GCS maintaining at 12.
	Monitor for seizure activity; institute seizure precautions. Administer ordered anticonvulsant.	Increased pressure on brain tissue may cause cellular irritability and seizure activity.	No sign of seizure activity. Precautions in place; padded side rails in place.
	Keep head of bed (HOB) at 30 degrees and body in correct alignment; turn side to side q2h if condition warrants.	Keeping head slightly elevated and in proper alignment helps promote venous drainage from the head.	HOB at 30 degrees; positioned in correct alignment with neck midline. Turned q2h.
	Administer diuretic as ordered.	Diuretic decreases vascular volume and intracranial volume, lowering ICP.	Mannitol administered.
	Keep room calm and softly lit; do not disturb more than necessary; talk to patient while giving care; allow rest periods between any invasive procedures; reorient patient frequently.	Invasive procedures and agitation raise ICP.	Room is tidy and softly lit; care procedures grouped at intervals, allowing rest.

PROBLEM STATEMENT/NURSING DIAGNOSIS

Altered self-care ability related to confusion and grogginess.

SUPPORTING ASSESSMENT DATA

Objective: Falls asleep during attempts at bath, etc.; confused about where he is and what activities are happening.

Goals/Expected Outcomes	Nursing Interventions	Selected Rationale	Evaluation
Patient will have adequate assistance with hygiene and dressing.	Provide assistance with all ADLs.	Patient with altered LOC may require temporary assistance with ADLs.	Assisted with morning care.
	Inspect skin when turning; place foam pad on bed.	Pressure-relieving device helps prevent pressure ulcer formation.	No signs of reddened areas on skin. Foam pad on bed.
Patient will resume self-care by discharge.	Encourage self-care as LOC improves.	Resolution of increased ICP improves ability to perform self-care.	Continue plan. Not ready for self-care yet.

PROBLEM STATEMENT/NURSING DIAGNOSIS

Altered family coping related to patient's decreased LOC and hospitalization.

Continued

Nursing Care Plan 22.1 Care of a Patient With a Head Injury and Increased Intracranial Pressure—cont'd

SUPPORTING ASSESSMENT DATA

Subjective: Mother states she is afraid son is going to die.

Objective: Mother keeps trying to rouse the patient when she is in the room.

Goals/Expected Outcomes	Nursing Interventions	Selected Rationale	Evaluation
Mother's anxiety will decrease as she gains information about her son's condition and prognosis.	Explain to family that confusion and grogginess are usual after head injury.	Knowledge decreases fear of the unknown.	Explained patient's condition to family and measures to keep ICP down. Mother seems less anxious. Discussed need for calm and positive talk in room.
	Explain that the danger is if the ICP keeps increasing; tell what measures are being done to minimize increasing ICP; explain all procedures; explain that calm, rest, and positive talk in the room will help.	Knowing the treatment plan decreases anxiety.	
	Call hospital chaplain or own minister if family desires.	Presence of spiritual advisor can decrease anxiety and promote coping.	
	Keep family informed of changes in patient's condition.	Families need to make informed decisions.	

CRITICAL THINKING QUESTIONS

1. Why would it be contraindicated for this patient to strain to have a bowel movement?
2. Why is it important to decrease stimuli and provide a calm, soothing environment for this patient? (Be specific.)

ADLs, Activities of daily living; *ICP,* intracranial pressure; *LOC,* level of consciousness.

Patient Teaching

Instructions for Care of a Patient With a Head Injury

Teach the family or significant other to do the following:

- Do not leave the patient alone until they are "back to normal."
- The patient should avoid bending, straining, or performing strenuous activity.
- The patient should not operate machinery or drive until cleared by the health care provider.
- The patient may complain of nausea, mild headaches, difficulty concentrating, or dizziness. The symptoms may continue for weeks.
- For 48 hours, watch for and report the following signs:
  - Change in LOC (e.g., becoming more groggy, difficult to awaken, confused, restless, agitated)
  - Projectile vomiting (vomit travels a distance) without nausea or persistent nausea or vomiting
  - Unusual dizziness, sleepiness, loss of balance, or fall
  - Change in vision (i.e., seeing double, blurred vision)
  - Seizures or weakness in an arm or leg
  - Clear or blood-tinged drainage from ears or nose
  - A change in speech or ability to find words or converse
  - Worsening headache
  - Behavior that is odd for the individual

Think Critically

Why are patients with a head injury positioned with the head of the bed elevated 20 to 30 degrees and with the head and neck in proper alignment?

Legal and Ethical Considerations

Documenting Patient Teaching

Because there are legal ramifications of inadequate patient and family teaching, document all teaching in the medical record and send home clearly written instructions with the patient. It is best to have the patient or family sign a form for the record that indicates that teaching and written instructions have been received.

excessive production of CSF; or tumors, abscesses, or any other space-occupying lesion within the skull presents a risk for increased ICP. Pressure against cerebral veins and arteries interferes with the flow of blood, producing local ischemia and hypoxia. Pressure against the cells themselves can interfere with their vital functions. If the ICP rises very high and remains high for very long, death can result from inadequate cerebral perfusion or cerebral herniation. Brainstem injuries or pressure on the brainstem from increased ICP causes respiratory depression from pressure on the medulla oblongata—carbon dioxide accumulates, causing vasodilation and further increases in ICP. Normal ICP is 0 to 15 mm Hg. Concept Map 22.1 shows the relationship between the causes and the pathologic occurrences of increased ICP.

SIGNS, SYMPTOMS, AND DIAGNOSIS

When the body can no longer compensate for the increase in volume in the cranial vault, decompensation begins and clinical signs of increasing ICP become

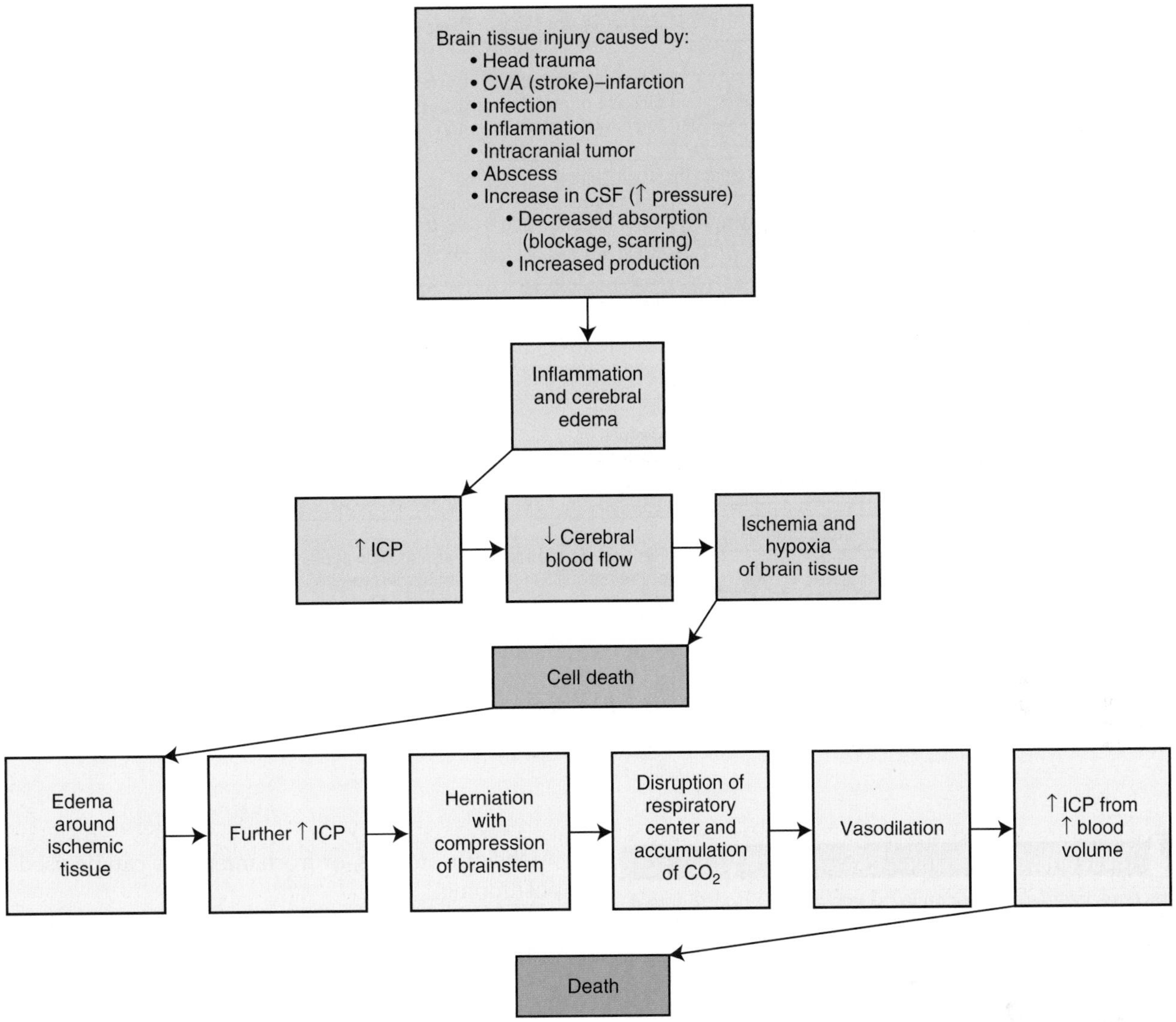

Concept Map 22.1 Pathophysiologic changes from a brain injury that increase intracranial pressure *(ICP)* and can lead to death. *CSF,* Cerebrospinal fluid; *CVA,* cerebrovascular accident.

apparent. **The earliest sign of increasing ICP is lethargy and decreasing consciousness, accompanied by a slowing of speech and delay in response to verbal cues.** **Papilledema** (swelling of the optic disc) viewed with an ophthalmoscope is a classic sign of increased ICP. Headache, nausea, and vomiting may also occur.

When ICP rises, it affects the oxygenated blood perfusion of the brain, and tissue hypoxia occurs. Extended periods of hypoxia cause brain cell death. The body tries to compensate for hypoxia by raising blood pressure, to force more oxygenated blood through the brain tissue. For blood to flow into the brain, blood pressure (mean arterial pressure) must be higher than the ICP pushing against flow into the brain. If ICP continues to rise, the brain tissue will herniate through the tentorial notch at the midline of the foramen magnum. This herniation results in pressure on the vital structures of the midbrain, pons, and medulla and causes changes in the vital signs and pupil reactions characteristic of increased ICP.

As brain tissue swells or fluid volume increases in the cranium, damage occurs or pressure is placed on the oculomotor or third cranial nerve. Pupils begin to react slowly; pupil size becomes unequal, progressing to dilation, and then the pupil size becomes fixed as reflexes disappear.

Clinical Cues

Abnormal pupillary responses can reverse to normal if the cause of increased ICP can be resolved in time.

The classic signs of increased ICP, the first three of which are called the *Cushing triad,* are:

- Rising systolic blood pressure
- Widening pulse pressure
- Bradycardia with a full, bounding pulse
- Rapid or irregular respirations (Fig. 22.7)

These signs tend to be late, as are pupil changes, and signal a severe emergency and the need for immediate action to try to prevent the patient's death.

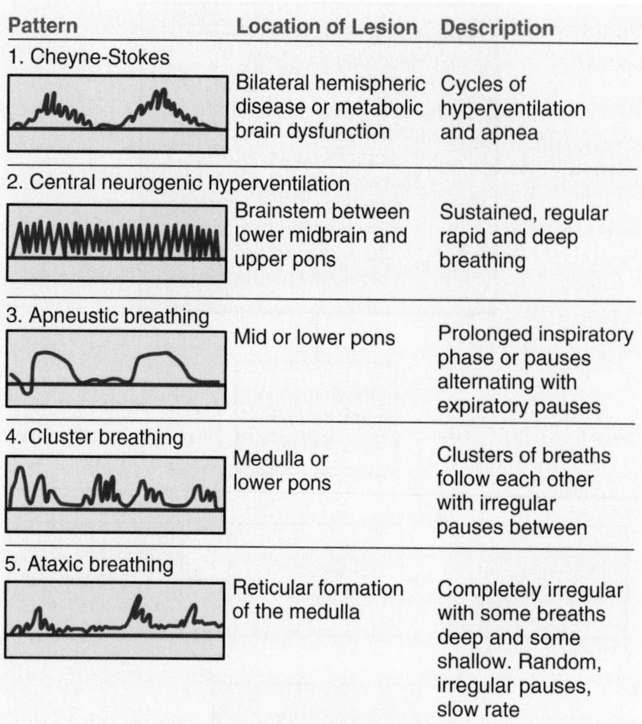

Pattern
Location of Lesion
Description
1. Cheyne-Stokes
Bilateral hemispheric disease or metabolic brain dysfunction
Cycles of hyperventilation and apnea
2. Central neurogenic hyperventilation
Brainstem between lower midbrain and upper pons
Sustained, regular rapid and deep breathing
3. Apneustic breathing
Mid or lower pons
Prolonged inspiratory phase or pauses alternating with expiratory pauses
4. Cluster breathing
Medulla or lower pons
Clusters of breaths follow each other with irregular pauses between
5. Ataxic breathing
Reticular formation of the medulla
Completely irregular with some breaths deep and some shallow. Random, irregular pauses, slow rate

Fig. 22.7 Common abnormal respiratory patterns associated with coma. (From Lewis SL, Bucher L, Heitkemper MM, et al.: *Medical-surgical nursing: assessment and management of clinical problems,* ed 10, St. Louis, 2017, Elsevier.)

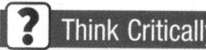

> **? Think Critically**
>
> Why does increasing intracranial edema cause a double threat to the brain?

TREATMENT

A patient with greatly increased ICP is usually placed in an intensive care unit. Increased ICP is treated with supportive care to keep the pressure from rising further and with interventions to decrease the cranial blood or CSF volume. Osmotic diuretics (mannitol, glycerol, urea) or hypertonic saline are administered to remove fluid from the body tissues, thereby reducing fluid in the brain. Dosage is determined by body weight, and electrolytes are monitored every 6 hours because mannitol and diuretic action can cause electrolyte imbalances. Furosemide (Lasix) is sometimes also given. An indwelling urinary catheter is inserted to monitor output. Electrolytes and fluid balance are watched closely.

Dexamethasone (Decadron) may be given to decrease the inflammatory response and cerebral edema if the ICP is caused by a brain tumor or abscess (Drappatz, 2018). Histamine-2 (H_2)–receptor blockers or proton pump inhibitors are administered to protect the gastric mucosa. With the head of the bed at 20 to 30 degrees, the head and neck must be kept positioned midline so that venous drainage into the body is not restricted. Hip flexion should be less than 90 degrees. Rolled washcloths, towels, or trochanter rolls can be used for positioning.

If ICP is dangerously high as indicated by a Glasgow Coma Scale score of 9 or less and an abnormal CT scan, the surgeon may insert an intraventricular catheter into the lateral ventricle, through which CSF can be drained in small amounts to relieve the pressure. Pressure can be monitored with the catheter or a separate probe positioned in the epidural area. Cerebral perfusion pressure (CPP) is maintained at 60 to 70 mm Hg or higher to ensure oxygenation of the brain tissue (CPP = Mean arterial pressure – Intracranial pressure) (Howells et al., 2018). Other devices may be used to monitor cerebral oxygenation and blood flow.

If the patient is on a ventilator and is extremely agitated, sedation may be used to prevent further increases in ICP. Continuous infusion of dexmedetomidine hydrochloride (Precedex) or propofol (Diprivan) may be used for sedation because they have a short half-life and can be cleared from the body quickly. Because carbon dioxide is a vasodilator in the brain and can increase blood volume within the cranial cavity, hyperventilation is sometimes used short term to combat the increased ICP. This is accomplished by increasing the rate of controlled respiration. A carbon dioxide level between 25 and 30 mm Hg will decrease ICP by causing vasoconstriction. Box 22.2 provides general guidelines for the care of patients with increased ICP.

Barbiturates are sometimes used along with continuous brain wave monitoring when patients do not respond

Box 22.2 Guidelines for Patients With Increased Intracranial Pressure (ICP)

DO

- Conduct neurologic checks at least once every hour unless more frequent monitoring is indicated.
- Report changes immediately.
- Maintain a patent airway and adequate ventilation to ensure proper oxygen and carbon dioxide exchange.
- Elevate the head of the bed 20 to 30 degrees to facilitate return of blood from the cerebral veins.
- Use measures to maintain normal body temperature. Elevations of temperature raise blood pressure and cerebral blood flow. Shivering can also increase ICP.
- Monitor intake and output. Restrict or encourage fluids according to the health care provider's order.
- Give passive range-of-motion exercises.
- Space activities apart.

DO NOT

- Allow patient to become constipated or perform Valsalva maneuver.
- Hyperextend, flex, or rotate the patient's head.
- Flex the patient's hips greater than 90 degrees (as in female catheterization).
- Place patient in Trendelenburg position for any reason.
- Allow patient to perform isometric exercises.

to the more common therapies for reduction of ICP. Their purpose is to induce heavy sedation and slow metabolism, thereby decreasing ICP. In general, the short-acting barbiturates are used (e.g., pentobarbital [Nembutal] and thiopental [Pentothal]). Anticonvulsant medications such as levetiracetam (Keppra) or phenytoin (Dilantin) may be used to prevent seizures for several months or years after injury.

Temperature control is achieved by placing the patient on a hypothermia blanket for cooling if increased ICP has affected temperature regulation by pressure on the hypothalamus and the patient is feverish. Fever increases cerebral metabolism and cerebral edema.

Warmed blankets and tepid baths can be used to raise the temperature of a hypothermic patient and prevent shivering. Deep vein thrombosis prophylaxis is started early. Intravenous insulin may be titrated to maintain the blood glucose level at 140 to 180 mg/dL.

Decompressive craniectomy may be performed to relieve pressure when medical measures are not adequate. A portion of the skull is removed, and the dura is opened to allow for expansion of the swollen brain without compression. The removed skull is stored in a freezer or in the patient's body, usually in a pouch created in the abdomen. The skull will be replaced after about 3 months of brain healing. During this time a helmet or other protective device should be worn to prevent further brain injury.

The interventions listed can all decrease ICP. Decrease of ICP does not mean increased survival or decreased disability for all patients.

Complications

Damage to brain cells from injury and during periods of increased ICP may cause residual scarring and seizures. **Hydrocephalus** (excessive accumulation of CSF) may occur (see Chapter 23), causing motor deficits, cranial nerve deficits, or decreased cognitive ability. Rehabilitation efforts are focused on eliminating or decreasing deficits and promoting as much cognitive and physical function as possible (see Chapter 9).

Diabetes insipidus. Diabetes insipidus may occur from injury or edema of the pituitary gland. Antidiuretic hormone is released in inadequate amounts, resulting in polyuria, and the awake patient may complain of **polydipsia** (excessive thirst). Intravenous or subcutaneous vasopressin and fluid replacement are the preferred treatments. Carefully monitor intake and output and electrolyte balance.

NURSING MANAGEMENT

ASSESSMENT (DATA COLLECTION)

Early recognition of increasing pressure is extremely important. Careful neurologic assessment with monitoring of the patient's LOC, pupillary reactions, level of neuromuscular activity, and vital signs is essential to accurately evaluate the patient's progress. "Neuro" checks are performed every 15 minutes to every 2 hours for acute patients (see Chapter 21). The following indications that ICP may be rising should be reported immediately:

- Extreme restlessness or excitability after a period of apparent calm
- Deepening stupor and decreasing LOC
- Headache that is unrelenting and increasing in intensity
- Vomiting, especially persistent, projectile vomiting
- Unequal size of pupils and other abnormal pupillary reactions
- Leakage of CSF from the nose or ear
- Changes in the patient's blood pressure, pulse, or respiration; widening pulse pressure; a slow, bounding pulse

? Think Critically

Why do you think an older adult is at greater risk when a head injury or other cause of increased ICP occurs?

NURSING DIAGNOSIS, PLANNING, AND IMPLEMENTATION

The appropriate problem statement is *Potential for altered cerebral tissue perfusion due to effects of increasing intracranial pressure.*

Goals of nursing care are to:

- Maintain cerebral perfusion
- Reduce ICP
- Maintain adequate respiration

- Protect from injury
- Maintain normal body functions
- Prevent complications

The expected outcome would be that the patient will not experience brain damage from increased ICP.

Maintaining an open airway and adequate respiration may require suctioning and possibly intubation with mechanical ventilation. A patient whose LOC is decreased and whose gag and swallowing reflexes are impaired is in danger of aspirating blood, vomitus, mucus, and other material into the air passages and requires intubation. **An unconscious patient requires care for all basic needs** (see Chapter 21, Table 21.9).

When positioning the patient, prevent a Valsalva maneuver, which could raise ICP. For this reason, instruct the patient not to grip the side rails or push with the feet or elbows against the mattress during repositioning. Plan uninterrupted rest periods between activities that cause an increase in ICP; preferably, plan rest for 1 hour at a time. Provide a soothing environment free of noxious odors and noise. Keep the room temperature adjusted to normalize the patient's temperature and to prevent shivering (Lennon, Ramdharry, & Verheyden, 2018).

Nutrition supplied early improves outcomes after brain injury and increased ICP because nutrition promotes healing (Carney et al., 2016). If the patient is unable to take food orally, supplementation begins within 3 days after injury. Full nutritional supplementation should be in place by day 7. Nutrition is planned according to determined metabolic needs and the fluid and electrolyte status. Metabolic needs are calculated based on age, weight, and height.

◆ EVALUATION

Data are gathered regarding the success of the nursing interventions. If the interventions are not helping the patient meet the expected outcomes, the interventions should be changed.

INJURIES OF THE SPINE AND SPINAL CORD

ETIOLOGY

A person may suffer from injury to the spinal cord in a number of ways. Injury in the cervical and lumbar areas is more common because these segments are more mobile. Automobile accidents, gunshot wounds, diving accidents, falls, and other forms of trauma often inflict severe damage to the spinal cord, but tumors, degenerative disease, and infections also can impair the functions of the spinal cord and its branches. Generally speaking, spinal cord injuries are classified according to their anatomic location—that is, cervical, thoracic, lumbar, or sacral (Fig. 22.8). There are 17,700 spinal cord injuries per year in the United States (National Spinal Cord Injury Statistical Center, 2018). Whatever the cause of spinal cord injury, motor and sensory losses may occur. The amount of loss of function and sensation depends on the level and extent of injury to the spinal cord.

PATHOPHYSIOLOGY

Fracture, dislocation, or **subluxation** (partial dislocation) of the vertebral column often results in spinal cord damage. Cord injury is caused by compression, pulling and twisting, or tearing of the cord, with two types of injuries occurring: complete and incomplete. Complete injuries result in loss of function below the level of the injury. Incomplete injuries result in various degrees of function and sensation. Penetrating trauma from gunshot or knife wounds or other types of accidents may cause severance, compression, or contusion of the spinal cord. Extreme flexion or hyperextension of the neck or falling on the buttocks (which causes flexion of the lower thoracic and lumbar spine) may cause spinal cord damage (Fig. 22.9). Tumor growth may compress or destroy spinal cord tissue. Whatever the cause of injury to the spinal cord, nerve transmission to the brain or from the brain may no longer occur below the level of the damage, resulting in various extents of paralysis.

Microscopic bleeding occurs in the gray matter immediately after spinal cord injury. Irritation of the cells causes edema to develop and spread along the next one or two cord segments. The edema peaks in 2 to 3 days and subsides about 7 days after injury. The edema causes temporary loss of function and sensation. Hemodynamic instability with drops in blood pressure may cause decreased blood flow, and hypoxia in the cord increases the initial damage. The inflammatory process may injure the myelin covering the axons, and the chemical and electrolyte changes interrupt nerve impulse transmission.

SIGNS, SYMPTOMS, AND DIAGNOSIS

A complete severance of the spinal cord, or damage to the cord's entire thickness, results in a total loss of sensation and control in the parts of the body below the point of injury. If the cord is damaged in the cervical region, the paralysis and loss of sensory perception may include both arms and both legs (*tetraplegia,* also called **quadriplegia**). Severe injury to the cord above the level of the fifth cervical vertebra often is fatal if emergency care is not immediate because the phrenic nerves that innervate the diaphragm originate in the third, fourth, and fifth cervical segments. Branches of these nerves play a major role in the control of respiration, and when they are severed, respiration must be maintained by artificial means. If the damage is only partial (incomplete), there will be some losses, but not all motor and sensory innervation is lost (see the Evolve website for the American Spinal Injury Association [ASIA] Impairment Scale).

Interruption of the thoracic spinal cord through L1 and L2 causes *paraplegia* (paralysis of both legs). Table 22.1 presents activities possible with varying levels of cord injury.

Injury to the spinal cord that does not involve complete severance of the cord may result in a temporary

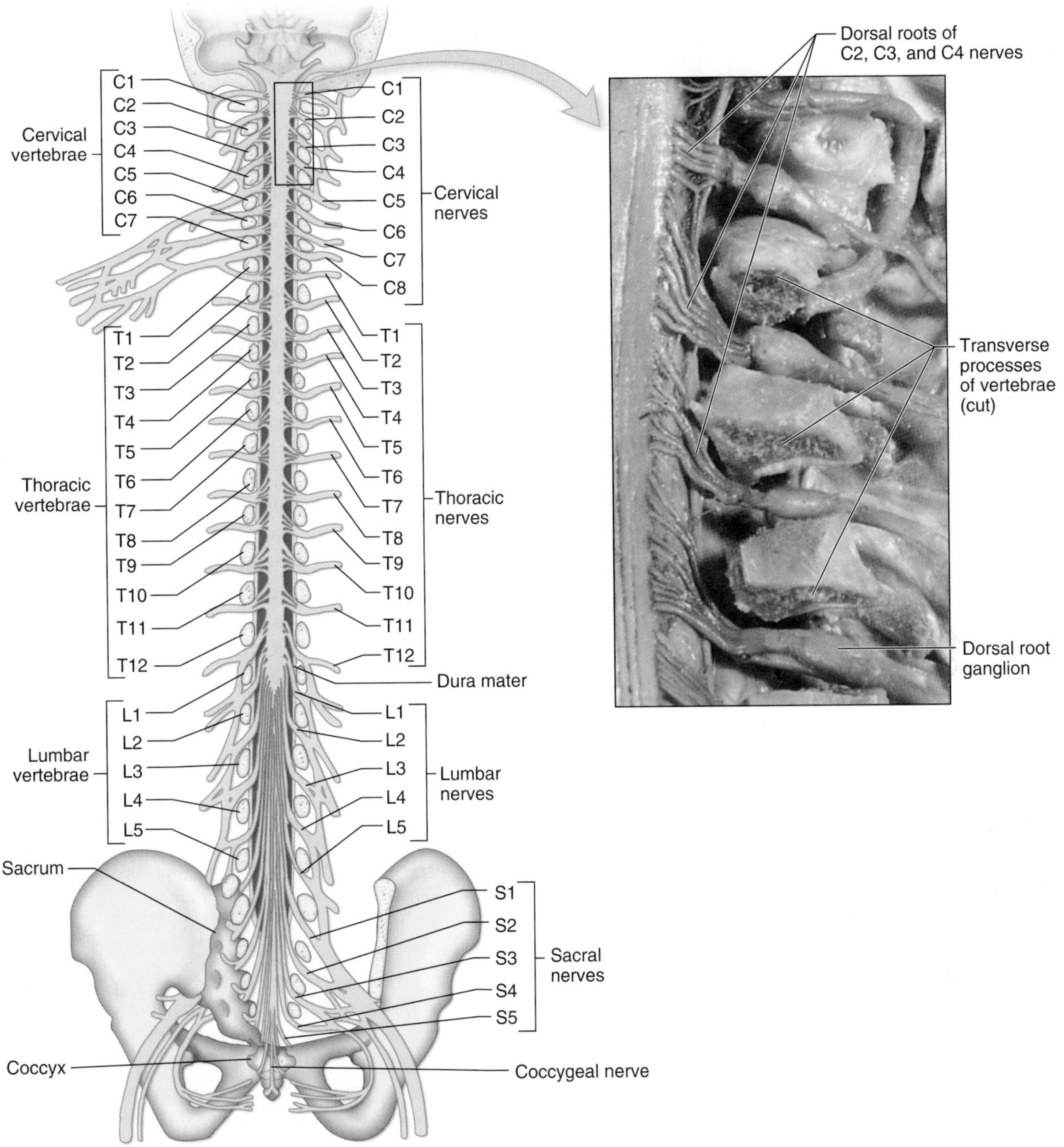

Fig. 22.8 Divisions of the spinal column and designations of spinal nerves. (From Thibodeau GA, Patton KT: *Anatomy and physiology*, ed 8, St. Louis, 2013, Elsevier. Photo courtesy Vidic B, Suarez RF: *Photographic atlas of the human body*, St. Louis, 1984, Mosby.)

paralysis, which may subside as the spinal cord recovers from the swelling and initial shock of the injury. Initial assessment of the damage is often one or two levels higher than the actual injury because of edema, resulting in decreased function until the edema subsides.

Diagnosis is made by physical examination and testing of reflexes. CT scan or MRI may be performed to determine the extent of the damage and to see whether the cord is completely *transected* (severed). This helps determine whether neurologic deficits are likely to be permanent. A myelogram may be performed in special circumstances.

TREATMENT

There are four main objectives in the treatment and nursing care of a patient with an injury of the spinal cord:

1. To save the patient's life
2. To prevent further injury to the cord by careful handling of the patient
3. To implement treatment to limit secondary damage to the cord
4. To establish a routine of care that will improve and maintain the patient's state of health and prevent complications, so that eventual physical, mental, and social rehabilitation is possible

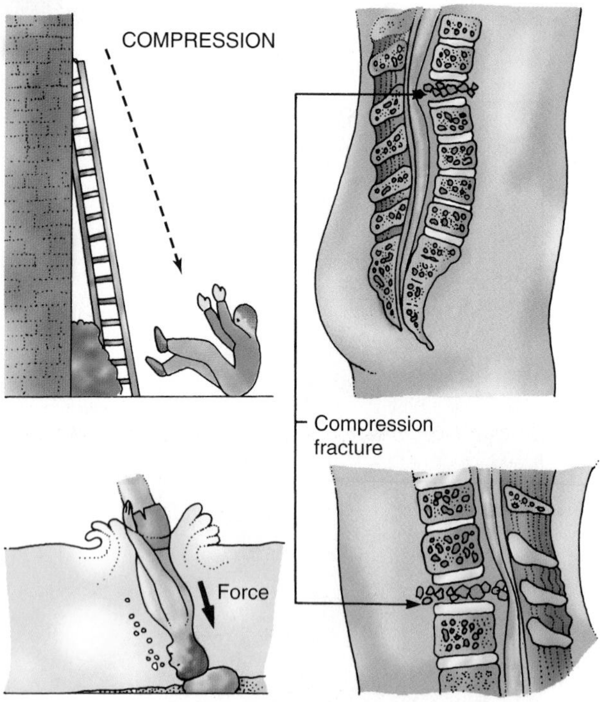

Fig. 22.9 Accidents can cause vertical compression of the cervical or lumbar spine. (From Ignatavicius DD, Workman ML: *Medical-surgical nursing: patient-centered collaborative care,* ed 8, St. Louis, 2016, Elsevier.)

As soon as an injury to the spinal cord occurs, the patient must be handled with extreme care.

Safety Alert

Prevent Further Spinal Injury

Anyone with a head injury is treated as if they have also suffered a spine injury until proven otherwise. The neck must be stabilized to prevent any movement. When no cervical collar is available, use a shirt, towel, coat, or other material rolled and placed around the neck as a collar to keep the neck as straight as possible, preventing it from flexing or hyperextending. If the patient must be moved to safety, they should be rolled like a log, as one straight piece, onto a flat surface, such as a board of plywood or a door removed from its hinges. Roll the patient as one piece onto their side, keeping the neck and shoulders in alignment; place the board behind them; and then carefully roll them back onto the board. This is done slowly and carefully to avoid twisting or bending the spinal column. The victim is kept still.

Because a nurse or health care provider may not be at the scene of the accident to supervise the moving of the patient, laypersons should learn the proper emergency care of such injuries. When an accident victim complains of neck or back pain or cannot move the legs or has no feeling in them, treat them as if they have a

Table 22.1 Level of Spinal Cord Damage, Function Present, and Activities Possible

LEVEL OF INJURY	FUNCTION PRESENT/NEUROLOGIC DEFICIT	ACTIVITY POSSIBLE
C1–C3	No respiratory function; usually fatal unless immediate emergency help is available to establish respiration Tetraplegia (quadriplegia)	Respirations supported by mechanical ventilation or stimulated with phrenic pacemaker. Can manipulate electric wheelchair with breath, chin, or voice control.
C4	Loss of diaphragm movement; breathe with assistance Tetraplegia (quadriplegia)	May live if assisted respiration is begun immediately. Can use a mouth stick to turn pages, type, or write.
C5	Partial shoulder movement; partial elbow movement	Can turn head. Able to feed self with special adaptive devices. Able to move wheelchair for short distances and move well with electric wheelchair. Can assist a bit with self-care.
C6	Retains gross motor function of arms; partial shoulder, elbow, and wrist movement possible Tetraplegia (quadriplegia)	Needs adaptive devices; may be able to propel wheelchair. Independent in feeding and with some grooming with adaptive devices. Can roll over in bed. Can drive a car with hand controls. Can assist in transfer. Can self-catheterize the bladder.
C7	Shoulder, elbow, wrist, hand partial movements possible Tetraplegia (quadriplegia)	Manipulates wheelchair with arms; transfers to and from chair; may drive specially fitted car. Excellent bed mobility. Independent in most ADLs.
C8	Normal arm movement; hand weakness Tetraplegia (quadriplegia)	Bed and wheelchair independent. Can perform most ADLs and may achieve vocational and recreational goals. Performs self-catheterization.
T1–T10	Normal arm movement and strength; loss of bowel, bladder, and sexual function	May achieve walking with braces. Able to perform ADLs and achieve vocational and recreational goals.
T11 and below	Loss of bowel, bladder, and sexual function	Wheelchair not essential. Able to perform ADLs, work, and recreational activities.

ADLs, Activities of daily living.

spinal cord injury. **To avoid flexion of the neck, no pillow or other kind of support is placed under the head. Do not move the patient unless life-threatening conditions require it.**

Transfer of the patient to the hospital should be done only by trained emergency medical technicians. In the ED of the hospital, the patient's condition is stabilized and a thorough examination is conducted to establish the extent of their injuries. Spinal injury is most commonly assessed with the American Spinal Injury Association (ASIA) scale (see the Evolve website). Methylprednisolone, a corticosteroid, is used by some providers with the hope of minimizing further damage to the cord from inflammation and swelling. Lack of clear evidence of benefit and the many side effects of the medication have made it a treatment option but not a treatment standard (Hansebout, 2018).

Clinical Cues

Drug metabolism is altered in patients with a spinal cord injury. Drug interactions are more common. Be vigilant in checking for signs and symptoms of drug interactions.

Normal saline is used for fluid replacement, and drugs such as dopamine (Intropin) may be given to sustain a blood pressure sufficient to prevent cord hypoxia. Pulmonary edema and increased ICP if a head injury is present are potential problems, and fluid balance is watched carefully.

Respiratory Management

Intubation and mechanical ventilation are often required to sustain life in patients with an injury at C5 or above. Patients who can breathe when they first arrive at the hospital may be intubated because as cord edema progresses, respiration may become impaired. Mechanical ventilation relieves the muscle work of breathing and conserves the patient's energy during the emergent phase of the injury.

Immobilization and Surgery

Surgery on the spine with removal of bone fragments is performed to relieve pressure, provide stabilization, and prevent further injury. **Cervical spinal cord injury with subluxation is usually treated with traction to immobilize the affected vertebrae and maintain alignment.** Traction can be accomplished by skeletal traction using Crutchfield or Gardner-Wells tongs with ropes, pulleys, and weights (Fig. 22.10), or with a halo ring and fixation pins with vest (Fig. 22.11). The halo is often used for cord injury not requiring surgery and allows for early mobilization.

Selecting the type of bed to be used for a patient with spinal cord injury depends on many factors. Some health care providers and nurses prefer placing the patient in a special lateral rotation bed that is designed to prevent the problems of immobility while maintaining traction (Fig. 22.12) if the patient will be bedbound for a prolonged period. Other mattresses and beds are available to meet

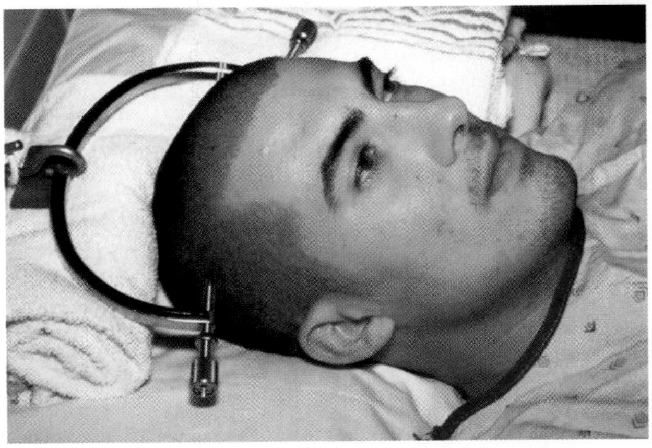

Fig. 22.10 Crutchfield tongs for cervical traction. (Courtesy Michael S. Clement, MD, Mesa, Ariz.)

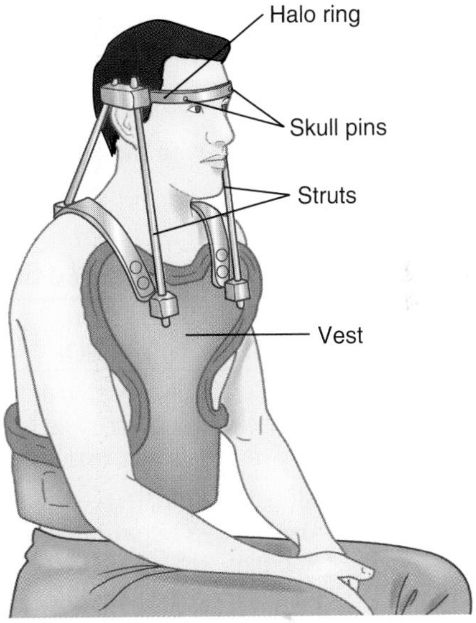

Fig. 22.11 Halo traction vest for cervical stabilization. The halo traction brace immobilizes the cervical spine. (Modified from Urden LD, Stacy KM, Lough ME: *Priorities in critical care nursing,* ed 6, St. Louis, 2012, Elsevier. In Lewis SL, Bucher L, Heitkemper MM, et al.: *Medical-surgical nursing: assessment and management of clinical problems,* ed 10, St. Louis, 2017, Elsevier.)

the needs of immobilized patients. If halo traction is used and the patient has an incomplete spinal cord injury, a standard hospital bed may be used. All measures to prevent the problems of immobility are instituted (see Chapter 9).

Urinary Management

An indwelling urinary catheter is inserted to prevent bladder distention and protect the skin from reflex bladder emptying. After the first week, a bladder management program will be initiated (see Chapter 21).

Psychological Care

The short-term and long-term psychological changes brought about by spinal cord injury and paralysis are difficult, if not impossible, to measure. Adjustment to such a drastic change in lifestyle is a continuous process that may well last a lifetime (see Chapter 9).

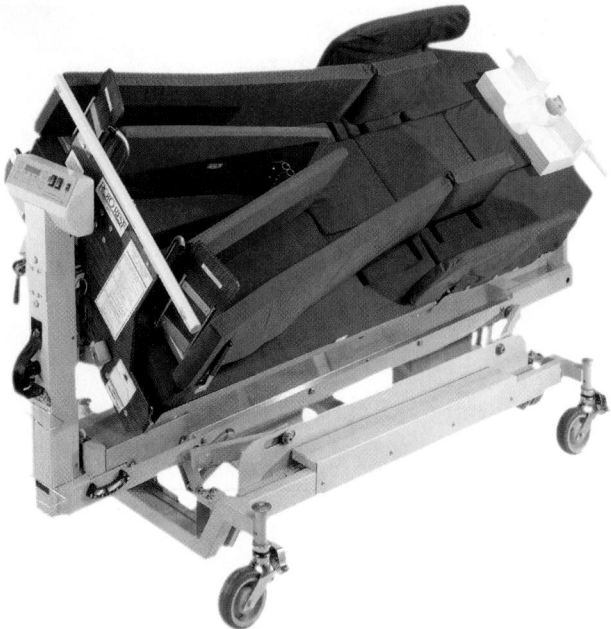

Fig. 22.12 RotoRest Delta Advanced Kinetic Therapy system. (Courtesy ArjoHuntleigh.)

Table 22.2 Stages of Grief and Associated Behaviors

STAGE OF GRIEF OR MOURNING	FREQUENT BEHAVIORS SEEN
Shock and denial	Complete dependence, withdrawal, excessive sleep, struggle for survival, unrealistic expectations
Anger	Hostility toward caregivers and family, manipulative behavior, abusive language, refusal to discuss paralysis and losses, decreased self-esteem
Bargaining	Bargaining with a higher power or fate: "If you'll let me walk again, I'll pray every day."
Depression	Sadness, "blue" mood, withdrawal, insomnia, agitation, refusal to participate in education for self-care, suicidal thoughts and comments
Adjustment	Begins active participation in therapy and education for self-care, planning for future, expresses hope for future functioning, finds meaning in whole experience of injury and therapy, return of usual personality

Grief and mourning response. Sustaining a spinal cord injury that causes permanent neurologic deficit brings with it many losses. Most patients experience grief and mourning of the losses experienced and the changes that such losses bring to their roles and lifestyle. Table 22.2 presents a review of the stages of grief and the behaviors that might be seen. In caring for these patients, use active listening, be supportive, and help the patient focus on positive strengths and the possibilities for the future.

Sexual Concerns

One area of concern to the patient and his family members that sometimes receives inadequate attention is that of sexual function and sexuality after spinal cord injury. Many individuals have difficulty discussing sexual matters. A nurse who wishes to help a patient deal with problems of sexuality must first come to terms with their own feelings and attitudes and clarify their own values. You should be open and honest in discussions about the patient's sexuality. The patient and their partner must be encouraged to verbalize concerns and questions and should be given guidance about alternative ways to express sexuality and meet sexual needs.

Complications

Spinal shock and neurogenic shock. The disruption in the nerve communication pathways between upper motor neurons and lower motor neurons causes spinal shock. Spinal shock is characterized by flaccid paralysis and loss of reflex activity and of sensation below the level of the injury. Spinal shock occurs immediately after injury and lasts 48 hours to several weeks.

Neurogenic shock may occur within 24 hours and is caused by loss of vasomotor tone caused by the injury; neurogenic shock is characterized by bradycardia, hypotension, venous pooling with decreased cardiac output, and occasionally paralytic ileus. Vital signs become labile. Treatment is aimed at maintaining adequate blood pressure and heart rate. Neurogenic shock may occur with a cervical or high thoracic injury.

Muscle spasms. Immediately after a spinal cord injury, the patient will usually have a flaccid type of paralysis due to spinal shock. Later, as the cord adjusts to the injury (a few weeks to a few months), the paralysis will become spastic, and there will be strong, involuntary contractions of the skeletal muscles. Proper positioning, braces, physical therapy, and medications can help control spasms that interfere with activities of daily living (ADLs) and other activities.

The patient and family may interpret these spasms as a return of voluntary function of the limbs and will have false hopes of complete recovery. You or the health care provider must explain to them that these spasms are common in patients with spinal cord injuries. To avoid stimulating the muscles when moving the patient and thereby precipitating a spasm of the muscles, avoid grasping the muscle itself. The palms of the hands are used to support the joints above and below the affected muscles. The administration of antispasmodic medications such as baclofen (Lioresal) orally may decrease the severity of the spasms (Table 22.3).

Autonomic dysreflexia (hyperreflexia). Autonomic dysreflexia (AD) is an uninhibited and exaggerated reflex response of the autonomic nervous system to some form of stimulation that occurs in 85% of all patients who have spinal cord injury at or above the level of the sixth

Table 22.3 Drugs Commonly Used to Treat Head and Spinal Cord Injuries

CLASSIFICATION	ACTION	NURSING IMPLICATIONS	PATIENT TEACHING
Corticosteroid			
Methylprednisolone (Solu-Medrol)	Decreases inflammation by suppression of leukocyte migration to injury site; decreases capillary permeability	Give as IV bolus and a continuous infusion for 23 h. May cause insomnia, increased susceptibility to infection, and GI distress. May delay wound healing. Monitor electrolyte levels. H_2-receptor blocker or proton pump inhibitor often given concurrently to prevent stress ulcer.	Advise to report heartburn or stomach pain.
Skeletal Muscle Relaxant			
Baclofen (Lioresal)	Inhibits synaptic responses in CNS by decreasing GABA, thereby decreasing frequency and severity of muscle spasms	Monitor for seizure activity. Observe for muscle weakness and fatigue. Assess for allergic symptoms: rash, fever, respiratory distress.	Advise not to drink alcohol because it increases CNS depression. Do not discontinue medication quickly or abruptly.
GABA Analog			
Pregabalin (Lyrica)	Neuropathic pain transmission from the spinal cord is reduced by pregabalins interactions with descending noradrenergic and serotonic pathways originating from the brain stem.	May cause somnolence and dizziness that can be interpreted as a change in LOC. May prolong INR.	Report any changes in mood or thoughts, as the medication can cause depression. Report side effects of blurred vision, muscle pain, or swelling in the extremities.
Gabapentin (Neurontin)		May cause somnolence and dizziness. May potentiate CNS depression when given with opioids.	Report any changes in mood or thoughts, as the medication can cause depression. Should not be discontinued abruptly.
Adrenergic Action Vasoconstrictor			
Dopamine (Intropin)	Acts on alpha receptors, causing vasoconstriction in blood vessels, thereby raising blood pressure	Monitor vital signs closely; assess for chest pain. Monitor I&O. Place patient on a cardiac monitor during therapy. May cause nausea, vomiting, or diarrhea. Be certain that IV access is patent because drug will cause necrosis if extravasation into the tissue occurs.	Explain purpose of drug is to raise blood pressure so that brain has adequate perfusion and oxygen. May cause headache.
Osmotic Diuretic			
Mannitol	Increases osmotic pressure of glomerular filtrate; promotes diuresis	Monitor vital signs closely. Track I&O; assess skin turgor and mucous membranes for signs of dehydration. Monitor electrolytes. Observe for nausea, backache, hives, and chest pain.	Explain that the drug will cause increased urine output and that this is its intended action.

Continued

Table 22.3 Drugs Commonly Used to Treat Head and Spinal Cord Injuries—cont'd

CLASSIFICATION	ACTION	NURSING IMPLICATIONS	PATIENT TEACHING
Sedatives			
Dexmedetomidine (Precedex)	Selective alpha-adrenergic agonist with sedative properties	At recommended doses, produces no evidence of respiratory depression but can cause hypotension and/or bradycardia. Administer in a continuous infusion and titrate for effect.	Report development of nervousness, agitation, or headache.
Propofol (Diprivan)	Sedative-hypnotic agent used for sedation; modulates the inhibitory function of the neurotransmitter GABA	Continuous infusion titrated for effect. Hypotension and respiratory depression may occur.	The family should be informed of the reason for the medication and the intended effect.

CNS, Central nervous system; *GABA,* gamma-aminobutyric acid; *GI,* gastrointestinal; H_2, histamine-2; *I&O,* intake and output; *INR,* international normalized ratio; *IV,* intravenous; *LOC,* level of consciousness.

thoracic vertebra (T6). The AD response is potentially dangerous to the patient because it produces vasoconstriction of the arterioles with an immediate elevation of blood pressure. The sudden hypertension can, in turn, cause a seizure, retinal hemorrhage, or stroke. Less serious effects include severe headache, changes in pulse rate, sweating and flushing above the level of the spinal cord lesion, and pallor and "goosebumps" below the level of injury.

AD occurs most often with spinal cord disorders at or above the T6 level. The problem can occur any time after a spinal cord injury after resolution of spinal shock; in some cases it has first appeared as late as 6 years after the injury.

Many kinds of stimulation can precipitate AD. Tight clothing around the waist may elicit an AD response. However, most stimulations are related to the bladder, bowel, and skin of the patient. For example, catheter changes, a distended bladder, the insertion of rectal suppositories, enemas, and sudden changing of position can provide the stimulation that results in AD (Stephenson, 2018).

Orthostatic hypotension. Vasoconstriction is impaired after spinal cord injury, and the lack of muscle function in the legs causes pooling of blood in the lower extremities. A sudden change in position from supine to sitting or sitting to standing may cause dizziness and fainting. Compression stockings, moving slowly, and use of a reclining wheelchair may help prevent this problem.

Deep venous thrombosis. Decreased blood pressure combined with lack of muscle movement slows venous return to the heart. Thrombosis may occur. Compression stockings, sequential compression devices, and/or low-molecular-weight heparin injections may be needed to prevent deep venous thrombosis. During the rehabilitation phase, oral anticoagulants are recommended.

Clinical Cues

Careful attention must be paid to keeping the bladder from becoming overdistended. If the patient is on bed rest, check the catheter and drainage tubing for the indwelling catheter every couple of hours. When voiding has not occurred, monitor output and time of voiding for patients who do not have an indwelling catheter, and palpate the bladder for distention every few hours.

When a patient exhibits symptoms of AD, an emergency exists. Efforts should be made to lower blood pressure by placing the patient in a sitting position or elevating the head to a 45-degree angle. If the cause of the stimulation is known—for example, an impacted bowel, overdistended bladder, or pressure against the skin—the stimulus should be removed as gently and quickly as possible. The health care provider should be notified immediately so that the appropriate medications can be prescribed and administered.

Infection. Impaired respiratory muscles with the resultant decreased cough and shallow respirations predisposes patients with a high spinal cord injury to respiratory infection. Mechanical ventilation with intubation provides an avenue for microorganisms to enter the lungs, so ventilator-associated pneumonia is a risk. Urinary catheterization for loss of bladder control is a risk factor for infection as well.

Skin breakdown. Lack of sensation and inability to move for repositioning places the patient at great risk for skin breakdown and pressure ulcers. Denervated skin is at higher risk of injury. Pressure-relieving devices, specialty mattresses or beds, meticulous skin care with regular inspection, and manual repositioning are essential to prevent this problem.

Renal complications. Urinary reflux from the bladder to the kidney often results from impaired bladder function. Catheterization and immobility predispose to bladder infection; the infection may travel up the ureters to the kidneys. Permanent kidney damage eventually may occur from such infections.

Think Critically

Name three care interventions that might trigger an episode of autonomic dysreflexia (AD). How could you possibly avoid causing this reaction?

Heterotopic ossification. Heterotopic ossification may occur with long-term immobility. Heterotopic ossification is bony overgrowth that may invade muscle. Assess for swelling, warmth, redness, and decreased range of motion of the extremities to detect ossification.

Neuropathic pain. As many as 40% of patients with spinal cord injury report neuropathic pain. Pregabalin and gabapentin are the primary medications used for neuropathic pain.

NURSING MANAGEMENT

There often is a tendency to treat a physically disabled patient as if they were less than a "whole" person with the same desires, hopes, and anxieties that all humans share. You can serve patients by reacting to and interacting with physically disabled patients in an open and honest manner. If unprepared to handle a certain problem, readily admit embarrassment, confusion, or lack of information, and seek assistance from other members of the health care team. Rehabilitation of patients with spinal cord injuries is discussed in Chapter 9.

ASSESSMENT (DATA COLLECTION)

Continued assessment for signs of altered respiratory pattern, decreased oxygenation, blood pressure instability, infection, skin breakdown, gastrointestinal or nutrition problems, and urinary problems is essential. Perform a daily review of systems and collection of data regarding physical status. Assess the tracheostomy tube, traction devices and pins, correct placement and use of sequential compression devices or compression stockings, indwelling catheter, IV cannula, feeding tube, and other equipment each shift.

NURSING DIAGNOSIS

Problem statements appropriate for a patient with a spinal cord injury may include:

- Altered gas exchange due to diaphragm paralysis, diaphragm fatigue, or retained secretions.
- Altered physical mobility related to vertebral column instability, disruption of the spinal cord, and traction.
- Altered cardiac output due to hypotension and decreased muscle action causing venous pooling.
- Altered nutrition due to increased metabolic demand from healing injuries, slowed gastrointestinal motility, and inability to feed self.
- Constipation due to lack of bowel enervation, decreased fluid intake, and immobility.
- Altered urinary elimination related to decreased innervation of the bladder.
- Pain due to muscle spasms.
- Potential for autonomic dysreflexia due to reflex stimulation of sympathetic nervous system.
- Potential for altered skin integrity due to immobility and loss of sensation.
- Altered coping ability due to loss of control over bodily functions and altered lifestyle secondary to paralysis.
- Altered body image due to paralysis and loss of control over bodily functions.
- Altered family function due to change in role within the family because of neurologic deficits.
- Grief due to neurologic deficits and to changes in roles and lifestyle.

PLANNING, IMPLEMENTATION, AND EVALUATION

Specific, individual expected outcomes are written for each problem supported by the data gathered. Long-term goals are considered, and planning for rehabilitation begins with hospitalization. The patient often will be transferred to a rehabilitation facility for intensive rehabilitation and retraining for ADLs.

Care for a patient with a spinal cord injury can be very complex, depending on the level of the injury. Often a head injury accompanies the trauma to the spinal cord. When a stabilization device is in place on the head, assessment and care of the pin sites are performed every shift and as needed. Sterile technique is used and is performed according to agency policy. Sterile normal saline is used for cleansing. No ointment is applied unless specifically ordered. Weights used for cervical traction must be kept hanging freely to be effective. Traction pull should never be interrupted. Tongs may stay in place for 4 weeks. If the patient is wearing a halo fixation device, skin care must be given frequently and the skin checked to see that the jacket is not causing pressure ulcers. One finger should be able to slip easily beneath the jacket to be sure it is not too tight. The patient is never moved or turned by holding or pulling on the halo device. **The halo jacket is never unfastened unless the patient is supine because head movement will immediately occur.** The jacket is unfastened only by trained technicians or providers for care and maintenance. In an emergency the front plate can be removed for cardiopulmonary resuscitation (CPR). Logrolling must be done with extreme care to avoid twisting the vertebral column and further damaging the spinal cord (Fig. 22.13).

All nursing measures designed to prevent the disabilities that may result from immobility, to promote healing, and to prevent complications are used to help the patient achieve the goals of rehabilitation. Bladder and bowel training programs, as well as instruction in

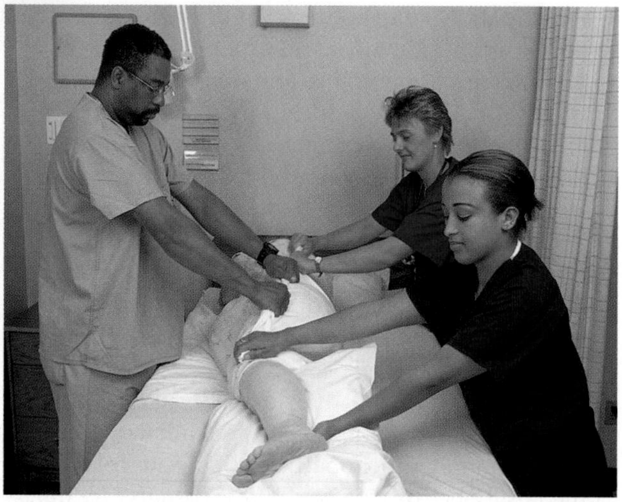

Fig. 22.13 Logrolling procedure using a lift sheet and three people. (From Williams P: *deWit's fundamental concepts and skills for nursing*, ed 5, St. Louis, 2018, Elsevier.)

moving from bed to chair—and other aspects of self-care—may be necessary. Realistic goals should be set for the patient and every effort made to achieve them.

Encourage the patient to do whatever they can for themselves as soon as is feasible. The overall goal is to promote as much independence as possible. A great deal of encouragement and praise are required. Evaluation is ongoing to determine whether the interventions have been successful in achieving the expected outcomes. If they have not been successful, the plan is revised.

Assignment Considerations

Inappropriate Delegation

Although many tasks may be delegated to certified nursing assistants (CNAs) or unlicensed assistive personnel (UAP), moving or positioning patients with neurologic injury or surgery should *not* be delegated. If given proper and complete instructions, the CNA or UAP may logroll the patient with your help and supervision.

Rehabilitation

A full team of professionals will be involved in the care and rehabilitation of patients with a spinal cord injury. The physical therapist, occupational therapist, psychologist, physician, respiratory therapist, pharmacist, and ancillary personnel will collaboratively plan the patient's care. The patient and family are often invited to participate in the planning process.

The use of robotics and computers is providing hope for some patients to walk again. A system called *functional electrical stimulation (FES)* is used to generate neural activity and overcome lost function. The system stimulates muscles to make walking motions. The patient is suspended in a harness to support body weight and is retrained to walk using a treadmill. The antidepressant escitalopram (Lexapro), a selective serotonin reuptake inhibitor (SSRI), has improved results of the therapy for some patients. Research is under way on a neuroprosthetic microchip implant that would help certain patients to walk again. The ReWalk brace support suit that is combined with computerized technology received U.S. Food and Drug Administration (FDA) approval for use at home and in the community in 2014 (ReWalk, 2018). It allows an otherwise healthy paraplegic to walk using Canadian crutches. It runs on a power pack carried on the back.

Communication between team members is crucial to the success of the individual plan. When the patient is discharged, all plans and specifics required for the patient's care must be shared with home caregivers and home care nurses who will be involved in care.

BACK PAIN AND HERNIATED DISK (BULGED, SLIPPED, OR RUPTURED DISK)

ETIOLOGY

Back pain is one of the most common reasons for missed work and is the third most common reason for a visit to the health care provider's office. In people younger than 45 years, back pain is the most common cause of work absence and is the most costly health condition for employers. On-the-job accidents and resultant trauma to the spine is one cause of injury, but simple sprains and strains can happen sometimes with simple movements. Obesity, lack of exercise, and poor lifting and moving techniques contribute to the stress placed on the back muscles and to the occurrence of injury or the severity and duration of pain. Other risk factors leading to back pain include lack of exercise (causing poor muscle tone), poor posture, cigarette smoking (which decreases oxygenation to the disks and predisposes to degenerative disease), and stress. Repetitive heavy lifting also may cause back pain. This is often a factor for health care workers. Causes of musculoskeletal back pain include:

- Acute lumbosacral strain
- Instability of lumbosacral spine
- Osteoarthritis of the spine
- Intervertebral disk degeneration and spinal stenosis
- Herniation of the intervertebral disk

Preventing back pain and disorders begins with proper posture and the use of correct lifting techniques. Maintaining one's weight within normal limits also helps decrease back strain. Sufficient physical exercise that maintains the condition of the back muscles and specific exercises to strengthen the abdominal and back muscles can greatly decrease the repeated incidence of injuries that lead to back pain.

PATHOPHYSIOLOGY

The bodies of the spinal vertebrae lie flat on one another like a stack of coins. Between the vertebral bodies there is a disk of fibrous cartilage filled with gelatinous substance (in the nucleus) that acts as a cushion to absorb shocks to the spinal column. This gelatinous disk may be ruptured by an injury, such as by the strain caused

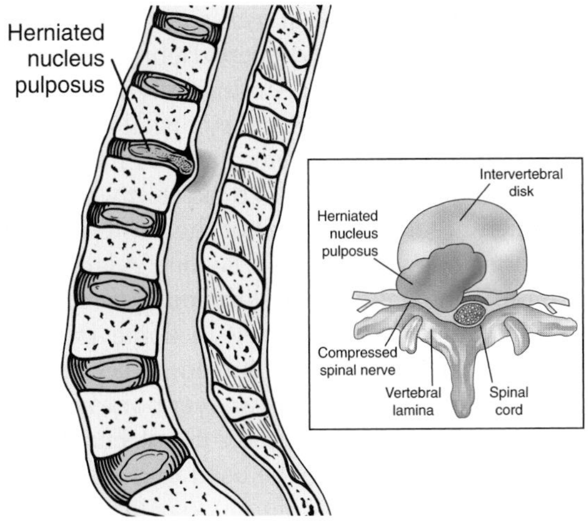

Fig. 22.14 Herniated disk (nucleus pulposus) with compression of spinal cord. (*Spine*, from Lewis SL, Heitkemper MM, Dirksen SR, et al.: *Medical-surgical nursing: assessment and management of clinical problems*, ed 7, St. Louis, 2007, Mosby. *Inset*, from McCance KL, Huether SE: *Pathophysiology: the biologic basis for disease in adults and children*, ed 8, St. Louis, 2019, Elsevier.)

when lifting a heavy object or by wrenching the spinal column or falling on the back. When the disk ruptures, part of the contents squeezes out from between the vertebrae, and disk fragments may lodge in the spinal canal. The disk compression on the adjacent nerve root causes the pain (Fig. 22.14). When protein from the disk content leaks out into the canal, the body perceives it as a foreign substance, causing an inflammatory response with pain. Thus the person suffers from what is sometimes called a *slipped disk*. Another name for this condition is *herniated nucleus pulposus*.

Older Adult Care Points

Older adults have decreased flexibility of the spine and, as age increases, degeneration of the spine. Many older adults suffer from osteoporosis and osteoarthritis. These factors make older adults more prone to back pain, especially if regular exercise is not performed to maintain flexibility and bone density.

Acute back pain usually occurs from activity that puts stress (hyperflexion) on the tissues of the lower back. Back pain that is a result of muscle spasm is usually self-limiting and often resolves within 4 weeks. Chronic back pain is pain that lasts for more than 3 months or is a repeat episode. Chronic back pain may be caused by degenerative disk disease or osteoarthritis, but lack of exercise, prior injury, and obesity are common factors. The most common sites of disk rupture are L4 to L5 and L5 to S1. Herniation may also occur at C5 to C6 or C6 to C7.

SIGNS, SYMPTOMS, AND DIAGNOSIS

Sometimes a lumbar herniated disk causes pain radiating down the sciatic nerve into the buttock and below the knee. Muscle weakness and paresthesias may occur. Cervical herniated disk causes pain in the neck and shoulder, radiating down the arm with numbness and tingling in the hand. Muscle tightening and spasm in the area of injury are common.

Diagnosis requires a history and physical examination. The straight leg raise test is often used for low back pain. While the patient is supine, the leg is raised off the bed or examination table with the whole leg straight. If low back pain occurs, the test confirms a disk problem. Reflexes may be decreased or absent. The patient may experience muscle weakness or paresthesias in the legs or feet.

If conservative therapy does not relieve the pain, diagnostic radiographs, MRI, or CT scanning is performed. An electromyogram may be ordered to determine the degree of nerve irritation and to rule out other pathologic conditions.

TREATMENT

The health care provider will treat back pain initially with conservative measures in the hope that surgical correction will not be necessary. If there is no sciatic pain, bed rest is not recommended because research has shown that walking provides a quicker recovery. When sciatic pain is present, lying down for short periods can help relieve the pain. Standing or lying is recommended instead of sitting, which puts pressure on the disks (Atlas, 2017). Ice packs are applied for 5 to 10 minutes at a time each hour for the first 48 hours to reduce muscle spasm in the back. After 48 hours, heat may be more helpful because heat relaxes strained muscles. Ultrasound treatments are often helpful. Heating pads, hot packs, and hot showers work well to relax the muscles.

Complementary and Alternative Therapies

Help for Pain

Acupuncture, acupressure, and massage therapy have all proven beneficial for back pain. Research from the National Institutes of Health has proven that acupuncture is effective for back pain. For those with chronic back pain, acupuncture is worth trying. Massage and acupressure help relieve muscle spasm, especially when heat is applied to the affected muscles first.

Studies show that wearing a portable heat wrap decreases pain moderately and more than ibuprofen (Qaseem et al., 2017). Transcutaneous electrical nerve stimulation may help relieve the patient's pain. Acupuncture has proven useful to help relieve back pain. Back strengthening exercises are prescribed as soon as acute symptoms subside; these exercises are initially supervised by a physical therapist. The exercises are encouraged for a lifetime because muscles need to be toned to prevent back strain. Specially designed corsets or back braces are sometimes used to maintain proper alignment of the spine. The patient is cautioned not to lift anything heavier than 2 to 5 lb and not to twist when reaching for things. The patient should be up and moving around frequently rather than sitting for long periods. High heels should not be worn.

Swimming or walking for short distances frequently is very beneficial for patients with back pain. Standing for long periods is to be avoided, and when standing the patient should shift weight from one foot to the other frequently. Adjustments and treatments by a chiropractor may also help relieve pain, although chiropractic treatment is not appropriate for all types of back injuries. Chiropractic treatment seems most effective if the pain has been present for less than 16 days. If pain continues beyond 3 to 4 weeks or if pain is worsening, there is evidence of neurologic deficit, and surgery may be indicated.

For many patients, gentle yoga movements have been more successful than prescribed back exercises for relieving pain. For others, core body stretching and muscle strengthening work well.

Surgical Procedures

Although the majority of patients recover with nonsurgical treatment, for the minority of patients who cannot find relief through conservative measures, surgical intervention may be an option. Spinal fusion is the most common surgery performed for low back pain. The disk between vertebrae is removed, and the vertebrae are "fused" using a variety of methods. Lumbar disk replacement is being done instead of fusion, replacing the damaged disk with an artificial disk. Studies show similar outcomes with both procedures. Long-term data for artificial disks are not yet available. A diskectomy is performed to decompress the nerve root. This is a microsurgical technique that uses a very small incision through which the herniated intervertebral disk material is dissected and extracted. A minimally invasive electrothermoplasty or radiofrequency diskal nucleoplasty may be performed. If the area cannot be handled with microsurgery, an open incision diskectomy or laminectomy, which involves removal of the posterior arch of the vertebra along with the disk, is done. A laminectomy may be done in conjunction with spinal fusion.

A spinal fusion is necessary in some patients to stabilize the spine. In a spinal fusion, a piece or pieces of bone from the iliac crest or cadaver bone are grafted onto the vertebrae to strengthen them. Fixation with metal rods and screws may be used to decrease spinal motion and irritability.

A laminectomy may be performed for conditions other than a ruptured disk—for example, for such degenerative diseases of the spine as Pott disease (tuberculosis of the spine), for fractures of the spine, and for spinal dislocation. Once a laminectomy with a fusion has healed, the fused vertebrae are immobile.

NURSING MANAGEMENT

Preoperatively, a baseline neurologic assessment is performed and documented. Other preoperative care is the same as for other types of general surgery. Postoperatively, the major concern after spinal fusion, laminectomy, or diskectomy is to keep the spinal column in alignment so that healing can take place and no further injury occurs to the spinal cord. Restrictions on lifting, bending, and twisting will be implemented. For outpatient surgical patients, physical therapy will instruct them on proper techniques before discharge. Inpatients will have the same movement restrictions and will ambulate several times a day.

Focused Assessment

Data Collection After Spinal Surgery

Immediately postoperatively, assess the patient every 15 minutes for 1 hour, every 30 minutes for 2 hours, and then as indicated by hospital policy. Assess the following areas and compare findings with the preoperative data.

SENSATION
- Check extremities for numbness and tingling.
- Check all anatomic surfaces of forearms and hands, upper and lower legs, and feet.

MOVEMENT
- Check for ability to move shoulders, arms, hands, legs, and feet.

MUSCLE STRENGTH
- Check each extremity for weakness by having the patient push against your hands while you apply downward pressure to the extremity.

WOUND
- Assess surgical site(s) for drainage, noting amount, color, and characteristics.
- Check carefully for signs of CSF leak at surgical site.

PAIN
- Assess for site of pain, characteristics of the pain, and degree of pain on a scale of 1 to 10, with 10 being the worst pain.
- Reevaluate pain after administering analgesia for effectiveness.
- Monitor respirations and vital signs.

SKIN PRESSURE POINTS
- Check for reddened areas on bony prominences when turning patient.

Clinical Cues

Postoperative patients who have been living with chronic pain may have been taking opioids for pain management preoperatively. Tolerance to the medications may require higher doses of the opioid to relieve surgical pain.

An IV opioid via patient-controlled analgesia pump may be ordered for pain control in the first 24 to 48 hours after surgery. Assess frequently for effectiveness of the pain medication. Nonopioid medications and nonpharmaceutical therapies may also be used for pain management. Once fluids are being taken, oral analgesia is started with acetaminophen with hydrocodone (Vicodin) or oxycodone (Percocet). Muscle relaxants may be given as well.

After spinal surgery when the patient is steady enough to be out of bed, a bedside commode (or for the male patient, standing at the bedside) is encouraged to promote complete bladder emptying. Reinforce teaching on using the logroll technique when getting up to the commode to prevent twisting and turning of the spine. Provide privacy for toileting activity. If difficulty with voiding occurs, intermittent catheterization or an indwelling catheter will be required

Interference with bowel function and paralytic ileus may occur after laminectomy or spinal fusion. Observe for constipation, nausea, abdominal distention, and return of bowel sounds. Stool softeners are used to help prevent constipation. Incontinence or difficulty with bowel evacuation may indicate nerve damage and should be reported to the surgeon.

Permitted activity varies according to the underlying pathology and the patient's progress. Be clear about activity orders, whether a brace or corset is to be worn, and whether it is to be put on while lying down, sitting, or standing.

If a bone graft has been performed, the donor site must be assessed regularly and care provided. Pain is usually greater at the donor site than at the spinal fusion site. If the fibula is the donor site, neurovascular assessments of the limb must be performed on a regular schedule, as edema can occur. Ice packs to the surgical sites can reduce pain and swelling. The skin and incisions must be protected with a barrier.

Depending on the type of spinal surgery performed, many weeks to months are needed for complete recovery. The patient must learn to perform activities without twisting the spine.

Patient Teaching

Guidelines for a Patient With Low Back Pain or Spinal Surgery

DO

- Bend knees, with back straight, and crouch to lift an item off the floor—no more than 8 pounds.
- Carry items close to the center of your body.
- Walk as much as is tolerated. Start with 10 minutes and slowly progress to 20 to 30 minutes three to four times per day.
- Maintain appropriate body weight; lose weight if overweight.
- Use a lumbar pillow or roll when sitting and particularly when driving for long distances.
- Do not sit longer than 1 hour at a time in the first 2 weeks.
- Consider how to safely perform a task before starting to do it.

DO NOT

- Lean over without bending the knees.
- Reach to lift items or lift heavy items higher than the elbows.
- Stand or sit for long periods.
- Sleep with legs out straight without pillow cushioning under the thighs or between the legs when on the side.
- Bend from the waist to pick up an item.
- Twist to the side to lift things (e.g., groceries or things in the car or trunk).

Get Ready for the NCLEX® Examination!

Key Points

- Head injuries can result in concussion, contusion, coup-contrecoup (acceleration-deceleration) injury, skull fracture, or tearing of cranial vessels.
- Subdural, subarachnoid, or epidural hematoma may result from a head injury; epidural hemorrhage is a life-threatening event.
- A significant head injury causes disruption in normal LOC.
- Drainage from the ear or nose should be evaluated to determine the presence of CSF.
- Any lesion or extra fluid that begins to take up space in the cranial vault causes an increase in ICP.
- The earliest sign of increased ICP is decreasing LOC.
- Treatment of increased ICP includes maintaining a patent airway, administering diuretic agents to decrease edema, monitoring neurologic signs for increased ICP, regulating temperature, maintaining adequate blood pressure, and instituting nursing measures to prevent further increases in ICP (see Chapter 21, Table 21.9, and Nursing Care Plan 22.1).
- Neurologic assessment is performed every 15 minutes to 2 hours for acute patients with injury to or surgery on the brain.
- For maintenance of a patent airway, intubation or a tracheostomy and mechanical ventilation may be necessary.
- Early nutritional support is very important for both head injury and spinal cord injury patients.
- Unconscious patients require care for all basic needs; the eyes must be protected from injury because the blink reflex may be absent.
- Complications of head injury and increased ICP include hydrocephalus and diabetes insipidus.
- The extent of permanent cord damage often cannot be assessed until many days after injury because of

edema and the resulting pressure that edema causes on the spinal cord.
- The degree of neurologic impairment and activities that the patient will still be able to perform depend on the level and extent of the injury (see Table 22.1).
- Autonomic dysreflexia is potentially very dangerous to the patient because it can severely elevate blood pressure.
- Traction provided by Crutchfield or Gardner-Wells tongs, or a halo ring and fixation pins, immobilizes the spine while healing takes place.
- Back pain can be caused by muscle strain or herniated or ruptured intervertebral disk.
- Back pain should be treated conservatively before surgery is considered.
- Treatment depends on whether a disk rupture is present and on the severity of the pain and disability.
- Conservative treatment includes rest, gentle exercise, ice or heat, analgesics, and muscle relaxants. Surgical procedures include minimally invasive procedures, microdiskectomy or laminectomy (with or without fusion), and spinal fusion.
- Postoperative care depends on the type of procedure performed.

Additional Learning Resources

SG Go to your Study Guide for additional learning activities to help you master this chapter content.

Go to your Evolve website (http://evolve.elsevier.com/deWit/medsurg) for the following FREE learning resources:
- Animations, audio, and video
- Answers and rationales for questions and activities
- Glossary with pronunciations in English and Spanish
- Interactive Review Questions and more!

Review Questions for the NCLEX® Examination

1. A 75-year-old patient who fell and hit his head a week ago is admitted for apparent personality changes, decreased level of consciousness, and irritability. The health care provider suspects a possible subdural hematoma. A family member asks about the condition. An accurate explanation would be:
   1. "It is the presence of bleeding in the brain parenchyma."
   2. "Bleeding occurs between the skull and the dura mater."
   3. "It is the collection of blood between the brain and the inner surface of the dura mater."
   4. "It is the intermittent blockage of circulation in various areas of the brain."

   NCLEX Client Need: Physiological Integrity: Physiological Adaptation
2. A nurse is admitting a patient with a possible basilar skull fracture. Which clinical finding(s) would likely confirm the diagnosis? *(Select all that apply.)*
   1. Battle sign
   2. Partial blindness
   3. Ecchymosis around eyes
   4. Rhinorrhea
   5. Swallowing difficulty

   NCLEX Client Need: Physiological Integrity: Physiological Adaptation
3. Which statement by a high school athlete being discharged after experiencing a concussion indicates a need for more teaching?
   1. "I can go to football practice tomorrow."
   2. "I need to report a worsening headache to the health care provider."
   3. "I need to rest and not overdo activities."
   4. "I can expect to be more fatigued for a while."

   NCLEX Client Need: Health Promotion and Maintenance
4. You keep a postcraniotomy patient's neck in midline position and ensure that there is no excessive hip flexion. The rationale for your action would be that this position:
   1. restores neutral position of the joints.
   2. prevents a further increase in intracranial pressure.
   3. promotes comfort and rest.
   4. prevents the formation of blood clots.

   NCLEX Client Need: Physiological Integrity: Reduction of Risk Potential
5. A nursing assistant is attending to the needs of a patient with a head injury who is lethargic and has increased ICP. Which action by the nursing assistant indicates a need for further instruction?
   1. Notifying the nurse of patient coughing
   2. Monitoring blood pressure every shift
   3. Keeping the patient NPO
   4. Reporting blood on the dressing

   NCLEX Client Need: Safe and Effective Care Environment: Coordinated Care
6. The classic signs of increased ICP include which of the following? *(Select all that apply.)*
   1. Rising systolic blood pressure
   2. Widening pulse pressure
   3. Bradycardia
   4. Positive Babinski sign

   NCLEX Client Need: Physiological Integrity: Physiological Adaptation
7. The surgeon inserts an intraventricular catheter into the lateral ventricle of a patient with increased ICP. When asked by a relative about the procedure, an accurate response would be:
   1. "The catheter allows direct visualization of the brain tissue."
   2. "The catheter is used to monitor brain waves."
   3. "The catheter is used to remove excess fluid inside the brain."
   4. "The catheter is used to infuse fluids and medications into the brain."

   NCLEX Client Need: Physiological Integrity: Physiological Adaptation

8. A 30-year-old man is admitted to the emergency department after a motor vehicle accident. After examination, the patient is diagnosed with a T6 spinal cord injury. He has flaccid paralysis, slowed heart rate, low blood pressure, and no bowel sounds. The patient must be developing:
   1. autonomic dysreflexia.
   2. muscle spasms.
   3. spinal shock.
   4. diabetes insipidus.

   NCLEX Client Need: Physiological Integrity: Physiological Adaptation
9. A 40-year-old man with a T4 spinal cord injury suddenly complains of severe headache, increased pulse rate, sweating, flushing above the level of the spinal cord lesion, and "goosebumps" below the level of injury. Which immediate nursing action(s) should be taken? *(Select all that apply.)*
   1. Place flat in bed.
   2. Identify the cause of stimulation.
   3. Administer ordered antihypertensives.
   4. Loosen tight clothing.
   5. Clamp indwelling catheter.

   NCLEX Client Need: Physiological Integrity: Physiological Adaptation
10. Postoperative pain management for the patient with lumbar surgery may include: *(Select all that apply.)*
    1. use of ice packs on the area of back pain for up to 20 minutes each hour while awake for the first 48 hours.
    2. NSAID medications given orally or IV.
    3. complete bed rest to prevent injury to the operative area and promote comfort.
    4. higher dosing of opioids delivered by PCA.
    5. massage and warm whirlpool baths.
    6. topical analgesic creams.

    NCLEX Client Need: Physiological Integrity: Pharmacological Therapies

Critical Thinking Questions

Scenario A

Mary is a 22-year-old college student who received a head injury in an automobile accident. She was healthy before the accident. The emergency medical services team brought her to the emergency department (ED). She is stabilized in the ED, cervical spine injury is ruled out, and she is admitted to the neurologic intensive care unit. She is confused and groggy and has leakage of CSF from one ear and irregular respirations.

1. What assessments would you perform?
2. What specific nursing measures would you include in your care plan concerning the leaking CSF?
3. What measures would you take to provide appropriate respiratory care?

Scenario B

Gus Berrini is a 40-year-old truck driver who received a severe spinal injury when he was shot in the back by a hitchhiker. The bullet severed the spinal cord at the sixth thoracic vertebra.

1. What kinds of activities should Mr. Berrini eventually be able to perform?
2. How would you plan his care during the acute stage of his illness so that efforts at rehabilitation might be successful?
3. Which other members of the health care team might participate in his care and rehabilitation?

Scenario C

Henry Jones, a 35-year-old construction worker, comes to the clinic with low back pain. He states that this is not the first time he has had a problem with back pain. He says that this time it is worse and that he can hardly move. He is unable to work.

1. What tests will the health care provider probably perform or order?
2. What is likely to be recommended in the way of treatment?
3. What should Mr. Jones be taught before he leaves the clinic?

23 Care of Patients With Brain Disorders

http://evolve.elsevier.com/deWit/medsurg

Objectives

Theory

1. Choose the appropriate nursing actions and observations to be carried out for a patient experiencing a seizure.
2. Explain why seizure may be a consequence of a stroke, tumor, or infection in the brain.
3. Compare the subjective and objective findings of ischemic stroke and intracerebral bleed.
4. Devise a nursing care plan for a patient who has experienced a cerebrovascular accident (CVA, or stroke).
5. Write nursing actions to assist a patient who has developed a complication after a CVA.
6. Summarize subjective and objective findings indicative of a brain tumor.
7. Illustrate the pathophysiology behind the symptoms of a brain tumor.
8. Discuss the mechanism by which infection in the brain may cause increased intracranial pressure (ICP).
9. Compare and contrast symptoms of meningitis and encephalitis.
10. Distinguish the assessment data that differentiate migraine headaches from cluster headaches.
11. Compare the signs, symptoms, and treatment of trigeminal neuralgia and Bell palsy.

Clinical Practice

12. Identify appropriate Transmission-Based Precautions to be used with meningitis caused by bacteria and viruses.
13. Teach a teenage patient recently diagnosed with epilepsy what they need to know about the disorder and their care.
14. Perform neurologic checks on a patient who is admitted with a suspected CVA.
15. Assist with the care of a patient who has had intracranial surgery.
16. Devise a teaching plan for a patient who has experienced a CVA and has right-sided hemiplegia.

Key Terms

ablation (ă-BLĀ-shĕn, p. 563)
agnosia (ăg-NŌ-zhă, p. 547)
aneurysm (ĂN-ūrĭ-zĭm, p. 545)
aphasia (ă-FĀ-zhă, p. 546)
apraxia (ă-PRĂK-sē-ă, p. 547)
ataxia (ă-TĂK-sē-ă, p. 546)
aura (ĂW-ră, p. 539)
automatisms (ăw-TŌM-ă-tĭsmz, p. 541)
dysarthria (dĭs-ĂHR-thrē-ă, p. 546)
dysphagia (dĭs-FĀ-j(ē-)ĕ, p. 551)
dysphasia (dĭs-FĀ-zhă, p. 547)
embolus (ĔM-bō-lŭs, p. 543)
epilepsy (Ĕ-pĭ-lĕp-sē, p. 539)
hemiparesis (hĕm-ĭ-pĕ-RĒ-sĭs, p. 546)
hemiplegia (hĕ-mĭ-PLĒ-j(ē-)ĕ, p. 546)
homonymous hemianopsia (hō-MŎN-ĭ-mŭs hĕ-mē-ă-NŎP-sē-ă, p. 547)
hydrocephalus (hī-drō-SĔF-ă-lăs, p. 549)
infarct (ĭn-făhrkt, p. 543)
nuchal rigidity (NŪ-kăl rĭ-JĬ-dĭ-tē, p. 558)
postictal (PŌST-ĭk-tĕl, p. 539)
ptosis (TŌ-sĭs, p. 562)
rhizotomy (rī-ZŎ-tĕ-mē, p. 563)
scotoma (skō-TŌ-mă, p. 561)
status epilepticus (STĂ-tŭs ĕp-ĭ-LĔP-tĭ-kŭs, p. 539)

Concepts Covered in This Chapter

- Functional Ability
- Family Dynamics
- Self-Management
- Intracranial Regulation
- Sexuality
- Infection
- Mobility
- Tissue Integrity
- Coping
- Patient Education
- Collaboration
- Care Coordination

SEIZURE DISORDERS AND EPILEPSY

ETIOLOGY

Seizures can be symptomatic of a large number of disorders, including brain injury from a stroke, pressure from a brain tumor, infectious diseases with high fever, end-stage renal disease with uremia, toxicity (such as that occurring in eclampsia during pregnancy or in drug poisoning), epilepsy, and tetanus. **Seizures also can occur any time the brain is deprived of oxygen.**

Seizures may be symptoms of an underlying illness. Metabolic disturbances such as acidosis, electrolyte imbalances, hypoglycemia, hypoxia, and water intoxication may cause seizures. Alcohol or barbiturate withdrawal can cause seizures. In children, a high temperature is a common cause of seizures. Many types of seizure disorders are linked to genetic defects. The World Health Organization (WHO, 2018) defines epilepsy as two or more unprovoked seizures. Epilepsy affects 3 million adults and 470,000 children in the United States (Centers for Disease Control and Prevention [CDC], 2018a). Incidence increases in those 60 to 80 years of age.

PATHOPHYSIOLOGY

Epilepsy is a chronic disturbance of the nervous system characterized by various types of persistent seizures that are the result of abnormal electrical activity of the brain. Epilepsy is characterized by recurring seizures thought to be caused by a group of abnormal neurons firing spontaneously, resulting in excessive excitation or loss of inhibition. The neurons involved have a low threshold for excitation. The excitation spreads to surrounding cells, spreading the activity to a small area or throughout the brain. A seizure classification system was developed by the International League Against Epilepsy (ILAE) in 2010 and further revised in 2017. Seizures are classified based on three key features: type of seizure at onset, awareness during the seizure, and motor or other symptoms present. Each seizure lasts a few seconds or a few minutes. The abnormal electrical activity generated can be captured by an electroencephalogram (EEG).

SIGNS AND SYMPTOMS

Seizure Classification

Classifying seizures into different types helps with diagnosis and appropriate treatment. The first step in seizure classification is to identify how the seizure begins in the brain. Focal seizures (previously called partial seizures) affect only one part of the brain, leading to localized clinical symptoms. Generalized seizures involve both sides of brain (bilateral) and usually the whole body if motor symptoms are present. The onset may be unknown if not witnessed, or the seizure may start as focal and progress to bilateral. Awareness during the event is assessed, as is motor movement and other symptoms. The classification system can be seen on the Evolve website.

Generalized seizures are divided into motor and nonmotor (absence) seizures. Generalized seizures include absence, myoclonic, clonic, tonic, tonic-clonic, and atonic seizures and infantile spasms (usually caused by increased temperature).

Generalized seizures are characterized by bilateral synchronous electrical discharges in the brain. The whole brain is affected, and there is no warning or **aura** (preceding sensation). The patient usually quickly loses consciousness and is unconscious for a few seconds up to several minutes.

The manifestations of epilepsy depend on the area of the brain where the abnormal firing occurs. **Absence seizures may last only a few seconds. The onset is sudden, with no aura or warning and no postictal symptoms.** Seizures of this type tend to affect children between 5 and 12 years of age and disappear during puberty. There usually is a twitching around the eyes and mouth. The person remains standing or sitting and appears to have had no more than a lapse of attention or a moment of absentmindedness.

With tonic convulsions, there is continued contraction of all muscles, and the body becomes rigid. Tonic-clonic seizures usually begin with bilateral jerks of the extremities. There is loss of consciousness with both tonic and clonic convulsions. The patient may be incontinent during the attack, and there is danger of biting the tongue. In the **postictal** (after a seizure) phase, the person is confused and drowsy.

Atonic or akinetic seizures are characterized by loss of body muscle tone that results in nodding of the head, weakness of the knees, or total collapse and falling ("drop attacks"). The person usually remains conscious during the attack.

Unknown onset seizures are those in which the beginning of the seizure was not witnessed and it cannot be determined if there was a focal or generalized onset.

Unclassified seizures simply indicate that not enough data have been obtained to determine which type of seizure the patient is experiencing.

Status epilepticus indicates prolonged partial or generalized seizure activity of 5 minutes or more, rather than one seizure, without recovery between attacks. Status epilepticus is a grave condition in which there is a rapid, unrelenting series of convulsive seizures without intervening periods of consciousness, and it may include an absence of respiration. **Irreversible brain damage can occur if the seizures are not controlled.**

DIAGNOSIS

Diagnosis of epilepsy is based on the history and the actual signs and symptoms observed during a seizure. A thorough physical examination and tests for underlying disease are ordered based on the history and physical findings. EEG and magnetic resonance imaging (MRI) can be helpful in identifying or ruling out a cause for seizures. The diagnosis is made when metabolic abnormalities, toxins, infection, or other reversible causes are ruled out and two unprovoked seizures occur more than 24 hours apart.

TREATMENT

When the cause of seizures is known, as in cases of high fever or drug toxicity, medical treatment is aimed at controlling or eliminating whatever is responsible for the seizures. For recurrent seizures, as in epilepsy, the condition usually is managed with anticonvulsant drug therapy. An implanted vagus nerve stimulator is

Box 23.1 Medications Commonly Used for Seizure Control

DRUGS FOR GENERALIZED TONIC-CLONIC AND FOCAL SEIZURES
- Carbamazepine (Tegretol)
- Diazepam (Valium)
- Felbamate (Felbatol)
- Fosphenytoin (Cerebyx)
- Gabapentin (Neurontin)
- Lacosamide (Vimpat)
- Lamotrigine (Lamictal)
- Levetiracetam (Keppra)
- Oxcarbazepine (Trileptal)
- Phenobarbital (Luminal)
- Phenytoin (Dilantin)
- Pregabalin (Lyrica)
- Primidone (Mysoline)
- Rufinamide (Banzel)
- Tiagabine (Gabitril)
- Topiramate (Topamax)
- Valproic acid (Depakene)
- Vigabatrin (Sabril)
- Zonisamide (Zonegran)

DRUGS FOR NONMOTOR SEIZURES
- Clonazepam (Klonopin)
- Divalproex (Depakote)
- Ethosuximide (Zarontin)
- Lamotrigine (Lamictal)
- Valproic acid (Depakene)

GENERAL NURSING IMPLICATIONS
- Educate the patient about the importance of taking the drug exactly as prescribed.
- All of these drugs cause some degree of sedation, drowsiness, and lethargy. Warn about driving or operating machinery when these effects are significant. Advise not to drink alcohol or use other central nervous system depressants.
- The patient should not stop taking an anticonvulsant abruptly without consulting the health care provider.
- Check interactions with other drugs before administering any of these drugs. Interaction with anticoagulants, oral contraceptives, digoxin, aspirin, certain antibiotics, antacids, folic acid, and other drugs are significant. Some anticonvulsant drugs interact with each other (e.g., phenobarbital).
- Periodic blood work, every 1 to 3 months, should be performed when taking an anticonvulsant. It may be used to check therapeutic blood levels or organ dysfunction.
- Dosages of each drug are based on therapeutic blood level of the drug.
- Anticonvulsants have a narrow therapeutic range; toxicity occurs if too much of the drug is taken.
- The patient should be under the close supervision of the health care provider.
- All anticonvulsant drugs can produce some unpleasant side effects, such as fever and leukopenia and, in the case of phenytoin, gingival hyperplasia and rash.
- Physical dependence can become a problem for patients taking either phenobarbital or primidone, which is largely converted to phenobarbital in the bloodstream.
- Toxic side effects such as ataxia, drowsiness, nausea, sedation, and dizziness are not uncommon.

proving helpful for generalized epilepsy in many patients with uncontrolled seizures.

The major antiepileptic drugs are presented in Box 23.1. Patient education is extremely important because the patient will need to report any untoward effects to the health care provider or nurse clinician so that the dosage can be adjusted or the drug changed. All anticonvulsant drugs cause some central nervous system (CNS) depression with grogginess, dizziness, fatigue, and cognitive changes.

A ketogenic diet is beneficial in younger patients with refractory (difficult to control) generalized seizures. A ketogenic diet provides sufficient calories from fats and proteins but produces a ketotic (acidotic) state that seems to prevent seizure activity. The diet is prescribed by the health care provider and is monitored by a dietitian.

Biofeedback techniques are geared toward teaching the patient to maintain a certain brain wave frequency that is not susceptible to seizure activity.

Uncontrolled seizures secondary to hypoglycemia (as in improperly controlled diabetes mellitus) can be relieved by intravenous (IV) administration of 50% dextrose. If the unrelenting seizures are caused by chronic alcoholism or withdrawal, treatment consists of IV administration of lorazepam.

Status epilepticus is a medical emergency usually caused by abruptly stopping antiseizure medications in a patient with epilepsy. Rapid assessment and treatment are needed. Preferable treatment in these cases involves administering benzodiazepines: IV lorazepam, intramuscular (IM) midazolam, or rectal diazepam. IV medications are preferred, but other routes can be used when IV access is not available. After seizure activity has been suppressed, an anticonvulsant medication should be given to help prevent the recurrence of seizure activity (Glauser et al., 2016). Care is focused on supporting vital signs and preventing injury. Intubation may be required for respiratory support. If seizures will not stop, an anesthetic agent may be required.

Surgical Treatment

Surgical procedures involve removing the epileptic focus or preventing the spread of epileptic activity by focal cortical resection. Extensive imaging and testing are done to localize and identify seizure focus. It is recommended that patients with drug-resistant focal seizures undergo surgical evaluation. These surgeries involve risk and are reserved for those patients with conditions in which surgical intervention has proven effective.

For intractable focal seizures, vagal nerve stimulation therapy can be effective. In a surgical procedure, electrodes are placed around the vagus nerve, and a connecting wire is tunneled under the skin to connect to the stimulator, which is placed under the skin in the chest. The device acts like a pacemaker and provides a small electric current for 30 seconds every 5 minutes that stimulates the brain to interrupt seizures.

NURSING MANAGEMENT

ASSESSMENT (DATA COLLECTION)

Patients with a known seizure problem usually are treated on an outpatient basis but may be encountered in a hospital or long-term care facility. Assess these patients carefully to provide optimal safety and care. Significant history information includes the kind of seizures they experience, whether they have any sensation just before the appearance of clinically observable signs, what medications they are taking, and what measures are known to be helpful either to prevent a seizure or to assist during a seizure and afterward. Assessment should include any factors that could have triggered the seizure (e.g., hyperventilation, bright lights [photosensitivity], alcohol and other drugs, fluid and electrolyte imbalances, lack of sleep, and emotional stress).

Focused Assessment

Observations to Make During a Seizure

Observe as much of the following as possible and document your findings.

- Time the seizure began and the time it ended
- What the patient was doing just before the seizure (e.g., was the patient picking at clothing?)
- Where in the body the seizure began; what parts of the body are involved
- Which way the eyes are moving; whether they constrict or dilate, deviate to the right or the left, or roll upward
- Which side the head turns toward
- Whether the patient cries out or screams as the seizure begins
- Whether there is evidence of **automatisms** or repetitive movements: lip smacking, chewing, grimacing, tapping, or "pill rolling"
- Whether movements are bilateral and symmetric
- Incontinence of urine or stool, vomiting, frothing at the mouth, or bleeding
- Whether the patient becomes apneic or cyanotic
- Level of awareness of the patient
- Changes in skin color or profuse perspiration

Postictal assessment, after a patent airway is ensured, includes determining the following:

- Length of time before regaining awareness
- Presence of lethargy or confusion
- Presence of headache
- Presence of speech impairment
- Presence of muscle soreness
- Whether there was an aura before the seizure began
- Effects of the seizure on the patient's vital signs

When caring for a patient who is likely to experience a seizure during an acute illness, periodically observe the patient for tremors, unexplained sensory or motor changes, mental changes that indicate confusion or disorientation, and restless or agitated behavior. In many cases, a change in the neurologic status of a patient can signal the possibility that a seizure might occur.

NURSING DIAGNOSIS, PLANNING, AND IMPLEMENTATION

The main problem statement for a patient who experiences seizures is *Potential for injury due to seizure activity.* Expected outcomes are written for the individual patient and the type of seizure disorder, possible triggers, and manifestations.

Maintaining therapeutic blood levels of anticonvulsant medications is extremely important in the prevention of seizures. Verifying what medications the patient is on at home and when the last dose was taken is information gathered on admission. If the patient is being admitted for a problem other than seizures, you should make sure that the admitting health care provider has complete information regarding seizure medications. If the patient is NPO (nothing by mouth), you should request that alternate routes of administration be ordered.

Nursing care of patients with epileptic seizures involves immediate care during and after a seizure, and long-term management and control of seizures and their psychosocial implications. Witnessing a seizure for the first time can be a frightening experience. Your first responsibility is to stay calm, remain with the patient, and call for assistance.

The environment of a patient at risk for seizure should be made as safe as possible. If the patient is very likely to have seizures, the side rails and headboard of the bed are padded. **Never try to pry open the patient's mouth or insert something into it once the jaw is clamping down because teeth may be broken and the airway may become obstructed.**

If a seizure comes on without warning and the patient drops to the ground, do not attempt to move them during the seizure. If they are on a hard surface, the head should be protected from injury by placing a rolled blanket or coat under it. The head should be turned to the side, if possible, to prevent aspiration of secretions. Remove glasses if present. Do not attempt to restrain the patient's movements. Loosen any garment around the neck that is causing restraint of breathing or airway. If supplemental oxygen is near, it should be administered, if possible. Call for help and provide privacy, if possible. When the seizure is over, turn the patient to the side and suction the airway if needed. Check oxygen saturation with a pulse oximeter. Check the glucose level, if possible, and assess for injuries. Stay with the patient until they are completely conscious. When consciousness is regained, reorient and reassure them. The patient should be allowed to rest or sleep after the seizure. Thoroughly document the event in the medical record with time, duration of the seizure, and observations of the seizure activity and any aura that occurred before its start.

Safety Alert

If a patient who is receiving phenytoin is receiving tube feedings, stop the tube feeding for 2 hours before and 2 hours after administering phenytoin to ensure proper drug concentration and absorption.

The long-term management of epileptic seizures is primarily focused on providing the patient with the information and support they need for self-care and to avoid recurring and debilitating seizures. Psychosocial support is necessary to encourage the patient to talk about their fears and concerns. Lifestyle changes will have to be made if they are not permitted to drive. Most states allow resumption of driving when a patient has been seizure-free for 1 year. A referral to the local epilepsy society for connection with a support group can be very helpful for both the patient and their family.

Most individuals who have epileptic seizures have normal mental function between seizures and are quite capable of being contributing members of society if only they are provided the resources and support to manage effectively.

Patient Education

Self-care for an epileptic patient requires that they understand the nature of their disorder, the purpose of the prescribed medications, their side effects, and the signs of toxicity that should be reported to the health care provider. The patient must understand the necessity for compliance with the prescribed regimen to prevent recurrent seizures. They will need assistance in developing coping mechanisms to deal with the psychosocial impact of having epilepsy.

◆ EVALUATION

Evaluation is based on whether the expected outcomes are being achieved. This includes whether the patient is seizure-free or whether the number of seizures has decreased. Patient compliance with the medication regimen and avoidance of triggers for seizure activity are evaluated as well. Patient teaching may need to be reinforced. If progress toward the achievement of outcomes is not occurring, the plan must be revised.

TRANSIENT ISCHEMIC ATTACK

Between 200,000 and 500,000 Americans experience **transient ischemic attacks (TIAs)** each year. TIAs are caused by a brief interruption in blood flow. Narrowed arteries and vascular occlusion, perhaps by small emboli or vasospasm, cause the interruption. Recreational drugs that constrict vessels are another cause of TIAs. TIAs are warnings that a more serious neurologic event may occur; 10% to 15% of patients who experience a TIA have a stroke within 90 days. During the TIA, the person may feel a sudden weakness or numbness on one side of the body, slurring of speech or inability to talk, visual disturbances such as blindness or double vision, confusion, diminished coordination or ability to balance, and a headache. Symptoms are similar to those of a stroke. These symptoms generally resolve within 24 hours without residual deficit. The definition of TIA has been changed to "a transient episode of neurologic dysfunction caused by focal brain, spinal cord, or retinal

Patient Teaching

Patients With Epilepsy

Cover the following points in the teaching plan:

- Treatment and side effects of anticonvulsant therapy
- Triggers for seizures and how to avoid them (lack of sleep, alcohol and recreational drugs, stress, photosensitivity)
- Necessity of taking medication daily and as close to the same time each day as possible
- That the greatest trigger for a seizure is not taking the medication
- Handling a missed dose or inability to retain medication
- Not using over-the-counter or prescription medications without consulting the health care provider who prescribed the anticonvulsants
- Schedule for laboratory work to determine drug therapeutic levels
- Need for medical alert bracelet, necklace, and wallet card listing the provider's phone number and drugs being taken
- Resources for assistance available in the community
- Need for proper nutrition; dangers of erratic meals
- Avoiding alcohol and excessive fatigue
- Relaxation therapy for stress reduction
- Danger of swimming alone
- Refraining from driving or operating dangerous machinery until seizures are well controlled
- Keeping follow-up appointments with the provider

FOR WOMEN

- Risk of seizure during menstruation
- Necessity of consulting the provider before becoming pregnant because some anticonvulsant drugs may cause congenital abnormalities

FOR THE FAMILY

- What to do in the event of a seizure
- How to protect the patient during a seizure:
    - For tonic-clonic generalized seizure: assisting to the floor, protecting the head, loosening clothing, turning to the side
- When medical assistance is necessary

Think Critically

What safety measures would you teach a 22-year-old man who has just been diagnosed with generalized motor seizures?

ischemia, *without* acute infarction" (Furie & Ay, 2018). It is known that there is risk of permanent brain injury as a result of ischemia lasting less than 1 hour, so the time frame has been removed from the definition. It is very important that the person be evaluated by medical personnel because the same symptoms may indicate an ischemic stroke (brain tissue infarction) that will not resolve without treatment.

Anyone exhibiting symptoms of a stroke should have immediate assessment according to the American Heart Association guidelines, which include assessment using the National Institutes of Health (NIH) stroke scale within 10 minutes of arrival, computed tomography (CT) scan performed within 25 minutes of arrival and interpreted within 45 minutes, and thrombolytic therapy (if indicated) administered within 1 hour of arrival. Many smaller hospitals without neurology specialists on staff use video technology to consult with larger centers, facilitating assessment and evaluation of the patient. The period to initiate treatment is within 4.5 hours of the onset of symptoms. One of The Joint Commission's (TJC's) Core Measures is that appropriately screened patients receive thrombolytic therapy for ischemic stroke (TJC, 2018).

CEREBROVASCULAR ACCIDENT (STROKE, BRAIN ATTACK)

ETIOLOGY

More than 795,000 first and repeat strokes occur in the United States each year. Stroke is the leading cause of disability and the fifth leading cause of death (CDC, 2017). The incidence is about 19% higher in males than in females. About 34% of cases occur in people younger than age 65 years (CDC, 2017). An increase in public education about the risk factors for and signs of stroke could result in decreased disability and death from stroke.

Control of high blood pressure, quitting cigarette smoking, decreasing intake of cholesterol and controlling blood lipids, maintaining a normal blood sugar level, avoiding excessive alcohol intake, getting sufficient exercise, preventing obesity, and living a lifestyle that helps prevent heart disease can help reduce the risk of stroke. Atherosclerosis is a major cause of stroke because it can predispose to thrombus formation in the brain vessels or plaque in other arteries that can break off and become emboli.

PATHOPHYSIOLOGY

A cerebrovascular accident (CVA) is the result of an interruption of blood flow to a specific area of the brain. Stroke can happen in two ways, hemorrhagic or ischemic. The most common cause of stroke is *cerebral ischemia*. Ischemia of cells directly causes cellular **necrosis** (death) and **infarct** (area of tissue that has become necrotic from lack of blood supply) (Fig. 23.1). Ischemia can be caused by cerebral thrombosis (formation of a blood clot in a cerebral artery) or an **embolus** (a traveling clot, fat, bacteria, or tissue debris that lodges in a vessel, occluding it). Vessel spasm or pressure on the vessel from a mass such as a tumor can reduce or stop blood flow, resulting in ischemia or infarct, but this happens infrequently.

> **Health Promotion**
>
> **Risk Factors for Stroke**
>
> Educate all patients about the risk factors for stroke and encourage measures to alter those factors that can be changed.
>
> **MODIFIABLE RISK FACTORS**
> - Cigarette smoking
> - Using cocaine or other recreational drugs
> - Drinking more than two alcoholic drinks (male) or one alcoholic drink (female) per day
> - Heart disease (especially atrial fibrillation)
> - Diabetes
> - Sickle cell disease
> - Unhealthy diet
> - High blood pressure
> - High cholesterol
> - Sedentary lifestyle
> - TIAs
> - Use of oral contraceptives or hormone replacement therapy
> - Obesity
>
> **NONMODIFIABLE RISK FACTORS**
> - Age older than 65 years
> - Heredity (family history of stroke increases individual risk)
> - Prior stroke
> - Race (African Americans, Hispanics, American Indians, and Alaska Natives have a higher risk rate)
> - Gender (incidence is higher in women)

> **Cultural Considerations**
>
> **Greater Incidence of Stroke in African Americans and Hispanic Americans**
>
> African Americans have about a 50% greater incidence of stroke than whites and are more likely to die of a stroke. A study at the University of Michigan found that Hispanic Americans have a far greater chance of having a stroke than non-Hispanic whites. Untreated hypertension may be the risk factor involved (CDC, 2018).

> **Health Promotion**
>
> **Dangers of Cocaine or Methamphetamine Use**
>
> Caution people about the dangers of using cocaine or methamphetamine. Both of these drugs can cause vasoconstriction and brain ischemia. Cocaine may also cause hemorrhage. Using these drugs causes a fivefold increase in the incidence of stroke. The incidence of this type of stroke has greatly increased in young adults (NIH, 2017).

The carotid arteries supply a major portion of the blood that goes to the brain (Fig. 23.2). If plaque forms in these arteries as a result of atherosclerosis, the person is at risk

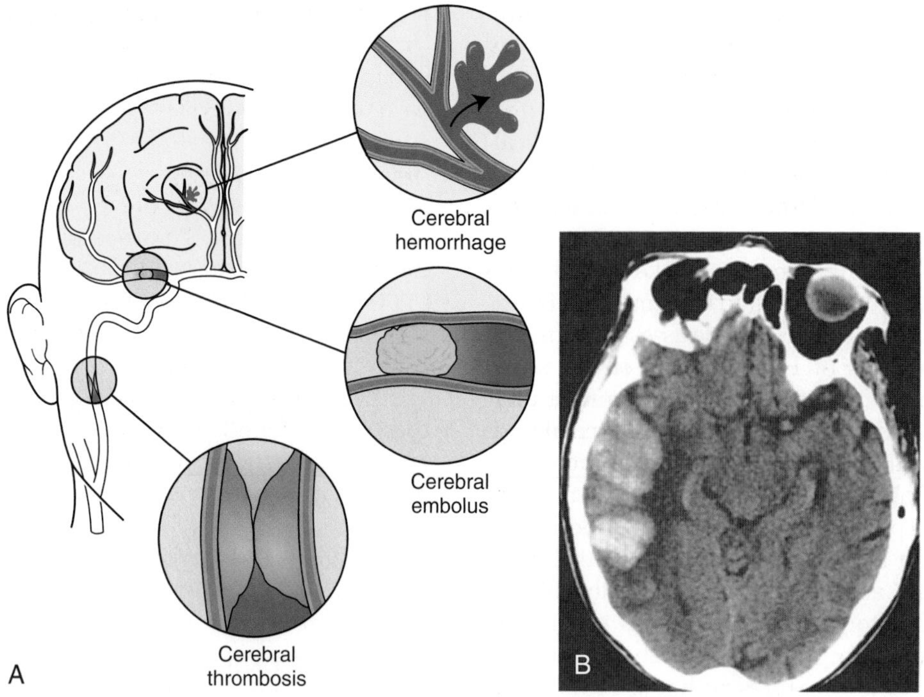

Fig. 23.1 **A,** Events that cause stroke. **B,** Magnetic resonance imaging showing hemorrhagic stroke in the left cerebrum.

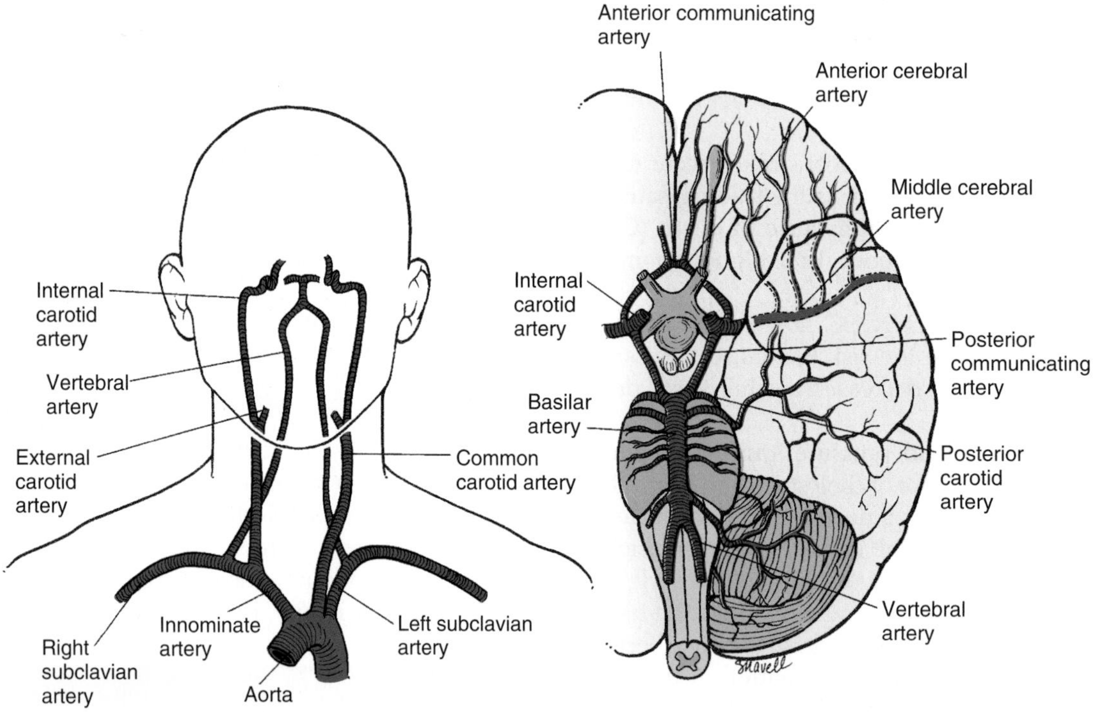

Fig. 23.2 Major arteries supplying blood to the brain. Blockage of any major artery precipitates a cerebrovascular accident (CVA).

for a stroke as blood supply to the brain is diminished or stopped. Atrial fibrillation is a common cause of embolic stroke. The atria are not contracting, allowing blood to pool and clot (see Chapter 19). If the clot becomes an embolus, it will leave the left atrium, travel through the left ventricle, and then be expelled out into the aorta. The carotid and vertebral arteries arise off the aorta, and it is a straight shot for the embolus to continue to travel upward to the brain. Less common causes of stroke are arterial spasms, compression of cerebral vessels by a tumor, local edema, or another disorder.

? Think Critically

How many risk factors for stroke are present for each member of your family?

The second mechanism of stroke is intracerebral hemorrhage (a blood vessel ruptures and leaks blood into brain tissue, or an aneurysm or arteriovenous malformation in the brain leaks or ruptures). Sustained hypertension can weaken blood vessels and lead to vessel rupture without aneurysm formation. The bleeding may be within the brain tissue or within the meningeal layers or both. Bleeds occurring within the brain tissue cause tissue damage, inflammation, and swelling, leading to increased intracranial pressure (ICP).

Structures that can cause an intracerebral hemorrhage are an aneurysm and an arteriovenous malformation. An **aneurysm** is an abnormal ballooning of an artery wall. It may be congenital or caused by a weakening of the artery wall from chronic hypertension. An **arteriovenous malformation (AVM)** is a congenital abnormality and is a tangled mass of malformed, thin-walled, dilated vessels that form an abnormal communication between the arterial and venous systems (Fig. 23.3). An AVM can leak, causing an intracerebral hemorrhage. Vasospasm often occurs after intracerebral bleeding, leading to ischemia of the brain tissue and more neurologic impairment. Resultant deficits are the same as for other kinds of strokes.

Subarachnoid hemorrhage, which refers to bleeding in the brain below the arachnoid, often causes rapid onset of neurologic deficit, severe headache, and loss of consciousness. The subarachnoid space is the location of cerebrospinal fluid (CSF) circulation. Bleeding into the subdural space results in blood being circulated throughout the brain and spinal dural sac, causing irritation and inflammation. A leaking cerebral aneurysm may cause a severe headache. However, sometimes bleeding is slower, producing a more gradual progression of headache, neck stiffness, and other neurologic signs, such as blurred vision.

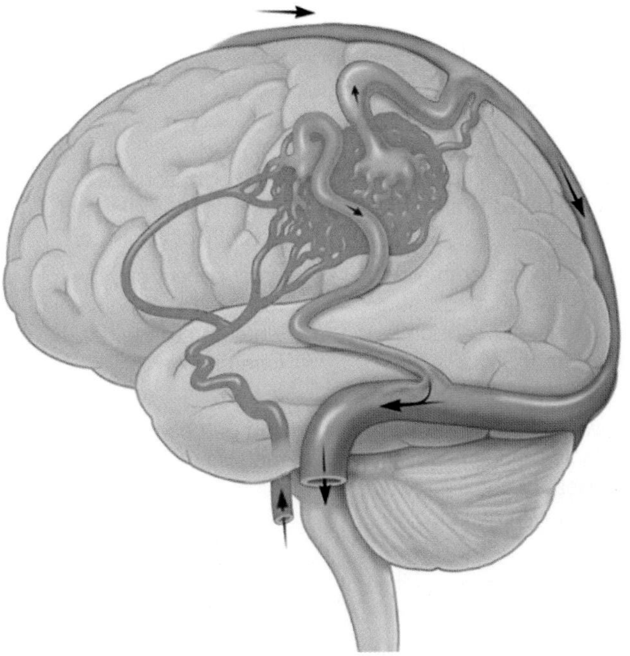

Fig. 23.3 Cerebral arteriovenous malformation (AVM). (From Kumar YK, Mehta SB, Ramachandra M: Computer simulation of cerebral arteriovenous malformation—validation analysis of hemodynamics parameters, *Peer J* 5:e2724, 2017.)

Stroke Prevention

Many strokes can be prevented either by surgical procedures or by medical management of diseases that predispose a person to a CVA. An angioplasty with stent placement is an option for opening occluded carotid arteries. Care for patients undergoing vascular surgery is presented in Chapter 18.

Aneurysms and AVMs can sometimes be surgically corrected, if found before rupture. Medical preventive measures are aimed at eliminating or managing some of the conditions that predispose a person to stroke. Management of atrial fibrillation is important in stroke prevention. Control of hypertension and the effective treatment of inflammatory heart disease, congenital heart defects, cardiac dysrhythmias, and atherosclerosis have significantly reduced the incidence of stroke. Teaching people to seek assistance immediately when signs of stroke occur may allow medical intervention that will decrease permanent neurologic deficit.

Patient Teaching

Warning Signs of Stroke

Teach people to seek immediate medical attention in an emergency department if any of the following warning signs of stroke appear.

- Sudden weakness, numbness, tingling, or loss of feeling in the face, arm, or leg
- Sudden trouble seeing in one or both eyes; double vision
- Sudden confusion, slurred speech, trouble talking, or difficulty understanding what others are saying
- A sudden, severe headache for no known reason
- Sudden trouble walking, dizziness, or a feeling of spinning around
- Loss of balance or coordination
- Blackouts

Should any of these signs occur, ask the person to:

- Smile (note any facial droop or asymmetry)
- Hold their arms out straight with palms up (watch for arm drift)
- Repeat a sentence or repeat what you say (note any abnormal speech pattern)
- These symptoms are known by the acronym FAST—**F**acial drooping, **A**rm weakness, **S**peech difficulty, **T**ime to call 911.

Clinical Cues

Valve disorders and arrhythmias such as atrial fibrillation predispose to stroke from emboli. Emboli form in the chambers of the heart when blood flow is abnormal, and these emboli can be ejected into the cerebral circulation.

Aspirin or another antiplatelet drug to reduce platelet aggregation and decrease the chance of thrombosis often is prescribed to prevent the recurrence of stroke from thrombosis (Table 23.1).

SIGNS AND SYMPTOMS

The neurologic effects of stroke can range from mild motor disturbances to profound coma. Fig. 23.4 shows selected control zones of the brain and motor and sensory functions likely to be affected by a stroke. Signs and symptoms will depend on the type of event that has caused the stroke and the location of the occlusion or bleed. There may be weakness (**hemiparesis**) or paralysis (**hemiplegia**), difficulty or inability to speak or understand (**dysarthria** or **aphasia**), difficulty with vision, loss of balance or poor coordination (**ataxia**), decreased level

Table 23.1 Drugs Commonly Used for Patients After a Cerebrovascular Accident[a]

DRUG	ACTION	NURSING IMPLICATIONS	PATIENT TEACHING
tPA (alteplase; tissue plasminogen activator)	Converts fibrin to plasminogen, causing lysis of thrombus or embolus of CVA	Frequent VS; monitor for dysrhythmias; frequent neurologic checks; assess for bleeding until 24 h after infusion. Monitor for hypersensitivity; monitor clotting/bleeding studies. Do not give concurrently with anticoagulants, antiplatelet aggregation drugs, or NSAIDs.	Explain that the IV infusion is for the purpose of breaking up the clot stopping blood flow to part of the brain.
Aspirin (Ecotrin)	Decreases platelet aggregation	Administer with food; observe for signs of intestinal bleeding, tinnitus. Monitor blood count and liver enzymes.	Instruct to take with a full glass of water and when in an upright position. Ask to report any blood in stool, bleeding gums, nosebleeds, or excessive bruising. Report ringing in the ears or skin rash. Caution not to crush the pill. Warn not to take OTC products containing aspirin or salicylic acid.
Nimodipine (Nimotop)	Inhibits calcium ion flux across cellular membrane; decreases or prevents cerebral vasospasm	Frequent neurologic assessment and VS; monitor liver enzymes; assess BP and apical pulse immediately before administration. Hold if systolic BP is <90 mm Hg. Monitor for hypotension. Should be held for heart rate <60 beats per minute.	Advise that the drug may cause hypotension and dizziness with movement.
Anticonvulsants	Prevention of seizures in post-CVA patients	Prophylactic administration is not recommended. Medications are given if seizures develop.	Take medications as prescribed and do not abruptly discontinue.
BP medications	Various categories of drugs have different mechanisms of action. The intent is to control BP.	Maintain BP within ordered parameters to prevent bleeding in hemorrhagic stroke and to maintain cerebral perfusion in ischemic stroke.	Instruct patient on how to monitor BP at home and when to call the health care provider.
Statins	To control cholesterol and prevent plaque formation	This may be a new medication for the patient. Side effects include headache, drowsiness, nausea, or vomiting, which are also associated with neurologic disorders.	Teach purpose of medication and side effects to report: muscle pain, memory loss, high blood sugar.
Antiplatelet/ anticoagulation	For ischemic stroke prevention	Other antiplatelet medications in addition to aspirin may be ordered. Anticoagulation is indicated if the stroke was embolic from atrial fibrillation.	Increased risk of bleeding with minor injuries. Follow up with any lab monitoring.

[a]See Chapter 19 for information on warfarin (Coumadin).

BP, Blood pressure; *CVA*, cerebrovascular accident; *IV*, intravenous; *NSAIDs*, nonsteroidal antiinflammatory drugs; *OTC*, over the counter; *tPA*, tissue plasminogen activator; *VS*, vital signs.

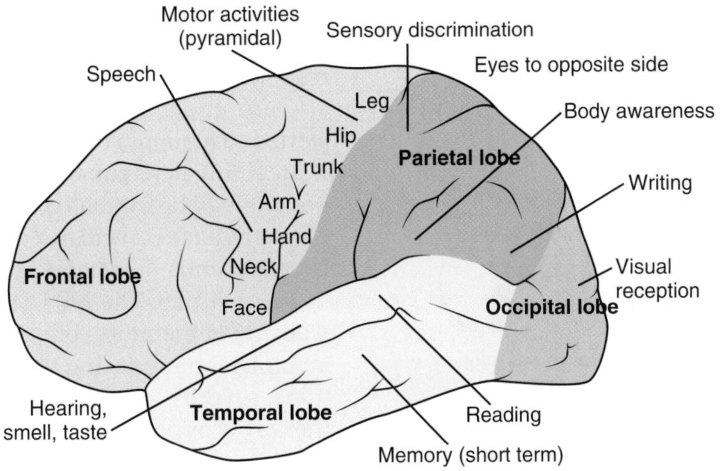

Fig. 23.4 Each area of the brain controls a particular activity.

of consciousness (LOC), and confusion. Incontinence may occur. Bleeding into the brain or edema around necrotic tissue causes ICP to increase (see Chapter 22 for information on increasing ICP).

Safety Alert

Swallow Evaluation

Patients should be kept NPO until swallowing can be evaluated, to prevent aspiration. A nursing bedside swallow evaluation can be performed to see if liquids and oral medications can be given safely. A speech therapist will perform a complete evaluation and determine the appropriate consistency of foods and any other guidelines.

Motor function deficits affect mobility, respiratory function, swallowing, speech, gag reflex, and self-care abilities. Because the pyramidal pathways cross at the level of the medulla, injury to brain cells in the right hemisphere affects the left side of the body, and damage to cells in the left hemisphere affects the right side of the body. There may be hemiplegia or hemiparesis. Muscle tone is usually flaccid at first, and then there may be spasticity and hyperreflexia. Keeping the body in good alignment to prevent contractures is very important.

Language disorders involve expression and comprehension of both written and spoken words. Aphasia or **dysphasia** (minimal speech activity) or a mixed type of aphasia may occur (see Chapter 21). Many stroke patients experience dysarthria (difficulty in speaking) because of lack of muscular control of the tongue. A speech therapist works with the patient to improve speech and swallow capability. Computer software programs for rehabilitation of patients with aphasia have been beneficial to many.

The frustration of trying to perform a function that was always easy before the stroke may cause the patient to cry. Alternatively, the patient may display an angry emotional outburst and sometimes use foul language.

Clinical Cues

When assessing the timing of the onset of stroke symptoms, the terminology used is "last known normal." This means the time that the patient was last seen at their baseline of function or "normal" for them. When a stroke happens during sleep or the onset is unwitnessed, this information is not readily available, which affects treatment options that are based on time.

Memory and judgment may be affected by the stroke. The ability to learn may be affected, which makes relearning activities to promote independence a slow process. A great deal of patience and encouragement is needed from the staff working with the patient.

Spatial-perceptual deficits may cause the patient to totally neglect input from the affected side of the body (*unilateral neglect*). They must be taught to attend to the body parts on that side of the body to protect them from injury. **Homonymous hemianopsia** (blindness in part of the visual field of both eyes) adds to the spatial-perceptual problems by making it difficult to judge distances (Fig. 23.5). The patient is taught ways to deal with the problems of the type of visual defect developed. **Agnosia** (inability to recognize an object by sight, touch, or hearing) makes it difficult to do ordinary tasks. **Apraxia** (the inability to carry out learned sequential movements on command) adds to the difficulty in regaining independence.

Bladder and bowel incontinence are often temporary after a stroke. Constipation does occur because of immobility, weakened abdominal muscles, dehydration, and diminished response to the defecation reflex. The patient's inability to express needs and their difficulty in managing clothing contribute to bladder and bowel incontinence and constipation. With time, these problems can be overcome.

DIAGNOSIS

A patient presenting with stroke symptoms will undergo a CT scan within the first 45 minutes of emergency

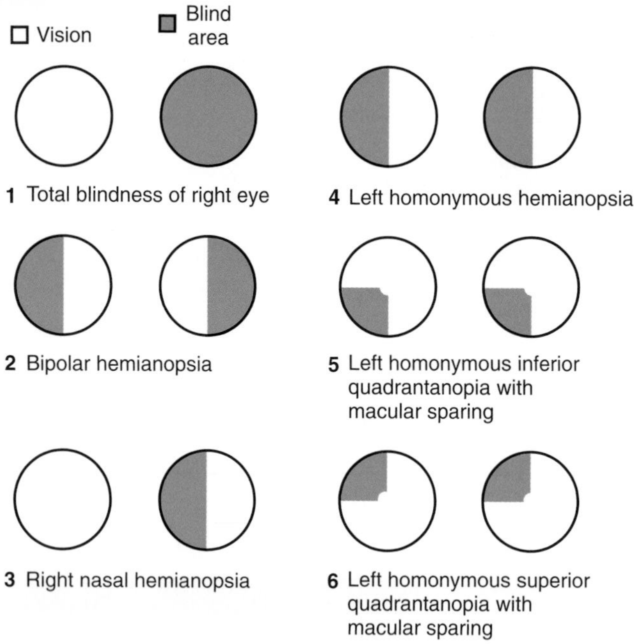

Fig. 23.5 Homonymous hemianopsia: visual field defects that can occur after a stroke. (Adapted from Black JM, Hawks JH: *Medical-surgical nursing: clinical management for positive outcomes*, ed 8, Philadelphia, 2009, Saunders.)

Clinical Cues

The 2018 Ischemic Stroke Guidelines recommend that all hospitals have an organized stroke response with stroke teams. Many facilities call a "code stroke" when a patient presents with stroke symptoms, to mobilize all necessary disciplines to promptly evaluate and treat the patient (Powers et al., 2018).

department arrival. The scan will rule out a hemorrhagic stroke. It does not confirm an ischemic stroke because the tissue changes are visible until after the time frame for treatment. If immediate treatment is not indicated, in addition to a complete physical and neurologic examination, the health care provider may order an MRI or cerebral angiogram to determine the specific cause of the stroke. An EEG is performed; brain scans or transcranial Doppler flow studies and carotid artery Doppler studies may also be ordered. Testing for blood levels of glutamate, which increases during a progressive ischemic stroke and damages brain tissue, may alert providers to patients whose condition is likely to deteriorate rapidly. Hemorrhagic stroke is diagnosed with CT scan or MRI.

TREATMENT

When a stroke is suspected, the first priority is to maintain an open airway. All constricting clothing around the patient's neck should be removed, and the patient should be turned to one side to prevent aspiration of saliva and obstruction of the air passages. When outside of the hospital, no attempt should be made to move the person until an ambulance has arrived. Reassure the patient, regardless of whether they are able to respond. Elevate the head slightly to reduce ICP.

Once under medical care, supplemental oxygen is started to maintain oxygen saturation greater than 94%. If breathing is impaired or the patient is comatose, the patient may be intubated and mechanically ventilated. Hypoglycemia is evaluated and treated if present because hypoglycemia signs and symptoms can be similar to those of stroke. The NIH Stroke Scale (see the Evolve website) is the most commonly used scoring tool and is implemented during the initial assessment to determine severity of deficits and whether thrombolytic therapy is appropriate. Two IV lines for drug and fluid access are inserted. In addition to the CT scan, an electrocardiogram (ECG) is obtained, and blood is drawn for laboratory testing to determine treatment options.

Clinical Cues

There is a fine line between keeping blood pressure high enough to perfuse the brain when an obstruction is present and keeping blood pressure low enough to prevent vessel rupture or increased bleeding from a rupture that has occurred.

Once the specific cause of the stroke has been determined, the health care provider is able to plan a more effective regimen of care. Recombinant tissue plasminogen activator (rtPA) is used to dissolve clots and emboli in ischemic stroke. It must be administered within 3 to 4.5 hours of the onset of symptoms (Powers et al., 2018). If the patient meets the criteria for thrombolysis, rtPA is administered IV with a bolus dose, and the rest of the dose is infused over 1 hour. Percutaneous mechanical thrombectomy may be considered within 6 hours of symptom onset, but its availability is limited to big centers with interventional specialists. Aspirin for platelet inhibition is given, and in specific conditions anticoagulants may be given to prevent further clot formation. If tPA has been given, no anticoagulants or antiplatelet aggregation drugs are given for 24 hours. **The drug is *not* administered to anyone with a known risk of bleeding or who has had an intracerebral bleed.** Antihypertensive drugs are prescribed as appropriate.

Nimodipine or nifedipine may be given to decrease arterial spasm if the stroke is from subarachnoid hemorrhage. Testing of new drugs continues in an effort to find a way to decrease the resultant damage from a stroke. Statins are being studied for their neuroprotective effect. The 2018 American Heart Association guidelines do not include any recommendations for use of neuroprotective medications due to lack of clinical evidence of their effectiveness. Hypertonic saline may be used in the place of mannitol in patients with hemorrhagic or ischemic stroke to decrease ICP. The patient is given sedation and analgesia for the headache and neck pain. Blood glucose levels are monitored and controlled.

Thrombectomy using devices inserted percutaneously to trap and remove the clot can be used up to 8 hours

> **Clinical Cues**
>
> Additional noninvasive imaging studies such as CT perfusion or angiography scans may be done to see if a patient who is not a candidate for rtPA therapy might benefit from mechanical thrombectomy. This intervention can happen from 6–24 hours of onset of symptoms.

after the onset of an ischemic stroke. A catheter is threaded up through the femoral artery to the brain, and a wire device is then guided through the catheter to the brain. In one device, the end of the wire resembles a corkscrew and ensnares the clot, which is pulled out through the catheter. Another device deploys like a stent, trapping the clot inside and allowing for removal. The interventional radiologist or neurologist performs this procedure during angiography. If successful, blood flow can be restored to the brain within 20 minutes. Clot aspiration is another retrieval method. Several methods of mechanical removal of a clot are undergoing trials. Risks of bleeding associated with these procedures must be considered.

Surgical Procedures

A cerebral aneurysm may be repaired during a craniotomy by placing a clip around the stalk of the aneurysm. The aneurysm may be wrapped with a material that prevents the wall from rupturing if it cannot be clipped or resected. An interventional radiologic procedure in which a small platinum wire is guided carefully into the aneurysm is another option. Coils of wire are curled into the aneurysm sac, filling it (Fig. 23.6). Thrombosis completes the solidification of the aneurysm, effectively eliminating it. AVMs are treated in much the same way but may be eliminated using radiosurgery. More than one type of intervention may be used.

About one third of all strokes can be traced to obstruction of any one of the four arteries in the neck that supply blood to the brain. These arteries are generally accessible, so the surgeon can open the artery and remove the obstruction, which is usually from plaque buildup. If there is near-total occlusion of the carotid artery, either an angioplasty procedure with stent implantation or a carotid endarterectomy is considered. If occlusion from plaque obstruction is less than 60%, medical treatment with diet and lifestyle modification and medication to prevent platelet aggregation (i.e., aspirin, clopidogrel [Plavix], dipyridamole [Persantine]) is prescribed. Carotid procedures are usually not done emergently as a treatment for stroke.

The blood from intracranial bleeding may be surgically removed if the procedure will reduce ICP and not cause more brain injury.

Neurologic assessments are performed often to monitor closely for signs of increasing ICP (see Chapter 22). Measures are instituted to prevent or alleviate a rise in ICP. Increased ICP occurs most commonly with subarachnoid hemorrhage.

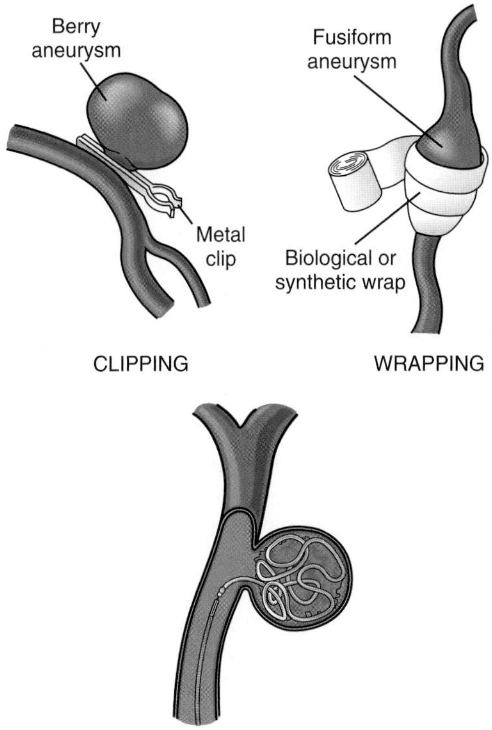

COILS CAUSE THROMBOSIS

Fig. 23.6 Techniques used for aneurysm repair.

> **Clinical Cues**
>
> If any change in the patient's thought processes or LOC occurs or if the patient becomes more restless, notify the health care provider immediately because this may be an early sign of increasing ICP. Treatment to decrease ICP may prevent disability and may prevent death from herniation of the brain.

COMPLICATIONS

Extension of Hemorrhage or Rebleed

If initial symptoms were caused by a leaking cerebral aneurysm, rupture is a danger until the aneurysm is repaired. Neurologic signs and LOC are watched closely to detect deterioration of the patient's condition because of further bleeding and a rise in ICP. The patient is kept as quiet as possible, with outside stimuli kept to a minimum.

Seizures

Seizures are a common complication of a stroke because neural pathways are interrupted when blood flow is blocked or there is irritation of the cerebral cortex from an intracerebral bleed. The type of seizure depends on the area of the brain involved and the extent of the intracerebral bleed or blockage of blood flow. Generalized seizures may occur. Prophylactic use of antiseizure drugs is not currently recommended. If seizures occur, they are treated with standard antiseizure medications.

Hydrocephalus

If blood has leaked into the ventricular system, it interferes with the resorption of CSF, causing **hydrocephalus**.

This is more common when a subarachnoid hemorrhage has occurred. It may be necessary to prevent increased ICP by shunting the fluid out of the brain; a catheter is placed into the lateral ventricle and then tunneled down to the right atrium or the peritoneal cavity to drain the excess fluid.

NURSING MANAGEMENT

When a patient is first admitted to the hospital after a stroke, the general state of health is assessed, as are the effects of the stroke. The American Heart Association and American Stroke Association have jointly issued clinical practice guidelines for poststroke rehabilitation. The guidelines cover recommendations for assessment and intervention for residual deficits (Winstein et al., 2016).

Care of patients who have had a stroke is described as occurring in phases: the initial hospital care, rehabilitation efforts begun in the acute care setting, transition to intensive rehabilitation as either an inpatient or an outpatient, and community-based rehabilitation. These are not phases in the sense that one begins only after another is finished. There is overlapping of activities in each phase. Because approximately 80% of all stroke patients survive the first or initial phase of their illness, rehabilitation and plans for self-care are of the utmost importance. Chapter 9 discusses concepts of rehabilitation.

Assess stroke patients for risk of falls and institute appropriate interventions to prevent falls. Assess pain regularly using an appropriate validated pain scale. A nutritional and dysphagia screening should be completed within 24 hours of the patient being awake and alert (Winstein et al., 2018).

Clinical Cues

Because of the damage to the nervous tissue, fatigue is another problem for stroke patients. When working with a patient to relearn walking, dressing, or other activities, keep the session short and allow for adequate rest periods between activities.

ASSESSMENT (DATA COLLECTION): ACUTE PHASE OF STROKE

Immediate assessment of breathing and respiratory rate is essential. LOC is assessed next. Initial care of stroke patients includes careful assessment to determine the extent to which neurologic functions have been affected. Use an established stroke scale to evaluate any deficits that are present. Complete hemiplegia is a common effect of stroke. Aphasia often indicates ischemia of the brain cells on the left side of the brain and is usually accompanied by right-sided hemiplegia. Fig. 23.7 illustrates deficits often experienced by damage to the left or right side of the brain.

After the acute stage of the stroke has passed and the patient is physiologically stable, an assessment of functional abilities is performed so that rehabilitation goals and plans can be devised. Assessment of and nursing intervention for patients with problems of immobility, incontinence of urine and feces, aphasia, delirium or confusion, and altered LOC are discussed in Chapter 21. Because a patient who has had a stroke is at risk for a second occurrence, assessment for new signs of neurologic impairment is ongoing.

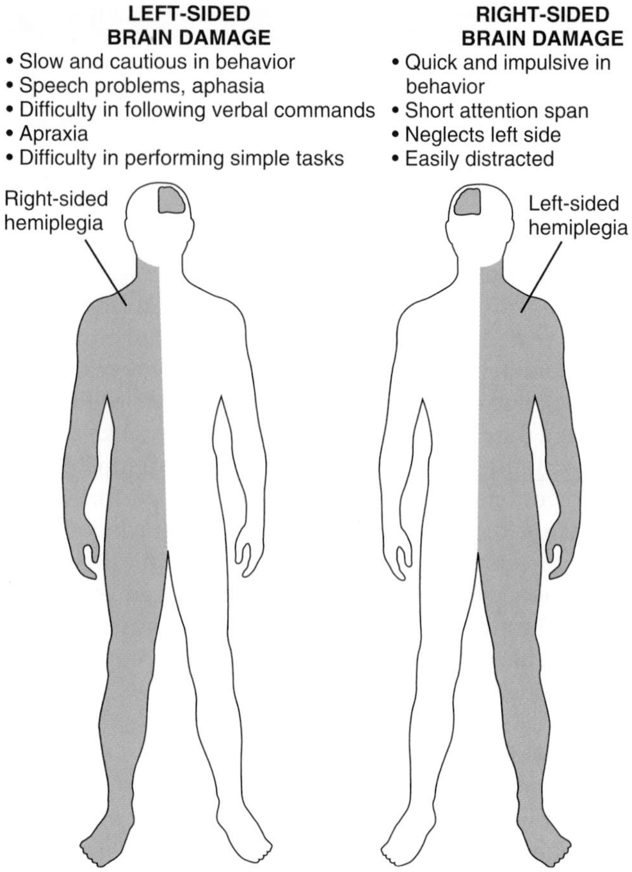

Fig. 23.7 Comparison of deficits and behavior related to damage to the left and right sides of the brain.

NURSING DIAGNOSIS AND PLANNING

Problem statements for a patient who has experienced a CVA commonly include the following:

- Potential for alteration in airway maintenance.
- Altered breathing pattern.
- Potential for injury due to weakness, paralysis, lack of sensation, confusion, decreased consciousness, or unilateral neglect.
- Altered physical mobility due to weakness or paralysis.
- Altered nutrition due to impaired swallowing and hemiparesis or hemiplegia.
- Altered self-care ability due to inability to perform activities of daily living (ADLs; feeding, bathing, grooming) without assistance.
- Altered urinary function due to neurologic deficits.
- Altered bowel function due to impaired mobility and neurologic impairment.

- Potential for altered skin integrity due to decreased mobility, paresis, or paralysis.
- Altered communication ability due to inability to clearly verbalize or inability to comprehend communication.
- Altered body image due to neurologic damage and hemiplegia.
- Altered sensory perception: visual—due to loss of vision in parts of visual field; kinesthetic—related to decreased sense of touch on one side of the body.
- Decreased self-esteem due to alteration in body image and to dependence on others.
- Altered coping ability due to loss of usual lifestyle, neurologic deficits, and dependence on others.

Planning for specific goals must take into account the patient's previous lifestyle, age, general health or illness status, and specific problems of care. An 80-year-old retired person will not have the same goals for rehabilitation and recovery as a 47-year-old mother of three who had been working full time as a schoolteacher before her attack.

Major nursing goals during the first phase of care are to:

- Maintain an adequate airway.
- Establish baseline data regarding vital signs, LOC, neuromuscular function, and neurologic status.
- Preserve joint and muscle function.
- Prevent complications that may interfere with rehabilitation.

Specific individual expected outcomes are written for each identified problem or nursing diagnosis (Nursing Care Plan 23.1).

◆ IMPLEMENTATION

The amount of activity permitted a stroke patient during the initial acute stage of their illness depends on the cause of the stroke. If there is danger of continued hemorrhage from a ruptured artery and resultant increase in ICP, physical activity will necessarily be limited. When there is no danger of further damage to the brain, the patient usually is encouraged to become active as soon as the condition has stabilized.

Many patients have **dysphagia** (difficulty swallowing) after a stroke. A speech therapist should be consulted for a swallowing study and to devise a plan to improve swallowing. Be certain the patient has had the evaluation

Nursing Care Plan 23.1 Care of a Patient Who Has Experienced a Stroke

SCENARIO

Mr. Lewis, age 68 years, was admitted 4 days ago for an ischemic stroke, or cerebrovascular accident (CVA). He woke up with weakness and facial drooping. His wife called an ambulance, and he was evaluated in the emergency department. Because his "last known normal" was 8 hours prior, he was not a candidate for thrombolytic therapy. He is currently experiencing left-sided paresis, decreased alertness, and difficulty swallowing.

PROBLEM STATEMENT/NURSING DIAGNOSIS

Altered cerebral tissue perfusion related to obstruction from a thrombus.

SUPPORTING ASSESSMENT DATA

Subjective: "What day did you say it was?"
Objective: Requires shaking his shoulder and calling his name to arouse him. MRI shows thrombotic ischemic CVA.

Goals/Expected Outcomes	Nursing Interventions	Selected Rationale	Evaluation
Patient will show no further decrease in LOC.	Monitor neurologic status q2h. Notify health care provider of decreasing LOC, pupil changes, change in respiratory pattern, widening pulse pressure, slowing of pulse, or increase in temperature.	Changes in neurologic signs may indicate rising intracranial pressure.	No changes in neurologic signs. Difficult to arouse but orients quickly.
	Monitor for seizure activity.	Seizure activity is common after a brain injury or CVA.	No signs of seizure activity.
	Administer medications to prevent clot formation as ordered.	Aspirin is effective to help prevent clot formation.	Managed to swallow the enteric-coated aspirin tablet.
	Monitor for bleeding gums, blood in urine or stool.	Antiplatelet medications may cause bleeding.	No signs of blood in urine or stool; gums not bleeding.

PROBLEM STATEMENT/NURSING DIAGNOSIS

Altered swallowing ability related to weakness of swallowing muscles.

Continued

Nursing Care Plan 23.1 Care of a Patient Who Has Experienced a Stroke—cont'd

SUPPORTING ASSESSMENT DATA

Subjective: "I almost choked on that capsule."
Objective: Coughing when trying to swallow capsule.

Goals/Expected Outcomes	Nursing Interventions	Selected Rationale	Evaluation
Patient will not aspirate food or pills.	Place in high Fowler position for meals, snacks, and oral medication administration.	Gravity will assist swallowing in this position.	Raised to high Fowler for oral intake.
	Instruct to tilt head and neck forward when attempting to swallow.	Facilitates elevation of the larynx and posterior movement of the tongue, allowing food to go into esophagus rather than trachea.	Is tilting head and neck forward when swallowing.
	Have patient swallow a sip of water before eating or taking an oral medication.	Ensure that patient can swallow.	Swallows sip of water without much difficulty now.
	Assist to choose foods for meals that are easily swallowed.	Custard, eggs, canned fruit, mashed potatoes, and other soft foods are more easily swallowed.	Choosing soft foods for tomorrow's meals.
	Encourage to take small bites of food.	Small amounts are more easily swallowed than large amounts.	Is taking small bites of food.
	Use a thickening agent in liquids if they are ordered by speech therapist.	Thickening makes liquids easier to swallow without aspirating.	Thickening agent not needed.
	Avoid putting foods of different texture in the mouth at the same time.	More than one food texture creates higher risk of aspiration.	Is eating one type of food at a time.
	Reinforce swallowing techniques/exercises recommended by speech therapist.	Muscle strengthening exercises may improve swallowing if done regularly.	Is practicing techniques suggested by speech therapist to improve swallowing.

PROBLEM STATEMENT/NURSING DIAGNOSIS

Potential for injury related to muscle weakness in left extremities.

SUPPORTING ASSESSMENT DATA

Subjective: "I can't put full weight on my left leg."
Objective: Left leg unable to push much against resistance; when trying to stand, left leg will not support full weight.

Goals/Expected Outcomes	Nursing Interventions	Selected Rationale	Evaluation
Patient will not fall or sustain injury before or after discharge.	Assist to stand and walk to the bathroom.	Assistance prevents falling.	Using front wheel walker to walk to bathroom.
	Instructed not to get up without assistance.	Assistance prevents falling.	Asking for assistance to go to the bathroom.
	Place call bell within reach each time he is repositioned.	Allows patient to call for help when wishing to arise.	
	Encourage ROM exercises and strengthening exercises taught by physical therapist.	Working the muscles may improve muscle tone.	Performing ROM and strengthening exercises three times per day.

PROBLEM STATEMENT/NURSING DIAGNOSIS

Altered self-care ability related to weakness and poststroke fatigue.

Nursing Care Plan 23.1 Care of a Patient Who Has Experienced a Stroke—cont'd

SUPPORTING ASSESSMENT DATA

Subjective: "I'm too weak to hold the razor properly to shave."
Objective: Hand shakes when trying to grip razor and shave.

Goals/Expected Outcomes	Nursing Interventions	Selected Rationale	Evaluation
Patient will resume some self-grooming by discharge.	Assist with bathing, dressing, and grooming.	Assistance prevents undue fatigue. Assistance helps accomplish daily hygiene activities.	Assistance with bathing, dressing, and grooming provided.
	Encourage patient to attempt to comb hair and brush teeth.	Small accomplishments provide hope of independence.	Attempted to comb hair with right hand; praise given.
	Praise for every successful attempt at self-care.	Praise reinforces desired behavior.	Patient attempted self-grooming activity.
	Help to practice shaving with electric razor using right hand.	New skills improve with practice.	Wife will bring in an electric razor for him tomorrow. Continue plan.

PROBLEM STATEMENT/NURSING DIAGNOSIS

Limited coping ability related to memory impairment, difficulty swallowing, and paresis of left extremities.

SUPPORTING ASSESSMENT DATA

Subjective: "I don't want to be a burden to my wife."
Objective: Tends to forget what wife or nurses have told him; eyes fill with tears at times.

Goals/Expected Outcomes	Nursing Interventions	Selected Rationale	Evaluation
Patient will express hope of meaningful recovery before discharge.	Assure that it is too early to tell what permanent disability might be present from the stroke.	Validates that the future is not known at this time.	Assurance given during bathing discussion.
	Help patient explore his fears and anxieties about his condition and his future.	Expressing fears decreases anxiety.	Spoke about fear of being dependent on wife for daily care.
	Actively listen with patience when patient shares his thoughts.	Actively listening establishes trust and provides emotional support.	Sat with patient, established eye contact, and listened to his concerns.
	Do not express negative thoughts or opinions about his condition or progress in his or his wife's presence.	Negative thoughts can destroy hope.	No negative comments made.
	Point out each small bit of progress in self-care, eating, and mobility.	Acknowledging progress toward recovery helps dispel fear of permanent dependence.	Acknowledged improvement in swallowing at noon meal. Continue plan.

CRITICAL THINKING QUESTIONS

1. How would you incorporate Mrs. Lewis into the care of her husband?
2. What might be accomplished with an occupational therapy consultation for this patient?
3. How could a social services consult be helpful for this patient and his wife?

LOC, Level of consciousness; *MRI*, magnetic resonance imaging; *ROM*, range of motion.

Safety Alert

Early Mobilization

"High-dose, very early mobilization within 24 hours of stroke onset can reduce the odds of a favorable outcome at 3 months and is not recommended" (Winstein et al., 2016, p. e7).

Think Critically

What interventions would you use to help a patient with unilateral neglect?

to ensure intact swallowing before feeding orally. When the patient has dysphagia, aspiration when eating is a real danger.

Measures to prevent complications, such as subcutaneous low-molecular-weight heparin injections (contraindicated in hemorrhagic stroke) and sequential compression stockings to prevent deep venous thrombosis, skin care to minimize the risk of skin breakdown, physical therapy and splinting to prevent contractures and spasticity, and measures to prevent falls, are included in the complete plan of care. To reduce the possibility of recurrence of a stroke, risk factors are identified and teaching is begun to modify them.

◆ EVALUATION

Evaluation is based on whether the interventions are effective in achieving the expected outcomes. Assess whether the overall goals have been met. If the outcomes are not being met, the care plan must be revised.

◆ REHABILITATION

Plans for rehabilitation should begin the moment the patient is admitted. This means proper positioning, range-of-motion exercises for affected limbs, adequate nutrition and fluid intake and output, prevention of pressure ulcers, use of devices to keep extremities in anatomic position, and all other nursing measures directed toward maintaining normal body functions until the patient is able to maintain them on their own.

If the patient has homonymous hemianopsia, they have a visual defect affecting the same half of the visual field in each eye. They will not be able to see past the midline toward the side opposite the lesion and must turn their head to scan that side (see Fig. 23.5). The problem may cause accidents when ambulating. The patient must be taught ways to deal with this visual problem. Teach patients with unilateral neglect to bathe both sides of the body. Demonstrate how to dress the affected side first. The weakened arm and/or leg must be positioned in correct alignment when the patient moves. A sling may be used to prevent shoulder subluxation of the affected upper extremity.

If disabilities from inactivity are prevented, rehabilitation has a much better chance of success. During the acute care inpatient phase, various members of the health care team collaborate with the patient and their family to help resolve both psychosocial and physical problems. The team members may include a physical therapist, speech pathologist, social worker, psychologist, and occupational therapist. The patient usually is transferred from the hospital to a rehabilitation facility. The patient is encouraged with physical therapy to strengthen muscles as well as their resolve to help themselves. Active muscle exercise is necessary to retrain them.

There are many ways to encourage the patient. Instead of feeding them every item on their tray, let them hold bread and other "finger foods," suggesting that they feed themselves these things. Chewing may be slow at first; the patient should not be hurried, nor should they be allowed to chew to the point of exhaustion. Eating often is difficult and messy, and privacy must be provided. If hemiplegia is causing the patient to "pocket" food in the folds of the mouth, the mouth should be checked after meals.

Combing and brushing the hair is good exercise for the arm and shoulder, as are brushing the teeth and washing the face and hands. The patient may not be able to carry all these procedures through to completion at first, but with occupational therapy and encouragement they can gradually improve until they are able to perform much of their own personal care. **The patient who has sustained a brain injury becomes fatigued very quickly, and this must be kept in mind when performing self-care activities.** Encouragement and praise for the smallest accomplishment can help the patient's tattered self-esteem. Be sure to deliver the message in an adult-to-adult communication style, not as if praising a child. Maintaining the individual's dignity and showing respect for them as an adult can help their resolve to keep trying.

Stroke patients can be prone to rapid mood swings and spontaneous weeping. All health care workers must be patient and accepting, and explaining to the patient and family that this is common after a stroke can ease the patient's embarrassment.

Nutrition Considerations

Patients With Dysphagia

To help prevent aspiration, tell the patient to:

- Sit up straight to eat and tilt your head slightly forward.
- Place only one teaspoon of food in your mouth at a time.
- Place the food on the unaffected side of your mouth if you have paresis from a stroke.
- Place your chin on your chest and swallow; wait a few seconds and swallow again.
- Refrain from taking liquids and solids at the same time.
- Sip from the cup or glass rather than using a straw.
- Remain in an upright position for 45 to 60 minutes after a meal.

Interventions to assist the patient to eat without aspirating include the following:

- Plan a 30-minute rest and relaxation period before each meal.
- Allow plenty of time for a relaxed meal.
- Serve food cold or well warmed; lukewarm foods are more difficult to swallow.
- Serve foods in the consistency ordered; some patients find semisolid food easier to swallow.
- Avoid serving peanut butter, syrup, and bananas because they are sticky and difficult to swallow.
- Avoid serving dry foods such as rice, popcorn, toast, or crackers because they tend to be more difficult to swallow and can stick in the throat.
- Keep the container for liquids more than two-thirds full so that the patient does not have to tilt the head back too far to drink. Tilting the head back tends to cause fluid to go into the trachea.

◆ CONTINUUM OF CARE

The acute rehabilitation phase starts in the acute care facility and transitions into the acute rehabilitation facility inpatient setting. The degree of rehabilitation needed will determine length of stay. Assessment in the acute care setting must indicate that a patient has rehabilitation potential, or other plans are made. Some patients may be cared for at home if the family can provide the needed care; others may be placed in long-term care facilities if care is complex or beyond the capability of the family.

After acute rehabilitation, plans are made for discharge and referral to individuals and agencies outside the facility that will help the patient and the family adjust to their new way of life. A visiting nurse often is assigned for a period to coordinate rehabilitation efforts, assist with teaching, and assess the patient's status. The patient continues rehabilitation as an outpatient under the health care provider's supervision. In some rural areas, TeleHealth services using the internet and telephone are available to provide continued speech therapy.

BRAIN TUMOR

ETIOLOGY AND PATHOPHYSIOLOGY

About 80,000 new primary brain tumors are discovered each year in the United States. More than 700,000 Americans are living with a brain tumor today (American Brain Tumor Association, 2018). Metastatic tumors from a different site of origin occur in 10% to 30% of adults with systemic malignancies (Loeffler, 2018). It is not known how brain tumors begin, and there are more than 120 different types. Most brain tumors are benign and not cancerous (American Brain Tumor Association, 2018). Malignant tumors are primarily (78%) those arising from the glial cells. Glial cells include astrocytes, ependymal cells, and oligodendroglial cells. Tumors are classified according to the type of cells that produce the malignancy (Table 23.2).

Neoplasms within the confines of the skull are space-occupying lesions and thus create problems of increasing ICP by compressing adjacent tissues. If the tumor arises from brain cells, the cranial nerves, or the pituitary gland, the neoplastic cells can infiltrate and destroy these structures; other types of tumor can destroy tissue through pressure. Many brain tumors, such as meningiomas and acoustic neuromas, are benign. However, because of the increased ICP that tumors cause and the way they can invade brain tissue, a benign tumor also presents a serious condition.

Intracranial tumors may begin in the brain itself, or they may begin in the meninges, cranial nerves, or pituitary gland. Primary malignant brain tumors rarely metastasize outside the brain. Tumors in the cerebral hemispheres are termed *supratentorial*, and those located beneath the tentorium (fold of dura mater) are termed *infratentorial*. This area of the cerebral hemisphere contains the structures of the brainstem and the cerebellum.

Table 23.2 Different Types of Brain Tumors[a]

TUMOR	LOCATION	CHARACTERISTICS
Benign		
Acoustic neuroma	Eighth cranial nerve	The growth is benign but can press on other nerves or the brain, causing hearing loss, ringing in the ear, loss of balance, and headache.
Meningioma	Most arise from the dura and are external to the brain tissue	A very small percentage are malignant. The tumors are usually slow growing, and symptoms occur from the pressure on surrounding structures.
Pituitary adenoma	Pituitary gland	
Hemangioblastoma	Usually found in the cerebellum	Are made up of blood vessels and may be contained within a cyst. Produce erythropoietin, leading to a high number of circulating red blood cells.
Malignant		
Gliomas		
Glioblastoma multiforme	Most commonly in the frontal and temporal lobes of the cerebral hemispheres	Rapidly growing and invasive. Resistant to usual therapy; disruption of tumor blood supply that makes it difficult to deliver drugs to the tumor.
Astrocytoma	Most commonly in the cerebrum	Most common glioma. Subdivided into four grades depending on how likely they are to spread.
Medulloblastoma	Cerebellum	More common in children. Alteration in balance and coordination.
Oligodendroglioma	Cerebral white matter in the frontal, parietal, temporal, and occipital lobes	Most common presenting symptom is seizure. Headache and focal neurologic deficits depending on the location.
Ependymomas	Form in the lining of the ventricular system	Intracerebral tumors are more common in children, and spinal tumors are more common in adults. Seizures are common, as are signs and symptoms of increased intracranial pressure.
Metastatic tumors		Mostly from lung, breast, kidney, thyroid, and prostate carcinomas.

[a]Primary brain tumors are classified by the type of tissue from which they derive.

SIGNS, SYMPTOMS, AND DIAGNOSIS

There can be as many symptoms of intracranial tumors as there are functions of the structures within the skull. The symptoms depend on location and may appear gradually, or—if the tumor is a highly malignant, fast-growing type—they may appear suddenly. In a slow-growing type of tumor, the patient may first show personality changes, disturbances in judgment and memory, loss of muscular strength and coordination, or difficulty in speaking clearly. Headache awakening the patient is a key sign. Vomiting, visual problems, and other signs of increased ICP also may occur. Approximately 20% to 50% of adults with brain tumors develop seizure activity. Diagnostic procedures to identify the site and extent of intracranial tumors include skull x-rays, MRI, and CT scans. Magnetic resonance (MR) spectroscopy gives information on the tumor's metabolic profile, and MR perfusion imaging examines the cerebral blood volume and patterns of perfusion that are altered in areas of the tumor. MRI can be used simultaneously with positron emission tomography (PET) to provide structural information correlated with physiologic activity.

TREATMENT

The three modes of therapy for intracranial tumors are the same as those for neoplastic diseases elsewhere in the body: surgery, radiation therapy, and chemotherapy. Radiation can be delivered as whole brain radiation therapy (WBRT), stereotactic radiosurgery (SRS), or brachytherapy. WBRT is just as its name implies; the radiation is applied to the entire brain. SRS is not a surgical procedure but uses a steel frame attached to the head with ports through which radiation is directed from several angles. Measurements are calculated by a computer to precisely locate the tumor, and the radiation is delivered only to the tumor, which spares surrounding tissue. These procedures also can be used for small recurrent tumor growth. Gamma knife and cyber knife are different techniques of radiosurgery therapy. With brachytherapy, tiny radioactive particles are inserted into the tumor tissue or the space from which the tumor was surgically removed. This treatment allows for radiation to be applied directly to the affected tissue and may be temporary or permanent. Radiation precautions may be needed during this period if multiple particles were implanted.

Most chemotherapy drugs cannot cross the blood-brain barrier. To get the drugs into the brain circulation, an Ommaya reservoir may be implanted between the scalp and the skull. An Ommaya reservoir consists of a port attached to a catheter that is placed in the lateral ventricle of the brain (Fig. 23.8). Chemotherapy drugs can be injected into the port and instilled into the CSF in the ventricle. In this way the chemotherapy drug is carried to the tumor cells in greater quantity than can be achieved by infusion of the drugs into the bloodstream. The U.S. Food and Drug Administration (FDA) has

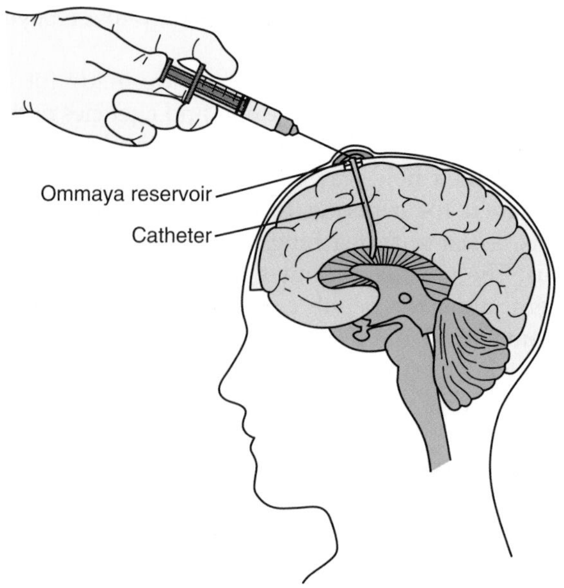

Fig. 23.8 Implantation of an Ommaya reservoir for chemotherapy of a brain tumor.

approved a wearable device that uses low-intensity, alternating electrical fields to disrupt tumor cell division. The electricity is delivered via electrodes placed on the scalp, which requires shaving the head. At this time glioblastomas are the only brain tumors being treated with this therapy (Batchelor, 2018).

In patients with gliomas, implantation of carmustine (BiCNU, Gliadel) wafers into a glial cell tumor site after resection slows growth. The drug is inserted into brain tissue after removal of the glioma, to fight the malignancy and slow or prevent regrowth. Temozolomide (Temodar) is an oral chemotherapeutic drug that crosses the blood-brain barrier. Trials with local hyperthermia, biological therapy, electrochemotherapy, and immunotherapy are under way. Molecularly targeted drugs include erlotinib (Tarceva), gefitinib (Iressa), and bevacizumab (Avastin). Treatments are discussed more thoroughly in Chapter 8. If there are signs of increased ICP, measures are instituted to try to lower the ICP and to provide supportive care (see Chapter 22).

Surgery

Surgery is used to remove intracranial tumors, then other modes of treatment are used to destroy remaining cells. Sometimes, however, the tumor has infiltrated vital parts of the brain that must not be traumatized by surgical procedures. If the tumor is in the cerebrum, a *craniotomy* is performed. A "window flap" of scalp and bone is cut and pulled down, the dura is opened, and the tumor is removed. Tumors in or near the cerebellum are removed through an incision under the occipital bone. If the tumor cannot be removed entirely, a portion may be removed to relieve compression of the brain against the skull. This procedure is only a temporary measure to relieve the patient's symptoms.

Care of patients after brain surgery is presented in Chapter 22.

Think Critically

How should a patient who has had a craniotomy for a supratentorial tumor be positioned?

NURSING MANAGEMENT

Routine neurologic assessments are performed, and the patient's ability to perform ADLs is evaluated. Pain assessment and control are important. Helping the patient and family to communicate fears and cope with the situation should be part of the care plan. Problem statements commonly used for a patient with a brain tumor include the following:

- Potential for altered tissue perfusion due to tumor pressure and cerebral edema.
- Pain due to cerebral edema and increased ICP.
- Altered self-care ability due to altered neuromuscular function, sensory deficits, or decreased LOC.
- Anxiety or fear due to diagnosis and prognosis.
- Potential for injury due to seizure activity caused by the tumor.
- Potential for injury due to increasing ICP from tumor growth.
- Altered memory due to damaged cells from pressure.
- Altered home maintenance ability due to physical impairments.
- Decreased self-esteem due to inability to work.

Specific outcomes appropriate for the individual are written and interventions are planned to help the patient meet the outcomes. Evaluation is based on data that indicate that the outcomes are being met. (See Chapter 21 for care for common problems and interventions for various problem statements related to neurologic conditions; see Nursing Care Plan 23.1 for further interventions.)

COMPLICATIONS

- *Hydrocephalus.* Obstruction of CSF flow may require placing a shunt to reduce CSF pressure and prevent increased ICP. A shunt is a tube placed in a ventricle of the brain and attached to a valve system that opens when the pressure from fluid rises to drain excess CSF from the ventricles to the peritoneal cavity or into the atrium of the heart, where it is absorbed (Fig. 23.9).
- *Intracerebral hemorrhage.* Bleeding in the brain may occur as the tumor erodes blood vessels. Depending on the condition of the patient, the size of the tumor, and prognosis, various measures to stop the bleeding and reduce ICP will be used.
- *Seizures.* Seizures are common in patients with primary and metastatic brain tumors. They are usually focal and are treated by anticonvulsant medications. They may be the first clinical sign of a brain tumor or occur during the course of the disease.

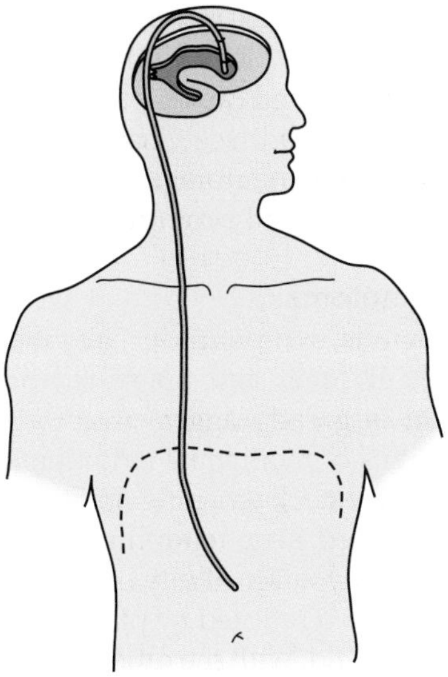

Fig. 23.9 Ventriculoperitoneal shunt to drain excess cerebrospinal fluid into the peritoneal cavity, where it is absorbed through the mucosa.

INFECTIOUS AND INFLAMMATORY DISORDERS OF THE NERVOUS SYSTEM

BACTERIAL MENINGITIS

Etiology and Pathophysiology

Meningitis is an inflammation of the membranes covering the brain and spinal cord and is caused by an infectious agent. Viruses, bacteria, and fungi can cause meningitis. Fungal meningitis occurs mostly in patients with acquired immunodeficiency syndrome (AIDS). The membranes can become infected in a number of ways because infectious agents can be carried through the bloodstream to the membranes, or brain tissue can become affected as an infection in a particular area of the brain spreads. Infection can spread from the spinal cord or sinuses to the brain. Two examples of how infectious organisms may enter the cranial vault other than via the bloodstream are (1) through an opening in the skull from a head injury or surgery or (2) by accidental introduction of infectious agents into the spinal canal during spinal puncture.

Many different strains of bacteria can cause meningitis, but the causative organisms are usually *Streptococcus pneumoniae* or *Neisseria meningitidis.* In children the causative organism may be *Haemophilus influenzae* type B. Bacterial meningitis commonly follows an upper respiratory infection. Immunization of all young adults against bacterial meningitis is recommended.

Health Promotion

Meningitis Immunization

Meningitis vaccine is required for many students entering college. The requirement varies by state. The CDC (2017) recommends vaccination for all adolescents and for others at increased risk for meningitis. It also should be encouraged for adults living in a communal situation. Meningitis can spread quickly when people are in proximity, such as in classrooms or dormitories.

The organisms that cause meningitis produce bacterial toxins that damage the blood-brain barrier, increasing vascular permeability and causing cerebral edema. Thus the ICP will be elevated (see Chapter 21). Meningitis can cause permanent neurologic damage or death if not identified and treated promptly.

Signs and Symptoms

The most obvious symptoms of meningitis are the **sudden onset of fever** and a **severe and persistent headache that is greatly aggravated by moving the head.** Other signs of meningeal irritation include pain and stiffness of the neck when flexing the neck (**nuchal rigidity**), exaggerated deep tendon reflexes, irritability, photophobia, and hypersensitivity of the skin. A positive Brudzinski sign can be elicited by placing a hand behind the patient's head and, with the other hand on the chest, gently flexing the patient's neck forward by moving their chin toward the chest. If there is flexion of the knees and hips when you try to flex the neck, the Brudzinski sign is positive and indicates meningeal irritation. To elicit a Kernig sign, position the patient supine and, with the hip and knee flexed at 90-degree angles, slowly extend the knee (Fig. 23.10). If there is pain, not just discomfort, behind the knee, the Kernig sign is positive, indicating meningeal irritation. Meningococcal meningitis commonly is accompanied by a petechial rash covering the chest and extremities. Seizures are also typical, as are nausea and vomiting. Quick medical attention is needed to prevent brain injury or death.

Diagnosis

When meningitis is suspected, a lumbar puncture (spinal tap) is performed, and the CSF is examined for the number and type of organisms present. A Gram stain identifies the causative organism. Prior to performing a lumbar puncture (LP), a CT scan may be done to rule out other causes of the symptoms and determine if there is evidence of increased ICP. In the presence of increased ICP, a LP can be dangerous and lead to brain herniation. Blood tests are performed to rule out other disorders that can mimic meningitis. Blood cultures will also be done.

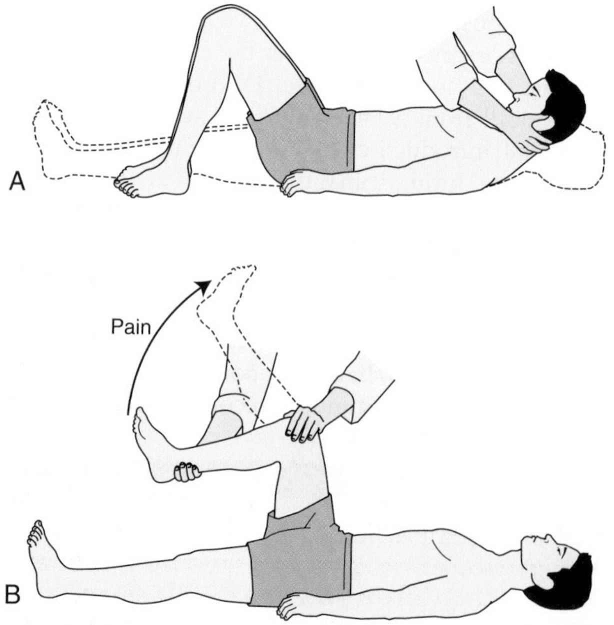

Fig. 23.10 **A,** A positive Brudzinski sign: passive flexion of the head and neck causes flexion of the thighs and legs. **B,** A positive Kernig sign: inability to extend the leg from a position of 90-degree flexion at the hip because of pain and spasms in the hamstring muscle.

> **Clinical Cues**
>
> When meningitis is present, the spinal fluid may appear milky as a result of the increased number of white blood cells suspended in the fluid. Other abnormal findings in the CSF include the presence of protein and decreased amounts of glucose.

Treatment

Successful treatment of meningitis and prevention of permanent disability depend on early recognition and prompt treatment. Antibiotics are started immediately for bacterial meningitis, and when the causative organism has been identified, specific antibiotics to which the organism is sensitive are administered. A combination of two antibiotics is common. The disease usually responds well to IV antibiotic therapy followed by oral doses given for 10 days. Dexamethasone along with the antibiotics has proven beneficial to decrease inflammation for many patients. The timing of the dexamethasone is important. It should be given prior to the first dose of antibiotics to prevent damage from the intense inflammatory reaction caused by substances released from the massive amount of bacteria killed (Hasbun, 2017). Anticonvulsant medications are administered if seizures occur, and acetaminophen is given for headache.

> **Clinical Cues**
>
> Narcotics are rarely used for pain control in patients with increased ICP because they cause sedation and prevent accurate neurologic assessment.

Prophylactic antibiotics are usually given to those in close contact with the patient to prevent the spread of the disease. Death occurs in about 25% of cases.

VIRAL MENINGITIS

Several viruses can cause meningitis; the most common are enteroviruses, arboviruses, human immunodeficiency virus (HIV), and herpes simplex virus. Viral meningitis tends to be milder than bacterial meningitis. The initial signs and symptoms include a headache, fever, photophobia, and stiff neck. Symptoms of brain involvement are not common.

The CSF is examined to confirm the diagnosis. A complete blood cell count will show increased lymphocytes (*lymphocytosis*). A polymerase chain reaction (PCR) test to detect virus-specific deoxyribonucleic acid (DNA) or ribonucleic acid (RNA) can diagnose CNS viral infection.

The disease is self-limiting and is managed symptomatically. Full recovery typically occurs within 7 to 10 days. Sometimes residual effects such as persistent headaches, mild mental impairment, and lack of coordination occur.

NURSING MANAGEMENT

ASSESSMENT (DATA COLLECTION) AND NURSING DIAGNOSIS

In addition to noting the specific signs and symptoms of meningitis, assess the patient for subjective and objective data relevant to each of the patient care problems that might accompany the disease. Examples include seizures, elevated body temperature, nausea and vomiting, pain, increased ICP, and fluid and electrolyte imbalances. Ongoing, vigilant neurologic assessment is a high priority in monitoring for signs of increasing ICP, changes in condition, and response to treatment. An ongoing assessment should be performed each shift.

Focused Assessment

Assessment of a Patient With Brain Infection

An assessment (data collection) should be performed each shift for the following areas:

- Neurologic check for increasing ICP (including headache and LOC)
- Stiff neck or paralysis
- Temperature and monitoring of temperature trend
- Assessment for electrolyte and fluid imbalance; skin turgor, mucous membranes, condition of lips; intake and output
- Gastrointestinal assessment: bowel sounds, distention, constipation, diarrhea, nausea, vomiting
- IV access site
- Skin condition
- Psychosocial concerns

Problem statements are written for the specific problems identified during data collection (see Chapter 21, Table 21.9, and Nursing Care Plan 23.1).

PLANNING, IMPLEMENTATION, AND EVALUATION

Expected outcomes are written for the problem statements chosen. Specific nursing interventions in the care of patients with meningitis are primarily concerned with measures to:

- Conserve the patient's strength
- Prevent seizures
- Promote healing

Preventing the spread of infection includes use of Standard Precautions and droplet precautions.

The patient's room should be quiet and dimly lit. Sudden noises or bright flashes of light can cause a seizure because the sensory input activates nerve impulses. Care and treatments are coordinated to allow as much rest as possible. Meningitis often produces mental confusion and delirium as well as the possibility of seizures.

Clinical Cues

The presence of herpes lesions, in addition to drying of the lips and mouth from fever and dehydration, requires special mouth care. Using Standard Precautions (see Appendix B), the lips and mouth should be cleansed and lubricated at least every 2 hours during the acute stage of the disease.

Fluid volume deficit is a common problem. Monitor the patient's intake and output and prevent dehydration. Report excessive vomiting or outward signs of early dehydration promptly so that IV fluids may be given to correct fluid volume deficits.

The patient will need support and reassurance because the severity of this illness is frightening. If confusion occurs, frequent orientation is necessary. The family needs information and reassurance as well.

Once the acute stage of the disease is over, the patient can gradually resume their former activities. Side effects of the disease, such as paralysis, deafness, and visual defects, sometimes occur, but these *sequelae* (results) of meningitis do not usually occur if the disease is diagnosed and treated in the early stages. Gather evaluation data regarding the effect of the interventions performed. Determine whether the expected outcomes are being met. If outcomes are not being met, the plan must be revised.

ENCEPHALITIS

Etiology and Pathophysiology

Encephalitis is less common than meningitis. It is an acute inflammation of the brain that is serious and sometimes fatal. Meningitis can progress to encephalitis when, in addition to the meninges, brain tissue is involved. Encephalitis can occur without meningeal irritation. If both the brain and meninges are affected, it is called meningoencephalitis. Some of the viruses responsible for encephalitis are associated with seasons of the year or with geographic locations. Ticks and mosquitoes are the vectors that transmit the disease. Examples of viruses in the United States that cause encephalitis are eastern equine encephalomyelitis, western equine encephalomyelitis, La Crosse encephalitis, St. Louis encephalitis, and West Nile viruses. Encephalitis may occur as a complication of the viral diseases chickenpox, measles, and mumps. Postviral encephalitis is an immune-mediated disorder and follows the end of the viral infection by 2 to 12 days. Herpes simplex virus 1 (human herpesvirus 1) is commonly the cause of non–vector-transmitted encephalitis. Cytomegalovirus encephalitis is a complication in patients with AIDS.

Health Promotion

Protect Against Mosquitoes and Ticks

During mosquito season, wear insect repellent and protective clothing. Prevent water from standing in containers around the home and property to discourage the breeding of mosquitoes. Avoid being out of doors for recreational purposes at dusk and at night, when mosquitoes are more likely to be out. Use insect repellent and protective clothing when out in wooded areas. Skin should be inspected for ticks after the outing.

Clinical Cues

Whenever a patient is admitted with symptoms of a brain infection, check the skin thoroughly and question the patient about a recent history of herpes lesions. If you find any herpes lesions or are told that they were present within the past several days, notify the health care provider immediately. Herpes encephalitis can be fatal if not treated early.

Once the virus crosses the blood-brain barrier and enters neural cells, disrupting normal neural function, hemorrhage and an inflammatory response occur in the gray matter. Different viruses have affinity for different types of cells, which explains the variation in symptoms produced by each virus.

The severity of the illness may be mild or fatal. The most common types of viral encephalitis in the United States are caused by herpes simplex virus 1, West Nile virus, and the enteroviruses (Said & Kang, 2018).

Neurologic impairment is caused by direct infection of neural cells. Western equine encephalitis is usually seen in June and July. Herpes simplex encephalitis spreads from neural tissue to the CNS. It can be a primary or secondary infection and can occur from reactivation of latent virus. **If treatment for herpes simplex encephalitis is not started before coma occurs, death is almost certain.**

Signs, Symptoms, and Diagnosis

The onset of encephalitis may be sudden or insidious. There may be behavioral and personality changes and a decreased LOC. **Stiff neck, photophobia, and lethargy are classic symptoms of encephalitis. Seizures, acute confusion, and flaccid paralysis may occur.** CNS signs usually appear 1 to 4 hours after the onset of other symptoms. Lethargy may progress to coma. A patient with herpes simplex encephalitis may exhibit flulike symptoms that rapidly progress.

Encephalitis symptoms differ from those of meningitis in that with encephalitis there is altered mental status, motor or sensory deficits, and speech or movement disorders.

Diagnosis is confirmed by the presence of the virus in the CSF or bloodstream. The CSF in herpes simplex encephalitis will show a slightly elevated white blood cell count, a small increase in protein, and normal glucose levels. PCR tests for herpes simplex virus DNA and RNA levels in CSF allow for early diagnosis. MRI, PET scanning, and an EEG may be performed to demonstrate inflammation and the disruption of normal neural impulses. A brain biopsy may be required to verify the responsible organism so that proper treatment can begin.

Treatment and Nursing Management

The treatment of encephalitis is primarily symptomatic, with general supportive measures to maintain cardiac and respiratory function, maintain the patient's strength, promote healing, and prevent complications. Herpes simplex type 1 encephalitis is treated with antiviral IV acyclovir. There is no specific drug treatment for other types of encephalitis.

Specific nursing measures are essentially the same as for any patient who is subject to seizures, high fever, delirium, or altered LOC (see Chapter 21, Table 21.9). The nursing care plan must be individualized to the patient's needs.

Complications

Permanent neurologic disabilities may occur, such as problems with walking, paralysis, cognition, memory, and self-care. About 65% of encephalitis survivors have long-term problems.

BRAIN ABSCESS

A brain abscess is a collection of purulent material in a cavity within the brain. A bacterial infection that has traveled from the gums or teeth, sinus, ear, or mastoid region to the brain usually is the cause. An abscess can form from bacteria introduced at the time of any type of head injury or cranial surgery. **Signs and symptoms are headache, fever, and progression to lethargy and confusion.** If the abscess is not treated, ICP will rise as the size of the abscess increases. Teach patients who experience sinus infections with purulent drainage to seek treatment if symptoms last for more than a few days. A combination of antibiotics is used to eradicate the abscess. Surgery may be required to drain the abscess or relieve ICP.

HEADACHES

Headaches are the most common cause of complaints of pain. Headaches are commonly caused by allergy and related sinus problems or by tension, or they are vascular in origin. Arthritis, cervical spondylitis, and temporomandibular joint syndrome may also cause headaches. The pain of a headache may be minor or severe. Persistent headache requires testing to rule out organic problems such as anemia, brain tumor, or cerebral aneurysm.

Treatment for severe, recurrent headaches begins with determining the cause, if possible, and identifying factors that seem to precipitate the headache. Mild headaches usually are relieved by rest and a mild analgesic.

MIGRAINE HEADACHES

Approximately 30 million Americans have at least one migraine headache a year. Women experience them more often than men. Multiple theories have been presented as to the cause of migraines, and advances in imaging and laboratory studies have produced more knowledge about the process. The actual mechanism is not known but is thought to arise in the nervous system itself, altering the constriction and dilation of cerebral vessels, producing the headache symptoms characteristic of migraine. Attacks usually occur irregularly and may begin with an aura such as visual disturbances or "spots before the eyes" (**scotoma**). Many patients with migraine do not have an aura preceding the attack. Pain usually begins on one side of the head and is described as throbbing in character. A migraine headache is often accompanied by nausea and vomiting. Symptoms may last for 4 to 72 hours. Light or sound causes irritation and sensitivity, and for some patients with migraine, certain types of light set off the headache. Frequent migraine headaches are very debilitating.

Safety Alert

Triptans and Antidepressant Use

Patients who are taking triptans as migraine medication should not also take antidepressant or mood disorder medications that are selective serotonin reuptake inhibitors (SSRIs) or selective serotonin-norepinephrine reuptake inhibitors (SNRIs). There is a greater risk of increased serotonin levels occurring if triptans are combined with SSRIs or SNRIs, and the resulting serotonin syndrome can be life threatening. Signs and symptoms of serotonin syndrome include restlessness, hallucinations, loss of coordination, tachycardia, rapid changes in blood pressure, hyperthermia, overactive reflexes, nausea, vomiting, and diarrhea. Consult with the health care provider rather than abruptly stopping the SSRI or SNRI medication.

Treatment involves preventive measures as well as intervention for acute pain. Lying in a darkened, quiet, odor-free room with eyes closed decreases the symptoms. Sometimes doing this at the very beginning of symptoms can prevent a full-blown migraine headache. Various behavioral treatments such as biofeedback, acupuncture, and relaxation therapy, combined with lifestyle adjustments and medication, seem to offer the best result. Prevention strategies help decrease sensitivity of the neurologic system, preventing new attacks (National Institute of Neurological Disorders and Stroke [NINDS], 2018).

Treatment consists of using one or more of the agents listed in Box 23.2. A cold compress to the temple, eye, and occiput areas is helpful. Identifying food or other substances that seem to trigger an attack is very important.

If migraine headache tends to occur around the time of menses, hormone therapy may be effective in preventing the headache.

Box 23.2 Medications Used for Migraine Headache Treatment

DRUGS THAT ABORT MIGRAINE SYMPTOMS

- Acetaminophen-isometheptene-dichloralphenazone (Midrin)
- Almotriptan (Axert)
- Dihydroergotamine (D.H.E. 45 injection, Migranal nasal spray)
- Eletriptan (Relpax)
- Ergotamine tartrate (Cafergot)
- Frovatriptan (Frova)
- Methysergide (Sansert)
- Naratriptan (Amerge, Naramig)
- Rizatriptan (Maxalt, Maxalt-MLT)
- Sumatriptan (Imitrex, Imigran)
- Zolmitriptan (Zomig, Zomig ZMT)

PREVENTIVE DRUGS (TAKEN DAILY)

- Level A: Established efficacy
  - Divalproex sodium (Depakote)
  - Frovatriptan (Frova)
  - Metoprolol (Toprol)
  - Propranolol (Inderal)
  - Timolol (Blocadren)
  - Topiramate (Topamax)
  - *Monthly injections*
    - Erenumab (Aimovig)
    - Fremanezumab (Ajovy)
- Level B: Probably effective
  - Amitriptyline (Elavil)
  - Atenolol (Tenormin)
  - Nadolol (Corgard)
  - Naratriptan (Amerge)
  - Venlafaxine (Effexor)
  - Zolmitriptan (Zomig)

Nutrition Considerations

Finding Foods That Trigger a Migraine Headache

Ask patients who have migraine headaches to keep a food diary to determine whether any of the following foods or additives are triggering the attacks:

- Alcohol
- Caffeine
- Chocolate
- Artificial sweeteners (aspartame, sucralose, saccharin)
- Monosodium glutamate (MSG)
- Citrus fruits
- Meats with nitrites (bacon, salami, etc.)
- Salt
- Foods containing tyramines: peanuts, raisins, vinegars, soy sauce, aged cheese, yogurt, sour cream, chicken livers, sausages, bananas, avocados, pickled herring, freshly baked breads, pork, beans

Noninvasive neuromodulation devices are available for preventative and acute symptom treatment. Transcutaneous treatment modalities include single-pulse transcranial magnetic stimulation, vagus nerve stimulator, supraorbital stimulation, and anodal transcranial direct current stimulation. Implanted devices are also used for patients with long-term chronic conditions who have not responded well to medications. OnabotulinumtoxinA (Botox) injected into neck and shoulder muscles has been shown to have a preventative effect (Blumenfeld, 2018).

Complementary and Alternative Therapies

Nutraceuticals

Food or dietary supplements taken for health benefits are known as nutraceuticals. Riboflavin (vitamin B_2), coenzyme Q10 (CoQ10), magnesium, butterbur root extract *(Petasites hybridus)*, and feverfew *(Tanacetum parthenium)* have all been shown to have some benefit in migraine prevention (Puledda & Shields, 2018).

CLUSTER HEADACHES

Cluster headaches have a higher incidence in men and are not as common as migraine headaches. A cluster headache causes the most severe headache pain. The pain has abrupt onset and usually lasts 30 to 90 minutes. It may start during sleep. The headache may recur several times a day, and the clusters usually last 2 to 3 months. The cause and pathophysiology are not clearly known, but the trigeminal nerve is implicated. Vasodilation occurs, causing the headache. It is believed that the disorder may be caused by dysfunction of the biological clock mechanisms of the hypothalamus. Alcohol can trigger this type of headache.

Signs and symptoms include severe unilateral orbital, supraorbital, or temporal pain along with one of the following: redness of the conjunctiva of the eye, tearing, nasal congestion, dripping nose, facial swelling, pupil constriction, or **ptosis** (drooping) of the eyelid. The person becomes restless, often paces the floor, and is sensitive to touch.

History usually is sufficient to diagnose a cluster headache, but CT, MRI, or magnetic resonance angiography may be performed to rule out tumor, aneurysm, or infection. Treatment for cluster headache includes a combination of analgesics and 100% oxygen by face mask, sumatriptan succinate (Imitrex) and other triptans, internasal lidocaine 4% aqueous solution, or oral ergotamine. Opiates are not generally used because they do not treat the cause of the headache and are not very effective in relieving neurologic pain.

TENSION HEADACHES

Tension headaches are quite common but are not as severe as migraine or cluster headaches. This type of headache usually also involves neck stiffness and limitation of range of motion of the neck. Analgesic medication, muscle relaxants, tension-reducing medication or relaxation techniques, massage, yoga, and biofeedback are often helpful. Biofeedback can be very effective in preventing or averting headaches for many people.

Safety Alert

Caution When Taking Analgesics

Fiorinal should not be used long term because it contains a barbiturate and is habit forming. Drugs containing acetaminophen should be used within the dosage guidelines and should not be used daily; acetaminophen can cause liver failure and impaired renal function. The guideline is to refrain from taking more than 4 g of acetaminophen per 24 hours. Remind patients who take acetaminophen not to combine it with alcohol because doing so can cause liver damage in some people. Those taking aspirin, ibuprofen, or a drug containing either should monitor themselves for peptic ulcer and gastric bleeding, as both aspirin and ibuprofen have an antiplatelet effect. Signs and symptoms to report are epigastric pain, dyspepsia, black stool, or vomiting of blood. Fatigue, headache, and dizziness may indicate anemia from a slow gastric bleed.

CRANIAL NERVE DISORDERS

TRIGEMINAL NEURALGIA (TIC DOULOUREUX)

Etiology and Pathophysiology

Trigeminal neuralgia is a relatively rare facial pain syndrome. The cause of trigeminal neuralgia is related to pressure on the nerve root. In rare cases this pressure is caused by a tumor or a lesion of the blood vessels. In 80% to 90% of cases the pressure is caused by an abnormal loop of an artery or vein. Multiple sclerosis can be a factor. In many cases no cause can be found, and the disorder is considered idiopathic. This disorder most commonly affects people older than 60 years.

Trigeminal neuralgia involves one or more branches of the fifth cranial (trigeminal) nerve. The three branches of this nerve are the ophthalmic, the mandibular, and the maxillary (Fig. 23.11). In most cases of trigeminal neuralgia, the ophthalmic nerve is not involved. The mechanism of pain production is controversial. It may be a result of demyelination caused by the compression

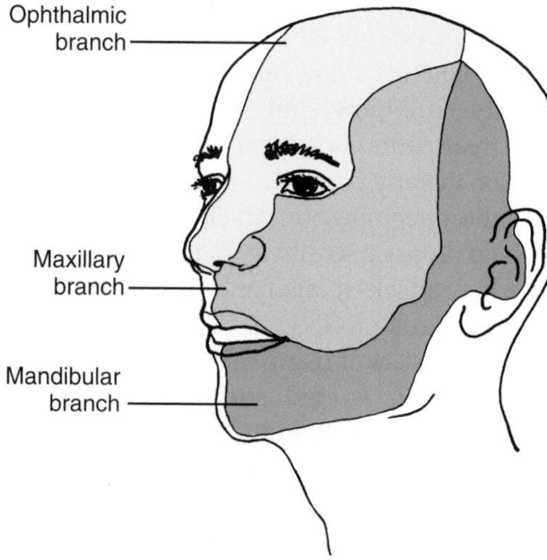

Fig. 23.11 Areas of innervation by each of the three branches of the trigeminal nerve.

of the nerve leading to "cross-talk" between nerves (Bajwa, Ho, & Khan, 2018).

Signs, Symptoms, and Diagnosis

The most notable symptom of trigeminal neuralgia is severe facial pain, which is described as sharp and intense, lasting for 1 to 2 minutes, and located along the pathway of one of the branches of the trigeminal nerve. The pain is localized on one side of the face, rarely affecting both sides. It can extend from the midline of the face across the cheek and jaw to the ear.

Attacks are usually triggered by exposure to drafts, light touch or vibration, drinking cold or very hot liquids, chewing, brushing the hair, shaving, or washing the face. The pain causes a brief muscle spasm of the facial muscles—the tic. Between acute flare-ups the patient may experience no pain or may report a dull ache. The pain during the acute phase is so severe that many patients live in constant fear that they will do something to provoke an attack.

Diagnosis is based on the patient's history and chief complaint and on tests to rule out a cerebellopontine angle tumor that is affecting the nerve. There is no test to confirm the diagnosis, and there are no observable pathologic changes.

Treatment

Medical management usually is preferred to surgical intervention. The drugs typically prescribed to prevent or relieve spasmodic pain are the anticonvulsant medications carbamazepine (Tegretol) and oxcarbazepine (Oxtellar), and the muscle relaxant baclofen (Lioresal). Medications listed as anticonvulsants such as gabapentin (Neurontin) and pregabalin (Lyrica) are used for neuropathic pain. Relief of severe pain may require surgical or interventional procedures. Microvascular decompression is a surgical procedure for those patients with a known compression of the nerve that can be surgically corrected. **Ablation** (removal or destruction of a body part or its function) procedures to destroy the nerve pathways delivering the pain messages can be done in a variety of ways. **Rhizotomy** (destruction of a spinal nerve root) can be performed with radiofrequency thermocoagualtion, mechanical balloon compression, or chemical injection. Radiosurgery, peripheral neurectomy, and nerve blocks may also be used.

❖ NURSING MANAGEMENT

◆ ASSESSMENT (DATA COLLECTION) AND NURSING DIAGNOSIS

Observing the patient between acute attacks can help identify clues to confirm the presence of trigeminal neuralgia. The patient may not want to wash their face (male patients may not want to shave), and the patient will guard their face or hold it immobile to avoid an attack. The patient is very sensitive to any contact with the face and will indicate the area of pain by pointing to but never touching it.

The problem for patients with trigeminal neuralgia is, of course, pain. Because chewing can provoke an attack of pain, the patient may be susceptible to nutritional deficit. Small, frequent feedings consisting of food that is moderately warm can help provide adequate nutrition while avoiding precipitating an acute attack.

◆ PLANNING, IMPLEMENTATION, AND EVALUATION

Specific expected outcomes are written for the patient regarding the control of pain and its triggers. Nursing interventions for a patient who is being treated medically include instruction about the expected actions and adverse side effects of the prescribed medications. Carbamazepine can damage the bone marrow and produce such hematologic reactions as leukopenia, aplastic anemia, and decreased platelet count. Skin eruptions also can occur as a reaction to carbamazepine or baclofen. The patient's blood count and liver function must be closely monitored to detect early signs of drug toxicity. Baclofen may cause transient drowsiness, nausea, weakness, or fatigue.

Surgical treatment of trigeminal neuralgia results in a potential for damage to the cornea when the ophthalmic branch is dissected. The patient must be taught to avoid rubbing their eyes or exposing themself to foreign objects because the normal protective corneal reflex is no longer functional. They should get into the habit of wearing protective goggles when there is the possibility of getting dust and debris in the eyes, and they should try to blink their eyes often to cleanse their surfaces.

Dissection of the second or third branches of the trigeminal nerve creates a risk of potential damage to the oral mucosa and teeth. The patient cannot feel hot liquids and foods and could be burned, could bite the inside of the mouth without realizing it, or may have dental caries that will not cause pain. Good oral hygiene and periodic dental examinations are particularly important when the body's natural warning system is not operative. Immediately postoperatively, an ice pack is applied to the cheek for 3 to 4 hours to prevent swelling.

Evaluation data are gathered to determine whether the specific expected outcomes are being met.

BELL PALSY

Bell palsy is weakness or paralysis of the muscles supplied by the facial nerve. It usually affects only one side of the face and usually occurs in people older than 30 years. The disorder affects about 23 in 100,000 people and typically affects the right side of the face. The etiology of Bell palsy is controversial. It is believed to be caused by edema and ischemia that compresses the facial nerve. The herpes simplex type 1 and herpes zoster viruses are believed to be a cause (Taylor, 2018). Stress can also be a factor. Exposure to cold is a risk factor. Sometimes the disorder occurs during pregnancy, most often in the third trimester. **Signs and symptoms are numbness and partial or total paralysis of the facial muscles suddenly or over a few days.** There may be taste disturbances. The eyelid on the affected side loses its blink reflex and the mouth droops, causing problems with drooling.

Diagnosis is by patient history and exclusion of other neurologic or muscular disorders and Lyme disease. If the patient is asked to raise the eyebrows, the eyebrow on the affected side will not move. When asked to smile, the face becomes distorted because the affected side of the mouth and face will not move normally.

Treatment consists of closing and patching the eye if it loses the blink reflex. Artificial tear eye drops also are used to prevent dryness of the cornea. Corticosteroids are given if they can be started right after the beginning of symptoms. They are ineffective if delayed for more than 7 days. Acyclovir may be prescribed as well because herpes virus may be a causative organism (Taylor, 2018). Recovery is individual; some patients with total paralysis may not achieve full recovery but will improve as inflammation declines. Between 80% and 90% of patients recover completely within 6 weeks to 3 months. Bell palsy recurs in 10% to 15% of patients.

Get Ready for the NCLEX® Examination!

Key Points

- Many conditions can cause a seizure. Epilepsy is a chronic condition in which abnormal electrical activity is triggered in the brain without an underlying metabolic cause.
- Seizures are classified as generalized or focal.
- Irreversible brain damage can occur if seizures are unrelenting and uncontrolled.
- Treatment of epilepsy is by drugs and/or surgery (see Box 23.1).
- Close observation of a seizure with documentation is very helpful (see Focused Assessment: Observations to Make During a Seizure).
- Patient education is extremely important for safety and for the prevention of recurrent seizures.
- A cerebrovascular accident is caused by a thrombus, embolus, or intracranial hemorrhage that interrupts circulation to an area of the brain.
- Risk factors for stroke are high blood pressure, atherosclerosis, cigarette smoking, excessive alcohol intake, insufficient exercise, high cholesterol, obesity, and diabetes.
- tPA is best given within 3 to 4.5 hours of the onset of symptoms to be effective for thrombotic stroke.
- Cerebral aneurysms and arteriovenous malformations may leak or burst and cause a stroke.
- Subarachnoid hemorrhage is a medical emergency.
- A thrombosis causes cerebral ischemia that may progress slowly; an embolus causes sudden neurologic deficits.
- Homonymous hemianopsia, hemiplegia or hemiparesis, agnosia, apraxia, aphasia, and dysphagia are some of the problems caused by a CVA.
- Fatigue and emotional lability with crying or outburst may be common after a stroke or other injury to the brain, depending on the area of the brain involved.
- Hydrocephalus may be a complication of several disorders of the brain; a shunt can be placed to divert the excess CSF to the peritoneal cavity or right atrium (see Fig. 23.9).
- Rehabilitation is extremely important for stroke patients and takes extensive work.
- Brain tumors may be benign or malignant; many are metastatic from a different malignant site (see Table 23.2).
- Brain tumors compress adjacent tissue, causing problems and increased ICP.
- Some common signs of brain tumors are personality change, disturbance in judgment and memory, loss of muscular strength and coordination, and difficulty speaking clearly. Headache, projectile vomiting, visual problems, and signs of increased ICP may be present.
- Depending on the site and type of brain tumor, treatment is by surgery, radiation, and/or chemotherapy.
- Viral and bacterial infections cause the inflammation of the membranes covering the brain and spinal cord in meningitis.
- Severe and persistent headache with nuchal rigidity are classic signs of meningitis, but a lumbar puncture is needed for diagnosis.
- Meningitis causes an increase in ICP.
- West Nile virus is a cause of encephalitis and is spread by mosquitoes.
- Encephalitis is most commonly the result of a viral infection or the toxins produced by viral organisms such as measles, chickenpox, and mumps.
- Stiff neck, photophobia, and lethargy are classic symptoms of encephalitis.
- Nursing care for encephalitis is focused on the problems of seizures, high fever, and delirium resulting from altered LOC (see Chapter 21, Table 21.9).
- A brain abscess can develop from a severe sinus, ear, tooth, or gum infection.
- Headaches are common, and approximately 23 million Americans get migraine headaches.
- Tracking triggers for migraine, avoiding them, and taking medication help prevent migraine attacks (see Nutrition Considerations: Finding Foods That Trigger a Migraine Headache).
- Migraine may be preceded by an aura and most often causes pain on one side of the head.
- Cluster headaches cause severe pain and tend to be periodic in nature.
- Trigeminal neuralgia is a painful disorder affecting the fifth cranial nerve and the muscles of the face. Only one side of the face is usually affected.
- Bell palsy is believed to be caused by edema and ischemia that compress the facial nerve. It causes weakness or paralysis of the muscles supplied by the nerve.

- Numbness and partial or total paralysis of the facial muscles, usually on one side, occur with Bell palsy.
- Corticosteroids and acyclovir are the drugs used to treat Bell palsy.

Additional Learning Resources

SG Go to your Study Guide for additional learning activities to help you master this chapter content.

Go to your Evolve website (http://evolve.elsevier.com/deWit/medsurg) for the following FREE learning resources:

- Animations, audio, and video
- Answers and rationales for questions and activities
- Glossary with pronunciations in English and Spanish
- Interactive Review Questions and more!

Review Questions for the NCLEX® Examination

1. You determine that the appropriate problem statement for a patient with status epilepticus is *Potential for injury due to seizure activity.* An appropriate expected outcome would be:
   1. Everyone will stay calm during the episodes.
   2. The caregiver will stay with the patient during the episodes.
   3. The patient will be free from any injuries associated with the seizures.
   4. Standing orders will be obtained to medicate acute seizure episodes.

   NCLEX Client Need: Safe and Effective Care Environment: Safety and Infection Control
2. Nursing care of a patient who *just* had a seizure includes which nursing intervention(s)? *(Select all that apply.)*
   1. Assess for injuries.
   2. Check the glucose level.
   3. Reassure and reorient the patient.
   4. Provide uninterrupted periods of sleep and rest.
   5. Provide a 24-hour sitter.

   NCLEX Client Need: Physiological Integrity: Reduction of Risk Potential
3. Which patient statement indicates a need for further teaching on the prevention of seizures?
   1. "I need to avoid situations that could potentially trigger a seizure."
   2. "Alcohol can lower the seizure threshold."
   3. "I must avoid becoming overly fatigued and should pace activities."
   4. "I am less likely to have seizures during menstruation."

   NCLEX Client Need: Health Promotion and Maintenance
4. A man and his wife are sitting in their pajamas in the living room when the man cries out. He attempts to rise from his chair, but he falls when he discovers that the left side of his body has become paralyzed. The left side of his mouth and his left eye are drooping. What should his wife do?
   1. Help him stand and walk to the car. She can drive him to the hospital because it is only 3 miles away. He will receive care more immediately than if the wife calls an ambulance.
   2. Sit with him for an hour to see if his condition resolves. If it worsens, she should transport him to the hospital.
   3. Call 911 immediately. The emergency team will be able to assess him, give supportive care, and transport him.
   4. Assess his pulse and breathing. If he is in no immediate cardiac distress, she can help him change into street clothes before driving him to the hospital.

   NCLEX Client Need: Health Promotion and Maintenance
5. Which are *true* regarding a stroke? *(Select all that apply.)*
   1. Timing of treatment is important.
   2. A fibrinolytic drug will be given.
   3. Clinical signs and symptoms determine if the stroke ischemic or hemorrhagic.
   4. A CT scan should be done within 20 minutes of arrival at the hospital.
   5. It may occur as a complication of atrial fibrillation.

   NCLEX Client Need: Physiological Integrity: Physiological Adaptation
6. A patient has had a cerebrovascular accident. You assess the patient's readiness for transfer to another level of care. The patient continues to have agnosia and apraxia. These clinical findings indicate that the patient would:
   1. require assistance with undertaking activities of daily living.
   2. demonstrate independence in performing ordinary tasks.
   3. prompt self to complete sequential tasks.
   4. not understand verbal communication.

   NCLEX Client Need: Physiological Integrity: Physiological Adaptation
7. Intracranial tumors may be treated by several modes of therapy. What types of therapy are you likely to see? *(Select all that apply.)*
   1. Insertion of tiny radioactive particles into the tumor
   2. High oral doses of iron for 5 days, followed by a selenium infusion
   3. Brain surgery where most or all of the tumor is removed
   4. Chemotherapy through a reservoir that is placed between the scalp and the skull to get past the blood-brain barrier

   NCLEX Client Need: Physiological Integrity: Physiological Adaptation

8. A 21-year-old man complains of a sudden onset of fever, severe headache, and stiffness of the neck. You note a petechial rash over the chest and extremities. Which nursing action(s) would be appropriate? *(Select all that apply.)*
   1. Institute Standard Precautions and droplet precautions.
   2. Administer antibiotics as prescribed.
   3. Maintain a quiet and dimly lit patient room.
   4. Encourage active range-of-motion exercises.
   5. Administer narcotic analgesics for headache and neck pain.

   NCLEX Client Need: Physiological Integrity: Basic Care
9. A patient is admitted to the urgent care center for complaints of an abrupt onset of severe headache. Clinical history indicates that symptoms started during sleep and recurred several times during the day. These symptoms suggest:
   1. brain tumor.
   2. migraine.
   3. cluster headaches.
   4. tension headaches.

   NCLEX Client Need: Physiological Integrity: Physiological Adaptation
10. You are providing care to a 60-year-old patient with trigeminal neuralgia, and you identify that pain is the priority problem. You anticipate:
    1. assessing the level of pain based on facial expressions.
    2. administering an anticonvulsant class of medication.
    3. placing warm cloths on the face.
    4. preparing the patient for surgery.

    NCLEX Client Need: Physiological Integrity: Pharmacological Therapies

Critical Thinking Questions

Scenario A

Jack Thompson, age 36 years, had a seizure while walking down the hall at work. He fell to the ground and demonstrated jerking motions of his body.

1. What type of seizure is this most likely to be?
2. What observations should be made if he has another seizure?
3. How would you care for Mr. Thompson after the seizure is over?
4. If Mr. Thompson is diagnosed with epilepsy, what patient teaching will he need?

Scenario B

Part I.

Bob Foster is a 77-year-old retired teacher who complained of a severe headache during dinner and then slumped over the table, unconscious. He was rushed to the hospital, and a tentative diagnosis of CVA was made.

1. What diagnostic tests might be appropriate for Mr. Foster?
2. What emergency care could you have given Mr. Foster if you had been present at dinner?

Part II.

Mr. Foster's diagnostic tests indicate a subarachnoid hemorrhage from a ruptured aneurysm. He is comatose; his pupils are equal and reactive to light; and he responds to pain with flexor posturing, opens his eyes at random, and seems to be paralyzed on the right side.

1. What are the priorities of care for Mr. Foster?
2. If Mr. Foster survives, what potential complications might he experience from the intracerebral hemorrhage?

Scenario C

Janice Pringle, age 19 years, has been experiencing headaches more frequently over the past 6 months. She comes to the student health center on her college campus to seek help. This headache is very bad, and she is nauseated.

1. What subjective and objective assessment data would you gather regarding this young woman and her headaches?
2. What are your priorities of care for Janice?
3. What interventions would you suggest at this time?

Care of Patients With Peripheral Nerve and Degenerative Neurologic Disorders

24

http://evolve.elsevier.com/deWit/medsurg

Objectives

Theory

1. Compare and contrast the pathophysiology of Parkinson disease and myasthenia gravis.
2. Examine treatments for Parkinson disease.
3. Discuss the nursing care needed for a patient with Parkinson disease.
4. Explain why multiple sclerosis might be difficult to diagnose.
5. Illustrate the differences between Huntington disease and amyotrophic lateral sclerosis.
6. Recognize the signs and symptoms of myasthenia gravis.
7. Compare and contrast the complications of Parkinson disease with those of myasthenia gravis.

Clinical Practice

8. Teach a newly diagnosed patient about the medications for Parkinson disease.
9. Teach a patient about the diagnostic tests that might be ordered if multiple sclerosis is suspected.
10. Write a nursing care plan for a patient with myasthenia gravis who is hospitalized with a respiratory infection.
11. Summarize a home care plan for a patient with multiple sclerosis.
12. Choose a nursing care plan for a patient with Guillain-Barré syndrome.

Key Terms

bradykinesia (brā-dē-kĭ-NĒ-zē-ă, p. 568)
chorea (kă-RĒ-ă, p. 579)
demyelination (dĕ-MĪ-ĕ-lĭ-nā-shŭn, p. 574)
diplopia (dĭ-PLŌ-pē-ă, p. 579)
hyperesthesia (hī-pĕr-ĕs-THĒ-zē-ă, p. 577)

Concepts Covered in This Chapter

- Functional Ability
- Self-Management
- Inflammation
- Mobility
- Sensory Perception
- Cognition
- Patient Education
- Collaboration
- Care Coordination

PARKINSON DISEASE

Parkinson disease (PD) is named after James Parkinson, who first described the syndrome in 1871. PD is considered a major health problem because of its crippling effects. It is a progressive disorder, beginning rapidly at first and then advancing more slowly. It affects more men than women and occurs most commonly after age 60 years. Approximately 7.5 million people in the world are affected with PD, and about 60,000 people in the United States are diagnosed with PD each year. The term *parkinsonism* is used to describe a clinical syndrome consisting of any combination of the following symptoms: bradykinesia, rest tremor, rigidity, and postural instability.

ETIOLOGY

The specific cause of PD is unknown, but it involves degeneration of the dopamine-producing neurons in the substantia nigra of the midbrain and the presence of Lewy bodies (cytoplasmic inclusions). Genetic susceptibility and environmental toxins appear to play a role. A history of head trauma increases risk (Jankovic, 2018). The most common type of PD is *idiopathic*—that is, the primary or specific cause is not known. Secondary PD can be drug induced, especially by reserpine-type antihypertensives such as methyldopa, phenothiazines, some tranquilizers such as the butyrophenones (e.g., haloperidol [Haldol]), some antiemetics, methamphetamine, and a few other drugs. These drugs block the uptake of dopamine at the receptors in the brain cells and therefore may induce PD symptoms. Pesticide and herbicide exposure is largely implicated as a cause of PD.

PATHOPHYSIOLOGY

PD affects the extrapyramidal system, particularly the motor structures in the basal ganglia. This is the part of the brain that controls balance and coordination. The basal ganglia are gray matter that is scattered throughout the white matter of the cerebrum beneath the cerebral

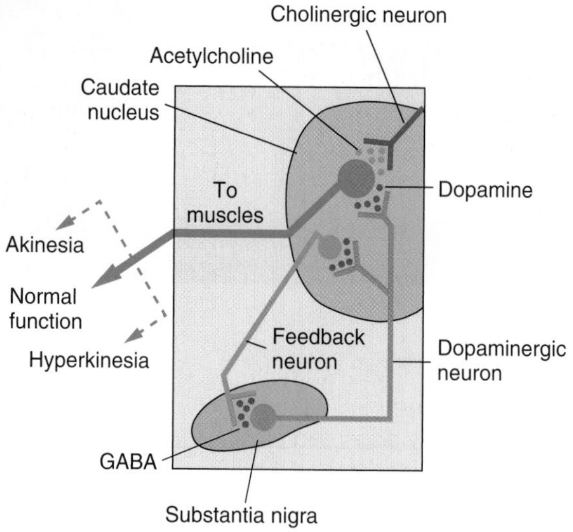

Fig. 24.1 Dopaminergic synaptic activity is mediated by dopamine. Cholinergic synaptic activity is mediated by acetylcholine. A balance between the two kinds of synaptic activity produces normal motor function. A relative excess of cholinergic activity produces akinesia and rigidity. A relative excess of dopaminergic activity produces involuntary movements. *GABA*, Gamma-aminobutyric acid. (From Lewis SL, Heitkemper MM, Dirksen SR, et al.: *Medical-surgical nursing: assessment and management of clinical problems*, ed 8, St. Louis, 2011, Elsevier.)

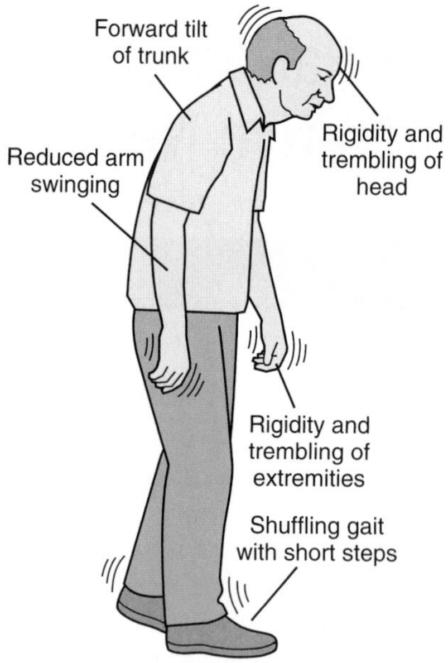

Fig. 24.2 Parkinson disease causes abnormalities of movement. Movements are jerky in nature.

cortex. Stimulation of the basal ganglia causes muscle tone in the body to be inhibited and allows refined voluntary movements. Two neurotransmitters accomplish this action: dopamine and acetylcholine (ACh) (see Chapter 21, Table 21.3, for the action of the common neurotransmitters). ACh-producing neurons transmit excitatory messages throughout the basal ganglia. Dopamine inhibits the function of these neurons to allow for control of voluntary movement (Fig. 24.1). There is usually a balance between these neurotransmitters. The degenerative changes in the basal ganglia that occur in PD lead to a decrease in dopamine. The ACh-secreting neurons remain active, creating an imbalance between excitatory and inhibitory neuronal activity. The excessive excitation of neurons prevents a person from controlling or initiating voluntary movements.

SIGNS AND SYMPTOMS

The onset of PD is gradual and may involve only one side of the body initially. A triad of symptoms is characteristic of PD: tremor, bradykinesia, and rigidity. The first, *tremor,* occurs when the body is at rest, decreases when there is voluntary movement, and is absent when the patient is asleep. The tremor is most often a "pill-rolling" motion of the thumb against the fingers (a circular rubbing of a finger or two as if rolling a piece of string or fuzz into a "pill"). When the patient experiences stress and emotional tension, the tremor becomes more pronounced.

Bradykinesia (a condition that causes slow movement and speech) produces poor body balance, a characteristic gait, and difficulty initiating movement. The gait is shuffling, with short steps that become quicker (Fig. 24.2). There is decreased swinging of the arms when walking. A foot may drag or may be stiff, producing a limp. Earlier in the disease process, the patient may lean slightly to one side, propel forward uncontrollably, or fall backward. In advanced stages there is a stiff, bent-forward posture when walking.

The third symptom is *rigidity* affecting the skeletal muscles and contributing to postural changes and difficulty in movement. Postural changes affect coordination and balance. The face becomes blank or masklike in appearance with little or no expression. Speech becomes low in tone, monotonous sounding, and slow; enunciation becomes difficult because of the decreased dopamine and the excitatory response from the increased ACh. Drooling may occur. The patient may experience decreased tearing, constipation, incontinence, excessive perspiration, heat intolerance, and decreased sexual ability. PD does not usually affect intellect; however, a percentage of patients do develop a dementia similar to that of Alzheimer disease. Mood disturbance does occur, and depression is a problem. Stress tends to make symptoms worse.

? Think Critically

A patient comes into the clinic complaining about hand tremors and "stiffness" of the joints that started recently, excessive sweating, and some urinary incontinence. You notice that their gait is abnormal. What would be a priority question you would ask as you start history taking?

DIAGNOSIS

The characteristic symptoms of the disease are used to diagnose the disorder. Laboratory tests usually reveal findings within normal ranges. However, magnetic resonance imaging (MRI) of the brain may be performed

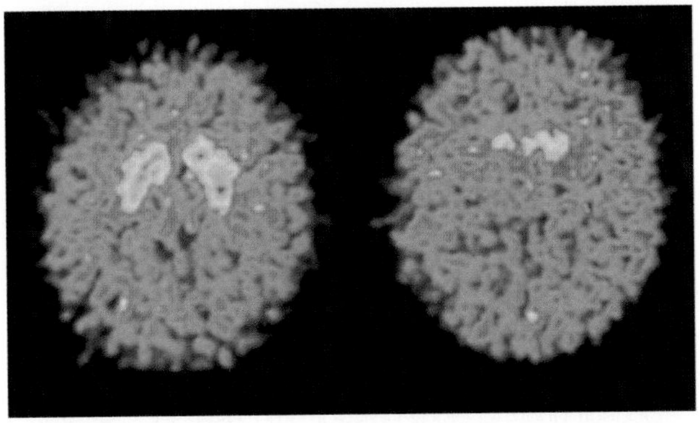

Fig. 24.3 Positron emission tomography scan showing reduced uptake of dopamine in a patient with Parkinson disease. (From Perkin DG: *Mosby's color atlas and text of neurology*, St. Louis, 2002, Mosby.)

to rule out other neurologic disorders. Single-photon emission computed tomography (SPECT) can display the reduced uptake of dopamine (Fig. 24.3).

TREATMENT

Treatment of PD usually includes drug therapy, physical therapy, and considerable emotional support. Currently, medications for PD all involve controlling symptoms, not slowing or controlling the disease (neuroprotective). Currently, no approved neuroprotective therapies are available. Drug therapy aims to provide dopamine to the basal ganglia and thus reduce symptoms. Anticholinergics, dopamine agonists, and monoamine oxidase inhibitors (MAOIs) are also used to control symptoms. MAOIs block the metabolism of dopamine, leaving more dopamine in circulation. Deep brain stimulation (DBS) is a surgical procedure used to treat many of the neurologic debilitating symptoms association with PD (National Institute of Neurological Disorders and Stroke [NINDS], 2018a). This procedure does not destroy tissue (as did previous PD surgeries) but serves to block transmission from certain targeted brain areas. Successful treatment usually involves a combination of these therapies.

! Safety Alert

Caution When Administering Monoamine Oxidase Inhibitors

When a patient with PD has been prescribed selegiline (an MAOI), caution them against eating foods containing tyramine, such as aged cheeses, anything fermented, smoked fish or meat, yeast extract, some imported beers, Chianti wine, dietary protein supplements, and soy sauce. Administering meperidine to someone taking an MAOI can cause **hyperpyrexia** (excessive elevation of temperature) and possible death. Many drugs interact adversely with MAOIs, and the health care provider or pharmacist should be consulted before a patient takes any other drug with an MAOI.

In the early stages of the disease when disability is not evident, selegiline (Eldepryl), a drug that increases dopamine's action, may be given. When disability is present, L-3,4-dihydroxyphenylalanine (L-Dopa or levodopa) or a combination of levodopa and carbidopa (Sinemet) is given. Sinemet is given in increasing doses until control of the symptoms is achieved; however, side effects can be troublesome (Box 24.1). Various drugs are used either alone or in combination with L-Dopa (Table 24.1).

Complementary and Alternative Therapies

Supplements Helpful for Parkinson Disease

Nutritional supplements that help slow the progression of PD include the enzyme NADH (nicotinamide adenine dinucleotide, 10 mg); coenzyme Q10 (100 to 200 mg); phosphatidylserine (200 to 300 mg); and the antioxidants ester-C (1000 mg twice a day), vitamin E as mixed tocopherols (400 mg), and alpha-lipoic acid (100 mg twice a day). Health care providers sometimes prescribe these supplements in addition to the treatment medications.

? Think Critically

What would be appropriate nursing interventions for a patient who is beginning to experience dysphagia?

Surgical Treatment

Stereotactic neurosurgery may be performed for implantation of DBS devices if the drug therapy fails to relieve a patient's PD symptoms.

DBS uses electrode implants to provide electrical shocks that control tremors by blocking them. The device that delivers the shocks can be adjusted as the patient's symptoms change or worsen (Slavin, 2018). There has been considerable success with DBS, but it is expensive: approximately $10,000 for the implant unit and another $8000 every few years for battery replacement. However, it has become the treatment of choice because it does not destroy brain tissue and it is reversible (Hauser, 2018).

Depression is common among patients with PD, but most respond well to a selective serotonin reuptake inhibitor (SSRI) antidepressant.

COMPLICATIONS

Dysphagia may develop, and mobility becomes severely limited as the disease progresses. Problems of immobility occur (see Chapter 9). Constipation, urinary incontinence, and insomnia are also common.

NURSING MANAGEMENT

ASSESSMENT (DATA COLLECTION) AND NURSING DIAGNOSIS

A thorough history is gathered, and a physical examination is performed for patients who have or are suspected to have PD. Nursing Care Plan 24.1 contains the common problem statements or nursing diagnoses, expected outcomes, and specific interventions for a patient with PD.

Box 24.1 Nursing Implications for Drugs Commonly Used for Parkinson Disease

WHEN GIVING A DRUG FOR PARKINSON DISEASE

- Pay close attention to dosage amount because therapy is individualized to each patient.
- Check other medications the patient is receiving for potential interactions with the antiparkinsonian drug, contraindicating administration of the drug.
- Administer the drugs as close to the time ordered as possible to maintain a consistent blood level of each drug.
- Carbidopa-levodopa may cause many neurologic disturbances, including psychiatric problems; discuss any onset of new symptoms with the health care provider.
- Administer anticholinergic medications with meals to decrease gastrointestinal irritation.
- Selegiline may increase the side effects of carbidopa-levodopa. If this occurs, seek an order to decrease the dosage.
- Monitor for effectiveness of each drug by observing for a decrease in symptoms, such as tremor, rigidity, or drooling; assess for decrease in side effects of carbidopa-levodopa when anticholinergic drugs are given for that purpose.
- Continually assess the patient for worsening of symptoms that may result from disease progression, side effects of medication, or failure of medication.

REGARDING POSSIBLE SIDE OR ADVERSE EFFECTS OF THE DRUG

- Monitor patients taking carbidopa-levodopa, amantadine, or bromocriptine for orthostatic hypotension and urinary retention.
- Assess patients who are taking carbidopa-levodopa for excessive or inappropriate sexual behavior.
- Bromocriptine may cause changes in mental status; report observed changes.
- Amantadine may cause insomnia and should not be administered at bedtime.
- Many of these drugs can cause nausea, dyspepsia, and abdominal pain.
- Anticholinergics are contraindicated in patients with acute narrow-angle glaucoma.
- Anticholinergics cause dry mouth and constipation; increase fluids to 3000 mL/day; treat constipation as needed per orders; add fiber to diet.
- Monitor blood pressure and pulse during initiation and adjustment of anticholinergic medication; report tachycardia.
- Consult pharmacology book or drug insert for specific side effects of each drug.

TEACHING FOR PATIENTS TAKING ANTIPARKINSONIAN DRUGS

- Selegiline may cause dizziness; warn patient to move cautiously during initiation of therapy.
- Orthostatic hypotension causes dizziness and can precipitate falls; it is important for the patient to allow the blood pressure to stabilize in a sitting position before standing, to rise slowly, and to ensure balance while holding on to something when standing before walking.
- Carbidopa-levodopa will turn the urine dark.
- Ropinirole (Requip) may cause drowsiness; advise the patient not to operate machinery or drive until adjusted to the drug.
- When taking a catechol-*O*-methyltransferase (COMT) inhibitor, it is important to have liver function checked regularly.
- Constipation is a problem with the anticholinergic drugs; increases in dietary fiber, plenty of fluid, and exercise can help control constipation; bowel movement frequency should be monitored to prevent impaction.
- Adjustment of dosages and combination of medications that will control symptoms with the fewest side effects may take weeks or months to accomplish.

Focused Assessment

Data Collection for a Patient With Symptoms of PD

Gather data regarding history by asking the following questions:

- Have you ever had a head injury, meningitis, encephalitis, or cerebrovascular disorder?
- Have you ever been exposed to metals, pesticides, or carbon monoxide for extended periods?
- What medications do you take? (Particularly important are major tranquilizers such as haloperidol [Haldol], phenothiazines, reserpine, methyldopa, and amphetamines.)
- Do you have a problem with fatigue?
- Have you noticed excessive salivation and problems handling secretions?
- Do you have any trouble swallowing?
- Have you been steadily losing weight?
- Do you experience constipation or urinary incontinence?
- Do you sweat excessively?
- Do you have difficulty initiating walking or other movements? Do you fall frequently?
- Has your dexterity decreased? Has your handwriting deteriorated?
- Do you have insomnia?
- Do you experience pain or cramping?
- Do you have mood swings? Are you depressed? Do you have hallucinations?

Points to cover in the physical examination:

- Presence of drooling
- Ability to swallow
- Facial expression or lack thereof
- Presence of ankle edema
- Evidence of postural hypotension
- Presence of tremor at rest; pill-rolling movements
- Rigidity of body and jerky movements of extremities
- Slow start, then quick, short steps when ambulating; shuffling gait with bent-forward posture
- Difficulty stopping once ambulating

Table 24.1 **Drugs Commonly Used for Patients With Parkinson Disease**

DRUG CLASSIFICATION	USE
Antiparkinsonian/Central Nervous System Agents	
Levodopa (L-Dopa) Carbidopa-levodopa (Sinemet)	Decrease presence of tremor, rigidity, and bradykinesia, and improve motor function.
Antiparkinsonian/Dopamine Agonists	
Bromocriptine mesylate (Parlodel) Pramipexole (Mirapex) Ropinirole (Requip) Rotigotine (Neupro) Apomorphine (Apokyn)	Decrease presence of tremor, rigidity, and bradykinesia, and improve motor function.
Antiviral	
Amantadine (Symmetrel)	Decreases presence of rigidity and bradykinesia.
Anticholinergic	
Trihexyphenidyl (Artane) Biperiden (Akineton) Benztropine (Cogentin)	Adjunctive therapy given with other antiparkinsonian, medications. Decreases tremor.
Monoamine Oxidase Inhibitor (MAOI)	
Selegiline (Eldepryl, Carbex)	Decreases presence of tremor, rigidity, and bradykinesia, and improves motor function.
Monoamine Oxidase Inhibitor B (MAOI-B)	
Rasagiline (Azilect) Selegiline (Eldepryl, Carbex) Safinamide (Xadago)	Used for motor symptom control, and have some neuroprotective effect.
Catechol-*O*-Methyltransferase (COMT) Inhibitor	
Tolcapone (Tasmar) Entacapone (Comtan)	Slow the breakdown of dopamine, thereby prolonging the action of levodopa. Are ineffective when given alone; used as levodopa extenders.

Assignment Considerations

Feeding a Dysphagic Patient

Unlicensed assistive personnel (UAP) should not be assigned to feed dysphagic patients if possible. If an aide must be used to help feed a patient with dysphagia, be certain that suction is turned on and at hand and that the aide has been trained in helping a dysphagic patient to eat. Remind the UAP that the patient should be positioned as upright as possible, to give small bites, to wait for that bite to be swallowed before offering another one, and not to rush the patient. Coaching the patient to drop the chin when swallowing helps prevent choking.

◆ PLANNING, IMPLEMENTATION, AND EVALUATION

Nursing care focuses on preventing complications of PD, drug therapy, enhancing voluntary movement, and safety. Constipation is a problem and requires the addition of fiber to the diet and an increase in fluids to at least 3000 mL per 24 hours. Grasping coins or other objects may help decrease tremors because it is an intentional action. Walking may be improved by having the patient think about imaginary lines across the pathway on which to walk. Imagining stepping over something helps prevent "freezing" when walking. Teach the patient to consciously assume correct posture. Not using a pillow when resting helps prevent flexion of the spine. Learning to sleep prone also is beneficial for posture correction. The physical therapist will institute an exercise program to help the patient maintain muscle function and promote joint mobility.

Remember that patients with PD need extra time to finish tasks. A warming tray can be used to keep food hot during meals so that the patient can take rest periods while eating. Considerable patience and understanding are necessary to help the patient cope with the frustration of deteriorating body control and inability to do things that they formerly could easily do. Degeneration of cognitive skills occurs in the late stages of PD.

Falls are common, and safety is a major factor. Using a cane or walker will increase stability and decrease the incidence of falls. Leg braces or foot braces may help maintain balance. Loose carpets should be removed from the home. Grab bars should be installed in the shower and tub; a raised toilet seat should also be installed. Patients with tremor must be cautioned against carrying hot liquids because spills may cause burns. Chapter 21 discusses measures to help with the problems typical of many neurologic disorders. Patient and family teaching is an important part of nursing care for patients with PD.

Nursing Care Plan 24.1 Care of a Patient With Parkinson Disease

SCENARIO

Henry Merkel, a 63-year-old man, is admitted to your unit because of increasing incidence of falling. He is diagnosed with Parkinson disease. He is beginning to have trouble swallowing, and his speech has slowed. He has a tremor in his left hand and upper extremity.

PROBLEM STATEMENT/NURSING DIAGNOSIS

Altered nutrition due to dysphagia.

SUPPORTING ASSESSMENT DATA

Subjective: "I can't chew and swallow very well. I've choked on food a few times."
Objective: Difficulty chewing; difficulty getting food to go down.

Goals/Expected Outcomes	Nursing Interventions	Selected Rationale	Evaluation
Patient will not aspirate food.	Monitor swallowing during drug administration and meals to assess degree of swallowing difficulty.	Allows assessment of swallowing ability.	Swallowing pills one by one without problem. No choking or difficulty during meal as long as eats slowly.
	Keep suction equipment at hand to remove pooled secretions and prevent aspiration; turn on before meal.	Readies suction and allows removal of secretions.	Suction on and at hand during meals.
	Maintain upright position for drug administration and meals.	Gravity helps food go down to the stomach and helps prevent aspiration.	Sitting fully upright for medications and meals.
	Provide semisoft foods and thickened liquids for diet.	Semisoft foods and thickened liquids are easier to swallow.	Has a semisoft diet. Thickener used for liquids.
	Obtain consultation with speech therapist for swallowing studies.	Detects dysphagia.	Consultation with the speech therapist is ordered.
	Reinforce teaching regarding methods to be used for swallowing.	Various maneuvers can assist with correct swallowing and prevent choking.	Teaching plan is in place, and teaching is ongoing.

PROBLEM STATEMENT/NURSING DIAGNOSIS

Potential for injury related to abnormal posture, rigidity, bradykinesia, and difficulty in initiating movements.

SUPPORTING ASSESSMENT DATA

Subjective: "I seem to have trouble with balance. I've fallen four times this month."
Objective: Rigidity of joints, jerky movements, shuffling gait, stooped posture.

Goals/Expected Outcomes	Nursing Interventions	Selected Rationale	Evaluation
Patient will ambulate safely without falling	Physical therapist to work with patient on joint mobility, muscle strengthening, and ambulation.	Physical therapy helps decrease rigidity and muscle weakness.	Physical therapist is working with the patient. Patient is performing prescribed exercises with spouse's help.
	Administer antiparkinsonian medication as ordered. Monitor for side effects and effectiveness of medication.	Decreases tremor, rigidity, and bradykinesia.	Receiving ordered medications with no signs of side effects. Rigidity slightly improved.
	Provide cane or walker if necessary.	Assistive device promotes safety.	Using walker when ambulating.
	Teach to perform active ROM exercises bid.	Techniques improve gait and movement.	Performing ROM exercises bid.
	Teach to walk as if over an imaginary line and to rock back and forth to initiate movement.		Physical therapist is coaching the patient in how to walk.

PROBLEM STATEMENT/NURSING DIAGNOSIS

Potential for altered nutrition related to eating difficulties and inadequate food intake.

Nursing Care Plan 24.1 Care of a Patient With Parkinson Disease—cont'd

SUPPORTING ASSESSMENT DATA

Subjective: "I haven't had much appetite lately."

Objective: Slight drooling, weight down 4 lb this month.

Goals/Expected Outcomes	Nursing Interventions	Selected Rationale	Evaluation
Patient will have no further weight loss.	Obtain consultation with dietitian.	Assists with nutritional problems.	Dietitian will come tomorrow.
	Offer six small meals per day.		Offering between-meal small snacks.
	Serve hot meals on warming tray and do not rush patient with eating.	Keeps food warm while patient rests during meal.	Reheating food as needed during meal.
	Offer nutritional supplements between meals if needed.	Increases caloric intake.	Taking a protein shake in the afternoon.
	Administer anticholinergic medication as ordered.	Decreases drooling.	Medication is showing effect in decreased drooling.
	Monitor for side effects and effectiveness of medication; observe for urinary retention.	Identifies side effects patient experiences.	No urinary retention or other side effects.
	Increase fiber intake and increase fluids to 3000 mL/day to prevent constipation.		Drank 2800 mL today. Fiber in diet increased.

CRITICAL THINKING QUESTIONS

1. What are the side effects of Sinemet?
2. What would you suggest be done around the house to help prevent falls?

bid, Twice daily; *ROM*, range-of-motion.

Patient Teaching

Patients With Parkinson Disease

Patients may benefit greatly from tips on how to cope with the illness. Be sure to keep individual teaching sessions short to avoid fatigue.

AIDS FOR DAILY LIVING

- Using adjustable tables may help reduce arm fatigue and increase comfort by providing increased support and stabilizing the arms.
- Reacher bars may be helpful in pulling items off shelves.
- Household chores such as folding laundry may provide gentle exercise.
- Music can provide relaxation or motivation for exercise.

HEALTHY EATING

- Take an adequate amount of time to be able to eat comfortably and without rushing.
- Eating foods high in fiber and getting adequate fluids can prevent problems with constipation.

TO PREVENT DROOLING OR SALIVATING

- Sit upright when eating.
- Close your lips and keep your chin up.
- Swallow often.
- Use a straw when drinking to strengthen the muscles of the lips, mouth, and throat.

WRITING TIPS

- Use big strokes when writing and use lined paper.
- Use a larger pen or marker and change writing position often.
- Try changing to a different pen if your hand tires.

BALANCE

- Change positions slowly.
- When turning around, do not pivot. Move forward and slowly walk in a circle.
- A sturdy, single cane with a wide rubber tip may help maintain balance.

EXERCISE

- Avoid moving quickly.
- Avoid moving in a backward direction.
- Be aware of shuffling: stop and check that your posture is upright before continuing.
- Look ahead, not down.

Evaluation includes gathering data about the results of the interventions implemented. Next, determine whether the expected outcomes are being met. If progress toward the outcomes is not occurring, revise the care plan.

MULTIPLE SCLEROSIS

ETIOLOGY

Multiple sclerosis (MS) is a chronic inflammatory disease that causes demyelination in the central nervous system

(CNS). The most common type of MS is characterized by periods of remission and exacerbation. Another type is progressive without remission periods. The cause of MS is not known, but the most widely accepted theory is that it begins as an inflammatory immune-mediated disorder. The inflammation may be a response to an environmental factor (bacteria, virus, or chemical) combined with a genetic predisposition for the disease. MS is considered an autoimmune disease, in which the immune system attacks healthy CNS tissue.

There is no cure. The disease is most common in people of northern European ancestry. It affects females two to three times more frequently than males. Symptoms typically appear between 15 and 50 years of age but can occur at any age. A genetic factor can be involved; the disease is sometimes seen in more than one family member. It is estimated that there are more than 1 million people with MS in the United States and 2.3 million around the world (Koskie & Kim, 2018).

PATHOPHYSIOLOGY

Lymphocytes and macrophages infiltrate the CNS; immunoglobulin G (IgG) levels increase in the cerebrospinal fluid (CSF), indicating a humoral response with B-cell activation. T cells become reactive to a single myelin protein. Myelin is a protective sheath that insulates axons and assists impulse transmission. Axons transmit electrical impulses from one neuron to the next. In patients with MS, plaques form along the myelin sheath, causing inflammation. When myelin is eroded by inflammation and replaced by scar tissue (**demyelination**), nerve impulses cannot travel along the damaged neurons (Fig. 24.4). Thus the muscles served by the affected nerves do not receive the impulses they need to perform in a well-coordinated and useful manner. When inflammation subsides, some remyelination occurs, but it is often incomplete, and nerve transmission is not normal. There are four clinical progressions of MS (Table 24.2).

SIGNS AND SYMPTOMS

Clinical signs and symptoms reflect the pathologic changes that occur as a result of inflammation and subsequent scarring of myelin covering the nerves. MS typically follows a course of unpredictable flare-ups that are followed by periods of partial or complete remission. The very nature of the disease affects a patient's life in terms of ability to make a living, maintain satisfying interpersonal relationships with family and friends, and maintain a positive self-image.

Because the disease can affect any CNS tissue, symptoms can be unpredictable and vary from person to person. The more common manifestations of MS are as follows:

- *Motor dysfunction* can include weakness or paralysis of limbs, trunk, and neck; diplopia caused by oculomotor weakness; and spasticity of the muscles.
- *Sensory dysfunction* may include numbness, tingling, burning, and painful sensations; patchy or total blindness or blurring of vision in one or both eyes; dizziness; ringing in the ears; and hearing loss.
- *Problems of coordination* include ataxia (unsteady gait), intention tremor of limbs and eyes, slurring of speech, and dysphagia (difficulty swallowing).
- *Mental changes* usually are limited to depression and cognitive problems such as impaired judgment,

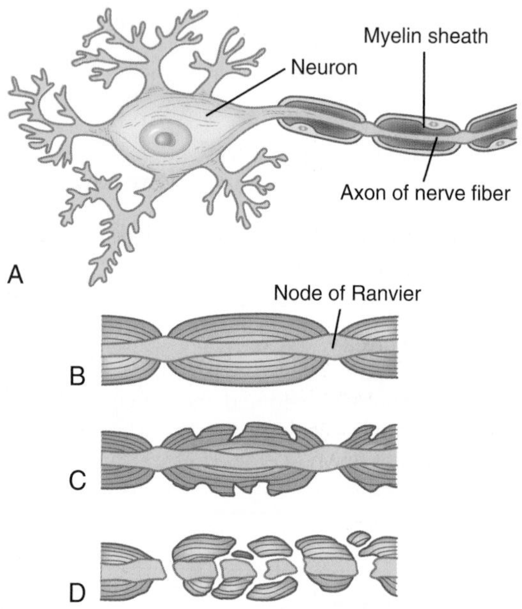

Fig. 24.4 Effects of multiple sclerosis. **A,** Normal nerve cell with myelin sheath. **B,** Normal axon. **C,** Myelin breakdown. **D,** Myelin totally disrupted; axon not functioning. (From Lewis SL, Bucher L, Heitkemper MM, et al.: *Medical-surgical nursing: assessment and management of clinical problems,* ed 10, St. Louis, 2017, Elsevier.)

Table 24.2 The Four Clinical Progressions of Multiple Sclerosis

TYPE OF PROGRESSION	CHARACTERISTICS AND CLINICAL COURSE
Relapsing-remitting (most common type)	Clearly defined relapses of acute worsening neurologic function. Partial or complete recovery occurs in remission period.
Primary progressive	Slow but almost continuous worsening, with occasional plateaus and temporary minor improvements.
Secondary progressive	Initial period of relapsing-remitting disease followed by a steadily worsening course. May or may not have occasional relapses, minor remissions, or plateaus.
Relapsing-progressive	Disease steadily worsens from onset, but there are clear acute relapses with or without recovery. Disease progresses between relapses.

decreased ability to solve problems, and memory loss, which occur late in the disease.

- *Fatigue* is a characteristic of MS and often is worsened by heat (e.g., a hot shower, hot weather, or high humidity may induce or worsen symptoms).
- Other problems that occur late in the disease are related to urinary and bowel incontinence and altered sexual function: loss of male and female self-esteem, physical impotence in men, and diminished sensation in women.

The neuromuscular dysfunctions characteristic of MS are unique to each person and can vary greatly from time to time in the same person. Symptoms may disappear for a while.

DIAGNOSIS

No laboratory test will definitively establish a diagnosis of MS, although most patients have elevated IgG levels in their CSF and oligoclonal bands (bands of IgG produced by electrophoresis of the CSF). An MRI study usually shows characteristic white matter lesions scattered through the spinal cord and/or brain, which confirms the diagnosis of MS. However, the clinical signs and symptoms presented by a patient usually are sufficiently characteristic of the disorder to allow the neurologist to make a diagnosis that the patient possibly or probably has MS. The clinical manifestations of the disease reflect the extent to which inflammation and scarring of the myelin have occurred (Fig. 24.5). In the past, diagnosis could take several years, occurring only after a second attack. In 2017 an international committee released guidelines that allow for diagnosis after one attack using clinical assessment with imaging and laboratory (CSF) studies (Carroll, 2018).

TREATMENT

Treatments fall into two categories, those that prevent attacks or modify the disease process and those that treat the symptoms of the disease. There has been an enormous amount of success with treatment from biological response modifier drugs, such as interferon beta-1b (Betaseron), which is effective for many ambulatory patients with relapsing-remitting MS. It is given by injection. It reduces MS attacks by one third and decreases the number of severe attacks. Disease-modifying drugs are very expensive and are used to prevent relapses. Autologous stem cell transplantation has shown to be effective in slowing the course of MS for those with relapsing forms of the disease. Patients with progressive MS did not do as well.

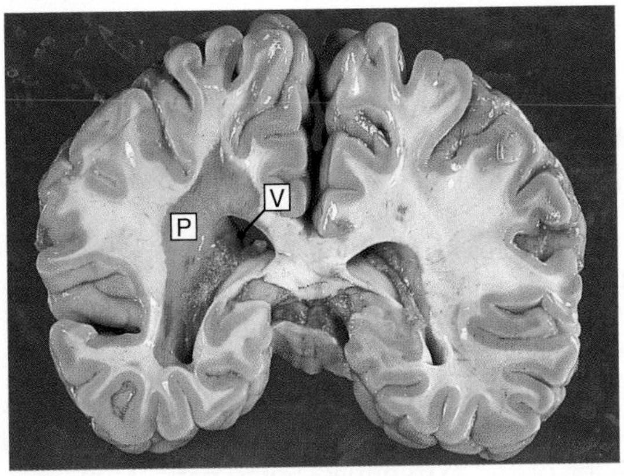

Fig. 24.5 Chronic multiple sclerosis. Demyelination plaque *(P)* at gray matter–white matter junction and adjacent partially remyelinated shadow plaque *(V)*. (From Stevens A, Lowe J: *Pathology: illustrated review in color,* ed 2, London, 2000, Mosby.)

Acute attacks are treated with intravenous (IV) methylprednisolone for 5 days, followed by oral prednisone in tapering doses. Emergent plasmapheresis may be implemented in place of IV steroids, if available at the facility. Adrenocorticotropic hormone (ACTH) may be given for its ability to suppress immune system activity. Most therapeutic efforts are centered on supportive measures to maintain resistance to infection; reduce muscle spasticity; and manage specific symptoms, such as diplopia, speech disorders, muscle weakness, fatigue, and depression. The drug regimen is geared to each patient's symptoms. CNS stimulants may be prescribed to combat fatigue. Sometimes the antiparkinsonian drug amantadine (Symmetrel) is used for fatigue.

The following medications have been approved by the U.S. Food and Drug Administration (FDA) for use in relapsing MS:

- Interferon beta-1a (Avonex, Rebif)
- Interferon beta-1b (Betaseron, Extavia)
- Peginterferon beta-1a (Plegridy)
- Glatiramer acetate (Copaxone)
- Natalizumab (Tysabri)
- Mitoxantrone
- Fingolimod (Gilenya)
- Teriflunomide (Aubagio)
- Dimethyl fumarate (Tecfidera)
- Alemtuzumab (Lemtrada)
- Daclizumab (Zinbryta)
- Ocrelizumab

An exercise program is very beneficial for patients with MS, to relieve spasticity and improve coordination (Harmon, 2016). Swimming provides considerable benefits because exercising in water is less fatiguing than exercising out of water. Because of fatigue, it is often difficult to convince patients with MS to exercise.

In addition, the patient should be provided with the support and physical and psychological means necessary to develop a positive and hopeful outlook. There is an understandable tendency to become depressed and pessimistic about the future when confronted with the realities of muscle weakness, incontinence, sexual impotence, and any combination of disabilities likely to be experienced during the course of MS. Antidepressants may be helpful. Disease-modifying agents can reduce disease activity, frequency of relapses, and possibly progression of MS.

NURSING MANAGEMENT

ASSESSMENT (DATA COLLECTION), NURSING DIAGNOSIS, AND PLANNING

A careful history can provide many clues to the possibility that the patient has MS. Testing extremity strength, looking for visual problems, and checking reflexes are part of the physical examination.

Problem statements are based on the assessment findings and may include the following:

- Fatigue due to improper transmission of neural impulses.
- Altered physical mobility due to muscle weakness, spasticity, or paresthesias (tingling or numbness).
- Altered self-care ability due to muscle spasticity and neuromuscular deficits.
- Altered urinary function due to sensory motor deficits.
- Altered sexual function due to neuromuscular deficits.
- Potential for altered skin integrity due to immobility.
- Altered family coping due to potential financial problems, changing roles, and fluctuating physical abilities.
- Decreased self-esteem due to loss of usual abilities and roles.

Expected outcomes are written for each problem statement or nursing diagnosis specific to the individual's problems.

IMPLEMENTATION AND EVALUATION

Appropriate care for a patient with MS depends on the severity of the disease and the symptoms. Care is individualized for each patient. During the diagnostic phase, the patient and family need a great deal of emotional support as they realize that MS is a chronic disease and there is no cure.

Ongoing care by an interdisciplinary team focuses on safety, prevention of complications, assistance with physical therapy, and emotional support. The patient should not be exposed to excessive heat or hot baths, which cause weakness to become much worse (Harmon, 2016). Care of the common problems of neurologic patients is covered in Chapter 21. The importance of proper nutrition with adequate fluids and fiber in the diet should be stressed to maintain proper bowel function and decrease the likelihood of urinary tract infections. Calcium and vitamin D should be included in the diet to help prevent osteoporosis that may result from the IV steroid treatments. Medications to decrease stomach acid and prevent ulceration from the steroids may be administered (histamine [H_2]-receptor blockers or proton pump inhibitors).

Help the patient and family establish a consistent daily routine that will promote optimum levels of functioning for the patient. The routine should include daily physical exercise balanced by rest periods to prevent fatigue. Patient teaching involves:

- Education about the unpredictability of the disease and the need to prevent stress, infections, and fatigue to maintain independence for as long as possible.
- Referral to the National Multiple Sclerosis Society and local support groups. (Additional information and local sources of help for the patient with MS and the family can be obtained at www.nationalmssociety.org or by writing to the National Multiple Sclerosis Society, 733 Third Avenue, 3rd Floor, New York, NY, 10017.)

Evaluation of care is based on whether the expected outcomes are being achieved. If they are not, the plan is revised.

ALZHEIMER DISEASE

Alzheimer disease, a form of dementia caused by pathologic changes in the brain tissue of the patient, is discussed in Chapter 46. Diagnosis is by history and examination because the specific diagnostic changes can be detected only at autopsy. The cause of Alzheimer disease is unknown, and considerable research is in progress to better define this disease. Much of this research centers around beta-amyloid and tau proteins (Lakhan, 2018). Alzheimer disease can occur during middle age or during the later decades of life and causes devastation to the patient and family. The disease has a slow onset, progresses at varying rates of speed through several stages, and is eventually fatal. See Chapter 46 for further information on Alzheimer disease.

AMYOTROPHIC LATERAL SCLEROSIS

ETIOLOGY AND PATHOPHYSIOLOGY

Amyotrophic lateral sclerosis (ALS) or motor neuron disease (MND), also called *Lou Gehrig disease*, is a progressive neuromuscular disease characterized by degeneration of the gray matter in the anterior horns of the spinal cord and the lower cranial nerves. After degeneration, electrical and chemical messages generated in the brain cannot reach the muscles to activate them. The incidence of ALS ranges from 2.7 to 7.4 per 100,000 people in the United States. It most often occurs between the ages of 40 and 70 years and affects men more than women. About 7000 new cases are diagnosed each year (Armon, 2018).

ALS is classified as being either familial (5% to 10%) or sporadic (90% to 95%) of unknown origin (idiopathic). Although some people with ALS can survive for many years, the disease usually progresses rapidly, resulting in death within about 3 years of the onset of symptoms.

SIGNS AND SYMPTOMS

One of the first clinical manifestations of ALS is weakness of the voluntary muscles, especially of the distal muscles of the extremities. Some patients may notice difficulty swallowing and speaking clearly because of oropharyngeal weakness. As the disease progresses, there is atrophy of the muscles. Until atrophy is complete, however, there may be spontaneous contractions or spasticity of the muscles and abnormal sensations *(paresthesias)*, such as tingling or prickling. The patient also may report pain, which is probably caused by strain on weakened muscles.

Only the motor neurons are affected in ALS; therefore the patient remains mentally alert and does not have sensory impairment. Depression is relatively common as a result of the unrelenting progression of muscle weakness and atrophy. Death typically results from respiratory infection and dysfunction as weakness and atrophy of the respiratory muscles impede normal respiration and mechanisms to clear bacteria and secretions from the lungs.

DIAGNOSIS AND TREATMENT

There is no laboratory test to confirm a diagnosis of ALS. Electromyography in combination with physical assessment and ruling out other neuromuscular disorders such as MS, myasthenia gravis, and progressive muscular dystrophy provide data for the diagnosis.

There is no cure for ALS. Eventually the muscle paralysis renders the patient totally dependent because of inability to move, swallow, speak, and ultimately breathe. Noninvasive ventilation (Chapter 14) can extend life and delay the need for an artificial airway. The drug riluzole (Rilutek), a glutamate antagonist, has been shown to slow the progression in certain patients (Armon, 2018). Eventually, impaired breathing requires a tracheostomy and mechanical ventilation.

NURSING MANAGEMENT

During the first contact with a patient with ALS, conduct a thorough neurologic assessment. As the disease progresses, periodic assessments can identify specific needs. The patient and family need to understand the progression of the disease to be able to make care decisions. While still able to function, the patient should make their wishes known to their family and health care provider. Problem statements likely to be associated with ALS are those related to difficulty with respiration, all problems of immobility, dysphagia, impaired ability to communicate, pain, ineffective coping, and depression.

In the later stages of ALS, the patient and family will need more assistance and guidance to maintain some level of independence and comfort for the patient. Rehabilitation includes obtaining equipment and devices such as a walker, wheelchair, hospital bed, suction machine, and nasogastric or gastrostomy tube feeding supplies.

Because of the nature of the disease, the patient and family will experience issues related to terminal illness, death, and the grieving process (see Chapter 8). Toward the end of life, the services of a visiting nurse or a hospice program can provide appropriate instruction and physical and emotional support. Support groups can be helpful in sharing information and in helping prevent caregiver burnout. Make sure that any advanced directive is available to caregivers.

GUILLAIN-BARRÉ SYNDROME

ETIOLOGY AND PATHOPHYSIOLOGY

Guillain-Barré syndrome (GBS) is one of several relatively rare immune-mediated polyneuropathy diseases that affects the peripheral nervous system, especially the spinal nerves outside the spinal cord. It also can affect the cranial nerves. The cause of GBS is not known, but it usually follows a simple viral respiratory infection or gastroenteritis in adults within 2 to 4 weeks. Other triggering events have been identified in a small number of patients. Some immunizations, surgery, trauma, and bone marrow transplantation are considered possible triggers. Authorities believe that the disease is a cell-mediated immunologic response preceded by stimulation from a viral infection, trauma, surgery, viral immunizations, human immunodeficiency virus (HIV), or neoplasm of the lymphatic system. Cytomegalovirus and Epstein-Barr virus are two viruses that have been linked to GBS.

Pathologic changes include demyelination, inflammation, edema, and nerve root compression. These changes bring about the paresthesia, pain, and progressive, ascending paralysis typical of the syndrome. Autonomic nervous system dysfunction with alterations in both sympathetic and parasympathetic systems may occur, causing orthostatic hypotension, hypertension, abnormal vagal responses, bowel and bladder dysfunctions, facial flushing, and diaphoresis. When the lower brainstem becomes involved, the cranial nerves are affected.

SIGNS AND SYMPTOMS

Objective and subjective symptoms of GBS include mild sensations of numbness and tingling in the feet and hands followed by muscle pain, tenderness, and aching, especially in the shoulder, pelvis, and thighs. There is progressive muscle weakness, usually starting in the lower extremities and moving upward over 24 to 72 hours. However, it also can affect the cranial nerves and facial muscles first and move downward. Symptoms peak in about 14 days. Sensory loss can also occur but is not as common as motor loss. If respiratory function is affected, ventilatory support may be needed.

Pain is common and may be evidenced as paresthesias, muscular aches and cramps, and **hyperesthesia** (abnormal sensitivity to stimuli). Pain often is worse at night when there is less distraction in the environment.

DIAGNOSIS

Diagnosing GBS is difficult because its characteristic signs and symptoms are similar to those of several other diseases. Analysis of the CSF is helpful. Typically there is an elevated CSF protein content that tends to rise as the disease progresses, peaking in 4 to 6 weeks. The number of leukocytes remains within normal limits, as does CSF pressure. Electromyography and nerve conduction studies show reduced conduction velocity. For the most part, the health care provider must depend on the clinical presentation to diagnose GBS.

TREATMENT

Medical treatment is mainly supportive. Within the first 2 weeks, plasmapheresis, in which the patient's plasma is removed and "washed" to remove antibodies, hastens recovery in some patients and decreases the time during which ventilatory support is needed. The use of IV immune globulin (IVIG) to hasten recovery is also effective (NINDS, 2018b).

Nutritional support via tube feedings may be required because of dysphagia. If paralytic ileus (halt to bowel peristalsis) occurs, parenteral nutrition will be necessary. Most patients with GBS recover and walk independently at 6 months, with full motor recovery within 1 year. Some patients have incomplete recovery after 18 months, and GBS has a 10% mortality rate. In older patients the main cause of death is dysrhythmia.

Clinical Cues

Signs and symptoms of paralytic ileus are absence of bowel sounds, abdominal pain, and considerable abdominal bloating with lack of passage of stool.

NURSING MANAGEMENT

ASSESSMENT (DATA COLLECTION), NURSING DIAGNOSIS, AND PLANNING

Assessment is the most important aspect of care during the acute stage. Monitor progression of ascending paralysis; assess respiratory function carefully; and assess gag, corneal, and swallowing reflexes closely. Monitor arterial blood gases and oxygen saturation. Observe vital sign trends and watch for orthostatic hypotension and cardiac dysrhythmia, which can indicate the degree of autonomic nervous system dysfunction.

Problem statements depend on the degree of nervous system involvement but may include the following:

- Altered gas exchange due to disease progression affecting respiratory nerves.
- Altered physical mobility due to paralysis of muscles from disease progression.
- Potential for injury due to dysphagia.
- Altered nutrition due to dysphagia and inability to feed self.
- Acute pain due to paresthesias, muscle aches and cramps, and hyperesthesias.
- Altered self-care ability due to inability to use muscles to accomplish activities of daily living.
- Fear due to seriousness of disease and unknown outcome.
- Altered communication due to paralysis of speech muscles or intubation.
- Potential for altered skin integrity due to immobility.

Expected outcomes must be written for each problem statement. Overall goals of care are as follows:

- Maintain adequate ventilation.
- Control pain adequately.
- Prevent damage from aspiration.
- Maintain communication.
- Maintain adequate nutritional status.
- Return patient to normal function.
- Prevent skin breakdown

IMPLEMENTATION AND EVALUATION

There are three phases of GBS: the acute phase, the static phase, and the rehabilitation phase. Each demands different kinds of monitoring and intervention. During the *acute phase,* the goals are to sustain life, prevent complications related to immobility, and promote rest and comfort. Respiratory problems are particularly troublesome and may require suctioning, tracheostomy care, artificial ventilation, and other life support measures.

Vital signs must be checked frequently. Alterations in the autonomic nervous system can cause drastic changes in blood pressure, particularly hypotension. Cardiac arrhythmias are also common, and the patient is continuously monitored.

The paralysis and loss of control that occur with GBS come on so suddenly and are so overwhelming that the patient becomes very frightened. Because the course of the disease usually extends for months with a very slow recovery, the patient begins to have feelings of hopelessness, despair, and isolation.

The *static phase* is a kind of plateau the patient reaches 1 to 3 weeks after the onset of the illness. During this time the motor loss and paresthesias no longer progress, and the patient's condition becomes somewhat stabilized; they get no better but no worse. This phase can last from a few days to months.

Think Critically

What problems requiring specific nursing interventions would you expect to encounter for a patient with GBS who is now stable but has paralysis of the lower extremities and paresis of the upper extremities?

During the static phase, nursing care is concentrated on preventing complications of immobility and helping the patient deal with feelings of anger, depression, and anxiety. Exercises are usually begun but are limited to passive and gentle range-of-motion and stretching exercises. There must be a balance of rest and exercise and no sudden changes in posture or position, in case blood pressure suddenly drops.

Meticulous skin care is essential because of immobility. Monitoring for thrombophlebitis is important because this is a common complication. Elastic stockings or sequential compression devices are applied to the legs, along with anticoagulant therapy, to try to prevent thrombophlebitis.

Clinical Cues

Signs of thrombophlebitis are warmth, swelling, and pain in the extremity. Temperature may be elevated.

The final phase, *rehabilitation,* is one of gradual recovery. The patient may become elated over the change in their condition and must be prevented from overexertion, which can lead to a relapse. As muscle function returns, the level of exercise and activity is slowly increased (Andary, 2018). It may take up to 2 years for maximal improvement with return to normal functioning. Approximately 80% to 90% of patients have little residual deficit.

POLIOMYELITIS AND POSTPOLIO SYNDROME

Poliomyelitis destroys the motor cells of the anterior horn of the spinal cord, the brainstem, and the motor strip located in the frontal lobe. It is caused by a virus and can be prevented by immunization with the Salk (killed virus) or Sabin (attenuated live virus) polio vaccine. It is rare in the United States, where immunization is given in childhood, but outbreaks still occur in other parts of the world. Some people who have had poliomyelitis develop postpolio sequelae or postpolio syndrome. A new onset of weakness, pain, and fatigue may occur in people who had the disease more than 30 years ago. Disability may be temporary or permanent. Treatment is geared toward making lifestyle modifications to preserve energy and physiologic function. Swimming in warm water has been found to promote comfort and help maintain flexibility.

HUNTINGTON DISEASE

Huntington disease or Huntington chorea is a rare, genetically transmitted degenerative neurologic disorder characterized by abnormal movements (**chorea**). It is accompanied by a decline in intellectual capacity and emotional disturbances. Signs of Huntington disease usually become evident during the fourth or fifth decade of life but may occur earlier. Women and men are equally affected. The disorder is progressive and causes disability and then death within 15 to 25 years after signs appear. Death is from neurologic degeneration affecting all body systems. Genetic transmission is by an abnormal gene on the short arm of chromosome 4. It is an autosomal dominant disorder, meaning that the children of a person who has the disease have a 50% chance of inheriting it. If a child does not inherit the disease, the gene is not passed on to the next generation.

A person with Huntington disease progresses from being fidgety and restless to a state of constant movement (chorea). Voluntary movement deteriorates until the patient is completely incapable of independent movement. Intellectual decline causes depression, suspiciousness, and eventual dementia. Genetic testing can confirm the diagnosis. Neuroimaging is not used for diagnosis but is helpful in ruling out other causes of symptoms. There is no known treatment to alter its course, but therapies are used to manage symptoms.

MYASTHENIA GRAVIS

ETIOLOGY AND PATHOPHYSIOLOGY

Myasthenia gravis (MG) literally means "grave muscle weakness." The disease is a chronic disorder. Skeletal muscles, respiratory muscles, and muscles enervated by cranial nerves are affected. The muscular weakness can be so mild that it causes a minor inconvenience or so severe that it is life threatening because of its effect on the muscles used for breathing and swallowing. In 15% of MG cases the weakness is localized to the muscles of the eye and is called ocular MG. Patients with weakness in all muscles have generalized MG.

Myasthenia gravis is an autoimmune disease in which a T cell–dependent immune attack is directed against the postsynaptic ACh receptors at the neuromuscular junction (the point at which nerve impulses are transmitted to muscle tissue) (Bird, 2018). The antibody reduces the number of functional receptor sites and restricts the neuron uptake of ACh. As a result, nerve impulses are not transmitted, and the muscle cannot contract properly.

There is a suggested connection between overgrowth of the thymus gland tissue and MG. Associations between MG and all types of thyroid disorders have been found in research studies.

SIGNS AND SYMPTOMS

Symptoms of MG include **diplopia** (double vision), difficulty chewing and swallowing, and ptosis (Fig. 24.6). The patient's voice tends to be hoarse or nasal in quality, and voice volume decreases toward the end of a sentence. Severe muscle weakness that improves with rest is the primary symptom of the disorder. Any of the skeletal muscles might be involved; intestinal, bladder, and heart muscles are not affected.

Ocular MG may occur first and be demonstrated by diplopia and ptosis. In a small percentage of patients, the disease progresses no further. If cranial nerves become more involved, bulbar myasthenia occurs, with facial and oropharyngeal muscle weakness causing a blank facial expression and a smile resembling a snarl.

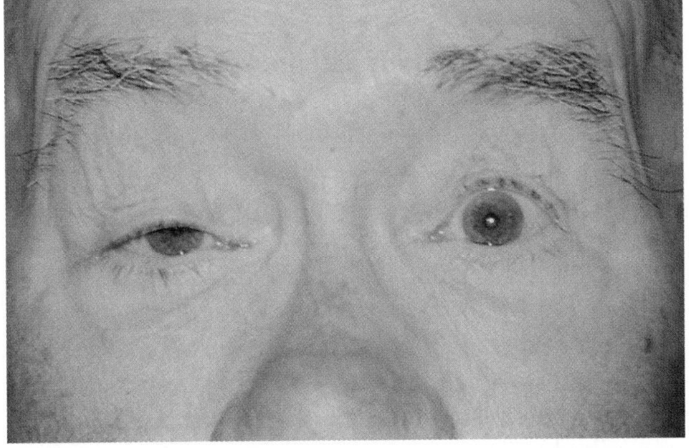

Fig. 24.6 Ptosis (drooping upper lid) characteristic of the muscle weakness of myasthenia gravis. (Courtesy Heather Boyd-Monk and Wills Eye Hospital, Philadelphia, Pa.)

Swallowing and speaking become difficult. Further progression to generalized myasthenia involves the muscles of the neck, shoulders, limbs, hands, diaphragm, and abdomen. The disease does not affect the level of consciousness. Muscles are strongest in the morning and become weaker with activity. Respiratory muscle weakness may require mechanical ventilation.

DIAGNOSIS

Diagnosis is established by history and physical examination, with confirmation from laboratory and electrodiagnostic testing. Blood tests for antibodies to ACh receptors and muscle-specific tyrosine kinase (MuSK) are ordered. Electrodiagnostic testing is performed to check muscle function. A chest radiograph and chest computed tomography (CT) scan will be ordered to check the thymus gland.

> **Clinical Cues**
>
> Edrophonium chloride (Tensilon) has historically been used to diagnose MG and to distinguish between cholinergic and myasthenic crisis. As of 2017 it is no longer available in the United States.

TREATMENT

There are two main modes of therapy: managing the disease by treating the specific symptoms and managing the underlying cause of the symptoms by inducing remission.

Because 80% to 90% of patients with MG have autoantibodies against ACh receptors, plasmapheresis (plasma exchange) can be an effective treatment for patients in crisis. It is particularly helpful in restoring muscle function when a patient is dependent on a ventilator. The purpose of the plasma exchange is to remove the circulating autoantibodies from the patient's blood. This mode of therapy may bring clinical improvement in some patients, but it is not a cure for MG.

Anticholinesterase therapy is the primary treatment for MG. Acetylcholine must be present at the point where nerve impulses are transmitted to the muscle for sustained repetitive muscle contraction to occur. Anticholinesterase agents inactivate acetylcholinesterase, a substance that prevents accumulations of ACh at the neuromuscular junction. Anticholinesterase agents temporarily increase muscle strength by allowing ACh to work, but they do not cure the problem. Two drugs commonly used as anticholinesterase agents are neostigmine (Prostigmin) and pyridostigmine (Mestinon). Pyridostigmine is more commonly used because it can be taken orally. Corticosteroids and immunosuppressant drugs such as azathioprine (Imuran), rituximab (Rituxan), or cyclosporine (Sandimmune) may be used to suppress the immune response. IVIG infusion is sometimes prescribed.

The dosage of anticholinesterase drugs is precisely calculated for each patient. The aim is to achieve a delicate balance between too much and too little ACh at the neuromuscular junction. Stress can quickly alter a patient's need for ACh; hence overmedication or undermedication can occur rather suddenly. Unfortunately, the symptoms of too much medication are quite similar to those of too little medication, so it is often difficult to adjust the dosage correctly.

Another method of treatment is to remove the thymus gland, which decreases the antibody production. Treatment with IVIG for 5 days may produce a favorable response for 30 to 60 days.

NURSING MANAGEMENT

ASSESSMENT (DATA COLLECTION), NURSING DIAGNOSIS, AND PLANNING

The severity of MG is assessed by asking about the degree of fatigue, what body parts are affected, and how severe the problem is. Observe for ptosis of the eyelid and inquire about diplopia. Knowledge of the disorder should be determined and the patient's coping abilities assessed. Assessment of respiratory function is a top priority. Assess muscle strength of the face, swallowing, speech volume and clarity, and cough and gag reflexes. Check the strength of the shoulder muscles and of the limbs.

> **Clinical Cues**
>
> When assessing the status of a patient with MG, have the patient look up at the ceiling. Watch to see whether the eyelids start to move downward. This is often an early sign of the disease or a sign that the medication is insufficient.

Problem statements will depend on the severity of the disease and may include the following:

- Altered breathing pattern due to diaphragm and intercostal muscle weakness.
- Altered airway clearance due to weakness of intercostal muscles and impaired cough and gag reflexes.
- Potential for injury due to difficulty swallowing and weakness of bulbar muscles.
- Altered nutrition due to impaired swallowing ability.
- Altered activity tolerance due to fatigue and muscle weakness.
- Altered communication due to intubation or weakness of larynx, mouth, and pharynx muscles.
- Decreased self-esteem due to inability to maintain usual roles and lifestyle.

Expected outcomes are written for each problem statement based on the specific problem the patient is experiencing.

IMPLEMENTATION AND EVALUATION

Infection, surgery, and other physical and emotional stresses can precipitate a myasthenic crisis and cause hospitalization. During the crisis, frequent monitoring

Patient Teaching

Patients With Myasthenia Gravis

Use your anticholinesterase medication correctly:

- Take the drug with food or fluid.
- Take the drug 45 minutes before meals to permit maximum effect for chewing and swallowing.
- Adjust drug dosage and times of administration as instructed according to your individual pattern of weakness and daily activities.
- Do not take over-the-counter or other prescribed medications without the approval of your health care provider or pharmacist.
- Report signs of cholinergic crisis to the health care provider quickly.
- Modify the diet for ease of chewing and swallowing; soft foods are easier to consume.
- Eat slowly in a calm environment and take small bites.
- Balance rest and activity throughout the day.
- Figure out ways to conserve energy while doing usual activities.
- Compensate with extra rest during periods of extra stress, illness, hormone swings during menstruation, and environmental temperature extremes.
- Wear a medical alert bracelet or necklace at all times; carry a card in your wallet stating that you have myasthenia gravis and list contact numbers for next of kin or significant other.
- Be aware of the signs and symptoms of myasthenic crisis and report them immediately.

is essential. The patient's ability to swallow and breathe on their own can be seriously compromised. Suctioning, intubation, and mechanical ventilation may be necessary to maintain life until the crisis is over.

Education of the patient and family must include instruction about the nature of the illness and the adverse effects of emotional upsets, respiratory infections, and similar stresses. Care focuses on the neurologic deficits and their effect on daily activities. Rehabilitation goals include education and support for the patient and family so that the patient remains as independent as possible.

Because patients with MG can become critically ill and need immediate medical attention at any time, they should at all times wear a medical alert emblem that identifies that they have the disease. The patient, as well as members of the family and the nurses who care for them in the hospital or at home, should know the symptoms of overdosage of anticholinesterase medication as well as the symptoms of myasthenic crisis caused by underdosage of anticholinesterase agents, a precipitating illness, or stress factors (Box 24.2). If any of these symptoms occur, the health care provider should be notified immediately.

Think Critically

What immediate action would you take if you found your patient in cholinergic crisis?

Box 24.2 Signs and Symptoms of Cholinergic Crisis and Myasthenic Crisis

CHOLINERGIC CRISIS

- Generalized weakness within 1 hour of the dose
- Dyspnea and increased bronchial secretions
- Poor tongue control, producing difficulty in chewing
- Difficulty swallowing and excessive salivation
- Restlessness, anxiety, and irritability
- Diaphoresis
- Abdominal cramps, nausea or vomiting, or diarrhea

MYASTHENIC CRISIS

Increase in myasthenia gravis symptoms after failure to take drug as prescribed or after a precipitating illness or increased stress:

- More difficulty swallowing
- Diplopia
- Ptosis
- Dyspnea

Notify the health care provider immediately if these signs and symptoms appear.

In addition to problems related to anticholinesterase drugs, patients with MG also can experience exaggerated and bizarre effects from a variety of drugs. These include steroids and thyroid compounds; sedatives and respiratory depressants, such as morphine; tranquilizers, such as the phenothiazines; many antibiotics; beta blockers; and some cardiac drugs, such as verapamil and procainamide. Because so many drugs are potentially dangerous to a patient with MG, it is imperative that you ensure that the health care provider ordering a medication is aware that the patient has MG. **Always check each drug the patient is to receive for interactions and contraindications.**

RESTLESS LEG SYNDROME

Restless leg syndrome (RLS) or Willis-Ekbom disease (WED) is a sensory-motor disorder that may affect up to 15% of the population, women more often than men (Ondo, 2018). It is marked by an uncontrollable urge to move the legs or arms, more often in the evening, and its cause is unknown. However, there does appear to be an underlying genetic component. RLS is classified as primary if no family history or other explanation is found and as secondary if they have a condition that is known to be linked to RLS. The latter is a more sudden onset and has been associated with anemia; Lyme disease; rheumatoid arthritis; chronic obstructive pulmonary disease (COPD); hypothyroidism or hyperthyroidism; fibromyalgia; and deficiencies of iron, folate, vitamin B_{12}, or magnesium (Ondo, 2018).

Patients with RLS usually have low iron levels, and iron replacement therapy is indicated. Nonpharmacologic therapies include exercise, avoidance of aggravating factors, leg massage, and decreasing caffeine intake. Drug therapies include pramipexole (Mirapex), ropinirole

(Requip), and rotigotine transdermal patch (Neupro), which are dopamine agonists. Alpha-2-delta calcium channel ligands such as gabapentin enacarbil (Horizant), gabapentin (Neurontin), and pregabalin (Lyrica) are also prescribed. Nurses should monitor medications closely and monitor patients taking dopamine agonists for orthostatic hypotension.

RLS is a frustrating complication for patients, but many benefit from available treatment. Foster an encouraging environment and provide education about the syndrome.

COMMUNITY CARE

After leaving the hospital, patients with neurologic problems often are cared for in long-term care facilities, rehabilitation programs, outpatient clinics, and the home. Nurses who work in long-term care facilities must be confident in caring for patients with PD because a large percentage of residents in these facilities have this disorder. Nurses who works with patients who have neurologic deficits that cause some degree of immobility must constantly try to prevent the complications of immobility and to achieve as high a level of function for their patients as possible.

Because older adult patients often have more than one chronic illness, it is essential that nurses be knowledgeable about medication interactions and side effects. Each patient's medications must be continually assessed for possible adverse effects and side effects, as well as for data indicating that each medication is producing a sufficient therapeutic effect to warrant continued administration. A close working relationship with the pharmacist can assist you in judging these matters. Collaborative care between the pharmacist, nurse, nurse aides, physical therapist, social worker, and others who interact with the patient is needed to provide the best plan of care for these patients who require complex care.

Home care nurses interact with entire families and need to continually offer support, as the difficulties of learning to live with someone who has a neurologic deficit are faced daily. Family roles often are altered and strained, and the period of adjustment for the patient and family is lengthy. It often is difficult for the family to cope with the personality changes that occur in patients with degenerative neurologic disorders. Referral to community support groups is often helpful for both the patient and family members.

Get Ready for the NCLEX® Examination!

Key Points

- The characteristic triad of symptoms of PD is tremor, bradykinesia, and rigidity.
- Treatment of PD is with drug therapy (see Table 24.1), physical therapy, and emotional support.
- When drug therapy for PD fails, surgical treatment may be warranted.
- MS is a chronic inflammatory disease that causes demyelination of axons in the CNS (see Table 24.2).
- Common manifestations of MS are motor dysfunction, sensory dysfunction, problems of coordination, mental changes, fatigue, bowel and bladder problems, and altered sexual function.
- MS is treated with biological response modifier drugs and drugs to treat the problems caused by the disease.
- Alzheimer disease is a form of dementia and is discussed in Chapter 46.
- ALS is a rare but devastating disease that usually results in death within 3 years after diagnosis.
- ALS affects the motor neurons and causes weakness of the voluntary muscles.
- Nursing care for patients with ALS focuses on preventing complications and dealing with the problems the disease has caused, particularly immobility, dysphagia, inability to communicate, pain, and depression.
- GBS affects the peripheral nervous system and the cranial nerves.
- GBS is a cell-mediated immunologic response to a stimulus from a viral infection, trauma, surgery, viral immunization, HIV, or neoplasm of the lymphatic system.
- GBS usually causes an ascending paralysis and considerable pain.
- Nursing care for GBS is directed at maintaining adequate ventilation, nutrition, and supportive care for immobility and activities of daily living.
- Postpolio syndrome is the reappearance of polio symptoms many years after the initial polio illness.
- Huntington disease is a genetic disease characterized by chorea.
- Huntington disease causes a decline in intellectual capacity, emotional disturbances, and total dependence, with death occurring in 15 to 20 years.
- MG is an autoimmune disease affecting the neuromuscular junction.
- MG is chronic and is manifested by fatigue and muscular weakness (both symptoms improve with rest).
- Ptosis, diplopia, a weak nasal-quality voice, a blank expression, and a smile resembling a snarl are signs and symptoms of MG.
- MG may affect the intercostal muscles and the diaphragm, causing inadequate respiration.
- Anticholinesterase therapy is the common treatment for MG.
- Nurses must know the signs of overdosage of anticholinesterase drugs.
- Restless leg syndrome, also known as Willis-Ekbom disease, disrupts sleep due to an uncontrollable urge to move in order to dispel discomfort. Movement may be of the whole body and not just the legs.

Additional Learning Resources

SG Go to your Study Guide for additional learning activities to help you master this chapter content.

Go to your Evolve website (http://evolve.elsevier.com/deWit/medsurg) for the following FREE learning resources:

- Animations, audio, and video
- Answers and rationales for questions and activities
- Glossary with pronunciations in English and Spanish
- Interactive Review Questions and more!

Review Questions for the NCLEX® Examination

1. The health care provider discusses the treatment options with a patient newly diagnosed with PD. The patient asks you, "What will happen to me?" An appropriate response would be:
   1. "You seem worried. Let's talk about your concerns."
   2. "Your provider can fully explain your condition."
   3. "You will be all right."
   4. "Your disease can be controlled."

   NCLEX Client Need: Psychosocial Integrity
2. A patient with PD has been taking carbidopa-levodopa (Sinemet) for 3 months and is being seen for follow-up. You would expect to observe which of the following? *(Select all that apply.)*
   1. Dark urine
   2. Bradykinesia
   3. Weight maintained
   4. Rigidity
   5. Walking without assistance
   6. Tremors

   NCLEX Client Need: Physiological Integrity: Pharmacological Therapies
3. You observe a nursing assistant feeding a dysphagic patient. Which action by the nursing assistant indicates a need for further instruction and guidance?
   1. The wall suction is turned on and readily available.
   2. The patient is propped up with one pillow.
   3. The food is cut into small, bite-size pieces.
   4. The nursing assistant coaches the patient to drop the chin.

   NCLEX Client Need: Physiological Integrity: Reduction of Risk Potential
4. A 45-year-old patient newly diagnosed with MS asks about their prognosis for the future. Teaching about the future might include stating:
   1. "The condition is a progressive neurologic disease, and you will likely end up using a wheelchair or scooter. You might start equipping your house to be wheelchair accessible."
   2. "With the new immune-modifying drugs available as treatment, you will not even be able to tell you have the disease."
   3. "MS may begin with exacerbations and remissions, but it will eventually develop into a progressive disease, affecting your entire neurologic system and thus your whole body."
   4. "The condition is a periodic demyelination of the central nervous system, often with periods of remissions and exacerbations. It is a manageable disease, and there are many patients who live active and rewarding lives. Use of the new immune-modifying agents will help reduce exacerbations."

   NCLEX Client Need: Psychosocial Integrity
5. A patient is admitted for progressive muscle weakness in the lower extremities. The patient complains of tingling and numbness in the hands. The patient recovered from the flu a week ago. Which intervention(s) should be anticipated in the care of this patient? *(Select all that apply.)*
   1. Medication for pain and discomfort
   2. Immediate need for physical therapy exercise
   3. Possible need for ventilatory assistance
   4. Need for airway suctioning
   5. Administration of muscle relaxants
   6. Seizure precautions

   NCLEX Client Need: Physiological Integrity: Physiological Adaptation
6. A female patient with MG may need additional teaching when she makes the following statement:
   1. "I should pace my activities to allow for rest periods."
   2. "I need to be careful when drinking liquids."
   3. "Pregnancy hormones will control my symptoms."
   4. "I must take my medications on a strict schedule."

   NCLEX Client Need: Health Promotion and Maintenance
7. You reinforce pharmacy instructions regarding safe use of pyridostigmine (Mestinon), an anticholinesterase, by a patient newly diagnosed with MG. Which patient statement indicates a need for further teaching?
   1. "I need to take the medication after meals on a full stomach."
   2. "I can adjust the drug dosage and times depending on daily activities."
   3. "I shouldn't take over-the-counter medications without health care provider approval."
   4. "I should balance rest and activity throughout the day."

   NCLEX Client Need: Physiological Integrity: Pharmacological Therapies
8. The priority nursing assessment of a patient with MG would be to:
   1. determine the degree of fatigue.
   2. assess the level of knowledge about the disease.
   3. monitor the adequacy of respiratory function.
   4. check the patient's swallowing, speech, and protective reflexes.

   NCLEX Client Need: Physiological Integrity: Reduction of Risk Potential

9. A patient presenting with numbness and tingling of the hands and feet, muscle pain, and weakness in the legs would be evaluated for:
   1. multiple sclerosis
   2. Guillain-Barré syndrome
   3. Parkinson disease
   4. Myasthenia gravis

   NCLEX Client Need: Physiological Integrity: Physiological Adaptation
10. Injury is a possible problem statement for patients with RLS. Which nursing intervention(s) would help prevent injury? *(Select all that apply.)*
    1. Educate the patient about daytime drowsiness, possibly severe, that may occur with the treatment for RLS. The patient should not drive or operate machinery until reaction to treatment is determined.
    2. Apply leg braces for the patient at night.
    3. Advise the patient to rise slowly to a standing position from a sitting or lying position.
    4. Install grab bars in the shower and tub.
    5. Use a two-wheeled walker for balance.
    6. Remove throw rugs from the environment.

    NCLEX Client Need: Safe and Effective Care Environment: Safety and Infection Control

Critical Thinking Questions

Scenario A

Guillermo Perez had a bout of the "flu" about a week ago. Today he noticed he was having trouble walking. When he got home from an errand, he had trouble pulling his sweater over his head. His wife brought him to the emergency department.

1. Which neurologic problem discussed in this chapter do you think he might have?
2. What might be done to establish a diagnosis?
3. What would be a top priority in his care at this time?
4. What further problems do you think could occur?

Scenario B

Mrs. Jones seems less animated than she has been over the past several months. Her husband tells you she has fallen three times since her last office visit. You notice that she seems more stooped over and her movements are "jerky." The health care provider examines her and, after a thorough history and physical examination, tells the couple that he thinks Mrs. Jones has PD. He prescribes Sinemet for her.

1. What can you anticipate that Mr. and Mrs. Jones will need to be taught?
2. What are the potential complications of PD?

Scenario C

A fellow student in your clinical group confides that she has MG. She takes Mestinon for control of the disease.

1. What factors could cause her symptoms to worsen?
2. What might happen if she forgets to take her medication before reporting for her clinical rotation?

Scenario D

A man comes to the clinic complaining of difficulty enunciating, having tingling and prickling in the extremities, and having increased difficulty walking. After diagnostic testing it is determined that he has ALS.

1. What is the focus of interdisciplinary care?
2. What is the prognosis for the patient?

The Sensory System: Eye

25

http://evolve.elsevier.com/deWit/medsurg

Objectives

Theory

1. Determine ways in which nurses can help patients preserve their sight.
2. Select nursing activities associated with assessing the eye.
3. Use the nursing process for patients with disorders of the eye.
4. Review errors of refraction and their treatment.
5. Devise nursing care for a patient who is undergoing a corneal transplant.
6. Compare measures used to provide assistance after a chemical eye burn with measures for an eye injury caused by a foreign object.
7. Summarize the signs and symptoms of selected disorders of the eye and appropriate medical treatment and nursing interventions for each.
8. Plan nursing interventions for a patient having a scleral buckle or a cataract extraction.

Clinical Practice

9. Provide teaching for a patient who is to undergo tests for a vision problem.
10. Perform focused assessments for disorders of the eyes.
11. Assist visually impaired patients to find resources to maximize their vision.
12. Provide appropriate preoperative care for a patient who is having eye surgery.
13. Properly administer eye medications to patients.

Key Terms

accommodation (ă-kŏm-ō-DĀ-shŭn, p. 597)
astigmatism (ă-STĬG-mă-tĭsm, p. 598)
cataract (KĂ-tĕ-răkt, p. 601)
drusen (drū-zĕn, p. 612)
ectropion (ĕk-TRŌ-pē-ŏn, p. 588)
enucleation (ē-nū-klē-Ā-shŭn, p. 601)
entropion (ĕn-TRŌ-pē-ŏn, p. 594)
exophthalmos (ĕk-sŏf-THĂL-mŏs, p. 593)
hyperopia (hī-pĕr-Ō-pē-ă, p. 597)
keratitis (kĕr-ă-TĪ-tĭs, p. 588)
myopia (mī-Ō-pē-ă, p. 597)
photodynamic therapy (fō-tō-dī-NĂM-ĭk THĔR-ĕ-pē, p. 613)
photophobia (fō-tō-FŌ-bē-ă, p. 593)
presbyopia (prĕz-bē-Ō-pē-ă, p. 587)
ptosis (TŌ-sĭs, p. 588)
refraction (rē-FRĂK-shŭn, p. 586)
xanthelasma (zăn-thĕ-LĂZ-mă, p. 593)

Concepts Covered in This Chapter

- Self-Management
- Sensory Perception
- Nutrition
- Health Promotion
- Safety

ANATOMY AND PHYSIOLOGY OF THE EYE

STRUCTURES OF THE EYE

- The eyeball is spherical in shape and 2 to 3 cm in diameter (Fig. 25.1).
- The sclera, which is part of the wall of the eyeball, is opaque white and covers the posterior five sixths of the eyeball.
- The transparent cornea is part of the wall of the eyeball and covers the anterior one sixth of the eyeball.
- The choroid is part of the middle layer of the eyeball. It is a highly vascular layer containing brown pigment located between the sclera and the retina.
- The ciliary body is part of the middle layer of the eyeball and contains fingerlike ciliary processes that produce aqueous humor. The ciliary body helps change eye shape for near and far vision.
- The iris is the third part of the middle layer of the eyeball; it is the colored portion of the eye and is a doughnut-shaped diaphragm with the pupil as the central opening. The iris contains two groups of smooth muscles that constrict and dilate the pupil to regulate the entrance of light.

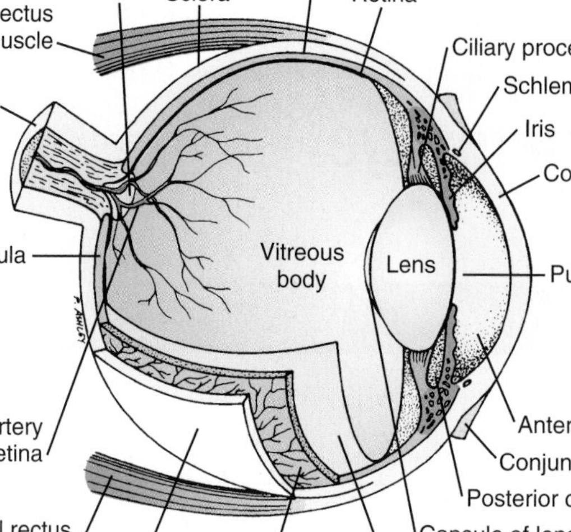

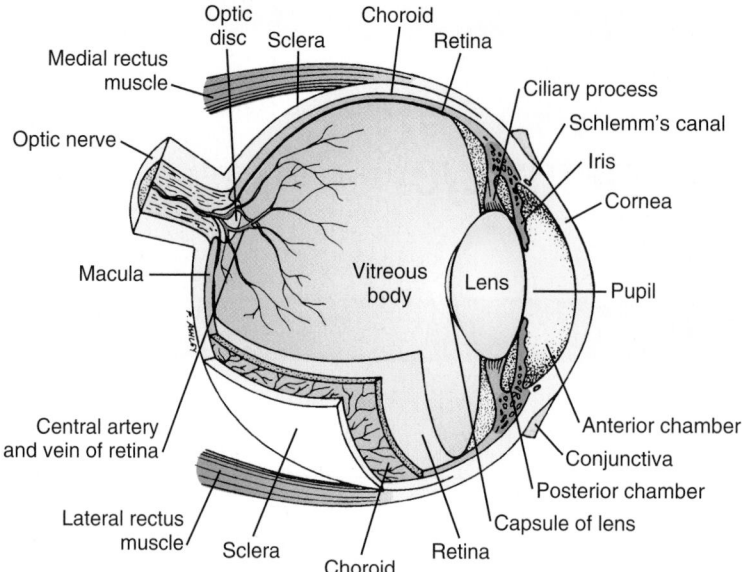

Fig. 25.1 Structures of the eye.

- The biconvex, transparent lens, together with the suspensory ligaments and the ciliary body, forms a partition that divides the interior of the eyeball into two chambers. The anterior chamber between the lens and the cornea is filled with aqueous humor. The posterior chamber, between the lens and the retina, contains vitreous humor.
- The suspensory ligaments connect the ciliary body to the lens.
- The retina is the inner layer of tissue of the eyeball and is found in the posterior portion of it. The retina contains several layers. The layer with rods and cones acts as the receptor for light images.
- The optic nerve carries messages from the nerve cells in the retina to the brain.
- The optic disc is formed by the axons of the ganglion cells of the retina.
- The macula lutea is a yellow spot just lateral to the optic disc that allows for visual detail.
- The fovea centralis is the area of the retina that produces the sharpest image.
- The eyelids are composed of skin, connective tissue, and conjunctiva. The conjunctiva is a thin mucous membrane that lines the eyelid and covers the anterior portion of the eyeball, except for the cornea.
- Eyelashes line the edge of the eyelid.
- Sebaceous glands are situated with the eyelashes.
- The lacrimal glands are in the upper outer area above the eyes. The lacrimal ducts and canals carry tears from the eye to the nose.
- Six muscles attach to the eyeball and allow for movement. The muscles come from the bones of the orbit and insert on the outer layer of the eyeball.

FUNCTIONS OF THE EYE STRUCTURES

- The bony orbit protects the eyeball.
- The eyelashes help trap foreign particles, keeping them from landing on the eyeball.
- The eyelids protect the eyes from foreign matter and help distribute moisture on the eye surface.
- The sebaceous glands secrete an oily fluid that lubricates the lids.
- Blinking of the eyelid 6 to 30 times a minute stimulates the lacrimal glands to produce tears.
- The lacrimal gland secretes tears that moisten, lubricate, and cleanse the surface of the eye. Tears contain an enzyme that helps destroy bacteria and prevent infections.
- The transparent cornea allows light to hit the lens. It assists with the bending of light rays (**refraction**), so that the rays will hit the retina in the right location for images to be transmitted to the brain.
- The choroid's brown pigment absorbs excess light rays that could interfere with vision.
- The ciliary processes secrete aqueous humor that helps maintain the shape of the anterior chamber; it also nourishes the structures in this part of the eye. The aqueous humor assists with refraction of light onto the retina. **The amount of aqueous humor present determines the internal pressure of the eye.** The aqueous humor is reabsorbed by the blood vessels located at the junction of the sclera and the cornea.
- Muscles in the iris control dilation and constriction of the pupil.
- The suspensory ligaments connected to the ciliary body and lens allow light to focus on the lens and retina, which is necessary for close vision.
- The retina's rods and cones are photoreceptors for light and color. The nerves of the retina transmit the images perceived to the brain.
- The optic nerve conducts nerve impulses from the retina to the brain.
- Visualization of the optic disc provides information about the pressure within the eye and within the skull. When intracranial pressure gets higher, the optic disc appears "swollen" or "choked."

Table 25.1 Muscles of the Eye

MUSCLE	CONTROLLING NERVE	FUNCTION
Extrinsic (Skeletal) Muscles		
Superior rectus	Oculomotor (CN III)	Elevates eye, or rolls it superiorly and toward the midline.
Inferior rectus	Oculomotor (CN III)	Depresses eye, or rolls it inferiorly and toward the midline.
Medial rectus	Oculomotor (CN III)	Moves eye medially, toward the midline.
Lateral rectus	Abducens (CN VI)	Moves eye laterally, away from the midline.
Superior oblique	Trochlear (CN IV)	Depresses eye and turns it laterally, away from the midline.
Inferior oblique	Oculomotor (CN III)	Elevates eye and turns it laterally, away from the midline.
Intrinsic (Smooth) Muscles		
Ciliary	Oculomotor (CN III): parasympathetic fibers	Causes suspensory ligament to relax, so lens becomes more convex for close vision.
Iris, circular muscles	Oculomotor (CN III): parasympathetic fibers	Decreases the size of the pupil to allow less light to enter the eye.
Iris, radial muscles	Sympathetic fibers from spinal nerves	Increases the size of the pupil to allow more light to enter the eye.

Adapted from Applegate EJ: *The anatomy and physiology learning system,* ed 4, Philadelphia, 2011, Elsevier.
CN, Cranial nerve.

- Visual impulses travel along the optic nerve to the optic chiasma just anterior to the pituitary gland; at this point some of the axons cross over to the other side. Images from the medial portion of the left eye and from the lateral portion of the right eye are carried by the right optic tract. Images from the medial portion of the right eye and from the lateral portion of the left eye are carried by the left optic tract (Fig. 25.2). Images are conducted to the visual cortex in the occipital lobe of the brain.
- Six muscles control movement of the eyeball. Table 25.1 lists these muscles and the nerves that control them.

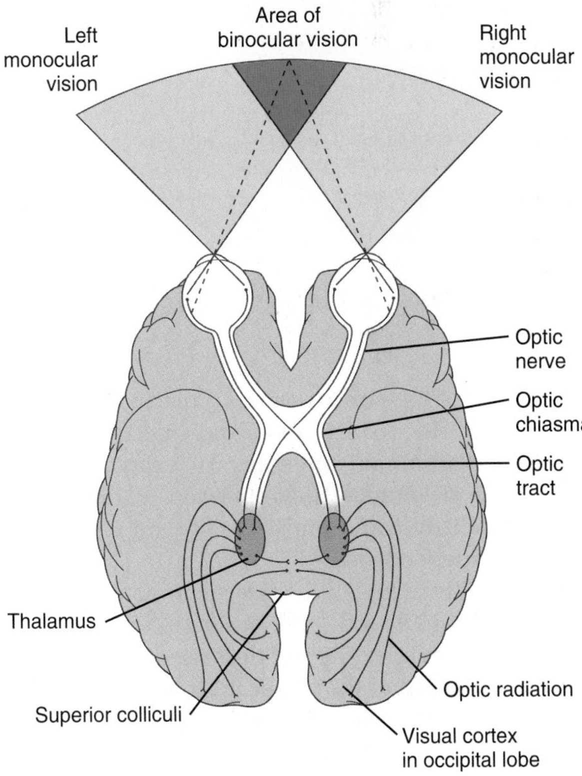

Fig. 25.2 Visual pathway.

AGING-RELATED EYE CHANGES

- Subcutaneous fat and tissue elasticity decrease, and the eyes appear to be sunken.
- *Arcus senilis,* an opaque ring outlining the cornea, sometimes results from the deposition of fatty globules (Fig. 25.3).
- The cornea flattens and develops an irregular curvature after age 65 years, causing astigmatism or making an existing astigmatism worse; vision becomes blurred. Cornea transparency also decreases.
- The sclera develops a yellowish tinge from fatty deposits; thinning of the sclera may cause a bluish tinge.
- The ability of the iris to dilate decreases, causing difficulty for the older person in going from a bright area to a darkened area.
- The lens of the eye changes after age 40 years, gradually losing water and becoming harder. Cataracts may form.
- The ciliary muscle has less ability to allow the eye to accommodate, a process responsible for the gradual extension of distance from the eyes at which an item to be read is held (**presbyopia**). This change usually begins around age 40 years.
- The farthest point at which an object can be identified decreases, and the visual field narrows.
- Pupil size becomes smaller, reducing the ability to see in dim light.
- Color discrimination decreases and may cause problems.

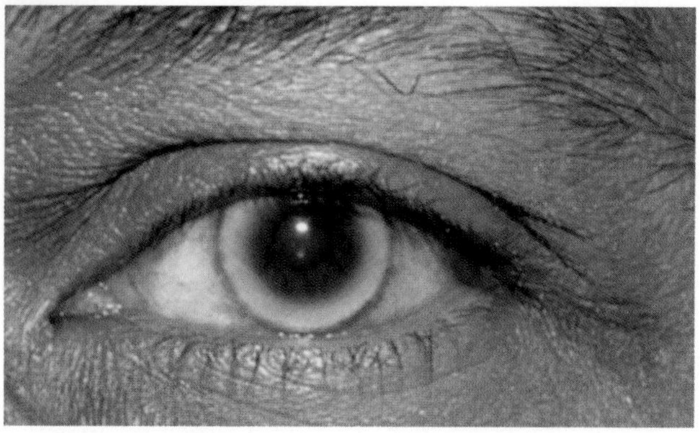

Fig. 25.3 Arcus senilis, a white ring around the cornea. (From Swartz M: *Textbook of physical diagnosis: history and examination*, ed 7, Philadelphia, 2014, Elsevier.)

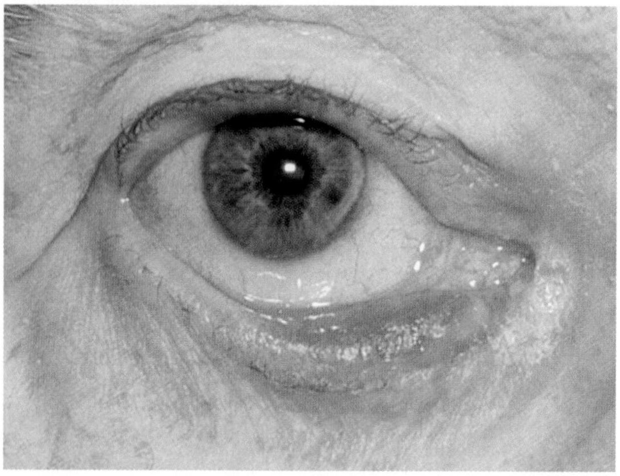

Fig. 25.4 Ectropion. (From Swartz M: *Textbook of physical diagnosis: history and examination*, ed 7, Philadelphia, 2014, Elsevier.)

- Moisture secretion decreases, placing the eyes at greater risk for irritation and infection. This is especially common after age 70 years. Repeated episodes of **keratitis** (inflammation of the cornea) may seriously compromise vision and can lead to loss of independence.
- Eversion of the lower lid (**ectropion**) occurs because of loss of muscle tone and elasticity (Fig. 25.4).
- Decreased muscle tone and decreased elasticity may cause drooping of the upper lid to a point where it interferes with vision (**ptosis**).

THE EYE

EYE DISORDERS

There are approximately 25.5 million visually impaired or blind people in the United States. Of those, 7.3 million are older than 65 years (American Foundation for the Blind, 2018). There are two general kinds of patients with impaired vision: those who were born blind and those who develop some degree of visual impairment later in life. This chapter focuses on the latter type of visually impaired patient.

Eye disorders are caused by injury or disease, or are disorders for which there is a genetic predisposition (such as retinitis pigmentosa). Diabetes mellitus and hypertension contribute greatly to visual loss in the United States. Stroke can cause altered vision or full or partial blindness. Untreated glaucoma causes blindness. Macular degeneration is another major cause of impaired vision. It is now known that smoking has a direct link to the incidence of macular degeneration. Cataracts eventually cause blindness if they are not removed.

Many new surgical techniques and medical treatments offer hope for eyesight preservation to increasing numbers of people. Efforts also have been made to educate the public about eye care, prevention of eye disease, and periodic examinations to detect eye disorders in their earliest and most treatable stages.

Acquired immunodeficiency syndrome (AIDS) can cause blindness as a result of opportunistic infections. Ocular problems common in patients with AIDS are discussed in Chapter 11.

Prevention

As health care providers, nurses share responsibility for preserving vision throughout the patient's life span. Three major nursing goals to promote good vision are:

- Health education to inform the general public about basic eye care
- Prevention of accidental injury to the eye
- Prevention of visual loss

Healthy People 2030 goals contain 10 objectives related to preventing vision loss and improving vision.

BASIC EYE CARE

To prevent eye strain, rest the eye muscles periodically when in front of electronic screens, whether working, watching or interacting, or performing any activity that demands intensive visual effort. If the eyes tire easily or if there is headache or burning, itching, or redness of the eyes, the eyes should be examined. A healthy lifestyle will help prevent vision problems. Good nutrition; staying active; not smoking; and controlling weight, blood pressure, and cholesterol will all contribute to better eye health.

Normal secretions of the conjunctiva and tear glands should be sufficient to lubricate the eye and wash away small particles of dust. **Accumulations of purulent material or excessive tearing usually indicate the need for an eye examination.** Dry eye syndrome in people younger than 60 years could be symptomatic of underlying disease.

Adults with no risk factors should have a baseline eye examination at age 40, every 2 to 4 years from ages 40 to 54, and every 1 to 3 years from ages 55 to 64. After age 65, eyes should be examined by an eye specialist every 1 to 2 years (American Academy of Ophthalmology [AAO], 2015). It is particularly important to test for glaucoma because this disease usually is asymptomatic until damage to vision has occurred. People with a

Nutrition Considerations

Vitamins and Antioxidants Beneficial to Vision

Vitamin A protects against night blindness, slow adaptation to darkness, and glare blindness. The carotenoids are the precursors for vitamin A and are found in green leafy and yellow vegetables. Carrots, greens, spinach, orange juice, sweet potatoes, and cantaloupe are rich sources of the carotenoids (Pazirandeh & Burns, 2018). Lutein and zeaxanthin, both antioxidants, may help prevent macular degeneration and cataracts. They are found in yellow fruits and vegetables, red and purple fruits, and greens. Lutein is particularly high in tomatoes, carrots, broccoli, kale, spinach, and romaine lettuce. Corn, cornmeal, kale, Japanese persimmons, and turnip greens have large quantities of zeaxanthin; corn contains the highest amount. Many vitamin supplements have added lutein to their formulation (National Eye Institute, 2018).

Older Adult Care Points

Older persons sometimes suffer from "dry eyes" as a result of decreased production of tears. This condition is treated by instilling "replacement tears," which are commercial preparations or prescriptions of solutions similar in composition to real tears.

family history of glaucoma should be especially careful to have their eyes tested frequently for increased pressure within the eyeball because this is the basic pathology of glaucoma and the disorder tends to be hereditary.

PREVENTION OF EYE INJURY

Accidental injury to the eye is a major cause of diminished or total loss of vision. Adults should be cautioned to wear protective eyewear when engaging in sports such as racquetball and squash in which small balls travel at high speeds. Protective eyewear should be worn when using machinery that might cause debris to fly into the eye, such as lawn mowers, weed trimmers, sanders, or power saws. Chemicals splashing into the eyes are another source of injury that can be prevented by protective eyewear.

The rate of occupational accidents has decreased since the establishment and enforcement of rules for wearing goggles and other protective devices by people working in a hazardous environment. The National Institute for Occupational Safety and Health (NIOSH) in Rockville, Maryland, provides information about eye safety and hazards in the workplace.

Cosmetics for the eyelids, eyelashes, and eyebrows can be a source of infection and allergy. Eye makeup should be discarded every 2 to 4 months to help prevent infection (U.S. Food and Drug Administration [FDA], 2018). Most dyes used for hair on the scalp are not intended for use on the eyelashes and eyebrows.

Saliva should not be used to moisten eye pencils, eye shadow, or mascara because it may contain organisms that can cause eye infection. Eye cosmetics should be applied with a steady hand to prevent accidentally scratching of the cornea and eyelids. Cosmetics should never be shared because this can transmit organisms.

Safety Alert

Contact Lenses

The Centers for Disease Control and Prevention (CDC) recommends the following for prevention of eye injury or infection: wash hands before handling contacts; do not sleep with contacts in place; keep water away from contacts (showering, swimming); clean contacts with lens disinfecting solution; never store lenses in water; replace contacts as recommended; clean contact case with lens solution—never water; replace lens case every 3 months.

Health Promotion

Danger Signals of Eye Disease

- Persistent redness of the eye. Infections and inflammations of the structures of the eye that are not treated may leave scars that can produce loss of vision.
- Continuing pain or discomfort, especially after an injury.
- Disturbance of vision. Although these symptoms may simply indicate a need for eyeglasses, blurred vision, loss of side vision, double vision, and sudden development of many floating spots in the field of vision may be symptomatic of more serious systemic diseases.
- Colored light flashes, or a feeling that a curtain has been pulled across the line of vision or a shade has been pulled down. This can indicate a retinal detachment and requires prompt attention.
- Crossing of the eyes, especially in children.
- Growths on the eye or eyelids, or opacities visible in the normally transparent portion of the eye.
- Continuing discharge, crusting, or tearing of the eyes.
- Unequal size of the two pupils or distorted shape.

PREVENTION OF VISION LOSS

Diabetes mellitus and hypertension are chronic diseases that—when uncontrolled—may cause vision loss. Patients with these disorders are more susceptible to retinopathy. Nurses should encourage good control over these diseases.

To help prevent infections that might cause corneal scarring and loss of vision, encourage people who experience an accident that causes a corneal abrasion to seek medical attention quickly. Promptly seeking medical attention when the eye is inflamed, is secreting purulent discharge, or is sore assists in treatment of infection that may cause a residual vision loss.

Assessing patients for the presence of cataracts and recommending regular periodic eye examinations should be a part of every nurse's practice. Cataract removal can greatly improve vision. Screening for glaucoma reduces the incidence of blindness from that condition. A handheld tonometer is used for measuring intraocular

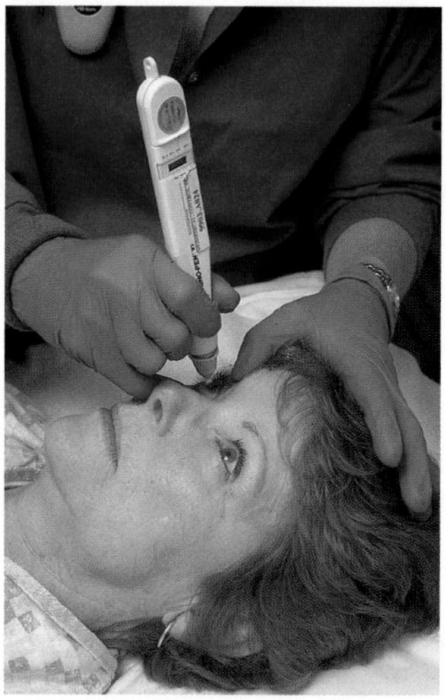

Fig. 25.5 A handheld tonometer is used to check intraocular pressure.

Cultural Considerations

Latinos and Eye Disease

The Los Angeles Latino Eye Study found that Latinos had high rates of diabetic retinopathy and of open-angle glaucoma. The study interviewed and examined 6300 Latinos age 40 years and older from the Los Angeles area. Many of the Latinos involved in the study were found to have previously undiagnosed diabetes. Almost half of the individuals in the study who had diabetes had diabetic retinopathy. Seventy-five percent of Latinos with glaucoma were undiagnosed before participating in the study (National Eye Institute, 2010). Further studies have identified that educational level, income, and mental health correlate with eye disease knowledge and exposure to health information. These findings are being used to improve health education to the Hispanic/Latino community (McClure et al., 2017).

Think Critically

Identify four specific ways in which you might help prevent eye disorders among your relatives and patients.

pressure (IOP) to identify glaucoma (Fig. 25.5). Free screening clinics often are available in communities. You can inform patients of when and where such screenings are available.

You must be aware that there are many types of vision loss. Some may affect only one area of the field of vision in one eye, whereas others may affect parts of the field of vision in both eyes. The degree of visual impairment varies greatly.

DIAGNOSTIC TESTS AND EXAMINATIONS

Diagnostic tests are performed to test visual acuity, prescribe prescription lenses, inspect the interior of the eye, check IOP, and assess the health of the retinal blood vessels (Fig. 25.6). Computed tomography, optical coherence tomography, and magnetic resonance imaging may also be used to diagnose eye disorders. Table 25.2 provides further information about diagnostic tests.

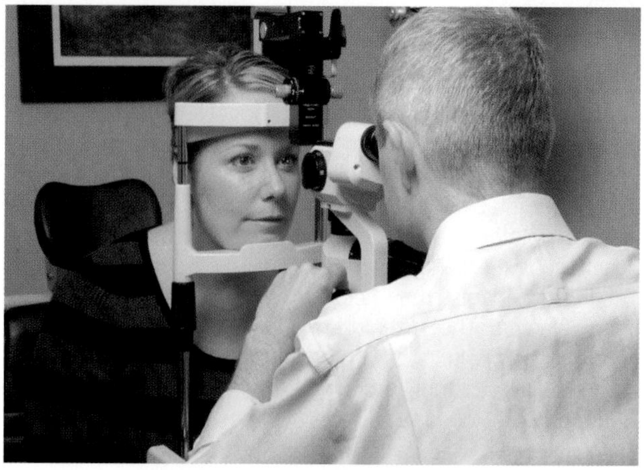

Fig. 25.6 Slit-lamp ocular examination.

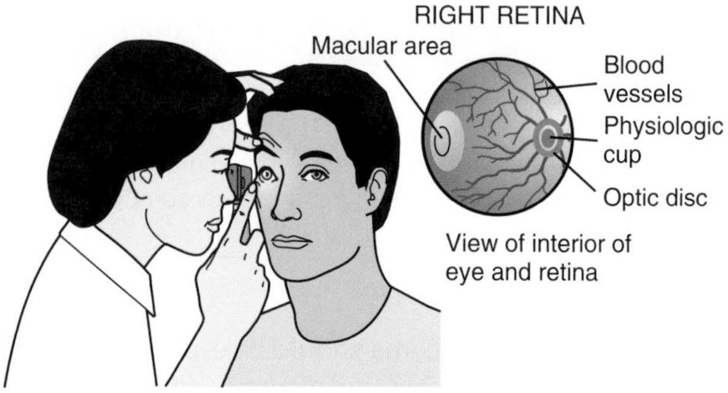

Fig. 25.7 Examination of the eye with an ophthalmoscope.

NURSING MANAGEMENT

The nursing care of patients with severe visual impairments demands a special awareness of the unique problems encountered by someone who has either a partial or a total loss of vision. You must be sensitive to these patients' special needs. Patient education is especially important to these patients' acceptance of their visual disorder, their participation in diagnostic and therapeutic measures, and their adjustment to their new surroundings when they are hospitalized or admitted to a long-term care facility.

ASSESSMENT (DATA COLLECTION)

All nurses should be able to perform a basic eye examination, inspecting the eye for signs of redness or discharge and checking visual acuity with a Snellen eye chart. Only nurses who have had special training are qualified to conduct a complete eye assessment (Fig. 25.7). Significant data can be obtained by nurses who lack specialized education by taking an adequate history.

Table 25.2 Diagnostic Tests for Eye Problems

TEST	PURPOSE	DESCRIPTION	NURSING IMPLICATIONS
Ophthalmoscopy (retinoscopy)	To inspect the fundus (back portion) of the eyeball to detect abnormalities of the retina, macula, optic disc, and retinal vessels	The examiner uses an ophthalmoscope (see Fig. 25.7) to focus light through the pupil onto the fundus.	The room is darkened before the examiner approaches the patient with the ophthalmoscope. Drops may be placed in the eye before this examination to dilate the eye and offer a wider area through which to view the fundus.
Visual acuity	To determine status of vision	The Snellen eye chart is used. It is placed 20 feet from the patient; first one eye is occluded, then the other eye is occluded. The person begins reading lines of letters that decrease in size. Visual acuity is expressed as a fraction for each eye. The numerator (first) figure indicates the distance between the patient and the chart. The denominator (second) figure expresses the distance at which the person with 20/20 vision could read the letters in the line correctly. Visual acuity of 20/20 in each eye is normal; vision of 20/200 (with correction) is legally defined as blindness.	Explain the procedure to the patient. Have the patient hold the occluding card close to the nose so that the entire eye is covered. Start with the third line. If the patient cannot read that, progress upward; if the line is correctly read, go to the next line down. Test the other eye. Record the findings.
Near vision test	To determine status of near vision	The patient is given a Jaeger Test Type card with different sizes of type on it. One eye is occluded while the patient reads the lines of type. Determination of vision status is made based on what a person with normal vision can read.	Explain that this is a simple test of vision to determine whether there are any problems that might require further testing.
Visual fields test (confrontation test)	To examine the patient's visual fields, detecting problems with peripheral vision	The examiner faces the patient and asks them to look directly into the corresponding eye of the examiner. The patient covers their left eye with their left hand and looks into the right eye of the examiner. Then the examiner's finger is moved from an area outside the peripheral vision into the line of vision. The patient indicates when the finger becomes visible. The examiner may also hold up a certain number of fingers to be distinguished. All four quadrants are tested. The test is repeated with the other eye covered.	Explain the test to the patient and remind them to keep looking directly into your eyes.
Extraocular muscle function test	To test the function of the extraocular muscles	Ask the patient to hold their head still and to move their eyes to follow a small object such as a pen to each of the six cardinal points: right; upward and right; downward and right; left; upward and left; downward and left.	Observe for parallel eye movements and any deviation of movement. Nystagmus is a normal finding for the far lateral gaze. Record your findings.
Color vision test	To determine whether the patient has any color blindness	Use the Ishihara chart book, which shows numbers composed of dots of one color within an area of dots of a different color. Ask the patient what they see on the page for each chart. Test each eye separately. Reading the numbers correctly indicates normal color vision.	Explain the purpose of the test. Tell the patient to tell you what number appears on the chart. Record your findings.

Continued

Table 25.2 Diagnostic Tests for Eye Problems—cont'd

TEST	PURPOSE	DESCRIPTION	NURSING IMPLICATIONS
Refraction	To determine amount of lens correction necessary to restore person's vision to as near normal as possible with eyeglasses	A series of glass lenses are placed in front of the patient's eyes to determine which lens provides the best vision correction. Each eye is tested separately.	A prescription for eyeglasses will be written depending on the findings of the refraction test. The test may be performed for both near and far vision.
Intraocular pressure test	To determine the amount of pressure within the eye; aids in diagnosis of glaucoma	After anesthetizing the cornea a tonometer is used to measure the pressure. Methods available: applanation tonometry—a tonometer tip is placed on an anesthetized cornea. Perkins tonometer—uses the same applanating prism but is portable. Noncontact tonometry—uses an "air puff" for measurement. Tono-Pen—handheld electronic device that contacts the cornea with a latex tip plunger. Icare—handheld device that measures an induction current.	Explain that this is a test to determine whether a patient might have glaucoma. More than one reading on different days is necessary to confirm a diagnosis of glaucoma. If a diagnosis of glaucoma is made, medication can be prescribed to help control the intraocular pressure and preserve vision. For Tono-Pen, verify no latex allergy. For Icare, no topical anesthesia is required.
Slit-lamp biomicroscopic examination	To examine the surface of the eye	A beam of light is reduced to a narrow slit that illuminates only a small section of the eye, allowing examination of a thin section of the eye structures at a time.	Explain that this device helps detect "floaters" in the vitreous humor and abnormalities of the cornea and other structures of the eye. The eyes may be dilated with mydriatic drops for this test.
Topical dye (corneal staining)	To detect abrasions of the cornea or the presence of a foreign body on the cornea	Fluorescein dye drops are administered to the affected eye. The dye remains on the injured tissue or surrounds a foreign body. Such areas usually appear as green spots.	Explain the procedure and the rationale for the test. Warn that the drops may sting slightly for a few minutes. Give the patient a tissue to absorb the excess drops because they may stain clothing.
Fluorescein angiography (retinal angiography)	To detect tumors of the interior of the eye and to help diagnose and measure the extent of retinopathy	An intravenous (IV) injection of sodium fluorescein is given. A short time later, photographs of the fundus are taken with a special camera.	An IV injection is necessary. A signed consent form is required to perform the procedure.
Indocyanine green angiography	To image the vasculature of the retina and choroid and to evaluate macular degeneration.	Similar to fluorescein angiography with indocyanine green used with an infrared-sensitive camera.	An IV injection is necessary. A signed consent form is required to perform the procedure.
Electroretinography	To test the functional integrity of the retina; evaluates degeneration of the photoreceptor cells	Electrodes embedded into a contact lens are placed directly on the anesthetized eye. A light stimulus is introduced. The change in electrical potential of the eye caused by the flash of light is measured.	Instruct the patient that they must fixate on the target and not move their eyes during the test.

Table 25.2 Diagnostic Tests for Eye Problems—cont'd

TEST	PURPOSE	DESCRIPTION	NURSING IMPLICATIONS
Optical coherence tomography (OCT)	To record images of retinal structures To differentiate the anatomic layers within the retina and allow measurement of retinal thickness To detect macular holes, epiretinal membranes, cystoid macular edema, and other pathologies	Focused beams of light that scan the structural features of the retina are directed into the eye. A cross-sectional image similar to a topographic map is produced.	The patient's eyes must be dilated. Tell the patient that they will be looking into a machine. The test takes 5 to 10 min.
Amsler grid test	To detect macular degeneration	Using a handheld card printed with a grid of black lines similar to graph paper, the patient fixates on a center dot and records abnormalities of the grid lines.	Test should be performed every week or two. Instruct the patient to record seeing wavy or missing lines or distorted areas.
Ultrasonography	To evaluate the characteristics of a lesion and its size and growth over time, or to determine the presence of a foreign body	A probe is placed directly on the eyeball. Sound waves are transmitted into the eye, bounce off the various tissues, and are collected by a receiver and amplified on an oscilloscope screen.	Explain the procedure to the patient.

History Taking

Many systemic diseases, including AIDS, hypertension, and diabetes mellitus, secondarily affect the eye and its functions. In the general assessment of any patient, you should be aware of the more obvious indications of an ophthalmic pathology, whether it is primary or secondary.

A history of neurologic disorders should be noted. Neuromuscular diseases are especially likely to cause diplopia, blurred vision, or inability to move the eyes. Endocrine disorders that secondarily affect the eyes include thyroid disease and diabetes mellitus. Acute hyperglycemia can alter the shape of the lens and temporarily cause blurred vision. **Prolonged hyperglycemia can adversely affect the blood vessels of the retina, causing dilation and blood flow changes leading to loss of vision.** Liver and kidney failure can produce pathologic changes in both neural and vascular structures within the eye. Retinal changes also can be caused by hypertension and atherosclerosis.

Some drugs can produce either transient or permanent ocular changes that lead to disturbances in color vision and visual acuity, and to the formation of cataracts, retinopathy, and glaucoma. Among common drugs that have possible ocular side effects are ethambutol, isoniazid, amiodarone, tamoxifen, isotretinoin (Accutane), and corticosteroids.

A family history of eye disorders can be significant because disorders such as strabismus, retinitis pigmentosa, glaucoma, and cataracts tend to run in families or follow a pattern of inheritance.

Sometimes patients are not aware of gradual changes in vision but have noticed that they have had more minor accidents lately, seem to be more easily fatigued, or are less interested in doing things that once gave them pleasure, such as reading, sewing, or some other hobby that requires close vision.

Physical Examination

Observe the patient's eyes and eye area for redness of the conjunctiva, swelling of the eyelids or in the periorbital space, excessive tearing, change in visual acuity, secretions and encrustations on the eyelids, abnormal position of the eyelid, and **exophthalmos** (protrusion of the eyeball). Abnormalities of lid position are described in Table 25.3. **Xanthelasma**, or soft, raised, yellow areas, sometimes appear on the eyelid after age 50 years (Fig. 25.8). Signs and symptoms of selected eye diseases are listed in Table 25.4. In addition to the more obvious signs of eye disease, visual impairment also can be assessed by noting the patient's head, hand, and eye movements. Tilting the head to one side to improve vision could mean that the patient has double vision or that one eye is much stronger than the other. Squinting could mean poor vision. Shading the eyes with the hands may indicate an increased sensitivity to light (**photophobia**).

Observation of the patient's ability to move the eyebrows and eyes can be helpful in diagnosing nerve

Focused Assessment

Data Collection for Eye Disorders

The following questions should be asked when gathering history regarding an eye disorder:

- Have you noticed a change in your vision?
- Do you have any pain or discomfort in the eyes? Itching? Burning? Stinging? Excessive tearing or watering?
- Have you had any episodes of blurred vision? Double vision? A loss in the field of vision? Blind spots? Floating spots?
- Do you have difficulty with vision at night?
- Is there any pain in your eyes when you are in bright light?
- Do you have headaches in the brow area?
- Do you see halos around lights?
- Have you ever injured an eye in any way?
- Do you experience frequent reddening of the eye (conjunctivitis)?
- Do you ever experience discharge or sticky matter in the eye?
- Do you find that your lids are crusty when you awaken?
- Do your eyes feel dry? Do you frequently use eye drops?
- Do you wear contact lenses? Use glasses?
- What medications do you take regularly?
- Is there any history of glaucoma in your family?
- Have you ever been told you have diabetes? Hypertension?
- When did you have your last eye examination?
- **For those patients who have a previous visual loss:** How do you cope with your loss of vision?

damage. Inability to raise the eyebrows indicates damage to the facial nerve. Movement of the eyeball to direct the gaze is controlled by six muscles, which are controlled by three cranial nerves: the oculomotor nerve (third cranial), the trochlear nerve (fourth cranial), and the abducens nerve (sixth cranial) (see Table 25.1).

◆ NURSING DIAGNOSIS

Problem statements or nursing diagnoses are based on the data obtained from assessment. The licensed practical/vocational nurse (LPN/LVN) collaborates with the registered nurse (RN) in formulating the nursing care plan and selecting the problem statements. Problem statements commonly used for patients with eye disease are as follows:

- Potential for injury due to decreased visual field.
- Fear due to visual loss.

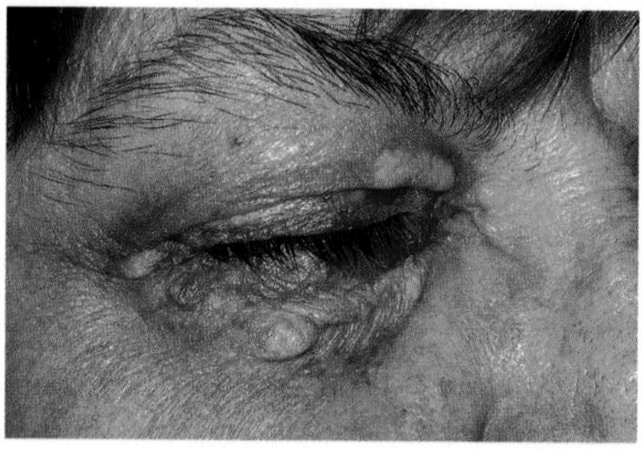

Fig. 25.8 Xanthelasma. (From Bolognia JL, Schaffer JV, Duncan KO, et al.: *Dermatology essentials,* St. Louis, 2014, Elsevier.)

Table 25.3 Abnormalities of Lid Position

ABNORMALITY	CAUSES	SYMPTOMS	TREATMENT
Entropion: Inversion of lid margin; eyelids are turned inward toward eyeball so that lashes rub against eyeball	Scarring and contraction of skin near eyelid (cicatricial entropion) or aging of skin with laxness of tissues supporting the lid and contraction of orbicularis muscle (spastic entropion)	Pain, tearing, redness, and corneal ulceration caused by lid margin and eyelashes rubbing against cornea	Splinting the lid, using a pressure patch, or taping lid into everted (turned outward) position Surgical correction by tightening musculature and everting lid margin
Ectropion: Eversion or outward turning of the lower lid	Aging and laxness of skin and muscle tissues, facial paralysis, edema of conjunctiva lining the lid, or contraction of scar tissue	Irritation of palpebral conjunctiva, spilling of tears down the cheeks because of a blocked outlet, irritation of skin of cheeks, symptoms of conjunctivitis	Usually responds to patching of the eye Surgical correction necessary if paralysis of orbicularis muscle is permanent, or if there is severe scarring and contraction of skin near the lid
Ptosis: Drooping of the eyelid so that it partially or completely covers the cornea	Congenital weakness of the levator superioris muscle or long-term presence of foreign body; one of first signs of myasthenia gravis	Obvious drooping of eyelid If not corrected in infants, can lead to blindness because light rays cannot enter and stimulate development of the eye Patient may be observed tilting head back or raising eyebrows to see from under eyelids	Surgical correction Removal of foreign body, if that is the cause

Table 25.4 Clinical Signs and Symptoms of Selected Eye Diseases, Medical Treatment, and Nursing Interventions

DISEASE	SIGNS AND SYMPTOMS	MEDICAL TREATMENT AND NURSING INTERVENTIONS
Blepharitis: Infection of glands and lash follicles along lid margin	Itching, burning, sensitivity to light Mucus discharge and scaling; eyelids crusted, glued shut, especially on awakening Loss of eyelashes	Warm compresses to soften secretions; scrub eyelids with baby shampoo; stroke sideways to remove exudate and scales. Antibiotic eye drops; systemic and topical antibiotics if skin is infected.
Chalazion: Internal stye; infection of meibomian gland	Astigmatism or distorted vision, depending on size and location of chalazion Small, hard tumor on eyelid	Chalazion may require surgical excision and antibiotics to prevent chronic state and cyst formation.
Hordeolum: External stye; infected swelling near the lid margin on inside	Sharp pain that becomes dull and throbbing Rupture and drainage of pus bring relief Localized redness and swelling of lid	Hordeolum usually resolves spontaneously. Warm compresses qid for 10–15 min to bring stye to a head and hasten rupture. Caution patient never to squeeze swelling because this could spread infection; poor health status can predispose a person to recurrence of styes.
Conjunctivitis: Inflammation of the conjunctiva; "pink eye" is a specific type caused by chemical irritants, bacteria, or virus	Varying degrees of pain and discomfort Increased tearing and mucus production Itching; sensation of a foreign body in the eye	Depends on type of infecting organism; antibiotic eye drops and ointments for bacterial infections. Not all bacterial infections need treatment; they are self-limiting. There is no role for glucocorticoid use in treatment. Special care when handling infective material.
Keratitis: Inflammation of the cornea	Varying degrees of pain and discomfort Photophobia; blurred vision if center of cornea is affected	Depends on specific causes; could be allergy, microbes, ischemia, or decreased lacrimation. Most superficial lesions are self-healing. Antibiotic eye drops or ointment used for bacterial infections. Steroids can reduce inflammation and discomfort; however, herpes infection can rapidly worsen keratitis unless an antiviral agent is given simultaneously. Patient is encouraged to use good personal hygiene, frequent hand hygiene.
Corneal abrasion or ulceration	Moderate to severe pain and discomfort aggravated by blinking History of trauma, foreign body, contact lens wear	Change or discontinue use of contact lens. Teach patient proper way to insert, remove, and care for contact lens. Caution patient not to moisten lens with saliva. Topical antibiotic ointment and cycloplegic drops for pain.

qid, Four times daily.

- Inadequate home maintenance ability due to impaired or lost vision.
- Potential altered activity due to visual limitation.
- Fall risk.
- Potential for altered role.
- Visual impairment.
- Altered sensory perception.
- Insufficient knowledge for instilling eye drops properly.

◆ PLANNING

Expected outcomes for these problem statements might be:

- Patient will compensate for decreased visual acuity and not suffer sensory deprivation.
- Patient will not experience injury.
- Patient will verbalize decreased fear as treatment begins to help condition.
- Patient will seek assistance with home maintenance within 7 days.
- Patient will explore means of diversion other than reading and watching television.
- Patient will demonstrate proper instillation of eye drops and will verbalize the schedule for the eye drops.

When a patient is visually impaired, plan extra time to assist with personal care, to allow the patient to perform as much self-care as possible. Planning also must incorporate patient teaching on the administration of medication and self-care instructions for a patient with decreased vision (see the Evolve website).

Box 25.1 Instillation of Eye Drops and Eye Ointment

Check the medication label and be certain which eye is to receive the medication. Follow the "Six Rights" of medication administration. Perform hand hygiene and apply gloves.

EYE DROPS

- Remove the cap and place it on the table on its side or upside down.
- With the patient sitting or reclining, ask the patient to look up at the ceiling and tilt the head slightly toward the eye receiving the drop.
- With a tissue beneath the fingers, retract the lower lid downward, exposing the conjunctival sac.
- Stabilize the eye drop container above the eye and drop the designated number of drops directly into the conjunctival sac. Do not place drops on the cornea.
- For systemically absorbed drugs, block the entrance to the lacrimal gland by placing a finger over it for 30 to 60 seconds.
- Carefully replace the cap on the container without contaminating the dropper tip.
- Ask the patient to close the eyelids gently for up to a minute to allow the medication to be absorbed by the eye.

EYE OINTMENT

Ointment rather than drops is sometimes used to aid in the process of treating rough, dry eyes and to introduce moisture to the surface of the eye. Also, ointment may include antibiotics.

- Remove the cap from the tube and place it on the table upside down.
- Expose the conjunctival sac.
- Apply a thin ribbon of ointment along the entire length of the conjunctival sac.
- To end the ribbon, twist the tube with a lateral movement of the wrist without touching the eye.
- Recap the tube.
- Ask the patient to gently close the eyelids and roll the eyes around under the lids to distribute the medication.

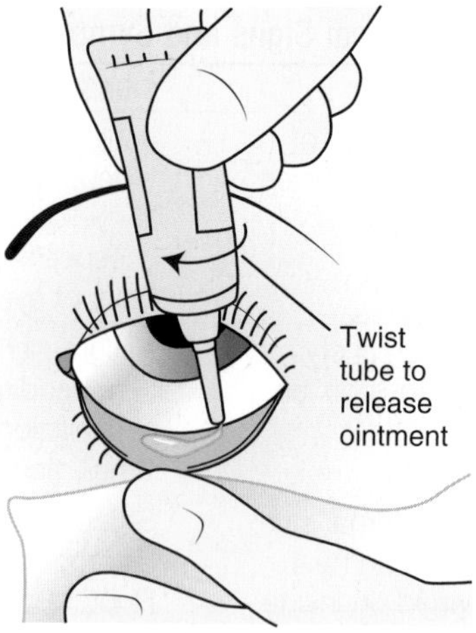

Fig. 25.9 Applying eye ointment.

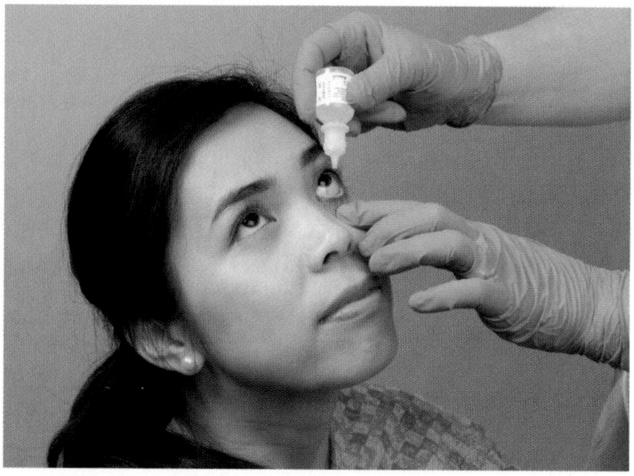

Fig. 25.10 Instilling eye drops.

◆ IMPLEMENTATION

Many eye problems require that eye drops or ophthalmic ointment be applied to the eye several times a day (Box 25.1; Figs. 25.9 and 25.10). A new contact lens delivery system is being tested to dispense a glaucoma drug directly to the surface of eye in a time-release manner. The lens stays on the eye for 1 month. Human trials began in 2019 (Ignotz, 2018). This will make it easier to deliver therapy to those patients who have difficulty self-administering eye medications.

Nursing Interventions for Visually Impaired Patients

Individuals with impaired sight must make considerable adjustments. People who have lost their eyesight may experience hopelessness and despair. Patients who are visually impaired go through stages of grief in much the same way a dying person does. A different lifestyle must be learned, but it is not necessarily less meaningful.

When communicating with these patients, remember that the person has a vision impairment; they are not deaf. Speak normally. Speak to the person and identify yourself as you enter the room, and do not touch the patient until after you have spoken to them—this prevents startling or frightening the patient if they did not hear you enter the room. Ensure that they are oriented to the room and can easily locate the call bell.

Prevention of accidents is an important part of the care of a blind person. Aside from the physical effects of bumping into objects or falling over them, a person who is visually impaired also may experience a loss of self-confidence and security if movement is not safe and independent. Doors should be kept closed or left completely open. They must never be left ajar. Always return things to their places when working in the room. If it is necessary to move any object in the room, ask for the patient's consent and state the object's new location. When you leave the room, tell the patient that you are going. This will prevent them from becoming frustrated by resuming a conversation, only to find that no one is there. When ambulating with a patient with a visual impairment, lead with the patient holding your arm as they follow.

Pity is neither expected nor appreciated by people with visual impairments. They want to be treated as other people and would prefer to ask for your help when they need it rather than have you do everything for them. If you are assigned to the care of a patient with a visual impairment, determine the amount of assistance the patient needs and wants by asking. Do not assume that the person is helpless, but do not neglect the patient when help is needed.

When a patient who is visually impaired is admitted, they will require special orientation to the room and surroundings. If there is total blindness, describe the size of the room and the placement of furniture, using the bed as the focal point. An ambulatory patient can be walked around the room and to the bathroom to develop familiarity with the location of the commode, bath, and sink. As with any patient, explain how to locate and use the call system, the TV, and the telephone (if there is one at the bedside). If the patient uses a cane or other aid, make sure it is where it can be easily located.

Most patients prefer to feed themselves if at all possible. However, it usually is necessary to set up the meal tray of patients who are visually impaired, using the "clock" method for placement of food on the plate. The patient is told what food is in which area (e.g., "The potatoes are at 2 o'clock."). Setting up the meal tray includes opening containers of milk and juice, pouring coffee or tea, and cutting meat into bite-size pieces, unless the patient is accustomed to doing these things.

> **Assignment Considerations**
>
> **Assisting Visually Impaired Patients**
>
> If a certified nursing assistant (CNA) or unlicensed assistive personnel (UAP) is assigned to help feed, ambulate, or care for a patient who is visually impaired, be certain that the aide understands what the visual impairment is and whether one or both eyes are affected. Ask that the aide announce their presence with a knock on the door and speak before touching the patient. Review how to assist with meals for a blind patient and how to aid with ambulation. Gently remind the CNA or UAP that the patient is blind and not deaf, unless deafness is also a patient problem.

Do not give a person who is visually impaired a straw or drinking tube unless you are asked to because it may be awkward to use. If you must feed the patient all of a meal, work slowly and calmly. Indicate about hot and cold foods on the tray, and ask the patient which foods they prefer next, altering as desired. Avoid talking too much, thus forcing the patient to either stop eating or answer you with a mouth full of food. Whenever possible, help the patient select finger foods such as sandwiches and raw fruit or vegetables from the menu. The goal is to help the patient maintain dignity and self-respect while meeting personal needs.

The Americans with Disabilities Act (ADA) allows for service dogs to stay with hospitalized patients. If a guide dog is present, do not interfere with it or pet it while it is working. Do not feed the dog; let the patient feed it at the appropriate time. Be sure the dog is near the bed on its own mat. Ask if the mat may be on the side of the bed that the staff are less likely to use.

> **Think Critically**
>
> Identify three specific ways in which you can assist a blind patient who is admitted to the hospital to maintain as much independence in this setting as possible.

◆ EVALUATION

Evaluation is based on reassessing data and determining whether expected outcomes have been met. This is an ongoing process. Some questions to be asked when gathering data for evaluation include: Is the patient compliant with the use of eye medications? Is an infection resolving? Is vision improving? If interventions have not been effective in helping the patient achieve expected outcomes, the plan of care should be altered.

COMMON DISORDERS OF THE EYE

ERRORS OF REFRACTION

The most common visual defects are those of refraction. This means that light rays entering the eye are not "refracted," or bent, at the correct angle (Fig. 25.11, *A*), and therefore do not focus on the retina. Errors of refraction may be caused by a number of structural defects within the eyeball itself. For example, if the distance between the lens and retina is too short, the light rays focus behind the retina. This causes difficulty in seeing objects close at hand and is called *farsightedness* (**hyperopia**) (Fig. 25.11, *B*).

If the opposite is true and the eyeball is too elongated, the light rays will converge and focus in front of the retina. The individual then has difficulty seeing objects at a distance and is referred to as being *nearsighted*. Nearsightedness is called **myopia** (Fig. 25.11, *C*).

Light rays from distant objects do not enter the eye at the same angle as light rays from near objects. When looking into the distance and then quickly looking down at a book, the eyes must make an adjustment to the difference in the light rays entering the eye. This adjustment, which is called **accommodation**, is accomplished by ciliary muscles and ligaments that change the shape of the lens, making it more rounded or flatter, thereby allowing light rays to fall on the retina (Fig. 25.12).

With increasing age, the ciliary muscles become less elastic and cannot readily accommodate the needs of distant and near vision. Hardening of the ciliary muscles occurs in many people older than 40 years and is known as *presbyopia*. Bifocal eyeglasses are usually prescribed

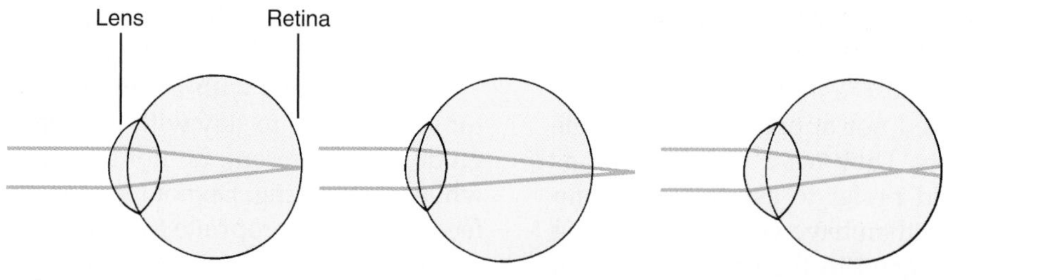
Lens
Retina
The lens bends light rays so that they focus directly on the retina.
A
Hyperopia. The lens is too close to the retina; light rays converge at a point beyond the retina.
B
Myopia. The lens is too far away from the retina; light rays converge before they reach the retina.
C

Fig. 25.11 **A,** Normal vision. **B,** Hyperopia. **C,** Myopia.

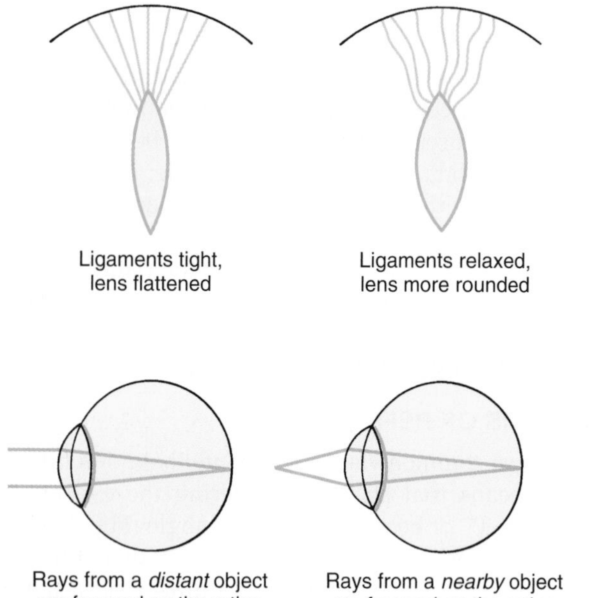
Ligaments tight, lens flattened
Ligaments relaxed, lens more rounded
Rays from a *distant* object are focused on the retina by a flattened lens
Rays from a *nearby* object are focused on the retina by a more rounded lens

Fig. 25.12 Flattening and rounding of the lens during accommodation.

for this condition because they allow for two sets of lenses in one pair of eyeglasses, one for viewing distant objects and one for seeing close objects.

Astigmatism is a visual defect that results from a warped lens or an irregular curvature of the cornea; either condition will prevent the horizontal and vertical rays from focusing at the same point on the retina. Very few people have perfectly shaped eyeballs, and thus there are very few who do not have some degree of astigmatism. If the astigmatism is very slight, the eye can accommodate for its imperfection by changing the shape of the lens. If there is a serious error of refraction, the eyes will tire easily or the person will have defective vision because the eyes cannot change the shape of the lens enough to compensate for the abnormality.

Serious errors of refraction are treated with prescription eyeglasses or contact lenses that are fitted so that the light rays are brought into proper focus on the retina. Advances have been made in refractive surgery that permits correction of refraction problems for some people. Those who are nearsighted (myopic) can undergo one of three procedures. In photorefractive keratectomy (PRK), an excimer laser is used to remove a thin layer of tissue from the cornea. This corrects the excessive curvature of the cornea that is interfering with the proper focus of light rays through the lens. The preparation takes 30 minutes, and the actual procedure takes less than 1 minute to perform; visual improvement is apparent within 3 to 5 days. Laser-assisted in situ keratomileusis (LASIK) is the most common procedure for nearsightedness in the United States. The middle layer of the cornea is reshaped with a laser after a very thin outer layer of the cornea is peeled back. The outer layer is replaced. Postoperative recovery is very rapid with little discomfort. The procedure takes about 10 to 15 minutes per eye and is performed as an outpatient procedure. Small incision lenticule extraction (SMILE) is a laser procedure in which the cornea is reshaped by excision of a small piece of corneal tissue, correcting myopia.

UVEITIS

The uveal tract consists of the iris, the ciliary body, and the choroid. Uveitis is inflammation of the uveal tract. Uveitis commonly results from other medical conditions, primarily systemic immune-mediated diseases causing inflammation or drug and allergic reactions. Infectious agents including herpes virus, syphilis, cytomegalovirus, toxoplasmosis, tuberculosis, and West Nile virus have all been implicated as a cause of uveitis. Signs and symptoms are tearing; blurred vision; photophobia; aching around the eye; a bloodshot sclera; or a small, nonreactive, irregular pupil. Treatment involves resting the ciliary body with a cycloplegic drug. The pupil is dilated to prevent adhesions of the involved structures. Analgesics, antibiotics, and oral or ocular steroid therapy may be used. Cool or warm compresses are used for discomfort. Sunglasses should be worn to reduce photophobia. Low light indoors is advisable.

DRY EYE

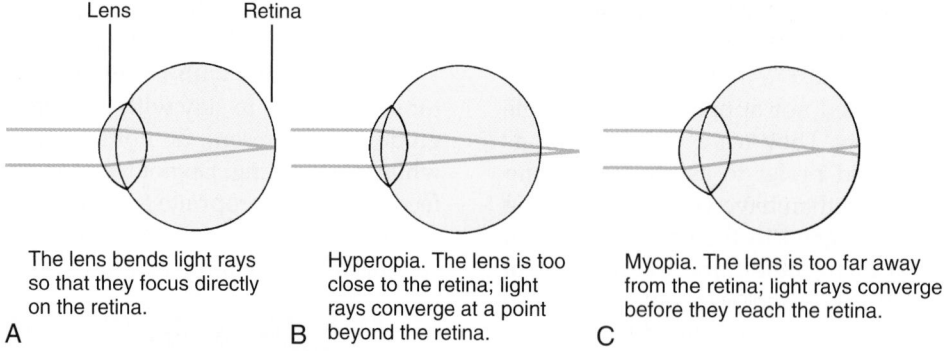

Dry eye is a common condition in people over 40 years old, especially in women after menopause. Because our population of older adults is growing, the incidence of dry eye is increasing. The symptoms of dry eye include tearing, soreness, and a gritty feeling in the eye. These symptoms can be treated with lubricating eye drops, but if the condition is left untreated it may lead to corneal ulcers.

Dry eye may be caused by a deficiency of tears, such as seen in Sjögren syndrome (see Chapter 11, Table 11.7), or it may be caused by evaporation, resulting from a dysfunction of meibomian glands that can be exacerbated by environmental conditions such as dust and wind (Foster, 2017).

Dry eye is managed by treating the underlying cause, such as meibomian gland dysfunction, and keeping the tear layer of the eye moist and functional. Patients with insufficient tears should use a solution of artificial tears that is readily available over the counter. Prescription eye drops and ointments are available for those conditions that do not respond to standard artificial tears (Shtein, 2018).

CORNEAL DISORDERS

Keratitis

Keratitis is an inflammation of the cornea caused by irritation or infection. Patients who have had a stroke may develop irritation of the cornea because the eyelid does not close normally. Keratitis may occur in a comatose patient who is not receiving proper eye care. Some people with exophthalmos (protruding eyeballs) develop this disorder. Bacterial infection is common among those who wear contact lenses. The eye becomes reddened, and there may be tearing along with a feeling of grittiness or pain. Discharge from the eye may occur. Treatment of irritation is instillation of artificial tears. Infection is treated by a medication to kill the organism. Drugs may be given topically, subconjunctivally, or by intravenous (IV) infusion.

Corneal Ulcer

A corneal ulcer may occur from irritation, infection, or injury. The ulcer is cultured to determine whether there is a causative organism when there is no history of injury. Antibiotic medication is usually prescribed. Scarring from corneal ulcers or severe infection is treated by keratoplasty.

Corneal Transplantation (Keratoplasty)

Corneal transplants replace corneas that have been damaged by genetic disorders, trauma, ulcers, or disease such as keratitis (inflammation of the cornea); transplants help restore corneal clarity. Two types of procedures are available: a full-thickness keratoplasty (corneal transplant) and a lamellar keratoplasty, which replaces only a superficial layer of corneal tissue. The full-thickness keratoplasty restores vision in approximately 95% of patients (Fig. 25.13, *A*). Corneas for transplantation are retrieved from donor cadavers soon after death. The transplantation is performed with regional anesthesia.

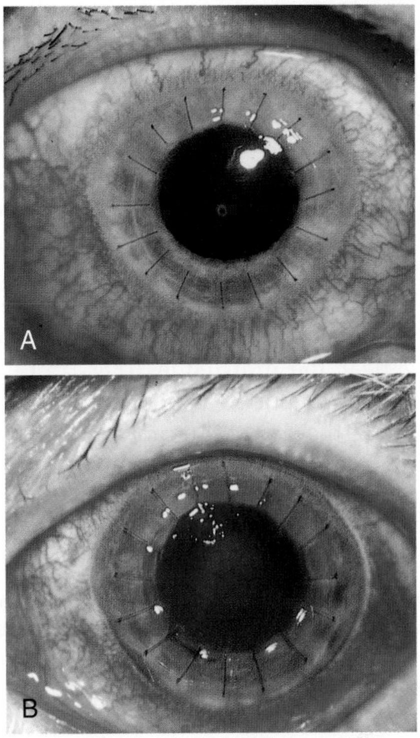

Fig. 25.13 **A,** Keratoplasty (corneal transplant). **B,** Acute transplant rejection. (Courtesy Ophthalmic Photography at the University of Michigan, W.K. Kellogg Eye Center, Ann Arbor, Mich.)

Descemet stripping endothelial keratoplasty (DSEK) replaces only the inside lining of corneal cells through a tiny incision and is currently the preferred technique. There are no sutures, and the cells are held in place for the first 24 hours by an air bubble. Vision is improved in a matter of weeks. DSEK is used only when disease is limited to the endothelial surface.

The patient must understand that it is difficult to predict when a donor cornea will become available, and therefore the procedure may be set up on short notice.

The surgery is an outpatient procedure. The patient must understand beforehand that it takes 1 to 2 weeks before any improvement in vision is noticeable and that improvement will continue for several months. Because the cornea does not have an abundant blood supply, healing is very slow and is not complete for about 1 year. **Prevention of infection is extremely important.** Preoperative care is much the same as for other eye surgeries.

! Safety Alert

Correctly Mark the Surgical Site

As part of the preoperative preparation, the surgeon clearly marks the operative site, verifying verbally with the patient that the site is correct. Document that this was done in the medical record and that all present agreed.

After surgery the patient is observed for 1 to 2 hours and then is discharged home. For some procedures a pressure dressing and eye shield may be applied in the surgical suite after the procedure and should be removed only by the health care provider the next day. The shield is then worn at night and when around small children or pets for at least a month. The pressure dressing helps keep the donor tissue in contact with the eyeball. Nursing actions focus on caring for the patient's disturbed visual sensory perception. Instructions regarding safety are provided before discharge. The patient may lie only on their back and nonoperative side postoperatively. Graft rejection is a possibility and is heralded by inflammation beginning near the graft edges (Fig. 25.13, *B*). This finding must be reported promptly. Should the first transplant fail, the procedure can be redone. Artificial cornea transplantation is evolving and gives patients another option; this procedure reduces the chance of rejection of human tissue.

Older Adult Care Points

An older adult patient who is temporarily or permanently visually impaired may experience a loss of independence and a change in self-perception. This patient will need specific suggestions on ways to maintain independence. After an outpatient eye surgery, the person will need someone to help at home for a few days at least.

Clinical Cues

Researchers are investigating using three-dimensional (3D) printers with a bio-ink mixture of alginate, stem cells, and collagen to produce corneas. Donor corneas are in short supply; using the stem cells from 1 donated cornea, 50 corneas can be "printed" (Isaacson, Swioklo, & Connon, 2018).

EYE TRAUMA

Eye trauma occurs from accidents and from debris in the air. Not using safety goggles or glasses when operating various types of power equipment accounts for most incidents of foreign bodies landing in the eyes. Windy weather can blow leaves, sand, or other debris into the eyes (Bashour, 2018). Penetrating injuries to the eye require prompt medical attention. Being struck in the eye by an object that does not penetrate, such as a baseball, can also cause injury.

Removal of Foreign Bodies From the Eye

If the foreign body is not deeply embedded in the tissues of the eye, it can easily be removed by irrigation. Irrigation with clear, lukewarm water (at home) or sterile water or saline is used to remove a foreign body sticking to the cornea. Continuous irrigation can be done with small tubing, and a bottle of solution or an irrigating syringe can be used. Be very careful not to touch the eye with the tip of the irrigating device. Sometimes a speck of foreign matter on the cornea can be removed with a moistened, sterile cotton swab. Have the patient tilt the head back. Hold the eyelids open to prevent blinking (Brady, 2018).

If a foreign body is sticking out of the eye, no attempt to remove it should be made. Both eyes should be patched to prevent further eye movement, and the patient should be transported to the emergency department or to an ophthalmologist. If the patient continues to complain of a sensation that a foreign body is in the eye after it appears to have been removed by irrigation, or complains of continuing pain, refer them to a health care provider immediately because there may be a corneal abrasion.

The provider will apply a stain to the eye to assess whether the cornea is abraded. If there is an abrasion, medicated ointment will be prescribed, and the eye may be patched (Box 25.2). The patient must be given instructions on how to instill the ointment. A thin line of eye ointment is applied from the inner canthus to the outer canthus along the lower eyelid inside the conjunctival sac (see Fig. 25.9). The patient closes the eyelid and moves the eyeball around in the socket to distribute the ointment. Excess medication is gently wiped away with a tissue, moving from the inner canthus to the outer canthus. If an eye patch is not applied, the patient is warned that the ointment may blur vision for a while. A corneal abrasion is painful; a nonsteroidal antiinflammatory drug may be used for discomfort.

Box 25.2 Applying an Eye Patch

- Perform hand hygiene and cleanse the skin of the patient's forehead and cheek with a skin preparation solution or pad.
- Prepare strips of nonallergenic paper or other tape to secure the patch.
- Ask the patient to close both eyes and position the patch over the lid of the eye to be patched.
- Secure the patch by placing strips of tape diagonally over the patch from the cheek to the forehead. Use several strips of tape to ensure adhesiveness.
- After surgery, a shield in addition to the patch is used for 2 to 6 weeks, depending on the surgeon's instructions.

FOR A PRESSURE PATCH

- Use two eye patches. Fold the first one in half; place it over the closed lid and then place the other patch on top of the folded one. Apply tape as instructed previously.

FOR SLEEPING

- A plastic or metal eye shield may be placed over the eye and secured to further protect the eye. In many cases, the patch can be left off when the shield is placed for sleeping.

Chemical Burns

Chemical burns should be treated by lengthy, continuous irrigation. If available, an IV bag of normal saline is the preferred solution; otherwise, tap water will suffice. Place the patient supine with the head turned to the affected side. With gloves on, direct the stream of fluid to the inner canthus so that the stream flows across the cornea to the outer canthus, holding the lids apart with your thumb and index finger. Water should be lukewarm. At intervals, stop and have the patient close their eyes to move secretions and particles from the upper eye to the lower conjunctival sac; then begin again. Continue for 30 to 60 minutes. The patient should be seen by a health care provider as soon as possible. All commercial businesses where exposure to chemicals is possible must comply with Occupational Safety and Health Administration (OSHA) standards and have an eyewash station within the facility as close as possible to the area where chemicals are likely to be used (Ventocilla, 2018).

Enucleation

If the eye is too damaged by trauma to be salvaged or is irreparably damaged by disease or tumor, **enucleation** (removal of the eye) is performed. An implant is created to maintain the orbital anatomy while a matching artificial eye is created. The implant is sutured to the muscle structures. When the artificial eye is placed over the implant, the muscle attachments allow for coordinated eye movement. The permanent prosthesis is placed about 6 weeks after the surgery.

Postoperatively, observe for signs of complications such as excessive bleeding, swelling, increased pain, elevated temperature, or displacement of the implant. Losing an eye is a devastating experience even when there has been a long period of painful blindness preoperatively. Understanding the emotional effects and supporting the patient are primary nursing responsibilities.

Care of an artificial eye. The procedure for cleansing and caring for an artificial eye is similar in many ways to the care of dentures. Both require basic principles of cleanliness, careful handling, and proper storage. An artificial eye is very expensive and must be handled very carefully.

The acrylic part of the prosthetic eye is cleansed by hand (no cloth is used) with gentle soap (mild hand soap or baby shampoo) and water, unless the patient, family, or health care provider directs otherwise. The frequency of cleaning is determined by the type of prosthesis in use. Scleral shells might have to be removed at night; other products can remain in place for months. Follow the manufacturer's instructions for cleaning. Use lubricating eye drops to moisten the prosthesis and use the plunger (if provided) to replace the prosthesis to the socket. When inserting or removing the prosthesis, have the head over a padded surface. The patient's upper lid is lifted, and the eye is inserted with the notched end toward the nose. After the prosthesis is placed as far as possible under the upper lid, the lower lid is depressed, allowing the eye to slip into place.

CATARACT

A **cataract** is opacity of the lens that produces an effect similar to one a person would experience when looking through a sheet of falling water. A cataract causes blurred vision because the lens, which is normally transparent, becomes cloudy and opaque.

Etiology and Pathophysiology

Congenital cataracts are most commonly caused by maternal infection with rubella or *Toxoplasma gondii.* Cataracts typically occur as a result of aging and are found in people older than 50 years (adult-onset [senile] cataracts).

Traumatic cataracts may occur from a physical blow, extreme heat, or chemical toxins. Cigarette smoking increases the risk of developing cataracts. Heavy drinking also is implicated. Chronic use of corticosteroids predisposes to the development of cataracts.

Health Promotion

Cataract Prevention

Encouraging the habit of wearing sunglasses that protect from ultraviolet light and a hat when outdoors can help prevent the development of cataracts. Cumulative exposure to ultraviolet light is the greatest risk factor for cataracts (American Optometric Association, 2018).

Think Critically

What would you teach a person with rheumatoid arthritis about eye care, if that person is on corticosteroids most of the time?

Signs, Symptoms, and Diagnosis

In addition to the blurred vision that is typical of opacity of the lens, with cataracts there may be decreased color perception. Uncomplicated cataracts are usually painless, but the patient may have photophobia (intolerance of light). Assessment may reveal the following symptoms:

- Hazy, blurred, or double vision *(diplopia)*
- Increasing complaints about glare
- Increasing nearsightedness
- Complaints that colors are faded or appear yellowish or brownish
- Desire for increased light by which to read
- Difficulty with night vision
- Frequent need for eyeglass prescription change

The loss of vision associated with cataracts is progressive and sometimes is partially caused by secondary glaucoma. As an untreated cataract progresses, the lens of the eye becomes cloudy or milky white, then may turn yellow, and eventually may become brown or black (Fig. 25.14).

Diagnosis of a cataract is confirmed by examining the dilated pupil with a slit lamp, which enables the

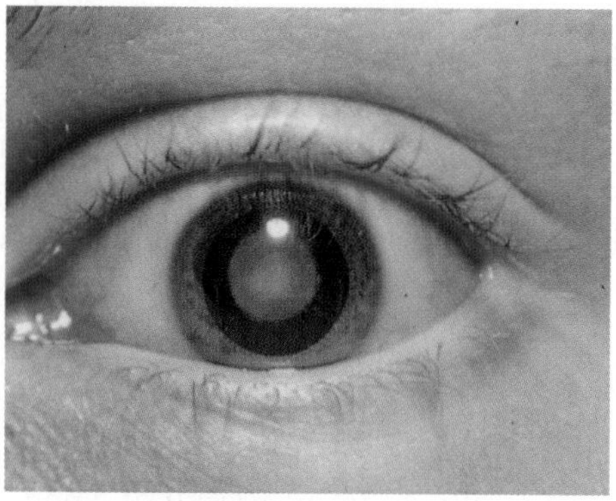

Fig. 25.14 Cloudy appearance of eye with cataract. (Courtesy Ophthalmic Photography at the University of Michigan, W.K. Kellogg Eye Center, Ann Arbor, Mich.)

examiner to see opacities more clearly. Glaucoma should first be ruled out as a possible cause of the symptoms. Tonometry is used to determine IOP, or the fluid pressure within the eye.

Treatment

Cataract surgery is performed when the loss of vision greatly affects the quality of the person's life. The only effective method of treating cataracts is surgical removal of the affected lens with clear lens implantation; cataract surgery is the most commonly performed surgical procedure in the United States. Surgical techniques are (1) **extracapsular extraction,** in which the lens is removed in one piece; and (2) **small incision cataract surgery,** in which the lens is removed in pieces after being broken up by ultrasound waves **(phacoemulsification)**. A small incision is made on the side of the cornea to extract the pieces. With either procedure, an intraocular lens is implanted. Lenses are available that allow for monofocal, multifocal, or accommodative vision rather than just monovision, in which vision is good at only one distance without glasses. If a monovision lens is chosen, vision is corrected for nearsightedness or farsightedness by the lens implant, and further correction of vision is achieved with regular eyeglasses or contact lenses. Multifocal or accommodative lenses are not typically paid for by health insurance, and this sometimes drives the lens choice. Vision is improved within 2 weeks and is usually fully recovered within 3 months of surgery (Nursing Care Plan 25.1). These outpatient surgical procedures are performed under procedural sedation and local anesthesia.

Nursing Management

The patient must be told that there is a period of visual adjustment after cataract surgery. The surgeon may prescribe miotic eye drops after surgery to constrict the pupil and decrease the danger of lens dislocation. **Patient adherence to the schedule for postoperative medications is critical to prevent complications and promote healing.**

Patient Teaching

General Care After Eye Surgery

Instructions for the patient and/or family caregiver:

- Always wash hands before instilling medication. Check the label of the container to be certain it is the right medication. Do not contaminate the applicator tip of the medication.
- Instill only the number of drops ordered; apply pressure at the inner canthus to prevent systemic absorption as appropriate; close the eye gently (do not squeeze the eye shut).
- Change the eye patch dressing (Fig. 25.15) at least once a day; change as needed to keep the area clean.
- Follow the medication schedule prescribed by the health care provider exactly. (Send home a written schedule.)
- Maintain designated head position and activity restrictions.
- Report signs of complications: sudden, increasing pain in the eye, which can indicate hemorrhage; purulent drainage; decreasing vision; or signs of increased IOP, such as brow headache.
- Keep the follow-up appointment with the surgeon.
- Use caution to prevent getting water in the eye.
- Protect the eye during the day with glasses; use sunglasses for outside wear; wear a protective eye shield at night.

Think Critically

Identify which patients should be carefully assessed for signs and symptoms of cataract.

GLAUCOMA

Etiology

The term *glaucoma* comprises a complex group of disorders that involve many different pathologic changes and symptoms but have in common an optic neuropathy that damages the optic disc, causing atrophy and loss of vision. The neuropathy often is caused by increased IOP (Boyd, 2018). Glaucoma may come on slowly and cause irreversible vision loss without presenting any other noticeable symptoms, or it may appear abruptly and produce blindness in a matter of hours. Glaucoma can be present at birth or can develop at any age. It can result from genetic predisposition, trauma, or another disorder of the eye. Glaucoma is commonly a manifestation of diseases and pathologies in other body systems. The amount of increased IOP that causes damage differs from one person's eye to another. **Blindness is preventable if the disorder is treated early.**

Think Critically

How can you include inquiries about family history or predisposing risk factors for glaucoma in your patient care?

Nursing Care Plan 25.1 Care of a Patient Undergoing a Cataract Extraction

SCENARIO

Mrs. Fort, age 79 years, is admitted to the outpatient surgery unit for extraction of a cataract of the left eye with lens implant. The vision in her right eye also is affected by a cataract, but the visual loss is not as severe in that eye. Mrs. Fort suffers from a crippling osteoarthritis of the hands, but her general health is good. She is well oriented, outgoing, and physically active. She lives alone in an apartment building for retired senior citizens. Her daughter and son-in-law live nearby and are in daily contact with her. Mrs. Fort has not been hospitalized since she was treated for pneumonia 20 years ago, and she is concerned about what to expect preoperatively and postoperatively.

PROBLEM STATEMENT/NURSING DIAGNOSIS

Insufficient knowledge related to preoperative and postoperative procedures and care.

SUPPORTING ASSESSMENT DATA

Subjective: "I have never had surgery before."

Goals/Expected Outcomes	Nursing Interventions	Selected Rationale	Evaluation
Patient will verbalize preoperative routine activities and postoperative procedures and expectations.	Teach patient and daughter about eye medications to be used at home and how to instill them; how to dress and shield eye properly; how to remove bandage without contaminating eye.	To comply with instructions, teaching must occur on how to instill drops, how to dress and shield the eye, and how to perform care needed.	Provided teaching for patient and daughter. Will ask for return demonstration before discharge. Left printed instructions.

PROBLEM STATEMENT/NURSING DIAGNOSIS

Potential for injury related to postoperative complications such as infection, trauma, and increased intraocular pressure.

SUPPORTING ASSESSMENT DATA

Objective: Undergoing cataract extraction; infection, trauma, and increased intraocular pressure are potential complications.

Goals/Expected Outcomes	Nursing Interventions	Selected Rationale	Evaluation
Infection, trauma, and increase in intraocular pressure will be prevented.	Teach signs and symptoms of complications that are to be reported to health care provider immediately: increasing eye pain, purulent discharge, decreasing vision, fever or chills, increasing brow headache.	Patient must know what to look for to report complications.	Gave instructions and left printed list. Will ask for feedback before discharge.
	Instruct to refrain from straining at stool; encourage to use milk of magnesia or stool softener to prevent straining as needed.	Preventing the Valsalva maneuver will help prevent an increase in intraocular pressure.	Verbalizes the ways to prevent raising intraocular pressure.
	Perform hand hygiene thoroughly before instilling eye medications or changing dressing; teach patient and daughter to wash hands before approaching eye area.	Aseptic techniques help prevent infection. Maintaining asepsis aids in protecting the surgical site from infection and prevents complications.	Patient and daughter state that they understand hand hygiene and aseptic techniques for postoperative eye care.
	Demonstrate how to put on eye shield for sleep.	Wearing a protective eye shield will protect the eye from bumps or scratches.	Instructed to clean the eye shield daily with 70% isopropyl alcohol.
	Instruct patient to avoid rapid or sudden movements and bending from the waist.	Bending from the waist increases intraocular pressure.	Instructed to crouch rather than bend at the waist and to avoid sudden movements.
	Instruct patient to take medication immediately for nausea and vomiting.	Quickly medicating for nausea may avert vomiting.	Instructions given and a written instruction sheet at bedside.
	Remind patient not to lie on affected side.	Sleeping on the affected side creates too much pressure on the eye.	Instruct to avoid sleeping on the operated side for at least 2 weeks.
	Encourage patient to seek assistance with ambulation while vision is blurred.	Walking alone with blurred vision increases risk for falls.	Instruct to seek assistance for ambulation.

Continued

Nursing Care Plan 25.1 Care of a Patient Undergoing a Cataract Extraction—cont'd

PROBLEM STATEMENT/NURSING DIAGNOSIS

Limited self-care ability related to disabilities imposed by osteoarthritis.

SUPPORTING ASSESSMENT DATA

Objective: Severe osteoarthritis of the hands with limited dexterity.

Goals/Expected Outcomes	Nursing Interventions	Selected Rationale	Evaluation
Assistance with administration of postoperative eye medications and eye care will be given by daughter.	Teach daughter techniques needed for postoperative eye care and give her a written schedule for that care.	Written instructions and a schedule reinforce the teaching and help care occur on time.	Daughter observed care and administration of eye medications today; will demonstrate postoperative eye care when meds are next due.

CRITICAL THINKING QUESTIONS

1. Why should you wait 5 minutes between instilling one type of eye drop and the next type of eye drop?
2. What is one of the most important things to teach someone who will instill eye drops or ointment postoperatively?

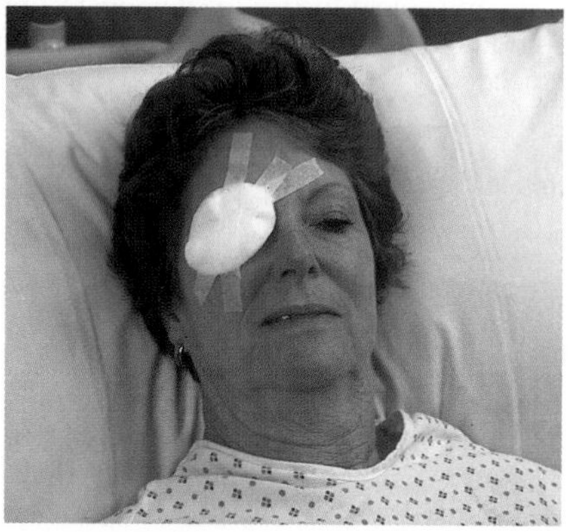

Fig. 25.15 Patient with eye patch to protect surgical site and prevent eye movement. The head is kept elevated in the immediate postoperative period.

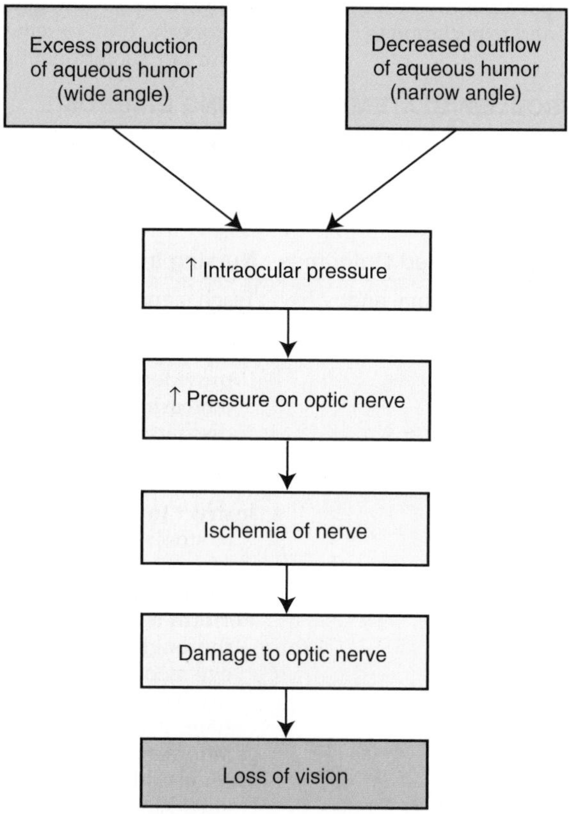

Concept Map 25.1 Pathophysiology of glaucoma.

Pathophysiology

The IOP is determined by the rate of aqueous humor production and the outflow of the aqueous humor from the eye. Aqueous humor is produced in the ciliary body and flows out of the eye through the canal of Schlemm into the venous system (Concept Map 25.1). An imbalance may occur from overproduction by the ciliary body or by obstruction of outflow. Increased IOP greater than 22 mm Hg requires thorough evaluation. Increased IOP restricts the blood flow to the optic nerve and the retina. Ischemia causes these structures to lose their function gradually. **The vision impairment from damage to the optic nerve or retina is permanent.** Glaucoma may be secondary to eye infection, trauma, eye surgery, or ocular tumor.

Glaucoma can be angle-closure glaucoma, open-angle glaucoma, developmental glaucoma, or mixed mechanism (Fig. 25.16). Open-angle and angle-closure glaucoma can be primary or secondary conditions, and each can be categorized as acute, subacute, or chronic. The terms *narrow angle* (angle closure) and *open angle* refer to the angle width between the cornea and the iris. *Acute* and *chronic* refer to either the onset or the duration of the problem. These two major types differ in their clinical signs and symptoms, treatment, and effects on vision. Secondary glaucoma may occur with diabetes mellitus, hypertension, or extreme myopia or after retinal detachment.

OPEN-ANGLE GLAUCOMA

Signs and Symptoms

Open-angle glaucoma, in which there is no angle closure, is a much more insidious and more common form of glaucoma, occurring in about 90% of people with glaucoma. It often is an inherited disorder that causes

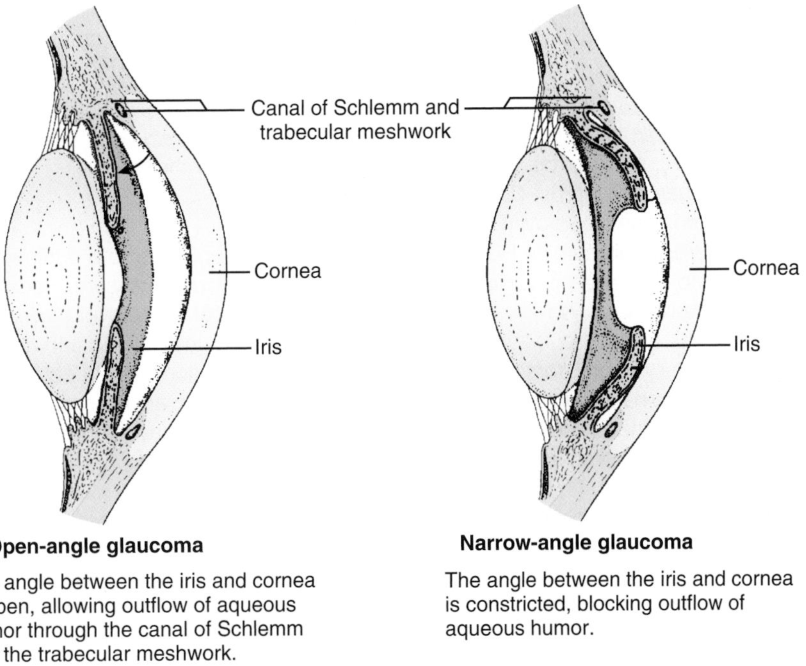
Canal of Schlemm and trabecular meshwork
Cornea
Iris
Cornea
Iris
Open-angle glaucoma
The angle between the iris and cornea is open, allowing outflow of aqueous humor through the canal of Schlemm and the trabecular meshwork.
Narrow-angle glaucoma
The angle between the iris and cornea is constricted, blocking outflow of aqueous humor.

Fig. 25.16 Comparison of open-angle (wide, chronic) and narrow-angle (closed, acute) glaucoma. (From Burchum JR, Rosenthal LD: *Lehne's pharmacology for nursing care,* ed 10, St. Louis, 2019, Elsevier.)

degenerative changes in the aqueous humor outflow tracts. It may be caused by a mixture of factors of overproduction of aqueous humor and anatomic problems within the eye. It usually is bilateral and can progress to complete blindness without ever producing an acute attack. Its symptoms are relatively mild, and many patients are not aware that anything is wrong until vision has been seriously impaired.

Health Promotion

Danger Signals of Glaucoma

The National Society for the Prevention of Blindness lists the following symptoms as danger signals of open-angle glaucoma:

- Eyeglasses, even new ones, that do not seem to clarify vision
- Blurred or hazy vision that clears up after a while
- Difficulty adjusting to darkened rooms, such as in movie theaters
- Seeing rainbow-colored rings around lights
- Narrowing of vision at the sides of one or both eyes

Encourage a complete eye examination if any of these signs is present.

Diagnosis

People at normal risk for glaucoma should be screened every 2 to 4 years before age 40, every 1 to 3 years from ages 40 to 54, every 1 to 2 years from ages 55 to 64, and every 6 to 12 months after age 65 (Glaucoma.org, 2017). Those with high risk factors should be screened every 1 to 2 years after age 35.

People at high risk for glaucoma are:

- Those with diabetes
- African Americans (at least four times as many African Americans as non–African Americans have glaucoma-related blindness)
- Individuals with a family history of glaucoma

A commonly used screening technique for early detection of glaucoma is to measure IOP with an air tonometer. A puff of air is directed at the cornea, which causes a momentary indentation while a pressure reading is taken (Glaucoma.org, 2017). The test is painless, and nothing but the air touches the eye. Verification of the diagnosis of glaucoma may require the use of a more complex instrument called an *applanation tonometer*. The cornea is flattened, and pressure is measured with a slit-lamp biomicroscope.

Treatment

The initial treatment of choice for chronic (open-angle) glaucoma is medication rather than surgery. If drugs are not effective or if they produce worrisome side effects, surgery is performed.

Drug therapy is intended to enhance aqueous humor outflow or decrease its production so that IOP is decreased (Table 25.5). Miotics cause blurred vision for 1 to 2 hours after use. Adjustment to dark rooms is difficult because of pupil constriction. Pilocarpine is available in an eye medication disk that resembles a contact lens. The disk is inserted into the conjunctival sac in a patient's lower eyelid, where it can remain for up to 7 days. The medication is slowly released. Use of the disk does not prevent the wearing of contact

Table 25.5 Drugs Commonly Used to Treat Eye Disorders

CLASSIFICATION	EXAMPLES	ACTION/NURSING IMPLICATIONS
Drugs Used for Glaucoma		
Miotics	*Prostaglandin analogs:* latanoprost (Xalatan), bimatoprost (Lumigan), travoprost (Travatan), unoprostone isopropyl (Rescula)	Increase outflow of aqueous fluid through the ciliary muscle by relaxation of the muscle.
	Cholinergics: pilocarpine HCl (Isopto Carpine), pilocarpine nitrate (Ocusert Pilo-20, Ocusert Pilo-40), carbachol (Miostat)	Constrict the pupil, promote outflow of aqueous humor, and reduce intraocular pressure. Reduce visual acuity in dim light; advise patient to avoid driving at night. Ocusert is placed in conjunctival sac and replaced weekly.
	Cholinesterase inhibitors: echothiophate iodide (Phospholine iodide), demecarium bromide (Humorsol)	Produce miosis, increase aqueous humor outflow, and decrease intraocular pressure. Avoid touching tip of bottle to eye; moisture may interfere with drug potency.
	Beta-adrenergic blockers: timolol maleate (Timoptic), betaxolol (Betoptic), levobunolol (Betagan), metipranolol (OptiPranolol), carteolol (Ocupress)	Reduce production of aqueous humor, thereby reducing intraocular pressure. Betaxolol reduces intraocular hypertension. Monitor pulse and blood pressure during initiation of therapy. Blurred vision decreases with continued use. Use beta blockers cautiously in patients with a history of asthma.
Carbonic anhydrase inhibitors	Acetazolamide (Diamox), dorzolamide (Trusopt), brinzolamide (Azopt)	Interfere with carbonic acid production, thereby decreasing aqueous humor formation and decreasing intraocular pressure. Taken orally or as eye drops (Trusopt). When taken orally, these drugs have a diuretic action; observe for dehydration and postural hypotension. Monitor electrolytes. Confusion may occur in older adults. Check for interaction with other drugs the patient is receiving.
Sympathomimetics	Epinephrine (Epifrin), dipivefrin (Propine), apraclonidine (Iopidine)	Reduce intraocular pressure by increasing aqueous outflow. May cause brow headache, headache, eye irritation, and blurred vision. Used for open-angle glaucoma only. May cause tachycardia and rise in blood pressure.
Alpha-2 adrenergic agonist	Brimonidine ophthalmic (Alphagan P)	Acts on alpha receptors in the blood vessels, decreasing the production of aqueous humor. Do not use with soft contact lenses. Contraindicated in heart disease.
Antiinflammatories	*Corticosteroids:* Pred Forte, Ocu-Pred, Ophtho-Tate *NSAIDs:* ketorolac (Acular), flurbiprofen (Ocufen) *Prostaglandin analog:* latanoprost (Xalatan)	Decrease inflammation and swelling; reduce miosis. Interact with contact lens materials.
Drugs Used to Facilitate Diagnosis and Surgery of the Eye		
Cycloplegic and mydriatic anticholinergic agents	Atropine (Atropisol), cyclopentolate (Cyclogyl), homatropine (Isopto Homatropine), scopolamine (Isopto Hyoscine), tropicamide (Mydriacyl)	Dilate the pupils and paralyze the muscles of accommodation, causing mydriasis and cycloplegia. Mydriasis facilitates observation of the eye's interior during an examination. Cycloplegia prevents movement of the lens during assessment of the eye.
Adrenergic agonist	Phenylephrine (Ocu-Phrin)	Induces mydriasis by action on the muscle of the iris. Causes blurred vision. Photophobia may be eased by using dark glasses.
Staining solution	Fluorescein	Turns corneal scratches bright green; a green ring surrounds foreign bodies. Dye will filter through the lacrimal duct into the nasal secretions.
Topical anesthetics	Proparacaine (Alcaine, AK-Taine), tetracaine (Pontocaine)	Anesthetize the eye. Caution patient not to rub the eye while it is anesthetized. Patch eye when patient leaves the office if medication is still in effect.

Table 25.5 **Drugs Commonly Used to Treat Eye Disorders—cont'd**

CLASSIFICATION	EXAMPLES	ACTION/NURSING IMPLICATIONS
Antiinfective Optic Medications		
Antibiotics	Gentamicin sulfate (Garamycin ophthalmic), erythromycin (Ilotycin), polymyxin B sulfate, neomycin sulfate, bacitracin, sulfonamides (Sodium Sulamyd, Gantrisin), ciprofloxacin (Ciloxan), chlortetracycline (Aureomycin), ofloxacin (Ocuflox)	Used to treat infection or for prophylaxis. Caution patient to use a clean washcloth and towel on the face each time to prevent reinfection.
Antifungal	Natamycin (Natacyn ophthalmic)	To treat *Fusarium*. Caution as for antibiotics.
Antivirals	Idoxuridine (IDV, Stoxil, Herplex), trifluridine (Viroptic) Vidarabine (Vira-A ophthalmic)	Store in refrigerator. Do not use with boric acid. If no improvement, discontinue after 1 wk. Effective against DNA viruses; used for keratoconjunctivitis.

DNA, Deoxyribonucleic acid; *NSAID*, nonsteroidal antiinflammatory drug.

lenses. Diuretics may be prescribed to reduce the production of aqueous humor fluid. Not all diuretics reduce IOP, and a substitute should not be used for the specific drug prescribed.

Whenever glaucoma is being managed by medication, the patient must continue the eye drops and oral medications on an uninterrupted basis. Patients admitted to the hospital for disorders other than glaucoma often are permitted to keep their glaucoma medication at the bedside if they can administer it themselves.

Complementary and Alternative Therapies

Marijuana and Glaucoma

Marijuana is known to decrease IOP. Many states have legalized use of medical marijuana, and patients are asking about its use for glaucoma. Research has shown that topical optic application of THC is not effective in reducing IOP. Smoking marijuana causes tachycardia and can decrease blood pressure, further reducing blood flow to the optic nerve. The drug also has a short duration, and maintaining decreased IOP would require that 8 to 10 marijuana cigarettes be smoked each day. Currently, the American Academy of Ophthalmology's Complementary Therapy Task Force statement indicates that there is no scientific evidence that there is greater benefit from marijuana than from effective medications that are already on the market and have fewer side effects (Grant, 2018).

When drugs do not control glaucoma and increased IOP persists, surgery is an alternative. The goal is to create openings so that excess fluid can escape. A laser is used to create evenly spaced openings in the collecting meshwork *(trabeculoplasty)* to facilitate aqueous humor drainage in open-angle or chronic glaucoma. Microsurgery filtering procedures create a drainage hole in the iris between the anterior and posterior chambers. A tiny shunt may be placed to drain excess aqueous humor if other surgeries do not produce the desired result. When surgical procedures fail, the ciliary body may be treated by applying a freezing probe tip *(cyclocryotherapy)*. This permanently damages cells in the ciliary body and decreases the production of aqueous humor.

Laser surgery is performed with local anesthetic, usually in the health care provider's office. The patient may experience a gritty sensation and blurring of vision during the first 24 to 72 hours. There is a possibility that IOP may increase because of an inflammatory response. **Increasing pain in the eye should be reported to the ophthalmologist immediately.** Elevated IOP may persist for a week or so in some patients. Glaucoma medications are continued to meet the patient's individual needs.

If a laser procedure is not effective, incisional surgical procedures may be performed, such as a microsurgery filtering procedure, which is an outpatient procedure using procedural sedation. Postoperatively the patient should be instructed to prevent increasing the venous pressure in the head, neck, and eyes by avoiding the Valsalva maneuver (straining with a closed glottis), not bending over, keeping the head up, and not making any sudden movements. A stool softener is given to prevent constipation. Strenuous exercise should be avoided for 3 weeks. The head of the bed should be elevated 15 to 20 degrees to decrease pressure within the eyes during sleep.

The patient must understand the importance of frequent checkups and the necessity of consistently following instructions; the surgical procedure does not always eliminate the need for medication.

Nursing Management

Education of the patient and the family is a major aspect of care. Failure to follow the prescribed treatment regimen to control glaucoma and neglecting to maintain regular follow-ups with the provider can result in progressive loss of vision and eventual blindness (Fig. 25.17).

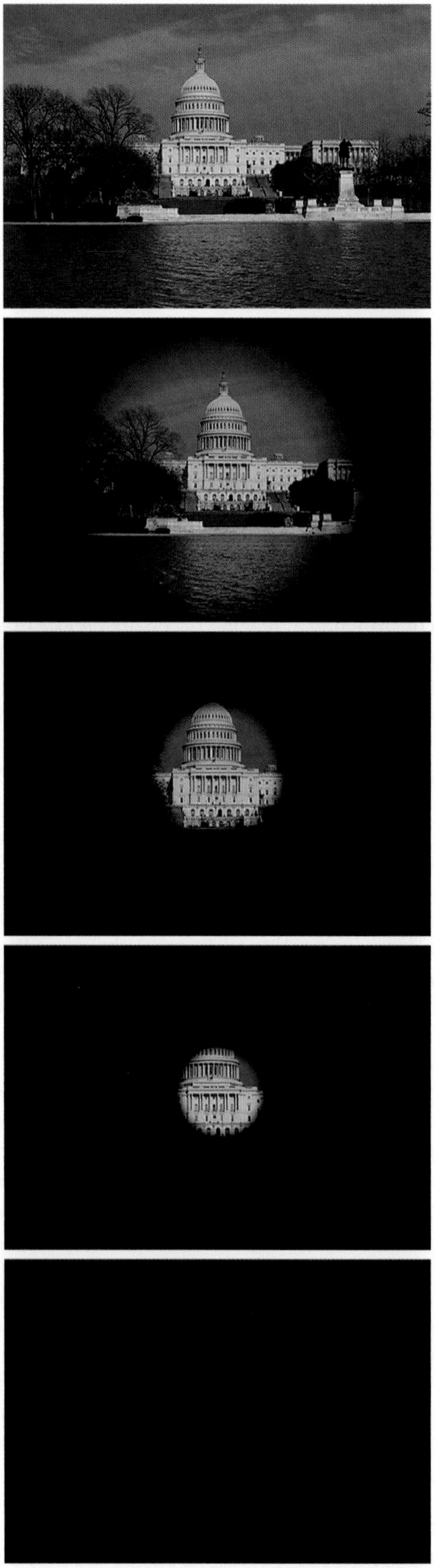

Fig. 25.17 Glaucoma causes a progressive loss of peripheral vision. (From Monahan FD, Neighbors M, Sands JK, et al.: *Phipps' medical-surgical nursing: health and illness perspectives,* ed 8, St. Louis, 2007, Mosby.)

Patients who have glaucoma need to be fully informed about the nature of this disorder, how it can affect vision, the treatments available, and the expected result of those treatments. An analogy that can be used to explain the nature of the disorder is to compare the eye to a sink with an open faucet (the ciliary processes), a drain (angle), and pipes (trabecular structures). As long as water flows into and out of the sink at the same rate, there is no problem. However, if something blocks the drain or the pipes, the water will fill the sink beyond its holding capacity. Treatment with miotics helps keep the pipes open so that drainage is possible; beta blockers and diuretics can slow down the rate at which water flows from the tap. If the medications do not work or if the sink suddenly is blocked by a clogged pipe, it may be necessary for the surgeon to clear the drainage system so that the water can drain from the sink.

In addition to learning about the nature of glaucoma and the expected results of prescribed treatments, the patient also must be made aware of the possibility of vision loss if the condition is not managed. **Teaching should emphasize that glaucoma medications prevent further vision loss, but medications cannot restore vision.** Teaching must be done with tact and sensitivity for the patient's feelings. The information should never be presented in such a way that the patient feels threatened or becomes so fearful that they are unable to participate in the management of their disorder.

Patient Teaching

Points to Cover in the Glaucoma Teaching Plan

- Signs of elevated IOP include pain in the eye, redness, tearing, blurred vision, halos around lights, and frequent need for change in eyeglasses.
- Measures to prevent increase in IOP include low-sodium (Furstenberg) diet, little caffeine intake, preventing constipation and Valsalva maneuver, and decreasing stress.
- Taking prescribed medications and refraining from taking over-the-counter or other medications without the health care provider's knowledge are important. Glaucoma medication must be taken regularly for life.
- Use good aseptic technique when instilling eye medication.
- Wear an ID tag or bracelet stating "Glaucoma," and carry a card in your wallet that states what medications are being taken.
- Keep an extra bottle of eye medication on hand. Carry eye drops.
- Maintain close medical follow-up with the provider.
- Practice safety habits; avoid night driving if possible.

ANGLE-CLOSURE (NARROW-ANGLE) GLAUCOMA

Signs, Symptoms, and Diagnosis

Narrow-angle glaucoma can be acute or chronic. Acute conditions are a medical emergency in which there is severe pain in the eye accompanied by the appearance of colored halos around lights, blurred vision, and pain in and around the eye. Nausea and vomiting may occur. The cause of narrow-angle glaucoma is the position of the iris, which lies too close to the drainage canal and bulges forward against the cornea, blocking the drainage of aqueous humor (see Fig. 25.16). The IOP rises suddenly, sometimes reaching a pressure of 50 to 70 mm Hg. Relief of the situation must be prompt or damage to the optic nerve will cause blindness in the affected eye. Diagnosis is by history, testing of IOP, and slit-lamp eye examination.

Treatment and Nursing Management

Emergency treatment in narrow-angle glaucoma consists of measures to reduce IOP as quickly as possible. During the attack, eye drops such as pilocarpine, timolol and apraclonidine, and IV acetazolamide are used. Surgery is performed as soon as inflammation subsides to relieve pressure against the optic nerve endings. *Laser iridotomy, trabeculectomy, laser trabeculoplasty,* or other procedures that allow filtering of the aqueous humor from the anterior chamber into the subconjunctival space are performed. If these procedures fail, sometimes *cyclocryotherapy* (the application of a freezing tip) may be used on the ciliary body to decrease the aqueous production.

Nursing management is the same as for other eye surgeries: teaching about activity precautions during healing, schedule for eye drops, symptoms to report to the surgeon, and aseptic handling of the eye drops and eye shield.

RETINAL DETACHMENT

Etiology

Retinal detachments occur most often as rhegmatogenous detachments where a hole, tear, or break in the neuronal layer allows vitreous humor to seep between layers. Traction or exudative mechanisms can also cause detachment. Congenital malformations, trauma, and metabolic disorder, such as diabetic or hypertensive retinopathy, can produce retinal detachment. Retinal detachments commonly occur in people with a high degree of myopia or in those who have had cataract surgery or direct trauma to the eye. The incidence of retinal detachment increases dramatically after 40 years of age and is most common between ages 40 and 70 years. Fifteen percent of people with retinal detachment in one eye develop detachment in the other eye.

Pathophysiology

Retinal detachment is not a detachment of the whole retina but a separation of the sensory layers of the retina from the pigmented epithelial layer, the choroid. Retinal detachment can cause vitreous fluid to leak under the retina, separating a portion of it from the vascular wall and thereby depriving the retina of its blood supply (Fig. 25.18).

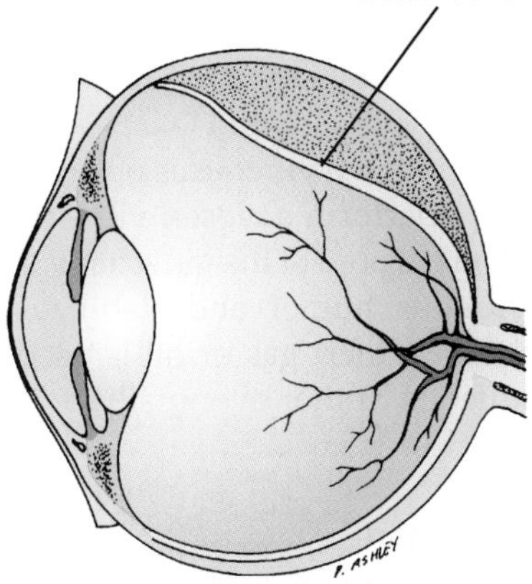

Fig. 25.18 Retinal detachment.

Signs, Symptoms, and Diagnosis

Onset can be either gradual or sudden, depending on the cause and extent of the detachment and the location of the area involved. The patient may see flashes of colored light accompanied by showers of floaters (black spots), or may feel as if a curtain has been drawn over a portion of the visual field. Later, cloudy vision or loss of central vision is noticed. In severe cases, there may be complete loss of vision.

? Think Critically

What would you say to your friend if you were having a meal together in a restaurant and he commented that he was seeing flashes of colored light in his left eye? What would you tell him to do?

Diagnosis of detached retina can be made with a direct ophthalmoscope, but diagnosis is greatly simplified by a stereoscopic indirect ophthalmoscope. This instrument permits visualization of the entire retina and produces an image of the retina with less magnification and distortion than the direct ophthalmoscope. Ultrasound can be used to detect retinal detachment when the eye is clouded by opacity from cataract or hemorrhage.

Treatment

Retinal holes and tears sometimes can be repaired on an outpatient basis with laser therapy that creates an inflammatory reaction, causing the layers to adhere during healing. Tears located in the posterior fundus can be coagulated and sealed with a laser beam or photocoagulator. Peripheral retinal holes through which no fluid has leaked can be closed by applying a freezing probe tip (cryotherapy). The frozen area scars over in a few days, and the hole is thus sealed. A third procedure, called *scleral buckling,* requires more extensive surgery. In effect, scleral buckling places the retinal breaks in contact with the pigmented epithelial layer. Adhesions are formed that bind the sensory and epithelial layers and the choroid together. Before the procedure, gas may be injected into the eye to apply pressure on the retina from the interior of the eye. This application of pressure helps hold the layers together during healing.

If hemorrhage into the vitreous is obstructing vision, the surgeon may perform a closed vitrectomy during retinal repair. The purpose of the vitrectomy is to remove the cloudy vitreous humor and stabilize the retina against the choroid. Inert gas or oil is used to fill the space until aqueous humor eventually refills the area (Mayo Clinic, 2018).

Nursing Management

Positioning of the patient and the level of activity allowed after surgery are prescribed by the surgeon. The head is positioned so that the area repaired is dependent, preventing the pull of gravity from disrupting the surgical site. The designated position for the head also is calculated to position the oil or gas bubble—if one was used—in the best place to apply pressure to the retina. Position the patient according to the surgeon's orders. IOP is monitored closely for at least 24 hours. Vision does not return immediately because of postoperative swelling and the effects of the dilating drops. Vision improves on a gradual basis over several weeks to months. The eyes may both be patched, or just the operative eye may be patched. Eye patches are changed at least once a day (see Box 25.2). A shield is worn when napping and at night. Several types of eye drops as well as an antibiotic ointment may be prescribed for postoperative use. Strict asepsis must be observed when instilling eye drops and ointment.

There usually is some degree of pain after all types of retinal surgery. Acetaminophen is usually sufficient to control the pain. Cold packs to the eye for 10 to 20 minutes at a time decrease swelling and inflammation, which helps control pain.

Flashing lights are common for the first few weeks after retinal surgery. These decrease over 2 to 6 months; if they worsen within several weeks of surgery, the surgeon should be notified. Light sensitivity is common in both eyes after surgery and may cause tearing. This gradually lessens over a period of 4 to 6 weeks. Wearing dark sunglasses when outdoors helps eliminate this problem. A moderate amount of discharge from the eye is not unusual; it should be yellowish or pink tinged. If the amount of discharge increases markedly or is accompanied by severe pain, or if discharge has a foul smell or a greenish tinge, infection may be present; notify the surgeon. Cleanse the eyelid with a gauze pad or cotton ball moistened with irrigating solution or tap water. Wipe from the inner to the outer area of the eye. A separate clean pad or cotton ball should be used for each eye.

The patient is permitted to shower and wash the hair as long as care is taken not to get water in the affected eye (see Home Care Considerations).

At discharge, the patient is cautioned to avoid heavy lifting, straining at stool, and vigorous activity for several weeks. Eyeglasses are worn during the day for protection, and the eye shield is worn at night after an eye patch is no longer necessary.

RETINOPATHY

Etiology

The two major causes of retinopathy are diabetes mellitus and hypertension. Years of elevated blood pressure cause retinal vasospasm, which damages and narrows the retinal arterioles, thereby decreasing the blood supply to the retina. Contributing factors are excessive use of nicotine and caffeine and high stress levels. Diabetes also affects blood vessels when blood glucose levels are poorly controlled over long periods.

Pathophysiology

Diabetic patients experience two different forms of retinopathy: proliferative and nonproliferative retinopathy. In the nonproliferative type of retinopathy, microaneurysms develop on the retinal blood vessels. These eventually swell and rupture, causing hemorrhage into the vitreous humor, which interferes with vision. The proliferative form of retinopathy occurs later in the course of diabetes. New blood vessels grow from the existing retinal vessels in a process called *neovascularization.* The new vessels are thinner and rupture more easily, causing hemorrhage. The blood from the hemorrhage causes scarring, which also interferes with vision. High blood pressure creates blockages in retinal blood vessels. Retinal hemorrhages and macular swelling may cause vision impairment.

Signs, Symptoms, and Diagnosis

It is important that patients with diabetes have regular, frequent eye examinations because the early stages of retinopathy present no symptoms. As the retinopathy progresses, there are alterations in vision such as blurring, missing areas in the field of vision, and seeing red or black lines or spots. These signs can be observed on ophthalmologic examination of the retina and by fluorescein angiography. When the macula is involved, there is a loss of vision that may progress to blindness. Retinal detachment may occur as a result of proliferative retinopathy.

Treatment

Tight control of blood glucose levels (100 to 115 mg/dL) is very important to prevent excessive diabetic retinopathy. There is no other known way to halt the process. The microaneurysms and the neovascularized vessels are treated with laser photocoagulation therapy to prevent hemorrhage and the consequent scarring and loss of vision. Vitrectomy also can be done if hemorrhage has caused serious impairment of vision. Hypertension must be kept under good control.

Nursing Management

Diabetic retinopathy is the leading cause of preventable blindness in adults of working age. Nationally

Home Care Considerations

Home Care Instructions for Retinal Surgery or Vitrectomy

Instructions will vary if the patient has a gas bubble that was injected intraocularly. Positioning and activity are more restricted for these patients.

ACTIVITY

- Restrict activity according to the health care provider's instructions. Bed rest with bathroom privileges for the first few days is common. The head may need to be positioned to the left or right most of the time. A head-down or semiprone position to the right or left will be required for most of the time if a gas bubble was injected into the eye.
- The following activities are allowed immediately after discharge, unless a gas bubble has been injected into the eye as part of the procedure:
  - Watching television from a distance of at least 10 feet.
  - Tub bath or shower, using extreme care not to get soap or water in the eyes. Take care to prevent a fall.
  - Walking outdoors with the guidance of a companion.
  - Reading for brief periods.
  - Gentle shampooing of hair with the head tilted backward and using care not to get soap or water in the eyes.
  - Riding in a car as a passenger.

EYE CARE

- The operative eye is to be patched at all times and protected by an eye shield or eyeglasses until you are told you may leave the eye uncovered. A patch or shield may still be recommended for use while sleeping. The eye patch is removed only to administer eye drops or ointment. The eyelid may be cleansed with cotton or gauze moistened with irrigating solution. Each time the patch is changed, check the movement of the eyeballs under the lids. Gently retract the upper lid and look down as far as possible. Next, look up while retracting the lower lid. This helps break adhesions of the eyeball to the lids.
- The following are expected and should not cause alarm: tearing, a small amount of blood on the eye patch, a scratchy sensation, blurred vision, unusual visual images, a few light flashes, and floaters. Call the provider if these symptoms increase *significantly* after discharge.
- Have someone else administer the eye medications. Assume a reclining position for eye drop or eye ointment placement. Pull down the lower lid and, with the patient looking up, place the correct number of drops into the center of the conjunctival sac. Let the lid gently close. The patient should try not to squeeze the eye shut or blink excessively. Wait 3 to 5 minutes between types of eye drops so that they do not wash each other out and dilute the intended effect. Patch the eye after each set of drops or ointment is administered. If a shield is to be used, it is placed on top of the taped-down eye pad.

COMFORT

- Take a prescribed analgesic or extra-strength acetaminophen to relieve pain. A cool washcloth or ice pack to the forehead may provide comfort. Report pain that grows markedly worse or is accompanied by nausea and vomiting.

PRECAUTIONS

- In case of cough, take cough syrup. Do not try to hold back sneezes. Do not strain at stool; take a stool softener or milk of magnesia if needed to prevent this.

RESTRICTIONS

- Avoid driving a car until visual acuity is 20/40 or better; your provider will tell you when you may resume driving.
- Avoid lifting heavy objects (those over 20 lb) for at least 4 months.
- Refrain from work for 2 to 6 weeks (depending on type of work); your provider will tell you when you may return to work. Light housework that does not require bending over or vigorous scrubbing may be resumed within 1 to 2 weeks depending on the type of surgery performed.
- Avoid vigorous or strenuous activity for 4 months.
- Do not bend with your head down; keep the head upright and bend at the knees.
- Avoid sports for 3 to 4 months.

Think Critically

How do the signs and symptoms of glaucoma and cataract differ?

and internationally the number of cases is expected to significantly increase in the next 15 years. Retinopathy can occur with type 1 or type 2 diabetes. You can be instrumental in promoting glucose control and regular eye examinations to help prevent and manage the condition. Nurses must encourage glucose testing in patients who have a family history of diabetes or who are in a high-risk category, so that the disease may be discovered early before vascular effects have occurred.

Think Critically

What would you teach a patient with diabetes about the prevention of retinopathy? What factors affect the development of retinopathy?

MACULAR DEGENERATION

Etiology

Age-related macular degeneration (AMD) occurs with aging and is the most common cause of visual loss in older adults. Its incidence is expected to increase with the longer life spans that Americans currently enjoy. The macular region of the retina provides color vision, acute vision, and central vision. Inflammation may be a factor; *Chlamydia pneumoniae* has been found in the eye tissue of some people with the wet form of AMD.

There is a genetic tendency for the disease, and diabetes and hypertension are associated risk factors. Wearing sunglasses regularly when outdoors may help protect against AMD. Certain vitamins, minerals, and antioxidants seem to help prevent or slow AMD.

Health Promotion

Tobacco and Alcohol and Macular Degeneration

Teaching people to quit smoking and to abstain from immoderate drinking (four or more alcoholic drinks a day) can decrease the incidence of AMD. Smoking is a risk factor for AMD and significantly increases the progression of the disease from early to advanced (Arroyo, 2018). In Britain there is a movement to add the warning about the risk of vision loss to the other warnings on cigarette packages.

Complementary and Alternative Therapies

Preventing or Slowing Progression of Macular Degeneration

Two major studies have shown that supplements can slow the progression of AMD. The formula includes vitamins C and E, zinc, copper, lutein, zeaxanthin, and omega-3 (National Eye Institute, 2018). The combination is available over the counter. Fish oil, which acts as an antiinflammatory, may protect the retina from AMD. If patients are on blood thinners, such as warfarin or aspirin, fish oil may increase the risk of bleeding.

Pathophysiology

There are two types of AMD: dry and wet. Exudative (wet) macular degeneration may occur at any age. In the dry (atrophic) form, gradual blockage in the retinal capillaries leads to death of rod and cone photoreceptors in the macula of the retina. This form accounts for 85% to 90% of cases. Dry AMD may progress to wet AMD. In the wet form, abnormal vessels develop in or near the macula. Central vision is affected. The fragile vessel network grows into the subretinal space and may bleed into the macular region, causing central visual impairment. Exudative macular degeneration is caused by a serous detachment of pigment epithelium in the macula. Central vision loss usually occurs rapidly.

Signs and Symptoms

Dry AMD is bilateral and progressive. Early symptoms may be an inability to see the vividness of colors or to see details. Blurred vision, presence of scotomas, or distortion of vision gradually occurs. Objects may appear to be the wrong size or shape, or straight lines may appear crooked or wavy. As central vision deteriorates, there may be a large dark spot or empty place over the center of what is viewed. The patient retains peripheral vision and can walk, dress, cook, and sometimes drive if impairment is minimal but cannot read when the disorder becomes severe. Exudative AMD usually starts in only one eye, but can progress to affect both.

Diagnosis

Ophthalmologic examination of the retina and macula is the first step in diagnosis. In dry AMD yellow exudates called **drusen** are found beneath the retinal pigment epithelium. Drusen represent extracellular debris. In wet AMD fluid and blood are detected by the examination. Patients at risk for macular degeneration, or extension of the problem, are taught to use an Amsler grid (a small card with lines in a grid formation) at home to assess progression of the disorder (Fig. 25.19). If macular degeneration is occurring, the lines appear wavy. Fluorescein angiography or optical coherence tomography shows the specific areas of the retina involved.

Clinical Cues

Researchers are investigating the possibility of diagnosing macular degeneration from a blood test. Lipid biomarkers are present in patients with macular degeneration and may help with diagnosis and treatment (Lains et al., 2018).

Treatment

Treatments available do not cure the disease but are intended to slow down the progression or improve vision. For both forms of AMD, smoking cessation is implemented to prevent progression of the disease. There is no specific treatment for dry AMD that restores vision, but a novel inhibitor of a protein involved in inflammation that contributes to vision loss is being developed and is in phase III trials. A combination of vitamins, minerals, and antioxidants is recommended to slow the progression of the disease. Several trials to slow or halt the progression of the dry AMD are under way, including needleless drug delivery systems. Stem cell and gene therapies are also being studied (AMD.org, 2019).

Wet AMD is treated with intraocular injections of vascular endothelial growth factor (VEGF) inhibitors. Several medications are in current use, and others are in clinical trials. Pegaptanib sodium injection (Macugen) was the first anti-VEGF medication approved by the FDA for the treatment of wet AMD. It is injected into the eye under local anesthesia once every 6 weeks. During clinical studies this drug has limited the progression to legal blindness by 50% compared with controls. Ranibizumab (Lucentis), bevacizumab (Avastin), and aflibercept (Eylea) are all delivered by intravitreal injection to block VEGF, preventing the progression of wet AMD. Injections are needed every 4 to 6 weeks, and the medications range from $1000 to $1500 per dose. Both eyes are usually injected, and annual costs can range from $10,000 to $20,000 depending on the number of injections. If a patient does not have Medicare Part B prescription coverage, treatment may not be available unless covered under private insurance (Baker-Schena, 2017). Researchers are testing the efficacy of certain drugs for use as eye drops to replace these injections.

A technique under investigation is transplantation of healthy stem cell–grown retinal pigment epithelium

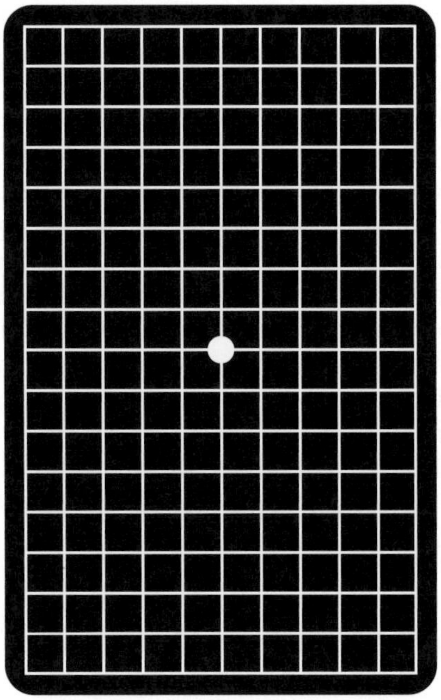
USE ONLY AS INSTRUCTED BY YOUR OPHTHALMOLOGIST
REMINDERS:
• Cover one eye; hold card directly in front of the uncovered eye
• Look at center spot
• Note any irregularities (e.g., wavy, gray, fuzzy)
• Rotate 90 degrees and repeat
• Test other eye
Contact your ophthalmologist as instructed, if necessary
Name
Address
Phone
The Yannuzzi Card (Modified Amsler Grid)
Copyright © 1981 BMI, A service from The Macula Foundation, Inc.

Fig. 25.19 Amsler grid used to check for macular degeneration. (Courtesy Macula Foundation, Inc., New York.)

cells to replace or enhance degenerating epithelium. It is hoped that transplantation of such cells before vision has greatly deteriorated will slow or eliminate the progression of AMD (National Institutes of Health [NIH], 2018).

A device for home use is available to monitor vision changes for those with dry AMD. The patient tests each eye daily, and the results are electronically transmitted to the health care provider's office. Treatment is most effective when changes in vision are detected early. A proprietary genetic test performed on saliva, Macula Risk PGx, is available for patients at increased risk of macular degeneration. The results of the test are used to identify those at risk for progressing to advanced AMD and to intervene in the modifiable risk factors. The test also helps identify which supplement therapy may be the most effective, based on the patient's genetic profile.

Photodynamic therapy using IV verteporfin (Visudyne), followed by a low-level laser (light) therapy that destroys only the cells that absorbed the dye, is another therapy for wet AMD. This therapy destroys abnormal blood vessels without permanent damage to the photoreceptor cells and the retinal pigment epithelium. Because direct exposure to sunlight or other intense forms of light can activate the dye in the cells, the patient must avoid those forms of light for 5 days, after which the remaining dye will have been fully excreted.

Multiple medications, devices, and interventions are under development for prevention, early identification, treatment, and someday a cure for AMD.

Nursing Management

Education on risk factors, early identification of vision problems, and encouragement to seek medical help can all assist patients in preventing vision loss. Help patients with permanent vision loss learn to use low-vision aids. A referral to a low-vision device specialist and low-vision support group commonly is needed. Devices are available to illuminate and magnify reading material. Books with large print are easier to read. Learning to turn the head and move the eyeballs to work around the central scotoma may help. Electronic magnification of a printed page on screen can be used for reading or doing crossword puzzles. Telescopic lenses can help for watching movies, attending the theater, reading street signs, and seeing traffic lights. A head-mounted low-vision enhancement system provides both distance and close-up enhancement. Easy-to-read watches with large numerals, television screen magnifiers, and guides that fit over checkbooks to assist with writing on them are some of the less expensive low-vision aids available.

> **Clinical Cues**
>
> Over-the-counter supplements are not controlled by the FDA in the same way as prescription drugs. Careful reading of the label contents is necessary. Many products claim to promote eye health and treat AMD. Only those products with the same ingredients in the same dosage as the Age-Related Eye Disease Study 2 (AREDS2) are recommended for AMD treatment.

NURSING CARE OF PATIENTS HAVING EYE SURGERY

PREOPERATIVE CARE

Most eye surgery procedures are done on an outpatient basis, unless the patient has other serious disorders such as cardiac dysrhythmias, severe diabetes, or a chronic disability. Therefore a large part of nursing care is directed at discharge teaching for home care. For at-risk patients, the procedure may be performed at a hospital as an outpatient. Inpatient status can be assigned if there are complications or the patient needs additional medical services.

Stool softeners may be started a day or two before surgery to prevent constipation and the Valsalva maneuver postoperatively. The Valsalva maneuver can increase IOP. Some health care providers direct the patient to wash the face with surgical soap several times on the evening and morning before surgery. The patient may be given instructions on the administration of eye drops on the night before and the morning of surgery.

After admission, the patient is fully oriented to the outpatient surgery unit and given instructions about the layout of the room and area and the ways in which help can be summoned. Side rails are usually necessary to prevent falls, and the patient should be cautioned against getting up without assistance. Preoperative eye drops and medications are instilled in the outpatient surgery center on the morning of surgery. Drugs must be given with extreme care and accuracy, especially if only one eye is affected. **Be sure that the medication is applied to the correct eye.** An IV infusion is started shortly before surgery.

Because most patients undergoing eye surgery are older adults and therefore are likely to have some additional chronic disease, remember to apply the principles of geriatric nursing in administering care. Fear, anxiety over the surgical procedure, and concern about the expected results of the surgery are all factors to be considered when preparing the patient for the operation. Instructions and information should be given both verbally and in writing. Measures to ensure patient safety are very important both preoperatively and postoperatively because the vision is impaired.

Safety Alert

Prevent Falls From Impaired Vision

An older adult who has a patched eye, has low vision, has been given procedural sedatives, and is in a strange environment is subject to falls. The patient may need to be reoriented to place, time, and surroundings frequently to decrease confusion and agitation.

POSTOPERATIVE CARE

In caring for a patient undergoing any type of eye surgery, the key word is *gentleness.* The patient's head should not be jarred when transferring from the operating table or stretcher to the bed. Remember to speak before touching a patient who is blind or who is wearing bandages over the eyes.

Patients are usually kept in the recovery area of the outpatient surgery department for 1 to 2 hours postoperatively. Nausea and subsequent vomiting can wreak havoc with delicate suture lines in the eye. **If the patient becomes nauseated, antiemetic medication should be administered immediately and all food and liquids withheld.**

An eye patch is often placed over the eye that was operated on (see Fig. 25.15). If it is necessary to restrict movement of the eyes, both eyes are patched.

Instructions regarding postoperative medications and how they are to be instilled are given before discharge (see the Evolve website). Different types of eye drop medications come with color-coded tops for easy identification. Eye drop bottles also can be "labeled" by wrapping one, two, or three rubber bands around them so that patients with a visual impairment can differentiate one type of drop from another.

Should the patient need to stay in the hospital because of other problems, you must be thoroughly familiar with their individual care needs. It should be known whether the patient can be turned on one or both sides or must remain flat on the back, whether pillows are allowed under the head, and how high the head of the bed may be raised. For certain types of retinal surgery, the head may need to be raised and positioned toward a particular side. If a gas bubble has been injected intraocularly, the patient is positioned prone or supine with the head toward one side or the other, according to orders. If the patient is allowed out of bed, care must be taken not to jar the head or move too suddenly.

Sexual activity usually can be resumed in 1 to 8 weeks postoperatively, depending on the procedure performed. The surgeon will explain this to the patient. Ensure that the patient understands the time of the next appointment with the ophthalmologist. The patient and family should be encouraged to follow the provider's directions faithfully during the healing period at home so that nothing will jeopardize the success of the surgery.

Discharge planning is of utmost importance. Refer to the earlier Home Care Considerations box for home care of a patient after retinal surgery or vitrectomy.

COMMUNITY CARE

Nurses in all settings should be conscious of eye safety for themselves and those around them. Public education on using sunhats, visors, and dark glasses when outdoors to protect the eyes from ultraviolet A and B (UVA and UVB) rays is another teaching opportunity for all nurses.

Nurses working in home care often find that patients have not had eye care in many years; prescriptions have not been changed, and patients' quality of vision has decreased. Arrange for referral to an appropriate agency to set up an eye examination when the patient cannot. Glaucoma testing should be encouraged every 2 to 3 years for all adults older than 40 years.

Both home care nurses and those working in long-term care should be alert to signs of progressing macular degeneration. The Amsler grid can assist in identifying this problem. Patients with known eye disorders should be assessed periodically to see how much their vision has deteriorated and how much their ability to perform activities of daily living and partake in usual hobbies is affected. You should be instrumental in helping patients obtain low-vision aids. The Library of Congress in Washington, D.C., lends records and recording machines without charge to people who are blind and maintains a wide selection of recordings. Recordings of required textbooks may be obtained free of charge from Recording for the Blind and Dyslexic.

Loss of vision need not be devastating for a person if support and encouragement are given for coping with the impairment. There are resources to help those with visual impairments learn to care for themselves, find employment, and enjoy educational and recreational activities. Many colleges provide special funds to enable blind students to hire readers and recording devices to help them with their studies.

All nurses have the opportunity to encourage the donation of corneas at death. Signing a donor card, as well as indicating "tissue donor" on one's driver's license, should be a consideration for all. You may be the person to approach a terminal patient or their family about the possibility of donating corneas after death and giving the gift of sight to another. Many facilities have professionals trained specifically to approach families, but nurses need to be knowledgeable about the process and able to answer questions.

Get Ready for the NCLEX® Examination!

Key Points

- Eye disorders are caused by injury, disease, or genetic predisposition.
- Everyone older than 40 years should have a complete eye examination.
- After age 65 years, an eye examination is recommended every 1 to 2 years.
- Control of diabetes mellitus and hypertension can help preserve vision.
- Obtaining a good history is important to data collection regarding vision.
- A problem with refraction is the most common eye disorder.
- Cataracts cause a blurring or loss of vision and usually develop slowly.
- Cataract surgery with lens implant usually restores vision.
- The increase in IOP that occurs with glaucoma will eventually cause blindness if untreated.
- Glaucoma medication typically must be used for the rest of the patient's life.
- Symptoms of retinal detachment include flashing colored lights followed by the appearance of "floaters."
- Unless treated quickly and successfully, retinal detachment causes vision loss.
- Positioning and restriction of movement are crucial after eye surgery.
- Retinopathy is a disorder that occurs most commonly in people with diabetes or hypertension.
- Strict glucose control helps prevent diabetic retinopathy.
- Retinopathy is commonly treated by laser.
- Keratoplasty may be performed to repair damaged corneas.
- Macular degeneration is a common problem in older adults but can occur at an earlier age.
- There is presently no cure for macular degeneration, but new drugs and treatments may be able to slow it or reverse some of the vision loss.
- Eye trauma should be treated promptly by a health care provider.
- Keep patients who have had eye surgery still and treat nausea immediately.

Additional Learning Resources

SG Go to your Study Guide for additional learning activities to help you master this chapter content.

Go to your Evolve website (http://evolve.elsevier.com/deWit/medsurg) for the following FREE learning resources:
- Animations, audio, and video
- Answers and rationales for questions and activities
- Glossary with pronunciations in English and Spanish
- Interactive Review Questions and more!

Review Questions for the NCLEX® Examination

1. A nurse evaluates the visual acuity of a patient using the Snellen chart. Which statement is true regarding the use of the Snellen chart?
   1. The chart is placed 40 feet away from the patient.
   2. The patient reads the letters using one eye at a time.
   3. The numerator (top number) indicates the smallest line that the patient could read.
   4. The denominator (bottom number) refers to the patient's distance from the chart.

   NCLEX Client Need: Health Promotion and Maintenance
2. While looking at a card with a geometric grid of identical squares, a patient is asked to focus on a central dot and to describe any distortions of the surrounding boxes. Which patient statement indicates a need for further diagnostic testing?
   1. "I get dizzy staring at these boxes for so long."
   2. "I am beginning to see color differences in the squares."
   3. "I can see all the boxes surrounding the dot."
   4. "There are wavy lines around the central dot."

   NCLEX Client Need: Physiological Integrity: Reduction of Risk Potential

3. During a health care provider visit, a 65-year-old man complains of pain in his right eye associated with excessive tearing. You note that the eye is red with lashes rubbing against the cornea. A likely condition would be:
   1. ptosis.
   2. ectropion.
   3. hordeolum.
   4. entropion.

   NCLEX Client Need: Physiological Integrity: Physiological Adaptation
4. Which nursing action(s) demonstrate(s) appropriate care of a patient who is visually impaired? *(Select all that apply.)*
   1. Introduce self before touching.
   2. Speak slowly with a loud voice.
   3. Keep the door ajar.
   4. Ensure ready access to the call button for assistance.
   5. Assist with feeding using the clock method.

   NCLEX Client Need: Psychosocial Integrity
5. A male patient was informed that he would need to wear a pair of corrective lenses for astigmatism. When asked about the condition, the patient demonstrates understanding when he states that:
   1. "Astigmatism is hardening of the ciliary muscles."
   2. "Astigmatism is an irregular curvature of the cornea."
   3. "Astigmatism enables focusing of light in front of the retina."
   4. "Astigmatism is an increased opacity of the lens."

   NCLEX Client Need: Health Promotion and Maintenance
6. Which instruction must be included in the discharge teaching of a patient who has undergone corneal transplant?
   1. Increase physical activity.
   2. Wear an eye shield when in close contact with children or pets.
   3. Remove the pressure dressing as needed.
   4. Lie only on the operative side.

   NCLEX Client Need: Health Promotion and Maintenance
7. An older adult is admitted for cataract extraction. Which sign or symptom is associated with this condition?
   1. Increased tearing
   2. Increasing farsightedness
   3. Increasing complaints about glare
   4. Bluish discolorations

   NCLEX Client Need: Physiological Integrity: Physiological Adaptation
8. People with diabetes may face several eye problems and diseases as a complication of their illness. Which of the following can cause severe vision loss or blindness in a person with diabetes? *(Select all that apply.)*
   1. Glaucoma
   2. Retinopathy
   3. Presbyopia
   4. Cataracts

   NCLEX Client Need: Physiological Integrity: Physiological Adaptation
9. After eye surgery, a patient is instructed to avoid movements that increase the venous pressure in the head, neck, and eyes. Which movement(s) increase(s) venous pressure? *(Select all that apply.)*
   1. Straining
   2. Bending over
   3. Keeping the head up
   4. Sudden head movements
   5. Strenuous exercises

   NCLEX Client Need: Physiological Integrity: Reduction of Risk Potential
10. A woman complains of eye itching, tearing, halos around lights, and decreased central vision. Which symptom most clearly relates to macular degeneration?
    1. Eye itching
    2. Tearing
    3. Halos around lights
    4. Decreased central vision

    NCLEX Client Need: Physiological Integrity: Physiological Adaptation
11. Before eye surgery, a patient is instructed to take stool softeners. When asked about the rationale for taking the stool softener, an appropriate response would be:
    1. "The medication reduces the possibility of straining at stool postoperatively."
    2. "The medication prevents constipation caused by anesthetic agents."
    3. "The medication cleanses the gastrointestinal tract."
    4. "The medication enhances surgical recovery."

    NCLEX Client Need: Physiological Integrity: Pharmacological Therapies
12. What advice may you give to an aging adult to help prevent macular degeneration? *(Select all that apply.)*
    1. Do not smoke or quit if you do smoke.
    2. Maintain a healthy weight; especially do not carry weight around the waist.
    3. Avoid bending or heavy lifting.
    4. Drink with a straw.

    NCLEX Client Need: Health Promotion and Maintenance

Critical Thinking Questions

Scenario A

Mr. Hartman comes to the ambulatory clinic because he "got something in my eye" while using the weed trimmer.

1. What type of examinations would you expect the health care provider to perform?
2. What would you teach Mr. Hartman about eye safety before he leaves?
3. What questions would you ask him about basic eye care while you are interviewing him before the provider sees him?

Scenario B

Mr. Lavant, age 52 years, and his wife, who has diabetes, have heard about a glaucoma screening clinic being held in their community. They are interested in attending the clinic but are very apprehensive about the kind of tests that will be done. They ask you about the tests and whether you think they should go to the screening clinic when they have no symptoms of glaucoma or any other eye disease.

1. How would you explain a test with a tonometer?
2. How would you explain glaucoma in terms that Mr. and Mrs. Lavant could understand?
3. Who are among the people at high risk for glaucoma?
4. What is the usual treatment for chronic, open-angle glaucoma?

Scenario C

Mr. Wilson, age 78 years, is scheduled for a right cataract extraction and intraocular lens implant. He has bilateral cataracts that have made him legally blind for years. He did not consult a health care provider until recently because he had always heard that cataracts had to be "ripe" before they could be treated, and he felt he could not afford frequent trips to a provider when nothing could be done for his condition. Mr. Wilson enters the outpatient surgery area, and you are assigned as his nurse.

1. How would you approach and orient Mr. Wilson to his surroundings?
2. What would you tell Mr. Wilson about the preoperative routine and medications at this time?
3. What problem statements would be appropriate for Mr. Wilson at this time?
4. What are the advantages of intraocular lens implants over cataract glasses and/or contact lenses?

26 The Sensory System: Ear

http://evolve.elsevier.com/deWit/medsurg

Objectives

Theory

1. Explore the effects of hearing loss on an individual and their family.
2. Summarize the anatomy and physiology of hearing.
3. Identify ways of preventing hearing loss.
4. Describe the testing that is done to identify which part of the hearing process has been affected by disease or trauma.
5. Compare the testing and interventions for conductive and sensorineural hearing loss.
6. Explain the signs and symptoms of selected disorders of the ear, appropriate medical or surgical treatment, and nursing interventions for each.

Clinical Practice

7. Teach a patient with tinnitus or vertigo measures that may decrease the symptoms.
8. Teach a patient to properly administer ear medication.
9. Provide appropriate care for a patient after ear surgery.
10. Instruct a spouse in ways to effectively communicate with a partner who is hearing impaired.

Key Terms

cerumen (sĕ-RŪ-mĕn, p. 618)
eustachian tube (yū-STĀ-shĕn tūb, p. 618)
myringotomy (mĭr-ĕn-GŎT-ĕ-mē, p. 633)
otorrhea (ō-tō-RĒ-ă, p. 625)
ototoxicity (ō-tŭ-tok-SĬ-sĕ-tē, p. 622)
presbycusis (prĕz-bē-KŪ-sĭs, p. 630)
sensorineural loss (sĕn-sō-rē-NŪ-răl lôs, p. 620)
tinnitus (tĭ-NĪ-tĕs, p. 622)
tympanoplasty (tĭm-pă-nō-PLĂS-tē, p. 633)
vertigo (VĔR-tĭ-gō, p. 621)

Concepts Covered in This Chapter

- Functional Ability
- Family Dynamics
- Self-Management
- Health Promotion
- Sensory Perception

ANATOMY AND PHYSIOLOGY OF THE EAR

STRUCTURES OF THE EAR

- The external ear consists of the pinna (auricle) and the canal (auditory meatus). The pinna is the fleshy part of the ear situated on the side of the head (Fig. 26.1).
- The auditory meatus is a tube approximately 2.5 cm long that extends from the pinna to the tympanic membrane.
- The meatus is lined with numerous hairs and glands that secrete a waxy substance called **cerumen** (earwax).
- The middle ear contains the auditory bones (ossicles) and opens into the eustachian tube.
- The auditory ossicles are three small bones: the malleus (hammer), the incus (anvil), and the stapes (stirrup).
- The malleus attaches to the tympanic membrane.
- The stapes attaches to the oval window.
- The incus links the malleus and the stapes.
- The tympanic membrane (eardrum) separates the middle ear from the external ear.
- The **eustachian tube** connects the middle ear with the throat.
- The oval window and the round window connect the middle ear to the inner ear.
- The inner ear is divided into the vestibule, the semicircular canals, and the cochlea.
- The inner ear contains a bony labyrinth with a membranous labyrinth lining; the inner ear is in the temporal bone of the skull.
- A clear fluid, endolymph, fills the membranous labyrinth.
- The cochlea contains the organ of Corti, which is composed of sound receptors.

FUNCTIONS OF THE EAR STRUCTURES

- The pinna collects sound waves and channels them into the auditory meatus.
- The hairs and cerumen in the canal help prevent foreign objects from reaching the tympanic membrane.
- The tympanic membrane vibrates when sound waves hit it; the sound vibrations are conducted to the malleus.
- The bones of the middle ear transmit the sound vibrations to the inner ear. The malleus transmits

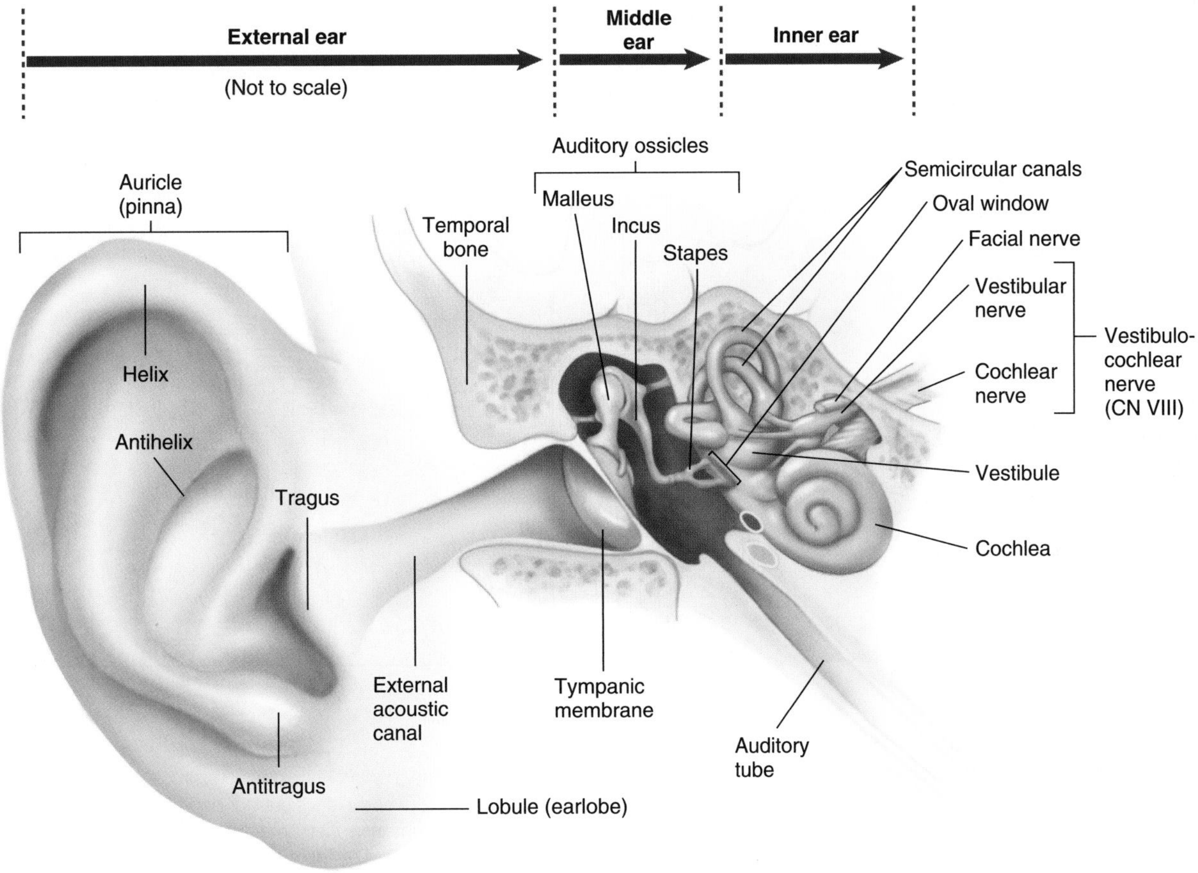

Fig. 26.1 Structures of the ear. (From Patton KT, Thibodeau GA: *Human body in health and disease*, ed 7, St. Louis, 2018, Elsevier.)

them to the incus, and the incus transmits sound vibrations to the stapes. The stapes transmits the sound vibrations to the oval window, which transfers the motion to the fluid in the inner ear.

- Fluid motion in the inner ear stimulates the sound receptors in the cochlea and the organ of Corti (Fig. 26.2).
- The organ of Corti transmits impulses to the cochlear branch of the vestibulocochlear nerve (cranial nerve VIII). This nerve carries the impulses to the medulla oblongata, the thalamus, and then to the temporal lobe of the brain, which contains the auditory cortex.
- The eustachian tube helps equalize pressure in the middle ear.
- Receptors responsible for equilibrium (balance) are located in the inner ear, within the bony vestibule and at the base of the semicircular canals.
- Impulses from the equilibrium receptors are transmitted to the brain via the vestibular branch of the vestibulocochlear nerve (cranial nerve VIII). The cerebellum is important in mediating the sense of equilibrium and balance (Fig. 26.3).

AGE-RELATED CHANGES IN THE EAR

- Cerumen becomes harder, containing less moisture, and its buildup within the ear may contribute to a hearing loss in the low-frequency range.
- The tympanic membrane loses elasticity.
- The joints between the auditory bones become stiffer; the stiffness interferes with the transmission of sound waves but is not clinically significant by itself.
- There is a gradual loss of the receptor cells in the organ of Corti after age 40 years.
- The number of nerve fibers in the vestibulocochlear nerve decreases, contributing to hearing loss and sometimes affecting balance and equilibrium.

THE EAR

The National Institute on Deafness and Other Communication Disorders (NIDCD, 2017) reports that 24% of adults ages 20 to 69 years in the United States show signs of noise-induced hearing loss, with those ages 60 to 69 having the greatest incidence. Social withdrawal is common when hearing becomes severely impaired. The inability to hear causes difficulty with communication. Approximately 2 in 1000 babies born in the United States have some form of congenital hearing problem. After age 75 years, about 50% of the population has some degree of hearing loss. It is believed that the trend of playing very loud music—which causes damage to the acoustic nerve—will result in considerably more hearing loss in the coming decades.

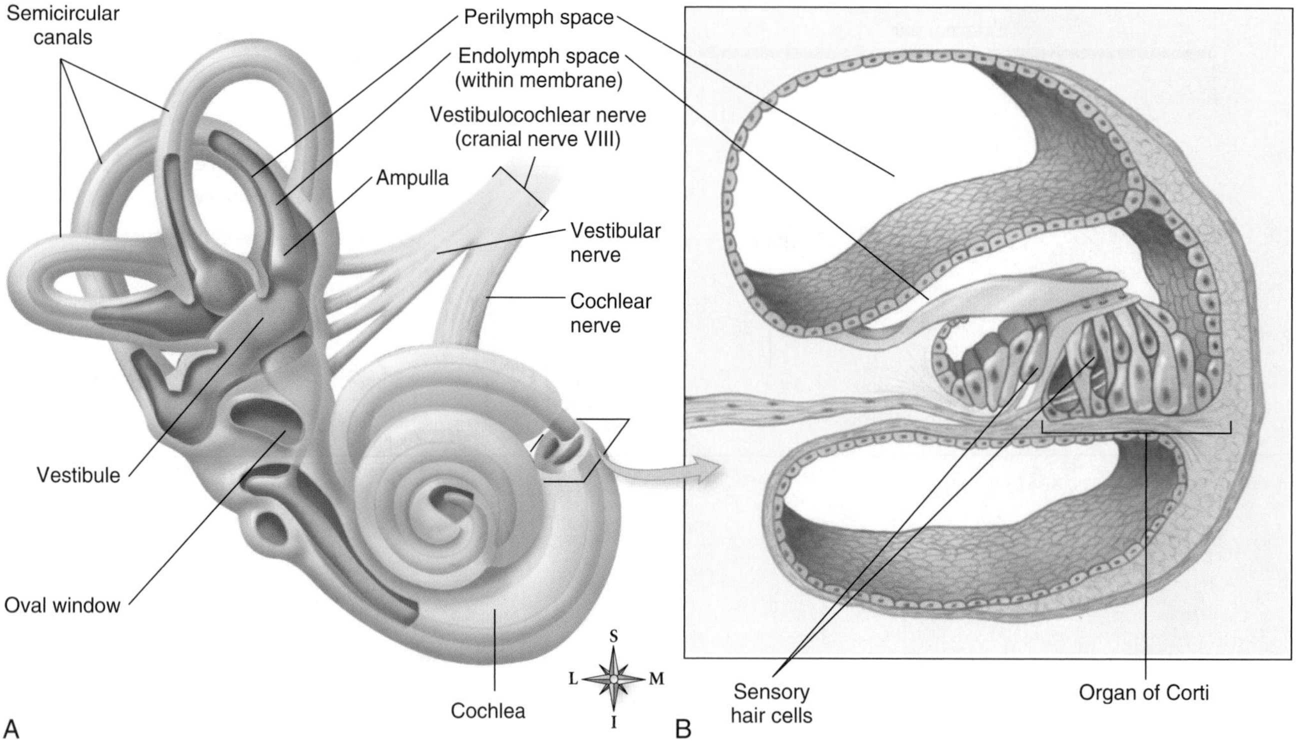

Fig. 26.2 Inner ear. **A,** The bony labyrinth is the hard outer wall of the entire inner ear and includes semicircular canals, vestibule, and cochlea. Within the bony labyrinth is the membranous labyrinth *(purple),* which is surrounded by perilymph and filled with endolymph. Each ampulla in the vestibule contains a crista ampullaris that detects changes in head position and sends sensory impulses through the vestibular nerve to the brain. **B,** The *inset* shows a section of the membranous cochlea. Hair cells in the organ of Corti detect sound and send the information through the cochlear nerve. The vestibular and cochlear nerves join to form the vestibulocochlear nerve, or cranial nerve VIII. (From Patton KT, Thibodeau GA: *Human body in health and disease,* ed 7, St. Louis, 2018, Elsevier.)

Health Promotion

Coping With Hearing Loss

The sooner a person with a hearing loss obtains and learns to use a hearing aid, the greater the hearing improvement. The brain is better able to integrate the hearing aid transmissions when hearing has not been impaired for a very long time. Encourage individuals with any hearing loss to be tested and to try a hearing aid if one is recommended. The person should be told that there is an adjustment curve with new hearing aid use and that it often takes several trips back to the hearing aid center for minor adjustments to the instrument to be made. The hearing aid does not restore normal hearing, so it takes practice in using the aid to achieve better hearing.

There are two types of hearing loss related to problems in the ear: *sensorineural* and *conductive.* Disorders of the hearing nerve (**sensorineural loss**) are the most common cause of hearing loss. Conductive hearing loss is caused by a problem transmitting sound impulses through the auditory canal, the tympanic membrane, or the bones of the middle ear. Causes of sensorineural and conductive hearing impairment are listed in Box 26.1. Both types of hearing loss may be present and called *mixed.* Auditory processing disorders occur in the brain as it tries to process the incoming information.

Box 26.1 Common Causes of Sensorineural and Conductive Hearing Loss

CONDUCTIVE LOSS

- Obstruction by impacted cerumen
- Infection with labyrinthitis
- Otosclerosis
- Trauma and scarring of the tympanic membrane
- Congenital malformation of the outer or middle ear

SENSORINEURAL LOSS

- Presbycusis
- Heredity with congenital loss
- Ototoxic drugs
- Loud noise exposure
- Tumor (acoustic neuroma)
- Ménière disease
- Severe infection such as measles, mumps, or meningitis
- Rubella in utero

These disorders are not a problem within the ear but need to be ruled out as a possible reason for symptoms.

Arteriosclerosis can cause decreased blood flow to the vestibulocochlear nerve (cranial nerve VIII), resulting in sensorineural hearing loss. This often contributes to hearing loss in older adults.

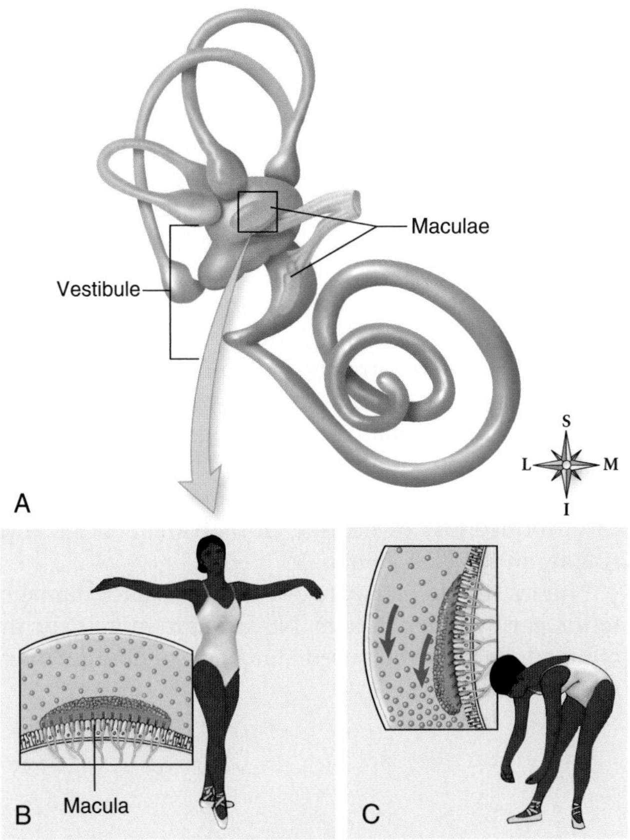

Fig. 26.3 Static equilibrium. **A,** Structure of vestibule showing placement of the maculae, which have mechanoreceptors that detect our "sense of gravity" or static equilibrium. **B,** Macula stationary in upright position. **C,** Macula displaced by gravity as person bends over. (From Patton KT, Thibodeau GA: *Human body in health and disease,* ed 7, St. Louis, 2018, Elsevier.)

A loss of hearing—like a loss of sight—burdens its victims with physical, emotional, psychosocial, and financial problems. Hearing allows for communication with others in everyday conversations, in the classroom, and in business transactions. Without the ability to hear, one can be deprived of many of the joys and pleasures of life: music, drama, exchange of ideas, and the thousands of sounds in one's environment. Because hearing warns one of danger, an inability to hear can cause anxiety and fear. Adults who have a hearing deficiency might lose jobs and alienate friends because of their communication handicap. Nurses must learn ways to help prevent hearing loss and to assist patients who already have such a loss.

Inner ear disorders can cause problems with balance. Dizziness, **vertigo**, and ataxia can greatly interfere with an individual's ability to work or to perform usual activities of daily living. Accidental injury and fractures from falls may occur.

HEARING LOSS

Causes and Prevention

A glance at the causes of hearing loss listed in Box 26.1 will help identify some of the ways nurses can help

Table 26.1 Range of Sounds Audible and Hazardous to the Ear

LEVEL IN DECIBELS (DB)	EXAMPLE
0	Lowest sound audible to the human ear
30	Quiet library, soft whisper
40	Living room, quiet office, bedroom away from traffic
50	Light traffic at a distance, refrigerator, gentle breeze
60	Air conditioner at 20 feet, conversation, sewing machine
70	Busy traffic, noisy restaurant; at this decibel level, noise may begin to affect hearing if exposure is constant
Hazardous Zone for Hearing Loss	
80	Subway, heavy city traffic, alarm clock at 2 feet, factory noise; these noises are dangerous if exposure to them lasts for more than 8 h
90	Truck traffic, noisy home appliances, shop tools, lawn mower; as loudness increases, the "safe" time exposure decreases; damage can occur in 2 h
100	Chainsaw, stereo headphones, pneumatic drill; even 15 minutes of exposure can be dangerous at this decibel level; with each 5-dB increase, the safe time is cut in half
120	Rock band concert in front of speakers, sandblasting, thunderclap; the danger is immediate; exposure of 120 dB can injure ears
140	Gunshot blast, jet plane; firecrackers; any length of exposure time is dangerous; noise at this level may cause actual pain in the ear
160	Rocket launching pad; without ear protection, noise at this level causes irreversible damage; hearing loss is inevitable

Adapted from Lewis SL, Heitkemper MM, Bucher L, et al.: *Medical-surgical nursing: assessment and management of clinical problem,* ed 10, St. Louis, 2017, Elsevier.

prevent hearing loss. Not all cases of hearing disability can be prevented, but education of the general public about causes of hearing loss can reduce its incidence. *Healthy People 2030* includes many objectives to prevent hearing loss and improve hearing among the American public. Adequate treatment of severe ear infections helps preserve hearing. Loud noise is a major cause of sensorineural hearing loss, and the use of headphones or earbuds contributes considerably to hearing damage (Table 26.1) (NIDCD, 2017). A large amount of hearing loss results from employment-related exposure to loud and continuous noise. Active and retired military personnel are experiencing hearing loss from exposure to loud noises.

Hairpins, the ends of pencils, cotton swabs, and other objects should never be used to relieve tickling or itching in the ear or to remove cerumen. Earwax normally moves on its own out of the ear canal to the outer ear, where it can be removed without danger of damaging the delicate lining of the ear canal or the tympanic membrane (eardrum). Obstructive cerumen should be removed by using drops that dissolve it or by using ear-irrigation devices, or by a health care provider or nurse skilled in removing impacted cerumen. Foreign objects, such as beans, peas, and other organic substances, also should be removed by someone who is experienced and aware of the potential for ear damage.

Conductive hearing loss most often occurs from stiffening of the bones of the middle ear or from scarring of the tympanic membrane. Continued exposure to excessively high levels of sound can produce sensorineural loss called *noise-induced hearing impairment.* This condition is particularly likely to occur in industrial settings where machinery operation creates loud noise. The standards of the Occupational Safety and Health Administration (OSHA) require the wearing of ear protectors in such settings.

Sustained exposure to noise levels of above 85 dB may result in hearing loss. Personal listening devices at high volumes can produce hearing loss with less than 5 minutes of exposure with dB levels of 105 to 110. The higher the sound level, the less time it takes to cause damage.

Many drugs can be toxic to the inner ear. This is especially true if a very high dose of the drug is given or if it is given incorrectly. Commonly administered drugs that can be ototoxic are many of the antibiotics, nonsteroidal antiinflammatory drugs (NSAIDs), chemotherapy agents, and potent diuretics, such as furosemide (Lasix) (Box 26.2). Aspirin and other salicylates can produce loss of hearing of high frequencies and ringing in the ears (**tinnitus**).

Nurses should be aware of the potential for damage to the ear by potent drugs. NSAIDs are more toxic in older adults and when used at maximum dosages over an extended period.

Box 26.2 Ototoxic Drugs and Environmental Chemicals

Ototoxicity (poisonous to the ear) is caused by drugs or chemicals that damage the inner ear or the vestibulocochlear nerve. There are more than 450 drugs that cause toxicity. The vestibulocochlear nerve sends balance and hearing information from the inner ear to the brain. Ototoxicity may result in temporary or permanent disturbances of hearing, balance, or both. Environmental chemicals can be toxic from inhalation of fumes or powder residue or from skin contamination.

DRUGS THAT MAY CAUSE OTOTOXICITY

Antibiotics

(Family history may increase susceptibility; may cause permanent damage.)

- Tobramycin
- Gentamicin
- Streptomycin
- Kanamycin
- Amikacin
- Neomycin
- Netilmicin
- Dihydrostreptomycin
- Erythromycin (IV)
- Vancomycin
- Chloramphenicol
- Minocycline
- Capreomycin
- Dibekacin
- Etiomycin

Antineoplastic Drugs

(May cause permanent damage.)

- Cisplatin
- Carboplatin
- Bleomycin
- Nitrogen mustard

Loop Diuretics (IV)

(Usually temporary damage.)

- Furosemide
- Torsemide
- Bumetanide
- Ethacrynic acid

Salicylates

(Usually temporary damage.)

- Aspirin

Nonsteroidal Antiinflammatory Drugs

(Usually temporary damage.)

- Ibuprofen
- Naproxen sodium
- Indomethacin
- Diclofenac

Narcotic Analgesics

(May cause permanent damage.)

- Hydrocodone
- Methadone
- Oxycodone
- Morphine

ENVIRONMENTAL CHEMICALS

- Metals (lead, mercury, gold, arsenic)
- Aniline dyes
- Toluene
- Carbon monoxide
- Trichloroethylene
- Xylene
- Povidone-iodine
- Nicotine
- Potassium bromate

IV, Intravenous.

Older Adult Care Points

The older the patient, the greater the chance of ototoxicity occurring from analgesic medications because many older patients have chronic conditions that cause chronic pain. Older adults' liver and kidneys generally have decreased function because of aging, so they cannot degrade and eliminate drugs as easily as those of younger people. This can cause drugs and drug metabolites to build up to toxic levels when medication is taken on a continuing basis.

Safety Alert

Dangers of Ototoxic Drugs

Know the toxic effects of the drugs you administer. Patients should be assessed frequently while receiving a potentially ototoxic drug. Any signs of ototoxicity, such as ringing in the ears, subtle changes in hearing ability, and difficulty in hearing, should be reported immediately. Ototoxicity commonly occurs because patients are taking more than one drug that can be toxic to the ear. Teach patients who are taking daily doses of aspirin or NSAIDs for arthritis or other chronic pain conditions to immediately report signs of ototoxicity.

Diagnostic Tests and Examinations

Visual examination of the ear. The two instruments most commonly used to examine the ear canal and tympanic membrane are the otoscope and the aural speculum. The otoscope is fitted with a light and a magnifying lens to facilitate inspection (Fig. 26.4). The aural speculum is used with a special circular, slightly concave head mirror that has a hole in its middle. The head mirror is positioned so that the central hole lies in front of the examiner's eye. A source of light, such as a lamp, is placed behind the examiner so that it shines on the head mirror and is reflected into the ear.

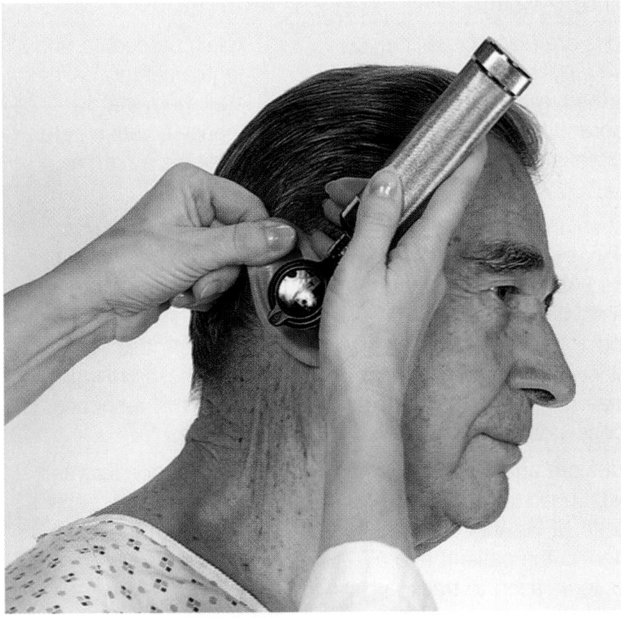

Fig. 26.4 Examination of the ear with an otoscope. (From Jarvis C: *Physical examination and health assessment*, ed 8, St. Louis, 2019, Elsevier.)

The simple speculum can be modified by attaching a special tube and inflatable bag (pneumatic otoscope), thereby creating an airtight system. This allows the examiner to determine whether the tympanic membrane responds to positive and negative pressure. The normal eardrum moves in response to pressure. Healed perforations and scars on the eardrum can be seen when the tympanic membrane is moved.

A simple hearing test is the *whisper test*. The examiner stands behind the patient and whispers a question to the patient, while having the patient place a finger on the tragus of one ear to mask hearing in that ear. If the patient hears the question, an answer is forthcoming. The examiner backs up a step and whispers another question, and so on. The other ear is tested in the same way.

Tuning fork tests. Tuning forks measure hearing by air conduction or by bone conduction (Weber test and Rinne test). A tuning fork is activated by holding it by the stem and striking the tines softly on the back of the hand (Table 26.2).

Test for nystagmus. To test for nystagmus (involuntary rhythmic jerking of the eyes), hold a finger directly in front of the patient at eye level. The patient is asked to follow the finger without moving the head. Move the finger slowly from the midline toward the right ear about 30 degrees. Then the finger is moved back to the midline and then slowly toward the left ear about 30 degrees. The patient's eyes are watched for any jerking movements. Nystagmus other than at the extremes of lateral gaze is abnormal and may indicate an inner ear problem, intracranial tumor, or paralysis of an eye muscle.

Romberg test. The Romberg test is a test of equilibrium. The patient stands with the feet together, the arms out to the sides, and the eyes open. Note the ability to maintain an upright posture without swaying. The patient is then asked to close the eyes, and posture is observed again. If the patient loses balance, it may indicate a problem with the inner ear or the cerebellum.

NURSING MANAGEMENT

ASSESSMENT (DATA COLLECTION)

Patients older than 60 years should always be assessed for hearing loss. If a patient has a known hearing impairment, assess how the patient is coping with it. Hearing and balance are subjective problems and require a good history from the patient.

Diagnosis of infection requires an otoscopic examination. It should be noted that the color, texture, and amount of cerumen varies among individuals. In whites and African Americans, cerumen tends to be moist and rust-brown colored. Native Americans and Asians have cerumen that is lighter in color and drier. There should be no secretions other than cerumen from the ear. Normally, the top of each pinna is aligned with the corner of the eye on each side of the head. Lesions on the pinna may indicate skin cancer, particularly in older adult patients. Ear pain may be referred from other parts of the head and neck and may occur from sinusitis, dental problems, or temporomandibular joint syndrome.

Table 26.2 Diagnostic Tests for Ear Problems

TEST	PURPOSE	DESCRIPTION	NURSING IMPLICATIONS
Weber test	To determine whether hearing loss is sensorineural or conductive	Tuning fork is struck, and then the handle is placed on the patient's forehead. Normal hearing or equal loss in both ears is demonstrated by hearing the sound in the middle of the head.	Explain purpose and procedure to patient.
Rinne test	To determine whether hearing loss is sensorineural or conductive	Tuning fork is struck, and then the handle is placed on the mastoid bone; the fork is removed and struck again and held beside the ear. The patient is asked in which position they heard the sound better or longer. If the sound lateralizes to the "good ear," sensorineural loss is suggested; if there is lateralization to the "bad ear," conductive loss is suggested.	Explain procedure to patient.
Audiometry—Pure tone	To determine degree of hearing loss in each ear	Earphones are placed on the patient's ears and, with the use of an audiometry machine, the audiologist channels sounds of different decibels and pitch into one ear and then the other. The patient signals when the tone is heard.	Explain procedure to patient.
Audiometry—Speech	To determine degree of hearing loss in each ear	Earphones are placed on the patient's ears and recorded or live speech is played. The patient is asked to repeat back words.	Explain procedure to patient.
Electronystagmography (ENG)	To assess for disease of vestibular system	Electrodes are placed near the patient's eyes. Caloric test is performed; movement of the eyes is recorded on a graph. Decreased response is abnormal.	Explain procedure and equipment to patient. Tell them that nausea, vertigo, etc., indicate a normal response.
Caloric test	To check for alteration in vestibular function in each ear	With patient in a seated or supine position, each ear is separately irrigated with a cold and then a warm solution to determine vestibular response. Normal response is nystagmus, vertigo, nausea, vomiting, falling; decreased response indicates abnormality.	Explain procedure to patient; tell patient they may experience nystagmus, vertigo, nausea, and vomiting, but these will indicate a normal response.
Evoked-response audiometry (ERA); auditory brainstem response (ABR)	To determine abnormality of nerve pathways between cranial nerve VIII and brainstem	Electrodes are attached to the patient's head in a darkened room; similar to EEG. Auditory stimuli are directed to the patient, and a computer is used to track and separate the auditory electrical activity of the brain from other brain waves.	Explain procedure and equipment to patient. Tell them the room will be darkened.

Table 26.2 Diagnostic Tests for Ear Problems—cont'd

TEST	PURPOSE	DESCRIPTION	NURSING IMPLICATIONS
Magnetic resonance imaging (MRI)	To detect tumor of cranial nerve VIII, acoustic neuroma	Huge electromagnet is used to detect radiofrequency pulses from the alignment of hydrogen protons in the magnetic field. A computer translates the pulses into cross-sectional images. Provides high-contrast views of soft tissue.	Explain to patient that their head will be placed in a machine that looks like a large tube. They will need to lie very still during the test; all metal must be removed before the test. Premedication may be required for patients with claustrophobia. The machine makes a very loud noise.
Rapid plasma reagin (RPR) blood test	To test for syphilis. Syphilis can cause problems with nerve transmission from the ear.	Blood is drawn and sent to the laboratory for determination of antibodies to syphilis.	Explain that a blood sample is needed.
Fasting blood glucose/ hemoglobin A_{1c}	Diabetic vasculopathy can cause cochlear ischemia	Blood is drawn to determine if complications of diabetes are the cause of hearing loss.	A fast of at least 8 h is needed for the blood glucose level.
Complete blood cell count with differential	To identify if anemia or infection are present	Anemia or infection may lead to sensorineural hearing loss.	Explain that a blood sample is needed.
Thyroid panel	To check if hyperthyroid or hypothyroid conditions are present	Hyperthyroidism or hypothyroidism can result in hearing loss.	Some medications affect test results; give a complete list of medications to the health care provider.

EEG, Electroencephalography.

Focused Assessment

Data Collection for Ear Disorders

Ask the following questions:

- Have you had any pain in the ear?
- Have you had a recent temperature elevation?
- Do you suffer from allergies?
- Do you have frequent upper respiratory infections?
- Have you ever been exposed to very loud noise? Do you work in an area that is noisy? Do you listen to loud music?
- Have you ever had a head injury?
- Do you scuba dive, hunt or shoot skeet, or fly in small airplanes?
- Do you ever have ringing, buzzing, or odd sounds in the ears?
- Do you feel your hearing ability has decreased? Do people you live with think that you do not hear as well as you used to hear? Do you frequently have to ask people to repeat things that have been said to you?
- Is there a history of hearing loss in your family?
- Have you ever had a very high fever?
- What medications are you taking regularly? Are there other medications that you have taken for an extended period in the past? Do you take aspirin?
- How do you clean your ears?
- Do you ever experience dizziness, vertigo, or loss of balance?

Focused Assessment

Physical Assessment of the Ear

- Compare the pinna on one side to the other for symmetry and placement.
- Palpate the pinna for the presence of nodules.
- Observe for the presence of lesions on the pinna.
- Check for drainage (**otorrhea**) from the ear; note color and odor.
- Observe the gait to detect any problem with balance.
- Observe for wavering when arising from a supine or seated position that might indicate dizziness or equilibrium problems.
- Observe for signs of bruising on the body from falls that may indicate problems with balance.
- Observe whether the person speaks in a voice that is louder than necessary.
- Observe whether facial expression indicates difficulty in understanding what is being said.
- Determine whether responses to statements are inappropriate.

Note: Someone qualified and experienced in using an otoscope should inspect the auditory meatus and the tympanic membrane.

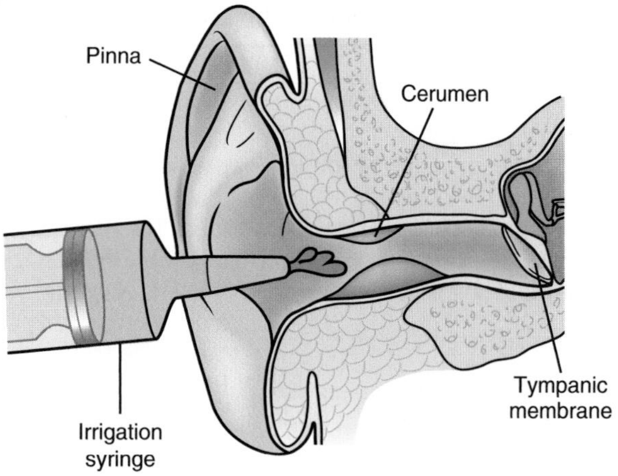

Fig. 26.5 Irrigating the external ear canal. Warm water is used to remove cerumen and debris from the canal. Aim the stream of water above or below the impaction to allow back pressure to push it out rather than farther down the canal.

The ears of older adults in long-term care facilities should be checked with an otoscope at regular intervals for cerumen. Many long-term care residents have a correctable hearing loss related to impacted cerumen. Cerumen can be removed by using cerumen softener drops and then irrigating the external ear canal (Fig. 26.5).

◆ NURSING DIAGNOSIS AND PLANNING

Problem statements or nursing diagnoses are chosen by considering the assessment data (Table 26.3). General goals for a patient with problems of the ear or hearing are:

- Promote knowledge to protect hearing
- Prevent infection and injury
- Promote effective communication
- Promote coping with hearing loss

Expected outcomes are written for each problem statement chosen for the patient's care plan. The outcomes should be written in collaboration with the patient and other health team members. In addition to the nurse and health care provider, an audiologist, hearing aid specialist, and speech therapist may be involved in the patient's care. Both long- and short-term goals for the patient should be considered.

When a patient is severely hearing impaired, communication with the patient for treatments and activities of daily living may take longer than with patients who hear normally. Take this into consideration when creating your daily work plan. If the patient does not have adequate aids for hearing, devise an acceptable method of two-way communication with the patient.

◆ IMPLEMENTATION

Interventions for patients with a hearing or balance problem are aimed at patient education, treatment of infection, preoperative and postoperative care and instructions, measures for communication (Box 26.3), and referral to resources. The hearing aid must be cared for properly (Box 26.4).

Box 26.3 Communicating With a Person Who Is Hearing Impaired

- If the person uses a hearing aid, encourage its use and see that it is situated, turned on, and adjusted before beginning speaking.
- Be certain you have the person's attention before speaking.
- Sit facing the person with the light on your face rather than from behind you.
- Ask permission to turn down the volume of or turn off the television or radio.
- The best distance for speaking to a hearing-impaired person is 2½ to 4 feet. Place yourself on eye level with the person. Do not speak directly into the person's ear because this prevents the person from obtaining visual cues while you are speaking.
- Do not smile, chew gum, or cover your mouth while speaking.
- Use short, simple sentences. If the patient does not appear to understand or responds inappropriately, state the message again using different words. Try to limit each sentence to one subject and one verb.
- Give the person time to respond to questions.
- Ask for oral or written feedback to make certain your message is understood.
- Avoid using the intercom system because it may distort sound.

Instillation of Ear Medication

Ear drops may be prescribed to dissolve cerumen, relieve pain, or combat infection in the auditory meatus (Box 26.5). The patient should be positioned in a supine lateral position so that the affected ear is uppermost. The medication should be at room temperature. Cold ear drops may cause discomfort or dizziness. For adults and children 3 years of age and older, the ear canal is straightened by drawing the pinna upward and toward the back of the head (Fig. 26.6). For a child younger than 3 years, the pinna is pulled down and back.

Communicating With a Patient Who Is Hearing Impaired

A patient who is hearing impaired has unique problems of communication when in the hospital or long-term care facility. If they cannot hear well and misunderstand or misinterpret the voices and sounds in the unfamiliar surroundings, they are likely to be frustrated, fearful, and anxious. Unless a special effort is made to have frequent contact with the patient, social isolation may occur.

When speaking to a patient who is hearing impaired, sit at eye level facing the patient. Gain eye contact and speak slowly and enunciate clearly. When trying to communicate with a person who is hearing impaired,

Table 26.3 Common Problem Statements, Expected Outcomes, and Nursing Interventions for Patients With Ear Disorders

PROBLEM STATEMENTS	GOALS/EXPECTED OUTCOMES	NURSING INTERVENTIONS
Insufficient knowledge about preventing hearing loss	Patient will verbalize ways to prevent further hearing loss. Patient will be free of ear infection within 10 days.	If cerumen is obstructing the auditory canal, irrigate as ordered; warm the irrigation solution to body temperature. If infection is present, instruct regarding antibiotic medication and encourage to take entire prescription. Instruct in use of hearing aid if one is prescribed. Advise of ways to prevent further hearing loss: avoid loud noise or wear ear protectors; seek treatment immediately for signs of ear infection.
Pain due to ear inflammation	Pain will be controlled with analgesia within 8 h. Pain will be resolved within 7 days.	Administer analgesics as ordered as needed. Warm analgesic ear drops to room temperature before administration. Have patient rest head on heating pad turned on "low" setting if this seems to decrease pain.
Altered communication ability due to hearing loss	Patient will assist in choice of methods to improve ability to communicate. Patient will try hearing aid for 2 wk if there is an indication that this device would help hearing.	Plan with patient the best way to communicate so that instructions and information are comprehended; explore tone of voice, level of volume, distance from patient when speaking, writing out communication, etc. Establish a routine procedure to confirm patient's understanding. Refer for evaluation by audiologist. Encourage daily use of hearing aid if one is prescribed. Explain that time and adjustments are necessary to obtain the optimum result. Give praise for efforts to use hearing aid.
Impaired safety or inability to perform well at work because of hearing loss	Patient will explore methods of maintaining safety within 2 wk. Patient will verbalize ways in which assisted hearing devices might help with performance in the work environment.	Encourage verbalization of fears. Use means to enhance communication. Advise of assisted hearing devices, hearing aids, and availability of "hearing ear" dogs. Introduce means of learning alternative communication methods, such as sign language and speech reading. Explore methods of enhancing attention to visual cues of dangers in the environment (e.g., close attention to signal lights or observing others at street crossings). Discuss problems of communication in social settings and explore possible solutions (e.g., masking devices for use in crowds, interacting with only one or two people at a time, avoiding noisy restaurants, or using hearing aid).
Potential for injury due to impaired equilibrium	Patient will verbalize methods to ensure safe ambulation within 3 days. Patient will not experience a fall or injury.	Administer medication for vertigo as ordered. Encourage a low-sodium diet. Instruct to change positions very slowly. Encourage to hold on to something solid or to someone when rising from a sitting to a standing position. If vertigo is present, instruct to not ambulate without assistance. Teach or reinforce vestibular/balance exercises as prescribed. Assist to identify any aura (presence of symptoms that precede an attack). Instruct to lie down and keep the eyes open and focused straight ahead when experiencing vertigo.
Altered self-care ability	Patient will verbalize ways to enhance safe self-care within 2 wk.	Describe measures to assist the person to adapt; refer to support groups and sources for information. Refer to community agencies and resources for the hearing impaired.
Potential for social isolation due to difficulty in communicating	Patient will establish an adequate social network within 2 mo.	Assist patient to consider possibilities for social contact despite hearing problems. Help patient obtain a telephone for hearing-impaired people. Encourage the use of email, texting, and other social media for contact with friends and family and social interaction with others.

remember that attempts to answer questions without fully understanding what is asked may occur. Past experience has taught many people with hearing loss that asking for repetition of questions irritates people and causes them to think the person is stupid. **For this reason, many people who cannot hear well commonly smile and say yes when such an answer is either incorrect or inappropriate.** Another problem is that the individual may fill in parts of sentences with similar-sounding words. For example, the words "Knott's Berry Farm" may be interpreted as "not very far." Some guidelines to help patients who are hearing impaired and improve nurses' ability to communicate are given in Box 26.3.

Box 26.4 Caring for a Hearing Aid

When a hearing aid does not work:

- Check that the switch is on.
- Examine the ear mold for attached wax or dirt; clean the sound hole.
- Check the battery to see that it is inserted correctly.
- Check the connection between the ear mold and the receiver.
- Replace the battery. Batteries last an average of 3 to 7 days depending on the type of aid.
- Check placement of the ear mold in the ear; it should fit snugly.
- Adjust the volume.
- If all else fails, take the hearing aid to an authorized service center for repair.

To clean the hearing aid:

- Turn the hearing aid off.
- If removable, wash the ear mold with mild soap and warm water; do not submerge in water.
- Use tools provided with the device to gently cleanse the opening or short tube that fits into the ear. Do not use toothpicks, as they can break off and lodge in the aid.
- Dry the ear mold completely before turning on the aid or before reattaching it to the hearing aid (if it is separate).

Think Critically

What three techniques of communication with a patient who is hearing impaired do you think would be the most helpful?

Box 26.5 Instilling Otic Medication

- Follow the "Six Rights" of medication administration.
- Read the order carefully to determine which ear is to receive the medication.
- Position the patient supine and in the lateral position so that the affected ear is uppermost.
- Draw medication into the medicine dropper by depressing the bulb and letting it go.
- Straighten the ear canal by drawing the pinna upward and toward the back of the head. For children younger than 3 years, draw the earlobe slightly down and back.
- Insert the tip of the medicine dropper into the external ear canal and depress the bulb to dispense the medication. Withdraw the dropper.
- Place cotton in the external meatus if ordered.
- Have the patient remain in the lateral position for 5 to 10 minutes.

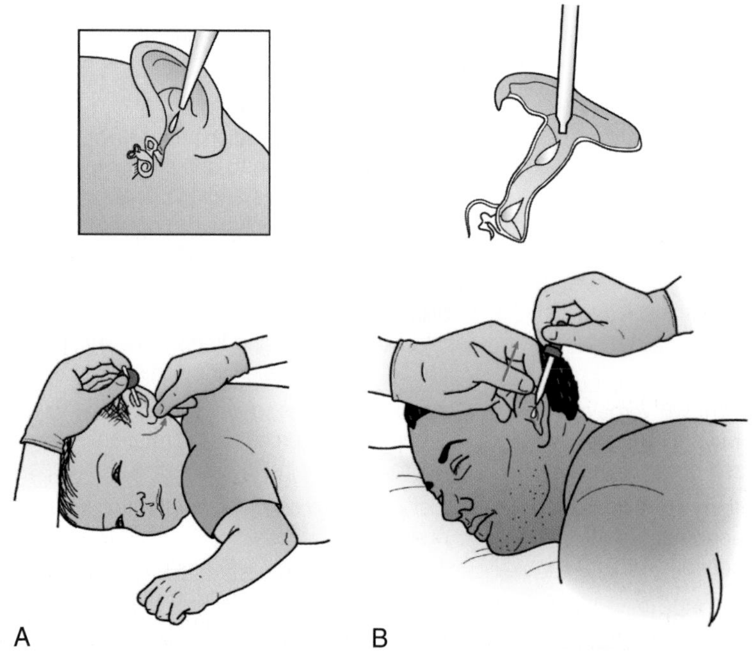

Fig. 26.6 Administering eardrops. **A**, Pull the lower earlobe downward and back for children who are less than 3 years old. **B**, Pull the upper earlobe upward and back for patients who are more than 3 years old. (From Willihnganz MJ, Gurevitz SL, Clayton BD: *Clayton's basic pharmacology for nurses,* ed 18, St. Louis, 2020, Elsevier.)

A note should be placed over the terminal on the central station intercom system that designates the room of a patient who is hearing impaired. This serves to remind the person answering the light to go to the patient's room rather than try to talk over the intercom system.

◆ EVALUATION

Evaluation involves reassessment to determine whether the expected outcomes are being met. Determining whether hearing has improved is the criterion by which effectiveness of treatment is evaluated. Improvement is verified by audiometry. Fading or resolution of dizziness and vertigo indicate that actions and treatments for these problems have been effective. Resolution of infection is determined by the appearance of the eardrum, absence of pain, and normal temperature. Determination of the effectiveness of communication will evaluate whether communication strategies were successful.

COMMON PROBLEMS OF PATIENTS WITH EAR DISORDERS

HEARING IMPAIRMENT

Hearing impairment ranges from difficulty in hearing certain ranges of tones or in understanding certain words to total deafness. Persons with sensorineural hearing loss typically have more difficulty hearing high-pitched tones than low-pitched ones; thus they commonly can understand the speech of men better than that of women. Another characteristic of sensorineural hearing loss is difficulty hearing softly spoken and poorly enunciated words. Speaking slightly louder to a person with sensorineural hearing loss may help, but it is especially important to speak slowly and clearly and to face the person when communicating with her. Because people with sensorineural hearing loss do not hear their own voices as well as a person with normal hearing, they tend to speak louder than necessary.

Assignment Considerations

Caring for a Patient Who Is Hearing Impaired

When assigning tasks for a patient who is hearing impaired to unlicensed assistive personnel (UAP) and certified nursing assistants (CNAs), remind them how to communicate effectively with the patient: face the patient and obtain their attention before speaking, then speak slowly and enunciate clearly in a normal voice. If the patient wears a hearing aid, it should be in the ear, and the patient should be reminded to turn it on before communication begins.

Hearing aids help some people with sensorineural hearing loss. Aids designed to amplify some pitches and block out others that do not need amplification are most helpful. Hearing aids are not always the answer to a problem of hearing loss, and for some people the most effective therapy is focused on rehabilitation to facilitate acceptance of the loss and learning new ways to communicate despite some degree of deafness. Most hearing aid professionals and companies will offer a 30-day money-back guarantee on any hearing aid so that the patient can try it. Most hearing aids function by air conduction. Other devices include bone conduction, cochlear implants, middle ear implants, and personal sound amplification products.

Many people have a combination of two or more types of hearing impairment. Often there is a combination of sensorineural and conductive loss. The appropriate device should be chosen based on the type of hearing loss present.

Clinical Cues

When a patient can benefit from a hearing aid, then the earlier it is obtained and used, the better the brain will adjust and the better the quality that can be achieved. Studies have shown improvement in cognition and decreased risk for falls, dementia, hospitalization, and depression with early use of technology to improve hearing (Hearing Industries Association, 2015).

Central hearing loss occurs in the brain as a result of a pathologic condition above the junction of cranial nerve VIII and the brainstem. Central hearing loss can result from a problem of transmission of stimuli in the brain, an inability to decode and sort signals received from one or both ears, or a failure in the transmission of sounds from one hemisphere of the brain to the other. Since the condition involves the processing of the sounds and not the acquisition of sounds, it is classified as a learning disability rather than a hearing disorder. Causes include brain tumors, vascular changes that suddenly deprive the middle ear of its blood supply, and cerebrovascular accidents.

Think Critically

How would you work with a patient who is hearing impaired and is a candidate for a hearing aid but adamantly refuses to consider trying one?

Dizziness and Vertigo

The sense of balance and equilibrium is governed by the vestibular system in the inner ear. Increases in fluid pressure in the inner ear, inflammations, and vascular disorders that interrupt blood supply to the cochlea can produce dizziness, loss of balance, and nausea and vomiting. Benign paroxysmal positional vertigo (BPPV) is the most common cause of vertigo and occurs as a result of small calcium crystals in the inner ear. Vertigo symptoms can range from mildly annoying to completely incapacitating and should always be assessed whenever a person has an ear disorder and loss of hearing. Ménière disease and labyrinthitis also cause vertigo.

A patient who experiences dizziness and positional vertigo should be cautioned to avoid suddenly turning the head or making other movements that aggravate the vertigo. They should be told to call for assistance whenever they need to move from the bed or chair. When helping the patient to their feet, move slowly and give them time to stand for a moment before beginning to walk. **Typically, patients with this kind of vertigo feel that the room is spinning around during an attack, and any motion exacerbates the sensation.** While the patient is having an attack of vertigo, they should lie in bed and remain as motionless as possible. Stabilizing the head with a pillow on either side may encourage immobility. Attacks can last from a few minutes to hours.

Medications to reduce motion sickness and nausea should be given precisely as prescribed. These are usually given every 3 to 4 hours or on a preventive basis *before* the patient's symptoms become severe. A series of head movements that can be done at home called *Epley maneuver, Brandt-Daroff exercise, Foster maneuver,* or *Semont maneuver* can be helpful in moving the calcium crystals causing BPPV.

When increased fluid pressure in the inner ear is suspected as the cause of dizziness, the health care provider may order a low-sodium diet and limit fluid intake. Patients with recurrent attacks of vertigo are encouraged to stop smoking if they are habitual tobacco smokers. Tobacco is vasoconstrictive and can affect the blood supply to the inner ear and nerves. Cardiac dysrhythmias can cause dizziness and must first be ruled out as a cause of the symptoms.

Stress may affect the frequency of attacks of vertigo in patients with inner ear disorders. Teaching the patient effective coping mechanisms to handle stress or adding rest periods to the work schedule may be helpful.

Tinnitus

Ringing, buzzing, or other continuous noise in the ear *(tinnitus)* can be mildly annoying or so severe that it interferes with activities of daily living and prevents the patient from getting sufficient sleep and rest. Tinnitus can be intermittent or continuous. Continuous cases are usually caused by an underlying medical problem. Common causes of tinnitus include **presbycusis** (hearing loss associated with aging), constant exposure to loud environmental noise, inflammation and infection in the ear, otosclerosis, Ménière disease, and labyrinthitis. Systemic disorders such as hypertension and other cardiovascular disorders, neurologic disease (including head injury), and hyperthyroidism and hypothyroidism also can cause ringing in the ears. **Tinnitus may be one of the first symptoms produced by an ototoxic drug.** Symptoms of tinnitus are subjective, and diagnosis is by patient history.

Medical treatment begins with efforts to determine the underlying cause and treat it. When the cause cannot be found, symptomatic relief is tried. The goal of treatment is to lessen the impact rather than eliminate the problem. However, some cases of intractable tinnitus resist all modes of conventional therapy. Identifying conditions that exacerbate tinnitus and providing treatment can indirectly help. Less traditional measures that have varying degrees of success include biofeedback training and "masking." Some patients have found drug therapies to be helpful. Carbamazepine shows benefit for those with tapping pulsatile tinnitus. Benzodiazepines, such as diazepam (Valium) or chlordiazepoxide (Librium), seem to help some people (Dinces, 2018).

> **Clinical Cues**
>
> Because of the overload of sensory input to the brain, a patient with tinnitus will become more fatigued than others when in a noisy location such as a social gathering or a restaurant. Family and friends should be informed of this situation.

Biofeedback training is especially helpful in those cases in which emotional stress and anxiety are believed to be the underlying causes of tinnitus. Through visual or auditory signals, the person learns to relax and exert some degree of control over the autonomic nervous system. This can lower blood pressure and pulse rate and relax muscles that are very tense.

Masking simply provides a low-level noise to block out, or "mask," the head noise heard by the person complaining of tinnitus. Some examples include playing soft music or a tape of sounds of nature, such as a waterfall, while the person is resting or sleeping; providing "white noise" in the working environment; using a hearing aid to amplify sound from the outside and overcome head noise; and wearing a special tinnitus instrument, which is a combination hearing aid and tinnitus masker for people who have both hearing loss and tinnitus. The therapeutic effect of masking is highly individualized. Some people find instant relief, some have partial abatement of the head noise, and some do not benefit from attempts to mask the sounds of tinnitus. Earplugs or ear protection should be worn when noise exposure cannot be avoided.

REHABILITATION FOR HEARING LOSS

Specific measures to rehabilitate a patient with hearing loss depend on the age and aptitude of the patient. Adults who have acquired the skills of speech and language before their loss of hearing occurred are better able to pick up language cues and understand what is being said to them, and therefore should have fewer problems with communication by language.

Lip-Reading (Speech Reading)

Instruction in reading lips is one mode of therapy for patients who are hearing impaired, but it is not a remedy for all difficulties. Only about 60% of the sounds in the English language can be identified by watching the lips. Most experienced lip-readers do not catch more than half of the words spoken to them. Communication by lip-reading is enhanced by other nonverbal clues, such as facial expressions and hand gestures. Learning to lip-read is difficult. It requires at least average intelligence, exceptional language skills, excellent eyesight, and much persistence and patience.

Sign Language

Many people who are deaf learn to communicate with sign language. American Sign Language (ASL) is the third most commonly used language in the United States. There are online dictionaries for ASL and several websites that provide tutorials. Most major hospitals have someone on staff who can act as an interpreter for ASL.

Hearing Aids

An evaluation by a reputable audiologist can lead to a prescription for a hearing aid designed to provide the best possible improvement of hearing. Hearing aids can improve hearing for various types of hearing loss. Hearing aids do not restore normal hearing but improve hearing. For people who do not have a defect in the middle ear, a hearing aid can transmit amplified sound from the receiver through the eardrum to the inner ear. This is accomplished by amplifying sound waves transmitted by air conduction and bone conduction. There are many types of hearing aids on the market. Newer digital types can amplify the tones needed while masking other levels of noise. It takes time to adapt to the use of a hearing aid, and the audiologist must make repeated adjustments to the device to achieve optimum function.

The design of a hearing aid varies. Some are worn in the ear, others are worn behind the ear, and still others are built into the frame of eyeglasses. Persons with binaural hearing loss (both ears are affected) must wear a hearing aid in each ear. Regardless of the type of hearing aid, it will have a microphone, an amplifier, a receiver, and a battery (Fig. 26.7).

The hearing aid should not be handled roughly or dropped. The ear mold, if removable, can be cleaned

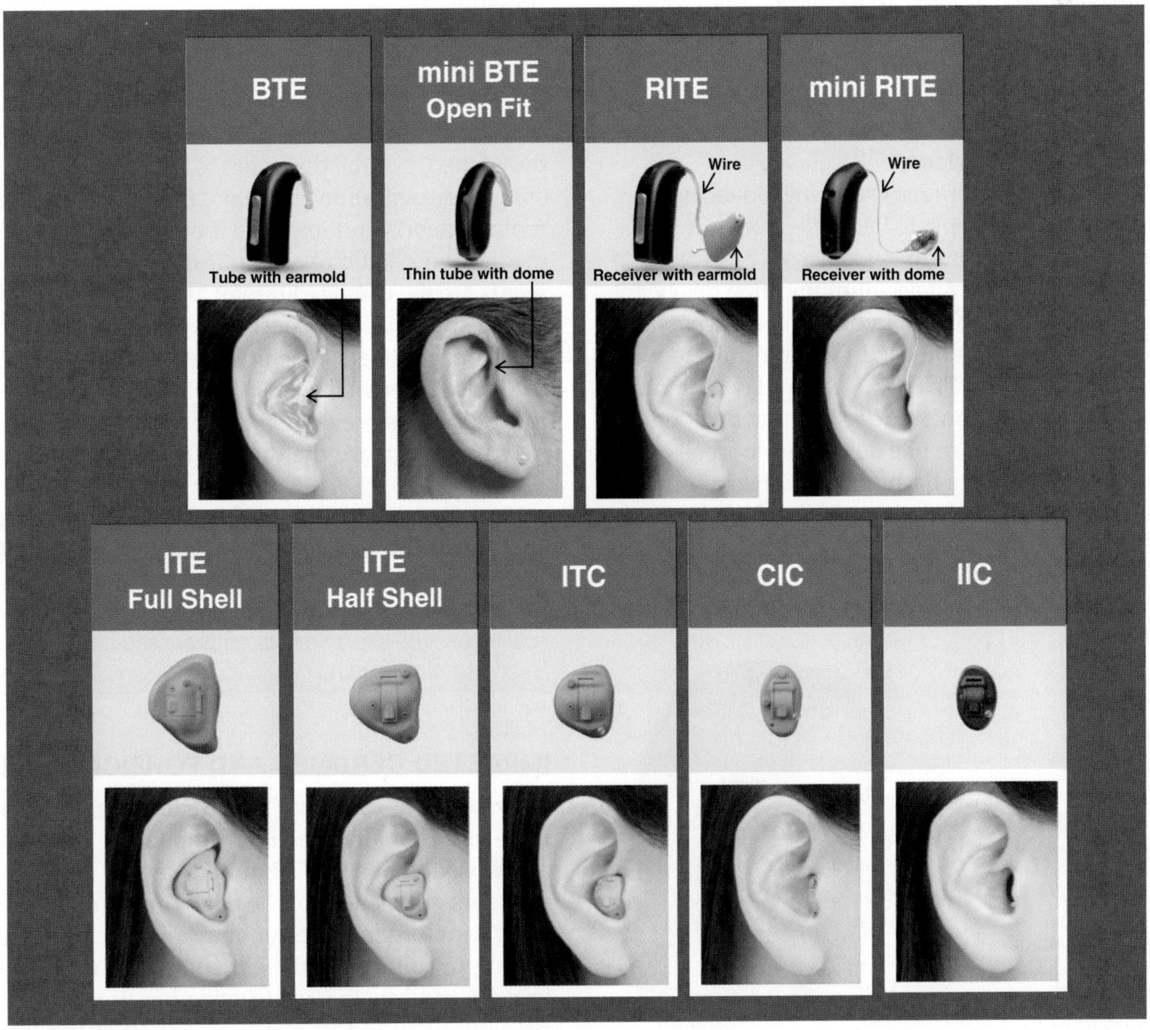

Fig. 26.7 Types of hearing aids. *BTE*, Behind-the-ear style; *CIC*, completely-in-the-canal style; *IIC*, invisible-in-the-canal style; *ITC*, in-the-canal style; *ITE*, in-the-ear style; *RITE*, receiver-in-the-ear style (also known as RIC, receiver-in-the-canal). (With permission by Oticon, Inc., Somerset, N.J. In Cifu DX, Lew HL, Oh-Park M: *Geriatric rehabilitation*, St. Louis, 2019, Elsevier.)

with soap and water, but the other parts of the aid should not get wet (see Box 26.4). Hair spray can damage the microphone of a hearing aid. Regular servicing by a dealer can keep the aid in good working order. When an incapacitated patient has a hearing aid, you are responsible for the security of the hearing aid.

Implantable middle-ear devices have become available for those who have limited success with conventional hearing aids and have severe sensorineural hearing loss (Weber, 2018). These are indicated for adults 18 years or older.

Cochlear Implant

Cochlear implants are available for patients who have moderate to severe bilateral or unilateral sensorineural hearing loss. The device is a small computer that changes spoken words into electrical impulses that are transmitted via an implanted coil to the nerve endings in the cochlea. Success with the surgical implant varies considerably from one person to the next (Fig. 26.8). Bone hearing devices and semi-implanted devices are also available. A speech therapist works with the patient once the cochlear implant is in place. The sounds transmitted are electronic and sound mechanical, but most patients adapt within 1 to 2 months. (See the Cochlear Implant section later in this chapter.)

Hearing Assistive Devices

Many devices on the market use hearing aid technology. These devices assist people to hear telephone conversations, television, and sound systems, such as those in church or at the theater. A telecommunication device for the deaf (TDD) is available. It is a combination typewriter and telephone, and can be used to communicate with someone else who has a TDD or to call a relay center that then communicates the message to the intended person. There are alarm clocks, smoke detectors, doorbells, and telephones that activate a flashing light when a sound is produced. "Hearing ear" dogs are trained to alert their owners to particular sounds and to keep their owners safe when around traffic.

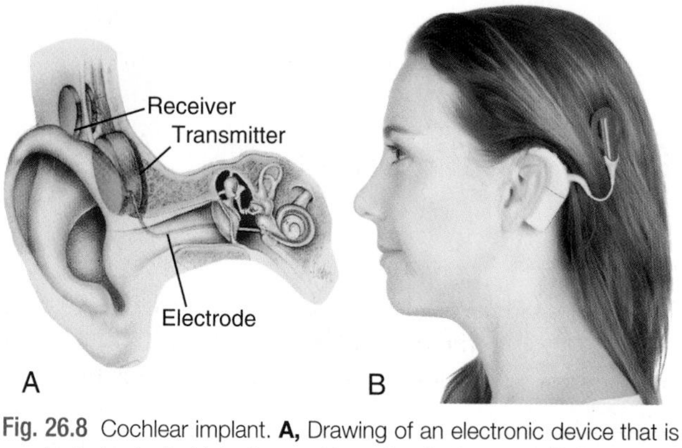

Fig. 26.8 Cochlear implant. **A,** Drawing of an electronic device that is surgically implanted into the cochlea of a deaf person. **B,** Young girl with a cochlear implant. (From Leonard PC: *Quick and easy medical terminology*, ed 9, St. Louis, 2020, Elsevier.)

COMMON DISORDERS OF THE EAR

EXTERNAL OTITIS

Etiology and Pathophysiology

Infection of the external ear is common and often occurs in swimmers. It is caused by either bacterial or fungal pathogens, with staphylococci being the most common cause. Other infections of the skin may affect the external ear (see Chapter 43). A moist environment or disruption of the skin from trauma provides a place for pathogens to grow. Cerumen protects the skin layers, and if too little is being produced or if it is washed away as in swimmers, the skin is exposed to infection. If too much cerumen is present, there can be retention of water and debris, which also increases the chance of infection.

Signs and Symptoms

Pain occurs with the infection. Itchiness of the ear canal and discharge of liquid or pus may occur. If swelling occurs in the ear canal, hearing may be impaired because sound waves cannot reach the tympanic membrane. The swelling may produce a feeling of ear fullness or pressure.

Diagnosis, Treatment, and Nursing Management

Redness is evident on otoscopic examination, and there may be drainage. A culture of the drainage may be performed, but the diagnosis is usually made based on clinical presentation. The ear canal may be irrigated to remove debris and improve the effectiveness of topical medications. Antibiotic or antifungal ear drops and ointments are the usual treatment. Drying agents or steroids may also be used. A severe infection may require oral antibiotics as well. Teaching patients to use drops of a drying solution in the ears after they have been exposed to water helps prevent external otitis. A mild analgesic may help decrease the discomfort during healing.

Clinical Cues

In nonswimmers with recurrent otitis externa, blood glucose testing should be done to see if undiagnosed diabetes is a contributing cause. Immunocompromised patients are more prone to otitis externa.

IMPACTED CERUMEN AND FOREIGN BODIES

Normally the ear canal is self-cleaning, but cerumen may occasionally become impacted. Impaction is diagnosed when the cerumen causes symptoms or prevents assessment of the ear. Foreign objects such as insects or organic matter may obstruct the canal. A feeling of fullness in the ear combined with a hearing loss can indicate that obstruction has blocked the canal, preventing sound waves from reaching the tympanic membrane. If otoscopic examination reveals hardened cerumen blocking the canal, it is removed by one of several methods. Wax softening drops may be used and work over hours to days. If the obstruction becomes complete or if the drops are ineffective, irrigation of the canal may be performed to remove it (see Fig. 26.5). Extreme caution must be used when irrigating so as not to damage the delicate inner ear structures. Visualization with an operating microscope provides depth perception to safely use suction or other instruments to remove the cerumen.

> **Older Adult Care Points**
>
> With increased age, the auditory canal narrows, and the hairs become coarser and stiffer. The cerumen glands atrophy, causing cerumen to be drier. This combination may result in impaction of cerumen that causes a conductive hearing loss and tinnitus. Older adults with this problem should be taught to use cerumen softening drops and an ear syringe to wash out the cerumen periodically. Those who are unable to cleanse the ears themselves should have regular ear checks performed by their health care provider.

OTITIS MEDIA

Etiology

This condition is an inflammation of the middle ear caused by various types of bacteria or viruses. Although it is mostly seen in infants and young children, it does occur in adults. It results in the accumulation of fluid behind the eardrum and some temporary impairment of hearing.

Pathophysiology

The inflammation and infection of otitis media usually follows an upper respiratory tract infection (URI) or trauma to the ear. It may be viral or bacterial in origin. Obstruction of the eustachian tube usually precedes the disorder and is caused by inflammation and swelling from URI or allergy. Middle ear inflammation occurs when the eustachian tube that usually drains that area becomes blocked. The obstruction changes the pressure within the middle ear due to retained fluid. The fluid provides an environment for *Streptococcus pneumoniae, Haemophilus influenzae,* or *Streptococcus pyogenes,* the most common bacteria associated with otitis media.

When the infection is sudden in onset and of short duration, it is called *acute otitis media.* The eardrum is retracted inward because of negative pressure from a closed eustachian tube. The pain can be severe. Otitis media sometimes is accompanied by an allergy and may be aggravated by enlarged adenoids. When the infection is repeated, often causing perforation of the eardrum and drainage, it is called *chronic otitis media.*

Fluid buildup in the middle ear without signs of inflammation or infection is called otitis media with effusion or *serous otitis media.*

Signs, Symptoms, and Diagnosis

Symptoms may be mild and may consist only of a feeling of fullness in the ear and evidence of impaired hearing and tinnitus. There may be pain in the infected ear. High fever, facial paralysis, or severe pain behind the ear are indications of unusual complications.

Diagnosis of otitis media is based on otoscopic examination showing redness and bulging of the eardrum, or pus behind the eardrum. Perforation may occur with drainage of the pus; this relief in pressure usually resolves the pain and pressure sensations.

Treatment

There is great controversy about using antimicrobials for otitis media because so many strains of pathogens are becoming antimicrobial resistant. If there is otitis media with fluid behind the eardrum and no acute systemic or local evidence of severe infection, antimicrobials are withheld. The condition is treated conservatively with antihistamines and decongestants. One quarter of otitis media infections are viral and resolve without treatment. Most of the studies on treatment protocols have been done on children. Adults with clinical evidence of infection are usually started on antibacterial medications to prevent complications such as mastoiditis, facial paralysis, and labyrinthitis. Severe complications include brain abscesses or otic meningitis.

For repeated episodes of otitis with fluid, or when the fluid will not resorb, a **myringotomy** (incision into the eardrum) is done, and a ventilating tube is inserted to drain the excess fluid in the middle ear and to equalize pressure while the eustachian tube is blocked. The tympanic membrane is anesthetized locally. The procedure is painless and takes about 15 minutes. The incision heals within 24 to 72 hours unless a tube is placed in the opening. Tubes remain in place for 6 to 18 months before they are expelled naturally. The hole then heals. If allergy is believed to be responsible for the fluid buildup, antihistamines are prescribed. Dilation of the eustachian tube with a balloon ("tuboplasty") has been tried with good results. There is limited experience with the procedure, and there are no long-term studies indicating outcome.

Acute otitis media occurs when pus-producing bacteria infect the middle ear. Treatment consists of systemic therapy with antibiotics for at least 5 to 7 days, topical therapy with ear drops, and oral analgesics to reduce pain and fever. With repeated episodes, **tympanoplasty** to repair a ruptured eardrum and damaged ossicles and, sometimes, mastoidectomy may be needed to eliminate all sources of infection and prevent further degeneration of bone.

Nursing Management

Keeping the patient comfortable at home, encouraging compliance with the medication regimen, and requesting return for an examination when medication is finished are usual nursing actions. Show a family member how to instill ear drops properly. Temperature should be taken each day during the course of acute otitis media to track improvement.

Infections in the middle ear always have the potential to spread to the meninges, causing meningitis, or to the mastoid bone, causing mastoiditis. Patients and families should be taught the signs and symptoms to watch for indicating that a more serious condition has developed. Although otitis media is a fairly common occurrence, it should always be treated immediately.

LABYRINTHITIS

Etiology and Pathophysiology

Labyrinthitis is an inflammation involving the vestibular portion of the labyrinth in the inner ear. Other terms for the condition include vestibular neuritis, vestibular neuronitis, neurolabyrinthitis, and acute peripheral vestibulopathy. It most commonly occurs from a viral respiratory infection but can be a complication of bacterial meningitis or chronic otitis media.

Signs, Symptoms, and Diagnosis

The symptoms include rapid onset of severe dizziness (vertigo) with nausea and vomiting and an unsteady gait. Nystagmus (abnormal jerking movements of the eyes) are a symptom used in diagnosis. Sensorineural hearing loss in the affected ear, or tinnitus, may also be present. Diagnosis is made from the symptoms and by ruling out tumor or other disease.

Treatment and Nursing Management

Treatment is aimed at treating the primary disease and controlling symptoms. Symptoms of vertigo and its associated nausea and vomiting are managed with antiemetics, antihistamines, and anticholinergics. Intravenous (IV) or transdermal (when available) routes are used instead of oral while nausea and vomiting are present.

Initially the patient is kept on bed rest to prevent falls and injury. The family is cautioned not to let the patient get out of bed without assistance. Nursing management consists of safety measures to prevent falling and instructions about the medications. Attention to hydration is important if the patient is nauseated to the point of repeated vomiting. Once symptoms are controlled, a vestibular rehabilitation program may be implemented to hasten long-term recovery of balance (Furman, 2018).

MÉNIÈRE DISEASE (MÉNIÈRE SYNDROME)

Etiology and Pathophysiology

The exact cause is unknown and is considered idiopathic, but Ménière disease occurs most commonly in females. It has been found in all age groups but is most common in those 40 to 60 years old. There is current speculation that there might be a relationship between migraine headache and Ménière disease (Moskowitz, 2018). If the symptoms occur as a result of a disease process, the condition is called Ménière syndrome.

An increase of endolymph within the spaces of the labyrinth (endolymphatic hydrops), with swelling and congestion of the mucous membranes of the cochlea, occurs. Resultant pressure in the labyrinth of the inner ear results in permanent damage to both the cochlear and the vestibular structures. The disorder is usually unilateral. Several theories have been offered as to the mechanism of the fluid buildup. Blockage of the endolymphatic duct, narrowing of the duct, genetic predisposition, viral infection, or vascular abnormality are all being investigated as possible causes. Without knowing a cause, treatment is symptomatic rather than preventative or curative.

Signs, Symptoms, and Diagnosis

The symptoms include intermittent attacks of dizziness, ringing in the ear (tinnitus), and unilateral sensorineural hearing loss. Poor balance makes walking difficult or impossible. **Any sudden movement of the head or eyes during an attack usually produces severe nausea and vomiting.** There is no specific test diagnostic for Ménière disease. The American Academy of Otolaryngology—Head and Neck Surgery (AAO-HNS) has proposed the following diagnostic criteria: two spontaneous episodes of vertigo lasting at least 20 minutes, confirmation of sensorineural hearing loss by testing (audiometry), and tinnitus and/or a reported sensation of fullness in the ear. A *caloric test* (electronystagmogram [ENG]) may be performed, which involves instilling very warm or cold fluid into the auditory canal. In a patient with Ménière disease, ENG testing is a very sensitive indicator of inner balance dysfunction. Magnetic resonance imaging (MRI) will be used to rule out central nervous system causes of the symptoms.

? Think Critically

How would you check for nystagmus when assessing a patient who has vertigo?

Treatment

Treatment of Ménière disease focuses on relieving symptoms; there is no cure for this condition, although the disorder does disappear spontaneously in some cases. For an acute attack, IV diazepam (Valium) provides vestibular suppression and nausea control. To prevent attacks, medical therapy is targeted to the causative disease or to dietary and environmental triggers. To control edema and reduce pressure in the inner ear, the patient may be placed on a low-sodium diet, their fluid intake may be restricted, and diuretics may be ordered. Loop diuretics have known ototoxicity properties and should be used with caution. Antiemetics act as vestibulosuppressants and are given to help control the vertigo and nausea. Antihistamines such as dimenhydrinate (Dramamine) and meclizine (Antivert) also act as vestibulosuppressants and help control dizziness. They should be used only for vertigo attacks and should not be taken routinely.

The patient is kept quiet and in bed to avoid aggravating symptoms. The patient may be very irritable and withdrawn, and may refuse to eat or drink because of fear of vomiting. Care should be taken to avoid increasing irritation by jarring the bed, turning on bright overhead lights, or making loud noises.

If attacks continue and are very severe despite medical treatment, the endolymph sac from the inner ear can be removed with microsurgical techniques, but this is reserved for medical treatment failures. When hearing loss is total on the affected side, surgical destruction of cranial nerve VIII may resolve the symptoms. Although this produces permanent deafness in the affected ear, the severe attacks are eliminated. In most persistent cases of Ménière disease, the patient will eventually suffer a serious or even total loss of hearing regardless of the treatment used.

For those with dizziness and unsteadiness who do not wish to undergo surgery, vestibular rehabilitation therapy, a home-based exercise, may decrease the dizziness and balance problems resulting from inner ear damage. A positive pressure device that is used at home applies pressure to the middle ear to improve fluid exchange. Studies have reported mixed results, but some patients have found it effective in decreasing vertigo symptoms (Moskowitz, 2018).

? Think Critically

What would you teach a patient with Ménière disease about a low-sodium diet?

Nursing Management

Encourage patients who use nicotine products to quit because nicotine constricts blood vessels and decreases inner ear circulation. If allergy seems to be a factor in the onset of attacks, encourage consultation with an allergist to obtain control of allergens. Decreasing stress is a helpful intervention when there has been a pattern of attacks after particularly stressful times in the patient's life. Dietary changes to limit caffeine, salt, alcohol, and monosodium glutamate (MSG) have proven helpful for some patients.

ACOUSTIC NEUROMA (VESTIBULAR SCHWANNOMA)

An acoustic neuroma is a rare benign tumor on cranial nerve VIII that is usually unilateral. It occurs in 1 in 100,000 people. Symptoms are gradual hearing loss and tinnitus. Unsteady gait, facial numbness, vertigo, and taste disturbances may also be found. The tumor is slow growing, and symptoms are dependent on the structures affected by the tumor and the tumor size. Neuromas that are identified early on imaging studies, without clinical symptoms, may be watched until symptoms appear. This tumor is usually curable with surgery, without recurrence in most patients. Stereotactic (gamma knife, CyberKnife) radiotherapy may be indicated for select patients. If untreated, acoustic neuroma causes deafness. Treatment is surgical, and nursing care is much the same as for other intracranial surgeries, using measures to decrease intracranial pressure.

OTOSCLEROSIS AND HEARING LOSS

Etiology and Pathophysiology

Otosclerosis is a hereditary degeneration of bone in the inner ear. It occurs twice as often in females and begins in the late teens or early 20s. It may become worse during pregnancy. Hearing is decreased if there has been damage to the tympanic membrane (eardrum) from trauma or infection.

The sense of hearing depends in part on the vibration of very small bones of the inner ear. The *stapes,* or stirrup, is particularly important because it conducts sound waves to the fluid in the semicircular canals in the inner ear. Otosclerosis is a disease process that causes the formation of excess bone. This causes the footplate of the stapes to be fixed so that it no longer vibrates to transmit sound waves received via the tympanic membrane.

Signs, Symptoms, and Diagnosis

The patient often complains of difficulty hearing the voices of others, yet their own voice sounds unusually loud. In response to this, they may lower their voice to the point that they can scarcely be heard by others. Diagnosis is by otoscopic examination, Rinne and Weber tests, and audiogram.

Treatment

The hearing loss of otosclerosis can sometimes be corrected by using a hearing aid. Care for a hearing aid is presented in Box 26.4. Microsurgical intervention can restore air-conductive hearing by providing a new movable pathway for the sound waves. During the operation, called a *stapedectomy,* the stapes is removed and is replaced with a prosthetic device. This device may be a steel wire and fat implant, a wire and a segment of vein, or a vein graft with polyethylene tubing. In any case, the prosthesis is attached to one end of the *incus* (anvil of the middle ear) so that sound can be transmitted to the inner ear. The surgical procedure is extremely delicate and would not be possible without the dissecting binocular microscope and other modern surgical instruments that allow visualization and manipulation of the very small structures of the middle ear. Outpatient surgery with local anesthesia is typical. Hearing improvement may not occur for about 6 weeks.

Tympanoplasty reconstructs the middle ear and improves conductive hearing loss. Tympanoplasty involves the surgical reconstruction of the tympanic membrane and ossicles to restore middle-ear function. There are several types of procedures, ranging from simple closing of a tympanic membrane perforation to extensive repair of the middle-ear structures. The procedure is performed with an operating microscope via the external auditory canal or through a postauricular incision. Although performed as an outpatient procedure, tympanoplasty requires general anesthesia.

Nursing Management

Postoperative care involves keeping the patient quiet and flat in bed for 4 hours. The head is turned so that the affected ear is uppermost. When the patient is allowed to move around, they must be warned that dizziness is likely to occur, especially if the head is turned suddenly. Position changes should be accomplished slowly. Coughing and sneezing should be prevented; if unavoidable, they should be accomplished with the mouth open to decrease pressure in the ear (Nursing Care Plan 26.1). Change the cotton in the ear as needed. Drainage may continue for about a week.

COCHLEAR IMPLANT

Adults who have severe hearing loss that occurred after development of language skills and whose hearing is

Nursing Care Plan 26.1 Care of a Patient Having a Tympanoplasty

SCENARIO

Miss Cook, age 38 years, is a high school teacher who has had progressive hearing impairment as a result of recurrent otitis media of the right ear. She is admitted to outpatient surgery for tympanoplasty. During her initial assessment, the nurse found Miss Cook to be well informed about the nature of her disorder but somewhat anxious about the outcome of surgery. Her physical health status is good; her only previous hospitalization was for an appendectomy when she was 19 years old. Care is for the postoperative period.

PROBLEM STATEMENT/NURSING DIAGNOSIS

Potential for injury related to graft displacement.

SUPPORTING ASSESSMENT DATA

Objective: Tympanoplasty.

Goals/Expected Outcomes	Nursing Interventions	Selected Rationale	Evaluation
No preventable injury will occur.	Position patient side-lying on nonoperative side.	Prevents collection of fluid behind graft and reduces pressure.	Positioned on nonoperative side or back with HOB raised 30 degrees.
	Reinforce preoperative instructions to remain in bed for 4 h and avoid sudden movements, blowing nose, or sneezing.	These measures help prevent graft disruption.	Compliant with instructions.
	Check vital signs for evidence of infection bid.	Elevation in temperature may indicate beginning infection.	Temperature within normal range. No sign of infection.
	Give analgesic or sedative as ordered.	Analgesic or sedative will promote rest.	Patient resting comfortably; pain at 2/10.
	Provide quiet environment.	A quiet environment will promote rest.	Instruct patient and family to limit activities.

PROBLEM STATEMENT/NURSING DIAGNOSIS

Fall risk related to vertigo and instability.

SUPPORTING ASSESSMENT DATA

Subjective: After tympanoplasty, states she is very dizzy and nauseated.

Goals/Expected Outcomes	Nursing Interventions	Selected Rationale	Evaluation
Falls will be prevented.	Up with assistance only. Repeat explanation for safety precautions.	Helps to prevent falls.	Asking for assistance when needs to get up.
	Caution patient to change positions and turn her head very slowly.	Abrupt changes in position are likely to cause vertigo and nausea.	Compliant with instructions.
	Provide well-lighted room when ambulating.	Good lighting prevents tripping over obstacles when ambulating.	Room lighting is adequate.
	Administer medication prescribed for vertigo.	Medication can help control vertigo.	Medication for vertigo is effective.

PROBLEM STATEMENT/NURSING DIAGNOSIS

Insufficient knowledge regarding postoperative care.

Nursing Care Plan 26.1 Care of a Patient Having a Tympanoplasty—cont'd

SUPPORTING ASSESSMENT DATA

Subjective: Asks about restrictions and self-care.
Objective: Cannot verbalize knowledge of medications.

Goals/Expected Outcomes	Nursing Interventions	Selected Rationale	Evaluation
Patient will verbalize knowledge of home self-care before discharge.	Instruct to avoid loud noises and pressure changes for 6 mo, especially avoiding flying and diving.	Loud noise and pressure changes can disrupt the graft.	Instructions reviewed verbally, and printed instructions left with patient.
	Stress importance of not blowing her nose for at least 1 wk and preventing upper respiratory infection; if at all possible, protect her ear against cold; and refrain from any activity that might provoke dizziness or disturb the graft (e.g., straining at stool, bending, and heavy lifting).	Preventing pressure changes helps protect the integrity of the graft.	Provided correct feedback on postoperative precautions.
Patient will demonstrate dressing change correctly before discharge.	Teach patient how to change dressing on the external ear.	Will prepare patient for self-care.	Patient has not changed bandage yet.
	Reiterate importance of taking full course of prescribed antibiotic and reporting to surgeon at scheduled times.	Taking the full course of antibiotics correctly will help prevent infection.	Acknowledges importance of taking antibiotics as directed.
	Reassure patient that because of swelling of tissues and presence of surgical pack, it may be several weeks before she can fully evaluate effectiveness of the surgery.	Inflammation at the surgical site will cause swelling that interferes with hearing initially.	Reassurance given. States she understands that it may be a while before hearing is as good as it will get.

CRITICAL THINKING QUESTIONS

1. Why can dizziness and vertigo occur after a tympanoplasty?
2. What level of noise would be considered "too loud"?

bid, Twice daily; *HOB,* head of bed.

not improved with conventional hearing aids may be candidates for cochlear implants. The hearing loss is related to injury that has damaged the hair cell system in the organ of Corti. The hair cells are necessary for normal hearing, and hearing aids augment the function of the hair cells. The cochlear implant uses the spiral ganglion neurons for sound transmission. Implants may be contraindicated in conditions where the nerve function has been altered.

An incision is made behind the ear, and an implant is placed. Electrodes are placed into a cochleostomy and extracochlearly. The device is secured, and the incision is closed. An audiologist will work with the patient and family for the initial stimulation and mapping, which occurs 3 to 5 weeks postoperatively. For the device to work, an external sound processor that rests behind the ear is added. The sound processor captures sounds and converts them to digital code, which is transmitted to the implant under the skin. The implant converts the digital code to electronic impulses and sends them to the electrodes. The electrodes stimulate the nerve, which sends the impulses to the brain, where they are interpreted as sound. The device does not restore "normal" hearing, and a period of adjustment is needed. Current recommendations include bilateral implants for improvement in hearing during noise, directionality, and speech perception. Technologies are being developed that allow for fully implantable devices and hybrid devices that preserve some intact hearing.

Postoperatively, the dressing will be removed in 2 to 3 days, and the wound is monitored for bleeding or infection. Pain medication and oral antibiotics are given. See Postoperative Care below.

Clinical Cues

After ear surgery, glasses should be taped and positioned so that they do not rest on the incision.

NURSING CARE OF PATIENTS HAVING EAR SURGERY

Most ear surgeries are performed as outpatient procedures. Nursing care is focused on the immediate preoperative and recovery periods and on instructions for home care.

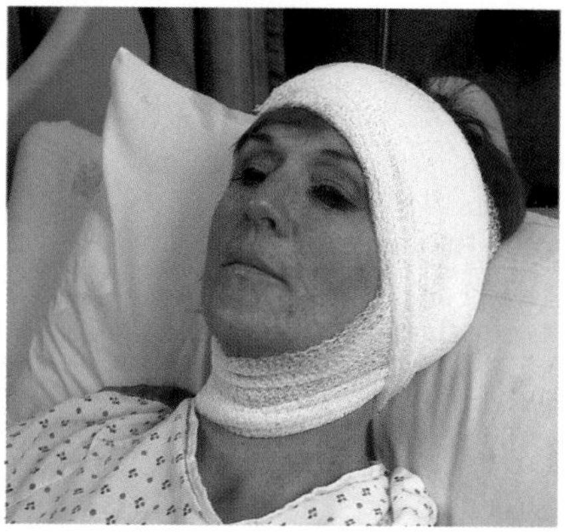

Fig. 26.9 An ear surgery dressing. The patient is positioned with the head elevated or side-lying on the unaffected side.

PREOPERATIVE CARE

Nursing care of patients during the preoperative period is routine, except for the administration of ear drops or other special medications. Male patients should be clean shaven on the morning of surgery. The external ear and surrounding skin should be thoroughly cleansed, preferably with a surgical soap. Female patients with long hair should have it braided or pinned back securely so that it will not become soiled by drainage from the ear or serve as a source of infection at the operative site.

POSTOPERATIVE CARE

The patient will often return from major ear surgery with an ear dressing (Fig. 26.9). If the dressing is wrapped under the chin, make sure the bandage is not pressing on the trachea. The full head bandage will be replaced by a headband-type covering after the first postoperative visit on the day after surgery. Positioning of the patient after ear surgery depends on specific instructions from the health care provider. Often the patient is placed flat in bed, and the head is supported so that it does not turn from side to side. In addition to noting the vital signs, watch for signs of injury to the facial nerve, including inability of the patient to close the eyes, wrinkle the forehead, or pucker the lips. The patient and family are advised to report such symptoms to the surgeon.

Safety precautions, such as raising side rails, should be taken to prevent injuries from dizziness and loss of balance during the recovery period. Balance is temporarily affected as a result of disturbance to the mechanism that maintains equilibrium. When the patient is allowed to get up and move around, assistance should be provided to prevent falls. The patient should arise slowly to a sitting position and sit for a few minutes. Then the patient stands while holding on to something or being supported by another person. Dizziness must pass before the patient attempts walking.

Because the ear is so near the brain, special effort must be made to prevent contamination of the surgical site. Dressings may be reinforced to keep them dry, but excessive drainage must be reported to the surgeon.

The patient should be instructed beforehand about what is to be expected from the surgery. Hearing is usually impaired immediately after surgery because of edema or bandages but is expected to improve in time.

Myringotomy (incision of the eardrum) with placement of tubes is a lesser outpatient procedure, and the only dressing may be a cotton ball in the ear. There is less occurrence of dizziness or nausea with this surgery.

Home Care Considerations

Instructions After Ear Surgery

The following instructions are given to the patient after ear surgery at the time of discharge:

- Sneezing, coughing, and nose blowing are all ways in which the operative site may be disturbed. Avoid nose blowing if possible. Cough or sneeze with the mouth open. Continue this for 1 week after surgery.
- Do not drink through a straw for 2 to 3 weeks. Avoid drinking directly from the mouth of a plastic bottle because negative pressure occurs if the bottle opening is sealed.
- Limit physical activity for 1 week after surgery. Refrain from exercising and sports for 3 weeks or until the surgeon discharges you.
- Avoid heavy lifting for 3 weeks. Avoid bending over from the waist or moving the head rapidly for 3 weeks.
- Keep the ear dry for 4 to 6 weeks after surgery by placing a cotton ball covered with petroleum jelly (such as Vaseline) in the ear canal when showering; refrain from shampooing hair with water for 1 week after surgery.
- After the initial dressing is removed, place a cotton ball loosely in the ear to keep it dry and protected; change the cotton ball as needed and at least daily.
- Avoid people with colds.
- Do not fly until the surgeon allows it.
- Wear ear protectors when exposed to a loud environment.
- A return to work is usually allowed after 3 to 7 days; strenuous work may not be resumed for 3 weeks.

The surgeon will explain the specific time limitations for each activity based on the type of surgery.

Although many disorders of the ear are treated on an outpatient basis, it is important for the nurse taking care of an inpatient to be aware of any vision or hearing problems that may affect care. Patients who adapt well in their home environment to sensory impairments may need help in a hospital setting. Find out what deficit is present and how the patient normally compensates. Facilitate measures for the patient to maintain their independence and dignity. Adjust teaching as needed to make sure that adequate communication has occurred and that the patient has the knowledge and information necessary to safely take medications and to perform self-care.

COMMUNITY CARE

Cautioning people about the dangers of listening to loud music through earpieces can help curb hearing loss. Teaching adults to seek prompt medical attention for symptoms of otitis media prevents damage to the tympanic membrane and preserves hearing ability.

A hearing assessment should be part of any thorough health assessment. Encouraging those who have any difficulty with hearing to have a thorough evaluation and to try a hearing aid, if the need is indicated, could help improve the quality of their lives. There is little economic reason for refusing to *try* a hearing aid. Veterans should be told that Veterans Health Administration clinics will perform hearing tests and supply a hearing aid. The Office of Vocational Rehabilitation and Employment may provide this service as well.

Nurses in home and long-term care settings should frequently assess the function of the patient's hearing aid. Older adults with arthritis or poor vision may have difficulty properly inserting the battery into a hearing aid. If the aid is not working, it may be that the battery simply is not inserted correctly.

Hearing ability changes with aging, and reassessment needs to take place at routine intervals.

Various accommodations are available for individuals who are hearing impaired. Assistance dogs can help keep a person with a hearing impairment safe both in the home and when out and about.

Get Ready for the NCLEX® Examination!

Key Points

- The tympanic membrane must be able to vibrate when sound is received for the sound waves to be transmitted to the middle ear.
- The bones of the middle ear transmit the sound waves to the inner ear.
- Sound is transmitted from the inner ear to cranial nerve VIII.
- Changes in the ear structures with aging may cause hearing impairment.
- Exposure to loud noise causes sensorineural hearing loss.
- A variety of drugs are ototoxic (see Box 26.2).
- There are several diagnostic tests and examinations for problems of the ear (see Table 26.2).
- Learning to communicate with people who are hearing impaired is important for nurses (see Box 26.3).
- Labyrinthitis and Ménière disease cause dizziness and vertigo.
- Decreasing stress often decreases dizziness and vertigo.
- Tinnitus is common with a variety of ear disorders.
- A variety of treatments are available to help patients with tinnitus; biofeedback and masking help many people.
- Lip-reading or speech reading is helpful to people with hearing impairments but is difficult to learn.
- Various types of hearing aids are available, but using one takes practice.
- Cochlear implants are available for patients who have severe hearing loss.
- Nurses should actively educate the community about ways to prevent hearing loss.
- Otitis media is a common malady that may be induced by allergy or upper respiratory infection.
- Impacted cerumen or foreign bodies in the ear interfere with hearing.
- Otosclerosis is generally hereditary.
- Tympanoplasty may be performed for otosclerosis or for tympanic membrane dysfunction.
- Labyrinthitis and Ménière disease cause vertigo and tinnitus.

Additional Learning Resources

SG Go to your Study Guide for additional learning activities to help you master this chapter content.

Go to your Evolve website (http://evolve.elsevier.com/deWit/medsurg) for the following FREE learning resources:

- Animations, audio, and video
- Answers and rationales for questions and activities
- Glossary with pronunciations in English and Spanish
- Interactive Review Questions and more!

Review Questions for the NCLEX® Examination

1. When a patient is receiving furosemide (Lasix) for a problem with edema, which side effect relative to this drug is important to the patient's health?
   1. Decreased rate of respirations
   2. Nausea
   3. Constipation
   4. Hearing loss

   NCLEX Client Need: Physiological Integrity: Pharmacological Therapies
2. A nurse applies a vibrating tuning fork to the middle of a patient's forehead. What response would indicate normal hearing?
   1. Hearing the sound in the back of the head
   2. Feeling a vibration but hearing no sound
   3. Hearing the sound in the middle of the head
   4. Feeling a vibration and hearing a sound in the temporal area

   NCLEX Client Need: Physiological Integrity: Physiological Adaptation
3. When administering ear drops to an adult, you would:
   1. draw the pinna upward and toward the front of the head.
   2. draw the pinna upward and toward the back of the head.
   3. pull the pinna downward and toward the front of the head.
   4. pull the pinna downward and toward the back of the head.

   NCLEX Client Need: Physiological Integrity: Pharmacological Therapies

4. A patient returns 1 week after receiving hearing aids and states, "I guess I may as well return these; I just cannot get used to them." What is an appropriate nursing response? *(Select all that apply.)*
   1. "Maybe a different type of hearing aid would be better for you."
   2. "You have not been able to hear well for a long time. Adjusting to the way you hear the sound through a hearing aid may take quite a bit of time, but it will be worth it!"
   3. "To adjust to the hearing aids, you must wear them most of the time. Are you able to keep them in most of the time, or do you spend most of your time without them?"
   4. "My daughter adjusted to hers in just a few days. Something is not right here."

   NCLEX Client Need: Psychosocial Integrity
5. When communicating with a patient who is hearing impaired, you should: *(Select all that apply.)*
   1. sit at eye level facing the patient.
   2. use a slightly higher tone than usual.
   3. enunciate clearly.
   4. speak directly into the patient's ear.
   5. use simple, short sentences.

   NCLEX Client Need: Psychosocial Integrity
6. While ambulating, a patient with Ménière disease complains of dizziness and vertigo. An immediate nursing action would be to:
   1. provide oxygen.
   2. have the patient sit down.
   3. administer nausea medication.
   4. notify the health care provider.

   NCLEX Client Need: Physiological Integrity: Physiological Adaptation
7. Older adults are more prone to conductive hearing loss and tinnitus because of:
   1. hypertrophy of the cerumen glands.
   2. hardened cerumen.
   3. widening of the auditory canal.
   4. hair loss in the auditory canal.

   NCLEX Client Need: Physiological Integrity: Physiological Adaptation
8. You emphasize safety precautions to an 80-year-old female patient with Ménière disease. An appropriate nursing approach would be to:
   1. use the patient's first name when addressing her.
   2. include family members in instructions.
   3. address decision making with the patient.
   4. set a specific schedule for providing instructions.

   NCLEX Client Need: Safe and Effective Environment: Safety and Infection Control
9. A 59-year-old patient with labyrinthitis is requesting to get up to go to the bathroom. What nursing interventions are appropriate? *(Select all that apply.)*
   1. Medicate for nausea
   2. Medicate for pain
   3. Assist patient with ambulation
   4. Keep the room lights dim
   5. Have the patient sit up slowly
   6. Have the patient close their eyes when moving the head

   NCLEX Client Need: Physiological Integrity: Reduction of Risk Potential
10. Which statement by the patient indicates that further teaching is needed regarding home instructions post ear surgery?
    1. "I should take it easy for the next week."
    2. "I need to keep my ear dry when I shower."
    3. "I will be able to fly to see my grandson this weekend."
    4. "I will keep my head elevated."

    NCLEX Client Need: Health Promotion and Maintenance

Critical Thinking Questions

Scenario A

Mrs. Como is admitted to the hospital for management of her hypertension. She has had sensorineural deafness for several years, and it is much worse in her left ear than in her right. Her inability to hear well causes additional stress for Mrs. Como, and she is especially anxious about being in the hospital among strangers. Mrs. Como also suffers from tinnitus, which adds to her stress and inability to relax and rest. Tinnitus and the stress of not being able to hear adversely affect Mrs. Como's hypertension.

1. What evidence would you expect to find that indicates Mrs. Como has a hearing impairment?
2. What can you do to improve communication with Mrs. Como and help allay her anxiety about being in the hospital?
3. Why could her hearing problem make her blood pressure rise?
4. What resources are available to Mrs. Como to address her hearing problem?

Scenario B

Mrs. Martinez is scheduled for a cochlear implant and states that she "really doesn't understand" how the device works.

1. What should she be told?
2. What should she expect she will need to do after the cochlear implant surgery?

Scenario C

Mr. Thompson is suffering from a severe attack of Ménière disease and vertigo. He is severely nauseated, and his vertigo prevents him from getting out of bed. The health care provider wants to rule out the possibility of tumor as a cause of Mr. Thompson's vertigo, so he is scheduled for an ENG with a caloric test and an MRI scan.

1. What nursing actions would be appropriate for Mr. Thompson?
2. How would you explain this disorder to him?
3. How would you explain these tests to him?

The Gastrointestinal System

27

http://evolve.elsevier.com/deWit/medsurg

Objectives

Theory

1. Explain the various functions of the gastrointestinal system.
2. Distinguish major causative factors in the development of disorders of the gastrointestinal system.
3. Summarize measures to prevent disorders of the gastrointestinal system.
4. Determine nursing responsibilities in the pretest and posttest care of patients undergoing diagnostic tests for disorders of the gastrointestinal system.
5. Develop a nursing care plan for a patient with diarrhea.
6. Correlate changes that occur with aging with alterations in gastrointestinal function.

Clinical Practice

7. Perform an assessment of gastrointestinal status.
8. Provide pretest and posttest care of patients undergoing tests of the liver, gallbladder, and pancreas.
9. Provide care for a patient who is experiencing vomiting.
10. Teach a patient strategies to alleviate constipation.

Key Terms

absorption (ăb-sŏrp-shŭn, p. 644)
adhesions (ăd-HĒ-shŭnz, p. 644)
anabolism (ă-NĂB-ō-lĭzm, p. 644)
anorexia (ăn-ō-RĔK-sē-ă, p. 654)
ascites (ă-SĪ-tēz, p. 652)
catabolism (kă-TĂB-ō-lĭzm, p. 644)
chyme (KĪM, p. 642)
flatus (FLĀ-tŭs, p. 656)
mastication (măs-tĭ-KĀ-shŭn, p. 642)
metabolism (mĕ-TĂ-bō-lĭzm, p. 644)
pancreatitis (păn-krē-Ă-TĪ-tĭs, p. 646)
peristalsis (pĕr-ēs-TĂL-sĭs, p. 642)

Concepts Covered in This Chapter

- Fluid and Electrolytes
- Glucose Regulation
- Nutrition
- Inflammation
- Pain
- Patient Education
- Health Promotion
- Care Coordination

ANATOMY AND PHYSIOLOGY OF THE GASTROINTESTINAL SYSTEM

ORGANS AND STRUCTURES OF THE GASTROINTESTINAL SYSTEM

- The organs of the gastrointestinal (GI) system are the mouth, pharynx, esophagus, stomach, small intestine, large intestine, rectum, and anus (Fig. 27.1).
- The accessory organs are the liver, gallbladder, and pancreas (Fig. 27.2).
- The gastroesophageal sphincter (cardiac sphincter) controls the opening from the esophagus into the stomach; it prevents reflux from the stomach into the esophagus.
- The stomach lies in the upper left portion of the abdominal cavity (see Fig. 27.1).
- The pyloric sphincter controls release of food substances into the small intestine (Fig. 27.3, *B*).
- The small intestine is divided into the duodenum, jejunum, and ileum and is about 6 m long.
- The ileocecal valve controls the progress of substances into the large intestine.
- The large intestine is divided into the cecum, colon, rectum, and anal canal; the colon is about 1.5 m long.
- The colon has four portions: the ascending, transverse, descending, and sigmoid colon.
- The appendix is attached to the cecum and has no known function in the digestive process.
- The walls of the digestive tract have four layers: mucosa, submucosa, muscular layer, and a serous layer called serosa.
- The peritoneum is a serous sac that lines the abdominal cavity and encloses the intestines, stomach, liver, and spleen, and partially encloses the uterus and uterine tubes.

FUNCTIONS OF THE GASTROINTESTINAL SYSTEM

- The teeth and tongue are instrumental in the chewing (**mastication**) process, and they help break down food into smaller pieces that can be acted on by various enzymes.
- Food moves from the mouth through the pharynx and down the esophagus through **peristalsis** (wavelike motions of involuntary muscles within the walls of the organs) to the stomach, where mixing movements occur.
- Mucus, hydrochloric acid (HCl), intrinsic factor, pepsinogen, and gastrin are secreted into the stomach from cells within its walls and are mixed into the food to break down further the particles for absorption. This mixture of partially digested semiliquid food is called **chyme**.
- The small intestine receives the chyme from the stomach, adds more digestive enzymes and fluids, receives bile and pancreatic enzymes from the common duct, and further digests the chyme into a more liquid state.
- Substances are moved along the intestinal tract by the peristaltic action of the intestinal smooth muscle.

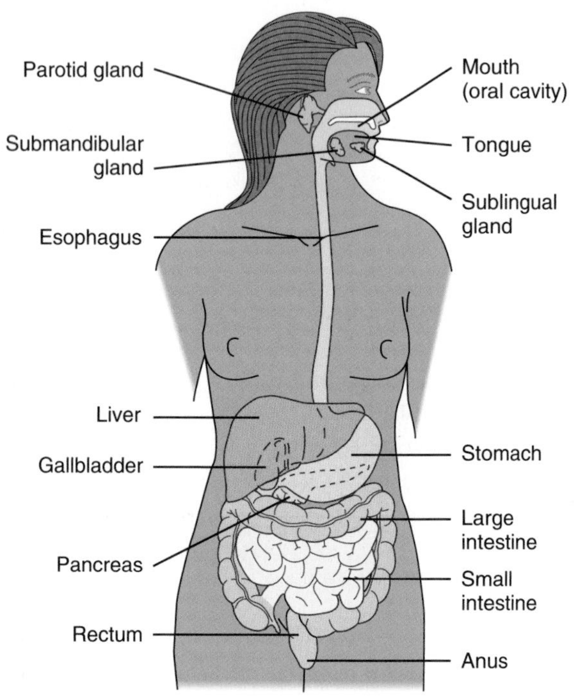

Fig. 27.1 Organs of the digestive system.

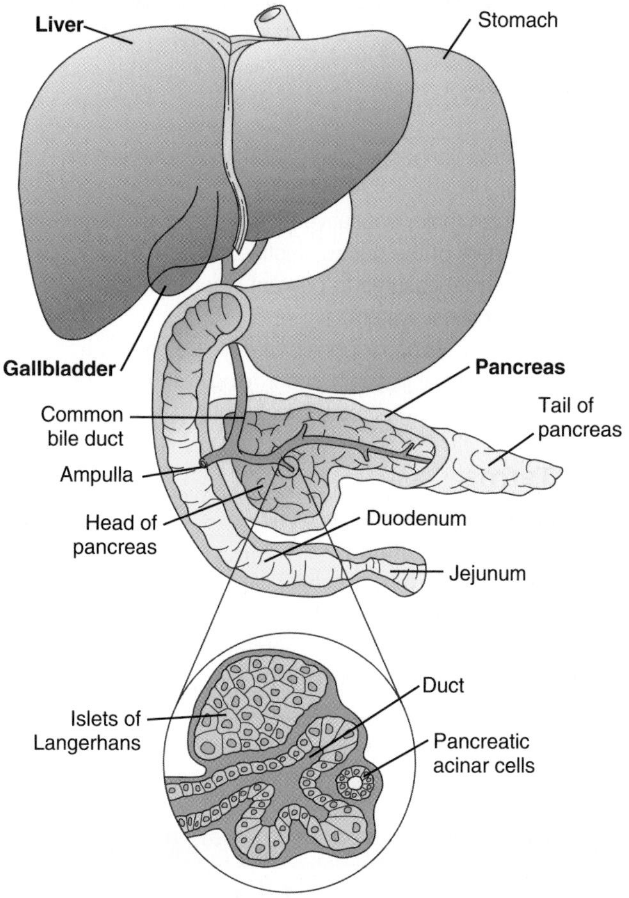

Fig. 27.2 Accessory organs of the digestive system.

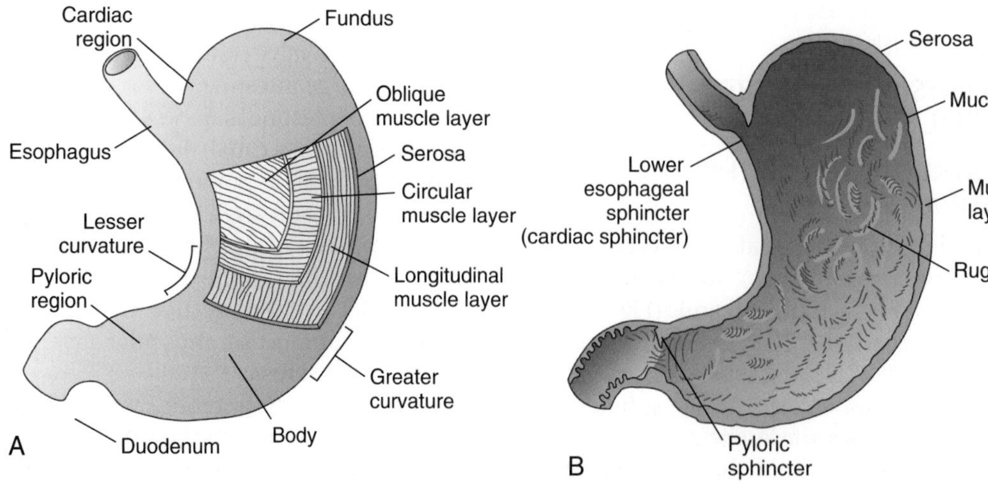

Fig. 27.3 The stomach. **A,** External view. **B,** Internal view.

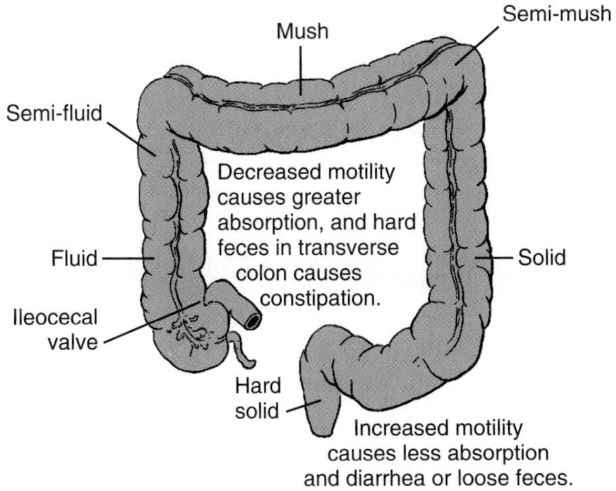

Fig. 27.4 Absorptive and storage functions of the large intestine.

- Digested food particles are absorbed into the bloodstream from the villi on the walls of the small intestine.
- The large intestine reabsorbs water and electrolytes, formulates some vitamin K, and eliminates waste products (Fig. 27.4).
- The large intestine is populated with bacteria that aid in the breakdown of waste products.
- The rectum stores fecal material until it is eliminated through the anus.
- The internal anal sphincter at the top of the anal canal is under involuntary control; the external anal sphincter at the end of the anal canal is under voluntary control.
- The gastrocolic reflex initiates elimination; it is stimulated by the ingestion of food. By tightening the voluntary anal sphincter, the reflex emptying of the rectum can be stopped.

CONTROL OF THE GASTROINTESTINAL SYSTEM

- The intestine is lined with various receptors that interact with the nervous and endocrine systems.
- These mechanisms help control the release of digestive hormones and enzymes as well as initiating peristalsis.

EFFECTS OF AGING ON THE GASTROINTESTINAL SYSTEM

- With advanced age, muscles used for swallowing may become weaker and less coordinated, and food particles are retained in the cheek pouches or pharynx.
- The esophageal sphincter becomes less efficient at opening and closing, and risk for aspiration increases.
- Taste buds atrophy, causing inability to distinguish between flavors, particularly between salty and sweet.
- After age 70 years, the parietal cells in the stomach decrease their secretion of HCl; enzyme and intrinsic factor secretion also decrease. The lack of intrinsic factor may cause pernicious anemia.
- The mucosa of the small intestine becomes less absorptive, and the large intestine may develop diminished motility.

STRUCTURES AND LOCATIONS OF THE ACCESSORY ORGANS

- The *gallbladder* is a small sac attached to the lower portion of the liver.
- The *liver* is a large, reddish-brown organ located in the upper right quadrant of the abdominal cavity under the diaphragm; it is protected by the rib cage.
- The portal vein transports all venous blood and nutrients absorbed from the small intestine to the liver.
- The *pancreas* is an elongated, flat organ that sits behind the stomach and consists of a "head" and a "tail" (see Fig. 27.2).
- The gallbladder connects to the common bile duct that leads from the liver to the duodenum.
- The pancreatic duct extends the length of the pancreas and connects with the common bile duct, conducting its secretions into the duodenum.

FUNCTIONS OF THE GALLBLADDER, LIVER, AND PANCREAS

- The gallbladder stores bile produced in the liver and delivers it as needed to the small intestine; the gallbladder can store up to 50 mL of bile.
- The liver manufactures and secretes bile and bile salts necessary to digest fat and fat-soluble vitamins.
- The liver synthesizes albumin, fibrinogen, globulins, and clotting factors.
- The liver is a storage area for glucose (in the form of glycogen); vitamins A, D, E, K, and B_{12}; and iron.
- The liver receives blood directly from the digestive tract via the hepatic portal vein. All nutrients and oral medications pass through the liver before being distributed to other parts of the body.
- The liver is responsible for how drugs are metabolized.
- The liver detoxifies and breaks down many compounds and drugs, preparing them for excretion; it alters ammonia, a by-product of protein metabolism, so that it does not harm the body.
- The liver helps break down and excrete hormones, drugs, cholesterol, and hemoglobin from worn-out red blood cells.
- The liver plays a major role in glucose metabolism, removing excess glucose from the blood, converting it to glycogen, and then, as glucose is needed, converting glycogen back to glucose.
- The liver plays key roles in lipid metabolism, breaking down fatty acids and synthesizing cholesterol and phospholipids, and in converting excess carbohydrates and proteins into fats.
- The liver is instrumental in protein metabolism, converting certain amino acids into different ones as needed for protein synthesis.
- The liver is a large filter containing phagocytic Kupffer cells that remove bacteria, damaged red blood cells, and other toxic materials from the blood.
- The liver may store between 200 and 400 mL of blood.

- The liver synthesizes the prothrombin needed for normal blood clotting.
- The islets of Langerhans, which are regions of endocrine tissue in the pancreas, secrete the hormones insulin and glucagon into the blood; insulin is essential to the metabolism of carbohydrates and maintenance of electrolyte balance.
- The pancreatic acinar cells secrete digestive enzymes into ducts that connect with the pancreatic duct.
- The major pancreatic enzymes are amylase, protease, trypsin, and lipase; these enzymes are essential to the digestion and absorption of nutrients from the small intestine.
- Secretion of pancreatic enzymes is controlled by secretin and cholecystokinin, two substances secreted by the intestinal mucosa.

EFFECTS OF AGING ON THE ACCESSORY ORGANS OF DIGESTION

- Gallstone incidence is higher in older adults, possibly because of an increase in biliary cholesterol related to diet and a tendency toward dehydration.
- Secretion of lipase from the pancreas decreases, altering fat digestion, and may contribute to a depressed nutritional state in older adults.

THE GASTROINTESTINAL SYSTEM

The intestinal tract and accessory organs of digestion perform the intake, absorption, and assimilation of food to provide nourishment for the body. The transfer of nutrients from the intestine into the blood is referred to as **absorption**. Food substances are moved along the intestinal tract by *peristalsis*. **Metabolism** is the sum of many physical and chemical processes of the absorbed nutrients. Metabolic activities involve the synthesis of substances needed to build, maintain, and repair body tissues (**anabolism**). Metabolism is also responsible for the breakdown of larger molecules into smaller molecules so that energy is available (**catabolism**).

GASTROINTESTINAL SYSTEM DISORDERS

Causes

The GI tract is subject to infection, inflammation, physical and chemical trauma, and structural defects. An intestinal tract problem may be caused by blockage of movement of food through the intestine (intestinal obstruction). Postoperative **adhesions** sometimes cause intestinal obstruction. Adhesions are bands of scar tissue that bind together two anatomic surfaces that are normally separate. Tumor may also cause intestinal obstruction. Obstruction of the bile or pancreatic ducts can cause interference with the flow of digestive juices and of the enzymes needed for digestion. Continued irritation and inflammation of the GI mucosa can lead to intestinal bleeding and to increased peristalsis, causing inadequate absorption of nutrients.

Psychological and emotional stresses greatly influence appetite and motility of the stomach and intestines. The secretion of digestive juices in amounts sufficient for the breakdown of food is regulated in part by the emotions regulated by the nervous system. The stress response may cause excessive GI secretions and decreased perfusion to the organs.

Think Critically

Why do you think health care providers frequently place hospitalized patients on GI prophylaxis medication?

Excessive stimulation of digestive acid and enzymes can cause a breakdown in the integrity of the mucous membrane lining the digestive tract. The damage to the mucous membrane can result in gastric or duodenal ulcers or chronic colitis.

Some disorders, such as Crohn disease and ulcerative colitis, are correlated with a genetic predisposition. Both disorders are more common among those of European Jewish heritage. Certain forms of colon cancer have been identified as having a genetic link, and there is a familial tendency for the occurrence of colon cancer. Esophageal and stomach cancer are linked to consumption of charred foods and those containing nitrites and cigarette smoking.

Patient Teaching

Foods That May Contribute to Colon Cancer

The patient should be taught that the following foods may contribute to the development of colon cancer.

NITRATES AND NITRITES

- Hot dogs
- Bologna and other luncheon meats
- Bacon
- Ham
- Smoked fish
- Some imported cheeses (check labels)

Nitrates and nitrites are used extensively as food preservatives. Check labels on deli products. Charred grilled foods and meat cooked at high temperatures also contain substances that are potentially cancer-causing.

Health Promotion

Maintaining GI Health

Research studies show mixed results on the cancer risk posed by processed foods with nitrates and nitrites. If other risk factors for GI cancer such as high-fat diet, obesity, excessive alcohol consumption, or smoking are present, it is best to avoid the possible nitrate-nitrite risk.

Autoimmune diseases often affect the GI system, causing inflammation or fibrosis of organs. Treatments such as drug and radiation therapy may cause GI problems as a side effect. Some people who have undergone chemotherapy for cancer develop a mechanical form of sprue, a malabsorption problem that remains even after chemotherapy is complete. Lactose intolerance, which is common among older adults, may cause continuous diarrhea and malabsorption.

Think Critically

Can you identify any GI problems that seem to run in your family? What measures can family members take to prevent such problems?

Prevention of Gastrointestinal System Disorders

Eating a normal-portioned, well-balanced diet aids digestion. Maintaining good oral health is important to the health of the rest of the body. Consuming sufficient bulk in the diet helps maintain a healthy colon by enhancing passage of waste. A diet lacking in fiber is one factor in the development of diverticulosis, in which pockets form along the colon where waste material can lodge. Maintaining hydration prevents constipation by helping to keep the stool moist.

Heeding the need to defecate promptly aids in keeping the gastrocolic reflex functioning well and prevents constipation and hemorrhoids. Straining at stool increases intra-abdominal pressure, which causes the hemorrhoidal vessels to engorge and contributes to hemorrhoid formation. Decreased mobility in older adults often leads to digestive problems; therefore ambulation is encouraged.

Health Promotion

Maintaining Abdominal Tone

Sufficient daily exercise maintains abdominal muscle tone and contributes to peristalsis and the ability to defecate normally. Defecating at around the same time each day aids the defecation process and helps promote the continued ability to control defecation.

Maintaining body weight within normal limits helps prevent hiatal hernia and esophageal reflux. Developing healthy coping mechanisms and keeping stress within acceptable limits may prevent ulcers and chronic irritability of the bowel.

Mechanical and chemical irritants that produce inflammation often can be identified by elimination diets to determine the foods that cause GI upsets. Once the offending foods are identified, the patient can learn to avoid those foods while maintaining adequate nutrition.

Following general rules of good hygiene and sanitation can prevent many infectious GI events: wash the hands before cooking and eating, and clean cooking and eating utensils properly. Food poisoning can be prevented by adequate refrigeration and by proper canning, freezing, and food-handling methods. Meats and foods containing mayonnaise or dairy products should be kept chilled. When not in the refrigerator, food should be kept covered.

Think Critically

How would you teach your family and friends about ways to decrease the risk of colon cancer? What would you recommend to your adult relatives regarding screening for colorectal cancer?

Causes of gallbladder disorders. The formation of stones within the gallbladder can cause irritation and create areas susceptible to inflammation and infection. Stones can lodge in the common duct, causing obstruction to the flow of bile. Very rapid weight loss associated with severe calorie and fat restriction or gastric bypass surgery appear to be associated with developing gallstones. Women develop gallstones more frequently than men. The incidence increases with age, obesity, and having several children because pregnancy causes stasis of bile. People who have diabetes mellitus or Crohn disease are at higher risk for the disorder. Gallbladder disease tends to run in families, and it appears that there may be a genetic link.

Cultural Considerations

Genetic Gallstone Risk

Native Americans secrete high levels of cholesterol in their bile. Most Native American men have gallstones by age 60 years, and 70% of the women of the Pima Indians in Arizona have gallstones by age 30 years. Mexican Americans of both sexes and all ages also have high rates of gallstones (Chemmanur, 2018).

Prevention of gallbladder disorders. Maintaining a normal body weight; eating a low-fat, low-cholesterol, high-fiber, and high-calcium diet; avoiding rapid weight loss diets; consuming alcohol moderately; and maintaining an active lifestyle all help prevent gallstones (Afdhal & Zakko, 2018).

Causes of liver disorders. The liver filters out many toxic substances and is constantly exposed to any infectious organisms circulating in the bloodstream. The hepatitis virus, in particular, attacks the liver, causing inflammation and damage to the tissue. Hepatitis B and C are the cause of liver cancer in 70% of cases (Schwartz & Carithers, 2018). *Healthy People 2030* objectives include reducing the number of hepatitis infections and increasing awareness of having a hepatitis infection.

Many drugs and chemicals are toxic to the liver, and nurses should always be aware of the drugs their patients are taking that may cause liver damage. Alcohol and other toxic substances are major factors in the development of cirrhosis of the liver (Box 27.1).

Liver trauma or laceration may cause massive internal hemorrhage. However, the liver is resilient and will regenerate if part of the liver remains functional and bleeding is stopped quickly.

Box 27.1 Drugs and Substances Toxic or Harmful to the Liver

HEPATOTOXIC DRUGS

- Acetaminophen (Tylenol)
- Amiodarone
- Atorvastatin
- Carbamazepine
- Erythromycin
- Ibuprofen
- Methyldopa
- Phenytoin
- Sulfonamides

Many more drugs can cause liver problems. Consult the nursing implications for each drug administered. Consider the adequacy of the patient's liver function when administering medications because the liver detoxifies all medications.

CHEMICAL SUBSTANCES

- Acetaldehyde
- Aerosolized paint
- Cadmium
- Ethyl alcohol
- Ethylene oxide
- Mercury
- Nitrosamines
- Paint thinner
- Polychlorinated biphenyls (PCBs)
- Many cleaning solvents and pesticides

Parasites may cause cirrhosis, cysts, or abscesses. Most parasites that damage the liver enter the body when people wade or swim in contaminated water in tropical countries or eat contaminated food.

Cancer in the liver may be primary or may be secondary to metastasis from a site elsewhere in the body.

Prevention of liver disorders. Obtaining immunization against hepatitis A and hepatitis B helps prevent these viral diseases. A vaccine against hepatitis C is currently undergoing clinical trials (Murphy, 2018). Adults should be tested for the presence of hepatitis C. Using Standard Precautions (see Appendix B) when handling any body fluids, particularly blood, greatly reduces the risk of infection with hepatitis B and C, which may decrease the chance of developing liver cancer. Refraining from consuming excessive amounts of alcohol decreases the risk of developing cirrhosis of the liver. Avoiding exposure to known toxic or carcinogenic chemicals and drugs helps prevent liver damage and liver cancer.

Health Promotion

Preventing Contraction of Hepatitis

Practicing good hygiene and avoiding contact with substances that harbor the hepatitis virus, such as raw oysters and shellfish from contaminated waters, may prevent infection with hepatitis A. Avoiding unprotected sex with people who are drug users, or those known to be carriers of hepatitis B or C, helps prevent the contraction of both types of hepatitis.

Causes of pancreatic disorders. **Pancreatitis** (inflammation of the pancreas) is associated with alcoholism, obstructive cholelithiasis, peptic ulcer, hyperlipidemia, and trauma. Pancreatic cancer incidence rises steadily with age. Although the cause of pancreatic cancer is not known, the incidence is higher in cigarette smokers. Obesity, chronic pancreatitis, and diabetes mellitus are also risk factors for this cancer. (See Chapter 37 for information on diabetes mellitus.)

Prevention of pancreatic disorders. Avoiding consumption of large quantities of alcohol may prevent pancreatitis. Removing a gallbladder that has gallstones can help prevent obstruction of the pancreatic duct with stones. Removal prevents backup of pancreatic enzymes that are believed to be a cause of pancreatitis. Elevated triglycerides may also precipitate pancreatitis. To prevent attacks, tryglycerides should be maintained below 200 mg/dL. Smoking cessation decreases the risk of pancreatitis and pancreatic cancer.

Diagnostic Tests, Procedures, and Nursing Implications

Diagnostic tests for disorders of the intestinal tract and accessory organs consist of x-rays, computed tomography (CT) scans, nuclear medicine scans, magnetic resonance imaging (MRI), ultrasound studies, endoscopy, biopsy, laboratory tests, tests of gastric secretions, and stool and urine studies (Table 27.1).

The patient often is scheduled for a series of tests, some of which use a contrast medium. Check the patient's allergies to verify that a particular contrast medium or injectable marker is not contraindicated. For women of childbearing age, a pregnancy test might be ordered. It is important that GI tests be performed in the correct order, so that the contrast media do not interfere with other tests. For example, if a patient is scheduled for an upper GI series, a gallbladder sonogram, and a barium enema, they should be done in this order: sonogram, barium enema, upper GI series.

CT colonography (virtual colonoscopy) is available for colon cancer screening. The procedure combines images from a high-tech spiral CT scan to create a computer-generated three-dimensional picture of the colon. The procedure is less costly than standard colonoscopy and requires no sedation. However, if a polyp or suspicious area is seen, the patient must undergo a regular colonoscopy for tissue specimens to be obtained (American College of Radiology, 2018). For screening, a yearly high-sensitivity fecal occult blood test, or fecal immunochemical test (FIT), is recommended starting at age 45 years. Stool DNA is recommended every 3 years (Wolf et al., 2018).

The patient needs specific instructions about preparing for a diagnostic test. Many of the studies require cleansing of the GI tract; inadequate bowel preparation may cause a delay or necessitate a repeat of the test. When laxatives are administered in liquid form, the patient can drink them more easily if they are chilled or poured over ice.

Older Adult Care Points

Older adults are especially at risk for problems of electrolyte imbalance, fluid overload, or dehydration when preparing for diagnostic tests that require a fasting state and/or bowel cleansing.

Assignment Considerations

Assisting With a Bowel Preparation

When an unlicensed assistive personnel (UAP) is assigned to care for a patient who is undergoing a bowel preparation for a diagnostic test, ask the UAP to be prompt in answering a call bell for assistance to the bathroom. The need to defecate may be urgent. When a patient is consuming large quantities of fluid, such as with GoLYTELY, ask the UAP to promptly report any degree of confusion, shortness of breath, extra weakness, or muscle cramping. Remember that delegation is never a substitute for good nursing assessment.

Clinical Cues

If a patient has trouble with nausea, sucking on an ice cube first and then using a straw to drink the solution for colon preparation helps decrease the taste sensation.

For many GI tests, the patient is kept on nothing-by-mouth (NPO) status the night before. In the hospital, mouth care should be offered in the morning, and the door of the room should be kept closed so that food odors do not enter and increase hunger. A food tray should be obtained immediately on return to the floor, as long as NPO status is no longer in effect. Provide juices, water, and coffee or tea while waiting for the meal tray to be delivered. Frequent assessment for signs of dehydration is necessary. Lack of oral intake can quickly dehydrate a patient who has already been ill with nausea, vomiting, or diarrhea.

Text continued on p. 652

Table 27.1 Diagnostic Tests for Gastrointestinal (GI) Disorders

TEST	PURPOSE	DESCRIPTION	NURSING IMPLICATIONS
Radiologic Examinations			
Upper GI series (UGI)	Radiographic examination with fluoroscopy to locate obstruction, ulceration, or growths in the esophagus, stomach, and duodenum	Patient drinks a contrast medium and is placed in various positions on the x-ray table.	Keep patient NPO for 8–12 h before the test. Explain what happens during test. After radiographs, increase fluids and give ordered laxatives to clear GI tract of contrast medium and prevent impaction. Stool may be white up to 3 days after test.
Barium enema (BE) (lower GI tract radiography)	Radiographic examination of the colon using fluoroscopy to locate tumors, obstruction, and ulceration	A radiopaque substance is instilled into the colon by enema. After evacuation of this substance, air may be instilled for contrast studies.	Keep patient NPO for 8 h before test. Give ordered laxatives and enemas. Bowel must be clear of stool. Explain what will happen during the test. Posttest care is same as for upper GI series.
Computed tomography (CT)—abdomen	To visualize soft tissue and density changes when sonography is inconclusive To detect tumors, abscesses, trauma, cysts, inflammation, and bleeding	Radiography is combined with computer techniques to provide a series of sectional pictures of the gallbladder, intestines, and other abdominal structures.	Patient is kept NPO for 4 h when oral contrast is to be used. Verify presence of signed informed consent form for this procedure. Assess for allergy to iodine or shellfish. Explain to patient that they will be positioned supine on a special, narrow table, and their body will be in the circular opening of the scanner. A safety strap over the waist will be used. Clicking noises will be heard from the machine. The test takes only a few minutes to obtain the images, but if oral contrast is ordered it needs to be ingested starting 2 h prior to the procedure.

Continued

Table 27.1 Diagnostic Tests for Gastrointestinal (GI) Disorders—cont'd

TEST	PURPOSE	DESCRIPTION	NURSING IMPLICATIONS
Virtual colonoscopy (CT colonography)	Noninvasive method of determining whether there are polyps or abnormalities in the colon Does not allow for biopsy of suspicious areas	Helical CT scan of the colon is performed. An oral contrast agent may be given 1 day before the scan.	Patient must lie still during the procedure. Remove all metal from the body surface. Usually takes about 10–15 min. Encourage large quantities of fluid after the procedure if barium contrast material was swallowed.
Magnetic resonance imaging (MRI) with or without contrast	To evaluate abnormalities in the liver or other abdominal structures.	Places the patient in a magnetic field. Uses radiofrequency signals to determine how hydrogen atoms behave in the magnetic field. Provides better contrast than CT between normal tissue and pathologic tissue. Administration of IV contrast may be used to provide better imaging.	Explain that there is no exposure to radiation. Antianxiety medication may be administered to those patients who are claustrophobic. There are no food or fluid restrictions before the test. The test takes 30–60 min. Remove all metal objects from the body, including dental bridges. Inform patient that they will be required to remain motionless during this study. A thumping sound will be heard during the test. There may be a tingling sensation in metal fillings.
Ultrasound Imaging			
Ultrasonography	To obtain images of soft tissue that indicate density changes To diagnose gallstones, tumor, cysts, abscess, etc.	Sonograms are produced with high-frequency sound waves that pass through the body. Echoes vary with tissue density.	Patient is kept NPO after midnight. Explain procedure: will be supine on table, lubricant will be applied to the skin surface, and a handheld metal probe is passed back and forth with light pressure. Test takes about 30 min. Patient needs to remain still.
Nuclear Imaging Scans (Scintigraphy)			
Hepatobiliary scintigraphy (hepatic iminodiacetic acid [HIDA] scan)	To determine bile flow distribution in the liver, biliary tree, gallbladder, and proximal small bowel To confirm acute cholecystitis	^{99m}Tc is injected. Patient is positioned under imaging camera, and images are taken as radioactive material is distributed.	Only traces of radioactivity are administered, and there is little radioactivity danger. Patient will lie flat during scanning. May take 60-90 min to complete.
GI scintigraphy	To determine site of active GI bleeding. Used primarily for lower GI bleeding.	Radioactive tracer is administered IV and attaches to red blood cells. Images of the abdomen are obtained at intermittent intervals.	Same as for hepatobiliary scan. The tracer remains visible for up to 24 h, and additional imaging can be obtained without reinjection of the tracer. The test helps determines if a surgical or interventional treatment would be beneficial.

Table 27.1 Diagnostic Tests for Gastrointestinal (GI) Disorders—cont'd

TEST	PURPOSE	DESCRIPTION	NURSING IMPLICATIONS
Endoscopic Studies			
Esophagogastroduodenoscopy	To visualize the esophagus, stomach, and duodenum with a lighted tube (endoscope) to detect tumor, ulceration, site of bleeding or obstruction Separate study of esophagus, stomach, or stomach and duodenum may be done. Interventions to obtain specimens or treat sites of bleeding can be done at the same time as the diagnostic procedure.	Patient is given IV sedation for the test. A local spray or gargle may be used to anesthetize the throat. The patient lies on a table with head extended, and the endoscope is introduced through the mouth.	Keep patient NPO for 8 h. Verify presence of signed informed consent form for procedure. Explain what they will experience during the test. Make sure an IV is in place. After procedure, keep patient NPO until gag reflex has returned. Take vital signs q15–30 min as ordered. Watch for signs of perforation: rising temperature, pain, changes in vital signs.
Endoscopic retrograde cholangiopancreatography (ERCP)	To identify obstruction and other pathologic conditions in the biliary and common ducts. To remove stones, place a stent, or facilitate bile drainage.	An endoscope is passed through the mouth into the duodenum with the use of fluoroscopy. A cannula is positioned in the common bile duct, and a contrast medium is injected. Radiographs are then taken. If obstruction is found, interventional procedures may be performed.	Verify presence of signed informed consent form for procedure. Patient is kept NPO after midnight. Explain the procedure to the patient (same as for esophagogastroduodenoscopy). Postprocedure care is same as for esophagogastroduodenoscopy.
Flexible sigmoidoscopy	To examine the lining of the rectum and sigmoid colon to detect polyps, tumor, obstruction, or ulceration	The patient is placed in the knee-chest position, often on a special table. A sigmoidoscope is introduced through the anus. Biopsies can be taken from areas of suspect tissue; polyps can be removed. The patient will experience some cramping during the procedure.	Give bowel preparation medications the evening before or as prescribed. Give clear liquids for dinner the night before, then keep patient NPO until after examination. Explain what they will experience. Encourage use of deep breathing and relaxation techniques to decrease cramping. Observe for rectal bleeding after biopsy or polyp removal.
Colonoscopy	To directly view the lining of the colon with a flexible endoscope	Patient is moderately sedated for this procedure, which takes about 30 min to 1 h. Polyps can be removed or biopsies taken.	Give clear liquid diet 1–3 days before test. Patient is kept NPO for 8 h before test. Give bowel prep as ordered. Explain procedure and what they will experience. Verify presence of signed informed consent form for procedure. After procedure, observe for rectal bleeding and signs of perforation: abdominal distention, pain, elevated temperature.

Continued

Table 27.1 Diagnostic Tests for Gastrointestinal (GI) Disorders—cont'd

TEST	PURPOSE	DESCRIPTION	NURSING IMPLICATIONS
Ambulatory pH monitoring	Determines presence and quantity of gastric reflux	A thin tube is placed transnasally with a pH sensor positioned 5 cm above the lower esophageal sphincter. pH is recorded for 24 h while the patient records symptoms, meals, and sleep. Another device placed endoscopically provides wireless pH monitoring. The capsule self-detaches within a week and is passed in the stool.	Explain the procedure to the patient and the role they play in monitoring. Verify presence of signed informed consent form for procedure.
Liver biopsy (percutaneous needle biopsy) Other methods of obtaining a biopsy sample of the liver include fine-needle aspiration, laparoscopic, and tranjugular	To remove a tissue sample for microscopic examination and diagnosis of various liver disorders	Under local or general anesthesia, a special biopsy needle is inserted through the abdominal wall into the desired area of the liver, and a tissue sample is aspirated.	Verify presence of signed informed consent form for procedure. Patient must be kept NPO 4–8 h before procedure. Place patient in supine or left lateral position. Patient will need to hold very still if performed under local anesthesia. The needle is introduced during sustained exhalation. Pain similar to a punch in the shoulder may be felt, lasting only 1 min or so. Procedure takes about 15 min. Take baseline vital signs. Assess for allergy to local anesthetic. Have patient empty their bladder before the procedure. Check coagulation studies for abnormalities. After biopsy, place a small dressing over puncture site; position patient on right side with support to provide pressure over biopsy site for 1–2 h. Observe for bleeding. Monitor vital signs q15min for 1 h; then q30min for 4 h; then q4h for 24 h. Assess for tenderness at biopsy site. Observe for respiratory problems, such as dyspnea, cyanosis, or restlessness, which might indicate pneumothorax. Instruct patient to avoid coughing or straining that might increase intra-abdominal pressure. They should refrain from heavy lifting or strenuous activities for 1–2 wk.

Table 27.1 Diagnostic Tests for Gastrointestinal (GI) Disorders—cont'd

TEST	PURPOSE	DESCRIPTION	NURSING IMPLICATIONS
Laboratory Tests			
Fecal analysis—stool examination Guaiac fecal occult blood test (gFOBT) or fecal immunochemical fecal occult blood test (iFOBT or FIT) Stool culture	The shape, odor, color, and consistency is observed, and the specimen is analyzed for presence of mucus and fat Tests for occult blood. Used as a colon cancer screening tool. Stool is examined microscopically for the presence of bacteria, fungi, viruses, or parasites	Stool specimen is obtained in clean container—bedpan or container in commode. For gFOBT, a small smear is made on special paper and tested with special solution for guaiac or with Hemoccult test. For iFOBT, a sample is returned to the health care provider for testing. To culture stool, a specimen is placed in container and sent to laboratory for testing.	Explain test to patient. Provide means for collection of stool. At home, a clean shallow pan, plastic bag, or plastic wrap may be used to collect the sample. Promptly retrieve stool, obtain sample for guaiac test (if done by nursing), place specimen in laboratory container, and dispatch to laboratory immediately (bacteria will multiply if specimen is left at room temperature for extended period; parasites may disintegrate). Patient must have red meat–free diet for at least 3 days before a stool guaiac test can be considered accurate. No dietary restrictions with iFOBT.
Serum bilirubin *Normal values:* Total: 0.3–1.0 mg/dL Direct (conjugated): 0.1–0.3 mg/dL Indirect (unconjugated): 0.2–0.8 mg/dL	To detect abnormal bilirubin metabolism Jaundice is present when bilirubin is >2.5 mg/dL	Collect venous blood. Protect sample from bright light.	Explain that a blood sample will be taken. Some laboratories require an 8-h fast.
Alanine aminotransferase (ALT) *Normal value:* 4–36 international units/L	An enzyme used to detect liver disease With viral hepatitis, ALT/AST ratio is >1.0 With other liver disease, ALT/AST ratio is <1.0	Collect venous blood. Injury of liver cells causes release of this enzyme.	Explain that a blood sample will be collected. No fasting is required.
Aspartate aminotransferase (AST) *Normal range:* 0–35 units/L	An enzyme found in heart, liver, and muscle tissue To detect acute hepatitis or biliary obstruction	Collect venous blood. Diseases affecting hepatocytes cause this enzyme to rise in the blood.	Explain that a blood sample will be drawn. Prevent hemolysis of sample. IM injection will affect level.
Alkaline phosphatase (ALP) *Normal range:* 30–120 units/L	Enzyme found in bone, liver, and placenta To detect liver tumor in conjunction with other clinical findings Rises when there is obstruction of biliary tree	Collect venous blood.	No fasting is required.
Ammonia *Normal range:* 10–80 mcg/dL	A product of protein metabolism To support diagnosis of severe liver disease with encephalopathy	Collect venous blood. May need to ice the specimen.	No fasting is required.

Continued

Table 27.1 Diagnostic Tests for Gastrointestinal (GI) Disorders—cont'd

TEST	PURPOSE	DESCRIPTION	NURSING IMPLICATIONS
Gamma-glutamyl transferase (GGT) *Normal range:* 8–38 units/L	To detect liver cell dysfunction, biliary obstruction, cholangitis, or cholecystitis	Collect venous blood.	Explain that a blood sample will be taken. Drugs that affect this test are alcohol, phenytoin, phenobarbital, clofibrate, and oral contraceptives.
Total protein *Normal range:* 6.4–8.3 g/dL	To detect altered protein metabolism Decreased in liver failure	Collect venous blood.	Explain that a blood sample will be drawn. No fasting is required.
Albumin *Normal range:* 3.5–5.5 g/dL	To detect altered protein metabolism	Collect venous blood.	No fasting is required.
Prothrombin time (PT) *Normal range:* 11.0–12.5 sec Many labs report INR instead of PT. International Normalized Ratio (INR) *Normal range:* 0.8–1.1	Protein produced by the liver and used in blood clotting Depends on adequate intake and absorption of vitamin K Reduced in patients with liver disease, causing a prolonged clotting time	Collect venous blood.	No fasting is required. Apply pressure to venipuncture site. INR used to determine therapeutic level of anticoagulant medication.
Partial thromboplastin time (PTT) *Normal range:* 60–70 sec	To detect deficiencies of stage II clotting mechanisms Prolonged in liver disease	Collect venous blood.	No fasting is required. Apply pressure to venipuncture site. Used to manage heparinization.
Activated PTT (aPTT) *Normal range:* 20–35 sec	Activators have been added to PTT test reagents: aPTT decreased in liver failure	Collect venous blood.	If patient is receiving heparin injections, draw specimen 30–60 min before next dose.
Helicobacter pylori antibody test *Normal:* none present	To detect antibodies to *H. pylori* bacterium in the stomach *H. pylori* is a risk factor for gastric and duodenal ulcers, chronic gastritis, or ulcerative esophagitis	Collect a sample of venous blood according to the laboratory's instructions.	Explain to patient that a blood sample will be drawn. No fasting is required.

IM, Intramuscular; *IV*, intravenous; *NPO*, nothing by mouth; ^{99m}*Tc*, technetium-99m.

NURSING MANAGEMENT

ASSESSMENT (DATA COLLECTION)

Assessment for problems of the digestive system and accessory organs begins during history taking. Ask questions about family history, diet, dietary intolerances, pain, bowel patterns, exposure to toxins or chemicals, and problems with blood clotting. Verify immunization status. Because of the many functions of the liver, assessment of a patient with liver disease must include all systems of the body.

Physical Assessment

Inspect the patient's teeth, gums, and oral mucosa for obvious problems. Examine the skin for color and lesions and note any discolorations on the abdomen. Assess for the presence of edema and **ascites** (fluid in the abdominal cavity) by observing for marked abdominal distention and taut, glistening skin. Check the contour of the abdomen, and note any outpouchings indicating a hernia.

Auscultate bowel sounds for each quadrant of the abdomen using the diaphragm of the stethoscope (Fig. 27.5). **Perform auscultation before palpation or percussion because palpation may cause peristaltic movement that otherwise would not have occurred. Bowel sounds are caused by air and fluid moving through the intestinal tract and are heard as soft gurgles and clicks every 5 to 15 seconds.** The normal frequency for these sounds is about 5 to 30 in 1 minute. Note

Focused Assessment

Data Collection for the Gastrointestinal System and Accessory Organs

When obtaining a GI history, ask the following questions:

- Have you gained or lost weight recently without trying?
- Do you have any difficulty chewing or swallowing?
- When did you have your last dental examination?
- Do you ever experience indigestion? Do certain foods disagree with you? Do you have known food intolerances?
- Do you drink alcohol? About how often do you drink? How many drinks do you average?
- Has your appetite changed in any way?
- Have you been experiencing any abdominal pain or nausea and vomiting? Do you experience any regurgitation or reflux? Is pain related to your eating patterns?
- Describe your usual diet. How much of each item do you eat? (Ask about what is eaten at each meal typically, and then ask about between-meal snacks and drinks.)
- What drugs do you take on a regular basis? (Aspirin, nonsteroidal anti-inflammatory drugs [NSAIDs], and corticosteroids are particularly important.)
- Are you able to shop and prepare meals? Is there any problem with obtaining sufficient food (if patient is known to have economic constraints)?
- Do you have any cultural preferences for food?
- What is the typical frequency of your bowel movements? Have you noticed any changes in color, frequency, or form of stools?
- How do you handle stress? How do you relax?

Additional questions pertinent to the accessory organs include the following:

- Does eating fatty or fried food give you pain or diarrhea?
- Does your blood take a long time to clot when you cut yourself?
- Have you had any rapid weight loss? Are you dieting?
- Have you been immobile for a long period of time?
- Have you been exposed to chemical toxins such as cleaning agents, pesticides, or industrial chemicals?
- Have you had hepatitis B and/or hepatitis A immunizations?
- Have you ever had a blood transfusion?
- Have you had any surgeries? If so, what were they and what year?
- Do you use recreational drugs?
- Do you have any tattoos or body piercings?
- Do you smoke? If so, how much do you smoke? How many years have you smoked?
- Have you experienced any abdominal trauma?
- Do you have a sexual partner? Are you monogamous? Has any sexual partner been a carrier of hepatitis B or hepatitis C?

both the character and the frequency of sounds. Loud, frequent sounds occur when there is excessive motility in the bowel. Although routinely performed, there is controversy about the usefulness or accuracy of bowel sound auscultation. It is agreed on, through research, that bowel sounds as an isolated clinical assessment have limited usefulness. Abdominal assessment findings may prompt the need for imaging studies if the findings indicate a change in condition (Elhardello & Macfie, 2018).

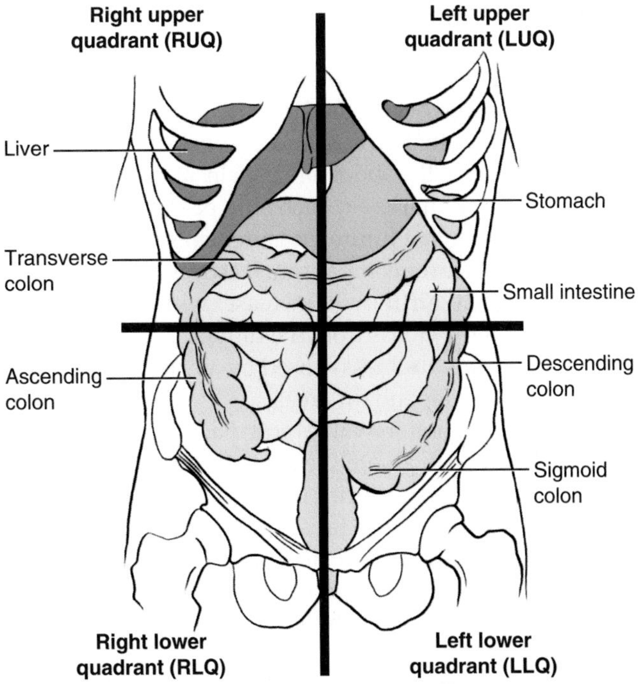

Fig. 27.5 Auscultate bowel sounds in all four quadrants. (From Williams P: *deWit's fundamental concepts and skills for nursing,* ed 5, St. Louis, 2018, Elsevier.)

Clinical Cues

For bowel sounds to be considered absent, it is necessary to verify that no sounds are heard after listening in each of the four quadrants for 5 minutes. Hypoactive bowel sounds can be noted in the medical record when no sounds are heard after listening in each of the four quadrants for 30 seconds. If hyperactive, high-pitched sounds are heard in one quadrant and decreased sounds are heard in another quadrant, assess for nausea and vomiting because the patient may have an intestinal obstruction.

Lightly palpate over each quadrant of the abdomen to detect areas of tenderness and any masses that might be present. Watch the patient's face during palpation to detect signs of discomfort. If a pulsating abdominal mass is present, do not perform palpation; this pulsation could signal an abdominal aneurysm with a potential danger of sudden rupture.

Percussion is performed by placing the middle finger of one hand on the abdomen and striking the finger lightly below the knuckle and listening for the pitch of sound produced. A resonant sound is heard over areas filled with air, and a dull, thudding sound is heard over solid organs. **Percussion detects excessive air in the intestinal tract, which occurs with irritation and inflammation.**

Assess ascites by placing the patient supine and exposing the abdomen. With the patient's arms at the sides and knees flexed, observe for bulging flanks, indicating fluid accumulation. If ascites is present, measure abdominal girth. Place a tape measure around the fullest part of the abdomen, usually at the umbilicus. Place small ink marks on each side of the tape on the axillary lines, so that future measurements may be taken at the same place for comparison. If ascites is continuous, the abdominal girth will increase with subsequent measurements. Percuss from the umbilicus to the flanks to detect shifting dullness caused by air rising and fluid shifting to the dependent areas.

Check the laboratory values and diagnostic test results (see Table 27.1). Evaluate the urine for presence of bilirubin, which makes the urine dark or tea-colored. Inspect stool for the presence of fat and urobilinogen. If undigested fat is present, the stool will float in the toilet bowl. If bile is not reaching the intestine, the stool will appear clay-colored or whitish.

Focused Assessment

Physical Assessment of the Gastrointestinal System and Accessory Organs

- Inspect the mouth for condition of teeth, gums, and mucous membranes.
- Assess swallowing ability.
- Inspect the skin for color, areas of discoloration, and presence of surface vessels and easy bruising.
- Inspect the sclera and mucous membranes for signs of icterus.
- Inspect the contour of the abdomen.
- Auscultate for bowel sounds in all four quadrants.
- Lightly palpate each quadrant of the abdomen.
- Percuss each quadrant of the abdomen if there seems to be a problem with intestinal irritation or inflammation.
- If there is evidence of ascites, measure abdominal girth.
- Inspect stool, if available, for characteristics; test for occult blood if indicated.
- Inspect color of urine.
- Inspect anus for presence of external hemorrhoids.
- If vomiting has occurred, inspect vomitus for characteristics; test vomitus for blood if indicated.

Older Adult Care Points

Medication reconciliation is extremely important in the older adult. Medications, both prescription and over the counter, are very important to consider when assessing the digestive system. Many drugs affect digestion, bowel motility, and appetite in these patients and can cause nausea, constipation, or diarrhea.

◆ NURSING DIAGNOSIS AND PLANNING

Problem statements and examples of expected outcomes for problems of the GI tract are listed in Table 27.2. More time is typically needed to care for a patient who has diarrhea or is incontinent of feces. It is important to consider the time it takes for toileting and cleaning up after loose bowel movements. A bowel retraining program takes patience and time. These time-consuming tasks are also assignment considerations for UAP. Patients may need to be treated using isolation precautions, which will increase time for care.

◆ IMPLEMENTATION

Institute nursing interventions to control and eliminate pain; maintain fluid and electrolyte balance; promote adequate nutrition, rest, and healing; and prevent complications (see Table 27.2). All nurses must ask each patient each day about bowel movements to prevent constipation and possible impaction in hospitalized patients.

◆ EVALUATION

Analyze laboratory values to see whether problems are resolving with treatment. Ideally the patient should demonstrate normalization of eating habits and bowel patterns; however, **continually evaluate whether the patient is experiencing adverse side effects of therapy or complications of the disease process.** For legal reasons and for continuity of care, your evaluation findings and your follow-up actions must always be documented.

COMMON PROBLEMS RELATED TO THE GASTROINTESTINAL SYSTEM

Anorexia

Anorexia is the absence of appetite. Physical causes for a diminished interest in eating include poorly fitting dentures, stomatitis, decaying teeth, halitosis, and a bad taste in the mouth. Pain or nausea or the presence of a mouth or GI infection or irritation decreases appetite. Diseases of the GI tract also can diminish appetite.

Appetite depends on complex mental processes having to do with memory and mental associations that can be pleasant or extremely unpleasant. Appetite is stimulated by the sight, smell, and thought of food. The physical and social environment in which a person is eating stimulates appetite. The enjoyment of eating can be inhibited by unattractive or unfamiliar food, by unpleasant surroundings, and by emotional states such as anxiety, anger, and fear. Mental depression also may cause anorexia.

Nursing management. Loss of appetite is to be expected when a person becomes ill. However, persistent anorexia must be addressed to prevent the consequences of inadequate nutrition. Because of the complex nature of anorexia, it may be necessary for you to talk with the patient, family, and significant others and to consult the medical record to learn why appetite has diminished.

Nursing interventions include mouth care before each meal to eliminate or minimize oral causes of poor appetite. Laboratory results regarding albumin and electrolyte levels should be monitored. The percentage of each meal eaten should be noted and documented.

Table 27.2 **Common Problem Statements, Expected Outcomes, and Interventions for Patients With Gastrointestinal Disorders**

PROBLEM STATEMENTS	GOALS/EXPECTED OUTCOMES	NURSING INTERVENTIONS
Fluid volume deficit due to nausea and vomiting or diarrhea	Vomiting will be controlled within 24 h; diarrhea will be controlled within 24 h. Fluid volume will be within normal limits within 48 h as evidenced by adequate skin turgor and urine output >50 mL/h.	Assess urine output for signs of fluid deficit. Provide mouth care after vomiting to decrease nausea. Medicate for nausea and vomiting as ordered. Provide quiet environment and rest. Medicate for diarrhea as ordered; keep patient clean and dry. Give only small sips of clear liquids by mouth until vomiting subsides. Continue clear-liquid diet until diarrhea is controlled.
Altered nutrition status due to anorexia, nausea, and vomiting	Patient will ingest at least 1200 calories per day after vomiting subsides.	Offer mouth care before meals. Provide six small meals a day plus small, high-calorie snacks between meals. Weigh every 3 days and record. Keep room odor free. Provide company and quiet atmosphere for mealtime.
Diarrhea due to intestinal infection or inflammation	Infection or inflammation episode will resolve within 72 h. Diarrhea will be controlled to prevent fluid imbalance within 24 h.	Medicate with antibiotics, antiinflammatories, and antidiarrheals as ordered. Rest bowel with clear-liquid diet or bland diet as ordered. Protect anal mucosa with barrier ointment. Keep anal area clean and dry. Provide warm sitz bath to soothe anal tissues as needed. Medicate for discomfort from abdominal cramping as ordered. Provide restful environment.
Constipation due to side effects of medication, loss of ability to initiate defecation, or improper diet	Patient will have normal bowel movements regularly within 2 wk.	Increase fluid intake to 2500 mL/day unless contraindicated. Add fruit juices to diet. Increase fiber in diet; add slowly to prevent excessive gas formation. Increase exercise on a daily basis. Encourage patient to heed gastrocolic reflex and not delay defecation. Administer stool softener or bulk laxative as ordered. Monitor for fecal impaction.
Incontinence due to lack of rectal sphincter control	Patient will use bowel training program. Continence will be achieved within 1 mo.	Institute bowel training program. Provide toileting opportunity after each meal. Provide privacy and comfort for attempts at defecation. Adjust diet to provide optimal fiber in diet. Keep patient clean, dry, and odor free.
Limited coping ability due to inability to handle excessive stress	Patient will identify desired ways of coping within 3 wk. Patient will learn new coping techniques within 2 mo.	Assist to identify present coping mechanisms. Assist to identify stressors. Instruct in ways to develop more effective coping mechanisms, such as relaxation techniques, alterations in perspective, exercise, or imagery. Refer for counseling as needed.

Older Adult Care Points

Both taste and smell sensation diminish with age. Sometimes this is because of a zinc deficiency. Older adults may lose teeth because of gingival or dental disease, making eating more difficult. Dental plates may not fit correctly, making eating painful. Many older adults take a variety of medications for various conditions. The combination of these medications may greatly affect appetite and digestion. *Polypharmacy* (taking many medications) is often a cause of anorexia in older adults.

If psychosocial or cultural factors are involved, you might try offering preferred foods if possible and not detrimental to health. Meals that include a variety of colors, textures, and tastes are more appealing and enjoyable than those that are monotonous and bland.

You, a family member, or a friend can provide companionship while the patient eats. If there is a patient cafeteria or a gathering place for patients to eat together and if the patient is able to go there for meals, this can sometimes alleviate or minimize anorexia.

Assignment Considerations

Assisting With Meals

Instruct the UAP who is assisting with meals to encourage patients to eat slowly and enjoy the meal. If it is necessary to feed the patient, this should be done cheerfully and in a manner that encourages the social aspect of eating.

Older Adult Care Points

If weight loss and loss of appetite occur in an older adult without evidence of any specific cause, the possibility of depression should be investigated. A depressed older adult may find it difficult to have any interest in preparing or eating food.

Any time a patient has continual problems with eating, a dental care history and an oral cavity examination should be performed. Some people may be embarrassed by physical limitations that cause them to be awkward with eating and so will eat very little in the company of others. Others who have difficulty swallowing and are afraid of choking are afraid to eat alone but are embarrassed when eating with others. It is essential to explore each patient's causes of anorexia and feelings about eating.

Food from home often is a welcome addition to institutional meals. The person bringing it will need to be advised of any restrictions on the patient's dietary intake and the importance of adherence to these restrictions.

Assignment Considerations

Oral Rehydration for Older Adults

Institutionalized older adults are at high risk for dehydration. Instruct the UAP to directly offer small amounts of fluid, especially water, to patients throughout the day (unless contraindicated) and to assist by opening containers and positioning fluids within reach. A variety of fluids, such as juice, milk, or low-sodium liquids, should be available. Commercial hydration beverages that are amino acid based are better at maintaining hydration status in the older adult than are glucose-based drinks (Clarke, Stanhewicz, & Kenney, 2018).

Nausea and Vomiting

Persistent nausea and vomiting interferes with eating and hinders nutrition. Nausea and vomiting may be related to illness, medication side effect, anesthesia, pain, effects of cancer treatment, or stress. Transient nausea is not treated, but when the disorder persists, medication with antiemetics and administration of intravenous (IV) fluids are necessary.

Accumulation of Flatus (Gas)

Surgical intervention, mechanical obstruction, and accidental injury to the intestinal tract can cause disturbances in the passage of gas and fecal material. Whenever ingested material cannot pass through the

Assignment Considerations

Smells Exacerbate Nausea

When caring for patients who are prone to nausea, all health care personnel should be instructed to avoid using self-care products with strong scents. Some very sensitive patients may be affected by the fragrance from common products such as laundry detergent, lotions, hair products, soaps, deodorant, or makeup.

Complementary and Alternative Therapies

Ginger for Nausea

Ginger has been used for centuries in Asia to combat nausea and vomiting, motion sickness, and dyspepsia. It stimulates intestinal tone and peristalsis. It is available candied; in capsules, fluid extract, and tablets; and as a tincture or as fresh gingerroot that can be grated and used to make tea. Ginger ale is a common remedy for an upset stomach. Ginger has antiplatelet properties and should be used with caution in patients taking anticoagulant or antiplatelet medications (Micozzi, 2019).

intestinal tract as it should, the material accumulates in the stomach and the intestines. Pressure and distention occur when peristalsis is decreased or the flow of chyme (semiliquid, partially digested stomach contents) is inhibited by an obstruction. **Flatus** (gas) is formed by the action of digestive juices and bacteria on the ingested material, resulting in bloating.

Nursing management. Assisting the patient to ambulate has traditionally been the nursing intervention for sluggish peristalsis or bloating. This works for some patients, but others continue to have discomfort. If the health care provider will permit it, a slight Trendelenburg position can be useful in speeding the expulsion of gas. Placing the buttocks and legs higher than the trunk and head causes gas to rise toward the rectum, making it easier to expel flatus. For patients who do not have abdominal incisions, massaging the abdomen gently is helpful. Work up the right side, across, and down over the left colon to move gas toward the rectum. Use both hands, placing the left hand behind the right after moving the gas along the bowel before lifting the right hand. This helps prevent gas from moving backward. Advise the patient to avoid chilled or hot drinks, which may create more gas. Antiflatulent medications that contain simethicone, such as Phazyme, are helpful if the patient is not NPO.

Constipation

When constipation occurs, the stool is hard, dry, and difficult to pass. There may be a bloated feeling, and defecation may be painful. Consistency of stool is greatly influenced by the type of food eaten and the quantity of liquid consumed. A diet low in fiber or inadequate

Patient Teaching

Exercise to Reduce Gas and Bloating

Teach patients experiencing bloating and excessive gas the following exercise unless contraindicated:

- Lie on your back with your legs extended and a pillow under your knees.
- Slowly raise your right leg, bend the knee, and bring the leg down toward the abdomen.
- Hold this position for a count of 10, then slowly lower your leg back down to the bed.
- Take three slow deep breaths and repeat the exercise with the left leg.
- When you feel the need to expel gas, do so; do not hold back.
- Repeat the exercise three or four times with each leg. Perform the exercise several times a day, with rest periods between the exercise periods.

Think Critically

Identify three ways to teach a patient prevention of excessive gas postoperatively.

fluid intake predisposes to constipation. Physical inactivity, ignoring the gastrocolic reflex, stress, and some neurologic disorders affecting the nerves in the intestinal tract also may contribute to constipation. Opioid medications can also contribute to constipation by slowing peristalsis. Methylnaltrexone bromide (Relistor), naloxegol (Movantik), lubiprostone (Amitiza), and naldemedine (Symproic) are all approved by the U.S. Food and Drug Administration for treatment of opioid-induced constipation in patients with noncancer pain who are receiving opiates for chronic pain conditions (Gregorian, Lewis, & Tsu, 2017).

In addition to not passing stool regularly, signs and symptoms of constipation include hypoactive bowel sounds, abdominal distention, a firm abdomen, and abdominal discomfort or pain.

Older Adult Care Points

Constipation is a problem among many people older than 60 years. Decreased GI motility, lack of exercise, limited fluid intake, and constipating medications taken for various conditions all contribute. In much older adults, difficulty getting to the bathroom and suppression of the defecation urge may also contribute to the problem. Reliance on laxatives is common among older adults and is to be discouraged. Counsel individual patients about ways to increase dietary fiber and encourage total fluid intake (including liquids in food) of at least 2500 mL/day, if not contraindicated by the presence of cardiac or renal disease.

Nursing management. The first step is to identify the cause of constipation. Initial treatment may include a rectal suppository to induce evacuation or the administration of a laxative. A stool softener may be prescribed. Fiber and liquids are increased in the diet. If this does not resolve the problem, the patient is placed on a bulk-forming laxative such as Metamucil, to be used daily, or on daily stool softeners. If the colon has become impacted with stool, digital extraction may be needed. The patient may be medicated with a mild analgesic 30 to 60 minutes before impaction removal to decrease the discomfort of the procedure, and an oil retention enema may be given. Then apply a lubricant, such as K-Y Jelly or the anesthetic lubricant lidocaine (Xylocaine) jelly, into the rectum and around the anus and, using a gloved finger, break up and remove the feces.

Nutrition Considerations

Hydration

Maintaining adequate hydration will help keep stool moist and easier to pass. The current recommendation for daily total water intake is 3.7 liters for males and 2.7 liters for women. Total water intake includes moisture in foods and liquid beverages other than water. Fruits and vegetables have a high liquid content. Increased activity and heat exposure increase daily fluid needs.

Counsel the patient to add a lot of raw fruits and vegetables to the diet, eat more whole-grain cereals and breads, add bran to the diet, and drink a lot of fluids. Fruit juices are particularly helpful because they contain fructose, which is a natural laxative. Help the patient design an acceptable exercise program, such as walking, bicycling, running, swimming, or active sports participation. Advise the patient to heed the urge to defecate without delay.

Think Critically

List six foods high in fiber that a patient might add to the diet to combat constipation.

Diarrhea

The frequent passage of liquid or semiliquid stool is called *diarrhea.* It occurs with a variety of illnesses, food poisoning, excessive stress, and inflammation of the bowel. Mild diarrhea is not treated. If diarrhea persists for more than 24 to 48 hours or if the number of stools is so excessive that great quantities of fluid are lost, treatment should begin. Signs and symptoms include multiple liquid or semiliquid bowel movements, hyperactive bowel sounds, and abdominal cramping.

Antidiarrheal agents such as diphenoxylate hydrochloride (Lomotil), loperamide hydrochloride (Imodium), tincture of opium (paregoric), or a combination product, such as Kaopectate, are administered (see Chapter 29, Table 29.1). If the diarrhea is severe, nothing is given by mouth until it subsides to prevent increased peristalsis triggered by ingestion of food or liquid. If diarrhea is moderate, only clear liquids are permitted by mouth. Severe, long-term diarrhea may require the use of total parenteral nutrition. When diarrhea is caused by infection, stool cultures and antibiotics may be necessary. As the condition improves, the diet is advanced.

Complementary and Alternative Therapies

Probiotics for Infectious Diarrhea

When probiotics ("friendly" bacteria that are normally present in the intestinal tract) are used in conjunction with rehydration therapy, risk for diarrhea and duration of diarrhea are reduced (WebMD, 2018).

Nutrition Considerations

Foods That Thicken Stool

When a patient has severe diarrhea and is permitted to resume solids foods, slowly introduce foods that help thicken the stool, including applesauce, bananas, rice, bread, beets, potatoes without skin, oatmeal, creamy peanut butter, pasta, tapioca, and yogurt.

Nursing management. For patients with diarrhea, monitor intake and output and assess the amount of fluid lost in the stool, measuring it if needed. Administer ordered medications and replace lost fluids. Monitor the patient for electrolyte imbalances and watch for signs of dehydration, such as decreased skin turgor, thick oral secretions, and decreased urine output. Taking small amounts of an electrolyte replacement solution, or Gatorade, helps prevent imbalances. Avoiding coffee or tea helps because caffeine is a gastric stimulant and increases peristalsis. Thorough hand hygiene is essential when caring for the patient, and Standard Precautions are followed (see Appendix B). When infection is the cause of the diarrhea, follow contact precautions to prevent spread of the infection. Antibiotics kill harmful bacteria, but they also eliminate normal intestinal flora. Patients taking antibiotics can develop a bacterial infection with *Clostridium difficile (C. diff.)* that causes severe diarrhea. Isolation precautions for *C. diff.* are not the same as contact precautions (see Chapter 6).

Warm sitz baths may relieve soreness and discomfort in the tissues; help the patient cleanse the area; and avoid excessive wiping. Keeping the patient clean and dry is a high priority. Odor in the room may be reduced with a deodorizing spray and by emptying and cleaning bedpans and commodes quickly.

Clinical Cues

Frequent, loose bowel movements cause rectal irritation. Instruct or assist the patient to apply a lubricant such as A&D ointment, Aquaphor, Desitin ointment, or petroleum jelly to protect the skin and promote comfort.

Bowel Training

Severe illness, trauma, neurologic damage, or prolonged bed rest may bring about bowel incontinence. This is very embarrassing for alert patients. Make every effort to keep the patient clean and dry. Tracking the time of incontinent movements and offering toileting after each meal may help eliminate the problem. Should incontinence be persistent, the cause should be identified and then a bowel training program instituted. For bowel training, the patient should be in a private environment 20 to 40 minutes after a meal and assume a normal sitting position for defecation if possible, or a side-lying position if bedridden. You or the patient performs digital stimulation by gently inserting and rotating a gloved, well-lubricated finger into the rectal sphincter. This action should be done on a regular basis to mimic the patient's normal bowel pattern. A warm drink with lemon or prune juice may also help stimulate the bowels. Suppositories, as well as a combination of the above interventions, may also be used. Consistency and patience are vital to the success of retraining the bowel. Encourage safety and instruct the patient to call for help in getting to and from the toilet. Reassure the patient that calling for help ensures safety and provides an opportunity to observe the progress of the training program.

Get Ready for the NCLEX® Examination!

Key Points

- Peristalsis moves food through the GI tract.
- The process by which nutrients are used in the body after digestion and absorption is called *metabolism.*
- *Anabolism* is the building of body tissues from the nutrients. *Catabolism* is the breakdown of larger molecules into smaller molecules so that energy is available.
- The gallbladder stores bile and can be removed without harm to the body.
- The pancreas provides enzymes for digestion and insulin, and daily replacement of these substances must occur if the pancreas is removed. The secretion of lipase from the pancreas decreases with age, altering fat digestion.
- Problems of the GI system include infection, inflammation, trauma, and structural defects. Continued irritation and inflammation of the GI mucosa can lead to intestinal bleeding and increased peristalsis with inadequate absorption of nutrients.

- Immunization for hepatitis A and B prevents liver disease. Hepatitis B and C are risk factors for liver cancer.
- Controlling alcohol consumption helps prevent cirrhosis of the liver and pancreatitis.
- If damage to the liver is halted before all tissue is affected, the liver can regenerate.
- Check urine color for darkness (color of tea) and check stool for whitish or clay color; these findings suggest that the bile ducts may be blocked.
- Taste and smell diminish with age, and the gradual loss of these senses may decrease appetite. Poor dentition may make eating difficult for the older adult.
- Medications can affect appetite and digestion.
- Ambulation and oral simethicone are helpful in reducing gas.
- Severe diarrhea can cause fluid and electrolyte imbalances and dehydration.
- Increasing fiber, fluids, and exercise helps prevent or relieve constipation.
- Bowel training is designed to mimic and restore the patient's normal bowel pattern.

Additional Learning Resources

SG Go to your Study Guide for additional learning activities to help you master this chapter content.

Go to your Evolve website (http://evolve.elsevier.com/deWit/medsurg) for the following FREE learning resources:

- Animations, audio, and video
- Answers and rationales for questions and activities
- Glossary with pronunciations in English and Spanish
- Interactive Review Questions and more!

Review Questions for the NCLEX® Examination

1. A common cause of liver toxicity is:
   1. daily hydrochlorothiazide administration for hypertension.
   2. regular consumption of a high-fat diet throughout life.
   3. long-term smoking of a pack of cigarettes per day.
   4. taking extra-strength acetaminophen at doses of 4500 mg per day.

   NCLEX Client Need: Physiological Integrity: Pharmacological Therapies
2. Measures used to teach patients to prevent gastrointestinal ulcers include:
   1. limiting the amount of routine alcohol consumption.
   2. refraining from the use of aspirin for a headache.
   3. taking an H_2 inhibitor to decrease stomach acid daily.
   4. eating hot, spicy food at least once each day.

   NCLEX Client Need: Health Promotion and Maintenance
3. You are planning care for several patients who had diagnostic testing. Which patient will require the most time for postprocedural care?
   1. Patient who had an ultrasound
   2. Patient who had hepatobiliary scintigraphy
   3. Patient who had a liver biopsy
   4. Patient who had a *Helicobacter pylori* antibody test

   NCLEX Client Need: Physiological Integrity: Reduction of Risk Potential
4. You are preparing a patient for a liver biopsy. Which nursing interventions should be included? (*Select all that apply.*)
   1. Attending to patient's fears and anxiety
   2. Checking for a signed consent form for the procedure
   3. Assessing for dehydration and electrolyte imbalance
   4. Positioning on right side
   5. Checking coagulation studies for bleeding problems
   6. Noting any allergy to local anesthetics

   NCLEX Client Need: Physiological Integrity: Reduction of Risk Potential
5. An 82-year-old patient is undergoing bowel preparation for a diagnostic procedure. What are potential complications of the bowel prep? (*Select all that apply.*)
   1. Constipation
   2. Rashes
   3. Dehydration
   4. Muscle cramps
   5. Chest pains
   6. Hypotension

   NCLEX Client Need: Physiological Integrity: Pharmacological Therapies
6. A decreased secretion of intrinsic factor is a physiologic change associated with the aging process; therefore, you suspect decreased intrinsic factor should assess for which behavior?
   1. A refusal to eat salty or sweet foods
   2. A change in stools after eating fatty foods
   3. Fatigue and activity intolerance
   4. Difficulties with mastication

   NCLEX Client Need: Physiological Integrity: Physiological Adaptation
7. Which laboratory values would you use to assess liver function?
   1. CBC, BUN, creatinine
   2. Lipase, amylase, WBC
   3. Troponin, CPK, myoglobin
   4. ALT, ammonia, INR

   NCLEX Client Need: Physiological Integrity: Reduction of Risk Potential
8. You emphasize the importance of eating natural sources of fiber to a patient who has frequent constipation. Which patient statement indicates effective health teaching?
   1. "I will consider eating more white bread."
   2. "I will drink fluids only while consuming meals."
   3. "I will add more milk to my morning cereal."
   4. "I will eat more fruits and vegetables."

   NCLEX Client Need: Health Promotion and Maintenance
9. A 30-year-old woman is admitted with complaints of severe nausea and vomiting over the past 2 days. On admission she is hypotensive and extremely weak. What is the priority problem?
   1. Altered breathing pattern
   2. Altered activity tolerance
   3. Deficient fluid volume
   4. Altered cardiac output

   NCLEX Client Need: Physiological Integrity: Physiological Adaptation

10. A nurse is discussing healthy lifestyle measures with a group of older adults during a senior seminar. What instruction(s) should you include as accurate information? *(Select all that apply.)*
  1. Consume sufficient fiber.
  2. Eat a normal, well-balanced diet.
  3. Exercise regularly.
  4. Drink at least three glasses of fluids a day.
  5. Take laxatives regularly.

  NCLEX Client Need: Health Promotion and Maintenance

11. An older adult woman of Puerto Rican descent is admitted for persistent anorexia and dehydration. There are no apparent underlying organic causes for loss of appetite. Which intervention(s) would be culturally appropriate? *(Select all that apply.)*
  1. Determine food preferences.
  2. Encourage family visits.
  3. Provide small amounts of food and fluid frequently.
  4. Consider parenteral nutrition.
  5. Consult a dietitian and speech therapy.

  NCLEX Client Need: Psychosocial Integrity

12. A patient who is dehydrated because of vomiting and diarrhea needs IV fluid therapy. The health care provider orders 1000 mL normal saline to infuse over 6 hours. The drop factor is 10 gtt/mL. You calculate the rate to infuse per gravity at ______________ drops per minute. *(Fill in the blank.)*

  NCLEX Client Need: Physiological Integrity: Pharmacological Therapies

Critical Thinking Questions

Scenario A

Mr. Achaba, 68 years old, was admitted with jaundice, abdominal distention, abdominal pain, and malaise. He is to undergo an ERCP. He is apprehensive and frightened about what may be wrong with him.

1. What is involved in an ERCP procedure?
2. Explain pretest care to help alleviate Mr. Achaba's apprehension.
3. What is included in post-test care?
4. What could be possible causes of his jaundice?

Scenario B

Ms. Hopgood is a resident in your extended care facility. She has been losing weight, has no appetite, and is becoming more withdrawn. Her daughter has a new job and is not able to visit as many times a week as she had been.

1. What assessments would you think appropriate for Ms. Hopgood at this time?
2. What nursing interventions could you institute that might improve her nutritional status?
3. What could you do to help her loneliness now that her daughter cannot visit as often?

Scenario C

You are making home visits to an older adult to check his blood pressure. During the visit he tells you that he is having trouble with constipation.

1. What questions should you ask to further assess the problem?
2. Why is constipation a common problem for people older than 60 years?
3. Would you recommend the use of an over-the-counter laxative? Why or why not?
4. What dietary and lifestyle recommendations would you make?

Care of Patients With Disorders of the Upper Gastrointestinal System

28

http://evolve.elsevier.com/deWit/medsurg

Objectives

Theory

1. Discuss management of patients undergoing bariatric surgery.
2. Compare the signs and symptoms of oral, esophageal, and stomach cancer.
3. Illustrate the cause of gastroesophageal reflux disease (GERD).
4. Explain the etiology and prognosis for Barrett esophagus.
5. Describe the pathophysiology, means of medical diagnosis, and treatment for gastritis.
6. Contrast the difference between the care of a patient with a nasogastric tube for decompression and the care of a patient with a feeding tube.
7. Determine reasons why total parenteral nutrition might be prescribed for a patient and describe necessary precautions to take during administration.

Clinical Practice

8. Implement a teaching plan for a patient who has GERD.
9. Provide appropriate care for a patient with dysphagia.
10. Plan postoperative care for a patient having gastric surgery.
11. Demonstrate proper care of a patient with a Salem sump tube for gastric decompression.
12. Manage a tube feeding for a patient receiving formula via a feeding pump.

Key Terms

achlorhydria (ă-chlŏr-HĪ-drē-ă, p. 679)
anastomosis (ă-năs-tŏ-MŌ-sĭs, p. 674)
bariatric (BĀ-rē-ĂT-rĭk, p. 663)
dumping syndrome (DŬM-pĭng SĬN-drōm p. 663)
dyspepsia (dĭs-PĔP-sē-ă, p. 668)
dysphagia (dĭs-FĀ-jē-ă, p. 665)
Helicobacter pylori (hĕl-ĭ-cō-BĂC-tĕr pī-LŌ-rē, p. 671)
hematemesis (hē-mă-TĔM-ĕ-sĭs, p. 673)
melena (mĕ-LĒ-nă, p. 678)
roux-en-Y (roo-ĕn-WĪ, p. 663)
stomatitis (stō-mă-TĪ-tĭs, p. 664)
vagotomy (vă-GŎT-ŏ-mē, p. 674)

Concepts Covered in This Chapter

- Fluid and Electrolytes
- Cellular Regulation
- Nutrition
- Inflammation
- Pain
- Stress
- Health Promotion
- Safety

EATING DISORDERS

ANOREXIA NERVOSA

Anorexia nervosa is classified as a psychological disorder (see Chapter 47), but it has serious nutritional consequences. In many contemporary cultures, the emphasis on a slim body has influenced young women's body image. A patient with anorexia nervosa refuses to eat adequate quantities of food and is in danger of literally starving to death. Although it is a psychiatric disorder, the patient may be admitted to the medical floor for treatment of malnutrition by enteral or parenteral therapy. Diagnosis requires extensive interviewing and treatment—including behavior modification and nutrition support—which may take months to years.

BULIMIA NERVOSA

Bulimia nervosa is another psychological disorder covered in Chapter 47. A person who has bulimia nervosa consumes large quantities of food and then induces vomiting to get rid of it so that weight is not gained. Laxatives may be taken to purge the system after an eating binge. Some patients with anorexia nervosa also have bulimia nervosa. Some individuals practice bulimia occasionally, without harm. When it is practiced frequently, it can lead to severe fluid and electrolyte imbalances, starvation, dental problems, and death. Treatment of bulimia includes psychotherapy, antidepressant medication, and behavior modification.

OBESITY

Obesity is a worldwide problem and is particularly prevalent in industrialized nations. More than 40% of adults in the United States are obese as defined by a body mass index (BMI) of 30 or above (Warren, Beck, & Rayburn, 2018). Obesity is a known risk factor for cardiovascular disease and associated death. Type 2 diabetes and certain cancers are also linked to obesity. Children are showing a continued trend for increasing obesity. There is an ongoing search to determine a possible genetic predisposition to this disorder. Preventing obesity and encouraging healthy and nutrition-dense foods are goals of *Healthy People 2030.*

Etiology and Pathophysiology

Several factors must interact for obesity to occur: a diet of foods high in calories and fat, lack of exercise, and overconsumption of food. There may be a genetic predisposition as well. Some medications increase appetite. Known contributors to obesity include readily available high-calorie prepackaged foods, the prevalence of high-fructose corn syrup in foods, consumption of sodas, and high-fat fast food and "supersized" portions available in restaurants.

For some people overeating is a reaction to stress; for others overeating is a substitute for absent pleasures. Some obese people seem to metabolize nutrients differently from others. The way a person develops fat cells and deposits fat is another factor in obesity. Family lifestyle is most likely a factor because obesity seems to occur among family members.

Signs and Symptoms

A person is considered obese if they weigh more than 20% above the ideal weight for their height, age, and body type. Approximately 3 million Americans are severely (morbidly) obese, meaning that they are 100% above their ideal body weight, or have a BMI greater than 40.

Obese patients should be counseled to lose weight to help prevent the many diseases in which obesity is a contributing factor. Complications of obesity include the following:

- Diabetes mellitus
- Hypertension
- Hyperlipidemia
- Coronary artery disease
- Obstructive sleep apnea
- Cholelithiasis
- Cancer
- Arthritis with back and/or knee problems
- Increased susceptibility to infectious disease and decreased wound healing.

? Think Critically

Your friend, who is overweight, asks your opinion about the effectiveness and safety of over-the-counter "diet" pills. How would you respond?

Diagnosis

To determine whether a patient is obese, the following measurements are used:

Table 28.1 Obesity Definitions

Underweight	BMI <18.5
Normal	BMI 18.5 to <25
Overweight	BMI 25 to <30
Obese	BMI ≥30
Classification of Obese	
Class 1	BMI 30 to <35
Class 2	BMI 35 to <40
Class 3	BMI ≥40

- Height and weight chart: if more than 20% above ideal body weight for age and body build, the patient is considered obese.
- Measure the waist and then the hip circumference. Calculate the waist-to-hip ratio (waist measurement divided by hip measurement). If the ratio is more than 1.0 in men or 0.8 in women, it indicates that the person is overweight. This is a more accurate indicator for obesity in the older adult.
- A BMI of more than 30 indicates obesity (Table 28.1) (see the BMI table on the Evolve website).

$$\text{BMI} = \frac{\text{Weight (kg)}}{\text{Height (m}^2\text{)}}$$

Thyroid function should be determined to confirm that hypothyroidism is not a cause of the weight gain.

Treatment

Dietary control and exercise are the main treatments for obesity. A general health assessment should be conducted before a patient is placed on a weight reduction diet. A health care provider will usually prescribe a lower calorie diet and exercise. The patient is taught ways to change thinking about food and weight. Those with a BMI greater than 40 may have surgery to achieve weight reduction if they meet established criteria. Participation in a support group and behavior modification with some sort of reward for weight loss are part of the total treatment plan. Teaching stress reduction and alternate ways of coping are essential to success. Medications that suppress appetite or block fat absorption may be used on a short-term basis. Orlistat (Xenical, Allī) inhibits lipase, causing fats to remain partially undigested and unabsorbed. Gastrointestinal (GI) side effects of orlistat include diarrhea (sometimes uncontrolled), abdominal cramping, and nausea. Lorcaserin (Belviq) can cause a 5% weight loss within 1 year for those for whom it works. It has a potential serious side effect of serotonin syndrome if taken along with selective serotonin reuptake inhibitor (SSRI) antidepressants or monoamine oxidase inhibitor (MAOI) medications. Phentermine-topiramate (Qsymia) has been found to be safe for 2 years of usage. A 12-week trial is used to determine whether it will work for the patient. Naltrexone ER/bupropion ER (Contrave) is an appetite suppressant that interacts with many depression medications. It is used as an adjunct to dietary modifications. Liraglutide (Saxenda) is also an appetite suppressant and is administered subcutaneously daily. These drugs are not to be used during pregnancy. The American Medical Association designated obesity as a chronic disease in 2013. This designation has helped speed up research studies for treatment and prevention (Garvey et al., 2016).

Older Adult Care Points

Older adults may become obese because of decreased mobility from arthritis or other joint disorders. Cooking and eating are less appealing if the person is living alone, and snacking on junk food may replace meals. Metabolic rate slows with age, and a decreased calorie intake is needed to maintain a normal weight.

Bariatric surgery. **Bariatric** surgery is considered when BMI is greater than 40 or BMI is 35 or greater with one or more obesity-related complications. The patient undergoes extensive counseling and assessment. The patient must agree to modify their lifestyle and follow the stringent regimen required to lose weight and keep weight off. Three common types of bariatric surgery are gastric restrictive, malabsorptive, and gastric restrictive combined with malabsorptive surgery.

Restrictive procedures. The most commonly performed restrictive surgical procedure is *laparoscopic sleeve gastrectomy* (LSG). A portion of the stomach is removed, leaving a banana-shaped pouch. This restricts the amount of intake. The removal of the stomach tissue also reduces the amount of ghrelin produced, which causes a decrease in appetite. *Adjustable gastric banding* is a laparoscopic procedure performed by placing an inflatable band around the fundus of the stomach. The band is inflated and deflated via a subcutaneous port to change the size of the stomach as the patient loses weight (Fig. 28.1, *A*).

Malabsorptive and combination procedures. The **roux-en-Y** gastric bypass (RYGB) limits the stomach size, and the duodenum and part of the jejunum are bypassed. This limits the absorption of calories (Fig. 28.1, *C*).

Biliopancreatic diversion with a duodenal switch creates a more tubular gastric "sleeve" with connection to a small part of the duodenum. Long-term problems can result from the decrease in the amount of food, vitamins, and minerals that can be absorbed (Fig. 28.1, *B,D*).

Complications. With the RYGB procedure, there is danger of leakage of stomach contents into the abdomen in the early postoperative period. Later, gastric stretching may cause the staple line to break and a leak to occur. Signs and symptoms include abdominal pain, nausea and vomiting, tachycardia, fever, and hypotension. An upper gastrointestinal (UGI) series or computed tomography (CT) scan can diagnose the problem. The band in the vertical banding procedure may erode into the stomach over time and cause leakage. RYGB patients are also at risk for **dumping syndrome**, which results in nausea, weakness, sweating, and diarrhea that occurs after meals. Other complications of major surgery may occur in the respiratory and cardiovascular systems (see Chapter 5 for complications of surgery). Patients who are obese have a greater risk of pulmonary dysfunction, thrombus formation, and death. Approximately one-third of patients who undergo bariatric surgery develop gallstones because of the rapid weight loss.

All bariatric surgery patients are at risk of nutritional deficiencies. Those who have the RYGB procedure are most likely to develop deficiencies of iron, vitamin B_{12},

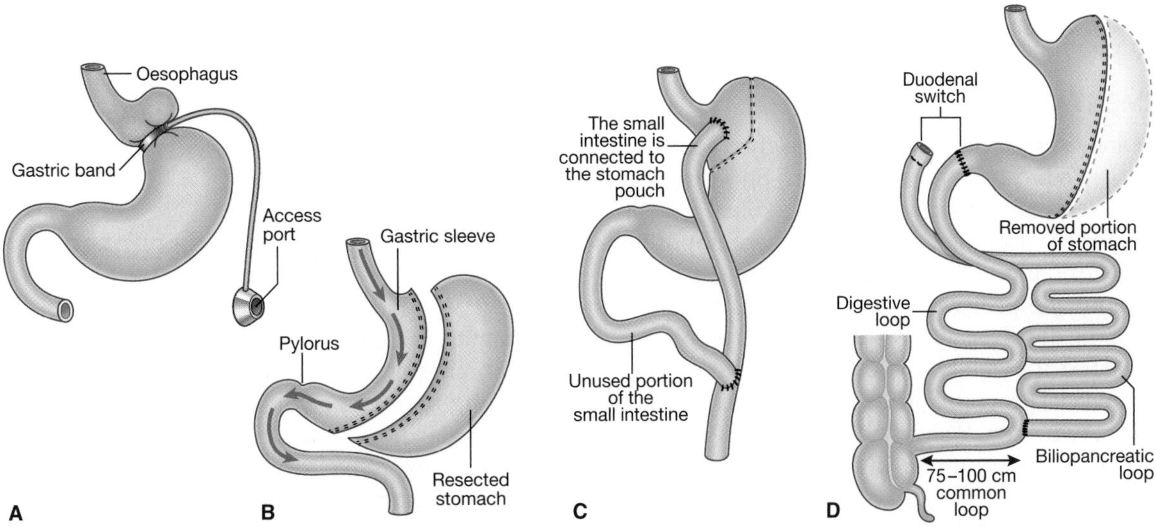

Fig. 28.1 Bariatric surgical procedures. **A,** Laparoscopic banding, with the option of a reservoir band and subcutaneous access to restrict the stomach further after compensatory expansion has occurred. **B,** Sleeve gastrectomy. **C,** Roux-en-Y gastric bypass. **D,** Biliopancreatic diversion with duodenal switch. (From Ralston SH, Penman ID, Strachan MWJ, et al.: *Davidson's principles and practice of medicine*, ed 23, London, 2018, Elsevier LTD.)

calcium, and folate. Supplements must be taken for life. Support by a dietitian is very important both preoperatively and postoperatively.

? Think Critically

What effect might a RYGB have on an individual's nutritional status? Why? What might be the physical long-term consequences?

NURSING MANAGEMENT OF OBESITY

ASSESSMENT (DATA COLLECTION)

Data collection includes establishing whether there is a family history of obesity, determining contributing factors, and obtaining an accurate record of eating patterns for a 7-day period. Physical assessment includes measuring weight and height, calculating BMI, and taking a skin fold thickness measurement. A general health assessment is performed.

NURSING DIAGNOSIS AND PLANNING

Examples of problem statements relevant to the care of patients who are obese include the following:

- Altered body image due to excess weight.
- Inadequate health management due to excess weight.
- Decreased self-esteem due to excess weight.
- Altered mobility due to excess weight.
- Potential for social isolation due to limited mobility.
- Weight above recommended BMI.

Goals should be long term, and expected outcomes might include the following:

- Patient will make positive statements about decreasing body size.
- Patient will consume less fatty food and more fruits and vegetables.
- Patient will verbalize feelings of self-worth.
- Patient will demonstrate understanding of treatment plan.
- Patient will increase physical activity as tolerated.

IMPLEMENTATION

The diet and exercise plan should be designed according to the patient's lifestyle and preferences. Encourage the patient to keep an eating and exercise diary. Weekly meetings for counseling and evaluation are important to provide guidance. Offer support by being available to talk about the positive aspects and frustrations of staying on the diet. Discourage fad diets and emphasize the importance of a well-balanced, nutritious, low-calorie diet. Commercial programs are available to assist patients with weight reduction. Weight Watchers and TOPS (Take Off Pounds Sensibly) are two commercial programs that have shown good long-term results with maintenance of normal weight.

Preoperative and postoperative care for a patient having bariatric surgery depends on the type of surgical procedure performed, but general principles are similar to those for other types of abdominal or abdominal laparoscopic surgery. Because of the weight and size of the patient, lifting apparatus and bariatric-size bed and chair must be available. Hospitalization may be for 1 to 5 days depending on the procedure and the patient. If a nasogastric (NG) tube is in place, do not reposition it because you might disrupt the suture line. Feedings are designed in consultation with a dietitian; you would anticipate feeding progression in the early postoperative period, then moving to multiple small meals, a balanced meal plan, and possibly parenteral nutrition (PN) in high-risk patients (Garvey et al., 2016). For example, feedings begin with 1 ounce of clear liquid at a time, advancing to pureed foods, thinned soups, and milk. Doses of multivitamins and other supplements are administered as needed per individual. The diet is increased in 1-ounce increments taken over 5 minutes until the patient's appetite is satisfied. The diet is maintained for 6 weeks and then progressed to regular foods. Nausea, vomiting, and discomfort may occur, especially if too many liquids are ingested. After hospitalization, the support of a registered dietitian is recommended, as this increases the amount of weight loss for most patients. Sugar in any form is avoided, as are concentrated sweets such as fruit juice; juice (if approved by the health care provider) should be diluted. In addition to being high in calories, concentrated sugar can cause dumping syndrome. For the first 2 months, calorie intake is between 300 and 600 calories a day; thereafter no more than 1000 calories a day should be consumed. The patient remains under medical supervision to monitor for vitamin deficiency or malnutrition. Supplementation with multivitamins, calcium, vitamin D, and vitamin B_{12} is taken routinely. The patient is monitored to ensure that adequate protein is being consumed.

EVALUATION

The patient's diet and exercise diary should be evaluated each week if possible. Weight is tracked on a graph to show progress in weight loss. If the outcomes are not being met, the plan's interventions must be reconsidered. Bariatric surgery patients do best with group support.

UPPER GASTROINTESTINAL DISORDERS

STOMATITIS

Stomatitis is a generalized inflammation of the mucous membranes of the mouth. Causes include trauma from ill-fitting dentures or malocclusions of the teeth, poor oral hygiene, and nutritional deficiencies. Excessive smoking, excessive drinking of alcohol, pathogenic microorganisms, radiation therapy, and drugs (especially anticonvulsants and those used in chemotherapy for malignancies) are other contributors to the problem.

Common symptoms of stomatitis include pain and swelling of the oral mucosa, increased salivation or excessive dryness, severe halitosis, and sometimes fever. Small crater-like aphthous ulcers, commonly called *canker sores,* may appear in the mouth.

Treatment of stomatitis is chiefly symptomatic unless a specific infectious causative agent is identified. Nursing measures to control the symptoms of stomatitis—including special mouth care, artificial saliva, and diet—are discussed in Chapter 8.

Complementary and Alternative Therapies

Lysine for Canker Sores

Canker sores from food sensitivities or stomach upset often can be healed more quickly by taking the dietary supplement lysine three or four times a day. This often helps reduce the length of time of a "fever blister" on the lips as well.

DYSPHAGIA

Dysphagia means difficulty swallowing. It is the most common symptom of disorders of the esophagus and varies from a mild sensation that something is sticking in the throat to a complete inability to swallow solids or liquids. Tumors, esophageal diverticula, inflammation, or motility disorders from a neurologic disorder may cause swallowing problems. If the patient is experiencing choking or difficulty with swallowing, they are kept on nothing-by-mouth (NPO) status, and swallowing ability is evaluated at the bedside by a nurse or a speech therapist. If additional information is needed, a modified barium swallow test may be ordered to determine the specific cause. Videofluoroscopy is used during the test to visualize the swallowing process.

Treatment and Nursing Management

Have the patient take some "practice swallows" before beginning a meal or giving oral medications for the first time. Watch to see that the larynx rises with each swallow. Observe the kinds of food the patient can tolerate and the conditions under which difficulties are experienced. Knowing the consistency and temperature of the foods most easily ingested by the patient is helpful. Some patients may choke on liquids but will tolerate soft and semisolid foods. Others may have the feeling that high-fiber foods are not moving past a certain point in the esophagus. Measures that may be helpful in relieving dysphagia include instructing the patient to chew food more thoroughly or to eat semisoft or pureed foods. Drinking liquids throughout the meal may help; however, **liquids will cause many patients to choke. If thin liquids are a problem, adding thickener to liquids makes them easier to swallow.** Sitting upright with the head forward and the neck flexed with the chin slightly tucked aids in swallowing. Head position may be altered, depending on the type of problem present. A speech pathologist should be consulted to design the most effective therapy for the patient.

Older Adult Care Points

Older patients who have experienced a stroke may have impaired swallowing ability. Swallowing pills is often difficult for this age group. Instruct older adults to take a drink of water, swallow, place the pill on the back of the tongue, take another drink of water, tuck the chin down slightly, swallow, and then drink at least 6 to 8 ounces of water.

The patient may be a candidate for neuromuscular electrical stimulation (NMES). One type of NMES device stimulates muscle at rest, to compensate for muscle wasting. Another NMES device is used for patients who have swallowing issues related to neurologic disorders such as stroke. Some helpful strategies to improve swallowing include licking lollipops to strengthen tongue movements, practicing vowel sounds to stimulate movement, and sucking or blowing through a straw to strengthen the soft palate. Meals should be served in a relaxing atmosphere with pleasant surroundings and relief from emotional stress.

Problem statements for the patient with swallowing problems include the following:

- Altered swallowing ability.
- Altered nutrition: less than body requirements.
- Aspiration risk.
- Potential for altered fluid volume.

Both acute and chronic dysphagia are likely to produce nutritional deficiencies and electrolyte imbalances. If the dysphagia is such that the patient cannot swallow enough food for adequate nutrition, tube feeding may be indicated. This sometimes is necessary when the dysphagia is the result of cerebral damage, as in cerebrovascular accident.

Clinical Cues

When your patient has a swallowing problem, the oral suction equipment should always be readily available. Aspiration of food or mucus can occur quickly. The patient or family should be taught how to quickly use the oral tonsil tip suction apparatus (Yankauer). Aspiration can cause pneumonia; the patient's respiratory status should be monitored after a choking episode.

If the patient cannot swallow anything because of a neurologic condition (see Chapters 21 and 23) or if the esophagus is obstructed and cannot be corrected surgically, the patient must have a gastrostomy tube placed. An opening in the wall of the stomach is created, and a feeding tube is sutured in place. Nursing interventions for feeding tubes are discussed later in this chapter.

CANCER OF THE ORAL CAVITY

Etiology, Pathophysiology, and Signs and Symptoms

Approximately 51,000 people will develop oral cancer in the United States annually, and 10,000 will die from oral cavity and oropharyngeal cancers (American Cancer Society, 2018b). Although the specific cause is unknown, oral or throat cancer is curable if discovered early. Oral cancers are primarily squamous cell carcinomas. Cell mutation occurs until an area of cells becomes neoplastic. A genetic factor is most likely present. Oral and pharyngeal cancer risks are cigarette smoking, use of smokeless tobacco, pipe smoking, and heavy alcohol use. The effect of using electronic cigarettes is not yet known. Infection with the human papillomavirus (HPV) is another risk factor. Although smoking is on the decline, HPV is on the rise. Leukoplakia, a precancerous lesion, may occur on the tongue or mucosa. Dental examinations should include inspection for this lesion. Sores or discolorations on the lips or in the mouth that do not heal within 2 weeks should be checked by a health care provider. The mnemonic RULE (red, ulcerated, lump, extending for 3 or more weeks) identifies the need for further testing.

Diagnosis and Treatment

Diagnosis is made by physical examination and biopsy. Oral cancer treatment varies depending on the structures involved. Surgery and/or radiation are the most common treatments. Targeted therapies are in use to treat the specific tissue involved and to avoid some of the side effects of conventional chemotherapy. *Mandibulectomy* (removal of the mandible), *hemiglossectomy* (removal of half of the tongue), or *glossectomy* (removal of the tongue) with resection of other parts of the mouth may be necessary. If the cancer has spread to the cervical lymph nodes, radical or modified neck dissection is performed. This surgery involves wide excision of the primary tumor with removal of the regional lymph nodes, the deep cervical lymph nodes, and lymph channels. A tracheostomy accompanies these procedures to protect the airway (see Chapter 13). A drain is placed to prevent fluid accumulation. Tube feedings are used for as long as swallowing is difficult.

Targeted modulated radiation and chemotherapy may be indicated depending on the degree of involvement of the lymph nodes and whether margins of the surgical specimen are clear of cancer cells. Chemotherapeutic agents used may include 5-fluorouracil, docetaxel, cisplatin, carboplatin, paclitaxel, and hydroxyurea singularly or in combination.

Nursing Management

Postoperative care includes close monitoring of respiratory status, airway, and oxygenation. Cold packs and elevation of the head prevent excessive swelling in the neck that might compress the airway, circulation, and nerves. Aseptic wound care and tracheostomy care are provided. Nutritional support is an ongoing concern and is very important in the healing process. Many of these patients are malnourished before surgery. See Chapter 8 for the specific care of a patient undergoing radiation and/or chemotherapy.

? Think Critically

You are caring for a young woman who was recently informed that she will need surgery and radiation treatment for oral cancer. What are the implications for her sense of body image and psychological well-being?

CANCER OF THE ESOPHAGUS

Etiology and Pathophysiology

Squamous cell carcinoma of the esophagus was the most common type of throat cancer, with cigarette smoking combined with heavy alcohol consumption as a major cause until the 1970s. Cigarette smoke and alcohol both irritate the mucosa of the esophagus. In the decades since the 1970s, reflux has replaced tobacco and alcohol as a primary irritant leading to adenocarcinoma of the esophagus. About 17,300 new cases were diagnosed in 2018 (American Cancer Society, 2018a). The cancer is usually well advanced when discovered. The tumor is either adenocarcinoma or squamous cell cancer.

Gastroesophageal reflux disease (GERD) is a cause of Barrett esophagus, which is a precancerous condition. The cellular changes caused by irritation of the stomach fluids may eventually become malignant. About 0.5% of patients with Barrett esophagus develop esophageal cancer each year. Care is focused on measures encouraging the prevention of GERD and on regular checkups. Periodic endoscopy and biopsy are performed for those who show dysplasia in the esophagus.

Signs, Symptoms, and Diagnosis

Signs and symptoms of esophageal cancer may include progressive dysphagia, hoarseness, regurgitation of foods, foul breath, and persistent cough. At first the dysphagia occurs only with solids such as meat, but then it happens with soft foods and eventually even with liquids. Pain occurs late in the disease; is substernal, epigastric, or in the back; and occurs with swallowing. Weight loss is typical. Barium swallow with fluoroscopy may show a narrowed esophagus. Definitive diagnosis is by esophagogastroduodenoscopy (EGD) and biopsy. Staging may be done by imaging studies such as CT scan or positron emission tomography.

? Think Critically

A 76-year-old Chinese man complains of progressive difficulty swallowing and fullness of the throat. When interacting with this patient, what would be the most effective approach to communicating important medical information?

Treatment

Appropriate treatment is decided based on the stage and type of cancer. Localized lesions can be removed with endoscopic mucosal resection. Other treatment options are endoscopic ablative therapy such as photodynamic therapy, radiotherapy ablation, or chemoradiation. An esophagectomy, or removal of sections of the esophagus and reconstruction with part of the stomach, is performed

Think Critically

A patient who smokes is awaiting surgery for esophageal cancer and wants to smoke. How would you approach the situation?

with extensive disease. Radiofrequency ablation uses bursts of radiofrequency energy to burn away abnormal cells. Photodynamic therapy uses a medication that causes damaged cells to be sensitive to light; a laser is used to destroy the damaged cells while preserving normal tissue. Endoscopic mucosal resection is a procedure in which a saline solution is injected under the lining of abnormal tissue, which makes it easier to suction away (Masab, 2018). For patients who have advanced-stage cancer, palliative care may include a combination of external beam radiation, chemotherapy, esophageal dilation, electrocoagulation, photodynamic therapy, and the insertion of expanding metal stents to relieve severe dysphagia (American Cancer Society, 2017).

Nursing Management

Postoperative care is the same as for any patient having gastroendoscopic, thoracic, or abdominal surgery, depending on the surgical procedure. Maintaining a patent airway is the top priority.

Nursing interventions focus on promoting adequate respiration, providing a way to adequately communicate, ensuring adequate nutritional intake to promote wound healing, and attention to pain and discomfort. Nutrition is initially supplied by parenteral fluids. Oral intake begins with small amounts of water every hour while the patient is awake, with gradual progression to small, frequent, bland meals. The patient should be upright when eating to prevent regurgitation. After esophageal resection, pain, increased temperature, and dyspnea may indicate leakage of the feeding into the mediastinum. Intolerance of food is evidenced by vomiting and abdominal distention. The patient may need a feeding tube for several weeks or a gastrostomy tube to sustain nutrition.

HIATUS (HIATAL) HERNIA (DIAPHRAGMATIC HERNIA)

Etiology and Pathophysiology

Loss of muscle strength and tone, factors that cause increased intra-abdominal pressure (such as obesity, ascites, or multiple pregnancies), and congenital defects contribute to the formation of a hiatal hernia. Hiatal hernia is the result of a defect in the wall of the diaphragm where the esophagus passes through; this creates protrusion of part of the stomach or the lower part of the esophagus up into the thoracic cavity. Hernias are classified as type I sliding and types II, III, and IV paraesophageal. In a type I hernia, the gastroesophageal junction is located above the diaphragm. Paraesophageal hernias have displacement of the fundus of the stomach or other abdominal contents into a hernia sac. Most hiatal hernias are type I.

Signs and Symptoms

Often there are no signs and symptoms of hiatal hernia unless there is reflux of stomach acid. Signs of reflux include indigestion, belching, and substernal or epigastric pain or feelings of pressure after eating caused by the reflux of gastric fluid into the esophagus. Regurgitation of a hot, sour liquid coming into the throat or mouth may occur. Nighttime coughing may awaken the patient. The symptoms are more severe when the patient lies down.

Diagnosis and Treatment

Hiatal hernia is diagnosed by a UGI series. Treatment includes weight reduction; avoidance of tight-fitting clothes around the abdomen; administration of antacids, histamine (H_2)–receptor antagonists, or proton pump inhibitors (PPIs); and elevating the head of the bed 6 to 8 inches. The patient is instructed not to eat within 3 hours of going to bed. Intake of alcohol, chocolate, caffeine, and fatty food is limited, and smoking should be avoided. Ingestion of fats relaxes the sphincter, allowing reflux. Occasionally a patient with reflux esophagitis, which is caused by the hernia, may bleed extensively. If bleeding or discomfort cannot be controlled, surgical correction of the hernia is required. Nissen fundoplication, Belsey fundoplication, or Hill repair are surgical treatments.

Nursing Management

Patients with hiatal hernia are taught ways to prevent pain and reflux. If weight is above normal, encourage weight reduction. Remind the patient to stay upright for 2 hours after eating and not to eat 3 hours before bedtime. Lifting or moving heavy items is to be avoided. If the head of the bed cannot be raised, a wedge pillow should be used to elevate the upper body; this position helps prevent reflux and assists gravity in maintaining the gastroesophageal junction and stomach in the abdominal cavity. Prescribed H_2-receptor antagonists or PPIs should be taken at bedtime to prevent reflux and damage from acid entering the esophagus. The patient should avoid foods that cause bloating, which increases abdominal pressure. Increased abdominal pressure may push the stomach upward through the diaphragmatic defect.

GASTROESOPHAGEAL REFLUX DISEASE

Etiology and Pathophysiology

GERD is a syndrome, not a disease. Ninety percent of patients with GERD have a hiatal hernia. GERD occurs equally in men and women. It is caused by transient relaxation of the lower esophageal sphincter and may accompany a hiatal hernia. The relaxation allows fluids or food to reflux into the esophagus from the stomach. Delayed stomach emptying is another factor. Certain foods and medications contribute to this mechanical problem. Being overweight is common among patients with GERD. GERD may contribute to bronchoconstriction and asthma symptoms because of irritation of the upper airway by gastric secretions. About 75% of patients with asthma have GERD (Harding, 2018).

Signs and Symptoms

Heartburn (**dyspepsia**) and reflux are the most common symptoms of GERD. Other symptoms may include chest pain, coughing, dysphagia, belching, flatulence, and bloating after eating. Symptoms are aggravated by lying down.

Diagnosis

GERD is diagnosed by the common clinical symptoms. If more alarming symptoms such as dysphagia, anorexia, or upper GI bleeding are present, EGD is performed. Other tests such as an esophageal manometry, ambulatory 24-hour pH monitoring, or radionuclide measurement of gastric emptying are used when the patient is not responding to medical therapy. Esophageal manometry measures pressures in the esophagus; pressures will be increased during episodes of reflux. For 24-hour pH monitoring, a tiny tube with a transducer is introduced into the esophagus to take measurements of the esophageal pH.

Treatment and Nursing Management

Diet therapy, lifestyle changes (particularly weight loss for those who are overweight), drug therapy, and education are the mainstays of GERD treatment. Drug therapy may include antacids, H_2-receptor antagonists, PPIs, and prokinetic drugs (Table 28.2). Check for interactions with other drugs the patient is taking. Verify that the patient can afford the drugs prescribed because some are very expensive.

Clinical Cues

Patients who are prescribed long-term use of PPIs are at risk for nutrient malabsorption, particularly of magnesium, calcium, and vitamin B_{12}. There is also risk of bacterial overgrowth because of the decreased stomach acid secretion. There have been links to pneumonia and possibly to more cases of *Clostridium difficile* in patients who are receiving these drugs. The studies indicating the possible adverse effects of the medications have been retrospective reporting of events. No formal studies have been done to show that PPIs cause the conditions that are listed as adverse effects. Most health care providers agree that PPIs used appropriately are safe and effective (Wolf, 2018).

If these therapies do not control the problem, endoscopic noninvasive therapies often are effective. Laparoscopic surgical fundoplication—in which the fundus of the stomach is wrapped around the esophagus to create a new valve junction (Fig. 28.2)—may be effective. It is not recommended for morbidly obese patients because it tends not to relieve symptoms in this group. This is the same procedure used to correct a hiatal hernia.

Patient Teaching

Measures to Decrease the Symptoms of Gastroesophageal Reflux Disease

DIETARY ALTERATIONS

- Avoid high-fat oils and spicy foods.
- Eat four to six small meals a day.
- Eat slowly, chew food thoroughly, and avoid using a straw for liquids to decrease belching and reflux.
- Avoid carbonated beverages because they increase bloating.
- Eliminate or limit alcohol, tomato-based products, caffeine, citrus juice, raw onions, chocolate, coffee, peppermint, and spearmint in the diet. These foods either relax the esophageal sphincter or increase acid production.

LIFESTYLE ALTERATIONS

- Wait 2 to 3 hours after eating before lying down.
- Do not wear clothes that constrict around the middle of the body.
- If overweight, lose the extra pounds; a 10% weight loss can decrease symptoms considerably.
- Sleep with the head of the bed elevated 6 to 8 inches with blocks or pillows.
- Take medications as directed in relationship to meals and bedtime.
- Stop smoking because it may stimulate gastric acid secretion.
- Participate in regular stress-reducing activities such as exercise, meditation, deep breathing, and laughter.

Think Critically

Many patients with GERD and hiatal hernia do not modify their diet and lifestyle over the long term; instead they rely on medications, which can be expensive, to decrease their symptoms. What measures could you use to show patients that lifestyle changes may control symptoms without medication?

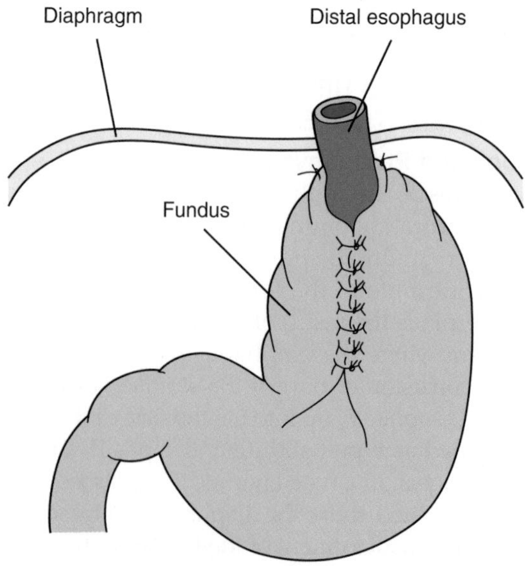

Fig. 28.2 Nissen fundoplication surgery for hiatal hernia or to treat gastroesophageal reflux disease.

Table 28.2 Drugs Commonly Used to Treat Upper Gastrointestinal Disorders

CLASSIFICATION	ACTION	NURSING IMPLICATIONS	PATIENT TEACHING
Antacids			
There are four antacid families consisting of compounds of aluminum, magnesium, calcium, and sodium. Gelusil, Maalox, Mylanta-II, Riopan, Di-Gel, Amphojel, Baselgel, Gaviscon	Neutralize stomach acid	Aluminum hydroxide compounds promote constipation, whereas magnesium hydroxide compounds promote diarrhea. Sodium compounds may adversely affect hypertension and heart failure. All antacids may adversely affect the dissolution and absorption of other drugs. One hour should be allowed between antacid administration and administration of another drug. Magnesium compounds are used cautiously in patients with renal insufficiency.	Antacids are used for relief of "heartburn" that occurs intermittently. Shake liquid preparations well before pouring from container. Chew antacid tablets thoroughly and follow with a glass of water or milk. Report problems of constipation or diarrhea to the health care provider. Take even after pain has disappeared; consult provider.
Histamine (H_2)–Receptor Antagonist			
Cimetidine (Tagamet) Famotidine (Pepcid) Nizatidine (Axid) Ranitidine (Zantac)	Suppress acid secretion by blocking H_2 receptors on parietal cells	Cimetidine may interact with many other drugs; check drug interactions for other drugs patient is receiving. Cimetidine may cause confusion and other CNS effects. Separate administration of these drugs and antacids by 1 h. Monitor for decreased abdominal pain and ulcer symptoms.	These drugs should be taken with meals and at bedtime. Once-a-day dose should be taken at bedtime. Advise patient to avoid cigarettes, aspirin, and other NSAIDs. Advise to avoid alcohol or only consume it in moderation and only in conjunction with food. Advise to use stress reduction techniques.
Proton Pump Inhibitors			
Omeprazole (Prilosec) Omeprazole and sodium bicarbonate (Zegerid) Lansoprazole (Prevacid) Dexlansoprazole (Kapidex)	Suppress secretion of gastric acid	May cause headache, nausea, vomiting, or diarrhea. Use is preferably limited to 4–8 wk.	Follow regimen of diet and stress reduction for ulcer healing.
Rabeprazole (Aciphex)	Same as above	Do not crush delayed-release tablets.	This is a slow-release preparation that acts throughout the day. Teach patient to wear sunscreen; drug may cause sun sensitivity.
Pantoprazole (Protonix)	Same as above	Do not crush tablets.	A slow-release preparation.
Esomeprazole (Nexium)	Same as above	Do not administer with digoxin, rabeprazole, or iron salts.	May affect absorption of digoxin, rabeprazole, and iron salts.
Misoprostol (Cytotec)	Prevents gastric ulcers caused by long-term therapy with NSAIDs	May cause diarrhea or abdominal pain. Not safe during pregnancy.	Is a synthetic prostaglandin. Report abdominal pain, diarrhea, or GI bleeding.
Miscellaneous			
Sucralfate (Carafate)	Provides protective coating barrier over ulcer crater	Monitor for constipation.	Take only as directed. Wait 30 min before taking any other drug.

Continued

Table 28.2 **Drugs Commonly Used to Treat Upper Gastrointestinal Disorders—cont'd**

CLASSIFICATION	ACTION	NURSING IMPLICATIONS	PATIENT TEACHING
Antimicrobials			
Clarithromycin (Biaxin)	Suppresses protein synthesis in bacteria Used to kill *Helicobacter pylori*	Assess for drug allergy. Report hematuria or oliguria. Administer every 12 h to maintain serum levels. Do not crush tablets. Monitor for diarrhea, abdominal pain, or signs of jaundice.	May cause diarrhea, anorexia, or nausea. Must be taken at regular intervals to be effective. Take the entire prescription. Taking acidophilus between doses may alleviate diarrhea. Increase fluid intake if diarrhea occurs.
Amoxicillin (Amoxil)	Causes cell wall of bacteria to swell and burst, preventing replication	Assess for drug sensitivity. Assess for side effects. Monitor renal function. Monitor for blood in stool and abdominal pain.	Take on an empty stomach with a full glass of water. Take at regular intervals around the clock to sustain blood levels. Take entire prescription.
Tetracycline	Bacteriostatic Inhibits protein synthesis in microorganism	Assess for drug sensitivity. Monitor CBC, liver, and kidney functions. Increases effect of warfarin and digoxin. Decreases effect of penicillin and oral contraceptives.	Do not take with dairy products or antacids; separate by 2 h. Avoid sun exposure. Supplies may be limited.
Metronidazole (Flagyl)	Kills amoebas and *Trichomonas;* degrades DNA in organism	Do not give during second and third trimesters of pregnancy. Increases action of anticoagulants. Decreases action of phenobarbital and phenytoin. May cause toxicity if administered with cimetidine or lithium. Patient should have vision examination before and after therapy. Monitor for neurotoxicity. Discontinue if fever, chills, rash, or itching occur.	Do not drink alcohol during or for 48 h after therapy has ended. May cause severe vomiting and prostration. Urine may turn dark brown. Notify provider of numbness or tingling. Dizziness may occur; avoid hazardous activities. May cause dry mouth; chew sugarless gum or sip water frequently.
Antispasmodics			
Dicyclomine hydrochloride (Bentyl, Antispas) Propantheline bromide (Pro-Banthine), hyoscyamine (Levsin) (not FDA approved) Hyoscine butylbromide (Buscopan)	Block acetylcholine, thereby decreasing smooth-muscle spasm and GI motility and inhibiting gastric acid secretion	These drugs interact with many other drugs; check each drug patient is taking for interactions. Most of these drugs are contraindicated in glaucoma, prostatic hypertrophy, myasthenia gravis, and other conditions; consult information on each drug individually. May predispose to drug-induced heat stroke. Monitor vital signs and urine output carefully.	Take 30–60 min before meal. Patient can suck on hard candy to relieve mouth dryness unless contraindicated. Drink 2500–3000 mL of fluid to prevent constipation. Avoid driving and hazardous activities if drug causes dizziness, sleepiness, or blurred vision. Report rash or skin eruption to provider.
Metoclopramide (Reglan)	Hastens gastric emptying and relaxes pyloric and duodenal segments of GI tract	Assess for neurologic or psychotropic side effects such as restlessness, anxiety, ataxia, or hallucinations. Not for long-term use.	Take before meals.

CBC, Complete blood cell count; *CNS,* central nervous system; *DNA,* deoxyribonucleic acid; *FDA,* U.S. Food and Drug Administration; *GI,* gastrointestinal; *NSAIDs,* nonsteroidal antiinflammatory drugs.

Complications

Irritation results when stomach contents containing hydrochloric acid, pepsin, and other enzymes are refluxed into the esophagus. Constant irritation may cause cellular changes, such as the precancerous lesions in Barrett esophagus. Reflux is also a risk factor for aspiration of stomach contents and pneumonitis. Acid reflux into the mouth, over time, may cause dental caries.

GASTROENTERITIS

Gastroenteritis is inflammation of the stomach and small intestine. It is caused by intake of food or water contaminated with a virus, pathogenic bacteria, or parasites. The norovirus is a common cause, as are *Giardia, Shigella,* and *C. difficile*. It is diagnosed by the clinical signs and symptoms of vomiting, diarrhea, abdominal cramping, mild abdominal tenderness, and distention. The diarrhea develops rapidly and lasts less than a week. Fever, elevated white blood cell count, and blood or mucus in the stool may occur. In healthy adults the disorder is self-limiting and does not require hospitalization. Young children, older adults, and chronically ill patients may need intravenous (IV) therapy to take in enough fluid to compensate for the fluid lost from vomiting and diarrhea.

A patient with gastroenteritis should be kept NPO until vomiting has stopped. When tolerated, fluids containing glucose and electrolytes should be started (e.g., Pedialyte, Gatorade), but fluids with high sugar content such as soft drinks and fruit juices should be avoided. If diarrhea continues beyond 3 or 4 days, stool studies for the causative organism should be performed. Therapy to eradicate the causative agent can then be started. Rest is important during the course of the vomiting and diarrhea. After 24 to 48 hours, medication may be prescribed for the vomiting, abdominal cramping, and diarrhea.

> **Nutrition Considerations**
>
> **Dietary Guidelines for a Patient With Vomiting**
>
> - Liquid diet for 12 to 24 hours. Frequent, small amounts of clear liquids are best.
> - Avoid milk, ice cream, pudding, cheese, yogurt, citrus juice, and cream soups.
> - Foods allowed on the liquid diet are electrolyte solutions, carbonated beverages, bouillon, unflavored gelatin, diluted apple juice, peach or pear juice, honey, sugar substitutes, and frozen Popsicles.
>
> When nausea and vomiting stop:
>
> - Add some of the following foods for the next 12 to 24 hours: soda crackers, toast and jelly without butter, tea, rice, pretzels, bananas, applesauce, cooked cream of wheat or cream of rice, and fruit or vegetable juice (BRATT diet: banana, rice, applesauce, tea, and toast).
> - If this diet is tolerated without further symptoms, add the following foods for the next 12 to 24 hours: potatoes (not fried), soups, soft eggs, custards, puddings, white turkey meat or white chicken meat, and cottage cheese.
> - If no further symptoms occur, resume a regular diet but avoid highly seasoned foods, greasy or fried foods, heavy fatty foods, excessively hot or cold foods, raw vegetables, coffee, colas, and milk products for 1 week after symptoms have stopped.

GASTRITIS

Etiology

The main cause of chronic gastritis is ***Helicobacter pylori*** bacteria, but other bacteria, viruses, or parasites can also be a cause. Contributors to acute gastritis and gastropathy are drinking excessive amounts of alcohol, infection from eating contaminated food, cocaine use, and ingestion of medications. Corticosteroids are very harsh on the stomach, as are nonsteroidal antiinflammatory drugs (NSAIDs) such as aspirin and ibuprofen.

Pathophysiology

Gastritis is not a disease; it is an acute or chronic inflammation of the mucous membrane lining the stomach causing changes in the tissue. Gastropathy is a similar disorder where changes to the lining of the stomach occur without the inflammation, usually a chemical process. Alcohol, NSAIDs, and cocaine can damage the lining of the stomach without causing acute inflammation. The clinical presentation is the same as gastritis, and visual inspection during EGD may be inconclusive. A tissue biopsy is needed to make the distinction. Untreated chronic gastritis may progress to ulcer formation and upper GI hemorrhage.

Signs, Symptoms, and Diagnosis

The main symptoms are anorexia, nausea, vomiting, pain and tenderness in the stomach region, hiccoughs, and sometimes diarrhea. A patient with chronic gastritis may have no symptoms but may suddenly experience massive hemorrhage from the stomach due to ulcers eroding blood vessels. Diagnosis is by history, physical examination, and endoscopic examination. Blood tests for *H. pylori* may be done if infection is suspected.

Treatment and Nursing Management

Acute gastritis usually is of very short duration. Treatment consists of withholding all foods by mouth and administering drugs that slow down the peristaltic action of the GI tract. If severe dehydration or nausea and vomiting occur, IV fluids may be given. Patients with gastritis must be watched closely for signs of fluid and electrolyte imbalance. Treatment for chronic gastritis consists of antispasmodics to decrease the pain of stomach spasms, antacids, an H_2-receptor antagonist such as ranitidine to decrease acid secretions and change pH, or a PPI to decrease the secretion of hydrochloric acid. All NSAIDs and substances known to cause gastritis are discontinued. When *H. pylori* is present, treatment is PPIs, amoxicillin, and clarithromycin for 7 to 14 days, with metronidazole substituted for amoxicillin if the patient is allergic to penicillin.

Older Adult Care Points

If an older adult experiences vomiting and is unable to retain fluids for 12 hours, IV fluids may need to be infused to prevent severe dehydration.

Chronic gastritis is not as easily treated as acute gastritis. Diet therapy is of primary importance; patients frequently admit to indiscretion in dietary and drinking habits and find it difficult to change. Patients with chronic gastritis should not eat any spicy or acidic foods. Tact and patience may convince the patient to follow the prescribed diet.

Think Critically

Food is an important part of any culture, ethnic group, or family. Most socialization and important events have food as a main component. What foods would you have difficulty giving up if medically indicated? What measures can you implement to help patients with diet restrictions?

PEPTIC ULCER

Etiology

About 4.5 million people in the United States have experienced a peptic ulcer. *H. pylori* infection with the use of NSAIDs is the major cause. Smoking, stress, and physiologic factors are other causes. *H. pylori* is rich in an enzyme that may cause corrosion of the coating of the upper GI mucosa, making it more susceptible to damage from gastric acid and pepsinogen. Duodenal ulcers and some prepyloric ulcers are associated with an increased amount or hyperacidity of the gastric juices, and 70% are associated with *H. pylori.* Gastric ulcers, by contrast, are characterized by normal or abnormally low levels of hydrochloric acid, but 90% have been associated with *H. pylori.* Colonization of the stomach with *H. pylori* is an important cause of gastric cancer and of gastric mucosa-associated lymphoid tissue (MALT) lymphoma (Anand, 2018).

Older Adult Care Points

By age 60 years, approximately 65% of the population in the United States is infected with the *H. pylori* bacterium. However, most people never have symptoms of gastritis, and few develop ulcers.

There is a weak genetic link for peptic ulcer that is not fully understood. Neither hot, spicy foods nor caffeine has been proven to be a risk factor for ulcers, but these substances make symptoms worse in many people. Gastric ulcers do occur in those who are poorly nourished because of poverty or poor eating habits. Despite the stereotype of the hard-driving executive suffering from an ulcer and ingesting antacid tablets, there is a greater incidence of ulcers in lower-income workers.

Stress does have a bearing on the progression of peptic ulcer. Tension, anxiety, and prolonged stress alter gastric function. Prolonged physiologic stress produces what is known as a *physiologic stress ulcer,* which is believed to result from unrelieved stimulation of the vagus nerves and decreased perfusion to the stomach. A stress ulcer is pathologically and clinically different from a chronic peptic ulcer. It is more acute and more likely to produce hemorrhage. Perforation occurs occasionally, and pain is rare. Stress ulcers are a hazard for patients who are severely ill and in intensive care units for prolonged periods. Patients with multiple trauma, burns, or multisystem disorders are subject to physiologic stress ulcers. Such patients often receive medication to prevent ulcer formation. GI prophylaxis has become commonplace in hospitalized patients, even those not critically ill or at high risk for bleeding. It is recommended that only those patients showing risk for bleeding should receive this therapy (Cook & Guyatt, 2018).

Drug-induced ulcers are most commonly caused by aspirin, NSAIDs, biphosphonates, alcohol, and glucocorticoids (Anand, 2018).

Pathophysiology

Normally the upper GI mucosa can resist corrosion; all areas exposed to hydrochloric acid and pepsin in gastric juices have an ample supply of mucous glands that secrete protective alkaline mucus. Ulcers develop when the mucosa cannot protect itself from corrosive substances, such as gastric acid, pepsinogen, alcohol, bile salts, and irritating food substances. A *peptic ulcer* is an ulceration with loss of tissue of the upper GI tract. The term includes both duodenal and gastric ulcers (Fig. 28.3). The most common site for development of a peptic ulcer is in the first few centimeters of the duodenum, just beyond the pyloric muscle.

Signs and Symptoms

Symptoms of uncomplicated ulcer include epigastric pain that might be described as burning, gnawing, cramping, or aching that usually comes in waves and

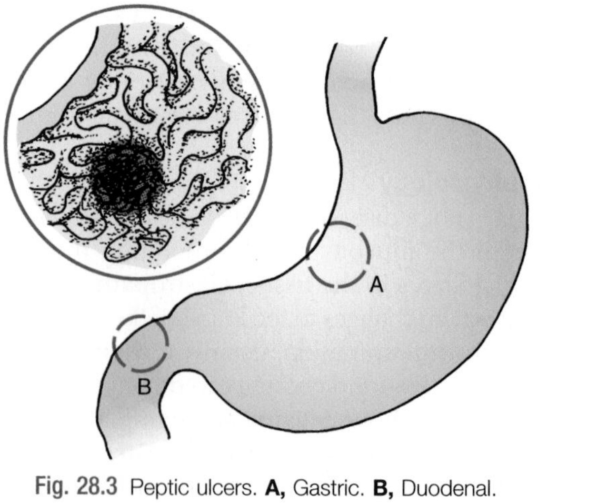

Fig. 28.3 Peptic ulcers. **A,** Gastric. **B,** Duodenal.

lasts for several minutes. The daily pattern of pain is associated with the secretion of gastric juices in relation to the presence of food, which can act as a buffer. **For example, with a gastric ulcer the pain is diminished in the morning when secretion is low and after meals when food is in the stomach, and pain is most severe before meals and at bedtime.** Discomfort often appears for several days or weeks and then subsides, only to reappear weeks or months later. Other subjective symptoms include nausea, loss of appetite, anemia, and weight loss. Spontaneous vomiting is more common with duodenal ulcers than with gastric ulcers.

Older Adult Care Points

Older adults may not display the typical ulcer symptoms. Pain may be poorly localized, or it may be described as lower chest discomfort or left-sided pain. Anorexia, weight loss, general weakness, anemia, nausea, and painless vomiting may occur; peptic ulcer is difficult to diagnose in this population.

Gastrointestinal bleeding. Signs of acute GI bleeding include complaints of weakness and feeling faint, nausea and vomiting, restlessness, thirst, and mental confusion. **Hematemesis** (the vomiting of bright red blood) indicates an active bleed; blood that has been sitting with gastric juices looks like coffee grounds. Diarrhea, decreased blood pressure, rapid pulse, and other signs of hypovolemic shock may occur. Blood in the GI tract acts as a cathartic and causes diarrhea. If bleeding from the upper GI system is profuse, maroon or bright red blood may appear in stool because of the rapid transit of the blood through the intestinal tract. Black stools almost always indicate the presence of digested blood, which means that the source of bleeding is in the upper GI tract.

Clinical Cues

Remember that iron salts can cause the stool to be black and that the ingestion of beets can cause the stool to be bright red.

Estimates of blood loss from the GI tract are based in part on blood pressure readings and pulse rates. Blood pressure and pulse rate should be monitored every 15 to 30 minutes when there is evidence of extensive GI hemorrhage.

Clinical Cues

Changes in the vital signs that signal hypovolemic shock do not appear until after the patient has lost 20% or more of the blood volume.

Hemoglobin and hematocrit levels are useful in determining the status of patients with GI bleeding. These levels can be normal or even slightly elevated at the beginning of a bleeding episode. It takes 4 to 6 hours for the body to shift fluids from other compartments to the intravascular compartment. The shift of fluid changes the ratio of formed elements to fluids in the blood. The white blood cell count may be elevated in massive GI bleeding due to the body's inflammatory response to injury. An elevated level of blood urea nitrogen (BUN) results from digestion of large amounts of blood (protein).

Diagnosis

Peptic ulcer is diagnosed by endoscopy, which can locate the site of ulceration and bleeding. It also allows for differentiation between benign and malignant ulcerations and between the esophageal ulcer and a *diverticulum* (pouching of the intestinal wall). EGD also allows for biopsy samples to be obtained and for treatments to be delivered. Angiography may be performed with massive bleeding. The source can be identified and needed therapies given.

Testing for the presence of *H. pylori* is essential. Testing can be done during an EGD, by blood sample or breath test. The urea breath test measures the gas released in the breath after ingestion of a radio-labeled urea isotope; when *H. pylori* is present, the test result is positive. Serum tests for *H. pylori* detect antibodies, indicating active or recent infection. A fecal antigen test for *H. pylori* is another option.

Think Critically

How do the symptoms of a gastric ulcer differ from those of a hiatal hernia?

When a patient is experiencing extensive GI bleeding, the patient's condition is stabilized, and diagnostic procedures are performed to locate the source of bleeding. These procedures include endoscopic examination of the esophagus, stomach, and small intestine.

Treatment

Peptic ulcer is initially treated with medication. Surgical treatment is used when conservative treatment is not effective. Medications to relieve pain from local irritation of the intestinal mucosa include antacids and PPIs, which decrease gastric secretions (see Table 28.2).

Endoscopy is routinely performed to identify the source of bleeding and, if indicated, to treat it. A tissue biopsy may be done. During the endoscopy, bleeding sites may be treated with thermal coagulation or placement of hemoclips. Injection therapy, usually with epinephrine, may be used with the coagulation and clip procedures. In July 2018 the U.S. Food and Drug Administration (FDA) approved a topical powder that promotes coagulation. The hemostatic nanopowder is sprayed onto the bleeding site through a catheter with endoscope guidance. When in contact with moisture, the powder forms a clot barrier (Saltzman, 2018).

PPIs are given IV or orally to decrease or stop acid secretion (see Table 28.2). These treatments are effective in stopping the bleeding 80% of the time; the other 20% will require surgery.

If there is major blood loss, transfusions of packed cells, platelets, or fresh frozen plasma may be necessary. Normal saline, Plasmanate (plasma protein fraction), or lactated Ringer solution may be administered until blood is available. Maintenance of fluid balance is extremely important. Intake and output must be measured and recorded accurately. Oxygen therapy is started to maximize tissue oxygenation. Adequate IV access must be maintained.

Eliminating *H. pylori* with antibiotics is first-line treatment; as well, gastric acid is reduced with PPIs. NSAIDS and other substances known to damage stomach mucosa are eliminated. Most ulcers heal without complications with this treatment.

! Safety Alert

Proton Pump Inhibitor Drug Interactions

Because PPIs slow the liver's ability to metabolize and clear some drugs from the bloodstream, they should be used with caution in patients taking diazepam (Valium), phenytoin (Dilantin), and warfarin (Coumadin). Patients taking a PPI along with any of these three drugs should be watched closely for signs of toxicity.

Complications

The three major complications of peptic ulcer are hemorrhage, perforation, and obstruction. Hemorrhage occurs when the ulcer erodes vessels, causing bleeding into the stomach. Signs of hemorrhage include vomiting of blood. If the hemorrhage is unchecked, hypovolemic shock may occur.

Perforation is erosion of the ulcer through all walls of the stomach or intestine. A spilling of the contents of the GI tract into the peritoneal cavity ensues; it constitutes a surgical emergency because of the danger of hemorrhage and peritonitis. **Perforation is characterized by a sudden and severe pain in the upper abdomen that persists and increases in intensity and sometimes is referred to the shoulders.** The abdomen is rigid and boardlike and extremely tender. In a short time the patient shows signs of shock.

Obstruction occurs as a result of scarring and loss of musculature at the pylorus, narrowing the stomach outlet, and is manifested chiefly by persistent vomiting.

Surgical Treatment

Surgical treatment becomes necessary when a chronic ulcer fails to respond to medical or endoscopic treatment; when complications such as perforation, obstruction, or hemorrhage occur; or when malignancy is present. All of the surgical procedures can be done laparoscopically or as an open procedure. The surgeon decides on the appropriate approach based on what is being treated and whether the surgery is elective or emergent.

In *pyloroplasty with truncal or proximal gastric vagotomy*, the pylorus, which has been narrowed by scarring, is widened. The branches of the vagus nerve (cranial nerve X) that stimulate acid secretion in the stomach are selectively severed (**vagotomy**) so that the stomach does not receive impulses from the brain and therefore does not secrete hydrochloric acid. A vagotomy is often done while a gastric resection is performed.

Subtotal gastrectomy (gastric resection) consists of removing a part of the stomach and then joining the remaining portion to the small intestine by anastomosis. **Anastomosis** is the joining of two hollow organs by suturing the open ends together so that they become one continuous tube. An *antrectomy*, in which the gastrin-producing portion of the stomach (the antrum) is removed, may be done in conjunction with a truncal vagotomy. When the fundus of the stomach is anastomosed to the duodenum, the procedure is known as a *Billroth I.* In the *Billroth II* procedure, the duodenum is closed, and the fundus of the stomach is anastomosed to the jejunum. *Total gastrectomy* is the surgical removal of all of the stomach. The esophagus is anastomosed to the small intestine (Fig. 28.4).

Nursing care of patients undergoing gastric surgery

Preoperative care. Patients having scheduled gastric surgery are restricted to a liquid diet on the day before surgery. On the day of surgery, the patient is kept NPO. An NG tube is inserted once the patient is in the operating room, and all stomach contents are suctioned out before surgery.

The patient undergoes the routine preparations necessary for all major abdominal surgery. Mechanical bowel preparation is rarely used prior to gastric surgery. If the patient has had a barium enema, look for and report stools that contain whitish material. The whitish material is barium, and it will become hardened if left in the colon, thus presenting the possibility of fecal impaction later. Make sure that orders have been obtained regarding which home medications are to be administered and which are to be held and that all preoperative teaching has been completed.

Postoperative care. Care of patients who have had gastric surgery is routine, with some exceptions. After surgery in which part of the stomach has been removed, care must be taken in handling the NG tube to prevent injury to the sutures and to prevent introduction of infectious agents. The surgeon will write specific orders about irrigating fluids and movement of the gastric tube.

After the tube is removed, the patient is given small amounts of liquid to determine tolerance. These liquids are gradually increased. The patient's ability to take them without nausea, vomiting, or abdominal distress is assessed. If the liquids are well tolerated, the patient progresses to small, frequent feedings. Within 6 months, most patients can take three regular meals a day. The

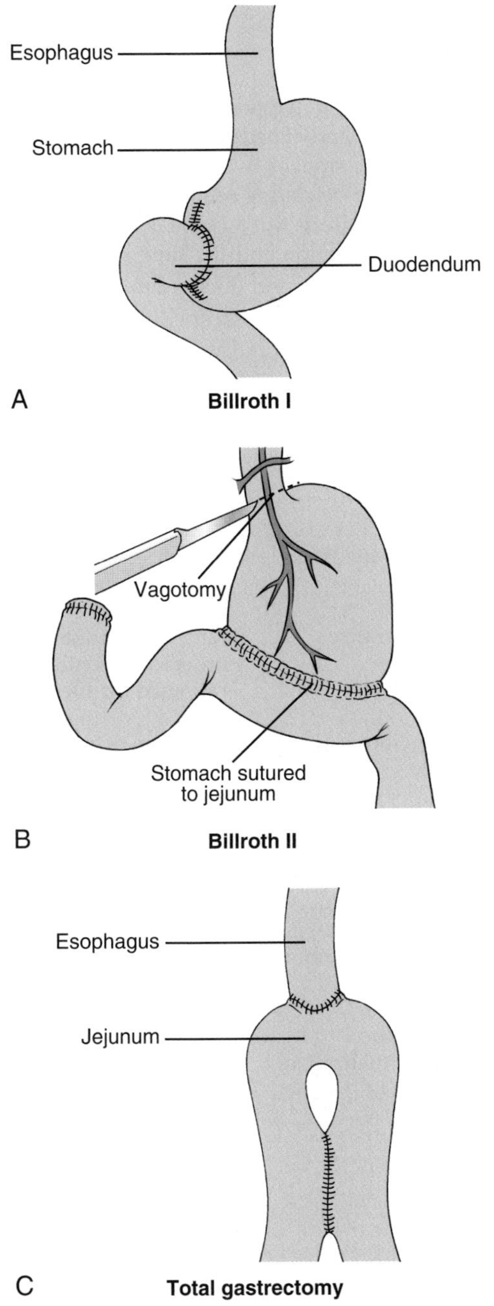

Fig. 28.4 Stomach surgical procedures. **A,** Billroth I. **B,** Billroth II. **C,** Total gastrectomy.

remaining portion of the stomach stretches to accommodate more and more food. Patients who have had a total gastrectomy have restricted diets. They are usually restricted to small, frequent feedings of easily digested semisolids for the rest of their lives. Before discharge, the hospital dietitian usually is called to help the patient and family learn about the special diet needed after undergoing gastric surgery. Medications may not be as effective due to altered absorption. The health care provider should be consulted on all medications.

Dumping syndrome. Some patients who have had a gastrectomy or who are started on full-strength tube feedings experience a complication known as *dumping syndrome*. The patient has nausea, weakness, abdominal pain, and diarrhea and may feel faint and perspire profusely or experience palpitations after eating. These sensations are caused by the rapid passage of large amounts of food, especially sugar and liquid, into the jejunum. This occurs because part or all of the stomach and duodenum has been surgically removed. The progress of the ingested foods and fluids is not slowed by passing through the upper portion of the GI tract. The patient with dumping syndrome should be taught to avoid eating large meals and to minimize fluids during the meal. Fluids may be taken in small amounts later, between meals. Refined sugar can cause or aggravate the condition, and the patient should try to avoid sugary foods or snacks. It also may be helpful for the patient to lie flat for 30 minutes after a meal.

For patients who require tube feedings, a dilute solution is started slowly, and concentration and volume are increased as tolerated. Initiating at full strength and full volumes may cause dumping syndrome with cramping and diarrhea.

❖ NURSING MANAGEMENT

◆ ASSESSMENT (DATA COLLECTION)

Begin by asking the patient to describe the chief complaint (patient's perception of the main problem).

Focused Assessment

Data Collection for Peptic Ulcer

Assess the following areas:

HISTORY

- Pain: where located, characteristics, what affects pain, what relieves it, when pain began
- Nausea or vomiting; presence of bright red or "coffee grounds" emesis
- Dark, "tarry" stool or maroon-colored stool
- Anorexia, weight loss

PHYSICAL ASSESSMENT

- Vital signs and changes from baseline
- Presence of restlessness, confusion, thirst
- Skin tone
- Appearance and amount of emesis
- Stool color, characteristics, frequency
- Abdominal tenderness, rigidity, guarding, bloating
- Bowel sounds

LABORATORY DATA

- Complete blood cell count (CBC)
- BUN
- *H. pylori* testing
- Coagulation panel

◆ NURSING DIAGNOSIS AND PLANNING

Common problem statements or nursing diagnoses, expected outcomes, and interventions for patients with a peptic ulcer are presented in Nursing Care Plan 28.1. Before a peptic ulcer can be successfully controlled, the

Nursing Care Plan 28.1 Care of a Patient With a Bleeding Peptic Ulcer

SCENARIO

Mr. Jackson is a 52-year-old long-distance truck driver admitted to the hospital with a diagnosis of bleeding peptic ulcer. He has had recurrent bouts of epigastric pain that is more pronounced before meals and at bedtime. Mr. Jackson states that he eats "whenever I can grab a bite." He eats mostly fried and spicy foods, and he smokes two packs of cigarettes a day. He went to the health care provider because of fatigue and discomfort that seemed to be getting progressively worse despite antacid use. He has been vomiting with blood in the secretions, and he is weak and dizzy. Mr. Jackson is the sole supporter of his wife and four children and is very concerned about the expense of hospitalization and the time spent away from work. He is scheduled for an urgent endoscopic examination of the esophagus, stomach, and duodenum.

PROBLEM STATEMENT/NURSING DIAGNOSIS

Pain due to irritation and possible ulceration of gastric mucosa.

SUPPORTING ASSESSMENT DATA

Subjective: Recurrent bouts of epigastric pain more pronounced before meals.
Objective: Epigastric tenderness increases with gentle palpation. Pain level 6/10 on admission.

Goals/Expected Outcomes	Nursing Interventions	Selected Rationale	Evaluation
Patient will verbalize pain level of 4/10 or below.	Assess location and severity of pain every shift.	Provides data on condition and need for medication.	Pain is epigastric at 3/10 on pain scale; now occurring between meals.
Patient will verbalize ways to prevent gastric pain.	Administer ordered antacids, antispasmodics, and H_2 inhibitors.	Medications neutralize stomach acid or decrease acid production.	Taking medications as ordered. Verbalizes rationale for medication.
	Give caffeine-free diet.	Caffeine causes more stomach acid production.	No caffeine drinks; bland diet. Verbalizes understanding of effect of caffeine on stomach pain.
	Encourage patient to quit smoking. Nicotine patch applied.	Smoking constricts blood vessels, decreasing perfusion to stomach. Decreased perfusion makes the stomach more susceptible to inflammation.	Patient said he would think about quitting smoking. Provided community resource information for smoking cessation.
	Give frequent feedings to neutralize gastric acid.	Keeping food in the stomach helps neutralize acid.	Eating a snack every 2 h between meals. Verbalizes understanding of how frequent meals or snacks can help control pain.

PROBLEM STATEMENT/NURSING DIAGNOSIS

Anxiety due to expenses, time off work, and worry about what is wrong with him.

SUPPORTING ASSESSMENT DATA

Subjective: "I'm the only one working"; expresses worry over hospital expenses; worried about blood in vomitus.
Objective: Self-treated with antacids and continued to work until symptoms progressed.

Goals/Expected Outcomes	Nursing Interventions	Selected Rationale	Evaluation
Patient will verbalize reduction in anxiety before discharge.	Encourage verbalization of concerns and fears.	Verbalizing fears may decrease their intensity.	Verbalizing specific concerns about finances and expresses fear that blood is a sign of serious illness.
Patient will devise plan to cover hospital expenses to decrease anxiety.	Advocate for financial consultation regarding hospital expenses.	A plan for meeting financial obligation will decrease anxiety somewhat.	Appointment with social worker to discuss financial situation.

Nursing Care Plan 28.1 Care of a Patient With a Bleeding Peptic Ulcer—cont'd

Goals/Expected Outcomes	Nursing Interventions	Selected Rationale	Evaluation
Patient will verbalize understanding of diagnosis and treatment of his condition.	Explain all diagnostic procedures and medications.	Decreases the fear of the unknown and reduces anxiety.	Brochure given about endoscopic procedures and test for *Helicobacter pylori;* reviewed purpose of each medication.
	Assess usual coping techniques and teach new ways to cope as necessary.	Establishes usual coping methods and provides data for other coping methods to be taught.	Uses smoking and television as relaxation.
	Reinforce wife's assurances that they can manage expenses at home.	Reinforcement of information helps patient remember.	Wife says he tends to be a "worrywart"; reinforced information about her ability to cope with expenses.
	Encourage relaxation techniques.	Relaxation techniques help decrease anxious feelings.	Taught relaxation exercise and encouraged to practice it.

PROBLEM STATEMENT/NURSING DIAGNOSIS

Potential for altered tissue perfusion due to increased bleeding (gastrointestinal) from irritation of gastric mucosa.

SUPPORTING ASSESSMENT DATA

Subjective: States has experienced blood-streaked vomitus; history suggestive of peptic ulcer; increasing fatigue.
Objective: Blood-tinged vomitus and blood in stool (positive guaiac test); pale conjunctiva; below-normal Hb and Hct.

Goals/Expected Outcomes	Nursing Interventions	Selected Rationale	Evaluation
Signs of intestinal blood loss will be promptly identified and reported to the health care provider.	Monitor CBC count for evidence of continued bleeding.	CBC count may indicate whether bleeding is occurring.	Hb 10.9 g/dL and Hct 30.
	Assess vomitus for blood.	Blood in vomitus indicates bleeding is still occurring.	No vomitus this shift.
	Check stool for occult blood as ordered.	Blood in stool indicates GI bleeding.	Stool positive for occult blood ×2.
	Monitor vital signs and assess for continued or rapid blood loss as ordered.	Active bleeding will be reflected by vital signs.	Pulse 92 and BP 138/86.
	Teach about foods high in iron (i.e., meat and green leafy vegetables) to correct anemia.	Eating foods high in iron helps correct anemia.	Agrees to try to eat more spinach, chard, and lean beef.
	Administer iron supplements as ordered.	Iron supplementation helps correct anemia.	Iron supplement not ordered yet.

POSTPROCEDURE

Mr. Jackson's health care provider found a bleeding duodenal ulcer on endoscopic examination, and it was treated with electrocoagulation. The provider has prescribed sucralfate (Carafate), 1 g orally four times per day before meals and bed, and pantoprazole 40 mg daily.

PROBLEM STATEMENT/NURSING DIAGNOSIS

Insufficient knowledge of factors that contribute to peptic ulcer and information about medications.

SUPPORTING ASSESSMENT DATA

Subjective: States was unaware that cigarette smoking contributed to ulcers; has never heard of the medications prescribed for him.

Goals/Expected Outcomes	Nursing Interventions	Selected Rationale	Evaluation
Patient will verbalize factors that contribute to ulcer formation.	Instruct in contributing factors of ulcer formation (i.e., explain how the eating behaviors of "grab a bite" and eating spicy or fried foods are contributing to ulcer formation).	Understanding how behavior affects health may help the patient make better choices.	Acknowledged that smoking, diet, and lifestyle contribute to his ulcer. States he will quit eating foods that cause pain (i.e., spicy foods).

Continued

Nursing Care Plan 28.1 Care of a Patient With a Bleeding Peptic Ulcer—cont'd

Goals/Expected Outcomes	Nursing Interventions	Selected Rationale	Evaluation
Patient will attempt to quit smoking within 2 wk.	Assist him to learn new ways to cope with stress.	Practicing relaxation and deep breathing helps decrease stress.	Taught deep-breathing exercise. Will begin exercise program for stress reduction.
	Discuss smoking cessation strategies (i.e., set a stop date, enlist help of family, use a prescribed nicotine patch, substitute an activity such as chewing gum).	Nicotine is very addictive, and having a formalized plan increases success.	Expresses interest in talking to doctor about continuing the nicotine patch after discharge.
	Discuss ways to manage proper eating when on the road (e.g., packing healthy snacks or choosing baked foods, not fried).	Knowing good food choices for his situation can help him eat properly when on the road.	Discussed food places that have appropriate choices. Wife agrees to pack fruits and whole-grain crackers.
Patient will verbalize reason for each medication, dosage schedule, and side effects.	Teach action, dosage, and side effects of sucralfate (Carafate), and pantoprazole. Obtain feedback for material taught.	Understanding how to take medications and what to expect, or report, helps with compliance and prevents toxic reactions.	Went over each medication and gave list with dosages. Discussed possible side effects and what to report to the provider.

CRITICAL THINKING QUESTIONS

1. How would you interact with this patient to try to help him quit smoking?
2. What does he need to know about taking a proton pump inhibitor if he is taking other medications?
3. Considering that he is a truck driver and on the road a lot, what can you do to help him change his diet?

BP, Blood pressure; *CBC*, complete blood cell count; *GI*, gastrointestinal; *Hct*, hematocrit; *Hb*, hemoglobin.

patient must understand how and why the ulcer developed in the first place. Once the predisposing factors are understood, it is easier to avoid them. Unless the patient can cooperate fully, there is a strong possibility that ulcers will develop again despite medical or even surgical treatment.

Think Critically

How can you increase compliance with the medication schedule prescribed for ulcers?

◆ IMPLEMENTATION

Measure blood pressure and pulse rate regularly. Observe skin color, observe for diaphoresis or thirst, and look for other signs of continued blood loss such as restlessness. Measure intake and output and note the character of vomitus, aspirated gastric fluid, and stools. Measure and record the patient's daily weight. **Melena** stools (black, tarry stools with digested blood) cause an unpleasant odor, and the room must be kept as free of odor as possible.

Diet counseling is a top priority once the patient is stable. Currently, most authorities believe that it is best to restrict only those foods that the patient identifies with the onset of symptoms. It is generally agreed that the kind of food is less important than when the food is eaten; therefore the patient is instructed to eat at frequent and regular intervals throughout the day rather than in two or three large meals. Meals should not be skipped. Alcohol and caffeine should be excluded.

◆ EVALUATION

You can point out signs of improvement that will help relieve the patient's anxiety. For example, as they can tolerate liquids and progress with their diet, they can see signs of improvement. After the bleeding has appeared to stop and the patient's vital signs have stabilized, there must be continuous monitoring for signs of persistent or renewed bleeding. If the patient had a surgical intervention, evaluation of the operative site and general postoperative assessments will indicate progress or identify potential problems so that they can be addressed.

GASTRIC CANCER

The American Cancer Society (2018c) estimates that 26,000 cases of stomach cancer are diagnosed annually, and 10,800 people in the United States die of stomach cancer each year. Stomach cancer is usually discovered very late because patients often lack symptoms. The 5-year survival rate is 90% if the disease is caught early and only 18% in those with advanced disease. Metastasis to surrounding organs is common in late disease.

Etiology

The cause of gastric cancer is unknown. For a small percentage of patents there is a genetic trait; for others environmental factors play a role. Pernicious anemia and **achlorhydria** (absence of hydrochloric acid) are often present as an outcome of autoimmune disease. It is believed that a diet high in smoked, highly salted, or preserved foods may be a contributor. The World Health Organization has classified *H. pylori* as a carcinogen. Alcohol use and tobacco smoking are both linked to gastric cancer. All of the causative factors alter the tissue lining the stomach and end up with the same result: abnormal cells that produce a cancerous growth.

Pathophysiology

Gastric cancer grows primarily from the mucous glands. Most tumors arise in the antrum or pyloric area. The lesion begins as an ulcerative crater with an irregular border and a raised margin. The tumor eventually spreads through the layers of the stomach and spreads to the lymph nodes, the liver, and the ovaries in women.

Nutrition Considerations

Prevention of Gastric Cancer

Refraining from eating a diet high in smoked and salted foods or pickled vegetables helps prevent gastric cancer. Eating a diet high in fruits and vegetables, particularly those high in betacarotene and vitamin C, decreases stomach cancer risk. People who eat a lot of red meat each week have double the risk of gastric cancer. Foods such as bacon and many "lunch meats" are high in nitrites, which are carcinogenic. When eating those foods, drinking orange juice reduces the absorption of nitrites. The ascorbic acid in the orange juice counteracts the nitrite concentration.

Cultural Considerations

Stomach Cancer Incidence

Stomach cancer has almost double the incidence in African Americans as in non-Hispanic whites. Native Americans and Hispanic Americans are also at an increased risk for stomach cancer. *H. pylori* is more common in Hispanic and African American individuals. Research with minority populations is under way to determine how *H. pylori* is transmitted in these populations in an effort to decrease the incidence of stomach cancer.

Signs and Symptoms

Gastric cancer is usually asymptomatic until the disease is far advanced. Signs and symptoms may include indigestion, loss of appetite, nausea and vomiting, and weight loss but may be limited to just intermittent abdominal distress. Belching and the use of antacids may relieve the distress. The patient may become pale and weak and complain of fatigue, weakness, dizziness, and sometimes shortness of breath. Anemia is the underlying cause of those symptoms. There is often blood in the stool.

Diagnosis

Diagnosis is by upper GI series and endoscopic examination of the stomach with biopsy. Anemia, verified with a CBC, is usually present. Tumor markers such as carcinoembryonic antigen and carbohydrate antigen (CA) 19-9 may be elevated but are not specific to gastric cancer. CT scans of the abdomen and pelvis may help with staging so that appropriate treatment is initiated.

Treatment and Nursing Management

Surgical intervention may relieve symptoms such as obstruction or may debulk the tumor. The same surgical procedures are used as for peptic ulcer; lymph node dissection may be performed. There is only a 40% 5-year cure rate with surgery for gastric cancer. A laparoscopic approach is used for early-stage tumors. Most centers use an open approach for more advanced conditions for better visibility. Radiation has proved to be of value only for palliation. Histology of the tissue and location of the lesion provide data for chemotherapy choices. Gastric cancers are usually adenocarcinomas. Human epidermal growth factor receptor 2 (HER2) and vascular endothelial growth factor (VEGF) are associated with adenocarcinomas and are the focus of some newer chemotherapy drugs. Cancer therapy and nursing care are discussed in Chapter 8. Nursing care after surgery is the same as for patients after surgery for a peptic ulcer but with excision of involved lymph nodes.

Clinical Cues

The incidence of gastric cancer has steadily fallen over the past 50 years. One contributing factor is thought to be the widespread use of refrigeration. This has allowed a mechanism for storage leading to the consumption of fresh fruits and vegetables rather than a diet high in preserved foods, which are usually preserved with salt.

COMMON THERAPIES FOR DISORDERS OF THE GASTROINTESTINAL SYSTEM

GASTROINTESTINAL DECOMPRESSION

Abdominal distention with increased pressure within the abdominal cavity is very uncomfortable. Excess fluids and gases also interfere with expansion of the lungs by pushing up on the diaphragm and with normal function of other nearby organs.

An NG tube to remove fluids and gas from the stomach may be inserted. Gastrointestinal tubes vary in length, design, and purpose. The Levin tube and gastric sump tube are shorter because they are intended to reach only as far as the stomach. The Miller-Abbott tube is a longer tube that can be directed past the stomach and into the small intestine.

Nursing Management

Observe the patient for continuing signs of abdominal distention during gastric decompression, which would indicate that excess fluids and gases are not being removed as intended. **Nausea, vomiting, complaints of feeling full or bloated, increasing shortness of**

Clinical Cues

Nasogastric (NG) is the route by which the tube is placed. *NG tube* is a generic term that you may see in health care providers' orders or in the nurses' or providers' notes, or you may hear that term in report; however, the purpose of the therapy for the NG tube dictates the type of NG tube. Make sure that you clarify the purpose of the therapy and the type of tube before starting the care of the patient.

breath, and increase in the girth of the abdomen are signs that the stomach and intestines are not being decompressed adequately.

Applying too much suction can pull the gastric mucosa into the drainage openings, or "eyes," of the tube, causing damage to the mucosa and traumatic ulceration.

Assignment Considerations

Caring for a Patient With a Salem Sump Tube

When assigning assisted ambulation of a patient with a Salem sump tube, remind the certified nursing assistant (CNA) or unlicensed assistive personnel (UAP) to keep the tube above the level of the stomach to prevent leaking of stomach contents from the pigtail. The main tube should be plugged for ambulation. The assistant can be instructed to reattach the tubing to the wall suction after ambulation is completed, but the nurse is ultimately responsible to follow up and verify that the tube and suction are functioning correctly.

Using a gastric sump tube (Salem, ventral) that has an air vent can help prevent damage to the mucosa. Sump tubes are usually attached to continuous "low" suction; Levin tubes function best with intermittent suction. **Unless ordered otherwise, use the low setting (80 to 100 mm Hg) for suction.** The connecting tubing leading to the suction machine works best if it is kept above the height of entry into the drainage container.

Clinical Cues

If there is leakage from the pigtail, it can be cleared by instilling a few milliliters of air; nothing but air should be instilled through it.

Irrigation of the tube with normal saline is usually ordered to keep the tube patent. The amount instilled should be added to the patient's intake count, and the amount of drainage is recorded as output for each shift. If the patient has had surgery on the intestinal tract, the irrigation procedure should be done with aseptic technique rather than clean technique.

The characteristics of the drainage are charted each shift. **If coffee ground–like material is noticed in the tube, the drainage should be tested for presence of blood** by using a Hemastix strip dipped into the secretions. If blood unexpectedly appears in the drainage, the health care provider should be notified. Fluid and electrolyte imbalance problems that can be caused by continuous suction and irrigation are discussed in Chapter 3.

An NG tube is uncomfortable for the patient. The naris must be checked for signs of pressure, and the tube may need to be repositioned in the naris to relieve the problem. Common complaints are sore throat, dry mouth, earache (from congestion of the eustachian tube), and dry lips and nasal mucosa. Frequent mouth care and application of a lubricant to the lips and nares will help. A room humidifier can also be helpful, but this requires a provider's order. The provider may allow the patient to have limited amounts of ice chips, hard candy, or chewing gum to decrease the problem of dry mouth.

After the tube is removed, the patient is monitored for nausea, vomiting, and abdominal distention. Sometimes it is necessary to insert the tube again.

ENTERAL NUTRITION

If a patient has long-term difficulty taking in food orally, as when in a coma or with dysphagia from a stroke, enteral feeding is indicated. A nasogastric or nasoduodenal tube (Fig. 28.5) will be used initially. If long-term feeding is needed, a gastrostomy tube (G tube) will be placed. Nasally placed tubes can also terminate in the jejunum, and percutaneously inserted tubes can also be placed so that the tube delivers feedings to the jejunum depending on the nutritional needs of the patient. Placement of feeding tubes other than in the stomach may also be indicated when a surgical procedure has altered the anatomy.

Small-bore, flexible tubes are inserted with a stylet and are usually positioned with the tip in the duodenum (nasoduodenal). In most states insertion of these tubes is restricted to the health care provider or a registered nurse. The tubes can easily be placed in the trachea in patients with a decreased level of consciousness, and fluoroscopy is sometimes used to ensure correct placement. Placement in the duodenum is confirmed by x-ray film before feedings are started. Thereafter the mark at the naris is checked to see that the tube has not slipped out of place before a feeding is begun. Because the tube is small and flexible, it is difficult to aspirate to check placement and residuals. The feedings can be given at specified times throughout the day or on a continuous basis. If continuous tube feedings are ordered, they are administered with a feeding pump.

Patients who require long-term nutritional support for problems such as inability to swallow may undergo percutaneous endoscopic gastrostomy (PEG). A feeding gastrostomy tube is placed endoscopically through the abdominal wall (Fig. 28.6). Use of endoscopy is not the only method of G tube insertion. The procedure may also be done as an interventional radiology procedure with the use of fluoroscopy. The tube is placed directly into the stomach through the abdominal wall. To ensure that the stomach is close enough to be cannulated, air

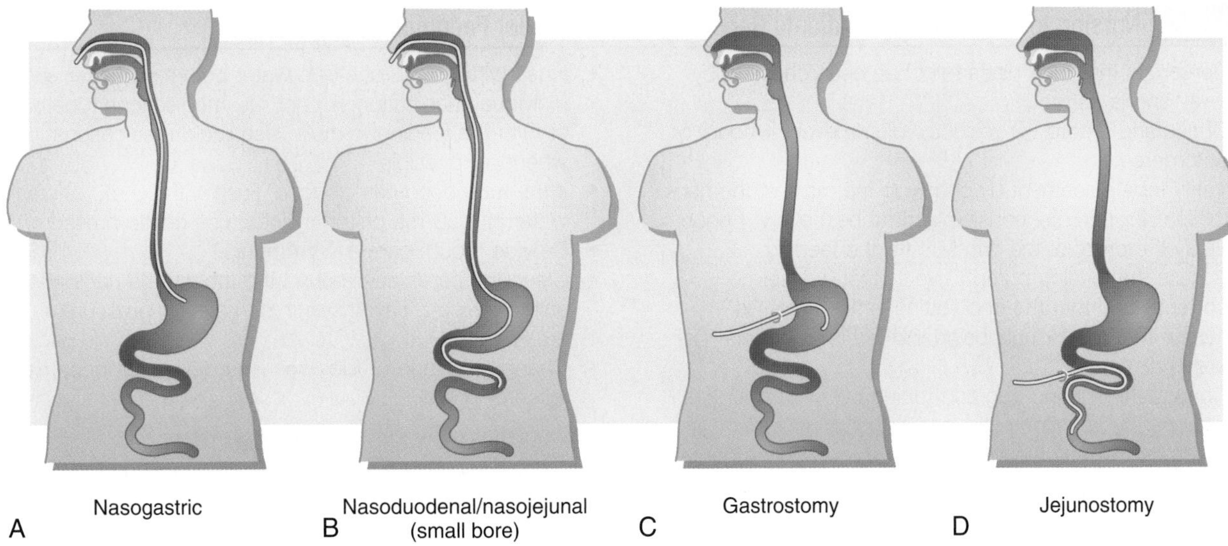

Fig. 28.5 Types of gastrointestinal tubes used for enteral feedings. **A,** A nasogastric tube is passed from the nose into the stomach. **B,** A weighted nasoduodenal/nasojejunal tube is passed through the nose into the duodenum/jejunum. **C,** A gastrostomy tube is introduced through a temporary or permanent opening on the abdominal wall (stoma) into the stomach. **D,** A jejunostomy tube is passed through a stoma directly into the jejunum. (From McCuistion LE, Vuljoin-DiMaggio K, Winton MB, et al.: *Pharmacology: a patient-centered nursing process approach,* ed 9, St. Louis, 2018, Elsevier.)

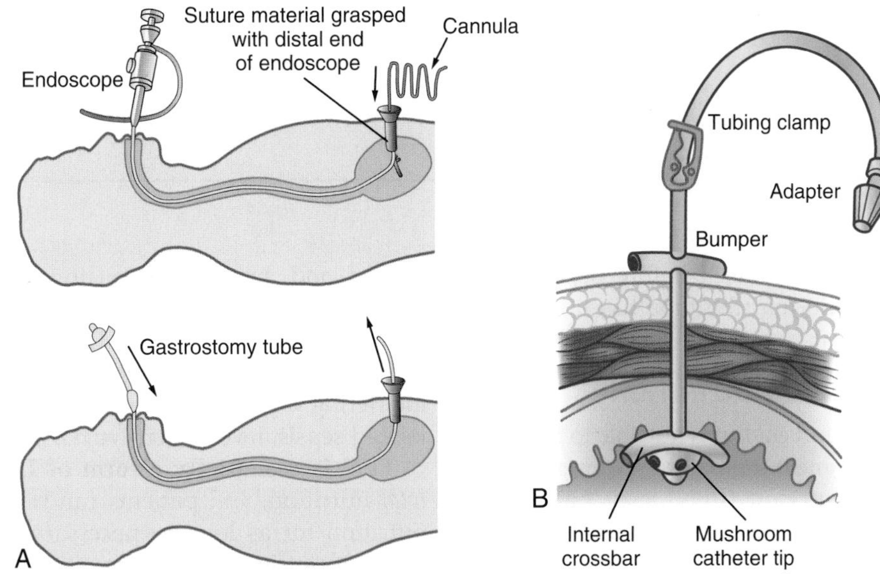

Fig. 28.6 Percutaneous endoscopic gastrostomy. **A,** Gastrostomy tube placement via percutaneous endoscopy. The gastrostomy tube is inserted through the esophagus into the stomach and pulled through a stab wound made in the abdominal wall. **B,** A retention disk on the inside of the stomach and a bumper disk on the outside secure the tube. (From Lewis SL, Bucher L, Heitkemper MM, et al.: *Medical-surgical nursing: assessment and management of clinical problems,* ed 10, St. Louis, 2015, Elsevier.)

is injected into the existing NG tube. This distends the stomach, allowing the health care provider to use a needle to gain access to the stomach. Prior to the procedure, verify which approach is being used so that appropriate patient preparation is completed. The patient then receives enteral feedings via the gastrostomy tube. The tube is marked with indelible ink at the point of exit so that correct placement can be checked daily. The area is observed for signs of infection and cleansed daily with soap and water until healing is complete. A 4 × 4 gauze dressing is used over the outside bumper while the area is healing. Box 28.1 presents nursing interventions for patients who are receiving tube feedings. **Adding a feeding when there is too much residual from the last feeding may cause regurgitation and aspiration.**

Sometimes the feeding tube is placed in the jejunum either during another surgical procedure or percutaneously. The tube is secured in place, and the spot where the tube enters the abdominal skin is marked.

Box 28.1 Nursing Interventions for Patients Receiving Enteral (Tube) Feedings

- Be certain that tube placement has been checked by x-ray and is correct.
- Check and record the residual volume every 4 hours or as ordered.
- Verify tube placement by checking the mark at the naris (or skin for percutaneously placed tubes) every 4 hours.
- Verify the order of the drip rate for the feeding.
- Assess the feeding pump to verify that it is set up correctly and that the drip setting is accurate. Be certain that the formula being instilled is what was ordered.
- Change the feeding bag and tubing every 24 hours. Change the irrigation set every 24 hours as well.
- When continuous feeding is ordered, add only 4 hours of formula to the bag at a time to prevent bacterial growth; a closed system may be used for 24 hours.
- Do not use food dye in the formula because it can cause complications.
- Keep the head of the bed elevated at least 30 degrees during the feeding and for 1 hour after an intermittent or bolus feeding. For continuous feeding, keep the patient in a semi-Fowler position.
- Monitor laboratory values: blood urea nitrogen, electrolytes, hematocrit, albumin, and glucose.
- Monitor for diarrhea or excessive gas.
- Monitor and record intake and output.
- Monitor and record the patient's weight at least weekly.
- Flush the tube with 30 to 60 mL of sterile water every 4 hours during continuous feeding and before and after each intermittent feeding. Give free water as ordered.
- Flush with 30 mL of sterile water before and after each individual medication; do not mix medications together or with the feeding formula. Use liquid medications whenever possible.
- If the tube becomes clogged, flush with 30 mL of sterile water in a 50-mL piston syringe; use gentle pressure.
- Provide mouth care every 4 hours.
- Clean the nares and around the tube in the naris each shift or twice a day. Inspect the naris for pressure areas.
- Change the tape or tube securing device if it becomes loose or soiled.

FOR GASTROSTOMY AND JEJUNOSTOMY TUBES

- Assess the insertion site for signs of infection or excoriation.
- Inspect the insertion site and change the dressing once a day. After the insertion site is healed, a dressing may not be necessary.
- Be certain that the tube is intact and that the mark on the tube is at the skin surface before starting or adding to a feeding. If it is not, stop the feeding and notify the health care provider.
- Gastrostomy tube only: Rotate the external bolster to reach all areas of the skin for cleaning. If the tube cannot be moved, report this to the provider because the retention disk may have become embedded in the tissue.
- Residuals are not checked on a jejunostomy tube.

The mark and suture are checked before beginning a feeding to make certain that the tube has not been dislodged.

PERIPHERAL PARENTERAL NUTRITION

If a patient can swallow and eat but is not able to take in enough nourishment to meet the body's requirements, peripheral parenteral nutrition (PPN) may be given to supplement the diet. As the name implies, PPN is delivered through a peripheral vein. The glucose content is no more than 10%, which is not enough to supply the calorie needs of the body. To increase calories, lipids may be given via a peripheral vein. Protein in the form of amino acids, vitamins, and trace minerals can be supplemented. The IV site needs to be monitored carefully to ensure that the components of the PPN have not caused inflammation. If infiltration occurs, soft tissue injury may result.

TOTAL PARENTERAL NUTRITION

Total parenteral nutrition (TPN) is indicated when the patient cannot ingest or digest foods normally or has a problem with malabsorption. If a patient has continued weight loss and a negative nitrogen balance, TPN is indicated. Conditions that could warrant TPN include severe trauma to the intestinal tract, as with a gunshot wound, and chronic inflammatory conditions. Regional ileitis that prevents absorption of nutrients is an example of an inflammatory condition. Other conditions not related to the intestinal tract but nevertheless capable of seriously interfering with normal nutrition over time include prolonged sepsis, fever, extensive burns, and cancer.

TPN is essentially a form of IV feeding. TPN is *total* nutrition, and patients can be maintained on IV nutrition for as long as necessary. The amounts and kinds of nutrients needed for total nutrition cannot be administered using peripheral veins, so the nutrient mix is given using a larger central vein through a central line. If long-term use is required, a long-term central catheter, such as a peripherally inserted central catheter (PICC) or an implanted port, will be placed.

Safety Alert

Do *not* confuse enteral feedings and TPN feedings. The solutions and routes are not interchangeable. **Infusing an enteral feeding into an IV site can result in death and *has* happened.** First, verify the solution and route. Trace the tube down to the patient's body to ensure that you are using the correct tube. The FDA is working with manufacturers to identify a solution to the problem of connections to enteral routes being the same as those for intravenous routes.

Care of the patient must be a team effort on the part of health care providers, pharmacists, dietitians, and nurses. Nursing care includes assisting with the insertion of the IV central line, changing the tubing with each new bag or bottle, changing the dressing, observing the insertion site, and removing the tubing when TPN therapy is discontinued. Day-to-day care includes monitoring vital signs, glucose levels, and fluid and electrolyte balance. The patient is weighed daily, and frequent mouth care is provided. The rate of TPN is slowly decreased to gradually lower the dextrose load before TPN is discontinued.

Get Ready for the NCLEX® Examination!

Key Points

- A calorie reduction diet combined with exercise and behavior modification are the initial treatments for obesity. Bariatric surgery may be considered for obese patients with a BMI over 40.
- Dysphagia may cause respiratory problems from aspiration.
- Oral cancer and esophageal cancer are associated with alcohol and tobacco use.
- Common symptoms of GERD include dyspepsia and reflux. Diet therapy, lifestyle changes, drug therapy, weight reduction, and education are the mainstays of treatment.
- A peptic ulcer (gastric or duodenal) is ulceration of the upper GI tract. Symptoms include epigastric pain before meals and during the night. Complications include hemorrhage, perforation, and obstruction.
- Monitor vital signs every 15 to 30 minutes when there is evidence of extensive GI hemorrhage. Replacement of blood and fluids may be required.
- Surgical procedures for peptic ulcer include pyloroplasty with vagotomy, subtotal gastrectomy, antrectomy, or total gastrectomy (see Fig. 28.4).
- *Helicobacter pylori,* autoimmune disorders causing pernicious anemia, and achlorhydria are all implicated in the development of gastric cancer.
- Symptoms of dumping syndrome are nausea, weakness, abdominal pain, diarrhea, faintness, palpitations, and diaphoresis.
- An NG tube is used for gastric decompression. After NG tube removal, the patient is monitored for abdominal distention, nausea, and vomiting.
- Various tubes can be used for enteral feedings when the patient is not able to take in food.
- When a patient cannot digest foods and liquids normally, total parenteral nutrition (TPN) may be required. The TPN solution must be sterile and administered at the ordered rate into a central blood vessel with high-volume blood flow.

Additional Learning Resources

SG Go to your Study Guide for additional learning activities to help you master this chapter content.

Go to your Evolve website (http://evolve.elsevier.com/deWit/medsurg) for the following FREE learning resources:
- Animations, audio, and video
- Answers and rationales for questions and activities
- Glossary with pronunciations in English and Spanish
- Interactive Review Questions and more!

Review Questions for the NCLEX® Examination

1. When working with an obese patient who wants to lose weight, which statement would indicate that the teaching has been understood?
   1. "Starting to exercise 2 hours a day is a good beginning for me."
   2. "Eating everything I want except for anything sweet will help me lose weight."
   3. "A program such as Weight Watchers will help me cut calories and keep on track."
   4. "Over-the-counter diet pills are a good way to jump-start my weight loss."
   NCLEX Client Need: Health Promotion and Maintenance

2. When screening for the presence of risk factors for oral and pharyngeal cancers, which questions would you ask? *(Select all that apply.)*
   1. How much alcohol do you consume?
   2. Have you had any oral lesions?
   3. Do you have family members who have cancer?
   4. Do you smoke?
   5. Have you been exposed to the hepatitis virus?
   6. Have you vomited blood?
   NCLEX Client Need: Physiological Integrity: Physiological Adaptation

3. You reinforce diet recommendations to a patient with GERD. Which patient statement indicates a need for further teaching?
   1. "I should avoid spicy Italian sauces."
   2. "Clothes should be loose around the waist and abdomen."
   3. "I need to wait 30 minutes after eating before lying down."
   4. "I need to consider removing caffeine from my diet."
   NCLEX Client Need: Health Promotion and Maintenance

4. A patient who has GERD for many years is diagnosed with Barrett esophagus. Etiologic factors for Barrett esophagus include:
   1. eating spicy foods and hot peppers on a regular basis.
   2. long-term gastroesophageal reflux causing mucosal irritation.
   3. previous history of oral cancer.
   4. moderate alcohol consumption during adult years.
   NCLEX Client Need: Physiological Integrity: Physiological Adaptation

5. A nurse is taking care of a patient who had a modified radical neck dissection surgery. The patient's spouse asks, "Why do you have to apply cold packs and elevate my husband's head?" Which response is the most appropriate?
   1. "These interventions decrease the need for opiates."
   2. "These interventions reduce neck swelling."
   3. "These interventions promote faster healing."
   4. "These interventions reduce the incidence of postoperative fever."

   NCLEX Client Need: Physiological Integrity: Reduction of Risk Potential
6. A nurse is reviewing signs and symptoms of esophageal cancer with people who are at risk. Which statement indicates that the participants have understood the information?
   1. "A feeling of fullness in the throat is an early sign."
   2. "Belching and indigestion are caused by cancerous lesions."
   3. "Common symptoms are halitosis and dryness of the mouth."
   4. "Choking or coughing while swallowing liquids is an early sign."

   NCLEX Client Need: Health Promotion and Maintenance
7. A patient reports a history of gastric ulcer. Which sign or symptom indicates the need for a priority action of health care provider notification?
   1. Epigastric pain that is described as a burning sensation
   2. Pain that is most severe at bedtime
   3. Vomit that "looks like coffee grounds"
   4. Discomfort that comes for several days and then subsides

   NCLEX Client Need: Physiological Integrity: Physiological Adaptation
8. While a nurse is obtaining a clinical history, a patient with a known history of peptic ulcers suddenly complains of severe upper abdominal pain of increasing intensity that spreads to the shoulders. The abdomen has boardlike rigidity. Which sign(s) and/or symptom(s) signal worsening condition related to the peptic ulcer? *(Select all that apply.)*
   1. Slow, deep respirations
   2. Decreased oxygen saturation
   3. Increased pulse
   4. Hot, dry skin
   5. Belching and flatulence
   6. Confusion and restlessness

   NCLEX Client Need: Physiological Integrity: Physiological Adaptation
9. A patient is receiving continuous enteral feedings. Which intervention will address the most serious problem associated with the feeding therapy?
   1. Assist the patient to ambulate several times a day.
   2. Raise the head of the bed.
   3. Place an emesis basin and tissues within close proximity.
   4. Offer water, other fluids, or ice chips frequently.

   NCLEX Client Need: Physiological Integrity: Reduction of Risk Potential
10. You are supervising a nursing student during the care of a patient with a gastrostomy tube. You should intervene if the student:
    1. aspirates for residual contents before feeding.
    2. flushes the tube after each feeding.
    3. changes the tubing and bag every 4 hours.
    4. cleans and dries the skin around the tube.

    NCLEX Client Need: Physiological Integrity: Reduction of Risk Potential
11. A family member tells you, "Dad seems to be having some trouble swallowing lately." What is your priority action?
    1. Notify the health care provider.
    2. Consult the speech therapist for advice.
    3. Initiate aspiration precautions.
    4. Observe during "practice swallows."

    NCLEX Client Need: Physiological Integrity: Reduction of Risk Potential
12. You are caring for a patient who is vomiting blood. The health care provider orders a normal saline IV fluid bolus of 500 mL to infuse over 30 minutes. The correct pump setting in mL/h is _______. *(Fill in the blank.)*

    NCLEX Client Need: Physiological Integrity: Pharmacological Therapies

Critical Thinking Questions

Scenario A

Ms. Olivera, age 56 years, is experiencing a lot of abdominal discomfort and reflux. She visits her health care provider, who believes she has GERD. She is 5 feet, 3½ inches tall and weighs 158 lb.

1. What measures would be recommended to decrease the symptoms of GERD?
2. What specific instruction would you give Ms. Olivera regarding her diet?
3. Why would losing some weight help her problem?

Scenario B

Mr. Eoyang, age 47 years, is admitted to the hospital because he has epigastric pain, is vomiting blood, and has a suspected gastric ulcer.

1. What tests might be done to establish a diagnosis for Mr. Eoyang?
2. What kind of information will help Mr. Eoyang prevent difficulty with his diet after he is discharged?
3. What would Mr. Eoyang need to know to keep his ulcer under control and eventually cure it?

Scenario C

The nursing assistant tells you that Mr. Yamamoto had an episode of coughing while he was eating breakfast. You check on him; he is not having any respiratory distress, but you notice that there are some food stains on his shirt. He says, "Sometimes water makes me cough." You decide to feed the patient his lunch so that you can observe him eating and inform the health care provider about your observations.

1. What position will you place him in before feeding?
2. Explain how to observe for problems with swallowing.
3. What dietary modifications can be made for patients who have difficulties with swallowing?

Care of Patients With Disorders of the Lower Gastrointestinal System

29

http://evolve.elsevier.com/deWit/medsurg

Objectives

Theory

1. Discuss the characteristics of irritable bowel syndrome.
2. Explain how diverticulitis occurs.
3. Identify the causes and signs and symptoms of a strangulated (incarcerated) hernia.
4. Illustrate how two types of intestinal obstruction occur and their symptoms.
5. Describe the pathophysiology, methods of diagnosis, and treatment for ulcerative colitis and Crohn disease.
6. Differentiate the signs and symptoms of appendicitis from those of peritonitis.
7. Plan nursing interventions for a patient having surgery of the lower intestine and rectum.
8. Discuss ways to help a patient psychologically adjust to having an ostomy.
9. Compare the characteristics of hemorrhoids, pilonidal sinus (cyst), and anorectal fistula.

Clinical Practice

10. Choose nursing interventions for a patient with inflammatory bowel disease.
11. Assess for the signs and symptoms of appendicitis.
12. Identify types of patients who are at risk for peritonitis.
13. Create a teaching plan for the prevention of colorectal cancer.
14. Write a nursing care plan for a patient with cancer of the colon and intestinal obstruction.
15. Evaluate a nursing care plan for a patient undergoing colostomy, considering the type of stoma and the effluent it produces.
16. Observe the equipment and procedure for changing an ostomy appliance.

Key Terms

anastomosis (ă-năs-tō-MŌ-sĭs, p. 698)
colectomy (kŏ-LĔK-tō-mē, p. 698)
colostomy (kŏ-LŎS-tō-mē, p. 698)
cryotherapy (krī-ō-THĔR-ă-pē, p. 709)
diverticulitis (dī-vĕr-tĭk-ū-LĪ-tĭs, p. 689)
diverticulosis (dī-vĕr-tĭk-ū-LŌ-sĭs, p. 689)
diverticulum (dī-vĕr-TĬK-ū-lŭm, p. 689)
hemicolectomy (hĕ-mē-kŏ-LĔK-tō-mē, p. 698)
hemorrhoidectomy (HĔM-rŏyd-ĔK-tō-mē, p. 709)
hemorrhoids (HĔM-rŏydz, p. 708)
hernia (HĔR-nē-ă, p. 691)
hernioplasty (hĕr-nē-ŏ-PLĂS-tē, p. 692)
herniorrhaphy (hĕr-nē-ŎR-ĕ-fē, p. 692)
ileostomy (ĭl-ē-ŎS-tō-mē, p. 699)
intussusception (ĭn-tŭs-sŭs-SĔP-shŭn, p. 690)
lysed (līzd, p. 691)
mucorrhea (mū-kō-RĒ-ă, p. 688)
paralytic ileus (păr-ă-LĬT-ĭk ĬL-ē-ŭs, p. 690)
peritonitis (pĕr-ĭ-tō-NĪ-tĭs, p. 696)
photocoagulation (fō-tō-kō-ăg-ū-LĀ-shŭn, p. 709)
pilonidal (pī-lō-NĪ-dăl, p. 709)
scleropathy (sklĕr-ō-pă-thē, p. 709)
steatorrhea (stē-ă-tō-RĒ-ă, p. 697)
volvulus (VŎL-vū-lŭs, p. 690)

Concepts Covered in This Chapter

- Self-Management
- Fluid and Electrolytes
- Cellular Regulation
- Nutrition
- Elimination
- Sexuality
- Inflammation
- Infection
- Pain
- Coping
- Patient Education
- Health Promotion

DISORDERS OF THE ABDOMEN AND BOWEL

DIARRHEA OR CONSTIPATION

Etiology

When a person maintains a consistent diet and activity schedule, bowel motility stays fairly constant. When illness or diet and activity changes occur, bowel motility is affected. Diarrhea, the occurrence of frequent loose or watery stools, can be caused by a number of disorders. Constipation is frequently caused by lack of fluid intake, medication side effects, or immobility but can be a symptom of a more serious medical condition.

Treatment and Nursing Management

A thorough general health assessment is conducted along with a focused assessment. Medications for symptom control are prescribed according to the patient's symptoms. Drugs that have been used include bulk-forming agents, antidiarrheals, antispasmodics, antidepressants, anticholinergics or sedatives, and mild analgesics to relieve discomfort (Table 29.1). A diet high in fiber also may be prescribed. Bulk-forming agents such as Metamucil or stool softeners may be recommended.

Gas-forming foods such as legumes and those in the cabbage family should be avoided. Avoiding onions, potatoes, cucumbers, coffee, tea, carbonated beverages, and alcohol can be helpful. Milk is restricted if the patient has shown evidence of intolerance to it. Lactase tablets may be used for lactase deficiency but are not indicated if an allergic sensitivity is present.

Wearing loose clothing is more comfortable if bloating or increased abdominal pressure occurs. Give instruction about medications and diet therapy.

IRRITABLE BOWEL SYNDROME

Irritable bowel syndrome (IBS) is a functional disorder of gastrointestinal (GI) motility. In the United States more people have IBS than diabetes or asthma, and IBS is a major reason for missing workdays. In North America, IBS is far more common in women than in men.

Etiology

The cause of IBS is unknown but is currently being researched. At this time, it is thought to result from a hypersensitivity of the bowel wall that leads to disruption of the normal function of the intestinal muscles. There is a familial predisposition. Stress, caffeine, and sensitivity to certain foods such as dairy and wheat products seem to trigger IBS in some people.

Pathophysiology

An altered bowel pattern and abdominal pain with bloating are caused by altered motility of the small and large intestines. IBS can occur after a bowel infection, possibly related to changes in intestinal cells and normal GI flora. There is evidence that with IBS there is an

Table 29.1 Drugs Commonly Used to Treat Gastrointestinal Disorders

CLASSIFICATION	ACTION	NURSING IMPLICATIONS	PATIENT TEACHING
Antidiarrheals			
Diphenoxylate hydrochloride (Lomotil) Loperamide (Imodium) Opium tincture (Paregoric) Kaolin-pectin combinations (Kaopectate) Bismuth subsalicylate (Pepto-Bismol)	Decrease motility, propulsion, and secretions. Decrease fluid in stool. Bind water; coat mucosa, absorb toxins.	Observe for effectiveness; should be effective within 48 h. Observe for signs of constipation. Use cautiously in patients with prostatic enlargement; may cause urinary retention. Warn that Pepto-Bismol will make stool black.	Warn that medication will cause dry mouth. Instruct not to take more than recommended dosage; toxicity can occur. With Lomotil, warn not to operate machinery until effect on central nervous system is known. Advise to contact health care provider if acute diarrhea does not abate within 2 days.
Antiflatulents			
Simethicone (Phazyme, Mylicon, Di-Gel)	Defoaming action disperses gas.	Warn that the drug does not prevent gas formation but will decrease bloating and discomfort. Gas is expelled via belching or flatus.	Instruct to chew tablets before swallowing.
Laxatives			
Bulk-Forming			
Methylcellulose (Citrucel) Psyllium (Metamucil, Konsyl)	Act like fiber, absorbing water in the bowel and hastening transit time through the bowel.	None specific; monitor effectiveness.	Instruct to take with an 8-oz glass of water to prevent esophageal or bowel obstruction.
Surfactants			
Docusate sodium (Surfak, Colace) Docusate potassium (Dialose)	Facilitate absorption of water by stool by decreasing the surface tension. Enhance secretion of fluid and electrolytes in the bowel.	Contraindicated for patients with signs of intestinal obstruction. Act in 24–48 h. Used to prevent constipation rather than treat it.	Instruct to take with a full glass of water. Not to be used for more than 1 wk without provider's knowledge.

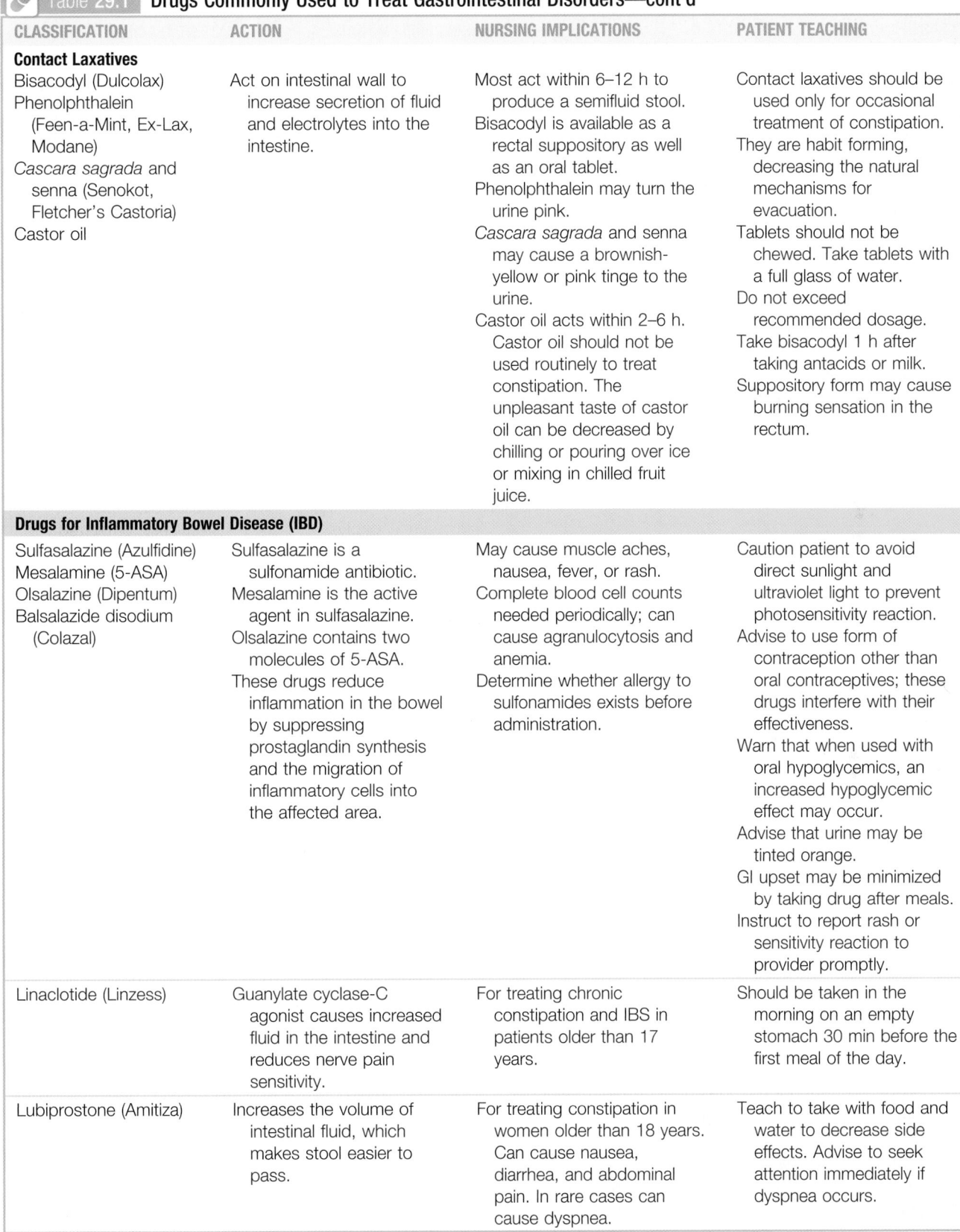

Table 29.1 Drugs Commonly Used to Treat Gastrointestinal Disorders—cont'd

CLASSIFICATION	ACTION	NURSING IMPLICATIONS	PATIENT TEACHING
Contact Laxatives			
Bisacodyl (Dulcolax) Phenolphthalein (Feen-a-Mint, Ex-Lax, Modane) *Cascara sagrada* and senna (Senokot, Fletcher's Castoria) Castor oil	Act on intestinal wall to increase secretion of fluid and electrolytes into the intestine.	Most act within 6–12 h to produce a semifluid stool. Bisacodyl is available as a rectal suppository as well as an oral tablet. Phenolphthalein may turn the urine pink. *Cascara sagrada* and senna may cause a brownish-yellow or pink tinge to the urine. Castor oil acts within 2–6 h. Castor oil should not be used routinely to treat constipation. The unpleasant taste of castor oil can be decreased by chilling or pouring over ice or mixing in chilled fruit juice.	Contact laxatives should be used only for occasional treatment of constipation. They are habit forming, decreasing the natural mechanisms for evacuation. Tablets should not be chewed. Take tablets with a full glass of water. Do not exceed recommended dosage. Take bisacodyl 1 h after taking antacids or milk. Suppository form may cause burning sensation in the rectum.
Drugs for Inflammatory Bowel Disease (IBD)			
Sulfasalazine (Azulfidine) Mesalamine (5-ASA) Olsalazine (Dipentum) Balsalazide disodium (Colazal)	Sulfasalazine is a sulfonamide antibiotic. Mesalamine is the active agent in sulfasalazine. Olsalazine contains two molecules of 5-ASA. These drugs reduce inflammation in the bowel by suppressing prostaglandin synthesis and the migration of inflammatory cells into the affected area.	May cause muscle aches, nausea, fever, or rash. Complete blood cell counts needed periodically; can cause agranulocytosis and anemia. Determine whether allergy to sulfonamides exists before administration.	Caution patient to avoid direct sunlight and ultraviolet light to prevent photosensitivity reaction. Advise to use form of contraception other than oral contraceptives; these drugs interfere with their effectiveness. Warn that when used with oral hypoglycemics, an increased hypoglycemic effect may occur. Advise that urine may be tinted orange. GI upset may be minimized by taking drug after meals. Instruct to report rash or sensitivity reaction to provider promptly.
Linaclotide (Linzess)	Guanylate cyclase-C agonist causes increased fluid in the intestine and reduces nerve pain sensitivity.	For treating chronic constipation and IBS in patients older than 17 years.	Should be taken in the morning on an empty stomach 30 min before the first meal of the day.
Lubiprostone (Amitiza)	Increases the volume of intestinal fluid, which makes stool easier to pass.	For treating constipation in women older than 18 years. Can cause nausea, diarrhea, and abdominal pain. In rare cases can cause dyspnea.	Teach to take with food and water to decrease side effects. Advise to seek attention immediately if dyspnea occurs.

Continued

Table 29.1 **Drugs Commonly Used to Treat Gastrointestinal Disorders—cont'd**

CLASSIFICATION	ACTION	NURSING IMPLICATIONS	PATIENT TEACHING
Infliximab (Remicade)	Monoclonal antibody that neutralizes the activity of tumor necrosis factor alpha found in Crohn disease; decreases infiltration of inflammatory cells.	Given IV over at least 2 h. Dose repeated at 2 wk and then q6wk from first dose. Observe for anaphylactic reaction.	May initially cause increased diarrhea. Advise to report nausea, vomiting, abdominal pain, itching, or rash to provider. Need periodic blood counts. Patient should not breastfeed while taking this drug.
Antispasmodics			
Dicyclomine hydrochloride (Bentyl, Antispas) Propantheline bromide (Pro-Banthine) Oxyphencyclimine hydrochloride (Daricon)	Block acetylcholine, thereby decreasing smooth-muscle spasm and GI motility and inhibiting gastric acid secretion.	These drugs interact with many other drugs; check each drug patient is taking for interactions. Most of these drugs are contraindicated in glaucoma, prostatic hypertrophy, myasthenia gravis, and other conditions; consult information on each drug individually. May predispose to drug-induced heat stroke. Monitor vital signs and urine output carefully.	Advise to take 30–60 min before meal. Patient can suck on hard candy to relieve mouth dryness unless contraindicated. Have patient drink 2500–3000 mL of fluid to prevent constipation. Warn to avoid driving or hazardous activities if drug causes dizziness, sleepiness, or blurred vision. Teach to report rash or skin eruption to provider.
Hyoscyamine (Levsin)	Inhibits action of acetylcholine at postganglionic receptor sites, decreasing spasm and abdominal pain.	May decrease absorption of antacids and antidiarrheals. May increase effects of anticholinergics. May cause urinary retention. Assess for dehydration; encourage adequate fluid intake.	May cause dry mouth. Instruct to inform provider of rash, eye pain, difficulty in urinating, or constipation. Advise to avoid hot baths and saunas. May initially cause dizziness or faintness; warn to not operate machinery until response is known.

5-ASA, 5-Aminosalicylic acid; *GI,* gastrointestinal; *IBS,* irritable bowel syndrome; *IV,* intravenously.

abnormality of nerve function in the intestine. The chemical mediator 5-hydroxytryptamine (5-HT), or serotonin, plays a role in bowel motility and visceral sensitivity, and medications altering 5-HT3 and 5-HT4 activity have been used in treatment (Zheng, 2017). Microscopic inflammation has been identified in patients and is opening new areas of therapy (Lehrer, 2018).

Signs and Symptoms

IBS is a group of symptoms that together represent the most common disorder in patients who consult gastroenterologists. The three characteristics typical of this disorder are (1) alteration in bowel elimination (either constipation or diarrhea or both); (2) abdominal pain and bloating; and (3) the absence of detectable organic disease. The bloating and abdominal pain usually have a sudden onset with production of flatus. The pattern of bowel dysfunction varies from case to case, and each patient seems to have a unique pattern.

Diagnosis

Diagnosis of IBS is based on clinical manifestations and ruling out the presence of organic bowel disease. Diagnostic criteria include the following:

- Abdominal pain or discomfort that is:
  - Relieved by defecation
  - Associated with a change in stool frequency and/or consistency
- **Mucorrhea** (mucus in the stool)
- Abdominal bloating

No diagnostic testing is recommended unless certain additional "alarm features" are present: weight loss, iron deficiency anemia, or family history of organic GI illness (Lehrer, 2018).

Treatment and Nursing Management

IBS is treated symptomatically to control the diarrhea or constipation experienced. Ongoing research is opening new ways of treating the disorder as the pathophysiology becomes better understood. Patients need reassurance and support; studies have shown that medical personnel tend to brush off the significant impact on quality of life that this condition imposes.

Gluten intolerance has been identified as a possible trigger for IBS symptoms. Ineffective coping patterns in response to stress may be present in these patients. Randomized, controlled trials have shown that cognitive therapy, psychotherapy, and hypnotherapy help improve overall symptoms (Lehrer, 2018). Consultation with a psychiatric nursing specialist can help the staff nurse develop more realistic goals and effective nursing interventions to improve the patient's coping skills.

Focused Assessment

Data Collection for a Patient With Suspected Irritable Bowel Syndrome

For a patient with symptoms suggesting IBS, gather the following data:

HISTORY

- When symptoms first began
- Stool pattern: frequency, character of stool
- Presence of bloating and flatus
- Incidence of pain or cramping: location, duration, character
- Pain that awakens the patient at night
- Precipitating factors for cramping or diarrhea
- Known food intolerances
- Methods of self-treatment
- Known stressors
- Methods of coping with stress

PHYSICAL EXAMINATION

- Presence and character of bowel sounds
- Degree of firmness and tenderness of abdomen
- Location of tenderness
- Appearance of stool

Complementary and Alternative Therapies

Peppermint Oil for the Relief of Abdominal Discomfort

Peppermint oil may provide some temporary relief of abdominal pain for patients with IBS; however, those with gastroesophageal reflux disease (GERD) who are taking acid-reducing medication should avoid this alternative therapy because it can worsen heartburn (Halas-Liang, 2018).

Clinical Cues

Having the patient keep a food diary can be very helpful in identifying foods that cause a reaction with bloating and inflammation. If the diary is kept over a period of weeks, a pattern may be established. Food intolerance symptoms may not be evident for up to 4 days after the food is eaten. Sometimes if one food is linked to the symptoms, that food can be simply left out of the diet.

DIVERTICULA

The term **diverticulum** refers to a small, blind pouch resulting from a protrusion of the mucous membranes of a hollow organ through weakened areas of the organ's muscular wall. Diverticula are most prevalent in older adults and occur anywhere in the intestinal tract but are found primarily in the colon. When diverticula are present, the patient is said to have **diverticulosis**. The exact incidence of diverticulosis is not known because most diverticula are asymptomatic. It is uncommon in people younger than 50 years and almost universal in those older than 90 years. Increases in intra-abdominal pressure from constipation and straining to defecate, obesity, and a low-fiber diet appear to be factors in the development of colon diverticula.

Etiology and Pathophysiology

Diverticulitis occurs when the diverticula become inflamed or infected; it occurs in about 20% of those affected by diverticulosis. Food particles accumulate in the diverticula, mix with the intestinal bacteria, and can irritate the mucosal wall. The intestinal wall may become infected, and if it is not treated, perforation and peritonitis may occur.

Esophageal diverticula occur when there is herniation of esophageal mucosa and submucosa into surrounding tissue. The disorder is more common in older patients.

Signs, Symptoms, and Diagnosis

A person with diverticulosis may initially be asymptomatic; however, symptoms will develop when inflammation or infection occurs because material has lodged in diverticula. For colon diverticula, there is usually a history of constipation. There may be rectal bleeding. **Diverticulitis of the intestine produces symptoms of diarrhea or constipation, acute left lower abdominal pain, bloating, nausea, and vomiting. The condition may be complicated by intestinal obstruction or by peritonitis if the intestinal wall ruptures.** If bleeding is massive, there will be hypotension and shock. Computed tomography (CT) of the abdomen with water-soluble colonic contrast is the preferred diagnostic test. Barium enema and colonoscopy should be avoided in acute cases because of the risk of bowel perforation (Ghoulam, 2018).

Esophageal diverticula produce symptoms of dysphagia, regurgitation, nocturnal cough, and **halitosis** (bad breath). There is a risk of esophageal perforation.

Think Critically

What is the difference between the signs and symptoms of diverticulitis and those of irritable bowel syndrome?

Treatment and Nursing Management

Diverticulosis often can be managed conservatively. A high-fiber diet, increased fluids and bulk laxatives, or stool softeners to control constipation may be all that are needed.

For acute uncomplicated diverticulitis, outpatient treatment may include clear liquids for 2 to 3 days with oral antibiotics. Mild pain medication may be used for abdominal discomfort in ambulatory patients. Diet can be advanced as tolerated. The role of the licensed practical/vocational nurse (LPN/LVN) is to reinforce education about the diet, fluid intake, and exercise. In acute complicated cases of diverticulitis or failed outpatient treatment, parenteral antibiotics with intravenous (IV) hydration and bowel rest by placing the patient on nothing-by-mouth (NPO) status for 2 to 3 days may be necessary. IV pain medication will be administered until the diet advances and patients can take solid foods and oral medications. Recurrent episodes of diverticulitis, or perforation and peritonitis, require surgical treatment. Perforation requires emergency surgical intervention. Urgent cases include obstruction and abscess not cleared by medical therapy. Patients who have had a complicated attack and wish to prevent further episodes may choose to have elective surgery to repair fistulas. The type of surgery performed and the approach are determined by the reason for the surgery. Laparoscopic surgery is done when possible with removal of the portion of diseased colon and reconnection of the bowel. In some cases, a temporary colostomy is needed to allow tissues to heal before reconnection. In other situations the colostomy is permanent.

Nutrition Considerations

Diet for Diverticular Disease

A high-fiber diet is encouraged for patients with diverticular disease. Eating whole-grain cereals and breads and fruits such as apples, berries, peaches, and pears adds fiber. High-fiber vegetables—squash, broccoli, cabbage, and spinach—and legumes, including dried beans, peas, and lentils, provide bulk that decreases constipation and speeds intestinal transit time. Drinking plenty of fluids helps regularity. This diet, combined with exercise to prevent constipation, can usually control diverticular disease.

INTESTINAL OBSTRUCTION

Intestinal obstruction is a sudden or gradual blockage of the intestinal tract that prevents the normal passage of GI contents through the intestines.

Etiology and Pathophysiology

Mechanical obstruction results in blockage of the lumen of the bowel. Examples include tumors, adhesions, strangulated hernia, twisting of the bowel (**volvulus**), telescoping of one part of the bowel into itself (**intussusception**), barium impaction, foreign bodies, and adhesions (Fig. 29.1). Abdominal adhesions are a common cause of intestinal obstruction. Adhesions form when inflammation from abdominal trauma or surgery has occurred, and fibrous bands of scar tissue hold together two segments of bowel that are normally separated.

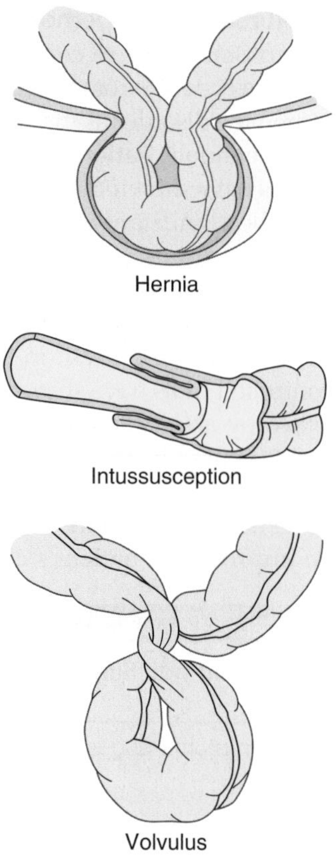

Fig. 29.1 Mechanical causes of intestinal obstruction.

Nonmechanical obstruction results from the absence of peristalsis. Nonmechanical obstructions may occur as a result of **paralytic ileus** (failure of forward movement of bowel contents) after abdominal surgery, infection, or hypokalemia. Poor intestinal perfusion, drug side effects (particularly narcotics), kidney disease, and infection can all interfere with normal peristaltic action and produce a nonmechanical obstruction.

Older Adult Care Points

Older adults are more prone to the occurrence of volvulus and consequent intestinal obstruction, partially because of decreased muscle tone. Suspect this disorder when an older adult complains of sudden abdominal pain with vomiting, has abdominal distention with a palpable mass, has increased bowel sounds on auscultation, and shows signs of dehydration.

When obstruction occurs, fluid and gas accumulate in the intestine, increasing intraluminal pressure. Peristaltic waves above the obstruction may occur as the intestine attempts to move material down the tract. These waves may cause severe pain.

Signs and Symptoms

The symptoms of intestinal obstruction vary according to the location of the obstruction. Obstructions occurring high in the intestinal tract are characterized by sharp, brief pains in the upper abdomen. Frequent, high-pitched bowel sounds are heard above the point of obstruction, and bowel sounds are absent below the obstruction. Other symptoms include vomiting, with rapid dehydration and only slight abdominal distention. An acute intestinal obstruction in the upper abdomen can cause respiratory difficulty because of the pressure of the distended abdomen against the diaphragm.

Obstructions of the colon are characterized by a more gradual onset, with marked abdominal distention as the bowel fills, possible vomiting (which occurs late in the process if at all), and **pains that last several minutes or longer and correspond to peristaltic waves.** Fecal odor or material in the emesis suggests a complete intestinal obstruction.

Diagnosis and Treatment

Abdominal radiographs are ordered to locate the obstruction. Abdominal CT scan may also be completed. Insertion of a nasogastric (NG) tube relieves symptoms by decompressing or removing gas, intestinal contents, and mucus. The long tube or Miller-Abbott tube has a balloon that is inflated after passage into the pylorus (Fig. 29.2). Peristalsis, which is preserved above the blockage, moves the tube to the point of blockage, allowing for removal of gas and liquids. Use of the long tube has not been shown to be more clinically effective than a standard-length NG tube (Bordeianou, 2018). Surgery is indicated for obstruction caused by adhesions, volvulus, hernia, or tumor. Adhesions are **lysed** (broken apart), a volvulus is untwisted, or a colectomy may be necessary if tumor is involved.

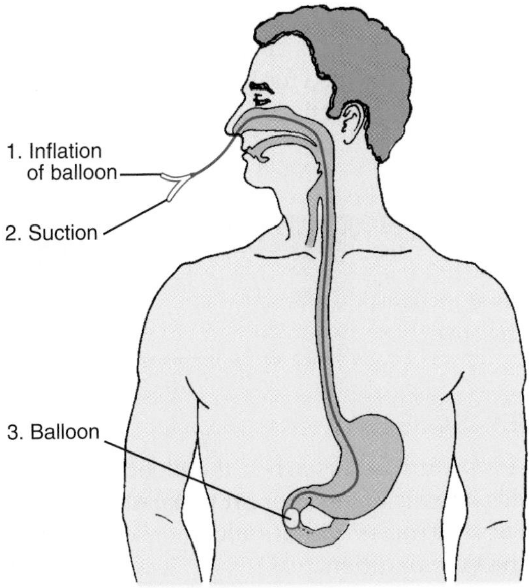

Fig. 29.2 Miller-Abbott intestinal tube used for decompression. It is advanced through the intestines to the prescribed point. The Miller-Abbott tube has a double lumen and is weighted with tungsten. *1,* Portion of the metal tip leading to the balloon. *2,* Portion of the metal tip leading to the lumen that can be suctioned. *3,* Balloon inflated with air.

Nursing Management

Placing the patient in a Fowler position helps relieve pressure and aids in removing gas and intestinal contents through the intestinal tube. Fluid and electrolyte status must be monitored closely. Measure abdominal girth every 2 to 4 hours by placing the tape at the same location on the abdomen each time. Pain control is essential, but worsening pain may signal an unresolved intestinal obstruction that can lead to rupture of the intestine, peritonitis, shock, and death. If the obstruction cannot be resolved, surgical correction must be done. Postoperative care is the same as for other abdominal surgery patients (see Chapter 5).

ABDOMINAL AND INGUINAL HERNIA

Etiology and Pathophysiology

If there is a defect in the muscular wall of the abdomen, the intestine may break through the defect. This protrusion is called a **hernia** or a *rupture.*

The most common locations for a hernia are areas where the abdominal wall is normally weaker and more likely to allow a segment of intestine to protrude (Fig. 29.3). These include the center of the abdomen at the site of the umbilicus and the lower abdomen at the points where the inguinal ring and the femoral canal begin. Hernias are identified by their location: ventral includes epigastric and umbilical; groin includes inguinal and femoral; pelvic includes sciatic and obturator; flank includes superior and inferior lumbar triangle. Hernias can be congenital or acquired. An acquired hernia may form at an old abdominal surgical incision (incisional hernia). The most common contributing factors in the development of a hernia are straining to lift heavy objects, chronic cough, straining to void or pass stool, and ascites. Inguinal hernias are more common in men. Hernias are classified as **reducible,** in which the protruding organ can be returned to its proper place by pressing on the organ, and **irreducible** or **incarcerated,** in which the protruding part of the organ is tightly wedged outside the cavity and cannot be pushed back through the opening. If the protruding part of the organ is not replaced and its blood supply is cut off, the hernia is **strangulated** or **incarcerated,** requiring prompt medical attention.

Signs and Symptoms

If the hernia is not incarcerated, there will be just an abnormal pouching, a "lump" or local swelling out from the abdominal wall or in the groin area (inguinal or femoral hernia). When pressure on the abdominal wall is removed by lying down, the swelling disappears. Lifting heavy objects, coughing, or any activity that puts a strain on the abdominal muscles may force the organ back through the opening, and the swelling reappears.

Some discomfort may accompany the hernia. Pain occurs when the peritoneum becomes irritated or when the hernia is incarcerated or strangulated. The flow of

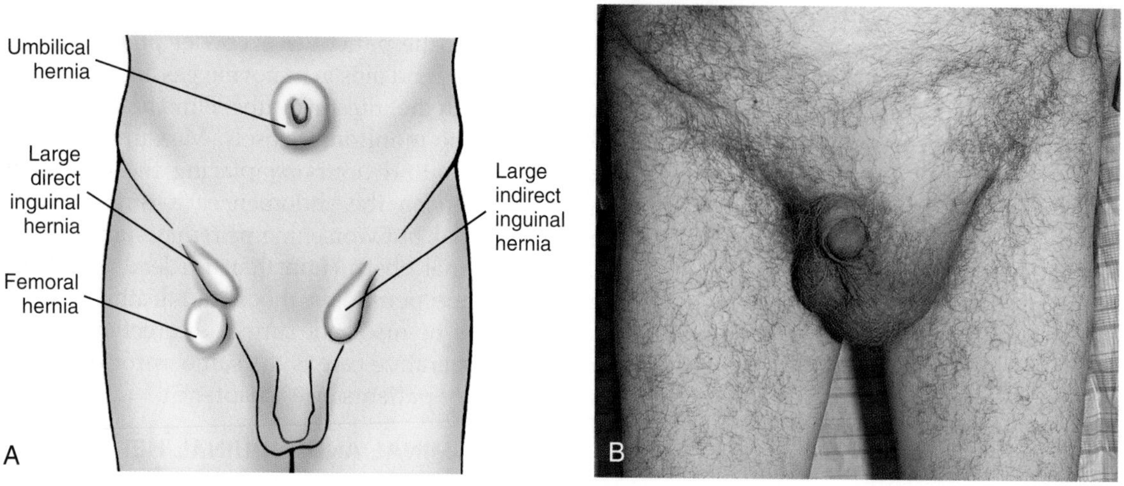

Fig. 29.3 **A,** Umbilical hernia. **B,** Indirect inguinal hernia. (**A,** From Lewis SL, Heitkemper MM, Dirksen SR, et al.: *Medical-surgical nursing: assessment and management of clinical problems,* ed 9, St. Louis, 2015, Elsevier. **B,** From Swartz MH: *Textbook of physical diagnosis: history and examination,* ed 7, Philadelphia, 2014, Elsevier.)

intestinal contents can be blocked by an incarcerated hernia, causing symptoms of intestinal obstruction. **This is an emergency because when the blood supply is restricted, part of the intestine may die.**

Treatment

The surgical procedure used in the treatment of a hernia is called a **herniorrhaphy**. The defect in the muscle is closed with sutures. If the area of weakness is very large, a **hernioplasty** is done. In this procedure, some type of strong synthetic material is sewn over the defect to reinforce the area. The material used is a mesh product; it has potential for complications because a foreign object is being implanted. Studies show that recurrence of a hernia is significantly decreased with the mesh implant. The procedure can be done on an outpatient basis as an open or laparoscopic procedure. Local or regional anesthesia is used instead of general anesthesia for uncomplicated and minimally invasive cases.

If surgery is not possible because of age or high surgical risk, the patient may be fitted with an appliance called a *truss,* which simply reinforces the weakened cavity wall and prevents protrusion of the intestines. The truss is put on in the morning before the patient gets out of bed because the hernia is more likely to be reduced at that time. It is only a symptomatic measure and does not cure the hernia.

Nursing Management

Care after hernia repair is directed at pain control and preventing recurrence of the hernia. The patient is cautioned not to do heavy lifting, pulling, or pushing that increases intra-abdominal pressure. Postoperative care is similar to that for other surgical patients (see Chapter 5).

Careful discharge instructions are given to the patient to prevent problems at the surgical site. Guidelines on signs and symptoms of complications are sent home with the patient, along with a written list of activities to avoid until healing is complete. Lifting restrictions are usually implemented for 1 to 2 weeks, and the patient is instructed to support the site with the hand if coughing or sneezing.

> **! Safety Alert**
>
> **Hernia Mesh**
>
> The U.S. Food and Drug Administration (FDA) regulates implantable medical products. In 2010 a recall of mesh labeled with the C.R.Bard/Davol brand name was found by the FDA to be counterfeit after investigation of reports of complications. Since that time other recalls have happened with hernia mesh products from various manufacturers. The recalls were not found to be counterfeit but have included products that did not perform as expected. Use of mesh in hernia repair continues to be the standard of practice.

> **? Think Critically**
>
> What would you say to a family member who mentions that they have a swelling in the groin area and think they may have a hernia?

BOWEL ISCHEMIA

Bowel ischemia occurs when the blood supply to the bowel is insufficient to support metabolic needs. It can be an acute process with a sudden onset of symptoms or a chronic condition.

Etiology and Pathophysiology

The problem may involve the arterial or the venous blood supply in the form of emboli, thrombosis, or the gradual narrowing and occlusion of vessels. Ischemia can occur as the result of a bowel obstruction or as the result of hypovolemic shock. In 95% of chronic conditions, diffuse atherosclerotic disease of the mesenteric vessels is the source of decreased blood flow. Chronic mesenteric ischemia (CMI) is a rare diagnosis. Most episodes of bowel ischemia result from an acute event.

Acute mesenteric ischemia can result from arterial emboli or thrombosis. Emboli can originate in the heart chambers or plaque inflammation in major vessels, leading to clot formation. Acute events not involving obstruction of blood flow include those that decrease blood flow, such as hypotension, sepsis, or severe liver or renal disease. When blood flow is limited, the gut is bypassed in favor of the brain, heart, lungs, and kidneys, so hypotension has more of an effect on blood flow to the intestines than to other organs.

Signs, Symptoms, and Diagnosis

A careful history is necessary because the symptoms are similar to those of many other abdominal disorders. The sudden onset of severe abdominal pain signals an acute condition. Nausea, vomiting, diarrhea, and abdominal cramps may also be present. The abdomen is tender to palpation, and the patient will exhibit guarding. Bowel sounds will be minimal or absent. The white blood cell count is likely to be elevated. CT angiography or magnetic resonance angiography is used to confirm the medical diagnosis.

Treatment and Nursing Management

The patient will be NPO, and an NG tube will be inserted to relieve distention. Intravenous hydration is usually ordered, and a Foley catheter may be used to monitor output in the acute phase. Ischemia from an obstructive cause, either thrombus or embolus, may be treated with intra-arterial infusions of a vascular smooth muscle relaxant at the site of the blockage, or thrombolytic therapy may be used. The standard treatment is IV heparin. Surgical exploration of the abdomen may be indicated if the low perfusion has caused bowel tissue to become necrotic.

INFLAMMATORY BOWEL DISEASE: ULCERATIVE COLITIS AND CROHN DISEASE

Inflammatory bowel disease (IBD) includes both ulcerative colitis (UC) and Crohn disease (regional ileitis). UC is an inflammation with formation of ulcers of the mucosa of the colon. It almost always involves the rectum and extends up the colon in a continuous manner. It frequently is a chronic disease, and the patient is usually asymptomatic between acute flare-ups. People with UC have a 40% higher incidence of some types of arthritis. Crohn disease is a chronic inflammatory disease that involves all layers of intestinal tissue and can involve any part of the GI tract, but most commonly affects the distal ileum and proximal colon. Both diseases are idiopathic, meaning that the cause is not known. There are theories, and research is being conducted, but there is no proof of a cause.

Etiology

Crohn disease and UC have a genetic predisposition; UC is three times more common than Crohn disease. Both disorders also have an ethnic correlation: they are more common among the Jewish population. Immunologic activity is thought to be involved as well because anticolon antibodies are often present in the blood. With UC, infections and emotional tension often bring about acute attacks. Smoking increases the risk for Crohn disease but not for UC. Smoking cessation in patients with UC actually increased the incidence of the disease and the frequency of attacks. Nicotine patches are being investigated as a possible treatment for UC.

Pathophysiology

The pathophysiology of IBD is being investigated. It is suspected that UC and Crohn disease are immunologic responses to the same (as-yet-unknown) etiologic agent. The result is inflammation of the mucosal lining of the intestinal tract, causing ulceration, edema, bleeding, and fluid and electrolyte loss. UC and Crohn disease share many of the same characteristics (Table 29.2). One difference is that the inflammatory changes in UC are nonspecific, whereas those in Crohn disease are granulomatous (a mass of inflamed tissue characterized by the presence of small granules). Patients with longstanding chronic UC are at 10 to 20 times greater risk for developing cancer of the colon than patients with Crohn disease. The constant inflammation disrupts normal cell function, and cellular mutations may occur. Crohn disease can affect any area of the intestine, although it more often affects the ascending colon and can affect the small intestine (Fig. 29.4). UC typically affects the rectosigmoid and left colon. Changes caused by UC tend to be continuous along the affected portion of the bowel, whereas changes caused by Crohn disease are segmental, leaving healthy sections of bowel between diseased portions ("skip lesions"). With Crohn disease, radiography reveals a cobblestone appearance to the mucosa.

Signs and Symptoms

Patients with IBD have attacks of diarrhea that may be bloody and contain mucus; abdominal pain with cramping; malaise; fever; and weight loss. Bloody stools are more often found in UC than in Crohn disease. The color of blood in the stool depends on the degree and rapidity of the bleed. Slow bleeding and oozing will show a black, tarry stool. If diarrhea is frequent, the blood may be more reddish. The stool color is also dependent on where in the intestine the bleeding is occurring. Blood tends to be redder when the bleeding location is lower in the intestine. The bouts of IBD symptoms often are precipitated by events that cause physical or emotional stress. An acute attack can last for days, weeks, or even months, followed by periods of remission extending from a few weeks to several decades. A few patients experience only one attack and

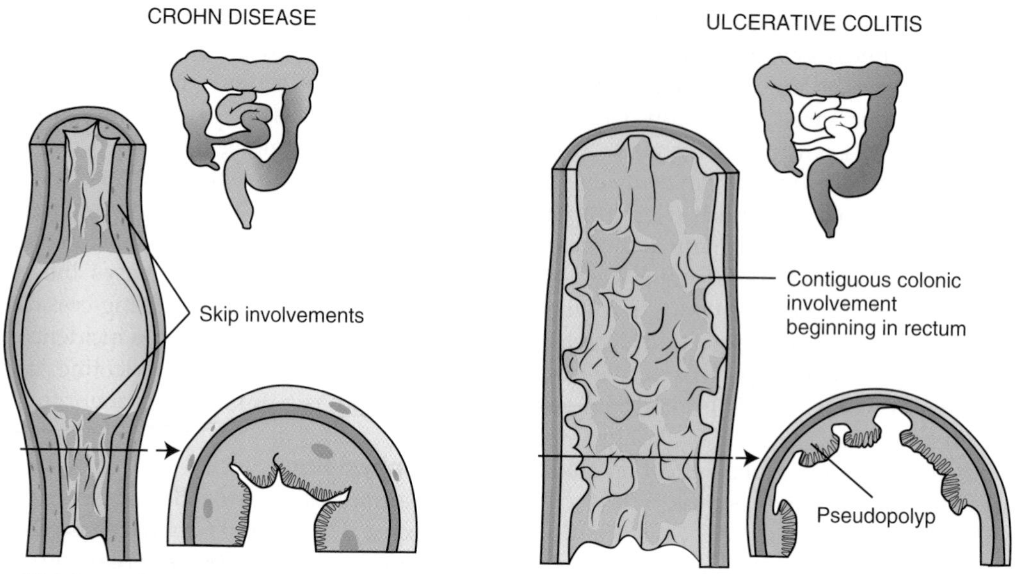

Fig. 29.4 Comparison of the distribution of disease and characteristics of lesions of Crohn disease and ulcerative colitis.

Table 29.2 Comparison of Ulcerative Colitis and Crohn Disease

	ULCERATIVE COLITIS	CROHN DISEASE
Area affected	Mucosa only; usually involves rectum and proceeds up the colon.	Full thickness of the intestine; most common in small intestine.
Characteristics	Mucosa is red; intestinal wall is edematous and friable, bleeding easily; pseudopolyps are present.	Edematous bowel wall, inflammatory cells, mucosal ulcerations, granulomas, and "skip" lesions (normal areas).
Signs and symptoms	Diarrhea, frequently bloody; abdominal cramping relieved by defecation; rectal bleeding.	Fever, malaise, fatigue, weight loss, intermittent diarrhea, cramping or steady right lower quadrant or periumbilical pain, postprandial bloating.
Complications	Massive hemorrhage; hypovolemia, toxic megacolon (rapid dilation of the intestines), cancer of the colon.	Fistulas, anal fissures, perianal disease, bowel obstruction or perforation.

then remain free of symptoms for the rest of their lives. Others have serious intestinal hemorrhage with fluid and electrolyte imbalances.

Safety Alert

Opioids and Anticholinergic Medications

If a patient has ulcerative colitis, opioid medications or anticholinergic medications should be avoided if there is fever, leukocytosis, or worsening symptoms because these medications will further reduce the tone of the colon (Peppercorn & Farrell, 2018).

Diagnosis

Medical diagnosis of IBD usually is based on the patient's medical history and symptoms. Colonoscopy, flexible sigmoidoscopy, mucosal biopsy, barium enema, and stool analysis may be performed to confirm the diagnosis.

Treatment

Treatment for UC and Crohn disease varies according to the severity and frequency of symptoms. Conservative approaches to medical treatment include administration of antidiarrheal drugs, long-term sulfasalazine therapy, and medications to relieve abdominal cramps. The recommended diet consists of low-fat, low-fiber foods that are high in protein and calories. Small, frequent feedings are best. Lactose avoidance helps some patients. During acute attacks, fluid replacement may be necessary. Blood transfusions are given when anemia is present. Medication therapy for Crohn disease includes a biologic agent (tumor necrosis factor inhibitor) with a drug to alter the immune response (azathioprine, methotrexate). Topical 5-aminosalicylic acid (5-ASA) medications given by enema or suppository have proven to cause remission of UC. Oral 5-ASA drugs, such as mesalamine (Pentasa) or olsalazine sodium (Dipentum), are useful for those patients who cannot tolerate rectal administration (see Table 29.1). Budesonide (Entocort) is used to help control disease in the ileum. Patients with advanced disease who are not surgical candidates may be given azathioprine, 6-mercaptopurine, methotrexate, levamisole, or cyclosporine to help control the disease (Rowe, 2017).

Infliximab (Remicade), a monoclonal antibody against tumor necrosis factor, has greater than 80% response rate for Crohn disease but only about a 50% success rate with UC. The drug is extremely expensive and is given IV by a set protocol. Certolizumab pegol (Cimzia) is a drug for patients with moderate to severe Crohn disease who have not responded to conventional treatments.

Surgical intervention is an alternative treatment for some patients. The surgical procedure usually involves removing the affected portion of the bowel, often by proctocolectomy, and creating an ileostomy. A patient with UC may be a candidate for an ileal reservoir (Kock pouch) or an ileoanal anastomosis rather than a standard ileostomy. Both procedures allow the patient control over the discharge of wastes from the reservoir, and consequently a collection pouch is not necessary. The patient uses a catheter to empty the reservoir after the Kock procedure. With an ileoanal anastomosis, the patient retains control over the anal sphincter with voluntary defecation. These procedures are not usually performed for Crohn disease because as the disease progresses, the area of the reservoir becomes involved.

NURSING MANAGEMENT

ASSESSMENT (DATA COLLECTION)

A complete health assessment is performed, with particular attention to nutritional, fluid, and electrolyte status. A thorough abdominal assessment is performed, identifying pain location.

NURSING DIAGNOSIS AND PLANNING

Problem statements or nursing diagnoses might include the following:

- Acute or chronic pain due to intestinal inflammation.
- Fluid volume deficit due to diarrhea fluid loss.
- Diarrhea.
- Altered nutrition due to altered GI absorption.

Expected outcomes might include the following:

- Patient's pain will be controlled with analgesia within 8 hours.
- Patient will regain fluid balance within 24 hours.
- Patient will experience decreased number of diarrhea bowel movements within 24 hours.
- Patient will show evidence of adequate nutrition by a normal nitrogen balance and no further weight loss.

Long-term goals are to help the patient adhere to the prescribed regimen, develop effective coping mechanisms, and participate in prescribed psychotherapy.

IMPLEMENTATION AND EVALUATION

For an acute attack of IBD, care includes monitoring the number and character of stools, periodic auscultation of bowel sounds, measurement of intake and output, and daily weight measurement. Check for signs of internal bleeding and monitor laboratory data for evidence of electrolyte imbalances and anemia. Indicators of successful therapy include a decrease in abdominal cramping and discomfort and return of typical bowel pattern.

> **Think Critically**
>
> Describe three key differences between Crohn disease and UC.

APPENDICITIS

Etiology and Pathophysiology

Appendicitis is an inflammation of the appendix, which is a blind pouch and is therefore easily infected by bacteria passing through the intestinal tract. Obstruction of the opening into the appendix traps fecal material, causing the inflammation.

Signs, Symptoms, and Diagnosis

Pain in the lower right side, halfway between the umbilicus and the crest of the ileum at McBurney point, is the best-known symptom of appendicitis. It is usually accompanied by muscle guarding. However, the location of the pain may—and often does—vary among individuals. The patient may rest with the right thigh drawn up. Extending the leg causes pain. **A slight temperature elevation (1° F), nausea and vomiting, and an increase in the white blood cell count also are characteristic of appendicitis.** IV contrast-enhanced CT scan or ultrasound is used for diagnosis. Radiation exposure concerns have made ultrasound the preferred imaging technique for children and pregnant women. Low-dose CT is used if available (Craig, 2018). Laboratory testing may be performed to rule out other causes of the presenting symptoms.

Treatment

Appendicitis is treated by surgically removing the appendix **(appendectomy).** This procedure may be performed laparoscopically or require an open laparotomy. Patients with nonperforated appendicitis should have surgery within 24 hours of diagnosis. Prior to surgery fluids can be replaced, electrolyte imbalances corrected, and antibiotics started. Before surgery, the patient is NPO. If the infection is widespread or the appendix has ruptured, immediate surgical intervention is indicated. **Under no circumstances should laxatives be given when appendicitis is suspected because of the increased risk for rupture.**

> **Safety Alert**
>
> **Cold, Not Heat, for Appendicitis**
>
> Never use heat to relieve abdominal pain if appendicitis is suspected. Heat might bring enough blood and fluid to the appendix to cause it to rupture and cause peritonitis. An ice bag may be placed on the abdomen to slow down the inflammation and thus prevent rupture of the swollen and inflamed appendix.

The patient is usually encouraged to be out of bed within several hours of surgery, if there are no complications. The patient undergoing an uncomplicated laparoscopic appendectomy may be discharged on the same day after an adequate anesthesia recovery period. The convalescent period is usually uneventful, and the patient may return to their former activities within 1 to 2 weeks. Recovery from an open laparotomy takes 2 to 4 weeks.

Nursing Management

Assess for nausea, determine pain level, take vital signs, and check the abdomen for rigidity that might indicate a ruptured appendix. A diet history for the previous 24 to 48 hours is obtained to help determine whether food poisoning is a cause of the symptoms. Date and character of the last bowel movement and usual bowel pattern are obtained. Common problem statements are listed in Chapter 27, Table 27.2. Preoperatively, *pain* is the primary patient concern, and you will monitor closely for signs of rupture. Postoperatively, pain control, mobility, and prevention of infection at the surgical site are nursing priorities.

> **Older Adult Care Points**
>
> Peritoneal inflammation does not necessarily cause abdominal rigidity in older adults. These patients often have only diffuse abdominal pain, malaise, and weakness. Confusion may be present, and older adults have an increased risk for falls.

PERITONITIS

Etiology

Peritonitis is an inflammation of the peritoneum. It usually occurs when one of the organs it encloses ruptures or is perforated so that the organ's contents (including bacteria) are spilled into the abdominal cavity. Examples of common causes of peritonitis are ruptured appendix; perforated duodenal or gastric ulcer; ruptured ectopic (tubal) pregnancy; diverticulitis with perforation; and traumatic rupture of the colon, spleen, or liver. Patients receiving peritoneal dialysis have a constant risk of developing peritonitis from pathogens entering the abdominal cavity via the dialysis catheter. Patients with cirrhosis can develop spontaneous bacterial peritonitis caused by translocation of gut bacteria to the ascites fluid.

Pathophysiology

As the peritoneum becomes inflamed, there is local redness and swelling of the membrane and production of serous fluid that becomes increasingly purulent as the bacteria multiply. Normal peristaltic action of the intestines slows or ceases, and symptoms of paralytic ileus occur.

Signs and Symptoms

The patient experiences nausea, vomiting, and severe abdominal pain and distention. Fever, chills, tachycardia, and pallor occur, and other symptoms of shock may emerge if sepsis is present. **Unless the condition is treated promptly and successfully, peritonitis can be fatal.** Early diagnosis and prompt treatment with antibiotics have improved survival rates for peritonitis.

Diagnosis and Treatment

Diagnosis of peritonitis is by history, physical examination, and results of a complete blood cell count (CBC). A CT scan of the abdomen may be performed to rule out structural problems or tumor. Broad-spectrum antibiotics are given IV, IV fluids and electrolytes are administered to restore a normal balance, and gastric or intestinal decompression is initiated to relieve distention. Surgical procedures needed to repair a ruptured organ are performed as soon as the patient's condition will permit. Complex situations may require multiple surgical interventions. The abdominal incision may be closed temporarily to protect from contamination. In some cases the wound may be left open with packing and dressings as the only covering.

Nursing Management

Frequent assessment and prompt and accurate reporting of unexpected changes in condition are required. The patient is usually placed in the semi-Fowler position to facilitate breathing, prevent respiratory complications, and aid in localizing the purulent material in the lower abdomen or pelvis. Vital signs are taken and recorded as frequently as every 15 minutes during the critical stage. If vomiting occurs, the characteristics and amount of vomitus are noted. Pain management is also important because this is one of the primary presenting symptoms.

A common complication of peritonitis is paralytic ileus. Auscultate at least once a shift for the return of bowel sounds. If the patient passes flatus or feces rectally, this should be recorded on the chart because it indicates return of peristalsis.

Because of the vascularity of the gut, bacteria are easily picked up by the circulatory system and spread throughout the bloodstream, causing sepsis. High fever and toxicity that accompany peritonitis may cause the patient to be disoriented, and they must be protected from self-injury. This includes putting side rails up, activating the bed alarm, or having someone at the bedside at all times. The patient should be turned *very gently* and moved in the bed with care because of extreme tenderness in the abdominal region. A high fever and the presence of a gastric tube demand frequent mouth care to protect the lips, prevent halitosis, and cleanse the mouth.

Antibiotics must be given as ordered and the IV site monitored so that rehydration with IV fluids and ordered medications can be delivered to relieve symptoms.

MALABSORPTION

Etiology and Pathophysiology

Many disorders interfere with the normal absorption of nutrients, water, and vitamins from the intestine.

Adult celiac disease **(sprue),** in which the patient cannot properly metabolize gluten (a protein found in all wheat products, barley, and rye), is one cause. Lactose intolerance is another cause because it results in diarrhea. Pancreatic disease with interference in secretion of pancreatic digestive enzymes also causes malabsorption. Some patients who have undergone chemotherapy for treatment of cancer experience alteration of the intestinal mucosa that causes malabsorption. **Whatever the cause, malabsorption creates a nutritional deficiency.** Pathophysiologically, there is irritation of the intestinal mucosa and consequent diarrhea. Both problems limit the ability of the intestine to absorb nutrients.

> **Cultural Considerations**
>
> **Lactose Intolerance**
>
> Lactose intolerance is most common in Native American, African American, Hispanic, and Asian populations, but it can affect people of any age and any ethnicity. It is caused by lack of the enzyme lactase, which is needed to digest lactose. Assess for bloating, flatulence, cramps, and loose stools or diarrhea after consuming milk or milk products.

Signs, Symptoms, and Diagnosis

A key sign of fat malabsorption is **steatorrhea**, or passage of stool that is bulky, frothy, and foul smelling and usually floats in the toilet. Other signs and symptoms include weight loss, weakness, and various signs of vitamin deficiency, depending on the type of malabsorption the patient is experiencing. Diagnosis is by history, upper and lower GI series, and endoscopy with biopsy. Gluten intolerance is diagnosed by blood tests for gluten antibodies and small bowel biopsy.

> **Clinical Cues**
>
> If your patient is to undergo testing for gluten intolerance, they must eat wheat and gluten products for a minimum of 2 weeks before testing. The gluten load should be the equivalent of two slices of bread per day; otherwise, the tests will not be accurate.

Treatment and Nursing Management

Treatment is directed at the underlying cause. Pancreatic insufficiency can be treated by administering pancreatic enzymes with meals. Celiac disease is treated by completely omitting gluten from the diet. Lactose intolerance is treated primarily by diet adjustment, limiting intake of lactose. Lactase enzyme preparations are available over the counter and relieve symptoms in some patients. Nursing management consists of supporting the patient through the diagnostic process and reinforcing teaching about diet and medications. The patient is often required to take supplements of vitamins and minerals as a lifetime therapy.

CANCER OF THE COLON

Cancer of the large intestine, also called colorectal cancer, is the third most common malignancy in both men and women in the United States. Certain forms of colon cancer have been identified as having a genetic link and show a familial tendency for occurrence. Approximately 97,220 colon cancer cases occurred in 2018 (American Cancer Society, 2018). Colorectal cancer is one of the most preventable and curable of all cancers if it is found in the early stages, and mortality rates have fallen over the last 30 years as detection has become easier. *Healthy People 2030* objectives include the reduction of deaths by colorectal cancer and a decrease in the incidence of invasive colorectal cancer.

> **Cultural Considerations**
>
> **Colorectal Cancer Incidence**
>
> Colorectal cancer incidence is highest in African American men and women. Mortality rates in African Americans also are higher than in the white population. It is not certain whether this is because of limited access to health care or other reasons. Always assess an African American older than 40 years for risk factors and signs and symptoms of colorectal cancer. Encourage annual screening after age 50 years. High-risk patients need individualized counseling for screening and follow-up (American Cancer Society, 2018).

Etiology

The cause of colorectal cancer has not been established but is generally believed to be a mutation of a naturally occurring process of colon tissue repair and replacement. The disease mainly occurs in people older than 50 years, although there is a type that occurs in young people. People most at risk include those with disorders of the intestinal tract, especially UC and inherited family cancer syndromes. Other risk factors are smoking, alcohol consumption, physical inactivity, obesity, and a diet high in saturated fat and/or red meat, as well as inadequate intake of fruits and vegetables (American Cancer Society, 2018a).

> **Nutrition Considerations**
>
> **The Colon and Conjugated Linoleic Acid**
>
> In research studies with animals, conjugated linoleic acid (CLA) was found to have a protective effect against inflammation in the colon. Human studies have found that the action of CLA in modifying the immune response decreased symptoms in patients with IBD. CLA is found in high-fat nonpasteurized dairy foods, grass-fed beef, and lamb with a diet supplemented by safflower oil (Bassaganya-Riera et al., 2012). Further study has shown that CLA prevents colitis but promotes colon cancer tumor growth (Moreira et al. 2019).

Pathophysiology

The cancerous tumor tissue may be polypoid, protruding into the bowel lumen, or it may be annular and extend

Health Promotion

Colon Cancer Preventive Measures

Preventive measures include a diet that is high in fiber and low in red meat and animal fat. Nutrients that offer protection against colon cancer are fiber, calcium carbonate, selenium, and vitamin C.

around the bowel, causing stricture. Most large bowel tumors are adenocarcinomas and are believed to arise from adenomatous polyps that visibly protrude from the mucosal surface of the bowel. The tumor may spread into adjacent structures or via the lymphatics or the bloodstream.

Complementary and Alternative Therapies

Aspirin, Folic Acid, and Calcium

Some studies suggest that polyp formation can be reduced by taking a baby aspirin or other nonsteroidal antiinflammatory drug (NSAID) each day and diet supplementation with folic acid and calcium. A diet high in fruits, vegetables, and whole grains and adequate exercise are still recommended for maintaining colon health (American Cancer Society, 2018a).

Signs and Symptoms

In the early stages, symptoms are typically mild and vague and depend on the location of the tumor and the function of the affected area. Weight loss may be the first sign. Later signs of colorectal cancer are the result of obstruction of the bowel and extension of the growth to adjacent structures. **Any change in bowel habits, either diarrhea or constipation, could be a sign of colon cancer** (American Cancer Society, 2018b).

Other symptoms include red blood in the stool, black tarry stools, change in stool shape (ribbonlike stool), abdominal distention without weight gain, sensation of incomplete evacuation after a bowel movement, and anemia resulting from intestinal bleeding. Abdominal pain and a sensation of pressure in the lower abdomen or rectum usually are present. Digital examination may reveal a mass in the anus.

Diagnosis

Screening tests include an annual stool guaiac test or fecal immunochemical test or stool DNA test (the ideal frequency for the DNA test is undetermined). Beginning at age 45 years, flexible sigmoidoscopy is recommended every 5 years, colonoscopy every 10 years, double contrast barium x-ray every 5 years, or CT colonography (virtual colonoscopy) every 5 years. Colonoscopy is recommended if any of the screening tests are positive (American Cancer Society, 2018b). If adenomatous polyps are discovered early and removed, colon cancer can be prevented. Tumors of the rectum or lower sigmoid colon are seen by proctosigmoidoscopy. Transrectal ultrasound may be used to determine the extent of a small rectal lesion. Carcinoembryonic antigen (CEA) is elevated in 70% of patients with colorectal cancer, but because it is nonspecific to this type of cancer, it is used mainly to monitor the effectiveness of treatment.

Treatment

Treatment of colorectal cancer usually involves surgical removal of the affected portion of the intestine. Reconnection of the remaining intestine portions (**anastomosis**) is done if the lesion is small and localized (**hemicolectomy**). Alvimopan (Entereg) may be used short term to speed the healing process of the bowel in cases where there is resection and anastomosis. Larger tumors are treated by excising the affected portion of the colon. Occasionally a surgically created opening on the abdomen (**colostomy**) is needed to provide for elimination of fecal matter. A permanent colostomy is rarely needed for cancer of the colon. After healing takes place, the colon is reconnected.

Most tumors are resected with an open approach, but laparoscopic surgery is an option for a small, localized tumor. Further treatment depends on the stage of the cancer—whether the tumor is through the bowel mucosa, through the bowel wall, or affecting lymph nodes or has metastasized to other organs.

Colectomy or hemicolectomy. **Colectomy** is the removal of the diseased portion of the colon. The remaining ends of the colon are reattached (anastomosed). **Hemicolectomy** is removal of one side of the colon.

Abdominoperineal resection. Abdominoperineal resection is performed for cancer in the rectum or low sigmoid colon. It is an extensive surgical procedure in which part of the colon and the entire rectum, anus, and regional lymph nodes are removed. Both an abdominal and a perineal incision are necessary for this procedure. Because of the nature of the surgery, a permanent colostomy is necessary.

Adjunctive treatment. Preoperative, intraoperative, or postoperative radiation and chemotherapy may be given for cancer of the rectum. Use of radiation or chemotherapy for colon cancer depends on the stage of the tumor and the presence of metastasis. These therapies may be used preoperatively to shrink a mass so that it is more easily addressed surgically. When metastasis is present, the patient is usually treated with 5-fluorouracil (5-FU) with or without leucovorin (folinic acid). Oxaliplatin (Eloxatin) is used with 5-FU and leucovorin for treatment-resistant tumors. Intra-arterial chemotherapy may be directed into the liver if metastasis has occurred. Two other drugs may be used as well. Bevacizumab (Avastin) is an antiangiogenesis medication that reduces blood flow to the growing tumor cells, depriving them of nutrients needed for replication. Cetuximab (Erbitux) and panitumumab (Vectibix) are monoclonal antibodies that bind to protein to slow cell growth. Both are used with other chemotherapy drugs. Irinotecan (Camptosar) is available to treat recurrent colon cancer. Capecitabine (Xeloda) is given orally when the tumor has not penetrated the colon wall.

Nursing Management

An abdominal assessment is performed. Questions are asked about bowel pattern and changes, diet pattern, and amount of red meat and charred or grilled food usually eaten. Determine the amount of alcohol consumption and the degree of cigarette smoking. Assess for a family history of colon cancer. Check diagnostic test results such as the CBC for anemia, liver enzymes, and amylase for signs of possible metastatic involvement of the liver or pancreas.

The patient is likely to be very anxious once a diagnosis of colon cancer has been made. Before surgery, focus on the preoperative care and what the patient needs to be taught. Cover what to expect and provide information about postoperative care. Nursing Care Plan 29.1 describes the postoperative care of a patient who has had abdominal surgery with a colectomy.

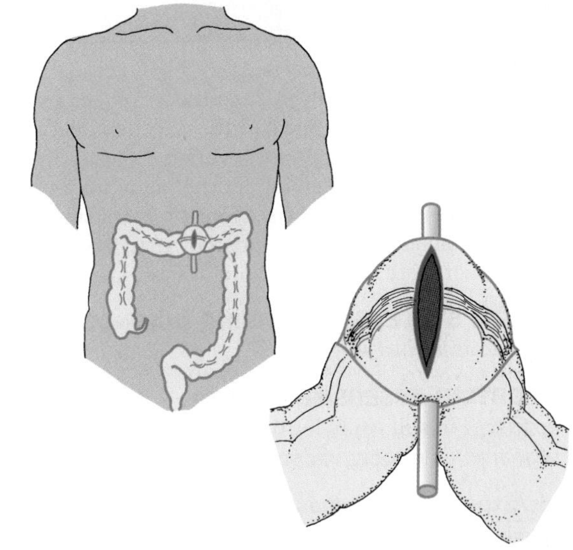

Fig. 29.5 First stage of loop transverse colostomy. A segment of transverse colon is brought out through the abdominal wall and supported by a bridge. A slit in the bowel allows feces to drain from the proximal colon. The support is removed 5 to 7 days after surgery or when the bowel adheres to the abdominal wall.

Health Promotion

Quadrivalent human papillomavirus (HPV) vaccine is FDA approved for use in prevention of anal cancer. HPV is associated with about 90% of anal cancer (Cagir, 2018).

Think Critically

What do you think the psychological concerns might be for a person who is to have a colostomy?

Common problem statements are located in Chapter 27, Table 27.2, but diagnoses specific to cancer (see Chapter 8) are also relevant. The patient will experience multiple physical and psychological challenges throughout the diagnosis and treatment process.

OSTOMY SURGERY AND CARE

In an ostomy procedure, an abdominal incision is made, and either the colon **(colostomy)** or the ileum **(ileostomy)** is brought to the outside to drain fecal material.

COLOSTOMY

A colostomy may be required after a colectomy. The colostomy may be permanent or temporary. For a temporary colostomy, the patient will have surgery later for anastomosis of the open ends.

Types of Colostomies

Colostomies are identified by their location and whether one or two lumens are visible. Transverse colostomies may be a **loop colostomy** or a **double-barreled colostomy.** Usually these techniques are used when there are plans for reversing the colostomy. Colostomies are also located on the ascending and descending colon and can be double lumen or single lumen. Single-opening colostomies are called *single-barreled* or *end colostomy.* **Sigmoid colostomies are the most common location.**

Loop colostomy. During surgery, a loop of the colon is brought through an abdominal incision and onto the surface of the body. An open or laparoscopic approach is used. The colon is transected, and the edges are sutured to the abdominal skin (Fig. 29.5).

An appliance for collection of fecal material is attached over the entire exposed colon.

Double-barreled colostomy. In a double-barreled colostomy, there are two separate stomas (Fig. 29.6). The loop of intestine is completely severed, creating a **proximal stoma** and a **distal stoma.** The proximal stoma is the one closer to the small intestine, so fecal material passes through it to the outside. The distal stoma leads to the rectum and should discharge only small amounts of mucus. The distance between the stomas varies; if they are too close together, it is difficult to get a good seal for the collection device around each one. Eventually the colon ends will be reattached.

Single-barreled or end colostomy. There is only one stoma in a single-barreled colostomy. The end is brought to the abdominal surface, **effaced** (cuffed over itself), and sutured to the skin, making what is called a *surgically mature stoma.* If the colostomy is temporary, the remaining portions of bowel and rectum are left intact. If the colostomy is permanent, an abdominal perineal resection may be performed to remove the freed bowel, anus, and rectum, or the end of the bowel is closed and

Nursing Care Plan 29.1 Care of a Patient Undergoing Colectomy for Probable Colon Cancer

SCENARIO

Mrs. Simpson, age 58 years, just returned from surgery and has a dressing over a colectomy site. She has a family history of polyposis of the colon. She had the colectomy because of a malignant lesion in the upper portion of the sigmoid colon. She was NPO before surgery for a variety of tests. She has an IV running at 125 mL/h and is on a clear liquid diet. She is experiencing pain and receiving morphine by PCA pump. She is very frightened because her father died of colon cancer. She dreads chemotherapy. Mrs. Simpson is a loan officer with a national bank, is very busy, and had put off having a physical examination and sigmoidoscopy until this month, when she noticed some blood in a loose stool. She had experienced some bouts of loose stools but thought these were a result of the stress she was experiencing on her job.

PROBLEM STATEMENT/NURSING DIAGNOSIS

Pain due to abdominal surgery.

SUPPORTING ASSESSMENT DATA

Subjective: "I'm still really hurting."

Objective: Colectomy, abdominal incision with wound drain; pain at 7/10.

Goals/Expected Outcomes	Nursing Interventions	Selected Rationale	Evaluation
Pain will be controlled to a level of 3/10 with analgesia during hospitalization.	Initially assess for pain q1–2h or PRN using pain scale and document location and characteristics.	Pain scale use provides more objective measure of pain. Frequency of assessment may be changed to q3–4h as condition improves.	Pain at 2–3 with use of PCA.
	Monitor use of PCA pump.	PCA allows patient better control over pain.	Using PCA appropriately.
Patient will use relaxation techniques to decrease pain before discharge.	Teach relaxation techniques to decrease anxiety.	Relaxation helps decrease pain.	Taught deep-breathing relaxation exercise.
	Provide comfort measures, such as a tidy, odor-free room and quiet environment.	Comfort measures help decrease the subjective experience of pain.	Lights dimmed and linens changed. Patient expresses appreciation.

PROBLEM STATEMENT/NURSING DIAGNOSIS

Potential for deficient fluid volume/nutritional intake due to prior NPO status and colon surgery.

SUPPORTING ASSESSMENT DATA

Objective: NPO for several days; on clear liquids; IV infusing.

Goals/Expected Outcomes	Nursing Interventions	Selected Rationale	Evaluation
Patient will not develop fluid or electrolyte imbalance as evidenced by good skin turgor, moist mucous membranes, and electrolyte studies within normal range.	Assess skin turgor and mucous membranes each shift. Monitor for adequate urine output.	Skin and mucous membrane assessment gives indication of fluid status. Adequate urine output indicates adequate intake.	Mucous membranes moist, good skin turgor. Urine output 600 mL this shift.
	Assess for signs of dehydration (i.e., poor skin turgor, decreased amounts of and concentrated urine).	If dehydration persists or worsens, the doctor must be notified so that therapy can be adjusted.	Voiding pale yellow urine; skin dry, but no tenting.
	Maintain IV fluid flow as ordered.	Provides fluid until the patient has adequate oral intake.	IV flowing at 125 mL/h.
	Evaluate tolerance of oral fluids, so that diet can be advanced to promote nutritional intake.	GI delivery of nutrition is the most effective and efficient.	Able to tolerate fluids without nausea or abdominal distention.
	Monitor electrolyte laboratory values.	Laboratory values indicate electrolyte imbalances if they occur.	Laboratory specimens to be obtained in A.M. No signs of electrolyte imbalance.

PROBLEM STATEMENT/NURSING DIAGNOSIS

Potential for infection due to colectomy and abdominal incision.

Nursing Care Plan 29.1 Care of a Patient Undergoing Colectomy for Probable Colon Cancer—cont'd

SUPPORTING ASSESSMENT DATA

Objective: Colectomy and abdominal incision with drain.

Goals/Expected Outcomes	Nursing Interventions	Selected Rationale	Evaluation
Patient will not experience wound infection as evidenced by temperature and WBC count within normal range at discharge and wound clean and dry without redness, pain, or purulent drainage.	Assess surgical wounds and adjacent tissues for redness, swelling, warmth, pain, and presence of odors or drainage.	Close observation is necessary to identify the beginning of infection in the early phase.	No redness noted in surrounding tissue. Denies pain or tenderness.
	Track temperature and WBC count.	Changes may indicate beginning infection.	Temp 98.8° F (37.1° C); WBC count 9400/mm^3.
	Reinforce dressings PRN; change q24h or PRN when ordered. Use strict aseptic technique for dressing changes. Clean skin around incision with ordered solution.	Maintaining sterile intact dressing decreases chance of infection.	Incision clean and dry without redness. Sterile dressing changed using sterile technique.
	Maintain patency of drain.	Draining excess fluids from wound site facilitates healing.	Drain in place; small amount of serous fluid noted.

PROBLEM STATEMENT/NURSING DIAGNOSIS

Potential of bleeding from surgical site.

SUPPORTING ASSESSMENT DATA

Objective: Fresh colectomy incision.

Goals/Expected Outcomes	Nursing Interventions	Selected Rationale	Evaluation
Patient will not have excessive blood loss as evidenced by stable vital signs and adequate urine output	Assess vital signs per postoperative routine: q30min for 2 h; q1h for 2 h; q2h for 4 h; then q4h until stable.	Vital signs can indicate hemorrhage.	P 86, R 18, BP 136/84.
	Notify health care provider if change of mental status, tachycardia with increased respirations, or BP 15–20 points below preoperative baseline level; unremitting pain.	Change of mental status is usually the first sign of decreased cerebral perfusion. Tachycardia with increased respirations and falling BP indicates hemorrhage.	Alert and oriented to person, place, and time. Skin is warm, pink, and dry. Vital signs stable.
	Monitor hourly urine output; report if <30 mL for 2 consecutive hours.	Decreasing urine output indicates decreased renal perfusion, which can lead to renal failure if prolonged and severe.	Urine output 125 mL over 2 h.
	Assess dressings for bleeding; check underneath patient.	Postsurgical patients have risk for hemorrhage, and blood can pool underneath the patient.	Dressings dry; no drainage under patient.
	Assess abdomen for increasing girth or rigidity.	Increasing abdominal girth or rigidity could signal internal bleeding.	Abdomen not rigid; girth not increasing.

PROBLEM STATEMENT/NURSING DIAGNOSIS

Anxiety due to fear of cancer, treatment, and possible death.

Continued

Nursing Care Plan 29.1 Care of a Patient Undergoing Colectomy for Probable Colon Cancer—cont'd

SUPPORTING ASSESSMENT DATA

Subjective: Father died of colon cancer; expresses fear of cancer and death; dreads chemotherapy.

Goals/Expected Outcomes	Nursing Interventions	Selected Rationale	Evaluation
Patient will openly discuss fears and concerns with nurse, family, or provider.	Establish trusting relationship with patient through active listening and attentive caring.	A trusting relationship helps patient express feelings.	Not wanting to talk yet; spent quiet time with patient.
	Assess mood and verbal and nonverbal behaviors that suggest readiness to talk.	Expressions of anxiety and fear will manifest differently for each patient; therefore therapeutic responses are based on assessment of the behavior (i.e., crying, yelling, demanding, rejecting, withdrawn, flat affect, sad expression).	Is withdrawn and quiet; does not wish to discuss situation until pathology report is back. Sat quietly with patient for 15 min.
	Reassure patient that you are available for future discussions.	Patient needs to know that you are willing to return and support her, regardless of how she initially responds to you.	Patient informed of hourly rounding schedule and that the nurse is available.
	Offer to contact a cancer organization that provides visits from survivors of similar cancers.	Talking with someone who has experienced the same situation allows the patient to be with someone who understands.	Name and telephone number of volunteer given to patient for contact when the patient is ready.
	Offer to contact hospital chaplain services or individuals of the patient's choice for spiritual support.	Many people seek faith-based support during times of crisis and find comfort and direction for decision making.	Patient requested her rabbi be asked to visit her.

PROBLEM STATEMENT/NURSING DIAGNOSIS

Potential altered breathing pattern due to anesthesia, analgesia, and postoperative pain.

SUPPORTING ASSESSMENT DATA

Subjective: "I don't want to cough."

Objective: Underwent general anesthesia; receiving morphine via PCA; shallow breaths.

Goals/Expected Outcomes	Nursing Interventions	Selected Rationale	Evaluation
Patient will not develop atelectasis or pneumonia as evidenced by normal breath sounds in all lobes of lungs.	Assist patient to turn, cough effectively, and deep-breathe at least q2h.	Coughing and turning assists with lung expansion.	Coughing and turning q2h. Decreased breath sounds in bases of lungs.
	Monitor for proper use of incentive spirometer.	Incentive spirometer helps prevent atelectasis.	Using incentive spirometer correctly q2h.
	Auscultate lungs every shift. Monitor pulse oximetry.	Auscultation tells whether all areas of the lungs are aerating.	Decreased breath sounds in bases bilaterally; no adventitious sounds. Spo_2 98%.
	Assist out of bed to sit in chair or ambulate as ordered.	Early mobility improves lung function and decreases complications such as pneumonia.	Able to move, stand, pivot, and sit in chair with one-person assist. Continue plan.

CRITICAL THINKING QUESTIONS

1. Why is it significant that Mrs. Simpson has familial polyposis?
2. What should other family members be told? What is your role in disclosing information?
3. Why is a patient such as Mrs. Simpson likely to have IV therapy ordered?

BP, Blood pressure; *GI*, gastrointestinal; *IV*, intravenous; *NPO*, nothing by mouth; *P*, pulse; *PCA*, patient-controlled analgesia; *PRN*, as needed; *R*, respirations; Spo_2, pulse oximetry; *WBC*, white blood cell.

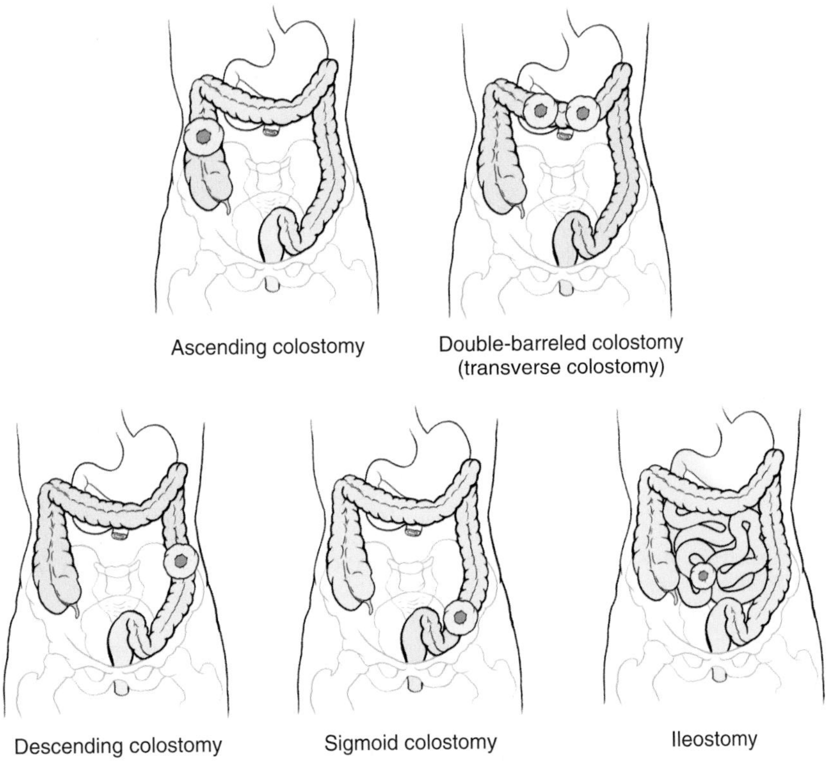

Fig. 29.6 Types of ostomies and intestinal diversions.

returned to the abdomen. It will continue to produce mucous and expel it from the anus.

Colostomy Locations

An ascending colostomy is one in which either one end or a loop of a portion of the ascending colon is brought to the surface of the abdomen to form a stoma. The stool from an ascending colostomy is watery and unformed.

An ascending colostomy usually is temporary and is performed to allow the bowel distal to the ostomy to rest and heal. This is sometimes necessary for patients with IBD, to reconstruct an intestinal birth defect, or for patients who have experienced an intestinal tear from trauma. After the rest and healing period, the surgeon will replace and reattach the intestine ends, and fecal material can be defecated normally.

A transverse colostomy is situated toward the middle of the abdomen (location of transverse colon). This kind of colostomy usually is temporary. The stool from a transverse colostomy is soft and is discharged unpredictably.

A sigmoid (descending) colostomy is located on the surface of the lower quadrant of the abdomen (see Fig. 29.6). It is the most common type of permanent colostomy and usually is done to treat cancer of the rectum. The stool from a sigmoid colostomy is more solid and well formed and may be discharged no more often than once a day or every 2 days. It is therefore much easier to establish a pattern of evacuation to control the flow of fecal material through a sigmoid colostomy.

ILEOSTOMY

An *ileostomy* is performed to drain fecal material from the ileum. It is indicated when disease, congenital defects, or trauma requires bypassing the entire colon. The most common indications for ileostomy are chronic IBD, such as UC and Crohn disease; malignancy; and the presence of many polyps in the colon (multiple polyposes). The latter disease is hereditary, and the polyps have a high potential for malignancy.

The site for the stoma of an ileostomy must be carefully selected so that it is not near any bony prominences, folds of skin, or scars and is in a place where the patient can see it and care for it (see Fig. 29.6). The stool from an ileostomy is liquid, and although digestion is completed by the time the fecal material reaches the stoma, it still contains digestive enzymes that are highly irritating to the skin. Skin protection is very important for long-term management.

Surgeons may choose from several techniques to create an ileostomy. The pouch ileostomy or continent ileostomy frees the ileostomy patient from the need to wear a collection device. A small segment of the ileum is looped back on itself to form a pouch (Kock pouch), and a nipple effect is created (Fig. 29.7, *A*). Pressure from the accumulating feces closes the nipple valve, preventing constant drainage through the stoma. The patient empties the pouch every 3 to 4 hours during the day by inserting a catheter into the stoma.

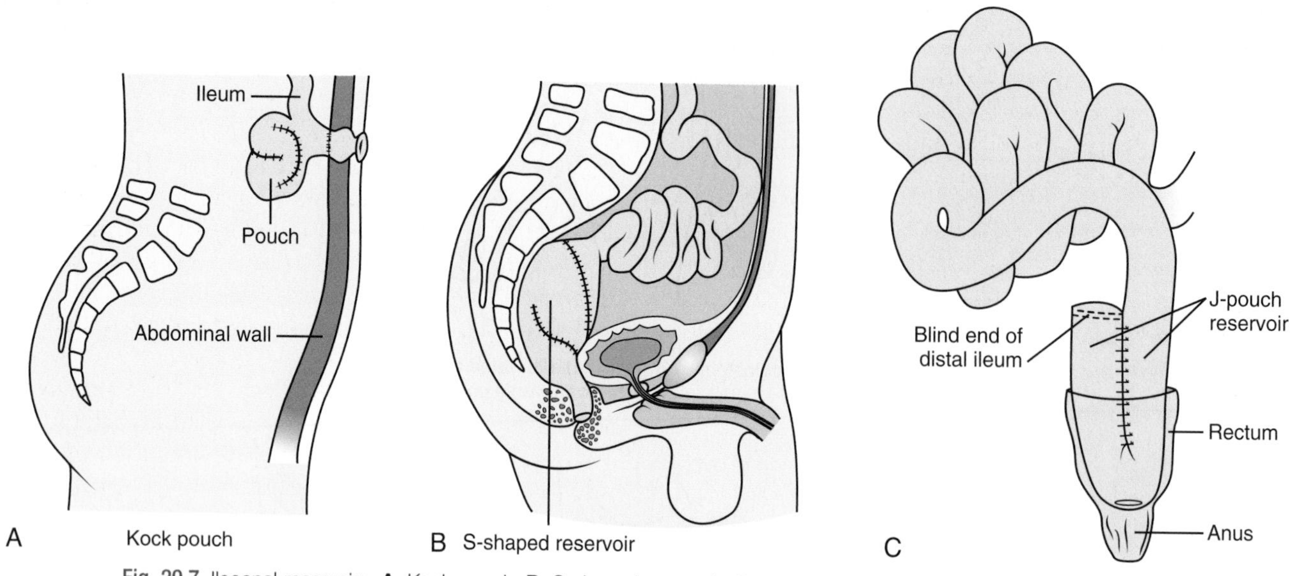

Fig. 29.7 Ileoanal reservoirs. **A,** Kock pouch. **B,** S-shaped reservoir. **C,** J-shaped reservoir. (From Williams P: *deWit's fundamental concepts and skills for nursing*, ed 5, St. Louis, 2018, Elsevier.)

Not every patient can be treated by this surgical technique. It has some disadvantages and must be performed by a surgeon skilled in the procedure. Among those who are not good candidates for a continent ileostomy are patients with chronic inflammatory disease, because the disease tends to recur. Another consideration is the patient's potential for self-care; a catheter must be inserted for periodic drainage of the Kock pouch, and the patient must be able to understand instructions and perform self-care. A third contraindication is related to previous surgery. Patients who have had a conventional ileostomy cannot have a continent ileostomy done if they have less than 29 mm of terminal ileum remaining. This much is needed to construct the nipple valve.

The preferred procedure for UC is the creation of a pouch from the terminal ileum; the pouch is sutured directly to the anus **(ileoanal pouch).** The anal sphincter is left intact and functional. It is a two-stage surgical procedure in which a loop ileostomy is performed and then is closed 3 or 4 months later, when healing is complete. The reservoir may be S-shaped or J-shaped (Fig. 29.7, *B and C*). Most patients then have three to eight bowel movements a day. Slight fecal incontinence may be a problem, particularly at night. This procedure is performed only on those patients younger than 55 years who do not have any anal sphincter deterioration. The mucosa is stripped from the small segment of the rectum that is retained to prevent recurrent UC. "Pouchitis" occurs in about 29% of patients and tends to be recurrent. A course of metronidazole (Flagyl) may adequately treat pouchitis. Otherwise, alternate antibiotics and/or steroids are used.

Although not every patient needing an ileostomy can have a continent ileostomy, it is a safe and effective procedure for many. It eliminates the need for an external appliance, is a more natural way to handle waste, greatly reduces fear of embarrassment from leakage of gas and feces, and minimizes peristomal skin problems.

PREOPERATIVE NURSING CARE

Before surgery of the large intestine, fecal material is removed from the colon. To accomplish this, the patient usually takes oral laxatives the night before surgery and ingests only clear liquids. An enema may also be indicated. In certain cases, oral antibiotics may be started.

The contents of the stomach are removed by inserting an NG tube and connecting the tube to a suction apparatus in the operating room. The tube may be left in place after surgery to remove accumulations of mucus and gas that may cause distention and strain on the sutures, but it is usually able to be removed in the operating room or recovery room. Postoperative ileus occurs in approximately 5% of patients, in which case the tube is replaced.

❖ NURSING MANAGEMENT

◆ ASSESSMENT (DATA COLLECTION)

The immediate postoperative care for a patient who has had intestinal surgery is the same as for other patients who have had major abdominal surgery. Frequent assessment of vital signs, surgical site, bowel sounds, and IV site is conducted. The patient is assessed for nausea and treated in the early postoperative period because vomiting places a strain on suture lines. Bowel manipulation during the procedure usually produces ileus for several hours to days. Pain is usually managed by opioid medications that contribute to decreased bowel motility. Intake and output are tracked, and fluid balance is assessed.

Psychosocial assessment postoperatively focuses on the patient's perception of their altered body image; the meaning of the altered body part; their usual and current coping skills, emotional state, support systems, and presurgery lifestyle; and their perception of physical prognosis and its effect on their life.

◆ NURSING DIAGNOSIS AND PLANNING

Problem statements or nursing diagnoses concerning the surgical procedure are similar to those for abdominal surgery (see Nursing Care Plan 29.1; see also Chapter 27, Table 27.2).

◆ IMPLEMENTATION

The patient is started on liquids when tolerated, and the diet is slowly advanced. Early feeding encourages peristalsis in the gut, decreasing ileus.

Complementary and Alternative Therapies

Chewing Gum Postoperatively

Several studies have shown that chewing gum helps decrease postoperative ileus (Kalff, Wehner, & Babak, 2018).

The passing of gas, liquids, or solids through the rectum (or stoma) is an indication of active peristalsis. Observe patients carefully for evidence of the return of peristalsis, and chart it in the medical record. The IV site, fluids, and electrolyte levels are monitored very carefully because the patient is especially prone to fluid and electrolyte imbalances. Pain assessment is ongoing, and the effectiveness of analgesia should be assessed after administering pain medication.

Think Critically

How does the effluent from a transverse colostomy, from a sigmoid colostomy, and from an ileostomy differ?

Care of the Stoma

The stoma is inspected for a normal pink or deep red color, which indicates adequate blood supply. It should look like healthy mucous membrane such as that inside the mouth. Later, the stoma will shrink in size and may be less highly colored. There may be slight bleeding around the stoma and its stem, but anything more than slight bleeding should be reported. Most collection devices are transparent, so checking for color and bleeding does not require removal of the appliance. Dark purple or black stoma color should be reported immediately. The skin around the stoma is assessed for irritation or signs of breakdown.

Observe the stoma for signs of edema. In the early postoperative period, the stoma will be slightly edematous and larger than it will be after complete healing has taken place. Stoma edema can be caused by a collection device whose opening is too narrow to accommodate the stoma. The opening of the collection device should be at least ⅛-inch larger than the circumference of the stoma. A variety of appliances are available, both one- and two-piece devices. The two-piece systems allow for changing the collection bag without removing the appliance from the skin. This allows for direct visualization of the stoma. Products that seal around the stoma to prevent leaks and that stretch to fit snugly around the stoma without compromising it are currently being used.

Fecal output from the colostomy stoma does not occur for 2 to 4 days because of the preoperative bowel evacuation, possible ileus, and clear liquid diet postoperatively. A surgical dressing may be in place immediately after surgery and is replaced with an appliance within 24 to 48 hours. If there is a perineal wound, the appearance, amount, and character of drainage are assessed and charted. Carefully inspect for signs of infection. Such a wound may be left open to heal by secondary intention, in which case it may be 3 months before it is completely healed. Initially there will be a drain in the wound. Antibiotic therapy is usually given for 24 hours postoperatively for antimicrobial prophylaxis or longer if there is a known infection.

A surgical dressing is never placed over an ileal stoma because output is continuous. If there is a significant decrease in ileal output accompanied by stomach cramping, the ileum may be obstructed. Such symptoms should be reported to the surgeon immediately. If the condition is not relieved, perforation or rupture of the intestine eventually may occur.

Older Adult Care Points

Older adults may require assistance with ostomy care because of poor vision or severe arthritis in the hands. In this case a family member must be taught the techniques of care. Older adults should be given easy-to-follow, large-print instructions for care.

Measurement of Intake and Output

Accurate recording of intake and output is especially important in the care of an ostomy patient. Total output of fecal material is calculated every 8 hours. If the stool is liquid, the accuracy of measurement is very important. When the patient's condition is stable, ostomy output is regular, and the patient's nutrition and hydration status are normal, intake and output recording is discontinued.

A patient who has had an ileostomy must always be watched for signs of dehydration and fluid imbalance. This is especially important during the immediate postoperative period but remains a concern for as long as the patient has the ileostomy. The function of the colon is to reabsorb water, sodium, and chloride and to secrete bicarbonate and mucus. Eliminating this step causes the ileostomy output to be liquid and acidic. To prevent dehydration, fluid intake should be sufficient to compensate for the loss of fluid through the feces.

Evacuation and Irrigation

Once the patient is eating again, ileostomy drainage is usually emptied five to eight times per day. The pouch should be emptied when it is one-third full. The patient sits on the toilet, unclamps the drainage device, and allows the effluent to drain into the bowl. The clamp is then closed, and the outside of the bag is cleansed of any debris. Ileostomies are not usually irrigated unless there is blockage by large particles of undigested food; then irrigation is done by a health care provider or enterostomal therapist.

A continent ileostomy with a Kock pouch has a drainage tube inserted, with gravity drainage maintained in the immediate postoperative period to prevent distention and allow the pouch to heal. In about 2 weeks, the patient is taught to insert a catheter into the pouch to drain the contents. As the pouch matures and its capacity increases, the time between drainings will lengthen. The pouch may be irrigated occasionally to remove fecal residue.

A sigmoid colostomy will usually expel formed stool on a relatively regular schedule. Irrigation of the colostomy gives the patient some control over when elimination takes place. The procedure is done daily or every other day at about the same time and takes close to an hour. A catheter with a cone tip is attached to a bag, which is filled with 500 to 1000 mL of warm (not hot) tap water. The bag is positioned 18 to 20 inches above the height of the stoma. The colostomy appliance is removed, and an irrigating sleeve is attached to direct the drainage into the toilet. The cone tip is lubricated and inserted gently into the ostomy stoma, and the water is infused slowly to prevent cramping and distention. The cone tip is removed, and the drainage flows through the sleeve into the toilet. When drainage is complete, the sleeve is removed, skin care is performed, and a clean appliance is secured in place. If the patient has a regular evacuation pattern, irrigation is not necessary. If the patient has a regular evacuation schedule whether irrigated or natural, they may be able to use a stoma cap and not need an appliance.

The major reason for irrigating a colostomy is to establish a pattern of predictable bowel movements at the patient's convenience. If the patient prefers not to irrigate, suppositories can be used to stimulate evacuation. Patients who do not irrigate must wear a drainable pouch because evacuation can be unpredictable.

Peristomal Skin Care

Drainage from an ileostomy contains enzymes and bile salts that are highly damaging to the skin. The area of skin around the stoma must be kept clean and protected; fecal material should not be allowed to seep around the opening of the collection device and pool on the skin. In the immediate postoperative period, the pouch should not be changed any more often than is necessary to prevent trauma to the skin.

The two major principles to follow to protect the skin are cleanliness and the provision of a protective barrier to prevent contact between the skin and the discharge from the stoma. If there is a proper seal to prevent seepage of feces around the stoma, irritation and breakdown of the skin occur much less frequently.

Appliances are generally changed every 2 to 3 days to maintain an effective seal. When the appliance is changed, it should be removed carefully and the skin washed gently with soap and water so that skin is not damaged by vigorous rubbing and scrubbing. The area should be rinsed thoroughly and dried by patting, not rubbing, the skin. In humid weather, a hair dryer on the low setting may be used to dry the skin. Possible causes of skin problems are allergic reactions, yeast infections, or irritation from changing the faceplate too frequently. After cleansing, a protective skin barrier paste, wipe, or spray—which serves to prevent contact between the skin and the waste being discharged through the stoma—is applied. This may or may not be used for a sigmoid colostomy stoma.

Protective barriers are available in a number of forms and types. The enterostomal therapist or surgeon will indicate which type of barrier is most effective for the

Cultural Considerations

Cultural Issues for Ostomy Patients

Be aware that cultural and religious considerations for hygiene and fasting may be important for your ostomy patient. For example, on the Jewish Shabbat, strictly observant practice may prohibit the use of running water or electricity; therefore hygiene must be accomplished before the start of Shabbat. A Muslim patient may observe a strict fasting practice for Ramadan that lasts 28 days, when no food or fluid is consumed between sunrise and sunset. An ileostomy patient could be at risk for dehydration, or a change of eating patterns could lead to diarrhea or constipation (Black, 2009).

Assignment Considerations

Ostomy Care

The care of a new postoperative ostomy should not be assigned to unlicensed assistive personnel (UAP) because assessments of the stoma, incision, and skin are essential. When ostomy care for a mature ostomy is assigned to a certified nursing assistant (CNA) or UAP, remind the person to note the color of the stoma and to immediately report if the stoma appearance is not rosy pink or if there is excoriation of the skin. Documenting the appearance of the stoma, the condition of the skin, and the type and amount of effluent is your responsibility regardless of whether the patient or assistive personnel does the actual cleaning and appliance change.

Clinical Cues

Gently placing a cotton tamponade into the stoma opening after removing the appliance will prevent ileostomy contents from getting on the skin and causing irritation while cleaning the skin and changing the appliance.

individual patient. Should the skin become highly irritated despite efforts to protect it, the health care provider will prescribe topical medications. Fungal infection of the skin sometimes occurs.

Older Adult Care Points

The changes related to aging reduce reaction time and manual dexterity, decrease visual and hearing acuity, and cause memory loss and fatigue. In addition, changes in body contour such as loss of supporting subcutaneous tissues, wrinkling, and fragility of skin may result in improper fit of appliances. An older adult may have been "educated" about self-care when the ostomy was first established; however, they may have had no follow-up because of transportation issues or because they "didn't want to bother anybody." You should advocate for regular follow-up appointments.

Changing the Collection Device

There are two kinds of pouches or appliances: drainable and closed-end. Each is attached to a faceplate that is secured to the skin around the stoma with a special adhesive. Drainable pouches are used when the flow of waste cannot be regulated and the contents must be emptied frequently (Fig. 29.8). Closed-end pouches are used only for security once bowel movements have been regulated. Either new appliance is trimmed to size using a template drawn from the dimensions of the stoma plus ⅛ inch if using cut to fit barriers. Barriers or wafers are also available in pre-cut and moldable options. The barrier should not be constricting to the stoma but must be tight enough so that skin is not exposed to effluent.

Psychosocial Concerns

Patients with an ostomy usually go through the stages of grief and loss (see Chapter 8). Your attitude toward the patient, the stoma, and care has a major effect on the attitude the patient develops about body image changes and self-care. Disposing of body waste is not a pleasant nursing task, but a matter-of-fact, efficient approach is best when caring for the stoma, the effluent, and the drainage device.

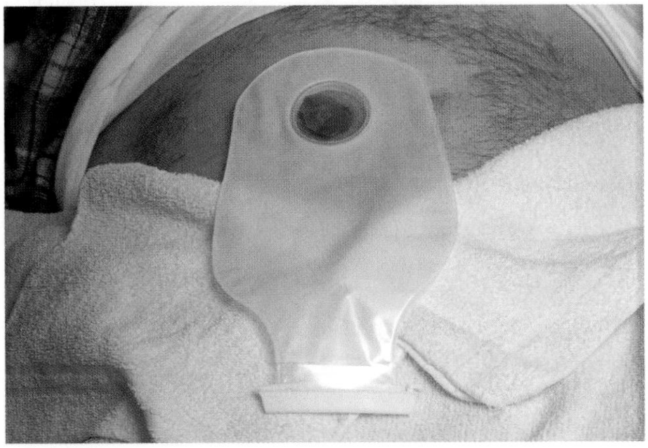

Fig. 29.8 Ostomy collection appliance in place and sealed around the stoma. (From Williams P: *deWit's fundamental concepts and skills for nursing*, ed 5, St. Louis, 2018, Elsevier.)

Encourage social interaction and contact available support groups. **As soon as postoperative pain is well controlled, it is best if the patient can talk with another person who has fully adjusted to their ostomy and is living a full and active life.** A series of such visits allows time to formulate and address questions. Such visits do require an order by the health care provider.

The patient should be guided to express their concerns about the physical and social problems they might encounter as a result of the ostomy. Most patients have concerns about odor, leakage, and noise from the passing of flatus. You and the patient should jointly explore changes in lifestyle and realistic alternatives. For example, a patient with a colostomy might be interested in trying a stoma cap or patch, which is a small, flat absorbent device that is placed directly over the stoma. The cap will absorb mucus but has no capacity to collect stool or fluids; thus irrigation must be done immediately before application. This option might be used for sexual relations or sports (Hooper, 2017).

You should indicate that concerns about sexual function are expected. Concerns should be addressed matter-of-factly, and the patient's sexual partner should be included in discussions. The enterostomal therapist is a good resource for specific information and suggestions in this area.

When the patient has prolonged dysfunctional grieving, becomes clinically depressed, or cannot accept their altered body image, referral for professional counseling is appropriate.

Patient Education

After teaching the patient about the physiology of the ostomy and the steps involved in taking care of the stoma and skin, teach the patient how to control odor. There will be odor when the drainage pouch is changed or emptied, just as there is with normal bowel movements.

Good basic hygiene is essential. Another measure used to control odor is to eliminate from the diet foods known to cause odor or gas. Such foods include eggs, fish, garlic, raw onions, cucumbers, radishes, sauerkraut, corn, broccoli, cabbage, cauliflower, asparagus, dairy products, beans and other legumes, soy, some spices, and chewing gum. Eating too quickly and not chewing food well can cause gas. Carbonated and alcoholic beverages also contribute to the problem.

Gas entering the pouch from the stoma will accumulate there until the pouch is opened and the gas is released (called "burping" the bag). To release gas, open the lower end of the pouch and gently press against its sides or, if using a two-piece device, slightly separate the pouch from the flange at the top; release gas; then reattach. If not released, the gas may cause enough pressure to make the device separate from the stoma. Other options include a charcoal-filtered valve that allows gas to escape. Deodorizing sprays and tablets can be put in the bag to reduce odor. A vent device can be added to the bag for easy removal of gas.

Patients with a colostomy slowly resume a regular diet. All ostomy patients are taught to prevent problems with diarrhea, constipation, and blockage. Dietary guidelines are more important for the ileostomy patient.

Patient Teaching

Measures to Prevent Intestinal Blockage for Ileostomy Patients

Teach the patient the following:

- Eat six small meals a day.
- Eat a soft diet during the healing period.
- Chew food very thoroughly.
- Add other foods to your diet gradually.
- Drink more than 8 cups of fluid per day.
- Avoid the following foods:
  - Dried fruits
  - Corn, including popcorn
  - Nuts
  - Sunflower and other seeds
  - Sausages and foods with casings
  - Apple peel
  - Oranges
  - Pineapple
  - Raw cabbage
  - Celery
  - Chinese vegetables
  - Coconut
  - Mushrooms
- If you experience a blockage in the intestine or of the ostomy:
  - Begin a liquid diet.
  - Cut the opening in your faceplate a little larger than normal because the stoma may swell.
  - Take a warm bath to relax the abdominal muscles.
  - Massage the abdomen and area around the stoma; this might increase the pressure behind the blockage and help it "pop out." Most food blockages occur just below the stoma.
  - Try different body positions, such as a knee-chest position, to move the blockage forward.
  - Take oral enzymes to encourage digestion.
- If you still have a blockage or have no stomal output for several hours:
  - Call your health care provider or enterostomal nurse and report the problems.
  - If you cannot reach your provider or the enterostomal nurse, go to the emergency department. Take all pouch changing supplies with you.
  - **Do *not* try to lavage the ileostomy.**
  - **Do *not* take a laxative.**
- Other pointers:
  - **Ileostomy patients should not take time-release capsules and enteric-coated tablets because there is not enough time for adequate absorption before the medication is expelled through the stoma.**
  - **Adequate intake of fluids is important for all ostomy patients, to prevent dehydration and electrolyte imbalance.**

Many sources of information are available for ostomy patients. These include the local branches of the American Cancer Society, ostomate clubs, enterostomal therapists, and other members of the health care team who have expertise in managing a stoma. Enterostomal therapists are wound care specialists (often with a master's degree but with certification in wound and ostomy care).

◆ EVALUATION

The patient should demonstrate an ability to perform ostomy care and an understanding of how to manage diet and prevent potential complications, such as fluid and electrolyte imbalance, skin breakdown, and blockage of the ostomy. In addition, the patient should demonstrate psychological adjustment to changes in body image. The plan is adjusted if goals are not being met.

ANORECTAL DISORDERS

HEMORRHOIDS

Hemorrhoids are varicosities of the veins of the rectum. They may be **internal** (inside the sphincter muscles of the anus) or **external** (outside the sphincter muscles) (Fig. 29.9).

Etiology and Pathophysiology

Venous congestion from interference with venous return from the hemorrhoidal vessels leads to the development of hemorrhoids. Constipation, obesity, prolonged standing or sitting, and pregnancy are predisposing causes of hemorrhoids. The habit of sitting on the toilet and straining at the stool for long periods is one of the primary factors responsible for many cases of hemorrhoids. Enlargement of the prostate, uterine fibroids, and rectal tumors are other contributing factors. Chronic liver disease with portal hypertension is another cause.

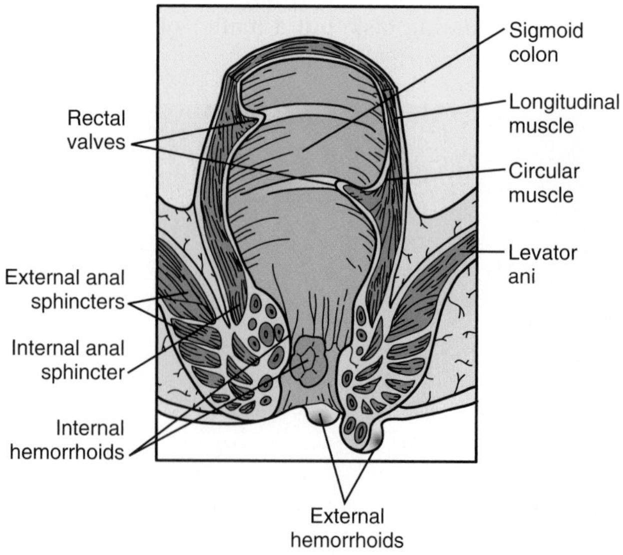

Fig. 29.9 Hemorrhoids. (From deWit SC, O'Neill P: *Fundamental concepts and skills for nursing,* ed 4, Philadelphia, 2014, Elsevier.)

Signs, Symptoms, and Diagnosis

Local pain and itching are the most common symptoms of hemorrhoids. Bleeding from the rectum at the time of defecation may also occur. Hemorrhoidal blood is usually bright to dark red and is located on the outside of the stool. External hemorrhoids are less likely to bleed, but they are more evident because they appear as tumorlike projections around the rectum. Diagnosis is by physical examination. If rectal bleeding has occurred, anoscopy and/or flexible sigmoidoscopy will be performed to rule out more serious causes of rectal bleeding and to diagnose internal hemorrhoids.

Treatment

The symptoms of external hemorrhoids may be relieved by correcting constipation, local applications of heat or cold, and sitz baths. The use of ointments that contain a local anesthetic helps relieve the itching and pain. Hydrocortisone ointment and suppositories help decrease the swelling. The patient also should be instructed to wash the anal region with warm water after each bowel movement to prevent infection at the breaks in the mucosa. Wipes not containing alcohol may be used for cleaning without the mucosal drying that soap causes. A high-fiber diet and adequate fluid intake can help decrease or eliminate symptoms.

Hemorrhoids that do not respond to conservative therapy can be treated by **sclerópathy** (injection of a solution that causes the vessel to dry up and disintegrate), **cryotherapy** (freezing), **photocoagulation** (burning), or infrared coagulation (IRC). **Hemorrhoidectomy** using a laser or standard surgical procedure may be performed. Another treatment method is rubber band ligation, in which a rubber band is slipped around the hemorrhoidal vessel, cutting off the blood supply. This causes the hemorrhoid to shrivel and disintegrate. All of these methods are usually done as outpatient treatments. Hemorrhoidectomy may occasionally be done as an inpatient procedure.

Nursing Management

Preoperatively, instruct the patient on rectal hygiene and the use of hydrocortisone suppositories or cream and sitz baths to decrease swelling. Teach the patient ways to prevent constipation and to promote regular bowel evacuation.

After surgery, the patient receives a prescription for analgesics. An air-filled or foam pillow may be used while the patient is sitting to decrease pain and pressure on the rectal area. The patient should not use a ring-shaped device because it increases stress to the surgical site. Sitz baths are usually ordered three times a day, and cold or warm compresses are a comfort measure. Mild, wet nonalcohol dressings also may be used on the surgical site. These dressings have a glycerin base and contain a mild astringent that reduces swelling and relieves pain.

Bowel movements after a hemorrhoidectomy will cause some pain, and the standard procedure is to administer a stool softener to make defecation less traumatic. The patient and family should be warned that the patient may become faint, and someone should stay close by.

A high-fiber diet is started right away because it is best if formed stool is passed regularly. A sitz bath after each bowel movement will offer relief and also cleanse the affected area, keeping it free from irritation. The patient should continue warm water cleansing after bowel movements until healing is complete.

PILONIDAL SINUS (PILONIDAL CYST)

Etiology and Pathophysiology

The word **pilonidal** means "having a nest of hair." A pilonidal sinus is a lesion located in the cleft of the buttocks at the sacrococcygeal region. It is sometimes called a *pilonidal cyst,* but it is believed to be a subcutaneous canal (sinus) with one or more openings into the skin (rather than a true cyst or fluid-filled sac). The condition occurs when the stiff hairs in the sacrococcygeal region irritate and eventually penetrate the soft skin in the cleft of the buttocks. Factors that can lead to development of such a sinus include local injury, improper cleaning of the area, and obesity. People who have more than the average amount of body hair are particularly susceptible.

Signs, Symptoms, and Diagnosis

A pilonidal sinus may cause no trouble until it becomes infected, and then the patient experiences pain in the area, with swelling and a purulent drainage. Diagnosis is by history and examination. Mild to severe pain, with a sudden onset while sitting or bending, indicates an acute flare-up and possible formation of an abscess.

Treatment and Nursing Management

When symptoms are severe or persistent, with abscess formation, the area must be incised surgically and the connecting canals opened and drained. Hairs and necrotic tissue must be removed so that the area can heal. This is usually performed as an outpatient surgical procedure. Packing is left in the cavity so that drainage can continue.

Postoperative care includes removal of wound packing, cleansing with warm water two to three times a day, and redressing the wound. Site care continues until the wound has closed. Good hygiene and shaving the site every few weeks may prevent future infections. Antibiotics do not heal a pilonidal cyst.

ANORECTAL ABSCESS AND FISTULA

Etiology and Pathophysiology

An abscess may form where there has been irritation with breaks in the skin or mucosa. Localized infection with a collection of pus forms an anorectal abscess. Tears in the mucosa of the rectum from hard, constipated stools may predispose to abscess and fistula formation. A fistula is a chronic granulomatous tract that travels in a line from the anal canal to the skin outside the anus or from an anorectal abscess to the anal canal or the area around the anus.

Signs, Symptoms, and Diagnosis

A discharge of pus from the fistula opening may be the first sign of an abscess or fistula. Both abscess and fistula are painful, and sitting or coughing aggravates the pain. If a fistula is accompanied by diarrhea, Crohn disease is suspected; 50% of patients with Crohn disease develop a rectal fistula. Diagnosis is by history and physical examination.

Treatment and Nursing Management

Antibiotics are usually not administered unless other conditions are present. Medication for pain is prescribed. Incision and drainage of an abscess may be necessary. A fistula usually requires surgical excision and repair. Nursing management involves teaching measures to prevent further incidence of constipation and infection and rectal hygiene measures. Sitz baths are used to decrease inflammation. Education about pain medication and possible complications is provided.

COMMUNITY CARE

Nurses in the community should teach self-care and habits that promote healthy function of the GI system. A healthy diet with appropriate quantities of fiber and fluid, counseling regarding exercise programs, and teaching about the warning signs of colon cancer are all appropriate nursing interventions, to be used whenever possible. Nurses should be a role model for a healthy diet and exercise program to maintain weight within normal limits.

Nurses who work in long-term care facilities and home settings must be vigilant to spot problems of the GI system. Monitoring nutritional and bowel status is standard practice for every patient. On a continuing basis it is important to assess bowel changes that might indicate colon cancer. Remember that patients who are under care for other disorders still need to have regular cancer screenings.

Get Ready for the NCLEX® Examination!

Key Points

- IBD includes UC and Crohn disease. An altered bowel pattern, abdominal pain with bloating, and diarrhea or constipation are typical. Problems include ulceration, edema, bleeding, and fluid and electrolyte loss. Drug therapy includes antidiarrheals, sulfasalazine, drugs to relieve abdominal cramping, and corticosteroids.
- Surgery for ulcerative colitis usually involves a proctocolectomy with ileostomy, a Kock pouch creation, or an ileoanal reservoir.
- A hernia can become incarcerated, trapping intestine, cutting off its blood supply, and causing intestinal obstruction.
- Diverticulitis produces diarrhea or constipation, left lower abdominal pain, fever, and rectal bleeding. Treatment of diverticulitis includes antibiotics, NPO status or a liquid diet, IV hydration, and surgical hemicolectomy.
- A high-fiber diet and a lot of fluid are prescribed for patients with diverticular disease.
- Mechanical bowel obstruction is mainly caused by adhesions, volvulus, intussusception, and strangulated hernia. Nonmechanical bowel obstruction may be a result of paralytic ileus after surgery, hypokalemia, infection, uremia, or heavy-metal poisoning.
- Appendicitis (inflammation of the appendix) classically causes right lower quadrant pain accompanied by muscle guarding. Nausea and vomiting, a slight temperature elevation, and an increase in the white blood cell count may also occur.
- Peritonitis is an inflammation of the peritoneum. Serous fluid is purulent, and normal peristaltic action slows or ceases.
- Malabsorption in adults is usually from sprue or lactose intolerance, radiation therapy, or chemotherapy. Malabsorption can also occur with IBD or diarrhea when transit through the intestines is too rapid.
- Ulcerative colitis, familial polyposis and other genetically transmitted GI diseases, smoking, alcohol consumption, obesity, physical inactivity, and a diet high in saturated fat or red meat are risk factors for colon cancer.
- Cancer treatment depends on tumor stage and may include surgery, chemotherapy, and radiation. Abdominoperineal resection may be performed for rectal cancer and includes a colostomy.
- An ileostomy drains fecal material from the ileum and is usually performed for IBD problems. Fluid and electrolyte monitoring is crucial when there is an ileostomy.
- A stoma should be a normal pink or red color. Protective powders, sprays, and skin paste and a proper fit of the appliance will help protect the skin. The opening should be cut ⅛-inch larger than the stoma.
- Hemorrhoids are caused by straining at stool for long periods while sitting on the toilet, prolonged standing, prolonged sitting, or pregnancy.
- Anorectal abscess or fistula may be treated with incision and drainage or surgery. Nursing measures include teaching to prevent further constipation and infection.

Additional Learning Resources

SG Go to your Study Guide for additional learning activities to help you master this chapter content.

Go to your Evolve website (http://evolve.elsevier.com/deWit/medsurg) for the following FREE learning resources:
- Animations, audio, and video
- Answers and rationales for questions and activities
- Glossary with pronunciations in English and Spanish
- Interactive Review Questions and more!

Review Questions for the NCLEX® Examination

1. You encourage a patient with IBS to keep a food diary. What is the best nursing response to the patient regarding the importance of keeping the diary?
   1. "The diary will monitor caloric intake."
   2. "The diary will help identify foods that cause bloating."
   3. "The diary will determine food preferences."
   4. "The diary will reinforce the need for better food choices."

   NCLEX Client Need: Health Promotion and Maintenance
2. A 68-year-old patient complains of mild left lower abdominal pain that is accompanied by frequent diarrhea, slight fever, and rectal bleeding. Which treatment measure should you anticipate?
   1. Administration of a bulk-forming stool softener
   2. Increasing fluid intake
   3. Encouraging solid foods
   4. Increasing physical activity

   NCLEX Client Need: Physiological Integrity: Basic Care and Comfort
3. A patient who was admitted with a bowel obstruction is complaining of severe pain. Their abdominal girth has increased by 4 inches in the past hour and the blood pressure is now 80/50 mm Hg. List your actions in priority order.
   1. Assess breathing.
   2. Notify the health care provider.
   3. Position to support blood pressure.
   4. Ensure IV patency.

   NCLEX Client Need: Physiological Integrity: Reduction of Risk Potential
4. During a home visit, you provide verbal instructions to a patient with a possible blockage of an ostomy. What would be an appropriate instruction to give?
   1. Massage the stoma.
   2. Try different body positions.
   3. Take a cold bath.
   4. Begin a high-fiber diet.

   NCLEX Client Need: Physiological Integrity: Physiological Adaptation
5. You are caring for a patient who is postoperative after an ileostomy. Which order should you question?
   1. Strict intake and output recording for 8 hours
   2. Clear liquid diet
   3. IV fluids 125 mL/h
   4. Occlusive dressing over stoma

   NCLEX Client Need: Physiological Integrity: Physiological Adaptation
6. In caring for a patient with an ostomy, which statement is true regarding medication administration?
   1. Time-release capsules can be given to patients with an ileostomy.
   2. Enteric-coated tablets are adequately absorbed by patients with ileostomy.
   3. Glycerin suppositories are readily evacuated in the distal colostomy stoma.
   4. An antiemetic suppository can be effectively absorbed when inserted in the distal colostomy stoma.

   NCLEX Client Need: Physiological Integrity: Pharmacological Therapies
7. A patient has a new colostomy. Which behavior is an early sign of acceptance of the change in body image?
   1. The patient allows you to empty the colostomy bag.
   2. The patient refuses to look at the ostomy site.
   3. The patient holds and examines a new appliance bag.
   4. The patient continues to ask for a bedpan to have a bowel movement.

   NCLEX Client Need: Psychosocial Integrity
8. A patient develops a paralytic ileus as a complication of peritonitis. Which patient comment suggests a return of peristalsis?
   1. "I feel thirsty; may I have some water?"
   2. "I would like to try to walk to the toilet."
   3. "When will I be allowed to have solid food?"
   4. "I am sorry to pass gas while you are here."

   NCLEX Client Need: Physiological Integrity: Reduction of Risk Potential
9. What would be included in the recommended diet for patients with IBD? *(Select all that apply.)*
   1. Low fat
   2. High fiber
   3. High protein
   4. Low calorie
   5. Lactose avoidance

   NCLEX Client Need: Physiological Integrity: Reduction of Risk Potential
10. You admit a 23-year-old patient with possible appendicitis. You anticipate which sign(s) and/or symptom(s)? *(Select all that apply.)*
    1. Increased red blood cell count
    2. Abdominal tenderness
    3. Anorexia and vomiting
    4. Mild fever
    5. Dark black stools

    NCLEX Client Need: Physiological Integrity: Physiological Adaptation

Critical Thinking Questions

Scenario A

Mrs. Blein, age 29 years, has had frequent bouts of diarrhea associated with physical and emotional stress since her early teens. She is admitted to the hospital with a diagnosis of UC. Her admitting health care provider, a gastroenterologist, feels certain that she will benefit from an ileostomy because previous efforts on the part of several other providers have brought no lasting relief from Mrs. Blein's symptoms. She is admitted to the hospital to rehydrate and improve her nutritional status for surgery. Mrs. Blein is 40 pounds underweight and is suffering from severe diarrhea and fluid deficit.

1. What questions would be relevant when taking Mrs. Blein's nursing history?
2. What should be included on Mrs. Blein's nursing care plan regarding observations, measurements, and nursing interventions?
3. Discuss some benefits of an ileostomy over the alternative of continued bouts of severe diarrhea.

Scenario B

Mr. Huang, age 52 years, was found to have occult blood in his stool when he underwent a physical examination for a new insurance policy. Fiberoptic flexible sigmoidoscopy revealed a small lesion in the sigmoid colon; the biopsy result was positive for malignancy. He is scheduled for a hemicolectomy.

1. What probable postoperative problem statements or nursing diagnoses should be on Mr. Huang's care plan?
2. What psychosocial concerns need to be addressed for this patient? What would be appropriate nursing interventions?
3. What further treatment will be necessary for Mr. Huang?

Scenario C

Mr. Frick has a history of diverticulitis. He reports that he has intermittent diarrhea and left lower abdominal discomfort. He is admitted to the hospital for symptoms of nausea, vomiting, and severe abdominal pain and distention. Mr. Frick is diagnosed with peritonitis.

1. What signs or symptoms should you observe for that may signal worsening of his condition?
2. What medical orders do you anticipate from the health care provider to treat Mr. Frick's peritonitis?
3. Discuss general nursing interventions that would be appropriate for Mr. Frick.

Care of Patients With Disorders of the Gallbladder, Liver, and Pancreas

30

http://evolve.elsevier.com/deWit/medsurg

Objectives

Theory

1. Explain the plan of care for a patient with cholelithiasis.
2. Describe treatment for a patient with cholecystitis.
3. Compare the ways in which the various types of hepatitis can be transmitted.
4. Identify signs and symptoms of the various types of hepatitis.
5. Devise appropriate nursing interventions for a patient with cirrhosis and ascites.
6. Summarize potential causes of liver failure.
7. Differentiate the signs and symptoms of acute and chronic liver failure.
8. Discuss the criteria used for selection of liver transplantation recipients.
9. Devise a nursing care plan for a patient with cancer of the liver.
10. Prepare a plan for adequate pain control for a patient with pancreatitis.
11. Compare the treatment options for cancer of the pancreas.

Clinical Practice

12. Perform preoperative teaching for a patient who is to undergo laparoscopic cholecystectomy.
13. Evaluate a nursing care plan, including psychosocial concerns, for a patient who has hepatitis with jaundice.
14. Implement a discharge teaching plan for a patient who has been in the hospital with a flare-up of chronic pancreatitis.

Key Terms

ascites (ă-SĪ-tēz, p. 725)
asterixis (ăs-tĕr-ĬK-sĭs, p. 728)
biliary colic (BĬL-ē-ăr-ē kō-LĬC, p. 714)
caput medusa (KĂP-ĕt mĕ-DŪ-să, p. 725)
cholecystectomy (kō-lĕ-sĭs-TĔK-tō-mē, p. 715)
cholecystitis (kō-lĕ-sĭs-TĪ-tĭs, p. 714)
choledocholithiasis (kō-lĕd-ō-kō-lĭ-THĪ-ă-sĭs, p. 713)
cholelithiasis (kō-lĕ-lĭ-THĪ-ă-sĭs, p. 713)
cirrhosis (sĭr-RŌ-sĭs, p. 725)
encephalopathy (ĕn-sĕf-ă-LŎP-ă-thē, p. 722)
esophageal varices (ĕ-sŏf-ă-JĒ-ăl VĂR-ĭ-sēz, p. 728)
fetor hepaticus (FĒ-tōr hĕ-PĂ-tĭ-kŭs, p. 728)
hematemesis (hē-mă-TĔM-ĕ-sĭs, p. 728)
hepatitis (hĕ-pă-TĪ-tĭs, p. 717)
icterus (ĬK-tĕr-ŭs, p. 726)
jaundice (JĂWN-dĭs, p. 714)
palmar erythema (PĂLHM-ĕr ĕr-ĭ-THĒ-mă, p. 725)
paracentesis (păr-ă-sĕn-TĒ-sĭs, p. 726)
prodromal stage (prō-DRŌ-măl STĀJ, p. 723)
pruritus (prū-RĪ-tŭs, p. 725)
pseudocyst (sū-dō-sĭst, p. 732)
spider angiomas (SPĪ-dĕr ăn-jē-Ō-măz, p. 725)
varices (VĂR-ĭ-sēz, p. 726)

Concepts Covered in This Chapter

- Fluid and Electrolytes
- Cellular Regulation
- Hormonal Regulation
- Nutrition
- Clotting
- Immunity
- Inflammation
- Infection
- Pain
- Patient Education

DISORDERS OF THE GALLBLADDER

CHOLELITHIASIS AND CHOLECYSTITIS

Etiology

Cholelithiasis is the presence of gallstones within the gallbladder or in the biliary tract. The stones may vary in size, from very small "gravel" to stones as large as golf balls. Tiny stones pass into the bile ducts, where they become lodged and obstruct bile flow (Fig. 30.1). When stones lodge in the common bile duct, the patient has **choledocholithiasis**. Cholelithiasis is more likely to occur in people with a sedentary lifestyle, a familial tendency, diabetes mellitus, and obesity. Cholesterol-lowering drugs increase the amount of cholesterol secreted in bile. This cholesterol secretion can increase the risk of gallstones.

Hemolytic disease, extensive resection of the bowel to treat Crohn disease, bariatric surgery, rapid weight loss, multiple pregnancies, and use of oral contraceptives or hormone replacement therapy also increase the risk for gallstones.

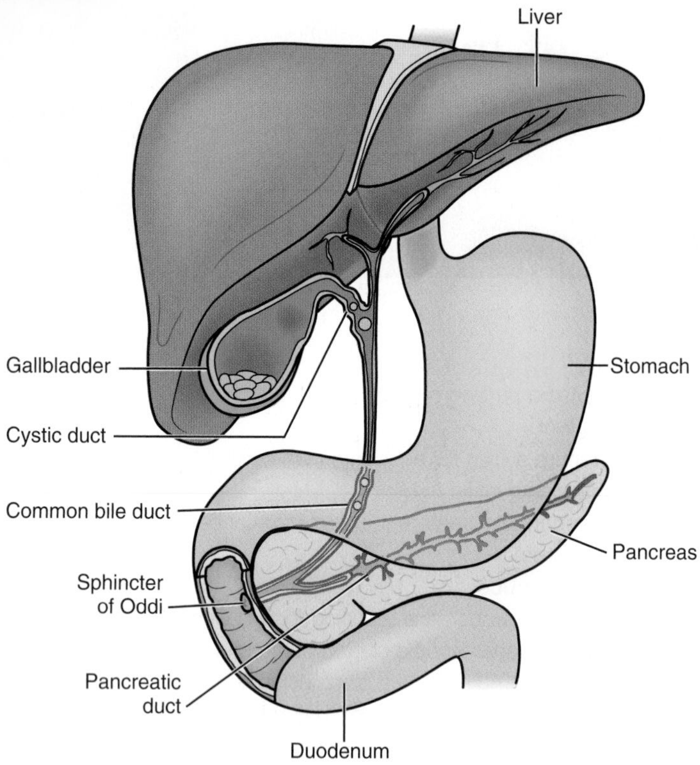

Fig. 30.1 Gallstones within the gallbladder with obstruction of the common bile and cystic ducts.

Cultural Considerations

Ethnic Predisposition to Gallstones

Native Americans are genetically more prone to develop gallbladder stones than any other group. Hispanic Americans have the next highest propensity to develop gallstones. Teaching dietary changes to decrease the amount of cholesterol and total fat in the diet may be an effective means of decreasing the incidence of gallstones in these populations (National Digestive Diseases Information Clearinghouse, 2017).

Cholecystitis is an inflammation of the gallbladder and is associated with gallstones in 90% to 95% of occurrences. Other causes include obstructive tumors of the biliary tract and severely stressful situations such as cardiac surgery, severe burns, or multiple trauma.

Pathophysiology

Cholelithiasis (gallstones) develops when the balance between cholesterol, bile salts, and calcium in the bile is altered to the point that these substances precipitate. When cholesterol precipitates, the nucleus of a stone can be formed. The stone grows as layers of cholesterol, calcium, or pigment accumulate over the nucleus. Immobility, pregnancy, and obstructive lesions decrease bile flow. Stasis of bile leads to changes in chemical composition and stone formation. The formation of stones within the gallbladder can cause irritation and areas of inflammation in the gallbladder wall (cholecystitis). Infection can occur from organisms such as *Escherichia coli*. The organisms enter the gallbladder through the sphincter of Oddi from adjacent structures.

Signs and Symptoms

Symptoms depend on the degree of obstruction to bile flow and the extent of inflammation of the gallbladder. The absence of bile in the intestine results in clay-colored stools that float because of undigested fat content. If a duct is obstructed by a stone, obstruction of bile flow by stones in the cystic or common bile duct causes strong muscle contractions that attempt to move the stones along; severe pain may be triggered by a fatty meal. Nausea and vomiting, fever, and leukocytosis occur with cholecystitis. Pain may be referred to the right clavicle, scapula, or shoulder. As bile backs up into the liver and blood, **jaundice** (yellow tint to skin and sclera) occurs. If obstruction is unrelieved, inflammation occurs and can progress to liver damage.

The symptom most often present in an acute flare-up of chronic cholecystitis is unbearable upper right quadrant pain (**biliary colic**). The pain sometimes is referred to the back at the level of the shoulder blades. Attacks can occur as frequently as daily or may appear only once every year or so. Vomiting may accompany acute flare-ups, along with chills and fever. If the inflammation is not corrected or if there is an infection, the gallbladder can become filled with pus and rupture. Rupture spills gallbladder contents into the abdominal cavity and causes peritonitis.

Chronic cholecystitis causes milder symptoms between acute attacks. Symptoms are indigestion after eating fatty foods, flatulence, nausea after eating, and some discomfort in the right upper quadrant. Table 30.1 compares signs and symptoms of gallbladder disorders.

Think Critically

What questions would you ask when assessing a patient who might have cholecystitis?

Older Adult Care Points

Cholelithiasis should be considered in any older adult with abdominal pain when another cause cannot be found. Symptoms may be atypical, and the presenting symptom of cholecystitis in this age group may be low-grade fever rather than pain.

Diagnosis

Gallstones usually can be diagnosed with ultrasonography or computed tomography (CT) of the gallbladder and biliary tract. Cholescintigraphy (hepatic iminodiacetic acid [HIDA] scan) diagnoses abnormal contraction of the gallbladder or obstruction. Liver function tests are helpful to diagnose gallbladder and biliary tract disease. Alanine aminotransferase (ALT) and aspartate aminotransferase (AST) will be slightly elevated. If there is common duct obstruction, gamma-glutamyl

Table 30.1 Comparison of Gallbladder Disorders

SIGN/SYMPTOM	CHOLELITHIASIS	ACUTE CHOLECYSTITIS	CHRONIC CHOLECYSTITIS
Pain/biliary colic	Sudden onset, acute	Waves of pain lasting 2–6 h	Intermittent during the year; pain commonly referred to back at shoulder blade
Nausea, vomiting	Often present	Frequent	During acute attack
Indigestion and flatulence	—	—	Common complaint
Low-grade fever	Present	Present, often with chills	Present
Jaundice	If duct is obstructed	May be present	May be present during attack

transpeptidase (GGT) is elevated. In biliary obstruction, both direct bilirubin and alkaline phosphatase levels are elevated.

The diagnosis of cholecystitis is aided by indicators of infection, such as elevated white blood cell count and sedimentation rate.

Treatment

Initially, a low-fat diet, loss of excessive body weight, and restriction of alcohol intake are recommended, and meals are spaced so that no large amounts of food are put into the intestinal tract at any one time. This prevents overstimulation of gallbladder activity. Treatment varies depending on whether the patient has symptoms. Medical treatment includes giving oral medications that dissolve the gallstones. If the patient does not respond to this therapy or if bile obstruction occurs, correction of the obstructed biliary tract is indicated. Endoscopic retrograde cholangiopancreatography (ERCP) may be performed to remove stones obstructing the common duct. The procedure combines endoscopy with fluoroscopy to visualize and treat obstructions. Gallbladder removal is indicated for patients with ongoing symptoms or complications. The procedure may be done laparoscopically or as an open abdominal surgery. Antibiotics are usually given only if peritonitis is present or as surgical prophylaxis.

The surgical procedure of choice is **cholecystectomy** (gallbladder removal). Laparoscopic cholecystectomy is the most common surgical procedure used. Three to four small incisions are made in the abdomen; abdominal muscles have less trauma from smaller incisions, and the patient experiences less pain and a quicker recovery than with an "open" cholecystectomy. A laparoscope with an attached camera and a dissecting laser are used along with grasping forceps. Carbon dioxide (CO_2) is instilled into the abdominal cavity to aid visualization. The gallbladder is removed through the incision at the umbilicus. The patient will have dressings over the incisions on the abdomen. In the United States, 90% of cholecystectomies are performed laparoscopically. Recovery time is shorter for the laparoscopic procedure compared with open procedures.

Monitor the patient closely for internal bleeding and watch for signs of increasing abdominal rigidity and pain and for changes in vital signs. Sometimes the retained CO_2 used during a laparoscopic procedure causes "free air" pain. Early and frequent ambulation helps the CO_2 gas dissipate. The patient is usually discharged after recovering from the anesthesia. Depending on age and condition, a longer stay may be indicated, and the patient must have careful discharge teaching about signs of complications.

Patient Teaching

Care After Laparoscopic Cholecystectomy

Teach the patient to:

- Remove the bandages from the puncture site(s) the day after surgery and shower, leaving the Steri-Strips intact. They will fall off in 7 to 10 days.
- Report the following signs and symptoms if they occur:
  - Redness, swelling, bleeding, or bad-smelling drainage from wound site
  - No bowel movement or gas for 3 days or watery diarrhea for more than 3 days
  - Bile-colored drainage or pus from any surgical site
  - Severe abdominal pain that is not relieved by medication or is getting worse
  - Nausea, vomiting, chills, or fever greater than 101° F (38.3° C)
  - Light-colored stool, dark urine, or yellow tint to the eyes or skin, which may indicate obstruction to the flow of bile
- Resume normal activities gradually.
- Expect that return to work is probable 1 week after surgery.
- Stick to a low-fat diet for several weeks, slowly introducing fattier foods to determine whether they cause unpleasant symptoms.

With an open abdominal cholecystectomy, a 2- to 4-day stay in the hospital is typical, and there is about a 6-week recovery period. Residual stones can lodge in the common duct after cholecystectomy. ERCP is usually used to remove residual stones.

Oral dissolution therapy is available and works best on small cholesterol stones. Ursodiol (Actigall) and chenodiol (Chenix) are prescribed for 6 months to 2 years to dissolve stones. This therapy may be tried in a patient who is a poor surgical risk. Although the medication may dissolve the stones, there is a high incidence of reoccurrence. Lithotripsy, or "shock wave" therapy, is rarely used for gallstones. The procedure involves using sound waves directed through the body to break up the stones. The treatment of choice is gallbladder removal.

Nursing Management

Preoperative care. Preoperatively, the patient will be kept on nothing-by-mouth (NPO) status. An analgesic may be ordered to decrease pain, and antiemetics are given for nausea. If nausea cannot be controlled with medication, a nasogastric (NG) tube may be placed to reduce vomiting.

> **Clinical Cues**
>
> In the recent past, morphine was not used because it was thought to cause spasm of the sphincter of Oddi; however, this is not supported by research (Bloom, 2014).

Intravenous (IV) fluids are begun to prevent dehydration. Coagulation times are monitored if jaundice is present, and vitamin K, if needed based on international normalized ratio (INR), is administered before surgery to improve clotting ability of the blood. The patient scheduled for gallstone surgery has needs similar to those of any patient having abdominal surgery. Teaching is adapted for the standard procedure or the laparoscopic procedure (see Chapters 4 and 5).

Postoperative care. The patient is placed in the semi-Fowler position after recovery from anesthesia. This position is more comfortable and decreases strain on the sutures. The patient will also be able to take deep breaths and cough more easily in this position.

A patient who has had open gallbladder surgery may have tubes or drains if continuing drainage is expected. In many cases, the surgery was performed to relieve an obstruction to the flow of bile through the bile ducts or to drain purulent material to the outside. The drain should be assessed with the dressing. The amount of drainage, color, and consistency are noted, and the collection container is emptied as needed. If the drain is a closed suction system, after emptying the drain is compressed to restore suction. The drain is left in for as long as necessary and is then removed by the surgeon.

When an obstruction of the common bile duct has occurred because of stones or tumors, the surgeon may insert a small T-shaped tube (T-tube) directly into the common bile duct during an open cholecystectomy (Fig. 30.2). This tube must be kept patent at all times and is connected to a small drainage bag (bile bag). The length of time the T-tube is left in place varies according to the condition of the patient. Only a small amount of bile will be going to the duodenum. No tension should be put on tubes or drains that have been inserted in the surgical wound. **Dressings must be changed carefully because T-tubes are sutured in place, and if they are accidentally pulled out, the patient must be returned to the operating room and the incision reopened to replace the tube.**

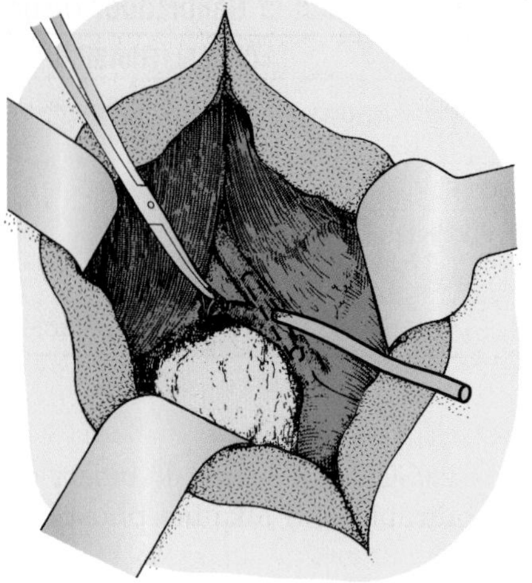

Fig. 30.2 T-tube inserted into the common bile duct and sutured in place.

The patient should be prepared to expect a greenish-yellow discharge (bile) on the dressings. The drainage bag is emptied when the dressing is changed and as needed. Patients may go home with the T-tube in place.

> **Patient Teaching**
>
> **Caring for a T-Tube**
>
> Teach the patient to:
> - Wear loose-fitting, older clothes.
> - Coil the drainage tubing and secure it to the abdomen with tape.
> - Take showers rather than baths.
> - Avoid heavy lifting and strenuous activity.
> - Carefully change the dressing every day, cleansing the skin around the tube.
> - Inspect for signs of infection: redness, swelling, warmth, pain, or pus.
> - Take their temperature every day and report to surgeon if it is greater than 100° F (37° C).
> - Empty the drainage bag at the same time each day.
> - Note the amount, color, and odor of the drainage.
> - Report any change in drainage, abdominal pain, nausea, or vomiting to the surgeon.
> - Return to the surgeon for the follow-up appointment.

Carefully observe the color of the patient's stools because a return of a normal brown-colored stool is an indication that bile is flowing and entering the small intestine. If the bile duct is obstructed, there will be signs of jaundice and stool will be light in color.

Patients who have had an open cholecystectomy may be reluctant to deep-breathe and cough because of pain in the operative area. Encourage these exercises with the use of an incentive spirometer, and auscultate lung sounds every shift to discover any signs of extra secretions or atelectasis. A patient-controlled analgesia (PCA) pump will help the patient cooperate with turning, coughing, and ambulating and thus prevent complications.

No specific diet is recommended for patients after gallbladder surgery, although it is wise to avoid excessive amounts of fatty foods.

? Think Critically

Explain the points to be covered in teaching a patient who is about to undergo a cholecystectomy.

Complications

Constant irritation of the gallbladder from inflammation and infection produces purulent material, and a fistula may form. Necrosis, gangrene, and rupture of the gallbladder causing peritonitis may occur. Choledocholithiasis may cause inflammation of the common duct and obstruct the pancreatic duct. This can lead to pancreatitis.

DISORDERS OF THE LIVER

The liver becomes inflamed when injured by trauma, toxins, or tumor invasion. Disruption of the normal functions of the liver occurs depending on how much of the liver tissue is affected. Chronic inflammation causes fibrosis of the liver cells and abnormal function.

HEPATITIS

Etiology and Pathophysiology

There are five types of viral **hepatitis** (Table 30.2) that cause physical problems. Liver cells are damaged either by direct action of the virus on hepatocytes or by cell-mediated immune responses to the virus. Hepatitis viruses cause extensive inflammation of the liver tissue. Liver cell damage results in necrosis of hepatic cells. The Kupffer cells proliferate and enlarge. Bile flow may be interrupted because of the inflammation. With severe inflammation, fibrous scar tissue may form in the liver.

Table 30.2 Comparison of Hepatitis-Causing Viruses

HEPATITIS A VIRUS (HAV)	HEPATITIS B VIRUS (HBV)	HEPATITIS C VIRUS (HCV)	HEPATITIS D VIRUS (HDV)	HEPATITIS E VIRUS (HEV)
Transmission Mode				
Fecal-to-oral route; poor sanitation and contaminated water and shellfish; often from infected food	Sexual contact, blood and body fluid contact; perinatal from mother to infant	Contact with blood and body fluids; sexual contact with carrier; contact with contaminated surgical, tattooing, and piercing equipment	Blood and body fluid contact; accompanies hepatitis B; close personal contact	Fecal-to-oral route; contaminated water or food
Incubation Period				
15–60 days (average 30 days)	6 wk–6 mo (average 12–14 wk)	6–7 wk	Same as hepatitis B, which precedes it; chronic carriers of hepatitis B are at risk throughout their carrier state	14–60 days (average 40 days)
Infective Period				
Most infectious 2 wk before onset of symptoms; not likely to be infectious after first week following onset of jaundice	Begins before symptoms appear and persists for 4–6 mo after acute illness; persists for lifetime of chronic carriers	Begins 1–2 wk before symptoms appear; continues throughout life for chronic carriers	Blood potentially infectious in active hepatitis B infection; may still be present in blood of chronic hepatitis B carriers even though undetectable	Shedding of virus starts during the incubation period and into the early acute phase of the disease
Signs and Symptoms				
Acute onset *Prodromal phase:* Malaise, fever, loss of appetite, nausea, fatigue, joint aching, skin rash, and upper abdominal discomfort May develop jaundice; malaise and fatigue	Slow onset May be asymptomatic	Slow onset May be asymptomatic until liver damage has occurred	Slow onset May be asymptomatic	Abdominal pain, anorexia, dark urine, fever, hepatomegaly, jaundice, malaise, nausea and vomiting

Scar tissue often obstructs normal blood flow, causing further damage from ischemia.

Liver cells do have the capacity to regenerate and resume their normal appearance. The cells can function for as long as there are no complications or added stressors.

Clinical Cues

Researchers believed they had discovered a new virus, hepatitis F, but the finding was not confirmed; when a valid discovery was made, hepatitis G (HGV) emerged. A virus that is a variant of HGV (virus type C) was cloned from a surgeon with the initials GB, and the virus has been labeled *GBV-C*. GBV-C and HGV are commonly found in the blood supply in the United States. Neither of the viruses cause hepatitis in humans (Chopra, 2018).

Hepatitis A and E viruses are transmitted primarily by the oral-fecal route. They are responsible for the epidemic forms of viral hepatitis. Hepatitis A virus can be transmitted by food handlers to customers or by mollusk shellfish from contaminated waters. Hepatitis E virus infection is primarily seen in less developed countries. It is transmitted through fecal contamination of water.

Hepatitis B, C, and D viruses may cause chronic inflammation and necrosis of liver tissue. A carrier state of hepatitis B, C, or D may occur, and asymptomatic individuals can transmit infection to others. **Hepatitis B and C viruses are transmitted by parenteral routes and sexually; they are present in the semen, vaginal secretions, and saliva of carriers. Sexual partners of patients who are carriers of hepatitis B or C virus are at high risk for contracting the virus.** Hepatitis D virus coexists with hepatitis B or C virus and is transmitted in the same ways.

Intravenous drug use is currently the primary cause of hepatitis C infection; therefore users are a target group for screening and counseling. The virus can also be transmitted by straws used to snort cocaine. Accurate numbers are hard to obtain because many infected individuals are asymptomatic and have not been tested. Since 1992 all blood products have been tested for bloodborne pathogens. Patients who received blood transfusions and clotting factors before that time may have been exposed and may be carriers. Hepatitis B and C viruses can be transmitted from mother to infant. **Hepatitis B and C are the most serious forms of hepatitis, often progressing to chronic hepatitis, cirrhosis, liver cancer, and death.**

Signs and Symptoms

The clinical signs and symptoms of hepatitis A tend to have an acute onset, whereas in hepatitis B, C, and D the onset is slower and more difficulty to identify. There are four phases of hepatitis A. In the first, the **viral replication phase,** individuals will have positive blood tests but display no symptoms. The second is the **prodromal phase,** in which symptoms such as nausea and fatigue and those that would likely be diagnosed as influenza begin (see Table 30.2).

The third phase, the **icteric phase,** is characterized by jaundice and lasts for 2 to 4 weeks. Urine becomes dark, and stools may become light if bile flow is obstructed. Pruritus may occur from the bile pigment deposited in the skin. The liver becomes tender and enlarged.

The fourth phase, the **convalescent phase,** begins when jaundice is disappearing. Convalescence may take 2 to 4 months. Major complaints are malaise and fatigue. Liver enlargement may continue, but if the spleen was enlarged, it returns to normal in this phase.

With chronic hepatitis B and C, patients are likely to be asymptomatic or have symptoms of chronic liver disease. Patients with acute hepatitis B or C could also be asymptomatic. Symptoms include fatigue, nausea, vomiting, poor appetite, right upper quadrant pain, dark urine, and light-colored stools.

Hepatitis D sometimes causes massive destruction of liver cells, liver failure, and death. Hepatitis B and D become chronic in 2% to 10% of infected patients. The patient is then a constant carrier of the virus. There are no currently known signs and symptoms of HGV or GBV-C, but many patients also have hepatitis B and/or C virus at the same time. GBV-C is diagnosed by laboratory tests.

Cultural Considerations

Hepatitis B Virus Among the Foreign Born

More than half of the hepatitis B virus infections in the United States occur in individuals born in Asia, the Pacific Islands, or Africa. It is the leading cause of liver disease and cancer among Asians (HHS.gov, 2017). Because of the high number of people who are unaware of their infection, the virus is passed from mother to child and within families.

Older Adult Care Points

Older adults who had several major surgeries and blood transfusions before 1992 are at higher risk for hepatitis B and C. These patients may be carriers of these viruses.

Clinical Cues

We often assume that liver disorders are associated with jaundice; however, be aware that viral hepatitis without jaundice (anicteric hepatitis) is two to three times more common than viral hepatitis with jaundice.

Diagnosis

Hepatitis is diagnosed by history, physical examination, and laboratory testing. Serologic assays or enzyme immunoassays (EIAs) detect specific antibodies to the various types of hepatitis. Molecular assays can detect viral nucleic acid. These assays do not measure the severity of disease or indicate prognosis. The genotype assay can be used to predict the response to and duration of therapy. Chronic hepatitis is determined by liver biopsy. Elevations in liver function tests (LFTs) are expected findings (Table 30.3). Abnormalities in the white blood cell count, platelets, alkaline phosphatase, albumin, and prothrombin time (PT)/international normalized ratio (INR) may also occur, depending on the severity of the disease.

Treatment

Hepatitis A is treated by rest and avoidance of any substances, including alcohol, that can cause liver damage. These measures help the liver regenerate. A well-balanced diet helps liver cells heal. Four to six small meals a day are tolerated more readily than three larger ones. Sucking on hard candy is recommended and adds to caloric intake. Nausea may be treated with ondansetron (Zofran) or over-the-counter medications. Phenothiazines are not used because of their hepatotoxic effects. Vaccines are available for those at risk for exposure. People who have been exposed to the patient should be notified so that they can receive prophylaxis.

For hepatitis B, drug therapy is used to decrease the viral load, thereby decreasing the disease progression (Table 30.4). Multiple medications are available for use in treatment of hepatitis B. Antiviral medications have been used successfully in treatment and cure of acute hepatitis C. Combinations of medications have proven the most effective.

Table 30.3 Laboratory Test Findings in Acute Viral Hepatitis

TEST	ABNORMAL FINDINGS
Aspartate aminotransferase (AST)	Elevated in prodromal phase up to 20 times normal; decreases as jaundice subsides
Alanine aminotransferase (ALT)	Elevated in prodromal phase; ALT/AST ratio greater than 1; decreases as jaundice subsides
Gamma-glutamyl transpeptidase (GGT)	Elevated
Bilirubin	Elevated unconjugated (direct) bilirubin
Alkaline phosphatase	Some elevation
Serum albumin	Normal or decreased
Serum bilirubin (total)	Elevated to about 8–15 mg/dL (137–257 µmol/L)
Prothrombin time (PT)/international normalized ratio (INR)	Prolonged

! Safety Alert

Drug Interactions

Most medications used for treating hepatitis have significant drug-drug interactions. When giving medications to patients being treated for hepatitis, make sure to check for dangerous drug interactions.

Nonpharmaceutical treatment is supportive to enhance the patient's natural defenses and promote healing of the liver. Hydration, sufficient rest, and adequate nutrition are the goals. Medication for nausea may be prescribed to encourage adequate nutrition.

Vaccines are available to provide active immunity against hepatitis A and B. The vaccine for hepatitis A is administered in two doses, 6 months apart. The vaccine for hepatitis B produces immunity in about 95% of vaccinated individuals and is administered in three or four doses for probable lifetime immunity (Samji, 2017).

Table 30.4 Drugs Commonly Used to Treat Liver Disorders

CLASSIFICATION	ACTION	NURSING IMPLICATIONS	PATIENT TEACHING
Diuretic			
Potassium-Sparing Diuretics			
Spironolactone (Aldactone)	Blocks action of aldosterone in the distal nephron, preventing sodium uptake in exchange for potassium secretion.	It is not necessary to supplement potassium for patients taking this type of diuretic alone.	Avoid foods high in potassium content: bananas, oranges, salt substitutes, dried apricots, and dates.
Amiloride (Midamor)	Potassium is "spared" (not secreted), and sodium is excreted.	Monitor potassium levels.	Alcohol consumption can worsen side effects of the medication.
Eplerenone (Inspra)	Blocks aldosterone.	If administered with ACEIs or ARBs, may increase risk of hyperkalemia.	Can take with or without food. May cause dizziness.
Triamterene (Dyrenium)	Inhibits the reabsorption of sodium in the distal tubule of the kidney.	Sensitive to light. Monitor potassium levels.	Take after a meal with a full glass of water.

Continued

Table 30.4 Drugs Commonly Used to Treat Liver Disorders—cont'd

CLASSIFICATION	ACTION	NURSING IMPLICATIONS	PATIENT TEACHING
Loop Diuretics			
Furosemide (Lasix)	Blocks reabsorption of sodium and chloride in the loop of Henle, promoting water secretion. Promotes powerful diuresis.	Give early in the morning. Monitor potassium levels and supplement potassium as needed. Monitor for hypokalemia, I&O. Weigh patient daily. Assess for hearing loss. Monitor for postural hypotension.	Warn that the drug will cause the need to empty the bladder frequently. Caution regarding dizziness when changing positions.
Bumetanide (Bumex)	Prevents the reabsorption of sodium in the ascending loop of Henle.	Monitor potassium. Can produce ototoxicity. Can react with NSAIDs, gentamycin, and digitalis.	Do not use if allergic to sulfa medications.
Ethacrynic acid (Edecrin)	Prevents the reabsorption of sodium.	Weigh patient throughout treatment to assess volume loss. Monitor potassium.	Do not take within 4 h of bedtime to avoid getting up to the bathroom during the night.
Torsemide (Demadex)	Increases urinary excretion of sodium, chloride, and water.	Onset of action is within 1 h, and action lasts 6–8 h. Use cautiously in patients with a sulfa allergy.	Report to health care provider if using aminoglycosides, NSAIDS, or digoxin. Drug interactions may occur.
Laxative: Ammonia Detoxicant			
Lactulose (Cephulac)	Prevents absorption of ammonia in the colon; increases water in the stool.	Assess stool amount and color. Monitor serum ammonia level, electrolytes, and I&O. Assess perineal skin frequently for excoriation from diarrhea.	Advise that this drug is intended to cause bowel evacuation and diarrhea is likely.
Antibiotic			
Neomycin (Mycifradin)	Decreases protein synthesis in bacterial cells, causing bacterial death.	Monitor renal function and hearing.	Explain the purpose of this drug.
Rifaximin (Xifaxan)	Decreases bowel flora. This prevents the breakdown of protein in the GI tract and helps prevent formation of ammonia.	May cause flatulence or headache. Observe for dehydration.	Taken twice per day with food.
Vasoconstrictor			
Vasopressin (Pitressin)	Causes vasoconstriction; stops bleeding of esophageal varices.	Monitor BP and I&O—may cause water retention.	Explain the purpose of the drug.
Vitamins			
Thiamine (vitamin B_1)	Corrects vitamin B_1 deficiency that occurs from excessive alcohol use.	Assess thiamine levels.	Explain purpose of the drug.
Vitamin K (AquaMEPHYTON)	Needed for hepatic formation of coagulation factors II, VII, IX, and X.	Monitor prothrombin time and INR.	Explain injection may cause discomfort.

Table 30.4 Drugs Commonly Used to Treat Liver Disorders—cont'd

CLASSIFICATION	ACTION	NURSING IMPLICATIONS	PATIENT TEACHING
Antiretrovirals			
Hepatitis B Lamivudine (Epivir)	Inhibits replication of HBV.	Monitor blood count, viral load, liver functions, amylase, lipase, and triglycerides. Watch for signs of lactic acidosis.	GI complaints and insomnia resolve after 3–4 wk. Drug is not a cure but will help control symptoms. Notify provider of swollen lymph nodes, fever, malaise, and sore throat. May still pass virus to others; maintain precautions.
Tenofovir alafenamide (Vemlidy)	Prevents virus replication.	May impair renal function. When discontinuing the drug, hepatitis B may reoccur.	Do not stop the medication without consulting the provider.
Adefovir dipivoxil (Hepsera)	Prevents DNA replication.	Monitor respiratory status; assess for skin rash.	Report any difficulty breathing or itching, swelling, or redness of the eyes.
Entecavir (Baraclude)	Prevents viral replication.	Monitor renal function.	May cause weakness.
Telbivudine (Tyzeka)	Prevents viral replication.	Monitor renal function and electrolytes.	May cause lactic acidosis and myopathy.
Tenofovir disoproxil fumarate (Viread)	Prevents viral replication.	Monitor renal function and electrolytes.	May cause lactic acidosis and severe hepatomegaly.
Hepatitis C Ribavirin (Rebetol)	Inhibits viral protein synthesis.	Ribavirin is used together with interferon alfa-2a to treat chronic HCV.	Drug may cause fainting or dizziness.
Glecaprevir/pibrentasvir (Mavyret)	Viral protein inhibitors, blocking RNA replication.	May cause headache, fatigue, nausea, or diarrhea.	Take with food.
Sofosbuvir/velpatasvir/voxilaprevir (Vosevi)	Direct-acting antivirals, interfering with RNA replication.	Severe bradycardia may occur in patients taking amiodarone.	May cause headache, fatigue, nausea, or diarrhea.
Sofosbuvir/velpatasvir (Epclusa)	Block an RNA polymer and a protein (NS5A) needed for RNA replication.	Proton pump inhibitors are not recommended for use with Epclusa.	May cause insomnia, irritability, weakness, and fatigue.
Elbasvir/grazoprevir (Zepatier)	Block viral RNA replication.	Genetic testing may be done to identify whether the drug will be effective. There are significant drug-drug interactions—check before administering medications.	Fatigue, headache, and nausea are the most common side effects.
Daclatasvir (Daklinza)	Direct-acting antiviral.	Taken with sofosbuvir. Several anticonvulsant medications are contraindicated.	Fatigue, headache, diarrhea, and nausea are the most common side effects.
Ledipasvir/sofosbuvir (Harvoni)	Blocks RNA replication.	Medications to suppress acid in the stomach may decrease absorption.	Fatigue, headache, and insomnia may occur.
Sofosbuvir (Sovaldi)	RNA replication inhibitor.	Antituberculosis medications are contraindicated.	Fatigue, headache, nausea, insomnia, and anemia are all side effects.

Continued

Table 30.4 Drugs Commonly Used to Treat Liver Disorders—cont'd

CLASSIFICATION	ACTION	NURSING IMPLICATIONS	PATIENT TEACHING
Immunomodulator			
Peginterferon alfa-2a (PEG-Intron, Pegasys) Interferon alfa-2b (Intron A)	Inhibits viral replication and increases phagocytic action of macrophages, augmenting specific cytotoxicity of lymphocytes.	Perform baseline assessments. Monitor for signs of depression; offer emotional support. Monitor for abdominal pain and bloody diarrhea. Monitor viral load.	Maintain hydration and avoid alcohol. May experience flulike symptoms. Can cause flulike symptoms, headache, and depression.
Octapeptide			
Octreotide	Off-label use for reducing splanchnic blood flow to decrease bleeding from esophageal varices by inhibiting the release of glucagon, which is a splanchnic vasodilator.	Alteration in glucagon release can affect blood sugar. Octreotide can also alter thyroid and cardiac function.	Side effects include headache, GI cramping, nausea, and vomiting.
Antimetabolite/Neoplastic Metabolite			
5-Fluorouracil (5-FU) and floxuridine (FUDR)	Antimetabolite that acts during cellular metabolism to prevent cellular division.	Perform baseline assessments with attention to temperature. Monitor blood count.	Avoid crowds and prevent exposure to infection. Promptly report fever, diarrhea, vomiting, bleeding, bruising, or redness and burning of the palms of hands or soles of feet.

ACEI, angiotensin-converting enzyme inhibitor; *ARB,* angiotensin II receptor antagonist; *BP,* blood pressure; *GI,* gastrointestinal; *HBV,* hepatitis B virus; *HCV,* hepatitis C virus; *I&O,* intake and output; *INR,* international normalized ratio; *NSAID,* nonsteroidal antiinflammatory drug.

Passive immunity to hepatitis A can be conferred by the administration of immune globulin (IG). IG is also recommended for those who have been exposed to someone infected with hepatitis B virus who was not immunized against this virus. There is no protective vaccine for hepatitis C virus.

Health Promotion

Healthy People 2030 **Goal for Hepatitis B**

Hepatitis is an occupational hazard for all people who have direct contact with patients or surgical and diagnostic equipment. Standard Precautions must be observed at all times. All health care personnel should be immunized with the hepatitis B vaccine. These practices will help meet the *Healthy People 2030* goal of reducing hepatitis B and the National Patient Safety Goal to reduce the risk of health care–associated infections.

NURSING MANAGEMENT

ASSESSMENT (DATA COLLECTION)

Data collection for a patient with hepatitis should include a nursing history of any previous contacts and whether the contacts have been notified and immunized. By law, viral hepatitis must be reported to the state department of public health. **Because the liver detoxifies many chemicals and metabolizes certain drugs, a complete list of recently taken or current medications is essential. It may be necessary to discontinue some drugs that are particularly toxic to the liver** (see Chapter 27, Box 27.1).

Assess for problems related to silent gastrointestinal (GI) bleeding, respiratory distress, and neurologic dysfunction. Mental confusion and coma associated with hepatic encephalopathy occurs from circulating toxins that result from liver failure. **Encephalopathy** is malfunction or disease of the brain.

NURSING DIAGNOSIS AND PLANNING

Problem statements specific to hepatitis infection might include the following:

- Altered nutrition due to anorexia, nausea, and vomiting.
- Fatigue due to disease process and malaise.
- Pain due to inflamed liver and pruritus.
- Insufficient knowledge due to disease process and self-care needed.
- Altered body image due to yellow discoloration of skin.

Expected outcomes might be as follows:

- Patient will maintain body weight within normal limits during illness.
- Patient will verbalize lessened fatigue after rest periods each day.

Focused Assessment

Data Collection for a Patient With a Liver Disorder

HEALTH HISTORY

- Have you ever had a parasitic infection?
- Do you have a history of cancer?
- How much alcohol do you drink?
- Do you have a history of hepatitis?
- Have you been exposed to hepatitis?
- What drugs do you take?
- Have you been exposed to pesticides or industrial chemicals? Which ones?
- Has your appetite decreased? Have you had nausea or vomiting?
- Are you more fatigued than usual?
- Have you noticed any fever?
- Have you noticed dark-colored urine?
- Have you had any light or clay-colored stools?
- Have you had excessive gas?
- Have you been bruising easily?
- Has your skin been itchy or made you feel uncomfortable?
- Has your abdomen increased in girth lately?
- Do you have abdominal pain? Where? Can you describe it?
- Have you gained weight recently?
- Do you take dietary supplements?

PHYSICAL ASSESSMENT

- Inspect the skin for signs of jaundice, scratch marks, and general condition.
- Inspect the sclera and mucous membranes of the mouth for signs of jaundice.
- Gently palpate the abdomen for masses and for liver enlargement.
- Auscultate bowel sounds.
- Measure abdominal girth for a baseline.
- Inspect extremities for signs of edema.
- Check liver function test values and urinalysis for bilirubin presence.

- Patient will maintain a pain level of 4 or less after pain medication and comfort measures.
- Patient will verbalize knowledge of disease process and self-care within 2 days.
- Patient will list personal strengths that compensate for altered appearance.

Older Adult Care Points

Older adults are at higher risk for drug-induced hepatitis if they have chronic conditions that require the administration of various drugs that can cause liver damage over a long period. With liver inflammation, the liver will not function well, and drug dosages will need to be lowered; otherwise drug toxicity may occur.

◆ IMPLEMENTATION AND EVALUATION

Nursing interventions include reviewing trends of serum liver enzyme levels and serum bilirubin values. Preventing the spread of infection is a major concern when caring for patients with viral hepatitis. The patient and family will need to be instructed regarding special precautions to prevent the spread of the infection, such as proper handling of body secretions, proper hand hygiene, and limiting contact with others.

Sedatives must be given with caution because a diseased liver cannot detoxify them very well. Alcohol is particularly damaging to the liver and should be avoided for 4 months after recovery from hepatitis.

The convalescence of patients with hepatitis is slow and long. A nutritious diet with supplements is prescribed. A variety of diversional activities that are not physically taxing, such as a new hobby or learning a new skill, computer games, puzzle books, and movies, should be planned. Nursing interventions for selected problem statements relevant to patients with hepatitis are found in Table 30.5 and in Chapter 27, Table 27.2.

Complementary and Alternative Therapies

Promoting Good Liver Function

Several supplements are known to be beneficial to promoting good liver function. *N*-acetylcysteine (NAC), glutathione (GSH), alpha-lipoic acid, milk thistle, licorice root, and antioxidants are helpful. NAC promotes detoxification pathways; GSH is an antioxidant and may reduce viral loads; alpha-lipoic acid may impede the development of fibrosis; milk thistle stabilizes hepatic cell membranes; and licorice root improves liver function. The health care provider should always be consulted before the patient takes supplements (Rakel, 2018).

Prevention

Transmission precautions. Both feces and blood of patients with hepatitis A contain virus during the **prodromal stage** (infected but asymptomatic) and early symptomatic stage. Consistent use of Standard Precautions will provide protection for health care personnel; the patient and family must use precautions at home.

Hepatitis B and D viruses are rarely transmitted by the fecal-oral route, but it is strongly recommended to be very careful when disposing of a patient's stool. Standard Precautions guidelines must be carefully followed for handling, sterilizing, and disposing of equipment contaminated with blood. Hepatitis viruses are transmitted by sexual contact, so the patient must be educated on that.

When a patient with viral hepatitis has been admitted to the hospital, the infection control professional must be notified. Hepatitis is on the Center for Disease Control and Prevention's (CDC's) National Notifiable Conditions list, and facilities and health care providers are required to report cases. It is important to familiarize yourself with the hospital's policies and procedures so that protection for others and follow-up for the infected patient are not overlooked. Infection with hepatitis A in a person who handles food on the job must be reported promptly. The CDC has published guidelines for the care of patients hospitalized with hepatitis. These

Table 30.5 Common Problem Statements, Expected Outcomes, and Nursing Interventions for Patients With Hepatitis

PROBLEM STATEMENT	EXPECTED OUTCOMES	NURSING INTERVENTIONS
Fluid volume deficit due to nausea and vomiting	Patient will cease vomiting within 24 h. Patient will establish fluid balance within 48 h as evidenced by moist mucous membranes, good skin turgor, adequate urine output, and stable blood pressure.	Administer antiemetics as ordered. Monitor IV infusion site and fluid rate. Encourage clear oral fluids if ordered and tolerated. Monitor electrolyte levels for imbalances. Monitor I&O. Provide mouth care q2h while awake.
Altered nutrition due to nausea, vomiting, and anorexia	Patient will ingest a 1200-calorie diet per day within 7 days after subsidence of acute vomiting. Patient will maintain present weight.	Keep door of room closed to keep odors out. Offer mouth care before mealtime. Provide six small meals a day plus small, high-calorie snacks between meals. Weigh daily and record. Keep hard candy at bedside for snacking.
Altered comfort due to jaundice and bile pigments in skin causing itching	Patient will verbalize that itching is decreased.	Assist to bathe with tepid water three times a day. Apply lotion q2h. Provide diversional activities. Teach relaxation techniques.
Insufficient knowledge due to ways in which HBV is transmitted, effects of hepatitis on the body, self-care measures, and measures to prevent transmission to others	Patient will verbalize ways HBV is transmitted, effects on body, self-care measures, and measures to prevent transmission to others before discharge.	Teach ways in which HBV is transmitted: parenteral routes, sexual contact, contact with blood and body fluids. Give explanation in understandable terms of what HBV does to the body. Reinforce teaching regarding self-care measures: hygiene, diet, rest, follow-up. Teach importance of not sharing personal articles (especially razor, toothbrush, etc.) with others. Instruct to inform health care workers of the presence of the virus until tests for it are negative. Inform that sexual partner(s) will need injection of special immune globulin for protection and then immunization.
Disturbed body image due to yellow skin color from jaundice	Patient will demonstrate acceptance of present body image by allowing visitors within 3 days.	Assure that jaundice is not permanent. Allow to ventilate feelings about the illness and present appearance. Encourage verbalization of positive aspects about self. Increase fluid intake to help flush bilirubin from blood during recovery.
Fatigue due to vague flulike symptoms	Patient will verbalize less fatigue before discharge.	Assess current level of energy. Assist with ADLs as needed. Suggest that visitors come when energy level is higher. Cluster care and allow for periods of rest. Help identify activities that require more energy and help patient prioritize accordingly.

ADLs, Activities of daily living; *HBV,* hepatitis B virus; *I&O,* intake and output; *IV,* intravenous.

Home Care Considerations

Preventing the Spread of Hepatitis Virus

HEPATITIS A

- Notify close contacts so that they can obtain immune globulin protection and hepatitis A vaccine.
- Practice extremely good hygiene, washing with warm water and soap (liquid soap is best).
- Wash hands after using the toilet, before eating, and after changing diapers.
- Avoid preparing food during the infectious period.
- Use separate bath and hand towels from other members of the family.
- Avoid sharing toothbrushes.
- Use gloves to disinfect the bathroom fixtures with a 10:1 bleach solution.
- Refrain from sexual contact until the health care provider states that the infectious period is over.

HEPATITIS B OR C

- Avoid sexual contact until there is no chance of transmission of the virus.
- Advise close contacts to obtain hepatitis B vaccine as indicated.
- Avoid sharing razors or toothbrushes because of the chance of blood transmission.

Safety Alert

Hepatitis C

Hepatitis C virus is transmitted by blood and saliva. Standard Precautions and careful handling of all body fluids are recommended. The first line of defense is scrupulous hand hygiene. Wear gloves when handling plasma-containing body fluids and use extreme caution when handling used needles, syringes, and IV tubing. Needle sticks; open wounds; and the mucous membranes of the eyes, nose, and mouth can serve as portals of entry. Dentists, health care providers, nurses, and other health care workers must be informed of a patient's carrier status, if known.

same guidelines can be modified for home care to prevent the spread of the infection.

Complications

A small percentage of patients with hepatitis can develop massive necrosis of liver cells that results in acute liver failure. *Acute liver failure* is the preferred term according to the American Association for the Study of Liver Diseases. *Fulminant hepatitis* or *necrosis* and *fulminant hepatic failure* are older terms. The only hope for recovery is a liver transplant; without transplant, death occurs in about 75% of these cases. Symptoms of liver diseases include mental confusion, disorientation, and drowsiness, which indicate hepatic encephalopathy. **Ascites** (abnormal accumulation of serous fluid within the peritoneal cavity) and edema accompany liver failure.

CIRRHOSIS

Etiology

Approximately 35,000 deaths are attributed to chronic liver disease and cirrhosis in the United States annually (Wolf, 2018). Hepatitis B and C, alcoholic liver disease, and nonalcoholic fatty liver disease are the leading causes of cirrhosis (Goldber & Chopra, 2018). Other less common disorders that alter liver function include **biliary cirrhosis (biliary cholangitis),** which results from chronic biliary obstruction and infection, and **cardiac cirrhosis (congestive hepatopathy),** which results from long-standing, severe right-sided heart failure in patients with cor pulmonale. Whatever the cause, in cirrhosis liver cells are damaged, causing altered function, blood flow, and structure.

Cultural Considerations

Regional Alcohol Consumption and Liver Disease

A University of Pittsburgh (2018) study found that people living in colder regions with less sunlight drink more alcohol and have a higher incidence of liver disease. Alcohol vasodilates blood vessels of skin, increasing the feeling of warmth. Alcohol consumption is also linked to depression, which can be exacerbated when there is less sunlight (seasonal affective disorder).

Pathophysiology

Cirrhosis is a progressive, chronic disease of the liver. Normal hepatic structures are destroyed and replaced with fibrotic tissue. Fibrous bands of connective tissue develop in the organ and eventually constrict and partition the liver tissue into irregular nodules. If this process is halted before too much liver tissue is damaged, the liver tissue will regenerate. Late cirrhosis is considered irreversible.

When liver cells begin to degenerate, the blood vessels within the liver also fail to function. This causes an obstruction to the flow of blood through the portal circulatory system, causing portal systemic hypertension. The altered vessel permeability and fluid leakage into the abdomen result in ascites. More fluid is contributed as the damaged liver obstructs flow through the lymphatic system and the protein-rich fluid collects in the abdomen. The damaged liver has a limited ability to synthesize albumin, which causes the osmotic pressure within the blood vessels to fall. The change in osmolality allows fluid to leak out of the vessels into the tissues, contributing to edema and providing more ascites fluid. Another mechanism contributing to ascites and edema is excess circulating aldosterone, which is not properly metabolized by the damaged liver. The excess aldosterone causes sodium and water retention (Concept Map 30.1).

Signs and Symptoms

Cirrhosis usually progresses without symptoms until severe liver damage is present. Subjective symptoms of liver cirrhosis include fatigue, weakness, headache, anorexia, indigestion, abdominal pain, nausea, and vomiting. The ascites fluid accumulation in the abdominal cavity causes increased abdominal girth and weight gain. Fluid retention in the right hemithorax or ascites can limit expansion of the chest and cause dyspnea. Objective symptoms of liver cirrhosis include excessive gas, skin rashes, and fever. Leg and foot edema and **palmar erythema** (redness of the palms that blanches with pressure) occur. Sometimes bluish varicose veins, called **caput medusa**, radiating from the umbilicus (indicating portal hypertension) are seen. Bleeding and bruising because of deficiencies in vitamin K, thrombin, or prothrombin interfere with clot formation. The liver often is enlarged and "knobby" and is palpable below the level of the right rib cage. Abdominal distention is present. The spleen also enlarges. Skin lesions, jaundice, **pruritus** (severe itching of the skin), bleeding disorders, endocrine disorders, and peripheral neuropathy occur in late disease. **Spider angiomas** (abnormal collection of blood vessels under the skin) may appear on the face, neck, upper trunk, and arms.

Urine may become dark and foamy, and stools turn clay colored, which indicates that bile is not reaching the intestine. Jaundice occurs either because the liver cannot metabolize bilirubin or because bile flow is obstructed. Excessively high levels of bile pigment **(bilirubin)** are present in the blood. The pigment is

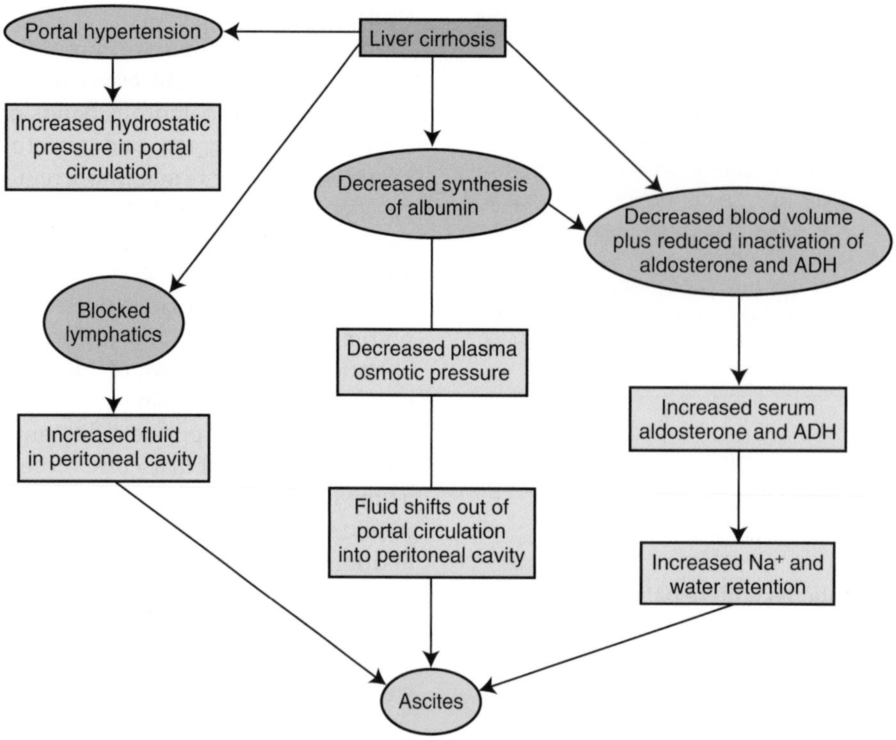

Concept Map 30.1 Relationship of systemic portal hypertension and ascites in liver cirrhosis. *ADH*, Antidiuretic hormone; *Na+*, sodium.

deposited in the skin, mucous membranes, and body fluids, causing a change in color ranging from pale yellow to golden orange. The first signs of jaundice are usually seen in the sclera of the eye (**icterus**), which takes on a yellow tint. Jaundice is not always a sign of liver damage. In **hemolytic jaundice,** there may be an increased level of bilirubin as a result of excessive destruction of red blood cells, with resultant release of the pigment into the bloodstream. Fig. 30.3 shows the signs and symptoms of cirrhosis. **Elevations in liver enzymes usually do not occur until 65% of liver function is gone.** The patient is likely to delay seeking medical attention until symptoms are pronounced.

Think Critically

List the ways in which you would collect data when checking a patient for signs of jaundice.

Clinical Cues

In people with dark skin, jaundice is best detected by checking the buccal mucosa, hard palate, palms, soles of the feet, sclera, and conjunctiva.

Diagnosis

A definitive diagnosis of cirrhosis of the liver is made by liver biopsy. Laboratory testing may show a low albumin level and elevated PT/INR, as well as elevated AST, ALT, ammonia level, and lactate dehydrogenase (LDH) values. Alkaline phosphatase and GGT will also be elevated. CT and liver ultrasound can help determine the size of the liver and the presence of any masses. They also outline the hepatic blood flow and any vascular obstruction. Magnetic resonance cholangiopancreatography—similar to ERCP but without the use of an invasive procedure—may be performed.

Treatment

Treatment is aimed at stopping the liver damage, preventing further damage, and managing the symptoms. Identifying and removing the cause of liver damage when possible is the primary treatment. Treating hepatitis, abstaining from alcohol intake, and managing diseases contributing to liver damage will stop progression of the condition. Since the liver is the primary detoxification center for all medications, dosages may need to be adjusted and current therapies examined to eliminate any hepatotoxic treatments. **Medical treatment of ascites includes restriction of fluid and sodium intake and administration of diuretics.** Abdominal **paracentesis** (removal of acites fluid) can be performed to remove accumulated fluid; however, this is a temporary measure that poses problems of rapid fluid shift, loss of protein, and the potential for introducing infectious organisms into the peritoneum. A transjugular intrahepatic portosystemic shunt (TIPS) may be used to decrease pressure between portal and hepatic veins in the liver and decompress **varices** (abnormally dilated veins). A catheter is inserted into the venous system and threaded to the hepatic vein and then directed to the portal vein. Stents that extend into both veins are

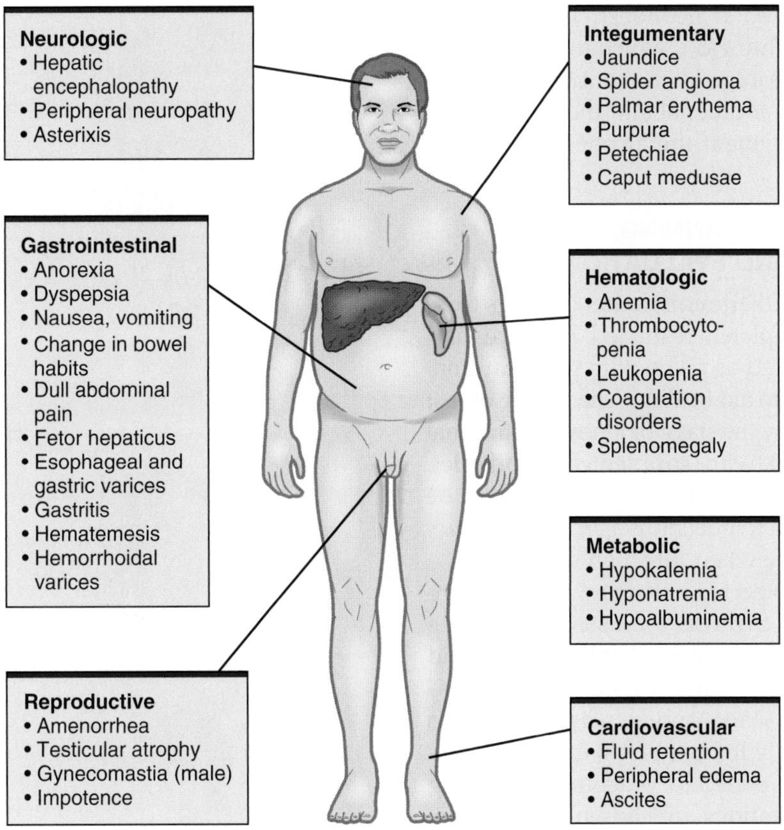

Fig. 30.3 Signs and symptoms of cirrhosis. (From Lewis SL, Bucher L, Heitkemper MM, et al.: *Medical-surgical nursing: assessment and management of clinical problems*, ed 10, St. Louis, 2017, Elsevier.)

placed through the liver, bypassing some of the portal circulation, thereby decreasing pressure. TIPS is performed to decrease risk of bleeding from esophageal varices and reduce accumulation of ascites.

! Safety Alert

Liver Inflammation

Patients with liver inflammation or cirrhosis should avoid taking large doses of vitamins and minerals. Vitamin A, iron, and copper can worsen the liver damage.

Traditionally, limitation of dietary protein intake was prescribed to decrease the nitrogen from protein breakdown available to form ammonia (NH_3); however, the current recommendation is to manage encephalopathy with medications rather than to restrict protein. Calorie and protein requirements are increased with cirrhosis, and most patients with liver disease are malnourished (Shergill et al., 2018).

Thiamine, zinc, and multiple vitamins are given to counteract vitamin deficiency, and enteral or parenteral diet supplementation may be implemented. Lactulose, an exchange resin, is given orally or by a feeding tube to induce diarrhea and prevent diffusion of ammonia out of the intestinal tract. Ammonia, a known neurotoxin, has been believed to be the origin of hepatic encephalopathy; however, many patients with cirrhosis have elevated ammonia levels without symptoms, and some patients with significant alteration in level of consciousness have normal ammonia levels. Research is focusing on the elevated levels of neurosteroids found in patients with cirrhosis and their effect on neurotransmission (Wolf, 2018). Kidney failure sometimes accompanies liver failure (hepatorenal syndrome).

Research continues on the use of cell-based and non–cell-based liver dialysis therapies to "bridge" patients who are waiting for a liver transplant or to support function while acute failure is resolving. Devices trialed so far have failed to show survival benefit with the therapy. Many patients with acute liver failure have potential for liver regeneration if function can be supported during the healing process (Goldberg & Chopra, 2018).

NURSING MANAGEMENT

ASSESSMENT (DATA COLLECTION)

A thorough assessment to identify specific patient care problems related to abnormal liver function is performed (see Focused Assessment). Assess for safety issues related to change in mental status. The patient may have signs of bleeding. Pay extra attention to ammonia levels, albumin, AST, ALT, and PT/INR results. Increase in ascites is determined by measuring and recording abdominal girth each day. Daily weight checks should also be initiated if fluid retention is observed. If alcoholism is an issue, be vigilant for signs of withdrawal, which may occur 6 to 12 hours after the last drink and can continue for 3 to 5 days (see Chapter 48 for additional information). Be sure to get an order to implement the alcohol withdrawal protocol if indicated.

◆ NURSING DIAGNOSIS, PLANNING, IMPLEMENTATION, AND EVALUATION

The intake of alcohol and administration of drugs toxic to the liver must be completely restricted. Sedatives and opiates are either avoided or given with great caution. Rest may be prescribed to aid healing. The degree of rest and activity is dictated by the stage of illness. Nutritional deficiencies are treated with supplements and diet. The patient is at great risk for infection and should be protected from exposure to infectious agents; antibiotics should be given quickly when infection occurs.

Nursing diagnoses, expected outcomes, and interventions for patients with cirrhosis are listed in Nursing Care Plan 30.1 (see also Table 30.5). Stabilization of fluid balance, normalization of vital signs, and progress toward baseline mental status and increasing ability to perform activities of daily living (ADLs) independently are indicators that the expected outcomes are being met; if not, new interventions are chosen for the plan.

? Think Critically

Identify signs and symptoms that you might find when assessing a patient with advanced cirrhosis of the liver.

Complications

Esophageal varices. Bleeding from **esophageal varices** (dilated, distorted, engorged veins) is a major complication of cirrhosis. They are the result of portal congestion and hypertension. In advanced cirrhosis, blood that normally flows from the intestines to the portal vein and on through the liver is shunted to other veins, including the veins of the upper stomach and lower esophagus. The added load of blood causes congestion of these veins, producing varicosities. When the vein walls rupture, bleeding occurs. The liver is no longer able to make vitamin K, which is an essential component of clotting, so bleeding can be substantial. Varices may rupture and produce **hematemesis** (vomiting of bright red blood) from increased blood pressure, coughing, vomiting, or mechanical irritation from poorly chewed food. More than 90% of patients with cirrhosis have esophageal varices, and 30% of those bleed (Carale, 2017).

Treatment options are administration of parenteral vasopressors such as vasopressin (Pitressin) to lower portal pressure, injection sclerotherapy, or ligation of the bleeding vessels (Fig. 30.4). Surgical intervention is used only when endoscopic treatment or medications have failed to control the bleeding. Vasoconstrictors such as somatostatin (Zecnil) and octreotide (Sandostatin) are used to reduce portal blood flow. A beta blocker may be given to lower blood

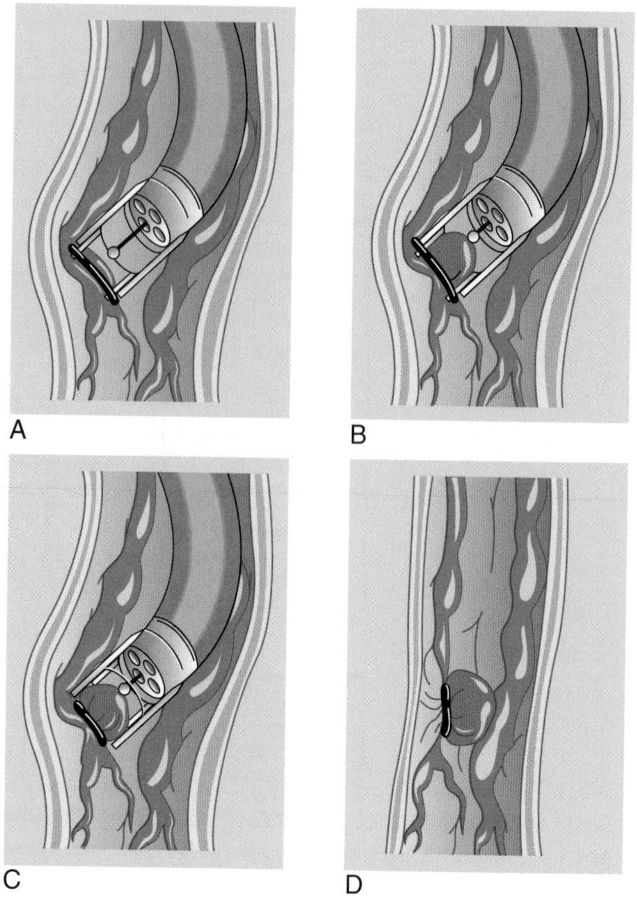

Fig. 30.4 Treatment for esophageal varices. **A,** Endoscope positioned over varix. **B,** Suction is applied to draw varix toward the endoscope. **C,** Ligation band is deployed around varix. **D,** Band in place. (From Good VS, Kirkwood PL: *Advanced critical care nursing*, ed 2, St. Louis, 2018, Elsevier.)

pressure. The patient is given vitamin K to help rectify clotting factor deficiencies. The treatment of hemorrhage of the upper GI tract is discussed in Chapter 28.

Encephalopathy. Portal systemic encephalopathy or hepatic encephalopathy is another dangerous complication of cirrhosis. Encephalopathy in this instance is directly related to liver failure and is believed to be caused by the buildup of ammonia and gamma-aminobutyric acid. Symptoms such as delirium, convulsions, **asterixis** (flapping tremors), and coma occur. Asterixis is identified by having the patient hold out the arms and hands and observing for rapid flexing and extension movements of the hands. There may be rhythmic movements of the legs with dorsiflexion of the foot and rhythmic movements in the face with strong eyelid closure. **Fetor hepaticus** (breath with a sweet, fecal odor) occurs as liver failure progresses.

LIVER TRANSPLANTATION

Liver transplantation is considered for patients with progressive and advanced liver disease that does not respond to treatment. It is most commonly done for nonalcoholic cirrhosis, chronic active hepatitis, sclerosing

Nursing Care Plan 30.1 Care of a Patient With Cirrhosis of the Liver

SCENARIO

A 62-year-old man with a 25-year history of alcoholism is admitted with hepatic encephalopathy caused by progressive alcoholic cirrhosis. His complaints include thirst, extreme fatigue, a swollen abdomen, edema of the feet and ankles, jaundice, itching, shortness of breath, nausea and indigestion, drowsiness, and confusion. Esophageal varices are present. All of his liver function test results and his ammonia level show elevation, and his PT and INR are prolonged. His hematocrit, hemoglobin, and serum albumin levels are low.

PROBLEM STATEMENT/NURSING DIAGNOSIS

Actual (or potential for) altered breathing pattern due to fluid accumulation in the chest (hydrothorax) or abdomen (ascites).

SUPPORTING ASSESSMENT DATA

Subjective: "I feel like I can't get my breath."

Objective: Shallow rapid breathing, RR 28–32/min; pauses to catch breath after slight exertion of moving in bed. Pulse oximetry 88% on room air.

Goals/Expected Outcomes	Nursing Interventions	Selected Rationale	Evaluation
Patient will maintain adequate oxygenation as evidenced by respiratory rate of 12–24/min and oxygen saturation greater than 95%.	Assess rate, rhythm, and quality of respirations and pulse oximeter readings at baseline and after interventions.	Changes in respiratory pattern or pulse oximeter suggest worsening, stabilization, or improvement.	Breathing is shallow and rapid if lying in supine position. If assisted to a sitting position, experiences temporary subjective relief.
	Place in semi-Fowler position and observe for relief.	Raising head of bed (HOB) usually alleviates dyspnea, but ascites or hydrothorax may restrict chest expansion.	Pulse oximeter 97% when coached to inhale deeply. Relief obtained with HOB at 30 degrees.
	Auscultate lung fields at the beginning of the shift and as needed (PRN) for worsening breath sounds.	Compare findings to your initial assessment to discover changes.	Diminished in the bases bilaterally, with fine crackles.
	Administer oxygen as ordered.	Oxygen is generally ordered if saturation falls below 93% (health care provider may set the parameter higher).	Currently pulse oximeter shows 95% when awake; however, level drops to 90% when asleep.
	Encourage use of incentive spirometer and teach deep breathing and coughing.	Chest expansion may be limited; therefore patient must be encouraged to make an extra effort to prevent pneumonia and atelectasis.	Willing to try spirometer but needs continuous reminding. Family members able to help by encouraging him.

PROBLEM STATEMENT/NURSING DIAGNOSIS

Potential for bleeding due to esophageal varices and decreased clotting factors.

SUPPORTING ASSESSMENT DATA

Subjective: "Every time they draw my blood, it leaves a really big bruise."

Objective: Elevated liver function test results; cirrhosis, spider angiomas, jaundice, ascites, and prolonged PT/INR.

Goals/Expected Outcomes	Nursing Interventions	Selected Rationale	Evaluation
Patient will not experience life-threatening hemorrhage while hospitalized. Any bleeding will be promptly recognized and reported.	Monitor stool and emesis for blood and other bleeding signs.	Alerts to bleeding.	No signs of bleeding.
	Feed only soft foods.	Prevents mechanical irritation of esophagus.	Eating soft foods; favors puddings and cooked cereals.
	Give vitamin K as ordered.	Vitamin K is needed for synthesis of clotting factors.	Vitamin K administered.
	Monitor vital signs q2–4h as ordered.	Vital sign changes, restlessness, and confusion may indicate bleeding.	BP 120/80, pulse 87/min, RR 24/min; is anxious.
	Observe for increasing restlessness and confusion.	Indicators of hypoxia secondary to bleeding.	Alert and oriented to person and place.
	Monitor PT and INR.	Prolonged clotting times contribute to rapid blood loss.	Laboratory test results pending.

Continued

Nursing Care Plan 30.1 Care of a Patient With Cirrhosis of the Liver—cont'd

PROBLEM STATEMENT/NURSING DIAGNOSIS
Acute confusion due to increased ammonia level caused by liver failure.

SUPPORTING ASSESSMENT DATA
Subjective: Confused as to month and why he is in the hospital.
Objective: Elevated serum ammonia and drowsiness.

Goals/Expected Outcomes	Nursing Interventions	Selected Rationale	Evaluation
Any worsening of cognitive status will be promptly identified and reported.	Mental status assessment done with each patient encounter.	Changes in mentation may signal a decrease in liver function.	Remains confused and drowsy but unchanged from admission.
Serum ammonia levels will not increase further during hospitalization.	Administer lactulose as ordered.	Lactulose decreases absorption of ammonia.	Lactulose administered; diarrhea occurring. A&D ointment applied to anal area after bowel movements.
	Monitor serum ammonia levels.	Assists in determining likelihood of coma.	Laboratory work to be drawn in A.M.

PROBLEM STATEMENT/NURSING DIAGNOSIS
Potential for injury due to confusion, drowsiness, and weakness.

SUPPORTING ASSESSMENT DATA
Subjective: "This room looks strange. I can't find the toilet."
Objective: Elevated serum ammonia and slight confusion.

Goals/Expected Outcomes	Nursing Interventions	Selected Rationale	Evaluation
Patient will not experience injury while hospitalized.	Monitor mental status every 2h.	Determines worsening of disorientation.	Oriented to person and place, can recall month with repeated coaching.
	Place call bell within reach and bed at lowest level. Activate bed alarm.	Prevents injury from accidental fall from bed.	Bed down, call bell within reach, alarm activated.
	Offer frequent assistance with toileting and other needs (i.e., hygiene, fluids).	Decreases incidents of wandering or falls if trying to meet own needs.	Offered toileting and mouth care q2–3h. No injury sustained. Continue plan.

PROBLEM STATEMENT/NURSING DIAGNOSIS
Altered self-care ability due to fatigue, drowsiness, and ascites.

SUPPORTING ASSESSMENT DATA
Subjective: "I'm so sleepy and weak."
Objective: Cannot perform ADLs; very drowsy, ascites present.

Goals/Expected Outcomes	Nursing Interventions	Selected Rationale	Evaluation
Patient will be able to assist with ADLs within 2 wk.	Have patient brush own teeth and wash face. Add in other self-care activities as energy level increases. Allow rest periods between activities.	Gradual increase in activity level allows for patient to participate and build strength.	Patient able to brush teeth, wash face, and wash perineal area.
Patient will be able to perform ADLs independently within 1 mo.	Offer mouth care q2h.	Mouth care improves appetite. Improved nutrition increases energy level.	Mouth care given q2h.
	Assist with meal trays, gradually decreasing assist.	May lack fine motor coordination to open packages.	Set up meal tray. Patient able to unwrap eating utensils and take lids off liquids.
	Assist with toileting. Gradually decrease assist.	Prevents falls and aids with elimination.	Assisted with toileting. Needed to be steadied upon standing, able to ambulate without assist.

PROBLEM STATEMENT/NURSING DIAGNOSIS
Fluid volume overload due to ascites and peripheral edema from portal hypertension.

Nursing Care Plan 30.1 Care of a Patient With Cirrhosis of the Liver—cont'd

SUPPORTING ASSESSMENT DATA

Objective: Ascites, pitting edema of feet and ankles, 6-lb weight gain in 2 days.

Goals/Expected Outcomes	Nursing Interventions	Selected Rationale	Evaluation
Patient will have no further increase in ascites this week.	Measure abdominal girth every shift.	Determines whether ascites is increasing or decreasing.	Abdominal girth down ⅛ inch.
Patient will have decrease in peripheral edema.	Administer diuretics as ordered and monitor I&O.	Diuretics remove excess fluid from the body. I&O tracks fluid removal.	Diuretic administered. Intake 400 mL; output 670 mL.
	Weigh daily and record.	Daily weight indicates whether diuretic therapy is effective.	Weight down 1.5 lb.
	Turn at least q1–2h. Provide good skin care.	Turning and skin care prevent pressure sores.	Turned q2h; skin care provided; no reddened or excoriated areas over pressure points.

CRITICAL THINKING QUESTIONS

1. Describe the correct way to measure abdominal girth.
2. Why is good skin care even more important when a patient has edema and ascites?
3. How high would a PT or INR level have to climb before you would report it to the health care provider immediately?
4. Why would it be important to monitor this patient for symptoms of alcohol withdrawal?

ADLs, Activities of daily living; *BP*, blood pressure; *I&O*, intake and output; *INR*, international normalized ratio; *PT*, prothrombin time; *RR*, respiration rate.

cholangitis, metabolic disorders, and biliary atresia in children. Some recovered alcoholics with cirrhosis are candidates. Between 70% and 80% of liver transplant recipients survive at least 3 years with good quality of life. Survival rates are 73% at 5 years after transplant (OPTN data, 2018). If the patient has encephalopathy preoperatively, an intracranial pressure monitor is placed to assess intracranial pressure (ICP). Every attempt is made to keep ICP within normal limits because increased ICP levels are correlated with decreased survival rates after transplantation.

Nursing Management

After surgery a T-tube and bulb reservoir drains will usually be in place. The patient must take cyclosporine for life to prevent rejection of the new liver. Other immunosuppressants such as azathioprine (Imuran), corticosteroids, tacrolimus (Prograf), monoclonal antibody OKT3, and interleukin-2 receptor antagonists such as basiliximab (Simulect) and daclizumab (Zenapax) may also be added. Strict infection control and prevention is necessary, and the patient is monitored closely for signs of hemorrhage or hypovolemia. Measures are instituted to prevent pneumonia, atelectasis, and pleural effusions. Liver function, serum potassium, serum glucose, and coagulation factors are monitored closely. Right quadrant or flank pain, increasing jaundice, fever, and changes in stool and urine color may indicate organ rejection. Close medical supervision is necessary after discharge.

CANCER OF THE LIVER

Etiology

Primary cancer of the liver is rare in the United States but is a common malignancy in Africa and Asia, where it is caused by a parasite called the *liver fluke*. Liver cancer may be triggered by aflatoxin, a mold that grows on spoiled peanuts, corn, and grains. Metastatic liver cancer is much more prevalent than primary liver cancer, but the end result is the same. Cirrhosis and hepatitis B or C increase the risk. Because of an increase in hepatitis C, there has been an increase in hepatocellular carcinoma. Three times as many men as women develop liver cancer.

Pathophysiology

There are two types of primary liver cancer: (1) hepatoma, which arises from the hepatocytes, and (2) cholangiocarcinoma, or bile duct cancer. Benign tumors also occur in the liver. Hepatoma usually develops in people who have cirrhosis. A rare disorder called *hemochromatosis*, which causes deposits of iron in the body, predisposes to the development of hepatoma. The cause of cholangiocarcinoma is unknown, but it occurs more often in people with inflammation of the bowel, such as ulcerative colitis.

Pathophysiologically, there is irritation and inflammation with disruption of the structure of normal liver cells. The cancer spreads throughout the organ and invades the portal vein and lymphatics. It may metastasize to the lungs, brain, kidneys, and spleen.

Signs, Symptoms, and Diagnosis

Symptoms may include right upper quadrant pain, fatigue, anorexia, weight loss, weakness, or fever plus signs of poor liver function. Pain may radiate to the back. Because symptoms often are vague, diagnosis of liver cancer occurs late, and death may occur within 6 to 18 months.

CT or magnetic resonance imaging (MRI) is used to determine the presence of tumor and the stage of the cancer and to find areas of metastasis. Fine-needle biopsy or brush biopsy during ERCP gives a definitive diagnosis for bile duct cancer.

Treatment and Nursing Management

If no distant spread is found and there is no lymph node involvement, surgical resection may be attempted. If the tumor is primary and has not metastasized, liver transplantation is an option. Treatment is combined radiation and chemotherapy that is infused intravenously or directly into the hepatic circulation. In chemoembolization, an interventional radiologist cannulates the main artery feeding the tumor and injects chemotherapy agents. The treatment may induce toxic hepatitis, which subsides after the end of therapy. Hepatocellular carcinoma does not respond well to chemotherapy as a curative treatment. Several medications that shrink tumors or halt their progression are available. Sorafenib (Nexavar) has improved the survival of patients with advanced cancer. Nivolumab (Opdivo) is approved for use in patients who have stopped responding to sorafenib, as is pembrolizumab (Keytruda). In August 2018 lenvatinib (Lenvima) was approved as a first-line treatment for lesions that cannot be treated surgically. Other drugs that inhibit tumor growth by interfering with the blood supply that feeds the tumor are being given in combination and singly; bevacizumab (Avastin) and atezolizumab (Tecentriq) are first-line treatment for advanced hepatocellular carcinoma. Sunitinib (Sutent) was also approved in August 2018 for first-line therapy (Cicalese, 2018).

Tumor ablation is used for tumors less than 5 cm in diameter. Ethanol or acetic acid is injected through the skin into the tumor. The liquid destroys the cancer cells. The procedure is carried out in the radiology department with the use of ultrasound.

Laser or radiofrequency ablation that uses heat to destroy cancer cells is performed with a local anesthetic. This procedure is used for cholangiocarcinoma. Cryotherapy may be used during surgery; a probe deposits liquid nitrogen to the tumor site. Cancer cells are destroyed by freezing.

Nursing care includes assessing for signs and symptoms of liver failure and blockage in the common bile duct. Additional care is directed at the associated problems, such as ascites and encephalopathy. Surgical care is provided as for other abdominal surgery patients (see Chapter 5). Care of patients undergoing chemotherapy and radiation for cancer is discussed in Chapter 8.

DISORDERS OF THE PANCREAS

ACUTE PANCREATITIS

Pancreatitis is an inflammation of the pancreas. It may be acute or chronic. Pancreatitis frequently accompanies obstruction of the pancreatic duct from gallstones or from the backflow of bile into the pancreatic duct.

Etiology

Most cases of pancreatitis are related to gallstones blocking the common duct. Viral infections, trauma, ERCP, penetrating ulcers, drug toxicities, metabolic disorders, scorpion stings, and a variety of other factors can also cause pancreatitis. Men tend to develop pancreatitis related to alcohol. In women, it is more commonly associated with gallstones.

Pathophysiology

In some types of pancreatitis, the severe inflammation and damage are caused by escape of pancreatic digestive enzymes. The enzymes act directly on the tissue, causing hemorrhage, autodigestion, and necrosis. It is unclear how the autodigestion is activated. Reflux of bile and duodenal contents into the pancreatic duct is a possible mechanism. A gallstone stuck in the ampulla of Vater can cause edema of the sphincter of Oddi, which might permit reflux of duodenal contents. Alcohol can cause spasm of the sphincter of Oddi, blocking secretion through the pancreatic ducts. This may lead to activation of the pancreatic enzymes within the pancreas.

Pancreatic abscess or pseudocysts may develop. An abscess may form from the purulent liquefaction of the necrotic pancreatic tissue. A **pseudocyst** is a saclike structure that forms on or around the pancreas (Concept Map 30.2).

Signs and Symptoms

Pancreatitis causes abdominal pain that is usually acute, but this can vary among individuals. The pain is steady and localized to the epigastrium or left upper quadrant. As it progresses, it spreads and radiates to the back and flank. Sitting and leaning forward may ease the pain. The severity of the pain may slowly decrease after 24 hours. **Eating makes the pain worse.** Nausea, vomiting, sweating, jaundice, and weakness often accompany pain.

> **Clinical Cues**
>
> A patient with acute pancreatitis may curl up in a tight fetal position (knee-chest) because this opens up the retroperitoneal space and decreases pain. Assuming a supine position for a procedure or assessment is likely to increase the pain; therefore acknowledge the patient's discomfort and help them resume the position of greatest comfort when the procedure is over.

Examination of the abdomen will reveal tenderness and guarding. If peritonitis is present, there will be distention and rigidity. Bowel sounds may be reduced or absent. A pseudocyst can be palpated as an epigastric mass in about 50% of cases. If retroperitoneal bleeding is present, there may be bruising in the flanks or a bluish discoloration around the umbilicus. There may

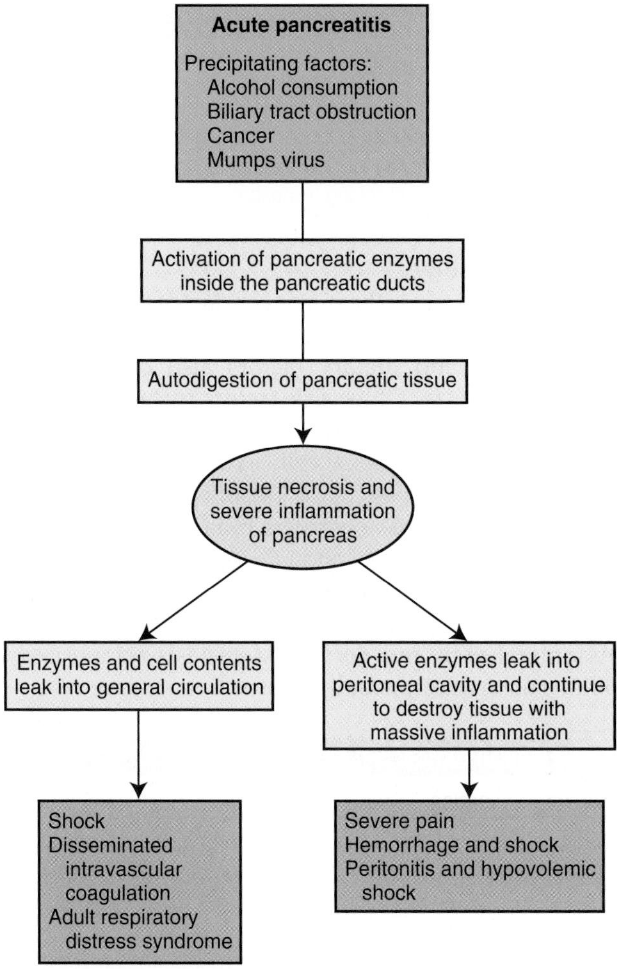

Concept Map 30.2 Pathophysiology of acute pancreatitis.

be signs and symptoms of respiratory distress (secondary to atelectasis, pleural effusion, or respiratory distress syndrome) or shock, tachycardia, leukocytosis, and fever. Serum amylase may be two times normal and will remain elevated for 72 hours. Serum lipase remains elevated for several days. If biliary obstruction is involved, mild jaundice may be present. Laboratory values will indicate hypoglycemia, hypocalcemia, and hypokalemia.

Diagnosis

Diagnosis is based on the symptoms, risk factors, and results of tests performed to rule out other disorders. An abdominal ultrasound, CT scan, and serum and urine amylase studies are usually ordered. Diagnosis is made when a patient presents with two of the following: (1) acute onset of severe epigastric pain, (2) lipase or amylase elevated three times normal, and (3) CT, MRI, or ultrasound findings consistent with pancreatitis (Swaroop, 2018).

Treatment and Nursing Management

Pain evaluation and control are primary nursing responsibilities. Vital signs are taken frequently, urinary output is measured, and the patient is monitored for signs of shock. IV fluids are given to maintain blood pressure and hemodynamic stability. Observe for signs of restlessness, use of accessory muscles for breathing, irritability, confusion, or dyspnea, which indicate respiratory distress, and administer oxygen as ordered. Monitor laboratory values and note changes. Administer fluids and observe for electrolyte imbalances. The patient is kept NPO during the acute phase until nausea and pain are controlled. Within 48 hours of admission, enteral feeding may be implemented via NG tube if the patient is unable to take in adequate nutrition. If gastric feedings are not tolerated, total parenteral nutrition (TPN) may be given. If the patient is receiving TPN, blood glucose needs to be checked regularly, and insulin may be necessary. As soon as tolerated, oral feeding with a low-fat solid diet may be provided. Nutritional support is important to healing (Uppal, 2018). Most patients with acute pancreatitis recover after receiving this type of treatment.

Assess for tolerance of the diet as the patient resumes foods. If abscess or pseudocyst are present, they may be surgically drained. IV hydromorphone or morphine via PCA pump may be needed to control pain. Histamine (H_2)–receptor antagonists or a proton pump inhibitor may be given to decrease the hydrochloric acid secretion that stimulates pancreatic activity. Administration of antispasmodics such as dicyclomine (Bentyl) or propantheline bromide (Pro-Banthine) is helpful.

> **Clinical Cues**
>
> When a powdered form of pancreatic enzymes must be taken, it should be mixed in nonprotein food, such as applesauce. Care must be taken not to let any of the medication remain on the lips or skin because it will cause irritation. Supplementation of pancreatic enzymes is used for chronic pancreatitis.

CHRONIC PANCREATITIS

Etiology and Pathophysiology

Alcohol abuse accounts for half of the chronic pancreatitis cases in men. It is the least common cause in women. There is some indication that there may be a genetic component that makes some people more susceptible to pancreatic injury from toxins such as alcohol. Cigarette smoking is also a risk factor and is dose dependent. Autoimmune conditions may also be implicated. Repeated bouts of inflammation cause progressive fibrosis of the gland, stricture of the ducts, and eventual calcification, leading to exocrine and endocrine dysfunction.

Signs and Symptoms

Abdominal pain is the major symptom. There may be periods of acute pain, but consistent chronic pain is more common. Nausea and vomiting may also be chronic. Other symptoms are related to pancreatic insufficiency as less and less pancreatic tissue is functional. Malabsorption with weight loss and steatorrhea, constipation, mild jaundice with dark urine, and diabetes mellitus develop.

Diagnosis

Determination of bicarbonate, protease, amylase, and lipase concentration and output in the duodenum after stimulation with secretin is a helpful test for chronic pancreatitis. This test is done in conjunction with magnetic resonance cholangiopancreatography (MRCP). Ultrasound may be used via the endoscope. Other helpful diagnostic tests are fecal fat determination, fasting blood glucose, arteriography, and radiographic examinations of the pancreas. Pancreatic cancer or a liver disorder can produce the same results on these tests. The differential diagnosis is difficult. Serum amylase and lipase may be elevated slightly or not at all. There may be increases in serum bilirubin and alkaline phosphatase. Leukocytosis and an elevated sedimentation rate are present. Advanced disease is best identified by CT scan.

Treatment and Nursing Management

Treatment during an acute episode of chronic pancreatitis is the same as for acute pancreatitis. The pain is caused by the inflammation and damage being done to the tissues. Minimizing the cause of the pain can reduce the pain. Obviously eliminating alcohol intake is essential. Small, low-fat meals and good hydration have helped some patients. Pancreatic enzyme supplements help suppress secretion of the enzymes that may cause further irritation. Amitriptyline and nortriptyline may help the neuropathic pain component. Nonsteroidal antiinflammatory drugs (NSAIDs) may also help. Long-term pain control presents problems. The patient is switched to non-narcotic pain medications to try to prevent addiction, but these are often insufficient for pain control. Complications such as diabetes mellitus must be addressed, and diet requirements and medications should be reviewed with the patient. Chronic pancreatitis interferes with the patient's usual lifestyle and often is accompanied by depression, so your patient should be periodically assessed for signs of depression, and appropriate referrals should be made. **A major nursing action is to be supportive of efforts to abstain from alcohol.** Table 30.6 presents problem statements and specific interventions appropriate for patients with pancreatitis.

CANCER OF THE PANCREAS

Etiology

The cause of pancreatic cancer is unknown. It is estimated that 55,440 new cases of cancer of the pancreas and 44,330 deaths will occur in the United States annually (American Cancer Society, 2018). It is more common in men than in women and occurs more often in people older than 55 years. Cancer of the pancreas is often fatal within 1 year. It is usually in an advanced state when discovered because it is asymptomatic in the early stages.

Cultural Considerations

Pancreatic Cancer Deaths

More African American men die of pancreatic cancer than do men from any other ethnic group. It may be due in part to having higher incidence of risk factors for pancreatic cancer such as diabetes and smoking (American Cancer Society, 2016).

Pathophysiology

Cigarette smoking is the major risk factor for pancreatic cancer; 2 to 3 of every 10 cases are linked to tobacco use. Obesity and dietary factors also contribute to pancreatic cancer. Other risk factors include diabetes, cirrhosis, and chronic pancreatitis. Adenocarcinoma arising from the epithelial cells in the ducts is the most common form of pancreatic neoplasm. Tumor in the head of the pancreas obstructs biliary and pancreatic flow. Cancer in the body and tail of the pancreas usually remains asymptomatic until it is well advanced and invades the liver, stomach, lymph nodes, or posterior abdominal wall and nerves. Metastasis occurs early. Biliary obstruction usually causes liver failure.

Health Promotion

Smoking Cessation

Most people are aware of the relationship between smoking and lung cancer; however, it is also necessary to teach patients the effects of smoking on other vital organs, such as the pancreas. Provide referral to community resources for smoking cessation and written materials with options on how to quit.

Signs and Symptoms

Epigastric pain and weight loss are the main symptoms of pancreatic cancer. Anorexia and vomiting may occur, and the patient may develop a dislike for red meat. When the disease is advanced, jaundice appears along with dark urine and clay-colored stools. There is glucose intolerance. There is a high incidence of clot formation with pancreatic cancer.

Safety Alert

Deep Vein Thrombosis

Because of the increased risk of clot formation in patients with pancreatic cancer, it is important to assess for signs and symptoms of deep vein thrombosis (DVT): pain, heat, or swelling in the calves. One leg may be swollen; measure the calf and ankle and compare to the other leg. Check for signs of pulmonary embolus as well: restlessness, apprehension, chest pain, decreased oxygen saturation, and shortness of breath. Should these signs and symptoms occur, report them to the health care provider immediately. The Joint Commission's National Quality Measures require rigorous prevention of DVT for all patients.

Diagnosis

Diagnosis is made by ultrasonography, imaging techniques, and fine-needle biopsy. Elevated carcinoembryonic antigen levels occur 80% to 90% of the time when

Table 30.6 **Common Problem Statements, Expected Outcomes, and Nursing Interventions for Patients With Pancreatic Disorders**

PROBLEM STATEMENT	EXPECTED OUTCOMES	NURSING INTERVENTIONS
Acute pain due to pancreatic inflammation	Patient's pain level will be maintained at 4/10 or below. Patient will state that pain is controlled within 8 h.	Medicate with analgesic as ordered. Instruct in use of PCA pump if ordered. Encourage relaxation techniques to decrease discomfort. Assess q2h for adequate pain relief. Administer adjunctive medications as ordered. Assist into knee-chest position for comfort. Maintain NPO status in early stages.
Potential for altered breathing pattern due to irritation or to diaphragm pressure from ascites or pancreatic abscess/ pseudocyst	Patient will maintain adequate oxygen levels as evidenced by oxygen saturation within normal limits.	Observe for signs of respiratory distress. Auscultate lungs for crackles or abnormal lung sounds. Monitor oxygen saturation with pulse oximeter. Administer supplemental oxygen as ordered. Encourage use of incentive spirometer as ordered. Place in semi-Fowler position as tolerated to promote better lung expansion.
Potential for bleeding due to potential autodigestion or rupture of abscess resulting in circulatory collapse	Patient will not experience shock symptoms while hospitalized.	Monitor laboratory values for liver enzymes, ammonia, albumin, sodium, potassium, calcium, and magnesium daily. Observe for subtle changes in mental status. Monitor vital signs closely. Observe stool for signs of bleeding. Monitor urine output. Report frank bleeding promptly.
Insufficient knowledge about pancreatitis and its treatment and prevention of recurrence	Patient will verbalize understanding of disease process within 2 wk. Patient will verbalize understanding of treatment regimen within 1 wk. Patient will verbalize ways to prevent recurrence of pancreatitis before discharge.	Instruct in patient-specific causes (i.e., alcohol, ulcer, gallstones) and disease process (i.e., eating triggers digestive enzymes that act directly on the tissues). Explain all aspects of treatment (e.g., NPO and possible NG decompression decrease the release of enzymes, and therefore pain is decreased) and reason for each medication (e.g., dicyclomine decreases GI tract spasms). Teach ways to prevent recurrence of pancreatitis (i.e., abstain from alcohol).
Fear due to possibility of disability or death	Patient will verbalize that fear has decreased before discharge.	Establish trusting relationship by attentive, caring attitude. Encourage verbalization of fears; actively listen. Encourage contact with minister, hospital chaplain, or spiritual advisor. Point out any encouraging signs of improvement.

GI, Gastrointestinal; *NG*, nasogastric; *NPO*, nothing by mouth; *PCA*, patient-controlled analgesia.

pancreatic cancer is present. However, serum beta human chorionic gonadotropin and carbohydrate antigen (CA) 72-4 are the strongest indicators of pancreatic cancer. The tumor markers CA 19-9 and CA 242 are used to monitor for potential spread or recurrence.

Treatment

High doses of opioid analgesics are usually required to keep the patient comfortable. Drug dependency should not be a concern. Treating or preventing malnutrition is a major goal. Enteral feedings may need to be given into the jejunum **(jejunostomy).** TPN may be needed to provide adequate nutrition (see Chapters 3 and 28).

Surgical treatment is appropriate for resectable tumor in about 15% to 20% of patients but has not been highly successful in curing the disease. It provides a 5-year survival rate of less than 5%. Surgery is used mainly to relieve symptoms of obstructive jaundice, severe pain, or other complications. A Whipple procedure, or radical pancreaticoduodenectomy, may be done for cancer of the head of the pancreas. The head of the pancreas, the gallbladder, the duodenum, part of the jejunum, and all or part of the stomach are removed. The spleen may also be removed. The remaining structures are anastomosed to the jejunum. Another option is total pancreatectomy. The patient will usually go to the surgical critical care unit after surgery. Nursing care is the same as for any abdominal surgery, but many complications can occur; vigilance is essential. The patient will need enteral feedings, perhaps for life. A stent may be placed in the pancreatic duct to promote exit of pancreatic secretions and enzymes.

Other treatments include radiofrequency ablation and microwave therapy, which use heat to destroy tissue, and cryosurgery, which uses cold. Embolization therapy can be used to cut off the blood supply to the tumor. Cyberknife treatment—an image-guided radiosurgery that helps target the pancreatic tumor without disrupting other tissue—is an option. Intensive external beam radiation therapy may offer pain relief, alleviate duct obstruction, and improve food absorption. Chemoradiotherapy may also be used. A radiation sensitizer substance (capecitabine or FU) is administered, which enhances the effect of the radiation. Radioactive iodine (^{125}I) seeds may be implanted in combination with systemic or intra-arterial administration of floxuridine.

Gemcitabine (Gemzar) and 5-fluorouracil (5-FU) are common for treatment of nonresectable or metastatic tumors (Ryan & Mamon, 2018). Outcomes for advanced cases are better when erlotinib is added. A combination of drugs has proven most effective, and other commonly used drugs include irinotecan (Camptosar), docetaxel (Taxotere), capecitabine (Xeloda), oxaliplatin (Eloxatin), and cisplatin (Platinol). Other drugs that may be used include the targeted-therapy drug sunitinib, which blocks the growth signal, and octreotide and lanreotide, which suppress the hormone release from the tumor. Ongoing trials are showing promise in new treatment options.

Nursing Management

Nursing care is geared toward managing the severe pain and managing the side effects of treatment. Postoperatively, observe for hyperglycemia, hemorrhage, bowel obstruction or paralytic ileus, wound infection, and intra-abdominal abscess. Monitor the NG tube for clear, bile-tinged drainage or frank blood with an increase in output because this may indicate leakage at an anastomosis site. Postoperative care is similar to that for any patient who has had abdominal surgery (see Chapter 5). Chapter 8 discusses care of patients undergoing chemotherapy or radiation for cancer.

COMMUNITY CARE

Nurses in the community should promote immunization against hepatitis B virus in all persons at risk. Teenagers and adults should be counseled about the possibility of transmission of hepatitis B virus by sexual contact and advised of measures for protection. The hepatitis A vaccine should be recommended for those traveling in areas where this disorder is prevalent and for those at risk of liver problems. Nurses should be aware of policies and procedures for reporting new cases of hepatitis to local health departments. All health care workers should be tested for the presence of hepatitis C virus.

Nurses in extended care facilities should be alert to signs of jaundice in patients. Dark-colored urine is a common early sign of a problem. Cancer and gallstones are both more prevalent in older adults, and when abdominal pain occurs these disorders must be considered. Home care nurses must be particularly alert to the possibility of liver or pancreatic problems caused by medications the patient is taking. Encourage regular laboratory work as recommended when the patient is taking a drug known to be potentially damaging to the liver.

Get Ready for the NCLEX® Examination!

Key Points

- Factors that are associated with cholelithiasis and cholecystitis include hemolytic disease, surgical treatment of Crohn disease, rapid-weight-loss diets or starvation, multiple pregnancies or hormonal replacement therapy, major trauma, burns, and cardiac surgery.
- Signs and symptoms of acute cholecystitis include acute pain, fever, anorexia, nausea and vomiting, dehydration, and mild jaundice.
- Typical symptoms of chronic cholecystitis are indigestion, flatulence, nausea after eating fatty foods, and intermittent pain referred to the back.
- There are five main types of hepatitis: A, B, C, D, and E (see Table 30.2). Hepatitis is treated by rest, a nutritious low-fat diet, and avoidance of substances that are harmful to the liver and antiviral medications for some types (see Chapter 27, Box 27.1).
- Signs and symptoms of liver disorders are fatigue, weakness, anorexia, abdominal pain, nausea and vomiting, skin rashes, itching, fever, dark urine, light-colored stools, peripheral edema, bruising, and jaundice.
- Chronic inflammation causes fibrosis and cirrhosis of the liver cells. Diagnosis of cirrhosis includes liver biopsy, liver function tests, prothrombin time, and albumin levels.
- Bleeding esophageal varices and hepatic encephalopathy are complications of cirrhosis.
- Chemotherapy, radiation, and ablation therapies are used for treatment of liver cancer.
- In acute pancreatitis, inflammation and damage are caused by escape of pancreatic digestive enzymes, causing hemorrhage, autodigestion, and necrosis. Symptoms include acute, steady pain in the epigastrium or left upper quadrant. Serum lipase and amylase are elevated. Treatment consists of pain control, reduction of pancreatic secretions, restoration of fluid and electrolyte balance, and treatment for complications such as shock or diabetes.
- Chronic pancreatitis is related to cigarette smoking, alcoholism, and autoimmune diseases. Long-term pain control is an issue.

- Signs and symptoms of pancreatic cancer are weight loss, anorexia, vomiting, and signs of pancreatic dysfunction. Not smoking reduces the risk of pancreatic cancer by 50%.
- Treatment of pancreatic cancer includes pain management and chemotherapy and radiation, which may improve food absorption, relieve pain, and alleviate duct obstruction.

Additional Learning Resources

SG Go to your Study Guide for additional learning activities to help you master this chapter content.

Go to your Evolve website (http://evolve.elsevier.com/deWit/medsurg) for the following FREE learning resources:

- Animations, audio, and video
- Answers and rationales for questions and activities
- Glossary with pronunciations in English and Spanish
- Interactive Review Questions and more!

Review Questions for the NCLEX® Examination

1. Before being discharged to home, a patient who had a laparoscopic cholecystectomy is given instructions regarding pain control. Which patient statements indicate successful teaching? *(Select all that apply.)*
   1. "I will stay mobile and change positions frequently."
   2. "Opioids are the best medication for relieving pain."
   3. "I will continue my swimming routine for exercise, and this will help my pain."
   4. "Passing gas will relieve my pain."
   5. "Pain will become less as the gas in my abdomen is absorbed."
   6. "I will take NSAIDs for pain control."

   NCLEX Client Need: Health Promotion and Maintenance
2. If the patient has a history of chronic cholecystitis, which comment is cause for the greatest concern?
   1. "I have back pain at the level of the shoulder blade."
   2. "I had nausea after eating a hamburger and fries."
   3. "I have generalized abdominal pain and fever."
   4. "I have discomfort in the right upper part of my abdomen."

   NCLEX Client Need: Physiological Integrity: Physiological Adaptation
3. You are caring for a 57-year-old patient with ascites resulting from liver disease. You anticipate that the health care provider will use which therapeutic regimen to reduce portal hypertension?
   1. Vascular shunting of the portal venous systems
   2. Repeated abdominal paracentesis
   3. Diet restrictions and nutrient supplementation
   4. Fluid replacement therapy

   NCLEX Client Need: Physiological Integrity: Reduction of Risk Potential
4. A patient with high levels of serum ammonia asks, "Why do I have to continue taking lactulose?" What is the best response?
   1. "It destroys ammonia-producing bacteria in the intestines."
   2. "It reduces intestinal absorption of ammonia."
   3. "It corrects vitamin B_1 deficiency."
   4. "It is used in preparation for a diagnostic test."

   NCLEX Client Need: Physiological Integrity: Pharmacological Therapies
5. You are caring for a patient who underwent a recent liver transplantation. You reinforce the teaching related to self-care. Which teaching topics are most important to address before discharge? *(Select all that apply.)*
   1. Reporting any kind of pain associated with fever and changes in stool color
   2. Location and meeting time of local support groups
   3. Use of strict hand hygiene in changing dressings
   4. The lifelong need to take antirejection medications

   NCLEX Client Need: Physiological Integrity: Reduction of Risk Potential
6. You are caring for a patient who underwent radical pancreaticoduodenectomy. Which postoperative complication would be the most likely to occur and cause the greatest concern?
   1. Hypoglycemia
   2. Adhesions
   3. Hemorrhage
   4. Anorexia

   NCLEX Client Need: Physiological Integrity: Reduction of Risk Potential
7. Which instructions should be given to a patient regarding preventing the spread of hepatitis A? *(Select all that apply.)*
   1. Bleach solutions must be used to clean the bathroom.
   2. Somebody else should be doing the cooking right now.
   3. No vaccination is available for hepatitis A.
   4. Good hand hygiene reduces the likelihood of passing the virus.

   NCLEX Client Need: Safe and Effective Care Environment: Safety and Infection Control
8. A patient has cirrhosis of the liver and ascites. You should question which order?
   1. Bed rest with bathroom privileges
   2. Discontinue furosemide (Lasix) 80 mg
   3. Give 2-g sodium diet
   4. Fluid restriction 1500 mL/24 h

   NCLEX Client Need: Physiological Integrity: Pharmacological Therapies
9. A patient with acute pancreatitis has a bluish discoloration around the umbilicus. What actions should you take? *(Place in priority order.)*
   1. Place head flat and feet elevated.
   2. Notify health care provider.
   3. Assess vital signs.
   4. Verify patency of IV line.

   NCLEX Client Need: Physiological Integrity: Physiological Adaptation

10. One goal of nursing care for a patient during the acute phase of pancreatitis is reduction of pain. Which nursing interventions help alleviate pain? *(Select all that apply.)*
1. Reinforce use of the PCA pump.
2. Maintain IV fluids as ordered.
3. Provide a soft diet with additional fluids.
4. Administer dicyclomine (Bentyl).
5. Give pancreatic enzymes.
6. Place the patient in a supine position.

NCLEX Client Need: Physiological Integrity: Physiological Adaptation

Critical Thinking Questions

Scenario A

Mr. Moser is admitted to the hospital with a diagnosis of cirrhosis of the liver. He is 59 years old and has been hospitalized several times for his condition. He has shortness of breath as a result of a swollen and enlarged abdomen, is anemic because of minimal but constant esophageal bleeding, and appears jaundiced. He has severe abrasions on his arms, legs, and abdomen from repeated scratching to relieve his pruritus. Mr. Moser is very depressed and will not converse with you when you enter the room with his breakfast tray on the first morning you are assigned to his care. He refuses to eat and indicates his attitude by pushing the tray away and turning on his side to face the wall.

1. What nursing measures might help relieve some of Mr. Moser's problems?
2. Why do you think he is depressed?
3. How would you go about helping him emotionally?
4. What special observations must you make while caring for Mr. Moser?
5. How would you explain a paracentesis to Mr. Moser if one were ordered for him?

Scenario B

Mrs. Lincoln, age 46 years, is admitted to the hospital for a laparoscopic cholecystectomy. She is extremely obese and enjoys eating rich, fatty foods, even though she knows this will add to her obesity and precipitate attacks of cholecystitis. You are assigned to care for Mrs. Lincoln when she returns from surgery.

1. How will you position this patient?
2. What would you need to assess to determine whether complications are occurring?
3. What would you need to teach the patient and family before discharge?
4. What problems might occur after discharge? What should be the diet for Mrs. Lincoln?
5. How soon will Mrs. Lincoln probably be able to resume most of her usual activities?

Scenario C

You are working in an employee health clinic and taking a health history from Mr. Austin, who is 52 years old. He reports that he has chronic pancreatitis.

1. What physical signs and symptoms should you ask about?
2. What questions should you ask about his diet and lifestyle?

31 The Musculoskeletal System

http://evolve.elsevier.com/deWit/medsurg

Objectives

Theory

1. Describe the normal anatomy of the musculoskeletal system.
2. Show how the musculoskeletal system provides the function of movement.
3. Discuss how the musculoskeletal system provides protection for the body.
4. Illustrate causes of disorders of the musculoskeletal system and ways to prevent them.
5. Compare the procedure and nursing care for the following diagnostic tests: bone scan, arthrocentesis, electromyography.
6. Distinguish ways in which older adults can increase musculoskeletal strength and protect bones.

Clinical Practice

7. Perform an assessment on a patient with a musculoskeletal disorder.
8. Assist in the development of a nursing care plan for a patient with a musculoskeletal disorder.
9. Use measures to reduce the chance of contracture for patients with musculoskeletal injuries.
10. Assist patients with musculoskeletal injuries with active or passive range of motion.
11. Teach a patient to properly use an assistive device.

Key Terms

ankylosis (ăng-kĭ-LŌ-sĭs, p. 752)
cartilage (KĂR-tĭ-lăzh, p. 739)
contractures (kŏn-TRĂK-chŭrz, p. 752)
crepitation (KRĔP-ĭ-tā-shŭn, p. 741)
isometric exercises (ī-sō-MĔT-rĭk, p. 749)
kyphosis (kī-PHŌ-sĭs, p. 746)
ligaments (LĬG-ă-mĕntz, p. 739)
orthopedic (ŏr-thō-PĒ-dĭk, p. 741)
ossification (ŏs-ĭ-fī-KĀ-shŭn, p. 741)
tendons (TĔN-dŏnz, p. 739)

Concepts Covered in This Chapter

- Functional Ability
- Self-Management
- Elimination
- Inflammation
- Mobility
- Tissue Integrity
- Pain
- Fatigue
- Coping
- Health Promotion
- Collaboration

ANATOMY AND PHYSIOLOGY OF THE MUSCULOSKELETAL SYSTEM

STRUCTURES OF THE MUSCULOSKELETAL SYSTEM

- The musculoskeletal system consists of the bones, joints, cartilage, ligaments, tendons, and muscles.
- There are three types of bone cells; osteoblasts are responsible for bone growth by making new bone cells and secreting collagen; osteocytes regulate mineral uptake and release; osteoclasts dissolve minerals for release into the bloodstream.
- A total of 206 bones make up the human skeleton (Fig. 31.1).
- Bone is either compact or spongy. Spongy bone contains red bone marrow (Fig. 31.2).
- Bones are classified as long, short, flat, or irregular.
- Each bone has markings on its surface that make it unique.
- The haversian system (or osteon) is a canal system that runs through the bone and contains the blood and lymph vessels.
- A joint is the articulation point between two or more bones of the skeleton. There are immovable, slightly movable, and freely movable joints (Table 31.1).
- **Ligaments** join the bones of a joint together.
- **Tendons** are connective tissues that provide joint movement.
- **Cartilage** is a type of connective tissue in which fibers and cells are embedded in a semisolid gel material. Cartilage acts as a cushion. The meniscus in the knee joint is a type of cartilage.
- A bursa is a fluid-filled sac that provides cushioning at friction points in a freely movable joint.

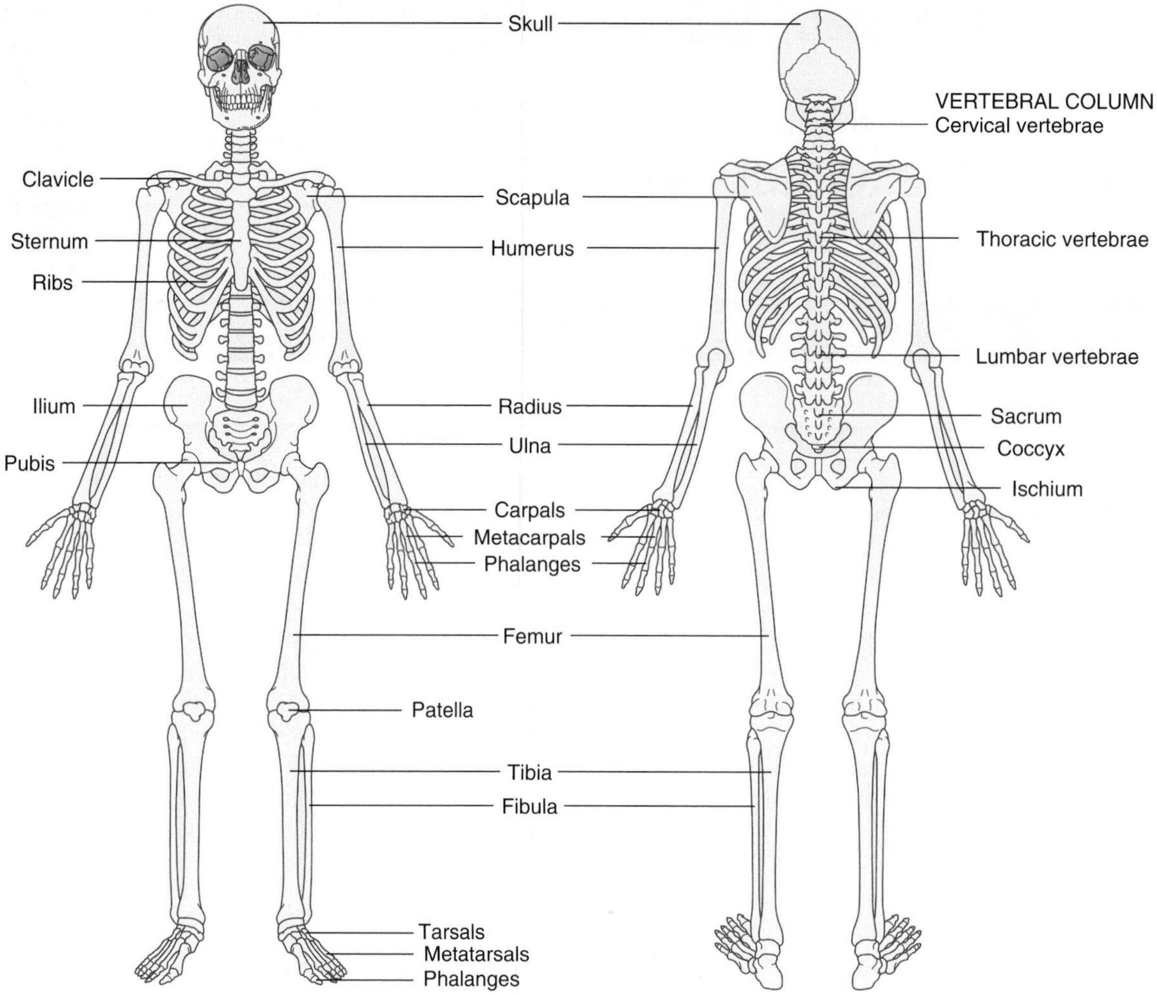

Fig. 31.1 Major bones of the human skeleton.

Table 31.1 Types of Moveable Joints and Examples

TYPE OF JOINT	EXAMPLE	MOVEMENT
Hinge	Elbow	Bidirectional to flex and extend
Pivot	Head of radius around ulna	Rotational to supinate and pronate
Saddle	Thumb	Circular clockwise and counterclockwise
Ball and socket	Shoulder and hip joints	Ball rotates within socket and moves up and down
Condyloid	Head to neck joint	Up and down and side to side
Gliding	Articulating surfaces of vertebrae	Lateral and up and down

- Skeletal muscle is made up of hundreds of muscle fibers bundled together and surrounded by a connective tissue sheath.
- Fascia is a connective tissue that surrounds and separates the muscles.
- The muscle coverings contain blood vessels and nerves.
- Muscle has properties that allow it to be electrically excited; cause it to contract, extend, or stretch; and provide elasticity.
- Skeletal muscles are attached to bones by tendons.

FUNCTIONS OF THE BONES

- Bones provide shape to the body.
- The skeleton provides a rigid framework that supports the internal organs and the skin.
- The skeleton protects the internal organs of the body.
- The skeleton provides attachments for tendons and ligaments and contributes to movement of the body.
- The red bone marrow in the spongy bones forms red blood cells, white blood cells, and platelets.
- The bones store and release minerals, such as calcium and phosphorus.
- The blood and lymph vessels in the canals transport nutrients to the bone cells and remove wastes.
- Bone is maintained by remodeling: existing bone is resorbed into the body and new bone is built by osteoblasts to replace it.

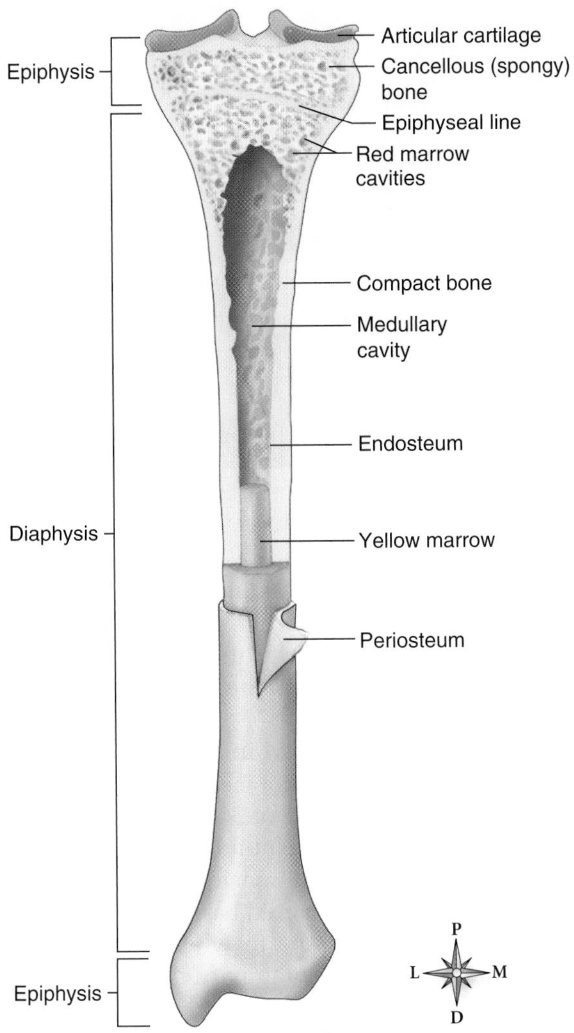

Fig. 31.2 Long bone. Frontal section (partial) of a tibia. (From Patton KT, Thibodeau GA: *The human body in health and disease*, ed 7, St. Louis, 2018, Elsevier.)

FUNCTIONS OF THE MUSCLES

- Contraction of skeletal muscles is produced by synchronized contraction of many muscle fibers.
- Skeletal muscles contract, thereby providing movement and joint stability, maintaining posture, and producing body heat.
- By shortening and stretching, opposing muscle groups provide movement of the joints.

AGING-RELATED CHANGES IN THE MUSCULOSKELETAL SYSTEM

- **Ossification**, or replacement of cartilage by more solid bony tissue, is not completed throughout the body until age 20 to 25 years.
- Bone density decreases in older adults because of the resorption of minerals.
- The loss of bone mass, or osteoporosis, occurs with aging and is more severe in women.
- The bones of older adults are brittle and less compact; thus they break easily.
- The bones of older adults do not heal readily after a fracture because the physiologic exchange of minerals decreases with advancing age, making the process of repair much slower.
- Thinning of the intervertebral cartilage and collapse of the vertebra result in kyphosis (dowager's hump). This is partially responsible for the decrease in height in older adults.
- Joint cartilage thins and erodes from years of use and results in stiffness and **crepitation** (a grating sound) of the joints.
- Joint motion may decrease, limiting mobility; swelling may occur.
- Ligaments become calcified and lose their elasticity.
- Older adults have a decrease in muscle mass; cells decrease in number, and the muscles atrophy. Consequently, older adults have less strength and endurance than younger people.
- Tendons shrink and become sclerotic, slowing muscle movement.
- Muscle cramping, especially at night, increases because of impaired circulation and accumulation of metabolic wastes.

MUSCULOSKELETAL DISORDERS

CAUSES

Disease, trauma, malnutrition, and aging all contribute to musculoskeletal problems. Trauma may cause bruising, strain, sprain, or fracture. Poor nutrition may deprive the body of sufficient calcium and phosphorus to build strong bones. Inadequate protein intake can cause muscle wasting. Malignant tumors place a large nutritional demand on the body, and nutritional imbalances that cause muscle wasting may occur. Tumor may invade bone as either a primary or a metastatic cancer. The decrease in estrogen production after menopause in women is believed to be a contributing factor to the occurrence of osteoporosis.

PREVENTION

Preservation of motion and mobility are important to prevent long-term **orthopedic** (refers to the function and structure of the musculoskeletal system) disability. Weight-bearing exercise throughout life is needed to maintain bone mass and can decrease the incidence of osteoporosis and increase muscle strength, mass, agility, balance, and coordination, thereby preventing falls and consequent fractures. A *Healthy People 2030* objective is to reduce hospitalizations related to osteoporosis-related hip fractures.

Complementary and Alternative Therapies

Benefits of Tai Ji Quan

Research in older community-dwelling adults has shown that tai ji quan balance training is beneficial in reducing falls (Li et al., 2018).

Lifting and moving objects correctly using large muscle groups helps prevent muscle strain and sprains. Seat belt use in an automobile reduces the incidence of trauma to bone and muscle during accidents. Wearing bicycle, motorcycle, and other sports helmets reduces the incidence of skull fractures. Consuming recommended amounts of calcium throughout the life span, obtaining sufficient vitamin D from sunshine or supplements, and maintaining adequate protein intake all help build healthy bone and muscle (Starkebaum, 2018). Refraining from using steroids on a long-term basis helps prevent osteoporosis and fractures.

Nutrition Considerations

Nutrition for Bone Growth and Density

Adequate amounts of calcium and phosphorus are essential for bone growth and density. Although green vegetables are a source of calcium, that calcium is not readily absorbed. Dairy products such as cheese, yogurt, and milk are better choices. Nondairy sources of calcium include canned sardines, salmon, tofu, figs, and dried apricots. Magnesium and vitamin K are required for healthy bones as well. These are provided by a healthy diet containing meat and green vegetables, such as spinach.

Health Promotion

Smoking and Musculoskeletal Health

Smoking has a significant effect on the bones and joints; smoking:

- Increases the risk of developing osteoporosis
- Increases the risk of a hip fracture with advancing age
- Increases the risk of developing exercise-related injuries
- Has a detrimental effect on fracture and wound healing
- Has a detrimental effect on athletic performance
- Is associated with low back pain and rheumatoid arthritis

Think Critically

What could you do now to promote healthy bones during your later years?

Diagnostic Tests and Procedures

Laboratory blood tests are performed on the minerals needed for bone growth (calcium and phosphorus), to detect bone disorders such as bone metastasis (alkaline phosphatase), detect muscle damage (creatine phosphokinase [CPK]), detect gout (uric acid), or diagnose rheumatoid arthritis or other connective tissue diseases (Table 31.2). Specific diagnostic tests of the musculoskeletal system are listed in Table 31.3.

Clinical Cues

Diagnostic tests for musculoskeletal disorders (and other disorders) often use contrast media or radiation. Before diagnostic testing, all patients should be assessed for allergies, and women of childbearing age may need a pregnancy test.

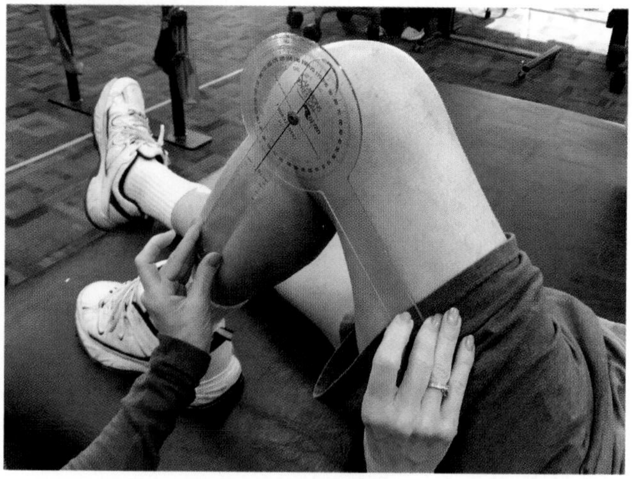

Fig. 31.3 Measurement of joint motion with a goniometer.

Range-of-motion (ROM) testing involves both active and passive maneuvers. In active testing, the part being measured must be moved by the patient. In passive testing, the evaluator moves the body part while the patient is relaxed.

The measurement of ROM in a joint is called *goniometry* (Fig. 31.3). One system of measurement commonly used is based on a full circle of 360 degrees. Each joint is evaluated in terms of the number of degrees it can be moved from the 0-degree position.

Muscle strength is measured based on the ability of a muscle to move the part to which it is attached, working against the force of gravity. A grading system is used, ranging from grade 5 (normal strength) to grade 0 (complete paralysis).

Other techniques used to evaluate musculoskeletal function include inspection, palpation, and tests for stability of a joint under stress.

Think Critically

How would you explain the difference between a bone scan and a dual-energy x-ray absorptiometry (DEXA) scan to a patient considering the purpose of each test and the difference in the procedures?

NURSING MANAGEMENT

DATA COLLECTION

History Taking

When reviewing the patient's past history, keep in mind the significance of disorders that primarily affect other systems but secondarily affect the bones and muscles. For example, sickle cell disease and hemophilia can cause bleeding into the joints and muscles, and psoriasis is sometimes the first sign of psoriatic arthritis, which is an inflammatory condition that affects the spine and the peripheral joints. Nutritional deficiencies can affect the mineral composition of bone and muscle, making them more susceptible to trauma and loss of function.

Table 31.2 Laboratory Blood Tests for Musculoskeletal Disorders

TEST	NORMAL VALUE	ABNORMAL SIGNIFICANCE
Calcium (total)	9.0–10.5 mg/dL 2.25–2.62 mmol/L	Elevated in extended immobilization and metastatic bone disease.
Phosphate (phosphorus)	3.0–4.5 mg/dL 1.0–1.5 mmol/L	Elevated when calcium level is high.
Alkaline phosphatase (ALP)	30–120 unit/L	Elevation may indicate Paget disease or bone metastasis.
Creatine kinase (CK) or creatine phosphokinase (CPK)	Male: 55–170 unit/L Female: 30–135 unit/L	Elevated levels of CPK isoenzymes may indicate muscle damage.
Myoglobin	<90 mcg/L	Elevation indicates muscle damage such as from trauma.
Uric acid	Male: 4.0–8.5 mg/dL 0.24–0.51 mmol/L Female: 2.7–7.3 mg/dL 0.16–0.43 mmol/L	Elevation indicates presence of gout.
Rheumatoid factor (RF)	Negative <60 unit/mL by nephelometric testing	>60 unit/mL may indicate rheumatoid arthritis or another autoimmune disease.
Antinuclear antibodies (ANA)	Negative at 1:40 dilution	Elevation may indicate rheumatoid arthritis or other autoimmune disease.

Table 31.3 Diagnostic Tests and Procedures for Musculoskeletal Disorders

TEST	PURPOSE	DESCRIPTION	NURSING IMPLICATIONS
X-ray films of the bones or joints	To detect fracture, avulsion, joint damage	Part to be x-rayed is positioned by technician, and x-ray films are taken.	Assess for pregnancy before testing.
Computed tomography (CT)	To detect musculoskeletal problems, especially of the spine and skull	The patient is placed on a hard table, and the part to be studied is positioned inside the machine; the procedure takes 10–15 min. Contrast material may be used. There is a clicking sound as the machine rotates to take the next view. A computer enhances the radiographic findings.	Patient must lie very still. Assess for allergies to contrast media.
Magnetic resonance imaging (MRI)	To diagnose musculoskeletal disorders	Magnetic fields and radio waves are used to visualize tissue densities by the density of hydrogen ions. Computer enhancement depicts normal and abnormal tissue.	There must be no metal on the body and no metal implants because of the strong magnetic fields used. The patient must lie still for 15–60 min.
Dual-energy x-ray absorptiometry (DEXA)	To measure bone density of spine, hip, femur, or forearm To monitor changes in bone density and to diagnose metabolic bone disease	Uses minimal radiation exposure. Patient will lie supine on the imaging table with the legs supported. The scintillator camera is passed over the patient and projected onto a computer screen.	Height is measured. All metallic objects must be removed. Test takes about 30 min.
Bone scan	To detect tumor, metastatic growths, bone injury, or degenerative bone disease	An IV injection or oral dose of a radioisotope is given, and after a specified time for the substance to be taken up by the bone, the area is scanned by scintillation camera.	Check for allergies and pregnancy. Patient will be asked to lie quietly for 30–60 min during the scanning. All metal must be removed from the area to be scanned. Assure patient that they will not be "radioactive." The isotope is eliminated from the body in 6–24 h.

Continued

Table 31.3 Diagnostic Tests and Procedures for Musculoskeletal Disorders—cont'd

TEST	PURPOSE	DESCRIPTION	NURSING IMPLICATIONS
Gallium/thallium scans	To detect bone problems, especially tumor invasion	The radioisotope gallium citrate (GA-70) or thallium-201 is administered 1–2 days before the scan.	The procedure takes 30–60 min, during which lying still is required; sedation may be given.
Arthrography (arthrogram)	To provide radiographic pictures of a joint showing the outline of the joint cavity and soft tissue structures not visible on routine x-ray films	Fluid may be aspirated from the joint space. A contrast agent, air, or both are aseptically injected into the joint after the area is anesthetized. The joint is manipulated to disperse the contrast agent. X-ray films are taken with the joint held in various positions. (May also use CT or MRI)	Informed consent is often required. There will be feelings of pressure and some discomfort. Administer an analgesic after the procedure, if needed. Observe for swelling; apply ice as ordered. Advise patient that crackling sounds may be heard or felt in the joint after the test and usually disappear in 1–2 days. Instruct patient to report any increasing pain or swelling to the health care provider.
Arthroscopy	To inspect the interior aspect of a joint, usually a knee, with a fiberoptic endoscope to diagnose problems of the patella, meniscus, and synovium; also used to evaluate the progress of arthritis or effectiveness of treatment	After injection of local anesthesia, an incision is made, and the arthroscope is introduced into the interior of the joint; instruments for tissue biopsy or surgical procedure may be passed through the arthroscope.	A sedative may be administered. Ambulation is encouraged when patient recovers from sedation but without overuse or strain of the joint for a few days. Observe for bleeding or swelling; ice packs may be used in the immediate postprocedure period. Assess for swelling, circulation, and sensation periodically to detect any complications.
Arthrocentesis	To extract synovial fluid for analysis or to reduce swelling	A needle is inserted into the joint space, and synovial fluid is aspirated. Depending on the joint, ultrasound or fluoroscopy guidance may be used. Corticosteroid may be injected after aspiration of fluid. The joint may be immobilized afterward. Ice packs are applied to relieve pain and reduce swelling.	Patient should avoid overuse of the joint until pain and swelling have subsided. Administer ordered analgesics PRN.
Culture of synovial fluid	To determine organism responsible for infection	Synovial fluid is aspirated and sent for culture and sensitivity to determine appropriate antibiotic for therapy. Results take 48–72 h to determine.	Have specimen of fluid transported to laboratory immediately in the appropriate container.
Biopsy	Bone: to detect tumor cells Muscle: to obtain tissue for cellular analysis	Under local anesthesia, a piece of bone or muscle is excised and sent for pathologic analysis.	Offer emotional support during the procedures. Afterward, medicate for discomfort as needed, apply ice packs to decrease swelling, observe for bleeding; perform circulation and sensation checks distal to the area biopsied.

Table 31.3 Diagnostic Tests and Procedures for Musculoskeletal Disorders—cont'd

TEST	PURPOSE	DESCRIPTION	NURSING IMPLICATIONS
Electromyelography (EMG)	To detect abnormal nerve transmission to the muscle and abnormal muscle function; helps determine rehabilitation progress	Needle electrodes are inserted in affected muscles, and, as the muscles are stimulated, the electrical impulses generated by the muscle contractions are amplified and displayed on an oscilloscope; tracings also are made on graph paper. The test usually takes about 1 h.	Obtain a signed consent form. Caffeine-containing drinks and smoking are restricted 3 h before the test. Withhold muscle relaxants, anticholinergics, and cholinergic drugs before the test as ordered. There may be slight discomfort when the electrodes are inserted; explain that they will be asked to relax and contract their muscles.

IV, Intravenous; *PRN,* as needed.

Family history may be significant because some bone and muscle disorders are either inherited or have a familial tendency. Muscular dystrophies, several motor neuron diseases, and metabolic diseases of muscle are all hereditary (Muscular Dystrophy Association, 2018).

Physical Assessment

Observe the patient for signs of joint pain, such as limping, poor posture, awkward gait, difficulty in arising or walking, and wincing on movement. Watch the patient during performance of activities of daily living (ADLs), noting problems of movement, and changes in facial expression to pick up signs of problems. If the patient is admitted with a fracture, obtain a history of the precipitating event so that an assessment can be made of other areas that may have been injured. Sometimes it is necessary to consult family members or someone who lives with the patient about the patient's true ability to perform the ADLs. **A self-care deficit is one of the primary issues for patients who have a problem with mobility.**

◆ NURSING DIAGNOSIS AND PLANNING

Caring for immobile patients requires careful planning. Making beds for bed-confined orthopedic patients is best done by two people. Bathing and grooming are more time consuming when the patient has an immobilized limb or has some other orthopedic device. **Planning for toileting needs at regular intervals is important for the well-being of a patient who is unable to get out of bed unassisted.** Neglecting such needs may cause incontinence and the time-consuming task

Focused Assessment

Data Collection for the Musculoskeletal System

- What do you see as your current problem?
- When is the pain the worst? What seems to bring it on? What relieves it?
- Do you have any pain in your wrists, elbows, knees, hips, or feet?
- Have you noticed any changes of sensation in your hands, feet, or elsewhere?
- Do you have any joints that are stiff, swollen, or painful?
- Do you have any restriction of movement in any joint?
- Do you have trouble sleeping because of muscle or joint pain?
- Do you have any joint deformity? Bunion? Hammer toe? Deformed knuckle?
- Have you ever had an injury to a bone?
- Have you ever experienced a severe muscle strain or muscle problem?
- Is there a history of osteoporosis or arthritis in your family?
- Do you have diabetes, sickle cell disease, psoriasis, systemic lupus erythematosus, or any other chronic metabolic disease?
- Are you taking any steroid medications regularly?
- Do you find that your fatigue level has increased?
- Do you have any problems with bathing, dressing, grooming, toileting, eating, ambulation, or going on social outings?
- Can you easily arise from a seated position?
- Do you have difficulty opening containers?
- What do you eat or drink that contains calcium? How much of it do you eat or drink?
- What is your daily (weekly) sunshine exposure? Do you take a vitamin D supplement?
- Do you use any alternative therapies or any other type of self-care measures? Are those self-care measures helping?
- Tell me about your work; do you lift, pull, or push? Are you sitting for prolonged periods or doing repetitive motions?
- Does your home have stairs or other features that are causing problems for you?
- Are you able to independently do home maintenance tasks (e.g., mow the lawn)?
- What type of physical activities or exercise do you routinely do (e.g., sports, gardening)? How often do you participate in these activities?
- Have you had surgery on any of your joints, bones, or muscles?

Focused Assessment

Physical Assessment of the Musculoskeletal System

Note the following points:

- *Posture:* Is there evidence of **kyphosis**, such as a rounded upper back, also called a *dowager's hump*? Are the knuckles swollen or deformed, indicating arthritis?
- *Gait:* Is it steady and even? Awkward?
- *Balance:* Is the patient able to sit, stand, and walk with a good center of balance?
- *Mobility:* Is any supportive device being used, such as a cane, brace, splint, or elastic bandage?
- *Range of motion:* Is the patient able to move the neck, shoulders, arms, and legs with full range of motion?
- *Strength:* Are grips in hands and push-pull in arms equal bilaterally? Is straight-leg raising against resistance equal bilaterally?
- *Spine:* Is there any tenderness of the vertebrae on palpation?
- *Appearance of joints:* Is there any redness, deformity, or loss of motion in elbows, hands, knees, ankles, and feet?
- *Skeletal muscle appearance in arms and legs:* Is there any degree of atrophy?
- *Ability to perform ADLs:* Is the patient independent or do they need assistance to dress, bathe, toilet, or eat?

Older Adult Care Points

Approximately 30% to 40% of inpatient safety incidents are related to falls, and older adults are particularly vulnerable because of changes related to aging, such as decreased strength, unsteady balance, loss of endurance, slow reflexes, gait disturbances and increased postural sway, and chronic diseases such as arthritis. Conduct a fall risk assessment (see Chapter 9, Box 9.4) and initiate fall precautions (Centers for Disease Control and Prevention, 2017).

Think Critically

After a hip replacement, can you trust the statement made by the patient, "I can shop, cook, clean, and do everything I need to do by myself"? If you cannot trust this statement, why not? How would you gather data about an older adult patient's ability to perform self-care activities at home before they are discharged?

of changing the bed and cleaning up the patient; incontinence is also demoralizing for the patient and increases the risk of tissue breakdown from the moisture and irritation of urine or feces. Repositioning the patient at 2-hour intervals is included in the daily work plan to prevent pressure ulcers.

Common problem statements and example outcomes and interventions for patients with musculoskeletal problems are presented in Table 31.4. Several other secondary problem statements may be appropriate for patients who are immobile. Constipation, altered tissue integrity, social isolation, potential for injury, and other

Box 31.1 Physiologic Consequences of Immobility

- *Cardiovascular system:* Decreased cardiac output with reduced force of cardiac contraction results from a lack of physical activity. Immobility causing decreased use of leg muscles leads to venous stasis and potential formation of blood clots.
- *Respiratory system:* Reduced lung expansion and consequent reduced gas exchange with potential for atelectasis and pooling of secretions occurs with immobility. Reduced cough effort along with pooled secretions predisposes to stasis pneumonia.
- *Musculoskeletal system:* Prolonged immobility leads to reduced muscle mass and atrophy. Demineralization of bones occurs with lack of weight bearing; osteoporosis may occur.
- *Integumentary system:* Skin breakdown may occur from a reduced flow of oxygenated blood from pressure on the skin resulting from immobility. Combined with lack of appetite from immobility and poor nutritional status, pressure ulcers may develop.
- *Gastrointestinal system:* Slowing of peristalsis and decreased muscle strength occur with decreased physical activity. Decreased appetite and an inability to assume an upright position for defecation also contribute to the constipation that can occur with immobility.
- *Urinary system:* Calcium from bone increases in the blood from immobility, bladder tone decreases, and more time in a supine position from immobility leads to urinary stasis. Infection, renal calculi, and urinary tract infection may occur.
- *Psychological effects:* Feelings of helplessness or hopelessness, boredom, depression, and disturbed body image may be accompanied by anger or anxiety and loss of self-esteem during extended periods of immobility. Social isolation may also occur.

problems caused by immobility may occur (Box 31.1; see also Chapter 9).

Interventions and outcomes are designed in collaboration with the patient and other members of the health care team. **The physical therapist and occupational therapist are especially important and act as resources for both you and the patient.**

◆ IMPLEMENTATION

Positioning

Patients with musculoskeletal problems must change their body position frequently and get up in a chair to prevent pressure ulcers, circulatory stasis, and respiratory and urinary complications. **It also is necessary to change joint positions to prevent joint deformity.**

When repositioning the patient, watch for early signs of muscle tightness and resistance to joint motion. Observe during routine ROM exercises; if any tightness or resistance to joint motion is noticed, position the joint extended so that muscles are stretched to normal limit to prevent the development of contractures.

Table 31.4 Common Problem Statements, Expected Outcomes, and Interventions for Patients With Musculoskeletal System Disorders

PATIENT PROBLEM	GOALS/EXPECTED OUTCOMES	NURSING INTERVENTIONS
Altered physical mobility due to immobilization, loss of limb, stiffness, pain, weakness, or inability to bear weight.	ROM of unaffected joints will be maintained. No signs of joint contractures will be present at discharge.	Active ROM at least tid for all unaffected joints while on bed rest. Passive ROM on affected joints as ordered. Ensure that joints are in correct alignment when at rest and after turning. Maintain body in proper alignment. Assess immobilizer for correct fit and positioning every shift; assess for signs of complications related to pressure or pins. Supervise exercise to prepare muscles for ambulation. Instruct in use of ambulatory devices as appropriate; supervise practice; assess for proper "fit" of device. Encourage use of prosthesis for ambulation; assist with practice. Assess for signs of complications in stump and assess that prosthesis is attached correctly. Maintain abduction pillow between legs if one is ordered.
Altered activity tolerance due to stiffness, pain, limited mobility, fatigue.	Patient will meet activity goals with increasing success and minimal discomfort.	Determine factors that increase fatigue. Space activities with rest periods throughout the day. Assist to set goals for slow, steady increase in exercise and activity during periods of remission of arthritis symptoms. Perform exercises after heat treatments to decrease discomfort; apply in safe manner. Apply cold as needed after exercise for discomfort. Administer medications to decrease inflammation and pain, allowing greater level of activity. Advise of assistive devices that might make ADLs easier and help conserve energy. Assist in obtaining needed devices. Supervise practice with assistive device.
Pain due to injury, surgery, or joint disorder.	Pain will be controlled as evidenced by patient verbalization of pain level 4/10 or less.	Assess for factors contributing to pain level, such as increased pressure, infection, positioning, or swelling. Assess pain in systematic, objective manner and track course of pain and effectiveness of pain control (see Chapter 7). Instruct in relaxation, distraction, and imagery techniques to decrease pain. Instruct in use of various heat and cold treatments to decrease pain. Administer analgesic, antiinflammatory, and steroid medications, as ordered, to decrease pain. Instruct in use and side effects of each drug. Assist to an anatomically correct position to enhance circulation and alignment. Advise of alternative methods of pain control, such as transcutaneous electrical nerve stimulation (TENS). Monitor patient-controlled analgesia (PCA) use for effectiveness of pain control.
Potential for infection due to trauma or surgical incision.	No signs of infection will be present, as evidenced by normal white blood cell (WBC) count and normal temperature; wounds will be kept clean and dry.	Follow Standard Precautions and strict contact precautions if indicated when performing patient care and use strict aseptic technique for wound or pin care. Assess for signs of infection every shift; assess wound for redness, swelling, and tenderness. Administer prophylactic antibiotics as prescribed. Assess temperature trends and trend of WBC values for signs of infection. Assess patient for subjective signs of malaise. Sniff around cast for signs of foul odor indicating infection.
Potential for altered tissue perfusion due to swelling and pressure.	Patient will have no evidence of seriously decreased circulation distal to site of trauma. No evidence of nerve compression from swelling will be present.	Perform neurovascular assessment hourly for 8 h, then q2h for 48 h. Question patient regarding sensation distal to site of trauma or surgery. Apply cold to area of injury or surgery, as ordered, to reduce swelling; elevate extremity to slightly above heart level. Immediately report signs of compartment syndrome (i.e., severe, unrelenting pain; numbness) to health care provider and obtain order for measures to relieve pressure.

Continued

Table 31.4 Common Problem Statements, Expected Outcomes, and Interventions for Patients With Musculoskeletal System Disorders—cont'd

PATIENT PROBLEM	GOALS/EXPECTED OUTCOMES	NURSING INTERVENTIONS
Altered self-care ability due to immobilization.	Patient will receive assistance for all ADLs, as needed.	Assess degree of inability to perform various self-care activities. Formulate plan to assist patient with ADLs. Answer calls for assistance with toileting promptly; do not leave on bedpan longer than necessary. Open food containers and cut food as needed for self-feeding with one hand. Do not serve extremely hot liquids to patients who have difficulty with coordination or with holding drinking containers or to immobilized patients. Provide assistive devices and help patient to be as self-sufficient as possible without incurring undue fatigue when performing ADLs. Caution patients about change in body's center of gravity when a limb is casted or amputated.
Altered body image due to change in appearance and/or loss of mobility or function.	Patient will begin adaptation to change in appearance or loss, as evidenced by verbalization of feelings of self-worth; maintenance of relationships with significant others; active interest in personal appearance; willingness to resume usual roles and participate in social activities; and making plans to adapt lifestyle to meet restrictions imposed by loss.	Assess degree of body image disturbance, noting verbal or nonverbal clues to negative response to changes. Assist to verbalize feelings about effect of loss on usual roles and lifestyle. Be present and supportive during initial dressing changes on stump after amputation. Assist patient to identify strengths and abilities and positive coping mechanisms. Clarify misconceptions about limitations on mobility and activity. Promote activities that require patient to confront the body changes that have occurred, such as bathing, ADLs, or dressing changes. Demonstrate acceptance of patient and encourage significant others to do the same with touch and affection. Encourage as much independence as possible; allow to do things for self. Assist patient to explore viable options for changes in lifestyle and career. Refer for vocational retraining if needed. Encourage maximum participation in planning of care and self-care to provide a sense of control over life. Encourage participation in social activities and in a support group. Refer for psychological counseling if adaptation does not occur within 6 mo and patient is depressed or in denial.
Decreased ability for home maintenance due to immobility or limited self-care ability.	Patient will obtain needed assistance with home maintenance.	Assess degree of self-sufficiency and ability to perform ADLs before discharge. Contact social worker for coordination of home care if needed. Obtain bathing and homemaker assistance as needed. Assess continued need for in-home services weekly. Instruct on home adaptations that could aid in efforts at self-care, such as grab bars in bathroom, alterations in counter spaces for food preparation, transportation options for grocery shopping and appointments, or assistive devices for self-feeding and grooming. Assess degree of assistance family members can provide for patient in home environment. Determine safety of home environment for patient.
Potential for disuse syndrome due to immobility or trauma.	Patient will not suffer permanent joint deformity or muscle atrophy.	Position joints as ordered; keep rest of body in correct alignment. Begin exercise of affected joint as soon as provider orders. Encourage active exercise of unaffected joints tid. Perform passive ROM as ordered tid. Use heat and cold treatments before and after exercising stiff or deformed joints. Assess joints for contractures and muscles for atrophy q24h. Encourage participation in ADLs to exercise joints.

ADLs, Activities of daily living; *ROM,* range of motion; *tid,* three times a day.

Patients with flaccid paralysis are not necessarily positioned in the same way as those with spastic paralysis. For example, foot splints are appropriate for proper positioning of the feet to prevent foot drop in a patient with flaccid paralysis. In contrast, putting the soles of the feet of a patient with spastic paralysis in contact with foot splints could trigger muscle contraction and aggravate the spasticity. Use a bed cradle or pillows positioned at the foot of the bed to relieve pressure of the bedclothes to help prevent foot drop in these patients.

Preventing ankylosis. Ankylosis is the result of injury or disease in which the tissues of the joint are replaced by a bony overgrowth that completely obliterates the joint. Proper positioning and movement of the joint passively can help prevent this. Sometimes it is extremely difficult to prevent this process (as, for example, in some types of arthritis). In these cases the joint may be braced in the position that will be most useful to the patient, even though there is no motion in the joint.

Lifting and turning the patient. When working with orthopedic patients, all movements must be *gentle* and *firm*. When moving or turning the patient, obtain sufficient help from adequately trained personnel. Each person involved, including the patient, should understand exactly what is to happen and how the move will be accomplished. If the patient can help without damaging the diseased joint or limb, encourage them to do so. If they are unable to help, explain the procedure and instruct them to relax completely. Many times the patient is afraid that moving and turning will cause pain. Explaining the long-term benefits, such as preserving skin integrity and decreasing respiratory problems, will increase cooperation.

Exercise

ROM exercises, both passive and active, are planned and carried out as soon as feasible after decreased mobility occurs as a result of disease, injury, or surgery. The exercises are done to maintain connective tissue within the joint and thereby ensure that every joint retains its function and mobility. **ROM exercises should be done three or four times a day.** Other kinds of exercises are planned according to each patient's needs and the amount of motion allowed by the health care provider. **Isometric exercises** involve generating tension between two opposing sets of muscles—for example, trying to flex the lower arm while using the opposite hand to try to extend it.

Safety Alert

Caution With Isometric Exercises

Isometric exercise may be contraindicated in patients with hypertension, increased intracranial pressure, or congestive heart failure because isometric exercise causes a significant increase in blood pressure and heart rate.

Gradual mobilization. Progressive mobilization involves assessing the patient's ability to move their limbs, turn in bed, transfer from bed to chair and back again, and stand and walk. These measurable signs of independent movement represent various stages to which the patient can gradually progress. According to The Joint Commission's National Patient Safety Goals, it is a nursing responsibility to recognize that these patients are at risk for falls while they are learning to regain mobility.

Clinical Cues

The health care provider's orders should include level of activity (i.e., bed rest, out of bed to chair, physical therapy); however, if this order is not included—or if your assessment finds that the patient either cannot accomplish the orders or has already surpassed the ordered level of activity—notify the provider so that a reevaluation of the patient's abilities and new orders occur.

Setting goals for progressive mobilization must consider the pathologic condition causing immobility, any contraindications to movement of a body part, and the ability of the patient to understand and take part in carrying out the rehabilitation activities. In some cases, passive exercises and positioning may be necessary until the patient is able to carry out exercises and positioning on their own. If the patient is to be cared for by family members once back at home, it is essential that they be included in planning and setting goals of intervention to prevent disability and promote mobilization.

Health Promotion

Gentle Stretch for Upper Back

Patients who are kyphotic (or those who hunch over their books while studying!) can develop discomfort and tension in the upper midback. Encourage periodic and conscientious attempts to sit upright with the shoulders pulled back. Another exercise is to stand in a corner, place palms on the opposing walls or use an open door frame and gently lean into the corner or the opening. This may feel uncomfortable at first, so encourage the patient to go slowly.

Patients suffering from intense joint pain as a result of rheumatoid arthritis will need proper timing of exercises to follow administration of analgesic and antiinflammatory drugs. If possible, the schedule for drug administration should be adjusted so that the patient receives their first dose of medication in the morning 30 to 60 minutes *before* beginning exercises.

Sometimes after a total knee replacement, the surgeon will order attachment of an apparatus to the affected limb that provides continuous passive motion (CPM) of the joint within set limits. The apparatus is driven by a motor and requires no effort on your part or on the part of the patient to move the limb (Fig. 31.4). It is used intermittently throughout the day. When this

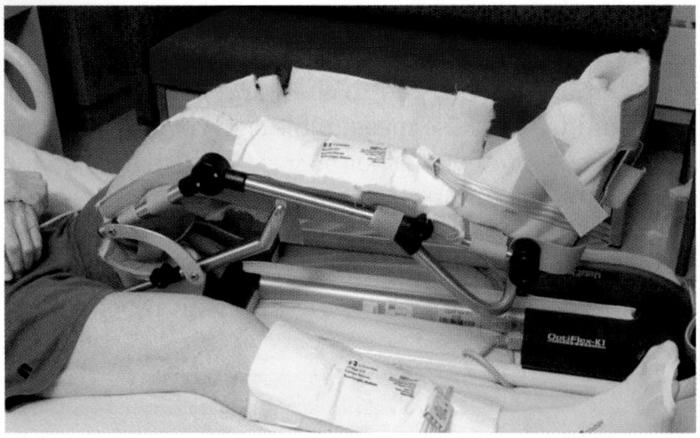

Fig. 31.4 A continuous passive motion machine encourages joint mobility.

type of apparatus is used, the nursing care plan should include specific instructions regarding its proper application and setting and regular assessment of adequacy of pain relief. Pain is helped by the continuous circulation of ice water through a pad placed on the knee or affected joint. The cold helps reduce swelling, inflammation, and pain.

Exercises to recondition muscles for ambulation after injury or immobilization include quadriceps setting and gluteal setting.

Teaching Ambulation With Assistive Devices

For convalescent patients or those who may always need support while walking, crutches can mean the difference between freedom to move about and confinement to one location or a wheelchair. Before attempting to walk with crutches, the patient should be instructed in their use and manipulation to ambulate safely and effectively.

Patient Teaching

Quadriceps and Gluteal Muscle Exercises

QUADRICEPS SETTING

- Instruct the patient to straighten the leg out while lying down and to tense the leg muscles and straighten the knee, while raising the heel slightly.
- The contraction is held for a count of five and released for a count of five.
- The exercise is done on each leg 10 to 15 times hourly while the patient is awake.
- Commercial breaks on television are a good reminder to do this.

GLUTEAL SETTING

- Instruct the patient to contract the buttocks and pinch them together for a count of four, then relax for a count of five.
- Repeat 10 to 15 times hourly.

Think Critically

You are working in a long-term care facility. Your patient is in a coma because of a head injury that occurred 3 months ago; her husband visits every day. How could the husband participate to prevent contractures?

The type of crutch to be used will depend on the extent of disability or paralysis and the patient's ability to bear weight and maintain balance. If the crutches are too short or too long, patients will have problems with moving and shifting their weight. When walking, the patient should straighten the elbow and the wrist during weight bearing. The muscles of the arms, shoulders, back,

Patient Teaching

Crutch Gaits

GAIT	SEQUENCE	PATTERN
Four-point gait	Advance left crutch. Advance right foot. Advance right crutch. Advance left foot. Advantages: most stable crutch gait. Requirements: partial weight bearing on both legs.	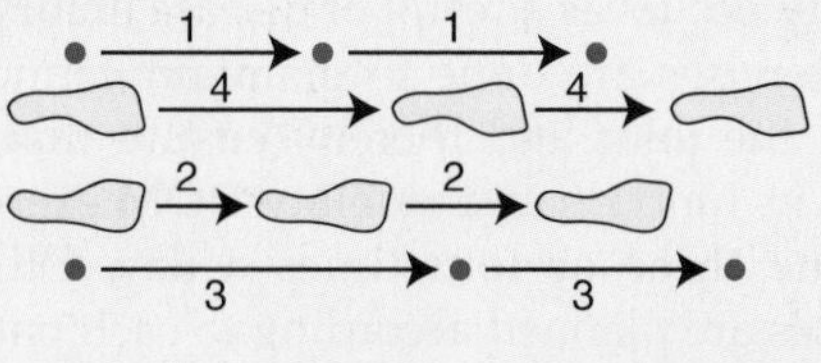
Three-point gait	Advance both crutches forward with the affected leg and shift weight to crutches. Advance unaffected leg and shift weight onto it. Advantages: allows the affected leg to be partially or completely free of weight bearing. Requirements: full weight bearing on one leg, balance, and upper body strength.	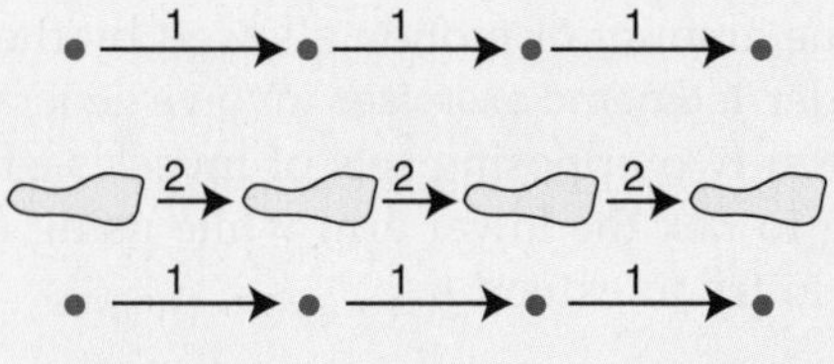
Two-point gait	Advance left crutch and right foot. Advance right crutch and left foot. Advantages: faster version of the four-point gait, more normal walking pattern (arms and legs moving in opposition). Requirements: partial weight bearing on both legs, balance.	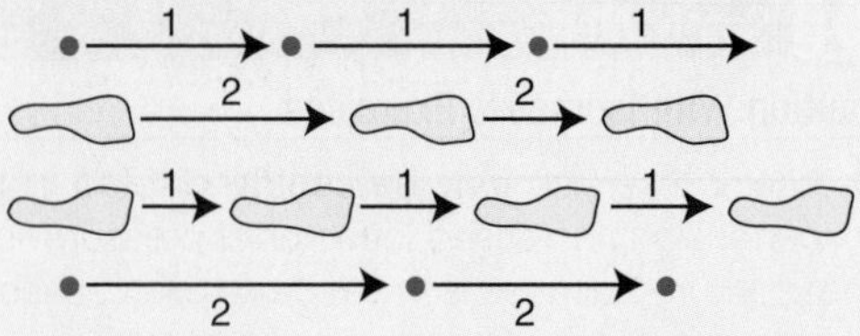

and chest are all used in the manipulation of crutches. Therefore many physical therapists start the patient on special exercises to strengthen these muscles several weeks before the patient begins to use the crutches.

Safety Alert

Crutch Safety

Height is considered when fitting crutches to the patient. When in the standing position with axillary crutches, the axillary bar should be two fingerbreadths below the axilla. The elbow should be flexed at a 30-degree angle when the palms of the hands rest on the hand grip. It is important that the patient not rest their body at the axilla on the top of the crutch; body weight should be borne by the arms on the hand rests of the crutches. If crutches are too long, pressure on the axilla will occur and can cause nerve damage.

To measure for crutches, the patient stands wearing shoes and positions the crutch tips at a point 4 to 6 inches (10 to 15 cm) to the side and 4 to 6 inches (10 to 15 cm) in front of the feet. Although the physical therapist supervises the preparation and instruction of patients before they start to use crutches and then evaluates their ability to use them correctly, you are sometimes responsible for assisting a patient with crutch walking while they are in the hospital.

When teaching a patient to ambulate with a cane, be certain that the cane has an intact rubber tip. The cane is the right length if the hand grip is at hip level and the elbow is bent at a 30-degree angle when weight is placed on the cane. **It should be used on the good side unless the health care provider orders otherwise.** The tip of the cane should be placed 6 to 10 inches (15 to 25 cm) to the side and 6 inches (15 cm) in front of the near foot when walking. The patient should look straight ahead, rather than down, when ambulating. **The cane is advanced at the same time as the affected leg.** "Go up the stairs with your stronger leg first, then your weaker leg, then the cane. If you are going down the stairs, start with your cane, then your weaker leg, then your strong leg" (Medline Plus, 2017).

Walker height is correct when the person's elbow is bent at a 15- to 30-degree angle while standing upright and grasping the hand grips. The walker is lifted or rolled on its wheels slightly in front of the patient while leaning the body slightly forward. A step or two is taken into the walker, and then it is lifted and placed in front of the person again.

Older Adult Care Points

Many older adults are hospitalized with injuries they sustain from inability to maneuver crutches, a cane, or a walker. It is essential that older adults be taught proper methods of using assistive devices and that they receive supervised practice before they are discharged.

Psychosocial Care

Unfortunately, many orthopedic conditions require prolonged periods of confinement to bed or, at best, immobilization of a part of the body and restricted physical activities. This leads to frustration and a feeling of hopelessness and despair on the part of the patient. When the patient is young and unaccustomed to depending on others for personal care, a reaction of anger and

Patient Teaching

Special Maneuvers on Crutches

MANEUVER	SEQUENCE
Walking up stairs	Stand at the foot of the stairs with weight on the good leg and crutches. Put weight on the crutch handles and then lift the good leg onto the first step of the stairs. Put weight on the good leg and lift the injured leg and crutches onto that step. Repeat for each step.
Walking down stairs	Stand at the top of the stairs with weight on the good leg and crutches. Shift weight completely onto the good leg and put the crutches down on the next step. Put weight on the crutch handles and transfer the injured leg down to the step with the crutches. Bring the good leg down to that step. Repeat for each stair step.
Sitting down	Crutch-walk to the chair. Turn around slowly so that the back is to the chair and the backs of the legs touch the seat of the chair. Transfer both crutches to the side with the injured leg and grasp both hand grips with that one hand. As weight is supported on the crutches and the good leg, reach back with the free hand and grasp the arm of the chair. Lower slowly onto the chair seat, using the support of both the crutches and the chair. Sit back in the chair and elevate the leg. Keep the knee slightly flexed when elevated because too much extension can decrease the circulation. To get up, bring both crutches along the side of the injured leg and grasp the hand grip firmly. Make sure the crutch tips are firmly on the floor. Place the other hand on the arm of the chair and push up. After becoming upright, transfer one crutch to the other hand for walking.

bitterness may occur. If the patient is a wage earner or a member of the family on whom others are dependent, there is the additional burden of financial and role problems. If there has been an amputation or extensive scarring from an injury, the patient's self-image may suffer.

◆ EVALUATION

Determining the effectiveness of interventions to treat pain is based mainly on subjective information given by the patient, but also be alert to nuances of body language. Observation of the patient's ability to accomplish ADLs gives clues to improvement in mobility and activity tolerance.

Diagnostic test data from radiographs and laboratory reports are used to determine the effectiveness of treatments. For example, radiographs show whether fractures are healing, whereas laboratory reports help determine how well rheumatoid arthritis is controlled.

Common Problems Related to the Musculoskeletal System

Common problems specific to musculoskeletal disorders are those related to immobility, pain, and self-care deficit.

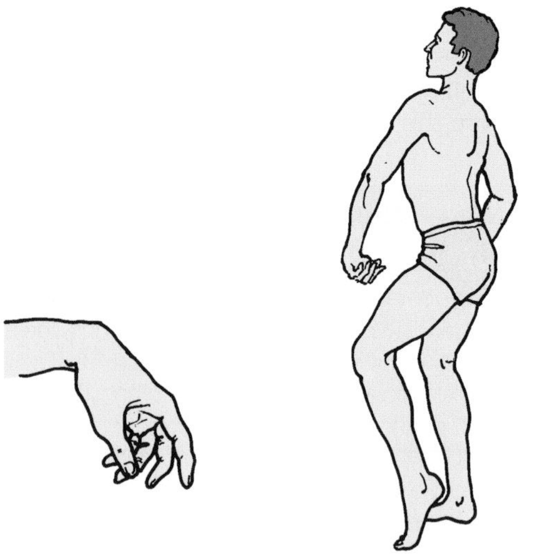

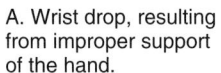

A. Wrist drop, resulting from improper support of the hand.

B. Flexion contracture of knee and hip force this patient to walk on tiptoe on the affected side. If both legs are involved, walking is impossible.

Fig. 31.5 Joint contractures.

Immobility. Many systemic responses and problems result from extended immobility (see Box 31.1). These problems are more common with neurologic injuries or disease that cause long-term immobility. For shorter periods of immobility that occur with sprains and strains, joint injury and replacement, fractures, back pain, or arthritis, the goals are quick ambulation and rehabilitation, with a return to an active lifestyle. Many interventions can prevent disability during the period of immobility.

Preventing Disability

The formation of **contractures** (shortening of skeletal muscle tissue causing deformity), loss of muscle tone, and fixation of joints can be prevented in most cases by consistent nursing intervention. The major components of the intervention are gradual mobilization, an exercise program, proper positioning, and instruction of the patient and family. **Within a matter of a few days, the structures of immobilized muscles and joints begin to undergo changes.** If no effort is made to prevent these changes, the patient will become permanently disabled. The pathologic changes most commonly associated with lack of motion include:

- Contractures
- Loss of muscle tone
- **Ankylosis** (permanent fixation of a joint)

Preventing contractures. Joint motion is the result of a shortening and stretching of opposing muscles. For example, when the flexor muscles of the leg contract and shorten, the opposing extensor muscles relax and lengthen. When skeletal muscles are not regularly stretched and contracted to their normal limits, they attempt to adapt themselves to this limited use by becoming shorter and less elastic. An "adaptive shortening," or **contracture,** begins to form within 3 to 7 days after immobilization of a body part, and the process usually is complete in 6 to 8 weeks. This means that planning and implementing nursing measures must begin immediately to prevent permanent and crippling disability. The most common contractures that occur in patients immobilized for long periods are foot drop, knee and hip flexion contractures, wrist drop, and contractures of the fingers and arms (Fig. 31.5).

Preventing loss of muscle tone. *Muscle tone* is defined as the readiness of the muscle to go to work—to contract and relax as needed. If a muscle is not regularly stimulated to action or if it is stretched beyond its normal limits for an extended time, it will lose its ability to contract and relax. For example, in foot drop, the calf muscles are shortened while the opposing flexor muscles are stretched. The result is loss of muscle tone and inability to produce motion. Performing ROM exercises helps prevent this (Fig. 31.6).

Pain. Pain occurs with most musculoskeletal disorders. Immobilization with slings, splints, and braces helps decrease pain by limiting movement of joints or muscles. Analgesics, muscle relaxants, heat, cold, topical pain-relieving substances, electrical stimulation, acupuncture, acupressure, massage, or chiropractic manipulation also are used to treat pain.

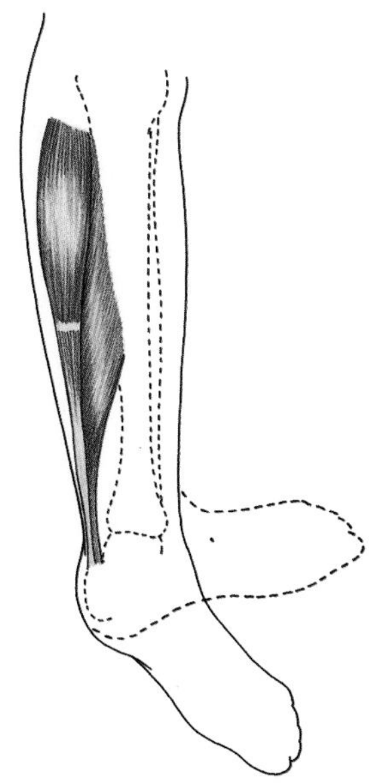

Fig. 31.6 Foot drop. Ankle is fixed in plantar flexion. (From Potter PA, Griffin A, Stockert PA, et al.: *Essentials for nursing practice*, ed 9, St. Louis, 2019, Elsevier.)

Clinical Cues

Alteration in Self-Care Ability

A patient with a musculoskeletal problem may need a little or a lot of help with activities of daily living. For those with a fracture, bathing help is typically needed. If an arm is immobilized, help with a meal tray and possibly with feeding will be required, particularly if the dominant hand is affected. Assistance may be needed for repositioning or transferring when the patient is in a leg cast, immobilizer, or external fixation device. A functional assessment should be performed to determine what assistance is necessary.

Common Therapeutic Measures

Special beds. Most hospital beds now have a built-in pressure-relieving mattress to help prevent skin breakdown. Another type of bed for patients who are on bed rest many hours each day has areas that inflate and deflate to deflect pressure from sequential areas of the body. An air-fluidized bed is used for various types of immobility and is very helpful in preventing pressure sores because it conforms to the body's weight, and the air shifts as the body's weight is redistributed.

With advances in technology, hospital beds have become more sophisticated. Beds that have built-in percussion and vibration for clearing lungs are available. Many critical care beds can be positioned into a chair shape, allowing the patient to sit up without having to move them out of the bed. Others have continuous lateral rotation by means of alternating pressure in the air mattress or by rotation of the whole bed (kinetic therapy). Built-in bed scales, exit alarms, and programmable control lock are features standard on most hospital

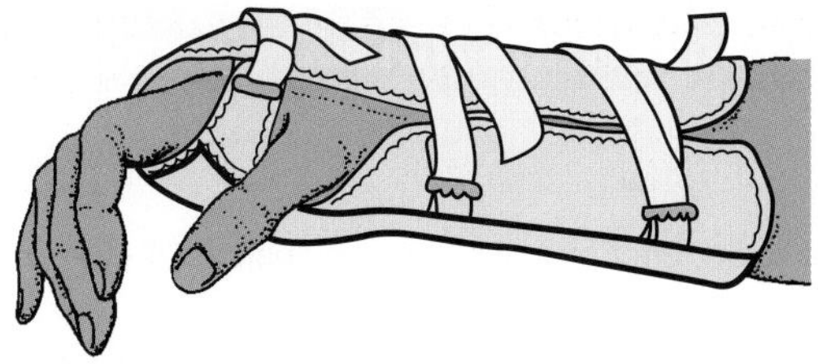

Fig. 31.7 Wrist splint.

beds. Wound care specialists are a good source for determining which type of bed would best help meet patient treatment goals.

Use of slings, splints, and braces. A sling used to support the wrist or elbow should support both joints of the arm. The sling should be positioned so that the fastening at the neck area does not rub the neck or press on a neck vessel. When a splint is applied to an extremity, it should support the joint that is to be immobilized, fit properly without impeding circulation or slipping out of place, and not cause increased pain (Fig. 31.7). If in doubt about how a splint is to be applied, seek help from an experienced nurse or the physical therapist.

A splint may be used on an extremity to limit motion while healing takes place in the bone, joint, tendon, or muscle. Be certain to check the instructions for application of the splint. Inspect the skin under the split each shift. Assess circulation after application of the splint.

A brace or immobilizer may be used on a leg during healing of an ankle injury or during the healing phase of a fracture. The device must be applied correctly, and the skin beneath it must be assessed for friction or injury each shift.

Physical therapy. Physical therapy sessions are often prescribed by the health care provider to assist the patient to regain mobility, increase strength after immobility, decrease pain, and prevent injury. In the acute setting, the physical therapist assesses functionality and rehabilitation potential. Recommendations are made to the provider. Specific exercises, ultrasound, electrical stimulation of muscles, massage, kinetic taping, and heat and/or cold may be used. The patient is to perform the exercises regularly at home between sessions and after a course of therapy is over. The proper way to use crutches, a cane, or a walker are taught and supervised until the patient is deemed "safe" to use the equipment.

Occupational therapy. The occupational therapist assists patients to perform activities of daily living using adaptive equipment or alternate movements. Learning new ways of getting out of a sitting position, getting in and out of a vehicle, moving in bed, cooking, eating, dressing, and other activities helps the patient regain or maintain independence.

Get Ready for the NCLEX® Examination!

Key Points

- The main functions of the musculoskeletal system are motion, support, and protection.
- Disease, trauma, disuse, malnutrition, and aging all contribute to musculoskeletal problems.
- Exercise and weight training throughout life can decrease musculoskeletal problems late in life.
- Using safety equipment for sports, during exercise, when driving, and while at work is very important in preventing trauma to the musculoskeletal system.
- You teach patients about diagnostic tests and procedures for the musculoskeletal system.
- Self-care deficit, impaired physical mobility, and pain are primary problems for patients with musculoskeletal injuries or disorders.
- You use many interventions to prevent disability during periods of immobility.
- Contractures can permanently impair a patient's ability to perform ADLs. Positioning must be performed correctly, and ROM exercises should be performed three or four times a day to promote function and preserve movement.
- You assist with supervising and teaching ambulation with assistive devices.
- Physical and occupational therapists are part of the collaborative team for musculoskeletal care and rehabilitation.

Additional Learning Resources

SG Go to your Study Guide for additional learning activities to help you master this chapter content.

Go to your Evolve website (http://evolve.elsevier.com/deWit/medsurg) for the following FREE learning resources:

- Animations, audio, and video
- Answers and rationales for questions and activities
- Glossary with pronunciations in English and Spanish
- Interactive Review Questions and more!

Review Questions for the NCLEX® Examination

1. When explaining the structure of the knee to a patient who has knee swelling, you state: *(Select all that apply.)*
   1. "Ligaments provide movement of the joint."
   2. "The meniscus in the joint acts as a cushion."
   3. "The tendons are needed for movement and can be injured."
   4. "The fascia may have deteriorated."
   5. "Muscles attach to the bones to help provide movement."

   NCLEX Client Need: Physiological Integrity: Physiological Adaptation

2. Which statement by the patient being taught about musculoskeletal health shows that teaching was effective?
   1. "I will use ice and cold therapy to maintain joint health."
   2. "I will exercise 3 to 4 hours a day to maintain mobility and muscle tone."
   3. "I will get 7 to 8 hours of sleep per night."\
   4. "I will quit smoking."

   NCLEX Client Need: Health Promotion and Maintenance

3. What action should you perform for the postprocedural care of a patient who just had an arthroscopy?
   1. Follow up on the results of the serum enzymes that were drawn before the test.
   2. Prepare an ice pack and obtain an elastic bandage.
   3. Verify muscle strength in the affected extremity.
   4. Encourage the patient to take fluids to decrease the swelling.

   NCLEX Client Need: Physiological Integrity: Reduction of Risk Potential

4. When a 76-year-old female patient complains of pain and soreness in the back, a first step in the assessment specific to this patient should include:
   1. family or personal history of osteoporosis or arthritis.
   2. physical examination of muscle strength of the extremities.
   3. history of fracture during the patient's lifetime.
   4. appearance of joints in the extremities.

   NCLEX Client Need: Physiological Integrity: Physiological Adaptation

5. You are teaching an older adult patient how to increase musculoskeletal and bone strength. Which interventions would be helpful? *(Select all that apply.)*
   1. Walk at least 30 minutes a day, 5 to 7 days a week.
   2. Eat more protein and vitamin C to build muscle.
   3. Walk up stairs as often as possible.
   4. Perform strength training exercises at least three times a week.
   5. Use 10-lb weights for various exercises at least three times a week.

   NCLEX Client Need: Health Promotion and Maintenance

6. You are working on a busy orthopedic floor. Which task(s) can be assigned to the unlicensed assistive personnel (UAP)? *(Select all that apply.)*
   1. Assist an older adult who has an arm sling to perform ADLs.
   2. Report the presence of contractures on a bedridden patient.
   3. Supervise a patient who is beginning to use crutches.
   4. Escort a patient in a wheelchair to the radiology department.
   5. Perform passive ROM on a patient who needs a bed bath.
   6. Instruct a patient to reapply a prescribed wrist splint to prevent contracture.

   NCLEX Client Need: Safe and Effective Care Environment: Coordinated Care

7. You evaluate a patient's ability to use a cane. Which action indicates proper use of the cane?
   1. The cane is advanced at the same time as the good leg.
   2. The hand grip is at the hip level.
   3. The cane is used on the affected side.
   4. The patient looks down while ambulating.

   NCLEX Client Need: Safe and Effective Care Environment: Safety and Infection Control
8. A 56-year-old man complains of joint pain, difficulty rising, and limping. He demonstrates poor posture and uncoordinated gait. You see the priority problem on his care plan as:
   1. limited ability for self-care.
   2. altered physical mobility.
   3. limited coping ability.
   4. altered activity tolerance.

   NCLEX Client Need: Safe and Effective Care Environment: Coordinated Care
9. You recruit the assistance of adequately trained personnel to turn an immobile patient. To prevent injury to the patient and the nursing staff, which measure should be taken before repositioning the patient?
   1. Encourage movement of all joints.
   2. Explain the details of the move.
   3. Discourage patient participation.
   4. Medicate the patient for anxiety.

   NCLEX Client Need: Physiological Integrity: Reduction of Risk Potential
10. To manage joint discomfort associated with movement for a patient with severe rheumatoid arthritis, you should:
    1. encourage deep-breathing exercises.
    2. administer pain medications immediately after exercise.
    3. schedule pain medication administration before exercise.
    4. provide a continuous infusion of pain medications.

    NCLEX Client Need: Physiological Integrity: Pharmacological Therapies
11. You assess the condition of a patient with a splint applied to the right arm. Which clinical finding is cause for the greatest concern?
    1. Warm skin under the splint
    2. Redness of skin under the splint
    3. Itching under the splint
    4. Palpable distal pulses

    NCLEX Client Need: Physiological Integrity: Reduction of Risk Potential

Critical Thinking Questions

Scenario A

Ms. Johnson has had trouble with her left knee for several years. She is scheduled for an arthroscopy and asks you about the procedure.

1. How would you describe the procedure to her?
2. What care is necessary after this procedure?
3. How long is she likely to be immobile after the procedure?

Scenario B

Mrs. Hamid has been experiencing muscle weakness in her right leg for a few weeks. Her health care provider has scheduled her for an electromyogram (EMG). She asks you about this procedure.

1. Is an informed consent needed for an EMG?
2. How would you describe the test to Mrs. Hamid?
3. What care is needed after the procedure?

Scenario C

Mrs. Green, age 67 years, sustained a fracture of the right humerus when she fell this morning. A cast has been applied.

1. What would you tell her she needs to do at home to keep her joints mobile?
2. What should she do to protect the muscle mass?
3. What nutritional teaching would you provide?

Scenario D

You are caring for Mr. Morgan, a 40-year-old self-employed carpenter. He is a large man with a heavy full-leg cast. He is having a lot of pain and expresses fear that moving will increase the pain.

1. Discuss some important considerations in turning, moving, bathing, and toileting for Mr. Morgan.
2. What is the psychosocial care for a patient such as Mr. Morgan who is immobile?

32 Care of Patients With Musculoskeletal and Connective Tissue Disorders

http://evolve.elsevier.com/deWit/medsurg

Objectives

Theory

1. Compare the assessment findings of a connective tissue injury with those of a fracture.
2. Determine the rationale for the "dos and don'ts" of cast care.
3. Outline the potential complications related to fractures.
4. Discuss the pathophysiology and implications of the six *P*s.
5. Contrast the preoperative and postoperative care of a patient with a total knee replacement with that of a patient with a total hip replacement.
6. Relate the special problems of patients with arthritis with specific nursing interventions that can be helpful.
7. Illustrate the process by which osteoporosis occurs, ways to slow the process, and how the disorder is treated.
8. Determine important postoperative observations and nursing interventions in the care of a patient who has undergone an amputation.

Clinical Practice

9. Gather data on a patient who has a connective tissue injury.
10. Instruct a patient going home with a cast about proper care of the cast and extremity.
11. Observe a physical therapist teaching quadriceps exercise and then assist the patient to practice.
12. Assess the skin of a patient who has a prosthetic device on an amputated limb.

Key Terms

arthroplasty (ĂR-thrō-plăs-tē, p. 769)
bivalved (BĪ-vălvd, p. 763)
compartment syndrome (kŏm-PĂRT-mĕnt SĬN-drōm, p. 763)
dislocation (dĭs-lō-KĀ-shŭn, p. 757)
fasciotomy (făsh-ē-ŎT-ō-mē, p. 763)
fracture (FRĂK-shŭr, p. 759)
nonunion (nŏn-Ū-nyŭn, p. 763)
orthoses (ŏr-thō-sēz, p. 769)
osteogenesis (ŏs-tē-ō-JĔN-ĕ-sĭs, p. 763)
osteomyelitis (ŏs-tē-ō-mī-ĕ-LĪ-tĭs, p. 762)
osteopenia (ŏs-tē-ō-PĒ-nē-ă, p. 777)
osteoporosis (ŏs-tē-ō-pō-RŌ-sĭs, p. 759)
sprain (SPRĀN, p. 756)
subluxation (sŭb-lŭk-SĀ-shŭn, p. 757)

Concepts Covered in This Chapter

- Functional Ability
- Self-Management
- Nutrition
- Elimination
- Inflammation
- Infection
- Mobility
- Tissue Integrity
- Pain
- Patient Education
- Collaboration
- Safety

CONNECTIVE TISSUE DISORDERS

SPRAIN

Etiology and Pathophysiology

A **sprain** is a partial or complete tearing of the ligaments that hold various bones together to form a joint. A sprain occurs during trauma when a joint is forced or twisted past its normal range of motion (ROM). The ankle, knee, and wrist are most the commonly sprained joints.

Signs, Symptoms, and Diagnosis

- *Grade I* (mild): Tenderness at site; minimal swelling and no loss of function; no abnormal motion. Slight stretching and microscopic tearing of ligament.
- *Grade II* (moderate): More severe pain, especially with weight bearing; swelling and bleeding into joint; some loss of function. Partial tearing of the ligament.
- *Grade III* (severe): Pain may be less severe, but swelling, loss of function, and bleeding into joint are more marked. Complete tear of the ligament producing instability of the joint.

Diagnosis is by physical and radiographic examination to rule out a fracture or other pathology.

Treatment and Nursing Management

RICE is the acronym used for treatment of sprains: **rest, ice, compression,** and **elevation.** Apply ice immediately after injury and for the next 24 to 72 hours. Apply the ice bag for 10 to 20 minutes every 1 to 2 hours during the day. Wrap the injured part snugly with an elastic bandage, being careful not to cut off circulation, and elevate. These measures can help minimize swelling and pain and stabilize the joint in proper alignment. The goal of treatment is to protect the ligament until it heals by scarring. Ligaments do not "grow" back together. Air casts, braces, or supports are used only until a joint has been strengthened. If a joint is immobilized too long and muscles are not exercised, muscle atrophy—which begins in a matter of days—can cause permanent disability. In some cases, surgical repair may be necessary. Grade III sprains often require a cast. Patients with grade II or grade III sprains need to rest the joint; crutches are needed for a lower extremity sprain. Nonsteroidal antiinflammatory drugs (NSAIDs) should be prescribed on an around-the-clock basis for the first couple of days to decrease pain and swelling. Care should be taken for longer use because there is evidence that NSAIDs may delay or suppress the body's ability to heal the injury (Vuurberg et al., 2018).

STRAIN

Etiology and Pathophysiology

A strain is a pulling or tearing of a muscle, a tendon, or both. A strain occurs by trauma, overuse, or overextension of a joint. The most commonly strained muscles are the back muscles. (See Chapter 22 for a discussion of the neurologic aspects of back problems.) Muscle strains also occur in other skeletal muscles. The most common sites are the hamstrings, quadriceps, and calf muscles. Joint strains are clinically very similar to sprains.

> **Complementary and Alternative Therapies**
>
> **Soothing Sore Muscles**
>
> Arnica applied topically is reported to soothe sore, tired muscles after extended hard work (Berry, 2018). Valerian or kava brewed as a tea is also believed to relax muscles. A little honey or apple juice will make the teas more palatable (Micozzi, 2019).

Signs, Symptoms, and Diagnosis

A history of overexertion or the presence of soft-tissue swelling and pain even at rest may indicate that a strain has occurred. Bleeding (ecchymosis, hemorrhagic area) will be present if a muscle is torn.

Treatment and Nursing Management

Ice and compression should be applied immediately, and the body part should be elevated and rested. The patient is taught to use ice for only 20 minutes each hour. When compression is used, the distal parts of the extremity must be checked for sensation and adequate circulation. Heat can be applied after 48 hours. Antiinflammatory medications are used for discomfort; when spasm is present, a muscle relaxant may be prescribed. Time is the greatest healer. The patient is cautioned against reinjury and is taught proper ways to lift and move. Surgical repair may be necessary.

> **? Think Critically**
>
> How would you assess for a circulation problem or nerve injury after an ankle sprain or strain?

DISLOCATION

Etiology and Pathophysiology

A **dislocation** is the stretching and tearing of ligaments around a joint with complete displacement of a bone. **Subluxation** is a partial dislocation. This occurs from trauma. The most common sites are the shoulder, knee, hip, ankle, and temporomandibular joint.

Signs, Symptoms, and Diagnosis

Dislocation often includes a history of an outside force pushing from a certain direction, severe pain aggravated by motion of the joint, muscle spasm, or abnormal appearance of a joint. A radiograph will reveal displacement of bone.

Treatment and Nursing Management

Reduction of displacement under anesthesia is used for most dislocations; sometimes manual reduction is used for the shoulder. Reduction can be very painful. Sometimes spontaneous reduction can be achieved. The goal is to stabilize the joint after reduction and then to rehabilitate to minimize muscular atrophy and strengthen the joint. Assess for adequate perfusion and movement of the affected part and distal to it, determine whether swelling is present, and assess the degree of pain. Nursing management is aimed mainly at pain control and at encouraging rest of the affected part. Heat or cold applications may be ordered.

ROTATOR CUFF TEAR

Rotator cuff injury usually results from repetitive activity, such as throwing or making overhead motions with the arm, and results in a degenerative tear. Falls and trauma may also cause acute injury. The rotator cuff is composed of four muscles. If the rotator cuff is torn, there is pain and the patient cannot perform abduction and external rotation of the injured shoulder. Treatment consists of rest, sling support for the shoulder, and NSAIDs for the discomfort. Some health care providers treat with injections of steroids or an antiinflammatory drug. When the acute episode is over, gentle, progressive exercise is prescribed. Heat is recommended before exercising the joint. If the tear will not heal, surgical repair is indicated.

ANTERIOR CRUCIATE LIGAMENT INJURY

Most anterior cruciate ligament (ACL) injuries of the knee occur from athletic activities, but falls and motor vehicle accidents also may cause such injuries.

Hyperextension, internal rotation, extremes of external rotation, and deceleration are involved. The ligament may be torn from the femur or tibia. Often a loud "pop" can be heard at the time of injury. There is swelling in the hours after the injury, and the knee feels unstable and can "give way." Full extension of the leg is difficult. Diagnosis is by physical examination, radiography, or magnetic resonance imaging (MRI). Arthroscopy is performed, at which time repair may be done. The ligament is repaired with a tissue graft.

After injury, the knee is immobilized, and measures are instituted to reduce swelling and pain. After repair, continuous passive motion (CPM) may be ordered to promote full mobility. A long-leg brace with fixed knee flexion may be used as well. Isometric exercises are prescribed in the recovery period, including quadriceps setting (see Patient Teaching: Quadriceps and Gluteal Muscle Exercises in Chapter 31), bent-knee leg exercises, and foot exercises.

MENISCAL INJURY

The meniscus is the shock absorber of the knee, and it lies on top of the tibia between the tibia and the femur. A meniscus tear may accompany an ACL injury. This type of injury often results from fixed-foot rotation in weight bearing with the knee flexed during sports activities, such as football, soccer, basketball, or skiing. After the injury, mild swelling occurs and there is joint pain. Popping, slipping, catching, or buckling of the knee can occur. Diagnosis is by physical examination to elicit a "click" and localized pain with particular movements of the joint. MRI is the most specific diagnostic test for a meniscal injury. Surgery for repair is done arthroscopically. Postoperatively, pain management is a priority. An exercise program is prescribed for muscle strengthening during recovery.

ACHILLES TENDON RUPTURE

The Achilles tendon attaches the soleus, plantaris, and gastrocnemius muscles to the calcaneus (heel bone). When overstretched, it can rupture. Sports injuries or a fall from a height are the usual mechanisms of injury. Arthritis, diabetes, and taking some antibiotics and other medications can predispose to Achilles tendon rupture. Injury most often occurs with bursts of jumping, pivoting, and running, such as occur in tennis, basketball, handball, and badminton. Symptoms include sudden pain at the back of the ankle or calf. There may be a loud "pop" or "snap" sound. A depression can be felt or seen 2 inches above the calcaneus. Pain, swelling, and stiffness, and then bruising and weakness, follow. There will be an inability to point the toes or stand on tiptoe. Diagnosis is by examination and squeezing the calf muscles while the patient is lying prone. The toes should point downward; if they do not, there is most likely an Achilles tendon injury.

Treatment may be by splinting, casting, or a combination of splinting or casting with surgery. Recovery takes 6 to 8 weeks, followed by physical therapy.

BURSITIS

Bursitis is an inflammation of the bursae, the saclike structures that line freely movable joints. It occurs from injury or overuse and often appears when a person has engaged in an unaccustomed activity, such as shoulder bursitis after digging up the garden plot in the spring. Bursitis may occur in any heavily used joint, but it most commonly occurs in the elbow, shoulder, hip, or knee.

Symptoms are localized tenderness and mild to moderate aching pain that is localized to the joint and is exacerbated by activity of the joint. Swelling may be present. Diagnosis is by history of injury and physical examination. Treatment is to rest the joint by altering aggravating activity and using antiinflammatory agents, ice, massage, and a compression wrap if there is soft-tissue swelling. If these measures—plus time—do not relieve the symptoms, an injection of cortisone into the bursa may be administered.

BUNION (HALLUX VALGUS)

A bunion, the most common foot problem, is a painful swelling of the bursa that occurs when the great toe deviates laterally at the metatarsophalangeal joint. It may be hereditary, or it may occur from ill-fitting shoes. Bunions are more common in women than in men. Wearing open-toed shoes of soft leather or athletic shoes that are wider in the toe area helps reduce pain. Metatarsal pads can relieve some of the pressure. Corticosteroid injections are given in the joint if active bursitis is present. Analgesics are used for discomfort. Bone realignment of the big toe, with removal of bony overgrowth, is performed when walking becomes too painful. Hammertoes are often fixed at the same time.

CARPAL TUNNEL SYNDROME

Etiology, Pathophysiology, Signs, and Symptoms

Carpal tunnel syndrome is a nerve problem that occurs when the median nerve is compressed as it passes through the carpal tunnel in the wrist. It produces pain, numbness, and tingling of the hand, particularly at night. Repetitive movements of the hands and wrists, particularly with constant flexion of the wrist, are contributing causes. Such movement occurs in certain types of factory work and in computer keyboarding. Sometimes there is no known cause.

Diagnosis, Treatment, and Nursing Management

Diagnosis is by physical examination, a compression test, and possibly electromyography to rule out other causes of symptoms. Treatment by rest, splinting, changing the angle of the wrist during repetitive movements, or steroid injection may solve the problem. If the symptoms are of long duration, muscle atrophy occurs; if sensory loss in the fingers and hands is progressive, surgery is indicated. Surgical decompression of the medial nerve by transection of the carpal ligament is performed, usually as an outpatient procedure.

Postoperatively, blood flow must be assessed hourly by checking color, warmth of the fingertips, and capillary refill. After anesthesia has worn off, sensation of the fingers is assessed. The wrist is immobilized in a splint, and the arm is elevated on pillows to reduce edema. The patient is warned to avoid heavy gripping and pinching for up to 6 weeks.

FRACTURES

Etiology and Pathophysiology

A **fracture** is a break or interruption in the continuity of a bone. Fractures occur mostly from trauma but result from a pathologic process in which bone has degenerated, such as in **osteoporosis** (metabolic bone disorder that causes a decrease in bone mass) or another metabolic problem. The **mechanism of injury,** or how the injury occurred, can provide clues about the type of fracture. For example, if a patient punches a wall or another solid surface, the fifth metacarpal commonly breaks, and the patient sustains a "boxer's fracture." Mechanism of injury is also important to help predict injury to the neighboring tissues. Damage varies according to the type of fracture, but there is always some degree of tissue destruction, interference with the blood supply, and disturbance of muscle activity at the site of injury.

Safety Alert

Proton Pump Inhibitors and Fracture Risk

In May 2010, the U.S. Food and Drug Administration (FDA) issued a warning that proton pump inhibitors (PPIs), including over-the-counter types, increase the risk for fracture of the hip, wrist, and spine. In epidemiologic studies, the risk was highest for people older than 50 years who had used PPIs for more than a year (Ault, 2010). Calcium and vitamin D supplements should be taken when a patient is taking a PPI long term. These findings were reaffirmed in 2018 (Nassar & Richter, 2018).

Signs, Symptoms, and Diagnosis

A fracture may cause minimal to severe pain depending on the type of fracture, the bone(s) involved, and the amount of displacement. Swelling usually occurs, and there may be bleeding into the tissues. Other symptoms of a fracture include pain, tenderness, deformity of the bone, ecchymoses, crepitation with any movement, and loss of function. Box 32.1 presents the most common types of fractures. Fig. 32.1 illustrates the characteristics of a variety of fractures. Diagnosis is by physical and radiographic examination.

Treatment

The emergency treatment and nursing care of fractures consists of preventing shock and hemorrhage and the immediate immobilization of the part to prevent unnecessary damage to the soft tissue adjacent to the fracture. An inexperienced person should never attempt to straighten or set a broken bone. The injured part

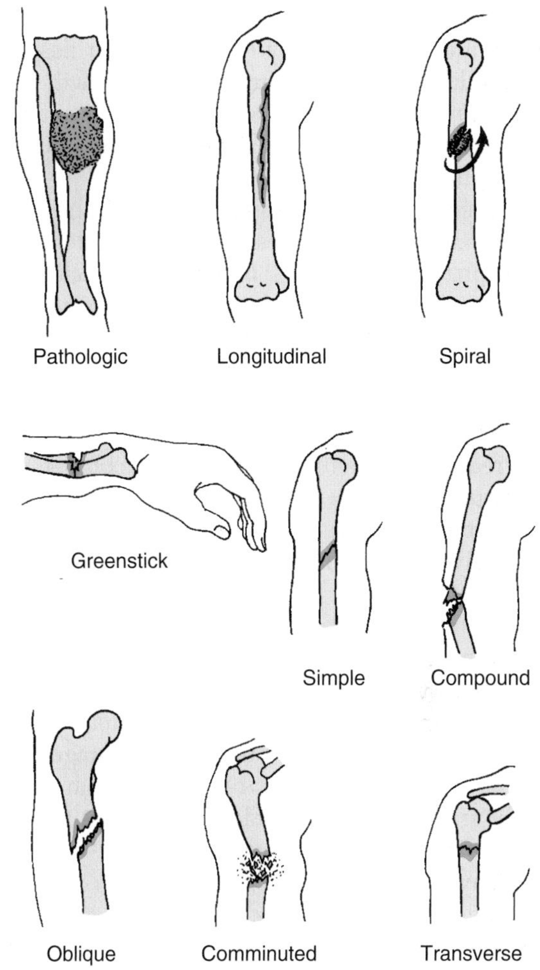

Fig. 32.1 Types of fractures.

Box 32.1 Types of Fractures

- **Complete fracture** is when a bone breaks into two parts that are completely separated.
- An **incomplete fracture** is when a bone breaks into two parts that are not completely separated.
- A **comminuted fracture** is one in which the bone is broken and shattered into more than two fragments.
- A **closed (simple) fracture** is one in which there is no break in the skin.
- An **open (compound) fracture** is one in which there is a break in the skin through which the fragments of broken bone protrude.
- A **greenstick fracture,** common in children, is one in which the bone is partially bent and partially broken.

Older Adult Care Points

Older adults are more at risk of sustaining a fracture because of decreased reaction time, failing vision, reduced agility, alterations in balance, and decreased muscle tone, all of which predispose to falls. You should assess for fall risk and initiate fall precautions as needed. Balance exercises can be very helpful in preventing fractures, as can the use of assistive devices.

should be immobilized in the position in which it is found at the time of injury: "splint it as it lies." The limb should be supported firmly so that it will not be jarred when the patient is being moved. If available, ice in a plastic bag can be applied to the fracture area to help minimize swelling.

In the emergency department or clinic, the patient will be examined by a health care provider, and a radiograph will be ordered if fracture is suspected. After a radiograph of the injured part has been made and the type of fracture and extent of damage have been established, a decision is made as to which method to use in reducing the fracture and providing immobilization. Surgery may be necessary to realign the bones and to reduce the fracture. If the skin was broken when the fracture occurred, tetanus immunization is given unless immunization is current. Prophylactic antibiotics are usually administered when a compound (open) fracture has occurred.

The primary goal in the treatment of fractures is to establish a sturdy union between the broken ends so that the bone can be restored to continuity. The healing and repair of a fracture begin immediately after the bone is broken and proceed through five stages:

1. Blood oozes from the torn blood vessels in the area of the fracture; the blood clots and begins to form a hematoma between the two broken ends of bone (1 to 3 days).
2. Other tissue cells enter the clot, and granulation tissue is formed. This tissue is interlaced with capillaries, and it gradually becomes firm and forms a bridge between the two ends of broken bone (3 days to 2 weeks).
3. Young bone cells enter the area and form a tissue called *callus.* At this stage, the ends of the broken bone are beginning to "knit" together (2 to 6 weeks).
4. The immature bone cells are gradually replaced by mature bone cells (ossification), and the tissue takes on the characteristics of typical bone structure (3 weeks to 6 months).
5. Bone is resorbed and deposited, depending on the lines of stress. The medullary canal is reconstructed during consolidation and remodeling (6 weeks to 1 year).

To facilitate the process of repair and ensure proper healing of the bone without deformity or loss of function, the health care provider must bring the two broken ends together in proper alignment and then immobilize the affected part until healing is complete. The procedure for bringing the two fragments of bone into proper alignment is called *reduction of the fracture.*

Reduction, surgery, and stabilization. There are two methods to reduce a fracture: closed reduction and open reduction. In **closed reduction,** the bone is manipulated into alignment; no surgical incision is made. A general anesthetic or heavy procedural sedation may be given before the fracture is reduced. An **open reduction** is performed after a surgical incision is made through the skin and down to the bone at the site of the fracture. In cases of open (compound) fractures and comminuted fractures, an open reduction is necessary so that the area can be adequately cleansed and bone fragments removed.

There are four methods of stabilizing a fracture after it has been reduced:

1. Internal fixation
2. External fixation
3. Casts, splints, or braces
4. Traction

Internal fixation. When a fracture has been reduced by an open procedure, to guarantee adequate union and stabilization of the bone fragments, the surgeon performs **internal fixation** of the bone. This means that pins, nails, screws, rods, or metal plates are used to stabilize the position of the two broken ends. Internal fixation is particularly necessary to treat fractures in older adults whose bones are brittle and may not heal properly (Fig. 32.2).

One of the most common internal fixation procedures is performed on a fractured hip: open reduction and internal fixation (ORIF). An incision is made, the fracture is realigned, and the bone is secured with pins, screws, nails, or plates. The portion of the femoral head affected by the fracture will determine whether fixation is adequate or an implantable device is needed

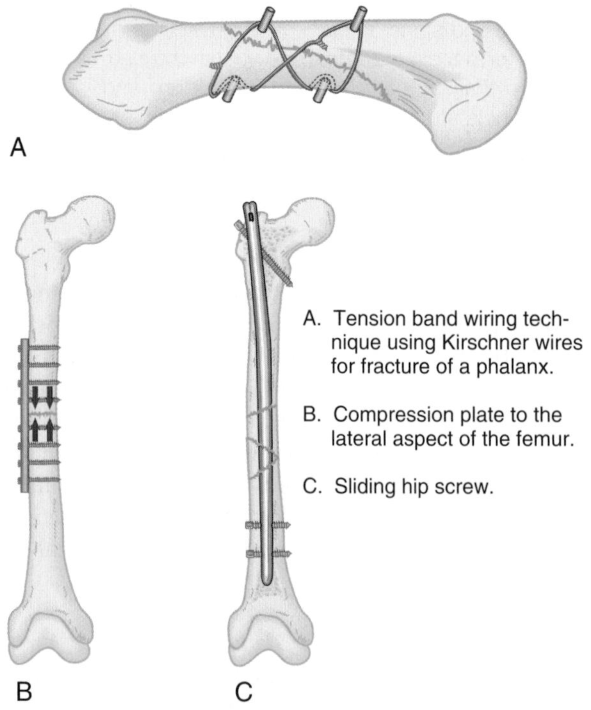
A
B
C
A. Tension band wiring technique using Kirschner wires for fracture of a phalanx.
B. Compression plate to the lateral aspect of the femur.
C. Sliding hip screw.

Fig. 32.2 Examples of internal fixation. **A,** Tension band wiring technique using Kirschner wires for fracture of a phalanx. **B,** Compression plate to the lateral aspect of the femur. **C,** Sliding hip screw. (From Black JM, Hawks JH: Medical-surgical nursing: clinical management for positive outcomes, ed 8, Philadelphia, 2009, Elsevier.)

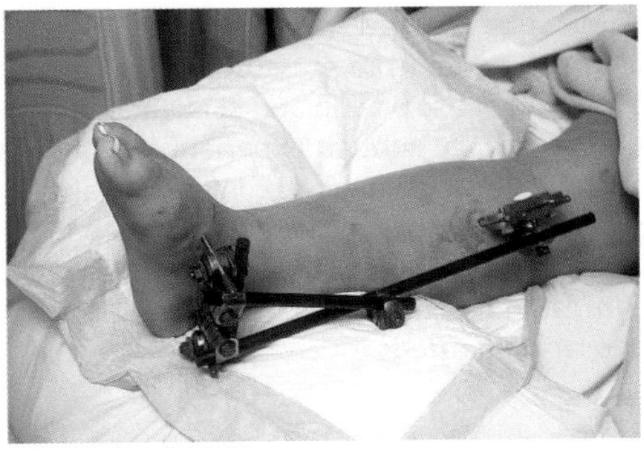

Fig. 32.3 External fixation.

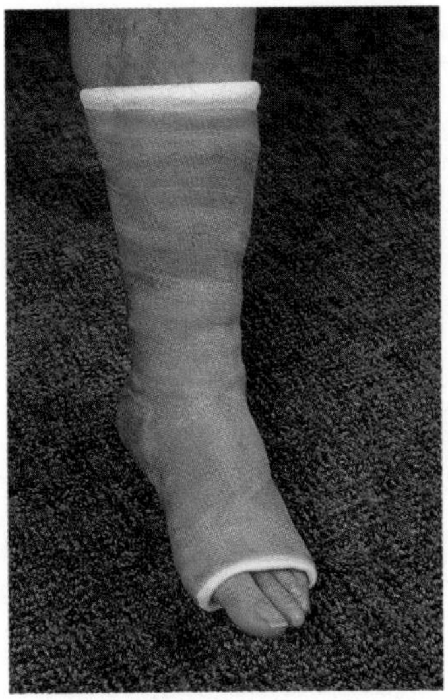

Fig. 32.4 Synthetic limb cast.

(arthroplasty). Administration of intravenous (IV) antibiotics to reduce the risk of infection is standard. Care includes maintaining good alignment of the affected leg, preventing complications of immobility, and keeping the patient comfortable with pain control measures.

External fixation. **External fixation** of fractures involves the use of a device composed of a sturdy external frame to which are attached pins that have been placed into the bone fragments. Fig. 32.3 shows a fixator that is applied by inserting heavy pins on either side of the fracture and then reducing the fracture by tightening nuts attached to the connecting rods.

External fixation is commonly used for fractures of an extremity or of the pelvis. Indications include the following:

- Massive open fractures with extensive soft-tissue damage
- Infected fractures that do not heal properly
- Multiple trauma with one or more fractures and other injuries, such as burns, chest injury, or head injury

External fixation has the advantage of allowing more freedom of movement than traction and usually is more comfortable. With good stability the patient may be able to get out of bed, although they must be assisted and advised not to bear weight on the affected limb. Physical therapy exercises will help the patient prevent many of the problems of immobility, and an occupational therapist can suggest ways to cope with activities of daily living (ADLs). Pin care should be performed regularly.

Particularly if the fixator must remain in place for months or years, the patient is likely to have problems with self-image and may feel embarrassed or frustrated about being out in public with an apparatus that is large and bulky.

Casts. Casts are used for stabilizing a fracture after a closed reduction. A cast is rigid and immobilizes the injured body part. Fiberglass and polyester-cotton knit casts are lightweight, dry quickly, and can bear weight within 30 minutes of application (Fig. 32.4). They are less bulky than plaster cases, do not crumble easily, and are less likely to be damaged by wetting. Fiberglass casts are less easily molded to a body part than are plaster casts, and synthetic casts are not suitable for immobilizing the fragments of severely displaced bones or for stabilizing serious fractures. Their rough exterior surfaces can damage the skin and tend to snag clothing and other soft materials. Synthetic casts are used mostly for upper-extremity fractures. Some health care providers still use plaster of Paris casts for lower extremities because plaster casts can bear more weight and last longer with weight bearing. A newly applied plaster cast usually is not dry for about 48 hours. A dry plaster cast is white, has a shiny surface, and will resound when tapped. A wet plaster cast is grayish and dull in appearance and will give a dull thud when tapped. The edges of plaster casts tend to crumble, with bits of plaster dropping inside the cast and causing the patient discomfort and skin irritation. This can be prevented by covering the rims of the cast with stockinette or applying tape in a "petal" fashion.

There are **long-leg** and **short-leg casts,** classified by how much leg they cover. A walking **cast shoe** is a canvas sandal with a thick sole that fits over the bottom of the leg cast; this shoe can be used once the patient is allowed to bear weight. When an arm cast is applied, a sling is often used to support the arm and provide extremity elevation. A **spica cast** (usually used in children) covers the trunk of the body and one or two extremities. There are long-leg and short-leg spicas that cover one or both legs and shoulder spicas that include the trunk and one arm.

When a surgical repair has occurred, casting is delayed for 1 to 2 weeks until the patient is seen in the office. Casts must be kept dry to prevent infection of the surgical wound. A wet cast must be changed as soon as possible.

Braces and splints. Braces provide support for fractures that have been reduced. The advantage of a brace is

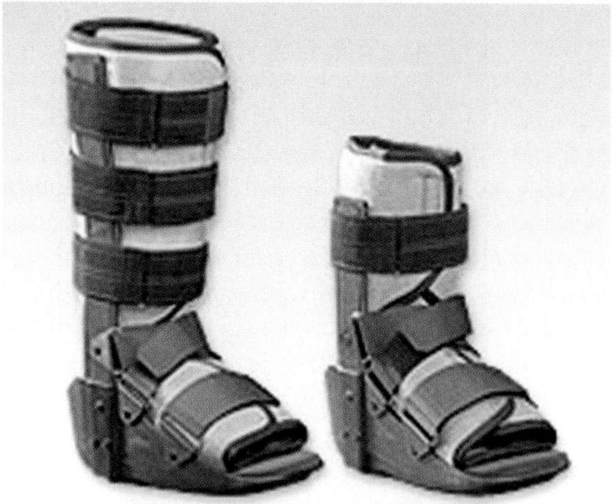

Fig. 32.5 Walking boot. (From Roberts JR, Hedges JR: *Clinical procedures in emergency medicine,* ed 5, Philadelphia, 2009, Elsevier.)

that it can be easily removed for assessment and care of the skin, and then reapplied. Examples include a commercial fracture boot to support the distal tibia, ankle, and foot (Fig. 32.5). A hinged brace is used for the elbow and knee, which allows for early motion of the joint. An adjustable dial allows for variations in flexion and extension during recovery. A knee immobilizer prevents motion and provides compression to reduce pain and swelling. Plaster of Paris can be used to create a "backslab" or splint (a slab of plaster that provides support but does not completely surround the injury). The slab is useful in the early phase because of the swelling that occurs after the injury (Garcia-Rodriguez et al., 2018).

Clinical Cues

Before cast application (especially plaster of Paris), advise the patient that they will feel warmth as the cast sets and dries. Never put a fresh cast over plastic; the heat generated may burn the skin because it cannot dissipate. A fresh plaster cast should never be covered; air circulation speeds drying.

Traction. Traction was used more commonly in the past and is now used for specific types of conditions.

Traction is the application of a mechanical pull to a part of the body for the purpose of extending and holding that part in a certain position during immobilization. The two general types of traction are **skeletal traction** and **skin traction.** In skeletal traction, the surgeon inserts pins, wires, or tongs directly through the bone at a point distal to the fracture so that the force of pull from the weights is exerted directly on the bone. Skeletal traction uses 10 lb or more of weight, and the body acts as the countertraction. With skin traction, a bandage (such as moleskin) or a foam traction boot is applied to the limb below the site of fracture, and pull is exerted on the limb. No more than 7 to 10 lb of weight is used for skin traction.

Skin must be checked regularly under skin traction because breakdown from pressure may occur. Because of the infrequent use of skin and skeletal traction, most nurses do not have enough experience with the setup and patient management to feel confident in assessments and the care needed. If you are caring for a patient with traction, make sure you review the facility policy and procedures and update your knowledge so that safe and appropriate care is given.

Clinical Cues

Skeletal traction (Buck traction) for hip fracture patients was common practice in the past. The rationale was to relieve pain and further injury by maintaining bone alignment while waiting for surgical correction. Multiple studies have shown that neither of these occur with use of traction. Use of a position splint controls pain better and results in less tissue injury (Tosun, Aslan, & Tunay, 2018).

Complications of Fractures

The sooner a fracture is fixed, the less likely complications become. Healing of a fracture can be impeded by improper alignment and inadequate immobilization. Continued twisting, shearing, and abnormal stresses prohibit a strong, bony union. Inadequate levels of serum calcium and phosphorus, vitamin deficiency, and generalized atherosclerosis—which deprives the healing site of adequate blood supply—also can complicate a fracture by delaying healing. Injury to blood vessels at the time of the fracture can further compromise blood flow. Nerves can also be injured, which may alter mobility.

Infection. Infection of the tissue at the fracture site is probably the most serious impediment to healing. Open comminuted fractures should be surgically addressed within 6 hours to decrease the chance of infection. Prevention of infection after surgery is a 2020 National Patient Safety Goal. Typically cefazolin (Ancef) is administered within 1 hour of incision, and two doses are given postoperatively. If the wound is grossly contaminated, additional antibiotics will be prescribed. It is important to monitor the patient's temperature and white blood cell (WBC) count for elevations and to assess the appearance of the area carefully for redness, swelling, heat, or purulent drainage.

Osteomyelitis. **Osteomyelitis** is a bacterial infection of the bone. The causative organism is most often *Staphylococcus aureus,* which enters the bloodstream from a distant focus of infection, such as a boil or furuncle, or from an open wound, as in an open (compound) fracture. It is usually found in the tibia or fibula, in vertebrae, or at the site of a joint prosthesis. Osteomyelitis has a sudden onset with severe pain and marked tenderness at the site, high fever with chills, swelling of adjacent soft parts, headache, and malaise. Patients with diabetes, with chronic renal failure, or on long-term steroid therapy are all at increased risk of infection and osteomyelitis. Diagnosis of osteomyelitis is made based on the following:

- Laboratory findings indicating an acute infection, such as high WBC count
- Radiographs, which may show bone destruction 7 to 10 days after onset of the disease
- History of injury to the part, open fracture, boils, furuncles, or other infections
- Biopsy, in which the bone sample exhibits signs of necrosis

The earlier osteomyelitis is diagnosed and treated, the better the prognosis. Intravenous antibiotics are often needed, and antibiotics are prescribed for 4 to 6 weeks; the abscess is incised and drained. Dead bone and debris are debrided from the site. The affected limb is immobilized for complete rest. Sometimes amputation is the only cure (see Chapter 6 for care related to infection).

Nonunion. **Nonunion** (failure to heal) of a fracture can be treated nonsurgically by an electrical bone growth–stimulating device, which uses electrical coils or electrodes to induce weak electrical current in the bone to stimulate **osteogenesis** (growth of bone cells). Use of such devices can prevent further surgery and bone grafting. This treatment is based on the fact that bone has inherent electrical properties used in healing.

Fat embolism. Fat embolism is a rare but serious complication of a fracture of a bone that has an abundance of marrow fat (e.g., the long bones, pelvis, and ribs). In the early postinjury period, patients with multiple fractures resulting from severe trauma are at risk for this complication. To form an embolism, the fat globules must be large enough or sufficient in number to partially or completely occlude a blood vessel. Rupture of small venules in the area permit entrance of fat globules into the circulation. **Signs and symptoms of fat embolism include a change in mental status, respiratory distress, tachypnea, crackles and wheezes on auscultating the lungs, rapid pulse, fever, and petechiae (a fine red rash over the chest, neck, upper arms, or abdomen).** Stay with the patient; put them in a high Fowler position, use a nonrebreather mask to give high-flow oxygen, and establish a peripheral IV line. Summon the health care provider immediately because there is an approximate 80% mortality rate from this complication. Anticipate hydration with IV fluids and correction of acidosis. Intubation and mechanical ventilation may also be needed if oxygen levels cannot be maintained with supplemental oxygen.

Older Adult Care Points

Older adults with a fractured hip are at high risk for fat embolism. Be especially vigilant and assess for this complication.

Venous thrombosis. The veins of the pelvis and lower extremities are very vulnerable to thrombus formation after fracture, especially hip fracture. Immobility and surgical procedures contribute to venous stasis. The Joint Commission's National Quality Measures call for aggressive prevention of thrombus formation. Compression stockings, sequential compression devices, and ROM exercises on the unaffected lower extremities are used to help prevent the problem. To meet the 2020 National Patient Safety Goals, you must be vigilant for the adverse effects of any prescribed prophylactic anticoagulant drugs, such as aspirin, warfarin, or low-molecular-weight heparin, and must be observant for instances of bleeding.

Compartment syndrome. **Compartment syndrome** is a restriction of blood flow that occurs in one or more muscle compartments of the extremities. Compartment syndrome is caused by external or internal pressure. External pressure can occur from dressings or casts that are too tight. Internal pressure occurs from IV fluid infiltration, inflammation, and edema (a shifting of fluid from the vascular spaces to the intracellular spaces). The increased fluid puts pressure on the tissues, nerves, and blood vessels, thereby decreasing blood flow.

Clinical Cues

Elevation is the key to preventing swelling and compartment syndrome; toes and fingers should be higher than the trunk.

The main sign of compartment syndrome is severe, unrelenting pain that is out of proportion to the injury and unrelieved by narcotics. Decreased sensation, numbness and tingling, paleness of the skin, and weakness of the extremity are other signs. Assess for the six *P*s: pain, pallor, paresthesia, pulselessness, paralysis, and poikilothermia (cold to the touch).

Recognition and immediate notification of the health care provider can prevent permanent loss of function. If a cast is in place, the cast can be **bivalved** (split through all layers of the material). Dressings will be cut or replaced. Surgical **fasciotomy** (linear incisions in the fascia down the extremity) may be necessary to relieve the pressure on the nerves and blood vessels if other measures do not relieve the problem. Fig. 32.6 shows the fascial compartments of the calf and forearm.

NURSING MANAGEMENT

DATA COLLECTION (ASSESSMENT)

Pretreatment

Ask the patient to describe the mechanism of injury. Physical assessment of a suspected fracture includes noting pain, swelling, discoloration, and deformity in the contour of the bone. With a possible extremity fracture, pulses should be bilaterally checked and compared. Nerve damage in a fractured leg is assessed by having

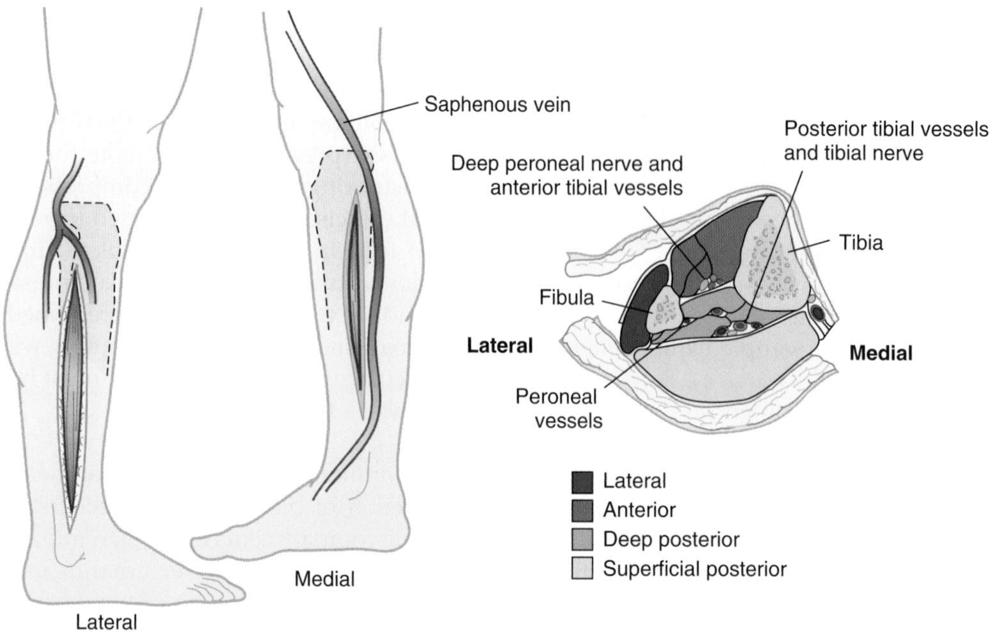

Fig. 32.6 Fascial compartments of the calf. (From Townsend CM, Beauchamp RD, Evers BM, et al.: *Sabiston textbook of surgery*, ed 20, Philadelphia, 2017, Elsevier.)

the patient flex and extend their foot. Next, obscure the patient's view and touch a toe with a sharp and then a dull object (e.g., the wooden end and then the cotton-tip end of an applicator, respectively); ask them to identify which toe was touched and to discriminate sharp and dull touch. To check nerve damage in the arm, have the patient wave their hand, have them grip your hand, and use the sharp/dull touch test on the fingers.

! Safety Alert

In-depth assessment and history must be delayed if a broken bone has pierced the skin and the bleeding is severe. Apply direct pressure over the wound. (Observe for shock and treat if necessary.) Prevent introduction of infectious agents into the wound and cover the open area with a sterile dressing (clean dressing if sterile supplies are not available).

Clinical Cues

In cases of fracture, assessment (six *Ps*) of extremities should be done bilaterally. Also remember to ask if the patient is left- or right-hand dominant; dominance can account for a weaker grip, and if the dominant hand is injured it will affect performance of ADLs.

Pain is not always present when a fracture has occurred. Numbness and tingling can also accompany a fracture. **If it is unclear whether a bone has been broken, it is best to treat the injury as if it is a fracture.** To prevent further trauma and pain, splint the area without moving or manipulating bone. Apply an ice pack, if available, and notify the health care provider of your findings.

? Think Critically

If you were in the park and you observed a child fall from a tree and obviously fracture a forearm, what would you do to assist?

Post-Treatment

Attention to pain control is important, especially when the patient is adjusting to fixation devices or a new cast. If elevating the limb, icing, or giving prescribed pain medication does not relieve the patient's complaints within 30 minutes, notify the health care provider.

Every immobilized patient should be routinely assessed for the various problems of immobility: skin breakdown, urinary tract infection, constipation, atelectasis, or deep vein thrombosis (DVT). Adequate nutrition and fluids are needed to promote healing and prevent the problems of immobility.

◆ NURSING DIAGNOSIS AND PLANNING

Problem statements for patients with fractures usually include the following:

- Pain due to disruption of bone and tissue.
- Altered physical mobility due to disruption of bone.
- Altered self-care ability due to inability to use an extremity.
- Potential for infection due to open fracture.

◆ IMPLEMENTATION

Traction devices must be assessed to ensure that they are in the correct position and that the weights are hanging free. The patient's body position should be assessed for proper alignment.

Focused Assessment

Physical Assessment of Neurovascular Status

Assessment should be performed at least once at the beginning of each shift to establish a baseline for any patient who has suffered a musculoskeletal injury and then performed as required. When a fracture is fresh, this assessment should be performed every 2 to 4 hours.

- *Skin color:* Is the skin pale (decreased blood), blue (decreased oxygenation), bruised (bleeding into surrounding tissues), or red (possible infection)?
- *Skin temperature:* Is the skin increasingly hot to the touch (infection) or cool (decreased blood flow)? Use the back of your hand to do the assessment.
- *Pulses:* Are pulses distal to the injury present and equal bilaterally?
- *Movement:* Can the patient actively move the affected area or the area distal to the injury? If active movement is not possible, passively move the area distal to the injury. How much discomfort is felt with movement?
- *Sensation:* Is numbness or tingling present (paresthesia)? Obscure the patient's view and gently touch a distal area with a paper clip. What and where does the patient feel?
- *Pain:* Where is the pain? What is the nature and intensity? Use a pain scale. Is pain increasing?
- *Capillary refill:* Does blanching occur when a nail bed distal to the injury is pressed? Assess by pushing on a nail bed, let up, and count the time it takes for color to return. Usual color should return in less than 2 seconds.

A thorough assessment of a patient in a cast should include the following:

- Complaints of numbness, a tingling sensation, increased pain with motion of the fingers or toes, or sharp localized pain, which can be caused by pressure from a tight cast. Notify the health care provider if the patient states that they can feel the bone fragments grating against each other (crepitation).
- Check frequently to determine whether the cast is properly supported or there is undue pressure on any underlying part of the body. A sharp, localized, burning pain could mean the beginning of a pressure sore. This should be reported so that the surgeon or orthopedic technician can cut a "window" in the cast to relieve pressure.
- Sniff at the edges of the cast to detect foul odors that are suggestive of infection.

Nutrition Considerations

Nutrition for Immobile Musculoskeletal Patients

Protein is essential to healing, and the diet should be designed to provide 1 g/kg of body weight. Vitamins D, B, and C and calcium are included in well-balanced meals to ensure optimal soft-tissue and bone healing; 500 mg of vitamin C will also help acidify the urine and prevent calcium precipitation that could form kidney stones. Fluid intake of 2000 to 3000 mL/day helps prevent bladder infection, kidney stones, and constipation. A high-fiber diet with a lot of vegetables and fruits promotes good bowel function and decreases the chance of constipation.

Think Critically

During a neurovascular assessment, the patient reports some decreased sensation and tingling in the fingers of the hand with a lower arm cast. What should you do?

The drainage from pin sites may occur for 48 to 72 hours after surgery involving external fixation. Meticulous cleaning of pin sites with sterile water should be performed daily. The goal is to reduce serosanguineous drainage and crusting that would support infection; also assess for pin loosening (U.S. National Library of Medicine, 2018). Your patient will appreciate a well-organized nurse with a gentle touch who remembers to premedicate 30 minutes before wound and pin care. For a body part with external pins, showering may be resumed 10 days after surgery.

When the patient is transferred from stretcher to bed, provide sufficient help; casts or external fixation devices can be heavy. Pillows for support should be placed on the bed *before* moving the patient onto them. Pillows are used to support the curves of large casts so that the weight of the body will not crack or flatten the cast. **Hardware of an external fixation device or brace bars between the legs of a cast are never used as handles for lifting and turning the patient.**

It is important to clarify with the health care provider how much weight the patient can bear on the affected extremity. Patients with some fractures should place no weight on the affected side, whereas other patients will be encouraged to move about without any restrictions.

Care of a Patient With a Cast

While the cast plaster is damp (grayish, dull appearance), use the palms of the hands or the flat surface of the extended fingers when touching the cast because fingertips can sink into the damp plaster and make impressions through the cast that rub against the tissue under the cast, predisposing to pressure sores. A plaster cast generates heat as it dries; assess the patient's subjective sensation of heat and pain because burns can occur. **During the first 24 to 48 hours after any cast has been applied to an extremity, the extremity should be elevated to minimize swelling.**

Whether fiberglass or plaster, the cast should be inspected every day for flattened areas, soft spots, cracking, and crumbling. The skin around the edges of the cast should receive special attention, including massage with lotion and close observation for signs of pressure or breaks in the skin. Patients must be instructed not to use sharp objects such as pencils or rulers to scratch under the cast. These can tear the skin, leaving an open break for the entrance of bacteria. To relieve itching, use a 60-mL plunger syringe and forcefully direct air under the cast. At home, the patient can use a hair dryer on the coolest setting to blow air into the cast.

A plaster cast will disintegrate if it becomes wet, so the patient will need assistance with bathing. Patients may have permission to shower with a synthetic cast; a plastic covering is secured over the cast and taped to the skin. Instruct the patient to avoid putting the casted area directly under the stream of water.

Depending on the injury or the type of cast, traction, or fixation device, moving or turning the patient for adequate back care may not be possible. Obtain an order for an overhead trapeze bar so that the patient can lift themself to enable back care to be given and the bottom sheet to be changed or tightened. Instruct the patient to lift themself straight up so that the amount of pull exerted on a limb in traction will not be altered. This same maneuver can be used when the patient is placed on a bedpan. A small "fracture" bedpan should be used and the lower back supported by a small pillow or folded blanket.

When a cast is removed, the underlying skin is usually dry and scaly. Scrubbing of the area must be avoided to prevent damage to the deeper layers of skin, especially because the cast is often reapplied after the health care provider does an examination. Nursing interventions for selected problems are summarized in Chapter 31, Table 31.4.

Clinical Cues

Ice bags can be used to help control swelling. However, because the weight of an ice bag could make an indentation in a wet plaster cast, the ice bags should be only about half full, and they should be laid against the cast and propped in position rather than set on top of it.

Think Critically

Your patient has an arm cast in place and is complaining of severe itching inside the cast. What could you do to help relieve the problem?

◆ EVALUATION

Your patient's pain should be under control, and they should be progressing toward independently accomplishing ADLs at their baseline level within a specified time. There should be no problems associated with immobility (i.e., skin breakdown or constipation, atelectasis, or DVT) or complications (i.e., infection, compartment syndrome). If the outcomes are not being met, the plan must be revised.

INFLAMMATORY DISORDERS OF THE MUSCULOSKELETAL SYSTEM

LYME DISEASE

Lyme arthritis occurs from a systemic infection caused by the spirochete *Borrelia burgdorferi*. The spirochete is transmitted by the bite of a blacklegged or western blacklegged tick. Most cases of this disease are in the New England and mid-Atlantic states, the upper Midwest, Northern California, and Oregon. The disease begins with flulike symptoms and a "bull's-eye" rash with pain and stiffness in the joints and muscles. Doxycycline, cefuroxime, or amoxicillin taken for 10 to 21 days can prevent the disease's progression. Diagnosis is based on clinical presentation and the possibility of being exposed to infected ticks. In the early stages, laboratory testing is not reliable and not recommended. If undiagnosed and/or untreated, stage II begins 2 to 12 weeks later with carditis and nervous system disorders such as meningitis, peripheral neuritis, or facial paralysis similar to Bell palsy. Intravenous antibiotics are necessary at this point. If undiagnosed and untreated, later chronic complications may occur. The patient may experience fatigue, cognition problems, and arthralgias. In some instances the only sign of Lyme disease is arthritis. Lyme arthritis can cause permanent damage to the nervous system and to the joints. Since the early stages of the disease have symptoms similar to those of flu, many cases are missed because patients do not seek examination from a health care provider. Many times Lyme disease is not identified until the later stages.

OSTEOARTHRITIS

Etiology and Pathophysiology

Osteoarthritis is a degenerative joint disease characterized by breakdown of cartilage in synovial joints, bone, joint capsule, surrounding tissues, and synovial fluid. This breakdown releases inflammatory molecules. Osteoarthritis has been called a "noninflammatory" disease, but now that more is known about the disease process, this label is no longer correct. The exact cause is not known, but risk factors include heredity, aging, female gender, obesity, previous joint injury, and recreational or occupational overuse of joints (Lozada, 2018). People with osteoarthritis seem to produce less collagen to strengthen cartilage and cover and protect joints in the body. With time and use, joints become thickened and withstand weight bearing poorly, with consequent damage to cartilage. The synovial cells then release enzymes that cause further cartilage degeneration.

Health Promotion

***Healthy People 2030* Goals Related to Arthritis**

The objectives aimed at reducing the disability caused by arthritis include the following:

- Reducing the mean level of joint pain, activity limitations, care limitations, effect on employment, and the proportion of those who find it "very difficult" to perform specific joint-related activities.
- Increasing health care provider counseling for weight and physical activity; increasing the proportion of those seeing a health care provider for joint symptoms and effective evidence-based arthritis education as an integral part of managing the condition.

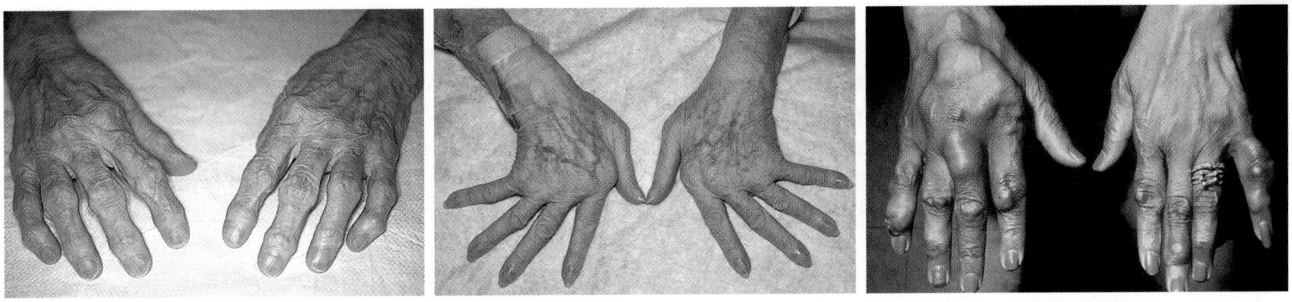

Fig. 32.7 Types of arthritis. **A,** Osteoarthritis. Note the presence of nodes in the proximal interphalangeal joints (Bouchard nodes) and distal interphalangeal joints (Heberden nodes). **B,** Rheumatoid arthritis. Note the marked ulnar (elbow-like) deviation of the wrists. **C,** Gouty arthritis. Note tophi (stones) containing sodium urate crystals. (From Swartz MH: *Textbook of physical diagnosis*, ed 7, Philadelphia, 2014, Elsevier.)

Signs, Symptoms, and Diagnosis

Secondary osteoarthritis occurs asymmetrically and typically affects only one or two joints. Secondary forms occur as a result of injury or other identifiable mechanism. Primary osteoarthritis, particularly of the hands, can occur symmetrically. Osteoarthritis is labeled primary when no cause can be identified. Clinically the signs and symptoms and treatment are the same. The chief symptoms are aching pain with joint movement and stiffness, with limitation of mobility. Joints may be deformed, and nodules may be present (Fig. 32.7).

Treatment

Treatment consists of pain management, strengthening and low-impact aerobic exercise, weight reduction if the patient is overweight, and maintenance of joint function. Salicylates, acetaminophen, or NSAIDs may be used. Acetaminophen in doses of 1000 mg, up to 3000 mg/day, is the standard for patients with mild to moderate chronic joint pain.

Safety Alert

Acetaminophen Usage

All other medications and over-the-counter drugs should be checked for acetaminophen so that overdose does not occur. Taking more of this drug than recommended (no more than 4000 mg/day in the short term or 3000 mg/day in the longer term) can cause irreversible liver damage. The drug should not be taken when drinking alcohol. For older adults, the lowest effective dose should be used. Encourage an adequate intake of water, at least 2000 mL each day, to promote excretion of the drug via the kidneys.

Older Adult Care Points

NSAIDs may not be recommended for older adults because of side effects and interactions with other drugs that those older adults may be taking. NSAIDs decrease the effectiveness of the angiotensin-converting enzyme (ACE) inhibitors used for hypertension and heart failure, and NSAIDs increase the effects of anticoagulants. Tramadol may be prescribed.

Corticosteroid injection into the arthritic joint may be performed if oral medication does not control the problem. Exercises for joint mobility are encouraged. Surgery or joint replacement may be performed to relieve severe pain and improve mobility. The hip and knee are the most common sites for joint replacement related to osteoarthritis.

Complementary and Alternative Therapies

Therapies for Pain Relief

Yoga and massage can help control and relieve the pain of osteoarthritis. Capsaicin cream, or ointment made from cayenne red pepper, blocks pain locally when applied topically to the inflamed joint. It can be used four times a day. It is available over the counter or by prescription.

Glucosamine and chondroitin have been shown in a research study to decrease the pain of moderate to severe osteoarthritis in some people. This substance may slow or halt the progression of osteoarthritis. Patients taking warfarin (Coumadin) should check with their health care provider before starting glucosamine (Rakel, 2018).

Injections of hyaluronic acid (HA) (Euflexxa, Orthovisc, Synvisc, Supartz, and Hyalgan) into the joint can act as a lubricant, decrease pain, and improve function for some patients with mild to moderate osteoarthritis. The intra-articular injections are given once a week for 3 to 5 weeks and may be repeated in 6 months. Stem cell treatments are another option being explored.

Another treatment for knee cartilage injury is the injection of autologous chondrocytes. Healthy articular cartilage cells are removed from the patient and sent to a special laboratory, where they are grown for 3 to 5 weeks and then reimplanted. Patients use crutches for 6 to 8 weeks after surgery. The procedure is successful in about 90% of cases. It works best in patients younger than 50 years with injury to a small focal area of cartilage (Ogura, Bryant, & Minas, 2017).

Nursing Management

Nursing interventions for osteoarthritis include teaching the patient to balance exercise and rest. Gentle exercise is very important in maintaining joint mobility. Walking, knitting, and swimming all help improve mobility and decrease pain. The patient should avoid placing stress on affected joints. Suggest the use of assistive devices to open containers and perform other household functions.

Instruct in moist heat application and encourage the patient to maintain weight within normal limits. Weight reduction decreases joint stress. Imagery, relaxation, and diversion are helpful to reduce pain. Quadriceps strengthening exercises may relieve pain and disability of the knee (see Patient Teaching: Quadriceps and Gluteal Muscle Exercises in Chapter 31).

> **Think Critically**
>
> Where would you suggest that a patient look for assistive devices available to those with arthritis?

RHEUMATOID ARTHRITIS

Etiology and Pathophysiology

Rheumatoid arthritis (RA) is an inflammatory disease of the joints caused by an autoimmune response to an external trigger. It can occur at any age but is most common among older women. The cause is not known, but hormonal, environmental, genetic, or infectious agents trigger an underlying autoimmune reaction. An abnormal immune response causes an inflammatory reaction of the synovial membrane. Vasodilation, increased permeability, and the formation of exudate cause red, swollen joints. Rheumatoid factor (RF), which is an antibody against immunoglobulin G, appears in the blood and synovial fluid in many patients.

There are remissions and exacerbations of the disease. As the disease progresses, pannus is formed. **Pannus** is granulation tissue derived from the synovium that spreads over the articular cartilage. Pannus releases enzymes and inflammatory mediators that destroy cartilage. The cartilage becomes eroded, and the pannus cuts off nutrition to the cartilage. Over time the pannus between the bone ends becomes fibrotic, causing ankylosis. Joint fixation and deformity become apparent (see Fig. 32.7). Along with these changes, exacerbations cause more damage, and there is atrophy of muscles around the joint. Tendons and ligaments stretch, and the joint becomes unstable. Muscle spasm draws the bones out of normal alignment. Contractures and deformity occur. Mobility becomes impaired if the knees or ankles are affected. Subcutaneous nodules may form over bony prominences, and nodules may occur in the pleura, heart valves, or eyes.

Signs, Symptoms, and Diagnosis

The signs and symptoms of RA are joint pain, warmth, edema, limitation of motion, and stiffness in multiple joints in the morning lasting more than 1 hour. The joints of the hands, wrists, and feet are most commonly affected by RA, and involvement is usually bilateral. Systemic symptoms of low-grade fever, anorexia with weight loss, malaise, and an iron deficiency anemia that is resistant to iron therapy may also be present. Joint deformity and consequent dysfunction can occur.

RA pain or immobility of joints interferes with self-care activities necessary to lead an independent lifestyle. Maintaining mobility and controlling pain with the least amount of side effects are the goals for the older adult. Table 32.1 presents a comparison of osteoarthritis and rheumatoid arthritis.

Diagnosis is by history of arthritis pain in three or more joints that lasts for more than 6 weeks, positive RF and/or anti-cyclic citrullinated peptide/protein antibody test (anti-CCP), elevated C-reactive protein or erythrocyte sedimentation rate, and exclusion of diseases that have similar clinical symptoms (Venables et al., 2018). Radiographs confirm the cartilage destruction and bone deformities.

Treatment

Treatment is aimed at relieving pain, minimizing joint destruction, promoting joint function, and preserving ability to perform self-care (Table 32.2). Rest and exercise, medication, immobilization with splints and use of other supportive devices during periods of severe inflammation, and hot and cold application are standard treatments. Surgical joint repair or replacement can reduce pain and improve mobility.

Rheumatoid arthritis pain is initially treated with NSAIDs. If diagnosed early, disease-modifying antirheumatic drugs (DMARDs) can be started to prevent joint delegation. Methotrexate is the first-line DMARD, if tolerated by the patient. Other medications include hydroxychloroquine, sulfasalazine, leflunomide, or a tumor necrosis factor (TNF) inhibitor. Long-term steroid therapy increases the risk for diabetes mellitus, osteoporosis, hypertension, acne, cataracts, and weight gain; therefore steroid preparations are reserved for controlling flare-ups (Cohen & Mikuls, 2018). DMARDs provide periods of remission, but they also have some serious side effects. Patients should be tested for tuberculosis (TB) before being started on TNF inhibitors because these drugs may exacerbate TB.

> **Complementary and Alternative Therapies**
>
> **Help Patients Evaluate the Safety of Complementary and Alternative Therapies**
>
> Some patients find symptom relief with dietary supplements such as omega-3 fatty acids, acupuncture, tai chi, and meditation. Research study results for various supplements have been mixed and have lacked conclusive evidence of efficacy. Patients with arthritis are particularly vulnerable to "miracle cures" or outright quackery; therefore it is the responsibility of all health care professionals to initiate a dialogue about complementary and alternative therapies or other methods that the patient is using, to evaluate their safety and to incorporate these self-care methods into the overall plan of care (National Center for Complementary and Integrative Health, 2019).

Table 32.1 Comparison of Rheumatoid Arthritis and Osteoarthritis

CHARACTERISTIC	RHEUMATOID ARTHRITIS	OSTEOARTHRITIS
Definition	A systemic disease in which pathologic changes and disability result from chronic inflammation of the joints	A progressive degenerative joint disease with some inflammatory features
Pathology	Chronic inflammation of synovial membranes and formation of chronic granulation tissue (pannus) in the joint; pannus is capable of eroding cartilage in joints and spreading to bone, ligaments, and tendons	Microscopic changes in the cartilage in the joint; eventually loss of cartilage, bony enlargement, and malalignment of joints
Etiology	Unknown; evidence that the pathologic changes are immunologic	Unknown; may be caused by "wear and tear" of aging
Rheumatoid factors (autoantibodies)	Usually present	Usually absent
Age at onset	30–40 yr most common but at any age	50–60 yr; rarely before age 40 yr
Weight	Normal or underweight	Usually overweight
General state of health	Varies; often anemic, "chronically ill," with low-grade fever and slight leukocytosis	Well nourished
Appearance of joints	*Early:* Soft-tissue swelling *Late:* Ankylosis, extreme deformity Joint involvement usually symmetric bilaterally and generalized	*Early:* Slight joint enlargement *Late:* Enlargement more pronounced, slight limitation of motion Joints typically involved are single-sided and weight-bearing: spine, hips, knees
Muscles	Pronounced muscular atrophy, particularly in later stages	Usually not affected
Other	Morning stiffness; pain on motion; swelling and tenderness of joints; subcutaneous nodules; typical rheumatoid changes seen on radiograph	Stiffness, relieved by moderate motion; joint malalignment; symptoms increase in cold, wet weather

The injection of steroids directly into a joint (intra-articular administration) has been used successfully in treating painful flare-ups, shortening the period of inflammation and relieving pain and other symptoms. When intra-articular steroid therapy is used, it is recommended that not more than two or three doses be injected into any joint within 1 year.

Use of opioids for RA pain management is not recommended. Decreasing the inflammation that is causing the pain and contributing to joint injury is a better approach. RA is a chronic disease, and chronic use of opioids is problematic. For acute flare-ups, short-term opioid use may be implemented.

Older Adult Care Points

Older adults must be taught to watch for side effects of medications and promptly report them to the health care provider or nurse. Dizziness, which predisposes to falls, can occur with analgesics for arthritis pain, particularly if the medication contains opioids. Advise patients to arise slowly, hold on to furniture until steady, use assistive devices, and wait for dizziness to pass before walking.

Surgical intervention and orthopedic devices. Casts or braces and splints (**orthoses**) may be used to immobilize an affected part so that it can rest during an active phase of arthritis. Devices that immobilize the affected joint should allow for motion of adjacent muscles to maintain them and improve strength and permit more independence. Braces help prevent deformities by maintaining an optimal functional position of the joints.

Surgical intervention for arthritis is used to provide pain relief and/or improve mobility for those patients who have not responded adequately to medical therapy. One such surgical procedure is **synovectomy,** which is the excision of the synovial membrane of a joint. The goal of synovectomy is to interrupt the destructive inflammatory process that eventually leads to ankylosis and invasion of surrounding cartilage and bone tissues. Tendon reconstruction is performed most commonly on the hand to restore function. For younger patients with osteoarthritis, **osteotomy** may be an option. In this procedure a wedge of bone is removed to allow for realignment.

Joint replacement. An **arthroplasty** (joint replacement) may be done for a knee, shoulder, elbow, finger, ankle, or hip. The hip and knee are the most commonly replaced joints. Uncemented press-fit prostheses are often used for young, heavier, and very active patients. The cement used for bone prostheses may last for 20 years or more.

Total hip replacement. The primary purpose of total hip replacement (THR) is to relieve chronic pain. Hip replacement for osteoarthritis can be performed with minimally invasive surgery and a shorter hospital stay for some patients (Fig. 32.8). A hip joint may be replaced

Table 32.2 Drugs Commonly Used to Treat Rheumatoid Arthritis

CLASSIFICATION	EXAMPLES	ACTION	NURSING IMPLICATIONS
Nonsteroidal antiinflammatory drugs (NSAIDs)	Acetaminophen, aspirin, ibuprofen (Advil, Motrin), naproxen sodium (Aleve), COX-2 inhibitors (Celebrex)	Reduce inflammation and pain	May take 2 wk to obtain results; give with food or a full glass of water, but some are best taken 30 min before a meal or 2 h afterward. May cause GI irritation. Monitor hematologic, renal, liver, auditory, ophthalmic functions; weight gain; and peripheral edema. Teach patient to report heartburn, dyspepsia, nausea, vomiting, diarrhea, or abdominal pain. Teach to avoid alcohol because of increased risk of GI irritation. Dosage in older adults may need to be reduced by half.
Corticosteroids	Prednisone, methylprednisolone (Medrol)	Reduce inflammation, decrease pain by suppressing the immune system	Usually rapid action. Instruct to take daily dose between 6 and 8 A.M. when natural steroids are released. Instruct not to stop taking this drug abruptly. Taper dosage downward as soon as symptoms improve. Monitor older adults closely for fluid retention, elevated blood pressure, and peripheral edema. Handle patients gently to prevent bruising; avoid using tape on skin. May cause osteoporosis, Cushing syndrome, mood changes, weight gain, cataracts, onset of diabetes, muscle weakness, and increased risk of infection.
Disease-modifying antirheumatic drugs (DMARDs)	Hydroxychloroquine (Plaquenil), sulfasalazine (Azulfidine), gold salts (Ridaura), D-penicillamine (Cuprimine, Depen), methotrexate (Rheumatrex), azathioprine (Imuran), leflunomide (Arava), others	Reduce inflammation and pain, suppress the immune system, and prevent joint and cartilage destruction	Plaquenil takes 6 mo to be effective; others take 1–6 mo. May cause rash, diarrhea, and retinal problems. Instruct that frequent eye examinations are necessary. Most of the drugs can cause GI symptoms and blood dyscrasias; monitor blood counts. Gold salts can cause liver toxicity; monitor liver functions. Methotrexate can cause pulmonary, renal, and liver toxicity. Imuran and leflunomide may cause birth defects or fetal death. Alcohol use increases chance of hepatic toxicity. Monitor blood and urine weekly. Check specific nursing implications for each drug.
Biological therapies (classifications include tumor necrosis factor inhibitors, interleukin antagonists, selective costimulation modulators, or targeted B-cell therapy)	Etanercept (Enbrel), infliximab (Remicade), certolizumab (Cimzia), rituximab (Rituxan), golimumab (Simponi), anakinra (Kineret), adalimumab (Humira), abatacept (Orencia), tocilizumab (Actemra)	Reduce inflammation by blocking the inflammatory response	1–2 wk for onset of action. Increased risk of serious infection and blood dyscrasias; monitor blood counts, temperature, and for malaise closely. May cause demyelinating disorders. Given IV or by subcutaneous injection; may cause injection site reaction. Do not immunize with live virus vaccines. Test for tuberculosis before starting these medications.

COX-2, Cyclooxygenase-2; *GI,* gastrointestinal; *IV,* intravenously.

either with a low-friction polyurethane socket for the acetabulum and a metallic replacement for the head of the femur or with synthetic materials combined with a porous bone implant (Fig. 32.9). The porous bone implant requires 6 weeks of healing. Patients with

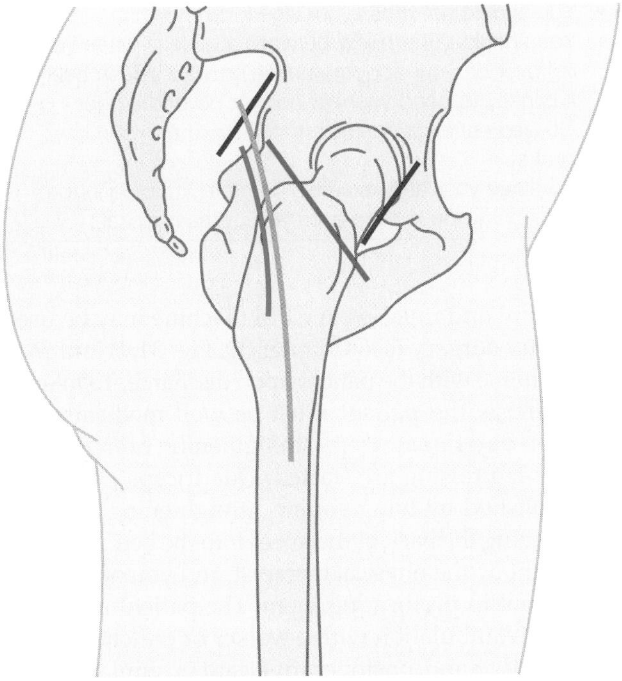

Fig. 32.8 Surgical approaches to hip replacement.

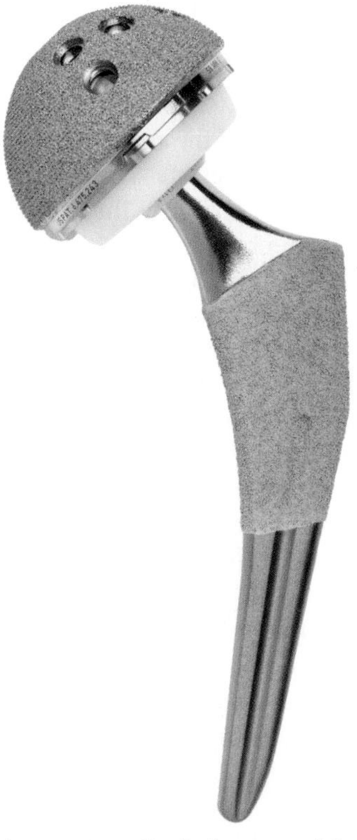

Fig. 32.9 Hip replacement prosthesis. (Image reprinted with permission from Stryker Corporation. © 2013 Stryker Corporation. All rights reserved.)

cemented prostheses can apply weight within a few days. For patients with uncemented implants, full weight bearing is avoided for at least 3 to 6 weeks. Crutches or a walker are used for ambulation, depending on the ability of the patient. The greatest dangers to successful replacement are infection and failure to function properly. Possible dislocation when the hip is rotated internally is an issue.

Hip resurfacing may be done for patients younger than 60 years. This procedure can help with pain, improve ambulation, and restore joint function. The procedure involves trimming the head of the femur and placing a metal cap over the end. The damaged bone in the socket is removed and replaced with a metal cup, and the capped end rotates in the cup (Bal, 2018). The advantage of this procedure is that there is greater range of hip motion than with a hip replacement, and dislocation is less of a risk.

There are multiple surgical approaches and techniques (see Fig. 32.8). Minimally invasive and robot-assisted surgeries usually result in shorter hospital stays, and the surgical approach determines movement restrictions. Make sure to find out the details of the surgical procedure so that you can provide appropriate teaching and answer patient questions.

Preoperative care. Specific instructions about the kind of surgery to be performed, the prosthesis to be used, the postsurgical procedures, and what is expected of the patient to help achieve the goals of rehabilitation are given. Instructions for postoperative exercises and the use of ambulation equipment, such as a walker, crutches, or canes, are provided. Some patients wish to donate blood several weeks before surgery in case a blood transfusion becomes necessary after surgery.

A surgical bacteriostatic scrub solution is prescribed for the shower on the night before and the morning of surgery, to decrease the chance of infection. Tell the patient that they will be placed in an orthopedic bed with an overhead trapeze bar attached after surgery. They may be transported to and from the operating room on the bed. Explain the use of an abduction pillow and turning procedures postoperatively.

Postoperative care. There may be a drain at the surgical hip replacement site, with a suction device attached to it. Intravenous fluids will be administered. A Foley catheter will usually be in place. Immediately after surgery, nursing intervention includes all the measures required to prevent respiratory and circulatory complications. However, extreme care must be exercised in positioning and repositioning the patient. To prevent dislocation, an abduction wedge or pillow may be secured between the legs (usually in the operating room) and is left in place when the patient is supine in bed until the surgeon requests its removal (Fig. 32.10). The wedge is positioned with the narrower end between the thighs, and the straps should not go over an incision, bony prominence, or drain. If an anterior surgical approach was used, the wedge may not be necessary.

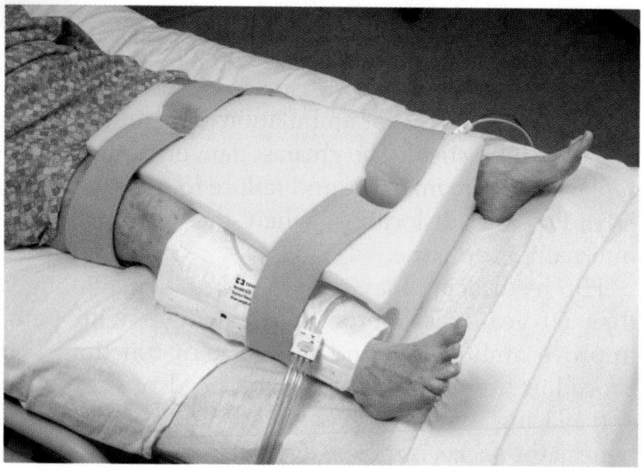

Fig. 32.10 Abduction wedge in place to prevent dislocation of hip prosthesis.

Make sure to find out what type of precautions are needed based on the surgical procedure, approach, and surgeon preference.

Safety Alert

Precautions With Hip Abductor Wedge

Circulation should be checked after each application of the wedge to be certain that the straps are not too tight. Skin should be assessed every shift on the surface of the legs, with particular attention to areas over bony prominences.

DVT is a possible complication of joint replacement. Low-molecular-weight heparin, enoxaparin (Lovenox), dalteparin (Fragmin), or tinzaparin (Innohep) is the drug of choice to prevent this problem. Patients may be sent home on enoxaparin, so instruction on self-administration of a subcutaneous injection or family instruction is needed. Most patients who have had a hip replacement are permitted to stand at the bedside on the operative day, supported by a walker and two people. Weight bearing on the operated joint is sometimes allowed, but there should be a specific written order about this from the health care provider. The patient will need instruction in transferring themselves from bed to chair, wheelchair, and toilet. Whenever seated, the chair seat should be adjusted so that the patient's hips are not flexed beyond a 90-degree angle. In addition to these instructions, the patient may be referred for outpatient or in-home physical therapy. Nursing interventions for selected problems related to THR are summarized in Nursing Care Plan 32.1 (see also Chapter 5 for general care of a postoperative patient). The rehabilitation team includes the patient, family, surgeon, nurse, physical therapist, and occupational therapist.

Total knee replacement. Chronic, uncontrollable pain from arthritis is the main indication for knee arthroplasty. Part or all of the knee joint may be replaced. For the best postoperative result, emphasis is placed on exercise

Patient Teaching

Total Hip Replacement Discharge Teaching

Before discharge, the patient who has undergone hip surgery should be given instructions for care at home. These include the following:

- It is okay to lie on your operated side.
- You should not cross your legs for 3 months.
- You should put a pillow between your legs when you roll over on your abdomen or lie on your side in bed.
- It is okay to bend your hip but not beyond a right (90-degree) angle (demonstrate); avoid sitting in low chairs.
- Continue your daily exercise program at home in the same way you did the exercises at the hospital.

of the joint and muscles. A CPM machine may be used soon after surgery (see Chapter 31, Fig. 31.4) and may be sent home with the patient upon discharge. To tolerate the exercise, the patient must be well medicated for pain. On day 1 quadriceps-strengthening exercises and straight-leg raising are started. Quadriceps exercise is accomplished by lying supine, straightening the legs, and pushing the back of the knees into the bed. Exercises are taught by the physical therapist, and you often assist the patient in performing them. The patient then progresses to ambulation with a walker or crutches. Other preoperative and postoperative care is similar to that for the patient undergoing any major surgery. After early release from the hospital, the patient continues physical therapy in the outpatient setting.

NURSING MANAGEMENT

ASSESSMENT (DATA COLLECTION)

Many patients who have arthritis live every day with pain, limited motion, and the chronic and incurable nature of arthritis; therefore carefully seek in-depth information about the patient's social history, their personal and family health history, current general health status, ability to do the things they want to do, and their experience of pain and how they have been dealing with it.

NURSING DIAGNOSIS AND PLANNING

Nursing problems for patients with arthritis depend on the degree of disability the disease is causing. Common problem statements might include the following:

- Chronic pain due to inflamed joints.
- Altered mobility due to pain, stiffness, and joint deformity.
- Altered body image due to joint deformities.
- Fall risk due to mobility issues.
- Fatigue secondary to chronic pain.

Expected outcomes for these problems and subsequent surgical or nonsurgical interventions might include the following:

- Patient's pain will be controlled with medications, heat, and exercise within 2 weeks.

Nursing Care Plan 32.1 Care of a Patient After a Total Hip Replacement

SCENARIO

Miko Yoshima, an 85-year-old woman, has just undergone a total hip replacement with a minimally invasive anterior approach for a hip joint damaged by osteoarthritis. She normally lives alone but has relatives within a 30-minute driving distance. She had been actively gardening and taking care of herself until pain severely limited her mobility over the past few months. (This care plan is specific to problems of hip replacement. All usual care for a postoperative patient [wound care, respiratory care, monitoring for complications, etc.] should also be included.)

PROBLEM STATEMENT/NURSING DIAGNOSIS

Altered mobility related to pain and activity restrictions after hip replacement.

SUPPORTING ASSESSMENT DATA

Subjective: "I'm quite uncomfortable."

Objective: Orders for non–weight bearing and up in chair tid; Pillow between legs when side lying.

Goals/Expected Outcomes	Nursing Interventions	Selected Rationale	Evaluation
Patient will regain sufficient mobility to completely care for self at home within 3 mo.	Teach use of walker.	Proper use of walker will help prevent falls and injury.	PT will instruct in use of walker tomorrow.
	Encourage ROM and exercises to improve muscle strength and joint flexibility.	ROM helps prevent joint problems in unaffected joints.	Assisted to perform ROM on shoulders, upper extremities, and other leg.
		Exercises decrease muscle atrophy and help strengthen muscles for ambulation.	Encouraged ankle rotations and foot exercises on affected leg with supervision.

PROBLEM STATEMENT/NURSING DIAGNOSIS

Acute pain related to surgical incision and rehabilitation therapy.

SUPPORTING ASSESSMENT DATA

Subjective: "My pain is at a 6 on a scale of 1 to 10."

Objective: Face appears pinched, and patient is not moving in bed at all.

Goals/Expected Outcomes	Nursing Interventions	Selected Rationale	Evaluation
Patient will experience pain control with PCA pump within 1 h.	Reinforce instructions on PCA use.	Knowledge of how to use pump provides medication for pain control.	Reinforced instructions; encouraging PCA use as needed.
Patient will have adequate pain control on oral analgesia before discharge.	Assess for pain when vital signs are taken.	Constant monitoring for pain can indicate need for more medication to keep pain from escalating.	Pain level is 2–6/10.
	Administer medication bolus per orders PRN.	Administering a bolus of pain medication can stop pain from increasing.	Bolus administered for pain level of 6/10.
	Monitor for excessive sedation, respiratory depression, decreased LOC, and confusion.	Excessive sedation, respiratory depression, decreased LOC, and confusion can indicate medication toxicity and danger for the patient.	No signs of problems of toxicity or CNS depression.
	Provide comfort measures: keep linens smooth and clean, reposition q2h and PRN, keep environment quiet and orderly. Keep warm with added warmed blankets. Put on socks if feet are cold.	Comfort measures and warmth help decrease pain perception.	Provided comfort measures. Replaced warm blankets q2h, as needed. Socks with slip-resistant soles applied.

PROBLEM STATEMENT/NURSING DIAGNOSIS

Insufficient knowledge related to precautions necessary after total hip replacement to prevent dislocation of operative hip.

Continued

Nursing Care Plan 32.1 Care of a Patient After a Total Hip Replacement—cont'd

SUPPORTING ASSESSMENT DATA

Subjective: "No one I know has had this surgery."

Goals/Expected Outcome	Nursing Interventions	Selected Rationale	Evaluation
Patient will verbalize movement restrictions to prevent hip dislocation within 24 h.	Explain positional restrictions: no flexion of the hip past 90 degrees, no internal rotation, limited abduction of the affected leg.	Extreme flexion or internal rotation of the leg may cause hip dislocation. Knowledge is necessary to comply with instructions.	Explained position restrictions.
	Advise not to cross the legs or to bend over from the hips to tie shoes or pick up something off the floor.	These maneuvers cause internal rotation and more than 90 degrees of flexion.	Advised about additional restrictions after discharge. Written instructions given.
	Instruct to only use a raised toilet seat for toileting.	Normal-height toilet seat may cause too much flexion.	States has raised toilet seat at home. Knows to use handicapped toilet stalls when out in public.
	Advise to report pain in hip, buttock, or thigh or continued limp.	Pain or continued limp may indicate dislocation.	Verbalizes understanding of symptoms to report.

PROBLEM STATEMENT/NURSING DIAGNOSIS

Potential for altered tissue perfusion secondary to DVT.

SUPPORTING ASSESSMENT DATA

Objective: Decreased mobility and total hip replacement.

Goals/Expected Outcome	Nursing Interventions	Selected Rationale	Evaluation
Patient will not experience DVT before discharge.	Encourage foot and calf exercises q2h.	Encourages circulation and helps prevent clot formation.	Performing exercises q2h while awake.
	Assist and encourage in prescribed physical therapy.	—	Working with PT.
	Administer low-molecular-weight heparin injections as prescribed.	Decreases ability of blood to clot.	Heparin injections administered into abdomen as prescribed.
	Assess for signs of thrombus formation, checking calf for warmth, swelling, and pain on foot dorsiflexion.	Finding a thrombus early aids in preventing further extension of clot and preventing embolus.	No redness, swelling, warmth, or pain in affected leg's calf.

CRITICAL THINKING QUESTIONS

1. Besides venous thrombosis, what other complications might occur in this patient?
2. If the patient is anxious about discharge, what could you specifically do to help dispel her anxiety?

CNS, Central nervous system; *DVT,* deep vein thrombosis; *LOC,* level of consciousness; *PCA,* patient-controlled analgesia; *PRN,* as needed; *PT,* physical therapist; *ROM,* range of motion; *tid,* three times a day.

Focused Assessment

Data Collection for a Patient With Rheumatoid Arthritis

During history taking, ask about:

- Pain pattern and pain medication use; other coping methods
- Degree of stiffness and duration after arising
- Family history of rheumatoid arthritis or immune disorders
- Diagnosis of accompanying disorders, such as interstitial lung disease, pericarditis, eye problems, and vasculitis
- Smoking history
- Fatigue level and degree of malaise and methods of coping
- Presence of fever
- Exercise pattern
- Ability to perform ADLs; ability to work; ability for home maintenance
- Adaptive equipment in use
- Usual roles at work, home, and community and social involvement
- Joint deformity or swelling of joints
- Symmetric involvement from one side of the body to the other
- Pain and degree of limitation with joint movement

- Patient's mobility will improve with the use of assistive devices and physical therapy within 3 weeks.
- Patient will demonstrate acceptance of self and appearance by maintaining a clean, neat appearance.
- Patient will not experience a fall.
- Patient will need adequate rest.

Plan extra time for patients with arthritis to perform self-care and to ambulate. Rushing the patient causes frustration and embarrassment. Even simple procedures will probably take longer because the patient may not be able to move and turn as easily as a person without arthritis.

◆ IMPLEMENTATION AND EVALUATION

Nursing interventions for arthritis are aimed at providing a balance of rest and exercise, providing freedom from pain, minimizing emotional stress, preventing or correcting deformities, and maintaining or restoring function so that the patient can enjoy as much independence and mobility as possible.

Rest and Exercise

The purpose of rest is to allow the body's natural defenses and healing powers to overcome the inflammatory process of arthritis. The more inflamed a joint is, the more rest is needed; this includes rest of the joint and the whole body. Fatigue is a common problem with arthritis and usually requires that the patient has rest periods during the day before they become too fatigued or exhausted. During periods of acute exacerbation of arthritis symptoms, the patient may need continuous bed rest. When the patient is lying down, they should maintain good body position and avoid pillows and other devices that support joints in a position of flexion. A firm mattress is recommended, with only one pillow under the head and neck.

It is necessary, however, even in the acute phase of arthritis, to balance rest with exercise. The patient should sit to do tasks whenever possible. Activities should be paced and interspersed with rest. An exercise program is prescribed based on assessment of the patient's status, the severity of inflammation, the particular joints affected by arthritis, and the patient's tolerance for activity. Because anemia and other blood disorders can accompany arthritis, the fatigue experienced by a patient may be somewhat alleviated by correcting underlying blood disorders.

Enlist the patient's cooperation to increase compliance with exercises that must be continued at home. Teach the patient how to perform specific exercises so that they do not increase pain. Each exercise should be done 3 to 10 times for each joint, with the lower number used on days when pain or fatigue is increased. When joints are inflamed, exercises should not be done. In many instances, doing the exercises in the right way can diminish discomfort. If pain persists for hours after exercises have been done, the patient's status should be reassessed and the exercise program revised. Precautions to prevent joint injury are always necessary for routine physical activities, general exercise, or a prescribed exercise program at home.

Patient Teaching

Instructions for Joint Protection

- Always stop an exercise at the point of real pain. Some discomfort can be expected, but it should be minimal. If your joints are still hurting 1 or 2 hours after exercise, you have done too much.
- Always use your biggest muscles and strongest joints. For example, push doors open with your arm instead of your hand; carry a shoulder bag instead of a hand purse.
- Try to do only those jobs that will allow you to stop and rest if you need to when pain develops. Conserve your energy for the things you really want to do.
- Exercise in a way that does not put strain on the joints. Exercising in water decreases joint strain.
- Slow down and move slowly and smoothly. Avoid rapid, jerky movements. Use the palms of the hands rather than the fingers to push up from a bed or chair when arising.
- Turn doorknobs counterclockwise (or clockwise if left-handed) to prevent extensive twisting of the elbow. Do not lift weights. Pick up heavier items with two hands.
- Let swollen, red, hot, and painful joints rest as much as possible. Do not use them any more than necessary.
- Change your body position frequently, alternating standing, sitting, and lying down.
- Set your own limits and compete with yourself, not with anyone else.
- Use assistive/adaptive devices, such as Velcro closures and built-up utensil handles, to protect joints of the hands. Use a long-handled hair brush.

Applications of Heat and Cold

Either hot or cold is suitable for treating arthritic joints, depending on the patient's preference and the effectiveness of each. The purpose of either hot or cold applications is to minimize pain, increase the joint's ROM, and improve exercise performance. In general, heat is better for subacute or chronic joint inflammation, and cold is more effective in the acute phase when joints are hot, red, and obviously inflamed.

Various forms of heat therapy can be used, including moist or dry heat and superficial or deep heat. For dry heat, a therapeutic infrared lamp is convenient and inexpensive for home use. For treatment of the hands, paraffin baths are effective. Wet heat can be applied by hot tub baths with the water temperature not exceeding 102° F (39° C) or by means of a towel dipped in hot water, wrung out, and applied to the joint. Whirlpool baths promote relaxation and motion with minimal pain, especially when prolonged treatment is indicated. However, immersing the whole body in warm water can cause physiologic changes in respiration and pulse rate and may be contraindicated in debilitated patients or older adults. The patient will need specific instructions on how to prevent injury to the skin and other hazards.

Safety Alert

Caution With Heat Application

Patients who have decreased sensation in a body part must be very careful when applying heat, or they may experience burns. Teach the family and patient to test the degree of heat being applied and to check the area after 5 minutes to make certain that burning is not occurring. A cloth should always be placed between the heat device and the skin.

Think Critically

If a patient asks about using a heating pad on a joint, what instructions would you give?

Diet

No special diet will cure or relieve arthritis, despite many claims to the contrary. However, some patients find that eliminating foods from the "nightshade" family, such as tomatoes, decreases their joint pain. The patient should eat an average, well-balanced diet with no excess or limitations in amount or types of foods. Explain that obesity can put additional stress on the weight-bearing joints and aggravate the arthritic condition; then help the patient review strategies for weight control.

Psychosocial Care

Chronic illness can be exhausting and depressing, causing social isolation. Evaluate the patient's coping ability and help with referrals to support groups, counseling, and social activities. As deformities occur, self-esteem can be affected. Encourage verbalization of feelings. Express acceptance of the patient's appearance. Suggest clothing options that may minimize visible changes. A support group sometimes helps reframe the disease's effects on the body. Encourage patients with arthritis to gain as much control over the disease as possible with appropriate coping mechanisms, pacing of activity, exercise, and medication.

Resources for Patient and Family Education

The Arthritis Foundation provides some excellent printed material written with the layperson in mind. Another source of information is the National Institute of Arthritis and Musculoskeletal and Skin Diseases (NIAMS) at the National Institutes of Health (NIH).

GOUT

Etiology and Pathophysiology

Gout is arthritis of a joint caused by high serum levels of uric acid. Uric acid crystals precipitate from the body fluids and settle in joints and connective tissue. Gout affects men more than women and generally occurs during middle age. It is more common among

Patient Teaching

Safe Application of Heat and Cold

HEAT

- Recommended for chronic or subacute inflammation.
- Heat should be used for 20 to 30 minutes at a time; repeat the application every 1 to 2 hours while awake.
- Use a shower massager for massage pulsation. Regulate water by turning on cold and adding hot water to desired temperature *before* entering the shower. Use a shower stool if balance is poor or fatigue is likely.
- Use a pad between the heat source and the skin to prevent burning.
- Use a heating pad that provides moist heat; it will penetrate best. Do not sleep on the heating pad. Use the low settings because heating pads often cause burns when turned up too high or used for too long.
- Reusable heat packs mold well to body parts because they are pliable. Follow directions explicitly, and test temperature by feeling the pack against the skin before applying it to the area in need. Use a light pad or thin dishtowel between the pack and skin. Heat in a microwave oven. Reheat as needed.
- Heat-producing ointments and gels containing menthol, camphor, capsaicin, or papain (extract from red peppers) may be applied to the sore muscle or joint as long as they do not produce skin irritation. Covering the area with plastic wrap after application helps hold the heat in longer. Wash hands thoroughly after application to prevent eye irritation.

COLD

- Recommended for acute phase of inflammation or acute pain.
- Do not apply to one area for more than 10 to 20 minutes at a time; apply no more than once an hour.
- Discontinue when numbness occurs.
- Not recommended for patients with impaired circulation.
- An ice water bath is useful for a hand or foot. The extremity can be exercised during treatment.
- An ice pack can be made by partially filling a double plastic bag with ice. Zip-type closures work best. A thin pad or dishtowel may be used between the pack and skin.
- Commercial cold packs mold to body parts better than do ice bags but do not stay cold for very long. Often two of these are needed to finish a 10- to 20-minute treatment. Commercial cold packs can be refrozen in the freezer. Disposable chemical packs that are activated when needed are also available. Bags of frozen peas make a good cold pack for some joints.
- Freeze ice in a paper cup; peel back part of cup to use as a hand grip. Wear a rubber glove or use a pad to protect the hand from the ice. Rub ice over the body part until skin feels numb but for no longer than 10 to 15 minutes at a time.
- Dry skin well after treatment.

populations that consume a high-protein diet. Two factors seem to be implicated: (1) a genetic increase in purine metabolism leading to overproduction or retention of uric acid and (2) consumption of a high-purine diet. Excessive alcohol consumption causes an increased production of keto acids that inhibit uric acid excretion, causing hyperuricemia. Deposits of urate crystals occur in joints and subcutaneous tissues and can cause kidney stones. The big toe is the most common site, but many other joints can be affected. Diuretic therapy may cause a secondary gout from fluid loss that increases the serum uric acid level in the body. Certain drug therapies interfere with uric acid excretion and can cause a secondary gout. Pseudogout is caused by calcium pyrophosphate crystals and is also called calcium pyrophosphate disease. The symptoms, pathophysiology, and acute treatment are very similar to those for gout, but the underlying causes are different.

Signs and Symptoms

Typical signs and symptoms are elevated serum uric acid and tight, reddened skin over an inflamed, edematous joint, accompanied by elevated temperature and extreme pain in the joint (see Fig. 32.7).

Diagnosis, Treatment, and Nursing Management

History and physical examination are usually sufficient to lead to a high suspicion of gout, but an arthrocentesis is needed to confirm the diagnosis. The aspirated fluid is examined for crystals, cultured, and analyzed. It is important to rule out septic arthritis as a cause of the symptoms because it can cause joint destruction within 24 hours without treatment. Serum uric acid level is usually ordered, but its elevation is not diagnostic for gout. Many patients with active gout have normal uric acid levels. Imaging studies are not helpful for diagnosis in the early stages of the disease. Renal function studies will be done prior to initiating drug therapies. Treatment during acute attacks consists of administration of NSAIDs for 2 to 5 days for the pain. Colchicine given orally may bring dramatic pain relief within 24 to 48 hours. Oral prednisone or cortisone injection into the joint may be used. Allopurinol (Zyloprim), probenecid (Benemid), lesinurad (Zurampic), or febuxostat (Uloric) may be prescribed to prevent further attacks. An IV infusion of pegloticase (Krystexxa) may be used in patients who do not respond to other therapies. Teach the patient about gout medication side effects and dosage. Advise that dietary management includes weight control and restriction of high-purine foods, such as anchovies, sardines, sweetbreads, liver, bacon, kidneys, and venison. Alcohol should be restricted. All forms of ingestible alcohol contain high levels of purine. Remind patients who take allopurinol that periodic liver function testing is needed because this drug can cause liver failure. Teach the patient that a fluid intake of 2000 to 3000 mL per day is needed to protect the kidneys from urate crystal deposits and to prevent kidney stones.

Older Adult Care Points

Older adults with decreased creatinine clearance should not take allopurinol. When the patient has both hypertension and gout, losartan (Cozaar) may be a good choice for therapy. Losartan promotes urate excretion.

OSTEOPOROSIS

Etiology and Pathophysiology

Osteoporosis makes the person more susceptible to fractures because of the decrease in bone mass. Fragility fractures are often **atraumatic** (occur without trauma). In the United States 10.2 million people have osteoporosis, and another 43 million have **osteopenia** (low bone mass) (Oleson, 2017). Osteoporosis causes more disability and the shortening of life than rheumatoid arthritis. In many cases it is underdiagnosed and undertreated (Chicea, 2018). There is a hereditary tendency for osteoporosis. Risk factors for osteoporosis include age, chronic disease (e.g., liver, lung, kidney), medications (e.g., steroids, anticonvulsants, anticoagulants, PPIs, selective serotonin reuptake inhibitors), long-term calcium deficiency, vitamin D deficiency, smoking, excessive caffeine or alcohol intake, and sedentary lifestyle. Eating disorders and inflammatory bowel disease lead to osteoporosis because they interfere with nutrition and absorption. The risk of osteoporosis increases considerably in women after menopause because estrogen production is reduced.

Older Adult Care Points

Public awareness of osteoporosis for older women has increased, in large part because the pharmaceutical industry has marketed drugs for prevention of osteoporosis and fragility fractures. However, older adult men have hormone changes around the age of 70 years; this increases their risk for osteoporosis. Older men should be assessed for risk factors and undergo diagnostic testing (NIH, 2015).

Signs and Symptoms

Osteoporosis is a silent disease, and there are no early signs or symptoms. Once the patient has developed osteoporosis, height loss, kyphosis (excessive curvature of the spine), and back pain may occur. Compression fractures of the spine may cause debilitating pain. Osteoporosis is commonly diagnosed after the patient sustains a fracture from little or no known trauma.

Older Adult Care Points

In a recent publication, the U.S. Preventive Services Task Force (USPSTF, 2018) stated that 21% to 30% of patients who experience a hip fracture die within 1 year of the injury. Women have higher rates of osteoporosis, but men have higher rates of death related to fractures.

Diagnosis

On radiographs the bone of the patient with osteoporosis appears porous. Dual-energy x-ray absorptiometry

(DEXA) and quantitative computed tomography (QCT) are used to assess bone density. DEXA is reported as a T-score. QCT of the hip produces measurements in g/cm^2 that are equivalent to T-scores from DEXA, but the correlation has not been validated.

- *Normal bone density:* T-score of greater than 1 standard deviation from a healthy young adult
- *Osteopenia:* T-score of –2.5 or more
- *Osteoporosis:* T-score below –2.5

Treatment

Treatment is aimed at stopping loss of bone density, increasing bone formation, and preventing fractures. Adequate dietary or supplemental calcium and vitamin D in combination with weight-bearing exercise are standard treatments.

Nutrition Considerations

Nutrition for Bone Growth and Density

Adequate amounts of calcium and phosphorus are essential for bone growth and density. Although green vegetables are a source of calcium, that calcium is not readily absorbed. Dairy products such as cheese, yogurt, and milk are better choices. Canned sardines or salmon also provide good amounts of calcium. Calcium supplementation is not recommended for the healing of fractures. It has proven not to be readily absorbed and tends to cause kidney stones.

Calcium supplements, if required, should be taken in divided doses during the day. Exposure to sufficient sunlight or vitamin D supplementation is necessary for the proper absorption and metabolism of the calcium. Current guidelines recommend 800 to 4000 units of vitamin D per day (ConsumerLab, 2019). Vitamin K is important to bone health as well, and most people obtain vitamin K by eating greens. Daily weight-bearing exercise can decrease the chance of developing osteoporosis. Walking down stairs seems to be especially helpful, but walking for 30 minutes three times a week is sufficient.

Salicylates and NSAIDs are prescribed to control back pain. A back brace may be ordered for a patient who has had vertebral compression fractures. The bisphosphonates (i.e., Fosamax or Boniva; Box 32.2), which are related to a bone resorption–inhibiting substance found naturally in the body, and hormone therapy are prescribed in addition to calcium and vitamin D supplements for those with osteoporosis. Treatment for 5 years with the bisphosphonates alendronate (Fosamax), risedronate (Actonel), zoledronic acid (Reclast), or RANKL inhibitor denosumab (Prolia) is recommended in women and men with known osteoporosis (Qaseem et al., 2017). Other classes of medications include parathyroid hormone, bone formation agents, and selective receptor modulators. Miacalcin or Fortical nasal spray, which contains calcitonin, slows the rate of bone loss. The spray is used with adequate calcium and vitamin D supplementation.

Box 32.2 Drugs Commonly Used to Treat Osteoporosis

HORMONES

- Raloxifene (Evista) (selective estrogen receptor modulator)
- Testosterone (men)
- Calcitonin (Miacalcin) (synthetic hormone; used only in patients who are not candidates for first-line therapies)
- Teriparatide (Forteo) (synthetic parathyroid hormone)
- Abaloparatide (Tymlos) (synthetic parathyroid hormone)

BISPHOSPHONATES

- Alendronate (Fosamax)
- Risedronate (Actonel, Atelvia)
- Ibandronate (Boniva)
- Zoledronic acid (Zometa, Reclast)
- Monoclonal antibody
- Denosumab (Prolia)

GENERAL NURSING IMPLICATIONS FOR BISPHOSPHONATES

- Monitor bone density test results.
- Must take regularly (weekly or monthly).
- Observe for hypercalcemia (paresthesias, twitching, colic, or laryngospasm).
- Take with 8 oz of plain water in A.M. 30 to 60 minutes before eating, drinking, or taking any other medication that day (timing depends on the drug).
- Swallow the tablet whole. Do not suck or chew on it.
- Remain upright for 30 to 60 minutes after dose to prevent esophageal irritation (timing depends on the drug). Do not eat or drink anything during these 30 to 60 minutes.
- Store medication in a cool location out of sunlight.
- If dose is missed, skip the dose; do not take it later in the day. For the weekly dose medication, take it the next morning after your scheduled dose. Skip the dose if it has been 2 days since it was supposed to be taken and resume the original schedule. If taking Boniva, take it the next morning after you remember you forgot to take it. Do not take two tablets in any 1 week; wait at least 7 days to take the next dose and then resume your original schedule.
- Take calcium and vitamin D supplements as recommended by the health care provider.
- Perform weight-bearing exercise to increase bone density.
- Advise the health care provider if pregnant or planning a pregnancy.

Intravenous zoledronic acid (Zometa) or denosumab (Prolia) may be used for prevention of osteoporosis and long bone fractures in patients with prostate cancer who are receiving radiation and hormonal therapy. The drug can also be used for men who do not tolerate oral bisphosphonates well (Liede et al., 2018).

Treatment of vertebral fracture. Vertebral compression fractures are common in patients with osteoporosis. These are often treated with pain medication, activity limitation, physical therapy, and bracing. There are two minimally

Safety Alert

Caution With Bisphosphonate Drugs

There have been some rare instances of jawbone necrosis in patients who have been taking bisphosphonate drugs. If a dental implant or extraction is planned prior to implementation of bisphosphates, delaying therapy is appropriate until healing is complete. There is also some concern that bisphosphonates increase the risk of femur fracture. Esophageal irritation or erosion can occur if the patient does not remain in an upright position for 1 hour after taking a bisphosphonate drug (Rosen, 2018). Patients should be reminded that adverse side effects are varied and any new onset of unusual signs or symptoms should be reported to the health care provider. These drugs should be stopped after 5 years.

invasive vertebral augmentation procedures for those who do not respond to the conservative therapies or whose pain cannot be controlled. **Vertebroplasty** involves the percutaneous injection of polymethyl methacrylate (PMMA), a bone cement, directly into an osteoporotic spinal area under fluoroscopy. This stabilizes the bone and helps reduce or eliminate pain. **Kyphoplasty** consists of the percutaneous insertion of an inflatable device into the fractured vertebral body under fluoroscopy. The device is inflated, elevating the end plates and restoring the vertebral body toward its original height. Thick PMMA is then injected under low pressure into the cavity. The device is deflated and removed. This provides pain relief and reduces kyphosis (Bethel, 2018).

NURSING MANAGEMENT

ASSESSMENT (DATA COLLECTION)

Assessment for risk factors for osteoporosis should be performed with every general health assessment. Data are gathered about family history of osteoporosis, use of steroid medication, diet, exercise pattern throughout life, and history of smoking and alcohol intake.

NURSING DIAGNOSIS AND PLANNING

The main problem is potential for injury due to possible fracture from thinning of the bone. The expected outcome would be "Patient will not experience a fracture during their lifetime."

IMPLEMENTATION AND EVALUATION

Nursing care is focused on promoting screening for osteoporosis and teaching about the benefits of a healthy lifestyle, the need for sufficient intake of calcium and vitamin D, and the advantages of weight-bearing exercise. Educating about the harmful effects of smoking and excessive alcohol intake is also important. For the patient with osteoporosis, teach about the medications prescribed for the disorder and their side effects and measures to halt or reverse the disease process. Teach the patient when to report medication side effects to the health care provider.

PAGET DISEASE

Paget disease is a problem of abnormal bone resorption followed by replacement of normal marrow with fibrous connective tissue. The abnormal bone is weak and prone to fractures. The cause of Paget disease is unknown, although it does occur in clusters in some families. Often the disease is found at the time a fracture occurs, when radiographs reveal the abnormality of the bone. Diagnosis is by radiograph and laboratory testing. A 24-hour urine collection for urinary pyridinoline collagen cross-link assay, which indicates osteoclastic activity, may be performed. Serum alkaline phosphatase is elevated if the disease is active. The main problem is pain. Miacalcin or a bisphosphonate may be given to slow bone resorption. Orthopedic care is given for fractures and necessary joint replacements. A firm mattress, wearing a corset or light brace to relieve back pain, and proper body mechanics are essential. The patient should avoid lifting or twisting.

BONE TUMORS

Etiology and Pathophysiology

Bone is subject to both benign and malignant tumors. Tumors arise from several different types of tissue, including cartilage (chondromas), bone (osteomas), and fibrous tissue (fibromas). Benign tumors often are found on radiograph or at the time of fracture.

Malignant bone tumors are either primary or secondary to metastatic disease. Diagnosing and treating cancer in other parts of the body early can prevent the occurrence of metastases to the bone. Primary malignant bone tumors are most common among people 10 to 25 years of age. The most common type is osteosarcoma, or osteogenic sarcoma. The tumors grow rapidly and metastasize. More than half of cases affect the knee area. However, the distal femur, humerus, and proximal tibia are other common sites of occurrence. Osteosarcoma may occur in men older than 60 years as a complication of Paget disease. Other types of primary malignant tumors include Ewing sarcoma, chondrosarcoma, and fibrosarcoma.

Signs, Symptoms, and Diagnosis

Signs and symptoms of malignant bone tumor include pain, warmth, and swelling. Metastatic bone tumors greatly outnumber primary bone malignancies. Malignancies of the prostate, kidney, thyroid, breast, and lung commonly metastasize to bone. Sites of metastases are usually the vertebrae, pelvis, ribs, and femur. Diagnosis of bone tumor is by physical exam, radiograph, bone scan, and biopsy.

Treatment and Nursing Management

Treatment for malignant bone tumors includes surgery, radiation, chemotherapy, and targeted therapy. Chemotherapy is given for about 10 weeks before surgery and then for up to a year after surgery. A combination of chemotherapeutic agents is used depending on the tumor size, location, and health care provider decision (American Cancer Society, 2018). Zoledronic acid (Zometa) may be used to treat hypercalcemia associated with bone tumors.

Nursing management includes helping the patient with the anxiety and fear that accompanies the diagnosis of a bone tumor. Care of surgical patients is presented in Chapters 4 and 5, and Chapter 8 discusses care of cancer patients. If a bone tumor is in an extremity, amputation may be part of the treatment.

AMPUTATION

About 80% of all limb amputations involve the lower extremities. The most common reasons for amputation of a lower limb are related to peripheral vascular disease, often associated with diabetes mellitus, and resultant gangrene. Other conditions necessitating lower-limb amputation include severe trauma, malignancy, and congenital defects. Military injuries from shrapnel and land mines often result in amputation.

About 70% of upper-extremity amputations are brought on by crushing blows, thermal and electrical burns, and severe lacerations, many from military action. Vasospastic disease, malignancy, and infection also can necessitate amputation of an upper extremity.

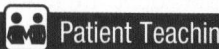

Patient Teaching

Care After Accidental Amputation

To care for a severed body part so that reattachment may be possible, do the following:

- Rinse the detached body part only enough to remove visible debris.
- Wrap the body part in a clean, damp cloth.
- Place the body part in a sealed plastic bag or in a dry, watertight container.
- Immerse the bag or container in a mixture of water and ice (3 parts water to 1 part ice). Do not let the body part get wet or freeze.
- Alternatively, place the container in an insulated cooler filled with ice.
- If no ice is available, keep the body part cool; do not expose it to heat.
- Tag the bag or container with the person's name and the name and location of the body part and take it to the hospital with the person.

With advances in technology, major improvements have been made in microvascular surgery, making reattachment or reimplantation of amputated parts possible. Teach the public what to do if an accidental amputation occurs.

Preoperative Care

If possible, the patient should participate in the decision to amputate a limb. They should understand the need for the amputation and what to expect postoperatively regarding pain, immobility, and readjustment to self-care. The patient needs to discuss realistic goals of rehabilitation with members of the rehabilitation team.

Although the loss of a limb can be very difficult for the patient and family to accept, it helps to know that the procedure is necessary and that every effort will be made to help the patient take full advantage of their remaining resources. The patient may experience stages of denial, anger, and so on, similar to those experienced with the dying process. In a sense, the patient must recognize the death of their former "self," work through the grief process, and move toward acceptance of a new body image.

"Phantom sensations" in the limb that has been removed are not unusual. The current hypothesis is that nerves in the spinal cord and brain "rewire" when the limb is lost and send pain messages to the brain (DerSarkissian, 2017). See Chapter 7 for further discussion of possible causes of phantom pain. The patient should be informed preoperatively that the sensations are not unusual and are not considered a psychiatric problem and that they should ask for help should the problem arise.

Physical preparation of the patient for amputation includes muscle-strengthening exercises to facilitate activity after amputation. These exercises are the first stages of the rehabilitation process, designed to help the patient achieve independence as rapidly as possible.

Postoperative Care

When the patient returns from the surgical suite, the two most immediate problems after amputation are hemorrhage and edema. To combat these problems, the stump is sometimes elevated for 24 to 48 hours. A lower extremity is not elevated for more than 24 hours because of the danger of hip contractures, which would prohibit rehabilitation efforts to achieve ambulation. The stump is checked at frequent intervals to determine whether bleeding is excessive. Fresh bleeding on the dressing should be reported immediately. When a ridged dressing has been placed over the incision, it is usually removable so that the surgical site can be assessed. Prophylactic antibiotics are given for 3 or 4 days, and wound drainage usually is handled with a wound drainage system. The incision should be dry, intact, and only slightly reddened along the suture line. The initial pressure dressing is removed by the surgeon 48 to 72 hours postoperatively (see Chapter 5).

Phantom limb sensations may or may not be painful. Intravenous infusion of ketamine early after amputation has been known to reduce or eliminate phantom pain in many patients. If the pain is severe or persists, various methods are used to control it. Another method is the use of transcutaneous electrical nerve stimulation (TENS). A device called a *stump stocking,* which is a silicone liner interwoven with an electromagnetic shield, works by blocking external electromagnetic impulses from outside sources. Those external impulses are believed to irritate nerve endings and trigger phantom

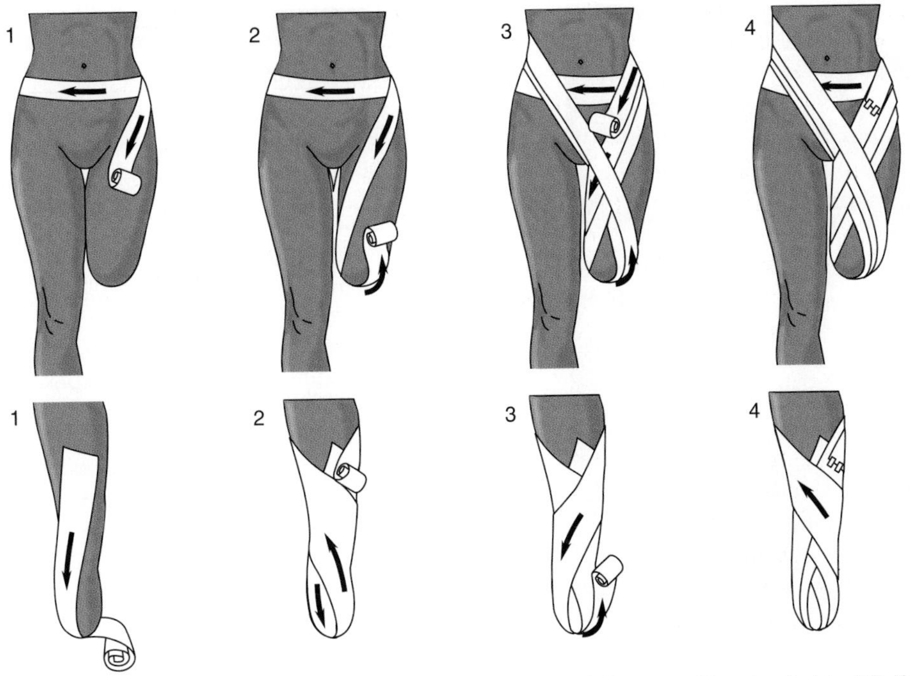

Fig. 32.11 A common method for wrapping a below-the-knee amputation (BKA) stump. (From Ignatavicius DD, Workman ML, et al.: *Medical-surgical nursing: concepts for interprofessional collaborative care,* ed 9, St. Louis, 2018, Elsevier.)

pain. A new treatment uses virtual reality goggles and a computer program to help visualize the limb as being whole (Mayo Clinic, 2018).

Three alternative modes for managing the stump after amputation are (1) soft dressing with delayed prosthetic fitting; (2) rigid plaster dressing and early prosthetic fitting; and (3) rigid plaster dressing and immediate prosthetic fitting. Each method has advantages and disadvantages. If a soft dressing is used, it is important that the stump be wrapped properly to control edema and ensure proper shrinkage of the stump for later fitting of a prosthesis. A pressure bandage wrapped in a figure-of-8 pattern is most common (Fig. 32.11). The bandage is anchored to the most proximal joint. It should be rewrapped three times a day, or whenever it is loose. A Jobst air splint may be used instead of the pressure bandage.

When the bandage is off, assess the skin for inflammation or breakdown. The skin should be pink in a light-skinned person and without discoloration. In a dark-skinned person, the skin should not be lighter or darker than other skin pigmentation. The skin should be warm but not hot. Skin breakdown on the stump is extremely serious because it interferes with prosthesis training and may prolong hospitalization and recovery. Patients with diabetes mellitus are particularly susceptible to skin complications because changes in sensation may obliterate the awareness of stump pain.

Many complications can be prevented if the patient is able to get up and about early in the postoperative period. However, weight bearing before the stump is adequately healed can cause weakening of the suture line and rupturing of the operative wound. A patient with a lower extremity amputation should lie prone for 20 to 30 minutes every 3 to 4 hours to prevent hip contracture until they are up and about regularly. The residual limb should be extended. Patients with amputations below the knee are better able to begin early walking and weight bearing than those whose limb has been amputated above the knee. The amputation of a limb displaces the body's center of gravity and interferes with the sense of balance. Adaptation to this change in the center of gravity occurs slowly, and the patient needs to be warned to move cautiously. When the prosthesis is off during the night, the patient may need assistance in turning until adjustment is made to the new center of gravity.

Proper positioning is required to prevent **abduction contractures.** ROM exercises are carried out with patients with an amputation as with any patient who must be protected from the disabilities resulting from immobility.

When a lower limb has been removed, the patient must learn how to balance on one leg, how to stoop and bend over without losing balance, and how to use the back muscles to maintain good posture while wearing an artificial limb. Teaching for self-care begins as soon as possible.

Rehabilitation

With the help of computer technology, prostheses that are a much better fit than ever before can be manufactured. Computerization has also provided a means of controlled movement of various parts of a prosthesis, allowing greater mobility and ease of performing ADLs. Usually both a physical therapist and an occupational therapist work with the patient who has suffered an

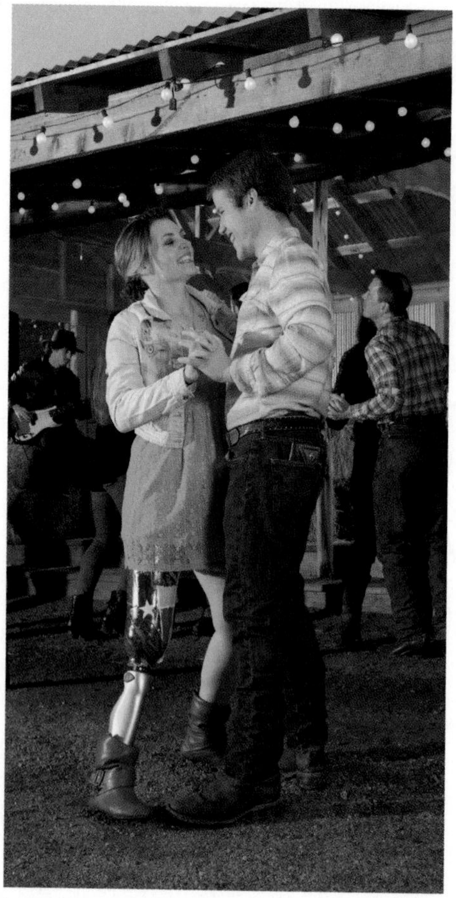

Fig. 32.12 C-leg prosthesis in action. (© Ottobock HealthCare LP, Minneapolis, Minn.)

Patient Teaching

Stump and Prosthesis Care

Instruct the patient in stump care as follows:

- Inspect the stump daily for redness, blistering, or abrasions.
- Use a mirror to examine all sides and aspects of the stump.
- Perform meticulous daily stump hygiene. Wash the stump with mild soap and water, then carefully rinse and dry it. Allow it to air-dry for 20 minutes. Apply nothing to the stump after it is bathed.
- During the healing process, protect the incision by wearing the removable rigid dressing (RRD).
- Put on the prosthesis immediately when arising and keep it on all day (once the wound has healed completely) to reduce stump swelling.
- Continue prescribed exercises to prevent weakness.
- Lay prone with hip extension for 30 minutes three or four times a day.
- For a lower extremity, replace shoes before wear becomes extreme because gait may be altered.

Care of the prosthesis includes the following:

- Remove sweat and dirt from the prosthesis socket daily by wiping the inside of the socket with a damp, soapy cloth. To remove the soap, use a clean, damp cloth. Dry the prosthesis socket thoroughly.
- Never attempt to adjust or mechanically alter the prosthesis. If problems develop, consult the prosthetist.
- Schedule a yearly appointment with the prosthetist.

Adapted from Lewis SM, Bucher L, Heitkemper MM, et al.: *Medical-surgical nursing: assessment and management of clinical problems,* ed 10, St. Louis, 2017, Elsevier.

amputation to help regain mobility, confidence, and the ability to handle ADLs. Assist with practice of bathing, shaving, dressing, and other ADLs.

Older adults and patients who are chronically ill can benefit from a positive yet realistic approach to problems related to amputation. The focus of attention should be on what the patient can do for themself and on what strengths they have. You can be of real assistance by helping the patient find short-range goals that can be accomplished without great difficulty and that indicate progress toward independence. For example, you can guide the patient toward devising ways in which personal needs such as bathing and grooming can be met. Later, give encouragement to sit up, exercise the other limbs, and assist with changing of the dressing. Finally, set a goal for wearing the prosthesis successfully and walking without assistance (Fig. 32.12; also see Chapter 9).

COMMUNITY CARE

Rehabilitation programs for patients with an amputation, arthritis, and other musculoskeletal disorders exist in most large cities and are being introduced into more communities through agencies such as the YMCA. The Arthritis Foundation has been instrumental in working with the YMCA to bring programs for exercise to local neighborhoods.

Outpatient rehabilitation programs through clinics work with patients who are regaining mobility and the ability to perform ADLs with a prosthesis. Rehabilitation is moving to a program "without walls," indicating a shift from an inpatient institute to rehabilitation in the home and community.

Home care nurses are particularly instrumental in preventing musculoskeletal injury in home care patients. The premises of the older adult are surveyed, and recommendations are made to make it safer for the patient. Flat, nonglare surfaces for walking, well-lit walkways, absence of loose rugs, installation of grab bars in showers and bathrooms, and use of communication systems to summon help are some of the measures instituted to protect older adults.

When a home care patient is on crutches, you should assess the patient's ability to go up and down stairs and to sit down and arise from the sitting position safely. Patient Teaching: Crutch Gaits in Chapter 31 presents the steps for performing these maneuvers correctly. Home care nurses must assess the capability and safety of older adults who are newly using assistive devices for ambulation and determine whether alterations in pathways in the home need to be made. Scatter rugs should be removed, and furniture may need to be rearranged to offer a path wide enough to allow the patient to move from one area to another.

Long-term care facility nurses survey patient units and group spaces daily to check for obstacles to ambulation and potential safety hazards. Slowly, our communities are becoming easier to navigate for older adults, and public places are becoming more accessible for individuals with handicaps and safer for frail older adults.

Get Ready for the NCLEX® Examination!

Key Points

- Sprains are treated with rest, ice, compression, and elevation (RICE).
- Bursitis occurs from injury or overuse.
- Carpal tunnel syndrome causes numbness, tingling, and pain in the hand.
- Fractures occur from trauma or metabolic disease. Signs and symptoms include pain, swelling, discoloration, and deformity in the contour of the bone. Complications include infection, osteomyelitis, fat embolism, venous thrombosis, and compartment syndrome.
- Compartment syndrome is an emergency situation. Signs and symptoms include edema, pallor, tingling, paresthesia, numbness, weak pulse, cyanosis, paresis, and severe pain.
- Osteoarthritis occurs asymmetrically and typically affects only one or two joints. Treatment consists of pain management, weight control, exercise, and maintenance of joint function.
- Rheumatoid arthritis is an inflammatory disease of the joints. Symptoms include joint pain, warmth, edema, limitation of motion, and joint stiffness and systemic symptoms, usually bilaterally. Treatment includes relieving pain, minimizing joint destruction, promoting joint function, and preserving the ability to perform self-care functions. Medications, rest, exercise, and applications of heat and cold are mainstays of treatment.
- Postoperative care after joint replacement is very important to prevent pain, prevent infection, prevent dislocation, and promote mobilization.
- DVT is a common complication of hip and knee joint replacement.
- Gout is caused by high serum levels of uric acid. Symptoms of gout are tight, reddened skin over an inflamed, edematous joint accompanied by elevated temperature and extreme pain in the joint.
- Calcium deficiency and estrogen depletion predispose to the development of osteoporosis, which increases susceptibility to fractures. Treatment includes calcium, vitamin D supplements, bisphosphonates, and other hormonal medications (see Box 32.2).
- The most common primary bone tumor is osteogenic sarcoma; many bone tumors are from metastasis of cancer elsewhere.
- Eighty percent of amputations involve the lower extremities. Hemorrhage and infection are complications of amputation. Proper stump care is essential to the success of rehabilitation.

Additional Learning Resources

SG Go to your Study Guide for additional learning activities to help you master this chapter content.

Go to your Evolve website (http://evolve.elsevier.com/deWit/medsurg) for the following FREE learning resources:
- Animations, audio, and video
- Answers and rationales for questions and activities
- Glossary with pronunciations in English and Spanish
- Interactive Review Questions and more!

Review Questions for the NCLEX® Examination

1. A young man is admitted to the emergency department after an injury to his left leg sustained playing football. He is complaining of pain around the knee and upper tibia. Which data from your assessment would indicate a fracture of the tibia rather than a connective tissue injury of the knee?
   1. Pain and soft-tissue swelling around the knee and an abrasion on the knee
   2. Pain, ecchymosis below the knee, and crepitation with any movement of the area
   3. Pain, swelling, and loss of function of the foot
   4. Limping when walking, facial grimace, and some swelling of the knee and lower leg

   NCLEX Client Need: Physiological Integrity: Physiological Adaptation
2. A 24-year-old woman limps into the emergency department after twisting her ankle during a soccer game. On examination, there is local swelling and difficulty maintaining balance. What immediate therapeutic measure(s) should you provide? *(Select all that apply.)*
   1. Application of elastic bandage
   2. Application of an ice pack
   3. Elevation of the ankle
   4. Ankle rest and limited weight bearing
   5. Application of a topical anesthetic

   NCLEX Client Need: Physiological Integrity: Physiological Adaptation
3. A patient with a plaster cast of the right arm complains of itching underneath the cast. What should you do to alleviate the symptom?
   1. Encourage deep breaths and scratch the other arm.
   2. Insert a cotton-tip applicator under the cast.
   3. Forcefully inject 50 mL of air underneath the cast.
   4. Administer pain medications.

   NCLEX Client Need: Physiological Integrity: Reduction of Risk Potential

4. You respond to a roadside emergency and find a middle-aged man with pain and tenderness over the left leg. You note a closed bone deformity with inability to move the leg. While waiting for the paramedics, what is the most important nursing action?
   1. Immobilization of the leg
   2. Realigning the bones
   3. Applying warm packs
   4. Elevating the extremity

   NCLEX Client Need: Physiological Integrity: Reduction of Risk Potential
5. A young adult patient has a fractured femur with internal fixation and a long-leg cast. Which signs of potential complications should you watch for? *(Select all that apply.)*
   1. Infection or osteomyelitis
   2. Compartment syndrome
   3. Pneumonia or stroke
   4. Pulmonary fat embolus
   5. Electrolyte imbalance
   6. Nonunion of bone

   NCLEX Client Need: Physiological Integrity: Reduction of Risk Potential
6. A difference in the postoperative care of a patient with a knee replacement compared with a patient with a hip replacement is that the patient with a hip replacement:
   1. has less chance of developing a deep vein thrombosis.
   2. has less difficulty with pain control.
   3. is allowed to stand at the bedside on the first postoperative day.
   4. has a CPM machine to exercise the joint.

   NCLEX Client Need: Physiological Integrity: Physiological Adaptation
7. You have just received shift report on four assigned orthopedic patients. Which patient should you check on first?
   1. A young trauma patient with a below-the-knee amputation who is having phantom pain
   2. An older adult woman with a total hip replacement who needs assistance with the bedpan
   3. A woman with an external fixation device who has a fever and foul odor at the pin sites
   4. A man with a full leg cast who reports persistent pain despite elevation and pain medication

   NCLEX Client Need: Safe and Effective Care Environment: Coordinated Care
8. You are assisting an older adult, in his or her home, who has rheumatoid arthritis in the hands and wrists. You would intervene to teach the patient about joint protection if the patient:
   1. turned the doorknob counterclockwise.
   2. used the palms of the hands to push up and off the bed.
   3. carried groceries into the house using both hands.
   4. pushed the door open with the arm.

   NCLEX Client Need: Physiological Integrity: Reduction of Risk Potential
9. You are caring for a 75-year-old female who is being treated for a new diagnosis of osteoporosis. What topics need to be included in discharge teaching? *(Select all that apply.)*
   1. Rationale for use and side effects of denosumab
   2. Diet recommendations for increased protein intake
   3. Calcium and vitamin D supplements
   4. Weight-bearing exercises
   5. Smoking cessation
   6. Heat and cold for symptom management

   NCLEX Client Need: Physiological Integrity: Pharmacological Therapies
10. A young patient returns from the operating room after a below-the-knee amputation and is alert and quiet. The stump is elevated, with the dressing dry and intact. What is the priority problem for this patient?
    1. Altered body image.
    2. Potential for bleeding.
    3. Altered mobility.
    4. Insufficient knowledge.

    NCLEX Client Need: Physiological Integrity: Reduction of Risk Potential
11. After sustaining a rotator cuff tear, a patient's arm is placed in a sling. The patient is instructed to rest and to take ibuprofen (Motrin) for pain. Which patient statement indicates a need for further teaching?
    1. "I will have less stomach upset if I take the pills with food."
    2. "I will not be able to play tennis for a while."
    3. "I need to rest in bed for the next 2 days."
    4. "The sling must be worn most of the time."

    NCLEX Client Need: Health Promotion and Maintenance
12. You are assuming recovery room care of a 52-year-old patient who had carpal tunnel repair. On receiving the patient, what is the priority nursing assessment?
    1. Sensation in the fingertips
    2. Color, warmth, and capillary refill
    3. Condition of the dressing
    4. Range of motion

    NCLEX Client Need: Physiological Integrity: Reduction of Risk Potential

Critical Thinking Questions

Scenario A

Mr. Patel, age 56 years, has been admitted to the hospital with a diagnosis of fracture of the left tibia. You have been told that when the patient returns from surgery, he will have an external fixation device in place.

1. How would you perform a neurovascular assessment?
2. How can you support the affected extremity?
3. What can you do to decrease swelling?
4. List the observations you must make while the fixation device is on Mr. Patel's leg.
5. What complications might occur?

Scenario B

Mrs. Hernandez, age 52 years, is a moderately obese woman who comes to the orthopedic clinic for treatment of arthritis of the knees and ankles. She has great difficulty walking and would use a wheelchair if she could afford one. Her daughter states that she is becoming more and more inactive and—though her mother says she does not want to become an invalid—she refuses to move about and do things for herself. Mrs. Hernandez lives alone and prefers not to live with her son because the grandchildren make her nervous. In fact, she prefers to be left alone because she feels that she cannot be of use to anyone. Her son feels that his mother could find many useful things to do in her neighborhood if she would only try.

1. How does obesity interact with arthritis in causing immobility?
2. What medications might decrease Mrs. Hernandez's pain?
3. What sort of exercise would be best for this patient?
4. How could you make Mrs. Hernandez feel more useful and motivate her to move about and get out of the house more often?

Scenario C

Mr. Gerhardt is a 78-year-old who is discharged home after a total hip replacement. You are assigned as his home care nurse to perform wound care, assess for complications, and monitor rehabilitation.

1. What teaching for self-care would you reinforce for Mr. Gerhardt on your first visit?
2. How would you determine whether the home environment is safe for Mr. Gerhardt?
3. Mr. Gerhardt is very depressed because he feels he will no longer be able to get out of the home to go fishing and visit with his friends. How would you approach the psychosocial aspects of his care?

Scenario D

During your daily run, you step on an irregular surface and twist your ankle. At home, you notice tenderness at the site, minimal swelling, and loss of function but no abnormal motion.

1. What first aid will you perform?
2. How will you know if you have a sprain or a fracture?

33 The Urinary System

http://evolve.elsevier.com/deWit/medsurg

Objectives

Theory

1. Illustrate the anatomy and physiology of the urinary system.
2. Differentiate the causes of urologic problems and disorders.
3. Discuss ways in which nurses can help patients prevent or cope with urologic disorders.
4. Examine the psychosocial effects of urinary incontinence.
5. Compare and contrast drugs for urinary incontinence with those for benign prostatic hypertrophy.

Clinical Practice

6. Identify nursing responsibilities in the preprocedure and postprocedure care of patients undergoing urologic diagnostic studies.
7. Perform initial and ongoing nursing assessment of a patient's urologic status, including laboratory data.
8. Describe five nursing responsibilities related to the care of a patient with an indwelling catheter.
9. Write a nursing care plan for a patient with urinary incontinence.

Key Terms

anuria (ă-NŪ-rē-ă, p. 797)
blood urea nitrogen (BUN) (blŭd ū-RĒ-ă NĪ-trō-jĕn, p. 789)
creatinine (krē-ĂT-ĭ-nēn, p. 787)
dysuria (dĭs-Ū-rē-ă, p. 797)
glomerular filtration rate (GFR) (glō-MĔR-(y)ĕ-lĕr fĭl-TRĀ-shŭn rāt, p. 787)
hematuria (hē-măt-Ū-rē-ă, p. 795)
micturition (mĭk-tū-RĬSH-ŭn, p. 788)
nephrotoxic (nĕf-rō-TŎK-sĭk, p. 795)
nocturia (nŏct-Ū-rē-ă, p. 797)
oliguria (ŏl-ĭ-GŪ-rē-ă, p. 797)
polyuria (pŏl-ē-Ū-rē-ă, p. 797)
proteinuria (prō-tēn-YŪR-ē-ă, p. 796)
residual urine (rē-ZĬ-dū-ăl Ū-rĭn, p. 797)
urinary frequency (Ū-rĭ-năr-ē FRĒ-kwĕn-cē, p. 797)
urinary hesitancy (Ū-rĭ-năr-ē HĔZ-ĭ-tăn-cē, p. 797)
urinary incontinence (Ū-rĭ-năr-ē ĭn-KŎN-tĭ-nĕns, p. 788)
urinary retention (Ū-rĭ-năr-ē rē-TĔN-shŭn, p. 797)
voiding (VŎYD-ĭng, p. 788)

Concepts Covered in This Chapter

- Self-Management
- Fluid and Electrolytes
- Acid-Base Balance
- Hormonal Regulation
- Elimination
- Inflammation
- Patient Education
- Collaboration
- Caregiving

ANATOMY AND PHYSIOLOGY OF THE UROLOGIC SYSTEM

STRUCTURES OF THE UROLOGIC SYSTEM AND HOW THEY INTERRELATE

- The kidneys, ureters, urinary bladder, and urethra are the structures of the urinary system (Fig. 33.1).
- The kidneys are bean-shaped organs positioned on either side of the vertebral column at the level of the first lumbar vertebra. The left kidney is slightly higher than the right one.
- The kidney consists of the cortex (outer layer), the medulla (inner layer), and the renal pelvis. The cortex contains blood vessels and nephrons, the medulla contains the collecting tubules, and the renal pelvis gathers the urine and directs it to the bladder (Fig. 33.2).
- The nephron is the functional unit of the kidney (there are 1 million nephrons in a kidney).
- The nephron consists of the glomerulus, which is a network of capillaries encased in a thin-walled sac called the *Bowman capsule,* and the tubular system.
- The tubular system of the nephron consists of the proximal convoluted tubule, the loop of Henle, the distal convoluted tubule, and the collecting duct (Fig. 33.3). Urine is carried by the ureters from the kidney to the bladder through peristaltic action.
- The bladder, a hollow muscular organ, serves as a reservoir for urine; the inner lining of the bladder is a mucous membrane.

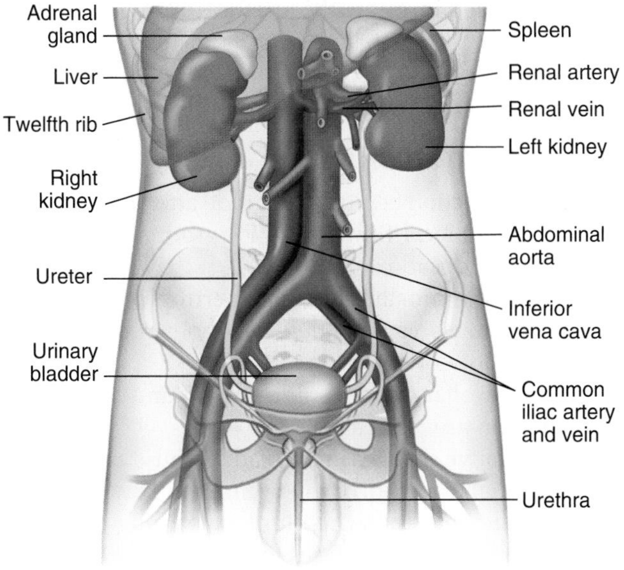

Fig. 33.1 Structures of the urinary system. (From Patton KT, Thibodeau GA: *Human body in health and disease,* ed 9, St. Louis, 2018, Elsevier.)

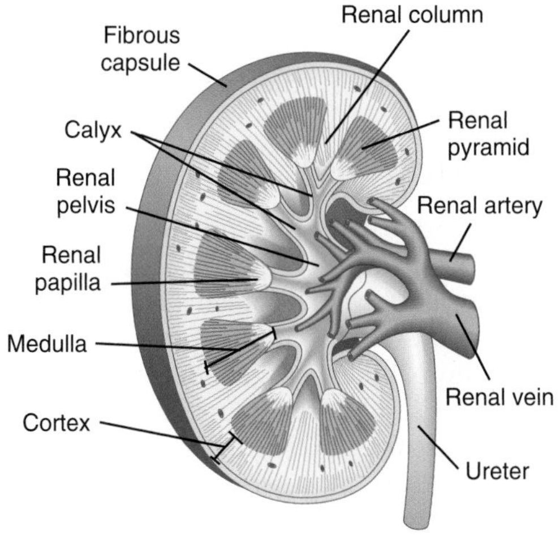

Fig. 33.2 Structures of the kidney. (From Lewis SL, Bucher L, Heitkemper MM, et al.: *Medical-surgical nursing: assessment and management of clinical problems,* ed 10, St. Louis, 2017, Elsevier.)

- The walls of the bladder are smooth muscle called detrusor muscle that expands to store urine and contracts to expel urine.
- The urine passes from the bladder down the urethra, which is approximately 3 to 5 cm long in women and 20 cm long in men.
- The internal, involuntary urethral sphincter is controlled by the detrusor muscle in the wall of the bladder.
- The external urethral sphincter voluntarily controls release of urine to the outside.
- Blood is brought to the kidney by the renal arteries that branch off the aorta. Blood is returned by veins to the inferior vena cava.

FUNCTIONS OF THE KIDNEYS

- The kidneys regulate serum electrolytes by filtration and reabsorption (Table 33.1).

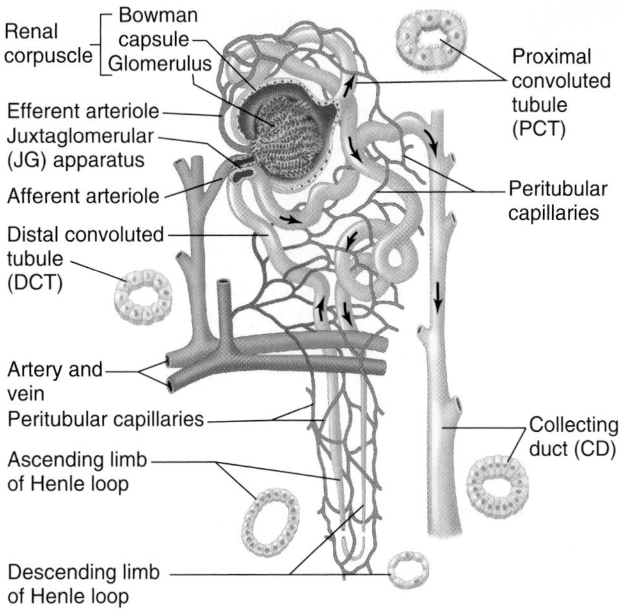

Fig. 33.3 The nephron. (From Patton KT, Thibodeau GA: *Human body in health and disease,* ed 9, St. Louis, 2018, Elsevier.)

- The kidneys eliminate metabolic wastes by filtration; 20% of the blood flowing through the glomerulus is filtered at any one time.
- Each nephron filters blood plasma through the semipermeable glomerular membrane.
- **Glomerular filtration rate (GFR)** is the amount of blood filtered by the glomeruli in a given time (average GFR is about 125 mL/min).
- The kidneys regulate fluid volume by filtration, reabsorption, and excretion.
- Most of the water and some of the electrolytes are reabsorbed into the bloodstream in the descending and distal convoluted tubules.
- The kidneys assist in maintaining acid-base balance by secreting hydrogen ions into the urine.
- Unwanted substances—urea, **creatinine** (waste products of protein metabolism and skeletal muscle contraction, respectively), and uric acid—are retained in the tubules along with some water.
- Approximately 200 L of liquid are filtered in a 24-hour period; 1.5 to 2 L are excreted as urine.
- The kidneys regulate blood pressure by secreting the enzyme renin.
- The kidneys increase red blood cell production by secreting erythropoietin.
- The kidneys metabolize vitamin D into an active form.

REGULATION OF FLUID BALANCE

- In response to low blood flow to the kidney, the juxtaglomerular cells release renin, which joins with angiotensin to form angiotensin I.
- Angiotensin-converting enzyme (ACE), produced by the lungs, changes angiotensin I to angiotensin II. Angiotensin II causes peripheral vasoconstriction, resulting in more blood flow to the kidney.

Table 33.1 Hormones and Metabolic Actions Associated With Kidney Function

HORMONES	ACTION
Circulating in the Blood to Influence Urine Volume and Concentration	
Aldosterone	Increases the reabsorption of sodium and excretion of potassium
Antidiuretic hormone (ADH)	Increases permeability in the tubules and reabsorption of water
Atrial natriuretic hormone	Increases the excretion of sodium
Brain or B natriuretic hormone	Increases the excretion of sodium
Produced by the Kidney	
Erythropoietin	Stimulates the bone marrow to increase red blood cell (RBC) production; increased production of erythropoietin is triggered by a demand for oxygen or when RBC level falls below normal
Calcitriol (active vitamin D)	Increases absorption of calcium and phosphorus
Renin	Assists in the regulation of blood pressure
Affecting Kidney Function	
Parathyroid hormone	Works in conjunction with calcitriol to increase absorption of calcium and phosphorus
Cortisol	Promotes sodium and water retention

- Angiotensin II also causes release of aldosterone from the adrenal glands, causing the kidneys to retain sodium and water and excrete potassium (see Chapter 17).
- Antidiuretic hormone (ADH) is released from the pituitary gland when fluid volume is low. It causes the kidney to conserve water.
- When adequate circulating volume is present, ADH is not released.

FUNCTIONS OF THE URETERS, BLADDER, AND URETHRA

- Each ureter is a small tube about 25 cm long; it carries urine from the renal pelvis to the bladder.
- The bladder holds the urine; normal capacity is 300 to 400 mL; maximum capacity may reach 1000 to 1800 mL.
- A feeling of bladder fullness and an initial signal to void (empty the bladder) occurs when the bladder contains 150 to 200 mL of urine.
- The **micturition** (voiding) reflex is then initiated and transmitted to the bladder. Urine then passes from the bladder through the urethra during urination (**voiding**).
- The flow of urine is controlled by the internal urethral sphincter and the external urethral sphincter.

AGING-RELATED CHANGES

- Kidney function begins to degrade after age 45 years, and renal blood flow and GFR gradually decrease with each decade.
- In men, the prostate gland hypertrophies with age and can cause varying degrees of obstruction to the normal flow of urine.
- Secretion of renin and aldosterone and vitamin D activation are decreased.
- Degenerative changes in the bladder muscles may lead to residual urine (incomplete emptying of urine) and **urinary incontinence** (involuntary passing of urine).
- Bladder capacity decreases to as little as 200 mL, and frequent emptying is needed.
- A decreased ability to concentrate urine leads to nocturia (urination during the night).
- Lowered estrogen levels in women result in tissue atrophy in the urethra, vagina, and trigone of the bladder (triangular portion at the base of the bladder), which predisposes to infection and incontinence.

THE UROLOGIC SYSTEM

The kidneys and urinary tract function to maintain the proper balance of fluids, minerals, and organic substances necessary for life. Problems in the heart, lungs, or circulatory system can arise from kidney disorders or kidney failure. Likewise, generalized diseases, such as atherosclerosis, other circulatory impairments, infections, or disturbances in the metabolic processes such as diabetes mellitus, may seriously impair the proper functioning of the kidneys.

DISORDERS OF THE UROLOGIC SYSTEM

Causes

The high volume of blood that is filtered by the kidney contains some bacteria. These bacteria can colonize the kidney, causing an infection. Also, bacteria can easily enter the urinary tract through the urethra, and the infection may spread up into the kidneys.

When an immune reaction occurs in the body, the glomeruli that filter the blood are exposed to antibodies and antigen–antibody complexes contained in that blood. These antibodies and antigen–antibody complexes can cause an autoimmune inflammatory reaction known as *glomerulonephritis* that damages the semipermeable glomerular membrane and interferes with normal kidney function.

Once urine is formed, the urinary system must be patent and unobstructed for urine to be excreted. Tumors may form in the bladder, ureters, or kidney and interfere with normal function by altering cell structure or impeding urine flow. Stones in the kidney or ureters may obstruct the flow of urine. In older men, an enlarged prostate may impede flow of urine through the urethra.

Tubular necrosis can be caused by lack of oxygen or bacterial or chemical destruction of cells, which affects the functional ability of the nephron and decreases kidney function. Many drugs can be toxic to the kidney, and heavy metals such as mercury can cause considerable damage.

Hypertension is a major cause of end-stage kidney disease; conversely, renal disorders can also cause secondary hypertension. Because so much of the kidney's function is directly related to the capillaries and arterioles, any disorder, such as atherosclerosis and diabetes mellitus, that systemically affects the blood vessels can affect the kidneys. When these vessels become **sclerosed** (hardened), blood flow through the kidney is decreased; kidney function diminishes, and eventually this leads to chronic renal failure. Reduced blood circulation related to decreased volume (e.g., hypovolemic shock) or decreased cardiac output (e.g., cardiogenic shock) puts the patient at risk for acute renal failure (ARF).

Patient Teaching

Kidney Health and Healthy Blood Vessels

For patients who have hypertension or diabetes mellitus, design a teaching session that will help them recognize that the atherosclerotic changes that occur in the blood vessels also cause decreased blood flow to the kidneys and eventually reduce kidney function. In accordance with the *Healthy People 2030* goals, emphasize that compliance with the treatment plan for hypertension or diabetes mellitus helps prevent kidney problems from occurring later in life.

Prevention

One of the best ways to prevent disorders of the urologic system is to drink an adequate amount of water. A minimum fluid intake of 2000 to 2500 mL/day is recommended to initiate good flow through the system. A healthful diet, exercise, and not smoking also promote urinary health.

Health Promotion

Bladder Health

Promote bladder and urinary tract health by encouraging patients to empty the bladder sooner rather than waiting to urinate. Emptying the bladder prevents urinary stasis and prolonged exposure of waste toxins on the bladder wall, which may contribute to cancer of the bladder. Delayed voiding also causes the bladder wall to stretch beyond normal capacity and places undue strain on the sphincters. Both can contribute to urinary incontinence later in life.

Controlling blood pressure and maintaining a normal serum glucose level can support healthy blood vessels. A good blood supply promotes good kidney function.

Carefully monitoring for adverse drug effects and avoiding the use of chemicals known to be harmful to the kidney help preserve optimal kidney function. Box 33.1 gives examples of substances that are toxic to the kidney. When drugs that can be harmful to the kidney—such as sulfa compounds—are prescribed, increasing the fluid intake to 3000 to 3500 mL/day reduces the risk of kidney dysfunction. (Increasing fluid intake must be carefully considered when the patient has other conditions, such as congestive heart failure or cirrhosis of the liver.)

Box 33.1 Examples of Potentially Nephrotoxic Substances

- Antiinfectives
  - Aminoglycosides (gentamicin, streptomycin)
  - Sulfonamides (trimethoprim-sulfamethoxazole)
  - Antifungals (amphotericin B)
  - Antitubercular (rifampin)
  - Cephalosporins (cefaclor)
  - Tetracyclines (doxycycline)
  - Miscellaneous (e.g., vancomycin, polymyxin B)
- ACE inhibitors (captopril)
- Antineoplastic agents (cisplatin, methotrexate)
- Immunosuppressants (cyclosporine)
- NSAIDs (salicylates, ibuprofen, indomethacin)
- Other drugs (acetaminophen, furosemide, phenazopyridine HCl, cimetidine)
- IV contrast media
- Heavy metals (lithium, gold salts, lead)
- Industrial (carbon tetrachloride for cleaning)
- Environmental (pesticides, snake venom)
- Recreational drugs (cocaine, heroin)

ACE, Angiotensin-converting enzyme; *IV,* intravenous; *NSAIDs,* nonsteroidal antiinflammatory drugs.

Patient Teaching

Over-the-Counter Drugs

Teach your patients to avoid routine use of over-the-counter drugs, such as nonsteroidal antiinflammatory drugs (NSAIDs) and acetaminophen, to decrease the possibility of hepatic or renal dysfunction through unnecessary exposure to chemicals. This is in accordance with National Patient Safety Goals—to actively involve patients in their own care to ensure safety.

Think Critically

What changes could you make in your dietary habits or lifestyle that might help prevent urologic problems?

Diagnostic Tests and Procedures

Patients experiencing problems with the urinary system undergo urine tests, such as a urinalysis and culture and sensitivity, and blood tests, such as a complete blood cell count (CBC), **blood urea nitrogen (BUN)**, serum creatinine, and creatinine clearance. Urea is produced when protein breaks down; it then combines with ammonia and is carried by the bloodstream to the kidneys for excretion. Creatinine is a by-product of skeletal muscle metabolism. BUN and serum creatinine are interpreted together, and laboratory values should be obtained before the use of radiologic contrast dyes. Creatinine clearance is a good measure of GFR. Cystatin C is a test used to evaluate GFR. Cystatin C is a low-molecular-weight proteinase inhibitor that is produced at a constant rate and filtered out by the glomerulus. During impaired kidney function, cystatin C levels will rise. Normal value is 0.70 to 0.85 mg/mL (depending on age). This test is more accurate for the assessment of GFR when measured with serum creatinine in patients with chronic kidney disease (Inker & Perrone, 2018).

Clinical Cues

BUN level and serum creatinine are the two most common tests used to screen for kidney problems. BUN can rise from dehydration and increased protein in the blood (nitrogen) from a high-protein diet or digestion of blood in the gastrointestinal (GI) tract with GI bleeding. To evaluate kidney function, the two values must be examined together. If BUN is elevated and creatinine is normal, the BUN elevation is not due to kidney problems.

Radiologic procedures range from a single view of the kidneys, ureters, and bladder (KUB) to interventional radiology, such as balloon angioplasty. A KUB is used to locate stones and detect structural abnormalities. Angioplasty is used to open blocked vessels and increase blood flow to the organs. Urodynamic tests, such as cystometrography, are used to measure flow volume and muscle function. Biopsies of the kidney or bladder are done in combination with radiologic examinations to locate lesions (Fig. 33.4).

Patient Teaching

Renal Biopsy

Teaching points for patients having a renal biopsy:

- *Explain purpose:* To diagnosis the cause of kidney disease, to detect cancer, or to evaluate kidney transplant rejection.
- *Explain procedure:* Local anesthetic is given. Needle is inserted through skin into the kidney to obtain a small sample under fluoroscopy or ultrasound. Total procedure time is 10 minutes.
- *Explain preparation:* Nothing by mouth (NPO) for 6 to 8 hours before procedure; blood tests will be performed before procedure (e.g., hemoglobin and hematocrit, prothrombin time, partial thromboplastin time).
- *Explain postprocedure care:* Must lie on back for 6 to 24 hours (time varies according to facility protocols and provider orders), avoid activities that increase abdominal pressure (e.g., sneezing, laughing), expect that urine will have blood for first 24 hours. Drink 3000 mL of fluid to flush urinary system (unless otherwise contraindicated).
- *Give home care instructions:* Avoid strenuous activity (heavy lifting or contact sports) for 2 weeks. Report bleeding (e.g., bright red or with clots) immediately. Report fever, malaise, or dysuria.

From Pagana KD, Pagana TJ: *Mosby's manual of diagnostic and laboratory tests,* ed 6, St. Louis, 2018, Elsevier.

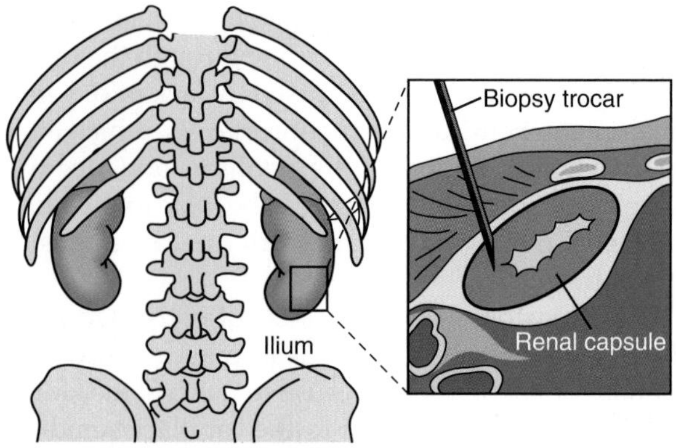

Fig. 33.4 Renal biopsy. A needle is inserted through the skin to obtain a tissue sample. (From Pagana KD, Pagana TJ: *Mosby's manual of diagnostic and laboratory tests,* ed 6, St. Louis, 2018, Elsevier.)

General nursing responsibilities for diagnostic testing include assessing for allergies to contrast media, verifying that a signed consent is present when indicated, and ruling out pregnancy before radiologic procedures and scans. Table 33.2 lists common diagnostic tests and procedures, along with nursing implications.

Think Critically

What is the rationale of having the patient use the clean-catch method rather than simply voiding into a collection container?

Older Adult Care Points

Older kidneys have less ability to concentrate urine. This predisposes the patient to dehydration when fluid intake is restricted for diagnostic tests. The contrast agents used for radiographic tests, in conjunction with dehydration, can cause acute renal failure in older adults. Older adults should be carefully rehydrated by encouraging several ounces of oral fluid (preferable to intravenous [IV] administration, if possible) every 1 to 2 hours and monitoring vital signs, urinary output, lung sounds, and respiratory effort to prevent fluid overload.

Clinical Cues

A 24-hour urine collection is usually started first thing in the morning. Have the patient void and discard the urine, note the time in the medical record, and then put each successive voiding into the collection container. At the time when the test is to end, have the patient void, and add this last urine to the collection bottle. Check with the laboratory as to whether the container must be kept on ice during the collection period. Place a sign on the patient's door and over the toilet stating "24-hour urine test in progress" so that everyone will save the urine properly.

NURSING MANAGEMENT

ASSESSMENT (DATA COLLECTION)

History and Present Illness

At the time of admission, obtain a personal history of previous disorders of the urinary tract, such as frequent

Text continued on p. 795

Table 33.2 Diagnostic Tests for Urologic Disorders

TEST	PURPOSE	DESCRIPTION	NURSING IMPLICATIONS
Urine			
Urinalysis	To detect bacteria, blood, casts, and other abnormalities of the urine	Normal urine is clear, is straw to dark amber in color, has a pH of 4.5–6.0, has a specific gravity of 1.010–1.030, and is negative for protein, glucose, ketones, and bilirubin. It should have only a rare RBC, no more than 0–4 WBCs, and an occasional cast.	Obtain a fresh 10-mL morning specimen. Send specimen to laboratory immediately. If vaginal bleeding is reported, health care provider may order a catheterized specimen. Presence of nitrites or leukocyte esterase usually indicates UTI.
Urine culture and sensitivity (C&S) (clean catch midstream)	To verify UTI and to determine the specific infectious organism and the sensitivity to specific antibiotics	Normally urine is sterile in the bladder. Several drops of urine are placed in a culture medium. After incubation (several days), the colonies are counted. If >100,000 organisms per mL are counted, there is a UTI. Sensitivity test: bacteria are exposed to various antiinfectives to determine which is most effective in killing the organism.	Instruct patient to perform the clean-catch method for specimen collection. A sterile specimen can also be obtained via urinary catheterization. Send specimen to laboratory immediately to prevent change in pH, which can affect bacterial growth. Check for results to verify that the patient is receiving the correct antibiotic therapy.
Urine osmolality	To determine whether the kidneys can concentrate urine; reflects hydration status	Normal findings for fasting specimen: >850 mOsm/kg. Increases in osmolality can indicate dehydration, azotemia, or chronic renal disease. Decreases in osmolality can indicate low-sodium diet, excessive water intake, or diabetes insipidus.	Give a high-protein diet for 3 days before the urine collection. Restrict foods and fluids for 8–12 h before obtaining fasting specimen. To collect a fasting urine specimen, have the patient empty bladder at 6 A.M., discard, then collect specimen at 8 A.M. Label as a fasting specimen and send to laboratory.
Uric acid	To check for renal failure, gout, kidney stones	Uric acid is an end product of protein metabolism. Normal findings: 250–750 mg/24 h (normal diet). Level is elevated in renal failure.	Take a diet history; specifically ask about purine-rich foods (e.g., organ meats or sardines). Patient needs to fast the night before specimen collection. Instruct on a 24-h urine collection. (Serum uric acid may be ordered.)
Creatinine clearance	To determine how well kidneys can excrete creatinine	Normal creatinine clearance: 15–25 mg/kg body weight in 24 h. Elevated serum creatinine with decreased urine creatinine indicates decreased kidney function.	Collect a 24-h urine specimen. A 5-mL venous blood sample is collected sometime during the 24-h collection period. Instruct patient to avoid rigorous exercise (according to laboratory protocol: avoid meat, tea, coffee, or drugs) during the collection period.
Urine cytology	Detects presence of bladder cancer noninvasively	Identifies cellular structures indicating bladder cancer.	Obtain a fresh urine specimen (not first morning specimen). Transport to laboratory within the hour.

Continued

Table 33.2 Diagnostic Tests for Urologic Disorders—cont'd

TEST	PURPOSE	DESCRIPTION	NURSING IMPLICATIONS
Blood			
Blood urea nitrogen (BUN)	To evaluate kidney function and hydration status	High BUN levels can indicate poor kidney function, dehydration, or increased breakdown of body protein (i.e., severe burns or excessive exercise). Lower BUN levels are found in severe liver damage, excessive hydration, and protein deficiency. Normal BUN levels average 7–20 mg/dL (depending on sex and age).	No fasting or patient preparation is required. Take a drug history; many drugs can alter results. Requires 5 mL of venous blood. When drawing specimen, make sure it is not hemolyzed.
Serum creatinine	To evaluate kidney function.	Creatinine is a waste product of skeletal muscle activity. It is produced in fairly constant amounts and is excreted through the kidneys. Normal serum creatinine is 0.8–1.2 mg/dL (depending on gender).	Meats, tea, or coffee may be restricted 6 h before the test. Cephalosporins may be stopped before the test. Record baseline height and weight. Instruct patient to avoid strenuous exercise before test. Requires 5–10 mL venous blood; may include a 24-h urine collection.
Cystatin C	To evaluate kidney function. Helpful in patients where creatinine may be misleading (e.g. obesity, cirrhosis, malnutrition)	Cystatin C is a small protein produced throughout the body and eliminated by the kidneys. Normal range 0.6–1 mg/L.	No special preparation needed. Requires a blood draw of 3 mL in lavender-top tube. Can be used instead of creatinine to evaluate kidney function.
Calculated Values			
BUN/creatinine ratio	To help distinguish between renal causes and nonrenal causes of abnormal values.	Levels of BUN in the blood are 10–20 times higher than creatinine. BUN levels change due to multiple conditions. Creatinine stays relatively constant. The BUN result is divided by the creatinine result.	Normal ratios are between 10:1 and 20:1. If serum creatinine is normal and BUN is elevated, dehydration, increased protein intake (GI bleeding), or other nonrenal cause is the reason. Any elevation in serum creatinine should be assumed to be an indicator of renal dysfunction until proven otherwise.
Glomerular filtration rate (GFR)	To measure the level of kidney function	GFR is calculated from creatinine, age, body size, and gender.	Normal value for adults is GFR >90 mL/min/1.73 m^2. GFR <60 indicates kidney damage.
Radiology Studies			
Kidneys, ureters, bladder (KUB)	To visualize the urinary structures or radiopaque stones	Single radiographic view of the lower abdomen done without contrast medium.	Patient needs an x-ray gown that has no radiopaque fasteners. Test for pregnancy before any radiologic study.
Intravenous pyelogram (IVP)	To visualize the kidneys, ureters, and bladder To detect obstructions related to stones or tumors Rarely used; CT and ultrasound more common	An iodine-based contrast is given via IV injection, then radiographs are taken at timed intervals, showing the flow of the contrast through the renal system.	Check for allergy to iodine; verify BUN and creatinine results; inform provider. Bowel preparation and NPO status may be required. After procedure, encourage PO fluids for rehydration.

Table 33.2 Diagnostic Tests for Urologic Disorders—cont'd

TEST	PURPOSE	DESCRIPTION	NURSING IMPLICATIONS
Retrograde pyelogram	To visualize the kidneys, ureters, and bladder during cystoscopy.	Catheters are threaded into the ureters during cystoscopy to inject the dye backward into the kidneys.	Check for allergy to iodine-based dye, verify BUN and creatinine results; inform provider. Bowel preparation and NPO status may be required.
Cystogram Can be done with contrast as a voiding cystogram. Can be done with radioactive material—radionuclide cystogram also called a bladder scan.	To visualize the contour of the bladder	Radiographs are taken before and after sodium iodide is instilled into the bladder through a urethral catheter. Or a radionuclide is instilled into the bladder through the catheter, and scanning is done with a scintillation scanner.	Check for allergies to iodine-based dyes. Give a clear liquid breakfast on the day of test. A Foley catheter is usually inserted before the procedure. Patient's bladder may feel very full during the examination, but bladder is drained after the radiographs are taken. Postprocedure, encourage PO fluids for flushing.
Magnetic resonance imaging (MRI)	To detect trauma or tumors in soft tissues	Noninvasive imaging uses a powerful magnetic field to scan radio wave frequencies and form 3D images. Can be done without contrast.	Considered relatively safe. Metal objects are forbidden during the procedure. Pacemakers and implants are contraindicated.
Computed tomography (CT) scan	To determine presence of a cyst, tumor, or renal calculi	A combination of radiologic and computer techniques yields cross-sectional information and indicates the density of tissues.	Contrast medium may or may not be given; check for allergy to iodine. Patient may need to be NPO before examination. Procedure lasts about 30 min; patient must remain quiet and cooperative.
Renal ultrasonography	To show size, shape, and location of kidneys, ureters, and bladder and obstructions to flow	A handheld transducer is passed over the skin, and high-frequency sound waves create visual images of the structures.	Patient may be asked to drink fluid to fill bladder before sonogram; other laboratories may require NPO for 8–12 h before the procedure. Test takes approximately 30 min.
Renal angiography	To assess renal arterial system function and identify areas of obstruction to blood flow	Under local anesthesia, a catheter is threaded through the femoral artery and up the aorta to the renal artery, and a contrast agent is injected. Fluoroscopy is conducted during the injection to observe for filling of blood vessels. Angiography is performed to detect complications in a transplanted kidney, to evaluate a mass, or to check the extent of kidney trauma.	Requires a signed consent. Check for allergy to iodine-based dye. A bowel preparation or NPO status for 6–8 h may be ordered. Postprocedure care includes monitoring femoral access site. If a closure device was used, 2–3 h of bed rest are indicated. Vital signs and popliteal and pedal pulses are checked q15min for the first hour and q2–4h, as ordered, for signs of bleeding or shock.
Radionuclide renal scan	To detect perfusion and function; can detect abnormal areas of kidney tissue (e.g., tumors or cysts)	A radioisotope is injected into the blood, and a scintillation scanner is passed over the area of the kidney. This yields a pattern of isotope uptake. Procedure may take 1–4 h to complete.	Explain that low-dose radiation is used and is quickly eliminated from the body and that the procedure is not painful, but patient must lie very still. There are no dietary restrictions, but the patient should drink 2–3 glasses of water before the test.

Continued

Table 33.2 Diagnostic Tests for Urologic Disorders—cont'd

TEST	PURPOSE	DESCRIPTION	NURSING IMPLICATIONS
Endoscopy			
Cystoscopy	To examine the interior of the bladder	Under short-acting or local anesthesia, a cystoscope is passed up the urethra into the bladder. The scope can be guided into a ureter to extract a stone or to biopsy lesions in the bladder. Depending on the extent of the procedure, general anesthesia or procedural sedation may be needed.	Requires a signed consent. Patient is usually NPO for several hours before the procedure. Give preoperative medication as prescribed. Postprocedure: burning, frequency, and pink-tinged urine may occur. Frank bleeding should be reported. Warm sitz baths and mild analgesics are given for voiding discomfort.
Urodynamics			
Cystometrography (CMG)	To measure bladder capacity, pressures, and sensations	A urinary catheter is inserted and attached to a cystometer. Fluid is instilled, and the patient reports when the need to void is first noted, then mild urgency, and finally when bladder feels very full. Readings of bladder capacity and pressure are recorded and plotted.	Sterile technique must be used for catheter insertion and bladder fluid instillation. The patient is monitored for signs of postprocedure infection.
Urethral pressure study	To determine urethral pressure needed to maintain urinary continence	A small catheter with pressure-sensing capabilities is inserted into the bladder. As the patient voids, the varying pressures of the smooth muscle of the urethra are recorded.	Sterile technique must be used for catheter insertion. The patient is monitored for signs of postprocedure infection.
Electromyography of the perineal muscles	To evaluate the quality of the voluntary muscles used in voiding	Electrodes are placed on the skin near the urethra and rectum or in the rectum and/or urethra to measure contraction and relaxation of the muscles involved in voiding.	Inform the patient that there is mild discomfort during electrode placement and nerve conduction testing. Analgesics may be given before or after the procedure to relieve discomfort.
Miscellaneous			
Bladder scan	Noninvasive method to measure postvoid residual volume or urinary retention	Portable handheld scanner uses ultrasound to create an image and calculate bladder volume. Can be done at the bedside (see Fig. 33.6).	Clean the probe. Palpate for the symphysis pubis and apply gel about 1 inch above. Ensure that the probe makes good contact with the gel-covered skin. Point the probe toward the coccyx. Press the scan button for the bladder volume readout.
Renal biopsy	To obtain tissue specimen to determine cause of renal disease, to check for malignancy, or to evaluate extent of transplant rejection	The patient is placed in the prone position, with a pillow under the abdomen at kidney level. A local anesthetic is given. CT or ultrasound is used to identify the position for biopsy needle insertion into the lower lobe of the kidney, below the 12th rib. The patient must hold breath while the needle is inserted and withdrawn. A tissue sample is extracted and sent to the laboratory.	Requires a signed permission form. Urinalysis, CBC, and coagulation studies should be completed. Patient may be NPO for 6–8 h before the procedure. After the procedure, a pressure dressing is applied, and the patient remains prone for 30–60 min and on bed rest for 6–8 h (time varies according to protocol). Vital signs are taken q5–15 min for 1 h and PRN until stable. Report signs of hemorrhage, back pain, shoulder ache, dysuria, or infection.

3D, Three-dimensional; *CBC,* complete blood cell count; *GI,* gastrointestinal; *IV,* intravenous; *NPO,* nothing by mouth; *PO,* by mouth, orally; *PRN,* as needed; *RBC,* red blood cell; *UTI,* urinary tract infection; *WBC,* white blood cell.

urinary tract infections (UTIs), illness or injury to any system, or problems that required surgery. A family history of diabetes, cardiovascular disease, or kidney stones is relevant to an assessment of kidney function.

Many substances can be toxic to the kidneys (**nephrotoxic**); obtain a patient history that includes use of prescription or over-the-counter drugs or illicit substances and any occupational exposure to hazardous materials. The complete drug history should be communicated to all health care professionals and conveyed if the patient is transferred to another facility; on discharge, the patient should receive a copy of the information in accordance with National Patient Safety Goals.

Clinical Cues

If the patient appears hesitant to disclose illicit drug use, use a matter-of-fact approach and explain that the information is important because of potential drug-drug interactions and adverse effects on organs such as the kidneys, heart, or liver.

Focused Assessment

Data Collection for the Urinary System

Ask the following questions when assessing a patient with a urologic problem:

- Do you or your family have a history of hypertension, cardiovascular disease, diabetes, kidney stones, frequent urinary tract infections, or other kidney problems?
- Have you ever had genital herpes or another sexually transmitted infection?
- Do you have any pain when urinating? Any abdominal or flank pain?
- Do you have any difficulty in starting the stream of urine?
- Do you feel as though you empty your bladder completely when you urinate?
- Have you noticed any change in the appearance or smell of your urine?
- Have you needed to empty your bladder more frequently than usual?
- Have you been experiencing any urgency, accompanied by dribbling or leaking urine?
- How many times do you need to get up at night to urinate? (Once a night is average.)
- Have you had any episodes of urinary incontinence?
- Has there been a change in urinary output, in voiding pattern, or in the characteristics of the urine?
- Do you have pain or discomfort in the bladder or kidney areas?
- Have you ever noticed blood in your urine (other than when menstruating [for women])?
- Do you have any problem with sexual dysfunction?
- Are you experiencing excessive fatigue?
- Have you noticed any itching of the skin?
- How much fluid do you drink in a day?

Clinical Cues

Collecting information about sexual health, sexually transmitted infections, and other genital and reproductive disorders is important because these may be a source of infection or blockage. You may find that it will be easier for you and the patient to talk about these issues toward the end of the interview, after a sense of rapport has been established.

Physical Assessment

Perform a general physical assessment, including a complete set of vital signs and a baseline weight. Observe for signs of generalized or facial edema. Gently palpate the abdomen and the bladder for distention or tenderness. Visually inspect the external genitalia, particularly if there are complaints of pain, discharge, bleeding, or prolapse or if there is an indwelling or recently removed catheter.

Focused Assessment

Physical Examination of the Urinary System

Physical examination should include the following:

- Inspect the abdomen for any visible abnormalities.
- Palpate all four quadrants for areas of tenderness.
- Palpate above the pubic bone for evidence of bladder distention.
- Inspect genitals as appropriate (e.g., reports of bleeding, discharge, presence of or recent discontinuation of indwelling catheter).
- Examine the urine for color, clarity, volume, and smell.

Nursing responsibilities in the daily assessment of urinary function include (1) measuring intake and output; (2) evaluating abnormal flow of urine; (3) noting the character of urine (i.e., color, odor, clarity); (4) noticing changes in the pattern of voiding; and (5) assessing pain and discomfort. Documentation includes objective observations of amount and characteristics of urine and the patient's subjective reports of pain, discomfort, and abnormalities.

Characteristics of urine. The color of urine can give helpful information about the status of the patient and the functioning of the kidneys. Table 33.3 lists color variations in urine and the significance of abnormal coloration.

Another characteristic that should be noted is **odor.** Normal urine develops an ammonia-like odor after it has stood for a length of time, but this odor should not be present in freshly voided urine. A foul smell may indicate infection. Acetone in the urine, which occurs during metabolic acidosis, causes it to have a sweet, fruity odor. Various supplements can affect urine odor, as can asparagus.

Hematuria means blood in the urine. Microscopic hematuria occurs when blood in the urine is not visible to the naked eye. Gross hematuria is a sign of bleeding

Table 33.3 **Common Causes of Variations in Color of Urine**

COLOR	MEDICATION	OTHER CAUSES
Colorless or pale yellow	Diuretics	Dilute urine because of diabetes insipidus, diabetes mellitus, overhydration, chronic renal disease, nervousness, alcohol
Bright yellow	Riboflavin (multiple vitamins)	None
Dark amber to orange	Phenazopyridine HCl (Pyridium) Nitrofurantoin (Macrodantin) Sulfasalazine (Azulfidine) Thiamine (multiple vitamins)	Concentrated urine because of dehydration or increased metabolic state (e.g., fever) Urobilinogen (a by-product of bilirubin normally excreted through stool and urine) Bilirubin (a component of bile normally metabolized and excreted via stool and urine) Foods: excessive carrots
Pink to red	Phenothiazines (e.g., Compazine) Docusate calcium (Surfak) Phenolphthalein (Doxidan) (in alkaline urine) Phenytoin (Dilantin) Rifampin Cascara (in alkaline urine) Senna (X-Prep, Senokot)	Fresh red blood cells Menstrual contamination Myoglobin (a by-product of excessive exercise or skeletal tissue damage) Porphyrin (porphyria is a hereditary metabolic disorder) Foods: beets, blackberries, red food dyes
Brown	Cascara (in acid urine) Metronidazole (Flagyl) (if left standing) Phenothiazines (e.g., Compazine)	Extremely concentrated urine because of dehydration or increased metabolic state Red blood cells (old blood) Bilirubin Urobilinogen Myoglobin Porphyrin
Blue or green	Triamterene (Dyrenium) Amitriptyline (Elavil) Methylene blue	Bilirubin Biliverdin (a blue-green pigment that occurs in bile) *Pseudomonas* infection
Dark brown to black	Nitrofurantoin (Macrodantin) Iron preparations (if left standing) Levodopa (if left standing) Methocarbamol (if left standing) Quinine Senna (X-Prep, Senokot) Methyldopa (Aldomet)	Melanotic tumors Addison disease Porphyrin Red blood cells (old blood) Large amounts of dietary fava beans, rhubarb, or aloe

from some point in the urinary tract. Red blood in the urine is not easily missed, but if the blood has been in the bladder or kidney for a long time, it will deteriorate and cause the urine to be a smoky gray or dark brown. If the blood is noticed as soon as voiding starts, it is likely that the blood is from somewhere in the urethra. If it is noticed at the end of urination, the site probably is near the neck of the bladder. Bleeding throughout voiding indicates that the blood is coming from a site above the neck of the bladder because the blood has been well mixed with the urine in the bladder.

Proteinuria is the abnormal presence of protein in the urine. Proteins are too large to pass through the structure of the glomerular membrane; therefore presence of protein is suggestive of damage to the membrane that occurs in renal disease, such as nephrotic syndrome or glomerulonephritis. Proteinuria is also seen in other conditions such as preeclampsia, multiple myeloma, and amyloidosis (Pagana & Pagana, 2018). Specialized assays are required to detect **microalbuminuria** (presence of albumin in the urine), which is suggestive of early kidney disease. This test could be considered essential for those at high risk for renal disease, such as persons with diabetes or hypertension. **Pneumaturia** means gas in the urine. This can occur if there is a fistula (abnormal passage) between the bladder and the bowel or vagina.

Changes in voiding pattern. Ask about or observe urinary frequency during the day and night. Other alterations include the size and force of the urinary stream, feeling of fullness even after voiding, and change in the amount urinated each time. Increased frequency can be a manifestation of some abnormality in the urinary drainage system, particularly in the bladder and urethra. The frequency with which a person feels the urge to urinate can be related to psychological as well as physiologic factors. Excitement, anxiety, and fear can produce increased frequency of urination. Caffeine and other diuretics found in foods and drinks and an increased intake of fluid can increase the number of times a person must urinate. Pathologic conditions that can cause increased frequency include inflammation of the bladder (cystitis) or urethra (urethritis).

Patient Teaching

Urinary Urgency

Urgency can be symptomatic of inflammation. *Urgency* refers to an almost uncontrollable desire to void. Incontinence sometimes occurs because the patient is not able to get to a toilet quickly enough after the urge to urinate occurs. Box 33.2 defines terminology related to changes in urine output and flow.

Pain and discomfort. In general, the locations in which the patient with a urinary problem is most likely to experience discomfort are either the bladder area or the region over the kidney.

Bladder pain can be caused by the stretching of an overfull bladder. Assessment of the size and location of the bladder is indicated when a patient reports pain in the bladder region. Normally the bladder cannot be felt. If a smooth, rounded mass is felt on palpation in the area above the pubic bone, the bladder is distended. Bladder pain can also be caused by spasms of the bladder musculature as it attempts to empty itself of clots, bits of tissue, and other cellular debris. This can occur postoperatively or when there is moderate to severe inflammation and bleeding in the urinary tract. Relief sometimes can be obtained by irrigating the bladder to remove the clots and debris.

Flank (side and back area of the body below the ribs and above the hips) pain can also be caused by obstruction and distention; in this case the affected organs are the ureters and kidney pelvis. Spasmodic peristaltic contractions along the ureter can be caused by stones, clots, a tumor, inflammatory swelling, or any other condition that prevents the flow of urine from the kidney to the bladder. When evaluating flank pain, note the location and assess for radiation of pain from the kidney or ureter to the genitalia and thigh.

Another kind of discomfort may be painful urination, or dysuria. **Dysuria** usually is caused by inflammation in either the bladder or the urethra. It often is described as burning and can range from mild to severe. Ask the patient when the pain occurs and whether it is felt immediately before, during, or after voiding.

Box 33.2 Terminology Related to Urine Output and Flow

- **Anuria**: Absence of urine. This rarely occurs but may be associated with acute renal failure. Some patients with chronic renal failure who are on dialysis are anuric.
- **Oliguria**: Diminished or abnormally decreased flow of urine; may result from dehydration, renal failure, or obstruction. Urine output less than 400 mL/day.
- **Polyuria**: Abnormally high and dilute urine output; the result of excessive solutes and increased excretion of water. Possible causes include hypercalcemia, diabetes insipidus, uncontrolled diabetes mellitus, and increased fluid intake.
- **Nocturia**: Urination that occurs during the night; may be related to the decreased ability of the aging kidney to concentrate urine.
- **Urinary frequency**: Voiding more often than every 2 hours. This can be the result of inflammation, decreased bladder capacity, psychological disorders, pregnancy, or increased fluid intake.
- **Urinary hesitancy**: A delay in starting the stream of urine; may be related to partial obstruction.
- **Urinary retention**: Retaining or holding urine in the bladder; various causes include neurologic, psychological, medication, obstruction, or anesthesia.
- **Residual urine**: Urine left in the bladder after voiding; related to poor muscle tone or partial obstruction.

Think Critically

What characteristics of a fresh urine specimen might indicate an infection? Why should UTIs be treated promptly?

◆ NURSING DIAGNOSIS

Problem statements commonly associated with urologic problems and disturbances in urinary flow include the following:

- Altered urinary function due to inflammation.
- Fluid volume overload due to inability of kidneys to produce urine.
- Pain due to ureteral spasm, bladder spasm, or inflammation.
- Fatigue due to effect of the accumulation of waste products.
- Insufficient knowledge due to prevention of UTI.
- Fear due to potential cause of hematuria or possibility of malignancy.
- Altered body image due to urinary diversion.

◆ PLANNING

Expected outcomes for these problems might include the following:

- Patient will void spontaneously, with decreased symptoms (e.g., urgency, dysuria, hematuria), within 48 hours after starting antibiotics.
- Patient will have no signs of fluid volume overload (e.g., weight gain, edema, or crackles in lungs) within 2 days.
- Patient will report bladder pain level less than 3/10 during this shift.
- Patient will have adequate energy to independently perform activities of daily living (ADLs) before discharge.
- Patient will identify four or five ways to prevent recurrent UTIs before leaving the clinic today.

- Patient will verbalize concerns or fears about signs and symptoms (e.g., hematuria) during this shift.
- Patient will demonstrate acceptance of stoma as evidenced by looking at stoma and handling ostomy equipment within 1 week.

Planning care for a patient with a disorder of the urologic system involves considering the effect of the disorder on the other body systems. **Fatigue and irritability are common when kidney function is impaired because of the buildup of waste products in the body and their effect on body cells.** In addition, educate the patient and the family to maximize participation in treatment goals and prevent complications. General nursing goals for addressing urologic disorders include the following:

- Absence of infection or pain
- Restoration of normal urinary output and fluid balance
- Assimilation of knowledge for appropriate self-care
- Promoting resolution of body image disturbance
- Prevention of complications

◆ IMPLEMENTATION

Caring for patients with urologic problems includes monitoring intake and output, body weight, and signs of edema. Monitoring drug combinations for potential nephrotoxicity and for possible urinary retention is also very important.

You must use strict aseptic technique when catheterizing patients, emptying drainage bags, handling drainage tubes and stents, and performing peritoneal dialysis or hemodialysis.

Care of Urinary Catheters

The catheter should be fastened to the upper leg with tape or a catheter-securing device (Fig. 33.5). Connecting tubing should be positioned so that there is no pulling on the catheter when the patient turns, moves in bed, or arises to ambulate; this prevents pulling on the balloon that holds the catheter in place, which would cause tissue irritation and predispose to infection. Irrigation of the bladder is not recommended unless there is an obstruction or a special solution needs to be instilled. Irrigation can be done with a closed system or by opening the indwelling catheter system. If open irrigation is performed, strict asepsis must be maintained. See Chapter 34, Table 34.3 for common urinary catheters and tubes used for urologic disorders. Box 33.3 reviews principles of catheter care.

Legal and Ethical Considerations

Urinary catheters are one of the common causes of health care–associated infection. In 2011 there were 93,300 UTIs in hospitalized patients, and 75% of those were catheter related (Centers for Disease Control and Prevention, 2018). Alternatives to catheterization should always be considered to prevent infection, and the care should be carefully documented. When a patient dies of a health care–associated infection, the death is investigated to determine how the infection developed and contributed to the death of the patient. The purpose of the investigation is to prevent future incidents.

Clinical Cues

Urine specimens from catheterized patients are obtained with a syringe from the sampling port using aseptic technique. Do not take the specimen from the drainage bag because the urine specimen must be fresh.

Measuring Intake and Output

The quantity of fluids entering the body, by whatever route, has a direct bearing on fluid balance (see Chapter 3). Patients with urologic disorders are very likely to suffer fluid imbalances, and therefore their intake and output should be measured and the totals recorded every 8 to 12 hours during hospitalization or acute illness. In critically ill patients, the urinary output is typically measured hourly. **Urine output should be at least 30 mL/h. For total output, measure all urine excreted, drainage from all tubes, any emesis, and watery stools.** An estimate of the amount of fluid lost through perspiration should also be considered if perspiration is excessive (e.g., sweating with fever). Any fluid used to irrigate catheters and tubing must be

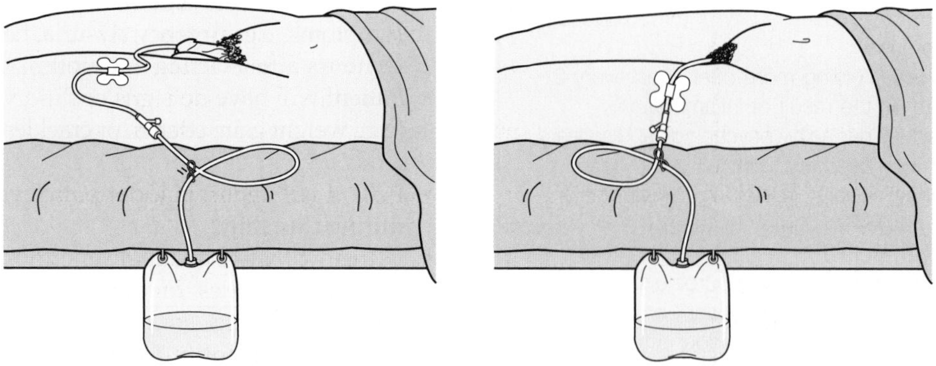

Fig. 33.5 Catheter tubing attached to a collection bag and secured to the thigh.

Box 33.3 Principles of Urinary Catheter and Tube Care

- Use aseptic technique and gentle handling when caring for any urinary drainage tube.
- Insert urethral catheters using sterile technique.
- Do not open a urinary drainage system unless there is no alternative (e.g., the drainage bag must be changed for some reason).
- Empty the drainage bag by opening the drainage port at the bottom of the bag; use aseptic technique and do not allow the drainage tube to touch the collection container. After reclamping the tube, wipe away residual urine from the tube with an antiseptic swab before securing it.
- Use the patient's individual collection container for draining the urine storage bag.
- Observe all tubes and level of drainage in the collection bag each time the patient is seen.
- Keep the drainage bag below the level of the catheter or insertion site (indwelling catheter drainage bags should have a backflow valve, but keeping the bag lower prevents backflow). If the bag must be raised above the insertion site, clamp off the tube briefly while repositioning the patient.
- Perform perineal care at least twice daily, cleaning the urinary meatus and catheter with soap and water; rinse well, just as the area would be cleansed if the patient were bathing normally (see agency's policy).
- Keep an intake and output record to help monitor kidney function.
- Encourage fluids of 3000 mL/day unless contraindicated.
- When irrigating, use the correct amount of sterile solution (according to agency policy or the amount of solution determined by the health care provider's order for nephrostomy tubes, ureteral tubes, or catheters).
- Use a steady, gentle stream to irrigate. Avoid exerting pressure that may traumatize or cause discomfort.
- Do not pull back forcefully on an irrigating syringe attached to a urinary catheter or tube; this creates negative pressure that may damage delicate tissues or collapse the tube.
- When discontinuing an indwelling catheter, never cut the catheter. Use a syringe to deflate the balloon.

measured, and the amount should be added to the total intake and subsequent output.

◆ EVALUATION

Compare intake and output data over time to determine clinical improvement or the presence of problems. The frequency of comparison will be hour-to-hour for critical patients or over a period of days for patients with chronic conditions. Laboratory data, such as BUN, creatinine, potassium, and urinalysis results, provide further information to evaluate the effectiveness of treatment. A decrease in subjective symptoms, such as flank pain or dysuria, also indicates resolution of the problem.

COMMON UROLOGIC PROBLEMS

URINARY INCONTINENCE

Etiology

In the United States, millions of adults experience transient or chronic incontinence. Accurate statistics are difficult to obtain because on average women wait 6.5 years to obtain a diagnosis and men are even more reluctant to talk about the problem or seek help. A large percentage of residents in nursing homes are incontinent, and it is the leading cause of admission to a long-term care facility (Vasavada, 2018). Women who have had several children may have anatomic changes that make incontinence more likely. Men may experience the problem because of an enlarged prostate. Other contributing factors include spinal cord injury, neurologic disorder (e.g., dementia), or functional disorder (e.g., difficulty manipulating clothing fasteners).

The first step in managing incontinence is to identify factors that may be contributing to the problem. Immobility; UTI; atrophic urethritis or vaginitis associated with menopause; stool impaction; prostate surgery; delirium or confusion; endocrine problems; and various types of medication, such as alpha-adrenergic agents, beta-adrenergic agonists, and calcium channel blockers, may contribute to the problem of incontinence. Obesity also is a factor because it causes increased pressure on the bladder.

Pathophysiology

Urine flow out of the bladder is controlled by two circular muscles called *sphincters*. The internal sphincter lies close to the lowermost part of the bladder, and the external sphincter surrounds the urethra. Many factors can cause loss of sphincter control. Unconsciousness, UTI, paralysis, interference with nerve transmission to and from the brain, and loss of muscle tone of the bladder and sphincters are some of the common causes of incontinence.

There are several types of incontinence: urge, stress, mixed, overflow, functional, or neurologic. **Urge incontinence** is the involuntary loss of urine when there is a strong urge to urinate (urinary urgency). **Stress incontinence** occurs when the urethral sphincter fails and there is an increase in intra-abdominal pressure, caused by such things as sneezing, laughing, coughing, or aerobic exercise. **Mixed incontinence** is a combination of different types, such as stress and urge incontinence. **Overflow incontinence** occurs when there is poor contractility of the detrusor muscle or obstruction of the urethra, as in prostate hypertrophy in the male or genital prolapse in the female. **Functional incontinence** is caused by cognitive inability to recognize the urge to urinate or a self-care deficit caused by extreme depression. Inability to reach the bathroom because of restraints, side rails, or an out-of-reach walker can also result in functional incontinence. **Neurologic incontinence** is caused by disorders of the neurologic system (e.g., multiple sclerosis or spinal cord injury).

Signs and Symptoms

The symptoms described by the patient will be helpful in identifying the type of incontinence being experienced. Unintended excretion of urine is the primary symptom. The circumstances under which it occurs are investigated and evaluated.

Diagnosis

Diagnosis of incontinence is based on a careful history, and the patient must be able to report symptoms accurately (Table 33.4). The patient may be asked to keep a bladder diary. Routine urinalysis is also performed. When conservative measures do not improve continence, the health care provider may choose to evaluate the condition with a series of diagnostic tests, including measuring the postvoid residual volume, stress testing, urodynamic studies, cystogram, or cystoscopy.

Treatment

Evidence-based practice indicates that stress incontinence that occurs with exercise, laughing, or coughing may be corrected by exercises to strengthen the pelvic floor muscles. Kegel exercises benefit men as well as women (Vasavada, 2018).

Vaginal weight training with a set of five small, cone-shaped weights that are used along with pelvic

Table 33.4 Common Problem Statements, Expected Outcomes, and Nursing Interventions for Patients With Incontinence

PROBLEM STATEMENT	GOALS/EXPECTED OUTCOMES	NURSING INTERVENTIONS
Altered self-care ability due to decreased muscular strength and fine motor coordination.	Patient will be able to physically get to the toilet (or commode chair) and accomplish toileting (i.e., undo clothing and sit on toilet) with assistance during this shift.	Assess abilities to stand, walk, and sit. Instruct patient to call for help when needing to go to the toilet. Offer assistance q2–4h. Obtain bedside commode as needed. Suggest clothing with elastic waistband or Velcro fasteners to eliminate zippers and buttons. Encourage independence as appropriate (consider strength and motor ability).
Urinary incontinence due to weak pelvic muscles.	Patient will increase control over incontinence within 8–12 wk.	Assess pattern of incontinence and identify actions associated with incontinence (e.g., laughing, coughing). Teach Kegel exercises. Teach to avoid bladder irritants such as coffee, nicotine. Refer to nutritionist for weight loss diet if overweight. Discuss use of incontinence pads or undergarments. Supply information about vaginal cone therapy.
Altered urinary function due to bladder spasms.	Patient will experience urge to void and be able to get to the toilet in time to prevent loss of urine.	Instruct patient to keep a voiding diary or observe for incontinence if unable to self-report. Help patient establish a voiding schedule (e.g., q3–4h). Give antispasmodic medications (e.g., tolterodine) as ordered. Teach patient about side effects of medication (e.g., possible urinary retention).
Altered self-care ability for toileting due to impaired cognition.	Patient will participate in a routine toileting schedule during hospitalization.	Assess cognitive deficits related to toileting (e.g., unable to remember to go to toilet; senses urge to go but cannot find the toilet). Observe for odors, stains, or wetness on clothing and linens. Assist (or remind) patient to go to the toilet q2–3h. Provide visual cues to prompt toileting (e.g., commode chair at bedside, large arrows pointing toward bathroom, picture of toilet on bathroom door). Give positive feedback for efforts.
Potential for altered skin integrity due to moisture and irritation of urine on skin.	Patient's skin will remain dry and intact without breakdown during hospitalization.	Assess for patterns of urinary incontinence (e.g., if patient cannot self-report, check q2–3h). Give fluids primarily during the day and space fluids (e.g., q2–3h) for predictability of voiding. Provide (or assist with) skin care (e.g., clean with mild soap and warm water; use skin barrier creams). Consult with enterostomal therapist (ET nurse) as needed (skin breakdown is progressive). Turn q2h if patient is bedridden or immobile. Ensure adequate nutrition for healing and skin integrity (e.g., high-quality proteins).

Table 33.4 Common Problem Statements, Expected Outcomes, and Nursing Interventions for Patients With Incontinence—cont'd

PROBLEM STATEMENT	GOALS/EXPECTED OUTCOMES	NURSING INTERVENTIONS
Disrupted sleep pattern due to nocturia.	Patient will rest and sleep at least 6 consecutive hours each night during hospitalization.	Assess for medication (e.g., calcium channel blockers) side effects that may be contributing to incontinence. Teach patient to avoid taking fluids in late evening hours. Assist (or instruct patient) to ambulate for at least 10 min 1–2 h before bedtime, then instruct to void before going to bed. Use incontinence pads or undergarments for women and condom catheters for men during the night.
Insufficient knowledge regarding management of incontinence.	Patient will verbalize two or three methods to manage incontinence before leaving the clinic today.	Teach patient about medication side effects (e.g., if on estrogen, patient should report vaginal bleeding or signs of deep vein thrombosis, calf pain, or swelling). Teach Kegel exercises; reinforce that results may take up to 3 mo. Teach bladder training; remind that accidents are expected during training period.
Potential for social isolation due to embarrassment.	Patient will maintain usual social contact with friends and family.	Encourage verbalization of feelings (e.g., shame or embarrassment). Assist patient to identify times, settings, and activities when incontinence may occur (e.g., during exercise). Help patient make a plan to deal with incontinence during social occasions (e.g., use of incontinence briefs, mapping out toilet locations, planning fluid intake around social occasions). Refer to support groups.

muscle exercise is another therapeutic option for incontinence. The lightest cone, which has a string attached, is inserted into the vagina and held in place by muscle tightening for 15 minutes twice a day. When there is no problem holding this cone in place, the next heaviest cone is used. This continues until the heaviest cone can be held in place for the 15-minute period. Maintaining normal weight and using topical estrogen therapy after menopause also decrease the incidence of this disorder.

Various medications have been found to be helpful in treating incontinence. Table 33.5 provides additional information about selected drugs for urinary incontinence.

A pessary, a stiff ring, that is worn in the vagina during the day to support the bladder is used as an assistive device to support the pelvic floor when treating vaginal prolapse and urinary incontinence.

Further treatment options for urinary incontinence include biofeedback therapy or an implanted sacral nerve electrical stimulation device used for treatment of overactive bladder (Abello & Das, 2018). Nonimplanted electrical therapies are also used. In transvaginal electrical stimulation (TES) (or transrectal for men), the nerves and muscles of the pelvic floor are stimulated by an electrically charged probe. Stimulation must be done in two 15-minute sessions twice a day for 12 weeks. Periurethral bulking is a procedure performed under local anesthesia in which collagen is injected into the urethra to increase resistance.

Surgeries to correct incontinence. A variety of procedures may be performed to correct the anatomic position of the bladder, by supporting the urethra. These surgeries are most often performed to correct urinary incontinence in women. Most often a vaginal approach is used to place either a midurethral or a bladder neck sling. If access through the abdomen is needed, a laparoscopic technique is used with or without robot assistance. An **artificial sphincter implant** is used in males to treat incontinence after a prostatectomy. A mechanical device is placed around the urethra to open and close it. After incontinence surgical procedures, monitor for UTI and difficulty voiding.

Patient Teaching

Kegel Exercises

- To locate the correct muscle, stop the flow of urine while urinating on the toilet by tightening the anus as if preventing a bowel movement.
- Practice for several days each time you urinate. Then begin the exercise program.
- While lying down, slowly count 1-2-3 while tightening the pelvic muscles.
- Release pelvic muscles slowly to the count 1-2-3. Do this 15 times.
- While sitting, repeat this sequence 15 times, tightening pelvic muscles while counting 1-2-3 and then slowly releasing to the count 1-2-3.
- Stand and repeat the sequence 15 times; tighten to the count 1-2-3 and slowly release to the count 1-2-3.
- Do the pelvic muscle exercises once a day. If you can do them twice each day, improvement in continence will occur more quickly.
- Improvement may be noted in 6 to 8 weeks but may take as long as 3 months.

Table 33.5 Drugs Commonly Used to Treat Urinary Incontinence and Retention

CLASSIFICATION	ACTION	NURSING IMPLICATIONS	PATIENT TEACHING
Urinary antispasmodics, antimuscarinics Oxybutynin (Ditropan), solifenacin (Vesicare), tolterodine (Detrol), trospium (Sanctura), darifenacin (Enablex), fesoterodine (Toviaz)	Used to relieve spasms of the bladder; treats overactive bladder and incontinence	Give mouth care as needed. Monitor I&O. Auscultate bowel sounds. Side effects include dry mouth, increased heart rate, dizziness, abdominal distention, and constipation.	Increase fiber-containing foods and fluids to prevent constipation. Do not drive if dizzy or drowsy. Use ice chips or hard candy for dry mouth. May need eye drops to moisten dry eyes.
Bladder stimulant Bethanechol (Urecholine)	Used to treat urinary retention	Monitor for orthostatic hypotension and bradycardia. Give 1–2 h after meals or with food for GI complaints. May cause diarrhea, cramping, or increased salivation.	Immediately report severe dizziness or difficulty breathing. Rise slowly from lying to standing position.
Medication for benign prostatic hypertrophy Tamsulosin (Flomax), doxazosin (Cardura), terazosin (Hytrin), alfuzosin (Uroxatral), silodosin (Rapaflo)	Relieves symptoms of urinary retention associated with obstruction from an enlarged prostate	May cause orthostatic hypotension. Side effects include back pain, chest pain, cough, diarrhea, nausea, dizziness, headache, weakness.	May take 6 mo for symptom relief. Do not crush, chew, or open the capsule. Immediately report a prolonged erection.
Tricyclic antidepressants Imipramine (Tofranil), amitriptyline (Elavil)	Reduce overactive bladder contractions; reduce sensory urgency and burning pain of interstitial cystitis	May cause dry mouth, blurred vision, or constipation.	Do not use within 14 days of MAOI drugs; observe for hypotension.

GI, Gastrointestinal; *I&O*, intake and output; *MAOI*, monoamine oxidase inhibitor.

When these measures do not solve the problem, incontinence is managed by intermittent catheterization, indwelling urethral catheterization, a suprapubic catheter, an external collection system (such as condom catheters and female external urine management systems), and protective pads and garments.

Clinical Cues

Your patient may develop leaking around the suprapubic catheter. If leaking persists and urine is continuously leaking onto the skin, this could mean that the tube is too small. If the tube has been there for a long time, the tissue contours may have changed since the initial insertion. Notify the health care provider for evaluation.

Nursing Management

Use a gentle and matter-of-fact approach when taking an incontinence history. National professional organizations have released guidelines for screening for urinary incontinence (O'Reilly et al., 2018). The patient experiencing urinary incontinence may be embarrassed by the symptoms but will likely welcome the help and suggestions. Observe the clothing for stains and odors and perform a general physical assessment that includes palpation of the bladder. Inspect the genitalia if there is reason to suspect a prolapse or if a catheter is present or recently has been removed.

Focused Assessment

Assessment for Urinary Incontinence

- What kinds of problems are you having with your bladder?
- Are you having trouble holding your urine (water)?
- When did the urine leakage problem start?
- How often do you leak urine?
- Are you soiling your clothing or bed linens?
- When do the leaks occur? Does it happen during the day or the night? Both?
- How often do you wear a pad or other protective device?
- What activities or situations are associated with leakage? For example, does laughing, coughing, sneezing, or exercising cause leakage?
- Are you having difficulty getting to the bathroom in time?
- Are there things about your house that are preventing you from getting to the bathroom in time? For example, do you have to climb stairs or walk a long distance?
- Do you have (or need) assistive devices (e.g., handrails) in the bathroom?

Older Adult Care Points

Assess older adults for gross motor strength, fine motor dexterity, and ability to balance and independently ambulate. An older adult may be having trouble walking to the bathroom or sitting on or rising from the toilet seat. In addition, clothing fasteners may be problematic.

When incontinence is not remedied by correcting an underlying cause, attempt to help the patient by setting up a voiding and fluid schedule. Assess when the patient is experiencing incontinence. Evidence-based practice suggests that a voiding diary is a useful tool for patients who can self-report (Lukacz, 2018). Box 33.4 provides guidelines for establishing a toileting schedule.

Toileting assistance can be offered at set times just before incontinence usually occurs. Getting the patient on a voiding schedule takes a great deal of patience and persistence on the part of both you and the patient. Accidents will happen during the retraining period, and patients need to be assured that this is expected. (See Chapter 22 for care of patients with incontinence related to spinal cord injury.)

Assignment Considerations

Bladder Training

When planning and implementing a bladder training program for a confused patient who is unable to self-report, there are several ways in which the unlicensed assistive personnel (UAP) can provide valuable help. Ask the UAP to record and report any fluids that are offered and consumed and the number of times that clothes, wet bed linens, or incontinence pads need to be changed. Once the schedule is established, direct the UAP to help the patient follow the schedule by assisting them to the toilet at the designated times.

Patients may experience transient incontinence or urinary retention after removal of an indwelling catheter that has been in place for several days. **Any bleeding, dribbling, or incontinence of urine or inability to void within 4 to 6 hours (maximum of 8 hours) after removal of the catheter should be reported to the health care provider.**

Box 33.4 Assisting Patients to Establish a Toileting Schedule

- Assess pattern of incontinence or instruct patient to keep a voiding diary.
- Assist (or remind) patient to go to the toilet at set times (just before the time when incontinence usually occurs).
- Space fluid intake and give most fluids during the day.
- Discourage intake of bladder stimulants, such as alcohol and caffeine.
- Help the patient ambulate at least 10 minutes an hour or two before bedtime because activity helps to mobilize fluid.
- Apply a condom catheter for males and external urine collection devices for women at night; it is not practical to continue a voiding schedule (every 3 to 4 hours) at night.
- Give positive reinforcement for any small successes.

Health Promotion

Drinks and Substances to Avoid

Advise patients that avoiding caffeine, alcohol, carbonated beverages, and aspartame may help bladder control. These substances may stimulate or irritate the bladder.

URINARY RETENTION

Urinary retention is retaining or holding urine in the bladder. It can be acute after a surgical procedure, after removal of an indwelling catheter, or with certain medications (e.g., atropine), or it may be a chronic condition related to anxiety, neurologic disorders, or obstruction of urine flow through the urethra, as in enlargement of the prostate gland. A straight catheter is used for a single "in-and-out" catheterization for temporary inability to empty the bladder. Also, patients who have permanent paralysis may use intermittent catheterization to empty the bladder.

Urinary retention will not cause the bladder to rupture, but urine will begin to dribble out of the urethra. Retention of urine stretches the bladder walls, causing extreme discomfort. Assess the degree of bladder distention using gentle palpation before and after intervention or, if available, bladder scanning will provide better data (Fig. 33.6). Assist the patient by providing privacy and adequate time for voiding efforts. A caffeinated drink, followed by a warm bath, may help. Instruct the patient to double void: void, sit on the toilet for several

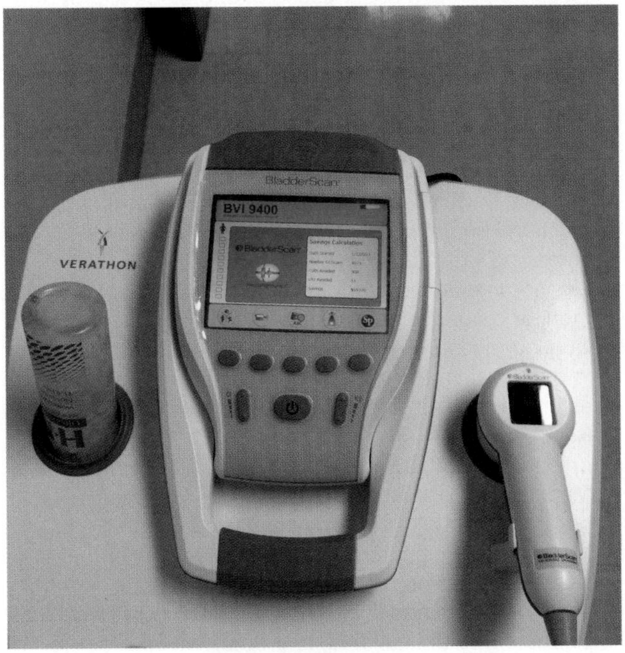

Fig. 33.6 Bladder scanner.

minutes, and void again. Schedule a trip to the toilet every 3 to 4 hours. Obtain an order for catheterization if other measures do not relieve the problem. A medication for urinary retention is bethanechol (Urecholine). See Table 33.5 for examples of medications that relieve the symptoms produced by benign prostatic hypertrophy (enlarged prostate gland).

Poor bladder tone or partial obstruction of the urethra can result in dribbling of urine or passing only the overflow, leaving the bladder partially full. During bladder retraining, residual urine can be measured by having the patient void as much urine as possible and then performing a bladder scan or immediately inserting a catheter (see Table 33.2). One hundred milliliters is considered a normal amount of residual urine. Any amount more than this can become stagnant and concentrated over time, predisposing the patient to bladder infection and the formation of stones.

? Think Critically

The health care provider ordered removal of an indwelling catheter. Three hours later the patient complains of bladder fullness with inability to void. What should you do?

Get Ready for the NCLEX® Examination!

Key Points

- The urologic system is responsible for maintaining proper balance of the fluids, minerals, and organic substances necessary for life.
- The nephron is the functional unit of the kidney. It consists of the glomerulus, which is a network of capillaries encased in a thin-walled sac called the Bowman capsule, and the tubular system.
- Kidney function, GFR, bladder capacity, ability to concentrate urine and secrete renin, and aldosterone all decrease with aging.
- Infection, immunologic disorders, metabolic disorders such as diabetes mellitus, and reduced blood flow secondary to shock or atherosclerosis can result in kidney damage.
- Stones, an enlarged prostate, or tumors may obstruct the flow of urine.
- Tubular necrosis affects the functional ability of the kidney. It can result from lack of oxygen or bacterial or chemical destruction of the nephron.
- Hypertension is a major cause of end-stage kidney disease; conversely, renal disorders can also cause secondary hypertension.
- To promote healthy kidneys, advise patients to drink plenty of water, to empty the bladder at regular intervals, to obtain prompt treatment for bladder infection, to practice good hygiene, to maintain normal serum glucose, and to take blood pressure medication as prescribed.
- BUN and serum creatinine are the most common screening tests for kidney function.
- Monitor intake and output, weight, and signs of edema; monitor drugs for nephrotoxic effects.
- Nursing measures for incontinence include assisting in determining and correcting the underlying cause, establishing a voiding and fluid schedule, coaching Kegel exercises, giving medications for incontinence as prescribed, and advising to decrease bladder irritants.
- Medications to treat incontinence, urinary retention, and benign prostatic hypertrophy are listed in Table 33.5.
- Many medications can affect the urinary system.
- Nursing measures for urinary retention include assessing for bladder distention, providing privacy, instructing to double void, and obtaining an order for catheterization as needed.

Additional Learning Resources

SG Go to your Study Guide for additional learning activities to help you master this chapter content.

Go to your Evolve website (http://evolve.elsevier.com/deWit/medsurg) for the following FREE learning resources:
- Animations, audio, and video
- Answers and rationales for questions and activities
- Glossary with pronunciations in English and Spanish
- Interactive Review Questions and more!

Review Questions for the NCLEX® Examination

1. What information should you give to a community group about prevention of urologic problems?
   1. Drinking orange juice every morning prevents urinary tract infection.
   2. Drinking several glasses of fluid a day helps preserve kidney function.
   3. Emptying the bladder prevents prolonged exposure to toxins.
   4. Eating spinach, chocolate, or strawberries may cause kidney stones.

   NCLEX Client Need: Health Promotion and Maintenance
2. You are planning care for four patients on the night shift. Which patient is most likely to have nocturia related to a decreased ability to concentrate urine?
   1. A patient with a high BUN
   2. A pregnant patient
   3. An older adult
   4. A patient who had a bladder scan

   NCLEX Client Need: Safe and Effective Care Environment: Coordinated Care
3. When starting a 24-hour urine collection, what is essential to ensure correct results?
   1. Include the first void of the 24-hour period.
   2. Record the time of initial void as the start time of the test.
   3. Discard the last void of the 24-hour period.
   4. Encourage fluid intake before starting the test.

   NCLEX Client Need: Physiological Integrity: Reduction of Risk Potential

4. A patient is scheduled to have a renal biopsy. What is included in the preoperative care for this patient? *(Select all that apply.)*
   1. Administer bowel preparation.
   2. Report abnormal coagulation studies.
   3. Enforce nothing by mouth (NPO) for 6 to 8 hours before the procedure.
   4. Check for allergy to contrast media.
   5. Insert indwelling urinary catheter.

   NCLEX Client Need: Physiological Integrity: Reduction of Risk Potential
5. You are trying to console an older adult who is embarrassed about wetting the bed. Which patient comment is consistent with functional incontinence?
   1. "I knew that I needed to go, but I couldn't get out of bed by myself."
   2. "Every time I laugh, cough, or sneeze I pass a little bit of urine."
   3. "When I need to pee, I really have to go right away!"
   4. "My doctor says that my enlarged prostate is causing the problem."

   NCLEX Client Need: Psychosocial Integrity
6. After placing an indwelling urinary catheter, you perform several interventions. Place the interventions in order of priority.
   1. Secure the drainage bag below the level of the bladder so that it hangs freely.
   2. Secure the catheter to the patient's leg.
   3. Check that the catheter tubing is unimpeded and is looped above the drainage bag.
   4. Use aseptic technique when emptying the drainage bag.
   5. Observe the amount of urine drainage in the bag whenever you are in the patient's room.

   NCLEX Client Need: Safe and Effective Care Environment: Safety and Infection Control
7. What is the first action you should take to assist a patient to develop a toileting schedule?
   1. Encourage use of condom catheters or incontinence pads
   2. Assess pattern of incontinence
   3. Schedule trips to the bathroom
   4. Provide positive reinforcement for small successes

   NCLEX Client Need: Safe and Effective Care Environment: Coordinated Care
8. When writing a nursing care plan for a patient with stress incontinence, what interventions should you include? *(Select all that apply.)*
   1. Instruct patient to keep a voiding diary.
   2. Teach patient Kegel exercises.
   3. Offer patient assistance every 3 to 4 hours.
   4. Obtain bedside commode as needed.
   5. Teach patient to avoid bladder irritants, such as coffee and nicotine.

   NCLEX Client Need: Physiological Integrity: Basic Care and Comfort
9. In determining the presence of stress urinary incontinence, what signs are characteristic?
   1. Involuntary loss of urine when the urge to urinate occurs
   2. Discomfort and burning frequently when urinating
   3. Inability to recognize the urge to urinate because of cognitive impairment
   4. Loss of urine when coughing, sneezing, or laughing or during aerobic exercise

   NCLEX Client Need: Physiological Integrity: Physiological Adaptation
10. Mirabegron (Myrbetriq) is prescribed for a patient with urinary urgency. Which statement by the patient indicates that the medication is having the intended effect?
    1. "My blood pressure is higher than it has ever been."
    2. "The burning feeling when I urinate has gone away."
    3. "The feeling of constantly needing to urinate is much less."
    4. "I have not had to urinate all day, which is great."

    NCLEX Client Need: Physiological Integrity: Pharmacological Therapies

Critical Thinking Questions

Scenario A

Mr. Jones, 65 years old, has a history of difficulty passing urine. The health care provider orders placement of a urinary catheter. You attempt to insert a 14-Fr Foley catheter, but you meet resistance and the catheter will not pass. The patient reports an uncomfortable sensation in his genital area during the attempt.

1. What is your initial action?
2. Based on your knowledge of pathophysiology, what would you suspect is preventing the passage of the catheter?
3. Why is it important to keep the drainage bag below the level of the bladder once the catheter has been successfully inserted?
4. How would you perform daily catheter care for Mr. Jones?
5. Discuss four or five general principles you would use while caring for Mr. Jones's catheter.
6. Which tasks would be appropriate to delegate to UAP? Select all that apply and give a rationale.
   a. Gathering the equipment for the catheterization procedure
   b. Inserting the Foley catheter
   c. Emptying the drainage bag at the end of the shift
   d. Checking the urinary meatus for complaints of bleeding

Scenario B

Mrs. Russlyn, a 56-year-old woman, reports that she must run to the restroom quickly when she feels the need to urinate. She makes a joke about needing to be close to a restroom when in public.

1. What type of incontinence is associated with losing urine when feeling the need to urinate?
2. What questions will you ask to collect additional data about Mrs. Russlyn's incontinence?
3. What kinds of treatment options are likely to be recommended for Mrs. Russlyn?

Scenario C

You are working in a long-term care facility and caring for Mrs. Mendez, an 86-year-old with Alzheimer disease. She has developed urinary incontinence.

1. What factors might be contributing to your patient's incontinence?
2. Explain how to develop a toileting and fluid intake schedule for Mrs. Mendez.

Care of Patients With Disorders of the Urinary System

34

http://evolve.elsevier.com/deWit/medsurg

Objectives

Theory

1. Examine the signs and symptoms of selected urologic inflammatory disorders (e.g., cystitis, urethritis, and pyelonephritis) and nursing interventions for these patients.
2. Explain nursing management for patients with acute or chronic glomerulonephritis.
3. Analyze types of patient conditions that create a risk for acute renal failure.
4. Compare the needs of patients on long-term hemodialysis with patients who use peritoneal dialysis.
5. Present the benefits and special problems associated with kidney transplantation.

Clinical Practice

6. Provide postoperative nursing care of patients after surgery of the kidney.
7. Select specific nursing responsibilities for the care of patients with kidney stones.
8. Provide postoperative nursing care of patients after surgery for urinary diversion.
9. Perform interventions to increase patient compliance in the treatment of chronic kidney failure.
10. Devise a nursing care plan for a home care patient with renal failure.

Key Terms

acute kidney injury (AKI) (ĕ-KYŪT KĬD-nē ĬN-jŭ-rē, p. 820)
acute renal failure (ARF) (ă-KŪT RĒ-năl FĀL-yŭr, p. 820)
anuria (ă-NŪ-rē-ă, p. 811)
azotemia (ă-zō-TĒ-mē-ă, p. 824)
chronic renal failure (CRF) (KRŎN-ĭk RĒ-năl FĀL-yŭr, p. 823)
cystitis (sĭs-TĪ-tĭs, p. 807)
end-stage renal disease (ESRD) (ĔND-stāj RĒ-năl dĭ-ZĒZ, p. 820)
glomerulonephritis (glō-mĕr-ū-lō-nĕ-FRĪ-tĭs, p. 811)
hemodialysis (hē-mō-dī-ĂL-ĭ-sĭs, p. 822)
hydronephrosis (hī-drō-nĕ-FRŌ-sĭs, p. 813)
lithiasis (lĭth-Ī-ă-sĭs, p. 814)
lithotripsy (LĬTH-ō-trĭp-sē, p. 815)
nephrectomy (nĕf-RŎK-tō-mē, p. 813)
nephritic syndrome (nĭ-FRĬ-tĭk SĬN-drōm, p. 811)
nephrostomy (nĕ-FRŎS-tō-mē, p. 813)
nephrotic syndrome (nĕf-RŎ-tĭk SĬN-drōm, p. 812)
oliguria (ŏl-ĭ-GŪ-rē-ă, p. 811)
peritoneal dialysis (pĕ-rĭ-tō-NĒ-ăl dī-ĂL-ĭ-sĭs, p. 822)
pyelonephritis (pī-ă-lō-nĕ-FRĪ-tĭs, p. 810)
renal stenosis (RĒ-năl stĕ-NŌ-sĭs, p. 813)
uremia (ū-RĒ-mē-ă, p. 824)
uremic syndrome (ū-RĒ-mĭk SĬN-drōm, p. 824)
urethritis (ū-rĕ-THRĪ-tĭs, p. 808)
urinary diversion (ūr-ĭ-NĂ-rē dĭ-VŎR-shŭn, p. 817)

Concepts Covered in This Chapter

- Self-Management
- Fluid and Electrolytes
- Acid-Base Balance
- Cellular Regulation
- Elimination
- Perfusion
- Inflammation
- Infection
- Patient Education
- Communication

The kidneys play a role in maintaining fluid balance, regulating the electrochemical composition of body fluids, providing protection against acid-base imbalance, forming red blood cells, regulating calcium levels, and eliminating waste products. The kidneys also help control blood pressure (BP), in conjunction with the endocrine system. Circulatory disorders, metabolic disorders such as diabetes mellitus, immunologic disorders, obstruction, bacterial infections, or toxic substances can all cause kidney dysfunction.

INFLAMMATORY DISORDERS OF THE URINARY TRACT

CYSTITIS

Etiology and Pathophysiology

Cystitis is an inflammation of the urinary bladder. It is one of the most common urinary tract infections (UTIs) in women because the female urethra is shorter and the urinary meatus is exposed to contamination from the vagina and anus. The *Escherichia coli* bacterium normally resides in the intestinal tract as a nonpathogenic microorganism; it accounts for about 80% of all UTIs in females. Cystitis can also be caused by nonbacterial pathogens, but this is less common. as is cystitis in men.

Cystitis and **urethritis** (inflammation of the urethra) are common in women after they have become sexually active. *Honeymoon cystitis* is a term sometimes used to refer to bacteria that have entered the urethra by way of friction during intercourse. In older women, the incidence of cystitis and urethritis increases as the decreased muscle tone in the urinary tract prevents complete emptying of the bladder. Urine that sits in the bladder (urinary stasis) provides a good medium for bacterial growth. The estrogen depletion that occurs with aging results in structural atrophy and urinary dysfunction.

Older Adult Care Points

The thirst sensation is usually reduced in older adults, resulting in less fluid intake. Older adults may choose to limit fluid intake due to incontinence issues and not wanting to use the restroom frequently when in social situations. Dehydration can result from these and other factors.

Fluid restriction may be needed to help control heart failure, renal failure, or other disorders that cause fluid retention. Restricting fluid intake decreases urine flow and makes the person more susceptible to UTI.

Signs, Symptoms, and Diagnosis

The most common symptoms of cystitis are painful urination, frequent and urgent urination, and low back pain. The urinary meatus may appear swollen and inflamed. Cystitis tends to recur, producing less acute symptoms such as fatigue, anorexia, and a constant feeling of pressure in the bladder region between flare-ups. The urine may appear cloudy or even bloody and have a foul smell. Urinalysis and urine cultures are used to establish a definite diagnosis and to identify the specific causative organism.

Older Adult Care Points

Confusion may be one of the first signs of cystitis or UTI in older adults. If a patient who is normally alert becomes confused, assess the urine for cloudiness, foul odor, or hematuria (blood in the urine), and check for signs of infection (fever, increased white blood cell [WBC] count).

Treatment and Nursing Management

Treatment and nursing care of cystitis and urethritis (see description of urethritis in the next section) are similar. First, specimens are collected for tests to identify the causative organism: urinalysis, urine culture and sensitivity, smear and Gram stain, or culture of the discharge. Specific antibiotics, such as trimethoprim-sulfamethoxazole (Bactrim), are used to combat infection and are combined with urinary analgesics such as phenazopyridine (Pyridium) to relieve discomfort.

Postmenopausal women may benefit from topical estrogen. Table 34.1 shows the most commonly used drugs and their nursing implications. The patient is encouraged to drink large amounts of fluids (eight to twelve 8-oz glasses unless contraindicated) to flush the bladder, and to continue the habit once the acute symptoms subside. Evidence-based practice indicates that cranberry-based products, which inhibit bacterial adhesion to the bladder wall, also have been used to prevent or treat UTIs (Rakel, 2018). Measures to relieve the discomfort include sitz baths and hot water bottles on the back or directly over the bladder region.

Patient Teaching

Preventing Urinary Tract Infections

The patient should be taught the following to prevent recurrence of urinary tract infections:

- Always wipe the anal area from front to back after a bowel movement.
- Avoid wearing any clothing that increases perineal moisture.
- Do not wash underclothing in strong detergents or bleaches; rinse clothing repeatedly until water is clear.
- Wear undergarments that do not retain moisture.
- Showering may be preferable over bathing for women.
- Do not use bubble bath, perfumed soap, feminine hygiene sprays, or over-the-counter vaginal douche products.
- Prolonged bicycling, motorcycling, horseback riding, or travel involving prolonged sitting can contribute to urethritis and cystitis.
- Drink at least eight full glasses of water each day.
- Do not ignore vaginal discharge or other signs of vaginal infection. *Candida* and *Trichomonas* infections should be treated promptly to prevent their spread to the bladder.
- Empty the bladder (urinate) promptly after sexual intercourse.

Complementary and Alternative Therapies

Vitamin C and German Chamomile

Vitamin C can help acidify the urine and decrease the frequency of cystitis. German chamomile is used topically for its antiinflammatory and antibiotic properties to soothe the inflamed genital area.

URETHRITIS

Urethritis is an inflammation of the urethra that can be caused by many different organisms. It is a common symptom of gonorrhea and should be investigated as soon as it is first noticed. Inflammatory involvement of the urethra from the herpes virus is found in males and females. Nonspecific urethritis (NSU) is a sexually transmitted inflammation of the urethra caused by a variety of organisms other than gonococci; although it may be sexually transmitted, it is not a reportable disease in the United States. NSU usually responds to treatment

Table 34.1 Drugs Commonly Used for Urinary Tract Infections

CLASSIFICATION	ACTION	NURSING IMPLICATIONS	PATIENT TEACHING
Sulfonamides			
Trimethoprim-sulfamethoxazole (Bactrim, Septra) Sulfisoxazole (Gantrisin) Sulfamethoxazole (Gantanol)	Active against gram-negative and gram-positive organisms	Assess for allergies to sulfonamides. Record I&O. Fluid intake is a minimum of 3000 mL daily. Monitor laboratory results and symptoms related to anemia, blood dyscrasias, and renal dysfunction (e.g., hemoglobin, hematocrit, WBCs, BUN). Sulfonamides can potentiate oral anticoagulants, methotrexate, and sulfonylureas (e.g., Glucotrol).	Drink at least 12 large glasses of water each day to prevent crystallization of urine. Immediately report rash, abdominal pain, blood in urine, confusion, difficulty breathing, or fever. Repeat urinalysis after course of medication.
Fluoroquinolones			
Ciprofloxacin (Cipro) Levofloxacin (Levaquin) Moxifloxacin (Avelox) Trovafloxacin (Trovan) Cinoxacin (Cinobac)	Bactericidal Considered second-line drugs; used as alternatives to other antibiotics	Can be taken with or without food; if antacids are ordered, wait 2 h after giving Cipro. Monitor WBCs for decreased leukocytes. Can potentiate warfarin and increase theophylline levels. Use cautiously in patients with history of seizure disorder or alcoholism.	Take all of medication. Drink at least 8 full glasses of water/day to prevent crystalluria. Fluoroquinolones may cause swelling and tearing of tendons. Report any pain, swelling, or bruising of joints.
Cephalosporins			
First Generation Cefazolin (Ancef)	Bactericidal; used to treat infections that do not respond to other, less expensive drugs	Use cautiously in those with allergy to penicillin. *Candida* (yeast) vaginitis is a common side effect.	Can cause dizziness or lightheadedness.
Second Generation Cefuroxime axetil (Ceftin) Cefuroxime sodium (Zinacef)	Bactericidal; inhibits cell wall mucopeptide synthesis Bactericidal; inhibits cell wall mucopeptide synthesis	Use cautiously in those with allergy to penicillin; caution if seizure disorder or renal impairment. Use cautiously in those with allergy to penicillin; caution if seizure disorder or renal impairment.	Increased vaginal *Candida* infections; increased diarrhea. Report excessive diarrhea, exhaustion.
Third Generation Ceftazidime (Fortaz) Cefixime (Suprax) Ceftriaxone (Rocephin)	Bactericidal; inhibits cell wall mucopeptide synthesis	May interfere with vitamin K metabolism; therefore may reduce prothrombin levels.	Immediately report rash, restlessness, gastrointestinal symptoms, confusion, or irregular heartbeat.
Fourth Generation Cefepime (Maxipime)	Bactericidal; used to treat infections that do not respond to previous cephalosporin-generation drugs	Monitor I&O, BUN, serum creatinine.	Avoid alcohol.
Aminoglycosides			
Tobramycin Gentamicin Streptomycin Amikacin Plazomicin	Effective against resistant infections; use cautiously because they are nephrotoxic and ototoxic and can cause agranulocytosis and thrombocytopenia	Monitor BUN, electrolyte, and creatinine levels. Older adults are especially vulnerable to problems with hearing, balance, and kidney dysfunction caused by aminoglycosides.	Use sunscreen and avoid direct exposure to sunlight. Report nausea, vomiting, tremors, or tinnitus. Take extra fluid unless contraindicated.

Continued

Table 34.1 Drugs Commonly Used for Urinary Tract Infections—cont'd

CLASSIFICATION	ACTION	NURSING IMPLICATIONS	PATIENT TEACHING
Penicillins			
Extended Spectrum Carbenicillin (Geocillin) Ticarcillin/clavulanic acid (Timentin) Piperacillin/tazobactam (Zosyn)	Bacteriostatic and bactericidal	Carbenicillin PO only. Ticarcillin/clavulanic acid IV only. Watch for signs of hypersensitivity (e.g., rash, itching, difficulty breathing). Do not give to patients with known allergy to penicillin. May decrease effectiveness of oral contraceptives and warfarin.	Take full course of prescribed medication. Take with water 1–2 h after meals to increase absorption. Immediately report abdominal pain, decreased urine, or watery or bloody diarrhea.
Miscellaneous Urinary Antibiotics			
Nitrofurantoin (Macrodantin, Furadantin)	Wide range of antibacterial action against gram-negative and gram-positive organisms, especially *Escherichia coli*	Monitor I&O. Liquid form can stain teeth; rinse mouth after administration.	Tints urine brown. Take with food and increase fluids. Can cause drowsiness; therefore avoid driving. Report numbness or tingling.
Fosfomycin tromethamine (Monurol)	Effective against most gram-negative and gram-positive organisms	Single-dose treatment. Not for use in children younger than 12 yr.	Can cause headaches and diarrhea.
Doripenem (Doribax) for complicated UTIs, including pyelonephritis	For serious infections caused by gram-positive and gram-negative bacteria	Injection only. Can reduce valproic acid levels to a subtherapeutic level, so level should be monitored.	The most common side effects include headache, nausea, diarrhea, rash, and phlebitis.
Urinary Analgesics			
Phenazopyridine (Pyridium)	Has analgesic effect on urinary mucosa	Is nephrotoxic and hepatotoxic and can cause gastrointestinal disturbance and anemia.	Colors urine orange and can stain fabric. Discontinue if sclera becomes yellow. Maximum 2 days' use.

BUN, Blood urea nitrogen; *I&O,* intake and output; *IV,* intravenously; *PO,* by mouth, orally; *UTIs,* urinary tract infections; *WBCs,* white blood cells.

with antibiotics. In women, trauma during childbirth and the proximity of the urethra to external genitalia and the anus predispose the urethra to infection and inflammation. Chemical irritation caused by use of spermicidal jellies, bath powders, feminine hygiene sprays, and bubble bath may also cause urethritis.

The chief symptoms of urethritis are burning, itching, frequency in voiding, and painful urination. There is a discharge that becomes increasingly more purulent if gonorrhea is present. The urinary meatus is swollen and inflamed. Diagnosis of urethritis is based on the presence of symptoms and a patient history that includes possible exposure to sexually transmitted infections (STIs). Culture and sensitivity of urine are obtained to identify causative organisms, and culture specimens are used to rule out STIs. The treatment and nursing management for urethritis are similar to those for cystitis. In addition, be especially aware of the possibility of a gonorrheal infection (until a definite diagnosis has been established) and carry out the necessary teaching to prevent spread of the infection to the eyes.

Think Critically

A young man is diagnosed with NSU. As you are handing him his prescription, he wants to know what he should tell his wife. What would you say to him?

PYELONEPHRITIS

Etiology and Pathophysiology

Acute **pyelonephritis** is an infection of the kidneys. It is thought to occur when bacteria (such as *E. coli*) from a bladder infection travel up the ureters to infect the kidneys. A common cause of pyelonephritis is an obstruction, causing stasis of urine and stones that cause irritation of the tissue. When bacteria enter the renal pelvis, inflammation and infection occur. After the infection is treated, the inflammation subsides; however, scar tissue is left in the place of healthy tissue. Chronic pyelonephritis is usually associated with congenital deformities in urinary anatomy and occurs primarily in children. With chronic infection and inflammation, more scar tissue develops, and eventually kidney function becomes impaired.

Signs and Symptoms

In acute pyelonephritis, symptoms include fever (often 103° F [39° C] or higher), chills, headache, malaise, nausea and vomiting, and pain in the flank (lateral abdomen) radiating to the thigh and genitalia. Eventually the urine becomes loaded with bacteria, blood, and pus.

Diagnosis

Diagnosis is based on manifestation of symptoms, physical assessment, and urine culture and sensitivity. Special diagnostic tests—such as a radiograph of the kidneys, ureters, and bladder (KUB), an intravenous pyelogram (IVP), or a renal computed tomography (CT) or magnetic resonance imaging (MRI)—may be obtained to determine the location of the obstruction if one is suspected or to rule out other causes of the symptoms.

Treatment

Prompt treatment of cystitis and prevention of recurrence can help prevent acute pyelonephritis. Bed rest, analgesics, and antipyretics are prescribed. Pyelonephritis is most commonly caused by gram-negative bacteria and less frequently by gram-positive bacteria. Sulfonamides such as trimethoprim-sulfamethoxazole (Bactrim) or a fluoroquinolone such as ciprofloxacin (Cipro) will be started because these drugs are effective against gram-positive and gram-negative bacteria. Once the culture report is complete and the sensitivity of the causative organism is known, the antibiotic therapy may be adjusted.

With chronic pyelonephritis, the patient may live for years without significant symptoms before renal damage leads to hypertension or kidney failure. Correction of obstruction, removal of stones, and prevention of stone formation are essential to correct chronic pyelonephritis and to prevent destruction and scarring of the kidney cells.

Nursing Management

Encourage fluid intake, record intake and output (I&O), monitor the urine for changes, and keep the patient comfortable. Intravenous (IV) fluids may be given to flush the kidneys, especially if the patient has nausea and vomiting. Ensure that the patient receives the appropriate antibiotics and understands the side effects to report and that the entire prescription should be completed.

ACUTE GLOMERULONEPHRITIS

Etiology and Pathophysiology

Glomerulonephritis is primarily seen in children and young adults and affects males more than females. It most commonly occurs about 2 to 3 weeks after a group A beta-hemolytic streptococcal infection, such as "strep throat" or impetigo; however, it can occur in response to bacterial, viral, or parasitic infections elsewhere in the body. It is an immunologic problem caused by an antigen-antibody reaction. Antigen-antibody complexes are deposited in the glomerular basement membrane, causing cell damage and altered permeability. Renal tissue becomes scarred, and function is impaired. **Nephritic syndrome** can occur as a result of the same conditions that cause glomerulonephritis. The damaged membrane allows large particles, such as red blood cells and protein, which normally would be retained in the bloodstream, into the urine.

Signs, Symptoms, and Diagnosis

A patient with acute glomerulonephritis usually becomes suddenly ill, with fever, chills, flank pain, widespread edema, puffiness around the eyes, visual disturbances, and marked hypertension. Diagnosis is based on physical findings and urinalysis. Presence of marked hypertension is a late manifestation. Diagnostic tests include creatinine, blood urea nitrogen (BUN), and complete blood cell count (CBC). The urine may be smoky, will contain red blood cells and protein, and will have an increased specific gravity. Serum creatinine and BUN levels rise above normal. If the condition is severe, hematocrit and hemoglobin will indicate anemia.

Treatment

Initial therapy includes IV methylprednisolone and cyclophosphamide. Management of symptoms may include a sodium-restricted diet if the patient has edema, and fluids may be limited if there is **oliguria** (diminished urine secretion in relation to intake) or **anuria** (absence of urine). A low-protein, high-carbohydrate diet also may be ordered. Antihypertensives may be needed.

Plasmapheresis is a blood cleansing procedure that may be used in autoimmune disorders such as acute glomerulonephritis or myasthenia gravis (see Chapter 24).

Nursing Management

Obtain a history of past illnesses, particularly infections, or autoimmune disorders such as lupus. Perform a general physical assessment, including vital signs and a baseline weight, and observe for fluid retention or edema. Edema that is obvious from external signs may be present in the internal organs. For this reason, mental status must be checked frequently for indications of cerebral edema with increased intracranial pressure. Cardiac failure or pulmonary edema may develop; therefore observe for extreme restlessness, increased respiratory difficulty, or cyanosis and be alert for sudden changes or worsening trends in BP, pulse, and respiratory rate.

Decreasing the work of the kidney is a primary goal in treating acute glomerulonephritis. **Absolute bed rest usually is ordered until the clinical signs of hematuria, proteinuria, and hypertension are gone.** If the patient responds quickly to treatment and wishes to be more active, you must emphasize the need for continued rest. Low-protein diets may be ordered if the BUN is elevated, to reduce nitrogenous waste by-products.

Patient Teaching

Sodium

Help your patient recognize that a low-sodium diet involves more than avoiding the salt shaker. Demonstrate how to read food labels to identify hidden sources of sodium in items such as catsup, canned soups and food, salad dressing, baked goods, and packaged meats.

If the patient has plasmapheresis therapy, you should monitor for bleeding at the puncture site every 2 to 4 hours. Also monitor for potential complications, such as hypovolemia or electrolyte imbalance. The prognosis for acute glomerulonephritis varies, depending on the extent of permanent damage done to the kidneys or other vital organs.

CHRONIC GLOMERULONEPHRITIS

Etiology and Pathophysiology

Chronic glomerulonephritis is the third leading cause of chronic kidney disease (CKD). All acute glomerulonephritis has the potential to become a chronic condition. Continued fibrosis within the glomerulus leads to reduction of the glomerular filtration rate (GFR) and retention of toxins, and the kidney atrophies; the number of functional nephrons decreases and eventually, kidney failure occurs. The prognosis for this disease depends on the cause of the glomerulonephritis, and the progression to renal failure varies with the individual.

Signs and Symptoms

Generalized edema, headache associated with hypertension, fatigue, dyspnea, weight loss, loss of strength, peripheral neuropathy, and tremors are symptoms of glomerulonephritis. Proteinuria, hematuria, and kidney failure occur as the kidney function becomes impaired. Some patients who develop chronic glomerulonephritis may have acute exacerbations.

Diagnosis

Diagnostic testing may be prompted by findings on a routine examination—for example, retinal hemorrhage discovered during an eye examination. Testing includes urinalysis, creatinine, BUN, CBC, and electrolytes. Abnormal laboratory values include proteinuria, urinary casts (protein plugs secreted by damaged tubules), elevated creatinine and BUN levels, anemia, hyperkalemia, hypermagnesemia, increased phosphorus, and decreased serum calcium and albumin.

Treatment and Nursing Management

The treatment for chronic glomerulonephritis in the latent stage is primarily symptomatic, with emphasis on avoiding fatigue and infections, particularly of the upper respiratory tract. When renal failure develops, dialysis (filtration of the blood) and possibly a kidney transplant are the only alternative therapies. Care of the patient with chronic renal disease is discussed in the Chronic Renal Failure section later in this chapter.

NEPHROTIC SYNDROME (NEPHROSIS)

Etiology and Pathophysiology

Nephrotic syndrome sometimes occurs after the glomeruli have been damaged by glomerulonephritis or some other disease. This damage results in increased membrane permeability and excretion of protein and decreased serum albumin (hypoalbuminemia). Hypoalbuminemia causes fluid to shift out of the vascular system into the body tissues, and the result is severe edema. Some patients recover without further incidence, whereas others experience repeated episodes and eventual kidney failure.

Clinical Cues

Nephrotic syndrome and nephritic syndrome are easily confused. Clinical symptoms are similar, although edema is more severe in nephrotic syndrome because of the loss of protein that would normally keep fluid in the vascular space. Proteinuria is found in nephrotic syndrome, and hematuria is the prominent finding in nephritic syndrome, causing tea-colored urine. Memory hint: Protein in urine causes foamy bubbles—nephr**O**sis—ocean foam. Hematuria—blood-red nephr**I**tis—inflammation.

Signs, Symptoms, and Diagnosis

Nephrotic syndrome is characterized by extensive proteinuria, hyperlipidemia (elevated blood lipids), hypoalbuminemia (low blood albumin), and severe edema. Facial edema, especially periorbital edema, may be present in the morning, whereas lower extremity edema is more evident at the end of the day. Ascites (accumulation of serous fluid in the abdominal cavity) may also occur because of fluid retention. The patient may be irritable, tired, or lethargic. Diagnostic tests include urinalysis and serum tests for protein and lipids. A renal biopsy may be used to verify the diagnosis or to evaluate the extent of kidney damage.

Treatment and Nursing Management

Treatment for nephrotic syndrome consists of an adequate-protein, low-fat, low-sodium diet; diuretics; supplemental multiple vitamins and minerals; and antibiotics if infection is present. Some patients are treated with cortisone and cyclophosphamide (Cytoxan).

Nursing care includes monitoring I&O, recording daily weight, encouraging rest, providing skin care, and encouraging compliance with dietary and medication regimen.

OBSTRUCTIONS OF THE URINARY TRACT

HYDRONEPHROSIS

Etiology and Pathophysiology

Whenever the normal flow of urine is obstructed (e.g., kidney stone, tumor mass, or enlarged prostate), there is a potential backward flow of fluid into the renal pelvis.

Hydronephrosis occurs if the obstruction is not resolved; the renal pelvis and ureters will become dilated and continue to fill with fluid. Soon the kidney cells will atrophy until all normal function ceases and the kidney becomes a thin-walled cyst. Hydronephrosis may be unilateral or bilateral (one or both kidneys). If it occurs on one side, the other kidney may enlarge and efficiently carry on the work of two kidneys. This is called *compensatory hypertrophy*.

Signs, Symptoms, and Diagnosis

Severe pain is present only if hydronephrosis develops rapidly. Otherwise there are no outstanding symptoms, and the patient may develop signs of kidney failure only after serious damage has occurred. A definitive diagnosis is obtained by extensive urologic examination and ultrasound. Detailed radiographic studies of the kidney and ureters, which usually reveal the site and cause of obstruction and distention of the renal pelvis, may be used to determine the best treatment.

Treatment

The primary goal of treatment for hydronephrosis is to remove the obstruction so that the kidney may drain properly. The ideal remedy is to drain the kidney in the early stages with a nephrostomy tube or ureteral stent. **Nephrostomy** is a percutaneous procedure that places a drainage tube into a kidney (Fig. 34.1). If a cause of the obstruction can be corrected surgically, the drainage tube may be placed during surgery to correct obstructions from large stones or strictures of the ureters. The nephrostomy tube stays in place to drain the kidneys while the surgical repair site heals. It is also used to drain purulent material from an infected kidney. If the damage is irreparable, surgery is necessary to remove the kidney (**nephrectomy**).

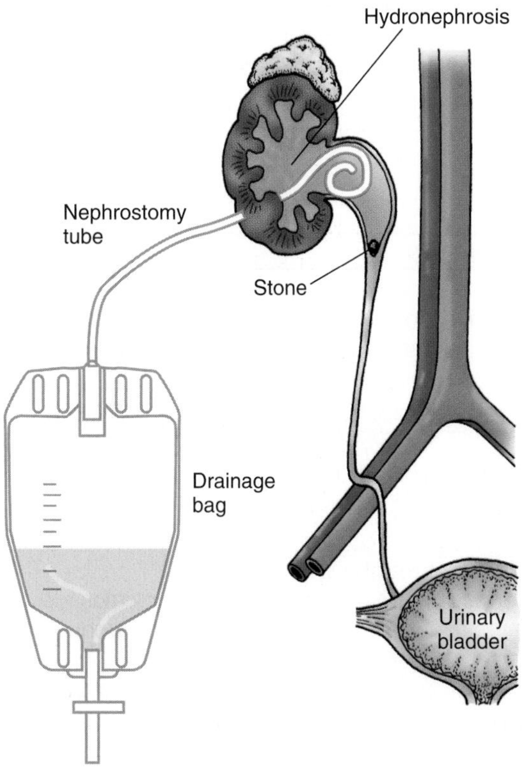

Fig. 34.1 Nephrostomy tube draining hydronephrosis caused by a ureteral stone. (Modified from Ignatavicius DD, Workman ML, et al.: *Medical-surgical nursing: critical thinking for collaborative care*, ed 9, St. Louis, 2018, Elsevier.)

> **Safety Alert**
>
> **Verify the Purpose and Type of Tube or Drain**
>
> **DO NOT confuse urinary drainage systems with gastrointestinal feeding or drainage systems!** They can look very similar. When working with tubes and drains, trace all tubes down to the patient's body surface *before* irrigation or instillation of fluids, feedings, or medications. Verify the purpose and type of tube or drain with the charge nurse if you are unsure.

Nursing Management

Postoperative nursing care. In nephrectomy the surgical incision(s) may be lumbar, transabdominal, thoracic, or laparoscopic. When the patient returns from surgery, you must carefully check for the location of the surgical wound(s) and the presence of any drains or tubes that may have been inserted during the operation. Nursing interventions focus on promoting unimpeded urine flow by properly caring for catheters and tubes.

> **Clinical Cues**
>
> A nephrostomy tube should never be clamped or irrigated without a specific health care provider's order that defines the circumstances and the amount of irrigation fluid.

Hemorrhage is a danger after surgery of the kidney because the kidneys have a very rich supply of blood directly from the aorta and vena cava. The vital signs are frequently monitored, and any indication of shock or hemorrhage is immediately reported.

Adequate drainage from the opposite kidney after surgery is of great importance. Urinary output must be measured very carefully and recorded. Fluids are adjusted based on the function of the remaining kidney. Adequate pain control and early mobilization can help prevent complications.

RENAL STENOSIS

The renal artery can become blocked or narrowed (**renal stenosis**) because of atherosclerosis or scarring. This blockage can result in hypertension or **chronic renal failure** (gradual loss of kidney function). The patient may be asymptomatic, but BP should be monitored. MRI, CT scan, or ultrasound may show a decreased kidney size. Anticipate that the patient will be prescribed antihypertensives to control elevated BP. Balloon angioplasty or stent placement can improve blood flow to the kidney. As long as blood flow is inadequate, the kidney will continue to produce renin in an effort to increase blood flow to itself. The continuous activation of the renin–angiotensin–aldosterone (RAA) system keeps the BP elevated until the obstruction is resolved.

RENAL STONES

A renal or kidney stone (**lithiasis**) is a crystalline mass that forms in the urinary system and, depending on the size and location, may obstruct the flow of urine. Stones can be as small as a grain of sand or large enough to fill the renal pelvis. This enlarged stone formation is called a *renal staghorn calculus*. Renal stones also vary in composition and in the environment in which they form. Some stones form more readily in acidic urine, whereas others occur in alkaline urine. There are four major types of renal stones, one of which is hereditary. Table 34.2 shows the risk factors and dietary interventions for each type of renal stone. Identifying the type and cause of stones can be very effective in preventing further formation and deciding the appropriate method of treatment for each patient. However, in about half of cases, the precise cause of stone formation cannot be identified.

Etiology and Pathophysiology

Certain conditions predispose a person to having renal calculi. Among the most common causative factors are (1) bariatric surgery, short bowel syndrome, or other conditions that decrease oxalate absorption in the gut; (2) inadequate fluid intake, which results in concentrated urine and inadequate flushing of the urinary tract; (3) sluggish flow of urine, as may occur with bed rest or immobility; and (4) diabetes, obesity gout, and hypertension. The most common type of stone is formed from calcium oxalate and less often calcium phosphate. Other types of stone are composed of uric acid, magnesium ammonium phosphate, or cysteine.

A small percentage of patients with calcium stones have a tumor of the parathyroid. This gland produces a hormone that raises the level of serum calcium and thus the level of calcium in the urine. Treatment of the parathyroid condition removes the cause of the stones. Risk factors for kidney stone formation include the following:

- Male gender
- A family history of renal stones
- Immobility for any reason, which contributes to urinary stasis and calcium loss from bones
- History of recurrent UTIs

Prevention

A continuous flow of dilute urine flushes the tract and removes substances that could form stones. **Ideally, adults must put out at least 2500 mL of urine every 24 hours to prevent stone formation; likewise, preventing urinary infections and maintaining adequate drainage through tubes and catheters is also necessary.** In those cases in which the urine pH is causing stone formation, changing the urine pH can prevent or reduce the incidence of renal calculi. Ascorbic acid or dietary modifications (e.g., cranberry juice, prunes, or lemon juice) can be used to alter urine pH.

Signs and Symptoms

Some renal stones do not cause noticeable symptoms and can be passed without the person being aware of

Table 34.2 Risk Factors and Treatments for Renal Stones

STONE TYPE	RISK FACTORS	INTERVENTIONS
Calcium oxalate (most common type)	An increased intake of protein, sodium; inadequate fluid intake, prolonged immobility	Increase fluid intake. Medications to bind oxalate (cholestyramine) or calcium (e.g., cellulose phosphate). Diuretics (e.g., hydrochlorothiazide) to encourage flushing. Avoid oxalate sources such as spinach, chard, parsley, peanuts, chocolate, and strawberries.
Calcium phosphate	An increased intake of protein, sodium; inadequate fluid intake, primary hyperparathyroidism	Limit intake of foods high in protein and sodium. Treat underlying hyperparathyroidism.
Uric acid	Excess dietary purine (e.g., organ meats, gravies, red wines, and sardines) Gout (primary or secondary)	Decrease intake of purine sources. Alkalinize urine with potassium citrate or lemonade. Administer allopurinol for gout (decreases production of uric acid).
Struvite (more common in women)	Urinary tract infections	Administer antibiotics for infection and acetohydroxamic acid, which inhibits the chemical action of bacteria that contributes to struvite stone formation.
Cystine	Hereditary cystine crystal formation	Encourage oral fluids, up to 3 L/day. Medications to prevent crystallization (e.g., tiopronin). Alkalinize urine with potassium citrate or lemonade.

them. Others may lodge in the renal pelvis and cause symptoms only after the destruction of kidney cells. The kidney stones that cause severe pain are those that are small enough to move along the ureter with the urine. As the stone rolls along, sharp little spikes scrape the ureteral lining, causing excruciating pain and bleeding. Pain is typically felt in the flank over the affected kidney and ureter and radiates downward toward the genitalia and inner thigh. Nausea and vomiting often occur because of the severity of the pain. **Moving stones can get trapped along the ureter, causing obstruction of flow and swelling of the ureter.**

Diagnosis

Diagnostic tests include a low-radiation-dose noncontrast CT of the abdomen and pelvis or an ultrasound. Urinalysis will identify whether blood, albumin, or other characteristics are present. Further studies of the blood and urine might be done to determine the levels of substances, such as calcium, uric acid, and cystine, that can contribute to stone formation.

Treatment

At first, the health care provider may try to flush the stone out by increasing the patient's IV fluids or oral fluid intake and managing pain by prescribing opioid analgesics or nonsteroidal antiinflammatory drugs (NSAIDs) and antispasmodics, such as propantheline bromide (Pro-Banthine) or oxybutynin chloride (Ditropan). If there is pus in the urine, an antibiotic is prescribed to deal with infection. To facilitate passing of stones that are small enough and in a suitable location, medical expulsive therapy (MET) is tried first with alpha blockers such as tamsulosin (Flomax).

When the stone is not passed spontaneously, cystoscopy or surgical intervention is necessary. Stones may be removed directly during ureteroscopy and ureteral stents placed if indicated. Other methods are used when stones cannot be accessed with ureteroscopy. Percutaneous nephrolithotomy (PNL; incision into the kidney to remove a stone) has largely replaced open surgery for stone removal. Less than 1% of patients require an open procedure. The PNL procedure is initially similar to nephrostomy tube placement, and a nephrostomy tube may be left in place post procedure. PNL is indicated when shock wave **lithotripsy** (SWL) has not been effective. SWL is performed in an operating room where high-energy sound waves are generated and focused on the stone, pass through a water-filled cushion, and break the stone. Sedation is used to help the patient remain calm and still during the 30- to 45-minute procedure, or the patient may be given general anesthesia. Ureteral stents or a nephrostomy tube that will help removal of the stones from the body may be placed (Dave, 2018).

MET therapy is used as an adjunct to SWL and increases the rate of stone passage.

If the stone is 5 mm or larger, the patient may also receive a ureteral stent (usually a soft, flexible silicone tube), which is inserted through a cystoscope or nephrostomy tube or during surgery. The stent runs the entire length of the ureter. One end is in the renal pelvis, and the other end is in the bladder. A stylet is used during placement to straighten the tube for insertion. Once the stylet is removed, the ends of the stent curl up—called a pigtail—holding the stent in place. The purpose of a ureteral stent is to maintain the patency of the ureter to allow stones to pass through. They are usually removed in 4 to 6 weeks in an outpatient setting. Table 34.3 provides additional information about common catheters and tubes used for urologic disorders.

> **? Think Critically**
>
> Based on your knowledge of anatomy and physiology, what is the difference between a **urethral** catheter and a **ureteral** catheter? (Note the spelling difference!) Why is it important to know the difference between these two catheter sites?

Nursing Management

During initial assessment of a patient with kidney stones, the patient may have extreme pain, so use concise questions to gather information about pain, changes in

Table 34.3 Common Catheters and Tubes Used for Urologic Disorders

TYPE	PURPOSE
Urethral catheter	Placed through the urethra to the bladder for one-time drainage or to obtain a specimen.
Foley catheter	Also a urethral catheter but indwelling and placed for continuous urine drainage from the bladder.
Suprapubic catheter	Continuous drainage of urine from the bladder; inserted in suprapubic area of abdomen through abdominal and bladder wall.
Ureteral catheter	Used in procedures to inject contrast for imaging or to access the ureter for intervention. Are removed when the procedure is complete.
Ureteral stent	Tube placed in ureter to hold it open during healing or to facilitate stone passage. One end is in the renal pelvis, and the other end is in the bladder.
Nephrostomy tube	Placed into the pelvis of the kidney through the skin to provide drainage of urine directly from the kidney to an external collection bag.

urinary output, and characteristics of the urine. Asking family about risk factors and history may be appropriate.

Attempts are made to have the patient pass the stone spontaneously, and all urine is strained to recover the stone or fragments for analysis. This is accomplished by having the patient void into a urinal or collection device and then pouring the collected urine through a fine mesh filter. Fluids are encouraged during this time to facilitate flushing of the stone.

After PNL a fluid intake of 3000 to 4000 mL/day is required to flush any residual stone fragments out of the kidney. The patient is monitored for infection, hemorrhage, and leakage of fluid into the retroperitoneal cavity.

After an SWL procedure, the patient may experience cramping pain and is given opioid pain medications. A fluid intake of 3000 to 4000 mL in the 24 hours following the procedure is necessary to help wash the stone fragments from the kidney.

After any invasive intervention, nursing actions include monitoring for infection, bleeding, urine output, and pain. Once stones have been removed, chemical analyses of urine, blood, and the stone itself are necessary to plan effective preventive measures.

Blood in the urine is expected after any procedure on the urinary tract.

UROLOGIC SYSTEM TRAUMA

TRAUMA TO KIDNEYS AND URETERS

Etiology and Pathophysiology

Accidental injury to the kidneys, ureters, bladder, or urethra should always be considered whenever there has been trauma to the abdominal cavity, lower back, or thoracic cage. Injury to the kidneys is usually caused by blunt trauma that is sustained during a motor vehicle, sports, or occupational accident. Damage can occur as a result of a direct blow, laceration from an adjacent rib or vertebra fracture, or sudden deceleration, which shears and tears the body tissue. Injuries include lacerations, contusions, and damage to blood vessels. Ureteral injuries are mostly associated with penetrating trauma; the right side is three times more likely than the left side to be involved. Trauma to the urinary system can range from minor contusion to severe hemorrhage that leads to hypovolemic shock.

Signs, Symptoms, and Diagnosis

Signs and symptoms characteristic of trauma to the kidneys include bruising, hematuria, abdominal or flank pain, and possibly an enlarged mass in the kidney area. Bleeding internally from kidney injury may not be evident by gross hematuria, but close monitoring of BP for hypotension is needed to identify the onset of shock. Diagnostic tests include serial urinalyses, hemoglobin and hematocrit tests, and measurements of electrolytes. Rising BUN and serum creatinine levels indicate diminishing renal function. Radiologic studies (KUB, IVP, or CT scan) can demonstrate the extent of damage to the urinary system. MRI or angiography is used in high-risk cases or if CT scan is indeterminate. Hourly measurements of urinary output and observation of the characteristics of the urine can help determine the type and extent of injury.

> **Clinical Cues**
>
> When a patient sustains significant trauma to skeletal muscle tissue, they may develop rhabdomyolysis. Damaged muscles release myoglobin into the bloodstream, and these large muscle proteins can cause *acute renal failure* (sudden loss of kidney function); however, the condition is reversible. Be alert for brown or tea-colored urine after trauma, strenuous exercise, or extensive burns, and report your findings to the health care provider.

Treatment

Bleeding in the kidney is often self-limiting. Lacerations and contusions without interruption of urinary function usually can be treated conservatively by bed rest. For this reason, the nephrologist may advocate a period of watchful waiting to see whether the kidney can be saved. If the kidney is severely damaged, the patient may undergo a nephrectomy. The remaining kidney then enlarges and is usually able to carry on the work formerly done by two kidneys.

Nursing Management

Preoperative nursing care. Patients with kidney trauma are likely to have damage to the colon, spleen, or pancreas. A comprehensive plan for dealing with problems associated with multiple trauma is necessary. Preoperatively the patient is monitored closely for signs of hypovolemic shock, cardiovascular changes, urinary output, and size of the flank hematoma. Grey Turner sign is bruising over the flank or lower back and suggests retroperitoneal bleeding. For most trauma patients, a urethral catheter is inserted into the bladder. An indwelling catheter allows for close observation of urinary output—for example, critically ill patients may need hourly urine output measurements, and a drainage bag with a urometer should replace the standard drainage bag.

Postoperative nursing care. Postoperative nursing care for nephrectomy or nephrostomy is described in the Hydronephrosis section earlier in the chapter.

TRAUMA TO THE BLADDER

Etiology and Pathophysiology

Any violent blow or crushing injury to the lower abdomen may result in rupture or perforation of the bladder wall, with resulting leakage of the urine into the pelvic tissues or peritoneal cavity. This results in severe inflammation (peritonitis). Bladder trauma is more likely to occur if the bladder is full at the time of an accident rather than if it is empty.

Signs and Symptoms

Early symptoms of bladder injury are painful hematuria or inability to void, marked tenderness and spasm in the suprapubic area, or development of a large mass in that area.

> **Clinical Cues**
>
> In cases of pelvic or perineal trauma, bleeding at the urethral meatus, inability to void, or a distended bladder may indicate a urethral tear. Notify the health care provider before inserting a catheter because catheter insertion can increase the damage by extending the tear.

Diagnosis and Treatment

Diagnosis is based on presence of gross hematuria, suprapubic pain, and difficulty voiding. Retrograde or CT cystography is obtained if bladder injuries are suspected. If the bladder has ruptured or is perforated, treatment consists of a suprapubic cystostomy to drain blood and urine.

Nursing Management

Patient care requires meticulous attention to drains and dressings to prevent infection and maintain good drainage. Cold applications to the surgical site both before and after surgery may be ordered. Observe the patient carefully for postoperative shock and hemorrhage. Any mass formation in the suprapubic area before or after surgery or any change in vital signs should be reported immediately.

UROLOGIC SYSTEM CANCERS

CANCER OF THE BLADDER

Etiology and Pathophysiology

It is estimated that approximately 80,000 new cases of bladder cancer will be diagnosed in 2019, resulting in death for 13,000 men and 4800 women (American Cancer Society [ACS], 2019). Bladder cancer is more common in men (ages 60 to 80 years) than in women. **Smokers have double the risk of developing this cancer.** People living in urban areas or with occupational exposure to nitrates, dyes, rubber, or leather processing (e.g., painters, hairdressers, or textile workers) are at higher risk. The bladder wall is exposed to these carcinogenic chemicals in the urine. Tumors of the bladder usually start in the superficial transitional cell layer and are considered papillomas (benign tumors on the epithelial tissue). Bladder tumors are removed—even though they are papillomas—because there is a high risk for invasion into the deeper tissues and metastasis.

Signs, Symptoms, and Diagnosis

The main symptom of a bladder tumor is hematuria. Frequency, urgency, or dysuria also may be present. Diagnosis is confirmed by examining the bladder wall with a cystoscope and biopsy of the tumor. Urine cytology and tumor marker testing can be helpful in the diagnosis and in follow-up after treatment.

Treatment

Treatment for bladder cancer is surgery, either alone or in combination with chemotherapy or radiation. The type of surgical treatment depends on the clinical stage of the tumor. Every effort is made to preserve the bladder if the tumor is confined to the mucosa or submucosa. In this case a partial cystectomy or transurethral resection of bladder tumor (TURBT) is performed and followed by intravesical immunotherapy (bacillus Calmette-Guérin [BCG] instillations [TheraCys]) or chemotherapy. The drugs that are used most often for intravesical therapy are mitomycin and thiotepa, but combinations of other drugs, such as valrubicin, doxorubicin, and gemcitabine, may be used (ACS, 2017). BCG was originally used as a vaccine against tuberculosis. It has helped patients with bladder carcinoma in situ (site of origin) by reducing tumor recurrence and by eliminating residual malignant cells after surgery. The solution is instilled into the bladder via a urinary catheter. The catheter is clamped for 2 hours, and the patient's position is changed every 15 to 30 minutes. Treatments are continued weekly for 6 weeks, with possible maintenance doses. Advise patients that BCG intravesical therapy is likely to cause future tuberculin skin tests to result in a false-positive result.

> **Safety Alert**
>
> **Precautions Following BCG Treatment**
>
> In addition to using Standard Precautions, for 6 hours following a BCG treatment the patient's toilet should be disinfected with bleach each time it is used for the disposal of the patient's urine. Take care that urine does not splash onto other surfaces, as BCG is a live vaccine.

Photodynamic therapy can be used for superficial tumors. In this therapy a solution of light-sensitive molecules is injected IV. These molecules adhere to cancer cells longer than they do to normal cells. A cystoscope with a red laser light can then be used to activate the photosensitizers that destroy tumor cells.

Surgeries for urinary diversion. Bladder surgery may be minor, such as removing polyps from the bladder interior using a cystoscope, or major, such as cystectomy (removal of the bladder) or partial cystectomy for bladder cancer. After cystectomy there is always the danger of hemorrhage and infection. There is also the need to devise a satisfactory arrangement for urine collection. When the bladder is surgically removed, the surgeon performs a **urinary diversion** to handle the excretion of urine and creates an artificial opening (stoma) on the skin surface. Diversions also can be performed for neurogenic bladder, congenital anomalies, strictures, or trauma. Diversions can be noncontinent or continent. Urinary diversion can be accomplished in several ways (Fig. 34.2), including by ileal conduit or ileal loop, ureterosigmoidostomy or sigmoid conduit, and ileal reservoir (i.e., Kock, Indiana, Mainz, or Florida pouch). The differences among these procedures are the segment of bowel that is used to create the conduit or reservoir and whether a valve mechanism has been added to achieve continence.

Cutaneous ureterostomy. In a cutaneous ureterostomy, the surgeon detaches one or both ureters from the bladder and brings them to the surface of the body, usually in the region of the flank. The patient may have one or two stomas. If the patient has a cutaneous ureterostomy with two stomas (one from each ureter), the continuous flow of urine from each stoma must be monitored and measured. Any urostomy bags or tubing leading from the ureterostomy should be kept open so that urine can flow freely.

Ileal conduit. An ileal conduit is also called *urinary ileostomy and ileal loop* or a *Bricker procedure.* A portion of the ileum is used as a tube or conduit through which urine flows to the outside. A section of ileum is removed, and the remaining ileum is rejoined by anastomosis (operative union of structures). One end of the ileal segment is sutured together, and the other is brought out through the abdominal wall, creating a stoma. The ureters are attached to the ileal conduit so that urine can flow through the conduit to the outside. This allows for one stoma instead of two.

Ureterosigmoidostomy or sigmoid conduit. A sigmoid or colonic conduit uses the sigmoid colon as the insertion site for the ureters, and urine is expelled with stool. No external stoma is needed. Due to potential for incontinence and other complications, currently the procedure is rarely performed, but you may care for patients who had the procedure many years ago.

Continent diversion (Indiana pouch). Typically, either ileum or a terminal ileum combined with ascending colon is used for continent urinary diversion. These segments are detubularized and then refashioned into a spherical shape and used as a reservoir. The spherical shape has an increased capacity and decreases the pressure inside by allowing the walls of the pouch to expand, preventing problems such as high-pressure reflux and eventual renal failure (Shariat et al., 2018). A one-way valve mechanism is created at the external stoma through which catheterization is performed intermittently throughout the day to empty the internal pouch. There is no external storage system.

> **Clinical Cues**
>
> If caring for a patient with an established urostomy, ask the patient their routine and what they need to maintain the ostomy. Get orders from the health care provider so that the patient can self-catheterize, irrigate, or perform needed self-care. If the patient is not physically capable, you should assist, using the patient's routine until they recover.

Orthotic bladder substitutes. Bladder substitutes or neobladders can be created using a portion of the patient's own intestine; they are used when the sphincter is intact and there is no cancer in the urethra or bladder neck. The advantage is normal micturition. Examples include Kock pouch, Indiana pouch, Mitrofanoff procedure, and ileal neobladder. Emptying of the surgically created bladders is accomplished by tightening the abdominal muscles.

Nursing Management

Postoperative nursing care. After surgery, observe for pain, abdominal rigidity, fever, and bleeding. Assess the amount and characteristics of the urine and mucus and record accurate output of urine every hour for the first 24 hours and then every 4 to 8 hours. During the healing process, a ureteral catheter will drain the newly constructed bladder. The bowel tissue used for construction of the bladder produces mucus, so irrigation of the catheter is necessary to prevent blockage of the catheter. If a noncontinent stoma is present, watch for swelling or clots that could obstruct flow. **Regardless of which surgical procedure the patient has had, the urine should never stop flowing.**

The urine should initially be light red or pink and progress to clear within 3 days or less. Bright red bleeding or clots should be reported immediately. The stoma should be pink or red. A pale, dark, or dusky stoma suggests decreased blood flow, which should be reported immediately. Skin irritation and breakdown can be a problem, and every effort is made to keep urine from touching the skin when the patient has an external stoma. A well-fitted and properly adhering collection appliance is essential. A thin gauze roll or tampon is placed into the stoma during appliance changing and cleaning to prevent leakage of urine onto the skin. For a permanent ostomy, the bag can be used for 3 to 7 days. The bag should be emptied when it becomes one-third to one-half full, to prevent the weight of the urine from pulling the bag loose. At night the bag can be connected to a larger urine container. The bag should be changed in the morning when there is less urine flow. The area is thoroughly washed with warm, soapy water, then rinsed and patted dry with a towel before a new bag is attached because any remaining moisture may interfere with the seal of the new appliance. A bath or shower may be taken with the bag on or off.

Most appliances contain an odor barrier; however, odor may be a problem because of poor hygiene; alkaline urine; normal breakdown of urine when it is exposed to air; and the ingestion of certain foods, such as asparagus. Dilute urine is also less odorous and can be accomplished by increasing fluid intake. Urine crystals that look like white, gritty particles are sometimes found on the stoma or skin if the urine is too alkaline.

Psychological care of a patient facing malignancy and an operation that will radically change their body image should be a primary nursing concern, and there

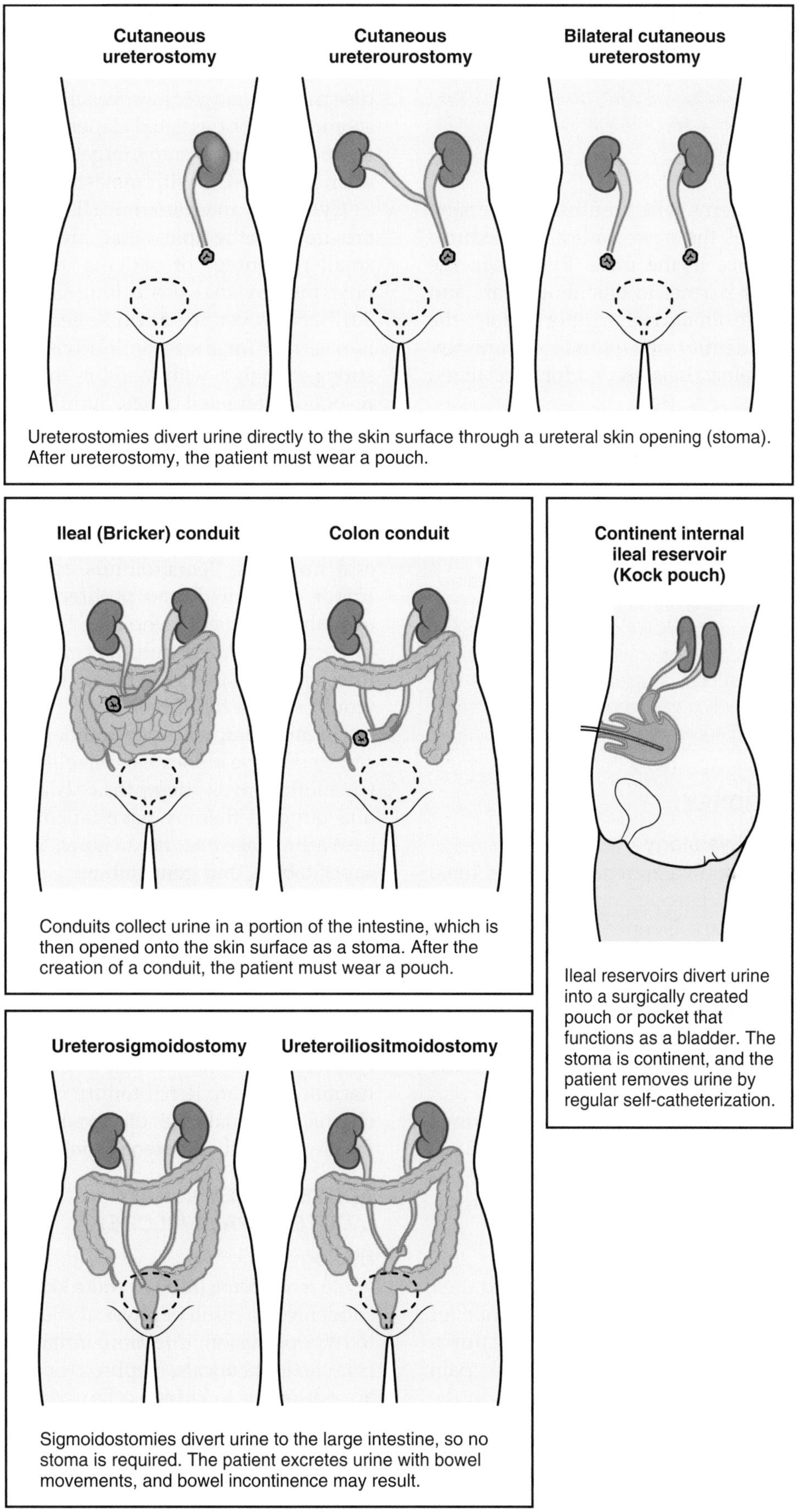
Cutaneous ureterostomy
Cutaneous ureterourostomy
Bilateral cutaneous ureterostomy
Ureterostomies divert urine directly to the skin surface through a ureteral skin opening (stoma). After ureterostomy, the patient must wear a pouch.
Ileal (Bricker) conduit
Colon conduit
Conduits collect urine in a portion of the intestine, which is then opened onto the skin surface as a stoma. After the creation of a conduit, the patient must wear a pouch.
Continent internal ileal reservoir (Kock pouch)
Ileal reservoirs divert urine into a surgically created pouch or pocket that functions as a bladder. The stoma is continent, and the patient removes urine by regular self-catheterization.
Ureterosigmoidostomy
Ureteroiliositmoidostomy
Sigmoidostomies divert urine to the large intestine, so no stoma is required. The patient excretes urine with bowel movements, and bowel incontinence may result.

Fig. 34.2 Urinary diversion procedures used in the treatment of bladder cancer. (From Ignatavicius DD, Workman ML, et al.: *Medical-surgical nursing: critical thinking for collaborative care,* ed 9, St. Louis, 2018, Elsevier.)

Complementary and Alternative Therapies

Reduce Odor of Urine

For patients with a urinary diversion, a diet that includes whole grains, nuts, plums, prunes, and cranberry juice will help acidify the urine and decrease odors.

are always sexual concerns when a urinary diversion is performed. Some of the more radical procedures will produce impotence in the male. Encourage the patient and spouse or partner to talk about fears and concerns and provide emotional support. Help the patient and family identify appropriate community resources and make referrals as needed for specialized counseling.

Clinical Cues

Clinical trials are in process for three-dimensional (3D) bio-printed bladders created from patients' own cells. One bladder has been in place and functional for more than 14 years (Belton, 2018). The neobladders created from intestine allow for continence, which greatly enhances quality of life, but the function of the intestine is to absorb substances, which means that some of what the kidney has filtered out may be reabsorbed. The laboratory-produced replacement bladders are showing promise in preventing this problem and functioning like the original bladder (Bagalá, 2018).

CANCER OF THE KIDNEY

Etiology and Pathophysiology

Cancer of the kidney, known as renal cancer or renal cell carcinoma (RCC), is relatively uncommon in people younger than age 45 years. Neoplasms of the kidney occur in men (ages 50 to 70 years) twice as often as in women. People with kidney cancer tend to be older and many times have other health problems, so treatment and predicting survival rates are complicated. Risk factors include smoking, obesity, hypertension, and exposure to cadmium, asbestos, or petroleum by-products.

The tumors usually begin growing in the proximal tubule. They can become very large before symptoms occur. As with other cancers, the stage at which RCC is diagnosed determines the treatment and prognosis.

Signs, Symptoms, and Diagnosis

More than 25% of patients are asymptomatic, and their cancer was found when imaging studies were done for some other reason. The classic symptoms of hematuria, palpable abdominal or flank mass, and flank pain (although pain and a mass may not be present in the early stages) are frequently not present. Other symptoms that may occur are fever, fatigue, weight loss, decreased appetite, and hypertension. Because of the lack of disturbing symptoms, RCC may not be identified until a late stage, making it harder to treat successfully. CT and MRI are the imaging studies most commonly used to identify RCC.

Treatment and Nursing Management

Surgical removal or partial removal of the affected kidney (nephrectomy) is curative in nonmetastatic disease. The surgical approach may be open, laparoscopic, or robot assisted depending on tumor characteristics. Immunotherapy, targeted therapy, and radiation are used for RCC with metastasis.

Cytokines interleukin-2 (IL-2) and interferon alfa are immunotherapies that are effective for only a small percentage of patients. Immunotherapy is the only therapy that has a long-lasting response (ACS, 2017). However, it can cause serious side effects, so it is reserved for those with advanced cancer who are strong enough to withstand this treatment or who do not respond to targeted drugs. Sunitinib (Sutent), sorafenib tosylate (Nexavar), temsirolimus (Torisel), everolimus (Afinitor), bevacizumab (Avastin), pazopanib (Votrient), cabozantinib (Cabometyx) lenvatinib (Lenvima), and axitinib (Inlyta) are targeted drugs for advanced kidney cancer. They act to deprive the tumor cells of blood and nutrients. Temsirolimus and everolimus inhibit tumor cell growth and proliferation; these drugs are available to patients who failed to respond to sunitinib or sorafenib. Pazopanib, cabozantinib, and lenvatinib interfere with the growth of new blood vessels that would supply the tumor.

Chemotherapy is not a standard treatment for renal cancer because kidney cancer cells are usually resistant. Chemotherapy is attempted only after immunotherapy and targeted therapy have failed. Drugs used in this case are vinblastine, floxuridine, 5-fluorouracil (5-FU), capecitabine, and gemcitabine.

Nursing care of patients with renal cancer after nephrectomy is the same as that for other cancer patients (see Chapter 8 for care of patients with cancer).

RENAL FAILURE

Renal failure is the inability of the kidneys to maintain normal function. Renal failure is classified as acute or chronic. The final stage of chronic and irreversible renal failure is called **end-stage renal disease (ESRD).**

ACUTE KIDNEY INJURY (ACUTE RENAL FAILURE)

Etiology

Acute renal failure (ARF) or **acute kidney injury (AKI)** occurs suddenly as a result of physical injury, usually secondary to hypoperfusion, infection, inflammation, or damage from toxic chemicals. Nephrotoxic agents are those that are poisonous to kidney cells and include many drugs, iodine substances used as radiographic contrast media, heavy metals, snake venom, or industrial chemicals. These toxins may inflict damage on the renal tubules, causing acute tubular necrosis (ATN) and loss of function. They can also indirectly harm the tubules by causing severe constriction of blood vessels that serve the kidney, producing renal ischemia. ATN is responsible for 90% of ARF. Other causes of renal ischemia include circulatory collapse, severe dehydration, and prolonged hypotension in compromised surgical or trauma patients.

Pathophysiology

Acute kidney injury is diagnosed when there is a sudden decline in GFR. The kidneys have decreased function but have not "failed." There are causes of AKI. **Prerenal AKI** is caused by decreased blood flow, such as in hypovolemia, or decreased cardiac output, such as in cardiogenic shock. **Intrarenal (or intrinsic) AKI** results from glomerular damage, ATN caused by toxins such as medications, or vascular disease that affects the vessels in the kidney (e.g., diabetes). **Postrenal (or obstructive) AKI** is caused by obstruction in the ureters, bladder, or urethra—for example, an enlarged prostate—that causes eventual backflow of urine into the kidney, which in turn leads to tissue damage. AKI is potentially reversible, especially if identified early; patients often regain kidney function. Concept Map 34.1 shows the pathophysiology of renal failure.

> **? Think Critically**
>
> During your clinical experience, which of your patients may have been at risk for AKI? What factors placed these patients at risk?

The course of AKI/ATN is divided into four phases: onset, oliguric, diuretic, and recovery phases. The onset phase lasts from hours to days and begins when the kidneys sustain injury due to one of the three mechanisms listed above. In the oliguric phase, the patient puts out 100 to 400 mL of urine in 24 hours. This phase

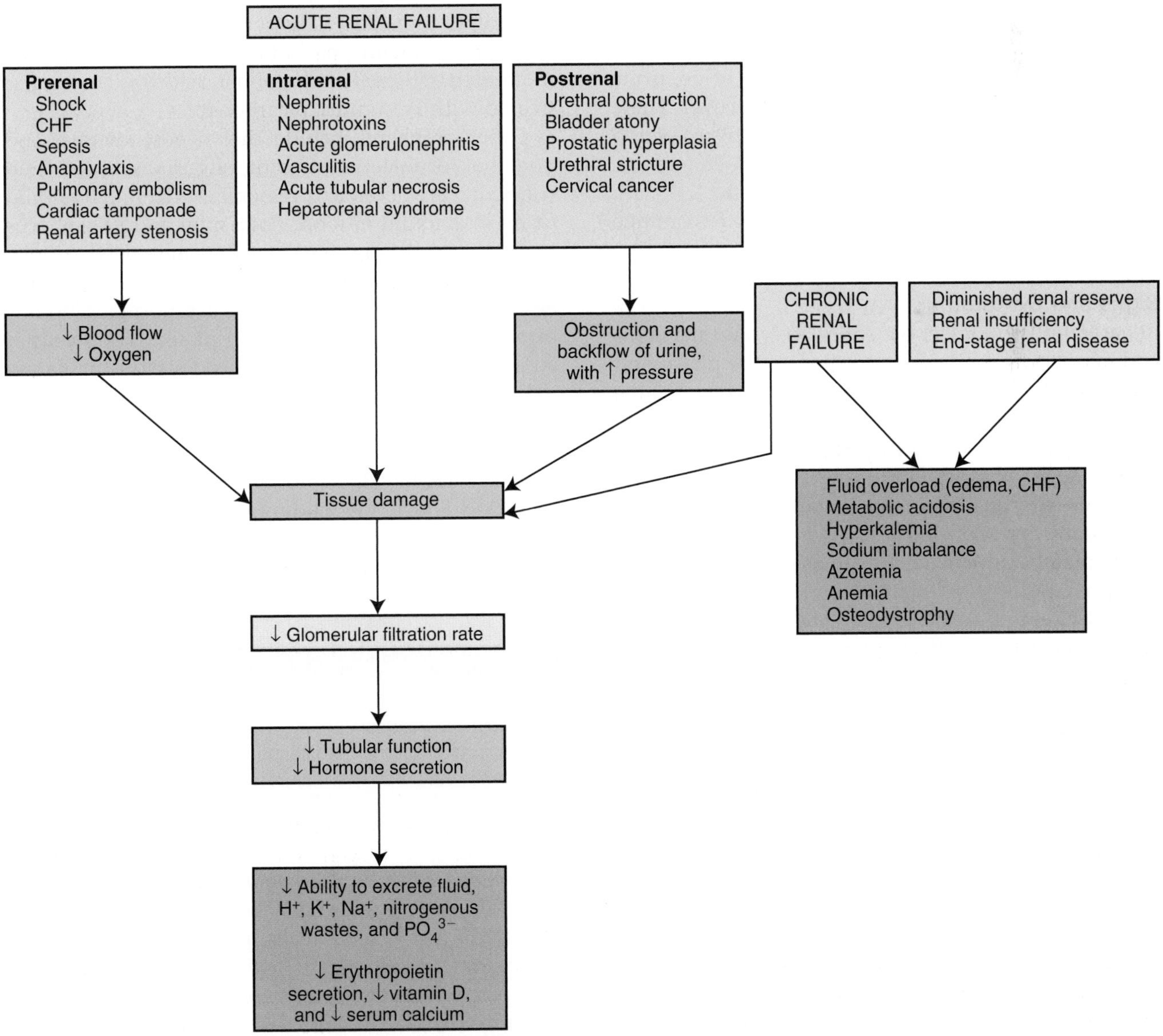

Concept Map 34.1 Pathophysiology of renal failure. *CHF*, Congestive heart failure.

usually occurs after the onset phase and lasts for an average of 10 to 14 days; however, it can go on for weeks to months, and prolonged oliguria worsens the prognosis. BUN and creatinine levels rise. When this occurs, there may be volume overload, which can precipitate heart failure, multiple electrolyte imbalances, metabolic acidosis, catabolism (destructive breakdown of body tissue), and ESRD; dialysis is needed.

> **Older Adult Care Points**
>
> Because of the overall decreased kidney function related to aging, older adult patients may experience oliguria even though urine volumes are as high as 600 to 700 mL/day.

The diuretic phase occurs only as the kidneys regain function. In this phase, the kidney is unable to concentrate urine, and output can be between 1000 and 2000 mL/day. With this increased output, there is a danger of dehydration, hyponatremia, and hypokalemia. Approximately 25% of deaths related to AKI occur during this phase.

The recovery phase begins as the kidney function starts to normalize. The concentration of urine, urine output, and electrolyte balance begin to recover. There are 1 to 2 weeks of rapid improvement and then a period of slower recovery lasting between 3 and 12 months. About one third of patients with AKI are left with residual renal insufficiency, and about 5% must continue dialysis.

Signs and Symptoms

Renal failure will affect the entire body, and the signs and symptoms will vary according to the phase and response to treatment. Carefully observe for any of the following:

- Changes in urine output and urine results (e.g., specific gravity, proteinuria)
- Electrolyte imbalances (e.g., hyponatremia, hyperkalemia, hypocalcemia)
- Fluid imbalance (e.g., hypotension, hypertension, edema, pulmonary edema)
- Acid-base imbalance (e.g., metabolic acidosis)
- Gastrointestinal effects (e.g., nausea, vomiting, anorexia, constipation)
- Mental status changes (e.g., lethargy, memory impairment)
- Anemia and platelet dysfunction (e.g., fatigue, bleeding signs, bruising)
- Impaired wound healing and susceptibility to infection (e.g., elevated WBC)

Diagnosis

Diagnostic testing includes urinalysis, creatinine, BUN, CBC, and electrolytes. Biomarkers of AKI are being studied, but no recommended practice has been published. Ultrasound can be performed if an obstruction is suspected. A renal biopsy may be obtained to assist in determining the cause or to evaluate the extent of kidney damage. There are several staging systems for AKI, with RIFLE being the most widely used to identify the degree of injury. The acronym stands for **R**isk, **I**njury, **F**ailure, **L**oss of function, and **E**SRD. Each stage is defined by GFR or urine output and/or the need for dialysis.

Treatment

Treatment of ARF is aimed toward correcting the underlying cause and preventing or controlling complications until the kidneys can recover and resume their normal functions. Symptomatic treatment includes correction of fluid and electrolyte balances, management of anemia and hypertension, and cleansing the blood and tissues of waste products with **hemodialysis** (filtration of blood across a semipermeable membrane) or **peritoneal dialysis** (filtration of blood across the peritoneal membrane). Volume overload is treated with diuretics and fluid restriction. Dialysis is also used to reduce volume overload if it cannot be reduced with drugs. Electrolyte imbalances (hyperkalemia, hypocalcemia, hyperphosphatemia, and mild hypermagnesemia) are monitored and treated. Metabolic acidosis, if severe, is treated with IV sodium bicarbonate.

Other problems include diet needs, anemia, and potential for infection. During oliguria, salt and fluid restriction are necessary; remember that much of fluid taken in is found in food. Potassium and phosphorus may also need to be restricted but may need supplementation once the diuretic phase starts. Anemia occurs because the kidney cannot produce normal amounts of erythropoietin. The life span of red blood cells is shortened because of both the toxic wastes circulating in the blood and the hemodilution from fluid overload. To treat this anemia, the health care provider may order epoetin alfa (Epogen, Procrit), a synthetic substance that stimulates red blood cell production. Infection is common with AKI and is the leading cause of death in these patients. You must be vigilant in monitoring for signs of infection that could be associated with IV access sites, drains and tubes, and a lowered immunity state.

> **Clinical Cues**
>
> Because the function of the kidney is to filter out waste products and then concentrate them for excretion, the highest concentration of any medication eliminated by the kidneys is found in the urine. This makes most medications potentially nephrotoxic.

Continuous renal replacement therapies (continuous hemofiltration). Renal replacement therapies consist of intermittent hemodialysis, peritoneal dialysis, and continuous hemofiltration. Continuous renal replacement therapies (CRRTs) can be used for patients in the intensive care unit (ICU) who have AKI and multisystem organ involvement or for those who are hemodynamically unstable. A double-lumen catheter is typically inserted into the subclavian or internal jugular vein. The blood is removed from the arterial lumen of the catheter, passed through a semipermeable membrane, and returned to the venous lumen of the catheter. The blood moves through the system by use of a pump. Continuous venovenous hemofiltration (CVVH) filters out wastes much more slowly than hemodialysis but does not cause such rapid fluid and electrolyte shifts because it runs continuously and not intermittently. Continuous venovenous hemodialysis (CVVHD) removes solutes and fluid. Slow continuous ultrafiltration (SCUF) is primarily used for fluid removal, such as for patients with pulmonary edema (Golper, 2018).

NURSING MANAGEMENT

ASSESSMENT (DATA COLLECTION)

When taking a patient's history, include questions that relate to fluid imbalance (e.g., changes in voiding patterns, weight gain, muscle cramps, cardiac arrhythmia or palpitations, vomiting, or edema) and potential risk factors (e.g., patient or family history of renal disease or hypertension; recent surgery, trauma, or anesthesia; and exposure to nephrotoxic substances or any medications). The patient should also be encouraged to describe specific symptoms (e.g., fatigue, lethargy, weakness, or pain).

All patients need a complete head-to-toe assessment and complete vital signs at the beginning of every shift. Acutely ill patients who are at risk for AKI need frequent reassessment for signs of fluid retention (e.g., skin turgor, edema, lungs sounds, weight, and strict I&O monitoring) and for imbalances in electrolytes (e.g., change of mental status or cardiac dysrhythmias).

NURSING DIAGNOSIS AND PLANNING

Examples of problem statements frequently associated with ARF include the following:

- Fluid volume overload due to decreased kidney function.
- Altered nutrition due to nausea and loss of appetite.
- Altered activity tolerance due to metabolic changes.
- Potential for infection due to indwelling urinary catheter.

Examples of expected outcomes include the following:

- Patient will have no signs of fluid overload (e.g., weight gain, edema, crackles in lungs, decreased urinary output) for the next 2 hours.
- Patient will metabolize sufficient calories (based on dietitian's calculation) to prevent catabolism (destructive breakdown of body tissue) during hospitalization.
- Patient will maintain bed rest and participate in activities of daily living (ADLs) as much as possible (e.g., brushes own teeth) during this shift.
- Patient will not have any signs or symptoms of infection (e.g., fever, cloudy urine) during hospitalization.

IMPLEMENTATION

Carefully monitor for signs of fluid imbalance. This includes physical assessment of edema, daily weights, and lung sounds. Strict measurement of I&O is essential. In the acute phase, hourly measurements of urine output are necessary.

Equipment, such as IV control pumps, should be used for accurate and safe delivery of IV fluids. In intensive care settings, arterial or central venous monitoring provides additional information about fluid status. Electrolytes should be monitored and may manifest as changes in the patient's mental status or cardiac dysrhythmias. The patient may be too ill to eat and may require enteral feedings. Even if the patient is unable to eat, make efforts to reduce noxious stimuli that exacerbate nausea and administer antiemetics. Assist with ADLs as needed during the acute phase and progressively provide opportunities for the patient to participate once fatigue resolves. To prevent infection, be vigilant for signs and symptoms of infection. Perform hand hygiene routinely and encourage others to do so. Surgical aseptic technique should be used for procedures such as Foley catheter insertion and central line dressing changes. Help the patient and the family cope with the stress of this serious condition by allowing them to express concerns and fears, by providing accurate information about AKI, and by making appropriate referrals.

EVALUATION

Evaluation of outcomes for acutely ill patients must occur often because the plan of care may need frequent revision. For example, **if there are sudden changes or if the hourly urine output drops below 30 mL/h, the health care provider must be notified immediately.** The patient should be assessed for signs of worsening, such as shortness of breath and lung crackles associated with pulmonary edema or decreased cardiac output associated with heart failure. The patient must be transferred from a general medical-surgical unit to the ICU if the condition becomes unstable.

CHRONIC RENAL FAILURE

Etiology

Chronic renal failure (CRF) is a progressive loss of kidney function that develops over many months or years. CRF is caused by destruction of the nephrons. All of the factors that can cause AKI may also cause CRF. Hypertension, diabetes mellitus, sickle cell disease, glomerulonephritis, nephrotic syndrome, lupus erythematosus, heart failure, and cirrhosis of the liver may also contribute to CRF.

The most common causes of CRF are diabetes and hypertension. **Nephrosclerosis results from hypertension and causes atherosclerotic disease of the small arteries in the kidneys.** Diabetes also affects the small blood vessels in the kidneys. As the blood supply decreases, the kidney cells degenerate and lose their ability to function, resulting in ESRD.

Health Promotion

Diabetes Mellitus

Diabetic nephropathy (kidney disease and dysfunction secondary to diabetes mellitus) is the most common cause of death in patients with diabetes mellitus. In keeping with the *Healthy People 2030* goal "to increase the proportion of adults with diabetes and chronic kidney disease who receive recommended medical treatment with angiotensin-converting enzyme (ACE) inhibitors or angiotensin II receptor blockers (ARBs)," help your patients understand the interrelationship between diabetes and kidney health.

Pathophysiology

In the early stages of the disease, the healthy nephrons compensate for the damaged or diseased nephrons. BUN and creatinine will start to increase after GFR has decreased to 50%. The patient does not experience symptoms until about 65% of the kidney tissue is damaged. In the final or end stage of renal failure, 90% or more of kidney function is lost. **Azotemia** is the accumulation of nitrogenous products, which is signaled by an increase in BUN and serum creatinine. The patient may experience nausea and vomiting and changes in mental awareness and levels of consciousness.

There are five stages of CRF, defined by GFR (normal 125 mL/min/1.73 m^2). In stage 1 GFR is greater than 90 mL/min/1.73 m^2; there is diminished renal reserve but no accumulation of metabolic wastes. In stage 2 GFR is between 60 and 89 mL/min/1.73 m^2; there is renal insufficiency, and more kidney damage has occurred. In stage 3 GFR is between 30 and 59 mL/min/1.73 m^2; BUN and creatinine elevate, edema may occur, and there is decreased urine output. In stage 4 GFR is between 15 and 30 mL/min/1.73 m^2; BUN and creatinine continue to elevate, anemia may develop, and discussions about dialysis or kidney transplantation should occur. In stage 5 GFR is less than 15 mL/min/1.73 m^2; this is ESRD. When circulating metabolic wastes accumulate in the blood, homeostasis cannot be maintained, electrolyte and fluid imbalances are serious, and dialysis or kidney transplantation becomes necessary to maintain life.

Safety Alert

Oliguria and Hyperkalemia

During oliguria the kidney is not able to excrete potassium; therefore be alert for high levels of serum potassium (greater than 6 mEq/L), which can adversely affect the heart, causing dysrhythmia and cardiac arrest.

Signs and Symptoms

The symptoms of CRF do not appear early in the disease. A high-normal elevation of creatinine is an early warning sign, and the patient is asymptomatic. There may be proteinuria, which does not produce clinical signs unless enough protein is lost in the urine to affect serum blood levels. In stage 3 kidney failure, symptoms of **uremia** or **uremic syndrome**, such as headaches, nausea, weight loss, and fatigue, occur. The loss of kidney function is not a slow, steady decline. Management of the underlying disease causing the injury to the kidney can slow down or halt the progression. Episodes of AKI may damage enough nephrons to move the patient from an early stage of kidney failure to ESRD. As renal failure progresses, the kidneys may not be able to produce much urine at all, and oliguria and eventually anuria occur. When the kidneys are not eliminating potassium, life-threatening hyperkalemia may develop.

Untreated uremia leads to dry, scaly skin, with a pallid yellowish gray color. Pruritus (severe itching) occurs. Uremic frost (a late sign) appears as evaporated sweat leaves urea crystals on the eyebrows, face, axilla, and groin. Calcium is not absorbed from the intestinal tract, and this leads to the loss of calcium from the body and a corresponding drop in serum calcium. If the hypocalcemia is not corrected, the patient will eventually suffer from muscle cramps, twitching, and possibly seizures. As kidney cells cease to function, they are progressively less able to secrete phosphorus in the urine. An elevated serum phosphate level (hyperphosphatemia) serves to exaggerate the problem of inadequate calcium absorption; phosphate binds with calcium, decreasing its absorption from the intestinal tract. The patient is hypertensive from fluid overload and the kidney sending out renin to try to increase blood flow. Pulmonary edema and heart failure may occur. Metabolic changes occur, including triglyceride elevation and carbohydrate intolerance. Anemia is present because of decreased production of erythropoietin. Anorexia, nausea, and vomiting occur because of gastrointestinal mucosa irritation from waste products circulating in the blood. Constipation from drug therapy and fluid restriction is common. Patients may complain about restless leg syndrome, and the leg discomfort may interfere with sleep. When circulating wastes are increased, the nervous system cells become irritated, and the patient can have an altered level of consciousness. Fig. 34.3 shows the manifestations of uremia in chronic kidney disease.

Diagnosis

Creatinine is a stable by-product of skeletal muscle activity that is excreted completely by the kidneys; therefore creatinine clearance (CC) is a good measure of GFR. Urine is collected for a 24-hour period. Serum creatinine and BUN are also evaluated. Based on GFR, creatinine and urine output, the diagnosis is made. Urinalysis with culture and sensitivity, hematocrit, and hemoglobin provide additional information. A renal ultrasound, renal scan, CT scan, and renal biopsy are additional diagnostic tests that do not confirm the diagnosis but help with identifying causes and contributing factors.

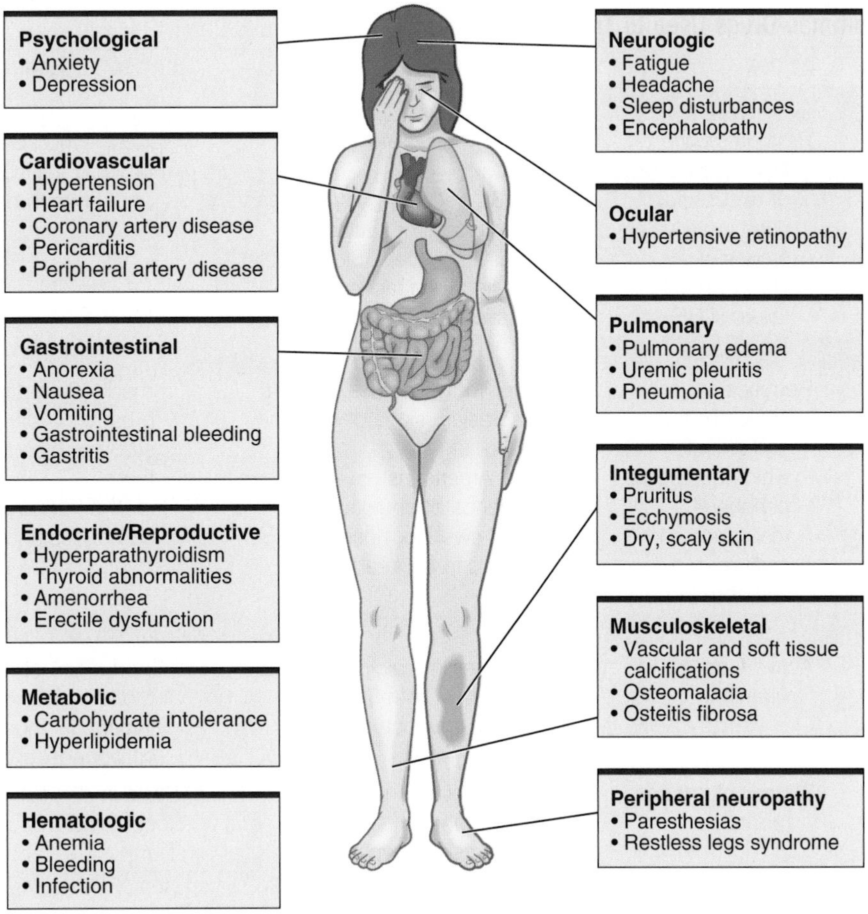

Fig. 34.3 Possible clinical manifestations of chronic kidney disease. (From Lewis SL, Bucher L, Heitkemper MM, et al.: *Medical-surgical nursing: assessment and management of clinical problems,* ed 10, St. Louis, 2014, Elsevier.)

Treatment and Nursing Management

Medical treatment and nursing intervention include measures to correct fluid and electrolyte imbalance and acid-base imbalance. Decreasing sodium and fat in the diet of patients with beginning renal insufficiency may help slow the disease process. Controlling diabetes, hypertension, or other underlying diseases can also slow progression of kidney injury. A variety of drugs, such as antacids, antihypertensives, antilipemics, epoetin alfa therapy, and vitamin and mineral supplements, are used to counteract the fluid and electrolyte imbalances, treat metabolic acidosis, and control complications (Table 34.4). Diuretics are used while there is some remaining kidney function (renal insufficiency) but are not useful during ESRD. Inotropic agents, such as digitalis or dobutamine, are used in severe cases of heart failure. Antiseizure medications, such as phenytoin (Dilantin) or levetiracetam (Keppra), also may be needed because uremic toxins can irritate the nervous system. Dialysis and kidney transplantation are the two treatments available for patients with ESRD.

Renal replacement therapy. Dialysis may be indicated for acute renal failure or for renal insufficiency when diet, medications, and fluid restriction have failed. It may also be used for patients with ESRD, drug ingestion or overdose (with a dialyzable drug), hyperkalemia, fluid overload, or metabolic acidosis (Mattiucci, 2018). Hemodialysis and peritoneal dialysis rely on diffusion and osmosis to remove waste elements normally excreted in the urine. The principle of **diffusion** states that solute molecules that are in constant motion tend to pass through a semipermeable membrane from the side of higher concentration to the side of lower concentration. In osmosis the fluid moves through the semipermeable membrane to equalize the concentration of particles on both sides.

Hemodialysis. During hemodialysis, blood moves from the arterial circulation through a dialysate bath and back to the venous circulation. A dialysis membrane separates the blood from the dialyzing solution. The molecules of waste pass through this membrane out of the blood and into the dialyzing solution until the two solutions are equal in concentration (Fig. 34.4).

A temporary access for hemodialysis can be achieved by inserting a jugular or femoral vein dialysis catheter. The jugular site has a low incidence of thrombosis; it can be used for 1 to 3 weeks and is preferred over the femoral site. Only trained dialysis staff should use these temporary access sites for medication administration

Table 34.4 Common Drugs Used to Treat Renal Failure

CLASSIFICATION	ACTION	NURSING IMPLICATIONS	PATIENT TEACHING
Diuretics			
Furosemide (Lasix)	Promotes urine flow; rids body of excess fluid; used in early stages of chronic renal failure (CRF)	Potentially nephrotoxic and ototoxic. Strict I&O recording is necessary. Monitor laboratory values for potassium levels. Side effects: vomiting, headache, constipation, and dizziness.	Report fever, sore throat, bleeding, bruising, difficulty swallowing, rash, or change in hearing.
Antihypertensives			
ACE inhibitors Enalapril (Vasotec) Benazepril (Lotensin) Captopril Quinapril (Accupril)	Reduces angiotensin II and aldosterone, which decreases peripheral resistance and sodium reabsorption	Monitor for hypotension, blood dyscrasias, signs of infection, or bruising. African Americans have a higher incidence of angioedema (facial swelling, hoarseness), which can be fatal.	Immediately report cough, difficulty breathing, rash, tremors, blood in stool, or bleeding after brushing teeth. Report persistent dizziness or numbness and tingling.
Vitamins			
Calcitriol (Rocaltrol)	Active form of vitamin D	Monitor serum calcium; normal level 8.4–10.6 mEq/L. Monitor for hypocalcemia.	Report signs of hypocalcemia (e.g., twitching of mouth, numbness of fingers, laryngeal spasm, carpopedal spasm).
Folic acid and vitamin B_{12}	For red blood cell formation	Give with food to promote absorption. Side effects not expected.	Store in dry, light-protected container.
Minerals			
Iron (ferrous sulfate)	Used to treat anemia	Give with water or juice to promote absorption. Do not give with milk products.	Take with food if gastric distress occurs. Sit upright for 30 min after taking. Stool may turn black; this is a harmless side effect.
Ferumoxytol (Feraheme)	Treats iron deficiency anemia of CRF	Administer by IV injection.	The most common adverse reactions are diarrhea, nausea, dizziness, hypotension, constipation, and peripheral edema.
Calcium Supplements			
Calcium carbonate	Prevents problems of calcium loss	Monitor serum calcium.	Constipation is a common side effect.
Calcium acetate (also binds phosphate)	Give with meals to bind phosphate	Monitor ECG changes for potential dysrhythmias.	Nausea, vomiting, drowsiness, or headache may occur.
Hematopoietic Growth Factors			
Epoetin alfa (Epogen, Procrit) Darbepoetin (Aranesp)	Treatment of anemia; promotes red blood cell formation	Can cause hypertension; monitor blood pressure. May need increased doses of heparin. Subcutaneous route is preferred.	Report nausea, vomiting, edema, fatigue, or chest pain.
Resins			
Sodium polystyrene (Kayexalate)	Treatment of hyperkalemia	Can be given mixed with food or in an enema. Monitor electrolytes. Side effects: nausea, vomiting, constipation, and anorexia.	Report any muscle weakness, irregular heartbeat, or stomach pain.

ACE, Angiotensin-converting enzyme; *ECG*, electrocardiogram; *I&O*, intake and output; *IV*, intravenous.

center. When a patient on dialysis is admitted to an inpatient facility, you should verify when the patient received their last treatment and when they are due for the next. Communication with the health care provider will facilitate the patient receiving their necessary dialysis sessions while they are an inpatient being treated for another problem.

Peritoneal dialysis. Peritoneal dialysis is an alternative procedure that can be used instead of hemodialysis to remove waste products or toxins that have accumulated as a result of ARF or CRF. During peritoneal dialysis, dialyzing fluid that is equal in osmolality and similar in composition to normal body fluid is introduced into the peritoneal cavity via a tunneled abdominal catheter by gravity (Fig. 34.6). Medications such as heparin, insulin, potassium, or antibiotics may be added to the solution. The solution is left in the peritoneal cavity for a specified time (dwell time), allowing the concentration of the solutions on either side of the peritoneal membrane to equalize.

After the fluid is infused, the patient can move about during the dwell time. At the end of the dwell time, the dialysate solution containing waste products is drained from the abdominal cavity. The drainage should be colorless or straw-colored unless the catheter was recently inserted (the drainage may be bloody for the first several treatments).

Peritoneal dialysis has several advantages: (1) treatment can be started more quickly than hemodialysis, (2) anticoagulants are not necessary, (3) maturation of the access site and canalization of blood vessels is not required, (4) there is less stress on the cardiovascular system because fluid exchanges occur more slowly, and (5) some patients with renal failure fare better on a gentler therapy. Peritoneal dialysis cannot be done when there is severe trauma to the abdomen; after multiple abdominal surgeries; if there are adhesions in the abdominal cavity; or if the patient has a severe coagulation defect, paralytic ileus, or diffuse peritonitis.

There are several types of peritoneal dialysis. The basic principles are the same, but the dwell times, schedule of frequency, and use of a control pump versus gravity flow will vary. The first type is **continuous ambulatory peritoneal dialysis (CAPD).** The CAPD process goes on 24 hours a day, 7 days a week. As a self-dialysis method, CAPD may be the easiest for the patient, and it requires no machinery. For CAPD, the bag of dialyzing solution is suspended above the level of the abdomen, and tubing is attached to the permanently implanted peritoneal dialysis catheter. The clamp on the CAPD tubing is opened and the dialysate solution runs into the abdomen by gravity flow. After the dwell time (4 to 8 hours), the fluid is drained. Automated peritoneal dialysis uses a machine to open and close clamps so that overnight peritoneal dialysis can occur. **Continuous cycler peritoneal dialysis** delivers three to six overnight exchanges. The machine is programmed to open the flow of fluid into the peritoneal cavity, then clamp for dwell, then open the outflow into the discard bag. It repeats the cycle as programmed. **Nightly intermittent dialysis** is also accomplished with the use of a cycler and is performed three to five times per week for 10 to 12 hours at night. This allows the patient to be free between treatment times. Intermittent or continuous peritoneal dialysis may be done in the acute care setting based on patient need.

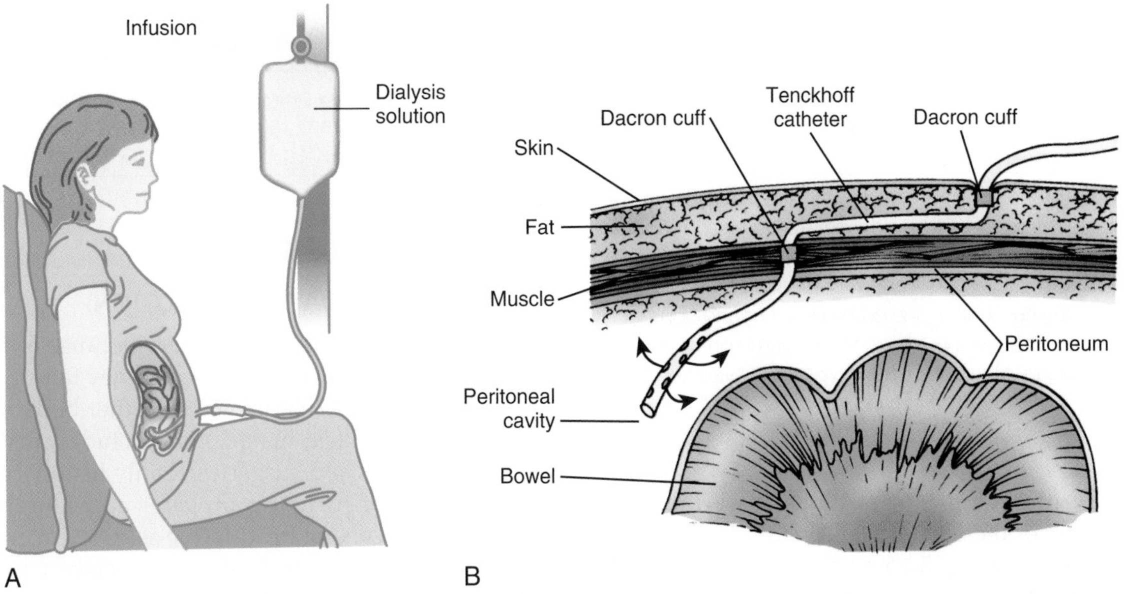

Fig. 34.6 **A,** Peritoneal dialysis through an abdominal catheter. **B,** Tunneled peritoneal dialysis catheter. The peritoneal membrane acts as the dialyzing membrane. (**A,** From Ignatavicius DD, Workman ML, et al.: *Medical-surgical nursing: critical thinking for collaborative care*, ed 9, St. Louis, 2018, Elsevier. **B,** From Ignatavicius DD, Workman ML: *Medical-surgical nursing: critical thinking for collaborative care*, ed 7, Philadelphia, 2010, Saunders.)

Complications. Potential complications of peritoneal dialysis include peritonitis, leakage, obstruction or other problems with the catheter, respiratory problems, and fluid overload or hypertriglyceridemia (disturbance of lipid metabolism).

Think Critically

What signs and symptoms might indicate that a patient undergoing peritoneal dialysis has peritonitis?

Nursing management. Nursing care for a patient undergoing peritoneal dialysis includes obtaining the patient's weight before and after the treatment; maintaining careful I&O records; maintaining strict aseptic technique in handling the dialysate bags, peritoneal catheter, and all equipment; monitoring vital signs; observing for complications such as peritonitis; and keeping the patient as comfortable as possible. The dialysate solution should be at room temperature or warmed if possible and must be instilled slowly. The patient and family are taught all steps of the procedure before discharge, to ensure safety and prevent infection.

Kidney transplantation. An alternative to dialysis is to transplant a kidney from a living tissue-compatible donor or from a cadaver donor whose kidney tissue is compatible with that of the recipient.

Tissue typing to determine donor–recipient compatibility is performed, along with extensive psychological assessment and counseling for both the live donor and the recipient. Transplant candidates must be free from medical problems that might increase the risks of the procedure or jeopardize the success of the transplant. Malignancy, IV drug abuse, severe obesity, active vasculitis, and severe psychosocial problems eliminate some candidates.

Legal and Ethical Considerations

Organ Donation

There are 58 organ procurement organizations (OPOs) in the United States. Medicare, Medicaid, and The Joint Commission mandate that the local OPO must be notified about brain death of a patient so that a well-trained representative of the OPO can evaluate the suitability of the potential donor and approach the family in a timely manner. Currently, research on increasing donation is being promoted, and grants are available (U.S. Department of Health and Human Services, 2018).

A significant factor in transplant therapy is the shortage of organs. In the United States, more than 100,000 people are on the waiting list for a kidney at any moment. Patients who are waiting for a transplant must be able to travel quickly to a transplant center when an organ becomes available. Hypertension is brought under the best possible control, any infection is treated, and the patient is dialyzed immediately before transplantation. One of the *Healthy People 2030* goals is to increase the proportion of patients who receive a kidney transplant within 3 years after being put on the waiting list.

There are four classes of immunosuppressive drugs commonly used to prevent organ rejection: (1) calcineurin inhibitors (e.g., cyclosporine [Sandimmune], tacrolimus [Prograf]); (2) antiproliferative agents (e.g., azathioprine [Imuran]); (3) mammalian target of rapamycin (mTOR) inhibitors (e.g., everolimus [Afinitor], sirolimus [Rapamune]); and (4) steroids (prednisone). The monoclonal antibodies basiliximab (Simulect), rituximab (Rituxan), and eculizumab (Soliris) may also be used in selected patients. Long-term problems for transplant patients are increased susceptibility to infection, toxicities from antirejection medications, and a higher risk of malignancy.

Renal transplant patients are transferred to critical care or specialty units after surgery, where they are closely monitored for signs of rejection: fever, increased blood pressure, and pain over the iliac fossa where the new kidney was placed (Fig. 34.7). Ongoing assessment includes watching for the signs of renal failure, particularly oliguria, anuria, and rising BUN levels and serum creatinine. Protection from sources of infection is a top priority. Once the new kidney is functioning properly, the primary health care provider may lift any previous dietary restrictions.

Renal failure and dialysis are very expensive for the patient and family. However, lack of funds does not exclude anyone from needed care. Since July 1973, an amendment to the Social Security Act allows Medicare to pay for most of the cost of treating ESRD, including dialysis and renal transplantation. Medical expenses continue after transplantation because the drugs needed to prevent rejection are very expensive.

Think Critically

You are caring for a patient admitted with pneumonia. One year ago, the patient received a kidney transplant. What precautions are needed when caring for this patient?

NURSING MANAGEMENT

ASSESSMENT (DATA COLLECTION)

The assessment findings will vary because of the slow but progressive development of kidney failure and the effect that kidney disease has on other body systems. Take a past medical history that includes medication, previous illness and surgeries, family history of illness, and a report of current complaints and concerns.

Perform a general head-to-toe assessment, including complete vital signs and a baseline weight. Observe for the following changes and symptoms:

- Neurologic changes (e.g., lethargy or irritability)
- Cardiovascular abnormalities (e.g., dysrhythmias or hypertension)

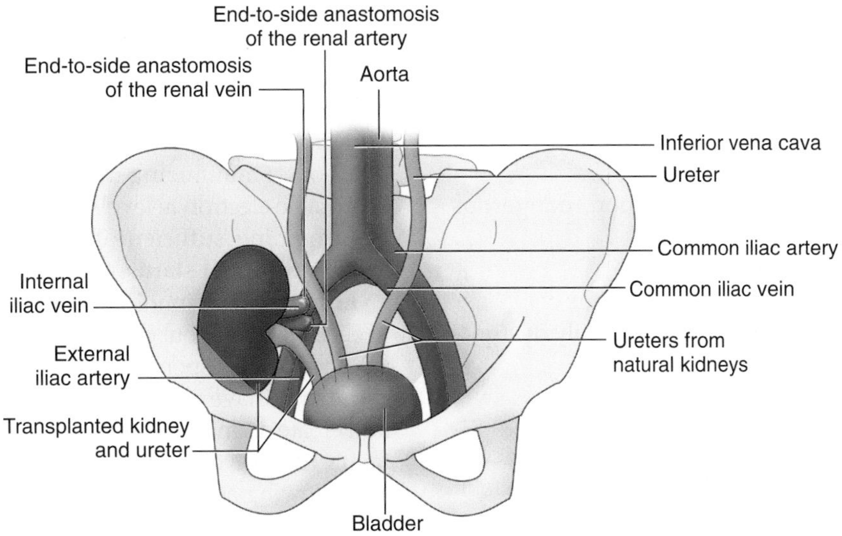

Fig. 34.7 Placement of a transplanted kidney. (From Ignatavicius DD, Workman ML, et al.: *Medical-surgical nursing: critical thinking for collaborative care,* ed 9, St. Louis, 2018, Elsevier.)

- Respiratory abnormalities (e.g., shortness of breath or fluid in lungs)
- Gastrointestinal distress (e.g., nausea, vomiting, or constipation)
- Musculoskeletal discomfort (e.g., muscle cramps, twitching, or restless legs syndrome)
- Skin changes (e.g., itching or uremic frost)

Monitor BUN, serum creatinine, electrolytes, and urinalysis. As the disease progresses, assess for impaired urine concentration, decreased output, and anemia.

In addition, assess patients for sexual difficulties or concerns. Patients may experience medication side effects, such as impotence. Weight gain, peripheral edema, or the presence of a dialysis access may alter body image or feelings of attractiveness. Fatigue caused by anemia or hormonal imbalance can result in decreased libido (sexual desire). Partners may fear that the patient is too ill to participate in sex or that the dialysis access will be damaged.

Clinical Cues

Help your patient verbalize concerns about sexual problems by using a matter-of-fact approach (e.g., "Mr. Smith, have you or your partner noticed any changes in your sexual relations since you started your new medication?"). You may not be able to directly solve the problem, but giving the patient the opportunity to talk about it is helpful. In addition, once you have assessed the problem, you can refer the patient to the appropriate resource if the problem is beyond your expertise (e.g., the health care provider may be able to change medication or the family may need psychological counseling).

◆ NURSING DIAGNOSIS

Patients with renal disease will have problems related to anemia, bleeding tendency, susceptibility to infection, nausea, vomiting, anorexia, gastrointestinal bleeding, and fluid overload that exacerbates conditions such as congestive heart failure. Examples of problem statements commonly associated with chronic renal disease and dialysis include the following:

- Altered nutrition due to dietary restrictions and loss of appetite.
- Fatigue due to anemia.
- Potential for infection from invasive procedures (e.g., dialysis access).
- Acute confusion due to accumulation of toxins.
- Altered sexual function due to stress and medication side effects.

Examples of expected outcomes include the following:

- Patient will eat at least 50% of all meals during this shift.
- Patient will have adequate energy to independently perform ADLs before discharge.
- Patient will not have any signs or symptoms of infection (e.g., fever, redness, or swelling at shunt site) during hospitalization.
- Patient will demonstrate ability to make safe judgments (e.g., calls for help as needed) and orientation to person, place, and time before discharge.
- Patient will verbalize concerns or fears about sexual dysfunction.

◆ PLANNING

In planning care for a patient with chronic renal disease, consider the stress of prolonged intensive treatment, the frustrations of dealing with an incurable illness, rigid dietary restrictions, fatigue, malaise, occasional limited mobility, and possible sexual difficulties, all of which take their toll on both the patient and the family. Consider the family's needs as well as the patient's when planning nursing intervention.

General nursing goals for care of patients with chronic renal disease include the following:

- Demonstrates understanding of therapeutic regimen (i.e., dietary and fluid modifications, dialysis)
- Prevention of fluid overload by adhering to fluid restriction
- Prevention of complications (infection, dangerous electrolyte abnormalities)
- Able to provide appropriate self-care
- Acknowledges acceptance of body image
- Prevention of caregiver role strain and family dysfunction related to chronic illness

? Think Critically

What kinds of behaviors would suggest caregiver role strain in the spouse of a patient who has ESRD?

◆ IMPLEMENTATION

Daily weight, measurement of I&O, determining the pattern of urination, and restricting fluid as ordered by the health care provider (generally calculated as intake of 500 to 700 mL plus the amount of output from the previous 24 hours) are essential to the well-being of a patient with renal damage. In addition to these basic procedures, there should be ongoing monitoring of electrolytes, BUN, and creatinine. Hyperkalemia and a sodium imbalance will occur, as will hypocalcemia and hyperphosphatemia (see Chapter 3).

Because of the buildup of nitrogenous wastes from protein metabolism, restriction of protein intake is necessary; only high-quality protein foods (e.g., meat and eggs) are encouraged (Fig. 34.8). Potassium is also restricted. Sodium intake often is restricted, especially if the patient is hypertensive. Previously, aluminum carbonate (Basaljel) was used as a phosphate binder; however, concern over elevated aluminum levels has prompted the use of calcium carbonate, which acts as a phosphate binder and a calcium supplement. The complexity of diet restrictions and modifications makes understanding and compliance very difficult for the patient and family (Table 34.5).

Assess the patient's health status and learning needs throughout the illness and provide information to manage symptoms and prevent further damage whenever possible. The expertise of other professionals, especially nutritionists, is needed to help accomplish the goals of (1) minimizing uremic toxicity; (2) maintaining acceptable electrolyte levels; (3) controlling hypertension; (4) providing sufficient calories; and (5) maintaining good nutritional status.

Encourage communication between patient and spouse to elicit feelings about changes in sexual activity, role reversal, and family responsibilities. Patients with kidney failure commonly have self-care deficits that affect self-esteem and create an increased caregiver burden. Encourage the family to achieve a balance between supporting the patient and allowing as much independence as possible.

◆ EVALUATION

For chronic renal failure, perform and compare data for daily physical assessments, weights, I&O, and laboratory reports. Monitor trends over a period of days to determine clinical improvement or the presence of problems. Daily fluctuations in subjective symptoms, such as fatigue or discomfort, along with ambivalent feelings toward the therapeutic regimen are expected; however, if symptoms are prolonged or ongoing, the care plan should be revised. Nursing Care Plan 34.1 includes problem statements or nursing diagnoses, interventions, and outcomes that are commonly used for patients with renal insufficiency and failure.

? Think Critically

Your patient with CRF is withdrawn and sullen at times but is sharp and demanding at other times. How will you respond to this? How will you help the family deal with this behavior?

COMMUNITY CARE

A major function of nurses in the community is to assist patients who have hypertension or diabetes to achieve good control of their disease, to help prevent damage to the kidneys. One *Healthy People 2030* goal is to reduce

Table 34.5 Dietary Restrictions for a Patient With Renal Failure

DIETARY COMPONENT	WITH CHRONIC UREMIA	WITH HEMODIALYSIS	WITH PERITONEAL DIALYSIS
Protein	0.55–0.60 g/kg/day	1–1.5 g/kg/day	1.2–1.5 g/kg/day
Fluid	Depends on urinary output, but may be as high as 1500–3000 mL/day	500–700 mL/day plus amount of urinary output	Restriction based on fluid weight gain and blood pressure
Potassium	60–70 mEq/day	70 mEq/day	Usually no restriction
Sodium	1–3 g/day	2–4 g/day	Restriction based on fluid weight gain and blood pressure
Phosphorus	700 mg/day	700 mg/day	800 mg/day

From Ignatavicius DD, Workman ML, et al.: *Medical-surgical nursing: critical thinking for collaborative care,* ed 9, St. Louis, 2018, Elsevier.

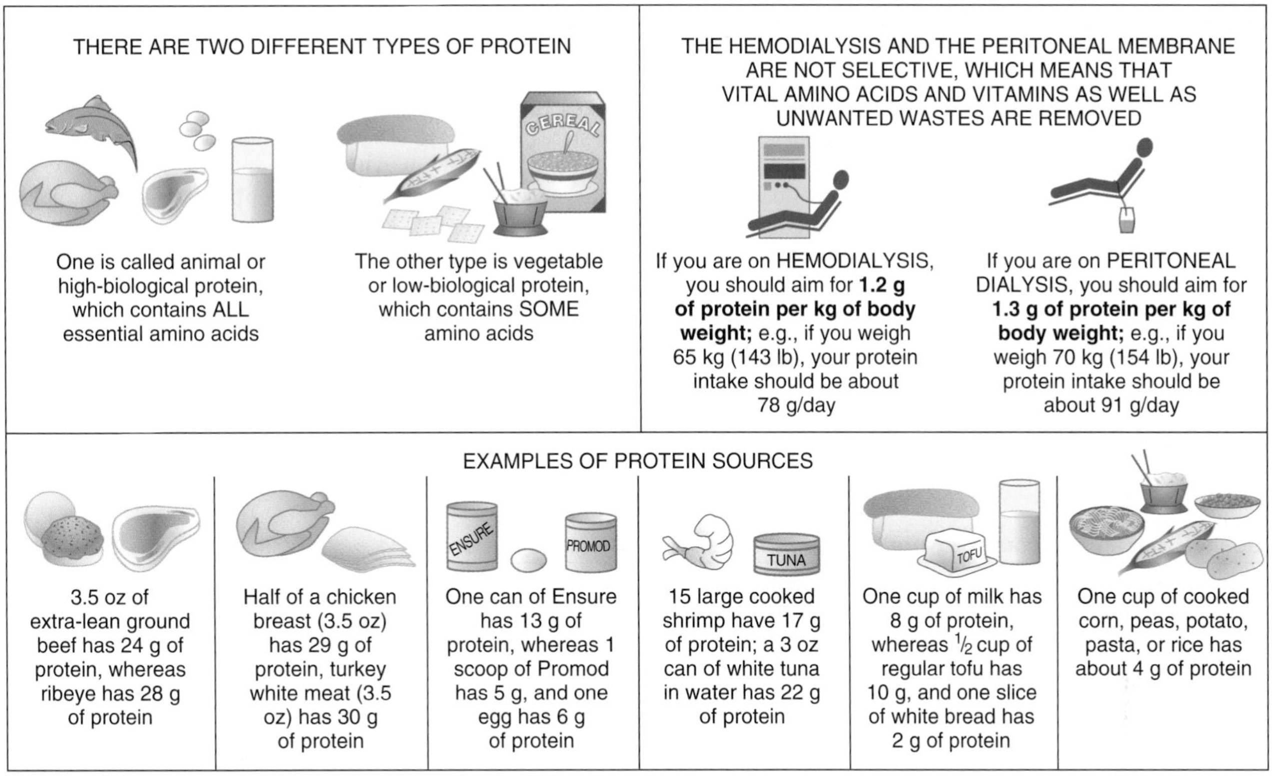
THERE ARE TWO DIFFERENT TYPES OF PROTEIN
CEREAL
One is called animal or high-biological protein, which contains ALL essential amino acids
The other type is vegetable or low-biological protein, which contains SOME amino acids
THE HEMODIALYSIS AND THE PERITONEAL MEMBRANE ARE NOT SELECTIVE, WHICH MEANS THAT VITAL AMINO ACIDS AND VITAMINS AS WELL AS UNWANTED WASTES ARE REMOVED
If you are on HEMODIALYSIS, you should aim for **1.2 g of protein per kg of body weight;** e.g., if you weigh 65 kg (143 lb), your protein intake should be about 78 g/day
If you are on PERITONEAL DIALYSIS, you should aim for **1.3 g of protein per kg of body weight;** e.g., if you weigh 70 kg (154 lb), your protein intake should be about 91 g/day
EXAMPLES OF PROTEIN SOURCES
ENSURE
PROMOD
TUNA
TOFU
3.5 oz of extra-lean ground beef has 24 g of protein, whereas ribeye has 28 g of protein
Half of a chicken breast (3.5 oz) has 29 g of protein, turkey white meat (3.5 oz) has 30 g of protein
One can of Ensure has 13 g of protein, whereas 1 scoop of Promod has 5 g, and one egg has 6 g of protein
15 large cooked shrimp have 17 g of protein; a 3 oz can of white tuna in water has 22 g of protein
One cup of milk has 8 g of protein, whereas ½ cup of regular tofu has 10 g, and one slice of white bread has 2 g of protein
One cup of cooked corn, peas, potato, pasta, or rice has about 4 g of protein

Fig. 34.8 Tips for protein intake. (From Black JM, Hawks JH: *Medical-surgical nursing: clinical management for positive outcomes,* ed 8, Philadelphia, 2009, Saunders. Modified from Darlene Michl, Victoria, B.C., Canada, www.personalhealthcoaching.ca.)

Communication

Hemodialysis Patient Nonadherance to Treatment Plan

John is a 48-year-old man who has end-stage renal disease and is on hemodialysis twice a week. He has not been compliant with his diet and fluid restrictions and has been increased to three dialysis treatments a week. He gained 5 lb over the weekend.

Nurse: "John, I see that you gained five pounds since Friday. Tell me about your weekend."

John: "I never have any fun or do normal things with my friends, so I went fishing with some buddies and we drank a lot of beer. We barbecued fish and some sausage. It was a real feast!"

Nurse: "How are you feeling today?"

John: "I feel rotten. I don't have any energy, and my thinking is slow. My legs are really swollen, and I'm having trouble breathing."

Nurse: "Do you think that might have something to do with the beer and food?"

John: "I suppose it does, but can't a guy have a little fun?"

Nurse: "John, I am concerned. You know that fluid and waste overload puts your whole body out of balance and causes damage in other organs. It's especially hard on the heart."

John: "Yeah, I know you've told me. It's just so hard. You don't understand what it is like."

Nurse: "You are right. I don't have kidney disease or the strict diet and fluid restrictions. I think it would be very difficult, but I would want to take care of myself for my family and friends."

John: "Well, you know that my wife left me and I don't see much of the kids, but I sure do enjoy my granddaughter. I really enjoy my times with the guys at the Lodge, too."

Nurse: "Do you have any friends who are in a similar situation who you can talk to?"

John: "No, none of my friends has kidney disease."

Nurse: "There is a young man who comes here for dialysis treatments who is always talking about fishing. Maybe the two of you could give each other some encouragement and support."

John: "Well, I don't know. I don't make new friends very easily."

Nurse: "He will be here on Wednesday. How about if we schedule your treatment for the same time? Perhaps you could get acquainted."

John: "Okay. That seems fine."

Nurse: "Next week we can talk again to see how you are doing with your diet, fluid restrictions, and medication schedule."

John: "Thanks. I will try to do better this week."

Nursing Care Plan 34.1 Care of a Patient With Chronic Renal Failure

SCENARIO

Mrs. Stevens, age 54 years, has had hypertension since her early 20s. She was diagnosed with chronic renal failure several years ago. Now she reports headaches, fatigue, and nausea. She states, "I have to sleep with three pillows, and I am just exhausted." She feels that "my doctor is keeping something from me," and she is withdrawn and sullen. Tearfully, she reports, "The renal diet is so complex, and my husband and son cannot manage the cooking and shopping." Her nephrologist conducted a series of diagnostic tests and recommended hemodialysis and eventual kidney transplantation when an organ is available. Laboratory results include hematocrit 25%, hemoglobin 9 g/100 mL, BUN 50 mg/dL, and creatinine 6 mg/dL; potassium 5.9 mEq/L; admission weight: 140 lb ("normal weight around 130 lb"); 3+ pitting edema, bilateral feet and ankles. She is admitted for ESRD with CHF and placement of a dialysis access.

PROBLEM STATEMENT/NURSING DIAGNOSIS

Altered activity tolerance related to anemia.

SUPPORTING ASSESSMENT DATA

Subjective: "I am just exhausted."

Objective: Hematocrit 25%; hemoglobin 9 g/100 mL, appears tired.

Goals/Expected Outcomes	Nursing Interventions	Selected Rationale	Evaluation
By discharge, patient will be able to perform ADLs independently without distress.	Check vital signs for changes when activities appear stressful or overtaxing.	Marked increase in pulse or respiratory rate during routine ADLs suggests activity intolerance.	Reported feelings of fatigue and mild dyspnea after walking to the nurses' station. Vital signs at that time were BP 145/90, P 120, R 32/min. Repeat vitals after 30 min of rest: BP 140/80, P 85, R 20/min.
	Have patient use rating scale (scale 1/10) for different types of activities, such as walking to the bathroom or climbing the stairs.	The exertional scale (1/10) allows the patient (and you) to rate and monitor performance and alter activities accordingly.	Ambulating in the hall was "too much"; reported an exertion level of 6/10.
	Adjust activities to allow for periods of rest.	Adequate rest facilitates recovery; activities can be increased or decreased according to the patient's level of tolerance.	Patient was assisted back to her room. Rested for 3 h.
	Assist with ADLs as required and keep personal articles within reach.	Patient's ability to do ADLs will wax and wane. Items close by and assistance as needed will help conserve energy.	Able to independently comb hair and apply makeup when personal items are within easy reach.
	Monitor for decreased hematocrit and hemoglobin values.	Normal range for hematocrit is 37%–47% (female). Normal range for hemoglobin is 12–16 g/dL (female).	7:00 A.M. hematocrit: 24%; hemoglobin: 9 g/100 mL.
	Give epoetin and monitor for side effects (e.g., increased BP, dyspnea, chest pain, seizures, headaches, calf pain). Give iron, multivitamins, and folic acid as prescribed. Instruct about foods that supply iron (e.g., lean meat and vegetables) and folic acid (e.g., whole wheat bread).	Nutritional supplements and epoetin are given to help the body with RBC production.	Epoetin given subcutaneously as prescribed. No adverse effects noted.

PROBLEM STATEMENT/NURSING DIAGNOSIS

Insufficient knowledge related to diet, nutrition, and plan of care.

Nursing Care Plan 34.1 Care of a Patient With Chronic Renal Failure—cont'd

SUPPORTING ASSESSMENT DATA

Subjective: "The renal diet is so complex, and my husband and son cannot manage the cooking and shopping." "My doctor is keeping something from me."

Objective: Appears overwhelmed at the amount of information and seems unsure how to use it effectively.

Goals/Expected Outcomes	Nursing Interventions	Selected Rationale	Evaluation
With help, the patient will create a sample diet that is within renal diet parameters within 2–3 days.	Assess readiness to learn, preferred learning styles, and barriers to learning. Include family in teaching.	Possible barriers for the patient include being upset, tired, uncomfortable, or anxious about her condition. Learning new information will be difficult under these conditions.	The patient identifies need for herself and her family to learn about her dietary restrictions. Patient also shows interest in attending a group class that will be conducted next month.
	Perform teaching in short sessions.	Complex information is best delivered in manageable pieces.	Limited teaching session to 10 min because of fatigue.
	Use language and terms that patient and family are able to understand.	Medical jargon and technical terms will not help the patient understand the basic dietary information.	Verbalized understanding of terminology related to health teaching (e.g., restricted protein).
	Obtain a dietary consultation and reinforce information provided by the nutritional expert.	A renal nutritionist must be consulted to create an individual diet plan based on laboratory values, nutritional requirements, and patient's eating preferences.	Nutritionist came to see the patient and discussed overall nutritional goals and plan. Arrangements have been made with the nutritionist to meet with the family next week.
	Ensure that the patient has verbal and written instructions.	Written material can be reviewed later and shared with the family.	Written information about diet and renal disease was provided.
The patient will be prepared for insertion of a tunneled dialysis catheter by stating the purpose of the catheter, stating that her questions have been fully answered, and signing the procedure consent without reservation.	After the health care provider explains the risks and benefits of the procedure, the nurse will verify patient understanding before obtaining consent.	You are responsible for verifying understanding before obtaining consent.	The patient states, "I am scared, but I understand that this procedure is necessary to be able to remove the extra fluid and toxins in my body with the dialysis machine. I feel my doctor told me everything I need to know for now."

PROBLEM STATEMENT/NURSING DIAGNOSIS

Fluid volume overload related to retention of sodium and water from inadequate kidney function.

SUPPORTING ASSESSMENT DATA

Subjective: "Sleeps with three pillows."

Objective: Admission weight: 140 lb (normal weight around 130 lb); 3+ pitting edema, bilateral feet and ankles. Crackles in lower lung fields.

Goals/Expected Outcomes	Nursing Interventions	Selected Rationale	Evaluation
Patient will not show signs of further increase of fluid load. O_2 saturation will be maintained above 92% and crackles will not increase this shift. Pitting edema will not increase.	Strict I&O. Daily weight. Patient will have restricted fluid intake of 500–700 mL for the day.	Discrepancies in I&O suggest fluid retention and overload.	Fluid intake 300 mL, no urine output. Weight unchanged from admission
	Assist with good oral care and discourage mouth breathing; rinse mouth frequently; space fluids throughout the day.	Patient's subjective feeling of moist oral mucous membranes will increase compliance with fluid restrictions.	Subjective relief obtained from periodic mouth care.

Continued

Nursing Care Plan 34.1 Care of a Patient With Chronic Renal Failure—cont'd

Goals/Expected Outcomes	Nursing Interventions	Selected Rationale	Evaluation
	Post a sign over the bed to alert visitors and health care team members about fluid restrictions.	Many persons can pass through a patient's room, and all should be aware of precautions to prevent inadvertently offering restricted foods and fluids.	Sign placed above bed for fluid restrictions.
	Check for signs of fluid overload: edema, crackles in lungs, orthopnea, and changes in mental status.	Peripheral fluid is observed in extremities and face. Edema within body organs (e.g., lungs or brain) manifests as functional impairment.	Fine crackles noted in base of posterior lung fields bilaterally. Reports some mild shortness of breath, especially with exertion or if lying flat in bed. Subjectively feels breathing is okay "when sitting in a chair." Resting pulse oximetry 94%. 3+ pitting edema noted bilaterally in feet.
	Restrict sodium to 2 g/day as ordered.	Decreasing solute load decreases fluid retention.	Compliant with 2-g sodium diet. Outcomes partially met.

CRITICAL THINKING QUESTIONS

1. What diagnostic tests do you think the nephrologist would have ordered for Mrs. Stevens?
2. Why is a tunneled catheter being used instead of an AV fistula?
3. If Mrs. Stevens does not agree to hemodialysis, what other alternatives are available to her?
4. What concerns do you anticipate that Mrs. Stevens's husband and son would have?

ADLs, Activities of daily living; *BP*, blood pressure; *BUN*, blood urea nitrogen; *CHF*, congestive heart failure; *ESRD*, end-stage rental disease; *I&O*, intake and output; *P*, pulse; *R*, respirations; *RBC*, red blood cell.

the rate of new cases of ESRD. All nurses can promote healthy kidney function by encouraging the intake of more water, the control hypertension and diabetes, and prompt recognition and treatment of urinary tract infections. In addition, nurses can participate in community education to increase awareness of organ donation programs.

Nurses in outpatient clinics assist with urologic procedures, such as cystoscopy and removal or destruction of renal stones. Clinic nurses will also have opportunities to teach patients how to manage problems of incontinence.

Home care nurses are constantly on the alert for signs of ARF or CRF among their patients. Many illnesses and the variety of drugs that these patients receive may cause kidney damage. Many home care patients have indwelling catheters that must be periodically replaced with new ones. Home health nurses also identify problems of incontinence and are able to see the environmental and social factors that must be addressed.

Nurses in long-term care facilities deal with a variety of urinary problems. Bladder training for incontinence is a prime consideration. Monitoring for drug toxicities in this population is imperative because drugs are not excreted quickly, and polypharmacy can have additive effects. Keeping residents dry and odor free is very important for physical and psychological reasons. Monitoring for urinary retention or obstruction to the flow of urine is another priority in the older adult population.

Nurses who work in dialysis centers are typically the primary nurses for patients in renal failure. These nurses must constantly assess patients for complications, watch for medication-related problems, and continue to reinforce diet and lifestyle modifications. Considerable psychosocial support and counseling may be necessary because patients undergoing dialysis commonly experience depression, hopelessness, sexual problems, role changes, and relationship problems.

Get Ready for the NCLEX® Examination!

Key Points

- Teach prevention of infectious disorders such as cystitis and urethritis (e.g., good hygiene, drinking plenty of water, and seeking prompt treatment for genital discharge or dysuria).
- Symptoms of pyelonephritis include fever, chills, headache, malaise, nausea and vomiting, and pain in the flank radiating to the thigh and genitalia.
- Acute glomerulonephritis is characterized by fever, chills, flank pain, widespread edema, visual disturbances, and significant hypertension. Nursing implications include encouraging bed rest; low-protein and low-sodium diet; and administering antihypertensives, corticosteroids, and diuretics as prescribed.
- Symptoms of chronic glomerulonephritis include edema, dyspnea, and headache associated with hypertension.
- In hydronephrosis the flow of urine from the kidney is obstructed; the kidney dilates and fills with fluid.
- In renal stenosis the renal artery becomes blocked or narrowed because of atherosclerosis.
- Renal stones are associated with frequent urinary infections, inadequate fluid intake and concentrated urine, urinary stasis, and urate in the urine.
- Symptoms of trauma to the kidneys, ureters, and bladder may include gross hematuria, pain, or an enlarged mass in the renal or bladder area.
- Risk factors for cancer of the bladder include male gender, smoking, and exposure to industrial toxins.
- Major symptoms of cancer of the kidney include hematuria and enlargement of the affected kidney.
- Prerenal ARF/AKI is caused by decreased blood flow, intrarenal AKI occurs from damage in the kidney, and postrenal AKI is caused by obstruction that causes backflow of urine into the kidney.
- ATN can be caused by decreased oxygenation or blood flow or nephrotoxic substances.
- The four phases of AKI are onset, oliguric, diuretic, and recovery.
- Nephrosclerosis (hardening of renal arterioles) caused by hypertension and diabetic nephropathy are the most common causes of CRF.
- Treatment of CRF includes diet management, fluid and electrolyte management, hemodialysis, or peritoneal dialysis and kidney transplantation.
- Hemodialysis is the use of diffusion to remove waste products normally excreted by the kidneys. Complications include fluid overload, electrolyte imbalance, anemia, platelet abnormalities, and infection.
- Nursing implications for peritoneal dialysis are to weigh the patient and take vital signs before and after treatment, measure I&O, use strict aseptic technique, and monitor for infection.
- Kidney transplant is another treatment for kidney failure. Signs of organ rejection include elevated blood pressure, fever, pain over the transplant area, fatigue, oliguria, and increased BUN and serum creatinine.

Additional Learning Resources

SG Go to your Study Guide for additional learning activities to help you master this chapter content.

Go to your Evolve website (http://evolve.elsevier.com/deWit/medsurg) for the following FREE learning resources:

- Animations, audio, and video
- Answers and rationales for questions and activities
- Glossary with pronunciations in English and Spanish
- Interactive Review Questions and more!

Review Questions for the NCLEX® Examination

1. Which patient statement indicates that your female patient needs additional teaching on the discharge instructions for urinary tract infection?
  1. "I will always wipe from back to front after a bowel movement."
  2. "I should avoid wearing tight slacks."
  3. "I won't wash my underclothing with strong detergents."
  4. "I will take a shower instead of a tub bath."
  NCLEX Client Need: Health Promotion and Maintenance

2. A patient with a history of throat infection becomes suddenly ill with fever, chills, flank pain, widespread edema, puffiness around the eyes, visual disturbances, and marked hypertension. You would anticipate which diagnostic test?
  1. Urinalysis
  2. CT of the abdomen
  3. Serum amylase
  4. Prothrombin time
  NCLEX Client Need: Physiological Integrity: Physiological Adaptation

3. A patient with nephrotic syndrome is admitted with severe generalized edema, ascites, and cloudy urine. The patient is irritable and tired. What is the priority nursing problem?
  1. Potential for infection
  2. Altered fluid volume
  3. Pain
  4. Fatigue
  NCLEX Client Need: Safe and Effective Care Environment: Coordinated Care

4. A 45-year-old man has a history of calcium oxalate stones, which can result in further renal calculi. What should you include about diet in this patient's education?
  1. He should increase his protein intake but restrict dietary calcium and sodium.
  2. He should increase intake of spinach and nuts.
  3. He should increase fluids and dietary calcium.
  4. He should increase sodium but decrease protein intake.
  NCLEX Client Need: Health Promotion and Maintenance

5. While caring for a patient who has received SWL (lithotripsy) for renal calculi, you would anticipate what possible actions that may be taken to help the patient increase the rate of stone passage? (*Select all that apply.*)
   1. Follow orders for MET.
   2. Increase oral fluid intake.
   3. Administer Vicodin for pain.
   4. Cystoscopy to retrieve the stones.
   5. Strain all urine.
   6. Low-salt and low-fat diet.

   NCLEX Client Need: Physiological Integrity: Basic Care and Comfort
6. You are assisting in administering BCG intravesically to a patient with bladder cancer. Place the steps in the correct order to accomplish this procedure.
   1. Clamp the urethral catheter for 2 hours.
   2. Change position every 15 to 30 minutes.
   3. Aseptically insert a urinary catheter.
   4. Drain urinary bladder.
   5. Instill the BCG fluid.

   NCLEX Client Need: Physiological Integrity: Pharmacological Therapies
7. A patient with CRF has a BUN of 120 mg/dL, creatinine of 9 mg/dL, and potassium of 6.9 mEq/L. What is the primary significance of these laboratory values?
   1. They are expected laboratory results for a patient with CRF.
   2. The values signify renal insufficiency.
   3. The results, in conjunction with uremic signs, indicates a need for dialysis.
   4. The patient should be referred as a good candidate for peritoneal dialysis.

   NCLEX Client Need: Physiological Integrity: Reduction of Risk Potential
8. What is included in the nursing care of a patient undergoing peritoneal dialysis? *(Select all that apply.)*
   1. Maintain aseptic technique when accessing a peritoneal catheter.
   2. Instruct the patient to remain supine until the dialysate is drained.
   3. Weigh the patient before and after dialysis.
   4. Monitor vital signs.
   5. Check color and volume of effluent.

   NCLEX Client Need: Safe and Effective Care Environment: Safety and Infection Control
9. You are sending a patient to the dialysis clinic. What predialysis nursing interventions should be included? *(Select all that apply.)*
   1. Withholding anticoagulants
   2. Administering antihypertensives
   3. Assessing dialysis access site
   4. Checking vital signs
   5. Monitoring laboratory values

   NCLEX Client Need: Physiological Integrity: Reduction of Risk Potential
10. A patient with ESRD is on dialysis and waiting for a kidney transplant. The patient says, "I am never going to be at the top of the list for a kidney. I wish I could just die and get it over with." What is the most therapeutic response?
    1. "I am sure you are going to get a kidney. A lot of people donate these days."
    2. "Are you thinking about hurting or killing yourself?"
    3. "I would be discouraged too, but I have never been very good at waiting."
    4. "You seem really down today. What's going on?"

    NCLEX Client Need: Psychological Integrity

Critical Thinking Questions

Scenario A

Mr. Jakes, 25 years old, complains of sudden onset of fever and chills, flank pain, and "feeling full all over and peeing dark smoke–colored urine." He tells you he had strep throat 2 weeks ago but is otherwise healthy.

1. Based on Mr. Jakes's history and complaints, what physical assessments should you perform?
2. Why is the history of strep throat 2 weeks ago significant?
3. The health care provider informs Mr. Jakes that he has glomerulonephritis and prescribes complete bed rest. How long must bed rest continue?

Scenario B

Mr. Mell, a 43-year-old interstate truck driver, complains of severe right lower back pain with nausea, vomiting, and pink-tinged urine. He relates a history of kidney stones and reports, "It always feels like this until the stone passes." The health care provider orders IV normal saline, morphine, routine laboratory tests to include BUN and creatinine, and a CT scan of the abdomen.

1. What are three or four risk factors for kidney stones that might apply to Mr. Mell?
2. His BUN result is 17 mg/dL, and his creatinine is 1.2 mg/dL. What do these results indicate? What is your responsibility in reporting these data?
3. What is the care for Mr. Mell after a lithotripsy?

Scenario C

Mrs. Diaz, 35 years old, has had a nephrostomy for treatment of hydronephrosis caused by a renal stone in the pelvis of the kidney. She returns from the interventional radiology department with a nephrostomy tube and a urethral catheter in place.

1. Explain the purpose of the nephrostomy tube.
2. What is the specific care for the drains and tubes?

The Endocrine System

35

http://evolve.elsevier.com/deWit/medsurg

Objectives

Theory

1. Identify the location of each endocrine gland.
2. Diagram the principal actions and target tissues for hormones of the hypothalamus and pituitary, parathyroid, adrenal, and pancreas glands.
3. Summarize the effects of the thyroid hormones.
4. Compare care for common diagnostic tests for the endocrine system.

Clinical Practice

5. Assess for specific age-related changes of the endocrine system in an older adult.
6. Teach patients about the diagnostic tests that might be performed for symptoms of endocrine disorders.
7. Perform a focused assessment on a patient who may have an endocrine disorder.
8. Distinguish appropriate problem statements or nursing diagnoses and interventions for problems common to patients with endocrine disorders.

Key Terms

adenohypophysis (ă-DEN-o-hī-POF-ă-sis, p. 839)
adrenocorticotropic hormone (ă-DREN-o-KOR-ti-kō-TRŌ-pik HŌR-mōn, p. 843)
endocrine (EN-do-krin, p. 844)
exocrine (Ek-so-krin, p. 844)
fructosamine assay (FRŬK-tōs-ăm-ēn ĂS-sā, p. 846)
glucocorticoids (glū-kō-KOR-ti-koydz, p. 843)
glucose tolerance test (GLŪ-cōs TŎL-ĕr-ĕns tĕst, p. 846)
hemoglobin A_{1c} (A_{1c}) (HĒ-mō-glō-bin, p. 846)
hormones (HOR-mōnz, p. 840)
hypersecretion (hī-per-SE-KRĒ-shun, p. 846)
hyposecretion (hī-pō-SE-KRĒ-shun, p. 846)
insulin (IN-sū-lin, p. 844)
mineralocorticoids (min-er-ăl-ō-KOR-ti-koydz, p. 843)
negative feedback (NĔ-gĕ-tĭv FĒD-băk, p. 845)
parathormone (păr-ă-THOR-mōn, p. 843)
pressor (PRĔS-sŏr, p. 843)
target cells (TĂR-gĕt sĕlz, p. 844)
target tissues (TĂR-gĕt TĬ-shū, p. 844)
thyrocalcitonin (thī-rō-KĂL-si-TŌ-nin, p. 841)
thyroid panel (THĪ-royd PĂN-ĕl, p. 846)
thyroxine (THĪ-rok-sin, p. 841)
triiodothyronine (trī-ī-ō-dō-THĪ-rō-nen, p. 841)

Concepts Covered in This Chapter

- Self-Management
- Fluid and Electrolytes
- Hormonal Regulation
- Glucose Regulation
- Reproduction
- Inflammation
- Stress
- Health Promotion
- Collaboration

ANATOMY AND PHYSIOLOGY OF THE ENDOCRINE SYSTEM

ORGANS AND STRUCTURES OF THE ENDOCRINE SYSTEM (Fig. 35.1)

- The pituitary gland connects to the hypothalamus via the hypophyseal stalk. The pituitary gland has two parts: the anterior pituitary (**adenohypophysis**) and the posterior pituitary (neurohypophysis).
- The thyroid gland has two lobes and lies below the larynx over the thyroid cartilage, in front of and on either side of the trachea.
- The parathyroid glands are four to six small glands that are located on the posterior surface of the thyroid gland.
- The adrenal glands are located on the anterior upper surface of each kidney; each is composed of the cortex and medulla.
- The pancreas sits in the upper left aspect of the abdominal cavity. Beta cells, which secrete the hormone insulin, and alpha cells, which secrete the hormone glucagon, are both found in the islets of Langerhans.
- The ovaries are located in the pelvic cavity in females.
- The testes hang suspended in the scrotum in males.
- The pineal gland is in the midbrain, in the cranial vault.

- The thymus gland lies at the base of the neck, in the front of the thoracic cavity.
- The heart is midchest and functions as an endocrine gland when it secretes the hormones atrial natriuretic peptide (ANP) and B-type (or brain) natriuretic peptide (BNP).

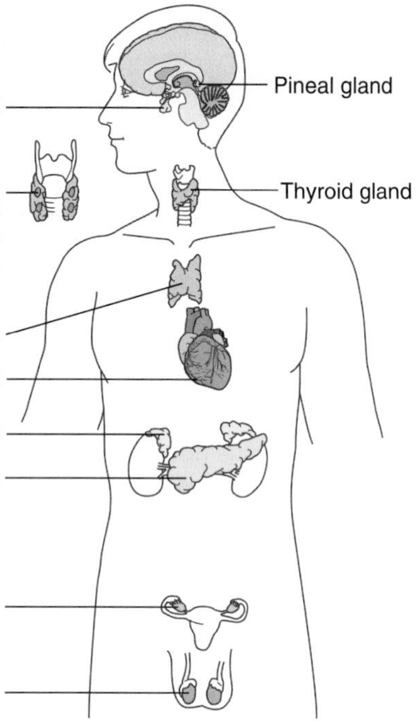

Fig. 35.1 Major endocrine glands.

FUNCTIONS OF THE ENDOCRINE SYSTEM

- When the muscle is stretched, the heart secretes hormones with a diuretic effect.
- The endocrine system alters chemical reactions and controls the rate at which chemical activities take place within cells.
- The hormones secreted change the permeability of cell membranes and select the substances that can be transported across cell membranes.
- The endocrine hormones activate a particular mechanism in a cell, such as the system that controls cellular growth and reproduction. The **hormones** produced by the endocrine system, the target organs on which they act, and the principal actions of each hormone are presented in Table 35.1.

EFFECTS OF THE PITUITARY HORMONES

- The effects of pituitary hormones when secreted are illustrated in Fig. 35.2.
- Any type of dysfunction of the pituitary gland will affect one or more of the hormones, as well as their target organs (Fig. 35.3).
- The posterior pituitary gland does not produce hormones; it stores and then releases oxytocin and antidiuretic hormone (ADH), which are produced in the hypothalamus.
- The anterior pituitary produces hormones that are secreted into the bloodstream as a result of "releasing hormones" from the hypothalamus.

Table 35.1 The Principal Endocrine Glands and Their Hormones

GLAND	HORMONE	TARGET TISSUE	PRINCIPAL ACTIONS
Hypothalamus	Releasing and inhibiting hormones	Anterior lobe of pituitary gland	Stimulates or inhibits secretion of specific hormones
Anterior lobe of pituitary	Growth hormone (GH)	Most tissues in the body	Stimulates growth by promoting protein synthesis
	Thyroid-stimulating hormone (TSH)	Thyroid gland	Increases secretion of thyroid hormone; increases the size of the thyroid gland
	Adrenocorticotropic hormone (ACTH)	Adrenal cortex	Increases secretion of adrenocortical hormones, especially glucocorticoids, such as cortisol
	Follicle-stimulating hormone (FSH)	Ovarian follicles in females; seminiferous tubules in males	Follicle maturation and estrogen secretion in females; spermatogenesis in males
	Luteinizing hormone (LH); called interstitial cell–stimulating hormone (ICSH) in males	Ovary in females, testis in males	Ovulation, progesterone production in females; testosterone production in males
	Prolactin	Mammary gland	Stimulates milk production
Posterior lobe of pituitary (storage only: ADH and oxytocin are synthesized in the hypothalamus)	Antidiuretic hormone (ADH)	Kidney	Increases water reabsorption (decreases water lost in urine)
	Oxytocin	Uterus; mammary gland	Increases uterine contractions; stimulates ejection of milk from mammary gland

Table 35.1 The Principal Endocrine Glands and Their Hormones—cont'd

GLAND	HORMONE	TARGET TISSUE	PRINCIPAL ACTIONS
Thyroid gland	Thyroxine and triiodothyronine	Most body cells	Increases metabolic rate; essential for normal growth and development
	Calcitonin	Primarily bone	Decreases blood calcium by inhibiting bone breakdown and release of calcium; antagonistic to parathyroid hormone
Parathyroid gland	Parathyroid hormone (PTH) or parathormone	Bone, kidney, digestive tract	Increases blood calcium by stimulating bone breakdown and release of calcium; increases calcium absorption in the digestive tract; decreases calcium lost in urine
Adrenal cortex	Mineralocorticoids (aldosterone)	Kidney	Increases sodium reabsorption and potassium excretion in kidney tubules; increases water retention
	Glucocorticoids (cortisol)	Most body tissues	Increases blood glucose levels; inhibits inflammation and immune response
	Androgens and estrogens	Most body tissues	Secreted in small amounts; effect is generally masked by hormones from ovaries or testes
Adrenal medulla	Epinephrine, norepinephrine	Heart, blood vessels, liver, adipose tissue	Helps cope with stress; increases heart rate and blood pressure; increases blood flow to skeletal muscle; increases blood glucose
Pancreas (islets of Langerhans)	Glucagon	Liver	Increases breakdown of glycogen to increase blood glucose levels
	Insulin	General but especially liver, skeletal muscle, adipose tissue	Decreases blood glucose levels by facilitating uptake and use of glucose by cells; stimulates glucose storage as glycogen and production of adipose tissue
Testes	Testosterone	Most body cells	Maturation and maintenance of male reproductive organs and secondary sex characteristics
Ovaries	Estrogens	Most body cells	Maturation and maintenance of female reproductive organs and secondary sex characteristics; menstrual cycle
	Progesterone	Uterus and breast	Prepares uterus for pregnancy; stimulates development of mammary gland; regulates menstrual cycle
Pineal gland	Melatonin	Hypothalamus	Inhibits gonadotropin-releasing hormone, thus inhibiting reproductive functions; regulates sleep and wakefulness
Thymus	Thymosin	Tissues involved in immune response	Immune system development and function
Heart	Atrial natriuretic peptide (ANP) B-type (or brain) natriuretic peptide (BNP)	Kidney	Increases sodium excretion, causing diuresis; inhibits release of renin

EFFECTS OF THE THYROID HORMONES

- The thyroid gland secretes the hormones **thyroxine** (T_4), **triiodothyronine** (T_3), and **thyrocalcitonin**. The *3* and the *4* indicate how many iodine atoms are attached.
- T_3 is the more potent form of thyroid hormone. T_4 is converted to T_3 by removing an iodine atom from the T_4 molecule.
- Intake of protein and iodine is needed to synthesize both thyroid hormones.
- Thyroid hormones activate the cellular production of heat; stimulate protein and lipid synthesis, mobilization, and degradation (breakdown); and stimulate the manufacture of coenzymes from vitamins.
- Thyroid hormones regulate many aspects of carbohydrate metabolism and affect tissue response to epinephrine and norepinephrine.

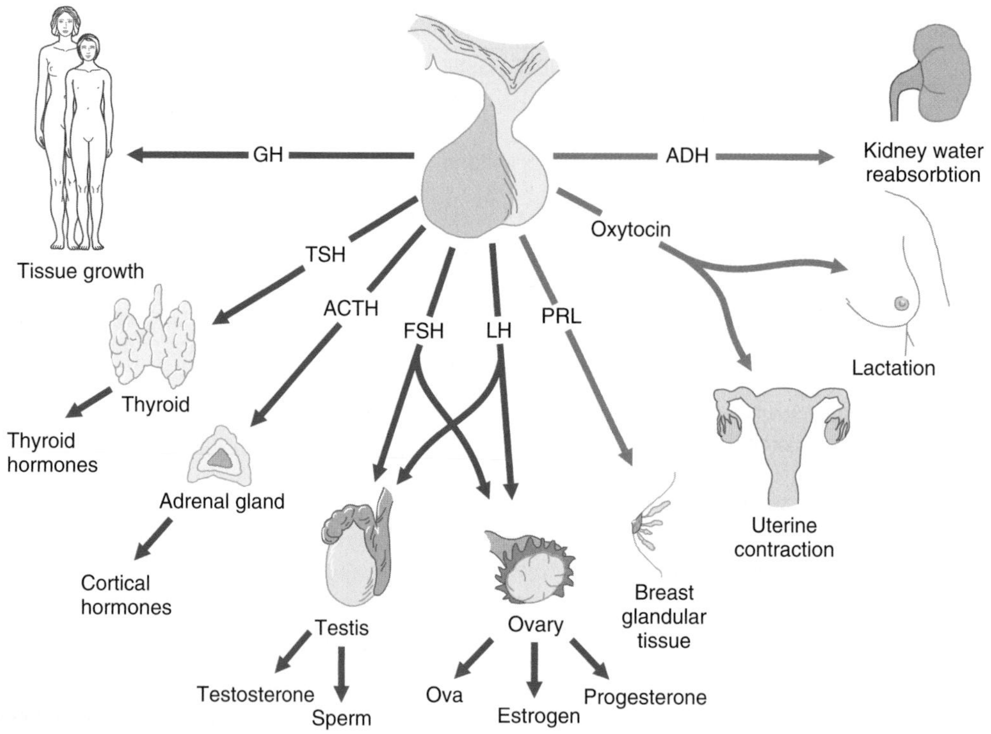

Fig. 35.2 Effects of hormones from the pituitary gland. *ACTH,* Adrenocorticotropic hormone; *ADH,* antidiuretic hormone; *FSH,* follicle-stimulating hormone; *GH,* growth hormone; *LH,* luteinizing hormone; *PRL,* prolactin; *TSH,* thyroid-stimulating hormone.

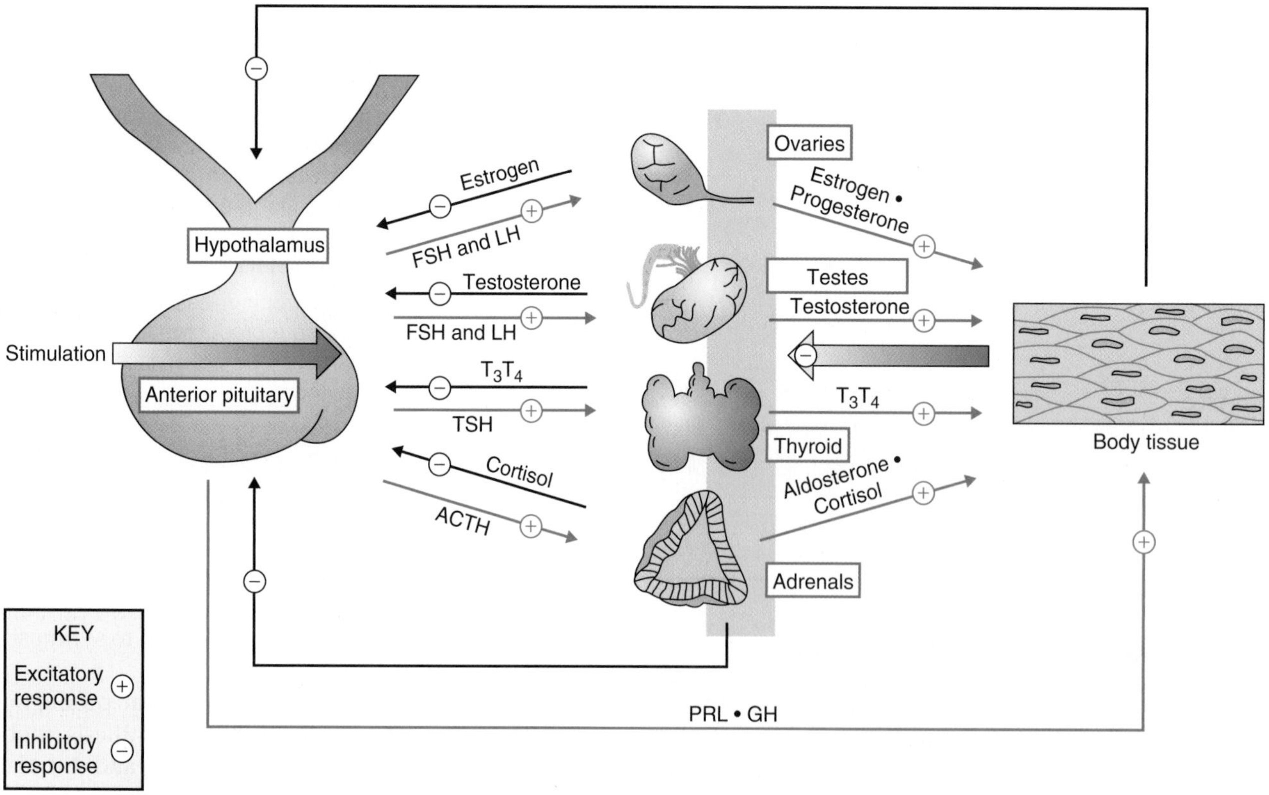

Fig. 35.3 Feedback system of the hypothalamus, pituitary, and target glands. *ACTH,* Adrenocorticotropic hormone; *FSH,* follicle-stimulating hormone; *GH,* growth hormone; *LH,* luteinizing hormone; *PRL,* prolactin; T_3, triiodothyronine; T_4, thyroxine; *TSH,* thyroid-stimulating hormone. (From Ignatavicius DD, Workman ML, Mishler MA: *Medical-surgical nursing: a nursing process approach,* ed 3, Philadelphia, 1999, Saunders.)

FUNCTIONS OF THE PARATHYROID GLANDS

- **Parathormone**, or **parathyroid hormone,** is produced and secreted by the parathyroid glands.
- A low calcium level will stimulate release of parathormone, which increases the plasma level of calcium. A high calcium level will inhibit the release of parathormone.
- Parathormone acts on the renal tubules to increase the excretion of phosphorus in the urine and to stimulate the reabsorption of calcium. It also stimulates the production of the active form of vitamin D, which enhances calcium absorption in the small intestine. Parathormone also acts on bone, causing the release of calcium from the bone into the bloodstream.
- Calcitonin (released by the thyroid gland) is the balance to parathormone that causes calcium to go into the bones and allows for renal excretion to reduce calcium levels in the blood.

Safety Alert

Parathyroid Deficiency

A deficiency of parathyroid hormone produces muscle cramps, twitching of the muscles, and in some cases severe convulsions because of hypocalcemia.

FUNCTIONS OF THE ADRENAL GLAND HORMONES

- The adrenal medulla (middle portion) secretes two hormones, epinephrine and norepinephrine (called catecholamines), in response to stimulation from the sympathetic nervous system.
- Epinephrine prepares the body to meet stress or emergency situations and prevents hypoglycemia (Fig. 35.4). Norepinephrine functions as a **pressor** (causing blood vessel constriction) to maintain blood pressure.
- The hormones secreted by the adrenal cortex are called *adrenal corticosteroids.* (The word *steroid* is sometimes used to designate an adrenal corticosteroid or a synthetic compound with similar properties.)
- The two major types of hormones secreted by the adrenal cortex are the mineralocorticoids (aldosterone) and the glucocorticoids (cortisol) (Fig. 35.5).
- The adrenal glands also secrete small amounts of androgenic hormones, which have effects similar to those of the male and female sex hormones.
- The **mineralocorticoids** affect the electrolytes, particularly sodium, potassium, and chloride. The primary mineralocorticoid is aldosterone, which promotes conservation of water by acting on the kidney to retain sodium in exchange for potassium. Water stays with sodium, and potassium is excreted in the urine.
- Without the mineralocorticoids, a person would die within 3 to 7 days because these hormones directly control fluid balance, blood volume, cardiac output, exchange of nutrients, and wastes in each cell; mineralocorticoids affect all chemical processes and glandular functions within the body.
- The **glucocorticoids** are essential to the metabolic systems for proper use of carbohydrates, proteins, and fats.
- The primary glucocorticoid is cortisol, or hydrocortisone. Cortisol acts to increase glucose levels in the blood. Cortisol also helps counteract the inflammatory response.
- Both aldosterone and cortisol are controlled by **adrenocorticotropic hormone** (ACTH)–releasing hormone from the hypothalamus and ACTH secreted by the anterior pituitary (see Fig. 35.3).

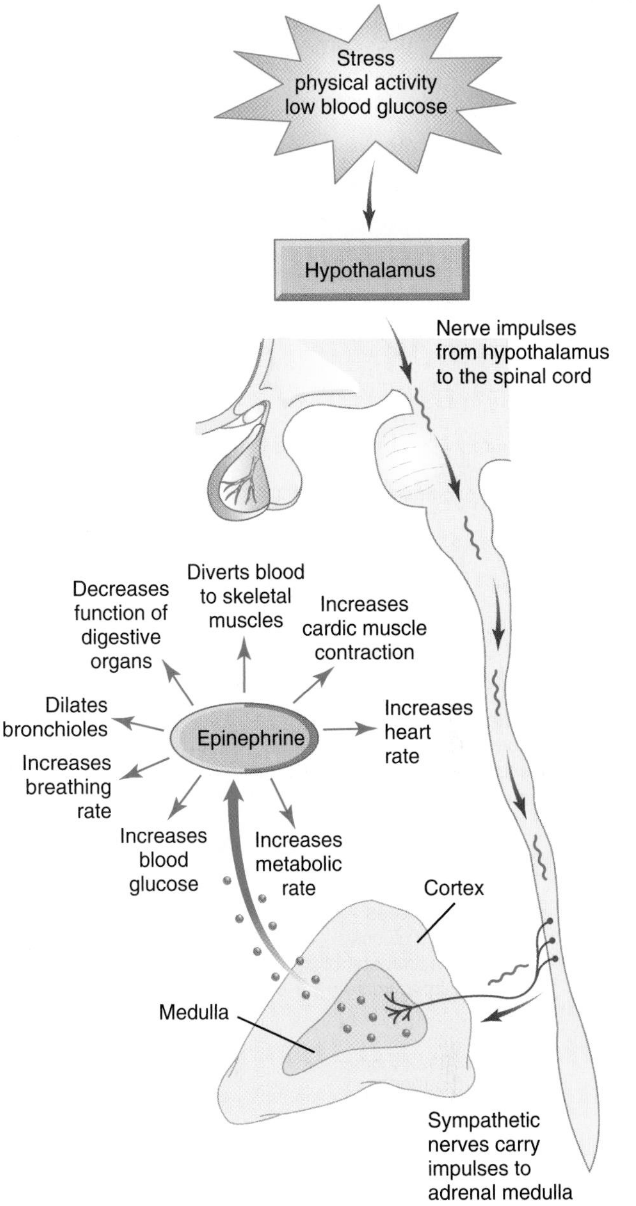

Fig. 35.4 Effects of epinephrine and control of its secretion. (From Applegate E: *The anatomy and physiology learning system*, ed 4, Philadelphia, 2011, Saunders.)

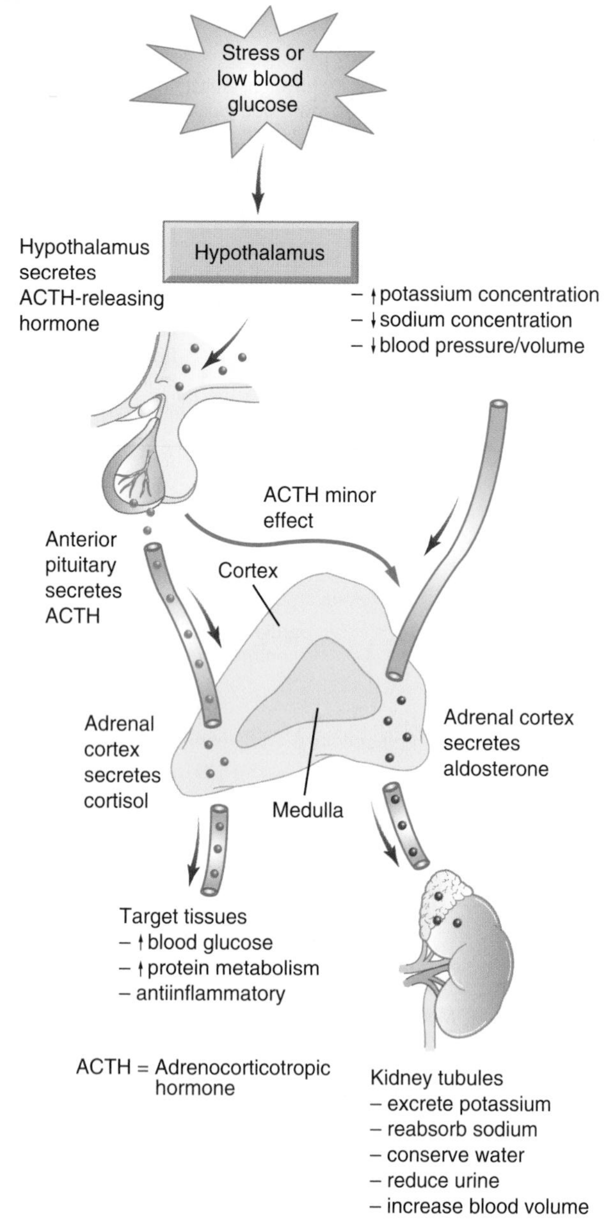

Fig. 35.5 Regulation of aldosterone and cortisol secretion. *ACTH,* Adrenocorticotropic hormone. (From Applegate E: *The anatomy and physiology learning system,* ed 2, Philadelphia, 2000, Saunders.)

HORMONAL FUNCTION OF THE PANCREAS

- The pancreas is both an **endocrine** (secretes into the bloodstream) and an **exocrine** (secretes through a duct to the target tissues) gland. Its endocrine function is to produce the hormones insulin and glucagon.
- The beta cells are responsible for producing and secreting insulin. **Insulin** is needed for the cells of the body to be able to use glucose as fuel. The alpha cells release glucagon, which stimulates the liver to change glycogen to glucose (Fig. 35.6).

EFFECTS OF AGING ON THE ENDOCRINE SYSTEM

- The pituitary gland becomes smaller.
- The thyroid becomes more lumpy or nodular; beginning around age 20 years, metabolism gradually declines.
- Hormones that usually decrease with older age include aldosterone, renin, calcitonin, and growth hormone; specific hormones decrease in older women (estrogen and prolactin) and older men (testosterone).
- Hormones that may increase with older age include follicle-stimulating hormone (FSH), luteinizing hormone (LH), norepinephrine, and ADH.
- Hormones that remain unchanged or are only slightly decreased with older age include thyroid hormones (T_3 and T_4), cortisol, insulin, epinephrine, parathyroid hormone, and 25-hydroxyvitamin D.
- Blood glucose levels rise with older age, with fasting levels climbing about 1 mg/dL for each decade after the age of 50 years and postprandial levels increasing 6 to 13 mg/dL.
- Although insulin levels remain unchanged with age, decreased glucose tolerance may occur because of changes in the cell receptor sites; older adults experience hypoglycemia more quickly than younger people and may progress to dangerously low levels of blood glucose before signs and symptoms are obvious. This decreased glucose tolerance because of cell receptor change can place older adults at risk for hyperglycemia and the onset of type 2 diabetes.
- Although thyroid hormone levels may decrease with aging, the body makes up for it by decreasing the rate at which thyroid hormone is broken down; therefore resting levels of thyroid hormone are usually normal in older adults. However, thyroid disorders are twice as common in older adults. Hypothyroidism is the most common thyroid disorder, especially in older women.
- The amount of hormones secreted by older adults changes, decreasing the individual's ability to adapt to stress and respond to environmental changes.
- Because of decreasing liver and kidney function in older adults, hormone replacement therapy must be done very cautiously to prevent hormone overdosage.

THE ENDOCRINE SYSTEM

The endocrine system regulates metabolism, growth and development, sexual function, and reproductive processes. A primary function of the endocrine system is to synthesize and release hormones directly into the bloodstream. The cells and tissues that are affected by a specific hormone are called its **target cells** or **target tissues.**

Some of the endocrine hormones, such as the thyroid hormones, affect practically every cell in the body. Others, such as the sex hormones, exert their special effects on only one organ system. Moreover, hormones from one endocrine gland can affect another endocrine gland. The pituitary gland, for example, secretes several different kinds of hormones that affect other endocrine glands. For this reason, the pituitary gland is often referred to as the "master gland" of the body.

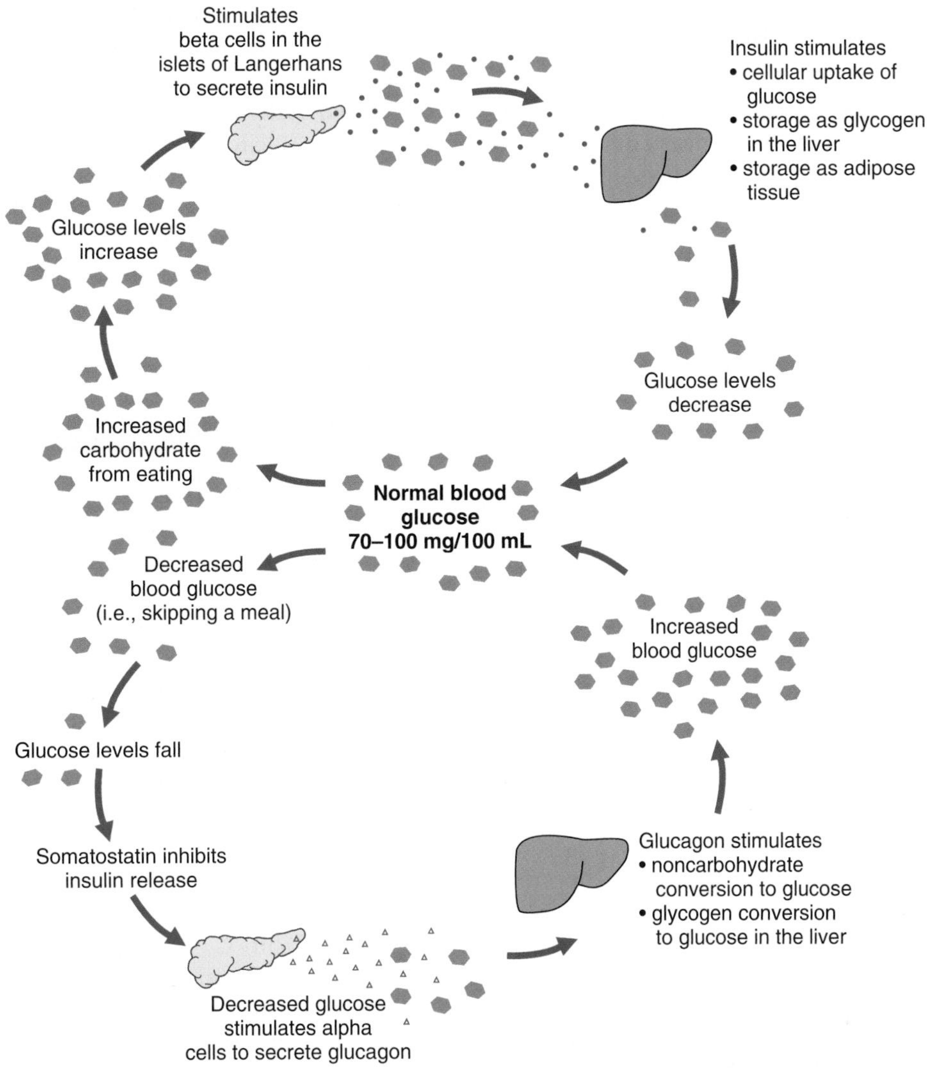
Stimulates
beta cells in the
islets of Langerhans
to secrete insulin
Insulin stimulates
• cellular uptake of glucose
• storage as glycogen in the liver
• storage as adipose tissue
Glucose levels increase
Glucose levels decrease
Increased carbohydrate from eating
Normal blood glucose 70–100 mg/100 mL
Decreased blood glucose (i.e., skipping a meal)
Increased blood glucose
Glucose levels fall
Somatostatin inhibits insulin release
Glucagon stimulates
• noncarbohydrate conversion to glucose
• glycogen conversion to glucose in the liver
Decreased glucose stimulates alpha cells to secrete glucagon

Fig. 35.6 Blood glucose regulation. (Adapted from Applegate E: *The anatomy and physiology learning system*, ed 2, Philadelphia, 2000, Saunders.)

The endocrine system and the nervous system are the two major control systems of the body, and their regulatory functions are interrelated. However, the endocrine system typically controls body processes that occur slowly, such as cell growth, whereas the nervous system controls body processes that occur more rapidly, such as breathing and body movement.

The secretion of a particular hormone normally depends on the need. If an endocrine gland receives a message that its hormone is in short supply, it will synthesize and release more of that hormone. If, on the other hand, the hormonal need of a target tissue is being satisfied, production or secretion of the hormone will be inhibited—a concept known as **negative feedback**.

Some glands, such as the adrenal medulla and posterior pituitary, receive their information about hormone levels in the body *directly* and respond only to stimulation of nerve endings within the glands themselves. However, the posterior pituitary gland *indirectly* receives notice to either release or inhibit hormones: stimulation comes by way of the hypothalamus and the anterior lobe of the pituitary (the adenohypophysis). The hypothalamus contains special nerve endings that produce releasing and inhibiting hormones; these hormones are then absorbed into capillaries of a portal system, which transports the hormones to the adenohypophysis (the anterior lobe of the pituitary). Thus the hypothalamus controls the secretion of hormones from the pituitary. The pituitary, in turn, controls the release or inhibition of hormones from other glands. Many of the hormones of the anterior pituitary are "tropic" hormones; that is, they tend to cause a change in the endocrine gland that is the target of the specific pituitary hormone. An example is ACTH, which acts on the adrenal cortex. (If you break down this term, you can easily see that the components *adrenal–cortex–tropic* tell you exactly where or what type of hormone this is and where it comes from.) The major endocrine glands are shown in Fig. 35.1; see Table 35.1 for the various tropic hormones and target tissues.

ENDOCRINE SYSTEM DISORDERS

Causes

Endocrine disorders are caused by an imbalance in the production of hormone or by an alteration in the body's ability to use the hormones produced. Dysfunction can occur at any point in the production-secretion-feedback regulation cycle.

Primary endocrine dysfunction means that an endocrine gland is either oversecreting or undersecreting hormone(s)—situations referred to as **hypersecretion** and **hyposecretion**, respectively. Tumor or hyperplasia of the endocrine gland may lead to hypersecretion. Hyposecretion is usually the result of destruction of endocrine glandular tissue by an inflammatory process or other destructive mechanism that interferes with normal endocrine function. Infection, mechanical damage, or an autoimmune response may cause such an inflammatory response in a gland.

Secondary endocrine dysfunction occurs from factors outside the gland itself. Medications, trauma, hormone therapy, and other factors may cause secondary dysfunction. Such dysfunction may be temporary or permanent; endocrine function often returns to normal if the cause is corrected (e.g., the medication is discontinued).

Prevention

Preventing most endocrine disorders is not possible through lifestyle changes; however, there are some dietary considerations regarding the thyroid gland that may be beneficial.

Health Promotion

Preventing Goiter

Goiter, an overgrowth of the thyroid, may be prevented by sufficient intake of iodine. Iodine is available in foods grown near the ocean and in seafood. Iodized salt is the major source for most people.

Think Critically

Why might a person with an endocrine disorder delay seeking medical care?

Diagnostic Tests and Procedures

Tests of the endocrine system are performed on blood samples; on urine samples; or by scans, ultrasounds, radiographs, or magnetic resonance imaging (MRI). Table 35.2 presents the various tests and procedures and their nursing implications.

Clinical Cues

Thyroid test results are altered by iodine-based contrast media for radiologic studies. Furosemide, phenytoin, heparin, aspirin, and other drugs may affect thyroid tests (Pagana & Pagana, 2018).

Abnormalities in thyroid gland activity are among the most common endocrine disorders. To detect abnormalities, a group of tests—called a **thyroid panel**—is performed. A thyroid panel measures TSH, T_4, T_3, thyroid antibodies, calcitonin, and thyroglobulin. These tests may also be ordered individually.

Laboratory testing for serum calcium and phosphate levels is usually performed to assess parathyroid function. Adrenal gland function is evaluated by laboratory testing, including electrolyte panels, glucose levels, and hormone levels; a 12-lead electrocardiogram (ECG) may be performed if cardiac dysrhythmias are suspected.

Think Critically

The health care provider has ordered laboratory tests to determine whether the patient has an endocrine disorder. The patient wants you to tell them the results of the tests. What will you do?

Diagnostic tests for detecting diabetes can be found in Table 35.3. According to the 2014 American Diabetes Association guidelines (American Diabetes Association, 2018), diagnosis of diabetes mellitus is based on one of four abnormalities:

1. Symptoms of diabetes mellitus (see Chapter 37) plus a random glucose level greater than or equal to 200 mg/dL
2. A fasting glucose level greater than or equal to 126 mg/dL
3. A hemoglobin A_{1c} level greater than 6.5%
4. A glucose tolerance test revealing a postprandial glucose greater than or equal to 200 mg/dL, 2 hours after 75 g of glucose is administered

In a **glucose tolerance test**, the patient is given a set amount of glucose to evaluate insulin secretion and ability to metabolize glucose.

The **hemoglobin A_{1c} (A_{1c})** test (formerly called the *glycosylated hemoglobin test*) measures blood glucose over a period of many weeks (Table 35.4). Glucose in the bloodstream attaches itself to the hemoglobin A (red blood cell) molecule and remains there for the life span of the red blood cell. Health care providers use A_{1c} test results to prescribe adjustments to a patient's treatment program for managing diabetes. One of the *Healthy People 2030* objectives is to reduce the proportion of adults with diabetes who have an A_{1c} value greater than 9 percent. Fructosamine assay is another test to monitor control of glucose over time. The **fructosamine assay** monitors blood glucose over a shorter time frame than the A_{1c} test because it measures sugar attached to the protein albumin, which has a shorter life span than hemoglobin.

NURSING MANAGEMENT

ASSESSMENT (DATA COLLECTION)

A full physical assessment and history are needed to evaluate a patient who is possibly experiencing an

Table 35.2 Diagnostic Tests and Procedures of the Endocrine System

TEST	PURPOSE	DESCRIPTION	NURSING IMPLICATIONS
Blood Tests			
Pituitary hormone levels: LH, FSH, GH, ACTH, TSH, prolactin	To detect oversecretion or deficiency of pituitary hormones	Sample of venous blood is drawn for immunoassay test; check laboratory procedure manual.	Monitor venipuncture site for bleeding; apply bandage or dressing.
Serum T_4 (total thyroxine) *Normal value:* 4.5–12 mcg/dL Serum T_3 (total triiodothyronine) *Normal value:* 70–190 ng/dL	To assess thyroxine in blood to evaluate thyroid function	Venous blood sample	Aspirin, iodine-containing medications, contrast media, and other drugs may affect result; check with laboratory.
TSH *Normal value:* 0.3–5 mcU/mL	To differentiate between pituitary dysfunction and primary thyroid dysfunction; assists with diagnosis of hypothyroidism	Requires a venous blood sample. Levels vary throughout the day, with lower levels at 10 A.M. and highest levels at 10 P.M.	Same as for serum T_3 and T_4.
Antithyroid antibody titer (antithyroglobulin antibody) *Normal value:* <116 international unit/mL	To detect the presence of thyroid antibodies and distinguish between autoimmune disorders and toxic thyroid adenoma	Requires a venous blood sample.	Radioactive iodine will interfere if given within 24 h of drawing the blood sample.
Calcitonin *Normal values:* Males: <19 pg/mL Females: <14 pg/mL	Used for differential diagnosis of cancer of the thyroid	Requires a venous blood sample.	If base level is within normal, the pentagastrin stimulation test may be administered by injection to test for calcitonin secretion. Blood samples are then drawn 1½ and 5 min after injection.
Cortisol *Normal values:* 8 A.M., 5–23 mcg/dL; 4 P.M., 3–13 mcg/dL	To assess cortisol production by adrenal glands	Requires sample of venous blood.	Explain that a specimen may be collected two or three times in 24 h to evaluate circadian effects on cortisol secretion. Keep stress to a minimum. Note time collected on laboratory slip.
Adrenocorticotropic hormone (ACTH) *Normal values:* Females: 6–58 pg/mL Males: 7–69 pg/mL	To assess ACTH production from pituitary gland	Requires venous blood sample. Place specimen in ice water immediately after drawing.	Note collection time on laboratory slip. Usually highest between 4 and 8 A.M. and lowest around 9 P.M.
ACTH stimulation test *Normal value:* after ACTH 24-h infusion, serum cortisol >40 mcg/dL	To assess adrenal response to ACTH To detect adrenal cortical insufficiency (Addison disease)	Baseline venous sample taken for cortisol determination. ACTH is administered IV infusion. Blood sample is withdrawn at 24 h.	Note time ACTH is administered; note time each specimen is drawn. Instruct patient to avoid strenuous activity on the day before the test. Check with laboratory regarding food restrictions.

Continued

Table 35.2 Diagnostic Tests and Procedures of the Endocrine System—cont'd

TEST	PURPOSE	DESCRIPTION	NURSING IMPLICATIONS
Dexamethasone suppression test Low dose overnight *Normal value:* after dexamethasone, serum cortisol <1.8 mcg/dL High dose overnight: decrease of more than 50% in serum cortisol	To diagnose Cushing syndrome To assess response to dexamethasone	Morning baseline serum cortisol levels are measured. Oral dexamethasone is administered at bedtime. Blood sample is collected the next morning to measure cortisol levels if an overnight test is ordered. A 24-h urine collection is done at the same time. A 3-day test may be done, which requires additional doses of dexamethasone and collection of all urine.	Explain the procedure to the patient. Check orders for drugs to be withheld. Both cortisol levels must be drawn at the same time each day. Note time specimens were drawn and patient medications on laboratory slips. Instruct patient to avoid strenuous activity the day before the test.
CRH stimulation test	To identify if an abnormality exists in the pituitary glands, hypothalamus, or adrenal glands. All of these play a role in cortisol secretion, and this test helps pinpoint the source.	Baseline serum cortisol levels are measured. An injection of synthetic CRH is given IV. Blood samples are taken at 30, 60, 90, and 120 min after administration of CRH.	Explain the procedure to the patient. The test may take up to 3 h to complete. The patient should have nothing by mouth (NPO) for 4 h before the start of the test.
BNP *Normal value:* <100 pg/mL BNP levels vary greatly by laboratory. Check normal for the reference lab used.	To identify elevated levels for evaluation of CHF and to monitor the effectiveness of treatment	Standard venous blood draw. No special instructions.	Levels >500 μg/mL are 90% predictive of CHF. Biotin affects results. Sample should be taken a minimum of 8 h after the dose.
Thyroid Scans			
Radioactive iodine uptake (RAIU) *Normal values:* <6% uptake in 2 h; 2%–25% in 6 h; 15%–45% in 24 h; 24-h urine: 40%–80% radioactive iodine excreted in 24 h	To assess function of thyroid gland To measure the rate of iodine uptake by the thyroid	Trace dose of radioactive iodine (RAI) is given orally. A gamma counter or scintillation counter is placed over the gland to measure the amount of RAI absorbed. Concurrent 24-h urine specimen may be collected to assess iodine secretion.	Test must not be performed during pregnancy or lactation. Explain that the amount of radioactive iodine used is small and will not make the patient "radioactive." Explain the procedure and the time it will take. Instruct how to collect 24-h urine specimen if required.
Thyroid scan	To determine size, shape, and activity of the thyroid gland To detect hyperactive "hot" spots and hypoactive "cold" spots	After administering RAI, a scintillation camera moves back and forth across the gland to obtain an image of iodine concentration and distribution in the thyroid gland. A computer may provide a three-dimensional image. Often done in conjunction with RAIU.	Same implications as for RAIU. Patient must lie perfectly still during the scanning. Scan takes about 20 min. Rescanning is performed at intervals of 6 and 24 h after RAI is administered.

Table 35.2 Diagnostic Tests and Procedures of the Endocrine System—cont'd

TEST	PURPOSE	DESCRIPTION	NURSING IMPLICATIONS
Urine Tests			
17-Hydroxycorticosteroids (17-OHCS) *Normal values:* Females: 2–8 mg/24 h Males: 3–9 mg/24 h	To determine levels of glucocorticoid metabolites	Collect a 24-h urine specimen in a container with preservative. Medications may interfere; consult with health care provider and laboratory about medications patient is taking.	Instruct patient in collection procedure. Note start and end time of collection on laboratory slip. Note medications patient is taking on laboratory slip.
17-Ketosteroids (17-KS) *Normal values:* Females: 6–17 mg/24 h Males: 6–20 mg/24 h Older than age 65: 4–8 mg/24 h	To determine amount of androgen metabolites in the urine	Collect 24-h urine specimen. Check with laboratory on need to keep specimen chilled.	Same as for 17-OHCS test.
Aldosterone *Normal value:* 2–26 mcg/24 h	To determine urinary aldosterone levels to assist in diagnosis of aldosteronism	Requires 24-h urine specimen with preservative; specimen must be kept chilled.	Instruct in dietary and medication restrictions. Record diet and medications on laboratory slip.
Fluid deprivation test	To detect diabetes insipidus	While patient is NPO, hourly urine output, specific gravity, and osmolality are measured, along with body weight and vital signs. Vasopressin is given subcutaneously; hourly measurements are continued for several hours.	Explain the procedure to the patient. Provide urine collection containers. Remind patient to void hourly.
Hypertonic saline test	To stimulate release of ADH to evaluate ADH secretion and detect diabetes insipidus	The patient is loaded with water. An infusion of hypertonic saline is administered. Urine output and urine specific gravity are measured hourly.	Tell patient to produce a urine specimen in the marked container every hour.

ADH, Antidiuretic hormone; *BNP,* B-type (or brain) natriuretic peptide; *CHF,* congestive heart failure; *CRH,* corticotropin-releasing hormone; *FSH,* follicle-stimulating hormone; *GH,* growth hormone; *IV,* intravenous(ly); *LH,* luteinizing hormone; *TSH,* thyroid-stimulating hormone.

Table 35.3 Diagnostic Tests for Detecting and Monitoring Diabetes Mellitus

TEST	PURPOSE	DESCRIPTION	NURSING IMPLICATIONS
Serum Tests			
Fasting blood glucose *Normal values:* 70–100 mg/dL Older adult: rises 1 mg/dL per decade of age	To determine level of circulating glucose; to detect hyperglycemia or hypoglycemia	Requires a fasting venous blood sample.	Explain importance of fasting state to the patient.
2-h postprandial blood glucose *Normal values:* 0–50 years: <140 mg/dL 50–60 years: <150 mg/dL 60+ years: <160 mg/dL	To determine need for glucose tolerance test; to determine need for change in diabetes therapy	Venous blood sample drawn 2 h after a meal.	Explain the importance of arriving for blood sampling exactly 2 h after finishing a meal.

Continued

Table 35.3 Diagnostic Tests for Detecting and Monitoring Diabetes Mellitus—cont'd

TEST	PURPOSE	DESCRIPTION	NURSING IMPLICATIONS
Glucose tolerance test *Normal values:* Fasting: <110 mg/dL 1 h: <180 mg/dL 2 h: <140 mg/dL 3 h: 70–115 mg/dL 4 h: 70–115 mg/dL	To detect abnormal glucose metabolism; to assist in diagnosis of diabetes mellitus	A venous blood sample is drawn after a 10- to 12-h fast; patient is given a glucose "load," usually a prepared liquid drink of 300 mL, that contains a specified amount of glucose. Venous blood samples are drawn at 30-min intervals for 2 h. Phenytoin (Dilantin), birth control pills, diuretics, and glucocorticoids will adversely affect results; consult health care provider regarding these medications.	Instruct patient to eat a balanced diet with at least 150 g of carbohydrate for 3 days before the test and maintain a normal level of physical activity. Instruct patient to fast for 10–12 h before beginning the test. Explain that during the test the patient cannot eat, drink, or smoke and must stay at rest for 2 h. During the test, instruct patient to report feelings of weakness, dizziness, nervousness, and confusion.
Hemoglobin A_{1c} (A_{1c}) *Normal values:* 4%–5.9% (of total hemoglobin) Good diabetic control: <7%	To determine degree of diabetic control of blood sugar over the preceding 2–3 mo.	A sample of venous blood is required. Fasting is not necessary.	Explain to the patient the need for this test to be done periodically to monitor effectiveness of diabetic therapy and determine degree of control over the disease process.
Fructosamine assay *Normal value:* 1.5–2.7 mmol/L	To determine degree of diabetic control of blood sugar over preceding 2–3 wk	A sample of venous blood is required. Fasting is not necessary.	Less influenced by age than A_{1c}. Serum albumin level will affect results.
C-peptide *Normal value:* 0.78–1.89 ng/mL	To evaluate endogenous secretion of insulin when the presence of insulin antibodies interferes with direct assay of insulin	A fasting sample of 1 mL of venous blood is used.	Caution the patient to fast for 8–12 h before the test. Water is permitted.
Urine Tests			
Ketone bodies	To determine presence of ketones in the urine, which indicates a state of ketoacidosis	A fresh urine sample is tested with a dipstick. Follow instructions on bottle of test material.	Instruct diabetic patient that ketone testing should be done whenever illness has interfered with normal eating and activity for more than 24 h and whenever signs of hyperglycemia are present.

Table 35.4 Average of Blood Glucose Based on Hemoglobin A_{1c} Levels

A_{1c} LEVEL	AVERAGE BLOOD GLUCOSE
4%	68 mg/dL
5%	97 mg/dL
5.7%–6.4%	Prediabetes
6%	126 mg/dL
Greater than 6.5%	Type 2 diabetes
7%	154 mg/dL

endocrine disorder. The patient's perception of the function of various body systems affected by the endocrine glands is essential.

? Think Critically

Why would it be important to assess the patient's past and current emotional status if you suspect an endocrine disorder?

◆ NURSING DIAGNOSIS

Table 35.5 presents the most common patient problems, expected outcomes, and nursing interventions for patients with endocrine problems. Additional problem

Table 35.5 **Common Problem Statements, Goals/Expected Outcomes, and Nursing Interventions for Patients With Endocrine Disorders**

PROBLEM STATEMENT[a]	GOALS/EXPECTED OUTCOMES	NURSING INTERVENTIONS
Altered fluid volume due to increased urine output (DI, HyperT, AD).	Patient will display balance between intake and output.	Monitor for dehydration and signs of decreased cardiac output. Measure and record intake and output q2h; maintain ordered IV fluid rate; encourage oral fluid intake.
Constipation due to loss of fluid from intestine, slowed intestinal peristalsis (DI, HypoT, AD).	Patient will display normal bowel pattern within 2 wk.	Provide high-bulk diet; encourage fluid intake; administer stool softener or laxatives as prescribed. Encourage exercise to promote better bowel function.
Altered body image due to changes in physical appearance (PT, HyperT).	Patient will verbalize acceptance of alteration in body appearance within 2 mo.	Allow time for verbalizing feelings. Assist to identify strengths and positive aspects of self and life. Focus on strengths and positive aspects. Give sincere compliments.
Altered sexual function due to decreased libido, amenorrhea, or impotence (PT, HyperT).	Patient will acknowledge need for patience until therapy improves the symptoms.	Help patient understand how therapy might help the problem. Assist patient to recognize and maintain personal worth as an individual. Assist to maintain roles within family or living unit. Help significant others understand patient's illness.
Insufficient knowledge due to illness and treatment (all endocrine disorders).	Patient will verbalize beginning understanding of concepts taught at end of 2 wk.	Teach patient and significant others about the disease and each aspect of treatment. Provide written instructions on medications, their side effects, and what should be reported to the health care provider. Provide instructions for "sick" days. Alert to signs and symptoms of too much or too little medication. Emphasize the importance of follow-up care. Stress the need for medical-alert tag or bracelet and wallet card.
Altered nutrition due to anorexia, constipation, increased metabolic rate (PT, HyperT).	Patient will regain and maintain weight within normal limits within 6 mo.	Weigh twice a week. Alter diet as needed to increase fiber and carbohydrate content. Provide small, frequent meals of preferred foods. Provide patient teaching about nutritional requirements.
Fatigue due to weakness, somnolence, lethargy (PT, DI, HypoT, CS).	Patient will verbalize decrease in weakness and fatigue within 1 mo; patient will demonstrate improved energy within 3 mo.	Provide periods of rest. Assist with ADLs as needed. Set slower pace for activities. Give patient time to respond to verbal communications. Encourage physical activity to highest level of tolerance.
Potential for injury due to possible increased intracranial pressure (PT), inability to think clearly (HyperT, HypoT), mental and physical sluggishness (HypoT).	Patient will not sustain injury.	Conduct regular checks of neurologic status. Monitor for signs of increased intracranial pressure. Continue hormone replacement therapy as needed to decrease symptoms from tumor or hypofunction.
Disrupted sleep pattern due to insomnia, hypermetabolic state (HyperT, CS).	Patient will report getting adequate rest within 1 wk of treatment.	Assist with rest periods during the day if fatigue is severe. Instruct in relaxation methods to help induce sleep. Provide noise-free, sleep-inducing environment.

Continued

Table 35.5 Common Problem Statements, Goals/Expected Outcomes, and Nursing Interventions for Patients With Endocrine Disorders—cont'd

PROBLEM STATEMENT[a]	GOALS/EXPECTED OUTCOMES	NURSING INTERVENTIONS
Limited coping ability due to emotional lability (HyperT, AD, CS).	Patient will devise plan to cope with mood swings until they resolve.	Encourage verbalization of feelings and concerns. Assure patient that as disease is controlled, moods will be more stable. Help patient identify strengths and focus on them. Teach relaxation techniques to handle stressful times. Explain physiologic causes of changes in mood.
Altered cardiac output due to fluid depletion (DI, AD), hypometabolic state (HypoT), hypermetabolic state (HyperT).	Patient will maintain adequate blood pressure.	Explain to patient how disease process is affecting heart function. Monitor for signs of dysrhythmia and hypotension. Assure that treatment of underlying disease should alleviate heart symptoms.
Potential for infection due to surgical incision (PT, HyperT), antiinflammatory effect of excess cortisol (CS).	Patient will not develop infection as evidenced by normal temperature, WBC count within normal range, and absence of visible signs of wound infection.	Maintain strict asepsis for invasive procedures and dressing changes. Monitor temperature, WBC, and subtle signs of infection; steroids can suppress usual signs. Advise to stay away from individuals who have colds or other infections.
Altered nutrition due to altered glucose metabolism (CS), hypometabolic state (HypoT).	Patient will regain and maintain weight within normal limits within 3 mo of beginning therapy.	Teach signs and symptoms of hyperglycemia and how to administer prescribed insulin; teach about correct diet for condition. Assist in designing diet according to food preferences. Teach to balance diet and exercise.

[a]Endocrine disorders to which these problem statements apply are in parentheses.
AD, Addison disease; *ADLs,* activities of daily living; *CS,* Cushing syndrome; *DI,* diabetes insipidus; *HyperT,* hyperthyroidism; *HypoT,* hypothyroidism; *IV,* intravenous; *PT,* pituitary tumors and hypopituitary syndrome; *WBC,* white blood cell.

Focused Assessment

Data Collection for the Endocrine System

Ask the following questions:

- Have you gained or lost weight over the past 6 months?
- Has your appetite increased or decreased?
- Have you noticed any changes in thinking? Any difficulty concentrating? Any difficulty with memory?
- Have you become more anxious or nervous? Do you cry a lot?
- Has your personality changed?
- Has your energy level changed?
- Have you experienced muscle cramping or numbness or tingling in your hands and legs?
- Have you been experiencing diarrhea or constipation?
- Have you had more gas or abdominal bloating?
- Have you noticed any facial or ankle swelling?
- Has your voice become huskier?
- Have you been thirstier than usual? Do you urinate more now?
- Have you had heart palpitations? Has your pulse rate changed?
- Has your sleep pattern changed? Do you need more sleep? Are you finding it difficult to sleep?
- Is there any history in your family of thyroid, pituitary, or adrenal disease or of diabetes?
- Have you noticed a difference in the way you react to the environmental temperature? Are you cold or hot when others are comfortable?
- Have you noticed any changes in the texture or thickness of your hair or eyebrows? What about your fingernails? Are they brittle?
- Has your skin become dry and rough?
- Have you ever had radiation treatments to the head or neck?
- *For women:* Have your menstrual periods altered?

statements or nursing diagnoses are included in Nursing Care Plans 36.1, 36.2, and 37.1.

◆ PLANNING

Planning care for a patient with an endocrine disorder will depend on the type of disorder the patient has. Stress has a direct effect on endocrine function. Therefore measures to help the patient decrease stress should be planned. General nursing goals for patients with an endocrine disorder are:

- Prevention of injury
- Maintenance of fluid and electrolyte balance
- Early identification of hormone imbalance
- Reduction of stress

- Use of effective coping mechanisms
- Knowledge of self-care
- Tolerance for physical activity
- Promotion of normal bowel function
- Improvement of mental-emotional status
- Integration of body image

◆ IMPLEMENTATION

Interventions vary depending on the type of endocrine problem and are discussed with specific disorders in Chapters 36 and 37 (see Table 35.5).

◆ EVALUATION

Evaluation is accomplished by determining whether symptoms are resolving and by laboratory testing to determine whether treatment of the endocrine problem is effective. Many of the symptoms of endocrine disorders are subjective, and you must collect reliable data from the patient about symptoms, such as levels of fatigue, feeling cold or hot, and paresthesias. Each patient is questioned about the symptoms and their improvement during the evaluation of care and treatment. In an effort to better evaluate changes in condition, several rating scales, much like the pain rating scale, are available for fatigue and paresthesias.

COMMUNITY CARE

Many patients with endocrine disorders are cared for in outpatient settings. Home care nurses frequently find that patients with heart disease, neurologic problems, diabetes, or respiratory problems also have a thyroid problem. Careful assessment by a clinic nurse may uncover a developing endocrine problem.

Get Ready for the NCLEX® Examination!

Key Points

- The endocrine system is made up of glands and hormones that regulate metabolism, growth and development, and sexual and reproductive processes.
- The primary regulatory activities of the endocrine system include altering chemical reactions, changing the permeability of the cell membrane, and activating a particular cell mechanism. The secretion of a particular hormone normally depends on the physiologic need for it.
- Any type of dysfunction of the pituitary gland will affect one or more of its numerous hormones as well as the target organ for that hormone.
- Age-related changes of the endocrine system include decreased size of the pituitary gland, decreased metabolic rate, decreases in some hormone levels, increases in others, and only slight changes in still others.
- Endocrine disorders are caused by an imbalance in the production of hormone or by an alteration in the body's ability to use the hormones produced. Primary endocrine dysfunction consists of either hypersecretion or hyposecretion; secondary endocrine dysfunction occurs from factors outside the gland.
- Endocrine system tests include examination of blood or urine, radiographs, ultrasound, and MRI scans.
- A thyroid panel may be ordered to evaluate thyroid function. Patients with primary hypothyroidism will have low levels of T_3 and T_4 and high levels of TSH.
- A full physical assessment and history are needed to evaluate the patient with a possible endocrine disorder.
- General goals for the patient with an endocrine disorder include prevention of injury, maintenance of fluid and electrolyte balance, maintenance of hormone balance, reduction of stress, and use of effective coping mechanisms.

Additional Learning Resources

SG Go to your Study Guide for additional learning activities to help you master this chapter content.

Go to your Evolve website (http://evolve.elsevier.com/deWit/medsurg) for the following FREE learning resources:

- Animations, audio, and video
- Answers and rationales for questions and activities
- Glossary with pronunciations in English and Spanish
- Interactive Review Questions and more!

Review Questions for the NCLEX® Examination

1. A patient is scheduled to have a RAIU thyroid scan. What important teaching points should be covered? *(Select all that apply.)*
   1. Thyroid medications should not be taken before the test.
   2. The radioactive iodine tracer will be given orally several hours before the actual imaging.
   3. The scanner may be donut shaped, and some patients experience claustrophobia.
   4. Diet intake has no effect on the test results.
   5. If other imaging studies using contrast are to be done, the RAIU should be done first.
   6. After the procedure, increase fluid intake for 24 hours.

   NCLEX Client Need: Physiological Integrity: Reduction of Risk Potential

2. A patient complains of muscle cramping and twitching. Based on knowledge of the endocrine system, which hormonal deficiency should be evaluated?
   1. Aldosterone
   2. Parathyroid hormone
   3. Estrogen
   4. Melatonin

   NCLEX Client Need: Physiological Integrity: Physiological Adaptation
3. You are taking care of a patient with a thyroid disorder. Which laboratory results would confirm the diagnosis of a primary thyroid problem rather than a secondary problem?
   1. Elevated serum calcium
   2. Decreased T_3 and T_4
   3. Elevated serum phosphate
   4. Decreased TSH

   NCLEX Client Need: Physiological Integrity: Physiological Adaptation
4. You are caring for several patients who have endocrine problems. For which patient are you most likely to perform a urine dipstick for ketone bodies?
   1. A patient with abnormal thyroid gland activity
   2. A patient with diabetes mellitus
   3. A patient with adrenal cortical insufficiency
   4. A patient with Cushing syndrome

   NCLEX Client Need: Physiological Integrity: Physiological Adaptation
5. A patient is on corticosteroid therapy for an acute exacerbation of a respiratory disease. The initial assessment confirms a patient problem of *fluid volume excess.* The underlying cause for this problem would be:
   1. suppression of normal corticosteroid secretion.
   2. artificial increase in corticosteroids.
   3. increased adrenocorticotropic hormone.
   4. mineralocorticoid insufficiency.

   NCLEX Client Need: Physiological Integrity: Pharmacological Therapies
6. You formulate a care plan for a postmenopausal woman who is admitted for hip fracture. Nursing assessments support the patient problem of *Potential for injury.* The most likely cause for the diagnosis would be:
   1. inadequate estrogen secretion.
   2. aldosterone deficiency.
   3. progesterone deficiency.
   4. inadequate parathormone secretion.

   NCLEX Client Need: Safe and Effective Care Environment: Coordinated Care
7. Older adults can have physiologic increases in circulating ADH. Based on knowledge of the function of ADH, which condition should you monitor for?
   1. Dehydration
   2. Fluid overload
   3. Decreased pulse
   4. Increased urine output

   NCLEX Client Need: Physiological Integrity: Physiological Adaptation
8. A patient is admitted with hyperthyroidism. The initial assessments suggest the patient problem of *Altered nutrition: less than body requirements.* An appropriate expected outcome would be:
   1. patient will identify causes of weight loss.
   2. patient will maintain weight.
   3. patient will have a balanced intake and output.
   4. patient will tolerate activities of daily living.

   NCLEX Client Need: Safe and Effective Care Environment: Coordinated Care
9. You are caring for a patient who had part of the thyroid gland removed. Based on knowledge of anatomy and physiology, which abnormal laboratory value is of particular concern for this patient?
   1. Blood glucose of 150 mg/dL
   2. Serum sodium of 149 mEq/L
   3. Serum calcium of 7 mg/dL
   4. Hemoglobin of 11 g/dL

   NCLEX Client Need: Physiological Integrity: Reduction of Risk Potential
10. You are preparing a patient for a glucose tolerance test. Which instructions must be included? *(Select all that apply.)*
    1. "Eat a balanced diet for 3 days prior to the test."
    2. "Maintain a normal level of activity."
    3. "Fast for 24 hours before the test."
    4. "No eating, drinking, or smoking during the test."
    5. "Report dizziness, nervousness, weakness, and confusion."

    NCLEX Client Need: Physiological Integrity: Reduction of Risk Potential

Critical Thinking Questions

Scenario A

Mrs. Kovash, a 64-year-old widow, comes to the endocrine clinic to be evaluated at the request of her nurse practitioner. She complains that in the past year she has "slowed down" considerably. She states, "I guess I'm just getting old." The nurse practitioner suspects that it may not be simply aging because Mrs. Kovash has always lived a healthy and active lifestyle.

1. What type of examinations would you expect the health care provider to perform?

2. What would you teach Mrs. Kovash about what to expect from the laboratory blood tests?
3. What questions would you ask the patient before tests for evaluation of thyroid function?

Scenario B

The health care provider tells you that a patient has a new-onset deficiency of ADH. You anticipate that the patient is likely to have dehydration, urinary frequency, constipation, fatigue, and knowledge deficit.

1. Use your knowledge of the endocrine system and explain to the patient why they are dehydrated and constipated.
2. What interventions could you use to address the patient's fatigue?
3. The provider orders intravenous fluid therapy, but the patient is reluctant to get "stuck with a needle." What patient teaching can you provide to help the patient understand the need for this therapy?

36 Care of Patients With Pituitary, Thyroid, Parathyroid, and Adrenal Disorders

http://evolve.elsevier.com/deWit

Objectives

Theory

1. Give examples of four major problems associated with hyposecretion of pituitary hormones and identify three nursing interventions appropriate for each problem.
2. Identify nursing problem statements and appropriate interventions for a patient with diabetes insipidus.
3. Plan appropriate nursing assessments and interventions for a patient who might experience complications of a thyroidectomy.
4. Compare and contrast the symptoms of hypoparathyroidism with those of hyperparathyroidism.
5. Identify six signs and symptoms of adrenocortical insufficiency (Addison disease).
6. Summarize four major causes of Cushing syndrome.

Clinical Practice

7. Individualize care for a patient with a pituitary disorder by choosing patient problem statements appropriate to the patient.
8. Select appropriate nursing interventions for a patient with adrenal insufficiency.
9. Implement patient teaching for a patient with hypothyroidism.
10. Plan postoperative assessment and nursing care for a patient who has had a hypophysectomy.
11. Evaluate the nursing care of a patient who has had a thyroidectomy.
12. Assist with the development of a teaching plan for a patient taking a corticosteroid.

Key Terms

ablation therapy (ăb-LĀ-shŭn THĔR-ă-pē, p. 864)
acromegaly (ăk-rō-MĔG-ă-lē, p. 857)
Addisonian crisis (ăd-ĭ-SŌ-nē-ĕn KRĪ-sĭs, p. 876)
anosmia (ăn-ŌS-mē-ă, p. 859)
autoimmune thyroiditis (ŏ-tō-im-YŪN thī-roi-DĪ-tĭs, p. 869)
benign pituitary adenoma (bĕ-NĪN pĭ-TŪ-ĭ-tĕr-ē ă-dĕ-NŌ-mă, p. 857)
catecholamines (kăt-ĕ-KŌL-ă-mēnz, p. 871)
Chvostek sign (VŎS-tĕks sīn, p. 870)
Cushing syndrome (KŪ-shĭng SĬN-drōm, p. 876)
diabetes insipidus (DI) (dī-ĕ-BĒ-tēz ĭn-SĬ-pĭ-dĕs, p. 859)
diuresis (dī-ŭr-RĒ-sĭs, p. 860)
exophthalmos (ĕk-sŏf-THĂL-mŏs, p. 863)
gigantism (jī-GĂN-tĭzm, p. 857)
Graves disease (grāvz dĭ-ZĒZ, p. 863)
Hashimoto thyroiditis (hă-shē-MŌ-tō thī-roi-DĪ-tĭs, p. 869)
hyponatremia (hī-pō-nă-TRĒ-mē-ă, p. 861)
hypothyroidism (hī-pō-THI-roi-dĭ-zĕm, p. 864)
lability (lā-BĬ-lĭ-tē, p. 877)
myxedema coma (mĭk-sĕ-DĒ-mŭ KŌ-mŭ, p. 869)
pheochromocytoma (fē-ŭ-krō-mŭ-ši-TŌ-mŭ, p. 871)
Sheehan syndrome (SHĒ-hăn SĬN-drōm, p. 858)
syndrome of inappropriate antidiuretic hormone (SIADH) (SĬN-drōm ŭv ĭ?-nŭ-PRŌ-prē-ăt ăn-tī-dī-yū-RĔ?-tĭk HŌR-mōn, p. 860)
tetany (TĔT-ă-nē, p. 867)
thyroid crisis (THĪ-royd krī-sĭs, p. 864)
thyroid storm (TS) (THĪ-royd, p. 867)
thyrotoxicosis (thī-rō-tŏk-sĭ-KŌ-sĭs, p. 867)
Trousseau sign (TRŪ-sō sīn, p. 870)

Concepts Covered in This Chapter

- Development
- Fluid and Electrolytes
- Thermoregulation
- Hormonal Regulation
- Cellular Regulation
- Glucose Regulation
- Nutrition
- Immunity
- Inflammation
- Infection
- Fatigue
- Stress
- Cognition
- Patient Education

DISORDERS OF THE PITUITARY GLAND

The pituitary is considered the "master" gland, controlling multiple functions in the body, and many syndromes can result from pituitary disorders. Hypersecretion or hyposecretion of hormones can be caused by various pathology. Pituitary tumors can stimulate the release of excessive amounts of a hormone, which can cause disorders such as Cushing syndrome, syndrome of inappropriate antidiuretic hormone (SIADH), or acromegaly. Damage to the pituitary may result in hyposecretion of hormones, resulting in conditions such as Addison disease, diabetes insipidus (DI), or dwarfism.

PITUITARY TUMORS

Tumors of the pituitary gland account for about 10% to 15% of all intracranial tumors. Local symptoms are more likely to occur when the tumor is large and creates pressure within the brain. Even smaller tumors can cause various systemic symptoms and endocrine dysfunctions, depending on whether they stimulate or inhibit the secretion of particular hormones.

Etiology and Pathophysiology

A tumor of the pituitary is usually a **benign pituitary adenoma**. The etiology is not clear, but these tumors tend to affect women more than men. Some tumors do not cause symptoms and may be identified during autopsy after death from other causes. If the tumor is large enough, there is increased pressure within the **optic chiasm** (the part of the brain where the optic nerve fibers cross), which if not relieved will damage the optic nerve.

Signs and Symptoms

Local symptoms of pituitary adenoma include headache from the pressure of the tumor and visual disturbance—with possible blindness—from pressure within the optic chiasm. Systemic symptoms may be vague and progress very slowly. Personality changes, weakness, fatigue, and vague abdominal pain can be present for years before the condition is diagnosed correctly.

Diagnosis

Diagnosis of a pituitary tumor begins with a complete history and physical examination. Magnetic resonance imaging (MRI) and high-resolution computed tomography (CT) with contrast media may be used to identify, localize, and determine the extent of the tumor. A thorough ophthalmologic examination will be performed to evaluate pressure on the optic chiasm or optic nerves. Laboratory studies will be done to see which hormones are affected.

Treatment

In some cases the health care provider may choose to treat the pituitary tumor conservatively with hormone therapy designed to reduce levels of hormone production. If the tumor continues to grow or presents serious hormonal imbalances, it may be treated surgically or by irradiation. Some specialists prefer to remove the pituitary tumor surgically and then treat the site with radiation to be sure that all tumor cells have been destroyed. **Hypophysectomy,** or surgical removal of the pituitary gland, is most commonly performed microsurgically. The usual approach is transsphenoidal via the nose or at the junction of the gums and upper lip (Fig. 36.1).

Nursing Management

After the surgery, the patient is kept in a semi-Fowler position. Closely monitor vital signs and the patient's neurologic status. It is important to note and communicate promptly any change in vision, mental status, level of consciousness, or strength. Also monitor for any complications, such as diabetes insipidus (discussed later in this chapter). A nasal drip pad is placed and is changed as needed. Expected drainage is bloody or mucuslike; clear, watery drainage should be reported. Because nasal packing will be in place for 2 to 3 days, the patient must breathe through the mouth. After surgery it is important that the patient not brush their teeth, cough, sneeze, blow their nose, or bend forward because these actions may interfere with the healing process. Assist the patient with mouth rinses and encourage hourly deep-breathing exercises to prevent pulmonary problems.

> **! Safety Alert**
>
> **Coughing**
>
> Coughing after a transsphenoidal hypophysectomy may lead to a cerebrospinal fluid leak.

> **? Think Critically**
>
> Considering the surgical approach used for removing a pituitary tumor, what postoperative complication is the highest risk?

HYPERFUNCTION OF THE PITUITARY GLAND

Excessive secretion of growth hormone (GH) results in **gigantism** in children, leading to excessively tall stature, because the bone growth plates have not yet closed. In adults the result is **acromegaly**. When prolactin or gonadotropin are excessive, alteration in fertility and sexual function may occur. Adrenocorticotropic hormone (ACTH) and thyroid-stimulating hormone (TSH) can also be secreted in excess. These are discussed in the adrenal and thyroid gland sections, respectively. Excessive antidiuretic hormone (ADH) causes syndrome of inappropriate ADH (SIADH; discussed later in this chapter).

Etiology and Pathophysiology

Pituitary adenoma may increase release of hormones. Stress and pregnancy are other causes of increased hormone release. Failure of the target organ can also create high levels of hormone because the gland is not responding and the stimulating hormone continues to be released.

Signs and Symptoms

Gigantism causes the adult's facial features to change: the lips thicken, the nose enlarges, and the forehead develops a bulge (Fig. 36.2). The hands and feet become enlarged in adults; the first sign may be that the patient's shoes no longer fit. Muscle weakness may occur with acromegaly, and osteoporosis and joint pain are common. Signs of prolactin excess include amenorrhea and milk secretion in females and loss of facial hair and impotence in males.

Diagnosis

Alterations in hormone levels can be detected by laboratory testing.

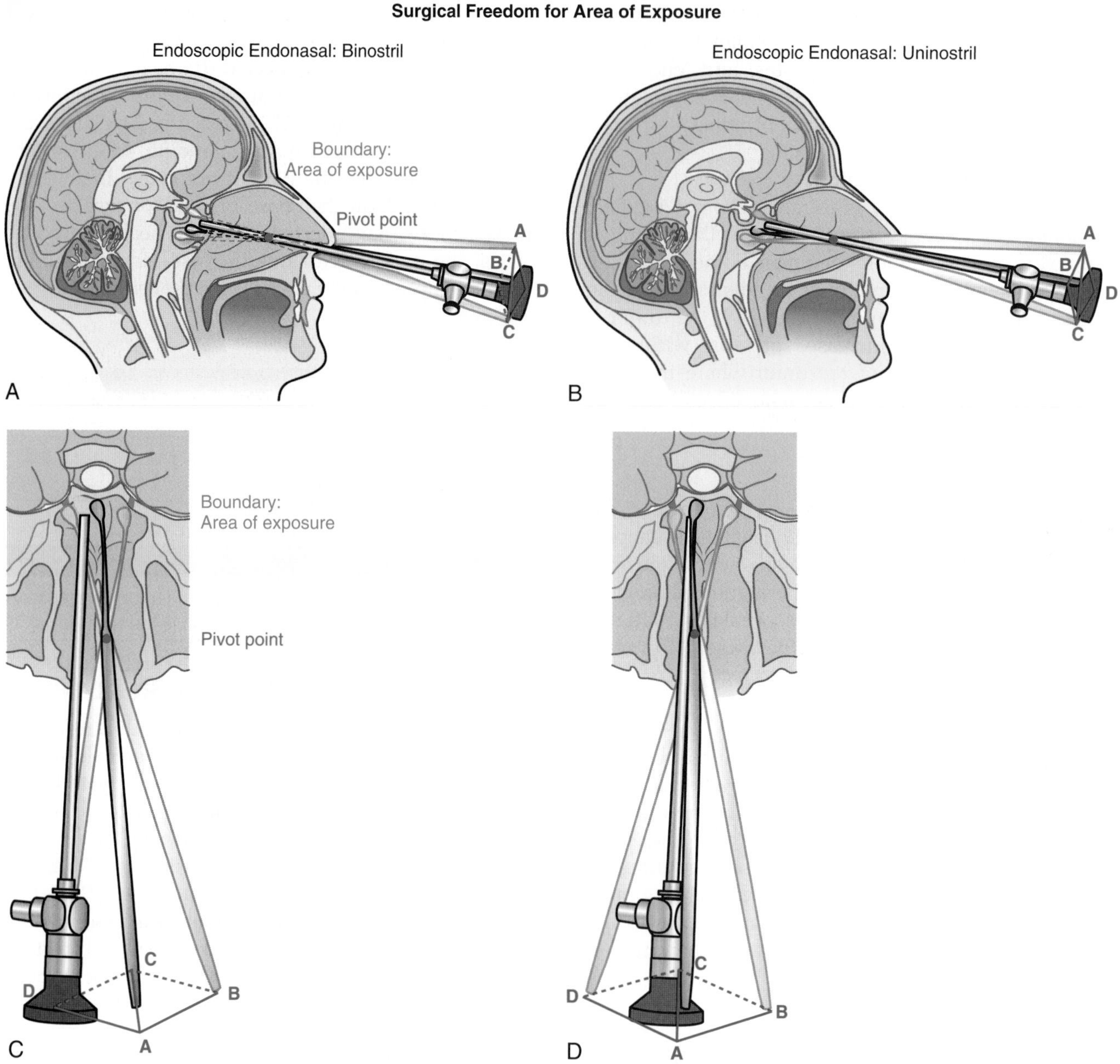

Fig. 36.1 Transsphenoidal surgical approach for hypophysectomy.

Treatment

Removal of the pituitary adenoma is indicated if a tumor is the cause. Medications that block hormonal effects may be used. Slow-release formulas of somatostatin are used for acromegaly.

Nursing Management

See the earlier discussion of hypophysectomy for postoperative management. Monitoring for effectiveness of medical treatment and patient teaching regarding new medications are nursing priorities.

HYPOFUNCTION OF THE PITUITARY GLAND

Hypofunction of the pituitary gland is a rare disorder characterized by a decrease in the level of one or more of the pituitary hormones.

Etiology and Pathophysiology

The most common cause of pituitary hypofunction is a tumor. Other causes include autoimmune disorders, infections, or destruction of the pituitary. A rare but serious postpartum complication, **Sheehan syndrome**, involves infarction of the gland secondary to postpartum hemorrhage.

The most common pituitary hormone deficiency involves a decrease in the amount of GH and gonadotropins. This decrease results in metabolic problems and sexual dysfunction. Decrease in GH will lead to short stature in children; in adults it leads to an increase in bone breakdown, resulting in increased bone fragility and risk for osteoporosis. The decrease in gonadotropins may lead to testicular failure in males and ultimately sterility. Ovarian failure, amenorrhea, and infertility

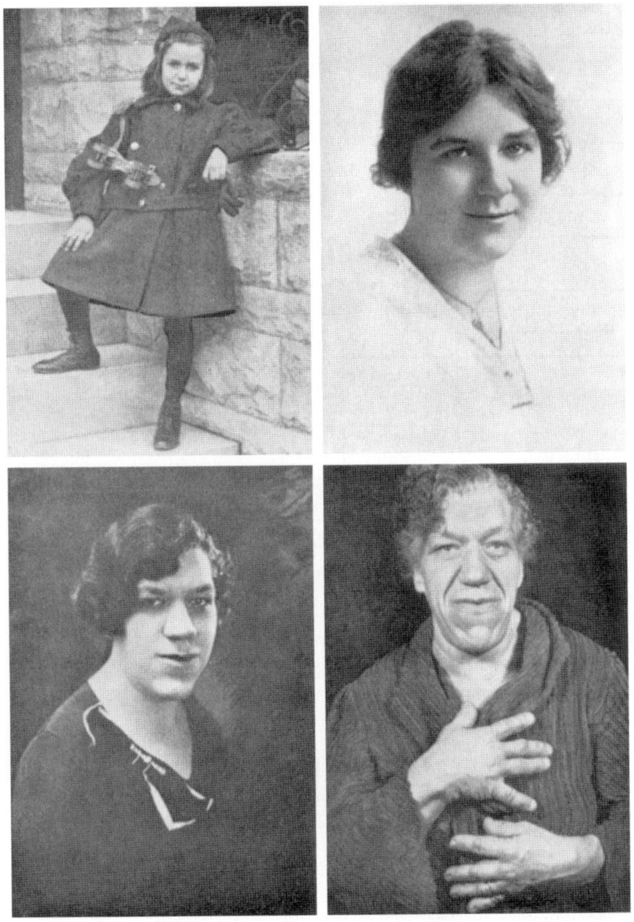

Fig. 36.2 The progression of acromegaly. (From Ignatavicius DD, Workman ML: *Medical-surgical nursing: critical thinking for collaborative care,* ed 6, Philadelphia, 2010, Saunders.)

Table 36.1 Decreased Hormones in Pituitary Hypofunction and Associated Clinical Manifestations

HORMONE DIMINISHED	ASSOCIATED CLINICAL MANIFESTATIONS
Growth hormone (GH)	Decreased muscle mass, reduced strength, pathologic fractures, depression
Follicle-stimulating hormone (FSH), luteinizing hormone (LH)	*Women:* Menstrual irregularities, diminished libido, decreased breast size *Men:* Testicular atrophy, diminished spermatogenesis, loss of libido, impotence, decreased facial hair, decreased muscle mass
Adrenocorticotropic hormone (ACTH), cortisol	Weakness, fatigue, headache, dry/pale skin, diminished axillary and pubic hair, postural hypotension, fasting hypoglycemia, decreased tolerance for stress, susceptibility to infection
Thyroid hormone	Similar to hypothyroidism, although milder: cold intolerance, constipation, fatigue, lethargy, weight gain
Oxytocin	Altered social interactions, depressive disorders

Adapted from Lewis SL, Bucher L, Heitkemper MM, et al.: *Medical-surgical nursing: assessment and management of clinical problems,* ed 10, St. Louis, 2017, Elsevier.

occur with decreased gonadotropins in women. Decrease in ADH release results in diabetes insipidus (DI).

Signs and Symptoms

Signs and symptoms of pituitary hypofunction depend on the cause of pituitary failure and the hormones involved. If the disorder is related to a tumor, the patient may experience headaches, visual changes, **anosmia** (loss of the sense of smell), or seizures. Other signs and symptoms depend on the hormones that are decreased and are outlined in Table 36.1.

Diagnosis

Diagnosis of pituitary gland hypofunction is made by history, physical examination, and diagnostic studies. Laboratory blood tests are performed to measure levels of pituitary hormones. MRI and CT are used to determine the presence or absence of a pituitary tumor.

Treatment and Nursing Management

The mainstay of treatment for hypofunction of the pituitary gland is lifelong replacement of the affected hormones. Somatropin, via subcutaneous injection, is used to replace GH. The patient experiences a feeling of increased energy and well-being, although there are side effects, such as edema, joint pain, and headache. Gonadal hormone therapy is usually offered, including testosterone for men and estrogen or progesterone for women, although associated risks may outweigh the benefits for some patients. If the disorder is caused by a tumor, surgery or radiation for tumor removal is usually performed, followed by hormone therapy.

Nursing management involves recognizing the signs and symptoms of hypofunction of the pituitary. Teach the patient about lifelong hormone replacement therapy, including the method and frequency of hormone replacements, side effects, and follow-up.

DIABETES INSIPIDUS

Etiology and Pathophysiology

Diabetes insipidus (DI) is characterized by the production of copious amounts of dilute urine. DI results from decreased production of antidiuretic hormone (ADH), which regulates reabsorption of water in the kidney tubules. When ADH is not present in a sufficient amount, the water is not reabsorbed from the tubule and is excreted as urine (Concept Map 36.1). The most common forms of DI are central and nephrogenic. Central DI most commonly occurs after trauma or surgery in the area of the pituitary or hypothalamus and may be temporary or

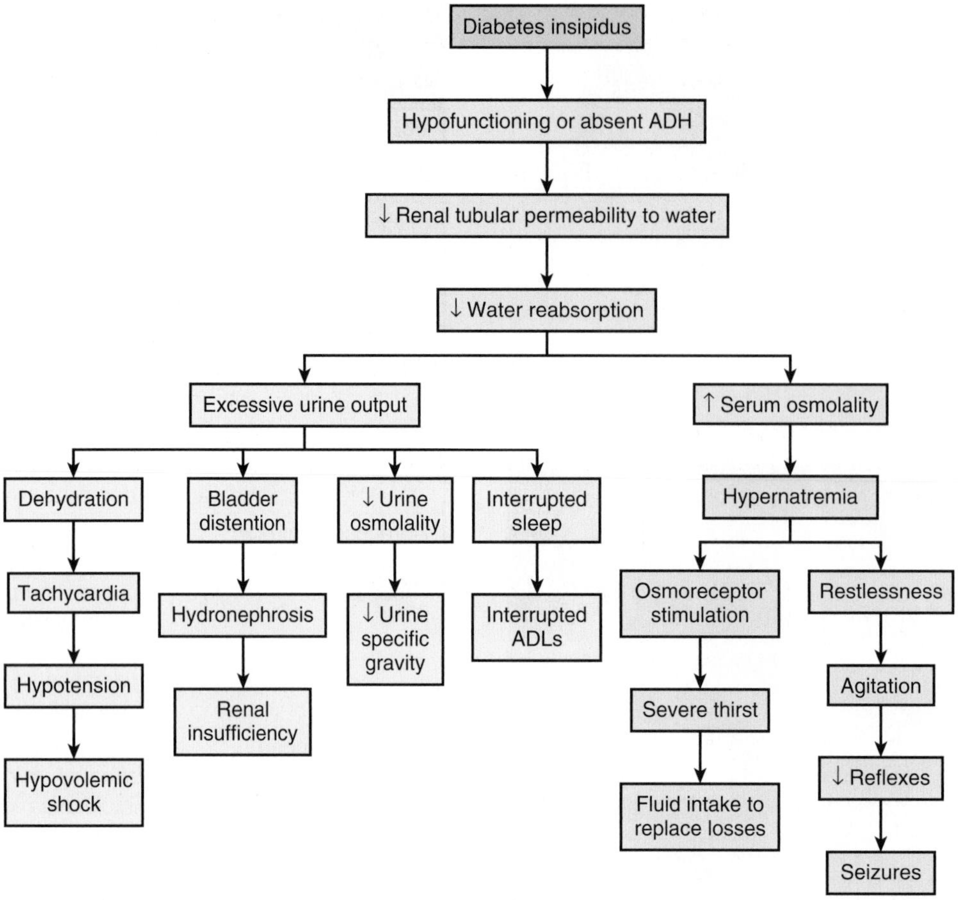

Concept Map 36.1 Pathophysiology of diabetes insipidus. *ADH,* Antidiuretic hormone; *ADLs,* activities of daily living.

permanent. Nephrogenic DI results from hypercalcemia or lithium toxicity, causing the kidney to be resistant to the effects of ADH. Two less common types of DI are gestational and primary polydipsia (dipsogenic DI).

Signs and Symptoms

The patient experiences profound **diuresis** (production of a large amount of urine), often as much as 3 to 20 L in every 24-hour period. Other signs and symptoms include thirst, weakness, and fatigue, often from *nocturia* (urination at night). The patient will exhibit signs of deficient fluid volume, such as tachycardia, hypotension, weight loss, constipation, and poor skin turgor. If untreated, the patient will demonstrate signs of shock and central nervous system manifestations, progressing from irritability to eventual coma from hypernatremia and severe dehydration.

> **Clinical Cues**
>
> Diabetes insipidus was named based on the polyuria that is similar to diabetes mellitus; however, DI has no effect on blood glucose levels.

Diagnosis

To diagnose DI a complete history is obtained, and a physical examination and laboratory tests are performed, including urine and plasma osmolality and urine specific gravity. A water deprivation test is performed to confirm a suspected case of central DI.

Treatment and Nursing Management

Replacement of fluid and electrolytes, along with hormone therapy, represents the basis of treatment of DI. Oral intake is encouraged to replace fluid losses and is supplemented with intravenous (IV) infusion as needed. In central DI, the hormone of choice to replace insufficient ADH is desmopressin acetate (DDAVP), available orally, IV, or nasally. Other hormone medication choices include vasopressin (Pitressin) via nasal inhalation or injection. For fluid replacement, hypertonic saline is used, titrated to match the patient's urinary output.

Nursing management focuses on early detection, maintenance of fluid and electrolyte balance, and patient education. Baseline vital signs and weight are important to accurately document and monitor throughout therapy. Strict (hourly) intake and output monitoring are essential to correct fluid losses and to titrate IV fluid replacement.

SYNDROME OF INAPPROPRIATE ANTIDIURETIC HORMONE

Etiology and Pathophysiology

Syndrome of inappropriate antidiuretic hormone (SIADH) is the opposite of DI. Excessive amounts of ADH are produced, resulting in fluid retention (Concept Map 36.2). Numerous factors can cause SIADH, including malignancies and tumors pressing on the pituitary.

Signs and Symptoms

Signs and symptoms of SIADH include confusion, seizures, and loss of consciousness accompanied by weight gain and edema. **Hyponatremia** from fluid excess, with serum sodium less than 120 mEq/L, occurs frequently. This causes muscle cramps and weakness. Urine output is diminished.

Diagnosis

SIADH is diagnosed by performing urine and serum osmolality tests simultaneously. Results will demonstrate a decreased serum osmolality (<280 mOsm/kg) and elevated urine osmolality (>100 mmol/kg), which indicates the inappropriate excretion of concentrated urine in the presence of a dilute serum. Other laboratory tests to support the diagnosis include a decrease in blood urea nitrogen (BUN), hemoglobin, hematocrit, and creatinine clearance secondary to hemodilution and elevated urine sodium.

Treatment and Nursing Management

Treatment of SIADH is aimed at correcting the underlying cause; restricting fluids to 500 to 1000 mL/day; and administering sodium chloride, diuretics, and demeclocycline (a tetracycline) to increase excretion of water. Tolvaptan (Samsca) is approved for the treatment of hyponatremia in SIADH. Tolvaptan improves serum sodium levels within 8 hours when given as an IV

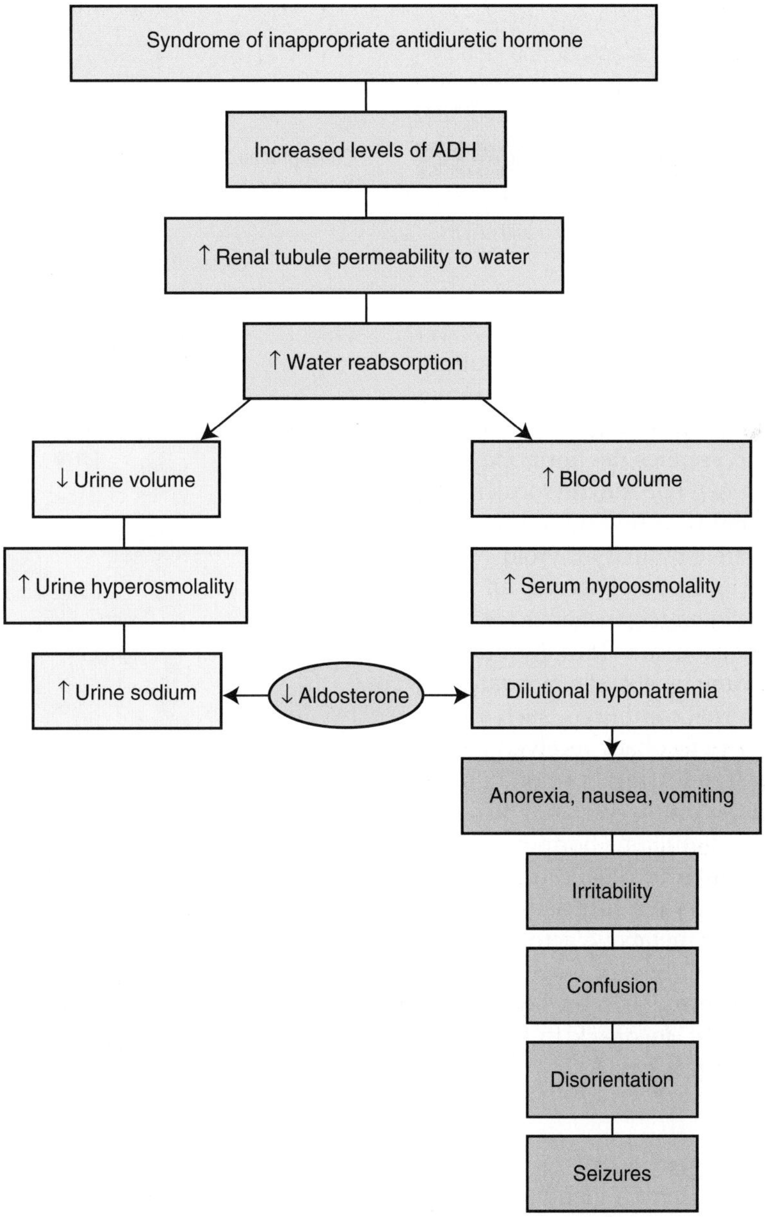

Concept Map 36.2 Pathophysiology of syndrome of inappropriate antidiuretic hormone (SIADH). *ADH*, Antidiuretic hormone.

infusion by blocking the action of ADH; however, there is a danger of overcorrection, and sodium levels need to be closely monitored.

Thorough nursing assessment and data collection are essential to monitor treatment and prevent complications of SIADH. Closely focus on the cardiovascular and neurologic systems and remain alert to the possibility of fluid shifts. Promptly notify the health care provider of any change in level of consciousness. Electrolytes are monitored closely (as often as several times per day), and daily weights are measured. Hyponatremia produces alteration in neurologic function and requires intervention. Too rapid correction can result in permanent neurologic deficit. Careful monitoring and implementation of ordered fluids and medications are critical to a good outcome.

Clinical Cues

Remember that ADH is ANTIdiuretic hormone. When it is present, it prevents diuresis. When it is absent, the kidneys release more urine.

Think Critically

Your patient has had nausea and vomiting for several days and is dehydrated. What response will the body make with ADH?

DISORDERS OF THE THYROID GLAND

Abnormalities in thyroid gland activity and resultant changes in the levels of thyroid hormones are among the most common disorders affecting the endocrine system. The thyroid gland secretes the hormones thyroxine (T_4), triiodothyronine (T_3), and thyrocalcitonin (see Chapter 35). The secretion of thyroid hormones is regulated by the hypothalamic-pituitary-thyroid control system (Concept Map 36.3). In other words, all three organs are involved in the closed-loop negative feedback system. Internal conditions, such as low thyroid and norepinephrine (NE) serum levels, can activate the hypothalamus, as can external conditions, such as low temperatures. In response to feedback received by the hypothalamus, thyrotropin-releasing hormone (TRH) is secreted. TRH acts on the pituitary gland, bringing about its release of thyroid-stimulating hormone (TSH). The TSH then acts on the thyroid cells, causing them to release thyroid hormones. When sufficient heat has been produced by increased metabolic activities (if a cold temperature was the stimulus), or when there are sufficient levels of thyroid hormone in the body fluids (if a deficit was the stimulus), feedback to the hypothalamus causes it to stop releasing TRH.

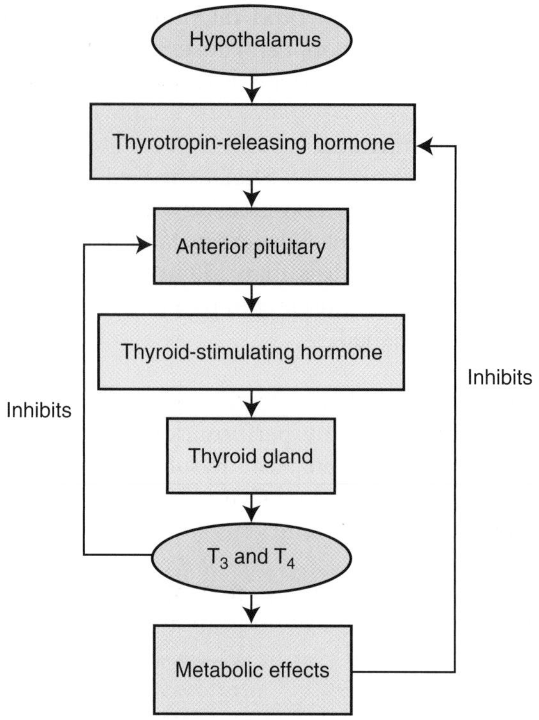

Concept Map 36.3 Regulation of thyroid hormone secretion by negative feedback control. T_3, Triiodothyronine; T_4, thyroxine.

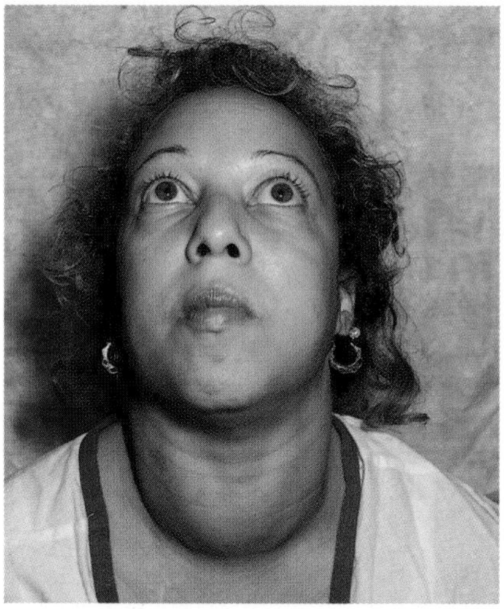

Fig. 36.3 Goiter. (From Ignatavicius DD, Workman ML, et al.: *Medical-surgical nursing: critical thinking for collaborative care,* ed 9, St. Louis, 2018, Elsevier.)

GOITER

Etiology and Pathophysiology

A goiter is a greatly enlarged thyroid gland (Fig. 36.3). One type of goiter is caused by a deficiency of iodine in the diet. Iodine deficiency can be prevented by increasing iodine intake—for example, by using iodized salt. Although the administration of iodine will not cure goiter, it will stop the continued enlargement of the gland. In the United States this is a rare cause of goiter; a more common cause is an increase of TSH from a lack of thyroid hormone production. Continuous TSH stimulation of the thyroid gland causes more tissue growth, resulting in the enlarged gland.

Signs, Symptoms, and Diagnosis

Because there may be no systemic symptoms or changes in the metabolic rate of a person with simple goiter, the first sign that is usually noticed is an enlargement in the front of the neck. Later, if the gland continues to grow bigger, it presses against the esophagus and causes some difficulty in swallowing. The goiter also can press against the trachea and interfere with normal breathing. The diagnosis of goiter is established by history, physical examination, and ultrasound imaging. Goiter can be associated with increased, normal, or decreased hormone production.

Treatment

If goiter resulting from iodine deficiency is treated early, the growth of the gland can be arrested, and in some cases the enlargement will eventually disappear. Medications prescribed include preparations containing elemental iodine (the iodide ion). If lack of thyroid hormone is causing increased tissue growth of the thyroid gland, supplemental thyroid hormone is given in the form of levothyroxine. A very large goiter that continues to grow and produces local symptoms of pressure—or one that presents the possibility of developing into a malignant growth or a toxic goiter—is surgically removed. Radioiodine may be given to destroy some of the thyroid tissue that is overproducing hormone.

Clinical Cues

Patients with goiter may develop toxic goiter when given iodine-based contrast media for imaging procedures. Premedication with beta blockers may help prevent the condition.

Nursing Management

Iodine preparations should be given well diluted and administered through a straw because they can stain the teeth. Adverse effects of iodine preparations can include gastrointestinal upset, metallic taste, skin rashes, allergic reactions, and epigastric pain. Patients receiving thyroid supplements should be monitored for signs and symptoms such as tachycardia, palpitations, nervousness, headaches, and fatigue, indicating overtreatment. Symptoms of inadequate treatment include weight gain, dry skin, hair loss, impaired memory, and cold intolerance.

HYPERTHYROIDISM

Etiology and Pathophysiology

Patients at greatest risk for hyperthyroidism are adult women between 30 and 50 years of age. **Primary hyperthyroidism** is the result of an abnormality of function involving the thyroid gland itself and causes excessive circulation of thyroid T_4 and T_3 hormones. However, it is possible for only the T_3 level to be elevated if the patient has **Graves disease** (toxic nodular goiter) or toxic adenoma of the thyroid.

High serum levels of T_4 can be caused by either overactivity of the thyroid gland or excessive doses of T_4 given in replacement therapy. Primary hyperthyroidism occurs within the thyroid gland. **Secondary hyperthyroidism** usually is the result of an abnormality in another gland, such as the pituitary gland producing too much TSH and therefore overstimulating the thyroid gland.

Primary hyperthyroidism can result from an autoimmune disorder such as Graves disease, also called toxic goiter. Medications containing iodine, such as amiodarone (an antidysrhythmic heart medication), can predispose to hyperthyroidism. Infections are another possible cause. In addition, smoking is a risk factor for developing hyperthyroidism (Ross, 2017).

Signs and Symptoms

The earliest symptoms of hyperthyroidism may be weight loss (despite a good appetite) and nervousness. Symptoms can vary from mild to severe and may include weakness, insomnia, tremulousness, agitation, tachycardia, palpitations, exertional dyspnea, ankle edema, difficulty concentrating, diarrhea, increased thirst and urination, decreased libido, scanty menstruation, and infertility. The condition sometimes is not diagnosed in its early stages because of the vagueness of the symptoms. In some cases hyperthyroidism is misdiagnosed as a cardiovascular disease because the symptoms are similar.

Older Adult Care Points

Older adults with hyperthyroidism may exhibit milder signs and symptoms or may exhibit an **atypical presentation,** such as shortness of breath, palpitations, or chest pain. Simple fatigue and slowing down may be the only presentation in this patient population.

If hyperthyroidism is not diagnosed correctly and continues untreated for any length of time, the patient can develop cardiomyopathy, heart failure, and cardiac-related death. The symptoms manifested by a patient with hyperthyroid are the result of an accelerated metabolic rate and a speeding up of all physiologic processes. Emotional upheaval occurs as a result of the action of thyroid hormones on the nervous system. The patient often reports episodes of emotional extremes with uncontrollable crying and depression followed by intense physical activity and euphoria. Patients with hyperthyroidism also exhibit an enlarged thyroid gland (toxic goiter) and abnormal protrusion of the eyeballs, or **exophthalmos** (Fig. 36.4).

Diagnosis

Medical diagnosis is based on clinical manifestations of hyperthyroidism and the results of laboratory tests for thyroid hormone levels. One indicator of hyperthyroidism is identified by assessment of the heart rate while the patient is sleeping. A rate that is consistently above 80 beats per minute could signify a toxic state resulting from excessive levels of thyroid hormone. The health care provider may also order an electrocardiogram (ECG) to evaluate cardiac dysrhythmias and a chest x-ray to determine heart size. A nuclear thyroid scan may be indicated.

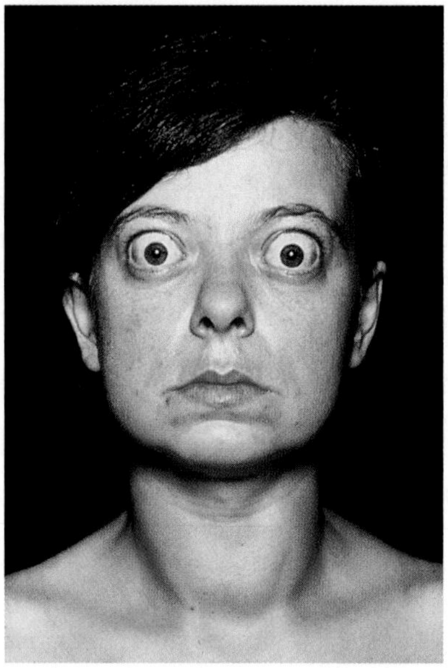

Fig. 36.4 Exophthalmos of Graves disease. (From Lewis SL, Heitkemper MM, Dirksen SR, et al.: *Medical-surgical nursing: assessment and management of clinical problems,* ed 7, St. Louis, 2007, Mosby.)

Treatment and Nursing Management

Hyperthyroidism may be treated medically by administering radioactive iodine and antithyroid drugs, mild sedatives, and beta-adrenergic blocking agents to control tremor, temperature elevation, restlessness, and tachycardia.

Antithyroid drugs are prescribed as the initial treatment of hyperthyroidism. Methimazole (Tapazole) is the main drug used. The patient must take the antithyroid drug at the prescribed time and strictly according to schedule. Propylthiouracil (PTU) is a second-line therapy because of its hepatotoxicity. These medications block the synthesis of thyroid hormone. Iodine preparations may be given to decrease thyroid hormone secretion.

Radioactive iodine (^{131}I), also known as **ablation therapy,** is the definitive treatment for hyperthyroidism; it destroys thyroid tissue. It is contraindicated in pregnant and nursing women because it can disable the thyroid gland in the fetus or infant. The main disadvantage of ablation therapy is the possibility of **hypothyroidism** (deficient activity of the thyroid gland) caused by overeffective treatment. The hypothyroidism can occur immediately after treatment or long after it is completed; thus the patient must have ongoing follow-up.

Dosage of the ablation therapy depends on the size of the gland and the thyroid's sensitivity to radiation. Most patients can be dosed and treated as outpatients. The same radioactive iodine is used for treatment of thyroid cancers, with the dosing being higher, requiring precautions that are more stringent. After treatment, all body fluids can be radioactive for a short time. Because the iodine circulates in the blood and is excreted by the kidneys, precautions must be taken when handling needles, syringes, and other equipment likely to be contaminated with blood and when handling bedpans, urinals, and specimen containers likely to be contaminated with urine.

All patients receiving radioactive iodine must be observed for signs of **thyroid crisis** resulting from radiation-induced thyroiditis (discussed later in this chapter).

> **! Safety Alert**
>
> **Aspirin Contraindicated in Thyrotoxicosis**
>
> Use of acetylsalicylic acid (ASA) is contraindicated in patients with thyrotoxicosis. Aspirin interferes with protein binding and increases the free forms of T_3 and T_4. ASA is used as an antiplatelet medication for cardiovascular disorders and is commonly found in combination analgesic medications.

Iodine preparations also may be given for 10 to 14 days before surgery of the thyroid to reduce the vascularity of the gland and hormone production, minimizing the danger of releasing large amounts of thyroid hormone into the bloodstream during surgery, and to decrease the risk of hemorrhage.

Because many of the signs and symptoms of hyperthyroidism mimic those of cardiac disease, when caring for an older adult be alert to the possibility that such signs may be indicative of an endocrine disorder rather than a cardiac disorder. Physical and mental rest is extremely important because physical stress and emotional upset can stimulate greater activity in the thyroid gland. Adequate rest is essential to conserve strength, but it is difficult for a person with hyperthyroidism to relax and get sufficient rest.

The diet of patients with hyperthyroidism should be sufficiently high in calories to meet metabolic needs. This will vary from person to person, but continued loss of weight is an indication that more high-calorie foods are needed. It may be necessary to refer the patient to a dietitian, who can develop a satisfactory diet that helps the patient maintain normal body weight.

Patients who are being treated medically for hyperthyroidism must understand that they have an illness that requires ongoing medication and frequent monitoring to assess the effectiveness of treatment. Sometimes it is difficult for the patient's family to accept and cope with the emotional outbursts and mood changes that occur when the disease is not under control. Once hormone levels return to the normal range, the mental and physical symptoms should subside.

Nursing interventions for selected problems of patients with hyperthyroidism are summarized in Nursing Care Plan 36.1.

THYROIDECTOMY

Patients who do not respond well to antithyroid drug therapy, who are unable to take radioactive iodine, or who have greatly enlarged thyroid glands are candidates for a subtotal thyroidectomy. Patients with thyroid malignancy undergo a total thyroidectomy. In the subtotal procedure, two thirds of the glandular mass

Nursing Care Plan 36.1 Care of a Patient With Hyperthyroidism

SCENARIO

Mrs. Jackson, age 35 years, has been having symptoms of hyperthyroidism. She complains of feeling "hot and soaked with perspiration all the time." She is 25 lb underweight, even though she reports a "ravenous" appetite. Her vital signs are P 110, bounding; RR 30 and somewhat irregular; BP 170/90. She had a physical examination at her health care provider's office, and her serum calcium level was 11.5 mg/dL. She was admitted for hypercalcemia and thyrotoxicosis. Mrs. Jackson is very apprehensive, agitated, and irritable.

PROBLEM STATEMENT/NURSING DIAGNOSIS

Potential for injury to heart (cardiac muscle) related to excess circulating thyroid hormone and excess serum calcium.

SUPPORTING ASSESSMENT DATA

Objective: Thyroid levels: T_3, 230 mg/dL; T_4, 16 μg/dL; calcium, 16 mg/dL.

Goals/Expected Outcomes	Nursing Interventions	Selected Rationale	Evaluation
Any abnormalities in cardiac function will be promptly identified and reported	Check vital signs q2h.	Increases in pulse and BP may indicate thyroid storm.	Patient's vital signs are BP 150/88, P 104, RR 28, T 100.6° F.
	Assess cardiac function each shift, including ECG monitoring, and watch for symptoms of worsening thyrotoxicosis, such as increased pulse, dyspnea, edema, and rising BP; report as needed.	Hyperdynamic vital signs can be taxing on the heart and must be monitored closely. Alterations in calcium can affect cardiac function.	Patient denies dyspnea.
Patient will have controlled calcium levels within 2 wk.	Medicate with calcium channel blocker as ordered; observe for side effects.	Beta-adrenergic blocking agents decrease sympathetic tone and decrease stimulation of the heart.	No dysrhythmias present. P now 70.
Patient will have normal serum calcium by discharge.	Give medication to decrease calcium levels (diuretic) and monitor electrolyte levels.	Loop diuretics increase calcium excretion in the urine.	Patient's calcium level is 9.0 mg/dL; A.M. thyroid levels are pending.

Goals/Expected Outcomes	Nursing Interventions	Selected Rationale	Evaluation
Patient will verbalize reduction of anxiety and agitation within 3 days of receiving prescribed medication.	Keep environmental stimuli at a minimum.	Excessive stimuli can worsen anxiety and agitation.	Patient exhibits decrease in agitated behavior.
	No visitors other than family as requested by patient. Approach in a calm and unhurried manner.	A calm approach can decrease patient anxiety.	Patient states that she feels "less anxious."
	Provide 30-min rest periods before lunch, in afternoon, and after supper.	Rest can promote sense of calmness.	Took a nap before lunch.
	Administer antianxiety medications as ordered.	Medications can reduce feelings of anxiety.	Goal met.

PROBLEM STATEMENT/NURSING DIAGNOSIS

Insufficient knowledge related to lack of information about disease and treatment.

SUPPORTING ASSESSMENT DATA

Subjective: States that she does not know anything about hyperthyroidism or its treatment.

Goals/Expected Outcomes	Nursing Interventions	Selected Rationale	Evaluation
Patient will verbalize basic understanding of disease and treatment before discharge.	Explain disease process; reinforce information about diagnostic tests and what to expect for each one.	Basic information about disease increases compliance and contributes to long-term self-management.	Patient verbalized basic understanding of hyperthyroidism.
	Stress importance of compliance and keeping appointments with provider.	Treatment of hyperthyroidism is lifelong.	Patient verbalized the importance of long-term follow-up.

Continued

Nursing Care Plan 36.1 Care of a Patient With Hyperthyroidism—cont'd

Goals/Expected Outcomes	Nursing Interventions	Selected Rationale	Evaluation
	Encourage questions and help the patient make a list. Reinforce options, as explained by the provider, for treatment.	Making lists is a self-management strategy that the patient can continue to use when talking to providers or others.	Patient verbalized correct rationale for treatment plan but decided to ask provider about options. Continue plan.

PROBLEM STATEMENT/NURSING DIAGNOSIS

Altered nutrition: less than body requirements related to increased metabolic rate.

SUPPORTING ASSESSMENT DATA

Objective: Lost 25 lb over past 6 months, although appetite has increased considerably.

Goals/Expected Outcomes	Nursing Interventions	Selected Rationale	Evaluation
Patient will gain 2 lb/wk when thyroid production is under control.	Weigh weekly; encourage high-calorie between-meal snacks (e.g., peanut butter, dried fruits).	Weekly weight is more reflective of true weight trends (daily weight tends to reflect water gains/losses).	Patient demonstrated 4-lb weight gain in 10 days but remains less than ideal body weight.
	Increase caloric intake to 3000 calories/day. Try to accommodate food preferences. Arrange dietitian consult.	High-calorie snacks can be helpful in "sneaking in" extra calories.	Eating peanut butter and wheat toast as a snack.

PROBLEM STATEMENT/NURSING DIAGNOSIS

Altered coping related to labile moods.

SUPPORTING ASSESSMENT DATA

Subjective: States she has been "very moody"; family says that she keeps changing her mind about things. Patient also states that she is very nervous and anxious.

Objective: Wringing her hands and fidgeting in bed.

Goals/Expected Outcomes	Nursing Interventions	Selected Rationale	Evaluation
Patient will return to her baseline emotional stability when thyroid production returns to normal.	Assure her that mood swings are manifestations of her thyroid disorder.	Knowledge that emotional lability is disease related can decrease anxiety.	The frequency of emotional episodes has decreased to approximately once per week.
	Help patient identify signals of mood change and suggest alternative coping strategies.	Early recognition of mood change allows patient to actively control behavior (e.g., feels irritable, so goes to a quiet corner to be alone).	Reports irritation whenever roommate turns on television; has asked the roommate to adjust the sound.
	Keep environmental stimuli at a minimum. Private room if possible.	Excessive stimuli can worsen anxiety and agitation.	Patient exhibits decrease in agitated behavior.
	No visitors other than family as requested by patient. Approach in a calm and unhurried manner.	A calm approach can decrease patient anxiety.	Patient states that she feels "less anxious."
	Establish trusting relationship; be accepting of behavior; spend uninterrupted time with her each shift; display acceptance of her and her behavior.	Acceptance of behavior and spending time with patient increases trust and self-esteem.	Spent 15 min with the patient. She apologized for being "moody." Reassured that this moodiness will pass after the condition is stabilized.

CRITICAL THINKING QUESTIONS

1. Considering Mrs. Jackson's nervousness and agitation, how would you proceed to implement a teaching session about her hyperthyroidism?
2. What specific nutritional suggestions might you offer Mrs. Jackson to help her gain weight?

BP, Blood pressure; *ECG*, electrocardiogram; *P*, pulse; *RR*, respiratory rate; *T*, temperature; T_3, triiodothyronine; T_4, thyroxine.

is removed. The remaining portion of the gland is left intact so that production and release of thyroid hormones can continue. For most patients, however, surgery is a treatment of last resort because of the potential complications of hemorrhage, hypoparathyroidism, and vocal cord paralysis. Many patients will be rendered into a state of hypothyroidism because of surgery or radiation therapy that alters thyroid function. It is then necessary to manage their illness with long-term thyroid replacement therapy.

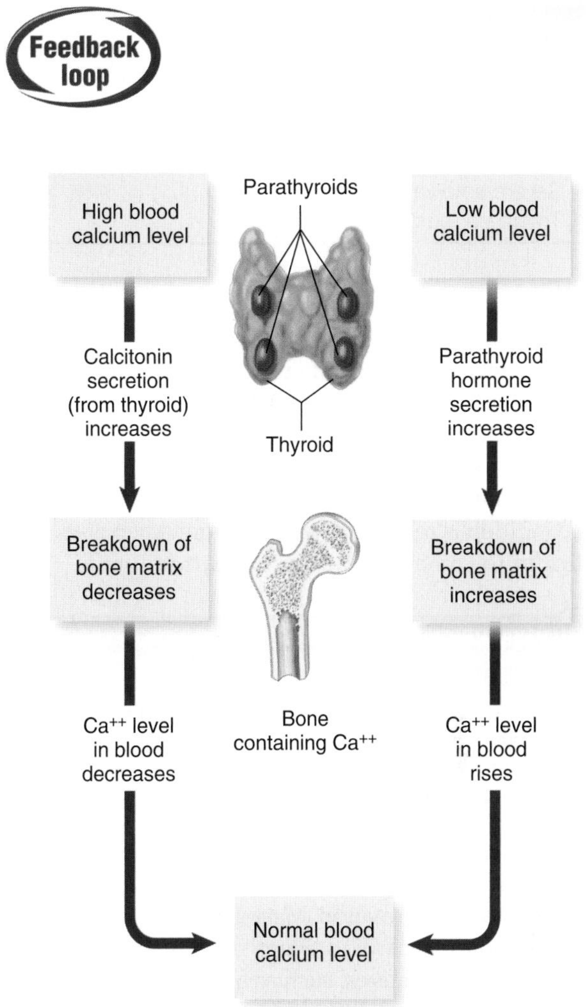

Fig. 36.5 Regulation of blood calcium levels. Calcitonin and parathyroid hormones have antagonistic (opposite) effects on calcium concentration in the blood. Both are negative feedback effects because they reverse a trend away from normal blood calcium levels. (From Patton KT, Thibodeau GA: *Human body in health and disease,* ed 7, St. Louis, 2018, Elsevier.)

Preoperative Nursing Care

Preoperative care is similar to that for any major surgery. If the patient appears nervous, tense, and apprehensive, this should be reported to the surgeon. These symptoms may indicate improper control of the thyroid gland and may predispose the patient to the postoperative complication of thyroid crisis (see the following section).

Postoperative Nursing Care

The patient is placed in Fowler position (sitting upright to at least 90 degrees) to facilitate breathing and reduce swelling of the operative area. The head is maintained in a neutral position to relieve tension on the sutures. The surgical approach may be a standard incision, minimally invasive video-assisted technique, or robotic-assisted technique.

The vital signs are checked every 5 to 15 minutes in the immediate postoperative period, progressing to hourly once the patient is considered stable. The patient is watched closely for signs of bleeding and swelling at the operative area, which may cause swallowing difficulty or airway compromise. Any rise in temperature, pulse, or respiration rate should be reported immediately because it may indicate a high level of thyroxine in the bloodstream. In some hospitals a tracheostomy set is kept at the bedside of postoperative thyroidectomy patients in case severe respiratory complications develop. Other symptoms to be reported are persistent hoarseness and loss of the voice, which may indicate damage to the vocal cords. **Tetany** (muscular twitching and spasms) and thyroid crisis are other possible complications. These are rare, but be alert for the beginning signs and immediately report observations. Thyroidectomy may be performed as an outpatient procedure for some patients. Patient discharge teaching should include the signs and symptoms of the previously mentioned possible complications.

Tetany results from injury to or accidental removal of the parathyroid glands. Parathyroid hormone is important in regulating body calcium and phosphorus levels, and a deficiency of parathyroid hormone produces muscle cramps, twitching of the muscles, and in some cases, severe convulsions from hypocalcemia (Fig. 36.5). These symptoms represent a medical emergency and must be reported to the health care provider at once. Treatment consists of IV administration of calcium gluconate during the emergency stage and doses of calcium and vitamin D to maintain calcium balance in the body. A prescription parathyroid hormone, Natpara, is available as a daily subcutaneous injection for a select group of patients who cannot be managed by calcium and vitamin D supplements. The drug was approved by the U.S Food and Drug Administration (FDA) in 2015 with a black box warning about possible increased risk for bone cancer (Gonzalez-Campoy, 2018).

Thyroid storm (TS), also known as *thyroid crisis* or **thyrotoxicosis**, is another possible complication of thyroidectomy. In the postoperative setting, the condition is caused by a sudden increase in the output of thyroxine caused by manipulation of the thyroid as it is being removed. Newer surgical techniques have made this a rare occurrence. Another cause of TS may be improper reduction of thyroid medication before surgery.

In a patient with hyperthyroidism, TS also can be triggered by other factors unrelated to surgery (Box 36.1); these patients can also develop TS as a result of consuming an overdose of levothyroxine.

Box 36.1 Causes of Thyroid Storm

- Administration of drugs or dyes containing iodine
- Pregnancy and childbirth
- Myocardial infarction or cardiac emergencies
- Infection
- Severe emotional distress
- Trauma or surgery

The symptoms of TS are produced by a sudden and extreme elevation of all body processes. The temperature may rise to 106° F (41.1° C) or more, the pulse increases to as much as 200 beats per minute, blood pressure (BP) elevates, respirations become rapid, and the patient exhibits marked apprehension and restlessness. Unless the condition is relieved, the patient quickly passes from delirium to coma to death from heart failure.

Assignment Considerations

Changes in Vital Signs

Remind the unlicensed assistive personnel (UAP) to report any sudden changes in vital signs (give specific parameters) or behavior (give examples) in patients with thyroid disorders.

Treatment of thyroid crisis must begin immediately after the first symptoms are noticed, rather than waiting for laboratory confirmation. Measures are taken to reduce the temperature; cardiac drugs are given to slow the heart rate; and sedatives, such as a barbiturate, are given to reduce restlessness and anxiety. Adequate fluids must be given to fuel the increased metabolic rate, or profound dehydration may occur.

Safety Alert

Use Caution With Radiology Contrast Studies

Radiocontrast agents have iodine as a base. Imaging studies routinely use these substances. Patients with iodine deficiency are at risk for iodine-induced hyperthyroidism (Surks, 2017).

Think Critically

What specific assessments would you perform on a patient who returned from having a thyroidectomy 4 hours ago?

HYPOTHYROIDISM

Etiology and Pathophysiology

Hypothyroidism can be caused by inflammation of the thyroid gland (thyroiditis) that damages tissue, iodine deficiency, decreased TSH secretion, hypothalamus dysfunction, atrophy of the thyroid gland, or treatment of hyperthyroidism that results in destroying too many thyroid cells and therefore a deficit of thyroid hormone. Genetic defects can cause congenital hypothyroidism, called *cretinism*. Cretinism is caused by a severe lack of thyroid hormone during fetal life and infancy and is characterized by growth failure and impaired neurologic function. Underactivity of the thyroid gland can also be caused by a pituitary or hypothalamus dysfunction that causes inadequate stimulation of the thyroid, inducing secondary hypothyroidism.

Signs and Symptoms

Children with hypothyroidism have delayed physical and mental growth and become very sluggish within a few weeks after birth. Adults who have **myxedema** (very low thyroid production) have a decrease in appetite but an increase in weight because of a slow metabolic rate. Other signs are bagginess under the eyes and swelling of the face. There is a tendency for patients with hypothyroidism to be lethargic and to sleep for abnormally long periods during the day and night. The speech may be slurred, and the individual will appear sluggish in both mental and physical activities. Other signs and symptoms of hypothyroidism are cold intolerance, constipation and abdominal distention, flatulence, impaired memory, depression, husky voice, thinning eyebrows, hair loss, brittle nails, easy bruising, fatigue, muscle cramps, numbness and tingling, dry skin, and nonpitting edema. Gastrointestinal symptoms are the result of decreased peristaltic activity and can lead to paralytic ileus if untreated.

Older Adult Care Points

Older adults who exhibit lethargy, slow thought processes, and lack of enthusiasm could be demonstrating signs of hypothyroidism rather than a brain disorder such as dementia. Hypothyroidism is particularly common in older women.

Diagnosis and Treatment

Medical diagnosis is based on clinical signs and symptoms and laboratory testing of serum levels of thyroid hormones and TSH. Hypothyroidism can be treated effectively with replacement of thyroid hormone. The dosage is gradually increased until a proper level has been reached, and then a delicate balance must be maintained so that the patient does not suffer from either hypothyroidism or hyperthyroidism. The results of treatment of hypothyroidism are striking, and most patients show a remarkable abatement of their symptoms. You may not see many cases of hypothyroidism in the hospital setting because treatment usually does not require hospitalization; however, many hospitalized patients are receiving thyroid replacement therapy. Consider how medications and diagnostic testing may alter their usual metabolic control.

Nursing Management

Patients with chronic hypothyroid have very rough and dry skin, and they will need massage with lotions and creams to prevent cracking and peeling of the skin. Provisions for extra warmth must also be made for those who have an increased sensitivity to cold. It is important that the patient receive thyroid medication every day.

Patient Teaching

Self-Care Management of Hypothyroidism

- Take levothyroxine on an empty stomach because many medications and foods, especially those rich in iron, fiber, calcium, or soy, interfere with absorption.
- Take levothyroxine at the same time each day; morning is usually recommended.
- It may take 6 to 8 weeks to feel benefit or improvement of symptoms.
- Levothyroxine is lifelong therapy; it should never be stopped by anyone except the practitioner who prescribed it.
- Contact your health care provider if you experience unusual bleeding, bruising, chest pain, palpitations, sweating, nervousness, or shortness of breath.
- Report signs and symptoms of myxedema (i.e., dizziness, respiratory distress, low blood sugar, or hypothermia) and hyperthyroidism (i.e., weakness, palpitations, agitation, increased urination, thirst, diarrhea, or insomnia).

Safety Alert

Thyroid Medications

In accordance with The Joint Commission's National Patient Safety Goals, you should increase awareness of look-alike, sound-alike products and help patients recognize the exact name and purpose of their medications. Thyroid medications should not be changed by the patient to the cheapest generic brand because even slight variations in the level of hormone can be dangerous. Prescriptions should be labeled "NO substitutions."

Do not rush patients with hypothyroid or give them the impression of being impatient about their sluggishness. Forgetfulness, inability to express oneself verbally, and physical inertia are mannerisms that are a direct result of the thyroid deficiency, and you must recognize them as unavoidable for as long as the condition is uncontrolled.

MYXEDEMA COMA

Although rare, **myxedema coma** is life threatening. It can be precipitated in patients with hypothyroid by abrupt withdrawal of thyroid therapy, acute illness, anesthesia, use of sedatives or narcotics, surgery, or hypothermia. Signs and symptoms are loss of consciousness along with hypotension, hypothermia, respiratory failure, hyponatremia, and hypoglycemia. Treatment is IV administration of levothyroxine sodium, fluid replacement, maintenance of an airway and respiration, IV glucose administration, corticosteroids, and warming measures.

THYROIDITIS

Etiology and Pathophysiology

Thyroiditis is an inflammation of the thyroid gland. There are three categories: acute, caused by a bacterial infection; subacute, caused by a viral infection; or chronic, the most common type, which is usually an autoimmune disorder. **Autoimmune thyroiditis**, also known as **Hashimoto thyroiditis**, is a chronic form that usually affects women between 30 and 50 years of age. The body produces antibodies against the thyroid, which in turn destroy the gland. The reasons behind autoimmune thyroiditis are not fully understood; however, there seems to be a genetic predisposition, and it is more prevalent in people with other autoimmune disorders, such as rheumatoid arthritis.

Signs, Symptoms, and Diagnosis

The patient will experience a painless enlargement of the thyroid gland and may have dysphagia caused by the inflammation. In the initial stages the inflammation will overproduce thyroid hormone, and the patient will display symptoms of hyperthyroidism. Tissue destruction occurs with the autoimmune response, resulting in a hypothyroid condition. Diagnosis is based on laboratory tests, including serum thyroid hormone levels, TSH levels, and radioactive iodine uptake. Needle biopsy of the gland may be performed.

Treatment and Nursing Management

Acute thyroiditis is treated with antibiotics. The subacute form is usually self-limiting, and treatment is symptomatic. The treatment for chronic thyroiditis is thyroid hormone supplementation to prevent hypothyroidism and suppress TSH secretion. Thyroid function in this disorder is usually normal or low rather than increased (as in acute thyroiditis). Left untreated, eventually hypothyroidism will develop. The goal of therapy is to decrease the size of the thyroid and prevent hypothyroidism. Surgery to remove part of the gland may be considered. Nursing management focuses on patient teaching and providing for comfort.

THYROID CANCER

Etiology and Pathophysiology

Not all thyroid nodules are cancerous. It is estimated that 2 or 3 nodules in 20 are carcinoma. Use of ultrasound for screening can help make the determination if further testing is indicated. The most common form of thyroid cancer is papillary carcinoma (80%), which occurs most often in younger women. This cancer is characterized by a slowly growing tumor that can be present for years before it is diagnosed. The cause of thyroid cancer is unknown, but exposure to irradiation for face, head, and neck conditions increases the incidence. Family history and genetic makeup are risk factors. Other thyroid cancers include follicular carcinomas, medullary thyroid carcinomas, and anaplastic carcinomas (Sharma, 2018).

Signs and Symptoms

The first sign of thyroid cancer may be a nodule found on a routine physical examination. Only 5% to 10% of nodules are found to be cancerous. If the nodule presses on the trachea or esophagus, voice changes, trouble breathing, or trouble swallowing may be present. Other signs and symptoms of thyroid cancer, such as fatigue, depression, and weight changes, can be easily missed or attributed to other causes.

Diagnosis

The diagnosis of thyroid cancer is made by examination and diagnostic tests. An ultrasound examination is used to assess thyroid size and to locate any nodules. Iodine uptake studies also may be used to check for nodules. TSH levels and other laboratory tests will be performed. **Fine-needle aspiration,** in which a specimen of tissue is taken and analyzed, is the definitive test.

Treatment and Nursing Management

The treatment for thyroid cancer is thyroidectomy. In some cases, radioactive iodine (ablation) therapy may be used in lieu of surgery to disable the gland (discussed earlier in the section on hyperthyroidism). Multiple drug therapies are available for patients who are not candidates for thyroidectomy. Most therapies are intended to control tumor growth and not to cure the condition.

DISORDERS OF THE PARATHYROID GLANDS

HYPOPARATHYROIDISM

Etiology and Pathophysiology

Hypoparathyroidism is most commonly caused by atrophy or traumatic injury to the parathyroid glands. **This can occur as a result of accidental removal or destruction of parathyroid tissue during a thyroidectomy,** irradiation of the thyroids or parathyroids, neck trauma, or idiopathic (having no known cause) atrophy of the glands. A deficiency of parathormone will result in a drop in serum calcium levels and an increase in phosphorus levels. Patients with chronic renal failure are unable to eliminate dietary phosphorus, and elevated phosphorus levels suppress parathyroid function and result in low calcium levels. There is an inverse relationship between phosphorus and calcium. High phosphorus levels decrease calcium levels.

Signs and Symptoms

Signs and symptoms of hypocalcemia include mild tingling, numbness, muscle cramps, and mental changes, such as irritability. **Chvostek sign** manifests as muscle irritability when the facial nerve is gently tapped. **Trousseau sign** manifests as a carpal spasm, elicited by inflating a BP cuff 20 mm Hg above the systolic BP (see Chapter 3). Tetany is a serious sign resulting from a lowered serum calcium level. In tetany, muscular twitching and spasms occur because of extreme irritability of neuromuscular tissue. If calcium levels continue to fall, the patient will suffer from convulsions, cardiac dysrhythmias, and spasms of the larynx.

Diagnosis

Medical diagnosis of hypoparathyroidism is established by clinical signs and laboratory data. An electrocardiogram (ECG) may demonstrate abnormalities that can lead to dysrhythmias, heart failure, and hypotension. A CT scan may reveal brain calcifications if the hypocalcemia is chronic. Changes in bone integrity may be seen on radiograph. Other laboratory tests that confirm the diagnosis include serum calcium, total protein, albumin, phosphate, magnesium, vitamin D, parathyroid hormone assay, and urine cyclic adenosine monophosphate (cAMP). Calcium is bound to protein, so alteration in protein levels can affect the serum calcium level.

Treatment and Nursing Management

Acute hypoparathyroidism with tetany is treated with IV calcium gluconate to raise serum calcium levels to normal range and with vitamin D. Oral or parenteral administration of calcium salts is used in the acute phase. In chronic hypoparathyroidism, treatment is aimed at restoring and maintaining normal calcium levels in the blood. This can soon be accomplished by parathormone replacement therapy, administration of vitamin D in massive doses to enhance absorption of calcium from the small intestine, and oral administration of calcium salts. Nursing care revolves around electrolyte replacement and patient teaching. Remind the patient that therapy for hypoparathyroidism is lifelong and advise the patient to wear a medical alert bracelet.

Nutrition Considerations

Dairy Products Are High in Phosphorus

You should teach patients with hypoparathyroidism to eat foods that are high in calcium but low in phosphorus. Milk, yogurt, and processed cheeses are high in phosphorus and therefore are not advised.

HYPERPARATHYROIDISM

Etiology and Pathophysiology

Hyperparathyroidism is an endocrine disorder in which excessive parathyroid hormone is released, unregulated by calcium levels. A benign enlargement of the parathyroid glands (adenoma) or hyperplasia of two or more glands is the main cause of primary hyperparathyroidism. Secondary hyperparathyroidism occurs because of hypocalcemia that is due to deficient vitamin D. This condition is common in patients with chronic kidney disease. Hypercalcemia (calcium level above 10.5 mg/dL) occurs with hyperactivity of the parathyroid glands because the hormone pulls calcium out of the bones. Other causes of hyperparathyroidism are outlined in Box 36.2.

Signs and Symptoms

Signs and symptoms of hyperparathyroidism may be mild or severe; are usually the result of dysfunction of other organs or tissues related to high calcium levels; and include dehydration, confusion, lethargy, arrhythmias, anorexia, nausea, vomiting, weight loss, constipation, thirst, frequent urination, and hypertension. If hypercalcemia exists, there may be skeletal changes, including

Table 36.2 Comparison of Hyperparathyroidism and Hypoparathyroidism

	HYPERPARATHYROIDISM	HYPOPARATHYROIDISM
Serum calcium levels	Increased	Decreased
Serum phosphate levels	Decreased	Increased
Bone resorption[a]	Increased	Decreased
Calcium and phosphate in urine	Increased	Decreased
Neuromuscular irritability	Decreased	Increased (may progress to tetany)

[a]Bone resorption involves taking calcium from the bone to increase serum calcium.

Box 36.2 Causes of Hyperparathyroidism

- Parathyroid tumor (benign or malignant)
- Congenital enlargement
- Neck trauma or irradiation
- Vitamin D deficiency
- Chronic renal failure with hypocalcemia
- Lung, kidney, or gastrointestinal tract cancers

Adapted from Ignatavicius DD, Workman ML, et al.: *Medical-surgical nursing: critical thinking for collaborative care,* ed 9, St. Louis, 2018, Elsevier.

thinning of the bone due to calcium being pulled out of the bone by parathyroid hormone and formation of bone cysts. A bone fracture often causes the patient to seek medical attention. The signs of hypercalcemia are manifested in virtually every major system in the body. Hyperparathyroidism and hypoparathyroidism are compared in Table 36.2.

Diagnosis

Clinical context is used for initial diagnosis. Laboratory testing for persistent elevated serum calcium and elevated parathyroid hormone is the best test for the initial confirmation. Serum albumin is also measured because serum calcium must be corrected for low albumin levels. Serum phosphorus levels will be low, and vitamin D levels are assessed.

Treatment

The treatment of hyperparathyroidism will depend on whether the condition has a primary or secondary cause and the severity of the symptoms. Primary symptomatic hyperparathyroidism will be treated surgically to remove the adenoma or tissue producing the excess hormone. A minimally invasive approach is used when imaging studies can isolate the involved gland. Asymptomatic primary conditions may be treated medically by infusions of isotonic sodium chloride and administration of loop diuretic agents that promote urine excretion of excess calcium; phosphate therapy and calcitonin is given to inhibit calcium release from the bone. Secondary forms of the disorder will be treated medically with vitamin D supplementation.

Nursing Management

Nursing management for patients on diuretic therapy includes accurate measuring of intake and output (every

! Safety Alert

Caution With Diuretics

Thiazide diuretics should be used cautiously in patients with hyperparathyroidism because they potentiate hypercalcemia by decreasing urinary calcium loss (Sterns, 2018).

2 to 4 hours), daily weight, monitoring of serum electrolytes, ongoing assessment for electrolyte imbalance, and appropriate nursing intervention. The patient may be placed on continuous cardiac monitoring, depending on the degree of the electrolyte imbalances. Postoperative management is similar to that for thyroidectomy. Assessment for signs and symptoms of hypoparathyroid within 24 hours of surgery is indicated.

DISORDERS OF THE ADRENAL GLANDS

PHEOCHROMOCYTOMA

Etiology and Pathophysiology

Pheochromocytoma is a rare tumor of the adrenal medulla that secretes **catecholamines** (epinephrine and norepinephrine). The tumor is usually benign but shows malignancy in about 10% of cases. It causes severe hypertension, and if left untreated it can lead to death. Research is demonstrating a genetic link to inherited gene mutations that predispose individuals to the tumor (Blake, 2018).

Signs, Symptoms, and Diagnosis

Signs and symptoms of pheochromocytoma are related to excess catecholamine release. Signs include tachycardia and severe hypertension (as high as 250/150 mm Hg) that can be intermittent or persistent. Profuse diaphoresis, severe headache, palpitations, nausea, weakness, and pallor may also be present.

Pheochromocytoma is diagnosed by measurement of serum catecholamines and 24-hour urine measurement of catecholamine metabolites. CT and MRI may be used to locate the tumor.

Treatment and Nursing Management

Treatment is surgical removal (often laparoscopically) of the tumor (adrenalectomy). Before surgery, the patient may be in hypertensive crisis and require close monitoring of vital signs and administration of IV antihypertensive medications. The patient should be monitored for signs and symptoms of side effects related to high doses of medication therapy.

ADRENOCORTICAL INSUFFICIENCY (ADDISON DISEASE)

Etiology and Pathophysiology

Addison disease is characterized by decreased function of the adrenal cortex, resulting in a deficit of all three hormones secreted by the adrenal cortex (cortisol, aldosterone, and testosterone). The major problems are related to insufficiencies of the mineralocorticoids and the glucocorticoids. The insufficiency of the androgenic hormones can be compensated for by the ovaries and testes.

Insufficient production of the adrenocortical hormones can result from a disorder affecting the adrenal cortex itself (primary insufficiency) or from a disorder affecting the pituitary gland that stimulates adrenal secretion (secondary insufficiency). Disorders causing a primary insufficiency include idiopathic atrophy, autoimmune disease, inflammation, infection, and nonsecreting tumors of the adrenal cortex. Secondary insufficiency occurs when the pituitary gland fails to secrete ACTH because the gland is underfunctioning or was surgically removed (hypophysectomy) or after abrupt withdrawal of steroid therapy.

? Think Critically

What signs and symptoms might you see in a patient who is developing Addison disease after stopping steroid therapy?

Signs and Symptoms

In the early stages of Addison disease, the clinical manifestations may be so vague as to be annoying to the patient but not serious enough to consult a health care provider. Hence Addison disease is easily missed or misdiagnosed. Later, as the hormone insufficiency worsens, there are severe symptoms associated with fluid and electrolyte imbalance and hypoglycemia. Considering the functions of the mineralocorticoids, a major problem is depletion of sodium (hyponatremia), which in turn causes depletion of extracellular fluid and potassium retention (hyperkalemia). The patient experiences generalized malaise and muscle weakness, muscle pain, orthostatic hypotension, and vulnerability to cardiac dysrhythmias.

Insufficiency of the glucocorticoids affects blood glucose levels and causes symptoms of hypoglycemia. There is also decreased secretion of gastrointestinal enzymes, which results in anorexia, nausea and vomiting, flatulence, and diarrhea. These symptoms, as well as anxiety, depression, and loss of mental acuity, have been correlated to absence of the peaks of cortisol output that normally occur every 24 hours.

Diagnosis

Diagnosis of Addison disease is made by laboratory testing. Blood cortisol and aldosterone levels are evaluated, and an ACTH stimulation test can determine whether the problem lies in the adrenal gland or in the pituitary. CT and MRI scans may be used to locate a tumor, calcification, or gland enlargement. Abnormal serum electrolyte levels (hyponatremia and hyperkalemia), decreased glucose tolerance, elevated white blood cell count (leukocytosis), and abnormally low levels of free cortisol are among the criteria used to diagnose Addison disease (Griffing, 2018).

Treatment

Replacement therapy to provide the missing hormones usually brings about a rapid recovery, but the patient must continue taking the hormones as lifelong therapy. Prednisone is given to replace glucocorticoids; fludrocortisone is a synthetic adrenocortical steroid to replace the mineralocorticoid aldosterone.

Nursing Management

Nursing management of patients with Addison disease includes:

- Intensive care and support during Addisonian crisis when the patient is in critical condition and in danger of death from fluid volume depletion, hypotension and shock, and impairment of cardiac function.
- Prevention of problems related to fatigue and orthostatic hypotension.
- Alleviation of gastrointestinal problems.
- Instruction of self-care.

Two important nursing measures are to provide both regular feedings throughout the day and adequate rest. The patient may feel well in the morning but may become progressively weaker and fatigued as the day goes on. If fasting is necessary for diagnostic studies or surgery, the patient with Addison disease probably will need IV glucose to prevent profound hypoglycemia. Maintenance doses of glucocorticoids are especially important whenever fasting is required.

Gastrointestinal problems bring on the possibility of altered nutrition due to anorexia, nausea and vomiting, and diarrhea. Specific fluid and electrolyte imbalances are covered in more depth in Chapter 3. Stress—even relatively mild physical or emotional stress—can quickly bring on an Addisonian crisis for a patient with Addison disease. The patient must avoid undue physical stress whenever possible and must learn effective coping mechanisms to deal with emotional stress (Nursing Care Plan 36.2).

ACUTE ADRENAL INSUFFICIENCY OR ADRENAL CRISIS

The presence of cortisol in the body allows the blood vessels to function properly in response to epinephrine and other catecholamines by constricting. Conditions that decrease the amount of circulating cortisol interfere with the ability of the blood vessels to constrict. Patients with Addison disease have a decrease in or absence of adrenal cortical secretions, primarily cortisol. Because cortisol is released in response to ACTH from the pituitary gland,

Nursing Care Plan 36.2 Care of a Patient With Adrenocortical Insufficiency (Addison Disease)

SCENARIO

Mr. Cox, age 49 years, is admitted with a diagnosis of adrenocortical insufficiency (Addison disease). He has recently experienced weight loss, weakness, poor coordination, vomiting, changes in skin coloration, and loss of body hair. During initial assessment, Mr. Cox is found to be confused, very irritable, and easily upset by questions. His family states that he has a "cold." His vital signs are BP 90/50, P 110 and slightly irregular, RR 16 and deep. He reports that he feels pretty good when he awakens in the morning but quickly becomes tired, and his muscles begin to ache. He is concerned about his weight loss and change in appearance and has noticed that he has been unable to "think straight." Admission laboratory data: blood glucose, 50 mg/dL; sodium, 90 mEq/L; potassium, 5.6 mEq/L; white blood cell (WBC) count, 12,000/mm^3. His family states that he became confused and agitated earlier that morning, which is not his normal, so they brought him to the hospital.

PROBLEM STATEMENT/NURSING DIAGNOSIS

Altered cardiac output related to decreased volume as evidenced by hyponatremia.

SUPPORTING ASSESSMENT DATA

Subjective: Feels very tired, weak, and uncoordinated.

Objective: BP 90/50. Altered level of consciousness.

Goals/Expected Outcomes	Nursing Interventions	Selected Rationale	Evaluation
Patient's BP and pulse will be within 10% of his normal baseline within 4 h of admission.	Obtain vital signs on admission and as required.	Nursing judgment will dictate the frequency of vital signs; unstable patients may need q15min.	BP continues between 90/50 and 100/60. Health care provider notified. Will repeat BP in 30 min.
	Monitor for signs of dehydration (i.e., thirst, dry mucous membranes).	Subjective and objective signs and symptoms of dehydration may occur before BP drops.	Reports thirst and dry sensation in mouth. Oral care given. Willing to take ice chips with subjective relief.
	Administer IV and oral fluids as ordered.	Fluid replacement will correct hypovolemia	IV infusing at 150 mL/h. Oral fluid offered but refused because of nausea; provider contacted for antiemetic order.
	Initiate I&O and track pattern over several days.	I&O should be balanced; however, in a hypovolemic state, output is likely to be less than input as the fluid balance recovers.	Intake for end of shift 1000 mL of IV fluid and 2000 mL of oral fluid; output 1000 mL of urine and 500 mL of emesis.

PROBLEM STATEMENT/NURSING DIAGNOSIS

Altered electrolyte balance related to insufficient production of mineralocorticoids and glucocorticoids.

SUPPORTING ASSESSMENT DATA

Subjective: Reports fatigue, weakness, mental acuity changes.

Objective: Blood glucose, 50 mg/dL; sodium, 90 mEq/L; potassium, 5.6 mEq/L.

Goals/Expected Outcomes	Nursing Interventions	Selected Rationale	Evaluation
Patient will have a stable glucose 70–100 mg/dL. Patient will have normal serum sodium and potassium within 24 h.	Observe for signs of hypoglycemia (i.e., shakiness, hunger, mental confusion); check fingerstick glucose and report promptly.	Hypoglycemia can be a warning sign of impending Addisonian crisis; brain tissue is very sensitive to low glucose levels.	Patient's blood glucose level is 110 mg/dL.
	Check to see that meals are served on time; provide snacks as needed.	Intake of nutritious foods is important to maintain adequate glucose and sodium levels.	Patient knows signs/symptoms of hypoglycemia. No problems noted at this time.

Continued

Nursing Care Plan 36.2 Care of a Patient With Adrenocortical Insufficiency (Addison Disease)—cont'd

Goals/Expected Outcomes	Nursing Interventions	Selected Rationale	Evaluation
	Monitor serum sodium and potassium. Watch for signs of hyponatremia (i.e., lethargy, muscle cramps or weakness, headache) or hyperkalemia (i.e., weakness, cardiac dysrhythmias).	Identifying problems with electrolytes in the early phase and acting quickly to restore balance prevents complications.	Since administration of D_5NS and 50 mg of IV hydrocortisone, patient is less confused.

PROBLEM STATEMENT/NURSING DIAGNOSIS

Impaired neurologic function related to cortisol deficiency, electrolyte imbalance, and hypotension.

SUPPORTING ASSESSMENT DATA

Subjective: "Unable to think straight."

Objective: Very confused, irritable and impatient; serum cortisol results pending.

Goals/Expected Outcomes	Nursing Interventions	Selected Rationale	Evaluation
Patient will maintain an adequate BP, normal-range blood sugar within 1 h of treatment. Electrolyte abnormalities will resolve within 6 h of treatment.	Vital signs q15min until stable.	Treatment should affect BP, and the effectiveness of treatment needs to be monitored.	BP now 110/70 and P 85.
	Administer IV fluids as ordered, monitoring IV site, lung sounds, and urine output.	IV fluids will restore volume. During fluid resuscitation it is important to monitor for fluid overload.	IV patent, no redness or swelling at site, no complaint of site discomfort from patient. Lungs clear. 500 cc clear yellow urine in past 2 h.
	Implement hypoglycemia protocol for fingerstick glucose below 50 or if symptoms are present.	Cortisol affects blood glucose regulation. Hypoglycemia should be managed to prevent complications.	Fingerstick glucose 98 after initial treatment.

PROBLEM STATEMENT/NURSING DIAGNOSIS

Insufficient knowledge related to illness, medications, and necessary changes in lifestyle.

SUPPORTING ASSESSMENT DATA

Subjective: States that he knows nothing about Addison disease, its diagnosis, or treatment; unfamiliar with corticosteroid therapy.

Goals/Expected Outcomes	Nursing Interventions	Selected Rationale	Evaluation
Patient will verbalize understanding of disease process, medications, and dosage schedule before discharge.	Answer questions and discuss Addison disease, medication purpose, side effects, and dose. Emphasize the importance of not suddenly stopping the medications.	Medication compliance is key to treating the disease and preventing complications.	Patient verbalized dosing schedule and the basic action of each medication. Wants a repeat teaching session about side effects and more information on how he might have gotten this disease.
Patient will verbalize plans for obtaining adequate rest before discharge.	Help him develop a balanced schedule that allows for periods of rest, work, social interaction, and recreation.	Once hormone levels are normalized, the patient with Addison can expect to resume normal activities as long as rest periods are integrated into the schedule.	Patient described his intention to integrate rest with desired activities.

Nursing Care Plan 36.2 Care of a Patient With Adrenocortical Insufficiency (Addison Disease)—cont'd

Goals/Expected Outcomes	Nursing Interventions	Selected Rationale	Evaluation
	Provide written instructions for symptoms of insufficient corticosteroid medication and those of excess medication.	Written instructions increase the retention of vital information. Patient must be able to self-identify and report problems.	Patient verbalized three signs and symptoms of insufficient hormone (weakness, fatigue, diarrhea) and excessive hormone (hunger, thirst, increased urination).
	Instruct him to report either set of symptoms to the provider promptly so that medication can be adjusted.	Patient must know when to contact provider so that problems can be prevented.	States that he is happy to know that medication can be adjusted to address stress and symptoms before things get out of control.
	Instruct to report periods of extra stress (minor illness such as a cold, emotional upset, or unusual physiologic or psychological stress) so that medication can be adjusted.	Patient must be aware that stress will have greater effect on his life because of Addison disease.	Asks family to help him recognize minor physical or emotional stresses he may overlook because those things are "part of my normal crazy life."
	Instruct him to wear a form of medical alert identification with data about steroid therapy.	Medical alert identification provides lifesaving information if he is ever unable to give health history.	States that he is a little embarrassed to wear jewelry that "publicly announces my problem," but agrees to seriously consider it.

CRITICAL THINKING QUESTIONS

1. In implementing the patient teaching plan for Mr. Cox, when would you perform your patient teaching, and why?
2. Mr. Cox has put together a proposed activity schedule for after he is discharged from the hospital. He lives in a rural community and must go to the post office to get his mail each day. He asks if you would look at the schedule and give him feedback on it. The schedule reads: *8 A.M. breakfast, 9 A.M. walk dog, 10 A.M. gardening, 11 A.M. walk to post office/get mail, 12 P.M. lunch, 1 P.M. nap, 2 P.M. watch television, 3 P.M. daughter over for visit.* What, if any, suggestions would you give Mr. Cox, and why?

BP, Blood pressure; *D_5NS*, 5% dextrose in normal saline; *I&O*, intake and output; *IV*, intravenous; *P*, pulse; *RR*, respiratory rate.

Patient Teaching

Managing Addison Disease

Teach the patient about the signs and symptoms of inadequate or excessive steroid levels, the importance of prompt reporting, and the following points:

- The nature of the illness and what can be done to control it.
- The purpose of each medication and the side effects to be reported.
- The importance of taking the medication every day and of never stopping corticosteroids suddenly; they need to be tapered off slowly.
- Signs and symptoms to report to the health care provider immediately (worsening weakness, hypotension, confusion, infection).
- The importance of contacting the provider so that medication dosage can be adjusted to combat the effects of stress.
- Diet adjustments to provide food throughout the day and a bedtime snack.
- The importance of following the prescribed diet to prevent gastrointestinal problems.
- Planned rest periods during the day and sufficient sleep at night, as well as prevention of physical stress.
- The need for a medical alert tag or bracelet stating that the patient has Addison disease and is on steroid therapy.

Think Critically

What specific interventions for a patient with Addison disease would you use to help teach the patient to decrease stress or to cope with stress?

abnormalities in ACTH release can also cause a reduction in circulating cortisol. Physical stress from the flu or other infection, or from surgery, can send a patient with Addison disease into **Addisonian crisis**. Steroids are given to treat many autoimmune diseases, and the body becomes dependent on this outside source of cortisol. If administration of the medication is stopped abruptly, acute cortisol insufficiency will occur. The body does not produce cortisol because enough is circulating from the medication therapy. If the medication is not given, the body does not have time to produce and release enough cortisol to maintain function, and a crisis situation is produced.

Decreased levels of cortisol result in decreased sensitivity of the blood vessels to sympathetic stimulation. It is the sympathetic stimulation that maintains vascular tone. Lack of vascular tone causes vasodilation, producing hypotension. Cortisol helps maintain BP and cardiovascular function, so the acute lack of it will decrease BP and produce typical signs and symptoms of shock. Other symptoms include severe abdominal, flank, or leg pain; tachycardia; nausea; and change in level of consciousness.

Treatment

Closely monitor vital signs, blood glucose, and sodium and potassium levels. Adrenal crisis requires immediate fluid replacement therapy to prevent irreversible shock. Intravenous hydrocortisone is given along with sodium, fluids, pressors, and dextrose until blood pressure becomes stable. Hyperkalemia must also be addressed with IV insulin and glucose, or calcium chloride (or calcium gluconate), and by monitoring arrhythmias and the patient's intake and output. Hypoglycemia is treated with IV glucose and with glucagon as needed; blood glucose is monitored every hour.

EXCESS ADRENOCORTICAL HORMONE (CUSHING SYNDROME)

Etiology and Pathophysiology

Cushing syndrome is a rare disorder. The symptoms typical of Cushing syndrome are manifestations of excess levels of the hormones from the adrenal cortex. The condition can be caused by:

- Excessive secretion of ACTH by the pituitary, which may result from faulty release of corticotropin-releasing factor (CRF) from the hypothalamus or a pituitary adenoma
- A secreting tumor of the adrenal cortex
- Ectopic production of ACTH by tumors outside the pituitary, such as lung cancer
- Iatrogenic Cushing syndrome from prolonged use of steroid therapy (the most common cause)

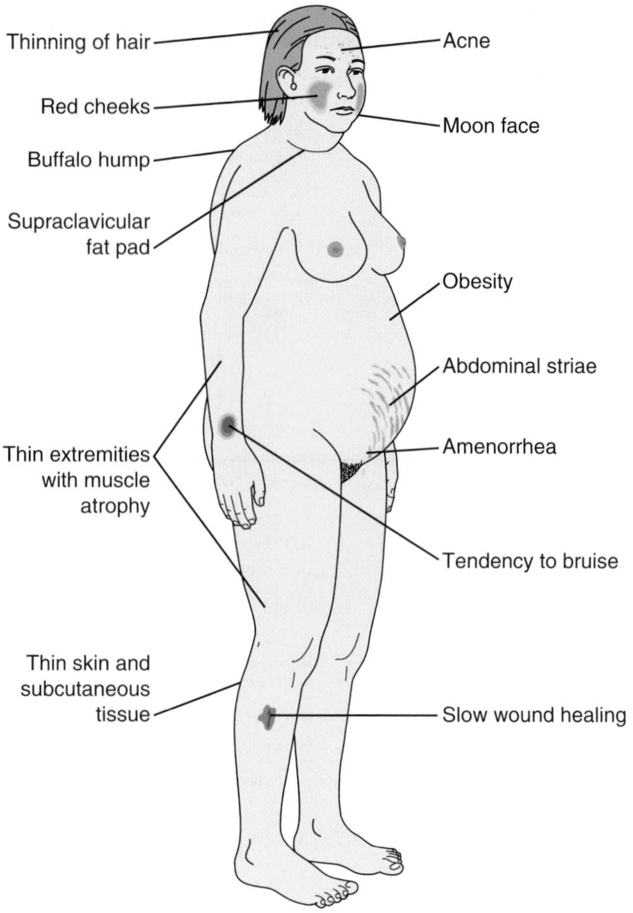

Fig. 36.6 Common characteristics of Cushing syndrome.

Signs and Symptoms

The signs and symptoms of Cushing syndrome are caused by excessive levels of cortisol (Fig. 36.6). They include painful fatty swellings in the intrascapular space (buffalo hump) and facial area (moon face), an enlarged abdomen with thin extremities, bruising after even minor traumas, impotence, amenorrhea, hypertension, and weakness from abnormal protein catabolism with loss of muscle mass.

Unusual growth of body hair (hirsutism) can occur in women with Cushing syndrome, and streaked purple markings in the abdominal area can occur because of collections of body fat. Patients with Cushing syndrome who have a familial predisposition to diabetes mellitus commonly develop type 2 diabetes from the anti-insulin, diabetogenic properties of cortisol.

Diagnosis

The diagnosis of Cushing syndrome is established by laboratory findings indicating consistently high levels of free plasma cortisol rather than the usual 24-hour fluctuations. A 24-hour urine test should be performed. If cortisol is elevated, a dexamethasone suppression test should be ordered: for the test, the patient is given a steroid at night, and blood and urine cortisol levels are then measured in the morning. Evening serum and salivary cortisol levels and a dexamethasone-suppression

Box 36.3 General Nursing Implications for the Administration of Corticosteroids

When giving a corticosteroid drug:
- Take baseline vital signs; steroids may elevate the blood pressure.
- Assess for signs of infection; steroids may mask the signs and symptoms of infection.
- Never stop steroid therapy abruptly; such abrupt withdrawal may cause death in a patient who has been on long-term therapy.
- Give oral doses with food to decrease gastrointestinal irritation; medications for gastrointestinal protection are indicated.
- Monitor older adults for signs of osteoporosis. Give vitamin D and recommend weight-bearing exercise to prevent osteoporosis.
- Watch for signs of depression in patients on high-dose steroid therapy.
- Monitor for signs of hypokalemia.
- Monitor blood sugar of diabetic patients closely; glucocorticoids may cause hyperglycemia.

Teach the patient to:
- Monitor weight because steroids may cause increased appetite and weight gain.
- Report slow healing of wounds to the health care provider.
- Schedule regular checkups for glaucoma and cataracts if on long-term steroid therapy.
- Take oral doses in the morning with food to decrease stomach upset. Take an acid-reducing medication to prevent stomach irritation.
- Not discontinue the drug abruptly but taper down the dosage before stopping it, and only with the approval of the provider who prescribed it.
- Watch for signs of hypokalemia, such as muscle weakness, fatigue, anorexia, and irregular heartbeat.
- Eat foods such as fresh and dried fruits, juices, potatoes, meats, and nuts that are high in potassium, particularly if on a potassium-wasting diuretic in addition to the steroid.
- Carry a medical alert card and wear a bracelet indicating steroid therapy when on long-term steroids.
- Avoid people with infections and stay away from crowds, especially during cold and flu season.
- Advise all other providers and dentists about their steroid therapy.
- Be aware that more insulin may be needed if they are diabetic.
- Be aware that antibody response from immunization may be reduced while taking steroids; live virus vaccines should not be used.
- Be aware that steroids alter the effect of other medications and the doses of these drugs may need to be adjusted.
- Have clotting time monitored closely when taking an anticoagulant at the same time as the steroid.

corticotropin-releasing hormone stimulation test help with the diagnosis.

Treatment

Pituitary Cushing syndrome can be treated by microsurgery on the pituitary gland. If Cushing syndrome is arising from an adrenal tumor, adrenalectomy is indicated. In this instance replacement of glucocorticoids is necessary. When surgical intervention does not restore normal cortisol levels, medications or radiation may be used.

Clinical Cues

Secondary Cushing syndrome produced by long-term cortisone therapy is often reversible if the medication is tapered off and stopped. However, most people taking cortisone are taking it for chronic health disorders and cannot discontinue it, so management of Cushing syndrome symptoms is initiated. Steroids should never be taken for a condition other than the specific health disorder for which they are prescribed (Box 36.3).

Nursing Management

The nursing care of patients with Cushing syndrome is primarily concerned with helping them cope with the many systemic problems caused by the disorder. Assist the patient with psychosocial concerns presented by emotional **lability** (continually changing) and depression when these occur. The patient needs assurance that, with proper treatment, the symptoms will improve within 2 to 12 months. In some patients, hypertension and glucose intolerance may continue to need management. Teach the patient about the immunosuppressive properties of cortisol and their increased risk for infection.

COMMUNITY CARE

Nurses in long-term care facilities must be alert for signs of adrenal dysfunction, especially among their older adult female patients. You often will be the one to notice subtle changes in the patient that have occurred over many months.

You can be instrumental in preventing secondary Cushing syndrome by cautioning patients to seek means of treatment other than long-term steroid therapy for arthritis or allergies. You must teach patients receiving a new prescription for steroids that this medication must be tapered, never stopped abruptly.

Get Ready for the NCLEX® Examination!

Key Points

- A pituitary tumor secretes GH and antagonizes the effect of insulin. Treatment consists of hormone therapy or surgery.
- Hypofunction of an endocrine gland typically mandates lifelong hormone therapy.
- Hypofunction of the pituitary gland is characterized by a decrease in pituitary hormones and metabolic and sexual dysfunction.
- DI can occur as a result of decreased production of ADH and can lead to hypernatremia, dehydration, and coma. Replacement of fluid, electrolytes, and hormones is required.
- In SIADH, excessive amounts of ADH are produced, resulting in fluid retention. Treatment includes correcting the underlying cause, restricting fluids, and administering medications. Cardiovascular and neurologic systems, electrolytes, and weight should be monitored.
- Signs and symptoms of hyperthyroidism are the result of an accelerated metabolic rate, although older adults may have milder or opposite symptoms. Ablation therapy and thyroidectomy are standard treatments.
- Hypothyroidism causes a decrease in appetite and an increase in weight. Myxedema coma can be precipitated by abrupt withdrawal of thyroid therapy, acute illness, or other stressors.
- The most common type of thyroiditis is autoimmune or Hashimoto. Treatment includes thyroid hormones or surgery.
- Thyroid cancer occurs most often in younger women. Treatment includes ablation therapy, thyroidectomy, or both.
- Hypoparathyroidism can occur from removal or destruction of parathyroid tissue. Treatment includes administration of calcium and vitamin D.
- Hyperparathyroidism is characterized by excessive synthesis and secretion of parathormone. Therapies include infusions of sodium chloride with diuretics, phosphate, and calcitonin; subtotal parathyroidectomy may be performed. Nursing care includes monitoring intake and output, weight, and electrolytes.
- Pheochromocytoma is a potentially fatal adrenal medulla tumor; treatment is surgical removal of the tumor.
- In Addison disease, there is decreased function of the adrenal cortex and a deficit of all hormones. Symptoms include severe fluid and electrolyte imbalances and hypoglycemia.
- Cushing syndrome involves excess levels of adrenal cortex hormones; it may be treated surgically.

Additional Learning Resources

SG Go to your Study Guide for additional learning activities to help you master this chapter content.

Go to your Evolve website (http://evolve.elsevier.com/deWit/medsurg) for the following FREE learning resources:

- Animations, audio, and video
- Answers and rationales for questions and activities
- Glossary with pronunciations in English and Spanish
- Interactive Review Questions and more!

Review Questions for the NCLEX® Examination

1. A 50-year-old man outputs 15 L of urine within a 24-hour period. He has poor skin turgor with low blood pressure and increased heart rate. You would plan to administer which medication?
   1. Furosemide (Lasix)
   2. Desmopressin acetate (DDAVP)
   3. Regular insulin
   4. Spironolactone (Aldactone)

   NCLEX Client Need: Physiological Integrity: Pharmacological Therapies
2. A 45-year-old man has muscle cramps and is weak and confused. Serum sodium is 115 mEq/L. You should report the condition and obtain an order to:
   1. give hypertonic (3%) IV saline.
   2. encourage fluid intake.
   3. infuse hypotonic intravenous fluids.
   4. administer vasopressin.

   NCLEX Client Need: Physiological Integrity: Physiological Adaptation
3. A 35-year-old woman reports episodes of emotional extremes, with uncontrollable crying and depression followed by intense physical activity and euphoria. She complains of dry eyes and difficulty swallowing. Her symptoms confirm a nursing problem of altered coping. What is a cause for this diagnosis?
   1. Parathyroid hormone deficiency
   2. Excessive thyroid hormone secretion
   3. Deficient estrogen production
   4. Growth hormone deficiency

   NCLEX Client Need: Physiological Integrity: Physiological Adaptation
4. A patient received large doses of radioactive iodine (I^{131}) for hyperthyroidism. Which nursing intervention(s) should be included? *(Select all that apply.)*
   1. Monitor vital signs.
   2. Restrict fluids.
   3. Encourage a low-fat, high-fiber diet.
   4. Properly handle contaminated materials.
   5. Encourage physical activity.

   NCLEX Client Need: Physiological Integrity: Reduction of Risk Potential
5. You are caring for a patient who has had a thyroidectomy. What should you monitor for? *(Select all that apply.)*
   1. Bleeding and swelling
   2. Hypothermia
   3. Increase in pulse
   4. Difficulty swallowing
   5. Difficulty breathing

   NCLEX Client Need: Physiological Integrity: Reduction of Risk Potential

6. A patient complains of severe muscle cramping and muscle twitching after a thyroidectomy. The following orders are obtained. Place the nursing actions in priority order.
   1. Seizure precautions.
   2. Administer calcium gluconate.
   3. High-calcium diet.
   4. Place on ECG monitor.

   NCLEX Client Need: Safe and Effective Care Environment: Coordinated Care
7. You are reviewing the medications that each of your patients will receive during the shift. Which patient is likely to receive levothyroxine?
   1. Patient who has Addison disease
   2. Patient who has hypothyroidism
   3. Patient who has hyponatremia
   4. Patient who has Graves disease

   NCLEX Client Need: Physiological Integrity: Pharmacological Therapies
8. A 25-year-old woman complains of amenorrhea with weakness, easy bruising, and painful, fatty swelling on the back. Which assessment question would be most appropriate to ask this patient?
   1. Have you been taking steroid therapy for a prolonged period?
   2. Have you been taking any medications that contain iodine?
   3. Have you been taking lithium for several years?
   4. Have you had a recent pregnancy with postpartum bleeding complications?

   NCLEX Client Need: Physiological Integrity: Pharmacological Therapies
9. You provide patient instructions on taking steroid medications. It is important for you to include which instruction(s)? *(Select all that apply.)*
   1. Take with food.
   2. May increase the risk of bone cancer.
   3. Watch for easy bruising.
   4. Do not stop the medication abruptly.
   5. May increase the risk of infection.

   NCLEX Client Need: Health Promotion and Maintenance
10. You are caring for a patient with adrenocortical insufficiency (Addison disease). Which set of laboratory values would be the primary interest for this patient?
    1. Serum sodium, white blood cell count, and blood glucose
    2. Serum calcium, serum phosphate, and vitamin D level
    3. Urine osmolality, plasma osmolality, and urine specific gravity
    4. Serum T_4, serum T_3, and thyroid-stimulating hormone

    NCLEX Client Need: Physiological Integrity: Physiological Adaptation

Critical Thinking Questions

Scenario A

Mrs. Timms has a tentative diagnosis of hyperthyroidism. She is 45 years old, 5 feet 7 inches tall, and weighs 102 lb.

1. What subjective and objective signs and symptoms would you expect Mrs. Timms to present during nursing assessment?
2. How would you prepare Mrs. Timms for diagnostic laboratory tests for thyroid function?
3. If Mrs. Timms's health care provider decides to treat her condition with large doses of radioactive iodine, what special nursing care will she require?
4. What other forms of therapy are used to treat hyperthyroidism?

Scenario B

Mr. Lau, age 37 years, is receiving adrenocorticoid hormones as replacement therapy for Addison disease.

1. What kinds of problems does insufficiency of the adrenal cortex hormones bring about?
2. What should be included in your instructions to Mr. Lau to help him manage his illness?

Scenario C

Mrs. Josten, age 48 years, is hospitalized for a cholecystectomy. She has Cushing syndrome, as well as gallbladder disease. She is 35 lb overweight and depressed.

1. What kinds of problems is Mrs. Josten likely to have as a result of her Cushing syndrome?
2. What would be your concerns in the immediate postoperative period?
3. What would you want to include in your discharge teaching plan?

Scenario D

A patient complains of fatigue, constipation, cold intolerance, flatulence, hair loss, and dry skin. You suspect that the patient may have a thyroid problem.

1. What other questions could you ask this patient?
2. What laboratory tests is the health care provider likely to order, and what are the normal values for those tests?
3. The patient is prescribed levothyroxine. What teaching points should you share about the medication?

37 Care of Patients With Diabetes and Hypoglycemia

http://evolve.elsevier.com/deWit

Objectives

Theory

1. Compare and contrast the two major types of diabetes mellitus.
2. Analyze the primary factors that influence the development of diabetes mellitus.
3. Explain the signs and symptoms of an insulin reaction (hypoglycemia) and discuss appropriate nursing interventions.
4. Summarize the acute and long-term complications of poorly controlled diabetes mellitus.
5. Identify sources of support and information for people with diabetes and their families.

Clinical Practice

6. Teach a person newly diagnosed with diabetes about the disease, treatment, and self-care.
7. Perform a focused nursing assessment and gather data for the management of type 1 and type 2 diabetes mellitus.
8. Interpret the results of laboratory tests used in the diagnosis and management of diabetes mellitus.
9. Assess for and gather data related to signs and symptoms that might indicate that a patient with diabetes is in early ketoacidosis.
10. Teach a patient how to recognize and self-treat hypoglycemia.

Key Terms

basal insulin (BĀ-sĕl Ī?N-sŭ-lĭn, p. 887)
bolus dose (BŌ-lĕs dōs, p. 887)
correction dose (kŭ-RĔK-shĕn dōs, p. 887)
diabetic nephropathy (dī-ĕ-BĔ-tĭk nĭ-FRŎ-pĕ-thē, p. 884)
diabetic neuropathy (dī-ĕ-BĔ-tĭk nŭ-RĂ-pĕ-thē, p. 894)
endogenous (ĕn-DŎJ-ĕn-ŭs, p. 881)
exogenous (ĕks-ŎJ-ĕn-ŭs, p. 881)
gastroparesis (găs-trō-pă-RĒ-sĭs, p. 894)
glucometer (glū-KĂ-mĕ-tĕr, p. 894)
glycemic control (glī-SĒ-mĭk, p. 883)
glycosuria (glī-cōs-Ū-rē-ă, p. 883)
hyperglycemia (hī-pĕr-glī-SĒ-mē-ă, p. 882)
incretin mimetics (in-krē′tin mĭ-MET-ĭks, p. 890)
insulin resistance (ĬN-sŭ-lĭn rĭ-ZĬ-stĕnts, p. 881)
insulin-to-carbohydrate ratios (ĬN-sŭ-lĭn tū kăr-bō-HĪ-drāt RĀ-shē-ō, p. 884)
ketoacidosis (kē-tō-ă-sĭ-DŌ-sĭs, p. 881)
medical nutrition therapy (MNT) (MĔ-dĭ-kĕl nū-TRĬ-shĕn THĔR-ŭ-pē, p. 884)
metabolic syndrome (mĕ-tĕ-BŎ-lĭk SĬN-drōm, p. 882)
neuroglycopenia (nū-rō-GLĪ-kŏ-PĒ-nē-ă, p. 900)
polydipsia (pŏl-ē-DĬP-sē-ă, p. 883)
polyphagia (pŏl-ē-FĀ-jă, p. 883)
polyuria (pŏl-ē-Ū-rē-ă, p. 883)

Concepts Covered in This Chapter

- Adherence
- Self-Management
- Fluid and Electrolytes
- Acid-Base Balance
- Hormonal Regulation
- Nutrition
- Immunity
- Infection
- Coping
- Patient Education
- Health Promotion
- Collaboration
- Safety

DIABETES MELLITUS AND HYPOGLYCEMIA

DIABETES MELLITUS

Diabetes mellitus is a group of diseases in which there is disturbance in metabolism and use of glucose. Type 1 diabetes is secondary to a malfunction of the beta cells of the pancreas. Beta cells are responsible for making insulin. Because insulin is involved in the metabolism of carbohydrates, proteins, and fats, diabetes mellitus is not limited to a disturbance of glucose homeostasis but alters other body functions as well.

Diabetes mellitus results in the body's failure to metabolize sugars and starch. Sugars accumulate in the blood and urine, and the by-products of alternative fat metabolism (ketones) disturb the acid-base balance of the blood, causing a risk of coma or death.

Nutrition Considerations

Type 2 Diabetes Prevention

The 2018 Standards of Medical Care in Diabetes from the American Diabetes Association (ADA) recommends increasing intake of nuts, berries, yogurt, coffee, and tea in an overall healthful diet to decrease the risk of type 2 diabetes (ADA, 2018).

Table 37.1 Clinical Categories of Diabetes Mellitus and Characteristics

TYPE	CHARACTERISTICS
Type 1	Little or no endogenous insulin is produced. New patients can be any age but usually are young. Patient must receive exogenous insulin and follow prescribed diet and exercise program. Renal, cardiovascular, retinal, and neurologic complications are likely if disease is not kept under tight control.
Type 2	Patients rarely develop ketosis but may develop hyperglycemic hyperosmolar state (HHS). Patients vary in need for exogenous insulin. Oral antidiabetic medications are given to help regulate blood glucose level. New patients are usually older than 30 years, and most are obese. Disorder often responds to diet and exercise.
Latent autoimmune diabetes in adults (LADA) (slow-onset type 1 diabetes or type 1.5 diabetes; type 1 diabetes, according to the World Health Organization)	Patients are typically not overweight, have no signs of metabolic syndrome, and may have a history of autoimmune disease. Patients demonstrate rapid failure of oral hypoglycemic drugs. Insulin should be started within 1 year of diagnosis.
Other specific types of diabetes with various causes	Types include drug- or chemically induced diabetes, diseases of the exocrine pancreas (cystic fibrosis), and genetic defects in the action of insulin or beta cell function.
Gestational diabetes	Occurs only during pregnancy. After pregnancy, women with gestational diabetes (2%–10% of pregnancies) have a 35%–60% chance of developing diabetes within 5–10 years.

Types of Diabetes Mellitus

Nearly 30 million Americans (approximately 9.4% of the population) have diagnosed diabetes mellitus, and millions more have diabetes and do not know it. The cost of treating diabetes in the United States is approximately $327 billion a year (National Diabetes Association, 2018a).

Table 37.1 summarizes the major characteristics of the two primary forms of diabetes mellitus. Type 1 diabetes—formerly known as *insulin-dependent diabetes mellitus (IDDM)*—accounts for about 5% to 10% of all cases. Type 1 diabetes occurs when the body's immune system destroys insulin-producing beta cells. There is no known way to prevent type 1 diabetes. People who have type 1 diabetes require injections of **exogenous** (from outside the body) insulin to maintain life because they produce little or no **endogenous** (inside the body) insulin on their own. In general, people with type 1 diabetes are more prone to a serious complication, **ketosis,** associated with an excess production of ketone bodies, leading to **ketoacidosis** (metabolic acidosis). Moreover, type 1 diabetes is more likely to develop early in life. In fact, type 1 diabetes was formerly called *juvenile diabetes* or *ketosis-prone diabetes* because of its typical early onset and potential for ketoacidosis.

Type 2 diabetes—formerly called *non–insulin-dependent diabetes mellitus (NIDDM)*—makes up 90% to 95% of all known cases of diabetes. Type 2 diabetes is believed to begin with **insulin resistance**, in which insulin interaction with glucose becomes less efficient, and therefore glucose metabolism is abnormal. More insulin is produced by the pancreas to maintain cellular metabolism. Type 2 diabetes tends to develop later in life than does type 1, and patients with type 2 rarely develop diabetic ketoacidosis. Box 37.1 lists the signs and symptoms of type 1 and type 2 diabetes. Factors associated with development of type 1 and type 2 diabetes are listed in Box 37.2.

Box 37.1 Symptoms of Type 1 and Type 2 Diabetes

TYPE 1
- Extreme thirst (polydipsia)
- Frequent urination (polyuria)
- Extreme hunger (polyphagia)
- Rapid weight loss
- Irritability
- Weakness and fatigue
- Nausea and vomiting

TYPE 2
- Possibly polydipsia, polyuria, and polyphagia
- More commonly excessive weight gain
- Family history of diabetes mellitus
- Poor healing of scratches, abrasions, and wounds
- Blurred vision
- Itching
- Drowsiness
- Increased fatigue
- Tingling or numbness in the feet

Cultural Considerations

Ethnicity and Type 2 Diabetes

Type 2 diabetes is being diagnosed more frequently in children and adolescents, particularly in American Indians, African Americans, and Hispanic/Latino Americans.

Latent autoimmune diabetes in adults (LADA) is a form of type 1 diabetes, according to the World Health

Box 37.2 Factors Associated With Development of Type 1 and Type 2 Diabetes

TYPE 1
- Family history: genetic predisposition
- Previous infectious disease
- Race: more common in whites, American Indians/Alaska Natives; less common in African Americans, Asians, Hispanics
- Presence of islet cell antibodies in the blood

TYPE 2
- Older age
- Obesity
- Family history of type 2 diabetes
- History of gestational diabetes
- Impaired glucose metabolism
- Physical inactivity
- Race/ethnicity (African Americans, Hispanic/Latino Americans, American Indians, some Asian Americans, Native Hawaiian/Pacific Islanders)

Data from U.S. Department of Health and Human Services (USDHHS), Centers for Disease Control and Prevention: *National diabetes fact sheet: general information and national estimates on diabetes in the United States*, Atlanta, 2018, USDHHS.

Organization. Other names for this condition are *slow-onset type 1 diabetes* or *type 1.5 diabetes.* It is believed that the presence of islet cell antibodies in the blood (which are not present in healthy individuals) will eventually destroy the beta cells, and insulin production will cease. Patients with LADA are usually not overweight, have no signs of **metabolic syndrome**, and may have a history of personal or familial autoimmune disease. The diagnosis is based on three criteria: (1) onset after age 30 years, (2) islet cell antibodies circulating in the blood, and (3) insulin is not required sooner than 6 months after diagnosis. Patients can be misdiagnosed as having type 2 diabetes. Rapid failure of oral hypoglycemic drugs suggests LADA. Evidence-based management suggests that metformin can be used in the early phase, and insulin should be started within 1 year of diagnosis; both may offer some protective effects against the destruction of the beta cells, whereas sulfonylureas may hasten destruction of beta cells and therefore are not recommended (Pozzilli & Pieralice, 2018).

Gestational diabetes may occur as a result of the stress of pregnancy. It may be treated with diet, oral hypoglycemia agents, or insulin. After pregnancy, the condition must be reevaluated; approximately 35% to 60% of women with gestational diabetes are diagnosed with type 2 diabetes in the years after delivery. The baby also carries an increased risk of type 2 diabetes later in life (ADA, 2018).

Etiology and Pathophysiology

At least four sets of factors influence the development of diabetes mellitus: genetic, metabolic, microbiological, and immunologic.

Genetic factors are included in the etiology of diabetes because diabetes tends to run in families. The risk of having some form of diabetes increases in proportion to the number of relatives who are affected, the genetic closeness of the relatives, and the severity of their disease.

Metabolic factors involved in the etiology of diabetes are many and complex. Emotional or physical stress can unmask an inherited predisposition to the disease, probably as a result of glucogenesis induced by increased production of hormones from the adrenal cortex (especially the glucocorticoids). Perhaps even more significant than metabolic factors is the association of type 2 diabetes and obesity. About 80% of patients with type 2 diabetes are obese (more than 20% above their ideal body weight), and there is a higher incidence of type 2 diabetes in people who lead a sedentary life and eat a high-calorie diet. **With weight reduction and increased physical activity, blood glucose can be restored to normal levels and maintained there—hence the importance of diet and exercise in the management of type 2 diabetes.** In type 2 diabetes there also seems to be a relationship to aging and a reduction in the function of the pancreatic beta cells and how they synthesize insulin.

Think Critically

What is one way in which you or your family members might decrease the risk of type 2 diabetes in later life?

Type 1 diabetes is classified as an autoimmune disorder. The immune system causes destruction of the insulin-secreting beta cells of the pancreas. When 80% to 99% of the cells have been destroyed, hyperglycemia develops. Some forms of type 1 diabetes may be related to the viral destruction of beta cells. It is not known if the viral infection initiates or accelerates autoimmunity causing beta cell damage (Richardson & Morgan, 2018).

Signs, Symptoms, and Diagnosis

The ADA recommends screening all adults, especially those who are overweight and have one or more additional risk factors, for type 2 diabetes, starting at age 45 years, to be repeated every 3 years. Hemoglobin A_{1c} (A_{1c} or HbA_{1c}), fasting plasma glucose (FPG), and 2-hour 75-g oral glucose tolerance test (OGTT) are appropriate screening methods (ADA, 2018).

In addition to laboratory tests (see Chapter 35), the health care provider depends on clinical signs and symptoms of diabetes mellitus to establish a diagnosis. The classic symptoms of diabetes mellitus, regardless of type, are related to an elevated blood glucose level, or **hyperglycemia**. Hyperglycemia increases the concentration of the intravascular fluid, raising its osmotic pressure and pulling water from the cells and tissues into the blood, causing cellular dehydration. The kidneys try to get rid of the extra glucose in the urine. Glucose is a large enough molecule to have osmotic properties and pulls water with it when eliminated in the urine. The loss of glucose (**glycosuria**) and water in the urine also causes electrolyte loss. Cellular dehydration causes thirst and a resultant increased intake of water (**polydipsia**), and the osmotic diuresis increases urination (**polyuria**). Hunger (**polyphagia**) is the result of the body's effort to increase its supply of energy, even though the intake of more carbohydrates does not meet the energy needs of the cells because insulin is not available or effective at allowing glucose into the cells.

Clinical Cues

Classic signs and symptoms of diabetes mellitus are polydipsia, polyuria, and polyphagia.

Fatigue and muscular weakness occur because the glucose needed for energy is not metabolized properly. Weight loss in patients with type 1 diabetes occurs for two reasons: (1) the loss of body fluid and (2) in the absence of sufficient insulin for use of glucose, the body begins to metabolize its own proteins and stored fat for energy. The oxidation of fats is incomplete, and fatty acids are converted into ketone bodies and acetone. When the kidney is unable to handle accumulated ketones in the blood, ketosis occurs. The overwhelming presence of the strong organic acids in the blood lowers the pH and leads to a severe and potentially fatal acidosis. The metabolism of body protein when insulin is not available causes an elevated blood urea nitrogen (BUN) level. People with diabetes are prone to infection, delayed healing, and vascular diseases. The increased risk for infection is thought to be partly a result of decreased normal function of leukocytes and abnormal phagocyte function, but is primarily from the hyperglycemic environment. Another contributing factor to infection and delayed healing may be decreased blood supply to the tissues because of atherosclerotic changes in the blood vessels. An impaired blood supply means a deficit in the protective cells brought by the blood to a site of injury.

Safety Alert

Immunizations

Because patients with diabetes are susceptible to infectious diseases, it is recommended that they regularly receive pneumonia and flu vaccinations.

Think Critically

If a friend complained of thirst, fatigue, and frequent urination, what questions would you ask? What would you suggest this person do?

Management of Diabetes

There is no cure for diabetes mellitus; the goal is to maintain blood glucose and lipid levels within normal limits and to control these factors to prevent complications. Studies have demonstrated that there are benefits of tight **glycemic control** (control of glucose in the blood) for people with both type 1 and type 2 diabetes. Patients attempting tight control follow an intensive therapy plan of blood glucose testing multiple times a day and insulin injections or an insulin pump. There are some risks associated with perfect control of blood glucose levels, and "tight control" is not indicated for every patient. The most serious control issue is hypoglycemia, or insulin reaction. Real-time continuous glucose monitoring (CGM) can be done through measurement of interstitial glucose, which is fairly close to plasma glucose. Some insulin pumps have CGM capabilities and can provide insulin as programmed to respond to changes in glucose levels.

Research has demonstrated that lowering A_{1c} levels to 6.5% is associated with decreased microvascular complications (eye, kidney, and nerve diseases) of diabetes. If the patient is older and very frail or if the life expectancy is short, the ADA recommends an A_{1c} of less than 8% to 8.5% (ADA, 2018).

The protocol for control of diabetes mellitus is highly individualized and depends on the type of diabetes a person has, age, general state of health, ability to follow the prescribed regimen, and acceptance of responsibility for managing illness, along with a host of other factors.

The overall goal of diabetes management is achieved when fasting blood glucose stays within normal limits, A_{1c} tests show that blood glucose has stayed within normal limits from one testing period to the next, the patient's weight is normal, blood lipids remain within normal limits, and the patient has a sense of health and well-being.

Older Adult Care Points

Older adults experience hypoglycemia more quickly than do younger people, and older adults are more prone to hypoglycemic episodes. Older adults may progress to dangerously low levels of blood glucose before signs and symptoms are obvious. Severe hypoglycemia in the older adult can precipitate myocardial infarction, angina, stroke, or seizures. For this reason, "tight" control may not be the best plan for older adults.

Diet. **Diet is the cornerstone of diabetic treatment.** Weight gain is common in persons with type 2 diabetes because of high caloric intake and decreased availability of endogenous insulin to fully use ingested food. Weight gain can make a patient with type 2 diabetes more insulin resistant. In many cases, people with type 2 diabetes can control their blood glucose by reducing caloric intake and increasing physical exercise. There is no such thing as a "typical" person with diabetes, and because diabetes is an unstable and changing process, each patient's needs will change from time to time. A person can eat the "perfect" breakfast 3 days in a row, which results in a "perfect" postprandial (after-meal) blood glucose value, only to eat the very same breakfast the next day and have a high blood glucose measurement. This can be frustrating for the patient. The strategies that are effective in managing diabetes can be altered by many factors (e.g., stress, illness, activity, health beliefs), and the strategies that are effective for one person with diabetes may not be effective for someone else.

Medical nutrition therapy (MNT) is recommended for all persons with either type 1 or type 2 diabetes. A registered dietitian (RD) or a certified diabetes educator (CDE) performs an in-depth assessment of the type of diabetes, height-to-weight ratio, usual dietary intake, food preferences, exercise level, and daily schedule. A range of interventions are considered when designing a plan that is individualized for the patient. These interventions include reduced fat intake, carbohydrate counting, simplified meal plans, healthy food choices, individualized meal planning strategies, exchange lists, **insulin-to-carbohydrate ratios** (adjusting insulin doses to match carbohydrate intake), physical activity, and behavioral strategies (ADA, 2018). In general, MNT is aimed at providing adequate nutrition with sufficient calories to maintain normal body weight and control of cholesterol and at adjusting the intake of food so that blood glucose is kept within safe limits.

Meal plans include diet guidelines consistent with recommendations for healthy adults. For patients with diabetes, distribution of calories is important for glycemic control. Breakfast calories should be 20% of the daily allotment, with lunch at 35%, dinner at 30%, and late evening snack at 15%. If the patient chooses to eat sweets and they are substituted for carbohydrates and do not exceed 10% to 35% of total energy intake, this does not have a negative effect. Proteins should make up 15% to 20%; for patients with **diabetic nephropathy** (kidney disease secondary to high blood glucose level), protein intake of 1 g/kg of body weight is recommended. Meals should include 14 g of fiber per 1000 kilocalories, which is the recommendation for the general public. Reduction of saturated fats, trans fats, and dietary cholesterol also improves cardiovascular outcomes (Klemm, 2019).

Clinical Cues

Emphasis should be placed on the positive aspects of the diet—on the foods allowed rather than those that are forbidden. A patient should not be made to feel guilty about having difficulty staying on the diet or the times when they "cheat" and eat foods that are not allowed.

Cultural preferences must be considered when devising meal plans. One of the most effective means of helping a person with diabetes follow the prescribed diet is by teaching about food values and how they affect diabetes. Initially, three or four teaching sessions performed by the RD or CDE and lasting 45 to 90 minutes are recommended, with annual follow-up as a minimum. The ADA and the American Dietetic Association have worked together to devise simplified methods of calculating a diabetic diet and planning meals for a person with diabetes. Organizations such as the ADA and the Joslin Diabetes Center, affiliated with Harvard Medical School, have instructive material available for patient teaching.

Older Adult Care Points

Weight loss is seldom a goal for older adults with type 2 diabetes unless weight is more than 1½ times normal for height and frame. Older adults are more susceptible to nutritional deficiencies from teeth problems, illness, and decreased appetite. Diet is typically managed by reducing concentrated sugars and by adhering to a meal schedule.

Think Critically

How would you obtain accurate data about what your patient with diabetes is eating each day?

Exercise. Physical exercise is an important part of managing diabetes. Muscular activity improves glucose use for energy and improves circulation. In addition to lowering blood glucose levels by "burning up" the glucose, exercise makes the insulin receptors on cells more sensitive to the hormone, and thus improves use of the available glucose. Exercise has been shown to improve glycemic control in type 2 diabetes. Diabetic control also considers blood lipid levels. Exercise contributes to that control by reducing triglyceride levels and increasing high-density lipoprotein (HDL) levels. People with type 1 diabetes may decrease their cardiovascular risk with regular exercise even though it does not contribute to control of blood sugar.

The exercise program should be designed for the individual patient. The plan should consider the age and overall physical condition of the patient, ability to carry out the exercises regularly, how well controlled the diabetes is, and baseline blood glucose. Exercise can rapidly lower blood glucose levels and cause serious hypoglycemia.

All exercise programs should begin with milder forms of exercise and gradually increase to the patient's level of tolerance or until the desired therapeutic effect is reached. A program should not be started until the blood glucose is under control. The exercise program should be planned so that the exercises are performed at the same time every day, preferably after a meal, when the blood glucose is highest. Blood glucose should be checked before beginning to exercise. The patient is encouraged to wear a medical alert bracelet (Fig. 37.1) and to exercise with a friend who knows the signs, symptoms, and treatment of hypoglycemia.

Glycemic control during exercise. General guidelines for exercise include practicing good foot care and wearing appropriate shoes and socks. This is very important if there is peripheral neuropathy resulting in decreased sensation. Some types of exercise can increase blood glucose by the release of epinephrine,

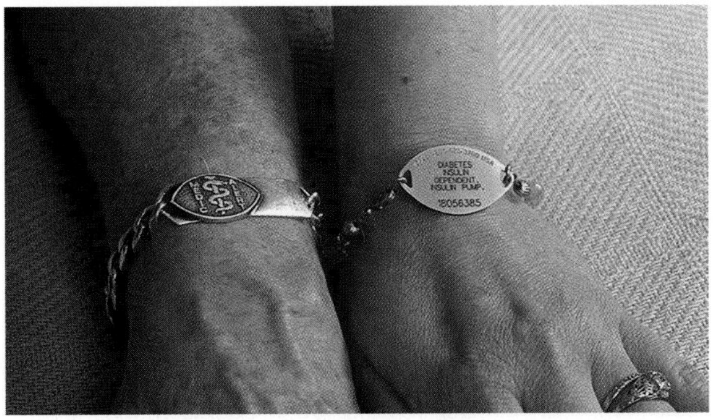

Fig. 37.1 Medical alert bracelets.

Patient Teaching

Home Treatment for Hypoglycemia

Patients should have an emergency plan and supplies for treating low glucose. When signs of hypoglycemia are present and the patient is able to swallow, give one of the following to provide 15 to 20 g of glucose or simple carbohydrates:

- ½ cup (4 oz) of juice or regular soda (not diet)
- 1 cup (8 oz) of nonfat or 1% milk
- 6 or 7 hard candies, such as Life Savers (not sugar-free)
- 1 small box (2 tablespoons) of raisins
- 3 glucose tablets
- 1 tablespoon of honey, sugar, or corn syrup
- 1 small tube (2 oz) of cake icing or glucose gel

Follow up with a longer-acting source, such as crackers and cheese or a meat sandwich.

If the patient is unable to swallow (groggy or unconscious):

- Turn the patient onto the side.
- Administer 1 mg of glucagon by injection after mixing the solution in the bottle until it is clear. Call 911 if unable to give injection.
- If the patient does not awaken within 15 minutes, give another dose of glucagon and immediately inform a health care provider.
- If a health care provider cannot be contacted, call 911 or the local emergency service.

Clinical Cues

Patients should be advised to check with their health care provider before starting an exercise program. Certain activities may not be advised if there are complications. For example, patients with neuropathy, retinopathy, or renal insufficiency may be unable to safely balance, see, or perform rigorous or strenuous activities.

Older Adult Care Points

Physical limitations may discourage older adults with diabetes from exercising. Older patients with diabetes are at risk of developing hypoglycemia up to 24 hours after exercising if the exercise is too strenuous. Walking, swimming, or stationary bicycle riding are among the safest activities for this group. Exercise should begin slowly and build up to 30 to 45 minutes, three or four times a week. The gradual increase helps prevent hypoglycemia, stress fractures, and cardiovascular complications.

but most will decrease blood glucose. Managing blood sugar during exercise is individualized to the patient and whether type 1 or type 2 diabetes is present. Gradual increase in activities and consultation with the health care provider are necessary for safe implementation of an exercise program. Key guidelines for safe exercise include knowing blood glucose before exercise. If blood sugar is low, a carbohydrate snack (20 to 40 g based on body weight) should be consumed before starting. Snacks during activity should be used to prevent hypoglycemia. The amount and frequency will be determined by the type and duration of exercise. A liquid or other readily absorbed source of carbohydrate is recommended.

Performing exercise when insulin or an oral antidiabetic agent is at its peak of action can bring on an acute hypoglycemic reaction. Eating a piece of fruit before even light exercise, if done between meals, also can help prevent hypoglycemia in people with type 1 diabetes. Once a patient begins to follow a regular exercise program, the insulin dosage and diet may need to be revised. In general, the patient may need to take less insulin and to increase caloric intake with regular exercise. Keeping a daily record of exercise, along with weight, insulin dosage, and blood glucose levels, can help motivate the patient to continue exercise.

Health Promotion

Insulin and Exercise

Advise patients to avoid injecting insulin into an area that will soon receive extra exercise (e.g., the leg). The abdomen is a good site for insulin injection because absorption is steady, rapid, and not affected by exercise.

Oral hypoglycemic agents. Oral hypoglycemic agents (OHAs) or antidiabetic agents may be prescribed for patients with type 2 diabetes to manage their blood glucose levels. These medications are not a form of oral insulin; pharmacologically, they are from completely different classes of medications. There are several major categories of OHAs that act in different ways to help achieve blood glucose control. Information about these medications can be found in Table 37.2. Many of these individual medications are combined and sold under a variety of brand names.

Safety Alert

Sulfa Drug Allergy

Because the sulfonylureas are from the same family of drugs as the sulfonamide antibiotics, they must be given with caution to persons known to have an allergy to sulfa drugs.

Patients receiving OHAs should know that these medications do not eliminate the need for following their diet and exercise program. Some may be under the impression that if they go off their diet and indulge

Table 37.2 Hypoglycemic Agents

GENERIC NAME (BRAND NAME)	MAIN SITE OF ACTION	HOW THEY CONTROL BLOOD GLUCOSE	OTHER CONSIDERATIONS
Biguanides			
Metformin (Glucophage) Also available in combination with other OHAs	Liver	Keep liver from releasing excessive insulin; make muscle cells more sensitive to insulin	Do not cause hypoglycemia or hyperinsulinemia Do not lead to weight gain Contraindicated in renal failure, liver disease, and acidosis
Alpha-Glucosidase Inhibitors			
Acarbose (Precose) Miglitol (Glyset)	Intestine	Reduce demand for insulin by slowing absorption of complex carbohydrates, resulting in less of a blood glucose "spike"	Contraindicated in people with inflammatory bowel disease or other intestinal diseases
Thiazolidinediones			
Pioglitazone (Actos) Rosiglitazone (Avandia) Also used in combination with other drugs.	Muscle cells	Make muscle cells more sensitive to insulin; decrease liver production of glucose	Contraindicated in people with congestive heart failure Actos and Avandia have a black box warning for cardiac risk
Sulfonylureas (Long-Acting)			
Glimepiride (Amaryl) Glipizide (Glucotrol) Glyburide (DiaBeta, Micronase, Glynase PresTab) Tolazamide (Tolinase) Tolbutamide (Orinase)	Pancreas	Stimulate pancreas to secrete more insulin	Quick action can cause hypoglycemia Contraindicated in advanced kidney or liver disease or for those with sulfa allergies
Meglitinides			
Nateglinide (Starlix) Repaglinide (Prandin)	Pancreas	Stimulate insulin secretion but shorter acting than sulfonylureas	Must be taken immediately before eating Lower risk of hypoglycemia than sulfonylureas
Dipeptidyl Peptidase-4 Inhibitors (DPP-4 Inhibitors)			
Sitagliptin (Januvia) Saxagliptin (Onglyza) Linagliptin (Tradjenta) Alogliptin (Nesina)	Endocrine system	Enhance a natural body system called the incretin system, which helps regulate glucose by affecting alpha and beta cells in the pancreas	May cause delayed gastric emptying (can affect absorption of other medications) Reduced dosage may be required in patients with renal impairment because medication is excreted via the kidneys
Sodium-Glucose Cotransporter-2 Inhibitors (SGLT2)			
Canagliflozin (Invokana) Dapagliflozin (Farxiga) Empagliflozin (Jardiance)	Kidney	Block reabsorption of glucose in the kidneys	Do not use in renal failure Can cause fluid loss from glycosuria
Glucagon-like Peptide-1 Receptor Agonists (GLP-1) (Incretin Mimetics)			
Exenatide (Byetta, Bydureon) Liraglutide (Victoza, Saxenda) Lixisenatide (Lyxumia) Albiglutide (Tanzeum) Dulaglutide (Trulicity) Semaglutide (Ozempic)	Gut, liver, pancreas	Slow gastric emptying and stimulate insulin release. Increase liver gluconeogenesis.	Medications require injection, and some are dosed twice daily, others daily, and the rest weekly. Contraindicated in patients with chronic renal failure on dialysis.
Dopamine-2 Agonists			
Bromocriptine (Cycloset)	Cells	Increases sensitivity to insulin	Not a first-line therapy. May be used alone or with other medications.

Table 37.2 Hypoglycemic Agents—cont'd

GENERIC NAME (BRAND NAME)	MAIN SITE OF ACTION	HOW THEY CONTROL BLOOD GLUCOSE	OTHER CONSIDERATIONS
Bile Acid Sequestrants			
Colesevelam (Welchol) Cholestyramine (Questran) Colestipol (Colestid)	Digestive system	Used for altering cholesterol levels. Also can decrease blood glucose levels, but the mechanism is poorly understood.	Can cause flatulence and constipation.
Synthetic Hormone			
Pramlintide	Pancreatic beta cells, gut	Decreases secretion of insulin and amylin in response to food. Delays gastric emptying.	Can cause severe hypoglycemia. Should not be given to patients on medications that alter gastric motility.

OHAs, Oral hypoglycemic agents.

themselves, they can just take more pills to compensate. Others who have been on a diet and exercise program for a time and then have an OHA prescribed for them think it is acceptable to stop planning their meals and exercising regularly. All OHAs can produce gastric irritation, nausea, vomiting, and diarrhea. Liver damage with jaundice, bone marrow depression, and allergic skin reactions may result in some patients. During illness and change in routine, insulin may be added to inpatient treatment. Most patients with type 2 diabetes controlled by OHAs can return to their usual medication regimen after the acute episode is resolved and will not need long-term injectable insulin.

Safety Alert

Insulin Concentration

Insulin is typically provided in 100 units per milliliter concentration (U100). The need for higher doses has led to the use of more concentrated drug. U200, U300, and U500 are now in use (Fig. 37.2). Be *extremely careful* in checking the concentration and using the correct syringe.

Clinical Cues

Metformin is the preferred drug for type 2 diabetes, so many patients take this OHA. Metformin should be held before surgery or a procedure requiring contrast media and for 48 hours afterward until renal function is verified.

Insulin therapy. Insulin therapy can be prescribed for patients with either type 1 or type 2 diabetes. The goal of insulin therapy is to closely mimic **basal insulin**, which is the amount of insulin that would normally be produced by the pancreas throughout the day to maintain a healthy blood sugar level between meals. The pancreas also produces extra insulin after meals **(postprandial).** The health care provider can use a variety of rapid-acting, short-acting, intermediate-acting, and long-acting

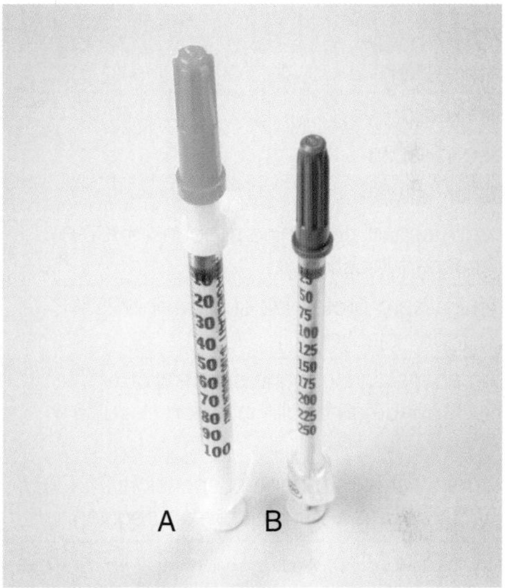

Fig. 37.2 Insulin syringes are available in **(A)** U100 and **(B)** U500 calibrations. (From Lilley LL, Rainforth Collins S, Snyder JS: *Pharmacology and the nursing process,* ed 9, St. Louis, 2020, Elsevier.)

insulins that best suit the individual patient (Table 37.3). A single daily injection of intermediate- or long-acting insulin, or a combination insulin (such as Humulin 70/30, which combines short- and intermediate-acting insulins), can be used for some patients. The multiple daily injection (MDI) regimen is frequently prescribed and offers the advantage of being more physiologically appropriate. MDI combines short- and intermediate-acting insulins, injected two or more times a day. The patient could also be placed on an intensified regimen. This regimen relies on the patient's ability to accurately perform blood glucose monitoring. The basal dose, again, would be intermediate- or long-acting insulin. A **bolus dose,** or **correction dose,** of short- or rapid-acting insulin is used to manage elevations in blood glucose and bring the next blood glucose measurement into range. Higher concentrations of insulin are used so that

Table 37.3 **Common Types of Insulins: Onset, Peak, and Duration of Action**

PREPARATION	BRAND NAME	ONSET (H)	PEAK (H)	DURATION (H)
Rapid Acting				
Insulin aspart injection	NovoLog	0.25	1–3	3–5
Insulin lispro injection	Humalog	0.25	0.5–1.5	5
Insulin glulisine injection	Apidra	0.3	0.5–1.5	3–4
Human insulin inhalation powder	Afrezza	0.25	1–1.25	2–3
Short Acting				
Regular human insulin injection	Humulin R Novolin R	0.5 0.5	2–4 2.5–5	5–7 8
Buffered regular human insulin injection	Velosulin BR	0.5	1–3	8
Intermediate Acting				
Isophane insulin NPH	Humulin N Novolin N ReliOn N	1.5 1.5	4–12 4–12	16–24+ 24
Insulin zinc suspension (Lente)	Novolin L	1	6–8	5.7–24
Insulin detemir injection	Levemir	1	6–8	5.7–24
Long Acting				
Glargine injection	Lantus	2–4	None	24
Detemir injection	Levemir	1	6–8	5.7–24
Degludec injection	Tresiba	0.5–1.5	9	3–4 days
Combination Insulin				
70% insulin aspart protamine suspension/30% insulin aspart injection	NovoLog Mix 70/30	0.25	1–4	24
75% insulin lispro protamine suspension/25% insulin lispro injection	Humalog Mix 75/25	0.25	1–2	16–20
70% human insulin isophane suspension (NPH)/30% human insulin injection (regular)	Humulin 70/30 Novolin 70/30 ReliOn 70/30	0.5	2–4	14–24
50% human insulin isophane suspension (NPH)/50% human insulin injection (regular)	Humulin 50/50 Novolin 50/50	0.5	3–5	24

Adapted from Ignatavicius DD, Workman ML, et al.: *Medical-surgical nursing: critical thinking for collaborative care*, ed 9, St. Louis, 2018, Elsevier.

large volumes of solution are not injected for those patients requiring high insulin doses. Regular insulin in U500 concentration has a longer duration and is used as a basal insulin rather than a bolus correctional dose.

Clinical Cues

If a patient is on a **sliding scale** of insulin based on fingerstick glucose results for nutritional coverage and receives **rapid-acting** insulin before meals, make sure the food tray is in front of the patient before giving the insulin to help prevent hypoglycemic events.

Insulin cannot be taken orally or given via a feeding tube because it is destroyed by gastric juices. Inhaled insulin was trialed in the late 1990s, on the market in the early 2000s, and then discontinued. An inhaled rapid-acting insulin is now available. The insulin is dispensed in a device much like the inhaled powders for lung disease. Insulin pens, filled with insulin, are another alternative to the traditional syringe-and-needle apparatus (Fig. 37.3, *A*). The patient selects the correct dose on a dial, and the insulin is delivered by a small needle at the end of the pen.

Clinical Cues

If regular insulin and longer-acting insulin are to be mixed in one syringe, the regular insulin is drawn up first to prevent any contamination of the regular bottle of insulin with the longer-acting variety. "Clear to cloudy" is an easy way to remember which insulin to draw up first. The clear (regular) insulin is drawn up first, followed by the cloudy (longer-acting) insulin. **Remember that every insulin dose must be verified by another nurse as it is drawn up, every time.** This habit will also help you meet the National Patient Safety Goal to increase the safety of administering medications.

Injectable insulin continues to be the most common delivery method, so it is critical that you be educated in all aspects of injectable insulin therapy. Insulin

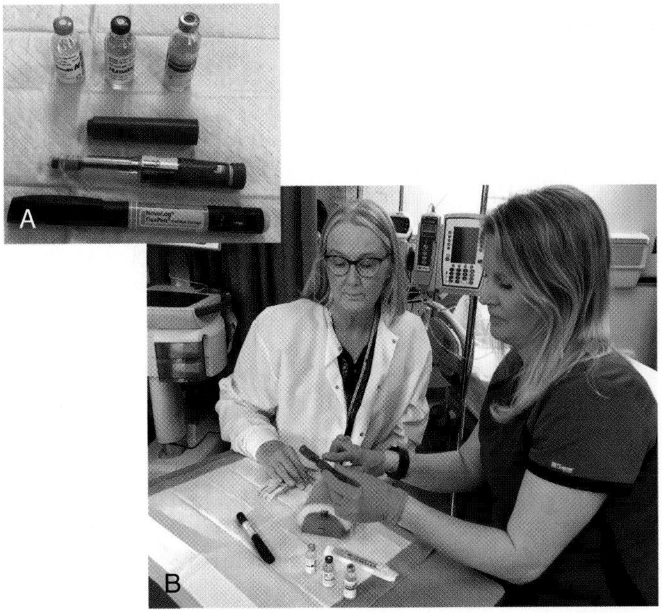

Fig. 37.3 **A,** Different insulin types and insulin pens. **B,** A nursing student performs a teaching demonstration for the instructor.

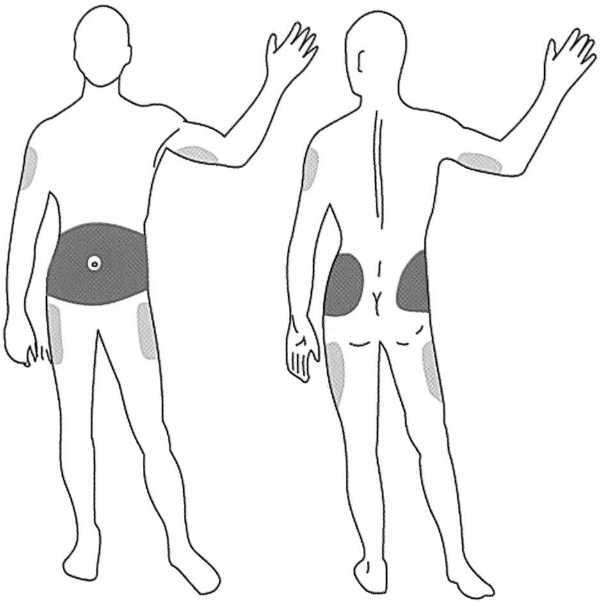

Fig. 37.4 Rotation sites for injection of insulin. (Courtesy ACCU-CHEK® is a registered trademark of Roche.)

Safety Alert

Insulin Pen Injectors

Patients must be careful when dialing the dose of insulin into a pen injector. If performed incorrectly, the numbers of the dosage will be transposed (e.g., 52 units instead of 25 units). This could happen if the pen is held in the left hand or if the number scale is held upside down.

injections are rotated within one body area to enhance absorption. Insulin enters the bloodstream at different speeds when given at different sites. The abdomen has the quickest absorption rate, followed by the upper arms. The thighs and buttocks have the slowest absorption, unless the injection is given before exercise when blood flow to those areas will be increased. Patients are given charts showing the places on the arms, legs, buttocks, and abdomen where insulin can be injected (Fig. 37.4). They are then encouraged to keep a daily record of injection sites to help remember which sites have been used and to prevent the problem of altered or erratic absorption.

Insulin requirements change as metabolic needs are altered by diet, exercise, age, and even changes in seasons. In the summer, for example, many people are outdoors and exercising more than during the winter months. Also, as a person grows older, the level of physical activity may decrease. Insulin requirements also are altered when the patient has an infection or illness or is under added stress.

Insulin pump. An alternative to insulin therapy by daily injections is the insulin pump. These pumps can deliver a continuous infusion of insulin through an automated system composed of a battery-driven electronic "brain," an electric motor and drive mechanisms, and a syringe (Fig. 37.5). The syringe is attached to plastic tubing and a subcutaneous needle, which is inserted into the abdomen or thigh. Pumps are helpful in managing diabetes because they allow for improved blood glucose control; people using pumps tend to have fewer episodes of and less severe hypoglycemia compared with MDIs.

The pump continuously delivers basal insulin to maintain blood sugar levels between meals and can be programmed to administer a bolus dose for meals or elevated blood sugar levels. CGM is possible via a small sensor inserted under the skin that monitors glucose in the interstitial fluid and not in the blood. CGM can be used to automatically deliver insulin based on changes in blood glucose. CGM devices can wirelessly send information to the insulin pump or other monitoring

Clinical Cues

Some patients can use the insulin-to-carbohydrate ratio method. The patient must receive extensive MNT and be taught to interpret blood glucose patterns, to count carbohydrates, and to calculate bolus doses based on carbohydrate intake. One unit of insulin will cover 15 g carbohydrate for most patients (weight and insulin sensitivity must also be considered). The diabetic educator should be contacted for assistance if a patient could benefit from this type of management system.

Think Critically

How would a patient know that their insulin requirement has changed?

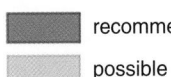

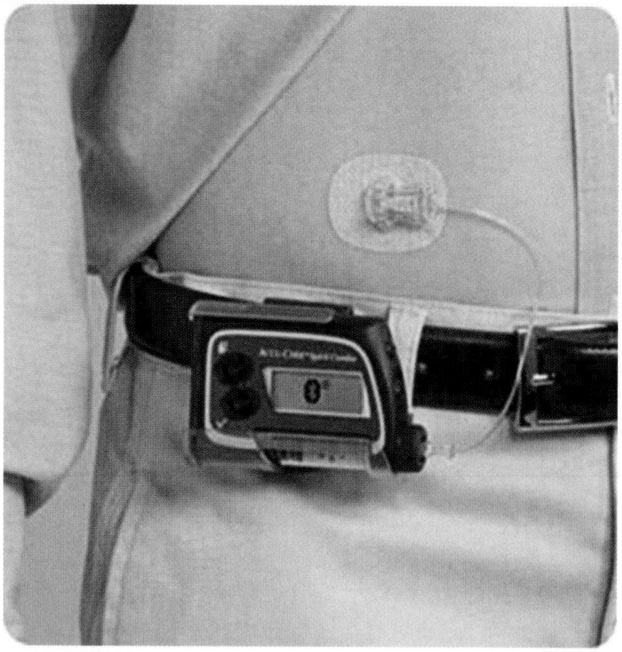

Fig. 37.5 Insulin pump. (Courtesy ACCU-CHEK® is a registered trademark of Roche.)

equipment. Insulin pumps are recommended for patients who are willing and able to monitor their blood glucose frequently during the day and who can understand the principles of basal and bolus insulin and carbohydrate counting. As the technology gets more sophisticated and easier to use, the popularity of insulin pumps is increasing.

Clinical Cues

The insulin pump will have to be disconnected for certain diagnostic tests, such as magnetic resonance imaging. Most patients can safely be without the pump for an hour, but blood glucose should be checked before disconnecting and after reconnecting (Umpierrez & Klonoff, 2018).

Other injectable agents. Historically, insulin was the only injectable medication for the management of diabetes; however, new injectable agents have been introduced. These medications do not replace standard diabetic medications but are used to enhance the effect of existing medications. One new category of medications is called **incretin mimetics** because they mimic the action of **incretins,** hormones released from the intestine. In type 2 diabetics they lower postprandial blood glucose levels in a number of ways (see Table 37.2). Other injectable medications to treat diabetes are synthetic hormones, such as pramlintide (Symlin), which can be used in types 1 and 2 diabetes. Although these medications are administered subcutaneously, none of these medications should ever be mixed in the same syringe with insulin, and the patient must be monitored carefully for hypoglycemia.

Safety Alert

Pramlintide

The medication pramlintide has a U.S. Food and Drug Administration (FDA) **black box warning** (a type of warning sometimes carried on prescription medications indicating the potential for serious adverse effects). This medication has the potential to cause severe hypoglycemia within 3 hours of administration. It is critically important that you observe the patient closely for any signs or symptoms of hypoglycemia.

Preoperative and postoperative insulin management. The emotional and physical stress of surgery can increase the blood glucose level and alter the amounts of medication needed for glycemic control. Patients with type 2 diabetes may be taken off OHAs up to 48 hours before surgery and started on insulin by injection to achieve adequate control of their diabetes during this stressful period. The patient should be reassured that the diabetes is not worse and that the insulin injections are only a temporary measure. A patient with type 2 diabetes will have bolus or correction dose orders (sliding scale) along with the usual insulin order. Blood sugar determinations are performed frequently.

For all patients with diabetes, intravenous (IV) fluids are begun as soon as the patient is ordered "nothing by mouth" (NPO) and are continued until the patient is eating again after surgery. During surgery, an insulin infusion of regular or short-acting insulin may be used, usually mixed in 5% dextrose or 0.9% NaCl solution, depending on hospital policy. Blood glucose is monitored closely during surgery and every 2 to 4 hours postoperatively; urine is checked for ketones when glucose levels are high. Patients well controlled on an insulin pump may continue to manage their blood glucose levels during hospitalization if their physical condition and hospital policy allow (ADA, 208).

Clinical Cues

Be especially alert for signs of hypoglycemia in patients who are receiving an insulin infusion. Blood glucose is monitored hourly. The rate of infusion is adjusted according to an algorithm.

Islet cell and pancreas transplantation. Clinical trials are under way for optimizing a procedure for treatment of type 1 diabetes by transplantation of insulin-producing islet cells. Cells are taken from the donor pancreas and injected into the hepatic circulation of the recipient, where the cells lodge and produce insulin. Lifelong immunosuppressive medications are still needed to prevent rejection of the cells. Whole organ transplantation of the pancreas is also done to replace insulin function. Many times a pancreas and kidney transplantation are performed together using organs from the same donor. Altered renal function is a complication of type 1 diabetes, and transplantation of both organs results in better outcomes (Thomas, 2018).

Table 37.4 Comparison of Hypoglycemia and Ketoacidosis

HYPOGLYCEMIA	KETOACIDOSIS
Etiology	
Overdosage of insulin Skipped or delayed meal Unplanned strenuous exercise	Failure to take insulin Illness or infection Overeating or too many carbohydrates Severe stress (surgery, trauma, emotional upset)
Symptoms	
Headache Weakness Hunger (polyphagia) Pallor Irritability Lack of muscle coordination Apprehension Shakiness Diaphoresis with cool, clammy skin Blurred vision Rapid heartbeat Confusion Coma (late)	Increased thirst (polydipsia) Increased urination (polyuria) Acetone breath odor ("fruity") Dry mucous membranes and sunken eyeballs (dehydration) Nausea and vomiting Deep respirations (Kussmaul respirations) Abdominal pain and rigidity Paresthesias, weakness, paralysis Hypotension Minimal urine output (oliguria) or none (anuria) (late sign) Stupor or coma (late sign)
Treatment	
If patient can swallow, give 3 glucose tablets or equivalent glucose gel, 6 oz of juice, 6 oz regular cola, 8 oz of 2% or skim milk, or 6–8 Life Savers candies. If patient cannot swallow, administer glucagon IM. If at the hospital, give $D_{50}W$ solution IV.	IV fluid and insulin with correction of electrolyte imbalances. Severe cases are hospitalized for stabilization.
Prevention	
Eat meals 4–5 h apart, plus prescribed snacks. Take correct dose of insulin. Test blood glucose level regularly and more frequently during illness. Eat extra food when exercising more than usual.	Take correct dose of insulin. Consult health care provider when ill (even for minor illnesses). Follow diet; do not overeat and do not overload with carbohydrates.

$D_{50}W$, dextrose 50% in water; *IM,* intramuscularly; *IV,* intravenously.

Complications

In general, people with diabetes are susceptible to two types of complications: short-term (acute) problems and long-term problems.

Short-term problems. Acute complications arise when the blood glucose suddenly becomes either too high (hyperglycemia) or too low (hypoglycemia) (Table 37.4).

> **! Safety Alert**
>
> **Hyperglycemia or Hypoglycemia**
>
> When there is doubt as to whether a patient is experiencing hyperglycemia or hypoglycemia, treatment is begun for hypoglycemia until a blood glucose determination is obtained to prevent brain damage from extremely low cerebral glucose levels. Caution should be used to not overtreat with glucose. Hyperglycemia can worsen neurologic conditions. Rapid determination of blood glucose is essential to proper management. Hyperglycemia usually develops slowly and does not cause immediate changes in level of consciousness. Hypoglycemia can occur rapidly.

When a patient is admitted to the hospital with hyperglycemia, decisions about the proper modes of therapy are based on the presence of objective and subjective symptoms. Type 1 diabetes is more likely to be complicated by ketoacidosis, whereas type 2 diabetes may cause hyperglycemic hyperosmolar state (HHS; previously called hyperglycemic hyperosmolar nonketotic syndrome, also abbreviated HHNC, HNKC, and HHNK).

Diabetic ketoacidosis. Diabetic ketoacidosis (DKA) is a serious condition caused by incomplete metabolism of fats resulting from an absence or insufficient supply of insulin. When insulin is not present in adequate amounts to meet metabolic needs, the body breaks down protein and fat for energy. This produces an abundance of the by-products of fat metabolism, which are potent organic acids called *ketones.* In an attempt to rid itself of acidosis produced by ketones, the body increases respiratory rate and depth (Kussmaul respirations). Acetone, a ketone body, is excreted in the urine, causing acetonuria or ketonuria, and from the lungs, which can be detected in the characteristic fruity odor to the breath.

As the kidney excretes excess glucose and ketones, it also eliminates large quantities of water and electrolytes. These pathologic changes are responsible for metabolic acidosis, dehydration, and electrolyte imbalances.

Signs and symptoms of DKA can be life threatening and are listed in Table 37.4. Intravenous fluids are administered first, then electrolyte imbalances are addressed in conjunction with an insulin drip. Electrolytes, especially potassium, and serum glucose, are monitored closely. In the absence of insulin, potassium comes out of the cells, and patients present with hyperkalemia. As IV fluids are given and insulin is administered, potassium returns to the cells, causing hypokalemia. These potassium shifts are very important to monitor and manage so that lethal cardiac dysrhythmias do not occur. **The goals of treatment are to restore the normal pH of the blood and other body fluids, correct the fluid and electrolyte imbalance, lower the blood glucose level gradually, and provide life support measures as necessary.** Infection is the most common cause of DKA; however, other causes include poor compliance with the prescribed regimen of diet and insulin therapy and insulin pump failure. After the patient is stabilized, the underlying cause must be determined and treatment or corrective measures implemented.

Nutrition Considerations

Ketogenic Diet

A popular diet for weight loss and overall health has long been used medically to treat refractory epilepsy in children. The ketogenic diet is high in fat and low in carbohydrates, causing the body to burn fat rather than carbohydrates for energy. Ketone bodies are by-products of fat metabolism. Ketosis in a person with normal insulin secretion does not result in acidosis. In addition to facilitating the entry of glucose into cells, insulin also regulates the amount of circulating ketones, preventing a buildup high enough to produce acidosis (Jockers, 2019).

Clinical Cues

If you suspect a patient is in DKA, immediately ensure that there is at least one patent IV access and anticipate an order for IV therapy.

Hyperglycemic hyperosmolar state. Hyperglycemic hyperosmolar state (HHS) occurs primarily in people with type 2 diabetes who experience high blood glucose levels because of illness or added stress, such as infection. Glucose levels greater than 600 mg/dL are common; in some cases the blood glucose can reach well over 1000 mg/dL. The extremely high level of glucose in the blood causes severe dehydration and circulating fluid volume depletion secondary to osmotic diuresis. Blood osmolality is considerably elevated (greater than 320 mOsm/kg). HHS is different from DKA because a small amount of circulating insulin remains available, resulting in the absence of ketosis and acidosis. Because ketosis and acidosis are absent, the gastrointestinal symptoms do not occur, and the patient does not seek medical care early in the course of illness. The patient's mental state may progress from confusion to complete coma. Also, in contrast to DKA, a patient in HHS may experience generalized or focal seizures.

Older Adult Care Points

Older adults are at greater risk for HHS because they become dehydrated more quickly than do younger patients. HHS may be the first indicator that the patient has diabetes. HHS most commonly occurs after a febrile illness or gastrointestinal flu, during which the patient has stopped eating properly and possibly has discontinued oral hypoglycemic agents.

Things that may precipitate HHS in a person with type 2 diabetes are (1) medications that increase serum glucose levels or cause dehydration, such as steroids, thiazides, phenytoin, and beta blockers; (2) acute illnesses, such as infection, myocardial infarction, and stroke; (3) chronic illnesses, such as congestive heart failure and renal dysfunction; and (4) treatments, such as total parenteral nutrition and peritoneal dialysis.

Treatment of HHS focuses on fluid replacement and correction of electrolyte imbalances. Because fluid replacement will initially be rapid, cardiovascular status and lung sounds must be assessed frequently. Small amounts of insulin may be used until the patient is stabilized. Blood glucose and intake and output must be monitored closely. The underlying illness that triggered the HHS must be identified and treated. HHS can be fatal, and mortality risk is directly correlated with higher elevations of blood glucose and the resultant severity of dehydration.

Rebound hyperglycemia. Rebound hyperglycemia, also known as the *Somogyi effect,* follows a period of hypoglycemia, often during sleep. When hypoglycemia occurs, the body secretes glucagon, epinephrine, growth hormone, and cortisol to counteract the effects of low blood sugar. The patient may report nightmares and night sweats along with morning elevated serum glucose; if the patient increases the insulin dose, it worsens the problem.

The Somogyi effect is diagnosed by checking blood sugars during the night; once verified, the usual treatment is to lower the insulin dosage or move the time of the intermediate-acting insulin to bedtime. Changing or increasing the bedtime snack also helps.

The **dawn phenomenon** is characterized by elevated blood glucose in the morning. It is caused by release of growth hormone, glucagon, and epinephrine during the night, as part of the body's natural circadian rhythm. These hormones act to raise the body's blood sugar. The dawn phenomenon is the reason why most people with diabetes do not tolerate carbohydrates well in the morning. The treatment is an intermediate-acting insulin at night.

Hypoglycemia. The word *hypoglycemia* means "low blood glucose." Hypoglycemia is a common complication of insulin administration in type 1 diabetes mellitus. Most often it is a response to either too large a dose of insulin or too much exercise in relation to the amount of food eaten. People with diabetes must be taught to monitor for the signs and symptoms of hypoglycemia: tremulousness, hunger, headache, pallor, sweating, palpitations, blurred vision, and weakness. Symptoms may progress to confusion and loss of consciousness. Individual reactions vary considerably. Some patients are alert with a glucose level of 40 mg/dL, whereas others are comatose at this level.

Treatment depends on the degree of hypoglycemia and level of consciousness. If the patient is alert enough to tolerate oral intake safely, glucose levels of 40 to 60 mg/dL respond to ingestion of food such as milk, crackers, or juice. Glucose levels of 20 to 40 mg/dL respond best to concentrated sugars, such as honey, table sugar, or juice. Patients must be taught how to self-treat hypoglycemia (see Patient Teaching: Home Treatment for Hypoglycemia). In the hospital, if the person is experiencing seizures or is not alert enough to tolerate oral intake safely or has a very low blood sugar, a solution of 50% glucose is given IV. When an IV access cannot be established, 1 mg of glucagon is administered intramuscularly. The injection is repeated in 15 minutes if symptoms are not resolved (see Table 37.4).

Long-term problems. The long-term consequences of diabetes mellitus are chiefly the result of damage to the large and small blood vessels, termed *macrovascular* and *microvascular*, respectively. Elevated blood glucose levels over a period of years seriously damage blood vessels and the organs they serve. Diabetes is the seventh leading cause of death in the United States for all age groups (Murphy et al., 2018). In addition, cardiovascular disease and other causes of death often can be attributed to diabetes. Damage to the mechanisms that control blood vessel health occurs when blood glucose is elevated over a long period. The alterations in the macrovascular system result in coronary artery disease, peripheral arterial disease, and stroke. Microvascular complications result from damage to the small vessels at the capillary level. This causes diabetic nephropathy, neuropathy, and retinopathy.

Patients who have had diabetes for more than 10 years are likely to develop one or more of the complications of the disease. The less closely the blood glucose has been controlled, the more likely is the development of cardiovascular, eye, and renal complications. **Improperly treated or untreated diabetes is the leading cause of new blindness, renal failure leading to dialysis, and nontraumatic lower limb amputations.** Although not every person with diabetes will suffer from long-term complications, many will periodically be hospitalized for diabetic-related conditions.

Cardiovascular disease. Two in three people with diabetes die prematurely from heart attack or stroke. In compliance with The Joint Commission's Core Measures, aggressive measures should be taken to prevent stroke in patients at risk. Tight glycemic control is the best strategy to prevent the vascular changes that cause myocardial infarction and stroke.

Peripheral vascular disease. Gangrene, which often leads to amputation, is far more common in people with diabetes. More than 60% of nontraumatic amputations occur among people with diabetes. Vascular changes typically cause very poor circulation in the feet and lower extremities. Healing of wounds in these areas is difficult because of poor blood supply. Because increased levels of glucose in the blood provide a good medium for bacterial growth and decrease the immune response, it is harder to eradicate infection. Learning and practicing excellent foot care are essential to prevent amputation. Multiple studies have identified early identification and intervention as tools to successfully prevent amputation.

Patient Teaching

Foot Care

- Inspect each foot daily for cuts, cracks, blisters, abrasions, or discoloration of the toes; report any abnormality to the health care provider. Use a mirror if unable to bend to see the bottom of the foot. Be certain to check between the toes.
- Wash the feet in warm (not hot) water, using mild soap; do not soak the feet because this can cause cracking of the skin.
- Thoroughly dry the feet after washing, paying special attention to drying between the toes. Rub in a nonscented, nonmedicated cream if the skin is dry; do not put the cream between the toes.
- Cut the nails along the shape of the toe and file the nails to remove sharp edges. Have corns, calluses, and ingrown nails managed by a podiatrist.
- Wear a clean pair of cotton socks each day.
- Wear properly fitted shoes with a firm sole that do not pinch or bind the foot; never walk barefoot.
- Break in new shoes gradually.
- Never wear open sandals or sandals with straps between the toes.
- Use socks and blankets to warm the feet; do not use a heating pad or hot water bottle near them.
- Test the temperature of bath water with wrist or forearm before stepping into the tub or shower.
- Elevate the feet whenever possible to improve circulation.

Nephropathy. Diabetic nephropathy occurs directly from changes in the renal blood circulation. Factors that influence whether a person with diabetes will develop kidney disease include genetics, blood glucose level, and blood pressure. After years of having to filter too much blood with elevated blood glucose, the filtering mechanism of the kidney begins to fail, allowing large particles that normally would have been filtered out (such as protein) to exit through the urine. In the early phase of albuminuria, there are small amounts of protein in the urine. If nothing is done to prevent further damage, increasing amounts of protein are excreted in the urine. Finally, the patient enters end-stage renal disease and requires either a kidney transplant or dialysis to perform the filtering for the kidneys.

Nephropathy can be delayed and possibly prevented by keeping tight control of blood glucose. Research has demonstrated that tight blood glucose control reduces the risk of developing albuminuria and the progression to renal failure. In patients with type 1 diabetes and early albuminuria and hypertension, angiotensin-converting enzyme (ACE) inhibitors have shown to be beneficial in slowing the elevation of albuminuria (ADA, 2018).

Retinopathy. Visual impairment and blindness are common sequelae of diabetes mellitus. The three most common visual problems are diabetic retinopathy, cataracts, and glaucoma. Retinal damage, which can cause visual impairment and blindness, occurs in most people with diabetes within 20 years of diagnosis. Changes in the retinal vessels lead to hemorrhages and to retinal detachment. A combination of laser intervention and medication has shown to be effective in reducing vision loss. Photocoagulation of destructive lesions of the retina with laser beams, coupled with use of ranibizumab to decrease retinal edema has shown the best outcomes (Bhavsar, 2018). Tight glucose control, frequent eye examinations, and treatment can help preserve vision.

Diabetic neuropathy. Approximately 60% to 70% of people with diabetes have mild to severe neuropathy. Pathologic changes in the nervous system cause symptoms such as paresthesia, numbness, and loss of function. **Diabetic neuropathy** primarily affects the peripheral nerves, causing sexual impotence in men, constipation, neurogenic bladder, and pain or anesthesia (lack of feeling) in the lower extremities. It is for this reason that foot care and daily inspection of the feet are so important. Because the patient often cannot feel cuts, blisters, or abrasions on the foot, there is great danger that a neglected sore might become infected. Although it may be mild at the beginning, eventually partial or almost total anesthesia of the affected part creates a potential for serious injury without awareness. In contrast, some patients experience debilitating pain and hyperesthesia; some lose deep tendon reflexes. No single therapy has been shown to effectively treat pain from diabetic neuropathy. Other problems related to diabetic neuropathies are the result of autonomic nervous system involvement. These include orthostatic hypotension, delayed gastric emptying or **gastroparesis**, diarrhea or constipation, and asymptomatic retention of urine in the bladder.

NURSING MANAGEMENT

ASSESSMENT (DATA COLLECTION)

Assess every patient for signs and symptoms of potential diabetes mellitus. Assess the skin for signs of poor wound healing or areas of infection. The feet should be inspected for signs of beginning sores. The patient should be weighed to determine whether weight is within normal limits.

Focused Assessment

Data Collection for Diabetes

The following questions should be asked to establish a database that indicates whether the patient may have diabetes, has poorly controlled diabetes, or has no signs of diabetes:

- Has anyone in your family ever been told they have diabetes? What about your parents and grandparents?
- Have you had any recent weight loss or weight gain?
- Have you become increasingly hungry over the past few months?
- Has your thirst increased? Are you drinking more fluids than you used to?
- Do you have to urinate (go to the toilet) more than you used to?
- Have you noticed that you are more tired than you were 6 months ago?
- Do you have any trouble with scratches and wounds healing or becoming infected?
- Have you noticed any numbness or tingling or "funny" sensations in your hands, legs, or feet?
- Is constipation becoming a problem?
- Are you having any sexual difficulties? Any impotence (men)? Any frequent vaginal infections (women)?

If the patient is known to have diabetes, ask these questions also:

- Do you feel that you can easily and correctly perform your blood glucose determinations? (Check the patient's performance using their own machine.)
- Are you having any trouble sticking to your dietary plan?
- How are you planning your meals?
- Are you taking your insulin or other antidiabetic medication(s) regularly?
- Are you having any problems related to the medication(s)?
- Are you keeping records of your blood glucose readings and your insulin injections? (Check records, if available.)
- Are you seeing your primary health care provider at regular intervals?
- Are you having your eyes examined regularly?
- Are you visiting the dentist regularly?

For a patient newly diagnosed with diabetes, you must assess whether the patient is a good candidate for using a **glucometer** (blood glucose–monitoring machine) (Fig. 37.6). The patient must have adequate peripheral circulation to easily obtain a drop of blood for the test. Manual dexterity is needed to perform the fingerstick to obtain a blood sample, place the blood in the right spot, and correctly read the meter. Patients with arthritis or visual impairment may have difficulty with these steps. The patient must be able to remember

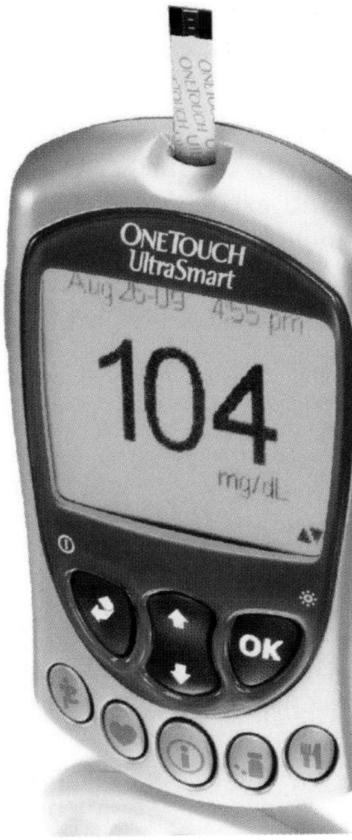

Fig. 37.6 Blood glucose monitor. (Courtesy OneTouch, part of Johnson & Johnson.)

the correct sequence of the steps and remember to do it at the designated times. Determining whether the patient can cope with learning the procedure and whether there is willingness to fit it into the daily routine are other assessment factors. Periodic assessment of glucose monitoring techniques, medication administration, and compliance with treatment regimen is essential. CGM can be used for those patients unable to manage a glucometer. The device can display the tissue glucose and signals a result that is too high or too low, alerting the patient to view the blood glucose value and to take corrective action (Peters, 2018).

◆ NURSING DIAGNOSIS

The following problem statements are common for patients with diabetes mellitus:

- Altered nutrition due to alterations in insulin availability or use.
- Insufficient knowledge due to newly diagnosed disease process, possible complications, and self-care needs.
- Potential for infection due to elevated blood glucose level.
- Limited coping due to needed lifestyle changes for disease management.
- Altered sensory perception due to effect of elevated blood glucose on vascular and nervous systems.
- Potential for injury due to decrease in tissue perfusion and sensation in feet.
- Pain due to nerve damage secondary to peripheral vascular disease.

There are many other nursing problems related to the various complications that patients with diabetes may develop. Nursing care plans must be carefully individualized to the problems and needs of each patient (Nursing Care Plan 37.1).

◆ PLANNING

When caring for a patient with diabetes, you should know the schedule for meal tray delivery and plan glucose testing and insulin injections for appropriate times. Fingersticks for blood glucose testing should be performed 30 minutes before breakfast. If 1 hour has elapsed without insulin being given after the reading was obtained, the test must be repeated before insulin administration. If rapid-acting insulin is ordered, it should not be given until the food tray is in front of the patient.

When a patient is NPO for tests or procedures, monitor for signs of hypoglycemia and obtain the patient's food tray immediately, when the patient returns from testing. The insulin dose should be adjusted according to health care provider order during the NPO period; insulin should not be withheld. Hyperglycemia must be anticipated and assessed for during hospitalization when the patient is undergoing the added stress of diagnostic testing, unknown diagnosis, unrelieved physical distress, new medications, or surgery.

To prevent delays, make certain that the patient's insulin, appropriate syringes, or oral medication are readily available. Examples of expected outcomes for a patient with diabetes mellitus include the following:

- Patient will demonstrate understanding of glucose monitoring and glucose-lowering medications.
- Patient will attain a body weight within normal limits within 6 months.
- Patient will demonstrate knowledge of disease process, possible complications, and self-care methods.
- Patient will consistently monitor for signs of infection.
- Patient will develop coping methods to perform self-care.
- Patient will verbalize ways to preserve and protect vision.
- Patient will demonstrate methods to prevent injury to feet.
- Patient will verbalize that pain is within acceptable limits (using pain scale) after medication and nonpharmaceutical measures are administered.

◆ IMPLEMENTATION

Intervention is geared toward assisting the patient with self-care, performing blood glucose determinations, administering medication when the patient is ill and cannot self-administer, observing for signs and symptoms of complications, assessing learning needs, and carrying out a teaching plan as indicated. Be sure to encourage others involved in the patient's care to be alert for signs and symptoms.

Assignment Considerations

Observations

Remind the unlicensed assistive personnel (UAP) to report any breaks in the skin observed while giving physical care to a patient with diabetes. Report excessive urination or changes in vital signs, such as increasingly rapid respirations.

Nursing Care Plan 37.1 Care of a Patient With Diabetes Mellitus

SCENARIO

Mr. Blackburn, age 49 years, is 5 ft 7 in tall and weighs 350 lb. He was to be admitted to the hospital for surgical repair of a hernia. During the preoperative evaluation, his blood glucose value was 420 mg/dL. On further examination by the health care provider, Mr. Blackburn reported symptoms of extreme thirst, hunger, and excessive urination. Surgery was rescheduled; further workup confirmed the suspected diagnosis of type 2 diabetes mellitus. Mr. Blackburn was extremely upset at learning the diagnosis and not being able to have his surgery. His response to the diagnosis was to ask the surgeon if he could be prescribed "some pills" and "get on with it." He has been admitted to the telemetry unit for dehydration and hyperkalemia.

PROBLEM STATEMENT/NURSING DIAGNOSIS

Excessive potassium and fluid deficit related to diabetes diagnosis.

SUPPORTING ASSESSMENT DATA

Objective: Potassium 6.2 mmol/L; poor skin turgor, BP 90/60, HR 102.

Goals/Expected Outcomes	Nursing Interventions	Selected Rationale	Evaluation
Patient will have fluid and electrolyte imbalance corrected without complications.	Continuous telemetry monitoring. Any abnormalities in cardiac rhythm will be promptly identified and reported	Dehydration and alteration in insulin effectiveness will cause elevated serum potassium, which can cause cardiac arrhythmias.	Sinus tachycardia on the monitor. No dyspnea, numbness, or tingling.
	IV fluids and medications as ordered, watching for signs of hypokalemia and fluid overload.	As fluids and antidiabetic medications are given, potassium may shift back into cells, producing hypokalemia. Large volumes of IV fluid may result in fluid overload.	Lungs clear, urine output 500 cc of clear yellow urine. No muscle cramping.

PROBLEM STATEMENT/NURSING DIAGNOSIS

Altered nutritional status/imbalanced nutrition: more than body requirements related to alteration in glucose use by cells.

SUPPORTING ASSESSMENT DATA

Objective: Blood glucose 420 mg/dL; weighs 350 lb.

Goals/Expected Outcomes	Nursing Interventions	Selected Rationale	Evaluation
Patient will develop meal plan that will assist in maintaining ideal body weight and blood sugar within normal limits.	Perform dietary assessment (i.e., typical intake, nutritional knowledge, cultural preferences).	Patient's current diet and general knowledge of nutrition and cultural preferences can be considered and modified.	Normally eats a lot of fast foods but likes fruits and vegetables and would like to improve diet.
Patient will demonstrate knowledge of correct meal planning within 3 mo.	Instruct in diabetic meal planning and carbohydrate counting. Consult with diabetic educator and/or dietitian.	The relationship of meal planning to control of chronic disease is new information.	States that he "doesn't get it" when asked about meal planning and carbohydrate counting.
	Assist with construction of an acceptable meal plan for attaining desired weight and to normalize serum glucose levels.	Any meal plan must be individualized for weight goals, lifestyle, and food preferences.	Able to correctly identify appropriate portion sizes of sample menu.
Hemoglobin A_{1c} and fructosamine assay levels will show compliance with dietary plan within 6 mo.	Reinforce health care provider's instructions to follow up for repeat laboratory tests and for additional dietary education.	Long-term goal is to achieve: Normal value A_{1c}: 3.9%–5.2% (of total hemoglobin) Normal value fructosamine assay: 1.5–2.7 mmol/L	A_{1c} and fructosamine assay level and reassessment of dietary success to be done at follow-up.

PROBLEM STATEMENT/NURSING DIAGNOSIS

Insufficient knowledge/deficient knowledge related to disease process, possible complications, and self-care.

Nursing Care Plan 37.1 Care of a Patient With Diabetes Mellitus—cont'd

SUPPORTING ASSESSMENT DATA

Subjective: Patient asks health care provider if he could be prescribed "some pills" and "get on with it."

Goals/Expected Outcomes	Nursing Interventions	Selected Rationale	Evaluation
Patient will verbalize basic knowledge about disease process within 1 mo.	Instruct patient about the disease process of diabetes using a variety of teaching methodologies based on the content and learning style.	Varied methods that target the patient's learning style (i.e., written material, demonstrations, videos) increase retention of information.	Patient verbalized basic knowledge of disease process.
Patient will verbalize ways to prevent the complications of diabetes within 3 mo.	Instruct on the potential complications of diabetes and how to decrease the risk of complications.	Knowledge empowers patient to achieve self-care and to take preventive measures.	Patient states, "I need to lose weight." Patient acknowledges complications of diabetes but states he needs more information.
	Instruct in oral medication or insulin administration.	Long-term self-management of medication is essential.	Very resistant to the idea of insulin injections but shows interest in learning about oral medications.
Patient will demonstrate proper foot care within 1 mo.	Instruct in proper foot care techniques (i.e., daily inspection, cleaning, foot attire).	Poor circulation and peripheral neuropathy can lead to infection or amputation.	Demonstrates proper foot care.
	Seek feedback on material taught by verbalization and demonstration of skills.	Provides opportunity for reinforcement or praise. Reteaching or redesign of materials might be necessary.	Expresses appreciation for time spent in teaching him about various topics; requests written information about foot care and medication side effects.

PROBLEM STATEMENT/NURSING DIAGNOSIS

Potential for injury/risk for unstable glucose level related to type 2 diabetes mellitus diagnosis.

SUPPORTING ASSESSMENT DATA

Objective: Admitting blood glucose 420 mg/dL.

Goals/Expected Outcomes	Nursing Interventions	Selected Rationale	Evaluation
Patient will have a premeal blood glucose of 70-140 mg/dL while in the hospital.	Monitor the blood sugar before meals and at bedtime or as ordered.	Illness and stress will affect blood sugar level and patient is newly diagnosed, so response to therapy must be closely monitored.	Blood glucose 230 mg/dL at 6:00 A.M. Health care provider aware, and order for correction dose of insulin obtained.
	Monitor for signs of hypoglycemia (i.e., hunger, sweating, confusion) and hyperglycemia (i.e., increased urination, thirst, rapid breathing).	Hypoglycemia must be treated immediately because brain cells need a continuous source of glucose. Hyperglycemia can cause long-term damage but can also be life threatening if ketoacidosis occurs.	Does not exhibit any signs of hypoglycemia (i.e., weakness, anxiety, palpitations) or hyperglycemia (i.e., nausea, acetone breath, or dry mucous membranes). "Feels pretty good, considering."
Patient will demonstrate blood glucose levels within acceptable limits within 1 mo.	Instruct in glucose monitoring technique appropriate to patient.	Proper instruction, including return demonstration, is important in ascertaining correct fingerstick values.	Able to perform fingerstick and check value. "I'm good with gadgets."
	Instruct to record blood glucose findings after testing.	Keeping a daily record is important in monitoring day-to-day fluctuations in blood glucose.	Likes to keep records. "It's good to have the data right where I can see it." Continue plan.

Continued

Nursing Care Plan 37.1 Care of a Patient With Diabetes Mellitus—cont'd

PROBLEM STATEMENT/NURSING DIAGNOSIS

Altered self-esteem/situational low self-esteem due to diagnosis of chronic disease requiring lifestyle changes or insulin injections for survival.

SUPPORTING ASSESSMENT DATA

Objective: Patient with newly diagnosed diabetes.

Goals/Expected Outcomes	Nursing Interventions	Selected Rationale	Evaluation
Patient will verbalize own strengths within 1 mo.	Encourage verbalization of feelings related to diagnosis of diabetes and need for lifestyle changes. Allow expression of frustrations.	Verbalization of feelings is an important first step toward identifying one's own strengths. Frustration is a normal human response to a real or perceived threat.	Initially very quiet; appears withdrawn and angry after health care provider informs of new diagnosis of diabetes mellitus. "I guess I am taking out my frustrations on you and the doctor." Reassured that frustration is normal.
Patient will express that control over the disease and life is possible.	Encourage exploration of strengths and positive measures of self-worth (i.e., roles, accomplishments).	Remembering past achievements can help patients realize their strengths.	States, "I am a hard worker. I own my own business—I can certainly learn to manage this too."
	Explain how control over disease and life is possible.	After feelings are expressed, patient will be more receptive to information. Knowledge and tools can help him achieve control.	"I think I am beginning to understand. Balancing food intake and insulin is like balancing a spreadsheet of expenditures at my business."
	Praise efforts at learning and practice of self-care techniques.	Positive reinforcement is a powerful tool for helping a patient accomplish acceptance of a situation.	Goal met. Reevaluate as needed.

CRITICAL THINKING QUESTIONS

1. The RN has planned the first teaching session for Mr. Blackburn, which you are to help implement. The topics planned for today include meal planning, short-term complications of diabetes, long-term complications of diabetes, foot care, and actions/side effects/interactions of OHAs. If the RN asked for your collaboration on the plan, what would you recommend?
2. Mr. Blackburn has visitors coming to see him. You greet them in the hallway and notice they are carrying bags from Dunkin' Donuts and cartons of Ben & Jerry's. How would you respond to this situation?

BP, Blood pressure; *HR*, heart rate; *IV*, intravenous.

Monitor the trend of blood glucose, A_{1c}, and fructosamine assay readings over time rather than focus only on the current reading. Assess how well the patient is eating and taking fluids. Intake and output recordings are appropriate if the patient is ill or having surgery. Any type of stress can alter the control of the patient's diabetes. Electrolytes also should be monitored, with particular attention paid to potassium levels, which can shift suddenly when insulin is insufficient.

Every patient taking insulin should be monitored for hypoglycemia after insulin injections. After injection of each type of insulin, you must know when hypoglycemia might occur and should assess the patient at that time. Patients are taught to report signs of hypoglycemia promptly, to prevent a crisis.

Monitoring for signs of ketoacidosis also is essential. Some of the earliest symptoms may be polyuria, fatigue, anorexia, abdominal pain, and a "fruity" smell to the breath. Look for beginning signs of dehydration with decreased tissue turgor, sunken eyeballs, and dry mucous membranes (see Table 37.4). Report such findings to the health care provider promptly.

Patient Education

The patient must be able to self-manage diet, medication, and progress. In addition, adjustments in lifestyle, recreational choices, and self-image will probably need to be made. The patient must be taught the correct steps for blood glucose monitoring (see Fig. 37.6).

Nonadherence to the treatment plan can be devastating to the patient's welfare and can mean the difference between leading a nearly normal life or becoming an invalid; eventually, not managing the disease may mean the difference between life and death for a person with diabetes. Many hospitals and clinics have developed standardized teaching programs for diabetes education because the task of diabetic teaching is very challenging and complex (see Fig. 37.3).

Major topics covered in a standardized program usually include the following:

- Pathophysiology of diabetes mellitus, including functions of the pancreas and contributing or precipitating factors in the development of diabetes
- How to manage a diet program
- Blood glucose monitoring at home
- Foot care
- Urine testing when blood glucose level is higher than 240 mg/dL to check for acetone
- Identification tag, identification card, and medical information (see Fig. 37.1)
- Information on what to do on "sick" days, especially when nauseated or vomiting and unable to maintain diet
- Community resources and help groups available to patient with diabetes and family
- Travel tips
- Devices that make insulin administration easier (especially for older adults, visually impaired patients, or patients with arthritis)

Patient Teaching

What to Do on Sick Days

A bad cold, flu, or minor gastrointestinal upset can create problems for diabetic patients.

MEDICATION

- Take insulin as prescribed. Adjust the dosage as directed, depending on blood glucose readings.
- If taking an oral hypoglycemic, take usual dose. Do not increase the dose unless ordered to do so by the health care provider. If vomiting and unable to take medication by mouth, the health care provider may temporarily prescribe insulin.

DIET

- Eat a normal diet on schedule.
- If nausea and vomiting occur, replace carbohydrate solid foods in the normal diet with liquids that contain sugar (fruit juice, regular soft drinks, or Jell-O).
- Take at least 1 cup of water or calorie-free, caffeine-free liquid each hour. If nauseated, take small sips to help prevent vomiting.

MONITORING

- Test blood glucose at least every 4 hours and record result. If severely ill, check blood glucose every 2 hours.
- Test urine for ketones if blood sugar level is higher than 300 mg/dL.

NOTIFYING THE HEALTH CARE PROVIDER

- Call the health care provider right away for vomiting, abdominal pain, or a temperature higher than 100.2° F (38.8° C).
- Notify the health care provider if blood glucose is higher than 200 mg/dL or if urine test shows ketones.
- Report to the health care provider if blood glucose level that was higher than 200 mg/dL does not come down with an additional dose of insulin.
- If unable to reach the health care provider, go to the hospital emergency department.

Patient Teaching

Instructions for Traveling

- Carry twice the medication or insulin you expect to need in case of travel delays. Take copies of prescriptions with you. Wear a medical alert bracelet or tag and carry a medical information card in a purse or wallet.
- Carry an emergency supply of fast-acting sugar at all times in case of a hypoglycemic episode. Also carry longer-acting foods, such as peanut butter and crackers.
- Pack dried fruit, nuts, and seeds as snacks. Because these are high in calories, measure portions in advance.
- Check your blood sugar frequently. Changes in time zones, eating, and activity level can affect blood glucose.
- If ill, seek medical attention immediately before a dangerous condition occurs.
- Stick to prescribed meal plans as much as possible, substituting available foods according to food group classification.
- Obtain sufficient rest and avoid stressful situations as much as possible to prevent stress-induced hyperglycemia.
- It is best to travel with someone who is familiar with diabetes and treatment. It is advisable to inform the airline or ship personnel about the diabetes.
- Obtain the usual amount of exercise or adjust food and medication accordingly.
- Drink a glass of water every 2 hours to prevent dehydration.
- Protect insulin from temperature extremes.
- Eat something at least every 4 hours.
- Call airlines and ship companies ahead of departure to request diabetic meals or take your own.
- Before departure, research food substitutions, so that personal meal plans are consistent.
- Remember time zones: going westward lengthens the day; take more insulin. Going eastward shortens the day; take less insulin.

The patient and significant others, staff nurses, health care providers, diabetic specialist, nurse educator, dietitian, podiatrist, and periodontist are all involved in the educational process. Because of frequent updates and changes in diabetes management, all persons responsible for the care of patients with diabetes should read and continue to study and learn about the current protocols.

◆ EVALUATION

For a patient with diabetes, the learning that has taken place and compliance with the treatment regimen are the essential components. Monitor A_{1c} and fructosamine assay levels to determine the degree of control of blood glucose. Question the patient about exercise and diet and give feedback. Observe demonstrations of learned skills for insulin injection, proper foot care, dietary planning, and glucose monitoring. If the expected outcomes are not being met, the nursing care plan must

Patient Teaching

Working With an Older Adult Who Has Diabetes

- Assess hearing and vision. Use aids as appropriate and ensure adequate lighting.
- Set a time for the teaching session that is agreeable to the patient.
- Arrange a quiet, nondistracting environment for the session.
- Be certain that the patient is comfortable before beginning.
- Keep the sessions short—no more than 15 to 20 minutes at a time.
- Limit information to a few major concepts per session.
- Go slowly and seek feedback that the patient has understood each point when finished presenting it.
- Allow time for the patient to jot down important points.
- Repeat key concepts frequently; if the patient does not understand, try rephrasing the concept.
- Use bold-type printed materials with a white or yellow background.
- Leave printed materials that are illustrated with simple drawings and that are not crowded with text.
- Printed materials should be written at a fifth- to tenth-grade reading level, depending on the patient.
- If the patient becomes frustrated or distracted, stop the session and reschedule it.
- Summarize what has been taught and what has been learned at the end of the session.

be revised. Collaboration with the health care provider and dietitian is necessary to design or redesign a plan that will be effective.

HYPOGLYCEMIA (NONDIABETIC)

Etiology and Pathophysiology

The organs involved in meeting the challenge of carbohydrate ingestion include the intestines, liver, and pancreas (specifically, the beta cells that produce insulin). Thus any condition affecting these organs and their systems can lead to hypoglycemia. Examples other than diabetes mellitus include gastrectomy and surgical bypass procedures. These types of surgery may restrict adequate glucose absorption. Tumors of the pancreas (insulinomas), liver disease, and disorders of the adrenal cortex and pituitary gland can also produce abnormally low blood glucose levels. People who abuse alcohol and other substances are also prone to hypoglycemia. Hypoglycemia related to diabetes is more common, has a different cause, and is treated differently.

Signs and Symptoms

Signs and symptoms of hypoglycemia include rapid heartbeat, tremulousness, weakness, anxiety, nervousness, and hunger. Symptoms can occur rather suddenly, within 4 hours after a meal is eaten. Some physiologic symptoms may be mistaken for indications of a psychiatric illness. These symptoms include irritability, personality change, temper tantrums, and other psychoneurotic manifestations.

Diagnosis and Treatment

Diagnosis of hypoglycemia is made with measurement of blood glucose values. A source of possible infection is investigated. The patient's insulin levels and C-peptide levels can also be measured. The diagnosis may be made using a glucose tolerance test or a medically supervised fast. Computed tomography (CT) scan, ultrasound, and other diagnostics may be used if an insulinoma (insulin-secreting tumor) is suspected.

Hypoglycemia is treated by modifying eating patterns. Smaller and more frequent meals that are relatively free of simple sugars are recommended. The diet should be high in proteins and low in carbohydrates, and carbohydrates should be complex ones, such as those found in whole fruits, vegetables, and whole grains. Refined sugar and white flour are omitted. Cases in which gastric surgery and intestinal bypass are believed to be the cause of hypoglycemia may be treated with drugs that reduce intestinal motility, allowing for greater absorption.

Complications

Untreated fasting hypoglycemia can lead to severe **neuroglycopenia** (shortage of glucose in the brain) and possibly death.

Nursing Management

In addition to information about the patient's physical and mental symptoms, assessment should include a detailed history of eating habits. Does the patient eat regularly? How often during each day? What kinds of foods constitute a typical meal? Are sweets craved? Have there been episodes of weakness, sweating, visual disturbances, and confusion or inability to concentrate? If these symptoms have occurred, when are they most noticeable (i.e., in a fed or fasting state)? Nursing interventions for patients with hypoglycemia include explaining the nature of the disorder and the need for diagnostic testing, objective observation and reporting of symptoms, and reinforcement of dietary instruction and restrictions.

COMMUNITY CARE

One major objective of *Healthy People 2030* is to "increase the proportion of persons with diagnosed diabetes who ever receive formal diabetes education." Nurses play a crucial role in home care and in teaching the older adult population who have diabetes. If nurses could follow the progress of these patients over the years with good assessments and implement ongoing patient education programs, the incidence of complications could certainly be decreased.

Long-term care nurses must be alert to the signs of diabetes. When a resident does not properly recover from a viral illness, in-depth assessment for signs of diabetes is proactive. Home care and clinic nurses must be persistent in assessing compliance with diabetic regimens and must also be instrumental in teaching the public about the signs and symptoms of diabetes and self-care to prevent complications. At present, diabetes is costing the United States more than $327 billion a year in health care expenditures. This is an area where nurses can be instrumental in cutting health care costs.

Get Ready for the NCLEX® Examination!

Key Points

- Diabetes mellitus involves a disturbance in glucose metabolism. Type 1 diabetes usually appears at a young age, and the patient requires insulin for life. Type 2 diabetes usually develops later in life but is now being diagnosed more frequently in younger people. Gestational diabetes may occur in pregnancy. Patients with LADA may be initially misdiagnosed with type 2 diabetes. The goal in diabetes is to maintain blood glucose and lipid levels within normal limits to prevent complications.
- The cornerstone of therapy for people with diabetes is diet and exercise. Insulin must be taken for type 1 diabetes; OHAs (and insulin) may be prescribed for type 2 diabetes.
- The diet plan provides optimal nutrition and calories to maintain normal body weight and allows adjustments to food intake to keep blood glucose within safe limits.
- The emotional and physical stress of surgery and illness can increase the blood glucose level and alter the amounts of medication needed.
- Basal insulin is the amount of insulin that would normally be produced by the pancreas throughout the day.
- A bolus or "correction" dose of short- or rapid-acting insulin is used to manage elevations in blood glucose and bring the next blood glucose into range.
- DKA is a serious condition caused by incomplete metabolism of fats as a result of the absence of insulin marked by metabolic acidosis, dehydration, and electrolyte imbalances.
- HHS occurs in people with type 2 diabetes because of illness or stress. Glucose levels are often between 600 and 1000 mg/dL, leading to severe dehydration.
- Hypoglycemia is often a response to either too much insulin or too much exercise in patients with diabetes. Monitor for hypoglycemia after insulin injections.
- If there is doubt whether the patient is suffering from hyperglycemia or hypoglycemia, treat for hypoglycemia until you obtain a blood glucose level.
- The long-term consequences of diabetes mellitus result from damage to large and small blood vessels. Cardiovascular disease, nephropathy, peripheral vascular disease, retinopathy, and neuropathy can all be reduced by strict blood glucose control.

Additional Learning Resources

SG Go to your Study Guide for additional learning activities to help you master this chapter content.

Go to your Evolve website (http://evolve.elsevier.com/deWit/medsurg) for the following FREE learning resources:

- Animations, audio, and video
- Answers and rationales for questions and activities
- Glossary with pronunciations in English and Spanish
- Interactive Review Questions and Exercises and more!

Review Questions for the NCLEX® Examination

1. A 30-year-old woman is admitted for urinary tract infection with sepsis. A urinalysis reveals presence of ketones, glucose, and nitrates. Which question would you ask to further assess possible diabetes mellitus?
  1. "Have you noticed an extra roundness to your face?"
  2. "Have you had more gas or abdominal bloating?"
  3. "Have you been thirstier than usual? Do you find you urinate more now?"
  4. "Have you experienced any pain or discomfort with urination?"
  NCLEX Client Need: Physiological Integrity: Physiological Adaptation

2. Which teaching technique(s) would be most useful for an older adult patient with diabetes? *(Select all that apply.)*
  1. Set a time for the teaching session that is agreeable to the patient.
  2. Invite the patient to join a teaching session for patients newly diagnosed with diabetes.
  3. Allow time for the patient to jot down important points.
  4. Use bold-type printed materials with white type on a dark blue or black background.
  5. Limit each session to 1 to 2 hours and give frequent breaks.
  6. Teach all necessary information in one session.
  7. Repeat key concepts frequently; if the patient does not understand, try rephrasing the concept.
  NCLEX Client Need: Health Promotion and Maintenance

3. A patient newly diagnosed with diabetes is given diet instructions. What should you do to effectively motivate the patient to comply with dietary recommendations? *(Select all that apply.)*
  1. Emphasize good food choices.
  2. Apply diet prescriptions to patient-preferred foods.
  3. Instill guilt to self-regulate when "cheating" occurs.
  4. Focus on the benefits of diet compliance.
  5. Involve meal preparers in diet teaching.
  NCLEX Client Need: Health Promotion and Maintenance

4. A 50-year-old woman was recently diagnosed with type 2 diabetes mellitus and wants to start a healthy lifestyle to control her disease. What initial recommendation should you make?
   1. Engage in brisk walking.
   2. Lose 10 to 15 pounds.
   3. Maintain adequate glucose control.
   4. Develop an exercise schedule.

   NCLEX Client Need: Physiological Integrity: Reduction of Risk Potential
5. You answer the call light for a patient with diabetes. The patient states that she feels shaky and weak. You note pallor and moist skin. List your nursing actions in priority order.
   1. Give patient 6 oz of juice.
   2. Document interventions.
   3. Check fingerstick glucose.
   4. Assess level of consciousness.

   NCLEX Client Need: Safe and Effective Care Environment: Coordinated Care
6. A patient who works as a personal trainer is diagnosed with insulin-dependent diabetes. What should you teach about self-administration of regular insulin?
   1. If you have a strenuous workout, skip your insulin for the day.
   2. Inject the insulin before moderate exercise.
   3. Exercise during the insulin peak of action.
   4. Use the abdomen as an insulin injection site.

   NCLEX Client Need: Physiological Integrity: Pharmacological Therapies
7. You are visiting an older adult patient who has successfully managed their type 2 diabetes for years. During the home visit, you note that the patient has severe arthritis; poor vision; and several dry, red areas on the lower extremities. What is the priority patient problem?
   1. Potential for noncompliance due to social circumstances.
   2. Potential for ineffective self-health management due to aging.
   3. Potential for infection due to poor peripheral perfusion.
   4. Potential for disturbed sensory perception due to degenerative changes.

   NCLEX Client Need: Physiological Integrity: Physiological Adaptation
8. You determine that the fingerstick blood glucose reading for a patient with diabetes is 750 mg/dL. What is your priority action?
   1. Immediately notify the registered nurse (RN) and the health care provider.
   2. Assess the vital signs of the patient.
   3. Check the record to verify whether the patient has type 1 or type 2 diabetes.
   4. Administer prescribed sliding scale insulin.

   NCLEX Client Need: Physiological Integrity: Reduction of Risk Potential
9. The nursing assistant tells you that a patient with diabetes has a blood glucose level of 60 mg/dL. What symptoms would you be most likely to observe with this glucose level?
   1. Confusion, tremulousness, pallor, sweating, and weakness
   2. Dry, flushed skin and mild irritability
   3. Deep, rapid breathing and abdominal pain
   4. Incoherent moaning, combativeness, and seizure activity

   NCLEX Client Need: Physiological Integrity: Physiological Adaptation
10. During a routine checkup, the health care provider tells a patient with diabetes that test results reveal albuminuria. Which long-term complication is specific to this test result?
    1. Metabolic syndrome
    2. Nephropathy
    3. Retinopathy
    4. Peripheral vascular disease

    NCLEX Client Need: Physiological Integrity: Reduction of Risk Potential

Critical Thinking Questions

Scenario A

Mrs. Lopez is 42 years old and has had type 2 diabetes mellitus for the past 10 years. She is admitted to the hospital for treatment of an infection of the great toe on her left foot, which is the result of improper care of an ingrown toenail. She is 45 lb overweight and admits to frequent binges of eating foods that are not on her diet. She does not exercise regularly because she says the housework she does gives her enough exercise. When asked about the OHA and diet that have been prescribed for her, she tells you that she takes her medicine and follows her diet "most of the time."

1. Describe the essential components of a teaching plan for Mrs. Lopez to help her manage her illness better. Why is foot care an important part of this plan?
2. What could you suggest to Mrs. Lopez to help her lose weight?
3. What do you think might motivate Mrs. Lopez to accept more responsibility for managing her illness?
4. What laboratory testing would be recommended to track Mrs. Lopez's compliance with the treatment regimen?

Scenario B

Mr. Tobin is a 22-year-old construction worker who has recently experienced fatigue, excessive thirst and urination, and weight loss. A routine urinalysis revealed glycosuria and a trace of acetone. His health care provider has arranged for him to have additional diagnostic testing to determine whether he has diabetes mellitus.

1. If Mr. Tobin is found to have type 1 diabetes mellitus, what kind of information will he need to manage his illness?

2. How would you explain the importance of good or tight control of his blood glucose levels to Mr. Tobin?
3. What criteria could be used to determine whether his diabetes is under control?

Scenario C

Mr. Smith is 76 years old and has recently been diagnosed with type 2 diabetes mellitus. It has been difficult to control his blood sugar, and his health care provider has added insulin to his treatment regimen. Mr. Smith was issued a glucometer by the hospital but says that the test strips are too expensive for him to buy very often. He lives alone, cooks for himself, and likes a glass of wine with dinner. Other than an occasional fishing trip, he does not exercise regularly.

1. How would you approach a teaching program for this patient?
2. What resources could you suggest that might assist him to purchase the test strips for the glucometer?
3. How can a glass of wine be incorporated into an acceptable meal plan for a patient with diabetes?
4. What sort of exercise program could you recommend to this patient?

Scenario D

You are making a home visit to a patient who normally administers her own insulin. On arrival you notice that she has tremulousness, is pale and sweating, and seems more irritable and distractible than usual. She reports taking her insulin, but she is unable to tell you when she took it or exactly how much she injected. She thinks her last food was during supper, last night, but she is unsure.

1. You check her blood glucose level with her home device and get a reading of 55 mg/dL. What does this value indicate?
2. Based on your assessment of the patient's symptoms and the blood glucose level, what is your next nursing action?
3. How will you determine that it is safe to leave the patient?

38 The Reproductive System

http://evolve.elsevier.com/deWit/medsurg

Objectives

Theory

1. Review the female and male reproductive organs and their role in overall health.
2. Compare methods of contraception.
3. Discuss normal physiology considering age-related changes to the female and male reproductive systems.
4. Explain assessment of the female and male reproductive systems.
5. Identify screening procedures recommended for maintaining reproductive health.
6. Explain how to provide culturally competent care for patients who are LGBTQ.
7. Distinguish the nurse's role during screening procedures, data collection, and education of patients concerning reproductive health.

Clinical Practice

8. Teach principles of breast and vulva self-examination to female patients.
9. Teach testicular examination to male patients.

Key Terms

androgens (ĂN-drō-jĕnz, p. 918)
climacteric (klī-MĂK-tĕr-ĭk, p. 906)
ejaculation (ē-jăk-ū-LĀ-shŭn, p. 918)
erection (ĕ-RĔK-shŭn, p. 918)
fibroids (FĪ-broydz, p. 914)
gonads (GŌ-năds, p. 916)
libido (lĭ-BĒ-dō, p. 919)
menarche (mĕ-NĂR-kē, p. 906)
menopause (MĔN-ō-păwz, p. 906)
menses (mĕn-sēz, p. 906)
menstruation (mĕn-strū-Ā-shŭn, p. 906)
prostate-specific antigen (PSA) (PRŎS-tāt spĕ-SĬ-fĭk ĂN-tĭ-jĕn, p. 920)
rugae (RŪ-jē, p. 916)
semen (SĒ-mĕn, p. 918)
spermatogenesis (spĕr-mă-tō-JĔ-nĕ-sĭs, p. 918)
vasectomy (vă-SĔK-tō-mē, p. 919)

Concepts Covered in This Chapter

- Development
- Hormonal Regulation
- Reproduction
- Sexuality

THE FEMALE REPRODUCTIVE SYSTEM

The female reproductive system depends on hormones produced by the endocrine system for correct development and reproductive function. A variety of hormones released in a specific order at specific times trigger the formation of internal and external sexual organs in the developing fetus. Puberty and sexual maturation are also dependent on accurate release of hormones at the appropriate time in the cycle. As the childbearing years draw to a close, hormone production slows until the reproductive cycle stops altogether.

Reproductive health can be disrupted by a variety of disorders, such as infertility; spontaneous abortion; premature labor; infection; and the growth of abnormal tissue, including cancerous and noncancerous tumors. Nursing care of patients with diseases of the female reproductive system, discussed in Chapter 39, is further complicated by the emotional effects of such disorders. The reproductive organs represent the biological aspect of sexual identity, and women may feel that their personal identity is compromised by disorders of this system.

ANATOMY AND PHYSIOLOGY OF THE FEMALE REPRODUCTIVE SYSTEM

PRIMARY EXTERNAL STRUCTURES

The **vulva,** or **pudendum,** is the external female genitalia. It is made up of the following structures:

- The **mons pubis** is a rounded mound of fatty tissue that protects the symphysis pubis. It is covered with pubic hair.

- The **labia majora** are two elongated, raised folds of pigmented skin that enclose the vulvar cleft. The pubic hair extends along these folds.
- The **labia minora** are soft folds of skin within the labia majora. They are soft, shiny, and made up of fat tissue and glands and have no hair follicles.
- The **clitoris** is located at the top of the vulvar cleft, above the urethral opening. It is made up primarily of erectile tissue and is highly sensitive to touch. It is a primary source of pleasurable sensation during sexual activity.
- The **urethral meatus,** or external opening of the urethra of the urinary bladder, is located below the clitoris within the folds of the labia minora.
- The **vaginal vestibule** is situated below the urethral meatus within the labia minora and is the entrance to the vagina.
- The **perineum** is the flat muscular surface between the vagina and the anus.

PRIMARY INTERNAL STRUCTURES

- The **vagina** is a muscular tube lined with membranous tissue with transverse ridges called rugae. It connects the external and internal female sexual organs (Fig. 38.1).
- The **uterus** (womb) is a hollow pear-shaped organ with a thick muscular wall. It lies at the upper end of the vagina. It can expand to many times its normal size to accommodate a growing fetus. The lower opening of the uterus is the **cervix,** which dilates during labor to allow for delivery of the infant.
- There are two **fallopian tubes** that branch outward from the right and left sides at the top of the uterus. They form the pathway for the **ovum** (egg) from the ovary to the uterus.
- There are two **ovaries,** one located near the end of each fallopian tube. These almond-shaped glands excrete estrogen and progesterone into the bloodstream. At birth, the ovaries contain all the eggs (**oocytes**—primitive ova or eggs) the woman will ever produce, approximately 2 million in each ovary (McCance & Huether, 2019), most of which will never mature for possible fertilization.
- The **bony pelvis,** located at the base of the body between the hips, supports the pelvic organs, including the growing uterus during pregnancy. It is assisted by the **pelvic floor,** a collection of strong muscles and supportive tissues that brace the pelvis and provide both support and protection for the pelvic organs.

ACCESSORY ORGANS

- The breasts or **mammary glands,** located on the upper chest, are the accessory organs. They are composed of fibrous, adipose, and glandular tissue and are responsible for **lactation** (milk production), which provides nourishment for the infant.

PHASES OF THE FEMALE REPRODUCTIVE CYCLE DURING THE CHILDBEARING YEARS

- The **ovarian cycle** has two phases:
  - *Follicular phase*: This is the first 14 days of a 28-day cycle. **Follicle-stimulating hormone (FSH)** and **luteinizing hormone (LH)** stimulate the maturation of ova in preparation for fertilization. Estrogen peaks when the ovum is released **(ovulation),** about 14 days before the next menstrual period. The ovum lives up to 24 hours after fertilization.
  - *Luteal phase:* This is days 15 to 28 of a 28-day cycle. LH and progesterone are the primary hormones

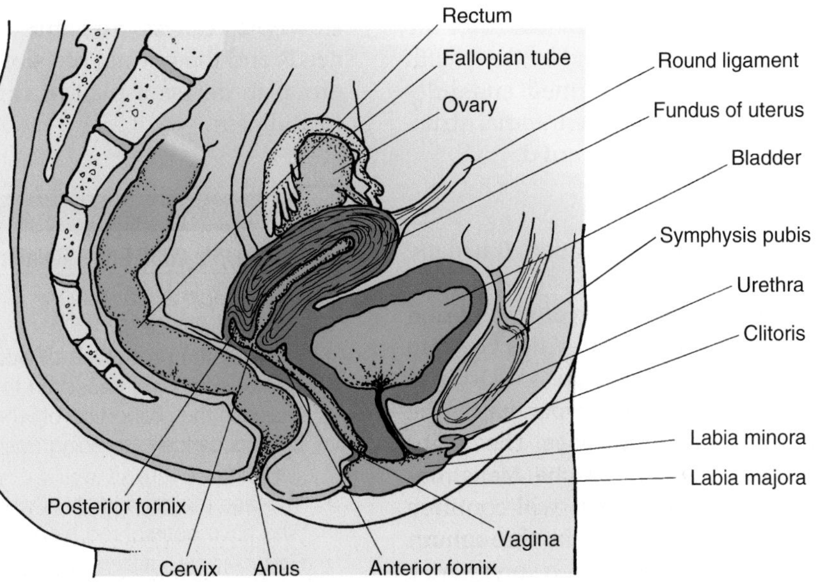

Fig. 38.1 Female reproductive organs.

Box 38.1 Stages of the Menstrual Cycle

DAYS 1 TO 5

Stage I: Menstrual Stage (Dismantling Stage)

1. Endometrium sloughs away as menstrual flow begins.
2. Progesterone and estrogen are no longer secreted.
3. New follicle starts to mature.

DAYS 6 TO 14

Stage II: Growth and Repair (Estrogen or Proliferative Stage)

1. Follicle grows, and egg matures.
2. Endometrium returns to normal state and then begins to thicken in response to estrogen.

Stage III: Ovulation

1. Ovulation occurs 14 days before menses, regardless of length of menstrual cycle. It takes place when the follicle ruptures and releases egg. If pregnancy does not occur, the corpus luteum deteriorates, estrogen and progesterone decline, and the thickened tissue on the endometrium of the uterus is sloughed off and is discharged via the vagina as a menstrual "period."

DAYS 15 TO 28

Stage IV: Secretory Stage (Postovulatory or Progesterone Stage)

1. Corpus luteum secretes progesterone.
2. Endometrium continues to thicken in response to estrogen and progesterone. Uterus prepares to receive fertilized ovum.

released in this phase. The blood supply to the uterus increases in preparation for possible implantation of a fertilized ovum. If fertilization and implantation do not occur, the lining of the uterus will degrade and be shed during menstruation, and the cycle begins again.

- The **menstrual cycle** has four phases (Box 38.1).

SEXUAL DEVELOPMENT IN THE FETUS

- During the first weeks of pregnancy, the male and female sexual organs are undifferentiated. After the seventh week, rapid changes occur, and by the twelfth week the external genitalia are formed and fully differentiated as male or female. The internal structures also are forming during this period.

SEXUAL MATURATION

- *Puberty* is the period of sexual maturation. It usually occurs between ages 9 and 17 years for girls; the average onset is 12 years of age. It involves a period of accelerated growth, after which the hips begin to widen and the breasts begin to develop. Axillary and pubic hair appears. Puberty is accompanied by the onset of the menstrual cycle, or **menses**. The beginning of menstruation is called **menarche. Menstruation** (shedding of the uterine lining) will continue at intervals of approximately 4 weeks throughout the childbearing years, except when pregnancy occurs.

MENOPAUSE

Toward the end of the childbearing years, women become **perimenopausal,** entering the phase known as the **climacteric** period. The menses become irregular in both pattern and flow and eventually stop altogether. **Menopause** has occurred when the menses have completely ceased for at least 12 months (Huether & McCance, 2019).

Signs and symptoms of the climacteric period and menopause include hot flashes (a sensation of warmth), hot flushes (a visible redness and moistness of the skin), and night sweats caused by vasomotor instability resulting from low estrogen levels. These symptoms usually decrease as the woman's body adjusts to the lower level of estrogen. Changes in the menstrual flow and menstrual irregularity require the woman to always be prepared for an unexpected menstrual period.

WOMEN'S HEALTH CARE

Women's health care involves the promotion of physical, psychological, and spiritual well-being.

Women continue to be increasingly economically independent and empowered to make health care decisions, although some do live alone with below-poverty-level income and lack caregivers or easy access to health care facilities. Health care education for adolescents includes information about puberty, menstruation, and sexuality. Teenagers and young women need information about safer sex, contraceptives, and choices concerning high-risk behaviors. Adult women require information about Papanicolaou (Pap) smears, breast self-examination, nutrition, exercise, and lifestyle management. Perinatal education is important. Older women require information about menopause, long-term illness, and disabilities that affect health care needs. Women of all ages need to be knowledgeable about the function of their bodies, health care needs, and signs and symptoms of wellness, as well as illness. You must understand all of these needs and the normal physiologic changes of each age group to devise a plan of care to maintain health or treat illness.

Clinical Cues

***Healthy People 2030* Goals Related to Women's Health Care**

Healthy People 2030 includes the following goals related to women's health care:

- Increase the proportion of women who receive a breast cancer screening based on the most recent guidelines
- Increase the proportion of women who receive a cervical cancer screening based on the most recent guidelines
- Increase the proportion of women of childbearing age who have optimal red blood cell folate concentrations
- Reduce pelvic inflammatory disease in women aged 15-24 years

NORMAL MENSTRUATION

During the first year after menarche, the menstrual cycle may be somewhat irregular, but by the second year, a regular cycle of approximately 28 days is normally established.

Attitudes and ideas regarding menstruation are formed early. They are based on the thoughts and beliefs expressed by other women and on personal experience. Incorrect perceptions about this normal process may increase physical discomfort or cause a young woman unnecessary embarrassment or fear. Although there has been significant improvement in communication with preadolescent young women about the changes they will experience, many still need further education. It is important for nurses to understand their own attitudes about sexuality and reproduction before attempting to provide information for women on these very personal issues. A healthy view of menarche as a natural physiologic process marking reproductive maturity should be encouraged.

Normal Menstrual Bleeding

Menstrual bleeding occurs about 14 days after ovulation and lasts between 2 and 8 days. Menstrual blood consists of endometrial tissue, blood, mucus, and vaginal and cervical cells. The amount of actual blood loss is only 30 to 80 mL (McCance & Huether, 2019). Blood flow may be heavy at first but gradually reduces to spotting. The color may change from bright red to brown, and the blood may have a musty odor. Once a menstrual pattern is established, a change from this pattern is reason to consult a health care provider. The length of the cycle can be influenced by stress, drugs, nutrition, and illness. Women should be encouraged to keep a calendar of their individual menstrual cycle to determine regularity and recognize deviations. Mild cramping may occur, and some mood swings may be associated with the hormonal changes. **Mittelschmerz** is a sharp pain in the right or left lower quadrant, sometimes felt at midcycle around the time of ovulation, and may last a few hours. Some women are sensitive to this phenomenon, and others never experience it.

Normal Vaginal Discharge

The vagina is a warm, moist, dark vault in which microorganisms can flourish. Normal vaginal secretions contain cervical mucus, endometrial fluid, exudate from the Bartholin glands and Skene ducts, and products of normal flora. The main line of defense against infection is lactic acid, which causes an acidic pH. Any change in this pH can result in infection. An increase in secretions normally occurs during pregnancy and at the midpoint of the menstrual cycle when ovulation occurs, and a decrease in secretions normally occurs after menopause.

Normal vaginal discharge has an off-white color and is odorless. If the vaginal discharge develops an odor, changes in color or consistency, or causes irritation or burning of the vaginal mucosa, a health care provider should be consulted.

THE NORMAL BREAST

Breasts are made of adipose tissue, milk-producing glands called lobules, ducts, and fibrous tissue that rest on the chest muscle. They may not be completely symmetric (one may be slightly larger than the other) and may feel a bit lumpy and tender, especially during the middle of the menstrual cycle. Age, pregnancy, medication, and diet can affect the way the breasts feel. As women age, the denseness and adipose tissue content decrease, whereas birth control pills, hormone replacement therapy, and pregnancy may cause the breasts to increase in size.

CONTRACEPTION

Many sexually active women of childbearing age are concerned about regulating, planning, or preventing pregnancy. Information about techniques of contraception is essential to provide to prevent unwanted, unintended pregnancies. With the assistance of a health care provider, women can select the birth control method best suited to their physical health; sexual activity; desire to have children at a future date; cultural, spiritual, and religious beliefs about family planning; and lifestyle.

Contraceptive Options

Women should make an informed decision concerning methods of reliable birth control, and you are responsible for providing comprehensive education concerning the advantages, limitations, and side effects of the various contraceptive drugs and devices available. Some methods of birth control provide protection against STIs, wheras others do not. Newer contraceptive regimens reduce the hormone-free interval, thereby decreasing the occurrence of menstrual periods. The most effective contraceptive methods for adolescents and young adults include abstinence, the use of planned contraception, the correct use of condoms to prevent STIs, and lifestyle counseling. In the United States, 41% of high school students reported sexual experience, 43% denied using a condom, and 14% denied using any form of protection (Centers for Disease Control and Prevention [CDC], 2016). *Healthy People 2030* goals include increasing condom use among sexually active unmarried males and females. Fig. 38.2 illustrates the correct application of a condom and a diaphragm. Table 38.1 reviews the various methods of contraception.

Natural Family Planning

Natural family planning, also known as fertility awareness, involves identifying signs of ovulation and abstaining from intercourse during periods of fertility. (The ovum is viable up to 24 hours after ovulation, and the sperm are viable up to 72 hours in the fallopian tube.) The **basal body temperature (BBT)** technique

HOW TO USE A MALE CONDOM

1. Apply condom before any contact with vagina because sperm are present in secretions *before* ejaculation.
2. Squeeze air from the tip of condom, and hold it while unrolling condom over erect penis. Leave a half-inch space at tip.

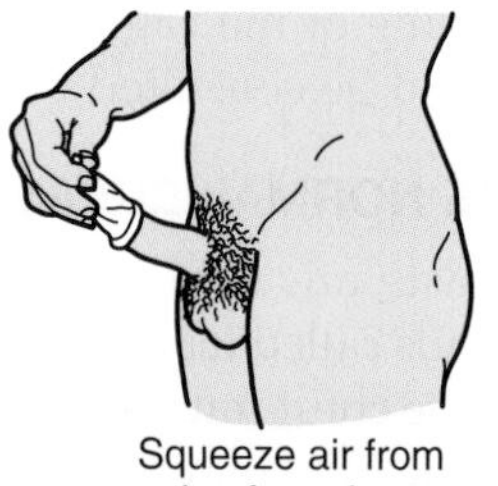

3. Use water-soluble lubricants, if needed.
4. To remove condom, hold it at the base of penis to prevent spillage as you withdraw from the vagina.
5. Dispose and use a new one each time. Be sure to check expiration date on condoms.

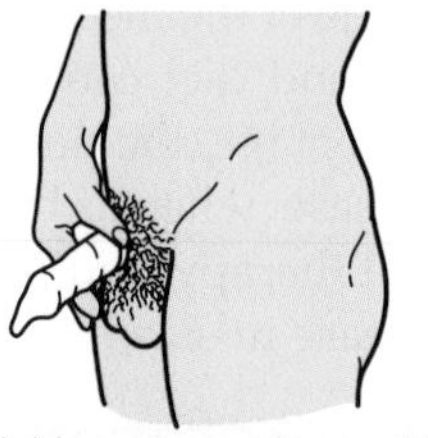

Hold condom at base of the penis to prevent spillage

A

HOW TO USE A DIAPHRAGM

1. The diaphragm can be inserted up to 4 hours before intercourse. Apply spermicide on the rim and inside the center of diaphragm.
2. Compress diaphragm using thumb and finger of one hand, and use other hand to spread the labia.

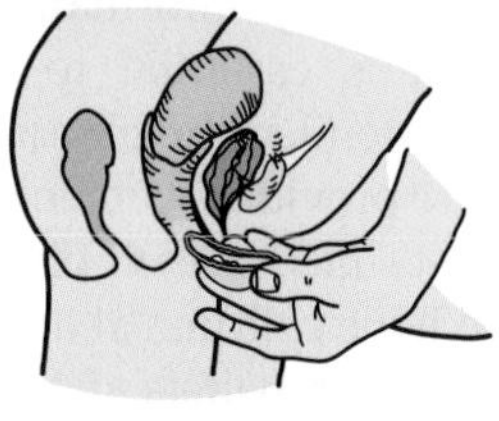

3. While squatting (or placing one foot on a chair), insert into vagina with spermicide toward cervix. Direct diaphragm inward and downward behind and below cervix.
4. Tuck the front rim of diaphragm into the pubic bone, and feel cervix through the center of diaphragm.
5. Leave in place at least 6 hours after intercourse.

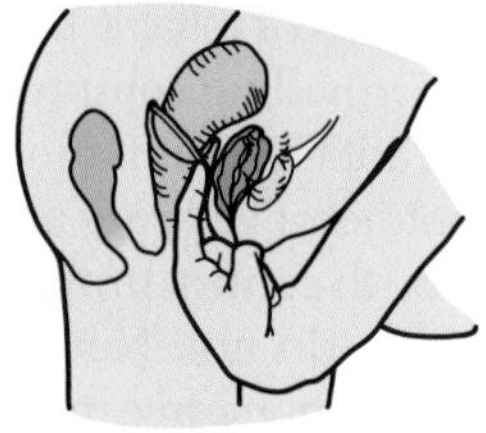

6. To remove, assume squatting position and bear down. Hook a finger over top rim, and pull diaphragm down and out.
7. Wash diaphragm with mild soap and dry after each use. Dust with cornstarch, if needed, and inspect occasionally for small holes.

B

Fig. 38.2 Proper application of **(A)** a condom and **(B)** a diaphragm. (Modified from Leifer G: *Introduction to maternity and pediatric nursing,* ed 7, St. Louis, 2015, Elsevier.)

involves monitoring the BBT each morning and noting a rise that occurs at ovulation. A cervical mucus test, called the *Billings Ovulation Method* (Billings Life, 2015), can also be used to track the occurrence of ovulation. The **calendar** or **rhythm method** is based on the knowledge that ovulation occurs 14 days *before* menstruation, and therefore keeping track of the woman's menstrual cycle can help predict the time of ovulation. The **Marquette Model** of natural family planning (Marquette University, 2018) incorporates the use of an electronic hormonal fertility monitor that tracks the levels of the urinary metabolites of estrogen and LH. Natural family planning requires the commitment of both partners and close, accurate monitoring during the menstrual cycle. Douching, withdrawal, and breastfeeding are unreliable methods of contraception.

Oral Contraceptives

Oral contraceptives (OCs) are the most popular method of reversible hormonal contraception in use. They are effective if used properly and offer some noncontraceptive benefits such as relief from breast tenderness, bloating, and symptoms of premenstrual syndrome (PMS), but they do have contraindications and cautions for users. You should counsel women on options and collect data that can determine which OC choice is best, if this is the method of birth control the woman prefers. The health care provider assists the woman in making the final choice. Traditional OC regimens are based on a 28-day cycle with a 7-day hormone-free interval that allows for menstruation and gonadotropin levels to rise and ovarian follicular growth to occur. When the OC cycle is not resumed on schedule, the risk of unplanned pregnancy occurs. Other OCs reduce the hormone-free interval, thereby reducing menstrual discomforts as well as decreasing the risk of contraceptive failure. Seasonale is an OC that provides delayed menstruation so that a woman has only four menstrual periods a year (U.S. Food and Drug Administration [FDA], 2018). Smoking increases the risk of complications related to OC therapy, especially in women older than 35 years (Martin & Barbieri, 2018).

Clinical Cues

It is important to tell patients that birth control pills and other birth control methods are not 100% effective in preventing conception. Abstinence is the only 100% effective method to prevent pregnancy.

Emergency Contraception

Known as the *morning-after pill,* emergency contraception may be considered after the woman has had unprotected intercourse. It was developed to decrease the number of unwanted pregnancies and elective abortions, yet is not meant to be used on a regular basis. Emergency contraception prevents pregnancy by preventing ovulation or fertilization or by slowing transport of the sperm and egg or altering the uterine lining to prevent implantation. Plan B One-Step, a tablet of levonorgestrel, is available over the counter in the United States and is to be taken within 72 hours of unprotected sex (Kaunitz, 2018). Ella, a prescription medication available in the United States and Canada that delays ovulation, should be taken as soon as possible after unprotected sex or failure of contraception and no later than 120 hours (5

Table 38.1 Methods of Contraception

HOW METHOD WORKS	SIDE EFFECTS/PRECAUTIONS	DEGREE OF EFFECTIVENESS/ USAGE NOTES
Abstinence		
Sexual contact is avoided.	Reliable method of preventing pregnancy and STIs.	100% if used consistently.
Fertility Awareness Methods		
Basal Body Temperature (BBT) BBT is measured and charted daily on awakening. Coitus is avoided on the day of temperature rise and for 3 subsequent days.	Temperature must be taken immediately before any activity, or it will rise above its basal level. The special thermometer should be kept at bedside.	Varies based on patient's compliance with technique. Can be moderately effective if practiced carefully.
Calendar or Rhythm Method Woman charts her monthly menstrual cycle on a calendar and avoids intercourse during fertile period.	Not effective for woman with irregular menstrual cycles. Several months of charting are necessary to establish clear pattern of menstrual cycle.	Fertility awareness methods that monitor multiple parameters (e.g., symptothermal method) may be more effective than the calendar or rhythm method, but the most important aspect of success is faithful adherence to the method.
Ovulation or Billings Method Cervical mucus changes are assessed. During ovulation, mucus is clear with high stretchability ("egg white" consistency). Degree of stretch is tested by pinching a small amount of cervical mucus between the thumb and forefinger and stretching it between them (called *spinnbarkeit*). During ovulation, mucus smeared on a glass slide will dry into a "fern" pattern.	Woman must feel very comfortable with her body and confident in her ability to detect and assess changes.	
Symptothermal Method Variety of parameters are recorded, including cervical mucus changes, BBT pattern, mittelschmerz (brief, sharp abdominal pain that may occur with ovulation), increased libido (sexual drive).	More effective for women with regular menstrual cycles. Requires significant accurate record keeping.	
Chemical Predictor Test A test kit that contains a chemically treated strip that will turn color when estrogen or luteal hormone levels are present in urine.	Increase in hormone levels occurs 12–24 h before ovulation.	
Mechanical or Barrier Contraception		
Intrauterine Device (IUD) A small, sterile, flexible plastic device that is inserted by a health care provider into the uterus. Can be a copper device (Paragard), which can provide 10 years of protection, or a device containing the hormone levonorgestrel (Mirena), which can provide 5 yr of protection.	May increase menstrual flow or cause cramping or low back pain. Increased incidence of PID in women with multiple sex partners, women whose partners have multiple partners, and women with previous incidence of PID. Patient must check placement by feeling for string once each month.	Up to 99% effective; must be removed by health care provider.

Continued

Table 38.1 Methods of Contraception—cont'd

HOW METHOD WORKS	SIDE EFFECTS/PRECAUTIONS	DEGREE OF EFFECTIVENESS/ USAGE NOTES
Male Condom		
A sheath commonly made of latex that is placed over the erect penis before intercourse. Oil-based lubricants such as petroleum jelly can cause latex to break down and reduce effectiveness. Some condoms, made of polyurethane, are compatible with oil-based lubricants.	Inexpensive, readily available, easy to use correctly. *Precautions:* (1) Leave space at tip for semen to collect to prevent it being forced upward out of the condom; (2) store in a cool place, and not for excessively long, to prevent breakage from aging of the latex or heat damage; (3) handle carefully to prevent spilling semen and possibly introducing it into the vagina.	82%–98% if used properly (CDC, 2017); use of spermicide increases efficacy.
Cervical Cap (e.g., FemCap)		
A one-size reusable, hormone-free, latex-free barrier that is held in place by the vaginal walls. Used with a spermicide and inserted before each intercourse act.	Effectiveness enhanced with use of spermicide. Should not be left in place for more than 48 h or used during menstruation. Woman should urinate before and after insertion.	92%
Female (Internal) Condom		
Sheath with retaining ring that is placed in the vagina before intercourse. Open end with large entrance ring extends outside the vagina. Can be inserted up to 8 h before intercourse.	The penis must remain inside the sheath, not between the sheath and the vaginal wall. Acceptance of the method has been slow because it is more expensive and more difficult and time consuming to place properly than the male condom. Effectiveness is enhanced with use of spermicide. Provides protection against STIs.	79%; failures can occur when the penis is withdrawn too far and reenters the vagina beside rather than within the condom.
Diaphragm		
A latex or rubber dome-shaped cup that fits snugly over the cervix. Spermicide is applied to the cervical side of the diaphragm, and it is inserted into the vagina so that the fitted ring holds it securely in place at the top of the vagina to wall off the cervix. The spermicide enhances effectiveness, should there be a leak around the edge or tear in the diaphragm.	A diaphragm must be fitted professionally and should be refitted annually, with a gain or loss of 7–10 lb, and particularly after pregnancy.	88%
Vaginal Sponge		
A nonprescription soft polyurethane sponge traps and absorbs semen and has spermicidal properties.	Sponge is moistened with 2 tablespoons of water and squeezed before insertion. Must remain in place 6 h after intercourse. Prolonged use can increase risk for toxic shock syndrome.	76%–88%
Spermicidal Methods		
Gels, Foams, Creams		
Work by killing sperm within the vagina. Must be applied before intercourse.	Available without prescription. More effective when used as an adjunct to condoms, diaphragms, and caps.	71%

Table 38.1 Methods of Contraception—cont'd

HOW METHOD WORKS	SIDE EFFECTS/PRECAUTIONS	DEGREE OF EFFECTIVENESS/ USAGE NOTES
Hormonal Methods		
Oral Contraceptives (OCs)		
"The pill" contains a combination of synthetic estrogen and progestin, hormones that prevent ovulation and thicken cervical mucus, making it difficult for sperm to travel upward (also true for injectable and timed-release hormonal methods). Traditionally based on a 28-day cycle with 7 hormone-free days that result in monthly menstruation. **Some formulations** are considered "low-dose regimens." **A formulation is available** that reduces menstrual periods to four times a year.	Prescription required. Must be taken faithfully to be effective. *Precautions:* Not recommended for women older than 35 years who smoke or women with a history of heart or liver disease, breast or uterine cancer, blood clots or venous inflammation, or unexplained vaginal bleeding. At least three regular ovulatory cycles should be evidenced before adolescents start OC use. May cause nausea.	91%
Injectable Contraceptives (Birth Control Shot; Depo-Provera)		
Synthetic timed-release progesterone is injected q12wk, preventing ovulation.	Injections given in clinic or office. Must be repeated q12wk to remain effective. *Precautions:* See oral contraceptives.	94%
Sustained-Release Implants (Nexplanon)		
A thin, flexible rod containing synthetic hormone is placed under the skin of the forearm in a minor surgical procedure. Effective for 3 yr.	Small incision required to place and to remove. *Precautions:* See oral contraceptives.	99%
Emergency Contraception		
Taken orally the day after unprotected intercourse, it induces menses and prevents implantation in the uterus.	Not to be used as a routine form of contraception. Women receiving the "morning-after" pill should also receive assistance in choosing an effective, ongoing method of contraception.	Varies depending on body mass index (BMI), conception probability based on cycle day, and further intercourse after use of emergency contraception
Vaginal Ring		
The NuvaRing (etonogestrel and ethinyl estradiol) is a flexible silicone ring inserted into the vagina for 3 wk and removed for 1 wk to allow for menstruation.	Leukorrhea and vaginal infection are possible side effects. Other side effects are similar to those for OCs, but fewer GI problems are experienced because it does not pass through GI tract.	91%
Skin Patch		
A transdermal skin patch containing norelgestromin and ethinyl estradiol applied to dry skin of back, buttocks, upper arm, or torso. Replaced weekly for 3 wk. Not applied in week 4 to allow for menstruation.	Some patients may have sensitivity to the adhesive used in the patch. Risk of thromboembolus may be higher than with OCs.	91%
Delayed Menstruation		
Seasonale is an OC that delays menstruation so that the woman experiences four menstrual periods a year. **Seasonique** is an OC that provides 84 days of combined hormones followed by a week of low-dose estrogen rather than a hormone-free interval. The four menstrual periods a year are lighter and accompanied by less discomfort.	A popular choice. Research continues regarding long-term effects.	97%–99.9%

Continued

Table 38.1 Methods of Contraception—cont'd

HOW METHOD WORKS	SIDE EFFECTS/PRECAUTIONS	DEGREE OF EFFECTIVENESS/ USAGE NOTES
Permanent Contraception		
Tubal Ligation (Female) (Surgical)		
Fallopian tubes are surgically cut or tied to prevent sperm from reaching ovum.	Sterilization procedures are considered permanent because reversal may not be effective.	99%
Vasectomy (Male)		
The vas deferens (sperm ducts) are cut and tied to prevent sperm from entering ejaculatory fluid.	Use another form of birth control until two sperm analyses are negative.	99%

GI, Gastrointestinal; *PID*, pelvic inflammatory disease; *STIs*, sexually transmitted infections.

days) after either event (Ulipristal: Drug Information, 2018). (See Legal and Ethical Considerations box.) The woman should be referred for counseling and follow-up care after use of any emergency contraception. Because emergency contraception is not effective if the woman is already pregnant, failure to menstruate by 21 days after initiation of therapy requires evaluation for pregnancy. There are no studies that specifically have investigated adverse effects of exposure to emergency contraception on the fetus in an early pregnancy (American College of Obstetricians and Gynecologists, 2018). Older evidence shows that there is no increased risk for complications to the pregnant woman or teratogenic risk to the fetus when taking OCs (American College of Obstetricians and Gynecologists, 2018).

Legal and Ethical Considerations

The "Morning-After" Pill

Although a form of the "morning-after" contraceptive pill is sold over the counter, there have been instances in which some pharmacists have been unwilling to provide it to customers, stating that the drug violates their religious principles. Is it ethical for pharmacists to withhold medication from a woman because of their own personal beliefs?

A copper intrauterine device (IUD) can be inserted up to 5 to 7 days after unprotected sexual intercourse to prevent implantation of the zygote in women who prefer long-term contraception (Kaunitz, 2018). A woman who seeks emergency contraception should be educated about methods of birth control and prevention of STIs.

Information on emergency contraception is provided at www.NOT-2-LATE.com.

MENOPAUSE

Hormonal changes and the cessation of menstruation signal the onset of menopause. Often referred to as the "change of life," the psychosocial implications of menopause can challenge some women's personal coping skills. Family support is helpful to maintain a sense of purpose in life. Other women feel a sense of freedom that results from the lack of need for contraception or medication for cramping.

Older Adult Care Points

Whether menopause is induced surgically or happens as a natural process of aging, the significant reduction in estrogen that occurs during and after this time causes a decrease in natural vaginal lubrication. Women may be prescribed vaginal creams containing estrogen to restore moisture and elasticity to vaginal tissues. Estrogen cream used as a lubricant for sexual intercourse is discouraged because the cream may damage latex condoms, and other methods of birth control should be used until full menopause occurs. Nonmedicated lubricants should be used for this purpose if necessary. Studies have shown that the estrogen contained in some vaginal creams can be systemically absorbed; therefore these products should be used with caution only after speaking with a health care provider.

Western culture values youth and beauty, and the onset of menopause may be seen by some women as a loss of attractiveness and the first step toward old age. In other cultural groups, the wisdom gained from life's experiences is valued. You must understand the perceptions of the woman and the family before designing and implementing a teaching plan that is patient centered.

HEALTH SCREENING AND ASSESSMENT

Primary prevention is designed to decrease the probability of becoming ill, such as by maintaining a health or nutrition history and providing immunizations. **Secondary prevention** involves screening for detection of specific diseases a patient is at risk for (such as through an annual mammogram) so that early treatment may be given. **Tertiary prevention** minimizes the impact of an already-diagnosed condition.

Adult women may be at risk for obesity, high cholesterol, high blood pressure, osteoporosis, and dental disease. Pregnant women or women who are planning pregnancy may be at risk for a folic acid deficiency that could result in a neural tube defect in the developing fetus; therefore prenatal vitamins, including folic acid supplements, may be prescribed.

Health screening begins with the woman's visit to her health care provider. It is your responsibility as the nurse to introduce yourself, ask pertinent questions, and document all information gathered. This phase is called *collection of data.* The data collected identify the patient and summarize her personal health history, the community in which she lives, and her available support system. Information on the woman's culture, lifestyle, and usual coping mechanisms will enable the health team to design an individualized plan of care. All data collection should include information regarding use of nonprescription as well as prescription medications and complementary and alternative medicine (CAM) therapy.

BREAST SELF-EXAMINATION

Breast self-examination (BSE) is optional and may be done monthly, about 1 week after menstruation begins, or on a specific date each month after menopause (Fig. 38.3). Research indicates that women are just as likely to find a lump by chance as they are via BSE (American Cancer Society [ACS], 2017). Mammography and magnetic resonance imaging (MRI) for women at high risk of breast cancer are other forms of screening tests. Tomosynthesis (three-dimensional mammography) is a more advanced form of traditional mammography. Testing for *BRCA1* and *BRCA2* gene mutations is offered to patients who have a high familial risk of breast cancer.

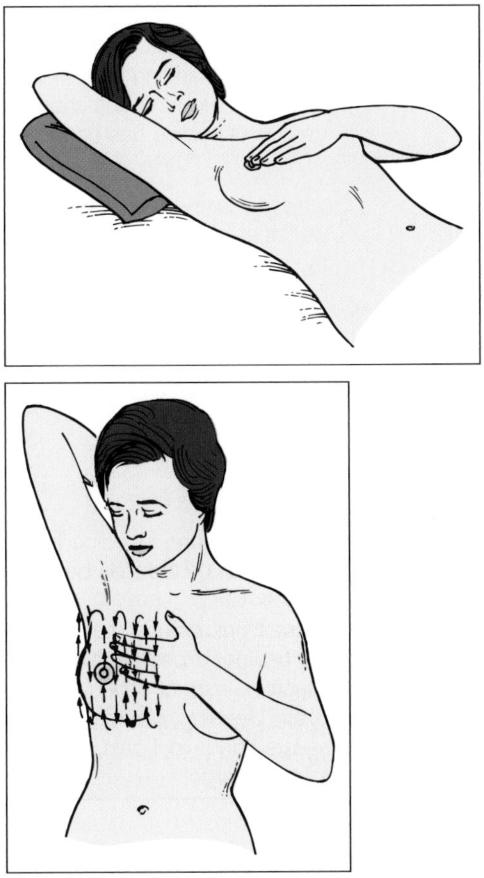

Fig. 38.3 Breast self-examination. (From Lowdermilk DL, Perry SE, Cashion K, et al.: *Maternity & women's health care,* ed 11, St. Louis, 2016, Elsevier.)

Clinical Cues

If a woman is reluctant to have a mammogram because of discomfort experienced during the procedure, suggest that she take acetaminophen an hour before the scheduled test (unless contraindicated). Also discuss the benefits of discovering breast cancer early versus the few minutes of discomfort experienced from breast compression that take place during the test.

VULVAR SELF-EXAMINATION

Many women are unaware of the importance of vulvar self-examination (VSE). Although serious lesions are less commonly found in this area than in the breast, early detection allows for rapid and often minimally invasive treatment. Delay in detection can lead to surgical disfigurement and even death. VSE should be performed monthly. It usually is done in a sitting position. One hand is used to hold a mirror, and the other separates the labia and exposes the area surrounding the vagina. Using both touch (to palpate for lumps or thickening beneath the skin) and visualization, the self-examination begins at the top of the mons pubis and works downward to the clitoris, the labia majora, the labia minora, the perineum, and finally the area around the anus. The woman should note any changes and report them to her health care provider. These include new moles, warts, or growths; new areas of pigmentation, especially white, red, or dark skin areas; ulcers or sores; and areas of continuing pain, inflammation, or itching. Most of these findings are not malignant and require little if any treatment. Treatment of malignancies that have been detected early can prevent surgeries such as **vulvectomy** (excision of the vulva) and prevent **metastasis** (spread of a malignancy to other areas of the body).

DIAGNOSTIC TESTS

You often are asked to assist with various diagnostic tests. Providing the woman with a clear explanation of what will be done and what she can do to minimize discomfort is essential. A consent may be required for certain procedures, and you are responsible for ensuring that the health care provider has obtained an informed consent. All patient questions should be answered clearly and accurately before the procedure begins. Table 38.2 describes common gynecologic diagnostic tests.

The Pelvic Examination

Assemble the equipment and direct the woman to take deep breaths and relax all muscles during exhalation (Box 38.2). The woman can be instructed to bear down as the speculum is being inserted. The speculum is gently

Table 38.2 Common Gynecologic Diagnostic Tests and Diagnostic Procedures

PURPOSE	DESCRIPTION	NURSING IMPLICATIONS
Pelvic Examination		
Visual inspection of the external genitalia, vagina, and cervix to obtain specimens such as a Pap smear.	*Equipment:* Gloves, vaginal speculum, lubricant, light, table with stirrups. *Process:* Inspection via the vaginal speculum; manual palpation of internal organs through abdominal wall, vaginally, and rectally.	Some discomfort during examination (decreased or eliminated if the patient remains fully relaxed). Nurse ensures that patient is appropriately draped and correctly positioned in the stirrups. Examination time is usually 5–10 min.
Pap Smear, Thin Prep		
To obtain samples of cells and fluids for pathology/cytology studies.	*Equipment:* Sterile specimen collection equipment. *Process:* Exudate, mucus, and cells obtained from surface of cervix with sterile swab or scraping tool and placed on laboratory slide or into preservative solution for pathology evaluation.	Cultures and smears of the cervix may cause mild bleeding and cramping.
Endometrial Biopsy		
To determine cause of postmenopausal bleeding, menstrual difficulties, infertility workup.	*Equipment:* Same as pelvic examination plus suction biopsy apparatus. *Process:* A suction biopsy of the endometrium is performed via the cervical opening.	Severe cramping may occur during procedure. Patient is usually premedicated. Normally some vaginal bleeding follows; flow should not be heavy.
Colposcopy		
Endoscopic examination of the vagina and cervix to evaluate abnormal cells and lesions, particularly after a positive Pap smear.	*Equipment:* Same as pelvic examination plus colposcope. *Process:* Area is visualized through the scope, with photos and possible biopsies of lesions requiring further study.	Patient is positioned as for pelvic examination. Procedure takes a few minutes. Biopsy may cause a small amount of bleeding and minor cramping. No tampons should be used until healing has occurred.
Hysteroscopy		
Endoscopic examination of the interior of the uterus; may also involve procedures such as biopsy or removal of **fibroids** (leiomyomas are benign tumors of the uterine muscle), adhesions, and septums. Endometrial laser ablation (destruction of areas within uterine lining) may also be performed.	*Process:* Hysteroscope is inserted vaginally, usually under local anesthesia. May also be done in combination with laparoscopy.	Occasional injury to cervix or uterine wall. If endometrial ablation is done, the woman will have difficulty becoming pregnant because the lining destruction is permanent.
Dilation and Evacuation (D&E)		
To detect cause of excessive bleeding; to remove hypertrophied uterine lining, retained placenta, or tissue remaining from incomplete abortion.	*Equipment:* Done in operating room. *Process:* The cervix is dilated, and the interior of the uterus is cleansed by scraping, suction, or both.	Mild cramping and bleeding for up to 1 wk. Next period may be either early or late. Complications include uterine perforation, excessive bleeding, infection. Instruct patient to report heavy bleeding, clotting, sharp/severe abdominal pain, abnormal or foul discharge.

Table 38.2 Common Gynecologic Diagnostic Tests and Diagnostic Procedures—cont'd

PURPOSE	DESCRIPTION	NURSING IMPLICATIONS
Mammography		
To screen the breasts for abnormal growths, particularly cancer.	*Equipment:* Done in the radiology department with special radiographic equipment. *Process:* A full-field digital mammography machine records images on a computer screen and can computer-enhance questionable images for increased accuracy.	Breast discomfort from compression of the tissue during the test; occasional mild bruising. Instruct patient to wear no deodorant or lotion on the upper body and to wear clothing that allows top to be easily removed.
Hysterosalpingography		
To detect uterine tumors, adhesions, or developmental anomalies; detect tubal obstruction preventing ova from reaching uterus.	Patient is placed in the lithotomy position on fluoroscopy table with a speculum in the vagina. Contrast media is injected through the cervix. Fluoroscopy is performed and radiographs are taken.	Have patient void before the procedure. Vaginal discharge may occur for 1–2 days after the test and may be bloody. Instruct patient to report fever, pain, or other signs of infection.
Ultrasound (Sonogram)		
Pregnancy: To determine gestation; screen for birth defects or placental abnormalities. *Gynecology:* To determine presence, location, and size of abdominal mass; determine whether a mass is **cystic** (fluid filled) or solid; locate intrauterine device; monitor ovulation in infertility.	*Equipment:* Ultrasound machine. *Process:* Sound wave transducer emits inaudible sound waves that record interior structures on the ultrasound screen. A video recording is made so that results can be restudied and evaluated. A "picture" of the fetus may be provided to the parents.	Some tests require a full bladder, which may be uncomfortable during the test. The nurse should assist the woman to empty her bladder immediately after the examination. Skin should be clean, dry, and free of lotions or powder. During pregnancy, two or more ultrasound examinations may be required. The use of independent three- or four-dimensional ultrasound procedures to provide mementos for parents is not recommended because the long-term effects of the extra energy used in these examinations on the fetus has not been researched.
Pelvic/Vaginal Ultrasound		
To detect thickness of uterine lining, size of uterus, presence of fibroids; size of ovaries; and presence of cysts or tumor.	*Process:* Ultrasound transducer is passed over pelvic area, or the transducer is inserted into the vagina and guided over areas of the surface.	Advise that there will be minor discomfort if vaginal transducer is used.
Breast Ultrasound		
To differentiate benign tumor from malignant tumor. Useful in women with dense breast tissue and fibrocystic disease.	*Process:* A noninvasive painless procedure.	An ultrasound will not detect microcalcifications that a mammogram can detect.
PET Scan		
To stage breast cancer and detect skeletal lesions.	*Process:* Performed in radiotherapy unit.	—
Breast MRI		
Used for women with dense breast tissue.	*Process:* Images are taken with an MRI machine.	Premedication to lessen anxiety for women with claustrophobia may be advised. Patient must not wear metal during test.

Continued

Table 38.2 Common Gynecologic Diagnostic Tests and Diagnostic Procedures—cont'd

PURPOSE	DESCRIPTION	NURSING IMPLICATIONS
Breast Biopsy		
To diagnose breast cancer. Usually performed when a suspicious breast lump is detected.	*Process:* A needle aspiration can be done on an outpatient basis under local anesthesia. An incisional biopsy can be done in a same-day surgery setting under local or general anesthesia. All removed tissue or fluid is sent to laboratory for analysis.	Check incision for bleeding. Encourage verbalization of fears. Schedule follow-up appointment for results of laboratory studies.

MRI, Magnetic resonance imaging; *Pap,* Papanicolaou; *PET,* positron emission tomography.

Box 38.2 Preparing a Woman for a Pelvic Examination

- The unit should provide privacy and good lighting.
- Assemble clean gloves and supplies.
- Orient the patient to the equipment and the purpose of the examination.
- Encourage the woman to void because a full bladder will make the examination more uncomfortable.
- Position and drape the patient appropriately.
  - Lithotomy
  - Side-lying
  - Knee-chest
- Stay with the woman, encouraging her with information to promote comfort.

placed into the vagina by the health care provider. The blades are then opened to view the cervix. Specimens may be collected for laboratory examination. A Pap smear may be obtained to determine the presence of abnormal cells. After the examination, assist the woman to a sitting and then a standing position. Disposable tissues may be provided to wipe lubricant from the perineum. The provider usually returns to speak with the patient after she dresses. Teaching may include review of the purpose of the tests performed and should include education about the need for routine checkups, Pap smear, and human papillomavirus (HPV) testing. The U.S. Preventive Services Task Force's (USPSTF, 2017) most recent draft recommendation includes screening for cervical cancer every 3 years via a Pap smear in women between ages 21 and 65 years. For women who wish to increase the length of time between screening, the USPSTF recommends screening with a Pap smear and HPV testing every 5 years.

Clinical Cues

Talking to the patient during the examination aids with distraction and enhances relaxation. If appropriate and the patient desires, you may use therapeutic touch by holding her hand or placing a hand gently on her shoulder to provide comfort and reassurance.

Older Adult Care Points

Older women may feel that they no longer need regular mammograms and Pap smears, particularly if they are not sexually active. The ACS (2017) recommends that screening mammography continue after the age of 55 every 1 to 2 years for as long as the woman is in good health and is expected to live 10 years or more (Fig. 38.4).

NURSING MANAGEMENT

ASSESSMENT (DATA COLLECTION)

Collect essential data regarding the patient's reproductive history and gynecologic concerns. This can be difficult for both the patient and you because it involves discussing intimate aspects of the patient's body and personal life. Collecting data about sexual health and sexual practices is an important part of routine data collection. Sexual health information should include the "5 Ps": **P**artners, **P**ractices, **P**rotection from STIs, **P**ast history of STIs, and **P**revention of pregnancy (CDC, n.d.). Also record information on the cultural and spiritual beliefs and attitudes regarding sexuality and sexual identity, reproduction, and body image, all of which affect the assessment process. Ask questions in a tactful and objective manner and appreciate that the patient has the right to choose not to answer.

ANATOMY AND PHYSIOLOGY OF THE MALE REPRODUCTIVE SYSTEM

STRUCTURES

- The male **gonads** (sex glands) are the testes; they are oval shaped and are encased in the scrotum, along with the epididymis, seminal vesicles, and vas deferens (Fig. 38.5).
- The scrotum is covered with wrinkled skin (**rugae**) and is very sensitive to temperature, pressure, touch, and pain.
- The **penis** is a cylindrical, erectile organ that hangs in front of the scrotum. It contains three columns of erectile tissue that can cause it to extend and enlarge in circumference, becoming stiff. The penis is covered with skin and includes a foreskin (unless circumcision

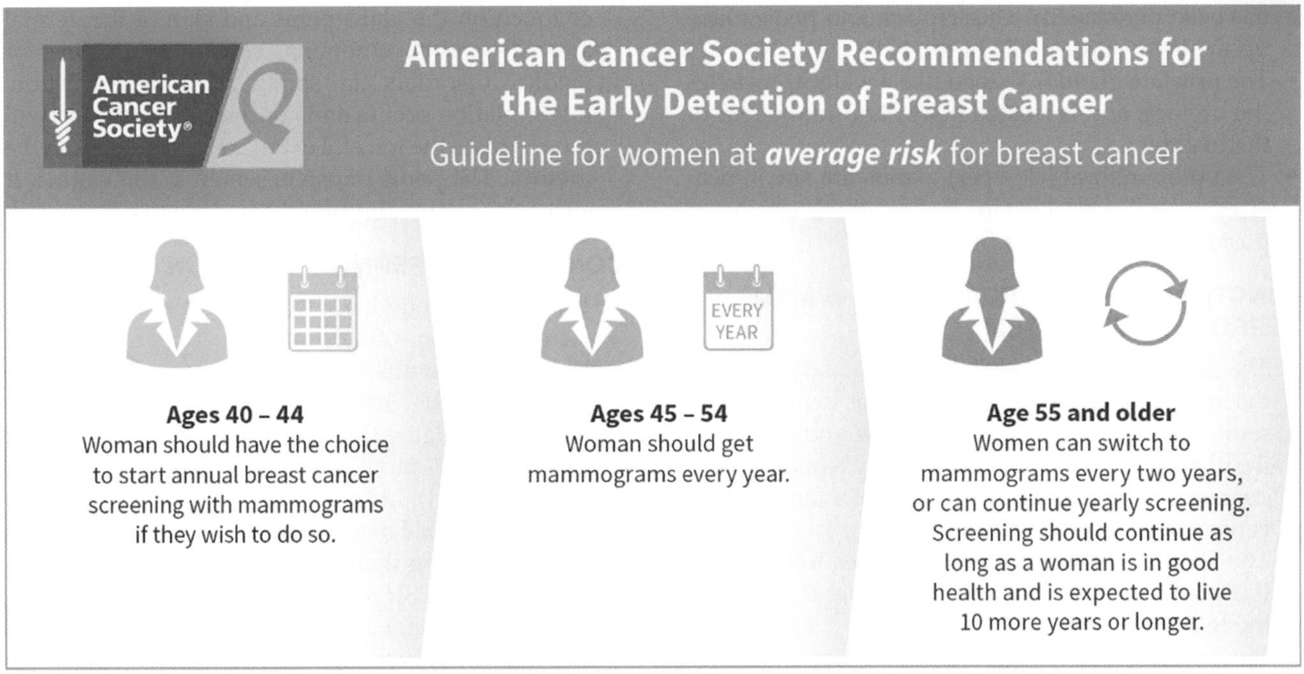
American Cancer Society®
American Cancer Society Recommendations for the Early Detection of Breast Cancer
Guideline for women at *average risk* for breast cancer
EVERY YEAR
Ages 40 - 44
Woman should have the choice to start annual breast cancer screening with mammograms if they wish to do so.
Ages 45 - 54
Woman should get mammograms every year.
Age 55 and older
Women can switch to mammograms every two years, or can continue yearly screening. Screening should continue as long as a woman is in good health and is expected to live 10 more years or longer.

Fig. 38.4 Breast cancer screening guideline. (© 2019 American Cancer Society, Inc. All rights reserved.)

Focused Assessment

Data Collection for Gynecologic History

Sample questions to use when collecting data from a patient with a gynecologic problem include the following:

- How old were you when you began menstruating?
- Are your periods regular? How often do they occur? How long do they last? (Or, if the patient has stopped menstruation due to menopause, ask when she had her last menstrual period.)
- How heavy is your flow? Do you ever pass clots or pieces of tissue? Do you have pain before or during your period?
- Do you have cramps, headaches, or abdominal or back pain at other times of the month?
- Do you have mood swings, depression, or periods of tearfulness associated with your menstrual cycle?
- Are you having any vaginal discharge or itching?
- Do you have bleeding or spotting between your periods?
- Do you have any problems urinating, including burning, pain, or incontinence?
- How many times have you been pregnant?
- Have you had any miscarriages?
- Have you ever had a pelvic infection?
- Do you perform breast and vulvar self-examination?
- When was your last Pap smear?
- When was your last mammogram?
- Are you taking any medications or supplements routinely?
- Are you currently using any method of birth control, and if so, which method?
- Do you feel comfortable with your method of birth control or have a desire to change methods?
- Do you have any specific concerns or questions that we have not talked about?

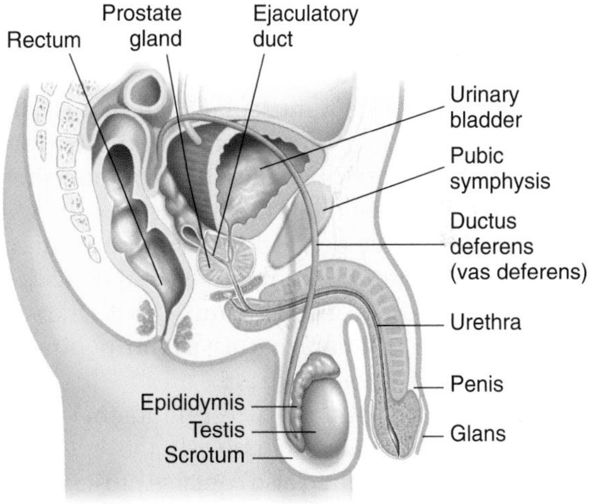

Fig. 38.5 Structures of the male reproductive system. (From Lewis SL, Heitkemper MM, Bucher L, et al.: *Medical-surgical nursing: assessment and management of clinical problems,* ed 10, St. Louis, 2017, Elsevier.)

Cultural Considerations

Culture and Women's Health

Cultural considerations can be particularly significant in the area of women's health care. Cultural and spiritual views regarding sexuality, reproduction, and the role of women in society will have a direct impact on the type of care sought and the amount and type of information the woman is willing and able to provide. You must not pass judgment based on your own cultural bias but must be culturally sensitive and supportive to the needs of women from diverse cultural backgrounds.

has been performed). The scrotum and penis make up the external genitalia of the male.

- The **prostate gland** is shaped like a walnut, encircles the urethra, and is located below and to the rear of the bladder.
- The bulbourethral (Cowper) glands are small, pea-sized glands located in the urethral sphincter, posterior to the urethra.

FUNCTIONS OF THE ORGANS OF THE MALE REPRODUCTIVE SYSTEM

- The **scrotum**—a thin-walled, muscular sac—holds the testes, the epididymis, and the vas deferens. The scrotum hangs from the pubic bone and suspends the testes outside the body, where they remain several degrees cooler than the body; the cooler temperature is needed to produce viable sperm.
- The spermatic cord attaches the testes to the body. It contains the blood vessels and nerves that supply the testes.
- The seminiferous tubules within the testes produce sperm (**spermatogenesis**). These tubules collect and transport the sperm to the epididymis. Testosterone also is produced in the testes.
- The **epididymis** is a long tube (almost 6 m if uncoiled) that conducts sperm from the testes to the vas deferens. Immature sperm mature as they travel through this tube. Mature sperm are stored in the lower portion of the epididymis.
- The **vas deferens** is a muscular tube that connects to the epididymis. It stores sperm and then carries it to the ejaculatory duct by peristaltic movements.
- The prostatic section of the urethra receives the sperm and carries it to the penile portion of the urethra for ejaculation. Secretions from the seminal vesicles and ducts of the prostate gland are mixed with the sperm in an alkaline solution that assists in neutralizing the acidity of the vaginal tract.
- The seminal vesicles produce a fluid that is thick and contains fructose to nourish the sperm and provide energy. The fluid also contains prostaglandins, which contribute to the motility of the sperm. This fluid mixes with the sperm to form seminal fluid, or **semen**. The average volume of semen ejaculated is 2.5 to 4 mL but may vary from 1 to 10 mL.
- The **prostate gland** produces thin, milky, alkaline secretions that contribute to the seminal fluid and enhance the motility of the sperm.
- The bulbourethral glands secrete an alkaline mucus-like fluid in response to sexual stimulation.
- The secretions of the bulbourethral glands neutralize the acid of residual urine in the urethra and provide some lubrication at the tip of the penis for intercourse.
- The penis is flaccid until sexual arousal causes the arterioles to the erectile tissue to dilate and the veins to constrict, engorging the penis with blood until it is enlarged and rigid. This is an **erection**. Erections are stimulated by anticipation, memory, visual sensations, or touch on the glans penis and skin of the genital area. Thoughts, emotions, some medications, or medical disorders can sometimes inhibit erection. If stimulation occurs and continues, **ejaculation** will occur. This is the forceful expulsion of semen from the urethra. The penis transfers semen to the vagina. It also carries urine through the urethra to be excreted.

CONTROL OF SPERM PRODUCTION

- The hypothalamus, the anterior pituitary, and the testes secrete hormones that control male reproduction.
- The hypothalamus secretes gonadotropin-releasing hormone (GnRH) in response to an unknown stimulus.
- GnRH stimulates the anterior pituitary to release luteinizing hormone (LH) and follicle-stimulating hormone (FSH). LH stimulates the testes to produce testosterone. FSH binds with cells in the seminiferous tubules, making them respond to testosterone. Testosterone and FSH stimulate the formation of sperm (spermatogenesis).
- The male sex hormones are called **androgens**.
- At puberty, testosterone levels rise and cause maturation of the male reproductive organs. Sperm take 70 days to mature and are constantly being produced once puberty has occurred.
- Normal sperm count is greater than 20 million/mL (Pagana, Pagana, & Pagana, 2017).

AGE-RELATED CHANGES

- The scrotum becomes more pendulous, and there are fewer rugae.
- Prostate enlargement may occur, with risk of urethral obstruction.
- Plasma testosterone and progesterone levels decrease.
- There is decreased sperm production, but fertility remains intact. Ejaculate volume decreases.
- After age 60 years, the cycle of sexual response lengthens. Arousal takes longer, and more direct penile stimulation may be needed; the firmness and/or duration of the erection may be decreased.
- Sexual activity in older men is closely related to their sexual activity in earlier years.
- Vascular problems are the major causes of impotence.
- Certain medical disorders, or the use of various medications, may have side effects that can affect sexual function.

THE MALE REPRODUCTIVE SYSTEM

The male reproductive organs are shared with the urinary tract, and disorders in functioning of one system typically affect the other. For this reason, men who have a disorder or dysfunction of the reproductive tract are commonly treated by a urologist.

FERTILITY

If the anatomy and physiology of the male reproductive tract are intact, sexual function is influenced by the functioning of the hypothalamus, pituitary, and testes; the metabolism and transport of sex hormones (such as GnRH and others); and the cognitive and sensory centers in the brain. A sexual desire (**libido**), the ability to respond to sexual stimulation with a penile erection, and the ejaculation of semen containing live sperm are necessary for fertility. Both the parasympathetic and sympathetic nervous systems influence the normal sexual response cycle.

> **Older Adult Care Points**
>
> As testosterone decreases with age, muscle strength, bone mass, libido, and erectile function can also decrease. This can affect the psychological sense of well-being. Testosterone replacement therapy is thought to decrease visceral fat and improve bone density, muscle strength, libido, and energy, but it may not improve erectile function. In men who have not had cancer, testosterone therapy has been used to improve sexual function; however, sufficient data are not yet available to demonstrate a clear benefit for this type of treatment (Dizon & Katz, 2018).

As a man ages, there is no abrupt cessation of gonadal hormone activity as there is in a woman. In the man, there is a gradual decrease in testosterone and other anabolic hormones, such as growth hormone and dehydroepiandrosterone (DHEA).

CONTRACEPTION

Contraception is a method of preventing unwanted pregnancy. The only 100% effective method of contraception is abstinence. Abstinence is encouraged for adolescents and young adults and is taught in some school programs. You must be able to provide contraceptive options for patients who prefer not to have children. Contraception is the responsibility of *both* the man and the woman. Methods of contraception are discussed in Table 38.1.

Reversible Contraception

Reversible contraception involves the use of spermicidal creams, gels, or foams applied before intercourse to kill sperm in the vagina. These are more effective if used in conjunction with a condom. A male condom is an effective reversible contraceptive technique if it is applied and used properly. The condom sheath is typically made of latex. Proper application includes timing of application and removal and providing a space at the tip for semen to collect. Oil-based lubricants such as petroleum jelly can cause latex to deteriorate, so these lubricants reduce the reliability of latex condoms. It is important to suggest the use of water-soluble lubricants such as jellies made for this purpose. Condoms made of polyurethane are compatible with oil-based lubricants. Latex condoms provide some protection against STIs.

Permanent Contraception: Vasectomy

Male sterilization by vasectomy is a popular method of permanent contraception. The term **vasectomy** refers to a surgical procedure performed on the vas deferens for the purpose of interrupting the continuity of this duct, which conveys the sperm at the time of ejaculation. This is considered a permanent procedure, but occasionally a vasectomy can be successfully reversed by vasovasostomy (microsurgery) if a man's life circumstances change. Some patients consider storing fertile sperm in a sperm bank before a vasectomy to father a child later.

A vasectomy is done on an outpatient basis in a clinic or health care provider's office with a local anesthetic. An incision is made into the scrotal sac on each side, and the vas deferens is lifted out. A segment of the vas deferens is cut out, the ends are bound, and the incision is closed.

The patient should be instructed to use ice applications and acetaminophen or ibuprofen for scrotal pain and swelling in the first 12 to 24 hours postoperatively. The patient should wear jockey shorts or a scrotal support for comfort. Sexual intercourse may be resumed in about 1 week, based on the provider's recommendation. Be sure to emphasize to the patient that *two* negative sperm counts are needed after vasectomy before the patient can be considered infertile and that some form of contraception should be used until then.

Because seminal fluid is manufactured in seminal vesicles and the prostate gland, there is no decrease in semen ejaculation after a vasectomy. However, the semen does not contain sperm. After vasectomy, the sperm cells produced by the vas deferens are reabsorbed by the body. Vasectomy has no effect on libido or sexual performance and provides no protection from STIs.

> **Clinical Cues**
>
> After a vasectomy, instruct the patient to use another method of birth control until *two* sperm counts are negative because active sperm are still present in the vas deferens. Another sperm count should be done 1 year later to verify that the vas deferens is not intact.

NURSING MANAGEMENT

ASSESSMENT (DATA COLLECTION)

Because some male reproductive disorders are more common in certain age groups, the age of the patient is relevant to nursing assessment. In men older than 50 years, the assessment is directed more toward detecting prostate problems, whereas younger men are carefully assessed for STIs and testicular cancer.

It may be awkward for new nurses to obtain a sexual and reproductive history, but with experience in interviewing male patients of all ages, they will soon become more comfortable and adept at obtaining necessary data. Because questions about urinary problems are usually less sensitive than those dealing with sexual dysfunction, it is best to begin with questions of this kind and then lead into more sensitive ones.

Open-ended questions that start out with "Tell me about..." or "When did you first notice..." give the patient room to discuss only those things he is comfortable talking about. Be sure to use terminology that the patient understands. It also is helpful to ask him to relate his problem to the impact it causes in his daily life. For example, tenderness and discomfort in the scrotal area could make sitting at a desk or walking very difficult and interfere with getting assigned work done. Frequent urination can cause distracting and sometimes embarrassing interruptions in his work schedule or recreational activities.

Focused Assessment

Data Collection for the Male Reproductive System

Ask the following questions:

- Have you noticed any changes in patterns of urination or any differences in the stream of urine?
- Do you ever have any discharge coming from the penis?
- Have you felt any masses or bumps in the scrotum or groin?
- Do you have any tenderness or pain in the scrotum or penis?
- Do you have any rectal or perineal pain?
- Do you perform regular testicular examinations?
- Have you had past infections of the reproductive system?
- What drugs and supplements do you take regularly?
- Do you have difficulty obtaining or maintaining an erection?

Health Promotion

Health Screening and Assessments

Regular self-evaluation of the testes, such as testicular self-examination for early detection of cancer, is encouraged. You can encourage the patient to perform self-examination and teach proper techniques and follow-up care (Fig. 38.6). (Privacy should be provided during examination and when obtaining specimens.)

Think Critically

Think of different populations that would benefit from learning about testicular self-examination. Would your teaching vary based on the different populations of men?

◆ DIAGNOSTIC TESTS

Tests for general state of health, such as complete blood cell count, urinalysis, chemistry profile, and thyroid tests, are often done initially when a patient has a problem concerning the male reproductive tract. Serum acid phosphatase is usually elevated in patients with prostate cancer. Serum alkaline phosphatase is elevated if malignancy of the prostate has metastasized to the bone. A kidney-ureters-bladder (KUB) x-ray, an intravenous pyelogram, and cystoscopy with uroflowmetry studies also may be performed (see Chapter 33 for more

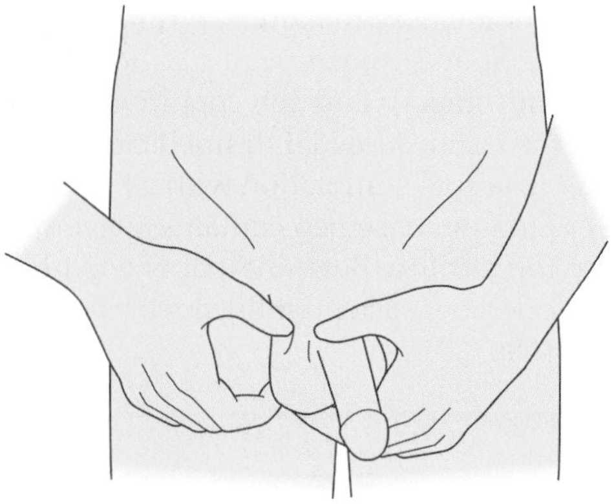

Fig. 38.6 Testicular self-examination. (Courtesy Coloplast Surgical Marketing, Minneapolis, Minn.)

information on these tests). Blood and urine tests are performed to detect a urinary tract infection (UTI).

Tumor protein marker studies are performed for patients with testicular cancer for follow-up to determine the success of treatment or recurrence of the disease. The primary tumor markers are alpha-fetoprotein (AFP) and the beta subunit of human chorionic gonadotropin (beta-hCG). A **prostate-specific antigen (PSA)** test detects levels of a glycoprotein produced by the prostate that is elevated in prostate cancer. Diagnostic tests that relate to the male reproductive organs are summarized in Table 38.3.

Think Critically

How would you begin your assessment interview with a 52-year-old man? What techniques will you use to obtain a thorough reproductive system history and information about present problems?

CARE OF PATIENTS WHO IDENTIFY AS LGBTQIA+

Nurses are called on to provide care with cultural congruence and compassion for all populations, respectfully upholding the dignity of each patient. Patients who identify as lesbian, gay, bisexual, transgender, questioning, intersex, asexual, or another designation must be afforded the same quality of care as those who identify as heterosexual male or female (Eliason & Chinn, 2018). Research shows that many individuals who identify as LGBTQIA+ avoid care, partially because of previous negative experiences within the health care system (The Joint Commission [TJC], 2014). Disparities within this community include the following (TJC, 2014):

- Less access to insurance and health care services, including preventive care (such as cancer screenings)
- Lower overall health status
- Higher rates of smoking, alcohol, and substance abuse
- Higher risk for mental health illnesses, such as anxiety and depression

Table 38.3 Diagnostic Tests for the Male Reproductive System

TEST	COMMENTS
Digital rectal examination	A lubricated, gloved finger is inserted into the rectum to evaluate the consistency and size of the prostate and detect any nodules.
Semen analysis	Through masturbation, the patient provides a specimen of semen, which is analyzed for volume and for sperm content and motility.
Testicular self-examination (TSE)	Monthly self-examination is encouraged.
Prostate-specific antigen (PSA) level	A sample of blood is examined for the level of glycoprotein produced only by the prostate. An elevated level is found in benign prostatic hyperplasia, and levels above 10 mg/mL may be indicative of prostate cancer. However, abnormal levels do not indicate a positive diagnosis. The United States Preventative Services Task Force recommends against routine screening for prostate cancer. The National Comprehensive Cancer Network recommends risk-stratified screening. The American Cancer Society recommends that men should make an informed choice.
Transrectal ultrasound	Recommended when PSA and/or digital rectal examination results are abnormal. May also be used to guide needle biopsies of the prostate.
Urography	Radiologically detects changes caused by ureter abnormalities and follows urine excretion pathway.
Uroflowmetry	Measures the volume of urine expelled from the bladder per second. Detects outflow tract obstruction. Patient voids into a urine flowmeter. Privacy is provided.
Prostate tissue analysis (biopsy)	Specimens of prostate tissue or fluids can be obtained by perineal or transrectal needle aspiration. If procedure is outpatient based, the patient is taught to report hematuria or change in urine flow after the procedure.
Cystoscopy	A lighted instrument is inserted through the urethra into the bladder. Used to detect prostate hypertrophy and bladder tumors. This is done as a sterile procedure.
Urethral smears	Used for laboratory microscopy study to identify pathogens. Prostate massage increases secretions in the urethra. A sterile swab is inserted into the urethra to obtain the specimen. Often used to diagnose some sexually transmitted infections.
Endocrine Studies	
Luteinizing hormone (LH) level	LH secreted by the pituitary stimulates Leydig cells in the testes to produce testosterone. High levels may indicate testicular failure.
Prolactin level	Prolactin, a hormone secreted by the pituitary, potentiates testosterone production.
Follicle-stimulating hormone (FSH) level	FSH is secreted by the anterior pituitary gland and stimulates the Sertoli cells in the seminiferous tubules to complete formation of mature sperm. Increased FSH levels indicate decreased spermatogenesis.
Testosterone level	Testosterone is secreted by the Leydig cells of the testes. High levels may indicate a testicular tumor. Low levels may occur in older men. Because testosterone levels are highest in the morning and lowest in the evening, it is important to obtain a morning sample.

- Higher rates of STIs, including human immunodeficiency virus (HIV) infection
- Increased incidence of some cancers

Care of patients who have undergone or are contemplating gender confirmation surgery should be approached from three important perspectives: the gender the patient identifies with; the type of surgery performed or to be performed (chest surgery, which is called "top surgery") and/or genital surgery (which is called "bottom surgery"); and the natal sex (the sex assigned at birth). You should ask the patient which name and pronouns are preferred and then use these as stated by the patient. Postsurgical intervention will vary based on which surgery has been performed ("top" and/or "bottom" surgery). Follow agency protocol for postoperative care that may include insertion of Foley catheters, drain care, and wound care. Following surgery, hormonal therapy will be prescribed or continued by the health care provider. Teach the patient how to take the medication and educate them about expected side effects as well as symptoms that need to be reported to the health care provider immediately. Remember to objectively teach patients about any health concerns that may remain based on natal sex. For example, a female-to-male transgender individual who has not chosen or yet undergone "bottom" surgery may still experience menstruation and need health teaching about routine Pap smears and pelvic examinations. A male-to-female transgender individual who has not chosen or yet undergone "bottom" surgery may still need teaching about monitoring for testicular and prostate cancer.

The most important support and interventions you can provide to all patients include compassionate care, acceptance, and knowledge. You can greatly affect disparities in care by becoming more self-aware, engaging in continuing education, and continuing to reach out to this community with objectivity, while providing excellence in care. Specific examples of nurse advocacy include the following (TJC, 2014):

- Ensure that the facility or agency is welcoming and safe for all patients
- Advocate for unisex or single-stall restrooms
- Avoid making assumptions about sexual orientation and gender identity
- Be aware of misconceptions, biases, and other communication barriers to care
- Recognize that self-identity and behaviors do not always align
- Honor and respect whatever information the patient shares with you about sexual orientation and gender identity
- Use neutral and inclusive language when talking with all patients
- Familiarize yourself with credible online and local resources for LGBTQIA+ patients
- Provide personalized care to all patients

Get Ready for the NCLEX® Examination

Key Points

- Women should keep a calendar of their individual menstrual cycles to determine regularity and recognize deviations from their normal cycle.
- Personal contraceptive techniques include fertility awareness methods, BBT, calendar and rhythm methods, ovulation or Billings method, and symptothermal method.
- Mechanical contraception methods include the use of a male condom, female condom, diaphragm, spermicide, cervical cap, or IUD.
- Hormonal contraception methods include the use of OCs, injectable contraceptives, transcutaneous patches, intrauterine and vaginal inserts, and sustained-release implants.
- Permanent contraception includes tubal ligation (female) and vasectomy (male).
- Emergency contraception may be indicated after unprotected intercourse but is not meant for regular use.
- BSE should be performed monthly 1 week after menstruation begins or on a specific date each month after menopause.
- School nurses can and should be a valuable resource to young women regarding issues of sexuality, reproduction, and disease.
- You must understand the perceptions of the female patient and family before designing a teaching plan.
- Menopause is described as cessation of menses for a 12-month period because of decreased estrogen production. The perimenopausal or climacteric period is the period around the actual cessation of the menstrual period. Common symptoms include irregular menstruation, hot flashes or hot flushes, fatigue, insomnia, emotional swings, depression, back pain, headache, irritability, and decreased libido.
- You can be instrumental in teaching and promoting use of monthly testicular self-examination and monitoring for prostate cancer by digital rectal examination and PSA testing.
- Nursing care is planned based on the patient's age, educational level, degree of comfort in discussing reproductive problems, and culture.
- You can greatly reduce health disparities in the LGBTQIA+ community by mindfully providing compassionate, nonjudgmental, personalized care.

Additional Learning Resources

SG Go to your Study Guide for additional learning activities to help you master this chapter content.

Go to your Evolve website (http://evolve.elsevier.com/deWit/medsurg) for the following FREE learning resources:

- Animations, audio, and video
- Answers and rationales for questions and activities
- Glossary with pronunciations in English and Spanish
- Interactive Review Questions and more!

Review Questions for the NCLEX® Examination

1. A female patient reports irritability, fatigue, mood swings, and feeling out of control several days before menstruation. Which teaching will you provide?
   1. "Avoid calcium-containing foods."
   2. "Exercise regularly."
   3. "Have occasional alcohol."
   4. "Consider a sodium-rich diet."

   NCLEX Client Need: Physiological Integrity: Reduction of Risk Potential
2. A 48-year-old female patient reporting irregular menses and hot flashes has been told by the health care provider that she has entered the climacteric period. When you find the patient crying, what is the appropriate nursing response?
   1. "Did you want more children?"
   2. "You seem sad. I am here to listen."
   3. "Everything will be all right."
   4. "Aging is not for the faint of heart."

   NCLEX Client Need: Psychosocial Integrity

3. You are discussing healthy lifestyle activities with a female patient. Which patient statement(s) require(s) further nursing teaching? *(Select all that apply.)*
   1. "I can use herbals such as evening primrose oil to decrease PMS symptoms."
   2. "I will focus on drinking caffeine-free soda to keep my fluid intake adequate."
   3. "I will douche regularly with an alkaline solution to maintain vaginal health."
   4. "I will wear form-fitting, nylon clothing and underwear for warmth and to prevent infections."
   5. "When I am 45 years old I should get an annual mammogram."

   NCLEX Client Need: Physiological Integrity: Reduction of Risk Potential
4. You are discussing contraception with a female patient who is in a monogamous relationship and wishes to prevent pregnancy. Which contraceptive methods will you teach that do not provide STI protection?
   1. Symptothermal method
   2. Billings method
   3. Water-soluble spermicidal lubricants during sexual activity
   4. IUDs
   5. Oral contraceptives

   NCLEX Client Need: Safe and Effective Care Environment: Coordinated Care
5. You are taking the gynecologic history of a postmenopausal patient. Which nursing actions develop rapport with the patient? *(Select all that apply.)*
   1. Establish firm eye contact.
   2. Involve spouse if the patient requests.
   3. Touch the patient.
   4. Use a polite tone of voice.
   5. Respect privacy.

   NCLEX Client Need: Psychosocial Integrity
6. A patient is discharged after having a vasectomy. Which patient statement(s) indicate(s) a need for further teaching? *(Select all that apply.)*
   1. "My spouse and I are not planning to have more children."
   2. "I will come back to the clinic to provide one semen sample."
   3. "There is a very slim possibility that this procedure can be reversed in the future."
   4. "I should use ice packs to the scrotum after surgery to reduce swelling."
   5. "I will wear boxer shorts until healing is complete."

   NCLEX Client Need: Safe and Effective Care Environment: Coordinated Care
7. You are caring for a 40-year-old male patient who reports wanting to talk to the health care provider about "my manhood." Which nursing actions are appropriate? *(Select all that apply.)*
   1. Establishing eye contact
   2. Demonstrating sensitivity to nonverbal cues
   3. Asking closed-ended questions
   4. Asking the patient's girlfriend to be present for an assessment
   5. Inquiring for more specificity about what the patient means by "manhood"

   NCLEX Client Need: Health Promotion and Maintenance
8. A 68-year-old male has come to the clinic stating that it is getting more difficult for him to urinate. Uroflowmetry has been ordered. How would you explain the test to the patient?
   1. The lab technician will draw a blood sample from your arm.
   2. The healthcare provider will palpate your prostate gland using a lubricated, gloved finger inserted into your rectum.
   3. Contrast will be infused IV and the pathway of urine will be examined by x-ray to identify obstructions.
   4. You will be asked to urinate in a device that will measure the volume of urine expelled from the bladder per second.

   NCLEX Client Need: Safe and Effective Care Environment: Coordinated Care

Critical Thinking Questions

Scenario A

A 70-year-old patient reports finding a lump in her right breast after doing a breast self-examination in the shower. She tells you that if the lump is malignant, she does not want it removed, nor does she want any treatment such as chemotherapy or radiation.

1. What are some possible reasons that the patient has already decided she does not want surgery or treatment?
2. Are there other types of treatment the patient may consider instead of surgery, chemotherapy, or radiation?
3. What types of resources are available to help the patient make this decision?
4. What is your role in supporting the patient's decision?

Scenario B

A 19-year-old is referred for further testing when he finds a lump in his testicle. You are the nurse preparing him for the diagnostic workup.

1. The patient states, if I had not said anything, none of this would be happening and I could go on with my life. I wish I had just ignored the lump. How do you respond?
2. What testing would you expect to be done?

39 Care of Women With Reproductive Disorders

http://evolve.elsevier.com/deWit/medsurg

Objectives

Theory

1. Discuss common menstrual disorders and nursing interventions for each.
2. Examine causes and treatment of infertility.
3. Describe changes associated with menopause, treatment options, and nursing interventions.
4. Articulate the role of robotic gynecologic surgery as an alternative to open surgery.
5. Compare benign and malignant disorders of the female reproductive system.

Clinical Practice

6. Use the nursing process in the care of a woman with a reproductive disorder.
7. Implement interventions for patients with common disorders of the female reproductive tract.

Key Terms

amenorrhea (ă-mĕn-ŏ-RĒ-ă, p. 931)
anovulation (ăn-ŎV-ū-LĀ-shŭn, p. 931)
cystocele (SĬS-tō-sēl, p. 929)
dowager's hump (DŎW-ĭ-jĕrz HŬMP, p. 927)
dysmenorrhea (dĭs-mĕn-ō-RĒ-ă, p. 925)
dyspareunia (dĭs-pă-RŪ-nē-ă, p. 927)
effleurage (ĕf-lū-RĂZH, p. 925)
endometriosis (ĕn-dō-mē-trē-Ō-sĭs, p. 932)
enterocele (ĕn-TĔR-ō-sēl, p. 929)
fibroids (FĪ-broydz, p. 931)
hirsutism (HĔR-sūt-ĭszm, p. 929)
hysterectomy (hĭs-tĕr-ĔK-tō-mē, p. 929)
lymphedema (lĭm-fĕ-DĒ-mă, p. 943)
menorrhagia (mĕn-ō-RĀ-jă, p. 931)
metrorrhagia (mĕ-trō-RĀ-jă, p. 931)
myomectomy (mī-ō-MĔK-tō-mē, p. 932)
oligomenorrhea (ŏl-ĭ-gō-mĕn-ŏ-RĒ-ă, p. 930)
polycystic ovarian syndrome (pŏ-lē-SĬS-tĭk, ōVĂR-ē-ăn SĬN-drōm, p. 929)
prolapse (PRŌ-lăps, p. 929)
pruritus (prū-RĪ-tŭs, p. 927)
rectocele (RĔK-tō-sēl, p. 929)
sentinel node biopsy (SĔN-tĭ-nĕl nōd BĪ-ŏp-sē, p. 940)
stress incontinence (STRĔS ĭn-KŎN-tĭ-nĕns, p. 929)

Concepts Covered in This Chapter

- Hormonal Regulation
- Reproduction
- Sexuality

MENSTRUAL DYSFUNCTION

PREMENSTRUAL SYNDROME AND PREMENSTRUAL DYSPHORIC DISORDER

Premenstrual syndrome (PMS), also known as *ovarian cycle syndrome,* is the presence of physical, psychological, or behavioral symptoms that regularly recur within the luteal phase of the menstrual cycle and significantly disappear during the remainder of the cycle. These signs and symptoms, which occur between ovulation and menstruation, include abdominal bloating, breast tenderness, irritability, appetite changes, fatigue, mood swings, and a fear of losing control. Management includes stress reduction, relaxation, and exercise interventions (Casper & Yonkers, 2018).

Premenstrual dysphoric disorder (PMDD), a more serious problem, is described officially in the *Diagnostic and Statistical Manual of Mental Disorders,* Fifth Edition (*DSM-5;* American Psychiatric Association, 2017). It is believed to be the result of abnormal serotonin responses to normal changes in estrogen levels during the menstrual cycle. The symptom criteria used to diagnose PMDD occur between ovulation and the onset of menstruation and begin to improve between the menstruation and ovulation phases; they are not present in the week after the menstrual period. Diagnosis is based on specific symptoms in a pattern throughout more than 3 months. Symptoms include depressed mood; anxiety; irritability; difficulty in concentrating; change in appetite and sleep; and physical symptoms such as breast tenderness, bloating, weight gain, and headaches. Symptoms may interfere with the normal lifestyle, social relationships, and/or work responsibilities.

Strategies for self-care include stress management exercises; some lifestyle changes; maintaining a healthy diet rich in complex carbohydrates and fiber; avoiding simple sugars, salty foods, and caffeine; and preventing hypoglycemia. Exercise may increase beta-endorphin levels, which results in relief of depression and mood elevation. Although eating chocolate has been shown to elevate depressed moods, consumption should be limited, as this mood elevation is brief and may not be helpful to maintaining a healthy weight. Peer support groups, psychological counseling, and prescribed medications can also be helpful. Medical management commonly includes oral contraceptives (low estrogen, progestin dominant), diuretics during the luteal phase of the menstrual cycle, and nonsteroidal antiinflammatory drugs (NSAIDs). Selective serotonin reuptake inhibitors (SSRIs), such as fluoxetine (Sarafem) or sertraline (Zoloft), or serotonin norepinephrine reuptake inhibitors (SNRIs), such as venlafaxine (Effexor), have been shown to be effective in longer term management (Casper & Yonkers, 2018).

DYSMENORRHEA

Dysmenorrhea is painful menstruation, a very common gynecologic concern. There are two classifications of dysmenorrhea.

Primary Dysmenorrhea

Primary dysmenorrhea usually occurs 6 to 12 months after the menarche (when the process of ovulation becomes established and regular menstruation occurs) and often affects adolescent girls (Mendiratta, cited in Lobo et al., 2017). It is believed be caused by the release of high levels of prostaglandins in the ovulatory cycle, causing uterine contractions and vasoconstriction that result in abdominal cramps that can be incapacitating in the first few days of menstruation (McCance & Huether, 2019). The most commonly reported symptom is pelvic pain that radiates into the groin. Backache, decrease in appetite, vomiting, diarrhea, syncope, insomnia, and headache are the most common symptoms reported. Pelvic examination results for patients with primary dysmenorrhea are normal.

A heating pad promotes vasodilation and often relieves cramps. Back massage and soft rhythmic massage of the abdomen (**effleurage**) can also relieve discomfort. Exercises such as the **pelvic rock** relieve discomfort by releasing endorphins, suppressing prostaglandins, and shunting the blood flow away from the pelvic organs, which results in less pelvic congestion. The pelvic rock is performed in the hands-and-knees position, alternating arching the back and contracting abdominal and gluteal muscles while exhaling and then hollowing the back and relaxing the muscles while inhaling. Several complementary and alternative medicine (CAM) therapies, such as aromatherapy and meditation, can also be helpful. A balanced low-fat diet with foods that are natural diuretics, such as cranberry juice, asparagus, and watermelon, may decrease edema. Medications such as NSAIDs are prostaglandin inhibitors and may relieve many discomforts. Health care providers may prescribe an oral contraceptive (OC), which provides relief from menstrual discomforts, along with the advantages of contraceptive protection. Seasonale is an OC that provides longer periods of pain-free amenorrhea by allowing only four menstrual periods per year. Lybrel (ethinyl estradiol 20 μg and levonorgestrel 90 μg) is a low-dose combination OC that prevents menstruation for 1 year (Kaunitz, 2017). Herbal preparations and over-the-counter CAM medications are available for self-treatment. You should be aware of the side effects and interactions of CAM therapies with prescribed drugs.

> **? Think Critically**
>
> Why should you ask patients about over-the-counter medications and herbal remedies they are taking and document their use in the electronic health record?

Secondary Dysmenorrhea

Secondary dysmenorrhea typically occurs after 25 years of age and is caused by pelvic pathology, such as endometriosis, endometritis (infection), adenomyosis, pelvic inflammatory disease, obstructive uterine or vaginal abnormalities, the presence of nonhormonal intrauterine devices (IUDs) or uterine polyps, fibroids, or cysts (McCance & Huether, 2019). Pain associated with secondary dysmenorrhea is characterized by a dull lower abdominal pain that radiates to the back or thighs. The pain may occur before the menstrual period and last throughout the days of menstrual flow.

Management involves treating the cause of the pelvic pathology. Temporary relief may be obtained with the same therapies used for primary dysmenorrhea (Table 39.1).

Sexual Disorders

In August 2015, the U.S. Food and Drug Administration (FDA) approved the first drug for female sexual dysfunction. This drug, flibanserin (Addyi) is for women with hyposexual desire disorder (HSDD), which develops in approximately 1 in 10 premenopausal women. An oral dose of 100 mg is taken daily, and if no improvement is seen in 8 weeks, the drug is discontinued (Sprout Pharmaceuticals, 2018). Because there is a potentially serious interaction with alcohol, the drug carries a black box warning, may be prescribed only by health care providers who have received specialized training, and is available only from certified pharmacies.

INFERTILITY

Some women wish to have children yet have difficulty conceiving. For these women, preconception guidance and perhaps infertility treatments may be helpful. Preconception guidance involves gathering data about the woman and her partner to provide information necessary to make an informed, individualized decision concerning conception or fertility assistance. Screening for genetic disorders may be advisable.

Table 39.1 **Drugs Commonly Used to Treat Dysmenorrhea**

CLASSIFICATION	SIDE EFFECTS	NURSING IMPLICATIONS
Nonsteroidal antiinflammatory drugs (NSAIDs) Ibuprofen, Motrin, Naproxen	Nausea, dyspepsia, itching, rash.	Contraindicated in hemophilia, bleeding ulcers, bleeding disorders. Should not be taken with aspirin. (Check labels on cold/allergy medications that may contain NSAIDs.) Should be taken around the clock when menses starts to treat discomfort. Patient should take with meals or milk and not consume alcohol.
Oral contraceptives	Women who smoke should not use hormone therapy. Risks and benefits should be discussed with health care provider.	Use with caution in women with blood clotting disorders, cardiovascular disorders, or cancer.

Cultural Considerations

Fertility

Symbols and rites that celebrate fertility are practiced by many cultures. In the United States, throwing rice at a bride and groom represents a wish for family growth. In some countries, rubbing the swollen abdomen of a statue of a fertility goddess is a popular practice for women seeking to conceive.

Primary infertility is the inability of a couple to conceive a child after at least 1 year of active, unprotected sexual relations without using contraceptives. **Secondary infertility** is the inability to conceive after having once conceived or to maintain a pregnancy long enough to deliver a viable infant. Approximately 1 in 8 couples in the United States have difficulty getting pregnant and/or sustaining a pregnancy (Resolve.org, 2018), and increasing numbers of couples are seeking medical intervention. Infertility services also assist individuals without a partner who wish to have a child.

The ability to conceive depends primarily on both partners having normal reproductive physiology, physiologically and psychologically sensitive interaction, and proper timing of intercourse. Factors in men that contribute to infertility include problems with the sperm, abnormal ejaculation, abnormal erections, and abnormal seminal fluid. Chapter 40 discusses problems that can occur in the male reproductive system. Factors contributing to infertility in a woman include the following:

- Ovulation problems
- An abnormality in the pathway between the cervix and fallopian tube
- An abnormality in the endometrium of the uterus or malformation of the uterus
- Tumors in the reproductive tract
- A vaginal or cervical environment that is inhospitable to sperm motility or viability

Repeated pregnancy loss can be caused by an abnormality in fetal chromosomes that results in spontaneous abortion, abnormalities of the cervix or uterus, disorders of the endocrine or immune system, infections, or environmental factors such as toxic agents. Preconception counseling helps the couple evaluate problems or risks related to conception (see the Communication box).

Diagnostic tests include a detailed health history and laboratory tests, such as serum prolactin levels and other endocrine evaluations, semen analysis, sperm antibody agglutination studies, and chromosome studies. Tests for tubal patency and other possible abnormalities in both the male and female reproductive tracts may also be needed.

Communication

Emotional Impact of Infertility

The emotional impact of infertility is intense. Some couples become almost desperate to conceive. Assess whether psychological intervention may be needed to assist the couple to deal with the stress of their situation. Indications that a referral may be needed include, but are not limited to, inability to focus on anything other than the desire to have a child and tension in the relationship of the couple, including blaming each other for the infertility.

ASSISTED REPRODUCTION

Assisted reproductive therapies (ARTs) are available but are associated with ethical and legal issues, such as the risk of having a multifetal pregnancy, freezing embryos for later use, and the use of a surrogate mother. Donor eggs or donor sperm can be used, making future legal challenges for custody a possibility. It is now possible for a child to have five technical parents: sperm donor, egg donor, gestational surrogate, and the parents who will raise the child. Success rates of ARTs vary, and the procedures are usually expensive and rarely covered by health insurance. Box 39.1 lists some types of ART procedures.

Box 39.1 Examples of Assisted Reproductive Therapy (ART) Procedures

- *In vitro fertilization and embryo transfer (IVF-ET):* Woman's eggs are collected from the ovary, fertilized in a laboratory, and transferred into the uterus at the embryo stage of development.
- *Zygote intrafallopian transfer (ZIFT):* After in vitro fertilization, the ovum is placed into the fallopian tube at the zygote stage of development.
- *Therapeutic donor insemination (TDI):* A donor's sperm inseminates the female.
- *Intracytoplasmic sperm injection:* Injection of one live sperm directly into the mature egg.
- *Surrogate mother:* The surrogate mother can be inseminated with one partner's sperm or be implanted with an egg fertilized by one partner's sperm in vitro. The egg is transferred to the uterus of the surrogate mother; she becomes a gestational carrier.

NURSING MANAGEMENT

DATA COLLECTION

A complete health history is needed as well as information regarding fertility. Lab testing will be completed on both partners.

NURSING DIAGNOSES

Patient problem statements that should be considered:

- Loss of power related to infertility
- Altered role performance
- Altered self concept
- Spiritual distress
- Altered family coping

TREATMENT

Interventions you can discuss with patients regarding infertility may include actions such as:

- Using water-soluble lubricants during intercourse because these do not have spermicidal properties.
- Having the male partner avoid environments that cause high scrotal temperatures, such as saunas, which can reduce sperm production as well as the life span of the sperm.
- Stress management, nutrition counseling, and lifestyle analysis.

Interventions for infertility can also involve medical therapy, such as the use of drugs that stimulate ovulation.

Complementary and Alternative Therapies

Herbal Products and Fertility

Because use of CAMs such as herbs and oils is common, women should be instructed that the use of these products should be avoided while trying to conceive and maintain a pregnancy (Saper, 2018). There is currently no scientific evidence that herbal products are effective in promoting fertility.

Box 39.2 Lifestyle Activities That Increase Risk of Osteoporosis

- **Inadequate lifetime intake of calcium and vitamin D:** Prevents reaching peak bone mass by age 30 years
- **Smoking:** Decreases estrogen production
- **Excessive alcohol intake:** Interferes with calcium absorption and depresses new bone growth
- **Excessive caffeine, cola, or soft drink intake:** Results in imbalanced calcium and phosphorus or demineralizes bone

MENOPAUSE

As noted in Chapter 38, menopause is the cessation of menses for 12 consecutive months because of a decrease in estrogen production. Although this is a normal progression within the life span of females, there are health changes and risks associated with menopause. The aging process and the decrease in estrogen levels can cause thinning of the vaginal walls **(atrophy)** as well as dryness and itching of the vagina (**pruritus**). These changes may result in painful sexual relations (**dyspareunia**) and can also lead to increased susceptibility to infections because the vaginal pH increases.

NURSING MANAGEMENT

DATA COLLECTION

The major health problems that occur at or after menopause include the development of osteoporosis and coronary heart disease.

Osteoporosis

Osteoporosis is a decrease in bone mass that increases the risk for bone fractures. The decrease in estrogen that occurs during menopause slows bone growth, and therefore bone deteriorates and thins before new bone growth occurs. Estrogen also enables vitamin D to assist in calcium absorption in the intestine, and a decrease in estrogen is associated with a decrease in calcium, which is essential to healthy bone tissue. Box 39.2 provides a list of some lifestyle activities that may increase the risk of developing osteoporosis. Denosumab (Prolia) is an FDA-approved used to increase bone density in the treatment of osteoporosis in menopausal women (FDA, 2017).

Older Adult Care Points

Older women who are on long-term estrogen replacement therapy are at increased risk for endometrial cancer and breast cancer; it is particularly important that these women have annual pelvic examinations and have regular breast cancer screenings.

The first signs of osteoporosis are loss of height, back pain, and the development of a **dowager's hump** in which vertebrae fail to support the upper body in an upright

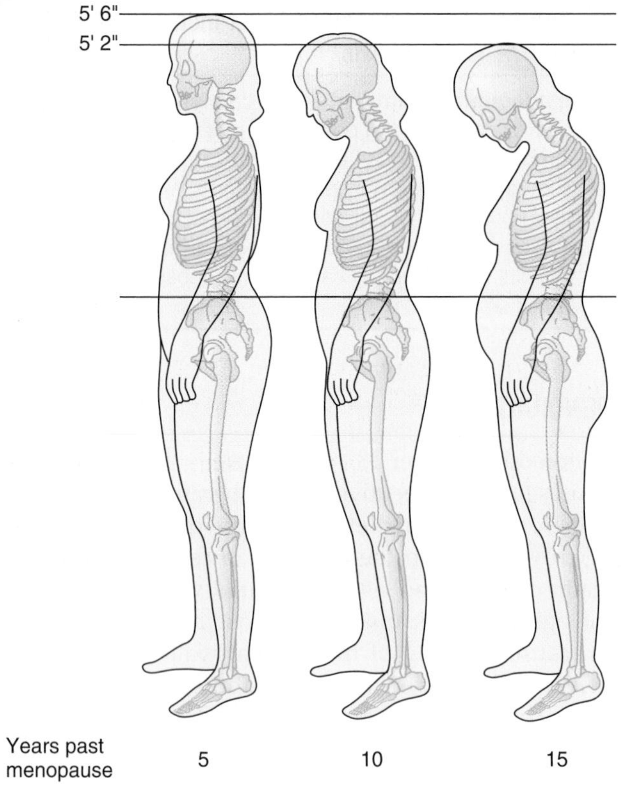

Fig. 39.1 With progression of osteoporosis, the vertebral column collapses, causing loss of height and back pain. *Dowager's hump* is the term used for this curvature of the back.

position (Fig. 39.1). The American College of Obstetricians and Gynecologists (ACOG) recommends bone density screening for menopausal women. Chapter 32 discusses osteoporosis in detail.

Postmenopausal women are at increased risk for coronary heart disease because of changes in lipid metabolism and a rise in total cholesterol. Diet and exercise can help minimize the effects of these risks. See Chapters 19 and 20 for details on cardiovascular diseases.

A physical examination, health history, lab testing, and bone density assessment can identify the presence or the risk for osteoporosis and coronary heart disease.

IMPLEMENTATION

Hormone Therapy

Hormone replacement therapy (HRT) (with estrogen and/or progesterone) was once the cornerstone of interventions that reduced the discomforts of menopause (hot flashes and vaginal atrophy) and protected women from developing coronary heart disease and osteoporosis. Research shows that HRT can slightly increase the risk of developing blood clots, stroke, heart attack, gallbladder disease, and uterine and breast cancer (ACOG, 2018). Therefore patients who are prescribed HRT must receive detailed education concerning the risks of therapy. A combination of estrogen and bazedoxifene (Duavee) was approved in 2013 to treat vasomotor signs and symptoms associated with menopause and may prevent postmenopausal osteoporosis in women who still have their uterus in place (Goldberg & Fidler, 2015).

Bioidentical Hormones

A bioidentical hormone such as oral estradiol, estradiol transdermal patches, or oral micronized progesterone (Prometrium) has a chemical structure identical to hormones produced in the human body but is clinically synthesized from steroidal molecules taken from wild yam or soy. It differs from "natural hormones" such as conjugated equine hormone (Premarin), which comes from the urine of pregnant mares and has a chemical structure different from the human hormone. Progesterone is a bioidentical hormone that has a different chemical structure from progestins. Both synthetic and bioidentical hormones interact with the same estrogen and progesterone receptors on target cells, but their physiologic side effects may differ. Bioidentical hormones are made (compounded) by individual pharmacies and are not regulated or approved by the FDA (ACOG, 2018). Bioidentical hormone drugs do not usually have package inserts. You should be alert to research findings that involve "hormone therapy" and inquire whether the hormones researched are bioidentical or synthetic FDA, 2018).

Minivelle, an estrogen-only transdermal patch, may be prescribed to treat vasomotor symptoms of menopause but may increase risk of dementia in women older than 65 years (RxList, 2018).

Alternative Therapies

Some CAM therapies have been helpful in relieving specific discomforts of menopause. Homeopathy, acupuncture, and certain herbs may offer relief, but each may have contraindications as well. Herbal therapy has not been fully researched or regulated, and side effects or interactions with food or drugs are possible. Phytoestrogens; soy products; and vitamins B, C, and E have been shown to be helpful in relieving menopausal discomforts. Soy isoflavones have been found to be very effective in relieving vasomotor symptoms of menopause but depend on specific bowel flora for activation. Soy should not be used by women with estrogen-dependent cancers or women taking tamoxifen (Nolvadex) (Zhang et al., 2017) or aromatase inhibitors. Medications such as alendronic acid (Fosamax) can be prescribed for women with osteoporosis, but side effects should be explained carefully. After taking alendronic acid, the woman must be able to sit upright for at least 30 minutes. Diet, yoga, and tai chi have remarkable value, and support groups are very effective in helping to manage menopause. Exercise has been shown to be of particular benefit in relieving menopausal symptoms (Pru, 2017).

DISORDERS OF THE FEMALE REPRODUCTIVE TRACT

PELVIC RELAXATION SYNDROME (CYSTOCELE, RECTOCELE, ENTEROCELE, AND UTERINE PROLAPSE)

When the muscles, ligaments, and fascia that support the pelvic floor weaken, the pelvic organs may descend toward the vaginal orifice. It can affect the bladder

Health Promotion

Using CAM Therapies for Menopause

Women should be encouraged to consult with a health care provider before using CAM therapies such as soy isoflavones, black cohosh, or other herbs. For some women with estrogen-dependent cancers, these substances may be contraindicated. Certain herbs may interact with other medications the patient is taking.

Nutritional Considerations

Managing Menopause

When phytoestrogens are recommended by the health care provider, teaching about these substances should be provided. Phytoestrogens are found in foods such as wild yams, cherries, dandelion greens, alfalfa sprouts, and black beans. Food sources of soy include tofu, soy milk, and roasted soy nuts.

(**cystocele**), rectum (**rectocele**), bowel (**enterocele**), or uterus (uterine prolapse).

Aging-Related Changes

After menopause, some atrophy of the female organs, loss of elasticity, dryness of the vaginal membranes, and reduction of bone mass occur because of the decrease in estrogen levels. Loss of natural tissue elasticity may allow internal organs to sag, or **prolapse**, into the vagina.

Etiology and Pathophysiology

Because the lack of estrogen results in weakening of tissue structures, pelvic relaxation syndrome is more likely to occur as women age. The bladder protrudes through the vaginal wall, forming a cystocele, or into the rectum, forming a rectocele. As expected life span has increased, these problems have also increased in frequency. Heavy lifting, constipation, and obesity contribute to the weakening of the pelvic floor muscles and tissues. Pelvic surgery and the strain of vaginal childbirth may also contribute to the development of pelvic relaxation syndrome.

Signs and Symptoms

Symptoms relate to the specific organs involved. In a cystocele, urinary frequency or incontinence is most common. A rectocele may result in constipation, soiling, or painful defecation. A uterine prolapse may result in dyspareunia. The uterus may protrude from the vaginal orifice. The woman often complains of general symptoms that include a sense of fullness in the pelvis and backache. **Stress incontinence** (loss of small amount of urine during coughing, sneezing, or lifting objects) may occur.

Diagnosis

Diagnosis is confirmed by history and physical examination. Obtain an obstetric history concerning the number of vaginal deliveries and the size of the infants, which may have contributed to the present problem. A history of stress incontinence or constipation may indicate how the problem may interfere with activities of daily living. A computed tomography (CT) scan may be required if other pelvic pathology is suspected. The patient and the health care provider determine whether a nonsurgical or surgical approach to management is most appropriate.

Treatment and Nursing Management

Nonsurgical management. Nonsurgical management includes teaching the woman how to perform Kegel exercises to strengthen the pubococcygeal muscles that support the pelvic floor (refer to Chapter 33, Patient Teaching: Kegel Exercises).

Lifestyle changes include increasing fluid intake and a high-fiber diet to prevent constipation and maintaining an optimal weight. Hormone therapy may be prescribed. A **pessary** (a hard rubber or plastic ring) can be fitted into the vagina by the health care provider to provide support to the pelvic structures.

Complementary and Alternative Therapies

Biofeedback and Transcutaneous Electrical Nerve Stimulation

Biofeedback and transcutaneous electrical nerve stimulation (TENS) may be performed by a licensed health care provider to help strengthen the pelvic floor muscles.

Surgical management. The procedure to repair a cystocele or rectocele is called an *anteroposterior repair (colporrhaphy)*. A **hysterectomy** (removal of the uterus) may be indicated (Table 39.2).

The management of pelvic prolapse includes minimally invasive surgery. Surgical repair may be accomplished laparoscopically, abdominally, or transvaginally. Research continues on the use of certain types of mesh to decrease the chance of postoperative complications. Surgical, anatomic, and functional outcomes using polyvinylidene fluoride (PVDF) and standard polypropylene (PP) mesh have been shown to have comparative outcomes, although use of PVDF has been associated with far fewer storage symptoms (i.e. frequency, urgency) and subsequent sexual dysfunction (Balsamo et al., 2018).

POLYCYSTIC OVARIAN SYNDROME

Polycystic ovarian syndrome is a congenital condition in which many cysts develop on one or both ovaries and produce excess estrogen. High levels of testosterone and luteinizing hormone (LH) and low levels of follicle-stimulating hormone (FSH) occur. Signs and symptoms include irregular menstruation, infertility, hyperinsulinemia, and glucose tolerance problems. Excessive hair on the body (**hirsutism**) is common.

Treatment involves use of OCs to inhibit LH and testosterone production. Surgical removal of the cysts may be indicated. If pregnancy is desired, ovulation-stimulating medications may be prescribed. Advise the patient on the importance of follow-up care to monitor the progress of this condition.

Table 39.2 Gynecologic Surgical Procedures

REASONS FOR PERFORMING	DESCRIPTION	NURSING CARE AND TEACHING POINTS
Dilation and Evacuation (D&E)		
Excessive vaginal bleeding; incomplete abortion; removal of placental fragments; therapeutic abortion.	Scraping away the inner lining of the uterus (endometrium) via the cervix.	Observe for excessive bleeding postoperatively.
Conization or Conical Excision		
Abnormal or early cancerous tissue; biopsy.	Removal of cone of tissue with scalpel or electrical cutting wire.	Office procedure. May cause some bleeding.
Fistulectomy		
Presence of rectovaginal fistula (channel between rectum and vagina) or urethrovaginal fistula (channel between bladder and vagina).	Surgical excision of the fistula and repair of the tissue to prevent passage of urine or feces into the vagina.	Observe for excessive bleeding or for vaginal fecal drainage postoperatively.
Hysterectomy		
Prolapse of pelvic organs; pain associated with pelvic congestion; endometriosis; excessive/debilitating uterine bleeding; fibroids; noninvasive uterine or cervical cancer.	Removal of entire uterus, vaginally or abdominally (open or robotic).	Observe for excessive bleeding; paralytic ileus can occur. Ends childbearing if premenopausal, which may have profound emotional effects.
Panhysterectomy		
Cancer; pain associated with pelvic inflammatory disease; recurrent ovarian cysts.	Removal of entire uterus, fallopian tubes, and ovaries.	See hysterectomy. Removal of ovaries induces menopause in premenopausal women.
Radical Hysterectomy		
Invasive cancer.	Removal of uterus, fallopian tubes, ovaries, upper third of vagina, and lymph nodes.	See hysterectomy and panhysterectomy. Vaginal alteration may affect ability to have sexual intercourse. Possible lymphedema from removal of nodes.
Anterior and Posterior Colporrhaphy		
Presence of prolapse of bladder and rectum into the vagina; may accompany a uterine prolapse.	Repair of the anterior and posterior wall of the vagina.	Observe for excessive bleeding.
Salpingectomy		
Tubal pregnancy; tumor; traumatic injury.	Removal of a fallopian tube.	Will not cause infertility if other tube/ovary is intact.
Oophorectomy		
Tumor; cystic disease; endometriosis; traumatic injury; severe hormonal disorder.	Removal of an ovary.	See salpingectomy. Only a portion of one ovary is necessary to provide normal hormonal balance before menopause.
Vulvectomy/Endoscopic Laparoscopy		
Malignancy.	Radical vulvectomy: surgical excision of the labia, clitoris, perineal structures, femoral and inguinal lymphatic tissues.	Major disfigurement; extreme supportive measures, including professional counseling, often required.

DYSFUNCTIONAL UTERINE BLEEDING

Dysfunctional uterine bleeding (DUB) is uterine bleeding that occurs at times other than the normal menstrual cycle or abnormal bleeding during menstruation. Uterine bleeding may be considered abnormal if the interval between menstruations is less than 21 days or more than 45 days, the duration of menstrual flow is more than 7 days, or the amount of blood loss exceeds 80 mL.

Oligomenorrhea (decreased menstruation) usually refers to menstrual periods that occur at an interval of 45 days or longer. The cause often involves a problem with the hypothalamus, the pituitary gland, or ovarian function. Hormone therapy is the treatment of choice, and the woman should be educated about the advantages and disadvantages of hormone therapy. The use of OCs can decrease menstrual flow. Structural abnormalities can cause obstructions or destruction of the endometrium, resulting in oligomenorrhea. The woman should be taught to keep close records of her menstrual cycle and associated symptoms.

Amenorrhea is the absences of menstruation. *Primary amenorrhea* refers to women who have not had a normal onset of menstrual periods (they never started to menstruate). *Secondary amenorrhea* applies to women who began normal menses that later ceased. Some causes include anatomic defects such as **imperforate** (closed) hymen, an endocrine dysfunction affecting female hormones, chronic disease, extreme weight loss or obesity, emotional disturbances, drug side effect, excessive exercise, or poor nutrition. Amenorrhea is a normal occurrence during pregnancy. Goals of treatment include progression of normal pubertal development; prevention of complications such as osteoporosis, endometrial hyperplasia, or heart disease; and promotion of fertility.

Metrorrhagia is bleeding between menstrual periods. Occasionally a brief episode of "spotting" occurs 14 days before the expected menstrual period (corresponding to the time of ovulation). This is known as "mittle staining" and is considered normal. Women who take OCs or have an IUD may have bleeding between menstrual periods, which is called *breakthrough bleeding*. The problem is usually resolved by adjusting the medication or dosage. Causes of abnormal metrorrhagia include leiomyomas, uterine polyps, trauma, foreign body, malignancy, infection, or an interrupted pregnancy. The treatment depends on the cause. Nursing responsibilities include providing reassurance, support, and education.

Menorrhagia is excessive menstrual bleeding or duration of the menstrual period. There are many causes, including hormone imbalances, malignancies, fibroids, infections, and the use of some drugs. One cause of heavy menstrual bleeding is von Willebrand disease, which is caused by a chromosome factor VIII dysfunction. Symptoms often include frequent nosebleeds and delayed postpartum hemorrhage. Blood tests should be taken during menstruation for accurate diagnosis. Treatment of menorrhagia depends on the cause. The hemoglobin and hematocrit should always be assessed to determine the seriousness of the blood loss. Tranexamic acid (Lysteda) is a drug approved for nonhormonal treatment of menorrhagia. This oral medication works by reducing clot breakdown in the uterus. Tranexamic acid should only be used with the most extreme measures of caution if given as adjunct to OCs because the risk for thrombus formation or stroke increases with the combination (Thorne, James, & Reid, 2018). Nursing interventions include education about follow-up care, an iron-rich diet, and information on the treatment options available.

ABNORMAL UTERINE BLEEDING

Abnormal uterine bleeding (AUB) is defined as uterine bleeding not related to the menstrual period. It is often caused by anovulation and a failure of hormonal changes during the menstrual cycle. It most often occurs at the beginning (menarche) or end (menopause) of the reproductive years. Bleeding from continuous estrogen production can also occur as a result of thyroid dysfunction, polycystic ovarian disease, infection, trauma, or neoplasm. Use of some herbal products that promote estrogen activity can also cause dysfunctional or abnormal uterine bleeding.

Older Adult Care Points

Vaginal bleeding in postmenopausal women is a possible warning sign of cervical or uterine cancer. An immediate pelvic examination is advised to determine and treat the cause of such bleeding. The incidence of these cancers increases with age.

Monitoring the hemoglobin and hematocrit is essential, and hospitalization may be required if the hemoglobin falls below 8 g/100 mL. Severe bleeding may be treated with intravenous conjugated estrogens (Premarin) until bleeding stops or slows significantly. A dilation and evacuation (formerly known as a *dilation and curettage*) and endometrial biopsy may be required. The woman may be given OCs for 3 to 6 months, after which the bleeding pattern will be reassessed.

Persistent **anovulation** (failure to ovulate) with continuous estrogen stimulation of the endometrium can cause abnormal tissue changes in the uterus. Nursing interventions include educating the patient about the use of unproven CAM therapies and proper use of OCs, providing support during treatments, and ensuring that the patient is aware of treatment options.

LEIOMYOMA

Commonly known as uterine **fibroids**, leiomyomas are benign tumors of the uterine muscle. Their growth is influenced by ovarian hormones, and they are common in women taking birth control pills. They spontaneously shrink during and after menopause. Common symptoms include backache, a sense of lower abdominal pressure, constipation, urinary frequency or incontinence, and abnormal uterine bleeding. A pelvic examination and ultrasound may help confirm the diagnosis.

Medical management depends on the size and location of the fibroids, the symptoms experienced, the desire for future pregnancies, and how near the woman is to natural menopause. In mild cases, monitoring and supportive care to relieve symptoms are indicated. NSAIDs or OCs may be prescribed. In severe cases, leuprolide (Lupron) or nafarelin (Synarel), which are gonadotropin-releasing hormone (GnRH) agonists that shrink the fibroids, and other hormones may be prescribed to suppress estrogen. These drugs may cause menopausal symptoms and bone demineralization, and their use is limited to a 6-month period to reduce the fibroids and prepare for surgery.

Uterine artery embolization involves the injection of special pellets into selected blood vessels that supply the fibroid, resulting in shrinkage of the fibroid. It is performed under conscious sedation by an interventional radiologist (a radiologist who specializes in invasive procedures not requiring general anesthesia). Cramping, nausea, fever, and malaise (postembolic syndrome) may occur postoperatively as the fibroid degenerates. Postoperative pain may require an overnight hospitalization and treatment with fentanyl or hydromorphone (Dilaudid) by patient-controlled analgesia. Maintenance of hydration and ambulation to prevent complications are encouraged postoperatively. After 6 weeks, magnetic resonance imaging (MRI) can be used to confirm the effectiveness of the procedure. Postoperative teaching includes avoiding anticoagulant drugs, including aspirin; avoiding douches, sexual intercourse, and the use of tampons for 4 weeks postoperatively; monitoring urine output; preventing constipation; and returning for follow-up care.

Myomectomy is the removal of the tumor from the uterine wall and can be accomplished by use of an endoscope via an abdominal incision **(laparoscopy)** or vaginally **(hysteroscopy).** It is performed in the proliferative phase of the menstrual cycle and does minimal damage to the uterine lining, allowing for positive pregnancy outcomes in the future. Fibroids can eventually return. **Hysteroscopic endometrial ablation** is a nonsurgical technique that involves resection of submucosal fibroids followed by scraping and burning of tissue. This procedure significantly reduces future fertility. **Myolysis,** laser or electrosurgical destruction of the fibroids, can also be done laparoscopically or vaginally and may preserve fertility. **Magnetic resonance–guided focused ultrasound surgery (MRgFUS)** is a mini-invasive procedure that has been shown to be a safe way to significantly reduce symptoms of premenopausal uterine fibroids with a rapid return to quality of life (Ferrari et al., 2016).

A **hysterectomy** (removal of the uterus) may be performed if the woman does not wish future pregnancies. A laparoscopic supracervical hysterectomy preserves the cervix and is less invasive, with fewer complications. However, for benign disease, the robotic or vaginal route for hysterectomy is preferred. Approximately 600,000 hysterectomies are performed within the United States annually, making this the second most performed surgery after cesarean sections for women of reproductive age (National Women's Health Network, 2018). Medical necessities for a hysterectomy include cancer, an unmanageable infection or bleeding, or a serious birth complication such as a ruptured uterus. Nursing responsibilities include providing education on the patient's options, clarifying misconceptions, and reducing patient anxiety. The postoperative teaching plan should include current information on the advantages and disadvantages of hormone therapy, comfort measures for pain relief, and when to resume normal activities. Nursing Care Plan 39.1 presents one example of managing the care of a postoperative patient after abdominal hysterectomy. The use of lubricants for vaginal intercourse and a plan for follow-up care should also be provided. Danger signs to report to the health care provider include bleeding or abnormal vaginal discharge.

ENDOMETRIOSIS

Endometriosis is a common disorder in which endometrial tissue (the inner lining of the uterus) is found outside the uterus, particularly on the ovaries, in the rectovaginal septum (wall separating the rectum and the vagina), and in the pelvis and abdomen (Fig. 39.2). It usually undergoes the same changes as the normal endometrium during the menstrual cycle and may bleed at the time of menses, which can cause irritation, pain, and the formation of adhesions. Other symptoms may include excessive menstrual flow, bleeding between periods, painful bowel movements, and painful coitus.

Continuous hormonal contraceptive therapy and drugs such as medroxyprogesterone acetate (Depo-Provera) or norethindrone suppress growth of the endometrial tissue. Danazol (Cyclomen, Danocrine) and GnRH agonists, such as leuprolide or nafarelin, create a "pseudomenopause" by interfering with hormones that stimulate ovulation and menstruation. Menopausal symptoms such as hot flashes, decreased **libido** (sexual drive), and reduced bone density may occur. Continuous hormonal contraceptive treatment may be continued for 3 to 6 months. Surgical treatment may include a laparoscopy to remove adhesions or laser ablation of the lesions, which may preserve fertility.

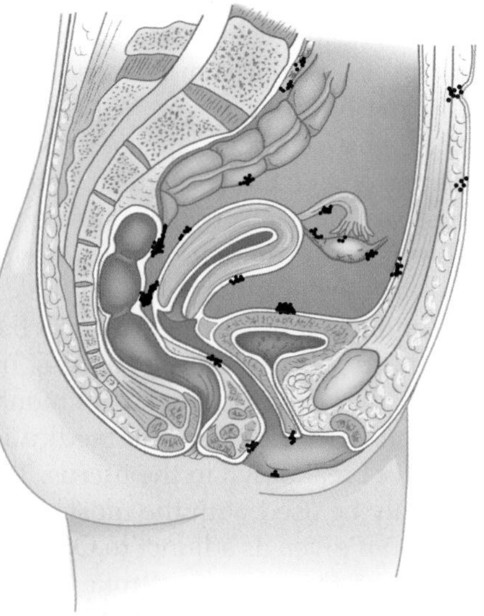

Fig. 39.2 Pelvic sites of endometrial implantation. Endometrial cells may enter the pelvic cavity during retrograde menstruation. (From McCance KL, Huether SE: *Pathophysiology: the biologic basis for disease in adults and children*, ed 8, St. Louis, 2019, Elsevier.)

Nursing Care Plan 39.1 Care of a Patient After Hysterectomy

SCENARIO

Marilyn Jariah, age 53 years, has just returned to the unit after abdominal hysterectomy for multiple fibroids, metrorrhagia, and greatly increased uterine size that caused abdominal pain. She has an IV infusion of 1000 mL normal saline in the left forearm, an indwelling urinary catheter, an abdominal dressing, and patient-controlled analgesia (PCA) pump containing morphine. Her vital signs are BP 140/84, P 84, R 18, T 98.2° F (36.8° C).

PROBLEM STATEMENT/NURSING DIAGNOSIS

Pain related to abdominal surgery.

SUPPORTING ASSESSMENT DATA

Subjective: Pain at 8/10 on pain scale: "It hurts to turn."
Objective: Abdominal hysterectomy incision.

Goals/Expected Outcomes	Nursing Interventions	Selected Rationale	Evaluation
Pain will be controlled by PCA, maintaining a level below 5/10.	Instruct patient in use of PCA pump. Administer booster medication as prescribed if needed.	When patient feels in control, anxiety is reduced and less pain medication may be required.	Analgesia via PCA pump provides adequate relief.
	Assess location, type, and quality of pain q2-3h using a pain scale.	Assessing location and quality of pain can alert nurse to developing complications.	Pain at 4/10 on pain scale.
	Assist with repositioning and support with pillows to attain comfort. Provide quiet, darkened atmosphere for rest and sleep.	Changing position prevents stasis of circulation; comfortable, supported position promotes relaxation.	Assisted to reposition q2h. Sleeping long intervals on side with pillow behind back and between knees for comfort.
	Monitor for side effects of analgesics, especially respiratory rate. Administer antiemetic as prescribed at first signs of nausea to prevent vomiting.	Morphine can depress respiratory rate.	Respirations 16–20. No nausea or emesis.
	Check Foley catheter and tubing for patency frequently to prevent bladder distention.	Bladder distention can increase pain and cause infection from stasis of urine in bladder.	Bladder not distended, Foley draining clear urine.

PROBLEM STATEMENT/NURSING DIAGNOSIS

Potential for fluid volume deficit due to possible hemorrhage.

SUPPORTING ASSESSMENT DATA

Objective: Abdominal hysterectomy.

Goals/Expected Outcomes	Nursing Interventions	Selected Rationale	Evaluation
Vital signs (VS) will remain stable and within normal parameters; no signs of shock or hemorrhage.	Monitor VS frequently per postoperative protocol routine.	A rapid pulse and decreasing BP can indicate development of shock.	VS are at baseline: BP 118/68, P 84, R 16.
	Check abdominal dressing and beneath patient for signs of bleeding with each set of VS; assess for bleeding from vaginal area.	Gravity can cause fluids to drain to a point beneath the patient.	Abdominal dressing clean and dry; no visible vaginal drainage.
	Assess for signs of intra-abdominal bleeding, such as increasing abdominal girth, decreasing bowel sounds, and increasing abdominal pain and rigidity.	Intra-abdominal bleeding is a complication of abdominal hysterectomy.	Abdomen soft; bowel sounds have returned; no evidence of intra-abdominal bleeding.

PROBLEM STATEMENT/NURSING DIAGNOSIS

Potential for altered breathing pattern due to pain.

Continued

Nursing Care Plan 39.1 Care of a Patient After Hysterectomy—cont'd

SUPPORTING ASSESSMENT DATA

Subjective: "It hurts to take a deep breath."

Objective: Abdominal hysterectomy.

Goals/Expected Outcomes	Nursing Interventions	Selected Rationale	Evaluation
Patient will have no signs of atelectasis or pneumonia as evidenced by clear breath sounds in all lung fields and afebrile status.	Assist patient to use an incentive spirometer, sit up to deep-breathe, and cough q2h while awake; give small pillow and instruct on splinting incision before coughing.	Cough and deep-breathing exercises can prevent development of atelectasis. Pain can prevent patient from taking deep breaths.	Able to deep-breathe and cough at 8 and 10 A.M. and 12 and 2 P.M. Sitting on side of bed at 8 and 10 A.M. and 12 and 2 P.M. while awake.
	Teach family or significant others to remind patient to deep-breathe.	Others can provide encouragement and support.	Family helping and reminding patient to do breathing exercises.
	Report adventitious, diminished, or absent breath sounds or crackles.	Abnormal breath sounds can be sign of developing complications.	Lung sounds clear bilaterally; all VS are WNL; T 98.0° F (36.7° C).

PROBLEM STATEMENT/NURSING DIAGNOSIS

Potential for infection due to surgery.

SUPPORTING ASSESSMENT DATA

Objective: Abdominal surgical incision.

Goals/Expected Outcomes	Nursing Interventions	Selected Rationale	Evaluation
Patient will remain free from signs and symptoms of infection throughout hospitalization and at discharge.	Administer prophylactic antibiotics as prescribed.	Antibiotics kill pathogens.	Tolerating prescribed medications.
	Monitor incision for signs of redness, swelling, purulent drainage, or hardness.	Redness, swelling, drainage, and pain at incision site may be signs of infection.	No incisional redness, swelling, hardness, or purulent drainage.
	Keep dressing clean and dry. Use careful aseptic technique when changing dressings.	A wound dressing must be kept clean and dry to prevent contamination that can cause infection.	Dressing clean and dry.
	Monitor WBC count and temperature.	—	WBC count WNL; afebrile.
	Assess vaginal drainage for signs of odor or change in character.	Odor or purulent appearance of vaginal drainage may indicate infection.	Vaginal drainage is minimal, serosanguinous, and without odor.
	Assess abdomen for signs of infection, increasing pain, localized tenderness, swelling, increased erythema (redness) around wound edges, decreased bowel sounds.	Tenderness, swelling, increased erythema, and decreased bowel sounds are signs of intra-abdominal infection.	Abdomen soft, active bowel sounds; no signs or symptoms of infection.

PROBLEM STATEMENT/NURSING DIAGNOSIS

Potential for injury (deep vein thrombosis) due to decreased activity level following abdominopelvic surgery.

SUPPORTING ASSESSMENT DATA

Objective: Abdominal hysterectomy and decreased activity level.

Goals/Expected Outcomes	Nursing Interventions	Selected Rationale	Evaluation
Patient will not exhibit signs of thrombophlebitis at time of discharge.	Encourage ambulation as soon as it is ordered; explain benefits of walking. Assist with leg and ankle exercises q2h.	Range-of-motion exercise and early ambulation can prevent the development of thrombus formation. Leg exercises increase circulation and prevent blood pooling.	Leg and ankle exercises q2h while awake and is tolerating ambulation.

Nursing Care Plan 39.1 Care of a Patient After Hysterectomy—cont'd

Goals/Expected Outcomes	Nursing Interventions	Selected Rationale	Evaluation
	Administer DVT prophylaxis medication as ordered	Heparin or low-molecular-weight heparin decreases the risk of DVT.	Platelet count unchanged from preop.
	Monitor SCDs every shift.	SCDs prevent pooling.	SCDs functioning properly.
	Encourage added fluid intake as soon as diet order allows.	Extra liquids keep blood more fluid and less likely to clot.	Presently NPO with IV fluids.
	Inspect lower legs every shift; check for positive Homan sign.	A positive Homan sign may indicate development of thrombophlebitis.	Homan sign negative.

PROBLEM STATEMENT/NURSING DIAGNOSIS

Alteration in body image due to removal of uterus.

SUPPORTING ASSESSMENT DATA

Subjective: "I wonder how this will affect the way my partner sees me."
Objective: Abdominal hysterectomy.

Goals/Expected Outcomes	Nursing Interventions	Selected Rationale	Evaluation
Patient will express concerns over loss of uterus before discharge. Patient will accept new body image within 3 mo as evidenced by lack of depression and engagement in usual activities.	Provide openings for conversation regarding patient's concerns over loss of uterus and its meaning to her. Explore her feelings regarding sexuality after hysterectomy. Encourage expression of positive aspects of having the hysterectomy and how she as a person is unchanged.	Enabling patient to verbalize and express concerns will make it possible to establish a patient-centered plan of care and teaching.	Patient is able to begin discussion about concerns; will continue tomorrow.

CRITICAL THINKING QUESTIONS

1. After having an abdominal hysterectomy, Ms. Jariah appears depressed and states that she is worried that her sexual relationship with her partner will "never be the same." What is the appropriate nursing response?
2. Which options for the treatment of uterine fibroids, in addition to abdominal hysterectomy, are available?

BP, Blood pressure; *DVT,* deep vein thrombosis; *IV,* intravenous; *NPO,* nothing by mouth; *P,* pulse; *R,* respirations; *SCD,* sequential compression device; *T,* temperature; *WBC,* white blood cell; *WNL,* within normal limits.

If the woman does not desire children in the future, a partial or complete hysterectomy and removal of all endometrial lesions is the most recommended treatment. Treatment for menopausal symptoms may be needed postoperatively.

Surgical Management

Robotic surgery is surgery performed by a surgeon's manipulation of robotic "hands" and electronic monitors. Benefits of robotic surgery include a shorter operative time, shorter hospitalization, more rapid recovery, and more sophisticated surgery. Robotic surgery is not indicated for very short procedures such as endoscopic sterilization. Urogynecologic reconstructive surgery, fistula repair, and hysterectomy are best accomplished by robotic approach. The application of robotic surgery to gynecologic cancer is growing. Robotic surgery may be preferred over minilaparotomy for tubal anastomosis or reproductive endocrinology.

INFLAMMATIONS OF THE LOWER GENITAL TRACT

Etiology and Pathophysiology

Inflammations or infections of the vulva, vagina, or cervix most often occur when the acid environment of the vaginal secretions changes, enabling the survival of pathogenic organisms. The acid environment of the vaginal vault is maintained by estrogen levels and the presence of *Lactobacillus.* Risk factors that alter the bacterial flora and pH environment within the vagina include aging; poor nutrition; the use of medications such as steroids, OCs, or antibiotics; and douching.

Organisms can also gain entrance to the vagina through contaminated hands, clothing, loss of skin integrity from trauma or surgery, or sexual intercourse. Vulvar infections typically occur as a result of skin trauma caused by itching and scratching. Although *Candida albicans* is normally present in low levels in

Table 39.3 Comparison of Two Types of Common Vaginal Infections

	BACTERIAL VAGINOSIS	YEAST INFECTION
Primary causative organism(s)	*Gardnerella* (most common).	*Candida* (formerly called *Monilia*).
Onset	May be asymptomatic.	Abrupt onset; may precede menstruation.
Odor	Fishy, most noticeable after intercourse.	None or mild "musty" odor.
Itching	Usually none (does not invade vaginal wall).	Severe; most prominent symptom.
Discharge	Thin, gray, may be frothy.	Thick, white, "cottage cheese" texture when colonization is heavy.
Sexually transmitted	Possibly; many women have this organism present in vaginal flora.	Possibly. Associated with high estrogen levels, diabetes mellitus, tight underclothing that increases warmth and moisture.
Vulvar signs	Absent.	Redness; excoriation from scratching; may have edema of labia.
Vaginal signs	Vaginal pH above 4.6. Little redness; discharge adherent to vaginal wall, normal cervix.	Normal cervix, no discharge. Lesions and edema from scratching.
Treatment	Metronidazole orally, sometimes vaginally; clindamycin in second trimester if pregnant (metronidazole associated with adverse pregnancy outcomes).	Miconazole, clotrimazole, or nystatin vaginally as directed. Oral treatment: fluconazole (Diflucan) 150-mg single dose. Over-the-counter treatment is available.

the vaginal area, a change in vaginal pH can lead to an overgrowth, resulting in vulvovaginitis (Table 39.3).

Signs, Symptoms, and Diagnosis

A history and physical examination usually reveal the nature of the problem. Lesions may be present, and **dysuria** (painful urination) commonly occurs because the acidic urine comes into contact with open lesions. An abnormal vaginal discharge that causes **pruritus** (itching discomfort) may occur. Women with cervicitis may experience bloody spotting after intercourse.

The diagnosis of the specific condition may be accomplished by culturing vaginal discharge or lesions, blood tests for specific infections, or a colposcopy or biopsy of the lesion. Drug therapy is prescribed based on the diagnosis.

Treatment and Nursing Management

Teach the woman about the risks and prevention of genital infections as well as the treatment protocol for the specific infection. Infections of the lower genital tract are typically treated with local creams, vaginal suppositories, or systemic antimicrobials. Hand hygiene is important. Wearing loose cotton underwear provides comfort and decreases irritation. Genital infections can cause the woman embarrassment, impair her self-image, and negatively affect relationships. Providing psychological support is very important. Because many organisms that cause lower genital tract infections are spread by sexual intercourse, prompt treatment is essential to prevent the spread of infection to the upper genital tract. The importance of recognizing symptoms and seeking health care should be stressed. Providing a nonjudgmental attitude will empower the woman to ask questions and seek advice. Ensure that the woman fully understands the directions for taking medication or applying creams and use visual aids whenever possible to ensure clarity of the directions.

TOXIC SHOCK SYNDROME

Toxic shock syndrome (TSS) is a rare and potentially fatal disorder most often caused by strains of *Staphylococcus aureus* that produce toxins that cause shock, coagulation defects, and tissue damage if they enter the bloodstream. It is associated with the trapping of bacteria within the reproductive tract for a prolonged time. Risk factors include the prolonged use of high-absorbency tampons, cervical caps, or diaphragms.

Symptoms of TSS include the following (Chu, 2018):

- Rapid onset of hypotension
- Sudden spiking fever
- Flulike symptoms, such as myalgias, weakness, and diarrhea
- Encephalopathy, evidenced by disorientation and confusion
- A diffuse, red, macular rash resembling a sunburn
- Peeling skin on the palms or soles (this is a very late sign of the condition)

Treatment includes hospitalization and intensive care with supportive treatments and intravenous antimicrobials. You have an important role in preventing TSS by teaching the woman hand hygiene when inserting tampons and the importance of changing tampons every 4 hours. Tampons should not be used when sleeping because they will likely remain in place for longer than 4 hours. Diaphragms and cervical caps should not be left in place for a prolonged time or used during menstruation.

CANCER OF THE REPRODUCTIVE TRACT

VULVAR CANCER

Vulvar intraepithelial neoplasia (VIN) refers to the growth of abnormal tissue on the vulva that may be precancerous. Cancer of the vulva is rare and occurs most commonly in older women. Symptoms include red, brown, or white patches on the skin of the vulva. Treatment includes surgical removal of the pathologic tissue. Some strains of VIN are associated with human papillomavirus (HPV). Incorporation of the HPV vaccine (Gardasil, Gardasil 9, or Cervarix) into the standard immunization regimen for all girls and young women further reduces the incidence of this condition. Melanoma may begin on the vulva as well, even though the vulva is not typically exposed to sunlight. Women should be encouraged to observe and report any changes in any moles or visible lesions in the vulvar area.

CANCER OF THE CERVIX

The risk factors for cancer of the cervix include having had multiple sex partners, sexual intercourse with uncircumcised males, starting intercourse at a young age (younger than 20 years of age), multiple pregnancies, obesity, and history of HPV infection or an STI. An approved HPV vaccine given to girls at or before puberty may prevent the type of HPV infection that causes cervical cancer. Regular pelvic examinations and Pap smears may enable early diagnosis and provide an opportunity for early and more successful intervention.

The U.S. Preventive Services Task Force (USPSTF, 2018) recommends screening for cervical cancer every 3 years for women ages 21 to 29 years. For women between 30 and 65 years of age, it is recommended that screening be performed every 3 years with cervical cytology, every 5 years if HPV testing is done alone, or every 5 years for HPV and cytology testing done together (USPSTF, 2018).

ACOG (2017a) recommends that testing take place as follows:

- Women ages 21 to 29 years should have a Pap smear alone every 3 years. HPV testing is not recommended.
- Women ages 30 to 65 years should have a Pap smear and an HPV test (co-testing) every 5 years (preferred). It also is acceptable to have a Pap smear alone every 3 years.

ACOG (2017a) also states that screening for cervical cancer can stop after age 65 years if:

- There is no history of moderate or severe abnormal cervical cells or cervical cancer, and
- The woman has had three negative Pap smear results in a row or two negative co-test results in a row within the past 10 years, with the most recent test performed within the past 5 years.

Treatment of cervical neoplasia may include cryosurgery, electrosurgical excision, or surgical conization of the cervix. Cervical cancer requires a hysterectomy with possible bilateral salpingo-oophorectomy (removal of the uterus, including the fallopian tubes and ovaries) followed by radiation and chemotherapy. See Chapter 8 for discussion of care of a patient receiving radiation or chemotherapy.

CANCER OF THE UTERUS

The most common malignant tumor of the female reproductive tract is endometrial cancer. It is a slow-growing cancer that most commonly occurs after menopause. The treatment of choice is a hysterectomy with bilateral salpingo-oophorectomy. Treatment is often complicated by the fact that many women with cancer of the uterus may be older or have chronic conditions such as diabetes. Surgery is commonly followed by radiation and chemotherapy. Chemotherapy agents may be used to augment treatment. See Chapter 8 for discussion of care of a patient receiving chemotherapy and radiation therapy.

CANCER OF THE OVARY

Most ovarian tumors are benign. However, ovarian cancer is known as a "silent cancer" because signs and symptoms are often nonspecific or vague, such as fatigue or abdominal distention with no detectable precancerous changes in the ovary. An important risk factor for the development of ovarian cancer is having a sister or mother with the disease or inheriting the *BRCA1* or *BRCA2* gene, which is also associated with breast cancer. Exposure to asbestos, talc powder, pelvic irradiation, or mumps has also been linked to the development of ovarian cancer. Women on hormone therapy should be informed about the risks for ovarian cancer. Factors that may prevent ovarian cancer include one or more term pregnancies, breastfeeding, tubal sterilization, and possibly the use of OCs. Ovarian cancer is classified according to the type of tissue within the ovary that is involved. Diagnosis is commonly made during a routine pelvic examination. An ovarian cancer tumor marker (CA-125), assessed by a blood test, combined with transvaginal ultrasound can detect ovarian cancer but often not at an early stage. In most cases, diagnosis of ovarian cancer is first established when the cancer is well beyond the ovary. Once diagnosis is established, a **panhysterectomy** (removal of the uterus, the fallopian tubes, and the ovaries) may be followed by chemotherapy and radiation. Usually a combination of agents is used; most commonly, cisplatin or carboplatin is paired with a taxane agent such as paclitaxel or docetaxel. CAM therapies may be helpful in managing the side effects of the cancer and the medications used to treat the cancer.

DISORDERS OF THE BREAST

Although the breast is not a reproductive organ, it is affected by hormonal changes related to the menstrual cycle and after pregnancy; therefore it is discussed in this chapter.

Health Promotion

Symptoms of Ovarian Cancer

The American Cancer Society has identified possible warning signs of ovarian cancer, which include the following:
- Bloating
- Abdominal or pelvic pain
- Difficulty eating or feeling full quickly
- Urinary frequency or urgency

BENIGN DISORDERS OF THE BREAST

Fibroadenoma

Fibroadenomas are commonly found in teenagers and young adults. Fibroadenomas are firm, rubbery, mobile nodules of fibrous and glandular tissue that may or may not be tender on palpation. They typically occur in the upper outer quadrant of the breast and do not change during the menstrual cycle. A fine-needle aspiration or biopsy can be performed to determine the presence of cancerous cells.

Fibrocystic Breast Changes

Fibrocystic breast changes (FBCs) are common during the reproductive years. An FBC is a palpable thickening of portions of the breast tissue associated with pain and tenderness. Multiple smooth, well-delineated cysts that are most painful during the premenstrual phase of the menstrual cycle may form. The "lumps" make breast self-examination (BSE) more difficult and cause anxiety when located. Women with FBCs can learn to recognize the size and shape of their normal lumps and should report any change in these findings, as well as other changes, to their health care provider. Treatment of FBCs is conservative and based on supportive care. Vitamin E and omega fatty acids (Mirhashemi et al., 2017), wearing a supportive bra, eliminating caffeine and alcohol, reducing dietary fat, and the use of NSAIDs can help control the discomfort associated with FBCs.

Intraductal Papilloma

Intraductal papilloma is the development of small elevations in the epithelium of the ducts of the breasts under the areola. The ducts erode, causing a serosanguineous discharge from the nipple. Treatment includes excision of the mass and analysis of the discharge to determine whether cancer cells are present.

Clarify and reinforce the explanations of diagnostic procedures to be performed and recognize the anxiety and apprehension that the woman feels until the final diagnosis is confirmed. The woman should be encouraged to express her concerns, and supportive care should be provided.

BREAST CANCER

In the United States, approximately 1 in 8 women (12%) will develop breast cancer in their lifetime (Breastcancer.org, n.d.). In 2018 more than 266,120 new cases of invasive breast cancer were diagnosed, in addition to 63,690 new cases of in situ breast cancer (Breastcancer.org, n.d.). Gender and aging are the highest risk factors. Early awareness via education, early detection available with new technology, and treatment advances have reduced the death rate associated with breast cancer. Although the risk of developing breast cancer increases with a woman's age, many other factors contribute to the risk (Box 39.3). Breast cancer is identified according to the structure affected and staged according to the size and degree of invasiveness (Table 39.4).

Box 39.3 Risk Factors for Breast Cancer

1. Family history of relative with breast cancer
2. Early menarche, late menopause
3. Late first pregnancy or no children
4. Dense breast tissue
5. Obesity or overweight
6. History of certain benign breast conditions
7. Consumption of alcohol
8. Not breastfeeding
9. Use of certain forms of contraceptives or hormonal replacement
10. History of chest radiation
11. History of exposure to diethylstilbestrol (DES)

Note that the absolute cause of breast cancer has not been established. It is thought to be caused by genetic factors combined with environmental factors, resulting in a cumulative risk level. Risk factors are listed at www.cancer.org.

Etiology and Diagnosis

The development of breast cancer is believed to be related to estrogen and progesterone. For example, women who start to menstruate at an early age (early menarche) and have late menopause are exposed to more estrogen spikes during monthly ovulation and are at higher risk of developing breast cancer. Conversely, women who have had multiple pregnancies have fewer monthly ovulating cycles and hormonal spikes and thus are at lower risk.

Genetic testing for *BRCA1* and *BRCA2* gene mutations continues because identifying high-risk women can result in specific interventions to prevent development of cancer, such as preventive mastectomy and reconstructive surgery. The current breast cancer risk assessment tool developed by the National Cancer Institute (NCI) is available at https://bcrisktool.cancer.gov/.

Since 2013 the USPSTF has not recommended that routine genetic testing be done. *BRCA* testing can be expensive and may not be covered by insurance. Instead, the USPSTF recommends that women who have at least one family member with *BRCA1*- or *BRCA2*-related cancers be screened for genetic testing using one of the following models:
- Ontario Family History Assessment Tool
- Manchester Scoring System

Table 39.4 Stages of Breast Cancer

CANCER STAGE	DESCRIPTION	5-YEAR SURVIVAL RATE
Stage 0	Carcinoma in situ	Nearly 100%
Stage I	Relatively small cancer that has not spread to the lymph nodes or has only a tiny area of cancer spread in the sentinel lymph node	Nearly 100%
Stage II	Larger than stage I cancer and/or has spread to a few nearby lymph nodes	Approximately 93%
Stage III	Larger than stage II cancer or growing into nearby tissues (the skin over the breast or the muscle underneath) or has spread to many nearby lymph nodes	Approximately 72%
Stage IV	Cancer that has spread beyond the breast and nearby lymph nodes to other parts of the body	Approximately 22%

Data from American Cancer Society: *Treatment of breast cancer by stage* (website): www.cancer.org/cancer/breast-cancer/treatment/treatment-of-breast-cancer-by-stage.html; and American Cancer Society: *Survival rates for breast cancer* (website): www.cancer.org/cancer/breast-cancer/understanding-a-breast-cancer-diagnosis/breast-cancer-survival-rates.html.

Legal and Ethical Considerations

BRCA1 and _BRCA2_ Genes

If all women are tested for the presence of the *BRCA1* or *BRCA2* gene, an ethical problem is raised regarding the action to take if the gene is present. Should the young woman have a prophylactic mastectomy? Should the woman be given prophylactic treatment with tamoxifen? Does the knowledge of the potential risk for cancer produce anxiety that may result in life changes that can have a negative outcome? Would there be health insurance implications?

- Referral Screening Tool
- Pedigree Assessment Tool
- FHS-7

The Referral Screening Tool (which can be found at www.breastcancergenescreen.org) and FHS-7 are the simplest and easiest to use. The USPSTF reports that no specific tool is better than another and makes no recommendation as to which tool to use.

Clinical Cues

Breast cancer in men is rare but does occur. It is usually diagnosed at a later stage because of lack of awareness that men can develop breast cancer and the lack of routine screening. Older age and liver disease are contributing risk factors.

Signs, Symptoms, and Diagnosis

Although many breast lumps are detected by women during BSE, most early breast cancer can be detected by mammography (x-ray examination of the breast) before it can be clinically palpated. Nipple discharge or change in the skin pattern, such as "dimpled skin" on the breast, may also be a sign of breast cancer. Any unilateral breast change should be reported immediately to a health care provider. Even a short delay in diagnosis can result in invasion of surrounding tissue and metastasis to other parts of the body. Fenretinide, a retinoid, and other agents continue to be studied as mechanisms to reduce the risk of breast cancer. Scintimammography (nuclear medicine breast imaging) involves injecting a radioactive tracer into a vein that attaches to a breast cancer cell and is detected by a camera for more accurate diagnosis than an MRI scan. This technology does not replace routine screening tests, such as mammography.

Prevention

A healthy lifestyle that includes exercise and a diet rich in antioxidants and phytoestrogens, such as vegetables, fruits, whole grains, and soy products, may protect against the development of many cancers. ACOG (2017) recommends the following as breast cancer screening guidance:

- Women at average risk of breast cancer should be offered screening mammography starting at age 40 years. If they have not initiated screening in their 40s, they should begin screening mammography by no later than age 50 years. The decision about the age to begin mammography screening should be made through a shared decision-making process. This discussion should include information about the potential benefits and harms.
- Women at average risk of breast cancer should have screening mammography every 1 or 2 years based on an informed, shared decision-making process that includes a discussion of the benefits and harms of annual and biennial screening and incorporates patient values and preferences.
- Women at average risk of breast cancer should continue screening mammography until at least 75 years of age. Beyond age 75 years, the decision to discontinue screening mammography should be based on a shared decision-making process informed by the woman's health status and longevity.

Tamoxifen is used to prevent recurrent breast cancer and is also recommended for women at high risk of developing breast cancer because it has been shown to have risk reduction benefits (Tamoxifen, 2018). However, this drug is not recommended for the general population because of potential side effects, such as increased bone pain, photosensitivity, headache, and increased risk for pulmonary embolism or uterine malignancies. Some literature indicates that third-generation aromatase inhibitors are more effective than tamoxifen in preventing recurrence of breast cancer in postmenopausal women with hormone receptor–positive invasive breast cancer (Carlson, 2016). Fenretinide, a retinoid, continues to be studied as a way to reduce the risk of breast cancer. Aromatase inhibitors, such as anastrozole (Arimidex) or exemestane (Aromasin), are other options that may be used.

Some women who have known genetic *BRCA1* or *BRCA2* predispositions have elected to have prophylactic bilateral mastectomies. The psychological implications and effect on self-image should be carefully weighed against preventive benefits. The decision is ultimately made by the woman after careful consideration and consultation with her health care provider.

Treatment

Treatment options are based on the type of breast cancer, stage of the disease, patient's age, physical and menopausal status, and other health factors that may affect the woman's ability to undergo the specific treatment. In general, the primary treatment depends on the size of the cancer and can be initial chemotherapy to shrink the tumor followed by surgical removal or simply surgical removal of a smaller tumor and varying amounts of surrounding tissue. The types of surgery include the following:

- **Lumpectomy** (removal of tumor only).
- Partial or **segmental mastectomy** (removal of tumor and a portion of the surrounding breast tissue and axillary lymph nodes).
- Simple or **total mastectomy** (removal of entire breast and axillary lymph nodes).
- **Modified radical mastectomy** (removal of breast, axillary lymph nodes, and lining over the chest wall muscles).
- **Radical mastectomy** (removal of breast, axillary lymph nodes, and chest wall muscles under the breast). Radical mastectomy was once very common, but high success rates with a reduction in disfigurement are now made possible by using appropriate staging of the disease when making treatment decisions.

A suggested nursing care plan for a woman undergoing a lumpectomy in a same-day surgery unit is presented in Nursing Care Plan 39.2.

If there is concern that cancer cells have invaded the lymph nodes, **sentinel node biopsy** may be performed, wherein the primary node is removed and, if laboratory results show no evidence of cancer, the remaining nodes are left intact. Alternatively, an axillary node dissection may be performed during breast surgery, in which the lymph nodes under the affected arm are removed and sent to the laboratory. This procedure may result in swelling of the affected arm.

Tamoxifen blocks estrogen by binding with the estrogen receptors. This drug is usually prescribed for 5 years. Nausea and anorexia may occur, and cholesterol and triglyceride levels should be monitored. Certain drugs interfere with the metabolism of tamoxifen and should be avoided, including some selective serotonin reuptake inhibitor (SSRI) and selective serotonin norepinephrine reuptake inhibitor (SNRI) antidepressants such as paroxetine, fluoxetine, and duloxetine; some antipsychotics such as pimozide, perphenazine, and thioridazine; some cardiac drugs such as quinidine or ticlopidine; some medications for infectious diseases such as terfenadine; and histamine (H_2)-blockers such as cimetidine.

Some women have a type of breast cancer tumor that manifests the human epidermal growth factor receptor 2 protein (*HER2*-positive breast cancer). Use of the monoclonal antibody trastuzumab (Herceptin) for 1 year as an adjuvant therapy is considered the standard of care (Piccart-Gebhart, 2016).

Radiation therapy commonly is performed after lumpectomy or segmented mastectomy to destroy micrometastases and decrease cancer recurrence rates. Radiation therapy options include whole-breast radiotherapy using external beam radiation weekly for 7 weeks; intensity-modulated radiation therapy (IMRT), which minimizes damage to surrounding tissue; accelerated partial breast irradiation (APBI), using a balloon catheter in the local tumor site; interstitial brachytherapy, with pellets inserted around the tumor site; or external beam radiotherapy (EBRT) after healing occurs (Fig. 39.3). Chemotherapy also may be considered as part of treatment, in combination with surgery and radiation. Aromatase inhibitors such as anastrozole; letrozole (Femara), currently in the tentative approval stage as an injected agent; or exemestane reduce the risk of recurrence by inhibiting the enzyme aromatase, which results in decreased estrogen production. Aromatase inhibitors are not used in premenopausal women with functioning ovaries (see Safety Note below). An estrogen receptor agonist such as fulvestrant (Faslodex) binds with estrogen receptors and can be used when

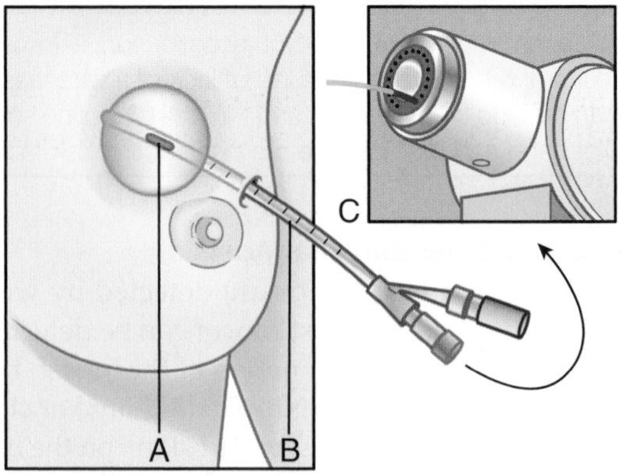

Fig. 39.3 High-dose brachytherapy for breast cancer. The MammoSite system involves the insertion of a single small balloon catheter **(B)** at the time of the lumpectomy or shortly thereafter into the tumor resection cavity (the space that is left after the surgeon removes the tumor). A tiny radioactive seed **(A)** is inserted into the balloon, is connected to a machine called an afterloader **(C),** and delivers the radiation therapy. (From Lewis SL, Heitkemper MM, Bucher L, et al.: *Medical-surgical nursing: assessment and management of clinical problems,* ed 10, St. Louis, 2017, Elsevier.)

Nursing Care Plan 39.2 Care of a Patient After Breast Lumpectomy

SCENARIO

A 33-year-old woman is ready for discharge from the same-day surgery unit after undergoing a breast lumpectomy for a suspicious breast lesion. She expresses concern about the amount of scar tissue that will form and that her breasts may no longer be the same size after the lumpectomy.

PROBLEM STATEMENT/NURSING DIAGNOSIS

Altered body image related to possible asymmetric breasts and scar tissue formation after breast lumpectomy.

SUPPORTING ASSESSMENT DATA

Subjective: Concern about scar tissue and that breasts will no longer be the same size.

Objective: Lumpectomy.

Goals/Expected Outcomes	Nursing Interventions	Selected Rationale	Evaluation
Patient will use positive coping strategies to adjust to changes in body image as evidenced by use of support system and available resources.	Assess for previous problem with self-esteem.	Previous coping strategies can be revealed by discussing previous experiences.	Patient discussed previous experiences and recognizes the stages of loss she experienced.
	Assess for signs of anxiety or inability to focus.	Anxiety is an expected result of a diagnosis that may involve a possible cancer.	Patient expressed understanding of prognosis as explained by health care provider.
	Encourage verbalization of feelings.	Verbalization can reduce anxiety and focus on the problem of altered body image.	Patient expressed concerns about scar tissue and alteration in breast symmetry.
	Involve family and interprofessional health care team in offering support.	Providing patient with broad support base and resources assists in adjustment.	Patient expressed understanding of healing process and resources available for assistance after discharge.
	Provide accurate information concerning prognosis.	Provides an opportunity to correct misinformation.	Patient expressed understanding of need for follow-up care.
	Encourage patient to help care for wound.	Looking at and touching wound indicates readiness to participate in self-care to achieve optimal wound healing.	Patient states will actively participate in wound dressing changes.

CRITICAL THINKING QUESTIONS

1. What factors influence a woman's perception of her body image?
2. What other problems or issues might exist for a woman sent home the same day after a breast lumpectomy?

tamoxifen fails. Ovarian ablation is the surgical removal or irradiation of the ovary to stop estrogen production. The use of goserelin (Zoladex) may be an alternative to chemotherapy. See Chapter 8 for care of a patient receiving chemotherapy or radiation therapy.

Safety Alert

A number of chemicals, such as parabens and phthalates, found in common cosmetic ingredients are being studied to determine their links to breast cancer (Breastcancer.org, n.d.). Individuals with breast cancer may wish to avoid products that contain these ingredients.

Breast Reconstructive Surgery

Plastic surgery of the breast may be performed to reduce breast size (reduction mammoplasty), enlarge breast size (augmentation mammoplasty), or reconstruct the breast after breast cancer surgery (reconstruction mammoplasty).

Reduction mammoplasty. Problems related to an excessively large breast include back and shoulder pain, pressure on nerves from brassiere straps, inability to buy clothing that fits, and psychological problems related to fear of ridicule or unwelcome sexual advances.

A mammogram may be necessary before surgery. The amount and degree of scarring should be discussed with the woman because the scar is determined by the technique of surgery. Although data suggest that breast reduction surgery does not interfere with successful breastfeeding, it is possible that milk production could be affected. Decreased nipple sensation or loss of part of the areola may also be a side effect of surgery that the woman should be aware of preoperatively. Information concerning successful breastfeeding after breast reduction surgery may be obtained from La Leche League International.

Augmentation mammoplasty. Breast augmentation may be initiated by patients who wish to improve their self-image. Breast augmentation can be accomplished by inserting a saline implant under the pectoralis muscle.

Reconstructive mammoplasty. Reconstructive mammoplasty creates a new breast when the natural tissue has been removed during mastectomy. A nipple or areola reconstruction provides a more natural appearance. Saline implants can be used, or skin and tissue may be taken from other parts of the body (autologous reconstruction). Tattooing of the nipple area provides natural-looking coloring. A pedicle flap tunnels body tissue to the breast area, keeping the blood vessels intact so that a microvascular surgeon is not needed. A free flap or muscle-sparing flap is another technique of reconstructive breast surgery in which blood vessels are harvested along with tissue and then reimplanted by a microvascular surgeon. Perforator flap surgery is a technique that spares muscle tissue but requires detailed surgical skill. Nursing responsibilities include frequent checking of the flaps for adequate perfusion, maintaining hydration to support flap perfusion, management of pain, and proper patient positioning as prescribed. Encourage deep breathing postoperatively. Range-of-motion exercises typically begin 1 week after surgery, and lifting 5-lb weights is prescribed for 6 to 8 weeks. The nipple is reconstructed 3 to 4 months after breast reconstruction surgery to ensure that swelling is minimal. Tattooing of the nipple is a popular option rather than construction of a new nipple.

Nursing Management for Breast Cancer Surgery

Preoperative care. Most women need extensive education before breast surgery. Many surgeons now provide educational programs for their patients, but it is important for you to determine whether the patient did in fact receive adequate information and whether she has a good understanding of what was taught. Women commonly are particularly concerned about the change in their appearance after breast surgery. Talking with a Reach to Recovery volunteer or a nurse with extensive professional or personal knowledge before surgery can be very helpful. Teaching points will vary depending on the amount of tissue to be surgically removed and whether a prosthesis will be implanted either during the initial surgery or at a later date (Fig. 39.4).

Postoperative care. Postoperative care includes pain management, observation for signs of infection, and continued supportive and educational measures. Because breast tissue is very vascular, bleeding may be a problem. Surgical dressings should be observed frequently during the first 48 hours after the procedure.

Body image issues, as well as societal focus on the breast as an identifier of femininity or sexual attractiveness, make treatment for breast cancer a highly

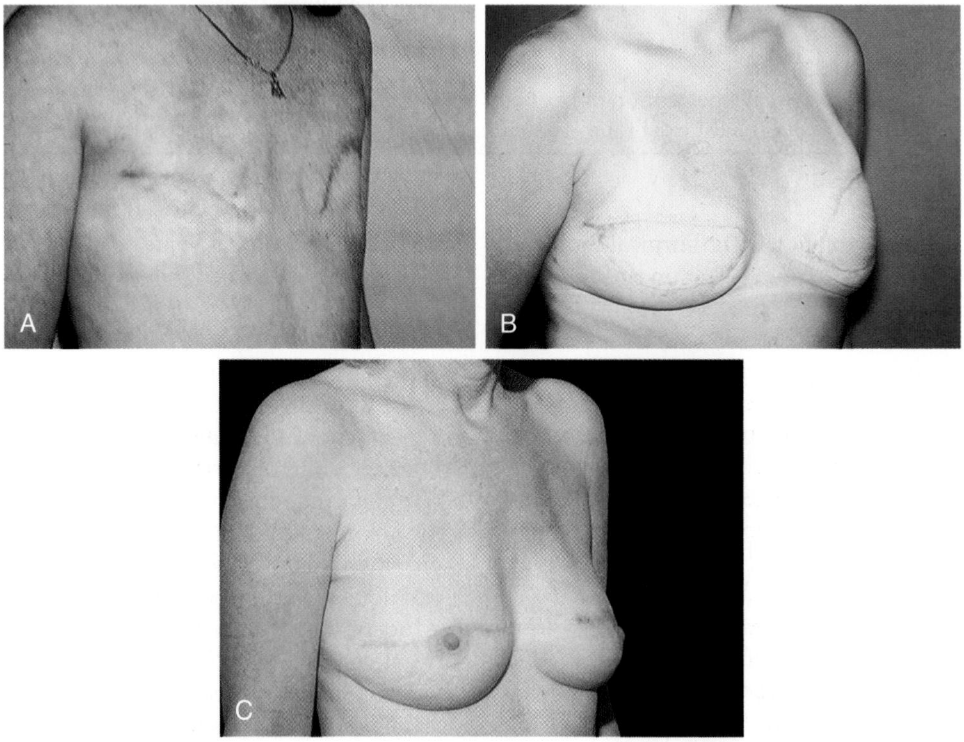

Fig. 39.4 Reconstructive breast surgery. **A,** Appearance of the chest after bilateral mastectomy. **B,** Postoperative breast reconstruction before nipple reconstruction. **C,** Postoperative breast reconstruction after nipple and areolar reconstruction.

emotionally charged experience. Women may wish to have ongoing supportive care, and many will benefit greatly from participating in a support group and from visits by American Cancer Society Reach to Recovery volunteers. These women have all undergone treatment for breast cancer and have been trained in peer counseling. The local chapter of the American Cancer Society can be contacted regarding Reach to Recovery visits.

Collaborative care. Collaborative care can help reduce anxiety and stress experienced by the patient. Provide emotional support and give accurate information. The woman and her partner may differ in how much information they want to discuss. Allow both to express their concerns openly.

Complications

Lymphedema. **Lymphedema** is swelling of the arm that sometimes occurs after breast cancer surgery because of the damage to and resulting congestion of the lymphatic tract. (It can also be idiopathic, or of unknown origin, or a congenital problem.) Approximately 9% of women who have undergone treatment for breast cancer develop lymphedema within 10 years (Nguyen et al., 2017). Lymphedema can become a chronic condition. The use of sentinel node biopsy, with removal of additional lymph nodes only if the sentinel lymph node is positive for cancer, has reduced the occurrence of lymphedema because of less damage to the lymph tissue and thus less chance of developing lymphedema. Postoperative nursing interventions that can reduce the risk of development of lymphedema after a breast node biopsy or breast cancer surgery include the following:

- Refraining from taking blood pressure in the affected arm
- Not giving injections or doing venipuncture in the affected arm
- Providing meticulous skin care
- Teaching the patient to wear gloves in the kitchen and when gardening to prevent skin irritation or injury
- Teaching the patient to avoid heavy lifting and to wear a compression garment during strenuous activities
- Teaching the patient to elevate and exercise the arm daily

Review exercises that may be helpful (Fig. 39.5). Discharge teaching should focus on the need for follow-up care, exercises to improve range of motion, prevention of infection, side effects of medical therapy, and community resources available.

Clinics that specialize in the care of patients with lymphedema are available in some states. The standard of care is complex physical therapy, which involves techniques that provide lymphatic drainage, specialized pressure bandaging, application of a compression garment, exercising, and skin care. More information can be obtained from the National Lymphedema Network website at www.lymphnet.org.

Patient Teaching

Measures to Prevent or Decrease Lymphedema

Teach the patient to:

- Elevate the extremity to the level of the heart. This reduces hydrostatic pressure within the veins.
- Apply elasticized stockings or gloves that do not have tight bands when up and active. This increases pressure on vessels and encourages venous return. (Garments may be removed when the extremity can be elevated.)
- Refrain from wearing constrictive clothing.
- Not cross the legs when sitting and not carry a heavy bag with the affected arm.
- Perform active exercise of the skeletal muscles to promote massage of the lymph vessels and the movement of lymph.
- Cleanse and dry the skin thoroughly and regularly and apply mild skin moisturizers to prevent cracking.
- Prevent minor trauma to the area (e.g., no blood pressure cuffs or blood draws on the affected extremity) and not use a heating pad.
- Wear gloves and sunscreen when gardening.

NURSING DIAGNOSIS

Problem statements commonly associated with gynecologic disorders include the following:

- Altered activity tolerance due to anemia from excessive blood loss, weakness, or disabling discomfort.
- Fluid volume overload due to premenstrual fluid retention.
- Altered skin integrity due to pruritus, genital lesions, and vaginal discharge.
- Pain due to menstrual cycle, decreased vaginal lubrication, or vaginal irritation.
- Altered sexual function due to dyspareunia (painful intercourse) or emotional issues.
- Limited coping ability due to negative attitude about human sexuality or menstruation.
- Altered body image due to surgery, fear of mutilating surgery, and loss of femininity.
- Insufficient knowledge about practices of personal feminine hygiene, normal anatomy and physiology of the female reproductive organs, or safe methods of contraception.
- Altered self-perception related to sterility, menopause, or surgery on a reproductive organ.

Expected goals or outcomes include the following:

- Patient uses energy conservation techniques while maintaining activity levels within capabilities.
- Patient maintains adequate fluid volume with appropriate management techniques.
- Skin remains intact with healing of existing wounds.
- Patient verbalizes an acceptable level of pain relief and ability to engage in normal activities.
- Patient expresses satisfaction with physical intimacy patterns and experience.

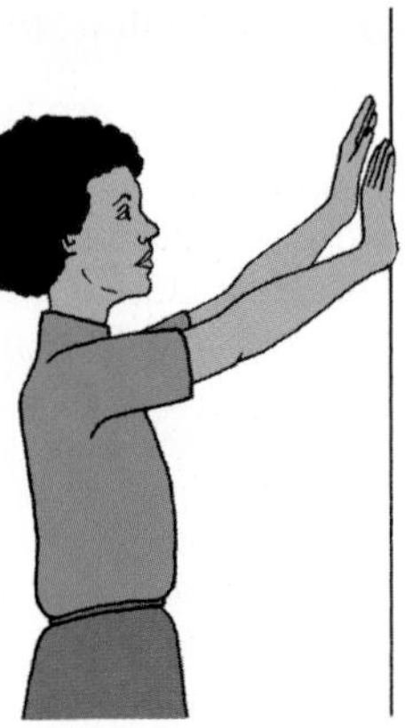

FRONT WALL CLIMBING

Patient stands facing the wall, elbows slightly bent. Palms are placed at shoulder level and fingers are flexed and unflexed as hands "walk" up the wall as high as possible. Hands are then walked back down to shoulder level. Patient moves toward wall as fingers climb higher and then away from wall as fingers move downward.

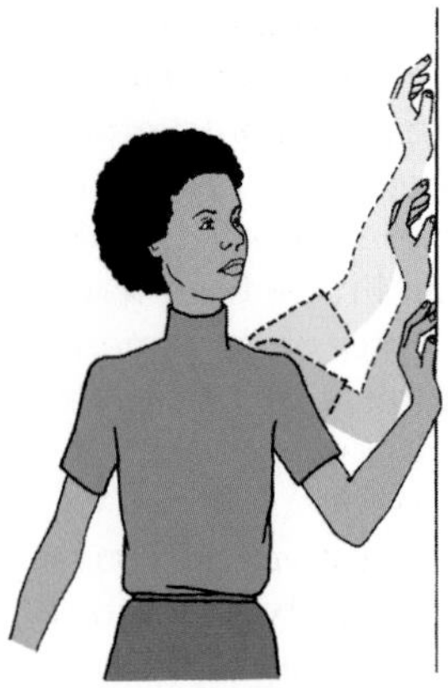

SIDE WALL CLIMBING

With operative side to wall, arm is extended until fingers touch wall. Patient moves toward the wall as fingers climb higher until body touches it. Maneuver is reversed as fingers climb back down wall.

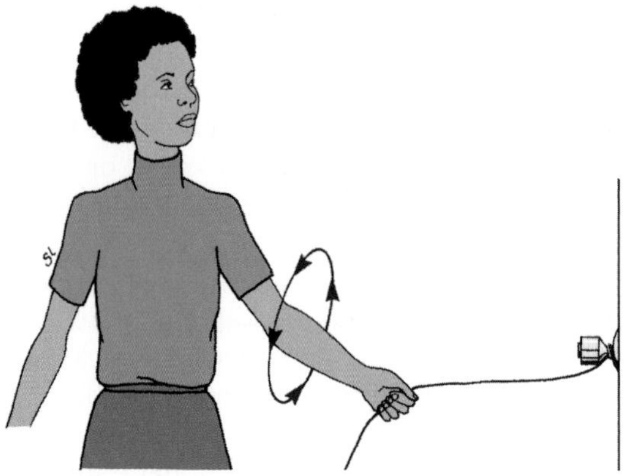

ROPE TURNING

One end of rope is tied to door knob. Patient holds other end of rope and swings it in a circular motion, being sure entire arm and not the wrist is in motion.

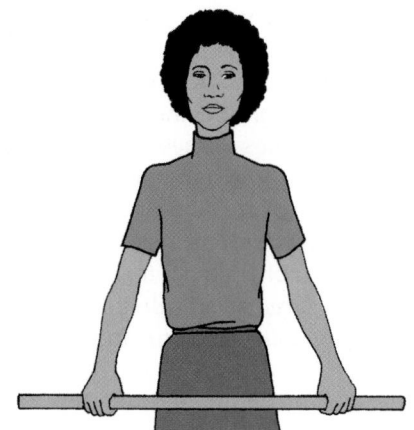

YARDSTICK OR BROOM LIFT

Holding a yardstick or broom handle with both hands, the back is placed against a wall. Arms are extended straight downward and, with elbows straight, the stick is raised by the straightened arms until knuckles touch the wall over the head.

Fig. 39.5 Postmastectomy exercises.

- Patient develops improved method of communication, problem-solving techniques, and positive attitude to enable effective coping with signs and symptoms.
- Patient evidences enhanced body image and self-esteem with ability to accept altered body part or function.
- Patient demonstrates motivation to learn and verbalizes understanding of female hygiene and safer sex practices.
- Patient recognizes and accepts positive aspects of self.

◆ PLANNING

Planning the care of a patient with a gynecologic problem depends on the specific disorder. However, prevention of infection, effective patient education, and emotional support are appropriate and consistent goals for the care plan for all patients with a gynecologic problem. The needs of a patient who will have gynecologic surgery include pain management, education regarding the procedure and follow-up care, infection prevention, and supportive care specific to the procedure. A woman who will be unable to bear children because of a hysterectomy performed early in life may have very different supportive needs from those of a postmenopausal woman undergoing the same procedure. Surgery for breast cancer brings fears of a major change in body image and the possibility of death if the disease is not controlled. These issues need to be addressed in the plan of care. The plan for a patient with an infection includes an appropriate medication schedule and monitoring for effectiveness of treatment (e.g., fever, swelling, pain resolving) and for signs of an allergic response to the prescribed antimicrobial agent.

In the outpatient setting, women may be seen for annual visits, reproductive or contraceptive counseling, treatment of infections or sexually transmitted infections (STIs), prenatal and postnatal care, and a variety of other reasons. If the facility uses standardized plans of care, they must be adapted to express the needs of the individual patient.

The plan of care must address education, pain management needs, emotional and physical care, family impact, cultural and spiritual influences, and financial concerns. Specific goals of care for any patient are based on nursing observation and assessment, prescriptions for medication and therapies, the patient's personal desires and goals, and input from other members of the health care team. The patient should agree to the goals, and they must be communicated clearly to other care providers through well-written care plans and documentation, as well as team conferences when appropriate.

◆ IMPLEMENTATION

The patient's needs must always be addressed when implementing various aspects of the plan of care. Various surgical and non-surgical procedures are used for gynecologic problems. Patient teaching should be an important aspect of each nursing contact. Education must be provided according to the patient's knowledge base and ability to learn new information.

◆ EVALUATION

Any nursing intervention requires evaluation of its effectiveness. This can be accomplished by asking the following questions: How effective were pain control measures? How is the patient tolerating the change in diet or new therapy? Have there been any adverse reactions to medications or treatments? A decision to continue the plan of care or revise the plan of care is the outcome of evaluation.

HOME CARE

As hospital stays continue to become progressively shorter, women go home very quickly after illness, surgery, or childbirth. Home health care can continue to provide care for these patients in the home setting.

Home health nursing responsibilities include pain management, observation of the surgical site for signs of infection (redness, swelling, pain, presence of exudate, foul odor, fever), or reopening of the surgical wound because of trauma or a poor healing response. If the procedure involves the pelvic reproductive organs, the home health nurse must also assess the amount and duration of bleeding, any increase in the volume of flow, and any change (e.g., purulence or foul odor) that indicates the presence of infection.

Continued patient education is a key role of the home health nurse. Even conscientious teaching by the hospital nurse needs ongoing follow-up, because the patient's learning ability in the hospital setting could have been impaired by immediate concerns such as acute pain, recovery from anesthesia, or emotional stresses associated with the diagnosis and the potential effects on daily living. The home health nurse can give accurate, detailed information on continued recovery and wellness as part of home care.

The home health nurse must be able to function independently within the appropriate scope of practice and needs to communicate with the other members of the care team by phone, electronic documentation, and group conferences. The nurse also is commonly the primary source of information about appropriate support groups and informational programs that can be of assistance to the patient and her family.

Patient Teaching

Teaching Older Adults

Older adults may need more time to process educational information. In any teaching plan, you should:

- Assess readiness and motivation to learn. The woman must sense that the information applies to her and is important.
- Provide brochures and a variety of teaching tools; reliable sources confer credibility of information.
- Include the woman's experiences and interests; personalizing teaching makes education more meaningful.
- Ask questions to confirm understanding.
- Provide socialization and opportunity to share. Use group sessions when possible.
- Provide short teaching sessions.
- Face the patient and speak clearly.
- Use a quiet, adequately lit environment.

COMMUNITY CARE

Community care can take many forms. In the area of general reproductive health, low-cost women's health care clinics and organizations such as Planned Parenthood offer pregnancy testing, counseling and instruction on contraception and prevention of STIs, programs concerning BSE and vulvar self-examination (VSE), and screening procedures such as pelvic examinations and mammograms. Instruction and low-cost screening may also be made available by local chapters of organizations such as the American Cancer Society. These outreach programs seek to make information and services available to all women at a reasonable cost. Such programs assist in the prevention and early detection of disease, reducing the long-term effects of potentially serious illness and the cost of intrusive health care.

Community care also involves educational public service announcements on radio and television, and in social media, newspapers, and magazines. These give the public valuable information on sexual health and disease prevention and treatment.

School nurses function as key educators regarding reproductive teaching and health maintenance. Drugs, alcohol, and early sexual activity are major health care concerns for adolescents. The school nurse is in a position to become a trusted source of accurate, nonjudgmental information for young people who need education in the realities of reproductive health.

A variety of programs exist for women at risk for serious diseases of the breast or reproductive organs. They may be sponsored by national organizations such as the American Cancer Society or by local groups or health care facilities and organizations. These programs provide both education and support groups for women undergoing treatment of serious health problems, such as breast or uterine cancer, infertility, fetal loss, and other health concerns specific to women. You can be very helpful in referring women to these community programs or by volunteering as a group facilitator or resource person.

Get Ready for the NCLEX® Examination

Key Points

- Reproductive health can be disrupted by many physical disorders that can also affect other body systems.
- Disorders of the female reproductive system can affect the woman's self-image.
- Modern technology can assist women who have fertility problems.
- PMS, also known as *ovarian cycle syndrome,* is the presence of physical, psychological, or behavioral symptoms that regularly occur in the luteal phase of the menstrual cycle.
- PMDD is a more severe type of PMS described officially in the *DSM-5*, a classification of disorders published by the American Psychiatric Association.
- A decrease in estrogen can increase the risk for the development of osteoporosis and increased blood cholesterol levels.
- Osteoporosis is a decrease in bone mass that increases the risk for bone fractures.
- Endometriosis is a condition in which endometrial tissue is found outside the uterus.
- Leiomyomas (fibroids) of the uterus are common among women between 25 and 40 years of age and may cause vaginal bleeding between menstrual periods.
- Pelvic relaxation syndrome can affect the bladder (cystocele), the rectum (rectocele), or the uterus (uterine prolapse).
- Robotic gynecologic surgery is an effective alternative to open surgery.
- Risk factors for cancer of the cervix include multiple sex partners, early sexual activity, multiple pregnancies, infection with HPV, and smoking.
- Screening measures such as mammography, BSE, VSE, and Pap smears allow early detection and treatment of cancer of the reproductive tract and accessory organs.
- Exercise to restore arm function is very important after mastectomy.
- Specific genes that can predict the risk of specific types of breast cancer have been identified.

Additional Learning Resources

SG Go to your Study Guide for additional learning activities to help you master this chapter content.

Go to your Evolve website (http://evolve.elsevier.com/deWit/medsurg) for the following FREE learning resources:

- Animations, audio, and video
- Answers and rationales for questions and activities
- Glossary with pronunciations in English and Spanish
- Interactive Review Questions and more!

Review Questions for the NCLEX® Examination

1. Which nursing intervention(s) will you recommend to a patient with dysmenorrhea? *(Select all that apply.)*
   1. Pelvic rocking exercises
   2. Cold compresses
   3. Effleurage
   4. Low-fat diet
   5. NSAIDs

   NCLEX Client Need: Health Promotion and Maintenance
2. Metrorrhagia is associated with which condition?
   1. Uterine polyps and leiomyomas
   2. Trauma and a foreign body in the vagina
   3. Cervical cancer
   4. All of these

   NCLEX Client Need: Physiological Integrity: Reduction of Risk Potential

3. A 67-year-old patient who has been menopausal for 13 years reports vaginal bleeding. Which are possible causes? *(Select all that apply.)*
   1. Postcoital bleeding from atrophic vaginitis
   2. Endometrial cancer
   3. Endometriosis
   4. Cervical polyp

   NCLEX Client Need: Physiological Integrity: Reduction of Risk Potential
4. You have provided a patient with specific instructions regarding postoperative right radical mastectomy care of the surgical site and surgical complications. Which patient statement indicates a need for further teaching?
   1. "Blood pressure cannot be taken on the right arm."
   2. "I can resume intense weight training soon after discharge."
   3. "No injections must be given in the right arm."
   4. "When gardening, I need to wear gloves."

   NCLEX Client Need: Safe and Effective Care Environment: Coordinated Care
5. A 42-year-old patient who had a left radical mastectomy expresses concerns about body image. What goal is appropriate?
   1. Participates in activities of daily living.
   2. Demonstrates acceptance of change in appearance.
   3. Performs aseptic wound care.
   4. States signs and symptoms of infection.

   NCLEX Client Need: Psychosocial Integrity
6. Which teaching will you include when educating a patient about how to manage lymphedema of the leg? *(Select all that apply.)*
   1. Elevate the affected extremity to heart level.
   2. Wear elastic stockings without tight bands.
   3. Wear restrictive clothing.
   4. Avoid crossing the legs while sitting.
   5. Do not engage in exercise.

   NCLEX Client Need: Safe and Effective Care Environment: Coordinated Care
7. You are caring for four patients. Which patient is at highest risk for development of ovarian cancer?
   1. 32-year old whose father died of colon cancer
   2. 40-year old who has *BRCA2* gene
   3. 53-year old whose mother had secondary dysmenorrhea
   4. 60-year old who delivered four children

   NCLEX Client Need: Physiological Integrity: Reduction of Risk Potential
8. A patient wishing to decrease her risk for breast cancer asks you what causes this disease. What is the appropriate nursing response?
   1. "Antiperspirants have been shown to cause breast cancer."
   2. "Researchers believe that genes and environmental factors cause this disease."
   3. "Age and weight are the most predictive risks for development of breast cancer."
   4. "There are no modifiable risk factors that you can control to prevent breast cancer."

   NCLEX Client Need: Health Promotion and Maintenance
9. A patient asks about options regarding reconstructive breast surgery. Which nursing response is appropriate? (*Select all that apply.*)
   1. "Nipple tattooing is an option."
   2. "Your surgeon will need to discuss possibilities with you."
   3. "Silicone implants can be used to reconstruct the breast."
   4. "It is wiser and healthier to refrain from reconstructive surgery."
   5. "Does your significant other want you to undergo reconstruction?"
   6. "Reconstruction can take place right after mastectomy."

   NCLEX Client Need: Safe and Effective Care Environment: Coordinated Care
10. You are assessing a patient with a suspected leiomyoma. Which assessment finding is anticipated? *(Select all that apply.)*
    1. Backache
    2. Lower abdominal pressure
    3. Diarrhea
    4. Urinary incontinence
    5. Abnormal uterine bleeding

    NCLEX Client Need: Physiological Integrity: Physiological Adaptation

Critical Thinking Questions

Scenario A

Mrs. Martinez is a 51-year-old college professor who is married with two grown children. She found a lump during BSE that was diagnosed as malignant. Mrs. Martinez states that she does not want to have the radical mastectomy recommended by her surgeon.

1. What are some possible reasons for Mrs. Martinez's hesitation about having a radical mastectomy?
2. Are alternative surgical procedures available to Mrs. Martinez?
3. What types of resources are available to help Mrs. Martinez make this decision?

40 Care of Men With Reproductive Disorders

http://evolve.elsevier.com/deWit/medsurg

Objectives

Theory

1. Discuss common disorders associated with the male reproductive system and nursing interventions for each.
2. Examine causes and treatment of male infertility.
3. Name the most common diagnostic tests and examinations associated with the male reproductive system.
4. Discuss surgical approaches to address male reproductive disorders.
5. Compare benign and malignant disorders of the male reproductive system.

Clinical Practice

6. Use the nursing process in the care of a male with a reproductive disorder.
7. Implement interventions for patients with common disorders of the male reproductive tract.

Key Terms

azotemia (ă-zō-TĒ-mē-ă, p. 952)
cremasteric reflex (krē-mă-STĔR-ĭk, RĒ-flĕks, p. 951)
erectile dysfunction (ED) (ĭ-RĔK-tĕl dĭs-FŬNK-shŭn, p. 948)
gynecomastia (jīn-ĕ-kō-MĂS-tĭ-ă, p. 953)
impotence (ĬM-pō-tĕnz, p. 948)
infertility (ĭn-fĕr-TĬL-ĭ-tē, p. 950)
orchiectomy (ŏr-kē-ĔK-tō-mē, p. 958)
premature ejaculation (prē-mă-TYŪR ĭ-jăk-yū-LĀ-shŭn, p. 949)
priapism (PRĪ-ă-pĭz-ĕm, p. 952)
PSA velocity (vĕ-LŎ-sĕ-tē, p. 959)
retrograde ejaculation (rĕt-rō-GRĀD ĭ-jăk-yū-LĀ-shŭn, p. 949)
tamponade (tăm-pŏn-ĀD, p. 954)
urodynamics (ū-rō-dī-NĂM-ĭks, p. 952)

Concepts Covered in This Chapter

- Reproduction
- Sexuality

DISORDERS OF THE MALE REPRODUCTIVE SYSTEM

Many diseases, disorders, and medications can affect the male reproductive system. The urinary system and reproductive system are so closely linked in the male that a disorder in one system is likely to affect the other.

Problem statements frequently associated with the male reproductive system may include the following:

- Elimination concerns due to urinary blockage.
- Anxiety due to failure to empty bladder totally or urine leakage.
- Pain due to pressure within the pelvis, bladder distention, surgical incisions, or bladder spasms.
- Altered sexual function due to decreased libido or erectile dysfunction.
- Self-image alteration due to changes in sexual function.
- Potential for infection due to urine stasis.

Additional problem statements may be appropriate for patients undergoing surgery or who have cancer (see Chapters 4, 5, and 8).

Specific nursing actions for selected problems of the male reproductive system are found within the sections on specific diseases that follow. Privacy should always be provided when assessing the genitals, performing catheter care, or doing dressing changes. The degree of modesty varies widely in men. You must be professional and display an objective, professional manner when providing care.

ERECTILE DYSFUNCTION

Erectile dysfunction (ED), also known as **impotence,** is the inability to consistently achieve or maintain an erection that is firm enough for sexual intercourse (Cunningham & Rosen, 2018). Impotence can also involve ejaculation problems. ED has psychological (called "psychogenic") and organic causes, including vascular, neurologic, cavernous, hormonal, or drug-induced origins.

Factors that interfere with the mechanisms of penile erection will cause ED. Any condition that impairs the blood supply to the penis, impairs nervous system function or hormonal supply, or impairs psychosocial

Clinical Cues

Sexual Activity Among Older Adult Men

Cultural factors can affect erectile function in older men. Some cultures may disapprove of sexual activity among older adults, and some older men may not seek guidance for ED.

responses can interrupt the process of penile erection. Anxiety and depression can affect achieving or maintaining an erection. Organic causes can include diabetes mellitus and other endocrine disorders, disorders of the urinary tract, neurologic disorders, and chronic illness (such as sickle cell anemia, hypertension, cardiovascular disease, liver disease, and cancer). Medications and drug and alcohol abuse can interfere with sexual performance. Some antihypertensive drugs, diuretics, tranquilizers, and medications used to prevent gastroesophageal reflux disease (GERD) can cause sexual problems. Antiparkinson medications have been shown to enhance sexual desire but not the ability to perform (Mireille et al., 2017).

A complete history and physical examination help in ruling out illnesses that may affect sexual performance. Sleep laboratories can monitor nighttime penile erections to detect organic causes of impotence. A Doppler probe can measure arterial flow in the penis essential for erections, and nerve conduction tests can rule out neurologic pathology related to impotence. Review the patient's medications for side effects affecting erectile function and conduct a complete evaluation for psychological causes of impotence before devising an individualized treatment plan.

Treatment

Treatment depends on the cause of ED. Medical conditions are treated, the medications prescribed are reviewed and adjusted, hormone therapy may be prescribed for hypothalamic-pituitary disorders, and vascular surgery may be indicated for penile blood flow obstruction.

The primary intervention for ED is modifying reversible causes of the problem. Drug therapy includes phosphodiesterase 5 (PDE5) inhibitors, taken as directed in a period before sexual activity. These drugs should not be taken with nitrate-based drugs because a serious drop in blood pressure can occur from the combination. If these methods fail to resolve ED, surgical interventions may include inserting a penile implant that can be rigid or flexible. One type of implant includes a pump, inflatable cylinders, and a reservoir for emptying after erection. The erection produced is usually firm enough to enable intercourse (Fig. 40.1). Complications of oral medication therapy include **priapism**, a persistent abnormal erection that can develop into a urologic emergency. Treatment options are presented in Table 40.1.

Be aware of relationship problems within the family unit that may contribute to ED. Asking open-ended

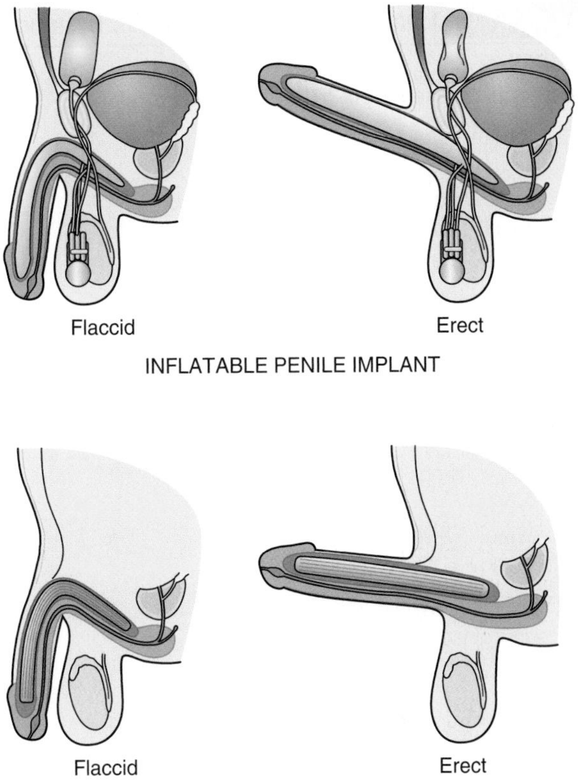

Fig. 40.1 Penile implants.

questions concerning sexual function or problems can provide information that will be helpful to the plan of care. Referral to a sex therapist may be indicated to help the patient integrate his sexual belief, practices, and abilities into a healthy lifestyle. Community support groups for patients with ED and their partners may be available.

Older Adult Care Points

Men can reproduce for as long as they can participate in intercourse. Older adults who have been consistently participating in intercourse throughout their adult life have the best chance of maintaining this capability. When abstinence has occurred over a considerable time, ED may become problematic. With patience and treatment, this problem may be treatable.

EJACULATION DISORDERS

Spinal cord injuries, neurologic disorders such as multiple sclerosis, diabetes mellitus, urologic surgery, or the side effects of various medications can cause problems with ejaculation. **Premature ejaculation** is the most common ejaculation problem in men; it occurs when the ejaculation reflex is not controlled, and the release of semen occurs before release is desired. Chemical, vibratory, and electrical stimulation can be used to treat premature ejaculation.

Retrograde ejaculation occurs when the semen travels toward the bladder rather than exiting the penis.

Table 40.1 Treatment Options for Erectile Dysfunction

OPTION	COMMENT
Medications Taken About 1 Hour Before Intercourse	
PDE5 inhibitors	Side effects can include headache, dyspepsia, and nasal congestion.
Sildenafil (Viagra) Vardenafil (Levitra): rapid onset Tadalafil (Cialis): longer lasting	Contraindicated in patients taking nitrates and patients with hypertension or retinopathy. Usually taken ½ to 4 h before sexual stimulation. Viagra can cause color vision disturbances and should not be taken more than once per day.
Yohimbine	Useful if organic disease is cause of ED.
Trazodone	Has sedation as side effect.
Intraurethral prostaglandin E_1 suppository (alprostadil)	Works locally on corpora cavernosa as a vasodilator.
Intracavernous injections of vasodilating drugs	Currently replaced by oral sildenafil therapy. May cause priapism.
Vasoactive drugs Papaverine gel Alprostadil (Caverject) Phentolamine (Vasomax)	Can be administered by topical gel, local self-injection, or insertion of medication pellet (alprostadil) into the urethra. Side effects can include pain, fibrotic nodules, and hypotension.
Complementary and Alternative Therapies	
Siberian ginseng	Believed to increase penile blood flow, but research-based evidence is lacking.
Ginkgo biloba Acupuncture Aromatherapy Sandalwood Rose Jasmine Ylang ylang oil Imagery Biofeedback Relaxation	These therapies may be used in conjunction with other options. Research-based evidence of effectiveness is lacking, but research is ongoing.
Other	
Sexual therapy	The psychosocial factors that may be causing ED are discussed with a qualified sex therapist. Counseling should include the partner.
Penile implants	Can be a semirigid rod or an inflatable prosthesis.
Negative pressure (vacuum constriction devices)	Used to induce erection by suction. A band is placed at base of penis to maintain erection. May be cumbersome to use. Injury can occur if constriction band is left in place longer than 1 h.

ED, Erectile dysfunction; *PDE5*, phosphodiesterase 5.

Determining the physical and psychological factors causing the retrograde problem is the priority for selecting appropriate treatment and planning care. Retrograde ejaculation may occur after prostatectomy.

If fertilization is desired, men with retrograde ejaculation may have sperm harvested from their urine for artificial insemination. When spinal injury is the problem, an electroejaculation device inserted into the rectum stimulates the prostate and enables sperm collection for artificial insemination.

INFERTILITY

Infertility is defined as failure of a couple to achieve a pregnancy after at least 1 year of active, unprotected intercourse. Approximately one third of infertility may result from factors in the male partner (U.S. Department of Health and Human Services, 2016). When taking a full sexual history, discussion with both partners concerning technique and timing of intercourse is important.

Hypothalamic-pituitary disorders and ED contribute to infertility, but testicular disorders are the most common organic cause of male infertility. Drugs, infections, systemic disease, and congenital disorders can cause testicular failure.

A semen analysis with sperm count and activity can be performed. Laboratory tests include follicle-stimulating hormone (FSH), luteinizing hormone (LH), and testosterone levels to determine whether hormone therapy is indicated. A postejaculation urine specimen may be examined to diagnose retrograde ejaculation of semen into the bladder. An ultrasound of the seminal vesicles may reveal dilated vesicles and obstruction of the vas deferens near the ejaculatory duct. Surgical resection of the ejaculatory duct may be indicated. A fine-needle aspiration or biopsy of the testicles may reveal pathology that can be treated.

Pathology may be corrected with medications, hormone therapy, or surgery. In vitro fertilization or intracytoplasmic sperm injection (ICSI) after sperm extraction is often successful.

The environment should be evaluated for toxins such as pesticides, lead, mercury, or radiation exposure—all of which can affect fertility. Occupational influences on fertility include exposure to organic solvents, oil products, chlorinated and fluorinated water, paint, irradiation, exhaust fumes, and heavy metals (Glaser, 2015). Patients seeking fertility should be instructed to prevent excessive heat around the scrotal area (Glaser, 2015), which could decrease sperm development. Hot tubs, using a laptop on the lap, and tight underwear should be avoided. Stress reduction techniques, information about timing and technique of intercourse, optimum nutrition, and health practices should be reviewed with both partners. When infertility is attributable to the man, his self-image may be affected; therefore objective, caring, and considerate family interactions are essential.

HYDROCELE

There is normally a small quantity of fluid in the space between the testis and tunica vaginalis within the scrotum (Fig. 40.2). A larger-than-normal amount of fluid accumulating in this space is known as *hydrocele.* The fluid accumulation may be caused by infection, such as epididymitis or orchitis, or accumulation may occur after trauma; hydrocele involves interference with lymphatic drainage of the scrotum. In many cases the cause is unknown. Hydrocele causes enlargement of the scrotum and usually is painless, but the weight and added bulk of the fluid can cause discomfort.

Treatment, when indicated, is aspiration or surgical incision and drainage of the sac. A pressure dressing and a drain are left in place postoperatively. Teach the patient to wear an athletic supporter for several weeks after treatment.

VARICOCELE

Dilation and clumping of the tributary vessels of the spermatic vein cause a painful swelling called *varicocele* (see Fig. 40.2). Varicocele typically occurs on the left side of the scrotum from retrograde blood flow from the left renal vein. The discomfort is rarely enough to warrant surgery. If infertility has been a concern, surgical correction via injection of a sclerosing agent or ligation of the spermatic vein may improve fertility.

Nursing measures to help the patient cope with fatigue, weakness, and fever are appropriate because these problems are commonly associated with urogenital infections and surgical procedures. Fluid intake should be increased to help prevent fluid deficit, reduce fever, increase urinary flow, and remove debris and bacteria. Teach the patient to wear scrotal support after any intervention.

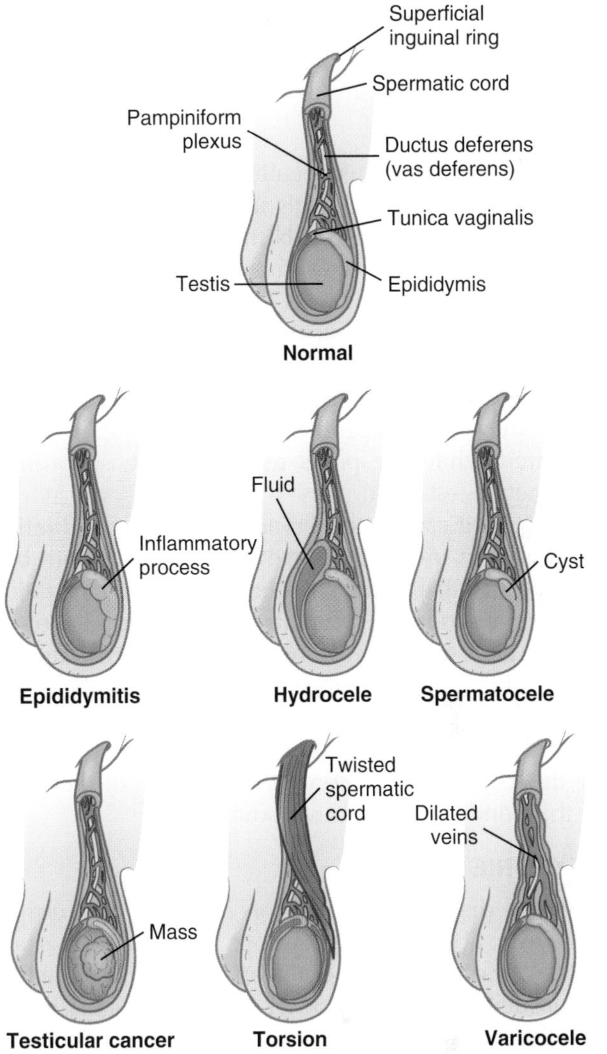

Fig. 40.2 Scrotal masses. (From Lewis SL, Heitkemper MM, Bucher L, et al.: *Medical-surgical nursing: assessment and management of clinical problems,* ed 10, St. Louis, 2017, Elsevier.)

TESTICULAR TORSION

Testicular torsion is a twisting of the testes and spermatic cord (see Fig. 40.2). It is commonly caused by elevated hormone levels in young adult men but can also result from scrotal trauma. Signs include sudden acute scrotal pain and an absence of the **cremasteric reflex** (retraction of the testicles when the inner thigh is stroked). Nausea and vomiting may also occur. A Doppler ultrasound scan may reveal diminished blood flow and confirm the diagnosis. To prevent testicular ischemia and necrosis, emergency surgery can be performed to secure the testicle within the scrotum or to remove the testicle if necessary. Provide routine postoperative wound care, with emphasis on providing support and relieving anxieties concerning the patient's self-image and future sexual performance.

PRIAPISM

Priapism is a prolonged penile erection resulting in a large, hard, and painful penis, unrelated to sexual desire or activity. The cause can be neurologic, vascular, or the result of medications such as those designed to increase sexual performance. The most common disease that causes priapism is sickle cell disease, which causes a local accumulation of erythrocytes that results in engorgement of the corporal bodies. Circulation to the penis may be compromised, and voiding may be impaired while the penis remains erect, so prompt treatment is essential.

Treatment can be conservative, to promote dilation of vessels in order to relieve pressure. Sedation, bed rest, warm baths or enemas, and urinary catheterization may be prescribed. Aspiration of the corpora cavernosa with a large-bore needle or a shunting procedure to divert blood may be necessary to prevent ischemia of the penis. Provide supportive care to the patient, who not only may be in pain, but also may be embarrassed by the loss of erectile control and fearful of the effect of this condition on future sexuality.

PEYRONIE DISEASE

Peyronie disease is a condition in which a plaque of nonelastic fibrous tissue develops in the tunica portion of the dorsal corpus cavernosum of the penis. The loss of elasticity in that section of the penis results in the inability to have a uniform erection of the penis. The penis will curve upward when erection occurs. Inability to penetrate the vagina may result, and the erection may become painful as well as embarrassing.

Conservative treatment includes local injections to dissolve the plaque. The size of the lesion and the level of ED may indicate a need for surgical intervention.

BENIGN PROSTATIC HYPERPLASIA

Etiology and Pathophysiology

Enlargement of the prostate, also known as benign prostatic hyperplasia (BPH), occurs when the prostate gland enlarges and extends into the bladder neck, causing obstruction of urine flow. An enlargement of the prostate often begins to develop before age 30 years. Prevalence of up to 60% has been noted by age 90 years (Lim, 2017).

Signs and Symptoms

BPH produces no symptoms until the growth becomes large enough to press against the urethra (Fig. 40.3). Then the patient begins to experience difficulty in urinating, evidenced by a decrease in the strength of the stream of urine, hesitancy, and dribbling after voiding. There may be frequency, nocturia, and urgency resulting from irritation of the distended bladder wall.

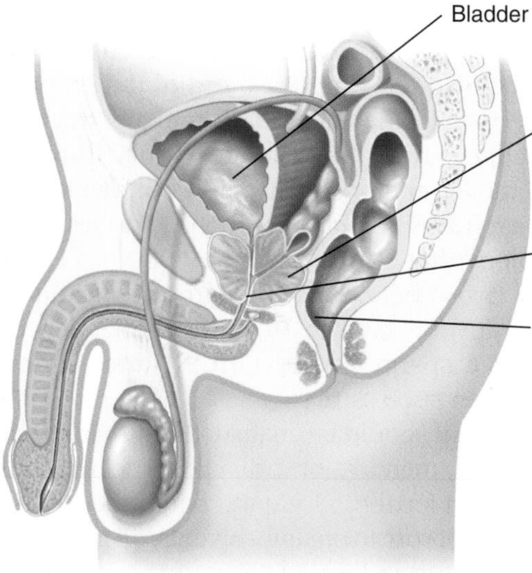

Fig. 40.3 Benign prostatic hyperplasia. (From Lewis SL, Heitkemper MM, Bucher L, et al.: *Medical-surgical nursing: assessment and management of clinical problems*, ed 10, St. Louis, 2017, Elsevier.)

In the later stages there may be complete obstruction of the urinary flow. Retention of urine (urinary stasis) is defined as more than 60 mL of residual urine after a void. Urinary tract infections can result from urinary stasis because the retained urine acts as a medium for organism growth. Gradual dilation of the ureter **(hydroureter)** and kidneys **(hydronephrosis)** can occur. Nitrogen products can accumulate in the blood (**azotemia**), and the back pressure into the kidney inhibits glomerular filtration, eventually causing renal failure if the urinary obstruction is not relieved. The American Urological Association Symptom Index (AUA-SI) is a tool used to assess symptoms related to urinary obstruction, which aids in clarifying the severity of the problem (American Urological Association, 2014). The tool gives a numeric score to the severity of each symptom of urinary retention. The total numeric score is used to determine appropriate treatment options.

Diagnosis

A digital rectal examination will reveal an enlarged prostate. The gold standard test for bladder outlet obstruction is increased bladder pressure relative to urinary flow. Pressure flow studies (**urodynamics**) can be performed. An ultrasound after urination or catheterization to determine residual urine volume is also a helpful diagnostic aid. A transrectal ultrasound differentiates BPH from prostate cancer, and a serum creatinine level can rule out renal insufficiency.

Treatment

If the patient cannot void, immediate catheterization will relieve the emergency problem, and follow-up care concerning the cause and severity of the prostate enlargement will then be completed.

Drug therapy. Drug therapy includes the following:

- **Alpha-adrenergic blockers,** which promote relaxation of smooth muscle and reduce blood pressure. Side effects of doxazosin (Cardura), terazosin, tamsulosin (Flomax), and alfuzosin (Uroxatral) include dizziness and orthostatic hypotension. These drugs offer prompt relief but may not reduce the prostate size. Silodosin (Rapaflo) also induces smooth muscle relaxation by selective action in the prostate, bladder base, prostatic capsule, and prostatic urethra.
- **5-Alpha-reductase inhibitors (5-ARIs)** are steroids and may take several months to work. Antiandrogen agents such as finasteride (Proscar) and dutasteride (Avodart) can decrease prostate size by reduced dihydrotestosterone (DHT) production. Side effects include decreased libido and increased breast size (**gynecomastia**). Finasteride has been approved for use to prevent prostate cancer in select patients when combined with doxazosin.
- **PDE5 enzyme inhibitors** are agents that inhibit the enzyme PDE5, thus producing increased vasodilation and inducing smooth muscle relaxation. Tadalafil (Cialis) requires sexual stimulation to activate the effect.
- Combination products recently have been shown to provide an improvement in symptoms and compliance. The most well known of these is a combination of dutasteride and tamsulosin (Jalyn), which is indicated for BPH with an enlarged prostate.

! Safety Alert

5-Alpha-Reductase Inhibitors and Cancer

A warning has been issued by the U.S. Food and Drug Administration (FDA) that individuals taking 5-ARIs may be at an increased risk for developing high-grade prostate cancer (Drugs.com, 2014).

Herbal therapy. Plant extracts such as saw palmetto (*Serenoa repens*) have been shown to be effective in minimizing symptoms associated with BPH (Ju et al., 2015). Patients wishing to use this herb should be referred to their health care provider.

Complementary and Alternative Therapy

Simple Lifestyle Changes for Benign Prostatic Hyperplasia

Urinating immediately when the urge occurs and going to the bathroom at regular intervals can relieve minor symptoms of BPH.

Surgery. Indications for surgical intervention include incontinence, hematuria, urinary retention, bladder stones, and urinary tract infections. Minimally invasive techniques such as balloon dilation, transurethral needle ablation, laser resection, and transurethral microwave thermotherapy are newer techniques that may help relieve symptoms. They are more effective than medications but less effective than surgery.

The most effective way to reduce symptoms is through surgery. This includes transurethral resection of the prostate (TURP), transurethral incision of the prostate (TUIP), laser photoselective vaporization of the prostate (PVP), and open prostatectomy. Ensure that the patient has a clear understanding of treatment options after the health care provider has explained them (Table 40.2).

Protein-specific antigen (PSA) is produced by the prostate tissue and is elevated in BPH, cancer of the prostate, and prostatitis and after prostate biopsy. Interpretation of PSA levels should take into consideration any diagnostic procedures involving the prostate gland. An elevated PSA is therefore not *always* indicative of cancer. The value of routine PSA screening continues to be evaluated (Pinsky, Prorok, & Kramer, 2017).

? Think Critically

A patient has been experiencing increasing difficulty in emptying his bladder and is diagnosed with BPH. Although surgery is recommended, the patient is reluctant. What other options that might prevent further organ damage are available to this patient?

Nursing Management

Preoperative care. Urinary drainage is accomplished by insertion of a catheter using sterile technique. If the obstruction is severe, a urologist may insert a special rigid catheter. A high fluid intake is encouraged, and antibiotics are routinely prescribed. Interview the patient to assess his understanding of the procedure to be performed and the impact on his lifestyle, self-image, and sexual function.

Preoperative teaching includes deep-breathing exercises; range-of-motion leg exercises; the general preoperative and postoperative routine; and explanation of care for the incision, catheters, and drains (see Chapters 4 and 5).

Postoperative care. Postoperative nursing care varies according to the type of prostate surgery performed (Fig. 40.4). The general principles of postoperative nursing care that apply to all patients having major surgery are necessary for the patient undergoing a prostatectomy. Potential postoperative complications are bleeding, urinary incontinence, and bladder spasms. Because hemorrhage always is a danger, vital signs are taken per agency protocol, then every 4 hours. The patient is monitored for pallor and rising pulse, which, along with blood pressure changes, may indicate excessive bleeding and shock. A high-fiber diet and a stool softener may be prescribed to prevent straining, which increases intra-abdominal pressure and can cause further bleeding.

Blood-tinged urine is normal for the first few days after the surgery. If the patient has a bleeding risk, an

Table 40.2 Surgical Interventions for Male Urogenital Problems

TREATMENT	COMMENTS
Minimally Invasive Treatments (Outpatient Surgery)	
Transurethral microwave thermotherapy (TUMT)	Heats and coagulates prostate tissue via a transurethral probe. A urinary catheter may be left in place for 1 wk after treatment to facilitate passing of necrotic tissue and prevent urinary retention. Antibiotics, analgesics, and bladder antispasmodics are prescribed after the procedure.
Transurethral needle ablation (TUNA)	Places radiofrequency needles directly into the prostate to coagulate specific tissue areas. Hematuria may occur for 1 wk after this procedure.
High-intensity focused ultrasound (HIFU)	High-intensity, low-frequency ultrasound waves destroy prostate tissue. Has been found to be effective in treatment of benign prostatic hyperplasia (BPH), but continued research on after effects are ongoing.
Surgery	
Open prostatectomy	Involves an external abdominal incision that allows complete visualization of prostate tissue. There is risk for infection and erectile dysfunction, postoperative pain, and a longer recovery period.
Suprapubic prostatectomy	Enters via the bladder.
Retropubic prostatectomy	Does not enter the bladder.
Perineal prostatectomy	The removal of the prostate via an incision in the perineum; has high risk for postoperative wound contamination, incontinence, and impotence.
Transurethral resection of the prostate (TURP)	TURP is the gold standard of treatment for BPH and is performed under spinal anesthesia. A resectoscope is inserted into the urethra to excise and cauterize obstructive prostate tissue. A large three-way catheter is inserted to provide hemostasis and allow urinary drainage. May be performed as outpatient surgery at many facilities.
Transurethral incision of the prostate (TUIP)	TUIP incises the prostate. May be performed as outpatient surgery at many facilities.
Laser prostatectomy	A modified TURP; uses a laser beam to destroy prostate tissue. Minimal postoperative bleeding occurs, but a catheter may be required for 1 wk postoperatively to prevent urinary retention from edema.
Transurethral electrovaporization of the prostate (TUVP)	Electrosurgical vaporization and desiccation destroy prostate tissue. Complications include hematuria and retrograde ejaculation.
Transurethral photoselective vaporization of the prostate (PVP)	Uses a green light laser beam to coagulate prostate tissue.
Urethral stent	A metallic stent is placed in the urethra to hold it open. This is usually a temporary measure because displacement is common.
Laparoscopic radical prostatectomy	Provides better visualization and fewer postoperative complications and has a shorter hospital stay.

irrigation system may be indicated to maintain patency of the catheter. To decrease clot formation, the bladder irrigation flow rate is adjusted to keep the urine diluted to a reddish pink, clearing to a pink tinge within 48 hours. Some pieces of tissue and small clots may be seen in the drainage. Additional intermittent irrigation with 20 to 30 mL of normal saline may be needed to clear the catheter of obstruction (Nursing Care Plan 40.1). Strict sterile technique must be used when irrigating the bladder, and the catheter should be connected to a closed drainage system to prevent infection.

Persistent bleeding turning the urine darker than cherry red or bright red, or viscous drainage with many clots, should be reported immediately to the surgeon. Traction may be applied to the catheter to supply pressure (**tamponade**) to prevent excessive bleeding.

Clinical Cues

When caring for a bladder irrigation system:

- Use sterile normal saline unless otherwise ordered.
- Monitor rate of irrigation.
- Monitor and record intake and output.
- Record the amount of irrigation fluid instilled and the amount returned. The difference equals the urine output.
- Check drainage tubes for kinks and clots.
- Observe for signs of bladder spasms and medicate promptly as needed.

The surgeon does this by pulling against the balloon and then taping the catheter to the thigh or abdomen. This pressure may cause the patient to have a sensation of a continuous need to void. Check frequently to see that the catheter and tubing are not kinked and that outflow is appropriate. The patient may have some urinary frequency and burning after catheter use is discontinued. Some blood in the urine may occur for several more days.

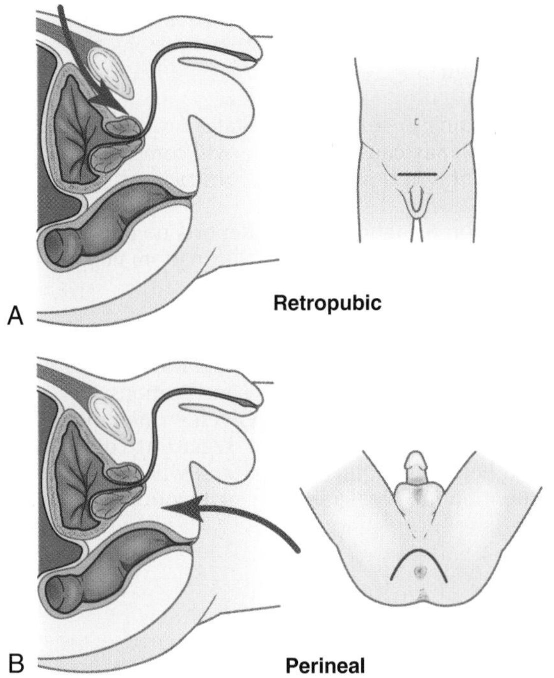

Fig. 40.4 Two approaches to perform a prostatectomy. **A,** The retropubic approach involves a midline abdominal incision. **B,** The perineal approach involves an incision between the scrotum and anus. (From Lewis SL, Heitkemper MM, Bucher L, et al.: *Medical-surgical nursing: assessment and management of clinical problems,* ed 10, St. Louis, 2017, Elsevier.)

The patient who has had a suprapubic prostatectomy may have a suprapubic catheter in addition to a urethral catheter. Each catheter is attached to a separate sterile drainage system. After the urethral catheter is removed (sometime after the third day), the suprapubic catheter is clamped, and the patient attempts to void. Residual urine is measured afterward by unclamping the suprapubic catheter. When there is no more than 60 mL of residual urine after voiding, the suprapubic catheter is removed. Dribbling of urine often occurs after prostatectomy because of decreased sphincter tone but usually stops within about 6 months. Patients who experience incontinence are taught perineal muscle strengthening (Kegel) exercises for this problem and are given instruction in bladder training (see Chapters 33 and 34). Teaching for this procedure should have been done preoperatively and exercises resume 24 to 48 hours after surgery. Kegel exercises and coping strategies should be taught to enable early return to a normal lifestyle.

When the urethral or suprapubic catheter is removed, the patient must be monitored carefully for ability to void. Intake and output are tracked closely. Any difficulty in voiding within 6 hours after removal must be reported to the surgeon promptly because a distended bladder may cause bleeding.

Monitor the incisional dressings and change them as often as necessary to keep the patient dry and comfortable. Urine is very irritating to the skin, and any area that is exposed to urine drainage is thoroughly cleansed before a new dressing is applied.

Prophylactic antimicrobials and analgesics are administered in the early postoperative period. Bladder

Nursing Care Plan 40.1 Care of a Patient After Prostatectomy

SCENARIO

A 70-year-old man who had a transurethral prostatectomy is admitted to the postoperative unit. His vital signs are stable, and his Foley is draining red urine with some clots. The patient is awake and oriented, and the health care provider has prescribed a diet as tolerated.

PROBLEM STATEMENT/NURSING DIAGNOSIS

Potential for fluid volume deficit due to postoperative hemorrhage and limited fluid intake.

SUPPORTING ASSESSMENT DATA

Objective: Transurethral prostatectomy.

Goals/Expected Outcomes	Nursing Interventions	Selected Rationale	Evaluation
Patient evidences normal fluid volume and stable vital signs.	Monitor vital signs.	A change in vital signs can indicate fluid deficit.	Vital signs stable.
	Monitor intake and output.	Encouraging oral fluids as tolerated and recording amount and type of output enable identification of fluid volume status.	Intake >3500 mL; output >3200 mL. Taking sufficient oral fluids.
Patient evidences clear to pink urinary drainage with no clots.	Assess skin turgor with vital signs	Decreased turgor is a sign of fluid deficit.	Normal skin turgor.
	Administer IV fluids as prescribed.	IV therapy can help maintain fluid balance.	IV infusion at 150 mL/h.

PROBLEM STATEMENT/NURSING DIAGNOSIS

Insufficient knowledge regarding self-care after discharge.

Continued

Nursing Care Plan 40.1 Care of a Patient After Prostatectomy—cont'd

SUPPORTING ASSESSMENT DATA

Subjective: "No, I've never had a catheter before. What do I have to do?"

Goals/Expected Outcomes	Nursing Interventions	Selected Rationale	Evaluation
Patient will list signs of infection, explain need for increased fluid intake, demonstrate care of catheter, and follow medication regimen.	Teach to report signs of infection: fever, chills, malaise, increased pain, purulent drainage, excessive swelling.	Early identification of infection is important to initiate timely treatment.	Provides accurate feedback on all instructions.
	Instruct to avoid heavy lifting, driving, and sexual activity until permitted by urologist.	Heavy lifting or sexual activity may cause disruption of tissue and bleeding.	States understanding and will comply with restrictions.
	Teach to report onset of burning on urination or cloudy urine after catheter is removed.	Burning on urination or cloudy urine may indicate bladder infection.	Reports no burning on urination; no cloudy urine.
	Explain what each medication is for and when and how to take it.	Helps with compliance with medication regimen.	States understands when and how to take the medications.
	Provide written information about signs and symptoms of urethral stricture or infection and teach to report these.	Written instructions can be reviewed at home and help to get quick attention for problems.	Given written instructions regarding complications and what to report to surgeon.

PROBLEM STATEMENT/NURSING DIAGNOSIS

Anxiety due to inability to achieve erection.

SUPPORTING ASSESSMENT DATA

Subjective: "Do you think my partner will leave me if I can no longer engage in intercourse?"

Objective: Prostatectomy

Goals/Expected Outcomes	Nursing Interventions	Selected Rationale	Evaluation
Patient will discuss concerns before discharge.	Encourage verbalization of problems and concerns.	Verbalization of concerns helps with identifying solutions.	Verbalizes concern about the possibility of not being able to obtain an erection.
	Provide information on alternative ways to achieve erection.	Gives the patient useful information in case of need.	Provided with information about alternate ways to achieve erection.
Patient will discuss concerns with his partner before discharge.	Counsel about other ways to achieve intimacy. Include partner in discussions.	Addressing individual needs of patient encourages learning and retention.	Agrees to include partner in discussions about his sexual concerns.
	Assist to make plan to meet sexual needs.	Provides tools to cope with sexual problems.	Patient and partner are collaborating on plan.

CRITICAL THINKING QUESTIONS

1. What are the priority nursing interventions if you notice that urinary outflow is less than intake?
2. Why is it important to address reports of bladder spasm pain as soon as possible? What medication is generally used for this type of pain?

IV, Intravenous.

spasms often are a concern after TURP or suprapubic prostatectomy. Before giving medication, check to see that the tubing is not kinked and the catheter is draining well because obstruction can cause bladder spasm. Abdominal distention may be a sign of catheter obstruction as well. A patient who has had a radical procedure may have a patient-controlled analgesia pump to control pain.

Discharge teaching includes care of the catheter, management of incontinence, maintaining hydration,

Clinical Cues

Belladonna and opium (B&O) rectal suppositories are effective for bladder spasms if they are given when the spasms first begin. Relaxation techniques and an anticholinergic drug, such as oxybutynin chloride (Ditropan XL), may be used to help relieve bladder spasms.

preventing constipation, observing for signs of infection, and management of anxiety related to impaired sexual function and self-image (see Patient Teaching: Discharge Instructions for a Patient After a Prostatectomy). Retrograde ejaculation (semen discharged into the bladder) may cause the urine to appear cloudy. Frequent planned urination and avoidance of irritating foods such as citrus, caffeine-containing products, and alcohol should be initiated. The patient should be taught to monitor output and contact the health care provider if unable to void. BPH can recur if not all prostate tissue was removed, so annual digital rectal examinations should be continued (see Nursing Care Plan 40.1).

INFLAMMATIONS AND INFECTIONS OF THE MALE REPRODUCTIVE TRACT

Many of the inflammations and infections affecting the male reproductive system are similar to those of the female reproductive system in cause and effect. For example, urethritis in men and women can be caused by common pyogenic and colonic bacteria and by *Neisseria gonorrhoeae.* Men also can be infected with *Trichomonas vaginalis* or *Chlamydia,* which are transmitted by sexual contact. Sexual partners may continue to reinfect each other until both are treated simultaneously.

Nonspecific genitourinary infections in men—including nongonococcal urethritis (NGU)—may be caused by various organisms, but these infections present substantially the same clinical picture. Among the symptoms of nonspecific urethritis are mucopurulent discharge from the urethra, painful urination of varying degrees of severity, and the occasional appearance of blood in the urine. A microscopic examination of a smear from urethral secretions may not show any specific organisms, but there may be an excessive number of white cells.

Epididymitis

Epididymitis is an inflammation of the epididymis and may result from an infection of the prostate or a urinary tract infection. A patient with epididymitis experiences groin pain and swelling and pain in the scrotum. In younger men, the major cause of epididymitis is *Chlamydia trachomatis,* a sexually transmitted organism. Symptoms include scrotal pain, swelling, induration of the epididymis, and eventual edema of the scrotal wall. The adjacent testicle may become involved. The urine may contain pus (pyuria), and chills and fever may follow. Antibiotics, ice packs, analgesics, sitz baths, and elevation of the scrotum are the prescribed treatment protocol. A local anesthetic may be injected into the spermatic cord to manage pain.

Orchitis

Orchitis is inflammation of the testicle and may affect one or both testes. It may be caused by local or systemic infection (viral or bacterial) or by trauma. Bilateral orchitis is serious and often causes sterility. **Mumps orchitis** occurs in about 3% to 10% of males who contract mumps (Centers for Disease Control and Prevention, 2018). Gamma globulin usually is given to decrease the possibility or severity of mumps orchitis. The symptoms and treatment parallel those of epididymitis.

Prostatitis

Prostatitis is an inflammation of the prostate that occurs from an infectious agent or other causes. The National Institutes of Health (NIH) uses the following classification system:

- *Type I:* **Acute bacterial prostatitis** with acute infection of the prostate gland
- *Type II:* **Chronic bacterial prostatitis** (CBP) with chronic or recurrent infection of the prostate
- *Type III:* **Chronic prostatitis/chronic pelvic pain syndrome** (CP/CPPS) with no demonstrated infection
  - Type IIIa: Inflammatory CPPS with white blood cells in semen and/or expressed prostatic secretions or voided bladder
  - Type IIIb: Noninflammatory CPPS with no white cells in semen, expressed prostatic secretions, or voided bladder
- *Type IV:* **Asymptomatic inflammatory prostatitis** with no subjective symptoms detected and inflammation shown via prostate biopsy or presence of white cells in expressed prostatic secretions or semen during evaluation for infertility or other disorders (Rees et al., 2015).

Symptoms include recurrent urinary infection, pelvic pain, and sexual dysfunction and are often mistaken for BPH. Because blood PSA levels are often elevated in prostatitis, misdiagnosis of prostate cancer can occur. Prostate massage, useful for diagnosis, presents a risk for bacteremia. The various types of prostatitis can be diagnosed with a segmented culture of initial stream urine, midstream urine, prostate fluid before and after massage, and postmassage urine specimen. Treatment includes bed rest, analgesia, bladder sedatives, sitz baths, and stool softeners to prevent straining. Antibiotics may be prescribed according to culture and sensitivity laboratory findings.

Antibiotics diffuse poorly into the prostatic fluid, so chronic prostatitis is commonly treated with alpha-adrenergic blockers (tamsulosin); fluoroquinolones may be prescribed. The patient is taught to recognize symptoms of urinary tract infection and to reduce retention of prostatic fluid by ejaculation. The patient should be taught to avoid foods that increase prostatic secretions, such as alcohol, chocolate, tea, and spices. Follow-up care to detect reinfection is essential.

CANCER OF THE MALE REPRODUCTIVE TRACT

Penile Cancer

Cancer of the penis is rare, occurring mostly in men with human papillomavirus infections or who were not circumcised (American Cancer Society, 2018c).

Cultural Considerations

Incidence and Mortality Rate of Penile Cancer

Penile cancer is very rare in industrialized countries (Pettaway, 2017). Testicular cancer is more common in Caucasian men (Michaelson & Oh, 2018); prostate cancer occurs most frequently in African American men (Sartor, 2018).

A nontender nodule may appear on the penis, and biopsy will show a squamous cell–type carcinoma. Laser resection of the lesion is the treatment of choice unless the cancer has spread. Radical resection of the penis followed by radiation and chemotherapy may be required. The shaft of the resected penis can respond to sexual stimulation and enable orgasm and ejaculation. After a total removal of the penis (penectomy) the patient may experience orgasm via stimulation of the scrotum and perineal area.

Testicular Cancer

Testicular cancer occurs most commonly in younger men and at a rate of 1 in 250 men; however, it is a highly treatable cancer (American Cancer Society, 2018b). Depending on the stage of cancer, the 5-year survival rate ranges between 73% (for distant) and 99% (for localized) (American Cancer Society, 2018d).

Men most at risk for testicular cancer are those who have had an undescended or partially descended testicle. Men who were exposed to diethylstilbestrol (DES) in utero also may be at high risk for testicular cancer, but evidence-based research is lacking. All males between ages 15 and 40 years should be taught to practice testicular self-examination on a monthly basis. (see Chapter 38, Fig. 38.6). Cancer symptoms appear slowly and involve painless enlargement of the testes, backache, and weight loss.

Health Promotion

Testicular Self-Examination

- Testicular self-examination should be performed monthly.
- Perform after bathing when scrotal skin is relaxed.
- Roll each testicle between thumb and fingers.
- Report lumps right away to your health care provider.

If a mass is found and thought to be malignant, diagnostic tests for tumor marker proteins such as elevated levels of alpha-fetoprotein (AFP), beta–human chorionic gonadotropin (beta-HCG), alkaline phosphatase, and lactate dehydrogenase are obtained to confirm diagnosis. Computed tomography (CT) scans and/or ultrasound should be performed to detect sites of testicular mass. Testicular cancer spreads rapidly via lymph and blood vessels. A microscopic tissue analysis is performed after surgical removal of the mass for definitive diagnosis.

There are three stages for classifying the malignancy of testicular cancer. In **stage I (localized),** the tumor is confined to the affected testis (American Cancer Society, 2018d). In **stage II (regional),** malignant cells have spread to the regional lymph nodes, usually on the same side as the affected testis (American Cancer Society, 2018d). In **stage III (distant),** there is metastasis to other organs, such as the lungs and liver (American Cancer Society, 2018d).

If the testicular tumor is limited to the scrotal sac and there is no metastasis, a laparoscopic surgical removal of the testis (**orchiectomy**) may be all that is necessary to cure the patient of his disease. A gel prosthesis can be implanted. Care is taken to preserve the nerves associated with ejaculation. The nursing care focuses on teaching and providing psychological support. Ice bags and scrotal support provide comfort, and the importance of follow-up care is stressed. Removal of only one testis will not affect the patient's ability to produce the male hormone testosterone or render him impotent because the other testis can carry on adequate testicular function.

Further treatment for stage II testicular cancer may include radiation. Chemotherapy is reserved for advanced stages of cancer and results in a high percentage of complete remission. See Chapter 8 for a detailed discussion of radiation and chemotherapy in the care of cancer patients.

Some men view an orchiectomy as a loss of masculinity. You can be instrumental in assisting the patient to verbalize his fears about the procedure and its implications. Time for questions and discussion of concerns should be provided for the patient and his sexual partner. Sperm banking before surgery is an option for patients who may face chemotherapy. Continued follow-up care is essential.

Prostate Cancer

Carcinoma of the prostate is the second most common cancer (next to skin cancer) that affects men (American Cancer Society, 2018a). The American Cancer Society predicted approximately 164,690 new cases for 2018 in the United States, with 29,430 men dying of prostate cancer (American Cancer Society, 2018a). Carcinoma of the prostate is usually a slow-growing cancer that is dependent on the hormone androgen. Some studies have identified an association with the prostate cancer antigen gene *(PCA3)*, which can be measured via urinary assay, as a significant risk factor. Studies continue to determine best preventative measures to avoid prostate cancer; current research focuses on the benefit of lycopenes and isoflavones, vitamin D, and 5-ARIs as potential means of prevention (American Cancer Society, 2018e).

Clinical symptoms and screening. If prostate cancer is detected early, the probability of cure is high. Early detection by digital rectal examination can reveal a hardened lobe of prostate early in the course of the disease. The United States Preventive Task Force (2018) recommends individualized decision making between a patient and health care provider about screening for men between the ages of 55 and 69 years and against screening for men over the age of 70 years.

> **? Think Critically**
>
> What sort of psychological support would the patient undergoing a prostatic biopsy need from you? What might be some of the patient's concerns?

An elevated PSA (about 4 ng/mL) may indicate prostate pathology but is not diagnostic for prostate cancer. The **PSA velocity** is a trend in PSA levels over time that may indicate a need for further tests to diagnose prostate cancer. A transrectal ultrasound may be performed, and bones may be scanned to detect metastasis. A ProstaScint scan combined with CT or magnetic resonance imaging (MRI) scans can detect prostate cancer cells when the PSA levels are low. A urine test to detect prostate cancer, PRoGensa PCA-3 assay, is closely related to biopsy outcomes. Transrectal, transurethral, and transperineal prostate biopsy and tissue analyses determine the severity or extent of prostate cancer (Fig. 40.5).

Treatment and nursing care. Because prostate cancer is relatively slow growing, conservative treatment may involve monitoring and follow-up care. Annual digital rectal examinations are performed, and PSA levels are monitored in high-risk patients. When surgical therapy is indicated, a laparoscopic radical prostatectomy is considered the most effective treatment for long-term survival before metastasis occurs. Other treatment options are listed in Table 40.3. Denosumab (Prolia) is a monoclonal antibody approved for treatment of bone loss (osteoporosis) in men who have had androgen deprivation therapy for prostate cancer.

An interprofessional approach integrates surgery, radiation, and androgen restriction. After surgery, PSA levels are monitored; a decrease may indicate treatment success. In the early stages, radiation therapy may be the treatment of choice. Gamma teletherapy (external) and brachytherapy (internal) are used for cancer of the prostate and provide greater preservation of sexual ability.

Chapter 8 presents a detailed discussion concerning care of patients receiving radiation and chemotherapy. Hormonal therapy is designed to suppress androgen stimulation of the prostate by decreasing plasma testosterone. Removal of the testes may be performed to cause prostate atrophy. An LH-releasing hormone (LHRH) agonist, such as leuprolide or goserelin, or androgen agents, such as flutamide, suppress androgen and may be used in combination with radiation therapy. Provide a sensitive, caring approach to the patient and family to help them cope with the diagnosis and make informed choices. Preoperative care involves restoration of urinary drainage, prevention of urinary tract infection, and understanding the options for treatment and their effect on sexual function. Complications of surgery may include bleeding, catheter obstruction, and sexual dysfunction. Impotence or retrograde ejaculation may occur. Options to enable erections and improve sexual function via prosthetic devices or medication should be discussed with the patient. The nursing care of a patient with a prostatectomy includes reducing anxiety, relieving discomfort, maintaining fluid balance, monitoring for bleeding or infection, catheter care, and teaching the patient self-care and the need for continued follow-up care.

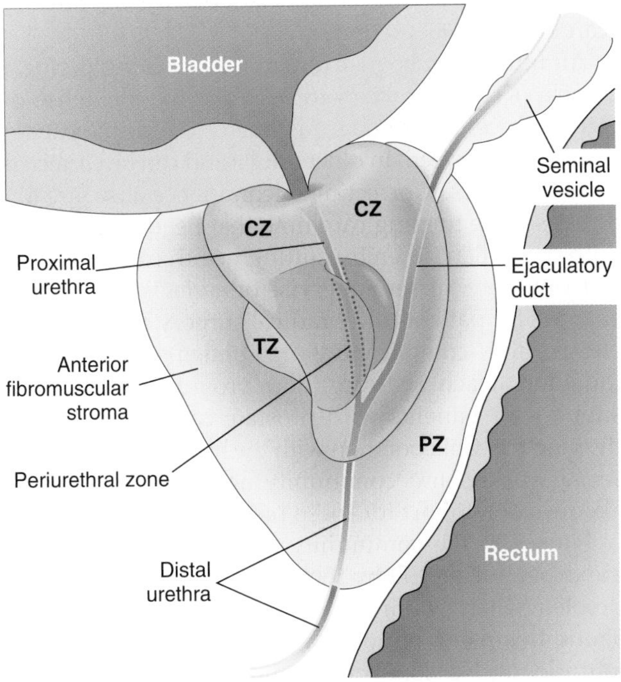

Fig. 40.5 Adult prostate. The normal prostate contains several distinct regions, including a central zone *(CZ)*, a peripheral zone *(PZ)*, a transitional zone *(TZ)*, and a periurethral zone. Most carcinomas arise from the peripheral glands of the organ, whereas nodular hyperplasia arises from more centrally situated glands. (From Kumar V, Abbas AK, Aster JC: *Robbins basic pathology*, ed 10, Philadelphia, 2018, Elsevier.)

> **Older Adult Care Points**
>
> For older adults undergoing chemotherapy or radiation therapy:
> - Monitor for infections.
> - Promote assisted ambulation.
> - Institute fall precautions.
> - Encourage use of an incentive spirometer.
> - Minimize pain.
> - Reorient to environment as needed.

COMMUNITY CARE

Nurses in the community can be instrumental in teaching and promoting testicular self-examination in men between ages 15 and 40 years. Educating all men older than 55 years about prostate cancer screening benefits and drawbacks will allow them to make a personal decision regarding PSA testing.

Table 40.3 **Treatment Options for Prostate Cancer**

TREATMENT	COMMENTS
Radical prostatectomy	The prostate gland, seminal vesicles, and portions of the neck of the bladder are removed. ED and incontinence are long-term complications. A laparoscopic approach provides fewer complications and shorter hospital stay. Robotic prostatectomy reduces risk of incontinence and impotence.
Cryosurgery	A freezing technique destroys prostate tissue. Complications include urethral damage, ED, and incontinence.
Radiation therapy	May be prescribed when the patient is not a candidate for surgery or may be offered in combination with surgery and hormone therapy.
External beam radiation	Most popular form of radiation therapy, given weekly on an outpatient basis for 2 mo. Side effects can include skin irritation, GI cramping and bleeding, ED, and bone marrow suppression. Cure rates for patients with localized cancer are comparable to radical prostatectomy.
Brachytherapy	The implantation of radioactive seeds into the prostate gland. It may be offered in combination with external beam radiation.
Hormone therapy	Designed to reduce androgens. Leuprolide (Lupron, Viadur), goserelin (Zoladex), and triptorelin (Trelstar) are common drugs used; produces a chemical castration.
Chemotherapy	Used for hormone-resistant cancer or late-stage cancer. The prostate has limited response to chemotherapy.
Bisphosphonates	Reduce bone complications in advanced stages of prostate cancer. Drugs may include zoledronic acid (Zometa), risedronate (Actonel), etidronate (Didronel), or alendronate (Fosamax).

ED, Erectile dysfunction; *GI*, gastrointestinal.

Patient Teaching

Discharge Instructions for a Patient After a Prostatectomy

The patient is instructed regarding the following points:

- Drink 12 to 14 glasses of water during the day to keep the urine flowing freely.
- Do not lift any object weighing more than 8 lb for 2 to 3 weeks after surgery (depending on health care provider's instructions), avoid strenuous activities.
- If blood is noticed in the urine, lie down and rest; drink more fluids and call the surgeon if the bleeding continues.
- Depending on the patient's occupation, it may be possible to return to work within 2 to 4 weeks. Consult the surgeon.
- Keep the catheter clean; cleanse the catheter and around the meatus daily with soap and water and rinse thoroughly.
- Report any cloudiness or foul smell in the urine.
- Report signs of infection such as fever, chills, or purulent wound drainage.
- After catheter removal, dribbling of urine may occur for up to 6 months. The problem usually will resolve. Perineal strengthening exercises help.
- After healing is complete, report any changes in the force or size of the urine stream to the surgeon.
- Report for annual checkups to detect recurrence of tissue growth or the development of prostate cancer.

Nurses in long-term care facilities must be watchful for urinary obstruction in older adult male residents. Alert men should be questioned regularly about problems with urination; men with cognitive impairment who do not have a normal urinary stream should be placed on intake and output recording to detect any problems with urinary obstruction. Palpation just above the symphysis pubis may reveal a distended bladder. Use of a bladder scanner can detect retention.

All nurses can be instrumental in teaching perineal muscle (Kegel) exercises to decrease the incidence of incontinence. Incontinence is one of the prime causes of loss of self-esteem in older adults and can be corrected in many cases. Correcting incontinence also greatly decreases the nursing care time that needs to be spent with the patient, thereby cutting health care costs.

Home care nurses supervise or assist with dressing changes for patients after radical surgery, monitor side effects and complications in patients undergoing radiation, teach self-care, and provide psychosocial support for patients with prostate cancer and sexual dysfunction. Collaboration with the health care provider, social worker, and community agencies can provide avenues of support for these patients.

Nurses in the community can assist patients who are experiencing ED by including assessment for this problem when working with male patients. Knowledge about treatment options, a matter-of-fact optimistic attitude, and a comfortable manner when speaking about this topic can provide hope and guidance. Sometimes ED is brought to light when speaking with the partner of a patient. Many times, a satisfying sexual life can be reinstituted for these people, providing added fulfillment and joy throughout the adult life span.

Get Ready for the NCLEX® Examination!

Key Points

- Anxiety, depression, various medications, and certain diseases can contribute to ED.
- Complications of treatment for ED can include priapism, which requires prompt intervention.
- Testicular cancer occurs most commonly in men ages 15 to 40 years, and the 5-year survival rate is ranges from 73% to 99%.
- Serum PSA levels become elevated when prostate disease (such as BPH or prostatitis) is present and therefore may not be a reliable marker indicating cancer.
- Treatment of BPH involves medications that relax the bladder and urethra (alpha blockers) and reduce prostate tissue through reduced DHT production (5-ARIs).
- Indications for surgical intervention for BPH include urinary retention, gross hematuria, bladder stones, and urinary tract infections.
- Patient education concerning disorders of the reproductive tract should include information about the effects on sexual activity.
- Older adults who have consistently participated in intercourse throughout adult life have the best chance of maintaining this capability into old age.
- Nurses in long-term care facilities must watch for signs of urinary obstruction in older men.

Additional Learning Resources

SG Go to your Study Guide for additional learning activities to help you master this chapter content.

Go to your Evolve website (http://evolve.elsevier.com/deWit/medsurg) for the following FREE learning resources:
- Animations, audio, and video
- Answers and rationales for questions and activities
- Glossary with pronunciations in English and Spanish
- Interactive Review Questions and more!

Review Questions for the NCLEX® Examination

1. A 25-year-old patient presents with severe groin pain, redness and swelling of the scrotum and fever with chills. You anticipate which of the following orders:
   1. Acetaminophen 500 mg po now.
   2. Acyclovir 400 mg po now and TID.
   3. Azithromycin 1000 mg po now.
   4. Benzathine penicillin G 2.4 million units IM now.
   NCLEX Client Need: Physiological Integrity: Pharmacological Therapies

2. A 23-year old patient reports sudden acute scrotal pain. Initial examination reveals absence of the cremasteric reflex. Doppler ultrasound reveals a diminished blood flow. Which condition do you anticipate?
   1. Varicocele
   2. Testicular torsion
   3. Hydrocele
   4. Priapism
   NCLEX Client Need: Physiological Integrity: Physiological Adaptation

3. A 26-year-old African American man was hospitalized for a prolonged penile erection unrelated to sexual desire or activity. For which condition do you assess?
   1. Diabetes mellitus
   2. Sickle cell disease
   3. Hemophilia
   4. Urinary infection
   NCLEX Client Need: Physiological Integrity: Physiological Adaptation

4. A postprostatectomy patient expresses concerns about his ability to have intimate relations with his partner. Which nursing interventions are appropriate? *(Select all that apply.)*
   1. Teach signs and symptoms of infection.
   2. Encourage him to verbalize personal concerns with his partner.
   3. Demonstrate appropriate aseptic wound care.
   4. Facilitate development of alternative coping strategies.
   5. Reassure him that the ability to have sexual intercourse will not be affected.
   NCLEX Client Need: Psychosocial Integrity

5. A 64-year old patient reports difficulty urinating, described as decreased strength of the urine stream, as well as hesitancy, dribbling, and urgency. Which nursing interventions are appropriate? *(Select all that apply.)*
   1. Teach to decrease caffeine and artificial sweeteners.
   2. Teach to limit spicy foods and alcohol intake.
   3. Apply a condom catheter.
   4. Restrict fluid intake.
   5. Plan a timed voiding schedule.
   NCLEX Client Need: Physiological Integrity: Basic Care and Comfort

6. A 30-year-old patient tells you that he located a lump on his testicle that he would like to have the health care provider check if it doesn't go away by his next visit. What is the appropriate response?
   1. "Most testicular lumps are not cancer; you can come back sooner if it does not go away."
   2. "Most testicular lumps are cancerous, so this should be checked immediately."
   3. "Most testicular lumps are benign, but we do not want to take a risk, so let's have it checked today."
   4. "Let's make an appointment on another day; this might go away without intervention."
   NCLEX Client Need: Physiological Integrity: Reduction of Risk Potential

7. You are taking care of a 40-year-old patient who had a bilateral orchiectomy and who expresses concern about how his sexuality will be affected in the future. What techniques will you use to demonstrate acceptance and a nonjudgmental attitude? *(Select all that apply.)*
   1. Establish eye contact.
   2. Demonstrate sensitivity to nonverbal cues.
   3. Ask repetitive questions.
   4. Involve nonessential family members.
   5. Encourage the patient to express his feelings.

   NCLEX Client Need: Psychosocial Integrity
8. A 40-year-old man requests a prostate examination and a PSA test, stating that he wants to start getting screened early. Which is the appropriate nursing response?
   1. "Screening for prostate cancer can begin at age 55 years; depending on the results, a screening prevention plan is devised based on risk."
   2. "You do not need to worry now. Prostate screening begins at age 50 years and then continues annually."
   3. "Prostate screening is done at the same time as your colon cancer screening and begins by age 50 years."
   4. "We only check PSA levels now. Prostate examinations have been found to be unreliable."

   NCLEX Client Need: Physiological Integrity: Reduction of Risk Potential
9. A patient who had TURP reports increasing bladder spasms. Which is the appropriate initial nursing action?
   1. Medicate with a B&O suppository.
   2. Check the urinary catheter tubing for kinks and obstruction.
   3. Teach relaxation exercises.
   4. Encourage use of patient-controlled analgesia.

   NCLEX Client Need: Physiological Integrity: Physiological Adaptation
10. A patient states that he was diagnosed with a hydrocele but is confused about what this means. How will you explain a hydrocele? *(Select all that apply.)*
    1. "A fluid collection within the scrotum that can be drained."
    2. "Sometimes caused by an infection of the testis that causes inflammation."
    3. "An inflammation of the testes and scrotum from an illness such as mumps."
    4. "Possibly occurred as a result of trauma."
    5. "An interference with lymphatic drainage of the scrotum."

    NCLEX Client Need: Physiological Integrity: Physiological Adaptation

Critical Thinking Questions

Scenario A

A 21-year old patient at the community health center reports that he has been diagnosed with testicular cancer and is scheduled for surgery. He states that he wants to have the surgery done but is afraid of how this will affect his "manhood."

1. What information could you give this patient to address his concerns?
2. How could you explain that removal of a testis does not render a man less masculine?

Scenario B

Mr. Heitz, a 70-year old patient, is 2 days postoperative from TURP. You notice that he is disoriented and restless, and he states that he needs to urinate. You check the catheter and find that it is not draining as it should.

1. What would you tell Mr. Heitz about his need to void?
2. What would you do about the catheter?
3. What further observations should you make while caring for this patient?
4. What special precautions should be taken for his safety?

Care of Patients With Sexually Transmitted Infections

41

http://evolve.elsevier.com/deWit/medsurg

Objectives

Theory

1. Differentiate prevention, signs and symptoms, treatment, and complications associated with common sexually transmitted infections (STIs) in male and female patients.
2. Explain the procedure for the various tests for STIs.
3. Illustrate the nurse's role in preventing, identifying, reporting, and treating common STIs.

Clinical Practice

4. Devise a teaching plan for a patient who has experienced a first incidence of genital herpes.
5. Instruct a female patient on ways to prevent contracting or transmitting human immunodeficiency virus (HIV).
6. Teach female and male patients ways to prevent STIs.

Key Terms

agglutination (ă-GLŪ-tĭ-NĀ-shŭn, p. 972)
bacterial vaginosis (băk-TĒ-rē-ăl vă-jĭ-NŌ-sĭs, p. 964)
chancre (SHĂNG-kĕr, p. 971)
gram negative (grăm ′NE-gə-tiv p. 972)
gram positive (grăm ′PÄ-zə-tiv, p. 972)
oophoritis (oof-ō-RĪ-tĭs, p. 964)
pelvic inflammatory disease (PID) (PĔL-vĭk ĭn-FLĂ-mă-tō-rē dĭ-ZĒZ, p. 963)
peritonitis (pĕr-ĭ-tō-NĪ-tĭs, p. 964)
salpingitis (săl-pĭn-GĪ-tĭs, p. 964)
sexually transmitted infection (STI) (SEK-sh(ə-)wəl-lē TRAN(t)s-′mit-tĕd, in-′FEK-shən, p. 963)

Concepts Covered in This Chapter

- Sexuality
- Infection
- Tissue Integrity
- Patient Education

The term **sexually transmitted infection (STI)** refers to specific infections spread by intimate physical contact. Modes of transmission include sexual intercourse and contact with the genitals (sexual organs), rectum, or mouth. STIs can also be transmitted via blood contact and to a fetus via the placenta or to a newborn during the birth process.

The incidence of STIs continues to rise throughout the world. Although all sexually active people must be considered potentially at risk, people with multiple sexual partners are at high risk for contracting an STI. The largest population groups affected by STIs are adolescents and young adults (Centers for Disease Control and Prevention [CDC], 2017b). Teens are engaging in sexual practices at early ages and often with multiple partners. They are often unaware of signs and symptoms of STIs and are reluctant or unable to access confidential health care. The risks of STIs do not disappear with age. People ages 50 years and older constitute 45% of Americans living with human immunodeficiency virus (HIV); older adults who are unaffected may have less awareness of their HIV risk factors (CDC, 2018b). Safer sex practices are essential at all ages.

Think Critically

What safer sex practices can help prevent the spread of STIs?

STIs have a major impact on reproduction, sexuality, and general health. Because STIs are communicable, these infections are of concern to the patient and to the general public health. Goals of *Healthy People 2030* include to increase access to resources that prevent STIs and to decrease the incidence of gonorrhea and syphilis. The progress in reaching these national objectives is monitored by the U.S. Department of Health and Human Services. One specific action that still reaches many people via social media was the creation of the CDC STD Facebook page, where clinicians, health departments, partners, and individuals can still come together to promote STI awareness and prevention.

COMMON INFECTIONS OF THE FEMALE REPRODUCTIVE TRACT

PELVIC INFLAMMATORY DISEASE

Pelvic inflammatory disease (PID) refers to any inflammation in the pelvic cavity. If the infection is in the fallopian tubes, it is called **salpingitis**. Infection of the ovary is called **oophoritis**; infection of the pelvic peritoneum is called pelvic **peritonitis**. The organisms causing the infection are usually introduced from the outside, traveling through the uterus to infect pelvic organs. PID is much more common in sexually active women, particularly women with multiple sexual partners (Ross, 2018). Most of these infections are caused by two sexually transmitted organisms, *Neisseria gonorrhoeae* and *Chlamydia trachomatis* (Ross, 2018), and the most common reproduction complication is infertility from damage to the fallopian tubes. However, PID can also result from an infection after pelvic surgery or childbirth and is not *always* an STI.

Symptoms of acute PID include severe abdominal and pelvic pain, fever, and chills, commonly accompanied by a foul-smelling purulent vaginal discharge. The patient usually appears acutely ill. Chronic PID usually causes backache, a feeling of pelvic heaviness, and disturbances in menstruation. However, mild cases may produce no symptoms but still cause significant reproductive damage. Acute PID usually is treated with intravenous (IV) antimicrobials, symptom relief, and patient support and teaching. See Chapter 39 for other common inflammations and infections of the female reproductive tract.

CANDIDIASIS

Candidiasis (moniliasis) is a yeast infection, and although it is not considered an STI, recurrent infections increase the risk for STIs in sexually active women. Candidiasis is caused by a change in the vaginal pH, which allows the yeastlike fungus *Candida albicans* to grow. The pH of the vagina can be altered by diabetes mellitus, oral contraceptives, some systemic antibiotic use, or frequent douches. Symptoms of candidiasis include itching; burning on urination; and a white, curdlike discharge. Treatment includes vaginal miconazole or clotrimazole for 3 to 7 days or oral fluconazole given in a single dose.

BACTERIAL VAGINOSIS

Bacterial vaginosis (BV) occurs when normal lactobacillus in the vagina is replaced by *Mycoplasma hominis* or anaerobic bacteria. Like candidiasis, it is not considered an STI because it does not have a single causative agent and there is no equivalent male diagnosis (Sobel, 2017). However, BV can increase the risk for STIs and does have serious consequences if it occurs during pregnancy. BV is associated with minor vaginal tissue trauma, often caused by frequent sexual activity or douching. Symptoms include a grayish-white discharge that has a characteristic fishy odor. Treatment includes metronidazole or clindamycin.

RISK FACTORS FOR TRANSMISSION OF SEXUALLY TRANSMITTED INFECTIONS

Although men and women are equally susceptible to STIs, **women ages 15 to 24 years are diagnosed with STIs at a much higher rate than men** (CDC, 2017a). Biologically, young, sexually active women have a large proportion of columnar epithelium lining the cervix and a vaginal pH that can be altered by frequent douching. An alteration of vaginal pH can place the woman at higher risk for an STI. During and after the sexual act, male secretions and semen are in contact with female mucous membranes for longer than female secretions are in contact with male mucous membranes; therefore women have an increased risk for STIs.

Cultural Considerations

Media Effects on Sexually Transmitted Infections

Custom and culture can affect the development of STIs. STI rates increase in societies in which the media (television, magazines, movies, and internet chat rooms) focus on sexuality and sexual experiences of people with varying behaviors and values, including greater sexual freedom.

The mucus plug in the cervix of women (which protects the upper genital tract) becomes more permeable around the menstrual period, which can result in an increased risk during this time for infections in the upper genital tract, such as PID.

Types of contraceptive used based on reproduction choices may influence a woman's increased risk of STIs because the use of oral contraceptives alters the cervical secretions, resulting in a more alkaline environment in the vagina and thus a more favorable setting for growth of organisms that cause STIs. The use of long-acting oral contraceptives may contribute to a reduced use of condoms, thus increasing the risk of exposure to STIs in both partners.

Cultural Considerations

Contraception Choices

Cultural or societal norms may influence whether partners share the dialogue about use of condoms or whether one partner makes the choice to use a condom or not. Nurses must be empowered with culturally appropriate ways of teaching people of all cultures about the benefit of condom use to decrease the spread of STIs.

Women may not seek medical care for an STI as quickly as men, particularly if symptoms are absent or vague. For example, vaginal discharge is usually considered a normal variance, and health care may not be sought until the infection spreads and symptoms of PID occur. In men, urinary tract infections associated with sexual activity may be the first sign of an STI. Men may seek earlier health care intervention because the signs and symptoms are more obvious and distressing. STIs can have long-term effects on reproduction in the form of sterility, complicated pregnancy, or neonatal infection. For that reason, health care screening services and easy access to health care are important in preventing the spread of STIs.

PREVENTION OF HUMAN PAPILLOMAVIRUS

The Advisory Committee on Immunization Practices of the CDC has recommended routine human papillomavirus (HPV) vaccinations for all girls and boys 11 to 12 years old through 18 years old (or 26 years old in special circumstances) (CDC, 2018c). Gardasil 9 provides protection against HPV types 6 and 11, which cause genital warts, and against HPV 16 and 18, the cancer-causing strains, as well as HPV 31, 33, 45, 52, and 58. Cervarix, another HPV vaccine, provides protection against HPV types 16 and 18 only. Both vaccines are highly efficacious against cervical, vaginal, vulvar, and anal cancers; are well-tolerated; and are considered safe. An HPV vaccine can be given to girls and boys as young as 9 years of age and to women up to 26 years of age. Three doses of either brand of vaccine are required; see the package insert for the specific dosing schedule.

LESIONS OF SEXUALLY TRANSMITTED INFECTIONS

In men, the lesions related to STIs may appear under the prepuce; on the head or body of the penis; or on the scrotum, perianal area, rectum, anus, or inner thighs. In women, lesions of STIs can appear on the vulva, vagina, cervix, perianal area, or inner thighs. Lesions around the mouth of either sex can occur in cases of oral sexual practices. Lesions can also be found far from the genital area. For example, lesions of syphilis include a classic rash on the palms of the hands and soles of the feet. Lesions of *N. gonorrhoeae* may spread and cause pustules on the extremities as part of an "arthritis-dermatitis" syndrome. Examples of common organisms involved in STIs are listed in Box 41.1.

Box 41.1 Causes of Sexually Transmitted Infections

BACTERIA
- *Neisseria gonorrhoeae*
- *Chlamydia trachomatis*
- *Treponema pallidum* (syphilis)
- *Haemophilus ducreyi* (chancroid)
- *Mycoplasma hominis*

VIRUSES
- Human herpesvirus 2 (herpes simplex virus type 2)
- Hepatitis B virus
- Human immunodeficiency virus (HIV)
- Human papillomavirus (HPV)

YEASTS AND FUNGI
- *Candida albicans*
- *Candida glabrata*
- *Candida tropicalis*

PARASITE
- *Trichomonas vaginalis* (trichomoniasis)

Data from Centers for Disease Control and Prevention: *Trichomoniasis* (website): www.cdc.gov/std/tg2015/trichomoniasis.htm.

REPORTING SEXUALLY TRANSMITTED INFECTIONS

STIs must be reported to the local public health agency in accordance with state and local statutory requirements. The CDC and local health authorities establish these regulations and provide regular updates and reporting forms to health care providers for monitored infections. Syphilis (primary, secondary, and congenital), gonorrhea, and chlamydia are examples of current reportable diseases, according to the public health guidelines from the CDC (2018a). The requirements for reporting other STIs differ by state, and health care providers must be familiar with their own state and local reporting requirements. This tracking information is used to determine community resource needs and is evaluated in terms of the national goals of *Healthy People*.

TRANSMISSION OF SEXUALLY TRANSMITTED INFECTIONS

STIs are primarily passed through some type of intimate contact: genital to genital, mouth to genital, or genital to rectum. They occur in all types of sexual relationships. Some infections, such as HIV or hepatitis B or C, also may be passed through blood contact, by the sharing of contaminated needles, or—though rarely—through transfusion with contaminated blood. Accidental transmission to health care personnel may occur via needle or sharps injuries or by direct exposure to open wounds or body fluids.

Bloodborne infections may be transmitted to a fetus before birth. Newborns are at risk for contracting any STI that may reside in the vagina at the time of birth. Depending on the organism, such exposure can lead to a variety of serious problems for the infant, including pneumonia and blindness.

? Think Critically

What are the four major modes of transmission for STIs?

In some states, screening for some STIs—particularly for syphilis—is required for a marriage license. However, it is expensive to screen for all STIs. The best approach to gathering control of STI transmission is public awareness and willingness to take responsibility for prevention and for treatment, should infection occur.

COMMON DIAGNOSTIC TESTS

Table 41.1 lists common STIs and contains information about modes of transmission, diagnosis, symptoms, treatments, and nursing responsibilities.

A variety of tests are used to detect STIs. Noninvasive diagnostic techniques that use urine samples have been developed. **Smears** and **cultures** may be taken directly from the site (e.g., vaginal, cervical, or urethral swabs).

Text continued on p. 972

Table 41.1 Common Sexually Transmitted Infections

INFECTION	MODES OF TRANSMISSION	SYMPTOMS	MEDICAL DIAGNOSIS	MEDICAL TREATMENT	NURSING INTERVENTIONS
Chlamydia trachomatis 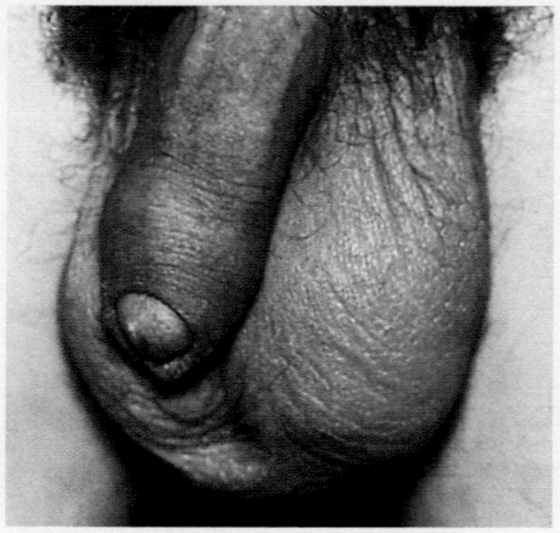	Direct sexual contact. May be transmitted to newborn during vaginal delivery. Very common STI in the United States.	*Male:* Often asymptomatic. Dysuria; frequency of urination; watery, mucuslike discharge. Causes about half the cases of epididymitis and nongonococcal urethritis. *Female:* Many females have no symptoms. Yellow vaginal discharge, urinary frequency, dysuria. May have unusual odor after intercourse. Can result in PID, ectopic pregnancy, and sterility. *Neonate:* Exposure can cause eye infections and pneumonia.	By cervical culture, DNA probe, enzyme immunoassay, ELISA, or nucleic acid amplification. *Screening protocol:* Test women ages 15–25 yr via self-obtained low vaginal swab (SOLVS) or first void urine (FVU). Test men seen in genitourinary clinic via urine sample. TMA, SDA, or PCR test; test for gonorrhea as well.	Azithromycin 1 g orally in a single dose. OR Doxycycline 100 mg orally twice a day for 7 days. *Alternative:* Erythromycin base 500 mg orally four times a day for 7 days. OR Erythromycin ethylsuccinate 800 mg orally four times a day for 7 days. OR Levofloxacin 500 mg orally once daily for 7 days. OR Ofloxacin 300 mg orally twice a day for 7 days.	*Education:* Encourage patients to seek attention for any unusual vaginal or penile discharge. Partner(s) must be treated concurrently. Encourage abstinence until course of treatment completed and condom use for prevention of future infection. Remind that patient must complete antibiotics to ensure effective treatment and prevent development of PID. CDC recommends screening all pregnant women and sexually active young women.
Human papillomavirus (HPV) *Condylomata acuminata* (genital warts) caused by HPV 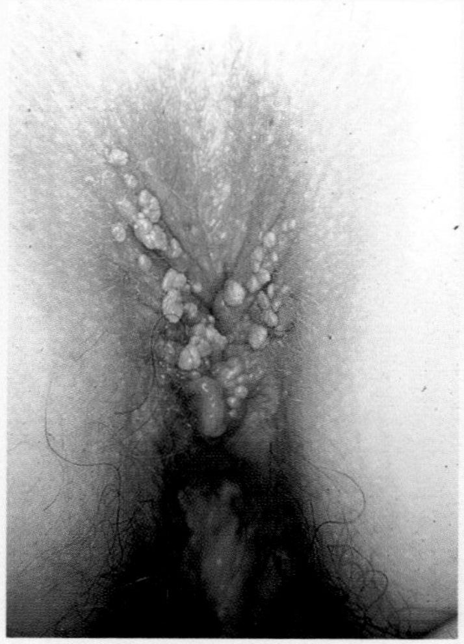	Spread during sexual contact. Highly contagious. Can be transmitted to newborn during vaginal delivery. Very common STI in the United States.	Warts are flat or raised, rough, cauliflower-like growths on the vulva, penis, perianal area, vaginal or rectal walls, or cervix. The flat variety is more likely to lead to tissue changes that contribute to cervical or penile cancer. *Neonate:* Laryngeal papillomas.	Biopsy, colposcopy, anoscopy, Pap smear.	Laser therapy, surgical removal, cryotherapy.	*Education:* Teach about mode of infection and use of condoms to prevent spread. Recommend regular Pap smears to female patients because of risk of cervical cancer. Vaccination is available and recommended for all girls and boys ages 9–26 yr.

Genital herpes 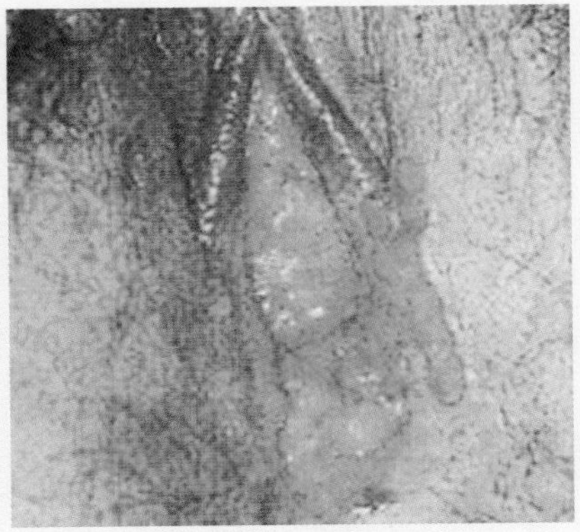	Caused by herpes simplex virus (HSV) types 1 and 2. Highly contagious, spread by direct contact; not limited to sexual contact. Self-inoculation also possible, for example, from lip ulcer (fever blister) to genitals. Invades nerve cells located near the site of infection. Lies dormant; flare-ups erratic and unpredictable. Some patients have frequent recurrence, others rarely or none. Neonate may be infected during delivery if mother has active disease (more common if initial episode occurs during pregnancy).	*Primary:* Fever, headache, malaise, myalgia, burning genital pain, dysuria (female), painful intercourse. Vesicles in genital area that ulcerate, crust over, and resolve spontaneously in about 2 wk. *Secondary:* Burning genital pain, possible numbness and tingling 24 h before lesions appear, vesicles. *Male:* Lesions may appear on glans penis, shaft of penis, prepuce, scrotal sac, inner thighs. *Female:* Vulva, vaginal surface, buttocks, cervix. Cervical lesions may be superficial with diffuse inflammation or a single, large, necrotic ulcer. Primary infection during pregnancy associated with high risk of premature labor and spontaneous abortion. *Neonate:* Local infections of eyes, skin, or mucous membranes to severe disseminated infection that can be lethal may occur.	Lesions usually easily identified by experienced clinician. Can be confirmed by viral cultures of fluid from vesicles.	No known cure. Treatment with acyclovir, valacyclovir, or famciclovir may reduce symptoms and accelerate healing. For individuals with frequent recurrence, continuous treatment may reduce frequency. Viral shedding may continue after lesions are healed.	Keep lesions clean and dry to prevent secondary infection. Increased fluids will dilute urine for greater comfort. Topical anesthetics and oral analgesics may help manage pain. Strict gloving and observation of contact precautions are necessary. *Education:* Encourage use of condoms with spermicide to help prevent spread, avoidance of sex if lesions present; scrupulous hand hygiene. If patient becomes pregnant while disease is active, infant will be delivered by cesarean section to protect it from exposure.

Continued

Table 41.1 Common Sexually Transmitted Infections—cont'd

INFECTION	MODES OF TRANSMISSION	SYMPTOMS	MEDICAL DIAGNOSIS	MEDICAL TREATMENT	NURSING INTERVENTIONS
Gonorrhea (GC) 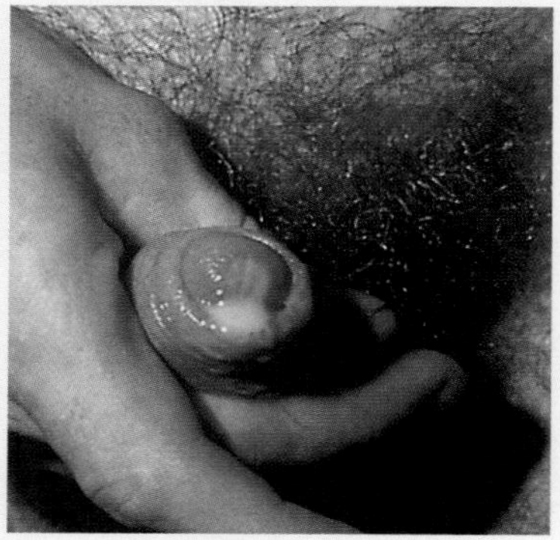	Easily transmitted by direct sexual contact. Transmitted to newborn during vaginal delivery if mother has active disease. Autoinoculation via fingers to eye possible. Occasionally becomes bloodborne.	*Incubation:* 2–6 days after exposure. May be asymptomatic. *Male:* Dysuria with frequency; scant to copious purulent discharge from penis, unilateral testicular pain. If untreated may develop urethral stricture and epididymitis; can cause sterility. *Female:* Vaginal discharge, burning on urination. Untreated, results in PID. May involve rectum, eyes, oropharynx. *Neonate:* If exposed at birth to mother's vaginal secretions, is at risk for ophthalmia neonatorum, which can cause blindness, and other infections within 2–5 days after birth. *Children:* Infection in children over 1 yr of age is likely the result of sexual abuse.	Confirmed by presence of the causative organism, *Neisseria gonorrhoeae,* in vaginal or urethral smear, rectal or pharyngeal culture. Nucleic amplification test using urine sample is accurate.	Single IM dose of ceftriaxone 250 mg plus a single dose of azithromycin 1 g orally.[a] *Alternatives:* If ceftriaxone is not available: Cefixime 400 mg orally plus azithromycin 1 g orally[a] If ceftriaxone cannot be given because of severe allergy: Dual treatment with single doses of oral gemifloxacin 320 mg plus oral azithromycin 2 g OR Single doses of IM gentamicin 240 mg plus oral azithromycin 2 g Hospitalize if PID or severe illness occurs.[a] Empirical treatment for chlamydia is recommended by CDC.	Observation of standard contact precautions and frequent hand hygiene. *Education:* Teach about prevention, treatment, and importance of completing treatment; naming all contacts for treatment; and having follow-up cultures to ensure that treatment has been effective. Encourage safer sex practices to prevent reinfection. Be sure patient understands how to take prescribed medication. Teach CDC recommendations for sexually active patients to be screened for GC infection.

Hepatitis B	Caused by hepatitis B virus (HBV). Transmission via sexual contact, blood contact, and to the fetus via the placenta in an infected mother.	May have anorexia, malaise, vomiting, abdominal pain, dark urine, jaundice, skin rashes, arthralgias, arthritis. Acute infection may be asymptomatic. Infection may be persistent and result in a chronic carrier state and may develop chronic active hepatitis, cirrhosis, hepatocellular carcinoma, hepatic failure, and death. Infants born infected are at high risk for chronic hepatitis B infection.	Serologic testing for HBV infection gives definitive diagnosis.	No specific therapy is available. HBIG is given prophylactically after known exposure. Hepatitis B vaccine (Hep B) is recommended for people at risk for exposure, including health care workers. Hep B vaccine is currently given as part of normal childhood immunizations with a three-dose regimen beginning at birth. Postexposure interval before vaccination administration should not exceed 7 days for needle-stick exposure and 14 days for sexual exposure.	Appropriate handling of all blood or body fluids to prevent transmission of infection. Prevention of needle-stick injuries. *Education:* Universal vaccination of newborns with single-antigen Hep B vaccine before discharge; routine screening of all women for HBsAg. Final dose of three-dose regimen should be given between 6 and 12 mo of age for infants from Alaska, Pacific Islands, Africa, and other endemic areas.

Continued

Table 41.1 Common Sexually Transmitted Infections—cont'd

INFECTION	MODES OF TRANSMISSION	SYMPTOMS	MEDICAL DIAGNOSIS	MEDICAL TREATMENT	NURSING INTERVENTIONS
HIV, AIDS, ARC	HIV is transmitted by intimate contact with body secretions of an infected person or exposure to infected blood or by perinatal transmission from mother to newborn.	Initially, flulike symptoms several weeks after HIV exposure. Antibodies appear in blood a few months to 1 yr later. A latent period follows with gradual reduction in CD4 cells. CD4 cell decline results in reduced immune function, resulting in opportunistic infections, such as Kaposi sarcoma, *Pneumocystis jirovecii* (formerly *Pneumocystis carinii*) pneumonia, and oral candidiasis. CD4 count below 200/mm^3 is diagnostic of AIDS.	Diagnosis of HIV infection based on reactive enzyme immunoassay (EIA) confirmed by a more specific assay (e.g., Western blot or immunofluorescent assay). ELISA and HIV-RNA tests are recommended by the CDC (Swan, 2009). AIDS and ARC may be diagnosed based on laboratory results and/or specific diagnostic criteria. The FDA has approved a rapid test for HIV screening that provides results in <1 h. A positive rapid HIV test requires further testing for confirmation.[a]	Currently there is no cure. Drug regimens interrupt reproduction of viruses. Numerous classes of antiretroviral drugs are tailored to individual patient needs. Postexposure prophylaxis (PEP) treatment should start within 72 h of exposure (CDC, 2018d).	Nurses should assess patients for individual risk factors and recommend HIV testing because many patients are unaware of their status. Patients who are HIV positive or who have been diagnosed with AIDS or ARC should receive specific professionally trained counseling on lifestyle practices, treatment protocols, and follow-up procedures. Provide support and information to improve general health. Safer sexual practices should be used to prevent spread. Patient should not breastfeed. Cesarean birth if pregnant.
Syphilis 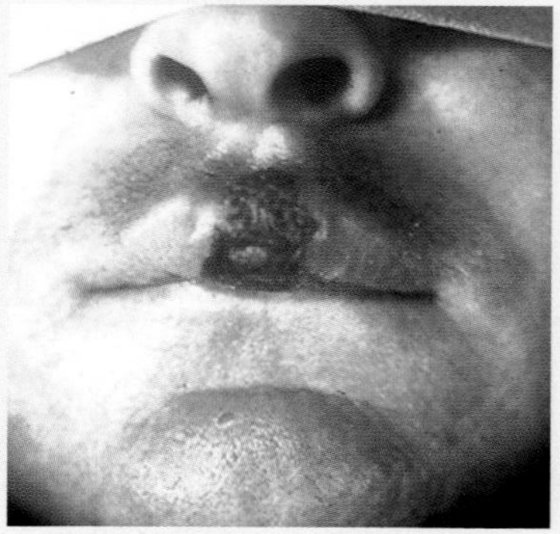	Direct body contact; organism (*Treponema pallidum*, a spirochete) requires warm, wet environment to survive; can be destroyed with plain soap and water. Can penetrate intact mucous membrane. Placental transmission to fetus in about 50% of women with active disease during pregnancy.	Syphilis has three stages. *Primary (after 3-wk incubation period):* **Chancre** (hard, painless sore) on the mucous membrane of the mouth or genitals, often unnoticed in women. Chancre teeming with spirochetes, very contagious at this stage.	*Screening:* VDRL and RPR tests, performed on blood or spinal fluid if neurosyphilis is suspected. May be negative in primary phase but always positive in secondary and tertiary phases. *Confirmation:* Dark-field microscopy of scrapings from chancre. FTA-Abs blood test.	Single-dose benzathine penicillin G 2.4 million units.[a] *Alternatively:* In the case of penicillin allergy: Doxycycline 100 mg orally twice daily for 14 days. OR Tetracycline 500 mg four times daily for 14 days.	*Education:* Caution patients not to ingest alcohol for 24 h before VDRL or RPR (may cause false-positive result). Remember that chancre is highly infectious (gloved contact only). Encourage naming of contacts so everyone can be treated. Encourage condom use to prevent reinfection.

		Spirochetes enter bloodstream 3–7 days after infection and begin to multiply rapidly (bacteremia). Symptoms disappear within 3–8 wk. *Secondary (6 wk later):* Symptoms vary. May have generalized skin rash. Serology test is positive. Symptoms may disappear as the disease enters latent period. *Tertiary (late: 1–20 yr after infection):* Spirochetes have had access to all body tissues. "Gumma," a soft encapsulated tumor, appears on any organ, causing symptoms (including neurologic). Congenital. Stillbirth, CNS damage.	Tests for other STIs should also be done.		Explain importance of follow-up (usually 3- and 6-mo VDRL) to ensure treatment has been effective. Follow-up usually at 1, 2, 3, 6, 9, and 12 mo for HIV-positive individuals.
Trichomoniasis	Sexually transmitted. The most prevalent nonviral STI in the United States (CDC, 2016).	Pruritus; frothy gray-green vaginal discharge; dysuria.	Laboratory observation of protozoa; ulceration on cervix or vaginal wall.	Metronidazole, single 2-g dose for patient and partner. OR Tinidazole 2 g orally in a single dose. *Alternative regimen:* Metronidazole 500 mg orally twice a day for 7 days[a]	*Education:* Educate concerning safer sex practices and importance of seeking early care for symptoms.

Chlamydia trachomatis and gonorrhea figures from Morse S, Moreland A, Holmes K, editors: *Atlas of sexually transmitted diseases and AIDS,* London, 1996, Mosby-Wolfe. HPV figure from Black JM, Hawks JH: *Medical-surgical nursing: clinical management for positive outcomes, ed 7,* Philadelphia, 2005, Saunders. Genital herpes figure from Morse SA, Holmes KK, and Ballard RC: *Atlas of sexually transmitted diseases and AIDS,* Philadelphia, 2011, Saunders. Courtesy Barbara Romanowski, MD. Syphilis figure courtesy U.S. Public Health Service, Washington, DC.

[a]2018 Centers for Disease Control and Prevention Treatment Guidelines.

AIDS, Acquired immunodeficiency syndrome; *ARC,* AIDS-related complex; *CD4,* T helper cell; *CDC,* Centers for Disease Control and Prevention; *CNS,* central nervous system; *DNA,* deoxyribonucleic acid; *ELISA,* enzyme-linked immunosorbent assay; *FDA,* U.S. Food and Drug Administration; *FTA-Abs,* fluorescent treponemal antibody absorption; *HBIG,* hepatitis B immune globulin; *HBsAg,* hepatitis B surface antigen; *HIV,* human immunodeficiency virus; *IM,* intramuscular; *Pap,* Papanicolaou; *PCR,* polymerase chain reaction; *PID,* pelvic inflammatory disease; *RNA,* ribonucleic acid; *RPR,* rapid plasma reagin; *SDA,* strand displacement amplification; *STI,* sexually transmitted infection; *TMA,* transcription-mediated amplification; *VDRL,* Venereal Disease Research Laboratory.

In some instances, organisms also can be cultured from the blood. **Biopsies** are microscopic tissue examinations performed on a sample taken from the affected area and are usually done to differentiate between benign and malignant tissues but can also provide a differential diagnosis for diseases that have specific cellular changes or organisms present.

Numerous types of blood tests can help detect STIs. They look for specific antibodies formed by the presence of certain microorganisms or for the effects of antigens (substances in the bloodstream that stimulate the production of antibodies). Such effects include the tendency for **agglutination**—the clumping together of cells in a variety of characteristic patterns.

Staining procedures differentiate organisms by using dyes that have been found to stain some bacteria in specific ways. An example of this would be a Gram stain, in which bacteria are first stained with crystal violet, then treated with a strong iodine solution, decolorized with ethanol or ethanol acetone, and then counterstained with contrasting dye. Those retaining the initial stain are considered **gram positive**; those losing the stain but accepting the counterstain are considered **gram negative**. Current development of noninvasive testing and screening procedures using urine samples will increase public acceptance of mass screening. See Chapter 6 for further discussion of testing for infectious agents.

NURSING MANAGEMENT

Identifying microorganisms is a complex procedure. When collecting or assisting with the collection of specimens, there are several specific responsibilities to ensure that the samples will allow accurate studies to be performed. These include the following:

- Ensuring that appropriate laboratory request slips have been prepared or entered electronically according to the health care provider's specific orders. If antimicrobials have been started, note this on the laboratory slip or in the electronic health record (EHR).
- Checking the laboratory manual for any specific restrictions or preparations for the tests ordered.
- Avoiding urethral swabs within 1 hour of the last void because organisms will have been flushed away.
- Avoiding douching before vaginal cultures or smears.
- Recognizing that some tests will give a false-positive reading if the patient is on specific medications or has other types of infection present. Check the patient's history.
- Understanding that antimicrobials may cause cultures to be negative even though the drug or the dose may not be sufficient to cure the infection. Document the medication history.
- Noting that stool present in the rectum can prevent good rectal swabs from being obtained.
- Using a **sterile** swab to collect cultures and smears that are sent to the laboratory.
- Preparing the patient. (See information on preparing the patient for a pelvic examination in Chapter 39.)
- Explaining what tests have been ordered and any specific home preparation. Answer all questions.
- Providing appropriate draping and privacy and remaining with the patient during the procedure.
- Providing emotional support as needed.
- Making sure that specimens are labeled appropriately and delivered to the laboratory with the corresponding laboratory slips.

ASSESSMENT (DATA COLLECTION)

Screening for potential STIs or risk for acquiring such an infection must be part of any patient history data collection. However, it may be challenging to get accurate information. Patients may not disclose symptoms such as inflammation, rash, or discharge if they fear it is related to sexual activity. Adolescents may fear parental disapproval, rejection, or disciplinary action if they admit to being sexually active and so may hide symptoms. Fear of finding a serious infection such as HIV also may make the patient reluctant to provide information.

Communication

Gathering Information

When someone is diagnosed with an STI, the public health department is responsible for collecting the names of sexual partners so that they can be contacted and treated. Many people do not wish to give out this information. Professionals who deal with these issues regularly, such as public health nurses, have special training in obtaining an appropriate history.

Obtaining a history from a patient seeking treatment for an STI requires tact, sensitivity, and an open and nonjudgmental attitude. Such a history involves asking very intimate questions and may involve a variety of cultural and personal issues.

Physical examination for STIs involves exposure of the most private parts of the anatomy. Such an examination is usually performed by both a health care provider and a nurse, particularly when there are gender differences between the health personnel and the patient. Provide appropriate draping and give the patient privacy when he or she is undressing for the examination.

Patients may request that a family member be allowed to remain with them, and they have this right. You should escort such individuals into the room and have them sit or stand by the patient in a manner that allows them to provide support. Make sure that any required equipment, supplies, specimen containers, and laboratory slips are ready in the examination room.

NURSING DIAGNOSIS

Problem statements for patients with an STI may include the following:

- Insufficient knowledge regarding modes of transmission, signs and symptoms, and treatment of STI.

Focused Assessment

Data Collection for Sexually Transmitted Infections

The following questions concerning sexuality are asked when assessing a patient with or at risk for an STI:

- Are you currently sexually active?
- At what age did you become sexually active?
- Do you currently have more than one sexual partner?
- Have you had other partners in the past?
- If yes to either of the last two questions: Do you understand the risks associated with having multiple sexual partners?
- If a sexually active female: Are you having regular gynecologic examinations with Papanicolaou (Pap) smears? If yes, when was your last examination?
- If a sexually active female: Are you currently pregnant or trying to become pregnant?
- Are you checked at least annually for STIs even if you do not have symptoms?
- If currently in nonmonogamous relationships: Are you using condoms to help prevent STIs?
- Have you ever had an STI? If yes, ask for specific information (what, when, how treated; was follow-up done?).
- Do you have symptoms or reasons to believe you might have an STI now? If yes, ask for specific information (symptoms, duration; partner[s] symptomatic?).

Think Critically

What factors make it challenging to take an accurate history or provide education for a patient with an STI?

- Pain due to inflammation.
- Anxiety due to intimate examination and personal information required.
- Fear of being HIV positive or having another STI.
- Absence of compliance related to repeated infection with STIs and refusal to use condoms.

◆ PLANNING

Expected outcomes for the patient with an STI may include that the patient will:

- Verbalize knowledge of self-care to prevent recurrence or other STI.
- Be free of pain after treatment.
- Cope adequately with history taking and physical examination.
- Have decreased fear of HIV or other STI diagnosis after examination and treatment.
- Comply with safer sex practices and treatment requirements.

In addition to managing the treatment protocol and any pain related to an STI, patient education and emotional support are primary aspects of providing care for patients with or at risk for STIs. Education may be interrupted by the patient's reluctance to discuss sexual issues. This may result from cultural or spiritual views or from more personal feelings. Patients of all ages may wish to protect themselves or their partners from possible judgment or embarrassment through disclosure of sensitive information. Maintain a nonjudgmental attitude and give assurance that information will be kept confidential within the health care system.

When planning education, consider the patient's existing knowledge and ability to understand the information provided. Select appropriate teaching aids, such as pictures, pamphlets, and three-dimensional models.

Emotional support is another important aspect of care for patients with an STI. Allow time in the teaching plan to listen to the patient's concerns and for answering questions. Be prepared with information on support groups, counseling services, and informational programs that may be of assistance. In the case of serious infections, such as HIV, support programs and professional counseling are particularly important for the patient.

◆ IMPLEMENTATION

Symptom Relief

STIs cause a variety of symptoms, some of which may cause mild discomfort or significant pain. Review Chapter 7 on pain management techniques and Table 41.1 for specific nursing interventions. Nursing Care Plan 41.1 gives specific nursing interventions for a patient with chlamydia.

Prevention of Spread

The spread of STIs is a major health concern in the United States. People often become sexually active at a young age, and it is not uncommon for individuals to have a variety of sexual partners over the years. Strategies for prevention and control of STIs are given in Box 41.2.

Box 41.2 Prevention of Sexually Transmitted Infections

The prevention and control of STIs are based on the following major strategies:

- Early education of adolescents on abstinence and safer sex practices.
- Education and counseling of people at risk on ways to prevent STIs through changes in sexual and lifestyle behaviors.
- Identification of asymptomatically infected people and of symptomatic people unlikely to seek diagnostic and treatment services.
- Effective diagnosis and treatment of infected people.
- Evaluation, treatment, and counseling of sexual partners of people who are infected with an STI.
- Pre-exposure vaccination of patients at risk for vaccine-preventable STIs such as hepatitis B and HPV.
- Follow-up of patients at risk or under treatment to ensure compliance.

HPV, Human papillomavirus; *STIs,* sexually transmitted infections.
Adapted from Centers for Disease Control and Prevention: *Human papillomavirus (HPV) infection* (website): www.cdc.gov/std/tg2015/hpv.htm.

Nursing Care Plan 41.1 Care of a Patient With Chlamydia

SCENARIO

A 21-year-old woman is admitted to the clinic and diagnosed with a chlamydia infection.

PROBLEM STATEMENT/NURSING DIAGNOSIS

Insufficient knowledge regarding new diagnosis of chlamydia infection.

SUPPORTING ASSESSMENT DATA

Subjective: "What is chlamydia?"

Objective: Positive test for chlamydia.

Goals/Expected Outcomes	Nursing Interventions	Selected Rationale	Evaluation
Patient will verbalize understanding of disease prevention, transmission, and treatment protocols.	Assess readiness to learn about chlamydia.	Readiness to learn is essential for successful learning to occur.	Patient asking questions about her diagnosis.
	Determine knowledge base concerning chlamydia.	Learning plan should build on existing knowledge.	Patient discussing her understanding.
	Identify barriers to learning.	Language barriers, cultural beliefs, and embarrassment can alter learning effectiveness.	Patient speaks fluent English and is willing to discuss illness.
	Teach the medication regimen.	Compliance with medication regimen is essential for successful treatment.	Patient verbalizes understanding of when and how to take medication.
	Review safer sex practices.	Safer sex practices can prevent exchange of body fluids and minimize risk of STI transmission.	Patient demonstrates understanding of safer sex practices.
	Schedule follow-up appointments.	Follow-up testing is an essential part of confirming successful treatment of chlamydia.	Patient promises to return for follow-up care.

PROBLEM STATEMENT/NURSING DIAGNOSIS

Altered tissue integrity due to chlamydia.

SUPPORTING ASSESSMENT DATA

Subjective: "I've had a small amount of vaginal discharge."

Objective: Chlamydia test positive.

Goals/Expected Outcomes	Nursing Interventions	Selected Rationale	Evaluation
Patient will show signs of successful treatment of chlamydia as evidenced by absence of symptoms and completion of medication regimen.	Assess for signs and symptoms of chlamydia such as vaginal discharge and dysuria.	Absence of symptoms may indicate successful treatment.	Patient does not evidence continued signs of the disease.
	Assess for risk factors for reactivation of disease.	Minimizing risk factors can prevent reinfection.	Patient states she is now in a monogamous relationship.
	Encourage woman to identify partners to enable treatment.	Treating sexual partners can minimize risk for reinfection and spread of infection.	Patient has contacted other partners, who have come in for examination.
	Teach safer sex practices and risk for recurrence.	Use of safer sex practices can minimize reinfection.	Patient evidences understanding of safer sex practices.

CRITICAL THINKING QUESTION

1. What are the long-term problems associated with untreated STIs such as chlamydia and gonorrhea?

STI, Sexually transmitted infection.

Health Promotion

Preventing Sexually Transmitted Infections

Although the only absolute prevention is abstinence, certain behaviors significantly reduce the risk of contracting an STI. These behaviors include using condoms with a spermicide containing nonoxynol-9, which acts as a barrier and has viricidal and bactericidal action; limiting sexual contacts, preferably to one partner (monogamy); and avoiding sexual contact if a partner is known to be infected or if lesions are observed in the genital, perianal, or oral regions. If the patient or the sexual partner is an IV drug user, education regarding not sharing needles is important.

◆ EVALUATION

Initially, each instance of patient teaching should be evaluated for effectiveness by reviewing information discussed to determine whether learning has occurred. Over time, evaluate whether the patient is following the recommendations. Negative follow-up cultures are a reliable indicator that treatments were followed as prescribed. During the follow-up interview, inquire about use of safer sex practices and evaluate retention of information previously taught.

COMMUNITY CARE

Most communities have clinics, often through the public health system, that provide screening and treatment for STIs. These services may be offered at low or no cost, and they provide a valuable service by assisting the community to control the spread of STIs.

Confidential screening and education on safer sexual practices are important services provided by community clinics. The health department and organizations such as Planned Parenthood are two of numerous community agencies that routinely provide pamphlets, posters, and classes on preventing and treating STIs. Public service announcements, such as the television spots on HIV/AIDS awareness, are another source of public education. In many areas, information and education are made available through schools and colleges and are directed both at students and their families and at the general community.

Get Ready for the NCLEX® Examination!

Key Points

- STIs are primarily passed through intimate contact with body fluids. Needle sticks or blood transfusions with contaminated blood can also spread STIs. An STI can also be transmitted to a newborn during the birth process.
- One objective of *Healthy People 2030* is to prevent infection, illness, and death related to HIV.
- STIs can be caused by bacteria, viruses, or protozoa.
- Contraceptive choice influences a woman's risk for STIs.
- A properly used condom offers protection from the transmission of STIs.
- STIs can cause sterility, complicate pregnancy, or cause neonatal infection.
- Certain STIs are reportable to the public health department.
- Awareness and reporting of symptoms of STIs can aid in early diagnosis, treatment, and education of patients.
- Nursing responsibilities include helping to identify, screen, and educate patients at risk for STIs.
- PID is an inflammation of the pelvic cavity commonly caused by STIs that can cause sterility.
- Candidiasis is a yeast infection caused by a change in vaginal pH that can be the result of frequent douching, use of oral contraceptives, or systemic antibiotic therapy.
- Bacterial vaginosis occurs when normal lactobacillus in the vagina is replaced by pathogenic organisms, and it increases the risk for STIs.
- Education on safer sex practices can prevent STIs.

Additional Learning Resources

SG Go to your Study Guide for additional learning activities to help you master this chapter content.

Go to your Evolve website (http://evolve.elsevier.com/deWit/medsurg) for the following FREE learning resources:

- Animations, audio, and video
- Answers and rationales for questions and activities
- Glossary with pronunciations in English and Spanish
- Interactive Review Questions and more!

Review Questions for the NCLEX® Examination

1. You are caring for four female patients. Which patient do you identify as most at risk to have an STI?
   1. 19-year old with urinary tract infection
   2. 31-year old who is eight weeks pregnant
   3. 40-year old with breast tenderness
   4. 53-year old who reports vaginal dryness

   NCLEX Client Need: Physiological Integrity: Reduction of Risk Potential
2. A mother brings her 12-year-old daughter in for an annual check-up. You recommend administration of one of the HPV vaccines. The mother replies, "My daughter does not need the vaccine because she is not sexually active." What is the appropriate nursing response?
   1. "You can bring her back when she becomes sexually active."
   2. "Studies have shown that the earlier the vaccine is given, the more effective it is. When she does become sexually active, the vaccine will be protecting her."

3. "If you wait until your daughter is sexually active, it will be too late. How will you know?"
4. "The vaccine must be given before your daughter is sexually active, or it will not work."

NCLEX Client Need: Health Promotion and Maintenance

3. You talk with the parents of a 9-year-old girl about the HPV vaccinations. The information session must include which statement(s)? *(Select all that apply.)*
   1. "The vaccine is a one-dose immunization."
   2. "The vaccine prevents genital warts."
   3. "The vaccine prevents some precancerous lesions of the cervix."
   4. "The vaccine protects against some other diseases caused by HPV."
   5. "The vaccine eliminates the need for routine cervical cancer screening."

   NCLEX Client Need: Health Promotion and Maintenance
4. An important nursing responsibility involves reporting certain sexually transmitted infections to the CDC and local health authorities. Which infection(s) should you prepare to report? *(Select all that apply.)*
   1. Gonorrhea
   2. Syphilis
   3. Bacterial vaginosis
   4. Candidiasis
   5. Chlamydia

   NCLEX Client Need: Safe and Effective Care Environment: Safety and Infection Control
5. A health care provider has ordered a Venereal Disease Research Laboratory (VDRL) test for a patient. Which condition do you recognize the provider is screening for?
   1. HIV
   2. HPV
   3. Syphilis
   4. Gonorrhea

   NCLEX Client Need: Physiological Integrity: Reduction of Risk Potential
6. You are assessing a patient for syphilis. Which will you document as classic signs and symptoms of syphilis? *(Select all that apply.)*
   1. An open ulcer on the genitals
   2. A red rash on the palms of the hands
   3. A cough and fever
   4. A red rash on the soles of the feet
   5. Abdominal pain accompanied by vomiting

   NCLEX Client Need: Physiological Integrity: Basic Care and Comfort
7. You are caring for a pregnant patient who has active genital herpes. When the patient asks about delivering her baby, which nursing response is appropriate?
   1. "You will receive antiviral medication to put the infection into remission before delivery."
   2. "A Cesarean section will be scheduled."
   3. "You can still deliver your baby vaginally because there is no risk to a neonate associated with genital herpes."
   4. "A nurse will bathe your baby immediately after delivery to reduce the risk of transmission."

   NCLEX Client Need: Safe and Effective Care Environment: Safety and Infection Control
8. You are caring for an adolescent who has been diagnosed with gonorrhea. When the patient refuses to notify recent sexual partners, what is your appropriate response?
   1. "Do you not feel responsible for infecting other people?"
   2. "You do not have to notify anyone that you don't wish to contact."
   3. "I am still accountable to report this disease through required channels."
   4. "It is considered a felony offense if you do not disclose names of your sexual partners."

   NCLEX Client Need: Health Promotion and Maintenance
9. You are teaching a female patient about a new diagnosis of genital herpes. Which patient statement indicates that further teaching is necessary?
   1. "Once my lesions are healed I am no longer contagious."
   2. "Primary lesions will resolve in about 2 weeks."
   3. "This infection can spread to other parts of my body."
   4. "A cesarean section may be necessary if the infection is active during delivery."

   NCLEX Client Need: Safe and Effective Care Environment: Coordinated Care
10. While inserting an indwelling urinary catheter, you notice raised, rough, cauliflower-like growths on the vulva and vaginal walls. Which causative agent do you anticipate?
    1. Herpes simplex virus
    2. Human papillomavirus
    3. *Treponema pallidum*
    4. *Neisseria gonorrhoeae*

    NCLEX Client Need: Safe and Effective Care Environment: Safety and Infection Control

Critical Thinking Questions

Scenario A

A patient tells you that she recently had intercourse for the first time and is fearful that she may have contracted a sexually transmitted infection.

1. What questions would you ask to assess whether the patient is situationally anxious or has physical symptoms that may be related to an STI?
2. What community resources may be helpful to this patient, regardless of whether she is diagnosed with an STI?

Scenario B

A patient states that he feels condoms are not necessary because he is almost positive that he and his partner are always faithful to each other.

1. What teaching will you provide to this patient regarding safer sex and the use of condoms?

The Integumentary System

42

http://evolve.elsevier.com/deWit/medsurg

Objectives

Theory

1. Describe the structure and functions of the skin.
2. Compare and contrast the various causes of integumentary disorders.
3. Analyze important factors in the prevention of skin disease.
4. Plan specific measures to prevent skin tears.
5. Interpret laboratory and diagnostic test results for skin disorders.
6. State nursing responsibilities in the care of patients with skin disorders.
7. Write outcome objectives for a patient with a problem of altered skin integrity.

Clinical Practice

8. Teach three patients to perform a self-assessment of the skin.
9. Analyze the changes that have occurred with aging that affect the skin barrier for one of your older adult patients.
10. Perform a focused integumentary assessment on a patient.
11. Provide skin care for an older adult with dry skin.
12. Implement a teaching plan appropriate for adolescents and young adults for the prevention of skin cancer.

Key Terms

biopsy (BĪ-ŏp-sē, p. 982)
erythrasma (ĕ-rĭth-RĂZ-mă, p. 982)
exudate (ĔKS-ū-dāt, p. 982)
keloid (KĒ-loid, p. 983)
keratoses (kĕr-ă-TŌ-sēs, p. 983)
macule (MĂK-ūl, p. 983)
papule (PĂP-ūl, p. 983)
plaque (plăk, p. 985)
pustule (PŬS-tūl, p. 985)
senile lentigines (SĒ-nīl lĕn-TĬJ-ĭ-nēz, p. 979)
senile purpura (SĒ-nīl PŬR-pū-ră, p. 985)
vesicle (VĔS-ĭ-kŭl, p. 985)
wheal (WĒL, p. 982)

Concepts Covered in This Chapter

- Self-Management
- Fluid and Electrolytes
- Cellular Regulation
- Nutrition
- Immunity
- Inflammation
- Infection
- Tissue Integrity
- Coping
- Health Promotion

ANATOMY AND PHYSIOLOGY OF THE INTEGUMENTARY SYSTEM

STRUCTURE OF THE SKIN, HAIR, AND NAILS

- The skin consists of two layers of tissue, the epidermis and the dermis (Fig. 42.1).
- The skin is attached to underlying structures by subcutaneous tissue.
- The epidermis consists of squamous epithelium and contains no blood vessels; cells receive nutrients by diffusion from vessels in the underlying tissue.
- Cell growth occurs from the bottom of the epidermis and pushes cells above to the surface, where they eventually die and slough off or are washed off. This layer is called the *stratum corneum.*
- The bottom layer of the epidermis contains melanocytes that contribute color to the skin.
- The dermis, also called the *corium,* is thicker than the epidermis and consists of dense connective tissue.
- The dermis contains both elastic and collagenous fibers that give it strength and elasticity.
- The dermis contains blood vessels and nerves, as well as the base of hair follicles, glands, and nails that are derived from the epidermis.
- A hair consists of a shaft and a root made up of dead keratinized epithelial cells.
- The hair root is below the surface of the epidermis and is enclosed in a hair follicle that is embedded in the dermis.

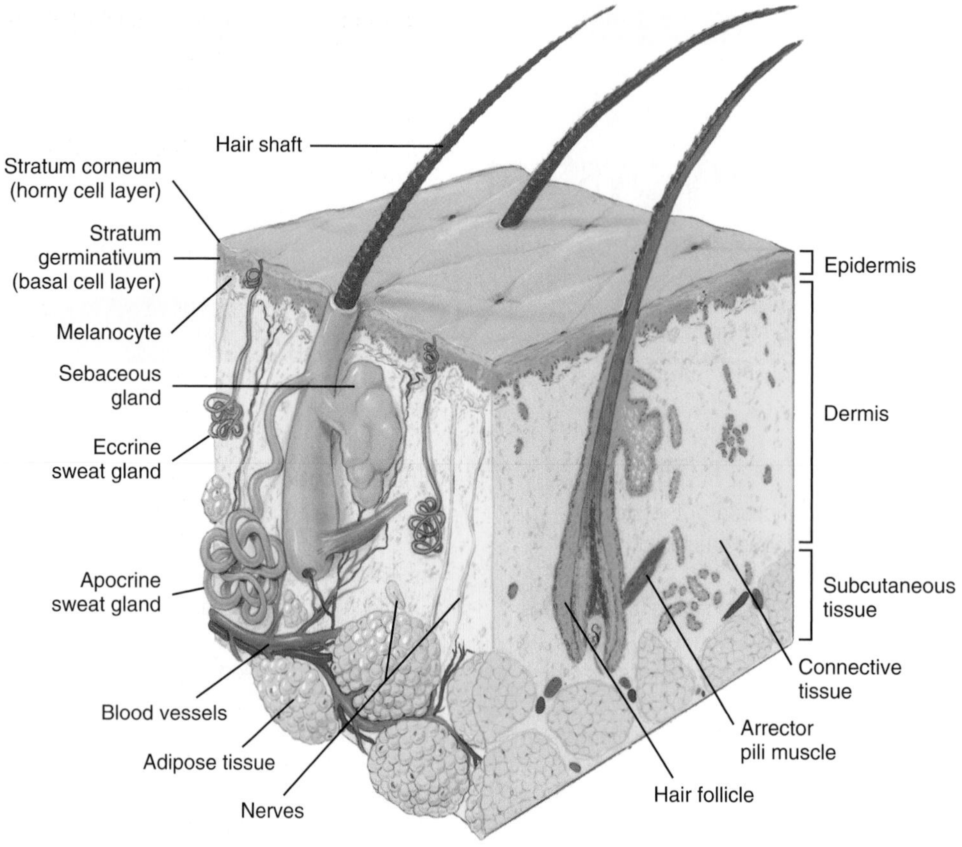

Fig. 42.1 Structure of the skin. (From Lewis SL, Butcher L, Heitkemper MM, et al.: *Medical-surgical nursing: assessment and management of clinical problems*, ed 10, St. Louis, 2017, Elsevier.)

- Fibroblasts that produce new cells to heal the skin are contained in the dermis.
- Glands contained in the skin are *sebaceous* (sweat producing) or *ceruminous* (wax producing).
- Nails are dead stratum corneum with a very hard type of keratin (Seeley et al., 2011).

FUNCTIONS OF THE SKIN AND ITS STRUCTURES

- The skin acts as a protective covering over the entire surface of the body.
- The keratin in the skin makes it waterproof, preventing water loss from the underlying tissues and too much water absorption during swimming and bathing.
- Skin provides a barrier to bacteria and other invading organisms.
- Skin protects underlying tissues from thermal, chemical, and mechanical injury.
- The skin helps regulate body temperature by dilating and constricting blood vessels and by activating or inactivating sweat glands.
- When the skin is exposed to ultraviolet (UV) light, molecules in the cells convert the rays to vitamin D.
- Melanin pigment absorbs light and acts to protect tissue from UV light.
- The nerve receptors in the dermis transmit feelings of heat, cold, pain, touch, and pressure.
- Hair follicles contained in the skin produce hair.
- Sebaceous glands secrete sebum that functions to keep hair and skin soft and pliable. Sebum also inhibits bacterial growth on the surface of the skin and, because of its oily nature, helps prevent water loss from the skin.
- Sweat glands act to excrete water and salt when the body temperature increases; sweat evaporates, producing a cooling effect.
- Sweat glands in the axillae and external genitalia secrete fatty acids and proteins as well as water and salts. They become active at puberty and are stimulated by the nervous system in response to sexual arousal, emotional stress, and pain.
- Hair color is produced by melanocytes in the skin and depends on the type of melanin produced.
- The shape of the hair shaft determines whether hair is straight or curly.
- Hair assists the body to retain heat.
- Nails cover the distal ends of the fingers and toes.
- Each nail has a free edge, a nail body, and a nail root that is covered by skin.
- The cuticle of each nail is a fold of stratum corneum.

AGING-RELATED CHANGES IN THE SKIN AND ITS STRUCTURES

- The number of elastic fibers decreases, and adipose tissue diminishes in the dermis and subcutaneous layers, causing skin to wrinkle and sag.

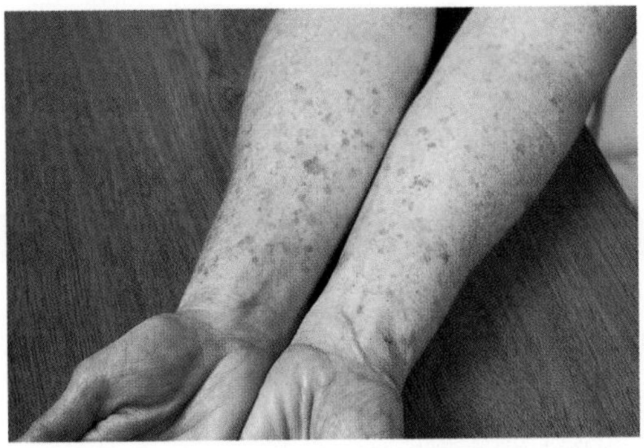

Fig. 42.2 Senile lentigines (age spots or liver spots).

- Loss of collagen fibers in the dermis makes the skin increasingly fragile and slower to heal.
- The skin becomes thinner and more transparent.
- Reduced sebaceous gland activity causes dry skin that may itch.
- Thinned skin and decreased sebaceous gland activity reduce temperature control and lead to an intolerance of cold and a susceptibility to heat exhaustion.
- A reduction in melanocyte activity increases the risk of sunburn and skin cancer.
- The number of hair follicles decreases, and the growth rate of hair declines; the hair thins.
- A decrease in the numbers of melanocytes at the hair follicle causes gradual loss of hair color.
- Nail growth decreases, longitudinal ridges appear, and the nails thicken; nails become more susceptible to fungal infections.
- Some areas of melanocytes increase in production, producing brown "age spots" or "liver spots," properly named **senile lentigines** (Fig. 42.2).

THE INTEGUMENTARY SYSTEM

The skin is the first line of defense against invasion by pathogenic bacteria living in the environment. When an area of the skin is destroyed by disease or trauma, its protective functions are immediately impaired. This impairment makes the body susceptible to infection. If very large areas of skin are destroyed, as in an extensive burn, fluid and electrolyte balance is disturbed. Protein and body heat are lost from burned areas. Skin diseases are common; they are often difficult to diagnose and cure and tend to recur. The physical effects of skin diseases are not often serious. However, when the disorder renders the patient unattractive, there is a psychological impact that threatens self-image and damages self-esteem. The skin also reflects systemic diseases.

DISORDERS OF THE INTEGUMENTARY SYSTEM

Causes

More than 3000 disorders of the skin have been officially named, and many more are not included in any official nomenclature. Most of the recognized and named skin disorders arise from some pathology in the skin itself. The remainder are manifestations of systemic disease. Skin disorders may occur from immunologic and inflammatory disorders, proliferative and neoplastic disorders, metabolic and endocrine disorders, and nutritional problems. Physical, chemical, and microbiological factors also can damage the skin.

Many patients with dermatologic disease are not hospitalized and are seen only in health care providers' offices and outpatient clinics. Others do not seek medical attention but treat their skin disorder themselves with home remedies and over-the-counter drugs. In some cases self-care measures are successful, but they also have the potential to aggravate the condition or only temporarily relieve more severe symptoms. This can lead to delay in treatment and allow the disease to progress to a chronic and sometimes untreatable state.

Prevention

Hygiene. The ritual of the daily bath is almost an obsession with the average American. Experts do not agree on what frequency of bathing is best for health, but most agree it does not need to be daily. People with healthy skin can usually bathe daily without damaging the protective layers of the skin, but those with skin disorders need to be careful not to worsen their condition. Hospitalized patients may be at risk for skin breakdown due to multiple factors. Keeping skin clean and dry is an important nursing intervention. Cleansing of skin can put patients at risk. Multiple studies have cultured *Escherichia coli* and methicillin-resistant *Staphylococcus aureus* (MRSA) from plastic bath basins routinely used in health care facilities. Some facilities are using a disposable basin liner to combat this problem (Muro et al., 2018). Other facilities have adopted disposable cleansing cloths to replace the individual bathing basin. Soap and water continue to have a place in hygiene, but beyond infection control, astute nurses assess for and consider skin type. Blondes and redheads with a fair complexion usually have very delicate skin that requires special care to prevent drying and irritation. If the skin appears dry and scaly, frequent bathing with soap and hot water only aggravates the condition. Oils and creams that cleanse the skin quite effectively and help replace the natural oils at the same time are available. On the other hand, people with dark hair usually have skin that is oilier and less susceptible to excessive drying and irritation. People with oily skin will need to clean the skin frequently with a liberal amount of soap and water and will need to apply fewer or no additional oils to the skin. When full bathing is not possible or impractical, cleaning of the axilla and perineal areas will prevent odors and irritation.

? Think Critically

You assist an older adult with a bath and notice that they have very dry skin. What interventions would you use?

Clinical Cues

Remember to dry areas where two skin surfaces touch, such as the axilla and under the breasts.

Diet. Even borderline deficiencies of vitamins and minerals will cause the skin to take on a sallow and dull appearance. Severe nutritional deficiencies lead to skin breakdown and the development of sores and ulcers. Dehydration causes loss of skin turgor and predisposes to pressure ulcers. People can be so concerned about their physical appearance that they refuse to eat properly for fear of gaining weight; however, a well-balanced diet will enhance appearance.

Age. Young people are not the only ones who should be concerned with the care of their skin. As we grow older, our skin undergoes certain changes that easily lead to irritation and breakdown if proper care is not given. The oil and sweat glands become less active, and the skin tends to become dry and scaly. It also loses some of its tone, becoming less elastic and more fragile. Frequent cleansing of the skin becomes unnecessary as the skin ages, and alcohol and other drying agents must be used sparingly, if at all. Assist older adult patients to establish a regular routine of massaging oil, cream, or oily lotion into the skin.

Older Adult Care Points

Older adults who have dry skin do not need a full bath every day; cleansing the axillae and genital-rectal area between bathing days should be sufficient. Older adults should use a mild lotion-based soap or body wash for bathing. After showering or bathing, a lotion or cream that helps seal in moisture should be applied while the skin is still damp. Moisturizing lotion or cream should be reapplied at bedtime.

Environment. Several environmental factors can have a direct effect on the health of the skin. These include prolonged exposure to chemicals, excessive drying from repeated immersions in water, very cold temperatures, and prolonged exposure to sunlight. Some of these are occupational hazards. A change of jobs may be necessary to eliminate contact with a factor that is causing a skin disorder. One of the *Healthy People 2030* objectives is to reduce occupational skin diseases or disorders among full-time workers.

Overexposure to the UV rays of the sun can seriously and permanently damage the superficial and deeper layers of the skin. The damage results in severe wrinkling and furrowing, as well as loss of elasticity, and the skin assumes a tissue-paper transparency. In addition to the potential for premature aging and degenerative changes, solar damage also can result in malignant changes. Ultraviolet rays from the sun have long been known to be carcinogenic. This is especially true for fair-skinned people who have subjected their skin to prolonged exposure to sunshine. Although sunburns are particularly harmful, it is the normal daily exposure of unprotected fair skin to sun that causes long-term damage.

Health Promotion

Sun Exposure Precautions

Health teaching to inform the public about the dangers of solar UV radiation should include the following information:

- Although fair-skinned people who freckle easily are more likely to suffer sun-damaged skin, people of all complexions and races can and do burn if exposed to sufficient sunlight.
- Although a good tan may be considered by many to be desirable, dermatologists say that there is no such thing as a “healthy tan.” Tanning causes damage to the skin. For those who insist on lying out in the sun, the initial exposure should be slow and gradual, and an adequate sunscreen with a sun protection factor (SPF) of at least 30, as well as ultraviolet A (UVA) and ultraviolet B (UVB) protection, should always be used. Too much sun too quickly only leads to blistering and peeling.
- Select a sunscreen preparation based on skin type and ability to tan, as well as its active ingredients and the amount of time to be spent in the sun. Remember that the sunscreen can be washed off by water or perspiration or rubbed off on sand and towels and must be reapplied periodically. Apply sunscreen liberally 15 to 30 minutes before sun exposure (U.S. Food and Drug Administration [FDA], 2018). Reapply every 2 hours. The ingredients in the sunscreen are used by the body and depleted within these 2 hours, so a higher SPF sunscreen will not last longer.
- The ingredients in sunscreen may be absorbed through the skin into the systemic circulation. Read the label carefully.
- Avoid exposure to the sun during the time its rays are most hazardous—that is, between 10 A.M. and 2 P.M. standard time or 11 A.M. and 3 P.M. during daylight saving time.
- You can become sunburned on a cloudy or overcast day.
- Light, loosely woven clothing will not give adequate protection from the sun’s rays.
- Remember that snow, water, and sand can reflect the sun’s rays and increase the intensity of exposure.
- Do not try to gauge how much you are being burned while in the sun. It may be 6 to 8 hours before a painful burn becomes obvious.
- Wear sunglasses and a hat when you go out in the sun, and when possible wear protective clothing.
- **Never use a tanning booth;** there is an eightfold increased risk of developing melanoma for persons under age 36 years who use tanning booths (Centers for Disease Control and Prevention [CDC], 2018).

INTEGRITY OF SKIN

Good nursing care includes protection of the skin and prevention of skin tears. A skin tear is a potentially preventable, traumatic wound that occurs primarily on

Complementary and Alternative Therapies

Ultraviolet Radiation Protection

An oral form of fern plant extract may help protect the skin from UV radiation. The fern extract is from *Polypodium leucotomos* and is a natural antioxidant with tumor inhibition properties. Initial studies showed that volunteer subjects could tolerate threefold to sevenfold longer sun exposure time.

Clinical Cues

It is estimated that 90% of people between 50 and 71 years of age are not getting adequate vitamin D. Adults with limited sun exposure are at especially increased risk of vitamin D deficiency, if their skin is dark. During spring, summer, and autumn, 5 to 15 minutes of sun exposure without sunscreen twice per week to the face, arms, hands, and back is sufficient for adequate vitamin D production (Drezner, 2019).

Think Critically

You are talking to a young woman who works as a ski instructor. She is fair-skinned and says that "on really sunny days, my hat is in my pocket and I never use sunscreen." Discuss some issues related to this woman's integumentary health.

the extremities of older adults because of age and debility. The wound occurs as a result of lack of caution when handling, friction alone, or shearing and friction forces that separate the epidermis from the dermis or separate both structures from the underlying tissue. Up to 90% of older adults in health care facilities sustain a skin tear injury each year (LeBlanc et al., 2018). The epidermis thins and becomes less elastic with age, making it susceptible to tearing with little trauma. Those individuals who require total care are at the highest risk. Risk factors for skin tears, other than age older than 65 years, are presented in Box 42.1.

The Payne-Martin, STAR Skin Care, and International Skin Tear Advisory Panel (ISTAP) classification systems identify skin tears as (LeBlanc et al., 2018):

- *Category I:* A skin tear without tissue loss in which the edges can be realigned
- *Category II:* A skin tear with partial tissue loss in which the edges cannot be realigned
- *Category III:* A skin tear with complete tissue loss in which the epidermal flap is missing

Nursing Management

Rigorous nursing care (Box 42.2) to prevent skin tears is obviously preferable to treating skin tears that could have been prevented. However, when a skin tear is discovered, steps for its management are as follows:

- Gently cleanse the skin tear with saline.
- Allow the area to air-dry or pat dry gently and carefully.
- If the skin tear flap has dried, remove it using scissors and sterile technique.

Box 42.1 Risk Factors for Skin Tears in Older Adults

Assess the patient for the following factors:

- Dry skin with dehydration
- Areas of ecchymosis
- Presence of friction, shearing, or pressure from bed or chair
- Impaired sensory perception
- Impaired mobility
- Taking multiple medications
- Prolonged use of corticosteroids
- Presence of renal disease, congestive heart failure, or stroke impairment
- Incorrect removal of adhesive dressings
- Rough handling when being bathed, dressed, transferred, or repositioned

Box 42.2 Measures to Prevent Skin Tears and Protect Fragile Skin

- Have patients wear long sleeves and long pants to protect the extremities or protect the fragile skin on extremities with stockinettes.
- Provide adequate lighting to reduce the risk of bumping into furniture or equipment.
- Maintain the patient's nutrition and hydration; offer fluids between meals.
- Lubricate the skin with cream or lotion twice a day, paying special attention to the arms and legs.
- Use an emollient soap for bathing and do not use soap every day on extremities if no soiling has occurred.
- Use a lift sheet to move and turn patients.
- Avoid wearing rings or bracelets that could snag the skin.
- Use transfer techniques that prevent friction or shear.
- Pad bed rails, wheelchair arms, leg supports, or other equipment where the patient might bump an extremity.
- Support dangling arms and legs with pillows or blankets.
- Use nonadherent dressings on fragile skin. Use gauze wraps or stockinettes to secure dressing. If tape must be used, use a paper or nonallergenic tape and apply it without tension.
- Mark the dressing with an arrow showing the direction in which it should be removed.
- Remove tape and dressing with extreme caution:
  - Use a solvent or saline to loosen the adhesive bond.
  - Slowly pull the skin away from the tape rather that peeling the tape off of the skin.
- If a thin hydrocolloid or solid wafer skin barrier is used as a protective barrier between the skin and the dressing, allow it to fall off naturally.

- If the skin tear flap is viable, gently roll the flap back into place using a moistened cotton-tipped applicator.
- If bleeding has stopped, silicone-coated net dressings are preferred; petroleum-based protective ointments are also used. Cyanoacrylate skin protectants are in

a liquid form that creates a barrier to protect damaged skin. The substance does not need to be removed because it will shed in approximately 1 week (LeBlanc et al., 2018).

- If bleeding continues, apply pressure and then dress with alginate and a secondary dressing.
- Manage in the same way as a skin graft. The flap should not be disturbed for about 5 days to allow the skin flap to adhere.
- Assess and measure the size of the skin tear.
- Document assessment and treatment.

A skin tear comprehensive assessment is essential to ensure that adequate attention is given to the wound. The dressing should (1) continuously cleanse the wound, (2) conform to the wound, (3) absorb exudates, and (4) keep the wound bed moist and reduce pain and discomfort. The wound must be watched for signs of infection. Extra padding for the involved extremity will help prevent additional injuries.

Clinical Cues

Best practice recommendations from ISTAP do not recommend use of transparent adhesive dressings for skin tears (LeBlanc et al., 2018).

Diagnostic Tests and Procedures

Skin biopsy. Removing a sample of tissue (**biopsy**) from a skin lesion usually is performed with a local anesthetic. It can be done by shaving a top layer off a lesion that rises above the skin line **(shave biopsy),** by removing a core from the center of the lesion **(punch biopsy),** or by excising the entire lesion **(excisional biopsy).**

Skin biopsy is used to differentiate benign from malignant lesions and to help identify the causative organism in bacterial and fungal infections. No special patient preparation is necessary beyond a simple explanation of the procedure and its purpose. If a local anesthetic is to be used, the patient is asked about any personal or family history of allergies. After the procedure, the patient is given instructions for the care of the biopsy site. After 12 to 24 hours the bandage is removed, the incision site is cleaned with soap and water twice daily, and a bandage is reapplied after each cleansing. The site may or may not be treated with a topical antibiotic solution or ointment. Sutures from an excisional biopsy will need to be removed in 3 to 5 days for the face; in 7 to 10 days for the scalp, chest, abdomen, and arms; and in 12 to 20 days for the back and legs (Alguire & Mathes, 2017).

Culture and sensitivity tests. When a bacterial, viral, or fungal infection of the skin is suspected, culture and sensitivity tests can be used to identify the causative organism and the drug most appropriate for treating the specific infection. A sampling of **exudate** (drainage) is taken from the lesion and sent to the laboratory for culturing. Once the organism has been cultured, colonies can be tested for sensitivity to certain antiinfective agents. Care must be taken when handling the specimen and its container to avoid contaminating people who will later be handling the specimen.

Safety Alert

Skin Drainage or Weeping

Whenever there is a question of a pathogenic process, weeping or drainage from skin lesions, or the suspicion of scabies, Standard Precautions should be used when touching the patient's skin to prevent self-contamination or transmission of an organism.

Microscopic tests. Various stains and solutions are used to prepare skin, hair, scales, or nail material for study. These tests can identify fungal, bacterial, and viral organisms. To check for organism infestations, scrapings are suspended in mineral oil and examined under the microscope.

Special light inspection. Inspection of the skin is one of the principal means by which skin lesions are diagnosed. To facilitate the diagnosis of certain kinds of skin disorders, special lights may be used by the examiner. A **cold light** is one in which the light is transmitted through a quartz or plastic structure to dissipate the heat. Because there is no danger of burning the skin, the cold light can be applied directly to the skin to illuminate its layers for visualization of malignant changes.

A **Wood light** is a specially designed UV light. The nickel oxide filter holds back all but a few violet rays of the visible spectrum. This special light is especially useful to diagnose fungal infections of the scalp and chronic bacterial infection of the major folds of the skin (**erythrasma**). Under a Wood light, fungal lesions and erythrasma are fluorescent. Erythrasma usually is seen on the inner thighs, scrotum, and axilla; under the breasts; and in the area between the toes.

Diascopy. Diascopy uses a glass slide or lens pressed down over the area to be examined, blanching the skin and thereby reducing the erythema caused by increasing blood flow to the area. The shape of the underlying lesion is then revealed.

Allergy testing. When a rash is suspected to be of an allergic nature, one of three methods is used to identify the responsible allergen. Test chemicals or substances are introduced to unaffected skin, usually on the forearm or back, by superficial scratches or pricks in the *prick testing*. In *patch testing,* the allergen is applied to the skin in the form of an adhesive patch and left for 2 days. The allergen can also be introduced by *intradermal* injection. If a localized reaction producing a **wheal** (smooth, slightly elevated area that is pale or reddened) occurs, the test is positive.

Nursing care for diagnostic tests. Check to see that the patient has signed an informed consent for any invasive procedure such as a biopsy. Reinforce what the health care provider has told the patient about the procedure and assess whether the patient understands or has additional questions. Check for allergies to the anesthetic or skin preparation solution. Properly label any specimens and send them to the laboratory. Apply a dressing and give both verbal and written postoperative instructions to the patient. Tell the patient approximately when the results will be back and that they will be notified of the results. Advise whether a follow-up visit is necessary.

NURSING MANAGEMENT

ASSESSMENT (DATA COLLECTION)

History Taking

Diagnosing skin disorders requires a thorough history to identify factors that predispose a patient to skin disease or factors that cause some types of skin disease.

Focused Assessment

Data Collection for Skin Disorders

The following questions should be asked when seeking data on a skin disorder:

- When did the rash or lesion first appear?
- Can you think of any event or different food you ate or substance you were using just before it appeared?
- What is your usual dietary pattern? What do you eat and drink?
- Have you noticed if anything makes it worse?
- What seems to make it better?
- Have you been using any chemicals lately for household cleaning or in pursuit of your hobbies?
- Have you been out in rural areas or in the woods lately?
- Have you been traveling? Did you visit a tropical area?
- Have you had any recent exposure to animals?
- What drugs are you taking? Do you take any over-the-counter medications?
- Are you using any street drugs? What route of administration?
- Have you ever had a drug reaction?
- Have you ever had radiation therapy?
- Do you have a history of any skin disorders in your family?
- Does anyone in the family currently have similar symptoms, such as a rash?
- Do you have any allergies?
- Are you experiencing itching? Pain? Fever?
- Have you had any gastrointestinal problems that began about the same time that the rash or lesion appeared? What about a runny or stuffed-up nose? Cough?
- Has the skin condition affected your social life or work?

Scabies, lice, and other parasites can be transmitted through close personal contact with infected persons at work, recreation, home, or school. It is important to know whether exposure has occurred, so that others can be notified and treated.

Many drugs can produce skin eruptions in certain individuals. Drug allergy or reaction can produce lesions and rashes that imitate those found in a long list of diseases, including measles, chickenpox, fungal infections, skin cancers, and psoriasis.

Itching and pain are the most common complaints. If the patient has recently been exposed to severe cold, their skin may be drier than usual, and they may complain of severe itching **(winter itch).** If the disorder is caused by an allergy, the patient also may complain of shortness of breath, cough, or some gastrointestinal symptoms. The patient also may be able to relate what other factors, such as stress or excitement, could be related to the appearance of the skin lesions.

Physical Assessment

A thorough inspection of the skin under good lighting is essential. Provide privacy and have the room at a moderate temperature so that the patient does not become chilled. The patient should don a gown that allows access to all areas of the skin.

Cultural Considerations

Coin Rubbing

Coin rubbing is a Southeast Asian folk remedy that is intended to draw illness out of the body. An oiled coin is rubbed over the skin surface and creates bruiselike marks or patterns of red lines or welts on the skin. The redness is interpreted as a sign that the remedy is bringing the illness to the surface (Giger, 2017).

Seborrheic **keratoses** are common in older adults. They appear as wartlike, greasy lesions on the trunk, arms, scalp, and sometimes the face. They are not a cause for concern.

Darkly pigmented people will have areas that are darker than other parts of the skin. This is caused by hormonal influences. The darker areas are the nipples, areola, scrotum, and labia minora. This is true among both African Americans and Asians. When the skin of a darkly pigmented person is damaged, scar tissue may hypertrophy, forming a **keloid** (a thick ridge of scar tissue that stands up from the surrounding skin) (Fig. 42.3).

The hair of African Americans differs in texture. It varies from being long and straight to being short, thick, and tightly curled. It is very dry and fragile and requires daily grooming with oil. Asians tend to have straight hair. If an African American child has malnutrition, sometimes the hair will turn a coppery red.

Clinical Cues

When trying to differentiate between a **macule** and a **papule**, shine a flashlight at a right angle to the lesion. A papule will cast a shadow. If there is no shadow, the lesion is a macule. To determine whether there is fluid in a lesion, place the tip of a penlight against the side of the lesion. If the light illuminates it with a red glow, it is fluid filled. If there is no light illumination, the lesion is solid.

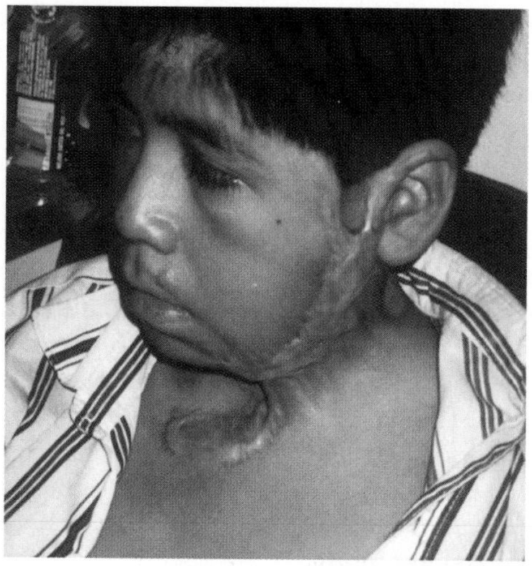

Fig. 42.3 A keloid scar. (From Damjanov I: *Pathology for the health professions*, ed 5, St. Louis, 2017, Elsevier.)

Clinical Cues

Pallor in a dark-skinned person presents as an ashen-gray tone to the skin. In a brown-skinned person, pallor gives the skin a yellow-brown color.

The skin should be lightly palpated to detect changes in texture and surface elevations. Palpation also is used to detect pain, areas of increased warmth, and tenderness. When checking the temperature of the skin, the back of the hand should be used. Skin turgor is assessed by lifting a fold of skin on the forearm, chest, or abdomen between two fingers and seeing how fast it falls back into place. Skin that takes longer than 1 to 2 seconds to return to place is called "poor skin turgor" and indicates dehydration.

Table 42.1 shows characteristics of various types of skin lesions. As you are performing your assessment you can simultaneously teach the patient about self-examination of the skin.

Assessing the Skin for Signs of Breakdown

Skin should be thoroughly assessed when the patient is admitted to your facility. Skin assessment is performed during every shift on immobile patients, noting the condition of skin over bony prominences. Findings must be documented accurately.

Once every 24 hours, usually during the bath, the skin is totally assessed. When a reddened area is found, it is checked for blanching by pressing gently in the center of the area to see if it turns from red to white or to a paler color on darker skin. **Blanching usually indicates that the redness is temporary and will resolve when pressure on the area is relieved.** (See Chapter 43 for additional information on pressure injury.)

◆ NURSING DIAGNOSIS AND PLANNING

Problem statements are based on the analysis of the data gathered from assessment. Problem statements

Focused Assessment

Physical Assessment of Skin

Perform a physical examination of the entire skin surface. Proceed from head to toe. Compare one side of the body to the other. Use the metric system when measuring lesions, and document all findings. Check the patient for the following:

- General appearance of skin surface: texture, elasticity, thickness
- Condition of areas between skin folds
- Type of lesions and distribution, size, and appearance; photograph or measure and document measurements
- Appearance of skin adjacent to lesions; note whether reddened areas blanch when mild pressure is applied
- Localized or generalized skin edema
- Characteristics of secretions: color, viscosity, amount
- Odor: description of odor; strong or faint; source—local or generalized
- Temperature changes: location of hot spots or cold areas of the skin

In addition:

- Check the back and the soles of the feet, including between the toes
- Observe patient for scratching, rubbing, or picking at lesions
- Observe patient for scratching of the scalp or pubic areas
- Inspect the hair for texture, brittleness, thinning, and cleanliness
- Inspect the nails for chipping, splitting, discoloration, and ragged or inflamed cuticles

Patient Teaching

Self-Assessment of the Skin

Teach the patient that the skin should be examined every few months. For the back or other areas, suggest that a family member or close friend examine that area of skin. If any changes have occurred, the patient should consult the health care provider right away. Advise that warts, moles, or discolorations of the skin should be checked each month for:

- Darkening or spreading of color or increasing unevenness of color
- Increase in size or diameter
- Change in shape; that is, has the lesion become elevated, or have its formerly regular edges become irregular?
- Redness or swelling of surrounding skin or any other noticeable change around the lesion
- Itching, tenderness, or other change in sensation
- Crusting, scaling, oozing, ulceration, or other change in the surface of the lesion
- When assessing for melanoma, check for the ABCDs: A = asymmetric, B = irregular border, C = color change, D = diameter change greater than ¼ inch

commonly associated with skin disorders are presented in Table 42.2.

Nursing goals for patients with skin disorders are to:

- Restore the skin to normal
- Decrease pain and itching

Table 42.1 Types of Skin Lesions

LESION	DESCRIPTION
Macule 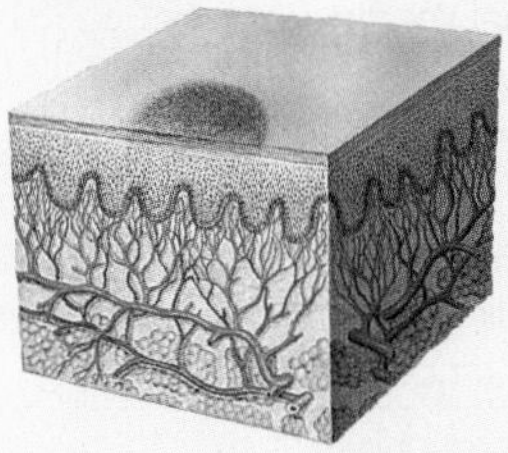	Circumscribed, flat area with a change in skin color; <0.5 cm in diameter. If >0.5 cm in diameter, it is a *patch*. *Examples:* Freckles, petechiae, measles, flat mole (nevus)
Papule 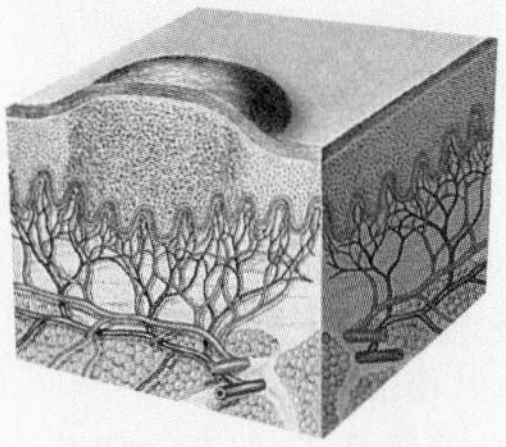	Elevated, solid lesion; <0.5 cm in diameter. If >0.5 cm in diameter, it is a *nodule*. *Examples:* Wart (verruca), elevated moles, lipoma, basal cell carcinoma
Vesicle 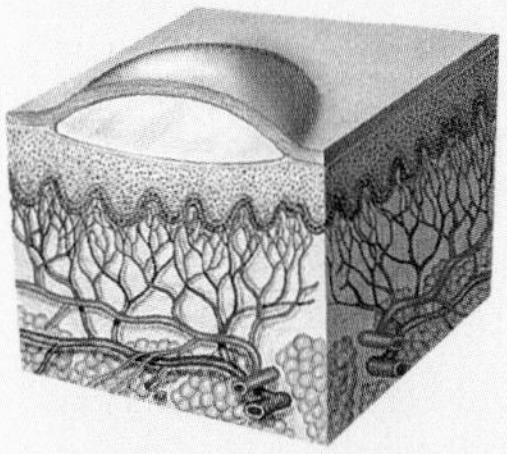	Circumscribed, superficial collection of serous fluid; <0.5 cm in diameter *Examples:* Varicella (chickenpox), herpes zoster (shingles), second-degree burn
Plaque 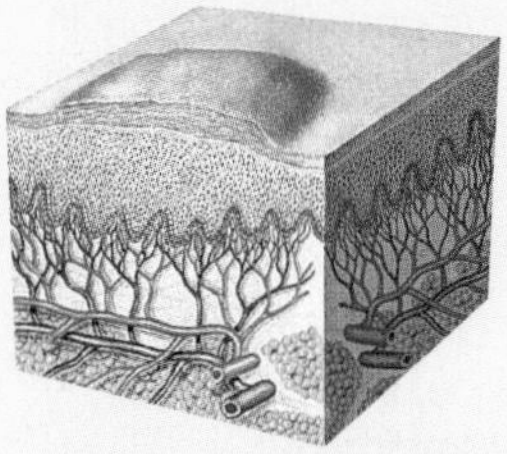	Circumscribed, elevated superficial, solid lesion; >0.5 cm in diameter *Examples:* Psoriasis, seborrheic, and actinic keratoses
Wheal 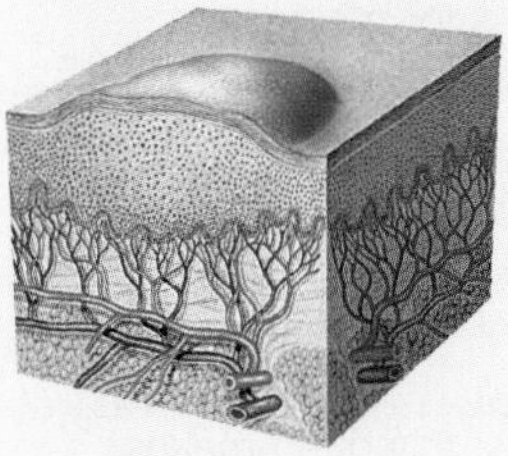	Firm, edematous, irregularly shaped area; diameter variable *Examples:* Insect bite, urticaria
Pustule 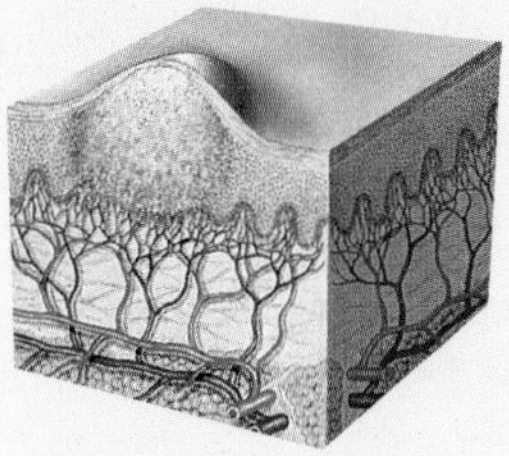	Elevated, superficial lesion filled with purulent fluid *Examples:* Acne, impetigo

From Lewis SL, Bucher L, Heitkemper MM, et al.: *Medical-surgical nursing: assessment and management of clinical problems,* ed 10, St. Louis, 2017, Elsevier. Figures from Patton KT, Thibodeau GA: *The human body in health and disease,* ed 7, St. Louis, 2018, Elsevier.

Older Adult Care Points

When checking skin turgor on an older adult, test the upper chest because the skin of the arms and hands of older adults may lose elasticity and is not a reliable index. Gently pinch a small amount of skin, lift it up, and let go. Note the time it takes for the skin to move back to its normal position. If the skin stays "tented" or takes more than 3 to 5 seconds to return to normal position, the patient is dehydrated. Older adults bruise more easily as the skin becomes thinner and collagen is lost. Patches of **senile purpura**, deep red areas, may occur even from minor injuries, so be gentle when testing skin turgor.

Legal and Ethical Considerations

Skin Lesion Documentation

All data gathered when assessing the skin and any lesions should be documented accurately, including location, size, appearance, and characteristics. Measure lesions using a ruler device and note the measurements in the chart. For pressure ulcers, many facilities take photos and enter those in the chart so that healing progress can be demonstrated.

Assignment Considerations

Observation While Bathing

Unlicensed assistive personnel are generally assisting with hygiene, and you should give specific instructions to report reddening, bruising, breaks in the skin, or new lesions. **Remember that total skin assessment cannot be delegated; this is your responsibility.**

- Protect the skin from further damage
- Prevent infection
- Prevent scarring as much as possible

Planning of the daily work schedule should include consideration of time necessary for dressing changes, soaks, special baths, and other skin treatments.

◆ IMPLEMENTATION

Some general rules when caring for patients with a skin disease may be helpful as a guide until specific orders are obtained:

- Bathing with soap is usually contraindicated in all inflammatory conditions of the skin.
- Dressings covering the skin lesions that have been applied by a health care provider should not be removed when the patient is admitted unless there are specific orders to do so.
- Do not attempt to remove scales, crusts, or other exudates on the skin lesions until the provider has had an opportunity to examine the patient.
- Observe the skin very carefully at the time of the patient's admission and record observations on the chart or report them to the nurse in charge.
- Avoid excessive handling or rubbing of the skin against the sheets and bedclothes when changing the bed.

Table 42.2 Common Problem Statements, Expected Outcomes, and Nursing Interventions for Patients With Skin Disorders

PROBLEM STATEMENT	GOALS/EXPECTED OUTCOMES	NURSING INTERVENTIONS
Altered skin integrity due to injury and treatment; excoriation or scaling; infectious process	Patient's skin will be intact within 2 wk (4 mo for burns). Number of lesions will decrease within 2 mo. Patient will exhibit no signs of infection within 3 mo.	Cleanse skin and apply topical medications as prescribed. Monitor for signs of adverse reaction to topical medication. Preserve integrity of grafted areas with aseptic dressing technique and splinting. Apply light treatments as prescribed.
Pain due to itching, soreness, or tenderness of lesions; exposure of denuded skin to air; or involvement of nerve tissue	Patient's pain will be controlled to less than 4/10 on the pain scale by medication and relaxation or distraction techniques.	Apply topical medication as prescribed. Administer analgesia as prescribed and as needed (PRN). Provide medicated baths as prescribed. Teach relaxation techniques. Provide distraction activities.
Decreased self-esteem due to disrupted skin surface and lesions	Patient will show increase in self-esteem by socializing with others within 3 wk.	Suggest ways to cover lesions. Help patient list positive aspects and achievements. Encourage socialization with others. Show acceptance and matter-of-fact attitude when dealing with patient's lesions.
Potential for infection due to loss of intact skin barrier	Patient will not experience skin infection before lesions are healed.	Cleanse skin carefully and gently. Use aseptic technique when attending to lesions. Apply prescribed topical medications. Encourage patient to keep hands off affected skin areas. Encourage hand hygiene for patient.
Anxiety due to chronic, recurring nature of skin disorder; reaction to diagnosis of cancer; slow healing	Patient will verbalize feelings within 3 wk. Patient will explore options for treatment of cancer. Patient will identify short-term and long-term goals that realistically match the slow healing process.	Provide atmosphere of acceptance. Allow patient time to verbalize feelings. Assist to recognize positive coping techniques by looking at ways patient has coped with anxiety in the past. Provide information on treatment and prognosis for skin malignancy.
Deficient knowledge regarding cause and treatment of skin disorder	Patient will verbalize knowledge of factors related to appearance of skin disorder. Patient will verbalize knowledge of treatment for disorder. Patient will demonstrate self-care techniques.	Explain the cause of the skin disorder and measures to prevent possible recurrence, if any. Instruct in various methods of treatment. Teach the side effects of medications. Instruct in self-care techniques for medication application, dressing changes, and so on. Obtain feedback of information and skills taught.
Disrupted sleep pattern due to itching or pain	Patient will obtain at least 7 h of rest per day.	Administer medication to relieve itching. Keep environment cool to decrease itching sensation. Caution patient to take cool or tepid baths or showers to decrease itching. Caution not to scratch lesions; this often makes itching worse. Suggest ways to use distraction (e.g., card or game playing, intense concentration on learning something, or reading an absorbing book) to decrease focus on itching. Administer hypnotic as prescribed. Administer analgesics as prescribed. Encourage use of meditation, relaxation, or imagery techniques to decrease pain. Provide restful, quiet environment. Use massage as appropriate to promote relaxation and sleep. Allow usual bedtime rituals that help patient induce sleep.

Table 42.2 **Common Problem Statements, Expected Outcomes, and Nursing Interventions for Patients With Skin Disorders—cont'd**

PROBLEM STATEMENT	GOALS/EXPECTED OUTCOMES	NURSING INTERVENTIONS
Potential social isolation due to long treatment process; disfigurement	Patient will maintain social contact with family and friends. Patient will reintegrate into community within 3–24 mo.	Encourage family and friends to send cards, call, and visit. Encourage patient to continue dialogue with family and friends. Refer to psychologist or social worker for grief work and reintegration of new body image. Refer to support group for expression of feelings and realization patient is not alone with such problems. Encourage return to employment or job training. Encourage return to church or community activities.

- Lotions or other skin products should not be used on the skin unless the provider has approved their use.

Once the provider has determined the type of lesions present, specific treatments will be ordered to relieve the patient's symptoms and promote healing. The two most commonly used treatments are special dermatologic baths and wet compresses or dressings. In addition, lotions, salves, or ointments may be applied locally at frequent intervals.

Although most skin diseases are *not* contagious, you should be careful to observe rules of cleanliness and Standard Precautions when caring for any patient with a skin eruption. **Special care is needed to prevent spreading infection from the fluid in all pustules and in the vesicles of fever blisters and cold sores.**

Giving Medicated Baths

Among the agents that may be added to the bath water are sodium bicarbonate, sodium chloride, cornstarch, oatmeal, medicated tars, oils, potassium permanganate, and special bath preparations.

Safety Alert

Prevent Falls

A nonslip bath mat should be used in the tub when giving medicated baths. The substances used for the bath can make the tub very slippery. Showers should have nonslip mats in them as well, especially when showering an older adult.

Patient Teaching

Easy Cleanup After an Oatmeal Bath

Put dry, uncooked oatmeal into an old sock to make an oatmeal sachet. Place the sachet in the tub and squeeze it repeatedly. After the bath is finished, discard the sachet.

During the bath, the patient must be protected from chilling because the bath usually lasts from 30 minutes to 1 hour, and most patients with skin diseases have a lowered resistance to cold. **When the patient is removed from the tub, the skin is dried by patting rather than by rubbing.** If medication is to be applied locally, it should be put on as soon as the bath is completed to keep **pruritus** (itching) at a minimum. **Medication is applied in a thin layer unless otherwise ordered.**

The medicated bath has a very soothing and relaxing effect on the patient and also helps relieve the itching and burning commonly associated with skin diseases. Encourage the patient to rest in bed and perhaps to take a short nap after each bath.

Laundry Requirements

The bed linens and gowns used for patients with severe skin diseases may need special laundering to eliminate all traces of soap. If the patient is to be cared for at home, vinegar may be added to the rinse water to neutralize the soap. One tablespoon of vinegar is used for each quart of water. Only detergent without perfume or other additives should be used. Dryer sheets should not be used because they contain chemicals that often cause skin problems. Residue from dryer sheets can remain in the dryer and affect laundry that has been washed separately for the individual with a skin sensitivity. New clothes should be washed before wearing when skin sensitivity is a problem. Washing removes chemical fabric-finishing products.

Application of Wet Compresses or Dressings

Wet dressings may be applied to the skin in various ways. The two general types used are **open dressings** and **closed dressings.** Open compresses must be changed repeatedly and are never allowed to dry. They usually need to be remoistened every 20 to 30 minutes. The solution used should be at room temperature or warmer. This type of dressing is used when the dermatologist wishes to have air circulating to the skin lesions. Closed dressings are thoroughly soaked with the prescribed solution and wrapped with an airtight, waterproof material. Obtain specific instructions from the dermatologist before applying wet dressings to any skin lesions.

Box 42.3 Guidelines for Applying Topical Medications[a]

POWDERS

- Dry the area thoroughly before applying powder to prevent caking.
- Do not apply to raw and denuded areas.
- Some powders, such as cornstarch, can serve as culture media for the growth of bacteria.

OINTMENT

- Use only a small amount and gently massage into the skin until a thin film covers the area. An exception is when ointment is used as an occlusive dressing, as for a burn.
- Ointments tend to leave a greasy feeling to the skin. They are best for chronic lesions because they help the skin retain moisture and natural oils.
- Avoid putting ointment on areas where the skin is creased and overlaps itself.

GELS

- A gel is a semisolid mixture that tends to liquefy when applied to the skin. It is absorbed into the skin and dries quickly, leaving a thin, nonocclusive film.
- If applied to abraded or sensitive areas, alcohol in the base can cause a burning or stinging sensation.

LOTIONS

- Lotions are powders suspended in water; they will leave a residue once the liquid evaporates from the skin. This residue should be washed off before a fresh dose is applied.
- Be sure that powder is uniformly dispersed in solution before applying, then use a firm stroke to distribute the medication evenly. Do not "dab" on lotions, as this can be irritating to the skin.

ALL TYPES

- Always apply topical medications sparingly and in a thin film that extends beyond the affected area by about ¼ inch. Thick layers of topical medications are wasteful, and some of these drugs, such as corticosteroids, are very expensive.
- Too much of some topical medications (e.g., antifungal agents) can chemically irritate the skin and delay healing. Thick layers also tend to soften the skin too much.
- If the skin condition appears to be getting worse after a topical agent is applied or if the patient develops eczema, suspect an allergic contact dermatitis caused by the drug.

[a]Allergies must be assessed before applying a topical medication.

Clinical Cues

When changing wet dressings, inspect the skin adjacent to the wound for signs of maceration from the moisture; this condition could cause the wound to enlarge.

Application of Topical Therapy

Many skin lesions are treated by directly applying medications to the surface of the affected area. This method is called *topical therapy.* Lotion, cream, ointment, powder, or gel may be used. The health care provider prescribes the kind of medication to be used and the way in which the drug is to be applied. Patients with skin conditions do not always consult a provider and sometimes choose to treat themselves at home. All patients should be instructed in the proper application of topical medications (Box 42.3). Occlusive dressings must not be applied over the area after application of the medication unless ordered by the health care provider (see Table 42.2 and Chapter 43).

Think Critically

If a patient has an order for a topical cream to be applied to an area of rash on the right upper thigh, how would you apply this cream?

◆ EVALUATION

Evaluation of treatment and nursing interventions for skin disorders is based on improved appearance of the skin, absence of signs of infection, relief from itching and pain, and signs of healing. Many skin disorders are slow to respond to treatment, and patience is required on the part of both the patient and you. Even a minor fungal skin infection may take 7 to 14 days to clear with topical medication. A fungal infection of a nail may take up to a year to clear. A major part of evaluation is to determine that treatment is not aggravating the condition.

Get Ready for the NCLEX® Examination!

Key Points

- The skin is essential for the maintenance of life; it is the first line of defense against pathogenic organisms. Skin has two layers, the epidermis and the dermis. New cells to heal the skin are contained in the dermis.
- Factors in the prevention of skin disorders include cleanliness, appropriate diet, proper skin care, limiting exposure to the sun, and careful handling of fragile skin.
- With increased age the skin becomes thinner and more fragile, less elastic, and drier.
- Fragile skin requires special attention: protective clothing (such as long sleeves), lubrication with creams or lotions, bed transfer techniques that prevent shear, padded side rails and assistive devices, use

of nonadherent tape, and use of solvent to loosen dressings and peeling them slowly.
- Several types of diagnostic measures are used: biopsy, culture, microscopic examination of scrapings or tissue, special light inspection, diascopy, and skin patch testing.
- A thorough health history is key in the diagnosis of skin disorders (see Focused Assessment: Data Collection for Skin Disorders).
- Teach self-examination of the skin, including the ABCDs: A = asymmetric; B = irregular border; C = color change; D = diameter greater than ¼ inch (see Patient Teaching: Self-Assessment of the Skin).
- Standard Precautions are used when touching patients with weeping lesions or when drainage is present.
- Treatments for skin disorders include medicated baths, special laundry precautions, application of compresses or dressings, and topical therapy.
- Systemic therapy may be used for some fungal infections and for serious bacterial infections.

Additional Learning Resources

SG Go to your Study Guide for additional learning activities to help you master this chapter content.

Go to your Evolve website (http://evolve.elsevier.com/deWit/medsurg) for the following FREE learning resources:
- Animations, audio, and video
- Answers and rationales for questions and activities
- Glossary with pronunciations in English and Spanish
- Interactive Review Questions and more!

Review Questions for the NCLEX® Examination

1. You note that a 55-year-old, light-skinned patient has dry, flaky skin. Which action by the patient should alert you to a problem?
   1. The patient always puts a moisturizing lotion on their hands after washing them.
   2. The patient takes daily showers with soap and hot water.
   3. The patient takes a daily multiple vitamin.
   4. The patient spends some time outdoors and uses sunscreen that they reapply every 1½ to 2 hours.

   NCLEX Client Need: Health Promotion and Maintenance
2. You are teaching teenagers about the importance of protecting the skin from UV rays. What information should you include? *(Select all that apply.)*
   1. Use a sunscreen with a sun protection factor (SPF) of at least 30.
   2. Apply sunscreen thinly.
   3. Wear light, loose clothing.
   4. Evaluate skin condition while in the sun.
   5. Wear sunglasses and a hat.

   NCLEX Client Need: Health Promotion and Maintenance
3. A patient with a suspicious skin lesion is scheduled for a punch skin biopsy. What is the most accurate explanation you would give about the procedure?
   1. "It is shaving a top layer off a lesion that rises above the skin line."
   2. "It is removing a core from the center of the lesion."
   3. "It is removing the entire lesion."
   4. "It is aspirating a tissue sample."

   NCLEX Client Need: Physiological Integrity: Reduction of Risk Potential
4. A patient has a rash of unknown origin. Which assessment question(s) would help determine the underlying cause of the lesion? *(Select all that apply.)*
   1. "When did the rash first appear?"
   2. "Can you think of any event or different food you ate or substance you were using just before it appeared?"
   3. "What drugs are you taking? Do you take any over-the-counter medications?"
   4. "Are you getting your usual amount of sleep?"
   5. "Is there a history of any skin disorders in your family?"

   NCLEX Client Need: Physiological Integrity: Physiological Adaptation
5. What physiologic changes in aging predispose older adults to skin breakdown? *(Select all that apply.)*
   1. Thickening of skin
   2. Loss of collagen
   3. Increased elastic fibers
   4. Decreased adipose tissues
   5. Reduced sebaceous gland activity

   NCLEX Client Need: Physiological Integrity: Physiological Adaptation
6. You need to apply a dressing to a patient who has fragile skin. Which intervention would you use to protect the patient from skin tears?
   1. Ask the health care provider to give specific orders for wound care.
   2. Gently clean and apply a sterile transparent dressing.
   3. Tape the dressing with paper tape and prevent tension.
   4. Allow any tape and gauze dressing materials to fall off naturally.

   NCLEX Client Need: Safe and Effective Care Environment: Safety and Infection Control
7. You are observing a nursing assistant who is providing skin care to an older adult patient. Which action by the nursing assistant indicates a need for further training?
   1. Using soap and hot water every day to clean the patient's body
   2. Alerting you about a wet dressing
   3. Reporting redness and blanching over the sacral area
   4. Applying lotion while the skin is still damp

   NCLEX Client Need: Safe and Effective Care Environment: Coordinated Care

8. You are supervising a new graduate nurse (GN) who is examining a new patient with skin lesions. You would intervene if the GN:
   1. gently handles the patient's extremities to prevent skin tears.
   2. observes the condition of the skin and measures the size of the lesions.
   3. removes the scales and crusts from the lesions to clean the skin.
   4. assesses for and documents any home remedies that the patient has tried.

   NCLEX Client Need: Safe and Effective Care Environment: Coordinated Care
9. You are taking care of a 75-year-old man who spends most of his time in bed or sitting. What steps should be taken to prevent a skin tear? *(Select all that apply.)*
   1. Have the patient wear long sleeves and long pants.
   2. Lubricate the patient's skin with cream or lotion twice a day.
   3. Massage the skin vigorously, especially over bony prominences.
   4. Never use a lift sheet to move or turn the patient.
   5. Pad bed rails, wheelchair arms, leg supports, or other equipment where the patient may bump an extremity.

   NCLEX Client Need: Physiological Integrity: Reduction of Risk Potential
10. You read in a patient's record that the health care provider observed "circumscribed, superficial vesicles with a collection of serous fluid." You anticipate that the health care provider will make which recommendation for the patient?
    1. A prescription for a topical application for acne
    2. Isolation precautions for herpes zoster
    3. Over-the-counter antihistamine for an insect bite
    4. Patient education to self-monitor the wart

    NCLEX Client Need: Physiological Integrity: Physiological Adaptation

Critical Thinking Questions

Scenario A

You have been asked to give a presentation to a ninth-grade class on skin care and prevention of skin cancer.

1. What specific information would you include about general skin care?
2. What would you say about lying out in the sun?
3. What information would you give regarding the use of indoor tanning?
4. What would you say about protection when out in the sun?

Scenario B

Mrs. Hess, an 83-year-old resident of a long-term care facility, has very dry skin. She asks you to look at spots on her hand that are brown and "ugly."

1. What could these lesions on Mrs. Hess's hand be?
2. What would you tell her?
3. Mrs. Hess asks you why she bruises so easily. She says she hates these reddish purple areas she gets on her arms and legs. What would you answer?
4. What nursing measures should be instituted for skin care for Mrs. Hess's dry skin?

Scenario C

You and a home health aide have been assigned to care for an older adult woman in the patient's home for several days. The patient has a noncontagious itchy rash, and the health care provider has suggested using oatmeal as a soothing bath and topical application of lotion and has ordered daily assessments to monitor the patient's condition. In addition, the patient's daughter has asked that the linens be washed daily.

1. Discuss which tasks you (i.e., the nurse) should perform.
2. Which tasks can be delegated or assigned to the home health aide? What specific instructions should be given to the home health aide about assigned duties?
3. During one of the home visits the daughter asks you to look at a mole on her back. "I can't see it very well, and of course my mother is not able to help me either." What would you do and say in this situation?

Care of Patients With Integumentary Disorders and Burns

43

http://evolve.elsevier.com/deWit/medsurg

Objectives

Theory

1. Describe the etiology of dermatitis.
2. Plan psychosocial interventions for a patient who has psoriasis.
3. Compare and contrast the treatment of fungal skin or nail disorders with the treatment of bacterial skin disorders.
4. Choose nursing interventions for a patient with herpes virus infection.
5. Examine the types of acne and their treatment.
6. Present the characteristics of the various types of skin cancer.
7. Analyze the important points of caring for an immobile patient to prevent pressure ulcers.
8. Construct a care plan for each stage of a pressure ulcer.
9. Summarize important assessment points for a patient who has sustained a burn.
10. Illustrate the nurse's role in emergency burn care.
11. Explain the psychosocial needs and interventions for burn patients.
12. Relate the process of rehabilitation for a patient with a major burn.

Clinical Practice

13. Teach a family about care for a patient and home when scabies is present.
14. Assess the skin of family members for signs of skin cancer.
15. Provide care for a patient with a stage III or stage IV pressure ulcer.
16. Apply Standard Precautions and sterile technique for the care of a burn.
17. Visit a burn intensive care unit and observe the wound care of a patient who is in the acute stage of a major burn.

Key Terms

allograft (ĂL-ō-grăft, p. 1014)
autograft (ĂW-tō-grăft, p. 1014)
autoinoculation (ăw-tō-ĭn-Ŏ-kū-LĀ-shŭn, p. 995)
biologic dressings (bī-ō-LŎJ-ĭk DRĔS-ĭngz, p. 1014)
biosynthetic (bī-ō-SĬN-thĕt-ĭk, p. 1014)
carbuncles (KĂR-bŭn-kŭlz, p. 995)
cellulitis (sĕl-ū-LĪ-tĭs, p. 995)
Curling ulcer ('kərliNG, 'əL-sər, p. 1009)
dermabrasion (dĕrm-ă-BRĀ-zhŭn, p. 993)
dermatophytosis (DĔR-mă-tō-fī-TŌ-sĭs, p. 997)
disseminated (dĭs-ĔM-ĕ-nāt-ĕd, p. 997)
eschar (ĔS-kăr, p. 1005)
escharotomy (ĔS-kă-RŎ-tō-mē, p. 1014)
furuncles (fyū-RŬN-kŭlz, p. 995)
mycoses (mī-KŌ-sēz, p. 997)
onychomycosis (ŏn-ĭ-kō-mī-KŌ-sĭs, p. 998)
purulent (PŪ-rū-lĕnt, p. 1008)
serosanguineous (SĔR-ō-săng-GWĬN-ē-ŭs, p. 1008)
shearing action (shər-iNG, AK-shən, p. 1003)
telangiectases (tē-lăn-jē-ĔK-tŭ-sēz, p. 992)
tinea pedis (TĬN-ē-ă pē-dĭs, p. 997)
xenograft (ZĒ-nō-grăft, p. 1014)

Concepts Covered in This Chapter

- Functional Ability
- Adherence
- Fluid and Electrolytes
- Thermoregulation
- Cellular Regulation
- Nutrition
- Perfusion
- Inflammation
- Infection
- Pain
- Stress
- Patient Education
- Collaboration

INFLAMMATORY INFECTIONS

Many skin diseases result from infection with bacteria, viruses, or fungi or from infestation with parasites. Diseases of this kind require special precautions to prevent spread of the infectious organism or the parasite. Hand hygiene is a first-line measure in the prevention of health care–associated infections and is mandated as one of The Joint Commission's National Patient Safety Goals. Infectious Disease National Centers, a division of the Centers for Disease Control and Prevention (CDC), recommends that contact precautions, as well as Standard Precautions, be implemented for a number of these diseases (Box 43.1). Some skin infections are not necessarily contagious; however, it can be difficult to quickly determine whether a condition is a contagious type at the initial examination. Therefore isolate the patient, perform hand hygiene, and use Standard Precautions (see Appendix B) if there is any doubt.

Box 43.1 Review of Contact Precautions

Specifications for contact precautions are as follows:

- A private room is indicated. In general, patients infected with the same type of organism may share a room.
- Gloves are worn when entering the room. Change gloves after contact with infective material, such as wound drainage or feces, and before treating a different location on the body. Perform hand hygiene before donning clean gloves.
- Remove gloves when leaving the room and perform hand hygiene using an antimicrobial agent.
- Gowns are indicated if soiling is likely, particularly if there is drainage from an uncovered wound or the patient is incontinent.
- Articles contaminated with infective material should be discarded in a biohazard waste receptacle or bagged and labeled before being sent for decontamination and reprocessing.
- Patient care equipment should be used only for the one patient and should be left in the room until no longer needed.
- Skin disorders that require contact precautions include:
  - Furunculosis, group A *Streptococcus*
  - Herpes simplex, disseminated, severe primary, or neonatal
  - Herpes zoster (varicella zoster) disseminated also requires airborne precautions
  - Impetigo
  - Infection or colonization by bacteria with multiple drug resistance (any site)
  - Pediculosis
  - Scabies
  - Skin wound or burn infection, major (draining and not covered by dressing, or dressing does not adequately contain purulent material), including those infected with *Staphylococcus aureus*
  - Vaccinia (generalized and progressive eczema vaccinatum)

DERMATITIS

Dermatitis is not contagious unless a secondary infection has occurred in the lesions.

Etiology, Pathophysiology, Signs, and Symptoms

Contact dermatitis is a delayed allergic response involving cell-mediated immunity. On contact with the skin, the allergen is bound to a carrier protein and forms a sensitizing antigen. T cells become sensitized to the antigen. Local skin irritation is evident within a few hours or days after exposure to an antigen. Erythema and swelling, pruritus, and the appearance of vesicular lesions follow. Many chemicals; cosmetics; soaps; latex; and poison ivy, oak, and sumac are contact irritants and can cause such a reaction.

Atopic dermatitis (also called eczema) affects about 10% of the population and is more common in infancy and childhood but does affect some adults. It results from a complex activation process that involves mast cells, T lymphocytes, Langerhans cells, monocytes, B cells that produce immunoglobulin E, and other inflammatory cells that release histamine, lymphokines, and other inflammatory mediators. Atopic dermatitis does seem to have a genetic, allergic association because it is more prevalent in families.

Stasis dermatitis generally occurs on the legs as a result of venous stasis and edema and is seen in conjunction with varicosities, phlebitis, and vascular trauma. Erythema and pruritus occur first, after which scaling, development of petechiae, and **hyperpigmentation** (excessive pigmentation) occur. Lesions may become ulcerated, particularly around the ankles and tibia.

Seborrheic dermatitis is a common inflammation involving the scalp, eyebrows, eyelids, ear canals, nasolabial folds, axillae, chest, and back. It is most common on the scalp. The cause is unknown. Lesions appear as scaly white or yellowish plaques with mild pruritus.

Diagnosis and Treatment

Dermatitis is diagnosed by inspection and by compiling a complete history, looking for possible exposure to causative substances.

In general, treatment is aimed at avoidance of the contact irritant or allergen, good skin lubrication, preservation of skin moisture, and control of inflammation and itching. Topical agents are often used. Corticosteroids may be used topically or sometimes orally or by injection to intervene in a severe episode of dermatitis.

Nursing Management

Teach patients to avoid contact irritants and to properly care for their skin. Instruct them in the proper way to apply topical agents. Caution any patient who is experiencing pruritus to avoid becoming hot, bathe in tepid water, and not puncture vesicles. The skin should be patted dry rather than rubbed dry.

ACNE

Etiology, Pathophysiology, Signs, and Symptoms

Acne is a disorder of the skin characterized by papules and pustules over the face, back, and shoulders. Some types of acne are related to cosmetics or to chemicals in the environment. For example, occupational acne is caused by prolonged contact with oils and tars.

There are many kinds of acne, but the two major types are **acne rosacea** and **acne vulgaris.** Acne rosacea usually begins between ages 30 and 50 years. It is characterized by erythema (redness), papules, pustules, and **telangiectases** (dilation of capillaries causing small red or purple clusters, also called "spider veins"). It occurs on the face over the cheeks and bridge of the nose. **Comedos** (dilated hair follicles filled with skin debris, bacteria, and sebum) do not occur. Factors that cause facial flushing precipitate worsening. Tea, coffee, alcohol (especially wine), caffeine-containing foods, spicy foods, sunlight, and emotional stress cause flare-ups.

Acne vulgaris is more common than acne rosacea. Factors that contribute to the development of acne include hereditary disposition, increased androgen levels, and premenstrual hormonal fluctuations. Use of heavy creams, use of certain drugs, and exposure to increased heat also contribute to the disorder. Acne vulgaris typically begins in early puberty, continues through the teens, and then begins to subside. Occasionally it persists, or it can recur several years later. The onset of acne vulgaris in adolescents is related to increased release of sex hormones, which stimulate activity of the sebaceous glands, causing increased production of sebum. Ducts leading from the sebaceous glands become plugged with sebum. It is not known why in some persons the ducts from these glands become plugged, but the increased production of sebum triggers the formation of blackheads and whiteheads. The color of blackheads results from particles of melanin, the skin's own pigment, combined with sebum and keratin. Accumulations of sebum, skin particles, and dead skin cells can cause an inflammatory reaction. Bacterial infection leads to the formation of pustules. An extensive inflammation can lead to the formation of cysts, with swelling above and below the surface of the skin.

There are many misconceptions about acne vulgaris and its treatment. It is not a contagious disease. It is not caused by uncleanliness or poor personal hygiene. Diet can contribute to the formation of lesions, but generally there is little or no relationship between the intake of certain foods and the appearance of the lesions of acne. Typically, chocolate, colas, and fried foods do not need to be eliminated from the diet in an effort to prevent or cure acne. A well-balanced diet is all that is recommended in the management of acne.

Diagnosis and Treatment

Diagnosis is by history and physical examination. Acne rosacea is treated by avoiding the triggers for flare-ups and with topical antibiotics, metronidazole (MetroGel), and retinoids. Sometimes oral antibiotics are prescribed.

Mild, noninflammatory cases of acne vulgaris respond well to efforts to remove blackheads and whiteheads by promoting dryness and peeling of the top layer of skin. The medication is applied directly on the skin. Nonprescription drugs, such as lotions, creams, and gels that contain sulfur, benzoyl peroxide, or sulfur combined with resorcinol usually are effective for noninflammatory acne.

Among the topical medications, retinoic acid (tretinoin [Retin-A]) is the best agent for **papular** and **pustular** acne problems. It should be used once or twice a day. Benzoyl peroxide is the most commonly used topical agent for acne and is available both by prescription and over the counter. Azelaic acid (Azelex) is applied topically twice a day. The U.S. Food and Drug Administration (FDA) has approved Veltin Gel, a water-based topical agent, for the treatment of acne vulgaris in patients 12 years and older (Drugs.com, 2018). It is expensive, but financial assistance is available.

Antibiotics such as tetracycline and erythromycin also are sometimes prescribed topically and orally for cystic acne to inhibit the growth of bacteria in the plugged ducts.

Isotretinoin (13-*cis*-retinoic acid) has been especially effective in controlling cases of cystic acne that are resistant to other forms of treatment. The drug was initially marketed under the trade name Accutane, but after black box warnings and increasing numbers of reports of adverse events, including gastrointestinal concerns, birth defects, and increased rates of suicide, Roche discontinued marketing Accutane in the United States in 2009. It is still available in generic form and by other trade names (FDA, 2018). Isotretinoin is taken by mouth daily for 2 to 4 months and inhibits activity of the sebaceous glands. Its effects are sustained for months to years after it has been discontinued. Almost all patients experience some adverse reaction to this drug. **Isotretinoin is used only for severe cystic acne that is resistant to all other treatment. There are serious adverse side effects, including organ damage and mental problems.** Laboratory testing includes hemoglobin, hematocrit, glucose, triglycerides, uric acid, alkaline phosphatase, and liver enzymes.

For larger areas, lasers or a light treatment called *photodynamic therapy* has been used with success. A photosensitive solution is applied to the skin and remains until absorbed. Light is then applied, which activates the chemicals, destroying the target cells. Photodynamic therapy was originally designed for treatment of cancer cells but has been shown to be effective for acne.

If the patient has deep scarring and pitting as a result of cystic acne, their appearance can be improved by **dermabrasion**. This dermatologic procedure involves mechanically scraping away the outer layers of skin and smoothing out its surface by applying motor-driven wire brushes or diamond wheels. Chemical dermabrasion is done by applying phenol or trichloroacetic acid to remove the scars.

Nursing Management

Teach the patient about the nature of their skin disease and give support while they are trying to cope with its physiologic and psychosocial effects. Acne can be particularly distressing to adolescents, who are often deeply concerned about their appearance and acceptance by their peers.

The face should be washed gently with a mild soap. Scrubbing the skin and using a harsh soap is damaging and contributes to inflammation. Special medicated soaps do not seem to be any better than a mild face soap. If the hair is oily, it should be shampooed frequently and kept off the face.

Squeezing pimples and pustules is not recommended. This can press the sebum and accumulated material more firmly into the clogged duct, increase the chance of inflammation, and spread an infection to other parts of the skin and body. Blackheads and whiteheads are best removed by applying a prescription medication that causes peeling of the skin. The hands should be kept off of the face.

Because the management of acne can go on for years and requires periodic evaluation by a dermatologist, patients and their families will need continued support and encouragement to follow the prescribed regimen. They will need to know the expected results of prescribed medications, any adverse reactions that might occur, and symptoms that should be reported immediately.

? Think Critically

What skin care measures would you recommend to a young teenager who is just beginning to experience face blemishes such as blackheads or whiteheads? The kids at school are calling them "scab face."

PSORIASIS

Etiology, Pathophysiology, Signs, and Symptoms

Psoriasis is a noncontagious, chronic, recurring skin disorder that typically appears as inflamed, edematous skin lesions covered with adherent silvery-white scales (Fig. 43.1). These scales are the result of an abnormally rapid rate of proliferation of skin cells. When the scales are removed, there is pinpoint bleeding. The plaques most often appear on the skin of the elbows, knees, and base of the spine. It also may affect the scalp, in which case it can be confused with **seborrheic dermatitis.** When the fingernails are involved, there can be pitting of the surface of the nails. The palms and soles also can be affected, making it difficult for the patient to carry out activities of daily living (ADLs).

In some cases the skin eruptions of psoriasis are accompanied by inflammation of the joints, especially those of the fingers and toes. This is called *psoriatic arthritis.* Psoriasis affects about 2% of the U.S. population. There is a genetic predisposition for the disease. It is likely that an immunologic event triggers the disorder because the first lesion commonly appears after an upper respiratory infection. T cells are mistakenly activated and trigger immune responses that speed up the growth cycle of skin cells. There is increasing evidence that the chronic inflammation of psoriasis may be a multisystem disorder. In addition to psoriatic arthritis, chronic kidney disease, cardiovascular disease, malignancy, and psychiatric disorders have all been linked to psoriasis (Korman, 2019).

Diagnosis and Treatment

Diagnosis is by history, physical examination, and ruling out other skin disorders. Each case of psoriasis is treated individually. The disease is unpredictable, tends to go into remission spontaneously, and sometimes will clear up temporarily with or without treatment.

Mild cases usually respond to steroid creams (triamcinolone acetonide [Kenalog]), but there is a possibility that eventually the disease will become resistant to steroids. Sunlight in moderate doses can help because the ultraviolet (UV) rays slow down the rate at which epithelial cells are produced. Extremes of UV radiation can have the opposite effect, resulting in an aggravation of the condition. Calcipotriene (Dovonex), a vitamin D analog cream, helps regulate skin cell production, decreasing the incidence of psoriasis plaques.

Tar preparations also act to impede the proliferation of skin cells and have long been used to heal psoriasis lesions. They may be administered in the form of baths, topical applications, or shampoos. Combinations of artificial UV radiation and a coal tar product commonly are prescribed for severe cases. This usually requires hospitalization so that the dosage of each component of therapy can be measured precisely. A form of therapy called *PUVA* combines application of one of a class of drugs called psoralens, which penetrates the skin, with exposure to ultraviolet light type A (UVA).

Antimetabolites have been used to treat severe psoriasis, helping to control the disorder by their antiproliferative action. Methotrexate is the most commonly used antimetabolite for this purpose. Acitretin (Soriatane) or cyclosporine is sometimes used. Brodalumab (Siliq) was FDA approved in 2017 as an injectable monoclonal antibody for use in psoriasis. It carries a black box warning regarding suicidal ideation and behavior. Other biologic agents shown to be efficacious include

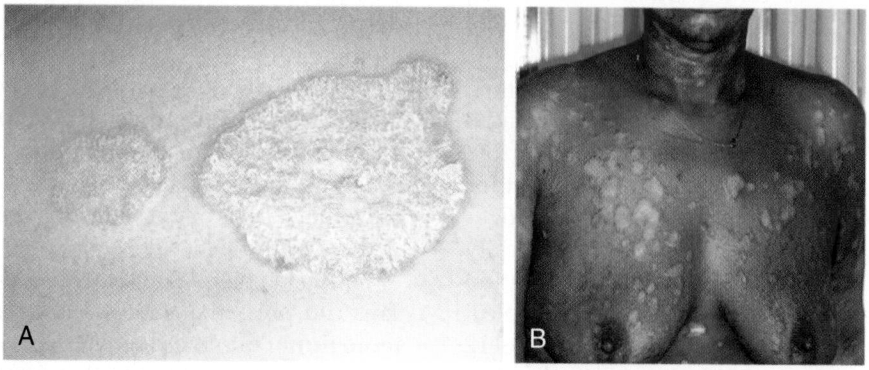

Fig. 43.1 **A,** Psoriasis vulgaris in a white patient. **B,** Psoriasis vulgaris in a patient with dark skin. (From Ignatavicius DD, Workman ML, Rebar CR: *Medical-surgical nursing: concepts for interprofessional collaborative care,* ed 9, St. Louis, 2018, Elsevier.)

infliximab (Remicade), etanercept (Embrel), efalizumab (Raptiva), and alefacept (Amevive).

Nursing Management

Patients with psoriasis will need instruction about the nature of their disease, teaching about the purpose of the prescribed treatment, and information about ways to avoid aggravating it. **The skin should be kept as moist and pliable as possible. Humidifiers to increase moisture in the environment are sometimes helpful.** Lubricating lotions and creams should be approved by the dermatologist before they are applied.

Minor scratches and abrasions and bacterial infections can trigger the formation of lesions at a new site. **Because any irritation or break in the skin seems to stimulate the growth of psoriatic plaques in a person susceptible to psoriasis, the patient should be cautioned to prevent injury of any kind.** This includes hangnails, damaged cuticles, blisters from poorly fitting shoes, scratches from pets, and potentially harmful agents in the environment such as radiation and chemicals.

STEVENS-JOHNSON SYNDROME

Stevens-Johnson syndrome (SJS) is an allergic reaction with skin manifestations. It can be caused by an infection, malignancy, or medication or be categorized as idiopathic. Medications that have been shown to cause the condition include the anticonvulsants carbamazepine (Tegretol) and phenytoin (Dilantin), the antimalarial sulfadoxine-pyrimethamine (Fansidar), and the antibiotic sulfamethoxazole-trimethoprim (Bactrim, Septra). However, over-the-counter medications can also cause SJS. Lesions that may be mistaken for chickenpox develop on the face, trunk, palms, extensor surfaces of joints, soles of the feet, and dorsum of the hands. The lesions have irregular borders and may have blistered, necrotic centers. There is evidence that a strong genetic predisposition may put patients at risk.

Treatment of SJS involves discontinuing the drug and providing supportive care with fluids and nutrition. Wound care is similar to that for a burn. The lesions are painful, and analgesia is provided. Sedatives may be necessary. If not treated early, SJS can cause death.

> **Clinical Cues**
>
> Assess the skin of every patient daily. Ask assistive personnel if they have observed any changes. If new skin lesions appear, seek an opinion from a health care provider. Check the medication profile and medication history to see what medications the patient has been receiving. Alert the provider if the patient has been taking a medication known to cause SJS.

BACTERIAL INFECTIONS

ETIOLOGY, PATHOPHYSIOLOGY, SIGNS, AND SYMPTOMS

Cellulitis is an infection of the dermis and subcutaneous tissue and is generally caused by *Staphylococcus*. It may occur as an extension of a skin wound, as an ulcer, or from furuncles or carbuncles. The area will be erythematous, swollen, and painful. It is treated with systemic antibiotics, and Burow soaks may be used to relieve pain. Burow solution is an astringent and topical antiseptic also called *aluminum acetate solution*.

Furuncles (boils) or skin abscesses are inflammations of hair follicles. The organism responsible is usually *Staphylococcus aureus*. Any skin area with hair can be affected. Initially there is a deep, firm, red, painful nodule 1 to 5 cm in diameter. The nodule changes to a large and tender cystic nodule accompanied by cellulitis. The lesion may drain large amounts of pus and necrotic tissue.

Carbuncles are a collection of boils that have multiple pus "heads," most commonly occur on the back of the neck, the upper back, and the lateral thighs. It begins as a firm mass and evolves into an erythematous, painful, swollen mass. It may drain through many openings in the mass. Abscesses may develop with fever, chills, and malaise.

DIAGNOSIS, TREATMENT, AND NURSING MANAGEMENT

Diagnosis is by history and examination. Treatment of any infected mass with pus is drainage of the lesion. If necrotic tissue is present, debridement should be performed. Antibiotics are given when indicated.

Nursing interventions are aimed at healing the infected areas and preventing recurrence. The patient is taught to avoid using cosmetic products and over-the-counter topical remedies on the affected areas. After incision and drainage, a dry absorbent dressing is applied and changed after 24 hours. Absorbent dressings are used until the wound stops draining, then a simple gauze covering is adequate. A clean washcloth and towel should be used for bathing each day until the wound is healed. Linens should be washed in hot soapy water and thoroughly dried before reuse.

VIRAL INFECTIONS

HERPES SIMPLEX

Herpes simplex virus type 2 (HSV-2) is most often associated with genital herpes, whereas herpes simplex virus type 1 (HSV-1) lesions are primarily orofacial (Fig. 43.2). Either type can cause lesions in the genital area as well as other regions of the body. **Autoinoculation** of the virus is possible by direct contact—for example, lips to fingers to genitals or lips to fingers to eyes.

> **Health Promotion**
>
> **Preventing Spread of Herpesvirus**
>
> Humans are the only species affected by HSV-1 and HSV-2, and the virus is spread by direct contact. The virus can be "shed" or transmitted even when symptoms are not present. Immunocompromised individuals are at greatest risk of acquiring the infection. If lesions are present, care should be taken to not have direct skin contact.

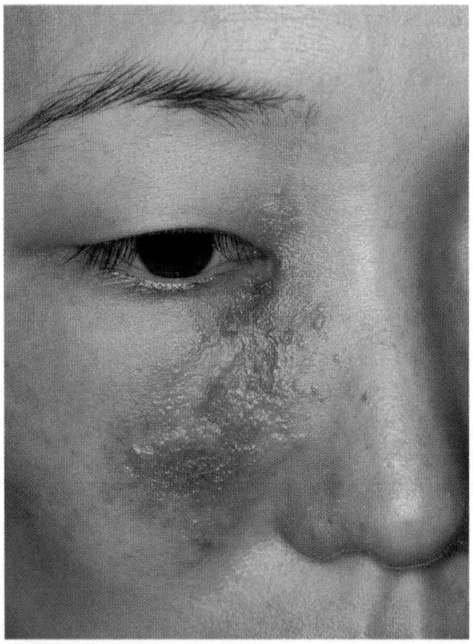

Fig. 43.2 Herpes simplex virus lesions. (From Bolognia JL, Schaffer JV, Duncan KO, et al.: *Dermatology essentials,* Philadelphia, 2014, Elsevier.)

Complementary and Alternative Therapies

Lemon Balm for Cold Sores

Lemon balm in a concentrated cream base has often been used to relieve the symptoms of **herpes labialis** (infection of the lips; commonly known as *cold sores* or *fever blisters*). In clinical studies it has been shown to shorten the healing period and prevent the spread of infection (Rakel, 2018).

Etiology and Pathophysiology

When initial infection occurs, the virus is imbedded in a nerve ganglion that innervates the site of the lesion. Reactivation of the virus causes new lesions to occur at the same site. The virus travels along the nerve to the site of the original infection. Reactivation is brought about by exposure to ultraviolet light, skin irritation, fever, fatigue, or stress.

Signs and Symptoms

An infection with HSV-1 appears as lesions on the lips and nares that are commonly called *cold sores* or *fever blisters.* The lesions are usually painful but do not cause systemic symptoms.

Diagnosis, Treatment, and Nursing Management

Diagnosis is by physical examination and history. Sometimes topical and oral acyclovir (Zovirax), famciclovir (Famvir), or valacyclovir (Valtrex), available by prescription, hastens healing. The symptoms of itching and burning that accompany oral herpes infection sometimes can be minimized by applying warm compresses to the sores, followed by local application of tincture of benzoin or spirits of camphor to aid drying and facilitate healing. The disease usually is self-limiting, which means that it does not progress and will subside on its own, but it can recur. Contagion is possible up to 5 days after appearance of the lesion. Docosanol cream (Abreva) sold over the counter is a helpful treatment for this disorder.

Patients should be cautioned to use good personal hygiene to prevent spreading the virus to the eyes and genital area and other body parts. Hand hygiene is a simple but essential part of preventing spread of the virus.

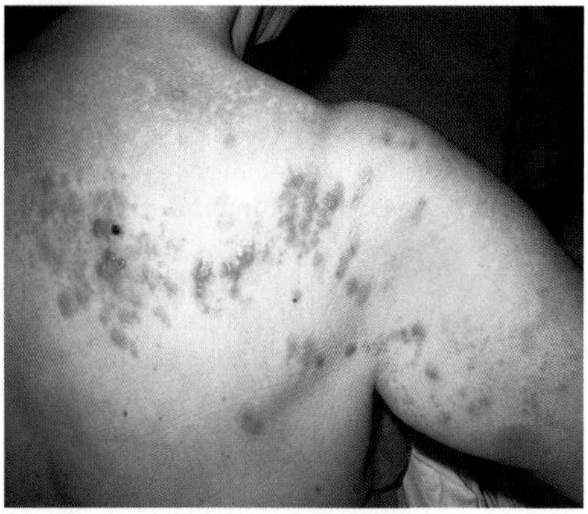

Fig. 43.3 Herpes zoster (shingles). (From Ignatavicius DD, Workman ML: *Medical-surgical nursing: concepts for interprofessional collaborative care,* ed 7, Philadelphia, 2017, Elsevier.)

HERPES ZOSTER

Etiology and Pathophysiology

Herpes varicella-zoster causes chickenpox (varicella), mostly in young children, and shingles (zoster) in all ages. In herpes zoster, the herpes viruses replicate in the peripheral nerve ganglia, where they lie dormant until reactivated by trauma, malignancy, stress, or local radiation (Fig. 43.3). Approximately 1 million cases per year occur in the United States, and about 1 in 3 people will be affected at some point in their lifetime (CDC, 2018). The risk is greater for immunocompromised individuals (those with cancer or human immunodeficiency virus/acquired immunodeficiency syndrome [HIV/AIDS]). The varicella vaccine is given in two doses to children to prevent chickenpox. The first is given at age 12 to 18 months and the second at age 4 to 6 years.

Older Adult Care Points

Approximately 50% of individuals who live past 80 years of age develop shingles. The CDC recommends use of Shingrix, a vaccine that boosts the immune response to the zoster virus. Zostavax is a live virus vaccine that is about 50% effective in preventing shingles; it appears to be effective in attenuating the disorder if it occurs and is effective for about 6 years. Zostavax is contraindicated in immunocompromised patients (CDC, 2018a).

Signs and Symptoms

Herpes zoster begins with vague symptoms of fatigue and low-grade fever and possibly loss of appetite. There may be only aching or discomfort along the nerve pathway with or without erythema. About 3 to 5 days after onset, small groups of vesicles appear on the skin. They usually are found on the trunk and spread halfway around the body, following the nerve pathways leading from the spinal nerve to the skin.

Safety Alert

Danger of Herpes Zoster Transmission

No health care worker or visitor should be in contact with a patient who has chickenpox or shingles if they have never had the disease or the two doses of the varicella vaccination. A pregnant woman should not care for a patient with chickenpox or herpes zoster. The virus is highly contagious and can harm a fetus.

The vesicles eventually change from small blisters to scaly lesions and are accompanied by pain and itching. The lesions usually affect only one side of the body or face. The pain of shingles often is quite severe. Pain can persist for several days or weeks after the skin lesions are completely healed. The pain of postherpetic syndrome is not easy to control.

Diagnosis and Treatment

Diagnosis is by history and physical examination. There is no cure for herpes zoster. The condition can persist for months, especially in older and debilitated patients. Herpes infections may be recurrent because complete immunity does not occur. **The earlier the condition is diagnosed and treatment begins, the better are the chances to decrease the amount and duration of the associated pain** (CDC, 2018a).

Symptomatic treatment typically involves administering an analgesic to relieve pain. Capsaicin, an over-the-counter analgesic that is applied topically five times a day, decreases pain for some patients. A paste made from aspirin and water placed on the lesions decreases pain for others. Antibiotics may be prescribed prophylactically against secondary bacterial infection of the lesions. Most health care providers prescribe oral acyclovir (Zovirax), famciclovir (Famvir), or valacyclovir (Valtrex) to diminish the extent or duration of the lesions. Valacyclovir is used only in otherwise healthy patients. Famciclovir, if given within the first 2 to 3 days of the outbreak, seems to shorten the duration of the chronic pain that typically follows shingles. Tricyclic antidepressants and gabapentin (Neurontin), an anticonvulsant drug, have been used with variable success at controlling pain.

Narcotic analgesics are avoided if possible because they can lead to addiction when used for an extended time. If the pain persists and is intractable, the provider prescribes a corticosteroid to reduce inflammation. Vidarabine, administered intravenously (IV), is sometimes given to patients who have an immune deficiency. It is usually effective in reducing, if not completely relieving, the pain.

Although shingles may be difficult to live with while the disease is running its course, the only lasting complication from the disease is postherpetic neuralgia. More serious but rare complications include outbreaks near the eye, in which case it can cause blindness or disseminated disease that can be life-threatening. The prognosis is less favorable in patients who have an underlying malignancy or who are immunocompromised.

Nursing Management

Care includes symptomatic relief from the pain and itching and prevention of a secondary bacterial infection.

Complementary and Alternative Therapies

Tai Chi Boosts Immunity to Shingles

Research has shown that practicing tai chi resulted in a level of immune response close to that of the varicella vaccine and that tai chi boosted the positive effects of the vaccine. The meta-analysis studied seven randomized, controlled trials, four controlled clinical trials, and five retrospective case-controlled studies (Ho et al., 2013).

Cold compresses (with Burow solution), calamine lotion, and diversional activities are sometimes helpful. Rest and adequate nutrition can promote healing and shorten the acute phase of shingles. Teaching imagery, deep muscle relaxation, or use of distraction activities may help decrease pain. Evidence supports initiation of isolation procedures based on symptoms rather than waiting for a confirmed diagnosis. If lesions are **disseminated**, meaning widely dispersed, or if the patient is immunocompromised, airborne and contact precautions are necessary until all the blisters are crusted. If the lesions are localized and can be kept covered and the patient is not immunocompromised, Standard Precautions are sufficient (CDC, 2018a).

FUNGAL INFECTIONS

Fungal infections are called **mycoses**; systemic fungal infections involving the lungs and other internal organs are called *systemic mycoses*. There are two groups of fungi that cause infections in humans: (1) fungi that are truly pathogenic to humans and (2) fungi that cause **opportunistic infections** (can cause an infection when the host has an altered immune system).

True pathogenic fungi can cause infection in an otherwise healthy person, but relatively few fungi are able to do this. Fungal infections are rarely fatal if they involve only the superficial tissues of the body. Nevertheless, mycotic skin infections can be exasperating because they are difficult to diagnose and often resistant to treatment.

The most common types of fungal infections involving the skin are **tinea pedis** (athlete's foot or **dermatophytosis**), **tinea cruris** (jock itch), **tinea capitis** (commonly known as *ringworm*), and **tinea barbae** (barber's itch). **Moniliasis**

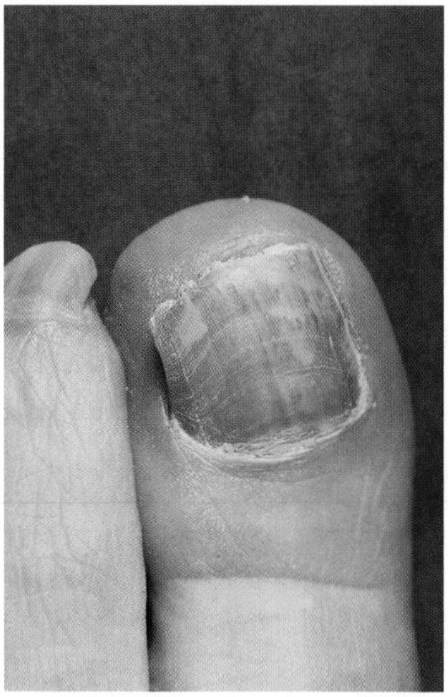

Fig. 43.4 Onychomycosis (nail fungus).

(thrush) is a fungal infection that can attack the mucous membranes of the mouth, rectum, and vagina **(candidiasis).** (This condition is discussed more fully in Chapter 11.)

The skin fungal infections produce itching, some swelling, and a breakdown of tissue. Because fungi thrive in warm, moist places, a tropical climate or other environmental factors that produce prolonged heat and moisture can encourage the development of fungal infections.

Older adults are prone to develop fungal infections of the fingernails or toenails (**onychomycosis**) (Fig. 43.4). Hands and feet should be thoroughly dried after becoming wet, with special attention to drying between the toes after the bath or shower. Nails should be cut straight across without rounding the edges. Wearing clean socks daily helps prevent fungal growth. In the toenails, the condition may become quite painful. Treatment requires oral antifungal medication daily for several months or topical agents daily for a year or more.

Complementary and Alternative Therapies

Treatment of Nail Fungus

Tea tree oil used topically daily on the nail and cuticle has been successful in treatment of yeast and fungal infection (Micozzil, 2019). It must be used regularly to be effective and may take weeks or months to cure the infection. Another inexpensive treatment that may work with consistent daily use is the topical application of Vicks VapoRub twice a day. This salve contains camphor, menthol, and eucalyptus. It seems to arrest the development of further fungal growth, allowing a fungus-free nail to grow. It takes about 6 months of treatment and is not effective for everyone.

There are many side effects of the oral antifungal medications. Liver function should be monitored during drug administration. Diagnosis of fungal infections is confirmed by microscopic examination of skin scrapings that have been treated with potassium hydroxide (KOH) solution. Fungal specimens generally show the typical filaments of fungal organisms. Patients should be taught how to prevent recurrence of fungal infections.

Patient Teaching

Preventing Recurrent Fungal Infection

Instruct the patient to do the following:

- Wear shoes that provide ventilation for the feet. Wear cotton socks when rubber-soled shoes or sneakers must be worn.
- Wash and dry the feet at least daily, being careful to completely dry the skin between the toes.
- Sprinkle an antifungal powder on the feet and between the toes if there is a tendency for athlete's foot. An antifungal spray may be used rather than powder.
- Change hose or socks daily; do not wear them more than 1 day without washing.
- Change underpants or shorts daily; do not wear them more than 1 day without washing.
- Use only clean towels, changing them at least every other day. Do not share towels or washcloths.
- Change bed linens at least once a week and wash in hot water.
- Do not use the combs, hairbrushes, hair clips, or hair ties of others and do not allow them to use yours.
- Inspect pets regularly for ringworm. Have a veterinarian check the animal if an infection is suspected.

TINEA PEDIS

Tinea pedis (athlete's foot) affects the feet, particularly between the toes. The infection may spread to the entire foot and cause blistering, peeling, cracking, and itching. If it continues unchecked, it can spread to other parts of the body. The condition can be complicated by a severe bacterial infection.

Etiology, Pathophysiology, Signs, and Symptoms

Most cases of tinea pedis are contracted and spread in swimming pools, spas, showers, and other public facilities of this type. *Trichophyton mentagrophytes* and *Trichophyton rubrum* are the usual infecting agents. These organisms may be normal flora that spread easily under conditions of excessive warmth and moisture. The skin between the toes becomes inflamed and develops cracks that become painful fissures. Intense itching is common.

Diagnosis and Treatment

Diagnosis is by physical examination. Treatment of tinea pedis consists of keeping the area dry, clean, and exposed to the air and sunlight as much as possible. Clean cotton socks should be worn every day, and the affected areas between the toes should be separated by gauze or cotton. Soaks of Burow solution help. Various topical antifungals, including ciclopirox (Loprox), miconazole, clotrimazole (Mycelex), econazole (Spectazole), ketoconazole (Nizoral), and naftifine (Naftin), can be prescribed. Most of the prescription medications are available over the counter in a lesser concentration. Some medicated powders, such as undecylenic acid–zinc undecylenate, work to keep the feet dry and also help control fungal growth. Systemic treatment for stubborn infection includes oral itraconazole (Sporanox) and terbinafine (Lamisil).

Nursing Management

Encourage the patient to keep the feet clean and dry and to wear clean cotton socks every day. Daily application of the topical agent must be done diligently to eradicate the problem. The patient should only use their own towel, and the shower or tub should be thoroughly cleaned and disinfected after bathing to prevent transmission to other family members. Personal footwear should be used in public places, such as the swimming pool and in the showers at fitness centers, and feet should be washed and dried thoroughly after using public facilities.

PARASITIC INFECTIONS

PEDICULOSIS AND SCABIES

Etiology and Pathophysiology

The parasites that cause **pediculosis** and **scabies** are found throughout the world in all types of climates. They can infest anyone. The parasites are particularly troublesome, however, where people live in crowded conditions and do not maintain their personal hygiene. The occurrence of pediculosis and scabies in the United States has recently increased significantly because of the growth of the homeless population and communal living. These parasites are often found among schoolchildren. The parasites are also found in nursing homes, dormitories, and sometimes hospitals.

Three basic types of lice that infest human beings are (1) the head louse, *Pediculus humanis capitis;* (2) the body louse, *Pediculus humanis corporis* (Fig. 43.5); and (3) the pubic or crab louse, *Phthirus pubis.* In addition, human beings also may be infested by *Sarcoptes scabiei,* the mange mite that produces scabies. The lice are oval and 2 to 4 mm long. All types are acquired by contact with infested people or their clothing, bed linens, and bedding. Pets have also been known to carry lice and the scabies mite.

Signs and Symptoms

The most prevalent symptom of louse infestation is severe itching. The resultant scratching can lead to excoriation of the skin and secondary infection causing impetigo, furunculosis, and cellulitis. Systemic infections are not commonly associated with louse infestation, but they carry bacteria that can cause epidemics such as louse-borne typhus, trench fever, and louse-borne relapsing fever (Guenther, 2018). If the lice infest the eyelids and eyelashes, the eyelids become red and swollen. Swelling may also occur in the lymph glands of the neck of a person heavily infested with head lice.

The scabies mites burrow under the top layers of the skin and live their entire lives there. They are more likely to be found in the skin between the fingers and toes, in the groin, and in other areas where there may be folds of skin. Excretions from the mites produce irritation with intense itching and blistering. Secondary infection is not uncommon with scabies, and some deaths have occurred when the scabies infestation has led to pneumonia or septicemia.

Diagnosis

Diagnosis is by body inspection and by examination of skin scraping of a lesion under the microscope. Lice eggs (known as nits) are deposited at the base of hair shafts and can be seen on close inspection. Scabies causes curved or linear white or erythematous ridges in the skin that are easily visible.

Treatment

The drugs most commonly used and considered most effective against lice and scabies are permethrin (Nix, Elimite), pyrethrins (RID), and malathion (Ovide). Some are available over the counter. These substances must be used carefully and the patient's liver function monitored because they can be very toxic. They are available as creams, lotions, and shampoos. A fine-toothed (nit) comb is then used to remove the nits (eggs) that may have remained on the hair. Benzyl alcohol lotion 5% (Ulesfia) is effective for head lice. It works by suffocating the lice. The amount required is based on the length of the hair, and a second treatment is required in 7 days (Guenther, 2018).

Nursing Management

Contact precautions are recommended. In addition, clothing, bedding, hats, stuffed animals, and other infested articles must be decontaminated to prevent reinfection. Laundering in hot water and machine drying using the hottest cycle is effective. Dry cleaning of nonwashable bed coverings or clothing can be effective. Mattresses, upholstered furniture, carpets, and other articles should be sprayed with a specific disinfectant. All combs and brushes should be soaked in very hot water for more than 5 minutes. For items that cannot be cleaned, such as some stuffed animals, sealing them in plastic bags with the air expelled for 14 days can be effective. All family members must receive instruction about the infection and ways to prevent reinfestation.

? Think Critically

How would you approach and instruct the parents of an 8-year-old who has scabies?

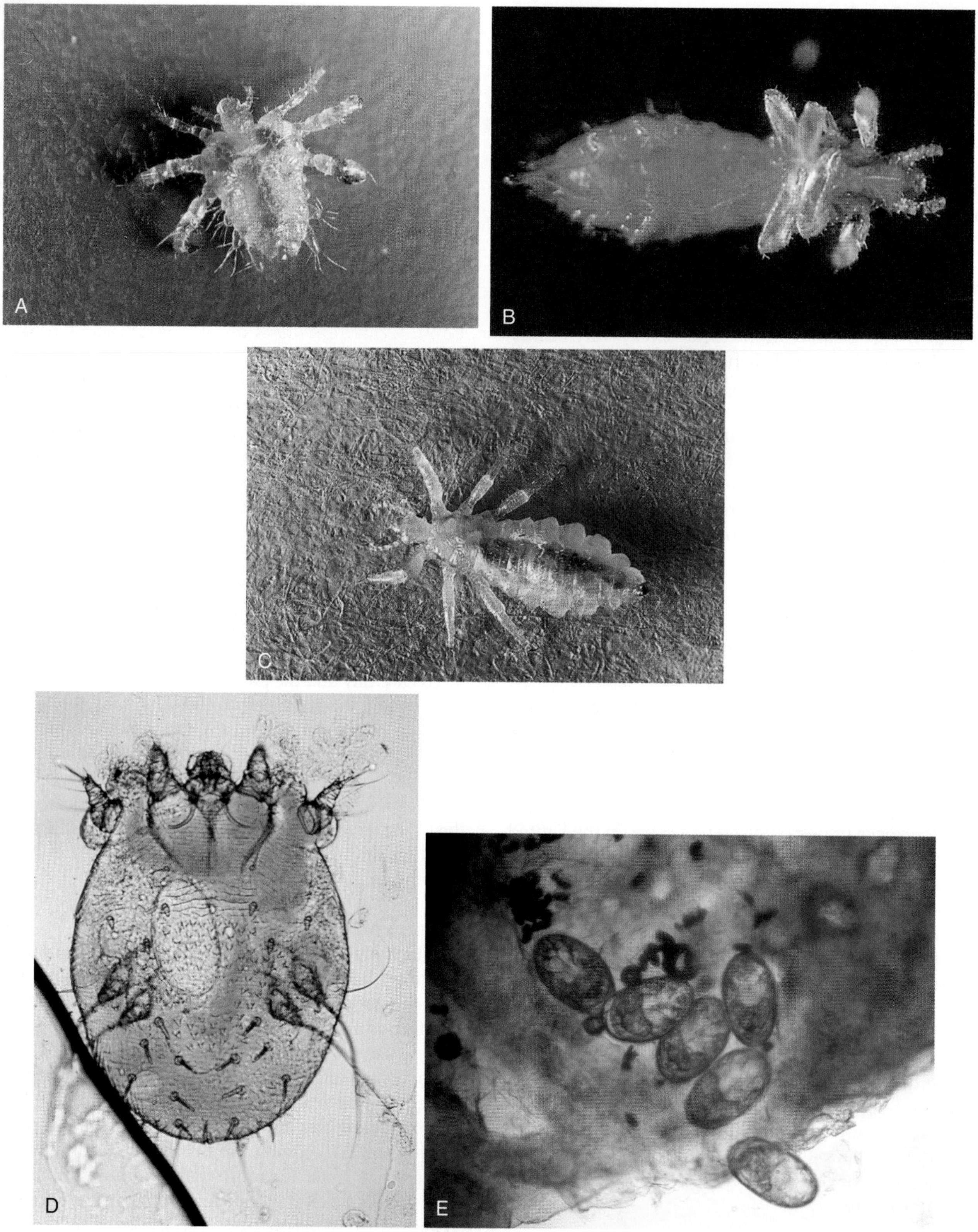

Fig. 43.5 Types of parasites that infest human beings. **A,** Pubic louse. **B,** Head louse. **C,** Body louse. **D** and **E,** Microscopic scabies. (**A and C,** From Habif TP, Dinulos JGH, Chapman MS, et al.: *Skin disease: diagnosis and treatment,* ed 4, Philadelphia, 2018, Elsevier. **B, D,** and **E,** From Zitelli BJ, McIntire S, Nowalk AJ: *Zitelli and Davis' atlas of pediatric physical diagnosis,* ed 7, Philadelphia, 2018, Elsevier.)

NONINFECTIOUS DISORDERS OF SKIN

SKIN CANCER

Skin cancer is often neglected because no pain is associated with it and patients fear that treatment will involve extensive or disfiguring surgery. More than 5 million cases of basal cell and squamous cell cancers occur in the United States each year. These are highly curable cancers. It is expected that 96,480 persons will have been diagnosed with melanoma, the most serious type of skin cancer, in 2019 and that 7230 deaths from melanoma will occur in that year (American Cancer Society, 2018). Most melanoma deaths could have been averted through early diagnosis and treatment. Kaposi sarcoma and T-cell lymphoma are discussed in Chapter 11.

Etiology and Pathophysiology

Several factors predispose an individual to developing skin cancer. Among these are internal changes in the cells that may be caused by hereditary factors and external influences such as chronic exposure to ionizing radiation, petrochemicals, or vinyl chloride or to other irritants in the environment. Sunburn as a child is a particular risk factor. Because characteristics are inherited, susceptibility to skin cancer tends to run in families. Blue-eyed blonds and redheads seem to be most susceptible, probably because they lack sufficient pigment to protect the skin cells from outside irritants. Those with a light complexion have a 24-fold greater risk of developing melanoma than African Americans, and before age 45 years the risk is higher for women than men (American Cancer Society, 2018).

Heavy exposure to UV radiation is a risk factor; this can be from alteration in the ozone layer inflicting much quicker damage to skin with much less sun exposure than in years past or long periods in the sun. Indoor tanning beds have been labeled "carcinogenic to humans" by the International Agency for Research on Cancer. The quickly proliferating skin cells of the younger generation are even more susceptible to this type of damage, and it is mostly the young who spend large amounts of time in the sun. You should instruct all people about the dangers of sunning without an appropriate protective sunscreen.

> **Think Critically**
>
> You and a friend are going on a beach vacation. How will you prepare? What advice will you give your friend for time spend on the beach?

Signs, Symptoms, Diagnosis, and Treatment

Signs and symptoms vary according to the type of lesion. Diagnosis is by examination, biopsy, and pathology study. The three main types of skin malignancy are basal cell carcinoma, squamous cell carcinoma, and melanoma. **Basal cell carcinoma** usually appears first as a small, scaly area and tends to become larger as the disease progresses (Fig. 43.6). It occurs most commonly on the face and trunk. As the scales shed, there is a small amount of bleeding, and a scab will form. When the scab is shed, the affected area becomes wider, and it is bordered by a waxy, translucent, raised area. **If such a sore has not healed within a month, it may be a basal cell carcinoma.** This spreading may continue very gradually during several months or years. Even though these malignancies do not metastasize, they can invade underlying tissues, and death can result from complications such as infection or hemorrhage from encroaching into a blood vessel. Small lesions can be removed under local anesthesia in a health care provider's office. Larger lesions respond well to radiation therapy.

Squamous cell carcinoma is caused by sunlight, affects the epidermis, and can become invasive and metastasize to other areas of the body. It appears on the head and neck most frequently. The tumor begins as a small nodule that rapidly becomes ulcerated (see Fig. 43.6). Treatment must begin early if the condition is to be relieved before the skin cells sustain extensive damage. Surgical procedures involve total removal or destruction of the lesions and the surrounding tissues that have been invaded. Cryotherapy, topical chemotherapy, laser surgery, and either topical or injected immune response modifiers are all used as therapies.

> **Older Adult Care Points**
>
> **Actinic keratoses** are very common among older adults. They appear on fair-skinned people as a small, scaly, red or grayish papule, particularly on areas of skin that are often exposed to the sun. These lesions should be removed because they can evolve into a squamous cell carcinoma that can grow rapidly and metastasize.

Malignant melanoma is the least common form of skin cancer but causes most skin cancer deaths. It arises from pigment-producing cells and varies in its course and prognosis according to its type (see Fig. 43.6). Causative factors are genetic predisposition, solar radiation, and steroid hormone influence. There are several types of melanoma, but the three major kinds of malignant melanoma are superficial spreading, nodular, and lentigo maligna melanoma. In general, the superficial lesions can be cured, but the deeper lesions tend to metastasize more readily through the lymphatic and circulatory systems. Characteristics of the three main types of skin cancer are shown in Table 43.1.

Malignant melanoma always requires surgical removal of the tumor and excision of adjacent tissues and possibly nearby lymphatic structures. Chemotherapy may be used to destroy tumor cells believed to have migrated beyond the tumor site. Radiation therapy usually is not indicated unless there is extensive metastasis. The radiation does not eliminate the disease, but it can relieve symptoms by reducing tumor size.

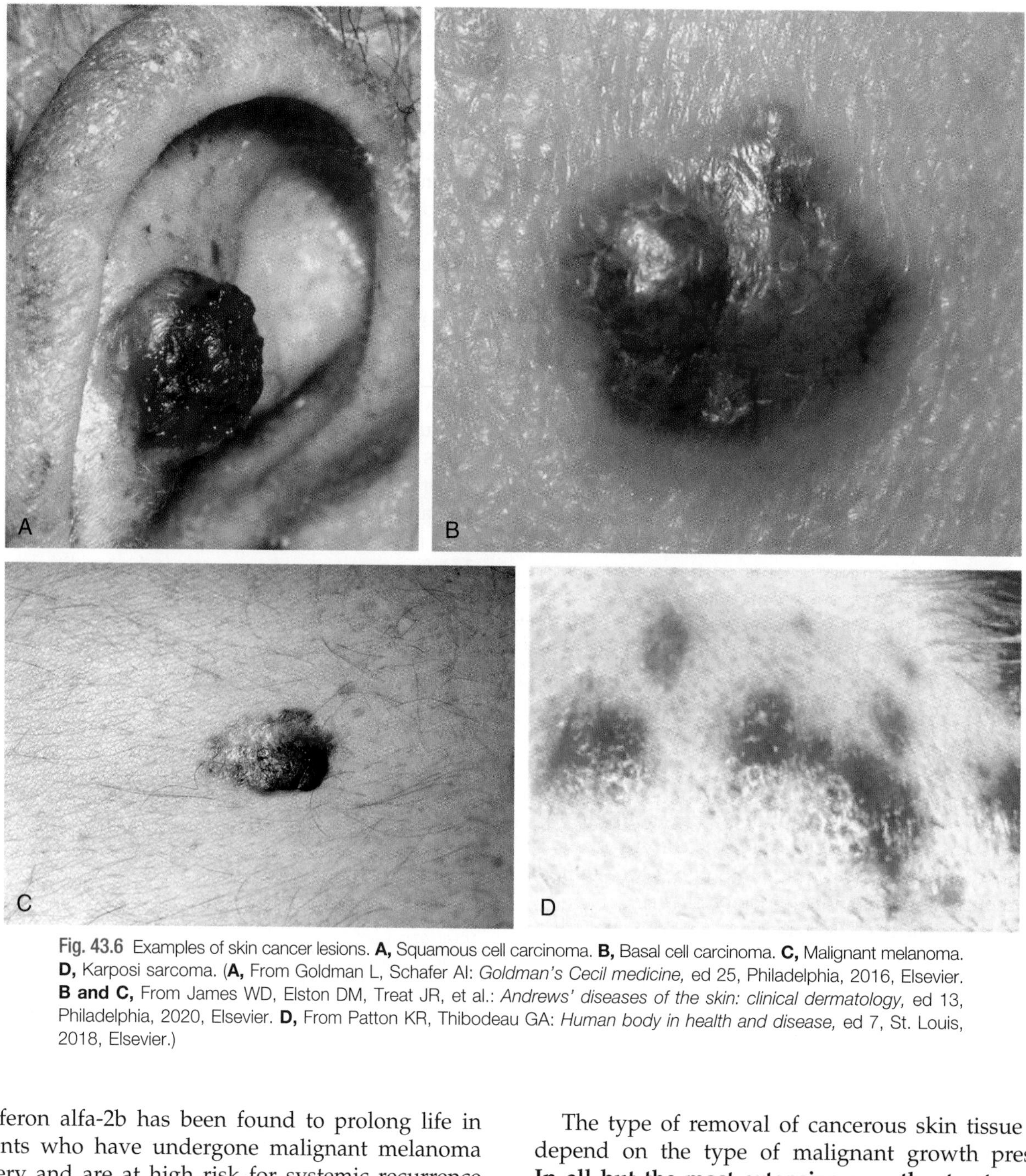

Fig. 43.6 Examples of skin cancer lesions. **A,** Squamous cell carcinoma. **B,** Basal cell carcinoma. **C,** Malignant melanoma. **D,** Karposi sarcoma. (**A,** From Goldman L, Schafer AI: *Goldman's Cecil medicine,* ed 25, Philadelphia, 2016, Elsevier. **B and C,** From James WD, Elston DM, Treat JR, et al.: *Andrews' diseases of the skin: clinical dermatology,* ed 13, Philadelphia, 2020, Elsevier. **D,** From Patton KR, Thibodeau GA: *Human body in health and disease,* ed 7, St. Louis, 2018, Elsevier.)

Interferon alfa-2b has been found to prolong life in patients who have undergone malignant melanoma surgery and are at high risk for systemic recurrence (American Cancer Society, 2018). In advanced cases, newer immunotherapy drugs are being used to enhance immune function. Ipilimumab (Yervoy), a CTLA-4 inhibitor, has been shown to prolong life. An oral agent, vemurafenib (Zelboraf), a *BRAF* inhibitor, is being used for late-stage melanoma and is the first drug approved that uses fragment-based drug discovery. In this method, small chemical fragments are grown or combined to produce a drug with a higher affinity for binding with the biological target. In patients with malignant melanoma and a known *BRAF* mutation, treatment with vemurafenib has a response rate of 50%. However, over several months the medication is less effective. Giving it with other medications that alter immune function is showing promising results (Dummer et al., 2018).

The type of removal of cancerous skin tissue will depend on the type of malignant growth present. **In all but the most extensive growths, treatment is relatively simple and completely successful if started early.** Although benign precancerous lesions do not inevitably develop into malignant lesions, the most advisable course of action is to remove them when they are first diagnosed. Removal is performed by surgery, **electrodesiccation** (tissue destruction by heat), **cryosurgery** (tissue destruction by freezing with liquid nitrogen), topical application of 5-fluorouracil (5-FU), interferon therapy, laser therapy, and molecular therapy. Radiation therapy is sometimes used to destroy the cancer.

Nursing Management

While performing daily care of patients, you often are in a position to notice these lesions in their early stages

Table 43.1 Three Major Types of Skin Cancer

TYPE	CHARACTERISTICS
Basal cell carcinoma	Slowly enlarging, firm, scaly papule. Crusted or ulcerated center that may be depressed; has pearly (semitranslucent) raised border. Dilated capillaries around lesion. Accounts for 70% of all skin cancers. Rarely spreads and is easily treated.
Squamous cell carcinoma	Appearance variable. Commonly seen as well-defined, irregularly shaped nodule or plaque. May be elevated, nodular mass, or fungated mass. Varying amounts of scale and crusting. May have ulcerated center. Predominantly on sun-exposed areas: head, neck, hands; 75% occur on the head. Spreads rapidly.
Malignant Melanomas	
Superficial spreading melanoma (SSM)	Appears in a variety of colors: white, red, gray, black, or blue over a brown or black background. Has irregular surface and notched border. Small tumor nodules may ulcerate and bleed. Horizontal growth can continue for years. Vertical growth worsens prognosis.
Nodular malignant melanoma (NMM)	Nodule with uniformly grayish black color; resembles a blackberry. May be flesh colored with specks of pigment around base of nodule. Itching, oozing, and bleeding may occur. Prognosis less favorable than superficial type.
Lentigo maligna melanoma (LMM)	Relatively rare. Arises from a lesion that resembles a large, flat freckle that is of variable color from tan to black. Has irregularly spaced black nodules on the surface. Typically located on the back of the hand, face, and neck. Develops very slowly; may ulcerate.
Acral lentiginous melanoma	Rarest type of melanoma. Located on the palms of the hands, on the soles of the feet, or under fingernails and toenails. Not related to sun exposure. Appears as a dark streak under the nail. On other areas presents as an odd-shaped black, gray, tan, or brown mark with irregular borders.

and should do your best to persuade the person with such a lesion to seek prompt medical attention. For hospitalized patients, notification of the health care provider is indicated. It is also helpful to teach assistive personnel the cues and clues that help recognize these developments.

Assignment Considerations

Report Different Skin Lesions

When assigning hygiene care to unlicensed assistive personnel, ask them to report any odd-looking lesions they find on the patient's skin. Skin cancers are often discovered on further assessment of suspicious lesions.

Because people who have skin cancer run a high risk of eventually developing another malignancy, either at the original site or elsewhere in the body, they should visit a provider at least once a year after the skin cancer has been cured. Although most skin cancers are easily curable, they should not be considered harmless and something to forget about after treatment (see Chapter 8).

Another nursing function is educating the patient about the type of cancer and helping to decrease fear. For many people, the diagnosis of "cancer"—even of an easily cured skin lesion—causes a change in body image and possibly in self-esteem. You can assist patients to talk about concerns and the future, point to community resources and support groups, and answer questions about treatment.

PRESSURE INJURY (ULCERS)

When a patient is on bed rest or constantly sitting because of paralysis, pressure against the skin in various areas interferes with circulation. Because cells die very quickly without adequate blood supply, pressure injury can develop. Depending on the patient's general condition, weight, and other factors, skin damage may occur within a few hours to a few days. Areas most prone to pressure injury are those over bony prominences. When the patient is placed in a position in which the bone is pressing on the skin where the skin is against the bed, the circulation to that area is compromised (Fig. 43.7). **Shearing action** (in which superficial layers of tissue are pulled and stretched across deeper layers of tissue) can cause damage to the skin if the patient is slid along the sheets for positioning, rather than lifted. The National Pressure Ulcer Advisory Panel (NPUAP) defines pressure injury as injury to the skin caused by pressure alone or in combination with shear. The term

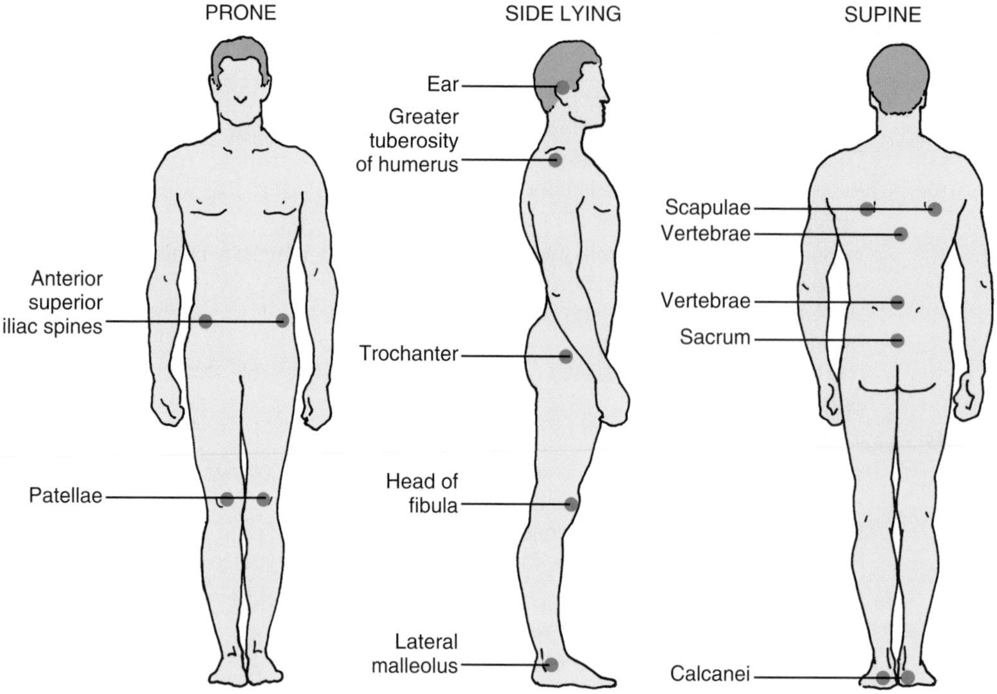

Fig. 43.7 Bony prominences most susceptible to skin breakdown depending on position.

ulcer has been replaced by *injury*, and the term *ulcer* is used only if an ulceration is present (NPUAP, 2014; Edsberg, 2016).

Risk Factors and Prevention

Every patient needs and deserves good skin assessment, but there are risk factors that make some patients more susceptible to problems, such as confinement, immobility, incontinence, malnutrition, decreased level of consciousness or confusion, obesity, diabetes mellitus, dehydration, edema, excessive sweating, and extreme age. Preventing tissue injury from pressure is far more desirable, more cost-effective, and less time-consuming than treating them. In fact, the importance of excellent nursing care is now a financial issue because Medicare and Medicaid levy penalties for hospital-acquired pressure injuries (Rondinelli et al., 2018). Pressure relief, positioning, padding, use of pressure-relief devices, adequate nutrition, and excellent skin care are the hallmarks of pressure injury prevention. Box 43.2 presents interventions for preventing tissue injury from pressure based on the Institute for Clinical Systems Improvement's health care protocol. Pressure injury can be very costly to the health care system, costing about $10 billion and 60,000 deaths annually (University of Michigan, 2018).

Nutrition Considerations

Nutrition and Wound Healing

Ongoing research is being conducted about the optimal amounts; however, increased energy (calories); protein; zinc; and vitamins A, C, and E have been shown to reduce pressure injury and promote healing of existing tissue injury (Saghalenini, 2018).

Signs and Symptoms

Once a patient has developed a pressure injury, treatment depends on the stage of the lesion. Several kinds of preprinted forms can be used to assess the risk of developing pressure ulcers. These assessment tools consider the general condition of the skin, control of urination and defecation, mobility, mental status, cleanliness, and nutritional status. They provide a more systematic approach to evaluate a patient's potential for pressure ulcer development. Many agencies use either the Braden scale system (Fig. 43.8) or the Norton system for systematic assessment of the skin.

The presence and stage of any tissue injury must be documented on admission to any health care facility or service. Classifying an ulceration or injury can also be helpful in evaluating the effectiveness of treatment and progress toward healing and repair. The NPUAP has updated pressure injury definitions for the prediction and prevention of pressure injury and a staging system for classification:

- *Suspected deep tissue injury:* Intact skin with a purple or maroon discoloration. Tissue may be firm, boggy, painful, cool, or warm.
- *Stage 1:* An area of intact skin that is reddened, deep pink, or mottled that does not blanch (Fig. 43.9).
- *Stage 2:* Partial-thickness skin loss involving the dermis and/or epidermis. The skin appears blistered or abraded or has a shallow crater. The area surrounding the damaged skin is reddened and probably will feel hot or warmer than normal (Fig. 43.10).
- *Stage 3:* The skin is ulcerated. There is a crater-like ulcer, and the underlying subcutaneous tissue is involved in the destructive process. The ulcer may

Box 43.2 Best Practice for the Prevention of Pressure Injury

- Assess the skin of all patients every 8 to 24 hours (interval depends on condition), paying particular attention to the bony prominences (see Fig. 43.7).
- Reposition patients on bed rest at least every 2 hours; use a written schedule for systematically turning and repositioning each patient.
- Use positioning devices, such as pillows, foam wedges, and padding, for patients on bed rest to keep body prominences from being in direct contact with one another.
- For patients on bed rest who are completely immobile, use devices that totally relieve pressure on the heels by raising the heels off the bed. Do not use donut-type devices.
- When the side-lying position in bed is used, avoid positioning directly on the trochanter.
- For patients on bed rest, maintain the head of the bed at the lowest degree permitted by the medical condition. Limit the time the head of the bed is elevated.
- Use lifting devices, such as a trapeze or bed linens, to move patients rather than dragging those who cannot assist during transfers and position changes.
- For patients with limited mobility, use a pressure-reducing device on the bed, such as a foam, static air, alternating air, gel, or water mattress.
- Minimize skin injury caused by friction and shear forces by proper positioning and correct transferring and turning techniques. Reduce friction injuries by using lubricants, protective films, protective dressings, and protective padding.
- Skin cleansing should occur at the time of soiling and at routine intervals based on patient need and preference. Do not use hot water and use a mild cleansing agent that minimizes irritation and dryness of the skin. Cleanse gently, minimizing the force and friction applied to the skin.
- Keep the environmental humidity above 40% and prevent exposure to cold. Treat dry skin with moisturizers.
- Do not massage bony prominences.
- Minimize skin exposure to moisture from incontinence, perspiration, or wound drainage. When sources of moisture cannot be controlled, underpads or briefs that absorb moisture and present a quick-drying surface to the skin should be used. Use an incontinence management program for incontinent patients. Check for incontinence at least every 2 hours.
- Correct inadequate dietary intake of protein and calories with nutritional intervention either by oral supplementation or enteral or parenteral feedings.
- For wheelchair-bound patients, use a pressure-reducing device such as those made of foam, gel, air, or a combination of items. Do not use donut-type devices.
- Positioning of wheelchair-bound patients should include consideration of postural alignment, distribution of weight, balance and stability, and pressure relief by device or repositioning.
- Any person at risk for developing a pressure ulcer when sitting in a chair or wheelchair should be repositioned, shifting the points under pressure at least every hour (every 15 minutes is preferable); patients who are able should be taught to shift weight every 15 minutes.
- If a potential for improvement of mobility and activity status exists, institute a rehabilitation program. Maintain current activity and mobility status with a range-of-motion exercise program.

or may not be infected. Bacterial infection is almost always present at this stage, however, and accounts for continued erosion of the ulcer and the production of drainage (Fig. 43.11).

- *Stage 4:* There is deep ulceration and necrosis involving deeper underlying muscle and possibly bone tissue. The ulcer can be dry, black, and covered with a tough accumulation of necrotic tissue, or it can be made up of wet and oozing dead cells and purulent exudates. Depth can be determined (Fig. 43.12).
- *Unstageable:* Full-thickness wounds with eschar and/or tissue that obscures depth determination.

Assignment Considerations

"On-Time"

The On-Time Quality Improvement for Long-Term Care was developed by the Agency for Healthcare Research and Quality (AHRQ). Part of the program includes assessment tools that can be completed by certified nursing assistants. The tools provide information about nutritional status, behavior, incontinence, and contributing factors. Data are then made available to health care providers, nurses, dietitians, and other care providers. The program fosters teamwork and communication and helps identify patients who are at risk for pressure ulcers (AHRQ, 2017).

A technology called *pressure mapping* helps identify areas of high pressure. The patient lies (or sits) on a sensor-filled mat, and the mat sends data to a computer, which creates a display of color-coded images. Red areas indicate higher pressures, and blue or green areas suggest lesser pressures. The patient can then be repositioned accordingly. The technology is an adjunct to, not a replacement for, good nursing assessment (Bader & Worsley, 2018). It is being used to identify best practice to prevent tissue injury from pressure and shearing.

Treatment and Nursing Interventions

Debridement. Removal of any **eschar** (dead, necrotic tissue) must occur for a pressure ulcer to heal. The exception is a heel ulcer with dry eschar that has no edema, erythema, drainage, or boggy tissue. **Debridement** can be done surgically with forceps and scissors or mechanically. Mechanical debridement is accomplished by whirlpool baths, wet-to-dry saline dressings, dextranomer beads sprinkled over the wound, or other proteolytic enzymes or chemical products that break down the dead tissue and absorb the exudate. Wet-to-dry dressings **are not recommended because of the damage that occurs to new granulation tissue when**

Patient's Name________	Evaluator's Name ________			Date of Assessment				
SENSORY PRECEPTION Ability to respond meaningfully to pressure-related discomfort	**1. Completely Limited:** Unresponsive (does not moan, flinch, or grasp) to painful stimuli, due to diminished level of consciousness or sedation. OR Limited ability to feel pain over most of body surface.	**2. Very Limited:** Responds only to painful stimuli. Cannot communicate discomfort except by moaning or restlessness. OR Has a sensory impairment that limits the ability to feel pain or discomfort over half of body.	**3. Slightly Limited:** Responds to verbal commands, but cannot always communicate discomfort or need to be turned. OR Has some sensory impairment that limits ability to feel pain or discomfort in one or two extremities.	**4. No Impairment:** Responds to verbal commands. Has no sensory deficit which would limit ability to feel or voice pain or discomfort.				
MOISTURE Degree to which skin is exposed to moisture	**1. Constantly Moist:** Skin is kept moist almost constantly by perspiration, urine, etc. Dampness is detected every time patient is moved or turned.	**2. Very Moist:** Skin is often, but not always moist. Linen must be changed at least once a shift.	**3. Occasionally Moist:** Skin is occasionally moist, requiring an extra linen change approximately once a day.	**4. Rarely Moist:** Skin is usually dry, linen only requires changing at routine intervals.				
ACTIVITY Degree of physical activity	**1. Bedfast:** Confined to bed	**2. Chairfast:** Ability to walk severely limited or non-existent. Cannot bear own weight and/or must be assisted into chair or wheelchair.	**3. Walks Occasionally:** Walks occasionally during day, but for very short distances, with or without assistance. Spends majority of each shift in bed or chair.	**4. Walks Frequently:** Walks outside the room at least twice a day and inside room at least once every 2 hours during waking hours.				
MOBILITY Ability to change and control body position	**1. Completely Immobile:** Does not make even slight changes in body or extremity position without assistance.	**2. Very Limited:** Makes occasional slight changes in body or extremity position but unable to make frequent or significant changes independently.	**3. Slightly Limited:** Makes frequent though slight changes in body or extremity position independently.	**4. No Limitations:** Makes major and frequent changes in position without assistance.				
NUTRITION <u>Usual</u> food intake pattern	**1. Very Poor:** Never eats a complete meal. Rarely eats more than a third of any food offered. Eats two servings or less of protein (meat or dairy products) per day. Takes fluids poorly. Does not take a liquid dietary supplement. OR Is NPO and/or maintained on clear liquids or IVs for more than 5 days.	**2. Probably Inadequate:** Rarely eats a complete meal and generally eats only about half of any food offered. Protein intake includes only three servings of meat or dairy products per day. Occasionally will take a dietary supplement. OR Receives less than optimum amount of liquid diet or tube feeding.	**3. Adequate:** Eats over half of most meals. Eats a total of four servings of protein (meat, dairy products) each day. Occasionally will refuse a meal, but will usually take a supplement if offered. OR Is on a tube feeding or TPN regimen that probably meets most of nutritional needs.	**4. Excellent:** Eats most of every meal. Never refuses a meal. Usually eats a total of four or more servings of meat and dairy products. Occasionally eats between meals. Does not require supplementation.				
FRICTION AND SHEAR	**1. Problem:** Requires moderate to maximum assistance in moving. Complete lifting without sliding against sheets is impossible. Frequently slides down in bed or chair, requiring frequent repositioning with maximum assistance. Spasticity, contractures, or agitation leads to almost constant friction.	**2. Potential Problem:** Moves feebly or requires minimum assistance. During a move, skin probably slides to some extent against sheets, chair, restraints, or other devices. Maintains relatively good position in chair or bed most of the time but occasionally slides down.	**3. No Apparent Problem:** Moves in bed and in chair independently and has sufficient muscle strength to lift up completely during move. Maintains good position in bed or chair at all times.					
				Total Score				

At risk = 15-18; Moderate risk = 13-14; High risk = 10-12; Severe Risk = 9.
Key: IV, intravenously; *NPO,* nothing by mouth; *TPN,* total parenteral nutrition.

Fig. 43.8 Braden scale for predicting pressure sore risk. (Copyright Barbara Braden and Nancy Bergstrom, 1988. Reprinted with permission. All Rights Reserved.)

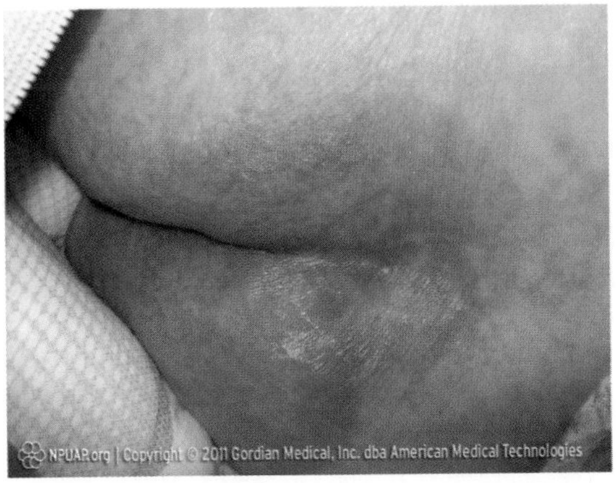

Fig. 43.9 Stage 1 pressure injury. (From the National Pressure Ulcer Advisory Panel and European Pressure Ulcer Advisory Panel: *Pressure ulcer prevention and treatment: clinical practice guideline.* Washington, DC: National Pressure Ulcer Advisory Panel, 2009.)

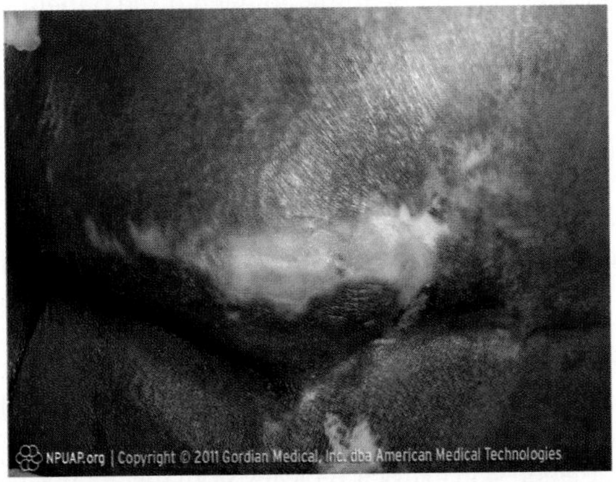

Fig. 43.10 Stage 2 pressure injury. (From the National Pressure Ulcer Advisory Panel and European Pressure Ulcer Advisory Panel: *Pressure ulcer prevention and treatment: clinical practice guideline.* Washington, DC: National Pressure Ulcer Advisory Panel, 2009.)

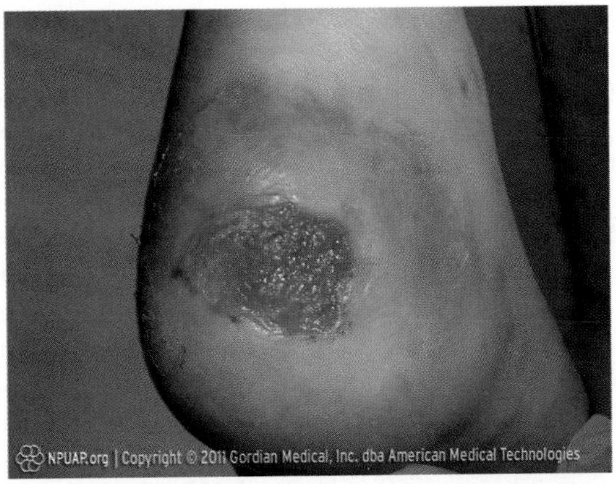

Fig. 43.11 Stage 3 pressure injury. (From the National Pressure Ulcer Advisory Panel and European Pressure Ulcer Advisory Panel: *Pressure ulcer prevention and treatment: clinical practice guideline.* Washington, DC: National Pressure Ulcer Advisory Panel, 2009.)

removed. Dressings that keep the wound moist should be used. Carefully read the instructions for whatever product is being used. Surgical debridement may be done in the patient's room, the health care provider's office, or the surgical suite depending on the depth

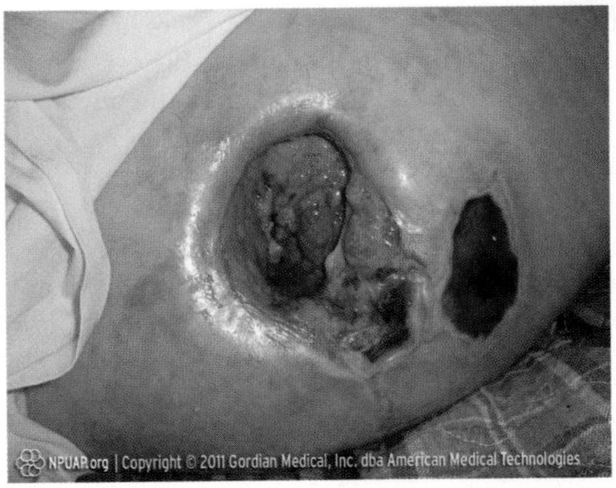

Fig. 43.12 Stage 4 pressure injury. (From the National Pressure Ulcer Advisory Panel and European Pressure Ulcer Advisory Panel: *Pressure ulcer prevention and treatment: clinical practice guideline.* Washington, DC: National Pressure Ulcer Advisory Panel, 2009.)

and extent of the wound. Surgical debridement may require a skin graft to cover the area exposed. Whenever surgical debridement, forceful irrigation, or whirlpool debridement is to occur, provide sufficient analgesia for the patient because the procedure is painful.

Cleansing and dressing. Many hospitals and larger long-term care facilities have a wound care nurse specialist who oversees wound treatment; you should consult these specialists for valuable advice about wound cleansing and dressing materials. After sharp debridement with bleeding, clean and dry dressings are used for 8 to 24 hours, then moisture-retaining dressings are applied. Ulcers are cleaned whenever the dressing is changed. Normal saline or other nontoxic solutions, such as Shur-Clens, and light mechanical action with sponges or irrigation equipment is a way of cleansing that prevents disruption of granulation tissue. At least 250 mL of solution and a 30-mL syringe with a small catheter or 18-gauge blunt needle attached is used to irrigate and to reach undermined areas and tunnels. A reddened wound bed requires gentle irrigation with a 30- to 50-mL needleless syringe to prevent damage to newly developing tissue.

Wound dressings are selected according to the characteristics of the wound. Common dressing materials include moisture retentive dressings, hydrogel dressings, hydrocolloid wafers, alginates, biologic dressings, and absorptive dressings. Use hypoallergenic tape when tape is necessary. Choose a dressing that keeps the ulcer moist and the surrounding skin dry. Prevent abscess formation by loosely filling all cavities with dressing material. Pressure must be kept off the wound for it to heal.

Other treatment methods. Application of electrical stimulation increases the rate of healing of pressure ulcers, venous leg ulcers, and diabetic foot ulcers (Nair, 2018). Application of an electrical current to the skin has been in clinical use for several decades. The therapy requires bulky equipment for generation and delivery of the electrical therapy. Researchers are currently developing a bandage that is wired to deliver the therapy. The electrical charge is generated by the movement of the chest wall during breathing from a band placed around the chest that contains nanogenerators (University of Wisconsin-Madison, 2018).

Negative pressure wound therapy (NPWT) is used effectively for chronic wounds, speeding healing time. NPWT can also be used on other types of wounds. A foam sponge is cut to fit into the open wound and an occlusive adhesive sheet is placed over the wound, extending past the wound edges. A hole is made in the adhesive, and a suction port is placed. Suction tubing is attached to the port and then to the vacuum source. The foam dressing facilitates suction applied to the full surface of the wound. The subatmospheric pressure stimulates the formation of granulation tissue and pulls away exudate from the wound (Gestring, 2018).

For an ulcer that will not heal using other methods, hyperbaric oxygen therapy may be prescribed if the equipment is available in the community. The patient is placed in the hyperbaric oxygen chamber for the treatments. Tissue becomes flooded with more oxygen than is normally available when breathing atmospheric-pressure air. This is an effective treatment for other difficult-to-heal wounds as well (Jones & Cooper, 2019).

Documentation. Pressure ulcers should be measured and documented when they are discovered and at least once a week thereafter. Document the characteristics of the wound and any exudate present. Exudate is usually **purulent** (containing pus) or **serosanguineous** (containing serum and blood). Serosanguineous exudate is amber colored and blood tinged. Purulent drainage may be one of several colors (Table 43.2).

All aspects of risk assessment, preventive measures instituted, objective description and measurement of pressure ulcers, treatment, and progress toward healing are documented regularly in the patient's chart. The Pressure Ulcer Scale for Healing (PUSH) tool is a good way to objectively document your findings. Photographs are usually taken of the ulcer on discovery and during treatment to document progress.

BURNS

Etiology and Pathophysiology

Burns are injuries to the skin caused by exposure to extreme heat, hot liquids, electrical agents, strong chemicals, or radiation. Inhaling smoke or fumes also causes injury. About 486,000 Americans seek care for burns each year. Most burns are relatively minor, but approximately 34,000 patients are hospitalized for burns each year. Fire and burns kill approximately 4000 people each year in the United States (American Burn Association, 2017). Thirty years ago most patients with burns to more than 50% of the body did not survive. Today, because of fluid resuscitation, burn wound excision and grafting techniques, new skin coverings, and nutritional supplementation, a patient may survive a 99% burn. Today, 96.7% of patients treated in a burn center survive. Many live with lifelong disabilities and scarring.

Electrical burns damage tissue deep within the body. The extent of damage is not always visible, and the entrance site and exit site may appear small. Cardiac monitoring should be initiated even if the patient does not complain of chest pain.

Chemical burns result from accidents in homes or industry. The severity of the injury depends on the duration of contact and the concentration of the chemical. The amount of tissue exposed to the chemical and the action of the chemical affect severity. Alkalis (e.g., industrial cleaners and fertilizers) cause greater injury and burn by liquefying tissue. Acids damage the tissue by coagulating cells and proteins. Chemicals for swimming pools, rust removers, and bathroom cleaners are acids. Organic compounds damage tissue by their fat solvent action.

Radiation skin injury is typically from therapeutic radiation treatment. In industries in which radioactive isotopes are used, the degree of injury depends on the amount and type of energy deposited over time. See Chapter 8 for care of skin damaged by radiation treatments.

Burns cause an acute inflammatory response (see Chapter 6). Serious burns have local and systemic effects. **All burns should be considered potentially life threatening until they are thoroughly assessed.** When a burn area is large, the inflammatory response can result in a massive shift of water, electrolytes, and protein into the tissues. This causes severe edema. Evaporation from denuded areas is four times that from intact skin. Hyperkalemia occurs when potassium is released from the damaged cells. Hyponatremia is caused by the stress response and potassium shifts. Metabolic acidosis develops. The loss of fluids from the vascular space leads to hypovolemia with low blood pressure and possible hypovolemic shock. Hematocrit will be increased because of concentration of the blood, which is missing the components that have shifted into the tissues. The increased viscosity of the blood causes slowing of blood flow in the small vessels, which in turn causes tissue hypoxia. There is danger of kidney failure from both the hypovolemia and the cellular debris that the kidneys must clear from the body. If the burn was caused by a fire, lung tissue injury from inhalation of heat and smoke may cause alveolar edema.

Table 43.2 Color of Purulent Exudate and Probable Pathogen

COLOR EXUDATE	MAY INDICATE
Beige with a fishy odor	*Proteus*
Brown with a fecal odor	*Bacteroides*
Creamy yellow	*Staphylococcus*
Green-blue with a fruity odor	*Pseudomonas*

The decreased perfusion to other organs causes changes in the gastric mucosa that impair its integrity. A type of ulcer called a **Curling ulcer** can occur within 24 hours.

The stress response to the trauma releases catecholamines, aldosterone, cortisol, and antidiuretic hormone. A hypermetabolic state results, and unless nutrition needs can be met, the body falls into negative nitrogen balance. A low-grade fever may develop as core temperature rises. Fluid replacement is essential.

Signs, Symptoms, and Diagnosis

Burn severity depends on the cause, the temperature and duration of contact, the extent of the burned area, and the anatomic site of the burn. Signs and symptoms vary from slight reddening of the skin to full loss of tissue down to bone with black, charred areas. Blisters may form. A dry, scablike crust forms over a superficial burn. Eschar is a hard, leathery layer of dead tissue that results when there has been a full-thickness injury. It is dark brown to black.

Diagnosis of the depth of the burn is made based on a classification system.

Classification of Burns

The classification of burns is based on the amount of the body surface that has been burned and the depth of the burn. The extent of a burn is roughly calculated outside of the hospital according to the "rule of nines" and is expressed as a percentage of total body surface (Fig. 43.13). The figures used in this method are fairly accurate for gross assessment in adults. The Lund-Browder classification or the Berkow chart can be used to compute the depth of the burn and the extent of the injury according to relative age, and the total burn estimate is used as the basis for treatment. Burns are a prevalent pediatric injury as well, and children cannot be assessed using the standard rule of nines. Similar charts with different percentages or charts specific to pediatric patients such as the pediatric Lund-Browder chart should be used.

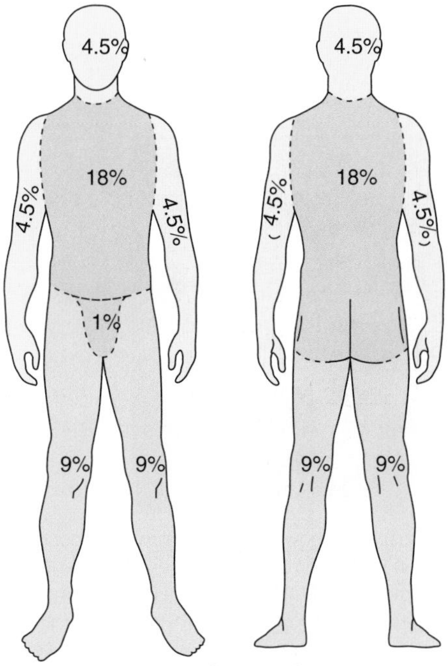

Fig. 43.13 Chart used for burn area estimate ("rule of nines").

The depth of a burn is more difficult to determine because various gradations of injury are sustained in a major burn. Some small patches may be more deeply burned than the areas adjacent to them. Burn depth originally was classified according to degrees, a first-degree burn being the most superficial and a fourth-degree burn being the deepest.

A more current method to evaluate the depth of burns is based on the layers of skin that have been damaged (Fig. 43.14). **Epidermal** or first-degree burns involve only the superficial epidermal layer and usually do not need treatment. **Superficial partial-thickness wounds** (second degree) (Fig. 43.15) are those in which the epidermal appendages (sweat and oil glands and hair follicles) are not destroyed and the wound will heal by itself if no further injury occurs from either infection or inappropriate treatment (see Chapter 5, Table 5.1 for the phases of wound healing). **Deep partial-thickness wounds** (second degree) include tissue through the lower layer of dermis and will require surgical treatment. **Full-thickness wounds** (third degree) (see Fig. 43.15) involve all layers of skin and the destruction of the epidermal appendages. Wounds of this type will require grafting for the wound to heal and for optimal function to be restored. Fourth-degree wounds involve underlying structures such as fat, muscle, or bone. Table 43.3 provides a guide for estimating the depth of a burn.

Emergency Treatment

First, all burn patients are treated as trauma patients. Establishment and maintenance of an airway is the first priority. The patient may have other life-threatening injuries besides their burns. Hemorrhage does not usually occur with burns. If a burned patient shows signs of bleeding, they must be checked for some other type of injury, such as a penetrating wound, fracture, or laceration that occurred at the same time they were burned.

Generally, patients are undressed and covered with a sterile or freshly laundered sheet; however, clothing that is stuck to the burn area is not removed before the patient is in the hospital. Rings, bracelets, and watches should be removed from injured extremities to prevent a tourniquet effect when swelling occurs. Salves, ointments, or any greasy substance should not be applied to a burned area because the removal of greasy substances is very painful and increases the possibility of infection. Blisters should not be disturbed initially because they serve as a protective covering over the wound. Box 43.3 outlines first aid for minor burns.

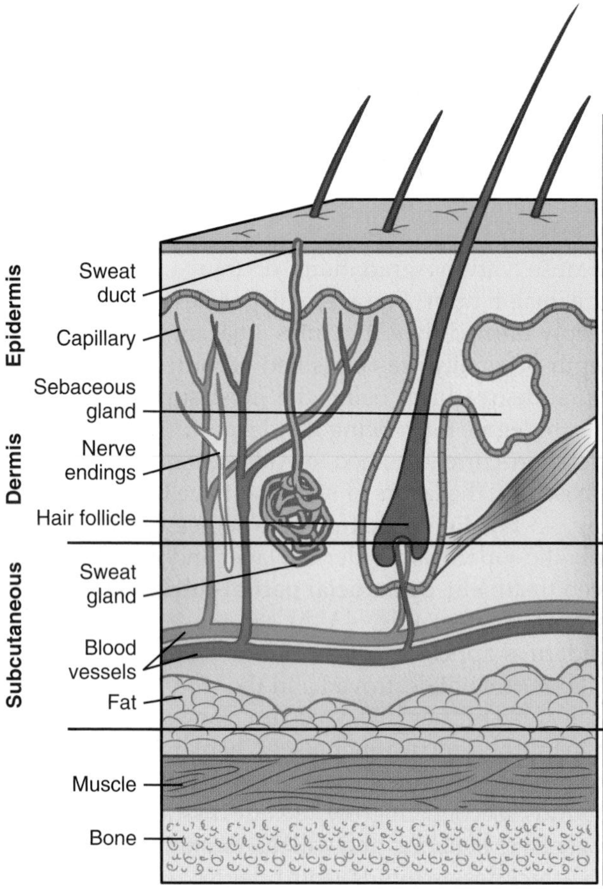

Depth	Degree	Wound appearance	Wound sensation	Course of healing
Superficial (epidermal)	1st degree	Epidermis remains intact and without blisters. Erythema: skin blanches with pressure	Painful	Discomfort lasts 48–72 hours. Desquamation in 3–7 days
Superficial partial-thickness		Wet, shiny, weeping surface Blisters Wound blanches with pressure.	Painful Very sensitive to touch, air currents	7–21 days. Healing rates vary with burn depth and presence/absence of infection.
Deep partial-thickness	2nd degree	Blisters (easily opened) Wet or waxy dry Variable color (patchy to cheesy white to red) No blanching	May be painful or reduced/absent sensation May sense pressure only	>21 days, usually requires surgical treatment
Full-thickness	3rd degree	Color variable (i.e., deep red, white, black, brown) Surface dry Thrombosed vessels visible No blanching	Insensate (↓pinprick sensation)	Autografting required for healing
Deeper injury	4th degree	Color variable Charring visible in deepest areas Extremity movement limited	Insensate	Amputation of extremities likely Autografting required for healing

Fig. 43.14 The tissues involved in burns of various depths. (Redrawn from Black JM, Hawks JH: *Medical-surgical nursing: clinical management for positive outcomes,* ed 8, Philadelphia, 2009, Saunders.)

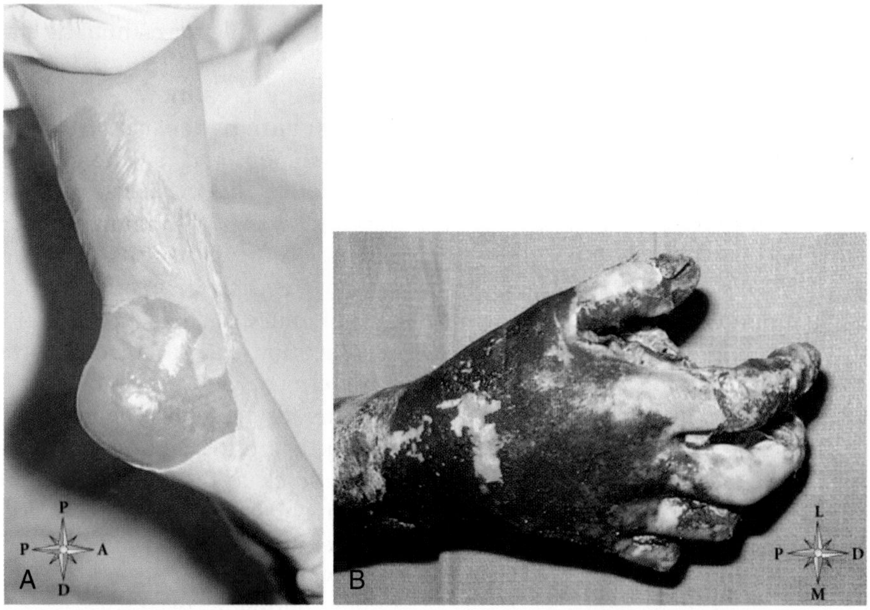

Fig. 43.15 Partial- and full-thickness burns. **A,** Second-degree (partial-thickness) burn showing a scald injury in a young child. **B,** Fourth-degree (full-thickness) high-voltage electrical burn resulting in underlying muscle and bone damage. (Courtesy Michael Peck, MD, University of North Carolina Burn Center, Chapel Hill, N.C. In Copstead LE, Banasik J: *Pathophysiology,* ed 5, St. Louis, 2013, Elsevier.)

Table 43.3 Classification of Burn Depth

CHARACTERISTIC	SUPERFICIAL BURN	SUPERFICIAL PARTIAL-THICKNESS BURN	DEEP PARTIAL-THICKNESS BURN	FULL-THICKNESS BURN	DEEP FULL-THICKNESS BURN
Color	Pink to red	Pink to red	Red to white	Black, brown, yellow, white, red	Black
Edema	Mild	Mild to moderate	Moderate	Severe	Absent
Pain	Yes	Yes	Yes	Yes and no	Absent
Blisters	No	Yes	Rare	No	No
Eschar	No	No	Yes, soft and dry	Yes, hard and inelastic	Yes, hard and inelastic
Healing time	3–5 days	Approximately 2 wk	2–6 wk	Weeks to months	Weeks to months
Grafts required	No	No	Can be used if healing is prolonged	Yes	Yes
Example	Sunburn, flash burns	Scalds, flames, brief contact with hot objects	Scalds; flames; prolonged contact with hot objects, tar, grease, chemicals	Scalds; flames; prolonged contact with hot objects, tar, grease, chemicals, electricity	Flames, electricity, grease, tar, chemicals

From Ignatavicius DD, Workman ML, et al.: *Medical-surgical nursing: patient-centered collaborative care,* ed 9, St. Louis, 2018, Elsevier.

Box 43.3 First Aid for Minor Burns

- Run cool water over the burn continuously for 10 to 15 minutes.
- Apply cool compresses if continuous water flow is not available.
- Do not apply ice, ice water, butter, or ointments.
- Do not pop blisters.
- Cover loosely with a sterile gauze bandage.
- Take ibuprofen or acetaminophen for pain.

Patients with serious burns are generally given nothing by mouth. Oxygen is administered if pulse oximetry indicates a problem with respiratory function or if inhalation injury is suspected. Assessment for carbon monoxide inhalation includes checking the mucous membranes for a cherry-red color. Intravenous fluid therapy and more extensive medical treatment are started as soon as possible. The American Burn Association has identified criteria for minor and major burn injuries. It recommends that all major burn injury patients be treated in a burn center. Every emergency department has guidelines that indicate criteria for transferring a victim to a burn center.

Emergent Phase of Burns

The emergent phase averages 24 to 48 hours but may last for as long as 3 days. It begins with fluid loss and edema formation and lasts until edema fluid is mobilized and diuresis begins.

The first hour of treatment after burning can be crucial to the eventual outcome of a serious burn. Other life-threatening injuries must be treated first.

If possible, details of the nature of the accident should be obtained so that a more thorough assessment can be made. Knowing the causes of the burn and whether there is any possibility of thermal damage to the respiratory tract can alert the team to the specific needs of the patient. The depth and extent of the burn area are estimated, and multiple IV lines are established. A tetanus toxoid injection is given in the emergency department; it is the only intramuscular injection given initially.

Respiratory support. There is a potential for respiratory obstruction if upper airway passages have been burned. Swelling will occur, and it will become increasingly difficult for the patient to breathe. Signs of respiratory distress such as increased respiratory rate, use of accessory muscles, nasal flaring, retractions, restlessness, and confusion may occur. Early intubation is recommended for an extensive upper airway injury.

Lower airway injury (damage to lung parenchyma) is caused by breathing in smoke and soot from the fire. This type of injury may also require intubation and ventilation and may be life threatening.

Patients who should be watched closely for signs of developing respiratory problems include those who have:

- Burns of the face and neck
- Singed nasal hair or darkened membranes in the nose and mouth
- Smoky-smelling breath
- Dark or black sputum
- Burning sensation in the throat or chest
- A history of having been burned in an enclosed space

Watch for increasing restlessness, coughing, hoarseness, rapid shallow respirations, *stridor* (high-pitched musical sound on inspiration), and falling oxygen saturation (below 95%). Humidified oxygen is given if the patient is experiencing respiratory distress, and bronchodilators may be given; intubation and mechanical ventilation may be required. Keep necessary equipment at hand and constantly assess the patient's respiratory effort. Use an incentive spirometer, coughing, turning, and early ambulation to maintain good respiratory function. Ongoing respiratory therapy treatments may be ordered.

Fluid resuscitation and prevention of shock. **A major concern in the care of a burn victim is to prevent shock from circulatory collapse.** The two most important measures used to relieve profound shock in a burn patient are:

- Replacement of lost fluids and electrolytes (fluid resuscitation)
- Enhancement of tissue perfusion

The loss of fluids and electrolytes results from the sudden capillary leak and shifting of the blood plasma and tissue fluids from their normal site to the area of the burn. This shift occurs in the first 24 to 48 hours after the burn. The fluids are then lost by movement from the vascular space to the interstitial spaces. Fluid resuscitation needs are based on one of several burn formulas. The Parkland formula for fluid resuscitation is:

$$4\text{ mL Ringer's lactate (RL)} \times \%\text{ burn} \times \text{weight in kg}$$

One half of the required fluid should be given within 8 hours of the time of the burn. The second half is given over the next 16 hours. After that, fluids are based on specific volume and electrolyte imbalances and response to treatment. **Fluid replacement is calculated from the time of injury, not from the time of arrival at the medical facility.** Important nursing functions are to keep IV access sites patent and secured in place and to ensure that the fluids are administered at the ordered rates.

Clinical Cues

In trauma patients, a Foley catheter is inserted to monitor hourly urine output and provide data to determine whether fluid resuscitation is adequate. The minimum acceptable urine flow for an adult is 30 mL/h. To obtain accurate hourly measurements, the drainage bag should have a urometer.

Unless fluids are replaced immediately, the cardiac output will drop, and the resultant profound shock may be fatal to the patient. The patient's vital signs must be checked hourly and recorded accurately. A blood pressure reading taken by cuff from an extremity may not be reliable. An arterial line may be inserted for more accurate monitoring of blood pressure changes. The state of sensorium or level of consciousness is another key observation in the assessment of tissue perfusion. Constantly assess the patient's level of alertness and clarity of thinking, asking the patient who they are, where they are, their age, what happened, and so on. There are significant dangers to fluid resuscitation; for example, excessive fluid potentiates adult respiratory distress syndrome, and extreme fluid deficit will cause acute renal failure. It is very important to monitor the signs of adequate fluid resuscitation and know when to increase or decrease the fluids based on clinical findings.

After the first 24 hours, 5% dextrose in water (D_5W) is given to maintain a serum sodium level of 135 to 145 mEq/L. Fluid intake and output and daily weights are measured for as long as the patient has open wounds. Laboratory data are checked frequently for evidence of either a deficit or a surplus of specific electrolytes.

Pain management. As soon as IV lines are established and fluid resuscitation is begun, pain control can begin. Measures to relieve pain include the administration of IV morphine or hydromorphone hydrochloride (Dilaudid). Doses of IV morphine may be higher than you are accustomed to seeing: 2 to 4 mg every 5 to 10 minutes is the standard starting dose, and the patient may require a much larger total dose because of the severe pain (Rice & Orgill, 2018). Fentanyl is another powerful opioid medication that can be combined with a benzodiazepine, such as midazolam, before painful wound care procedures. Ketamine and propofol are anesthetic agents that are used for control of pain during procedures. The massive fluid shifts that occur after a burn injury make absorption from an intramuscular site unpredictable in the first 24 hours after the burn.

For chronic pain, gabapentin and methadone can be prescribed. Nonsteroidal antiinflammatory drugs (NSAIDs) work to control pain but may not be used if ongoing grafting is necessary or because of stress ulcers.

Gastrointestinal management. To prevent gastric distention secondary to mesenteric vasoconstriction a nasogastric (NG) tube may be placed. Within 24 hours of injury, tube feedings may be initiated to help provide needed nutrients for healing and to counter the hypermetabolic burn response. Some patients may require medications to reduce gastric acid to prevent ulceration (Curling ulcer).

Acute Phase of Burns

The acute phase extends from the time of fluid mobilization and diuresis to when the burned area is completely covered by skin grafts or when burns are healed. Goals during this phase include management of pain and anxiety, prevention of wound infection, promotion of nutritional intake, and rehabilitation therapy.

Prevention of infection. Although wound infection is no longer the major cause of death in burn victims (the main cause of death is pneumonia), its prevention is important to recovery. Today patients are taken to the operating room very early after the burn. Burn eschar is excised away from the wound, and the area is covered with a biologic or biosynthetic skin. During the granulation stage of repair, the wound should look slightly pink and somewhat shiny. Healthy granulation tissue does not emit exudates. **A very wet wound that has a foul odor indicates infection.** A greenish blue wound exudate is a sign of *Pseudomonas* infection. Signs of inflammation, such as redness and swelling of the tissues adjacent to the wound, may indicate **cellulitis** (acute inflammation of the subcutaneous tissues). Signs of infection should be reported to the health care provider. If wound sepsis occurs, IV antibiotics specific to bacteria in the wound are given and topical antibacterial soaks are applied to the wound.

Critically burned patients have a high risk for pneumonia. Chan and colleagues (2018) identified that pneumonia in hospitalized patients may be ventilator-associated hospital-acquired pneumonia (V-HAP) or nonventilator hospital-acquired pneumonia (NV-HAP). Their study showed that burn patients were at higher risk for either type of pneumonia than similar patients that did not have burns (Chan et al., 2018). Examples of Core Measures for patients in intensive care units (ICUs) include protocols to prevent deep vein thrombosis and ventilator-associated pneumonia.

Wound treatment. General principles for the care of burn wounds include keeping the subendothelial layers moist, preventing infection, promoting healing, and minimizing pain. Antimicrobial ointments are used topically to prevent colonization of the wound. Superficial burns may then be covered with a nonadherent dressing, such as Xeroform, Adaptic, or Mepitel. Most burns have several thicknesses of burn, are not uniform, and may require different dressings. If healing tissues are normally in a moist environment, they will heal best if kept moist and not allowed to dry out. Surface skin that is normally dry should be allowed to dry for healing. Deep wounds will need surgical debridement and graft or flap coverage. If surgical intervention has not yet occurred, silver-containing dressings or ointments may be used to keep the wound moist and the dressing nonadherent. If the tissue is not ready for a skin graft but has been surgically cleaned, dressings with allografts, biologics, and biosynthetic coverings may be used (Tenenhaus & Rennekampff, 2018).

Burn wounds are cleansed with sterile saline using sterile technique at least once daily. Prior to wound care, analgesics should be given. The goal is to remove excess exudate and drainage and to minimize the danger of infection. Wounds of the face or ears are left undressed. After the wounds are cleaned, a topical ointment such as bacitracin is usually applied every 8 hours to prevent infection and promote healing. Burns on the hands, extremities, or trunk may be cleansed at the bedside, on a shower table in the burn unit treatment room, or in a whirlpool bath. Cleansing is done at least once a day, and these wounds are dressed. Dressings are composed of layers of sterile gauze saturated with topical medications, biologic dressings, synthetic dressings, or artificial skin. The wound is then wrapped with stretch gauze, such as Kling, or with elastic mesh webbing. Table 43.4 lists the most common topical medications and their nursing implications.

Table 43.4 Topical Medications Commonly Used to Treat Burns

MEDICATION	ACTION	NURSING IMPLICATIONS
Silver sulfadiazine (Silvadene, Flamazine)	Interferes with DNA synthesis by binding to bacterial cell membrane.	Assess for allergy to sulfonamides. Observe for rash, itching, or burning, which may indicate allergic reaction. Observe for leukopenia. Not effective against *Pseudomonas* infections. Cream must be removed and reapplied once or twice per day.
Mafenide acetate (Sulfamylon)	Bacteriostatic agent; effective against both gram-positive and gram-negative organisms.	Assess for allergy to sulfonamides. Observe for signs of allergic reaction. May cause metabolic acidosis; monitor blood gases and electrolyte levels. Application may cause pain for 30–40 min; medicate before applying. Penetrates eschar and is effective against *Pseudomonas*. Very effective for electrical burns.
Silver nitrate	Antimicrobial action.	Dressings must be kept continually wet with 0.5% solution. Stings on application; stains fabric. Monitor electrolyte levels; may cause imbalances. Penetrates wound only 1–2 mm.
Chlorhexidine gluconate	Antimicrobial.	Long lasting. Does not interfere with the ability of the wound to epithelialize. Only used on superficial burns.
Collagenase (Santyl) with polymyxin B (Polysporin) powder	Digests collagen in necrotic tissue; powder prevents infection.	Monitor for wound infection.
Polymyxin B–bacitracin	Wide-spectrum antibiotic action.	May cause itching, burning, and inflammation. Will not penetrate eschar. Must be applied q2–8h.

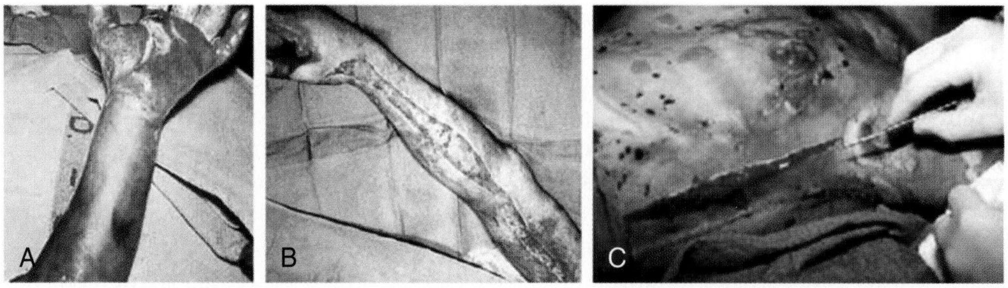

Fig. 43.16 Escharotomy to release circumferential burn eschar and improve circulation to a distal extremity. **A,** Tight circumferential eschar restricting swelling as edema forms in the tissue beneath the eschar. Edema compresses blood vessels, which inhibits blood flow to the distal extremity. **B,** An escharotomy incision allows outward swelling of edematous tissues. The restricted blood flow to the distal extremity is relieved. **C,** An anterior axillary incision is made bilaterally to relieve respiratory distress. (From Ignatavicius DD, Workman ML, et al.: *Medical-surgical nursing: concepts for interprofessional collaborative care,* ed 9, St. Louis, 2018, Elsevier.)

Escharotomy. Eschar is a source of infection, and it impairs healing. Removal of eschar and necrotic skin (**debridement**) is usually done within 24 to 72 hours after the burn (Fig. 43.16) as long as the patient is stable enough to tolerate general anesthesia. If removal of eschar is not possible, tissue perfusion or quality of respiration can become compromised because of circumferential eschar constriction, and **escharotomy** is performed. **An incision into the burn eschar with a scalpel or electrocautery relieves pressure caused by circumferential burns that encircle an extremity or that constrict movement of the chest.** The incisions extend into the subcutaneous tissue. If the pressure is not relieved, arterial blood flow in the extremity will be compromised, possibly causing necrosis; nerve damage from the pressure also may occur. An escharotomy on the chest improves lung expansion and oxygenation. The procedure does not cause discomfort because the nerve endings have been destroyed by the burn. No anesthesia is required. Early removal of eschar and necrotic tissue is the goal and prevents complications of eschar constriction.

Be alert for compartment syndrome, which occurs when increased pressure within a compartment (e.g., arm, leg) causes compromise of circulation to the area. Fluid accumulation from edema can cause compartment syndrome in burn patients. Monitor for increasing pain, paleness and tenseness of the tissue, numbness or tingling, discoloration in the distal portion of the extremity, and decreased sensation **(paresthesia).**

Debridement. Debridement may need to be an ongoing process as the full depth of the burn is realized. Mechanical techniques such as soap and water, moistened gauze, or chlorhexidine surgical scrub brushes may be used if irrigation with sterile saline is ineffective in removing dead tissue. Proteolytic enzymes may also be applied to chemically debride the wound. New tissue growth is promoted with a clean wound bed and moist sterile environment. Large wound debridement is done in the operating room.

Grafting. Surgical removal of eschar and applications of biologic dressings are done within the first few hours after the burn injury. **Biologic dressings** are materials obtained from cadavers or from animals. It is most desirable to graft the patient's own skin (**autograft**), but when this is not possible, a **homograft** (the skin of another person [**allograft**], obtained from a cadaver), a heterograft (**xenograft**, usually obtained from a pig), or artificial (**biosynthetic**) skin, such as Biobrane, can be used as a temporary measure. Biobrane is a nylon fabric with a silicone film that allows exudate to pass through. The many synthetic dressings available consist of silicone, plastics, or alginate (brown seaweed combined with other substances) and remain in place for 1 to 14 days. **The patient's own skin is the only permanent graft material.** Some success has been achieved in growing skin cells harvested from the patient in cultures, but this is a slow, expensive process. The epithelial sheets grown are then used for grafting.

When autografting is performed, there is a donor site from which a split-thickness piece of skin has been removed. That piece of skin may be used intact, or it may be cut into a mesh pattern (Fig. 43.17). It takes longer for a mesh graft area to heal because the skin cells need to grow into the holes between the links of skin. Artiss is a fibrin sealant used for adhering skin grafts for burn patients. Recovery time from a split-thickness skin graft is rapid, commonly less than 3 weeks (Ambardekar, 2017).

Donor sites may be covered by a film dressing to hasten healing and decrease pain. The donor site is often more painful than the graft site. Once the donor site has healed completely, skin may be harvested from that site again.

Pressure dressings are worn as soon as grafts heal to decrease scarring that can inhibit mobility. The pressure dressing may be an elastic wrap or a custom-fitted, elasticized piece of clothing that provides uniform pressure over the burned area (Fig. 43.18). These pressure dressings must be worn 23 hours a day, every day, until the scar tissue is mature. Scar maturity takes 12 to 24 months. Daily exercise and splint applications are used to prevent contracture formation. After burns are fully healed and the scar tissue has matured, plastic surgery may be performed to try to rebuild lost structures, such as the nose or an ear, or to enhance appearance.

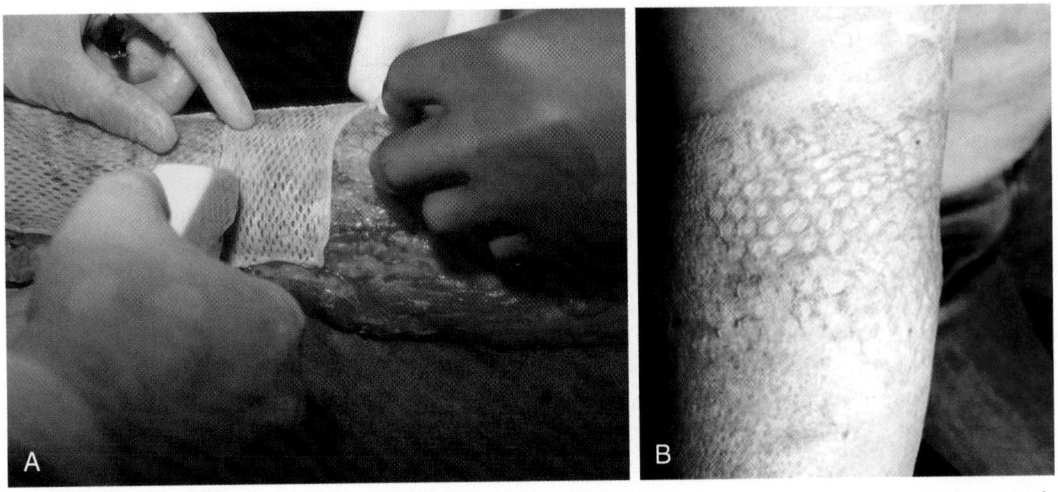

Fig. 43.17 Typical appearance of meshed autografts. **A,** Appearance during application of meshed autograft. **B,** Appearance of meshed autograft after healing. (From Ignatavicius DD, Workman ML, et al.: *Medical-surgical nursing: concepts for interprofessional collaborative care,* ed 9, St. Louis, 2018, Elsevier.)

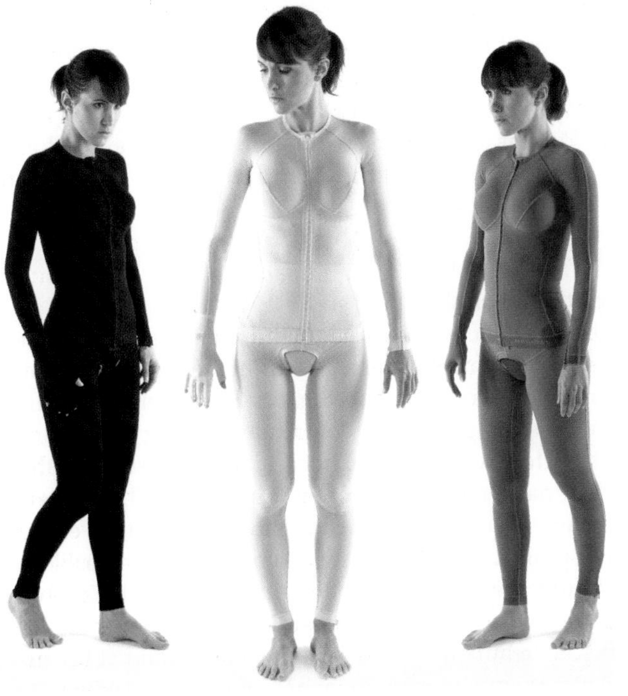

Fig. 43.18 Pressure garments are individually fitted. (Courtesy Medical Z, Houston, Tex.)

Complications

When a sizable burn occurs, blood flow is shifted to the brain, heart, and liver because of the fluid changes that occur. The gastrointestinal tract receives decreased blood, and gastric motility is impaired. Monitor peristalsis and be alert to signs of paralytic ileus. Severe abdominal distention may occur. A Curling ulcer may develop, inducing gastrointestinal bleeding. Stools are monitored for signs of occult blood. A histamine (H_2)–receptor antagonist, such as cimetidine (Tagamet), ranitidine (Zantac), famotidine (Pepcid), or nizatidine (Axid), may be administered IV to prevent this complication.

Contractures always are a threat with major burns and sometimes with minor burns. Proper positioning and regular exercise are essential to prevent musculoskeletal deformities after a burn. Although the motion of physical therapy exercises may be painful, the muscles and skin must be exercised and stretched every day for normal motion to be maintained. Sometimes it is necessary for the patient to continue visiting the physical therapist for several months after discharge from the hospital. Ambulation two or three times a day is begun as soon as the fluid shift has stabilized for patients who have no fractures or serious injuries to the feet or legs.

Rehabilitation Phase of Burns

A patient who has experienced a major burn is transferred to a rehabilitation facility. The rehabilitation phase begins with wound closure and ends when the patient reaches the highest level of function possible. This phase may last for years. The phases of burn rehabilitation have been referred to as the first 2 minutes, the first 2 hours, the first 2 days, the first 2 weeks, the first 2 months, and the first 2 years. Continued physical therapy and psychological care are essential to help the patient achieve their optimal level of function. Some patients must learn to use adaptive devices or alter the way they formerly accomplished tasks.

When the patient is ready and able to accept some responsibility for self-care, preparation for release from the hospital begins. Teach the patient how to apply topical agents without contaminating the wound and how to change dressings if these are used. A family member, if available, is included in burn care education.

Maturing scars usually appear red, hard, and raised before they eventually begin to fade and soften. Pressure garments and masks help prevent thick and disfiguring scars but are uncomfortable. The patient may resist wearing them unless there is understanding of their intended purpose. Your encouragement and reinforcement of the purpose can help.

Reintegration into roles, community activities, and employment takes time. Participation in a support group of burn victims is sometimes helpful. In this way the patient and family realize that they are not alone in their struggles with the many problems that the injury has brought. Assessment of the home environment and family interaction is essential before discharge. Knowing how the patient formerly coped with stressful situations helps the professional personnel involved support that patient. Having friends visit and making short trips out in public is helpful in dealing with the reactions of others to burn scars and disfigurement. Referral for job retraining may be required if the patient will be unable to return to a former occupation because of residual physical deficits. See Chapter 9 for rehabilitation goals and principles.

NURSING MANAGEMENT

Care of a burn patient is interdisciplinary and includes the services of the health care provider, surgeon, nurses, dietitian, respiratory therapist, physical therapist, occupational therapist, psychologist or psychiatrist, and social worker. Other health professionals are added to the team as needed. Collaborative planning meetings are scheduled at least once a week initially. Input for the plan of care is contributed by all members of the team.

ASSESSMENT (DATA COLLECTION)

A thorough assessment of all body systems and psychological response is performed on admission and continues throughout because of the potential for complications. The patient's vital signs and pain level must be checked and recorded at regular intervals. The condition of the wounds also should be assessed systematically to determine whether healing is taking place as it should and infection is being prevented. Wounds are carefully assessed at each dressing change. Signs that indicate infection include the following:

- Strong odor
- Color change to dark red or brown
- Redness around edges extending to unburned skin
- Texture change
- Exudate and purulent drainage
- Sloughing of graft

Such signs should be reported because a culture or biopsy should be performed.

> **Think Critically**
>
> What would you do if, when taking vital signs, you find that the pulse on the burned arm is weaker than that on the other, unburned extremity?

NURSING DIAGNOSIS

Care of a burn patient is extremely complex. The plan of care must be frequently revised and updated. Problem statements or nursing diagnoses commonly used for burn patients are included in Nursing Care Plan 43.1. Additional problem statements include the following:

- Altered nutrition due to increased caloric demands and inability to orally ingest sufficient calories.
- Anxiety due to pain, guilt associated with injury, financial concerns, appearance, treatment, and prognosis.
- Altered body image due to disfigurement secondary to burn injury.
- Altered family coping due to alteration in roles.
- Insufficient knowledge due to home care.

PLANNING

Examples of appropriate expected outcomes are written for the individual patient, such as the following:

- Patient will regain nutritional balance by no further weight loss and signs of wound healing.
- Patient will state that there is a decrease in anxiety.
- Patient will integrate the altered body image by expressing positive statements regarding their appearance.
- Patient will demonstrate new coping mechanisms.
- Family will state ways in which they are coping with caring for patient at home.
- Patient and family will learn to provide good care at home evidenced by continued recovery without complications.

IMPLEMENTATION

Managing Pain

Use gentleness and care in handling the patient as they are turned or treatment is administered. This reduces the amount of pain, and the less the patient is handled, the less danger there is of contaminating the wounds. **Despite advances in burn care, research studies show that pain continues to be undertreated, and even experienced clinicians tend to overestimate the efficacy of opioids.** Morphine or hydromorphone hydrochloride should be administered with a patient-controlled analgesia pump when possible. Boluses are necessary before treatments or surgical procedures and at bedtime. Antianxiety agents such as lorazepam (Ativan) or antipsychotics such as haloperidol (Haldol) or quetiapine (Seroquel) should be used along with analgesia. Burn pain can be distressful for years after the burn occurs (Wiechman & Sharar, 2018).

Pain continues even after the wound appears to have healed completely. Exercises to prevent contractures can cause pain because they stretch the skin while it is very tender. Splints to prevent musculoskeletal complications can also cause discomfort. Analgesics will allow the patient to get sufficient rest, but they should be given judiciously as the pain becomes less acute. If a patient begins to depend too much on one kind of analgesic, alternative drugs should be given.

Preventing Infection

An aseptic environment is needed for burn care. Stringent cleaning standards must be implemented and

Nursing Care Plan 43.1 Care of a Patient With a Burn

SCENARIO

Mr. Young, age 33 years, sustained partial- and full-thickness burns over both legs when a container of gasoline he was carrying ignited and he dropped it, splashing it onto his legs. In the emergency department, his wounds were cleaned and a topical agent was applied; no dressings were applied. Intravenous lines were established, and fluids were administered to prevent potential fluid and electrolyte imbalance. He received morphine for pain and on admission to the unit was fairly comfortable, conscious, and oriented. He is in the emergent phase.

PROBLEM STATEMENT/NURSING DIAGNOSIS

Fluid volume deficit related to fluid shift and loss of fluids via open burn wounds.

SUPPORTING ASSESSMENT DATA

Objective: Partial-thickness burns and full-thickness burns on legs; burn areas becoming edematous.

Goals/Expected Outcomes	Nursing Interventions	Selected Rationale	Evaluation
Patient will have adequate circulating blood volume as evidenced by blood pressure (BP) >100 mm Hg systolic and urine output >30 cc/h.	Monitor vital signs q1h.	Falling BP and rising pulse can indicate hypovolemia.	BP 120/80. Pulse 78/min. Respirations 24/min. Temperature 98.6° F (37° C).
	Monitor urine output, report drop below 0.5 mL/kg/h.	Urine output may also indicate hypovolemia because kidneys will be less perfused.	Urine output at 45 mL/h.
	Monitor laboratory values for electrolyte imbalances.	Changes in fluid volume may alter electrolyte balance.	Potassium 4.5 mEq/L. Sodium 140 mEq/L.
	Maintain IV fluids on schedule.	Adequate fluid resuscitation prevents hypovolemia.	IV fluids on schedule.

PROBLEM STATEMENT/NURSING DIAGNOSIS

Potential for infection related to burn damage to skin.

SUPPORTING ASSESSMENT DATA

Objective: Skin on both legs damaged by burns.

Goals/Expected Outcomes	Nursing Interventions	Selected Rationale	Evaluation
Patient will not experience infection of burn wounds as evidenced by normal vital signs and normalization of WBC count.	Assess for medication allergy.	Medication prescribed may be contraindicated.	No allergies to medication.
	Use strict aseptic technique for wound care.	Infection is the greatest cause of burn wound depth.	Strict aseptic technique provided to wounds.
	Do not submerge catheters or insertion sites during cleansing.	Invasive catheters are potential portals of infection.	Peripheral IV catheter and site covered with plastic for cleaning process.
	Assign private room and use contact precautions. Use Standard Precautions, including hand hygiene.	Major burns generally require contact precautions (follow facility procedures). Hand hygiene is a first-line measure to prevent infection.	Contact precautions initiated. Isolation supplies gathered and placed outside the door. Sign posted for isolation procedures and instructing visitors to see the nurse before entering.
	Apply topical antibiotic ointment to wounds bid.	Suppresses bacterial growth and promotes healing.	Wounds cleansed, antibiotic applied, and wounds redressed.
	Monitor WBC count for signs of infection; assess and cleanse wounds bid.	Cleansing wounds helps prevent infection and promotes healing.	Results for WBC count pending. No signs of wound infection.
	Encourage adequate nutrition.	High caloric intake with sufficient vitamins and minerals is needed for healing.	Taking fluids and sipping at supplemental protein shakes.

PROBLEM STATEMENT/NURSING DIAGNOSIS

Pain related to burn wounds and cleansing procedures.

Continued

Nursing Care Plan 43.1 Care of a Patient With a Burn—cont'd

SUPPORTING ASSESSMENT DATA

Subjective: States is in constant pain at an 8/10 level.

Objective: Grimacing and holding body rigid.

Goals/Expected Outcomes	Nursing Interventions	Selected Rationale	Evaluation
Patient's pain will be controlled to 4/10 with analgesia and nonpharmacologic methods.	Assess for quality, location, and intensity of pain every hour.	Pain is subjective, and patient must report own experience.	Reports pain at 4/10 currently; medicated 3 h ago. Acceptable level is 4/10, but requests additional medication before dressing change.
	Assess for and control noxious social or environmental stimuli.	Perception of pain is affected by various noxious stimuli, such as loud noise, visitors, dirty sheets, and bad odors.	Reports that visitors are laughing loudly in the stairwell; would like to have door closed.
	PCA IV initiated as ordered, giving boluses as appropriate before procedures and at bedtime.	IV narcotic analgesia is best for burn pain control initially. Patient-controlled medication delivery is most effective.	Bolus given for pain of 4/10 before dressing change.
Patient's pain will be controlled with oral medication before discharge.	Teach relaxation and imagery techniques to assist with pain control.	Relaxation and imagery techniques have proven helpful in pain control.	Began instruction on relaxation technique.
	Supply diversionary activities to diminish pain awareness.	TV, card games, visitors, computer games, and reading help divert attention from pain.	Is watching TV; not ready for greater activity yet.

PROBLEM STATEMENT/NURSING DIAGNOSIS

Altered self-care ability: toileting, dressing, related to inability to stand and walk.

SUPPORTING ASSESSMENT DATA

Objective: Burns on legs treated and grafted; unable to use legs for self-care activities.

Goals/Expected Outcomes	Nursing Interventions	Selected Rationale	Evaluation
Patient will assist with self-care activities within 3 mo.	Assist with hygiene and toileting as needed.	Assistance as needed must be provided to prevent infection and increase well-being.	Requires full assistance with ADLs today.
	Allow him to make decisions as much as possible to lessen feelings of helplessness.	Participation in care decreases feelings of dependency and increases feelings of control.	Choosing time for bath.
	Allow him to do as much as he is able to do.	Gradual resumption of activities can occur with encouragement and time.	"At least I can feed myself."

PROBLEM STATEMENT/NURSING DIAGNOSIS

Decreased self-esteem related to burns and worries about role in family as "breadwinner."

SUPPORTING ASSESSMENT DATA

Subjective: "With my legs burned, I won't be able to work anymore. I'm not much of a man anymore if I can't take care of my family."

Objective: Unable to use legs because of burns.

Goals/Expected Outcomes	Nursing Interventions	Selected Rationale	Evaluation
Patient will verbalize a plan of action to address his concerns before discharge.	Establish trusting relationship, actively listen to concerns and frustrations.	A trusting relationship helps him freely verbalize concerns and facilitates acceptance of treatment plan.	Expressed concerns about helplessness.
	Help him establish active role in recovery of use of legs.	Collaboration helps improve his self-esteem.	States wants to recover self-sufficiency.
	Allow him to do whatever ADLs are possible for him.	Performing self-care helps increase self-esteem.	Unable to ambulate or sit in chair.

Nursing Care Plan 43.1 Care of a Patient With a Burn—cont'd

Goals/Expected Outcomes	Nursing Interventions	Selected Rationale	Evaluation
	Praise him for his efforts with PT exercises and use of splints.	Praise encourages his actions.	Passive PT thus far.
	Help him establish small, accomplishable goals on a weekly basis.	Accomplishing small goals increases self-esteem.	Is thinking about goals for next week.
	Review past successes in overcoming obstacles.	Reflecting on past strengths helps patient envision transferring success to current challenges.	Recalls having a broken arm as a child and remembers learning to adapt and function with a cast in place.
Patient will discuss possible job retraining if needed.	Refer for job retraining if needed.	Extensive burns may affect ability to perform in current employment role.	Need for job retraining unknown at this time.

CRITICAL THINKING QUESTIONS

1. With partial-thickness burns on his legs and being unable to stand for long periods, do you think Mr. Young will be able to work as a mechanic again?
2. Because he has burns related to gasoline, what specific assessments should be made to determine whether there has been an inhalation injury?
3. Will he probably need skin grafting? If so, where? Is it likely that autografts could be used?

ADLs, Activities of daily living; *bid*, twice a day; *IV*, intravenous; *PCA*, patient-controlled analgesia; *PT*, physical therapy; *WBC*, white blood cell.

Complementary and Alternative Therapies

Helping Patients Cope With Pain

Proper body positioning, distraction therapy, music, television, games, and virtual reality technologies may help burn patients cope with pain. These adjunctive interventions do not replace medication or attentive nursing care.

monitored. Standard Precautions are used for all burn care, and private rooms are recommended. Meticulous hand hygiene is essential. Those in attendance wear caps, gowns, and gloves while caring for the patient as a protective measure. Contact precautions are used for infected wounds. Gloves are worn for all contact with open wounds and are changed when handling wounds on different areas of the patient's body and between handling soiled and sterile dressings. Hand hygiene is performed between glove changes. **Patient care items are not shared, and great attention is paid to maintaining asepsis for all patient care.** Bed linens are changed daily and whenever soiled, and a bed cradle or some other device is used to support the weight of the top covers to keep them off the burned areas.

Managing Itch

Multiple layers of tissue are involved in a deep burn. The treatment of postburn itch is a complex issue requiring trial of various treatments. Oral antihistamines are effective in many patients. Nonpharmacologic measures to reduce itching, such as massage, transcutaneous electrical nerve stimulation (TENS), music therapy, and botulinum toxin are used along with medication such as gabapentin. Therapeutic touch may prove helpful. Acupressure and acupuncture may assist with pain and itch relief. Topical antihistamines or local anesthetics have also shown effectiveness (Nedelec & LaSalle, 2018).

Nutritional Support

Enteral feedings are started within 24 to 28 hours after injury. Early feeding helps prevent ileus and provides needed nutrients. If enteral feedings are not tolerated, parenteral nutrition is provided.

A diet high in protein and calories is necessary for healing. The patient has increased metabolic needs directly proportional to the size of the burn area. Nutritional needs may be increased 50% to 150% above normal, and increased requirements can continue for 9 to 12 months. Caloric needs are calculated to include the patient's weight, age, and percentage of burn over total body surface as well as presumed energy requirements (Cochran, 2018). Only high-calorie liquids are given to drink. Free water intake is restricted. Dietary supplements include vitamins, especially vitamins A, C, and D. Minerals such as zinc and copper are supplied because deficiencies are seen in burn patients. Consultation with a nutritionist is essential because of the dietary issues that can occur for burn patients. There appears to be a maximum glucose load, and high carbohydrate intake can lead to hyperglycemia, dehydration, and respiratory problems. Excessive lipid intake has been associated with impaired wound healing, and ability to tolerate protein is related to renal function and fluid balance.

Psychosocial Support

Burn patients may face loss of mobility and independence or disfigurement involving the face or other parts of

Complementary and Alternative Therapies

Helping Burn Patients Relax

It was found that the use of immersive virtual reality in the form of video games was effective in reducing anxiety and pain in burn patients (Scapin et al., 2018).

the body usually visible to others. Many experience post-traumatic stress syndrome, and others may feel guilt, anger, or depression. Strive to develop an attitude of acceptance of the patient, a calm approach to dressing changes and discussions of scar formation, and an optimistic emphasis on what the patient can do and will be able to do in the future. When a patient has difficulty coping with the physical and psychosocial effects of a severe burn, effective nursing intervention can help the patient deal with their fears, anxieties, and sense of loss. Facility chaplains, counselors, social workers, and other team members can help the patient work through feelings. Assist the patient through the grief process and encourage them to relate what is experienced and their feelings about what has happened or is happening. Encourage the patient to ask questions and to verbalize their concerns about the care and the treatment plan. You can reinforce the patient's self-esteem by emphasizing the strengths you have noticed when the patient was coping with pain, inconvenience, or some other unpleasant situation. Involving the patient in performing self-care as much as possible and giving some sense of control over the situation are helpful. Clinical psychologists and psychiatrists may be needed if progress is not made.

The patient's body image may have been severely disrupted. Assist the patient to grieve over the loss and integrate the present body image. If the burns were caused by a suicide attempt or a risky behavior, psychiatric therapy will probably be necessary to deal with feelings of guilt. Although males and children younger than 4 years are more likely to experience burns, female patients tend to have greater adjustment difficulty with altered body image. A psychiatric clinical nurse specialist should be consulted to help the staff and the patient work through the complex psychological issues. Referrals to a psychologist, psychiatrist, social worker, or religious leader may also be necessary.

Clinical Cues

It is not uncommon for burn-injured patients to have post-traumatic stress disorder (PTSD). Be alert for symptoms: easily startled, irritable, short tempered, restless, avoidance of friends and interactions with others, and flashbacks of event. Notify the health care provider and request professional help from a clinician with specialized training in treating PTSD.

Patient and Family Education

The patient and family are taught about daily skin and wound care before discharge. They must be familiar with dressing instructions, lubrication of grafts, and donor site care. Moisturizing with an alcohol-free skin moisturizer is necessary at least three times a day. Pressure dressings or garments must be worn for 23 hours daily. Direct sunlight should be completely avoided for 1 year after injury because of increased sensitivity to UV rays.

Information about medication dosages, precautions, and potential side effects are sent home with the patient. Nutritional needs and diet recommendations are discussed. Adequate protein and calories are very important to full recovery. Referral is made to support groups or peers and counseling as needed for readjustment to life after the burn incident. The need for follow-up care is stressed, and appointment dates and times are established. See Nursing Care Plan 43.1 for interventions for selected problems in a burn patient.

◆ EVALUATION

Although the health care provider chooses the type of medication to be applied topically or administered systemically for pain, infection, and wound healing, you are responsible for continued assessment of the burn wounds to evaluate the effectiveness of the prescribed treatments. A systematic and ongoing assessment of scar tissue formation should be performed and evaluated to determine whether the patient is making an adjustment to the fact that burn scars may take as long as 12 to 24 months to mature completely. If outcomes are not being met, interventions are changed.

COMMUNITY CARE

Nurses in the community can do much to educate the public about the dangers of unprotected sun exposure and the signs of skin cancer. Nurses vigilantly assess changes in skin lesions that may indicate cancer. Skin self-screening is taught at every opportunity.

School nurses perform assessments for signs of lice and scabies. They teach families how to deal with these problems and how to prevent their spread.

One of the objectives for *Healthy People 2030* is to reduce the number of hospitalizations for older adults that result from pressure injury; therefore nurses employed outside the hospital setting are tasked with the challenge of prevention. Long-term care nurses must promote good skin integrity in all residents, handling older adults with special care to prevent tearing of the skin. Patients who are immobile are turned diligently to prevent pressure injury, and skin is inspected regularly. Home care nurses can encourage older adult patients to use skin emollients to moisten and protect the skin.

Teaching fire safety to children and parents and to workers in various occupational settings helps decrease fire injury. Home care nurses must continually assess patient homes for fire dangers and reinforce teaching to prevent home fires.

Get Ready for the NCLEX® Examination!

Key Points

- Dermatitis causes erythema and itching; a thorough history is necessary to locate the offending agent. Teach patients to avoid causative factors and how to apply topical medications.
- Acne often occurs at puberty; there is an accumulation of sebum and dead skin cells, which causes an inflammatory reaction. Drying agents that cause peeling work best to rid the skin of blackheads and whiteheads.
- There is a genetic predisposition to psoriasis, which appears as inflamed, edematous skin lesions with adherent silvery-white scales. It can be controlled but not cured.
- SJS is a potentially life-threatening allergic reaction usually triggered by medication.
- Hospitalized patients with bacterial skin infections require contact precautions.
- Viral skin disorders are caused by herpes viruses.
- Herpes zoster lesions follow nerve pathways; it is a very painful condition, and postherpetic neuralgia can occur. Anyone who has not previously had chickenpox or the immunization should not care for a patient with herpes zoster.
- Fungi prefer warm, moist places; for example, tinea pedis is one of the most common fungal infections and occurs on the feet.
- Treatment of pediculosis and scabies requires treating both the patient and objects that may harbor the parasites.
- Exposure to UV radiation (sunlight) is a major cause of skin cancer. Encourage use of a hat and sunglasses and sunscreen with UVB protection and an SPF of at least 30.
- Skin cancer has increased in incidence but is highly curable if treated in the early stages. All patients should be screened for skin cancer lesions and taught prevention measures and self-screening.
- Basal cell, squamous cell, and melanoma are the usual carcinomas arising from the epidermis.
- Actinic keratoses are a premalignant lesion common on the skin of older adults.
- If squamous cell carcinoma is not treated early, it can become invasive and metastasize.
- Melanoma is the most aggressive of the skin cancers and needs to be treated early to prevent metastasis.
- Pressure tissue injury is a potential problem for all immobile patients. Assessment includes risk factors and staging. Pressure injury should be measured and documented on discovery and then measured and documented regularly to show progress in healing. Treatment depends on the stage and location.
- Burns are caused by extreme heat, hot liquids, electrical agents, strong chemicals, or radiation. Treatment is based on classification.
- Burn care is divided into phases: emergency care, emergent care, acute care, and rehabilitation. Pain control is a major concern in every phase.
- Burn patients must be assessed for signs of respiratory problems. Suspect an inhalation injury if there are burns on the face or neck, singed nasal hair, darkened membranes in the nose or mouth, or a history of burn in a small space.
- With a major burn, fluid shifts can cause hypovolemic shock. Early fluid resuscitation is essential to prevent death.
- Burn care is aseptic. Eschar must be removed, and wounds must be debrided. Debridement can be very painful but is essential for healing and prevention of infection. Contracture prevention begins at the time of admission; special splints and positioning are used to preserve anatomic alignment.
- Early grafting with biologic or synthetic substances helps burn wounds heal more quickly. When skin grafts are healed, pressure dressings or garments are used to prevent excessive scarring.
- Burn patients can have problems with body image and also experience grief, loss, anger, or depression.

Additional Learning Resources

SG Go to your Study Guide for additional learning activities to help you master this chapter content.

Go to your Evolve website (http://evolve.elsevier.com/deWit/medsurg) for the following FREE learning resources:
- Animations, audio, and video
- Answers and rationales for questions and activities
- Glossary with pronunciations in English and Spanish
- Interactive Review Questions and more!

Review Questions for the NCLEX® Examination

1. In managing dermatitis, you should provide which instruction(s)? *(Select all that apply.)*
   1. “Avoid the irritant or allergen.”
   2. “Provide adequate skin lubrication.”
   3. “Wash skin frequently with germicidal soaps.”
   4. “Maintain skin moisture.”
   5. “Apply steroid-based preparations.”

   NCLEX Client Need: Health Promotion and Maintenance
2. A major type of skin disorder is acne rosacea. What information may be valuable for the patient education plan? *(Select all that apply.)*
   1. Acne rosacea usually occurs in adolescence and then begins to subside during adulthood.
   2. Diet is important, and flare-ups may be caused by caffeine-containing foods, spicy foods, sunlight, and alcohol.
   3. Comedos may occur on the face, upper shoulders, and back.
   4. The primary location for occurrence is on the face over the cheeks and bridge of the nose.
   5. Treatments may include metronidazole, retinoids, and occasionally antibiotics.

   NCLEX Client Need: Health Promotion and Maintenance

3. A male patient has inflamed, edematous skin of the elbows and knees accompanied by swelling of the joints of the fingers and toes. On examination, the skin is found to be covered with adherent silvery-white scales. Which question would provide more information about the patient's condition?
   1. "What do you do for a living?"
   2. "How much do you smoke?"
   3. "Have you had an upper respiratory tract infection recently?"
   4. "Have you recently changed your laundry detergent?"

   NCLEX Client Need: Physiological Integrity: Physiological Adaptation
4. A patient has skin lesions on the face, trunk, palms, extensor surfaces of joints, soles of the feet, and dorsum of the hands. On inspection, the lesions are found to have irregular borders and blistered, necrotic centers. The health care provider makes the medical diagnosis of SJS. What is the priority problem for this patient?
   1. Altered body image
   2. Altered self-care ability
   3. Potential for infection
   4. Acute pain

   NCLEX Client Need: Safe and Effective Care Environment: Coordinated Care
5. A school-age girl with evidence of severe itching in the scalp is checked for pediculosis. The problem of insufficient knowledge regarding management of the disease is identified for the child and the parent. What instructions would you include? *(Select all that apply.)*
   1. "Machine wash clothes and bedding using the cold cycle."
   2. "Share combs and hairbrushes with family members but not with friends."
   3. "Soak all combs and brushes in very hot water for more than 5 minutes."
   4. "Seal items that cannot be washed in air-expelled plastic bags for 14 days."
   5. "Reinfestation is unlikely if all family members are treated."

   NCLEX Client Need: Health Promotion and Maintenance
6. You are developing a plan of care for a wheelchair-bound patient. To prevent development of pressure tissue injury, which nursing interventions must be implemented? *(Select all that apply.)*
   1. Maintain postural alignment.
   2. Use pressure-relieving devices.
   3. Teach to shift weight every 15 minutes.
   4. Use donut-type devices.
   5. Reposition in the chair every hour.

   NCLEX Client Need: Safe and Effective Care Environment: Coordinated Care
7. Place these patients in order from 1 to 4 (1 being the patient at the highest risk, 4 being the patient at the lowest risk) for their risk for developing a pressure ulcer based on the Braden scale.
   1. Older adult who is NPO (nothing by mouth) for a procedure; able to independently ambulate and accomplish ADLs
   2. Patient who is paraplegic, well nourished, with strong upper body strength to self-transfer to wheelchair
   3. Thin older adult patient who walks occasionally but has limited mobility and cognitive impairments; reluctant to eat
   4. Patient who is comatose and unresponsive after a near-drowning accident; receives enteral feedings and is incontinent.

   NCLEX Client Need: Safe and Effective Care Environment: Coordinated Care
8. You note a reddened area on a patient's sacral area and check for blanching. What is the best rationale that supports this nursing action?
   1. Blanching suggests that the redness is probably temporary and will resolve when the pressure to the area is relieved.
   2. Checking for blanching is part of the daily routine for assessing any patient who is at risk for pressure injury.
   3. Evidence of blanching indicates that the patient is at high risk for pressure injury according to the Braden scale.
   4. Occurrence of blanching indicates that the redness is associated with a localized skin infection.

   NCLEX Client Need: Physiological Integrity: Reduction of Risk Potential
9. You make a home health visit 1 year after a patient was burned on more than 30% of their body. What problem may the patient be experiencing at this stage? *(Select all that apply.)*
   1. Concern with body image due to extensive scarring.
   2. Chronic pain due to contractures and nerve compartmentalization.
   3. Continued risk for infection due to reconstruction wounds.
   4. Increased risk for falls due to joint contractures.

   NCLEX Client Need: Physiological Integrity: Physiological Adaptation
10. While you are performing an initial assessment, a patient with extensive burn injuries suddenly develops increasing hoarseness and stridor. Pulse oximetry is 86%. What is the priority nursing action?
    1. Encourage the patient to take deep breaths.
    2. Provide humidified oxygen.
    3. Administer respiratory treatments.
    4. Suction respiratory secretions.

    NCLEX Client Need: Physiological Integrity: Pharmacological Therapies

Critical Thinking Questions

Scenario A

Mrs. Nash, age 32 years, has been assigned as your patient. She has severe dermatitis, which is probably allergic in origin. Her health care provider has ordered a topical lotion, dermatologic baths twice a day, and an antihistamine to relieve itching.

1. What kinds of data would you include in your ongoing assessment of Mrs. Nash's skin disorder?
2. What nursing care problems is Mrs. Nash likely to present?
3. What objectives and nursing measures to meet them would you include in Mrs. Nash's nursing care plan?
4. What would you teach Mrs. Nash about the application of topical agents when she returns home?

Scenario B

Ms. Moore, age 22 years, was badly burned when her clothing caught fire while she was grilling hamburgers on her patio. She has partial-thickness and full-thickness burns over her abdomen and down the front of both upper legs.

1. What is the priority of care after assessment when Ms. Moore reaches the emergency department?
2. What nursing measures should be taken to prevent infection of her burns?
3. What nursing measures would be included in the patient's nursing care plan to ensure that she did not suffer from an undetected fluid and electrolyte imbalance?
4. How is Ms. Moore's pain treated? Why?
5. List some specific things you and the other nurses could do to help her handle her sense of loss and altered self-image as a result of the appearance of the burns and scars.

Scenario C

Mrs. Chaco is an older adult who was admitted to your unit for dehydration and malnutrition. She responds to verbal commands but seems somewhat confused by your questions. She will quietly sit in a chair, with some movement of her arms, but makes no attempts to walk or stand. She can feed herself, but her appetite and food and fluid intake are very poor. She has had one episode of incontinence with a scant amount of dark yellow urine.

1. Rate this patient's risk for pressure ulcers using the Braden scale.
2. Discuss interventions that you will use to address her positioning and apparent lack of spontaneous mobility.
3. Discuss interventions that you could use to address her nutritional issues.
4. What instructions will you give to the nursing assistant about cleaning the patient's skin?

UNIT XV Emergency and Disaster Management

44 Care of Patients in Disasters or Bioterrorism Attack

http://evolve.elsevier.com/deWit/medsurg

Objectives

Theory

1. Analyze differences between an emergency situation and a disaster.
2. Discuss an emergency preparedness plan for a health care facility.
3. Compare the stages of psychological response that occur with a disaster.
4. Compare and contrast the parameters used in the triage system for victims after a disaster versus the routine triage that occurs in hospital emergency departments.
5. Identify responsibilities and duties of nurses in the care of disaster victims.
6. Explain safety measures to be used for a chemical emergency.
7. Demonstrate knowledge of measures to be taken in the event of a nuclear disaster.
8. Explain warning signs that suggest a bioterrorism attack has occurred.
9. Differentiate the signs and symptoms of the various agents that could be used for a terrorist attack.
10. Recognize the importance of debriefing of health care personnel after a disaster.

Clinical Practice

11. Participate in a disaster drill.
12. Gather supplies for a "bug out" bag and other disaster preparedness items.
13. Teach a group of adults how to prepare safe water after a disaster has disrupted the water supply.
14. Identify the measures you would take for your own safety when assisting others after a disaster has occurred.

Key Terms

bioterrorism (bī-ō-TĔR-ĕr-ĭ-zĭm, p. 1037)
debriefing (dē-BRĒ-fĭng, p. 1044)
decontamination (dē-kŏn-tăm-ĭ-NĀ-shŭn, p. 1036)
disaster (dĭ-ZĂ-stĕr, p. 1024)
mass casualty (măs KĂ-zhĕl-tē, p. 1032)
pandemic (păn-DĔ-mĭk, p. 1043)
surge capacity (sĕrj kĕ-PĂ-sĕ-tē, p. 1025)
triage (TRĒ-ăhzh, p. 1026)

Concepts Covered in This Chapter

- Self-Management
- Nutrition
- Immunity
- Infection
- Stress
- Coping
- Leadership
- Communication
- Collaboration
- Safety
- Care Coordination
- Health Care Organizations

DISASTER PREPAREDNESS AND RESPONSE

An extraordinary event, such as a multivictim incident involving an explosion or a train crash, requires a rapid and skilled response to manage the wounded. There may be walking wounded, critically wounded, and fatally wounded victims. This type of event usually can be handled by the community's emergency medical services (EMS) and the hospital emergency departments.

A **disaster** **exists when the number of casualties exceeds the resource capabilities of the area;** thus the community's existing emergency resources may be overwhelmed. Natural disasters include epidemics, earthquakes, explosions, hurricanes, tornadoes, fires, and floods. Intentional terrorist attacks or accidental human-made disasters may result from transportation incidents or events involving chemical, biological, or nuclear materials. A disaster causes mass casualties, psychological as well as physical trauma, and permanent changes within the community.

The governmental agencies responsible for disaster planning are the Department of Homeland Security, Center for Domestic Preparedness, Federal Emergency Management Agency (FEMA), and U.S. Public Health Service. The American Red Cross is a voluntary organization that traditionally provides the basic essentials of shelter, food, and first aid during a natural disaster (Fig. 44.1). In most communities the local Office

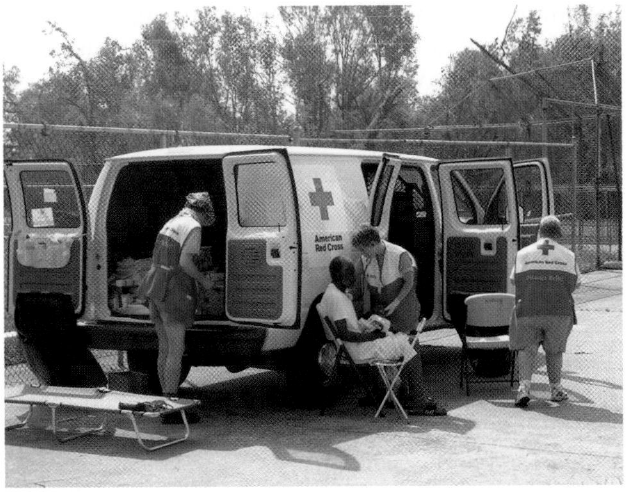

Fig. 44.1 A Red Cross volunteer checks on a resident affected by the extreme heat in Algiers, Louisiana, after Hurricane Katrina. (Courtesy the American Red Cross, printed with permission. Copyright The American Red Cross.)

of Emergency Services (OES), the Red Cross, and the Salvation Army work together to formulate disaster plans. They coordinate their services with each other and with other agencies in planning essential services, such as shelter, transportation, communication, and welfare. The Centers for Disease Control and Prevention (CDC) has a website with information on all types of disasters, weather events, and mass casualty events (http://emergency.cdc.gov/disasters/alldisasters.asp).

Special courses in civil defense and disaster nursing are offered by the OES, the Red Cross, and professional organizations. These courses help nurses and volunteer workers to understand the function and coordination of agencies involved in particular types of disaster. To increase availability of volunteer health care professionals, registries such as the Emergency Systems for Advance Registration of Volunteer Health Professionals (ESAR-VHP) have been designed to proactively verify credentials; provide disaster response training; and coordinate deployment of professionals in conjunction with local, state, and national response plans. In response to the increase in weather-related incidents, the U.S. Department of Health and Human Services has launched a website that serves as a "healthcare emergency preparedness information gateway." The Technical Resources, Assistance Center, and Information Exchange (TRACIE) can be found at https://asprtracie.hhs.gov and provides information and links to a wide variety of disaster information.

HOSPITAL PREPAREDNESS

The Joint Commission requires that hospitals have an emergency preparedness plan in place. There are guidelines for emergency preparedness by type of facility. Emergency department health care providers undergo formal training for disaster events. Emergency department nurses are encouraged to obtain certification in emergency preparedness. You should **proactively** (take action in preparation) seek out disaster training at your work setting and advocate for sufficient emergency supplies and support. Health care systems must self-evaluate **surge capacity**, which is defined as the maximum services a facility can offer when every resource is mobilized (TRACIE, 2019). This was also called *crisis capacity* by the Institute of Medicine (IOM) in a 2012 report. The emergency plan should be tested with drills at least twice a year.

Hospitals must plan for many possible scenarios from trauma to chemical contamination. Plans also must be in place for an incident that affects the physical functioning of the facility. If a storm or earthquake damages the hospital building or eliminates power or water sources, decisions on evacuation of patients will have to be made. If the hospital is intact and functional, the focus moves to management of a large volume of patients. Hospital disaster plans outline the command and decision-making structure in addition to details of communication and triage.

The emergency preparedness plan identifies who will be in charge and the chain of command for the facility. The designated communications officer is responsible for internal communication, such as keeping the staff informed, and for external communication, such as contacting other agencies for help or reporting data about infection or chemical contamination that could have widespread effects. There will be a hospital incident commander (health care provider or administrator) who assumes responsibility for launching the emergency preparedness plan. This person's role as commander is to view the entire situation, bring in needed human and supply resources, and facilitate the flow of patients through the system. Usual hospital routine will be altered to accommodate care for high numbers of patients. Departmental roles will be changed. Physical therapy and other departments may close their usual operations and become the minor treatment area for nonurgent patients. The concept of "reverse triage," or sending relatively stable patients home, can be used to free up beds. Reports from actual disaster events have shown that inpatients discharged a day earlier than planned showed no adverse outcomes.

A medical command provider will focus on determining the number, acuity, and medical needs of the casualties arriving from the scene of the disaster. This person will organize the emergency health care team response to the injured or ill patients. Specialists trained for the type of disaster that has occurred will be called in to help as the need is foreseen. Decisions will be made about who is to be evacuated to a facility with specialty care not available at the sending facility.

A triage officer, usually a health care provider, with the assistance of triage nurses, will rapidly evaluate each patient at the hospital and send the patient to the appropriate area for immediate or eventual treatment. The emergency department supervisor or charge nurse collaborates with the medical command provider and triage officer to organize nursing and ancillary personnel to meet patient needs. The disaster call list will be activated to call in off-duty staff as needed. In addition to these personnel, there will be a supply officer, communications officer, infection control officer, and public information officer. The public information officer will manage the media. Hospital staff, at all levels, will be called on to assist with whatever care is needed. Long-term care facilities may need to evacuate residents, or they may need to take in people from other facilities or the community.

Crisis standards of care (CSC) were developed by the IOM at the request of the U.S. Department of Health and Human Services. The publication outlines preparation for a crisis surge response and decision-making guidelines for delivering the best possible medical care to patients when there are not enough resources to provide the level of care normally given. This document is being used as the framework for organizations and communities in creating policies and procedures for disaster response (IOM, 2012).

TRIAGE

After a disaster, prehospital care of victims is prioritized according to a **triage** system that is different from regular emergency department triage (Table 44.1). Those with life-threatening conditions and a good chance of survival are cared for first. **When there are more victims of a disaster than medical personnel to treat them, those who are likely to survive are treated first; these patients are given red, yellow, or green tags (some classification systems may also include white tags). The mortally wounded and those who are not expected to survive are attended to later, and these patients are issued a black tag** (Fig. 44.2). The choices involved in issuing tags are difficult for most nurses, but in a disaster the good of many must prevail over benefit to the few.

Even though triage may have been done in the field, triage is performed again at the emergency care facility. Green-tagged patients usually comprise the greatest number in large-scale disasters. Patients need to be managed until they can be treated. If not managed, patients can become a health hazard by walking around with infection, radioactivity, or chemical contamination. A special bracelet with a disaster number may be applied to tagged patients.

Nursing Roles and Responsibilities During Disaster

Your nursing skills will be called into play under disaster conditions; for example, you could be asked to:

- Perform emergency nursing measures
- Evaluate the environmental and physical risks and shortages (e.g., no electrical power)
- Know measures for prevention and control of environmental health hazards (e.g., hand hygiene and food and water safety)

There are many variables to be managed in a disaster setting. Preparation and training are key to effective treatment of large volumes of patients. You are held accountable to practice within the scope of practice of your licensure and training when in your work setting. You may be called on to provide care that you have not performed since your initial training but is within your scope of practice. You should ask for help when needed and focus on delivering the best possible care. The Uniform Emergency Volunteer Health Practitioners Act (UEVHPA) provides immunity from lawsuits when nurse volunteers are providing care within the scope of practice of the state of licensure.

During emergency care, you will perform needed procedures such as inserting catheters, nasogastric tubes, and possibly intravenous (IV) lines and drawing blood. Basic principles of nursing apply in a disaster, but adaptation to "crisis standards" is necessary if there is a disparity between need and availability of equipment, supplies, or personnel. Performing nursing procedures in a disaster situation demands skill and judgment to provide for the good of the greatest number of people. You may be asked to help cook, serve food, pass out water, or do whatever else is a priority need at the time. Observing, recording, and reporting information about patients to appropriate authorities must be done in an organized manner. General physical and mental conditions of patients and signs and symptoms that

Table 44.1 Disaster Triage System

CLASSIFICATION	TRIAGE TAG	TYPICAL CONDITIONS	TREATMENT
Class I: Emergent	Red tag	Immediate threat to life, such as airway compromise or hemorrhagic shock	Immediate
Class II: Urgent	Yellow tag	Major injuries, open fractures, large wounds	Within 30 min to 2 h
Class III: Nonurgent	Green tag	"Walking wounded" (closed fractures, sprains, strains, contusions)	Wait for more than 2 h
Class IV: Minor	White tag	Minor injuries not requiring health care provider care (abrasion, bruises)	Dismiss
Class V: Dead or expected to die	Black tag	Dead or imminently dying with little chance of survival	None

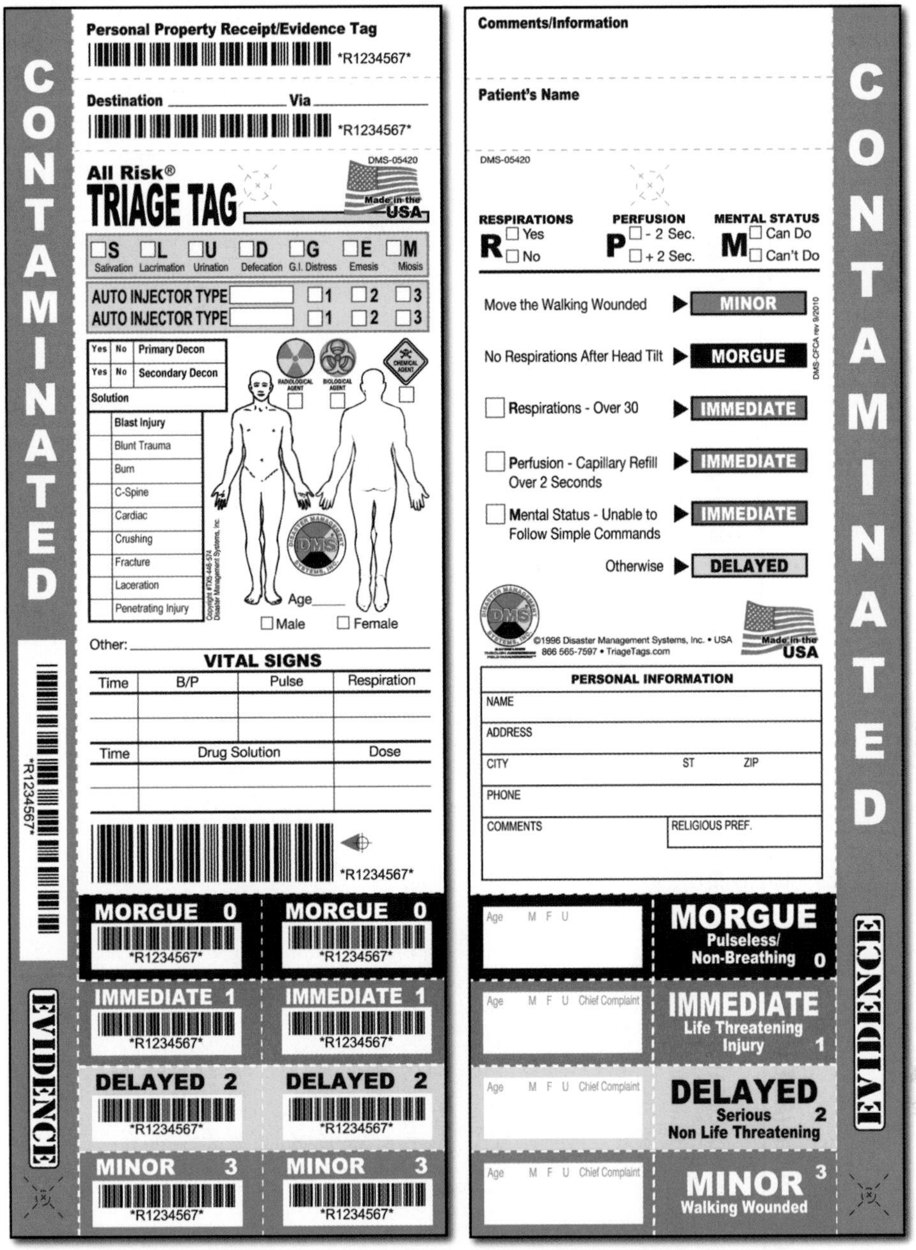

Fig. 44.2 Example of triage tags. (Courtesy Disaster Management Systems, Inc., Pomona, Calif.)

may indicate changes in condition must be quickly identified. During a disaster, preventing the spread of infection is a primary nursing concern. Table 44.2 identifies the communicable diseases that can become epidemic after a disaster. Infection control is a top priority when large groups of people are together in a shelter because the incidence of communicable disease is much greater. Although the National Patient Safety Goals are intended to prevent health care–related infections under normal circumstances, hand hygiene has an even greater potential as a basic infection control measure to protect large groups of people who may gather together after a disaster.

The emotional and physical comfort and safety of large numbers of disaster victims must be attended to with limited supplies, equipment, utilities, and personnel. You must understand the emotional stress caused by fear, problems of displacement and separation of families, personal and material losses, crowded living conditions, increasing anxiety, and continuing danger. You will need to help people of different cultural backgrounds and religious beliefs to accept and adapt to temporary living conditions in crowded and often adverse situations. People should be encouraged to verbalize their concerns and fears. **In a disaster situation, you should provide basic instructions about appropriate self-care within the current environment and encourage people to provide for their own needs. The prepared nurse will:**

- Be prepared for self-survival (i.e., stock your own household with emergency supplies)

Table 44.2 **Communicable Diseases With Epidemic Potential (All Except Tetanus) in Natural Disasters**

DISEASE	TRANSMISSION	AGENT	CLINICAL FEATURES	INCUBATION PERIOD	DIAGNOSIS	TREATMENT	PREVENTION/CONTROL
Waterborne							
Cholera	Fecal/oral, contaminated water or food	*Vibrio cholerae* serogroups O1 or O139	Profuse watery diarrhea, vomiting	2 hr–5 days	Direct microscopic observation of *V. cholerae* in stool	Intensive rehydration therapy; antimicrobials based on sensitivity testing	Hand hygiene, proper handling of water/ food and sewage disposal
Leptospirosis	Fecal/oral, contaminated water	*Leptospira* species	Sudden-onset fever, headache, chills, vomiting, severe myalgia	2–28 days	*Leptospira*-specific IgM serologic assay	Penicillin, amoxicillin, doxycycline, erythromycin, cephalosporins	Avoid entering contaminated water; safe water source
Hepatitis	Fecal/oral, contaminated water or food	Hepatitis A and E viruses	Jaundice, abdominal pain, nausea, diarrhea, fever, fatigue, and loss of appetite	15–50 days	Serologic assay detecting anti-HAV or anti-HEV IgM antibodies	Supportive care; hospitalization and barrier nursing for severe cases; close monitoring of pregnant women	Hand hygiene, proper handling of water/ food and sewage disposal; hepatitis A vaccine
Bacillary dysentery	Fecal/oral, contaminated water or food	*Shigella dysenteriae* type 1	Malaise, fever, vomiting, blood and mucus in stool	12–96 hr	Suspect if bloody diarrhea; confirmation requires isolation of organism from stool	Antibiotic treatment is usually not necessary. If treated, fluoroquinolones, or ceftriaxone; hospitalization of seriously ill or malnourished; rehydration	Hand hygiene, proper handling of water/ food and sewage disposal
Typhoid fever	Fecal/oral, contaminated water or food	*Salmonella typhi*	Sustained fever, headache, constipation	1–3 days	Culture from blood, bone marrow, bowel fluids; rapid antibody tests	Fluoroquinolones, ceftriaxone, ciprofloxacin	Hand hygiene, proper handling of water/ food and sewage disposal; mass vaccination in some settings

Acute Respiratory							
Pneumonia	Person to person by airborne respiratory droplets	*Streptococcus pneumoniae, Haemophilus influenzae,* or viral	Cough, difficulty breathing, rapid breathing	1–3 days	Clinical presentation; culture respiratory secretions	Treatment is pathogen driven. Macrolides for outpatient. Beta-lactam for inpatients. Combination therapy is most common	Isolation; proper nutrition; if cause is *Streptococcus,* polyvalent vaccine to high-risk populations
Direct Contact							
Measles	Person to person by airborne respiratory droplets	Measles virus *(Morbillivirus)*	Rash, high fever, cough, runny nose, red and watery eyes; serious post-measles complications (5%-10% of cases)—diarrhea, pneumonia, croup	7–21 days	Throat or nasopharyngeal swab. Tested for measles-specific IgM antibody and measles RNA	Supportive care; proper nutrition and hydration; vitamin A; control fever; antimicrobials in complicated cases with pneumonia, dysentery; treat conjunctivitis, keratitis	Rapid mass vaccination within 72 hr of initial case report (priority to high-risk groups if limited supply); vitamin A in children 6 mo–5 yr of age to prevent complications and reduce mortality risk
Bacterial meningitis (meningococcal meningitis)	Person to person by airborne respiratory droplets	*Neisseria meningitides* serogroups A, C, W135	Sudden-onset fever, rash, neck stiffness; altered consciousness; bulging fontanel in patients younger than 1 year	10–12 days	Examination of CSF—elevated WBC count, protein; gram-negative diplococci	Penicillin, chloramphenicol, ampicillin, ceftriaxone, cefotaxime, co-trimoxazole; supportive therapy; diazepam for seizures	Rapid mass vaccination
Wound-Related							
Tetanus	Soil	*Clostridium tetani*	Difficulty swallowing, lockjaw, muscle rigidity, spasms	2–10 days	Entirely clinical	Tetanus immune globulin	Thorough wound cleansing, tetanus vaccine

Continued

Table 44.2 Communicable Diseases With Epidemic Potential (All Except Tetanus) in Natural Disasters—cont'd

DISEASE	TRANSMISSION	AGENT	CLINICAL FEATURES	INCUBATION PERIOD	DIAGNOSIS	TREATMENT	PREVENTION/CONTROL
Vector-Borne							
Malaria	Mosquito (*Anopheles* species)	*Plasmodium falciparum, P. vivax*	Fever, chills, sweats, head and body aches, nausea and vomiting	7–30 days	Parasites on blood smear observed using a microscope; rapid diagnostic assays if available	Chloroquine phosphate, hydroxychlorquine	Mosquito control; insecticide-treated nets, bedding, clothing
Dengue fever	Mosquito (*Aedes aegypti*)	Dengue virus-1, -2, -3, -4 (Flavivirus)	Sudden-onset severe flulike illness, high fever, severe headache, pain behind the eyes, and rash. Severe cases can become hemorrhagic.	4–7 days	Serum antibody testing with ELISA or rapid dot-blot technique	Intensive supportive therapy	Mosquito control; insecticide-treated nets, bedding, clothing
Japanese encephalitis	Mosquito (*Culex* species)	Japanese encephalitis virus (Flavivirus)	Quick-onset, headache, high fever, neck stiffness, stupor, disorientation, tremors	5–15 days	Serologic assay for JE virus IgM-specific antibodies in CSF or blood (acute phase)	Intensive supportive therapy	Mosquito control, isolation of cases, mass vaccination
Yellow fever	Mosquito (*Aedes, Haemogogus*)	Yellow fever virus (Flavivirus)	Fever, backache, headache, nausea, vomiting; toxic phase—jaundice, abdominal pain, kidney failure	3–6 days	Serologic assay for yellow fever virus antibodies	Intensive supportive therapy	Mosquito control, isolation of cases, mass vaccination

From Waring SC, Brown BJ: The threat of communicable diseases following natural disaster: a public health response, *Disaster Manag Response* 3(2):44-45, 2005 with permission from the Emergency Nurses Association. All information verified as current via Centers for Disease Control and Prevention website, 2019.

CSF, Cerebrospinal fluid; *ELISA,* enzyme-linked immunosorbent assay; *HAV,* hepatitis A virus; *HEV,* hepato-encephalomyelitis virus; *IgM,* immunoglobulin M; *JE,* Japanese encephalitis; *RNA,* ribonucleic acid; *WBC,* white blood cell.

- Know the disaster plan for your workplace and identify your duties accordingly
- Know the meaning of warning signals of disaster and the action to be taken
- Know the measures for protection against radioactive, chemical, or biological contamination
- Know the community disaster plans and community health resources
- Know and interpret the community resources for citizen preparedness, such as first aid and medical self-help courses

Think Critically

You have just started your new nursing job. During your orientation and preceptorship, you do not receive any training about the hospital's disaster plan or what your role would be as a staff nurse. What should you do?

COMMUNITY PREPAREDNESS

Whether the disaster is natural or human-made, it will involve physical injuries, loss of property, and interruption of the normal activities of daily living. People often will need food, water, clothing, shelter, medical and nursing or hospital care, and other basic necessities of life.

Preparedness by health care professionals involves both personal and employment-related responsibilities. Disaster supplies, with all recommended items, should be prepared by every household.

Every family should have a contact person outside the immediate geographic area who extended family members can call to receive information about the welfare of their relatives. Communication into and out of a disaster region is often cut off. Each member of a family living together should know whom they are to call if separated from one another. Even if telephone communication is functional, the service is usually overwhelmed with activity. Texting and social media use a different bandwidth and may be more successful modes of communication.

Think Critically

If a disaster occurred in your community and you were not injured, where would you call or go to see how you could help?

Most people know about these recommendations, but few are truly prepared. According to an annual report by FEMA, preparedness has improved in the time since the September 11, 2001, terrorist attacks. There is still much more to be put in place on the federal and state levels. Natural disasters, including tornados, flooding, wildfires, hurricanes, and earthquakes, are frequent and seasonal in some areas. Knowing that such events are likely means that preparation is prudent and responsible. In addition to the standard disaster supplies, items specific to the event may be needed. The CDC website at www.emergency.cdc.gov gives instructions on how to prepare, what to do if the event occurs, and what resources are available. All nurses must encourage people in the community to prepare.

The local law enforcement agency, the city or county emergency management department, and the state public health department are responsible for coordinating efforts to assist people when a disaster happens. The American Red Cross may disperse personnel and supplies to assist with essential needs and medical care. If the state requests assistance, the Department of Homeland Security determines whether FEMA is to be called. If so, FEMA brings personnel and aid to the

Health Promotion

Disaster Preparedness

Community members should be encouraged to prepare for a disaster. Preparations should include a minimum of 3 days' supplies. At a minimum, have the basic supplies listed here. Keep supplies in a kit that you can use at home or take with you if you must evacuate.

- Water in plastic containers (1 gallon per person per day). Change the supply every 6 months.
- Nonperishable food that requires no refrigeration, preparation, or cooking and little water. Disposable dishes and eating utensils, a camping or military "mess kit," and a manual can opener are ideal.
- Flashlight.
- Battery-operated or hand-crank radio (National Oceanic and Atmospheric Administration [NOAA] Weather Radio, if possible).
- Extra batteries.
- First aid kit containing an assortment of bandages, scissors, tweezers, gloves, antiseptic, antibiotic ointment, thermometer, and moistened towelettes.
- Supply of essential prescription medications and nonprescription drugs: pain relievers, antacids, vitamins, laxatives, antiinflammatory agents.
- Sanitation and personal hygiene items (e.g., hand sanitizer, soap, disinfectant wipes).
- Extra set of clothing.
- Copies of personal documents (medication list and pertinent medical information, proof of address, deed or lease to home, passports, birth certificates, insurance policies, copies of insurance cards and official identification).
- Cellphone with chargers.
- Family and emergency contact information.
- Extra cash or traveler's checks.
- Emergency blanket.
- Maps of the area.

Add to the kit any items specific to the types of disaster common to your geographic area. Also include any items specific to individual family members such as infants or people with special needs.

A 3- to 6-week supply of food and water is recommended. In a disaster situation, it may take several days for rescuers to arrive. Food items should be used and replaced every 6 months to maintain freshness.

Data from American Red Cross: *Be Red Cross ready.* Retrieved from http://www.redcross.org/prepare/location/home-family/get-kit.

area. If a disaster is of major proportions, a Disaster Medical Assistance Team (DMAT) may be activated at the state or federal level. These units bring medical, paraprofessional, and support personnel along with medical equipment and supplies to sustain an operation for a minimum of 72 hours. The team provides **triage** (sorting casualties by priority of need for treatment), evacuation, primary health care, and assistance to local health care facilities that are overwhelmed. The emergency management team sets up a communications system, and the EMS personnel at the scene notify the emergency departments at the hospitals of the situation. Essential personnel are notified of a disaster or **mass casualty** (many-victims incident). If electronic communication systems are functional, alert messages are sent via telephone, computer, pagers, and other devices. Community residents are instructed about what to do if an earthquake, wildfire, hurricane, tornado, or flood occurs in their area. In the event of communication failure, amateur radio operators can provide essential communication services. The Amateur Radio Emergency Service (ARES) organization has formal agreements with FEMA, the Department of Homeland Security, the Salvation Army, and other agencies to provide communication services when standard communication methods are not functional.

! Safety Alert

Fire

In the event of a fire, if told to evacuate, leave quickly. If at home and the smoke detector goes off, do not wait to dress or gather belongings—get out of the dwelling. If fire or smoke is evident, drop to the floor and crawl to the exit. Cover your mouth and nose with a moistened cloth if smoke is present. Feel any door before opening it. If it is hot, find another way out. If clothes catch on fire, drop to the ground and roll to suffocate the fire. Keep rolling until the flames are out.

! Safety Alert

Tornado, Hurricane, and Flood

Choose ahead of time where you could go if evacuation is necessary. Evacuate when you are told to do so. Listen to a NOAA Weather Radio or local radio or television stations for evacuation instructions. Keep road maps handy because you may have to take unfamiliar routes and your electronic devices may not be functional. Bring the following with you:

- Prescription medications and medical supplies, glasses, hearing aid, and other assistive devices
- Bedding and clothing, including sleeping bags and pillows
- Bottled water, battery-operated radio and extra batteries, first aid kit, and flashlight
- Documents, such as driver's license, Social Security card, proof of residence, insurance policies, wills, deeds, birth and marriage certificates, and tax records, if they are readily available within the home

If advised to evacuate the area, residents should gather essential belongings, medications, pets, and keepsakes and leave immediately. If tornado sirens are sounded, people should take refuge in a basement or in an inner room without windows, such as a closet or a bathroom, to avoid flying debris. Getting into the bathtub and covering oneself with cushions or a mattress can also protect a person from flying debris. If outside, it is best to lie in a culvert or ditch below ground level.

? Think Critically

Consider your current level of nursing knowledge and your personal circumstances at home, including your family members, pets, and any preparations you have (or have not!) made for a disaster event. What would be your reaction if your instructor called you and asked you to help because of a local environmental disaster?

PSYCHOLOGICAL RESPONSES TO DISASTER

Any intense event results in an emotional response. Natural disasters or massive injuries from a human-made event have both physical and emotional effects. The phrase "they are in shock" is used to explain the emotional state of the victims after one of these events. Although emotions can trigger physical signs and symptoms, the condition is usually not life threatening unless the individual affected has a preexisting condition that puts them at risk.

Signs and symptoms of emotional shock include headaches, nausea, and chest pain. Preexisting medical conditions may worsen because of the stress. Remaining calm and seeing to immediate physical needs can reassure the patient that someone is in charge and has control over the situation. Severe emotional trauma, such as posttraumatic stress disorder, may take years of therapy to process.

After a major disaster, psychological events occur in stages. The stages are not always linear, and people progress through them at different rates (CDC, 2018):

- *Impact stage.* Survivors are stunned, apathetic, and disorganized. For several hours after the initial event, they may have difficulty following directions and will need strong support and firm guidance.
- *Heroic stage.* Individuals want to be helpful and may minimize or ignore their own injuries and demonstrate rescue behavior that is risky to self.
- *Honeymoon stage.* Survivors are grateful they are still alive. There is a strong sense of brotherhood and community spirit.
- *Disillusionment stage.* Reality of loss occurs. Ongoing physical and emotional fatigue can result in substance abuse and discouragement. Survivors feel abandoned and ignored by the larger community because of the gap between resources and need.
- *Reconstruction stage.* This stage may continue for years as people rebuild their lives and even begin to see the crisis, in retrospect, as a growth and opportunity period.

Individuals in communities that are affected by a disaster will need time to cope with events. Ineffective coping requires follow-up. Signs and symptoms that should prompt a mental health referral are severe anxiety, suicidal thoughts, inability to care for self, abuse of alcohol or drugs, depression, or domestic violence.

Think Critically

Are you and your family prepared for a disaster? Do you have a disaster kit on hand? If you have children, do you have measures in place for their care by others if you are unable to reach them? Is there an out-of-state contact person for family members to call to inform of their status?

Care of Special Populations

Ideally, there should be a community database that includes the needs of vulnerable groups (older adults, disabled persons, and immunocompromised persons) that require special assistance because a delay can result in death. Loss of electrical power is a serious issue for those who require oxygen or other life-sustaining mechanical equipment. Patients requiring hemodialysis may need to be temporarily relocated to areas with intact power and water resources. Older adults may be without their prescriptions for chronic or other serious health conditions. Eyeglasses or hearing aids may be lost, and many older adults cannot see or hear well without these aids. Developmental concerns should be considered; for example, infants need diapers, bottles, and formula or powdered milk. Infants are especially vulnerable to diarrhea and dehydration related to contaminated water sources.

Individuals with disabilities may need a means of mobility if they are separated from their belongings. They may need assistance with bathing, eating, and general activities of daily living. Immunocompromised people need special attention and care to prevent infection when in large crowds.

Water and Food Safety

Disruption or contamination of the water supply is probable when a disaster occurs. Floodwater or storm water should not be used to wash dishes, brush teeth, wash and prepare food, wash hands, make ice, or make baby formula. People will need to be taught how to purify water.

Healthy People 2030 objectives include improved food and water safety; during a disaster, special attention is required to safeguard food and water supplies. If there is a power outage and people can stay in their homes, they will need to know how to keep their food supply safe to eat (CDC, 2019) (Box 44.1).

Nursing Management in the Reconstruction Stage

Working toward restoring community and family life after the disaster—according to available resources—involves you and other members of the health care team.

Health Promotion

Preparing Safe Water

When the normal water supply is disrupted, water may be purified by:

- Bringing it to a rolling boil for 1 minute (3 minutes for elevations above 6500 feet). Let the water cool before drinking it. Store water in a clean, sanitized container.
- Adding household liquid bleach containing 5% to 6% sodium hypochlorite. Add 8 drops of bleach (or 0.5 mL) to 1 gallon of water and let stand for 30 minutes.
- Distilling the water. To distill, fill a large pot halfway with water. Tie a cup securely to the handle on the pot's lid so that the cup will hang right side up when the lid is upside down. Set the lid upside down on the top of the pot so that the cup hangs down into the pot below the lid (the cup should not dangle in the water). Boil the water for 20 minutes. The water that drips from the lid into the cup is distilled. This method frees water of microbes that may remain after bleach treatment.

Data from Centers for Disease Control and Prevention: *Making water safe in an emergency*. Retrieved from https://www.cdc.gov/healthywater/emergency/drinking/making-water-safe.html.

Box 44.1 Keeping Food Safe to Eat

Perishable foods should not be kept warmer than 40° F (4.4° C) for more than 2 hours. A closed refrigerator ordinarily will keep food chilled to below 40° F for 2 to 4 hours during a power outage. It is wise to have a quick-response digital thermometer on hand. If a power outage occurs, do the following:

- Keep the refrigerator and freezer doors closed. A freezer that is half full will keep food safe for up to 24 hours; a full freezer will keep food safe for 48 hours.
- If it appears that the outage will last more than 2 to 4 hours, pack refrigerated milk, dairy products, mayonnaise, meats, fish, poultry, eggs, gravy, stuffing, and leftovers into coolers and surround them with ice.
- When uncertain as to how long the power has been out, check the internal temperature of foods in your refrigerator with the quick-response thermometer. If the internal temperature is higher than 40° F, throw the food away.
- Throw away food that may have come into contact with floodwater or storm water.
- Throw away food that has an unusual odor, color, or texture.
- Food containers with screw-on caps, snap-on lids, crimped caps (beer bottles), twist-off caps, and snap-open caps, as well as home-canned foods, should be discarded if they have come into contact with floodwater or storm water because they cannot be disinfected.
- If cans have come into contact with floodwater or storm water, remove the labels and wash them with hot, soapy water or dip them in a solution of 1 cup bleach in 5 gallons of clean water. Relabel the cans with a marker.

Data from American Red Cross: *Food safety guidelines* (website): www.redcross.org/prepare/disaster/food-safety; Centers for Disease Control and Prevention: *Keep food and water safe after a disaster or emergency* (website): http://emergency.cdc.gov/disasters/foodwater/facts.asp.

Individual self-help and work therapy are encouraged, as are activities of daily living, with adaptations designed to attain and maintain a clean and healthy environment. Existing community facilities and resources must be used as much as possible for continued patient care.

You can promote the effectiveness of the health service agency in disaster preparedness by knowing and helping to implement the agency's disaster plan. You should understand the relationship among the plans of health agencies, local government, and community agencies. Trying to maintain and restore community health by controlling environmental health hazards is an important responsibility for every nurse.

PREPARING FOR CHEMICAL, NUCLEAR, OR BIOLOGICAL DISASTERS

CHEMICAL DISASTER

A chemical emergency can occur from a transportation accident or an explosion at a chemical plant. Chemical agents can be inhaled gases, liquids, or solids that are toxic to humans. Awareness of a chemical attack or accident is difficult because most chemical agents vaporize quickly from their liquid form. A lesson learned during the 1995 Tokyo subway sarin attack is that chemical agents are difficult to identify, and front-line staff are not always informed.

Many chemical agents give off no odor or have a familiar odor such as that of newly mown grass or bitter almonds or a fruity odor (Madsen, 2018). Indications that a chemical attack has occurred might include the following:

- Foglike or low-lying cloud suddenly appearing in the atmosphere
- Many dead birds, domestic animals, or insects within an area
- Many dead, dying, or sick people within an area or downwind from a suspicious cloud or fog
- An atypical, unexplained odor for the location

Chemical agents (Table 44.3) that might be used in a terrorist attack include pulmonary/choking agents, blood agents, vesicant (blistering) agents, incapacitating agents, and nerve agents (Madsen, 2018). These agents may be delivered through aerosol sprays, in explosive devices, or through food or water, depending on the action of the substance.

The public should be informed of what to do in the event of a chemical disaster.

Chemicals are dispersed as a gas or liquid or are aerosolized and may contaminate skin, clothing, and any object they touch. The vapor from a liquid or solid toxic chemical also is harmful. Those exposed to toxic chemicals should be decontaminated in the field before transport to a medical facility. Decontamination is usually done with running water and scrubbing. Most emergency departments have an isolated decontamination area in which the water from the shower area goes into a special holding tank. If multiple victims need decontamination, a portable tent may be placed outside the facility (Fig. 44.3).

! Safety Alert

Chemical Disaster

When a chemical disaster has occurred in your neighborhood, you should do the following (unless you are told to evacuate immediately):

- Close all windows and doors to the dwelling.
- Turn off all fans, heaters, and air conditioning systems.
- Close the fireplace damper.
- Wet some towels and jam them in the cracks under the doors. Use plastic garbage bags or plastic sheeting and duct tape to cover doors, windows and skylights, electrical outlets, exhaust fans or vents, window air conditioners, and heat registers.
- Go to an above-ground room with the fewest windows and doors.
- Take your emergency kit and a portable radio with you.
- Stay inside until you are told all is safe or you are asked to evacuate.

The importance of decontamination to protect staff and preserve the hospital environment was illustrated in the Tokyo subway attack, after which 110 staff members as well as 10% of the ambulance staff developed signs and symptoms of sarin exposure (TRACIE, 2019a). Chemical warfare agents can produce immediate respiratory distress if inhaled; therefore respirator masks are essential. First responders must use personal protective gear and have training to respond to chemical emergencies. Recognition that a chemical attack has occurred is the first step in adequate protection for the patient, first responders, and emergency department personnel.

Depending on the chemical agent, there may be an antidote that can be used (see Table 44.3). Each hospital should have a set of protocols in place. Symptomatic

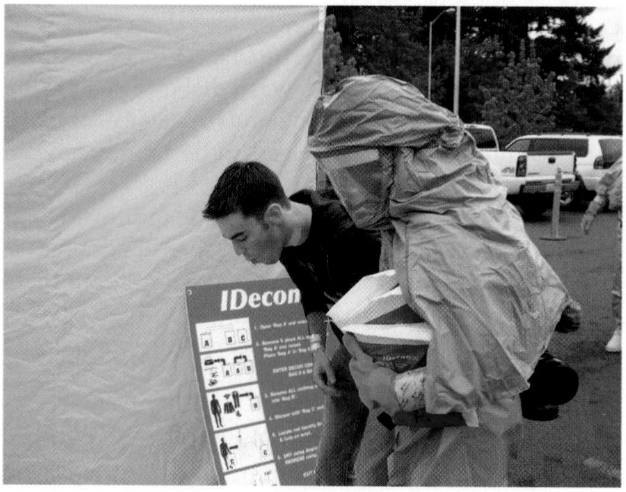

Fig. 44.3 Inflatable decontamination shower for ambulatory victims. (Courtesy PeaceHealth Southwest Medical Center, Vancouver, Wash.)

Table 44.3 Chemical Agent Symptoms and Care

CLINICAL PRESENTATION	DECONTAMINATION PROCEDURES	TREATMENT
Vesicant Agents (e.g., Phosgene, Mustard, Lewisite)		
Ocular: Eyelid swelling and inflammation, severe pain, conjunctivitis, and keratitis. *Dermal:* Pain, erythema, blisters, and burning followed by necrosis. *Respiratory:* Immediate upper airway irritation; burning of mucous membranes, laryngitis, shortness of breath, productive cough; inhalation and systemic absorption may cause pulmonary edema and death. *Gastrointestinal:* Nausea and vomiting, diarrhea, and abdominal pain. *Cardiovascular:* High-dose of lewisite exposure may cause capillary permeability and subsequent intravascular fluid loss, hypovolemia, and organ congestion. *Renal:* High levels of lewisite may cause renal failure caused by hypotension. *Hepatic:* High levels of lewisite may cause hepatic necrosis and hypoperfusion.	Decontamination for eyes must begin immediately by flushing eyes with water for 5–10 min and washing skin to minimize tissue damage. Decontaminate before bringing into health care facility. Negative-pressure room if available. All clothing is removed and skin washed with soap and water. If showers are available, showering with water alone is adequate. Place contaminated clothing and personal belongings in biohazard bag. Contain decontamination runoff. Patients whose clothing or skin is contaminated can contaminate health care providers by direct contact or through off-gassing vapor.	*For phosgene:* Restrict fluids. Obtain chest radiographs and blood gases. Oxygen/PEEP. *For mustard:* Possible tracheostomy. Establish IV: do not push fluids as with thermal burns. Drain vesicles and large blisters and irrigate with topical antibiotics. Antibiotic eye ointment. Morphine as needed (PRN). *For lewisite:* Treat affected skin with British anti-lewisite (BAL) ointment, if available. Treat affected eyes with BAL ointment, if available. Treat pulmonary symptoms. BAL deep IM; repeat q4h × 3. Morphine PRN. Severe poisoning: shorten interval for BAL injections to q2h.
Nerve Agents (e.g., Sarin)		
Respiratory: Bronchial constriction and spasm; severe respiratory distress or apnea; miosis; rhinorrhea. *Gastrointestinal:* Do not induce emesis.	Decontaminate before bringing into health care facility. Negative-pressure room. Contain decontamination runoff. Patients whose clothing or skin is contaminated with liquid or solid nerve agents can contaminate health care providers by direct contact or through off-gassing vapor. If exposed to liquid nerve agent, irrigate eyes for 5–10 min with water or saline within minutes of exposure to limit injury. If exposed to liquid nerve agent, cut and remove all clothing and wash skin immediately with soap and water. If shower is not available, wash with 0.5% bleach solution. If exposed to vapor only, remove outer clothing and wash exposed skin with soap and water or 0.5% bleach solution. Place contaminated clothing and personal belongings in biohazard bags.	*Nerve agent protocol:* Intubate and ventilate as needed. Atropine. Pralidoxime chloride (2-PAM C1). Diazepam for seizures. Reevaluate q3-5m for worsening.

Continued

Table 44.3 Chemical Agent Symptoms and Care—cont'd

CLINICAL PRESENTATION	DECONTAMINATION PROCEDURES	TREATMENT
Blood Agents (e.g., Cyanide)		
Dermal: Possible cherry red color to skin. *Respiratory:* Respiratory distress from cellular hypoxia, tachypnea, dyspnea, bradypnea, apnea.	Decontaminate before bringing into health care facility. Negative-pressure room. Contain decontamination runoff.	*For cyanide:* Administer antidotes: cyanide poisoning antidote kits containing amyl nitrite perles and infusion, sodium thiosulfate, and hydroxocobalamin are available.
Cardiovascular: Dysrhythmias caused by acidosis. *Neurologic:* Syncope, seizures, lethargy, confusion, coma.	Patients whose clothing or skin is contaminated with cyanide can contaminate health care providers by direct contact or through off-gassing vapor. Patients exposed only to vapor require no decontamination. Prevent dermal contact with gastric contents that may contain ingested cyanide-containing materials. Remove contaminated clothing and wash with soap and water.	Amyl nitrite, sodium nitrite, sodium thiosulfate. Hydroxocobalamin. Sodium bicarbonate for acidosis.
Pulmonary/Choking Agents (e.g., Chlorine)		
Acute exposure to gas can cause immediate coughing, eye and nose irritation, tearing. *Dermal:* Skin irritation, burning pain, inflammation, and blisters. Treat as thermal burns. Liquefied, compressed chlorine can cause frostbite. Treat by rewarming affected areas in a water bath of 102°–108° F (38.8°–42.2° C) for 20–30 min. Continue until flushing has returned to affected area. *Ocular:* Do not irrigate frostbitten eyes; if exposed to vapor, irrigate for at least 15 min; check for corneal damage. *Respiratory:* Airway constriction, pulmonary edema, and hemoptysis may occur.	Health care providers are at minimal risk of secondary contamination from patients who have been exposed to chlorine gas. Remove contaminated clothing and wash with soap and water. Flush exposed skin and hair with plain water for 2–3 min; then wash twice with soap and water. Clothing or skin soaked with industrial-strength bleach or similar solutions may be corrosive to personnel and may release chlorine gas.	*For chlorine:* Dyspnea. Oxygen by mask. Chest radiograph. Bronchodilators. Give supportive therapy and treat other problems.

IM, Intramuscular; *IV,* intravenous; *PEEP,* positive end-expiratory pressure.

supportive care is supplied with oxygen, IV fluids, and comfort measures.

NUCLEAR DISASTER

A nuclear disaster may be the result of an accident at a nuclear power plant, a disruption of a nuclear power plant by terrorists, or a nuclear bomb or "dirty bomb" (one containing radioactive substances). The amount of damage to each person depends on the type of radiation, the dose received, the length of time of exposure, and the route of the exposure. **Time, distance, and shielding are key to the quantity of radiation an individual will receive.** The shorter the time of exposure, the farther away from the radiation source, and whether the person was shielded by materials that are impermeable to radiation are details pertinent to radiation risk (World Nuclear Association, 2018) (see Chapter 8). Some types of radiation produce particles, and other types produce rays. Particles will adhere to airborne dust particles; may be inhaled; and will settle on clothes, crops, water supplies, and other surfaces.

Decontamination is done with showering and scrubbing the skin to remove particles. Radiation exposure to rays does not require decontamination, although rays can cause serious health effects or death because they do internal damage to tissues. However, if the exposure is from a terrorist attack, it would not be immediately known if the exposure to radiation was in the form of particles or rays. Therefore everyone exposed, or suspected of being exposed, will need to be decontaminated. Personnel

Patient Teaching

Removal and Disposal of Contaminated Clothing

If you are in an area where a chemical spill has occurred and the liquid or solid comes into contact with your clothing, you will need to (1) remove and bag contaminated clothing and (2) decontaminate your skin. Chemicals will penetrate the clothing and contaminate your skin. If the exposure to a chemical was by vapor (gas), you will only need to remove your clothing and the source of the toxic vapor. Up to 90% of the contaminant can be eliminated by removal of clothing (Williams & Sizemore, 2018). Perform the following steps:

- Quickly take off clothing that has a chemical on it. Any clothing that must be pulled over the head should be cut off instead of pulling it over the head.
- When helping others remove clothing, be careful not to touch any contaminated areas. Remove clothing as quickly as possible.
- As quickly as possible, wash any chemicals from your skin with large amounts of soap and water. If the eyes are burning, rinse with plain water for 10 to 15 minutes.
- If contact lenses are worn, remove them and place them with the contaminated clothing.
- After washing yourself, carefully place all contaminated clothing and contact lenses into a plastic bag. Avoid touching contaminated areas; use tongs, a stick, or a tool to place the clothing in the bag. Place the implement within the bag as well when finished using it.
- Thoroughly wash eyeglasses worn at the time of chemical contamination before wearing them again. Wash hands thoroughly again after cleaning glasses.
- Carefully seal the bag, place it within another plastic bag, and seal the outer bag.
- Dress in clothing that has not been contaminated (i.e., clothes that have been in the closet or dresser drawers).
- When health department or emergency personnel arrive, have them handle the bags and arrange for disposal.

Adapted from Centers for Disease Control and Prevention (CDC): *Chemical agents: facts about personal cleaning and disposal of contaminated clothing* (website): https://emergency.cdc.gov/planning/personalcleaningfacts.asp.

performing triage and decontamination must be protected from radioactive particulates and contaminated dust.

Usually, specially trained units supply personnel to handle decontamination. Minimal protective equipment includes protective gear for clothes and shoes (Tyvek suit), double gloves (one under clothing and taped to the skin and one over the clothing cuffs), and a high-efficiency particulate air (HEPA) respirator mask with a full facepiece. If no such mask is available, a fit-tested N95 respirator mask such as those used for tuberculosis precautions is better than no mask. Radiation detection badges are worn underneath the protective clothing. After disposing of the protective gear in specially marked biohazard containers, each person will be assessed to make certain radiation contamination has been eliminated (Radiation Emergency Medical Management, 2018).

Exposure to high doses of radiation rays that penetrate the body even for a few minutes may result in acute radiation sickness syndrome. Three subsyndromes may occur, depending on the dose of radiation received: hematopoietic syndrome, gastrointestinal syndrome, and cerebrovascular syndrome. Bone marrow tissue is affected first, preventing new cell production; then with increased dosage, the gastrointestinal lining is affected, destroying stem cells. A person who receives a high enough dose of radiation to cause cerebrovascular syndrome will experience effects on the bone marrow and gastrointestinal system as well, but the high-dose exposure may cause death. The effects of radiation are progressive as the dosage increases. Signs and symptoms may include nausea, vomiting, diarrhea, leukopenia, signs of bleeding or hemorrhage, lethargy, confusion, ataxia, convulsions, hair loss, and respiratory complications with fever and pneumonia (Table 44.4). Treatment of life-threatening injuries takes precedence over the radiologic damage (Pae, 2018).

Once injuries are managed and decontamination is complete, nursing care is supportive, with strict infection control procedures in place. Maintaining an accurate record of the onset and duration of the clinical symptoms is essential for the health care provider to decide on treatment strategies. Record hair loss, inflamed mucosa, and locations of erythema hourly and, if possible, record skin symptoms with a camera. Serial blood counts will be performed. Nausea is treated with antiemetics. Blood problems may be treated with blood component transfusions.

When the radiation exposure is in the form of particulates that have entered the body, treatment depends on the type of radiologic substance. The four types of agents used to reduce the radiation damage by reducing exposure to the radiologic substance are chelating agents, isotope-specific blocking agents, excretion agents, and diluting agents.

Chelating agents bind with the radioactive material and allow it to be excreted without being absorbed into the tissues. Radioactive iodine exposure is treated with potassium iodide, an isotope-specific blocking agent, to prevent the thyroid cancer this type of radiation causes. Excretion agents are used when radioactive material has been ingested; these reduce the time the radiologic material is in the gastrointestinal tract. Diluting agents reduce the concentration of the radioactive material. Water is the best example of a diluting agent. Special precautions need to be used when administering a mobilizing or diluting agent because the fluids produced could be radiologically contaminated.

BIOLOGIC DISASTER

Bioterrorism involves the deliberate release of microorganisms or toxins derived from living organisms that cause disease or death to humans or to the animals or plants on which we depend for food. The CDC lists more than 40 pathogens that have potential as biologic

Table 44.4 Acute Radiation Syndrome

SIGNS AND SYMPTOMS[a]	TIME OF ONSET[a]	DURATION	TREATMENT
Initial or Prodromal (Dose Dependent)			
Nausea, vomiting, diarrhea Progressive cognitive impairment at high doses	Minutes to hours after exposure	May last for several days	Serial CBC (for lymphocyte count) obtained every 2–3 hr for 8–12 hr; then every 4–6 hr for 2–3 days. Record all symptoms and time of onset (vomiting is correlated with prognosis). Fluids and antiemetics. Chelating, blocking, excretion, or diluting agents.
Latent			
Feels and appears relatively healthy	Hours to weeks after prodromal phase	May last several weeks	Patient education about significance of latent stage, need for infection control, and possible progression to phase of manifest illness. Continue to monitor for symptoms and CBC.
"Manifest Illness" (Obvious Illness)			
Signs and symptoms of leukopenia purpura, hemorrhage Pneumonia Hair loss Diarrhea, fever, electrolyte disturbance Convulsions, ataxia, tremor, lethargy	Hours to weeks	Hours to months	Supportive and symptomatic treatment. Isolation for leukopenia as needed. Possible stem cell replacement.
Recovery or Death			
Death	Days to years Death may occur within 1–2 days at >3000 rads; death occurs 3 wk–6 mo at >200–600 rads	Recovery lasts from several weeks up to 2 years.	Educate those who recover about increased future risk for cancers and advise to have frequent health checkups.

From Radiation Emergency Medical Management: http://www.remm.nlm.gov/index.html.
[a]Progression through phases and symptoms depends on the dose and type of radiation received.
CBC, Complete blood cell count; *rads,* unit of absorbed radiation dose.

weapons. Even pathogens that are readily found in the environment can be used as weapons. These organisms that cause a high death rate and are easily transmitted are labeled as category A. Public panic and fear is likely to accompany any breakout. The organisms are invisible to the naked eye and are easily transported without detection.

Recognizing a Bioterrorism Event

Many of the likely bioterrorism agents do not produce symptoms right away. Certain signs or events may present a warning that a bioterrorism attack has occurred. Some of the signs are as follows (Williams & Sizemore, 2018):

- Large numbers of patients with similar symptoms of disease
- Higher than expected illness and death incidence with common disease
- Unusual disease presentation
- Large numbers of patients with unexplained symptoms, diseases, or deaths
- Disease typical to the area with a sudden unexplained increase in incidence
- Atypical incidence of disease in patients not usually affected
- Sudden death of many animals in the community

Biologic Agents

Biologic agents (Table 44.5) are divided into three groups (CDC, 2017):

- *Category A agents:* Easily disseminated, and some may be transmitted from person to person as well. These could cause mass casualties, disrupt society, and require a well-organized and extensive health care system response for management.
- *Category B agents:* Moderately easy to disseminate. May be delivered through water and food sources. These produce moderate amounts of illness and low death rates. Public health department action is needed for management. Examples are Q fever, brucellosis, glanders, ricin toxin, epsilon toxin of *Clostridium perfringens,* and *Staphylococcus aureus* enterotoxin B.

Table 44.5 Category A Agents of Bioterrorism

PATHOGEN AND DESCRIPTION	CLINICAL MANIFESTATIONS	TRANSMISSIBILITY	TREATMENT
Anthrax *(Bacillus anthracis)*			
Inhalational Bacterial spores multiply in the alveoli Toxins cause hemorrhage and destruction of lung tissue High mortality rate	Incubation period: 1–2 days to 6 wk Abrupt onset Dyspnea, diaphoresis, fever, cough, chest pain, septicemia, shock, meningitis, respiratory failure, widened mediastinum (seen on chest radiograph)	No person-to-person spread Found in nature and most commonly infects wild and domestic hoofed animals Spread through direct contact with bacteria and its spores Spores are dormant, encapsulated bacteria that become active when they enter a living host	Antibiotics prevent systemic manifestations Effective only if treated early Ciprofloxacin (Cipro) is the treatment of choice Penicillin Doxycycline Postexposure prophylaxis for 30 days (if vaccine not available) Vaccine has limited availability. Antitoxins can be administered if available.
Cutaneous 95% of anthrax infections Least lethal form Toxins destroy surrounding tissue	Incubation period: up to 12 days Small papule resembles an insect bite Advances to a depressed, black ulcer Swollen lymph nodes in adjacent areas Edema	Spores enter skin through cuts or abrasions Handling of contaminated animal skin products	Oral doxycycline or quinolones are the antibiotics of choice
Gastrointestinal Intestinal lesions in ileum or cecum Acute inflammation of intestines	Nausea, vomiting, anorexia, hematemesis, diarrhea, abdominal pain, ascites, sepsis	Ingestion of contaminated, undercooked meat	Penicillin, doxycycline, or ciprofloxacin may be prescribed
Botulism *(Clostridium botulinum)*			
Spore-forming anaerobe Found in soil Seven different toxins Lethal bacterial neurotoxin	Incubation period: 12–72 h Abdominal cramps, diarrhea, nausea, vomiting, cranial nerve palsies (diplopia, dysarthria, dysphonia, dysphagia), skeletal muscle paralysis, respiratory failure	Spread through air or food No person-to-person spread Improperly canned foods Contaminated water Contaminated wound	Antitoxin given immediately Mechanical ventilation Penicillin Trivalent equine antitoxin (serotypes A, B, E) available from the CDC should be administered immediately after diagnosis Toxin can be inactivated by heating food or drink to 185° F (85° C) for at least 5 min
Plague *(Yersinia pestis)*			
Bacteria found in rodents and fleas *Forms:* Bubonic (most common) Pneumonic Septicemic (most deadly)	Incubation period: 2–4 days Hemoptysis, cough, high fever, chills, myalgia, headache, respiratory failure, lymph node swelling	Direct person-to-person spread Transmitted through flea bites Ingestion of contaminated meat	Antibiotics effective only if administered immediately Drug of choice: gentamicin or fluoroquinolones Vaccine under development Hospitalization Isolation for containment

Continued

Table 44.5 Category A Agents of Bioterrorism—cont'd

PATHOGEN AND DESCRIPTION	CLINICAL MANIFESTATIONS	TRANSMISSIBILITY	TREATMENT
Smallpox			
***Variola Major* and *Minor* Viruses**			
United States ended routine vaccination in 1971 Global eradication declared in 1980	Incubation period: 7–17 days Sudden onset of symptoms Fever, headache, myalgia, malaise, back pain Lesions progress from macules to papules to pustular vesicles	Highly contagious Direct person-to-person spread Transmitted in airborne droplets Transmitted by handling contaminated materials (i.e., linens)	No known cure. Vaccinia immune globulin (VIG) is first-line therapy Cidofovir (Vistide) may be used under an investigational drug protocol. Tecovirimat, cidofovir, and brincidofovir are antivirals that are FDA approved Isolation for containment Vaccine available for those exposed
Tularemia *(Francisella tularensis)*			
Bacterial infectious disease of animals Mortality rate about 35% without treatment	Incubation period: 3–10 days Sudden onset Fever, swollen lymph nodes, fatigue, sore throat, weight loss, pneumonia, pleural effusion, ulcerated sore from tick bite	No person-to-person spread Aerosol or intradermal route Spread by rabbits and ticks Contaminated food, air, water	Gentamicin treatment of choice Streptomycin, doxycycline, and ciprofloxacin are alternatives Vaccine not available in the United States. Has not shown to be helpful in ill patients
Hemorrhagic Fever			
Caused by several viruses, including Marburg, Lassa, Junin, and Ebola Ebola virus is life threatening	Fever, conjunctivitis, headache, malaise, prostration, hemorrhage of tissues and organs, nausea, vomiting, hypotension, organ failure	Carried by rodents and mosquitoes Direct person-to-person spread by body fluids Virus can be aerosolized	No intramuscular injections No antiplatelet drugs Isolation for containment Ribavirin (Virazole) effective in some cases No FDA approved treatment available

Adapted from Lewis SL, Heitkemper MM, Dirksen SR, et al.: *Medical-surgical nursing: assessment and management of clinical problems,* ed 9, St. Louis, 2014, Elsevier; Kellerman RD, Rakel DP: *Conn's current therapy 2019,* Philadelphia, 2019, Elsevier; updated from Centers for Disease Control and Prevention website: https://emergency.cdc.gov/agent/agentlist-category.asp, 2019.
CDC, Centers for Disease Control and Prevention; *FDA,* U.S. Food and Drug Administration.

- *Category C:* Agents that have yet to be weaponized but have the potential for high morbidity and mortality. These agents are plentiful and easy to produce and disseminate. Examples include hantavirus, H1N1 influenza, Nipah virus, and SARS corona virus.

Symptoms from exposure to a biologic agent are not immediate. There are various incubation periods. Therefore unless someone knows that they have been exposed to a strange powder or substance, decontamination does not take place. You particularly need basic knowledge about category A agents because they are easily disseminated and spread from person to person.

Anthrax. Anthrax is a category A agent caused by the gram-positive bacteria *Bacillus anthracis,* which forms spores. It is primarily a disease of sheep and cows. Animal vaccination programs have controlled naturally occurring anthrax in the United States. There are three forms of the disease: cutaneous (95%), gastrointestinal (<1%), and inhalational (5%). Aerosolized inhalable anthrax is most likely to be used for a terrorist attack. The greatest chance of inhaling the spores after aerosolization is during the first day after the event, before the particles hit the ground. Symptoms in those who have inhaled the spores will resemble a nonspecific influenza at first. A rapid downhill progression is then seen with respiratory failure, shock, and possibly death over a 2- to 5-day period. Features that differentiate anthrax illness from flu are shortness of breath, a nonproductive cough, chest discomfort, myalgia, and fatigue. The lack of a sore throat and rhinorrhea and the appearance of nausea and vomiting may be present and are also flu symptoms. Treatment is with ciprofloxacin (Cipro) or doxycycline (Vibramycin) for 14 days. Antibiotics are adjusted after culture and sensitivity results are known. Treatment continues for 60 days if infection is confirmed because the disease can continue to develop from germinating spores up to that time. Postexposure prophylaxis is also recommended for 60 days. Raxibacumab or obiltoxaximab monoclonal antibodies and Anthrasil, a human immune globulin, may be used with antibiotics for treatment of inhaled anthrax. Other care is supportive for respiration, fluid and electrolyte balance, and comfort. Extended precautions are not necessary because anthrax is not transmissible from person to person. An attenuated virus vaccine is available for prevention and for postexposure use.

Botulism. Botulism is a category A agent caused by the botulinum toxins produced by *Clostridium botulinum.* There are five forms of botulism described by how they are obtained—foodborne, wound, iatrogenic, adult intestinal, and infant botulism—which are acquired in a similar manner. Foods can become contaminated with botulism spores when canned or processed under conditions favorable for toxin production (e.g., insufficient heat). Botulism is not contagious, and the organism is destroyed by the addition of chlorine to water supplies or by boiling foods for 10 minutes (CDC, 2019). Organisms are naturally present in the soil and can cause wound infection. Inhalational botulism does not occur naturally and would most likely indicate a terrorist attack.

Double vision, drooping eyelids, and difficulty swallowing and speaking may be the early symptoms of botulism. A triad of symptoms is classic for the disorder:

- Symmetric descending flaccid paralysis progressing to respiratory weakness
- Absence of fever
- Alertness and orientation without sensory deficits

Respiratory support may require intubation and mechanical ventilation. If large numbers of persons are infected, the community health care resources would be taxed to provide adequate care for all. Treatment is with botulinum antitoxin if the toxin type is A or B. The CDC and public health departments stock these antitoxins. Early treatment is required because the antitoxin does not reverse the muscular paralysis that has already occurred. Supportive therapy may be needed for several weeks until new synapses can grow to replace those damaged by the toxins.

Plague. Plague is a category A agent caused by a gram-negative bacillus, *Yersinia pestis.* The bubonic form starts as a skin infection and spreads to the lymph nodes; it is naturally transmitted by infected fleas that bite rodents or people. Pneumonic plague is the most likely type to be spread by a terrorist attack with aerosolized plague organisms. Fortunately, plague bacilli are killed by sunlight and remain viable in aerosolized form for only about an hour after release. Clinical signs include abrupt onset of pneumonia with bloody sputum **(hemoptysis)** that follows a rapidly progressive course. Disseminated intravascular coagulation (DIC) can develop and lead to multiorgan system failure. Death is likely within 24 hours of infection if treatment is not started.

Gentamicin (Garamycin) is the IV drug of choice for this organism. Streptomycin given intramuscularly can be used as initial treatment. Ciprofloxacin and doxycycline are used to treat pneumonic plague and are given for 7 to 10 days. If treated early, the infection is usually not fatal. Plague can be transmitted from person to person, and respiratory droplet precautions along with Standard Precautions are necessary until 48 hours after treatment has been initiated. Researchers are currently working on a vaccine and have completed animal trials for a dual vaccine against anthrax and plague (American Society for Microbiology, 2018).

Smallpox. Smallpox is caused by *Variola* virus. It is communicable, it has a high mortality rate, and very few people have been vaccinated. The disease was declared eradicated worldwide in 1980, but laboratory strains of the virus still exist. Because it is so lethal and highly contagious, it is listed as a category A agent.

Smallpox has an average incubation period of 12 to 14 days. Symptoms begin with fever for 1 to 4 days, and then a rash occurs. High fever may be accompanied by headache, backache, malaise, vomiting, and delirium. The rash contains firm, deep-seated vesicles or pustules that are all in the same stage of development on any one area of the body (Fig. 44.4). The rash starts on the buccal and pharyngeal mucosa; spreads to the face, hands, and forearms; and then spreads to the rest of the body over several days. A cough may develop. Lesions progress from macules to papules to vesicles to pustules to scabs, with each stage lasting 1 or 2 days. It must be differentiated from chickenpox. With chickenpox, the lesions appear before illness symptoms and are usually concentrated on the trunk. Chickenpox lesions are usually more superficial and are "flimsy" rather than firm as in smallpox. Chickenpox lesions do not usually occur on the palms of the hands and the soles of the feet; smallpox lesions do occur in these areas (Fig. 44.5). Chickenpox lesions are often in various stages of development within the same area of the body,

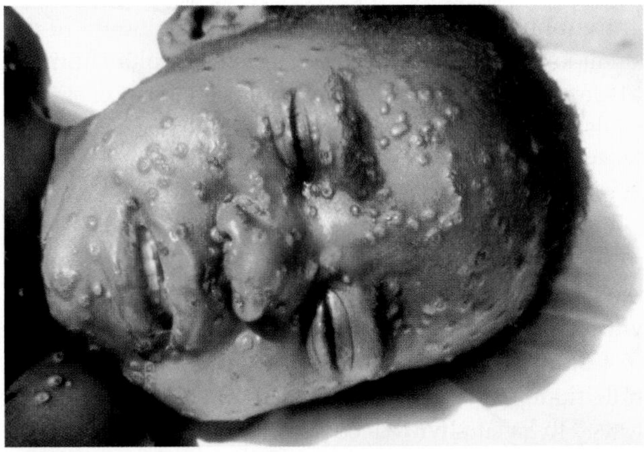

Fig. 44.4 Face lesions on a boy with smallpox. (Courtesy Centers for Disease Control and Prevention, Public Health Images Library.)

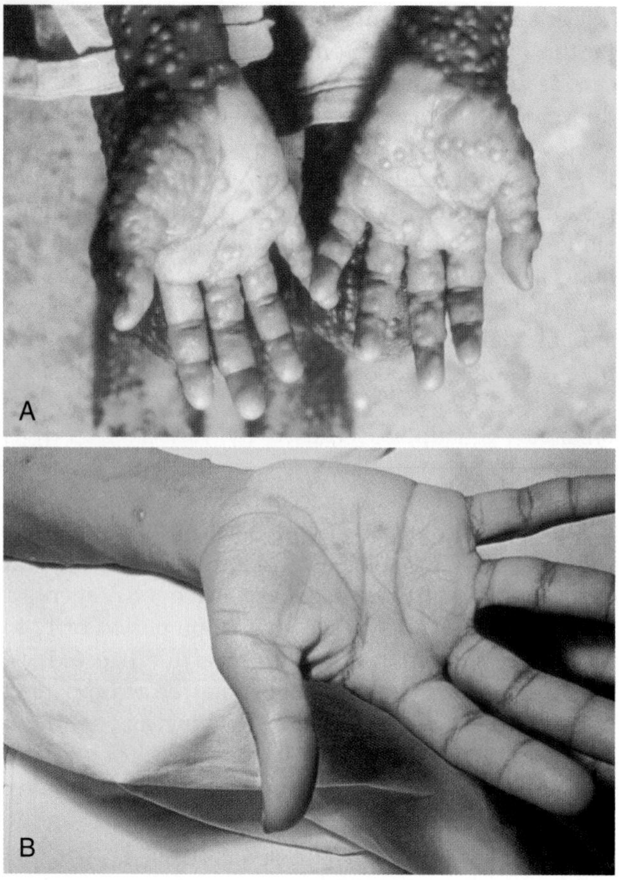

Fig. 44.5 Comparison of smallpox and chickenpox lesions. **A,** Smallpox. **B,** Chickenpox. (Courtesy Centers for Disease Control and Prevention, Public Health Images Library.)

whereas smallpox lesions are all in the same stage within an area.

Smallpox is communicable from the onset of rash until all scabs have separated from the skin. Patients should be treated with strict airborne precautions and contact precautions and be placed in a negative-pressure room with a HEPA-filtered exhaust system. All linens should be placed in biohazard bags and autoclaved before being laundered or incinerated.

Receiving the smallpox vaccine within 4 days of exposure can reduce the severity of the disease. Two antiviral medications are available for treatment of the smallpox virus. They have been tested in healthy humans to identify side effects but have not been through clinical trials since the disease has been eradicated. The CDC has stockpiled the medications, and they can be made available if needed (CDC, 2019). If health care workers are to be vaccinated, they will receive all necessary information about the vaccine and how to take care of the vaccination site. Medical management is supportive, with antimicrobial drug treatment for secondary infection of lesion sites, fluid and electrolyte replacement, and nutritional therapy. The first dose of smallpox vaccine lasts 3 to 5 years with decreasing immunity. Those who had multiple vaccinations may have longer-lasting immunity.

? Think Critically

Explain to someone how to distinguish smallpox lesions from those of chickenpox.

Tularemia. Tularemia is a category A agent caused by a gram-negative coccobacillus, *Francisella tularensis.* It is a vector-borne illness that is transmitted by an infected tick, mosquito, or deer fly bite, by direct exposure to contaminated animal tissues and fluids, or by ingestion of contaminated food or water. A variety of small mammals are natural reservoirs of the organism. It is seen throughout the United States except in Hawaii. If aerosolized, it could be inhaled, and this is the most likely form for a terrorist attack. The disease is not spread by person-to-person contact.

Tularemia occurs in six different forms: ulceroglandular, glandular, oculoglandular, oropharyngeal, pneumonic, and typhoidal. The pneumonic form is the one most likely to occur in a terrorist attack. The pneumonia caused by the inhaled form is difficult to differentiate from other pneumonias. Symptoms include abrupt onset of fever, chills, headache, muscle aches, nonproductive cough, and sore throat. Laboratory testing can establish the correct diagnosis.

Treatment is with streptomycin and gentamicin, the drugs of first choice. Doxycycline and ciprofloxacin may also be used but are not approved by the U.S. Food and Drug Administration (FDA) for this use. The course of treatment should extend through 10 to 14 days depending on the drug used. Tularemia is fatal if not treated with the proper antibiotics. Standard Precautions are used, but the inhalational form is not transmitted by person-to-person contact, and no other extended precautions are necessary. A vaccine previously available for protection from tularemia is under review by the FDA.

Viral hemorrhagic fevers. The hemorrhagic fevers are a group of illnesses caused by four families of viruses: arenaviruses, filoviruses, flaviviruses, and bunyaviruses. The viruses, which are within the category A agents, cause Ebola, Marburg, and Lassa hemorrhagic fevers. Junin, Machupo, Guanarito, and Sabia hemorrhagic fevers are more common in the Southern Hemisphere. No vaccines are available for these diseases, which occur in different geographic parts of the world. Reservoirs for the viruses are rodents and arthropods. Human infection usually occurs by being bitten by an infected arthropod, by contact with infected animal carcasses, or by inhaling aerosolized rodent excreta. Once contracted, the virus can be transmitted from person to person by blood and body fluids. Contact precautions and airborne precautions are necessary. The CDC (2018b) has guidelines on personal protective equipment (PPE) for caregivers. Only special biosafety laboratories can test for the viral hemorrhagic fevers. Such tests are performed at the CDC. It is thought that an aerosolized form of Ebola or Marburg virus might be used for a terrorist attack. Travelers from a region experiencing an outbreak could also carry the virus into other countries (CDC, 2018c).

The incubation period is between 2 and 42 days, depending on the virus, and there is a prodromal syndrome that lasts less than a week. Signs and symptoms are marked fever, fatigue, dizziness, muscle aches, and loss of strength. Symptoms may progress to abdominal pain, nonbloody diarrhea, weakness, and exhaustion. Later, bleeding begins, starting with bleeding under the skin causing petechiae and progressing to spontaneous bleeding and DIC. Many body systems are affected. Hypotension, conjunctivitis, pharyngitis, and skin rash may reflect increasing capillary permeability. Shock, nervous system malfunction, seizures, delirium, and coma may occur. Mortality rates can be very high with Ebola but are not always as high with the other viruses.

There is no specific treatment for these hemorrhagic fevers; treatment is supportive. Early identification is essential for supportive treatment to be effective. Two point-of-care fingerstick tests for Ebola are currently FDA approved (Global Biodefense, 2018). The antiviral ribavirin may be useful in treating Lassa fever. Expanded contact precautions and airborne precautions are essential. Double gloves, impermeable gowns, leg and shoe coverings, face shields, eye protection, and an N95 mask are required for patient contact. A negative-pressure room is desirable.

Prevention measures include use of insect repellant, bed nets, window screens, and proper clothing and the eradication of rodents from living spaces. Mosquito abatement is performed in areas of outbreak when possible. Vaccines are available for yellow fever and Argentine hemorrhagic fever but not for the others. All linens should be treated as infectious and either carefully disinfected or incinerated.

Pandemic influenza infection. **Pandemic** infection is an international outbreak of a new influenza A virus causing disease. Most people have had firsthand experience with the flu, but the H1N1 (swine) flu episode in 2009 heightened awareness of how readily a disease moves back and forth across international borders. The severe acute respiratory syndrome (SARS) outbreak in China made health care professionals feel particularly vulnerable to airborne respiratory infections (see Chapter 14). Flu is seasonal, and there are always fatalities associated with influenza. Unless the death rate is significantly elevated with international epidemiology, it is not labeled a pandemic.

Preparations for pandemic flu include teaching people to be prepared to stay at home for at least 2 weeks. You also need to reassure people that basic measures for prevention of respiratory infection can be effective. These include a healthy lifestyle to support the immune system, hand hygiene, covering the mouth during coughing or sneezing, disposing of tissues, and staying away from public places if possible.

Your Role in Preparedness and Response

In addition to learning about hospital protocols, community resources, and specific knowledge related to disaster care, you should explore your feelings about professional participation in a disaster event. Under normal circumstances, such as caring for infectious patients, your duty to care is high because the risk of harm to self is low; however, when the danger to nurses is unclear or apparent—such as occurred in the SARS outbreak—you could decide that preservation of self is reasonable. Studies have shown that nurses do not feel prepared to function in a disaster situation. Education and hands-on training are recommended to increase nurse preparedness (Labrague et al., 2018). In an epidemic, disaster setting, or terrorist event when you may be in danger while rendering care, your "duty to treat" is less clear than in a controlled health care setting. Professional organizations provide standards of practice, state boards of nursing outline scopes of practice, and employers have policies. You must decide for yourself what is ethically right in a given situation. Arming yourself with knowledge, preparing your own household, and having ethical discussions with colleagues will help you in your decision-making process.

Your role during a bioterrorism event includes the following:

- Recognizing clusters of cases or unusual cases suggestive of a biologic event
- Promptly evaluating and assisting with medical management
- Promptly communicating with the local public health department and infection control department
- Working closely with law enforcement, emergency management, public health, and other government agencies

Nursing management. When such patterns are discovered, you should implement the hospital and community response plan. **All staff must strictly adhere to infection control procedures and policies.**

If your assessment has aroused suspicion of a biologic event, ask these questions:

- Was there a sudden onset of severe respiratory or gastrointestinal problems?
- Has the illness progressed rapidly?
- Has the patient been healthy otherwise?
- Are the patient's family members, friends, or colleagues ill?

If the answers indicate that an infectious agent is present, immediately take the following steps:

- Notify your supervisor and the infection control department of the situation.
- Put a surgical mask on any patient who is coughing.
- Pay strict attention to Standard Precautions and hand hygiene, and encourage the patient and family to do the same.
- Wear an N95 or P100 respirator mask (one certified by the Occupational Safety and Health Administration [OSHA]).

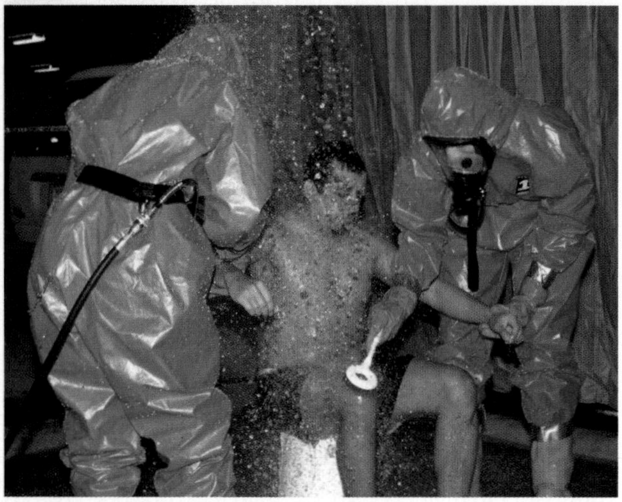

Fig. 44.6 Personnel wearing biohazard suits perform a decontamination scrub during a hospital bioterrorism drill. (Courtesy AP/Wide World Photos.)

- If indicated, isolate the patient in a negative-pressure room; obtain specimens for laboratory testing.
- Use all recommended PPE when caring for the patient and pay strict attention to Standard and Expanded Precautions.

When a known terrorist airborne event has occurred and victims are triaged to hospitals and emergency field medical units, victims will need to be decontaminated before being brought into the medical facilities. Outside shower areas will be set up to accomplish this decontamination. Whether the agent used in the attack is biologic or nuclear, the outside of the body must be thoroughly scrubbed. Personnel in biohazard suits handle this task (Fig. 44.6). Clothing must be removed and sealed in plastic biohazard bags to prevent contamination of others. The skin should be scrubbed in every area with warm, soapy water for at least 30 seconds. The hair should be soaped and shampooed several times.

In a crisis situation, firm directions should be given with a kindly tone. People need to know what will happen next. Active listening and assisting with problem solving provides needed psychosocial support. If a family has been separated, health care workers can help locate children and other family members. You should direct people to available support services to meet physical and psychological needs.

ACTIVE SHOOTER

Other critical incidents that require a trained response from the health care team may occur in a public or health care setting. One that is rare but can be deadly is an active shooter. First responders are trained and law enforcement officers are armed to manage a shooting situation. When it happens in a health care setting, there is much less preparation. The Joint Commission and OSHA require hospitals to address an active shooter scenario in their workplace violence plan. Some facilities have an overhead page to notify staff of the situation. Many hospitals are using the designation "Code Silver."

The general guidelines include to first be aware of potential violence based on behaviors, actions, and speech. Security or community law enforcement should be called as appropriate. Potential violence may come from patients, staff, or visitors. If a firearm is seen, health care workers should evacuate if possible, hide in a location not visible to the shooter, lock the doors, and silence their pagers and cellphones. A call to 911 should be made when it is safe to do so. As a last resort and if life is in imminent danger, incapacitating or acting with physical aggression and throwing items at the shooter may be attempted. Even more important is what to do when law enforcement arrives. They know someone is using deadly force, but they do not know who the perpetrator is. Bystanders should immediately raise their hands and spread their fingers to show that they are not holding a weapon, remain calm, and follow instructions. They should avoid making quick movements, pointing, or yelling. If there are shooting victims, law enforcement will determine when it is safe to render aid while maintaining the integrity of the crime scene; if there are fatalities, the area becomes off limits to health care personnel, and regular hospital activities may need to be relocated.

DEBRIEFING

Critical incident stress **debriefing** (CISD) teams provide sessions for small groups of personnel to help with effective coping strategies. After the turmoil and emotional impact of the disaster or critical incident, including its aftermath, personnel may find it difficult to return to their normal routine. Without intervention, some may develop post-traumatic stress disorder (see Chapter 47). There is strict confidentiality and unconditional acceptance of any information shared during the sessions. Participants are encouraged to bond by talking about where they were and what they were doing when they first heard about the disaster and to describe what they saw, heard, or smelled during the event. They are asked to share how they felt during the event, discuss how they feel now, and describe physical symptoms that have occurred since the incident. Facilitators reassure participants that strong reactions are normal, and they offer coping strategies. These coping strategies may include avoiding the use of alcohol or drugs, making sure to eat a well-balanced diet, watching for obsessing or fixation, taking time off from work, socializing with friends and coworkers, and getting professional help if necessary.

Get Ready for the NCLEX® Examination!

Key Points

- A disaster exists when the number of casualties exceeds the resource capabilities of the area.
- You should be proactive in being familiar with your facility's disaster plan, encouraging people to stock a disaster kit at home, and teaching the public about what to do when a disaster occurs (see Health Promotion: Disaster Preparedness).
- A chain of command is set in place when a disaster occurs, and it must be followed to ensure that appropriate notification and information is provided to the Office of Emergency Services.
- The stages of psychological response include impact, heroic, honeymoon, disillusionment, and reconstruction.
- Triage for a disaster is based on treating those with life-threatening conditions who have a likelihood of survival and identifying those whose treatment can be delayed.
- Reverse triage can be used to increase surge capacity.
- First aid, safety measures, and prevention and control of health hazards are priorities.
- Special populations such as older adults, infants, people who have disabilities, and individuals who are immunocompromised need help to stay safe and meet basic life requirements.
- People must be taught how to purify water (see Health Promotion: Preparing Safe Water).
- Knowledge of food safety when there has been a power outage or a flood is essential (see Box 44.1).
- Warning signs that a bioterrorism event has occurred include large numbers of patients with similar symptoms; illness and death rates higher than expected for common diseases; unusual disease presentation; increase in unexplained symptoms, diseases, or deaths; and sudden death of animals.
- Decontamination of individuals affected by a chemical, radiologic, or bioterrorism event is performed before they are allowed into the health facility.
- Debriefing by a trained team after a disaster helps prevent long-term psychological problems among the personnel involved in caring for people affected by the event.

Additional Learning Resources

SG Go to your Study Guide for additional learning activities to help you master this chapter content.

Go to your Evolve website (http://evolve.elsevier.com/deWit/medsurg) for the following FREE learning resources:
- Animations, audio, and video
- Answers and rationales for questions and activities
- Glossary with pronunciations in English and Spanish
- Interactive Review Questions and more!

Review Questions for the NCLEX® Examination

1. A large number of patients are arriving at the hospital from the scene of a chemical disaster. What is the priority action?
   1. Take vital signs to determine which patients are in distress.
   2. Call poison control for assistance in determining antidotes.
   3. Decontaminate all patients outside the hospital by showering.
   4. Instruct all caregivers to don personal protective equipment.

   NCLEX Client Need: Safe and Effective Care Environment: Safety and Infection Control
2. At a disaster scene, you notice that a person who has respiratory distress and severe total body burns has been triaged with a black tag. What should you do?
   1. Immediately obtain a portable oxygen tank and apply an oxygen mask.
   2. Seek out emergency services personnel to transport the patient to the hospital.
   3. Try to locate family members so that they can be present when the person dies.
   4. Stay with the person for as long possible to give support and comfort.

   NCLEX Client Need: Safe and Effective Care Environment: Coordinated Care
3. You are participating in a disaster drill. A mock victim with a green tag asks, "What does this tag mean?" What is the best response?
   1. "You can go home because you no longer need health management."
   2. "You potentially pose a health hazard, so you must sit in the green area."
   3. "You will have to wait for care because your injuries are not life threatening."
   4. "You will be seen and treated immediately by a health care provider."

   NCLEX Client Need: Health Promotion and Maintenance
4. While admitting a young, previously healthy patient with a severe respiratory illness, you become suspicious of a bioterrorism event. Which question would you ask to confirm the suspicion?
   1. "Have you been washing your hands frequently?"
   2. "Has the illness progressed rapidly?"
   3. "Do you have a fever?"
   4. "Are you a local resident?"

   NCLEX Client Need: Safe and Effective Care Environment: Safety and Infection Control

5. A patient is tentatively diagnosed with chickenpox. During skin assessment, what are you likely to find that confirms the diagnosis?
   1. Skin lesions are firm.
   2. Skin lesions are found on palms and soles.
   3. Skin lesions occur in various stages.
   4. Skin lesions occur with other signs and symptoms.

   NCLEX Client Need: Physiological Integrity: Physiological Adaptation
6. You are teaching a group of people about water and food safety after a disaster. Which comments by the learners indicate successful teaching? *(Select all that apply.)*
   1. "Contaminated water should be boiled for at least 20 minutes."
   2. "Eight drops of bleach to a gallon of water will purify the water."
   3. "A full freezer will keep food safe for 48 hours."
   4. "Any food that has an unusual odor, color, or texture should be thrown away."
   5. "Tightly sealed containers of food are safe to use even if in contact with flood waters."

   NCLEX Client Need: Health Promotion and Maintenance
7. Which patient needs to be put into isolation immediately?
   1. Diagnosed case of botulism poisoning
   2. Probable case of inhalational anthrax
   3. Known exposure to a high dose of radiation rays
   4. Suspected smallpox but probable chickenpox

   NCLEX Client Need: Safe and Effective Care Environment: Safety and Infection Control
8. Which behavior by a nurse indicates that there is a need for additional counseling beyond the counseling offered through a critical incident stress debriefing?
   1. Talks openly about the incident but is not ruminating
   2. Avoids coworkers and friends for a prolonged period
   3. Takes extra vacation time away from the city
   4. Attempts to resume a healthy lifestyle but is not sleeping well

   NCLEX Client Need: Psychosocial Integrity
9. In the event of a disaster requiring evacuation of homes, what items should be in a "go bag"? *(Select all that apply.)*
   1. All personal valuables
   2. Water and medications
   3. Flashlight and batteries
   4. Camp stove and eating utensils
   5. Clothing and important documents

   NCLEX Client Need: Health Promotion and Maintenance
10. There is a power outage, and the IV pumps are no longer functional. You must deliver a fluid bolus of 500 mL over 20 minutes. The drip factor for available IV tubing is 10 gtt/mL. What is the drip rate in drops/minute? _____

    NCLEX Client Need: Physiological Integrity: Pharmacological Therapies

Critical Thinking Questions

Scenario A

A hurricane has hit the town in which you live. There is widespread wind damage in much of the town, many streets are flooded, and a lot of people are injured. The power is out, and the phones are dead. Your neighbor has a gash in his lower leg and is bleeding.

1. Describe how you would stop the bleeding.
2. How would you transport your neighbor to a health care facility? What precautions would you take on the journey?
3. If teenagers want to go out and wade in the flood water to see if they can rescue stranded people or animals, what would you tell them?

Scenario B

You and several other health professionals have been asked to teach a community group about what to do in the event of a disaster or bioterrorism attack.

1. Outline what should be included in the teaching plan.
2. If questions arise about a nuclear disaster, what would you say about measures the community members could take?

Scenario C

You are working in a busy walk-in clinic. You recognize that emergency departments and clinics are likely to be the first places where infected people will show up if there is a biologic event. You must be vigilant for clusters of cases or unusual cases that may suggest that a bioterrorism event has occurred among the population that the clinic serves.

1. What signs or events would suggest that a bioterrorism event has occurred?
2. What assessment questions would you ask if you suspect a patient has been exposed to a bioterrorism agent?
3. If you determine that an infectious agent is likely, what should you do?

Care of Patients With Emergent Conditions, Trauma, and Shock

45

http://evolve.elsevier.com/deWit/medsurg

Objectives

Theory

1. Evaluate how your personal attitudes, experiences, beliefs, and values affect your ability to care for victims of abuse.
2. Explain the basic principles of first aid.
3. Summarize the importance of mechanism of injury and index of suspicion in caring for patients with traumatic injury.
4. State the key components of assessing a trauma patient.
5. Discuss prevention of injuries from extremes of heat and cold.
6. Determine specific interventions appropriate in the emergency care of accidental poisoning by ingestion and inhalation.
7. Describe emergency care of victims of insect stings, tick bites, and snakebites.
8. Review the appropriate nursing actions and care needed for a patient who has experienced a respiratory or cardiac arrest.
9. Identify signs and symptoms of shock.
10. Compare and contrast the treatment of cardiogenic, hypovolemic, and distributive shock.

Clinical Practice

11. Role play with fellow students, practicing techniques to calm a combative patient.
12. Observe how the triage nurse in the emergency department sets priorities for patient care.
13. Observe how the emergency team works together on a major accident victim.

Key Terms

anaphylaxis (ă-nă-fă-LĂK-sĭs, p. 1061)
angioedema (ăn-jē-Ō-ĕ-DĒ-mă, p. 1068)
automated external defibrillator (AED) (ĂW-tō-mā-tĕd ĕks-tĕr-năl dē-fĭb-rĭ-LĀ-tŏr, p. 1063)
C-A-B (chest compressions, airway, breathing) (chĕst kŏm-PRĔ-shĕn, ĔR-wā, BRĒ-thĭng, p. 1063)
flail chest (FLĀL CHĔST, p. 1054)
hands-only CPR (hăndz Ōn-lē sē-pē-ŏr, p. 1063)
hypovolemia (hī-pō-vō-LĒ-mē-ă, p. 1065)
index of suspicion (ĬN-dĕks ŭv sŭ-SPĬ-shĕn, p. 1052)
mechanism of injury (MĔ-kĕ-nĭ-zĕm ŭ?v ĬNJ-rē, p. 1052)
multisystem organ dysfunction syndrome (MODS) (MŬL-tē-sĭ-stĕm ŌR-gĕn dĭs-FŬNK-shŭn SĬN-drōm, p. 1068)
perfusion (pĕr-FŪ-zhŭn, p. 1063)
poison control center (POI-zĕn kŭn-trōl SĔN-tĕr, p. 1059)
push hard, push fast (pūsh hărd pūsh făst, p. 1063)
shock (shŏk, p. 1063)
systemic inflammatory response syndrome (SIRS) (sĭ-STĔ-mĭk ĭn-FLĂ-mĭ-tŏr-ē rĭ-SPŎNS SĬN-drōm, p. 1068)
triage (TRĒ-ăhzh, p. 1052)
vasoactive (vă-zō-ĂK-tĭv, p. 1068)

Concepts Covered in This Chapter

- Fluid and Electrolytes
- Thermoregulation
- Intracranial Regulation
- Glucose Regulation
- Nutrition
- Perfusion
- Gas Exchange
- Clotting
- Inflammation
- Infection
- Mobility
- Pain
- Stress
- Clinical Judgment
- Collaboration

PREVENTION OF ACCIDENTS

HOME SAFETY

Accidents in the home and community rank sixth as a leading cause of death for all age groups (Dowell, 2018). People younger than 5 years and older than 65 years are the principal victims of fatal mishaps occurring in the home. Attention to home safety for the very young and the older adult could potentially prevent many of these fatalities and injuries (Box 45.1).

HIGHWAY SAFETY

Thousands of people in the US are killed in motor vehicle accidents each year. An additional 2 million are injured. Improper driving, which is responsible for almost 90% of all accidents, can be caused by the influence of alcohol and/or drugs, distractions, fatigue, excessive speed, or emotional instability. Emphasis on using seat belts, better enforcement of laws against impaired driving, and discouraging use of cellphones have helped to decrease accidents and injury. According to the Centers for Disease

Box 45.1 Home Safety

KITCHEN
- For a gas, coal, or wood-burning stove, use the vents or flues; keep windows open a crack. Never light the stove with kerosene or gasoline. Turn off all flames after cooking. Repair any gas leakage.
- Use potholders. Keep handles of pots and pans turned away from edge of stove.
- Keep matches, sharp instruments, and poisons such as bleach and household cleansers out of children's reach. Place child safety locks on storage cabinets.
- Wipe up spills on floor.
- Keep electrical appliances in good working order.
- Place broken glass in a heavy paper sack to prevent cuts through plastic bags.

STORAGE AREAS
- Always keep cellars, attics, and garages neat.
- Clean and disinfect the area where garbage is kept and dispose of garbage frequently.
- Never place poisonous substances in drinking glasses, cold drink containers, or other containers that have been used for food or drink.
- Always label poisonous compounds; read labels of poisons and store the containers out of reach.

LIVING ROOM
- Be sure floors are not slippery. Use rubber mats under rugs to prevent slipping.
- Replace frayed or torn carpets.
- Cover electrical sockets.
- Replace frayed electrical cords. Keep electrical cords off floor where people walk.
- Place heaters a safe distance from walls. Use screens around fireplace.
- Pad sharp edges on furniture as necessary.
- Check ashtrays for lit matches or cigarettes when going to bed or leaving the house.

FURNACE
- Have a professional check and maintain the furnace every year, especially for leaks.
- Change filters monthly.

BATHROOM
- Use a rubber mat in the tub.
- Store medicines out of children's reach. Keep all medicines capped and labeled. Throw out old medicines. Keep phone number of poison center close to telephone.
- Be cautious in using appliances plugged into a wall plug near water.
- Keep hot water heater set at 120° F (48.8° C) or lower.

BEDROOM
- Do not smoke in bed.
- Use rubber mats under scatter rugs.

STAIRWAYS
- Cover with carpeting or rubber safety treads.
- Replace torn or frayed carpeting. Keep stairs clear of toys and cleaning equipment.
- Install handrails and proper lighting.
- Use gates at top and bottom for young children and confused older adults.

GENERAL AREAS
- Install smoke and carbon monoxide alarms throughout the house.
- Make sure candles are away from flammable materials. Never leave a lit candle unattended.

Control and Prevention (CDC), about 90 people per day die in a motor vehicle crash in the United States. Motor vehicle crashes are the leading cause of death for Americans in the first three decades of life (CDC, 2016).

WATER SAFETY

Water safety rules include selecting safe swimming areas, ensuring supervision of children and adults who are not strong swimmers, diving where the water is sufficiently deep and is free of rocks or obstacles, never swimming alone, and never swimming distances beyond one's ability. Every day about 10 people die of unintentional drowning (CDC, 2016a). **The victim of a diving injury preferably should not be removed from the water until emergency medical services (EMS) arrives because of possible neck and spinal cord injury. Bystanders should immobilize the head and neck, keeping the victim's face out of the water. If the victim is not breathing and rescue breathing cannot be performed in the water, remove the individual from the water and start rescue breathing. If pulseless, start cardiopulmonary resuscitation (CPR)** (American Red Cross, 2012). Techniques for rescuers have been modified since 2012, but the bystander instructions are current. Bystander intervention makes a critical difference in the survival of drowning victims. First, the rescuer should call for help. If possible, try to reach the victim without going into the water. After the rescued person is brought out of the water, they must be given CPR and rescue breathing if they are not breathing and are pulseless. If they are breathing, they should be placed on their side (Fig. 45.1) and the head should be turned to one side to prevent aspiration. Near-drowning victims should be transported to a medical facility. Although they

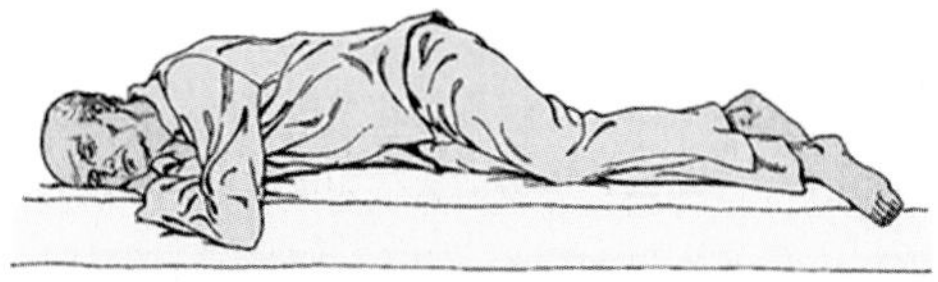

Fig. 45.1 Recovery position. (From Perry AM, Potter PA, Ostendorf WR: *Nursing interventions and clinical skills*, ed 6, St. Louis, 2016, Elsevier.)

may appear to be uninjured, they may have aspirated water, and pulmonary edema may occur. Bacterial or fungal pneumonia may follow aspiration of fresh water. There is danger of delayed cardiac irregularities for any victim who struggled in the water. Hypothermia has a protective effect, especially in young children, and can increase survivability; however, prolonged immersion negates this effect.

FIRST AID AND GOOD SAMARITAN LAWS

All states and the District of Columbia have adopted some form of "Good Samaritan" laws that protect medical personnel and nonmedical civilians from liability when rendering emergency medical care for victims of accidental injury. These laws guard against liability for care as long as medically trained individuals act in good faith and to the best of their ability. Such laws cannot prevent lawsuits from being filed but do provide legal protection to persons rendering care. Individuals who offer help are held to the standard of care consistent with their level of training. If a nursing assistant stops to provide emergency care, they will be held to a different standard than a health care provider who stops at the same accident scene. Both are expected to do the best they can in the circumstances. A bad outcome is not proof of improper care. Malpractice suits of this kind very rarely occur. Table 45.1 shows guidelines for first aid. Some states require medical personnel to render aid if they witness or come upon an accident scene. You should know the laws in your state.

The Cardiac Arrest Survival Act is a Good Samaritan law covering the use of automated external defibrillators (AEDs) in the event of a cardiac arrest. Each state has specific guidelines for implementation.

? Think Critically

You come upon a motor vehicle accident in which several people were involved and stop to render aid. How would you assess the situation for safety for yourself and the victims? How would you act to ensure safety at the scene?

PSYCHOLOGICAL AND SOCIAL EMERGENCIES

THE COMBATIVE PATIENT

Half of all health professionals have been verbally assaulted, and one quarter have been physically assaulted. Patient factors associated with an increased incidence of attacks on health care personnel include paranoid schizophrenia, personality disorders, dementia, substance abuse, and a history of abuse or violence. There are initiatives at the national level to encourage reporting of incidents, levy stiffer penalties, and increase education on de-escalation techniques (Ladika, 2018). Patients who are not diagnosed as mentally ill can also become violent when nurses and other health care personnel fail to respect their rights and needs or when they feel threatened. Pain, cognitive impairment, and being under the influence of mind-altering substances can contribute to a patient's lashing out. Signs and symptoms that usually precede an attack include increasing agitation or resistance, aggressive behavior, pacing, frowning, hyperalertness, increasing demands, and glaring. Families may also become verbally or physically aggressive. Health care workers should approach such patients and families in a nonthreatening manner, use a calm tone of voice, and remain calm (Box 45.2). Language barriers and hearing difficulties need to be considered as possible contributors to an escalating situation. It may be necessary to help the patient by exerting control. Physical force should be used only when there is threat of physical danger and verbal intervention is ineffective. One may simply tell the patient to stop screaming, to sit down, or to put down a weapon-like object. If physical restraint becomes necessary, enough people must be available to control the patient. If you have safety concerns, security personnel should be summoned if available. If the hospital does not maintain on-site security staff, local police should be notified.

Box 45.2 Strategies for Approaching a Combative Patient

- Offer help on a one-to-one basis. Several people trying to simultaneously talk to or subdue the patient may add to their fear and disorientation.
- Establish eye contact.
- Use the person's name frequently.
- Explain who you are and what you are trying to do.
- Express genuine concern about the situation.
- Use a soft voice.
- Make sure the patient can hear and understand what is being said.
- Observe for signs of drug or alcohol use.

! Safety Alert

The Occupational Safety and Health Administration (OSHA) requires employers to provide a workplace "free from recognized hazards that are causing or are likely to cause death or serious physical harm." Patient violence toward health care workers falls in this category. Workplaces are required to have a violence prevention program. The CDC offers an online Workplace Violence Prevention for Nurses program that can be accessed at http://www.cdc.gov/wpvhc/Course.aspx/Slide/Intro_1.

DOMESTIC AND INTIMATE PARTNER VIOLENCE

Annually, domestic and intimate partner violence results in 1500 deaths in the United States. In the 18 years and older population, 1 in 10 men experience domestic violence and 1 in 3 women do. The incidence is thought to be much higher but is difficult to quantify due to lack of reporting on the part of the victims (Huecker & Smock, 2019).

Table 45.1 General Principles of First Aid

ACTION	REASONING
Before attending to the victim or victims of an accident, quickly survey the accident scene to determine whether there are further hazards to yourself and the victims.	Spillage of gasoline after a motor vehicle accident can cause a fire or explosion, or there may be danger to the victim, yourself, and onlookers from oncoming traffic and secondary collisions. In both highway and home accidents, live electrical wires may be in the vicinity. Whenever there is a high risk of death from hazardous conditions in the immediate environment, the victims should be moved at once, regardless of the nature of their injuries. Victims may receive severe burns from lying on a sunbaked street or sidewalk while waiting for the ambulance. Although it may not be safe to move the victim to a shaded area, it is advisable to place clothing, newspaper, or some other protective covering between skin and the hot pavement.
If there are several victims of an accident, make a quick check on each one before beginning treatment.	The most serious and life-threatening injuries must be treated first; those victims who do not seem to be in immediate danger can be attended to by someone else who is capable of watching them and reporting any change in their condition.
Use a calm tone and short sentences to explain what you are doing. You must sound as if you are in control of yourself and the situation.	Giving reassurance to the victim will decrease anxiety and promote cooperation. Using short, simple explanations facilitates understanding during duress. Forcing yourself to remain calm can increase your own ability to function in an emergency.
Do not move a victim unless they are in immediate danger or until you have immobilized injured parts.	This is particularly true if spinal injury is suspected. Moving the victim can cause further injury if precautions are not taken.
Do not remove an object that has penetrated a part of the body and is still in place.	A knife, piece of metal, or sliver of wood that is protruding from the chest or abdomen should be left as is until it can be removed in a controlled situation by trained professionals. Removal of the object can cause further damage and make bleeding worse. Bandages are applied around the object to stabilize it and control bleeding as necessary.
Look for a MedicAlert bracelet or necklace.	If the victim is wearing one or has some other identification showing specific medical needs, bring this to the attention of the ambulance or hospital personnel.
Try to determine the mechanism of injury.	This will give clues about the type of injury sustained and the treatment required. When evaluating the victim, begin at the head and work downward to the toes (see Focused Assessment: Evaluation of Accident and Emergency Patients).
Do not try to give anything by mouth to a person who is unconscious or has a decreased level of consciousness or has injuries that might require surgery.	Aspiration of the material into the air passage may occur, causing breathing difficulty or complete airway obstruction.
Give an organized and chronologic report to the emergency medical services (EMS) or health care provider, including details of the incident (if you were a witness), assessment of injuries, and care rendered.	Any details of events leading to the incident, mechanism of injury, baseline assessment data, and care rendered will be useful in the emergency care at the hospital. Being brief and organized is important because the EMS personnel must simultaneously intervene and take a history if the victim is in critical condition.

Nurses are mandated reporters in most states and need to recognize signs of physical and psychological abuse. Physical signs include bruises, swellings, lacerations, fractures, hematomas, blackened eyes, abdominal injuries (especially during pregnancy), burns, and open wounds that do not match the description of how they occurred. Bruises or fractures in various stages of healing and signs of old lacerations and wounds in the presence of new ones indicate a need for a thorough assessment for abuse. Often the victim may explain all injuries as the result of logical accidents rather than disclose that battering by an intimate partner has occurred.

Psychologically the person may display signs of depression, low self-esteem, anxiety, and stress. Box 45.3 presents the types of questions that might be asked to elicit more information. Asking these questions after establishing rapport with the patient may encourage honest sharing of thoughts and feelings. Research shows that women welcome the opportunity to talk about domestic violence, but health care personnel do not

Box 45.3 Questions to Detect Abuse

- Have you been hit or hurt in any way in the past year?
- Who injured you? Has it occurred before?
- Are you afraid of anyone?
- Do you feel safe at home?
- Does your partner use drugs or alcohol? How does their behavior change after using them?

routinely ask about it unless there is a high index of suspicion. If battering is revealed, the person is referred to an appropriate shelter and community resources, and the incident is reported to the appropriate agency. **Most states have laws requiring health care providers to report domestic violence.**

Clinical Cues

Financial concerns, fear of reprisal against children or pets, lack of social support, and limited work experience may all prevent a woman from permanently leaving her abuser. You may feel frustrated, astonished, or helpless as you meet women who repeatedly return to their abusers. Understanding that leaving the abusive relationship does not guarantee safety can help you provide the needed resource referrals so that the victim can escape safely. Although statistically women are more likely to be abuse victims, annually 1 in 10 men are victimized and need referrals and support.

Child Abuse

If a child and caregiver make frequent trips to a clinic or emergency department (ED) for unexplained or questionable injuries, abuse could be occurring. Suspicion increases when the mechanism of injury reported by the caregiver (or child) does not match the injury pattern. **The law requires that child abuse or suspicion of child abuse must be reported.**

Think Critically

A caregiver reports that a child reached for a hot surface; there is a perfectly round burn in the middle of the palmar surface. What might you conclude about the caregiver's explanation?

Elder Abuse

The population of people older than 65 years is the fastest growing demographic. Just by virtue of sheer numbers alone, elder abuse will increase. Underreporting of events makes it difficult to get a true picture of the extent of the problem. It is estimated that 7% to 10% of older adults are affected (Nursing Home Abuse Center, 2018). Neglect is the most common form of elder abuse, but also assess for physical, emotional, sexual, psychological, or financial abuse. Older adults should be assessed for signs of fear, withdrawal, anxiety, or evasiveness. The caregiver should be assessed for a hostile, critical, or unsympathetic attitude or for burnout. The same signs of physical abuse listed for domestic abuse should be assessed for, as should signs of malnutrition, uncleanness, or severe depression. **The law requires that signs of elder abuse must be reported.** Immediate safety must be established, but referrals to support groups, counseling, respite care, Meals on Wheels, and transportation services can alleviate stress for caregivers. Older adults with dementia are at higher risk for abuse. Older adults also may have self-neglect due to diminishing capabilities, finances, or depression. Evaluation of the situation and providing resources may allow the older adult to safely remain at home.

EMERGENCY CARE

You may need to give emergency care in a variety of community, clinic, or hospital settings, but emergency nursing is generally associated with care of patients in the ED of a hospital. In a survey of hospital ED directors, 90% said that overcrowding and long wait times are an issue. One of the *Healthy People 2030* objectives is to reduce the proportion of patients who wait beyond the recommended time frame to see an emergency health care provider. A Joint Commission Core Measure holds hospital facilities accountable for the time patients wait in the ED for transport to an inpatient bed, the time from assessment to treatment, and the efficiency of the throughput process. A variety of conditions contribute to overcrowding, which leads to decreased patient satisfaction, frustration for health care personnel, and increased risk for poor outcomes (The Joint Commission, 2018). Lack of beds for admitted patients, nursing staff shortages, increased patient volume, and increasing complexity and acuity of patients requiring more time and resources are some of the factors that contribute to overcrowding. This causes delays in treatment of time-sensitive conditions such as acute coronary syndromes, antibiotic administration, and pain management.

Emergency nurses need excellent assessment and clinical decision-making skills and the ability to prioritize care under stressful conditions. Emergency nurses routinely follow protocols to initiate diagnostic testing or to start therapy, such as oxygen administration or peripheral intravenous (IV) access. Clinical decisions, prioritization, and use of protocols are based on (1) events or incidents that preceded the emergency visit, (2) mechanism of injury, and (3) index of suspicion. For example, two patients arrive at the hospital in an unresponsive state. For the first patient, friends report, "She was drinking and taking a lot of drugs for fun, and then we found her passed out with vomit on her mouth." For the second patient, bystanders report hearing him complain of chest pain and needing his heart medication and then finding him unresponsive in the parking lot. Both patients are unresponsive, but preceding events suggest that the first patient is experiencing an overdose with possible aspiration, whereas the second is more likely to have an acute cardiac problem.

Mechanism of injury refers to how the injury occurred; an experienced clinician may use this information to predict damage and complications. For example, toddlers commonly sustain dramatic-looking "goose eggs" on the forehead by falling against a coffee table, but these incidents are usually more traumatic for the parents than the child. A high **index of suspicion** is required to detect problems that are not initially obvious. For example, a patient reports being kicked and punched several times in the abdomen. At first the patient appears to be stable with minor abrasions; however, this patient will require a series of abdominal assessments to detect slow hemorrhage or internal tissue damage. Maintaining a high index of suspicion is important in a busy emergency setting because everyone (including the patient) is anxious for discharge or transfer to make room for others in the waiting room.

TRIAGE: INITIAL (OR PRIMARY) SURVEY

The process of setting priorities for treatment is known as **triage**. One of the most common methods for triage of patients uses ABCDE as a memory trigger for the sequence of assessment. *A* is airway, *B* is breathing, and *C* is circulation. *D* is assessment of neurologic disability. *E* is exposure: all areas of the body should be exposed so that injuries are not missed underneath clothing. The *E* can also mean environmental controls, such as decontamination and warming. This is a good systematic method for assessing inpatients who have had a change in condition so that critical assessments are not overlooked. Identified abnormalities that are life threatening should be addressed before moving on to the next assessment.

AIRWAY

A patent airway and adequate oxygenation are priorities. A simple way to assess airway is to ask the person to tell you their name and to ask how they are feeling. If the airway is partially obstructed, the voice quality may sound muffled or coarse. With severe shortness of breath, a person cannot complete full sentences. A confused answer suggests possible decreased cerebral perfusion and oxygenation. If the patient is unconscious, look for the rise and fall of the chest.

The most common cause of airway obstruction in an unconscious person is the tongue. The head tilt–chin lift maneuver repositions the trachea and tongue and opens the airway. Be sure to place fingers on the jawbone and not the throat to prevent narrowing the airway. The jaw thrust method should be used if a spinal injury is suspected. For this, the clinician positions themself at the head of the victim, placing their hands on either side of the patient's head and the thumbs on the patient's lower jaw near the corners of the mouth and pointing toward the feet; the fingertips are positioned around the bone of the lower jaw, which is then lifted (Fig. 45.2). (Note: Jaw thrust is not taught to lay rescuers; however, health care professionals must learn this maneuver.)

BREATHING

After ensuring that the airway is patent, assess chest rise and effort of breathing, noting rate and any respiratory distress. A pulse oximetry reading is taken and oxygen provided as needed; respiratory rate and effort are monitored. Emergency equipment for resuscitation and intubation should be checked every day, and use of the equipment should be reviewed periodically. If the patient is not breathing, the bag valve mask resuscitator should be used to ventilate the patient. End-tidal carbon dioxide (CO_2) monitoring via the nasal cannula or face mask can help complete the breathing assessment by evaluating adequacy of ventilation.

> **Clinical Cues**
>
> During emergency situations, "verbal orders" may appear to be the norm to inexperienced bystanders; however, the health care team members are working off well-established algorithms, such as Advanced Cardiac Life Support (ACLS). You are responsible for seeking clarification of orders; even under extreme circumstances, the excuse of misunderstanding a verbal order is not acceptable. The health care provider is responsible for writing or entering orders as soon as the crisis has passed.

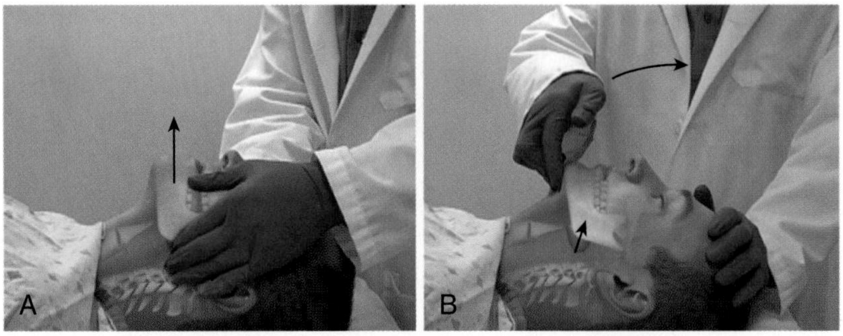

Fig. 45.2 Opening the airway. **A,** Jaw thrust. **B,** Head tilt–chin lift. (From Roberts JR: *Roberts and Hedges' clinical procedures in emergency medicine and acute care*, ed 7, St. Louis, 2019, Elsevier.)

Focused Assessment

Evaluation of Accident and Emergency Patients

AREA OF ASSESSMENT	MODE OF ASSESSMENT	RATIONALE
PRIMARY SURVEY	ABCDE	A systematic approach is needed for assessment.
A: Airway	Assess for signs of breathing and respiratory distress, gasping, wheezing, **stridor** (high-pitched sound made by partial airway obstruction), choking. Check mouth for easily removable foreign body.	Adequate air exchange is necessary for the body's oxygen needs. The tongue may block the airway in an unconscious patient.
	Do not tilt head and hyperextend neck; immobilize cervical spine (C-spine) as needed for suspected injury.	Any patient with an unknown degree of trauma is at risk for C-spine injury. Movement may worsen the injury.
B: Breathing	Quickly assess breathing. Watch chest and abdomen for rhythmic rise and fall. Note rate and quality of respirations. Look for tracheal deviation or asymmetric chest rise.	Normal breathing requires no intervention. Abnormal breathing should be further evaluated and assisted as needed.
C: Circulation/ hemorrhage	Feel for pulse in carotid or femoral artery; note rate and quality. Check blood pressure Check for bleeding. Control bleeding if present.	Absence of a pulse indicates cardiac arrest or obstructive shock. A rapid, bounding pulse may indicate fright hypervolemia. A rapid, thready pulse may indicate blood loss, leading to shock.
D: Disability (neurologic status)	Note if alert, oriented to time, place, person. Note response to verbal stimuli. Check for MedicAlert identification. Assess ability to move all extremities.	Additional assessment of trauma patients helps identify injuries.
E: Exposure/ environmental controls	Remove clothing to look for injuries that may be covered, especially if the patient is not alert or cannot communicate. Look for life-threatening injuries. Provide decontamination as needed. Keep patient warm.	The only way to verify whether there are other injuries is to look. Protect patient privacy, prevent hypothermia.
SECONDARY SURVEY	Head to toe assessment and history.	Initiated after life-threatening injuries are addressed.
Head, face, neck, neurologic status	Look for bleeding, bruising, abrasions. Inspect pupils, assess level of consciousness. Note and record Glasgow Coma Scale score for baseline.	Alterations in level of consciousness can be caused by a variety of conditions such as head trauma, stroke, hypoglycemia, or drug overdose.
	Maintain C-spine precautions, assess for neck injury.	Neck injuries may be hidden by the cervical collar.
Chest	Listen to breath sounds. Look for equal chest expansion.	Tension pneumothorax can develop after a chest injury.
Abdomen/ genitourinary system	Auscultate for bowel sounds. Palpate for tenderness, guarding, and fullness. Look for bloody urine.	Abdominal trauma can result in ruptured spleen or bladder, or liver damage.
	Note bruising or abrasions, such as Grey Turner or Cullen sign.	External trauma may indicate internal damage.
Limbs	Assess adequacy of circulation in all extremities.	Dislocations or fractures can compress nerves and blood vessels.
Log roll	Using at least four people, stabilize the neck and head and gently log roll the victim to assess the back of the head, neck, back, and buttocks.	Bleeding and fractures may obscure additional injuries that are located on the back. In penetrating injuries observe for entrance and exit wounds.

CONTROL OF BLEEDING

Severe bleeding can rapidly lead to irreversible hypovolemic shock. Arterial blood is bright red and gushes in spurts at regular intervals. Blood from a severed or punctured vein leaks slowly and steadily and is dark red.

Even major bleeding can usually be stopped by **applying pressure directly** over the wound. When in a health care work setting, CDC and OSHA requirements mandate use of personal protective equipment that includes barrier devices such as gloves when in contact with body fluids. In a community setting, adapt available material.

Safety Alert

Protective Gear

In a community setting, personal protective equipment may not be present where needed. If gloves are not available, create a barrier with plastic or multiple layers of cloth. Hands and any other skin in contact with blood should be washed as soon as possible.

National guidelines published by the National Association of State EMS Officials in 2017 recommend that for prehospital control of bleeding, direct pressure be held on the area of bleeding. If this is ineffective or impractical, a tourniquet may be implemented. If available, a topical hemostatic agent may also be used. Elevation of an injured extremity is no longer recommended.

Clinical Cues

Many patients are on antiplatelet drugs such as aspirin, clopidogrel (Plavix), prasugrel (Effient), or ticagrelor (Brilinta) or on anticoagulants such as warfarin (Coumadin), dabigatran (Pradaxa), rivaroxaban (Xarelto), or apixaban (Eliquis) to treat heart and vascular conditions. If there is injury, bleeding will be significant and may be difficult to stop.

If bleeding is copious and cannot be stopped with pressure and a tourniquet, occlusion of the arterial input may help stop or slow the bleeding. It is not always possible to compress the artery at the needed location, so this is not a first-line intervention. Pressure points for control of arterial bleeding are shown in Chapter 15, Fig. 15.4. If compression of the pressure point is successful, the distal pulse will be absent, and the patient will notice a tingling and numbness in the area. Compression of pressure points on the neck and head should not be used unless there is no other choice because this will interfere with the blood supply to the brain.

NECK AND SPINE INJURIES

Neck or spine injury should be suspected in any situation in which the individual has sustained multiple injuries, has fallen, or is unconscious. Examples of accidents that would increase the index of suspicion for spinal injury include motor vehicle collisions, diving, biking, or any situation in which the neck receives significant force. In emergency or accident situations, the rescuer may be distracted by severe bleeding or other life-threatening conditions and thus overlook the possibility of a spinal cord injury.

If a victim must be moved to safety before EMS arrives, the neck may be immobilized with a coat or towel rolled into the shape of a collar. The goal is to keep the neck as straight as possible, preventing it from flexing or hyperextending. Applying a cervical collar or other commercial device and maintaining traction on the head requires advanced training (Fig. 45.3). A cervical collar is not particularly comfortable for the patient, and it partially obscures assessment of the neck, jaw, and upper midchest, but removal of the collar is strictly at the discretion of the health care provider (see Chapter 22).

Safety Alert

Cervical Spine Immobilization

In any traumatic injury, spinal injury must be considered. Cervical spine immobilization is implemented as indicated. Regardless of the mechanism of injury, if the patient is awake, alert, conversant, and without significant distracting injury or intoxication, spinal immobilization is not necessary. A consensus statement has been released by the American College of Surgeons Committee on Trauma, American College of Emergency Physicians, and National Association of EMS Physicians regarding the use of spinal precautions called spinal motion restriction (SMR). Once in place, SMR is maintained in the health care facility until spinal injury is ruled out (Fischer et al., 2018).

CHEST TRAUMA

Penetrating thoracic trauma is less common but is more likely to be fatal than blunt chest trauma. Any of the structures located in the chest may be involved in the injury. There can be contusion of the myocardium, puncture of lungs, rupture of the aorta, diaphragm rupture, and tracheobronchial injuries in addition to bone fractures. Communities with access to a trauma center and shorter transport times have increased survival rates for all types of chest trauma (American College of Surgeons, 2018).

Fractured ribs are very painful because breathing causes movement at the site of injury. The treatment goal is to decrease pain so that the patient can breathe adequately. Nonsteroidal antiinflammatory drugs (NSAIDs) and ice to the injury are first-line pain interventions. Intercostal nerve block with local anesthesia may be used to control pain. Narcotic drug therapy is used cautiously because it can depress respirations. **Binding the ribs is not used as treatment because it impairs the ability to take deep breaths, causing atelectasis and possibly pneumonia.**

When three or more ribs are broken in two or more places, the chest wall becomes unstable. This condition is called **flail chest**, which produces **paradoxical chest movement.** When the patient breathes in, the fractured portion of the chest is drawn inward instead of expanding outward as the rest of the chest does; with exhalation, the flail portion expands outward as the rest of the chest collapses normally. This process interferes with oxygenation because the lungs cannot expand normally. Emergency treatment consists of turning the patient onto the affected side so that the ground or bed will act as a splint and reduce the pain of breathing. The patient is observed for signs of external and internal bleeding, pneumothorax, and shock; the force needed to break multiple ribs in multiple locations will also

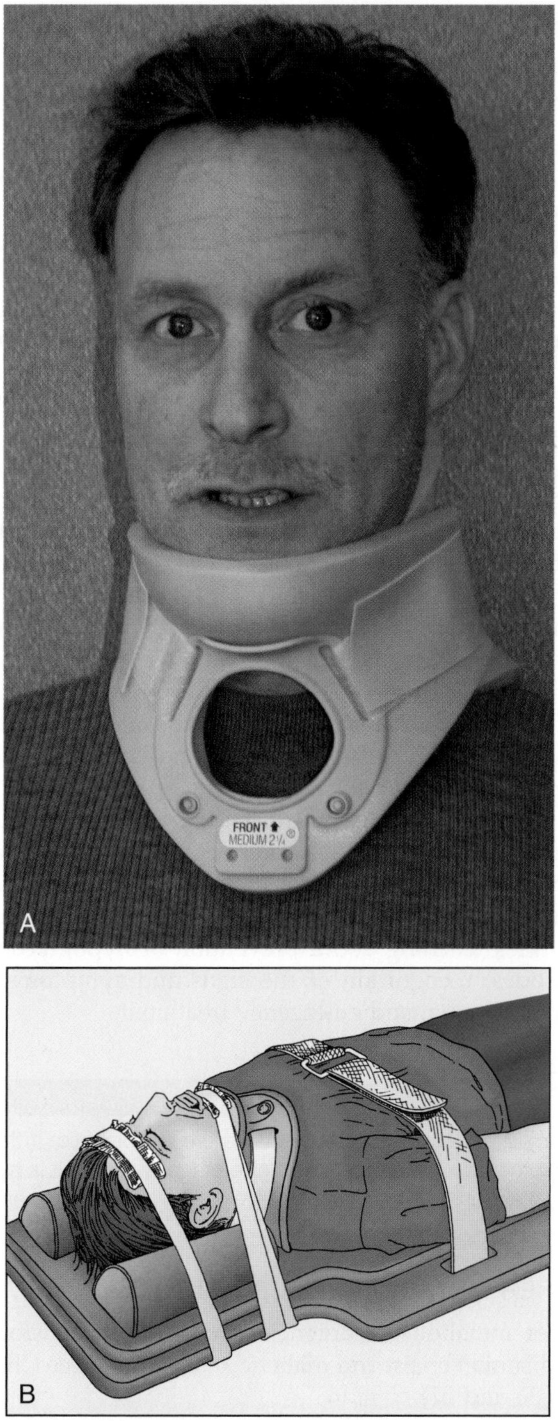

Fig. 45.3 Spinal immobilization. **A,** Philadelphia collar. **B,** Proper spine immobilization. (**A,** From Garfin SR, Eismont JF, Bell GR, et al.: *Rothman-Simeone and Herkowitz's the spine,* ed 7, Philadelphia, 2018, Elsevier. **B,** From Auerbach PS, Cushing TA, Stuart Harris N: *Auerbach's wilderness medicine,* ed 7, St. Louis, 2017, Elsevier.)

injure the underlying structures, which may result in bleeding.

Once the patient is in an emergency facility, flail chest is treated by intubation and mechanical ventilation while the ribs heal. The patient is usually given sedatives and pain medications to prevent fighting the action of the ventilator. Intermittent dosing or continuous infusion may be used depending on the needs of the patient. Surgical fixation of the flail segment has been shown to reduce length of stay in the intensive care unit and ventilatory requirements (de Campos & White, 2018).

Pneumothorax, Hemothorax, and Tension Pneumothorax

An open, or "sucking," chest wound is one in which pneumothorax (accumulation of air) or hemothorax (accumulation of blood) results from external penetration of the pleural cavity. Symptoms of pneumothorax or hemothorax include labored, shallow respirations that cause bubbling of blood at the site of the wound, lack of movement on one side of the chest when the person inhales and exhales, and chest pain. The patient should be placed in a semi-Fowler position if possible. Once the patient is in an emergency facility, treatment includes chest tube insertion with closed-system drainage (see Chapter 14).

Tension pneumothorax develops when air enters the pleural space on inspiration but remains trapped there rather than being expelled on expiration. It can occur from trauma, mechanical ventilation, or rib fracture during CPR. The air in the pleural space increases with each breath, and the pressure within the chest builds, which gradually collapses the lung. If unrelieved, this increasing pressure will cause a **mediastinal shift:** The structures in the mediastinum—the heart, great vessels, trachea, and esophagus—are all shifted to the unaffected side of the chest. This shift puts pressure on the heart, so it cannot fill with blood. Decreased cardiac output results, causing a decrease in blood pressure (obstructive shock). Emergent treatment is a needle thoracostomy. A chest tube with a drainage device or Heimlich valve may be placed to remove the air from the pleural cavity.

CARDIAC TRAUMA

Blunt chest trauma often causes myocardial contusion, but it also can cause tears in the great vessels and massive bleeding. Blunt force trauma directly on the sternum can cause cardiac arrest. Contusion may result in cardiac dysrhythmia. Symptoms may mimic those of a myocardial infarction (MI) because cardiac tissue has been damaged. Treatment is much the same as for an MI. The patient's cardiac rhythm is monitored closely when such trauma has occurred.

Penetrating trauma usually causes a hemothorax. Cardiac tamponade can occur from blunt force or penetration if bleeding into the pericardial sac occurs. Blood collects in the pericardial sac, which will not stretch, compressing the myocardium; the heart cannot fill or pump effectively. Heart sounds become muffled and distant, and hypotension occurs along with increased central venous pressure evidenced by neck vein distention. Shock (obstructive) and death will result if the bleeding is not stopped and the fluid removed. Surgical repair may be necessary.

ABDOMINAL TRAUMA

Penetrating abdominal trauma is usually the result of a knife or gunshot wound. Particularly with gunshot injuries, exit and entrance wounds are anticipated; thus all clothing must be removed by EMS or ED staff, and the anterior and posterior body surfaces must be examined. Patient management depends on the means of injury, location, associated injuries, and hemodynamic and neurologic status of the patient (Offner, 2017).

Blunt trauma is less dramatic but can result from improperly worn seat belts or physical assault. Rapid changes in speed, crushing, or shearing actions result in hemorrhage and damage to internal organs. The overall prognosis for blunt abdominal trauma is good, but the patient must be observed closely for symptoms of shock, and serial abdominal assessments must be performed. A bluish tinge around the umbilicus may indicate abdominal hemorrhage (Cullen sign). Ecchymosis or bruising along the flank can be a sign of retroperitoneal or intraperitoneal bleeding (Grey Turner sign).

Focused assessment with sonography for trauma (FAST), peritoneal lavage, or computed tomography may be performed to diagnose intra-abdominal bleeding. Additional diagnostic tests include serial hemoglobin and hematocrit, blood chemistries, and urinalysis. Treatment includes two large-bore IV lines, nasogastric tube, Foley catheter, and type and crossmatch for blood. Hemodynamically stable patients may not need immediate surgical intervention even if the FAST is positive (Legome, 2019).

MULTIPLE TRAUMA

The most common cause of multiple trauma is motor vehicle accidents. Among older adults, falls are the most common cause. Head injury, fractures, and chest and abdominal injuries are anticipated. Airway management is always the priority (see Focused Assessment: Evaluation of Accident and Emergency Patients). In head trauma, ventilation and oxygenation may be compromised because of decreased level of consciousness, and cervical spine precautions must be observed when performing airway interventions. Threats to breathing may include injuries such as pneumothorax, rib fractures, or open chest wounds. A patient with multiple trauma has a high risk for hypovolemic shock. Tension pneumothorax and cardiac **tamponade** (compression) can also compromise circulation and lead to shock. To manage these critically ill patients, evidence-based practice protocols are implemented based on Advanced Trauma Life Support, developed by the American College of Surgeons. More information can be found at http://www.facs.org/trauma/atls/.

> **Think Critically**
>
> What do you have available at home or in your car that could be used to hold pressure on a bleeding wound? Are you prepared to respond to an emergency?

METABOLIC EMERGENCIES

INSULIN REACTION OR SEVERE HYPOGLYCEMIA

Brain cells need a constant supply of glucose. If glucose levels drop, level of consciousness is altered, and blood vessels dilate from lack of function of the vasomotor center in the brain. The classic clinical picture of a patient who has received too much insulin includes an altered level of consciousness; cold, clammy skin; and hypotension, dizziness, and tachycardia. Most but not all patients experiencing hypoglycemia have diabetes.

Treatment

A glucose reading should be obtained first, if possible; if glucose monitoring equipment is not available but hypoglycemia is suspected, treatment should be initiated without delay. If the patient is awake, they should be given a glass of juice or milk. Glucose tablets or hard candy may also be used. Alteration in level of consciousness often results in impaired swallowing. Attempts to give glucose by mouth could result in aspiration. If a patient has a decreased level of consciousness, IV glucose may need to be given. If an IV line is not in place, intramuscular glucagon can be given by medical personnel or trained family members. Mental status should improve within minutes of receiving glucose. The patient should be given a protein meal, such as a meat sandwich, as soon as they are alert enough to eat. Follow-up care includes teaching about prevention of hypoglycemic episodes, recognition of the signs and symptoms of hypoglycemia, and emergency treatment.

> **Clinical Cues**
>
> Many patients with chronic renal failure are diabetic. If they become hypoglycemic, do not give orange juice, as it is high in potassium. Give apple, cranberry, or grape juice instead.

OTHER METABOLIC EMERGENCIES

Other metabolic emergencies include thyroid storm, Addisonian crisis, and diabetic ketoacidosis (see Chapters 36 and 37).

INJURIES CAUSED BY EXTREME HEAT AND COLD

HEAT ILLNESS

The body responds to heat exposure in various ways. Initially rash and edema may occur, progressing to cramps and syncope with nausea and vomiting. These symptoms are diagnosed as heat exhaustion. This may progress to heatstroke, which is the most severe heat illness and is identified by a body temperature higher than 106° F (41.1° C) with neurologic dysfunction. Heatstroke is the result of a serious disturbance of the heat-regulating center in the brain and can be exertional or nonexertional. Exertional heatstroke tends to occur in young, healthy individuals who engage in prolonged physical activity in a hot environment. The very young, the very old, those with chronic disabilities, those on medications such as anticholinergics, and those with weight or alcohol abuse problems are at risk for non-exertional heatstroke (Helman, 2018). Normally the body is able to regulate body temperature even with increased activity or changes in environmental temperatures by increasing perspiration and using other internal mechanisms. In heatstroke, these mechanisms fail to function properly, and the patient's temperature rises, the skin becomes dry and hot, and there may be convulsions and collapse. Alteration in neurologic function is common with both types of heatstroke. Other symptoms include visual disturbances; dizziness; nausea; and a weak, rapid, irregular pulse.

Prevention

Precautions are necessary in hot weather or when active in warm weather. Drinking plenty of fluids that are nonalcoholic, noncaffeinated, and low in sugar content (the wrong fluids can increase fluid loss) is important, as is not waiting until thirsty to drink fluids. Staying indoors during extremely hot weather or, if air conditioning or adequate cooling is not available in the home, going to a public place with air conditioning should be encouraged (CDC, 2018).

Lightweight, light-colored, loose-fitting clothing should be worn in the heat. Limiting outdoor activities to morning and evening hours and using sun protection such as wide-brimmed hats, sunglasses, and sunscreen will help prevent heat-related illness. Those out in the heat should rest often in shaded areas and limit exertion if possible.

Treatment

A person suffering from heatstroke should be placed in the shade and cooled immediately by sprinkling with water and fanning until EMS arrives. Active cooling measures at the hospital include removal of extra clothing or coverings, wiping the skin with cool wet towels or applying ice packs to the groin and axillae, use of a cooling blanket, and infusion of cold fluids. Active cooling measures are discontinued when the rectal temperature reaches 102.2° F (39° C); this prevents rebound hypothermia (Helman, 2018).

HYPOTHERMIA

People most at risk for hypothermia are older adults, very young and thin children, the mentally ill, the homeless, and others unable to alter their ambient environment. Hypothermia is a serious lowering of the total body temperature caused by prolonged exposure to cold. The extremities can withstand lower temperatures (20° to 30° F). When the core (central) temperature drops even 2° or 3° F, fatal cardiac dysrhythmias or respiratory failure can occur.

Symptoms of hypothermia range from mild shivering, complaints of feeling cold, and loss of coordination to eventual loss of consciousness and a deathlike appearance. Mild or moderate hypothermia may be difficult to identify in some patient populations. The symptoms of confusion, dizziness, chills, and shortness of breath may be misdiagnosed. In severe hypothermia, the body's protective mechanisms drastically slow the metabolic processes and require less than half of the normal oxygen. Pulse and respiration are barely detected, reflexes are absent, and the person is unconscious.

Prevention

Prevention of hypothermia includes eating high-energy foods, exercising, wearing layers of clothing, and covering the head. Between one half and two thirds of the body's heat is lost through the head. Hypothermia in older adults can easily be misdiagnosed because the symptoms resemble those of many diseases to which older adults are most susceptible. Mild hypothermia (90° to 95° F [32° to 35° C] body temperature) is usually well tolerated. Moderate hypothermia (84° to 90° F [29° to 32° C] body temperature) results in a mortality rate of about 21%. Severe hypothermia (core temperature below 82° F [28° C]) has an even higher mortality rate.

Most oral clinical thermometers used in hospitals and clinics do not register temperatures below 94° F (34.5° C). In the ED, rectal, bladder, or esophageal probes are used to monitor true core temperature throughout the warming process.

Older Adult Care Points

With aging, the body's ability to withstand the cold decreases. Older people may also be less active, thus generating less body heat. Older adults are at risk for accidental hypothermia after exposure even to mild cold weather or a small drop in temperature (Box 45.4).

Box 45.4 Prevention of Hypothermia in Older Adults

- Room temperature should not be lower than 65° F (18° C). An indoor thermometer should be kept in the house and checked daily during the cool seasons.
- An energy audit with suggestions from the utility company can prevent heat loss from the home.
- Suggest heating one or two rooms and closing off the other rooms of the house.
- Suggest aids such as a throw or quilt, extra socks, and warm hats to be worn indoors.
- Recommend wearing several loose layers of clothing to retain body heat.
- A head covering should be worn even while sleeping to prevent heat loss.
- Advise against using fireplaces in extremely cold weather because a substantial amount of heat is lost through the flue.
- Arrange for someone to check in daily with older adults who live alone.
- Suggest that an early alert system be installed, allowing the individual to call for help by pressing a button if unable to get to the phone.

Treatment

Once hypothermia is diagnosed, the core must be rewarmed first and continuous monitoring implemented. The goal is to prevent lactic acid or cold blood that has pooled in the extremities from being rapidly shunted to the heart, which can cause ventricular fibrillation. **The heart is extremely sensitive when cold, and the patient must be handled carefully to prevent dysrhythmias.** Rewarming outside a health care facility should be more gradual by wrapping the patient in a blanket and moving them to a warm location.

FROSTBITE

Frostbite is a localized injury to tissue caused by freezing. Exposure of the tissues to extreme cold constricts the blood vessels, damages vessel walls and tissue cells, and leads to the formation of blood clots. Frostbite is most common in the fingers, toes, cheeks, and nose, where exposure usually is greatest and blood supply is most easily hampered. Frostbite can be categorized by four degrees of severity much like burns. The full extent of injury cannot be detected on first examination. The appearance of a first-degree injury (superficial) includes reddened skin, swelling, waxy appearance, hard white plaques, and sensory deficit. Second-degree injury (superficial) also has redness and swelling and blisters filled with clear or milky fluid that form within 24 hours of injury. In third-degree injury (deep), the blisters are blood filled, and black eschar forms over several weeks (Fig. 45.4). Fourth-degree injury (deep) involves full-thickness damage affecting muscles, tendons, and bone, resulting in tissue loss (Zafren & Mechem, 2018).

Prevention

Like hypothermia, frostbite can be prevented by wearing protective clothing and avoiding exposure to extreme cold. Those who are intoxicated or under the influence of drugs may not realize they are suffering from frostbite; likewise, when a person is significantly hypothermic, cognition and judgment are impaired. Friends, family members, and bystanders must take the initiative to direct impaired individuals toward shelter and warmth.

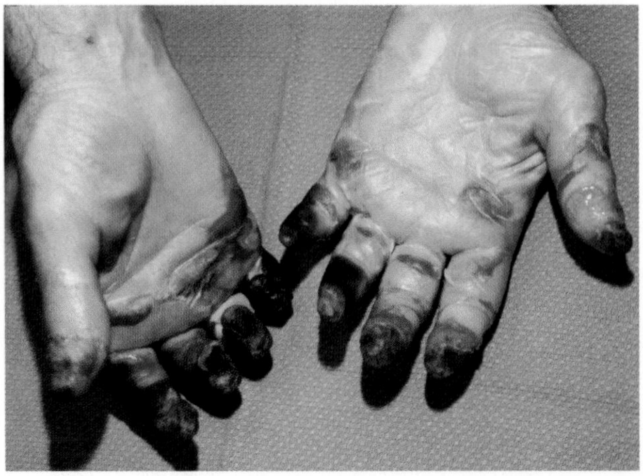

Fig. 45.4 Frostbite. (From James WD, Elston DM, Treat JR, et al: *Andrews' diseases of the skin: clinical dermatology*, ed 13, St. Louis, 2020, Elsevier.)

Treatment

Once the patient is removed from the cold, the affected area should be warmed in the field by forced warmed air; however, the **rewarming process should not be started if there is a chance of refreezing. Refreezing of thawed tissue is more damaging than prolonged freezing** (Zonnoor, 2018). After the patient arrives at the health care facility, rewarming is accomplished in a whirlpool bath with water at 40° to 42° C for 15 to 30 minutes for superficial injuries and up to 1 hour for deep injuries. Health care workers must handle the frostbitten part gently. Skin that has been frozen should never be rubbed or massaged. Rubbing snow or ice on the frostbitten part is dangerous and can cause further damage to the fragile tissues. The affected area should be wrapped in bulky clean or sterile bandages, separating skin areas such as between the fingers, and elevated. The patient should not be given alcohol or sedatives, which tend to further depress function. A tetanus immunization is given if not up to date. Debridement of dead tissue and skin grafting or amputation will be necessary if the deeper tissues have been destroyed. Extent of tissue injury may be unknown for several months. Burn centers are a good resource for management of severe frostbite injuries.

! Safety Alert

Frostbite

Do not try to hasten the warming process by using water that is hotter than recommended because this can add to the damage.

POISONING

ACCIDENTAL POISONING

According to the CDC, the incidence of opioid drug overdose has steadily increased and has now become the leading cause of injury and death in the United States, the rate exceeding that of motor vehicle–related accidental injury and death. Prescription and illegally produced opioid addiction and overdose have become a national epidemic (CDC, 2018b). Most states have passed laws or are in the process of doing so to further control prescribing and dispensing Schedule II medications, and the federal government has also implemented restrictions. With the regulation of prescription opioids, other medications have shown an increase in use and overdosage. Gabapentin and loperamide may be combined with opioids to potentiate the opioid effect. Some states are now also regulating these medications (Perrone, 2018). Naloxone is an opioid reversal agent and is carried by many first responders for immediate injection if an opioid overdose is suspected.

Children younger than 5 years old are at risk of accidental poisoning. Children age 12 years and older more commonly have an intentional ingestion. Prescription medications of family members are the most common poisoning emergency in the 5 years and younger age group. Substances ingested by children may include cosmetics, personal care products, cleaning substances, insecticides, and plants. Children explore their environment by sight, touch, smell, and taste; thus children are at risk for ingestion of a variety of substances, including poisonous mushrooms, plants, or toxic berries. Older adults are also at risk for accidentally taking too much prescribed medication because of forgetfulness, confusion about dosage or frequency, or inability to read small print on a medication bottle. The Joint Commission requires medication reconciliation for patients in an effort to prevent duplication of medications from different health care providers that could contribute to overdose.

Older Adult Care Points

If medications have not been adjusted as a patient has aged, dosages that were appropriate when prescribed may later lead to overdosage. Metabolic changes with aging include decreased liver and kidney function, both of which are responsible for drug metabolism.

Prevention

Prevention of accidental poisoning begins with a realization that there are literally thousands of poisonous substances in an individual's environment. Every home has a variety of poisons in the medicine cabinet; under the kitchen sink; or in the laundry room, utility room, and garage. Encourage families to look at their environment through the eyes of their children and older adults to discover potential poison sources. Make sure that adequate teaching has been done for use of prescription medications and their potential complications, including proper disposal of transcutaneous drug patches. National programs are being implemented to help prevent and educate about opioid addiction and overdosing. Nurses touch the lives of patients during vulnerable times when the individual might be open to reaching out for help. Teachable moments should be used to full advantage and could possibly save a life.

Symptoms

The symptoms of poisoning vary according to the substance ingested and the time that has elapsed since it first entered the body. Poisoning should be suspected if the victim becomes ill very suddenly and there is an open poison or drug container nearby. A peculiar odor to the breath may be present; for example, a garlic smell is associated with organophosphate poisoning. Other symptoms of poisoning include pain or burning sensation in the mouth and throat, an increase or decrease in pulse or respiratory rate, nausea, vomiting, disorientation, visual disturbances, loss of consciousness, or a deep unnatural sleep. Opioid overdose produces pinpoint pupils, unconsciousness, and respiratory depression.

Treatment

The health care team must first ensure circulation, airway, and breathing. You should listen carefully to the patient, family, or EMS personnel because they provide invaluable information as to **what** was taken (or inhaled) and **when** the event occurred. Availability of the container and any of the contents may help in identifying the poison. The **poison control center** (at 1-800-222-1222) should be consulted immediately, and the caller should be prepared to give the patient's age; weight; medical and medication history; allergies; what, when, and why the substance was taken; current signs and symptoms with vital signs and laboratory results; and any treatment rendered. Poison control gives advice about the severity of toxicity and treatment options.

Health Promotion

Poison Prevention

- Dispose of all medicines that are no longer being used by delivering them to an approved collection location. Many pharmacies and health care facilities will accept medications for disposal. Some drugs undergo chemical changes with age and become toxic compounds.
- Store poisons and inedible products separate from edible foods.
- Do not transfer poisonous substances from their original container to an unmarked one. **Never** place a poison in a container that is normally used for edible solids or liquids (such as a soft drink bottle).
- Never tell children that medicine is candy. Explain that medicine will make the child feel better and that it must be taken only as the doctor has directed.
- Always read the labels of chemical products before using them.

Safety Alert

Never dispose of unused or outdated medications in the sewage or water system. Measurable amounts of prescription medications have been found in drinking water. The U.S. Food and Drug Administration (FDA) has issued guidelines on drug disposal (see http://www.fda.gov/ForConsumers/ConsumerUpdates/ucm101653.htm).

Treatment of ingested poisons. Remember to ask about first aid measures that were initiated before arrival at the hospital. Syrup of ipecac is not recommended as a home remedy. However, if ipecac was given at home, initiate aspiration precautions because vomiting is likely to occur. A sample of vomitus should be saved for analysis and identification.

Treatment in the ED is targeted to the specific substance. Treatment for drug ingestion may include activated charcoal to decrease absorption of poison, gastric tube insertion (a sample of stomach contents should be saved for analysis), irrigation to remove stomach contents, sorbitol to enhance bowel excretion, and antidotes that are specific to the poisons. If a caustic substance was ingested, evacuation of stomach contents by a nasogastric tube may be helpful if done quickly. Lavage, activated charcoal, and other standard interventions are contraindicated (Kardon, 2018). If the nonmedication substance can be identified, the safety data sheet (SDS) will provide treatment recommendations.

INHALED POISONS

When a person has inhaled a poisonous substance, emergency help is necessary. Do not attempt to rescue a person without notifying someone of your location. If it is safe to do so, the person can be removed from the danger of the gas, fumes, or smoke. Windows and doors should be opened to remove the fumes. The rescuer should take several deep breaths of fresh air and then hold their breath when entering, holding a wet cloth over the nose and mouth. Lit matches or lighters should not be used as a light source because some gases can catch fire.

After rescuing the person from danger, clothing around the neck and chest should be loosened. The person's pulse, airway, and breathing should be checked and monitored. If necessary, CPR or rescue breathing should be initiated (see American Heart Association recommendations for rescue breathing and CPR).

Symptoms that may indicate inhaled poison include excessive coughing; shortness of breath, wheezing, and a burning sensation of the nose and throat; pale or bluish color to skin; dizziness, headache, nausea, and vomiting; and chest pain or tightness. Carbon monoxide (CO) is the most commonly inhaled poison and results in a **cherry red color of the mucous membranes.** A carboxyhemoglobin level should be obtained, and the patient should be treated with 100% oxygen until the carboxyhemoglobin level is less than 10%. In CO poisoning, the readings of pulse oximetry and the values of arterial blood gases can appear normal despite significant toxic exposure. Hyperbaric oxygen (HBO) therapy eliminates CO from hemoglobin more rapidly than just oxygen administration. HBO is not available at many facilities, and studies have not shown a clear benefit in patient outcomes. Current CO poisoning treatment guidelines do not include HBO therapy; however, it is frequently implemented at facilities with HBO capability (Shochat, 2018).

> **! Safety Alert**
>
> In addition to smoke alarms, carbon monoxide detectors are required in certain residential buildings in most states.

BITES AND STINGS

HUMAN BITES

A human bite that breaks the skin is called an *occlusive bite.* When a tooth meets the skin and muscle of a clenched fist, it is aptly named a *clenched-fist injury.* Infection occurs in 10% to 15% of human bite injuries and can be severe because of delay in seeking treatment. Occlusive bites are of concern because of the potential disruption of tissue, tendons, bones, and structures underlying the area of bite injury. Copious irrigation is required to clean the wound, which may or may not be closed. Prophylactic antibiotics are indicated (Barrett, 2018).

ANIMAL BITES

Family pets, especially dogs and cats, are the most common source of animal bites. Dog bites are more common than cat bites and occur most frequently in adults. However, children tend to sustain bites to the head and neck, which warrant more intensive medical care (Doud Galli, 2018). When a wild animal, such as a squirrel or fox, attacks and bites a human being without provocation, rabies should always be suspected as the cause of the animal's unusual behavior.

Treatment

Bite wounds should be cleaned immediately with soap and rinsed with warm running water for 5 to 10 minutes. The affected area is then treated with antibiotic ointment, covered with a clean bandage, and immobilized. Medical attention includes copious irrigation; suturing may be done if the wound is on the face or hand. Puncture wounds on the arms or legs are typically left unsutured and allowed to drain. If the patient has not had a tetanus shot in the past 5 years, a booster will be given.

The possibility of rabies infection must always be considered in an animal bite. The local animal control agency should be contacted to catch the animal if necessary. If it has been killed, animal control will take the body for examination. If a diagnosis of rabies in the animal has been confirmed or if there is no proof that the animal has been immunized against rabies, the victim is given rabies immune globulin (20 units/kg infiltrated around the wound and the remainder given intramuscularly). A series of intramuscular injections of human diploid rabies vaccine is given at the time of injury and on postinjury days 3, 7, and 14. Antibiotics are given for deep puncture wounds, particularly cat bites (Doud Galli, 2018).

SNAKEBITE

In the United States, approximately 8000 snakebites occur annually; approximately 2000 of these are from poisonous snakes. Fatalities are rare. From 1960 to 1990, 12 fatalities were identified (Daley, 2018). There are four kinds of poisonous snakes in the United States: copperheads, rattlesnakes, coral snakes, and cottonmouths (or water moccasins). Copperheads, rattlesnakes, and cottonmouths are all called pit vipers because they have pits or depressions behind their nostrils; coral snakes are small snakes with characteristic red, black, and yellow bands. Coral snakes have shorter fangs and smaller mouths than the pit vipers, and their venom injection resembles a chewing motion.

A venomous snakebite usually can be distinguished by two fang marks (though there may be only one on a small surface, such as a toe or finger), severe pain and swelling in the area, discoloration at the site of injection of venom, nausea and vomiting, respiratory distress, changes in vision, and increased sweating and saliva production. If prompt intervention is not taken, shock may occur. Nonpoisonous snakebites usually appear as either small scratches or lacerations.

Treatment

Nonpoisonous snakebites are treated as simple wounds and require only a cleansing of the wound with soap and water and the application of a mild antiseptic. First aid for a poisonous snakebite includes washing the wound, lowering the extremity or area and immobilizing it, keeping the victim calm so that the venom does not circulate as quickly, and seeking medical attention as soon as possible. Getting a description of the snake can help with treatment. In the field, rescuers should *not* apply suction, make incisions over the wound, apply ice, or give alcoholic beverages or stimulants. Prehospital care is centered on supporting the ABCs and prompt transport to a medical facility.

When a snakebite victim reaches a hospital or clinic, the victim is treated based on evaluation of the extent of the envenomation, whether it is localized or systemic, and whether coagulation abnormalities exist. A scale is used to determine the severity of the envenomation to make treatment decisions. Newer antivenins are recommended earlier in the treatment with more liberal dosing. Prevention of compartment syndrome has been noted with earlier administration. Most victims are admitted for observation for up to 24 hours and provided with a tetanus immunization, antibiotic prophylaxis, and symptom management (Daley, 2018).

BUG BITES AND STINGS

Systemic reactions to the bites and stings of insects and bees account for more deaths each year in the United States than do snakebites. A systemic reaction is caused by hypersensitivity to the venom of bees, wasps, hornets, fire ants, harvester ants, puss caterpillars, scorpions, or spiders. Symptoms of a systemic reaction include hives, swelling, general weakness, tightness in the chest, abdominal cramps, constriction of the throat, loss of consciousness, and possibly death from severe **anaphylaxis**. When the interval between the sting or bite and the development of symptoms is short, the possibility of death increases. Most bug bites result in local reactions and are not reported. Symptom relief is provided, and medical help is sought only if there are complications to the bite or sting.

The black widow and the brown recluse spiders are the best-known spiders that have a potentially serious bite. The symptoms of a black widow spider bite may not be obvious initially; the bite may feel like a pinprick with some slight redness and swelling. Within a few hours abdominal pain and muscle cramps occur. Other symptoms include nausea, vomiting, chest pain, and respiratory distress. A brown recluse spider bite usually goes unnoticed initially. Symptoms usually develop 2 to 8 hours after the bite and include severe pain and itching at the site, nausea, vomiting, fever, and muscle pain. The tissue may heal without problems, or blistering and development of necrotic tissue may occur, requiring surgical intervention.

> **! Safety Alert**
>
> A severe local reaction to a bug bite or sting puts the patient at risk for a systemic reaction with a subsequent exposure.

> **Older Adult Care Points**
>
> Anyone older than age 65 years should seek medical attention if bitten by a brown recluse or black widow spider. Older adults are more at risk for developing complications related to the bite.

Treatment

Treatment for a systemic reaction is to subcutaneously or intramuscularly inject aqueous epinephrine (1:1000 solution) in dosages of 0.5 mL for adults and 0.15 mL for children. An antihistamine, such as diphenhydramine (Benadryl), is given. An ice pack may be applied to reduce swelling and relieve pain. Patients who appear to be in shock should be kept warm and should remain lying down with the legs elevated and the head flat. If symptoms persist after 20 minutes and the patient has not yet reached a medical facility, a second injection of epinephrine should be given. Many patients who have a known allergy carry autoinjectable epinephrine in a prefilled syringe device that delivers a measured dose of medication when activated.

The female worker honeybee injects a venom sac that may remain embedded in the victim's skin. **The "stinger" should be removed as quickly as possible.** Do not use tweezers to remove an insect stinger, as this may cause squeezing of the venom sac and increase the severity of the symptoms. Use a credit card or any rigid item with a smooth, flat edge to scrape out the stinger.

An emergency kit that contains drugs, syringe, tourniquet, towelette, and tweezers is available by prescription and is used for treatment of systemic reactions to stings and bites. Individuals with known hypersensitivity to insect and bee venom should carry medical identification and an emergency kit and be thoroughly familiar with its use *before* the need arises. Persons who have systemic reactions or even severe local reactions with swelling beyond two joints should be referred for hyposensitization therapy.

Applying a paste of baking soda and water or household ammonia and a cold compress treats less serious stings of bees, wasps, yellow jackets, and hornets. Meat tenderizer also has been found to be effective in relieving the symptoms of minor insect sting reactions. Topical cortisone cream can relieve inflammation and itching.

Bites from venomous spiders, scorpions, and other poisonous insects are treated in the same manner as poisonous snakebites. Antivenin specific to the spider, scorpion, or other poisonous creature is available at hospital EDs and clinics that serve rural areas.

Ticks can carry Rocky Mountain spotted fever or Lyme disease. The tick is removed by grasping it as close to the skin as possible with tweezers and pulling it straight out without twisting. Applying turpentine, mineral oil, petroleum jelly, nail polish, or insecticide on the tick is not recommended because the tick may regurgitate stomach contents into the skin (CDC, 2019). After the tick is removed, the area should be washed with soap and water and a mild disinfectant applied. A health care provider can be consulted for possible infection or disease symptoms.

ELECTRICAL INJURIES AND BURNS

When an electrical current passes through the body, it can cause severe damage to the entire body, including cessation of breathing, circulatory failure, and serious burns. The current travels along the path of least resistance, which is usually the fluid-filled blood vessels, and may be conducted through the heart. The amount of voltage and current involved, the length of time in contact with the electricity source, and the condition of the skin all play a role in how much damage may occur as a result of an electrical shock.

Emergency treatment of electrical shock involves CPR if breathing has ceased or the heart has stopped and treatment of burns or other concurrent injuries. The proper procedure for separating a victim from a live conductor of electricity is shown in Fig. 45.5. **Remember that water serves as a conductor of electricity, and wet objects can transmit a fatal electric current to a person trying to rescue the victim of electrical shock.** All electrical shock victims, including those struck by lightning, must be observed for cardiac dysrhythmias and evidence of internal injury.

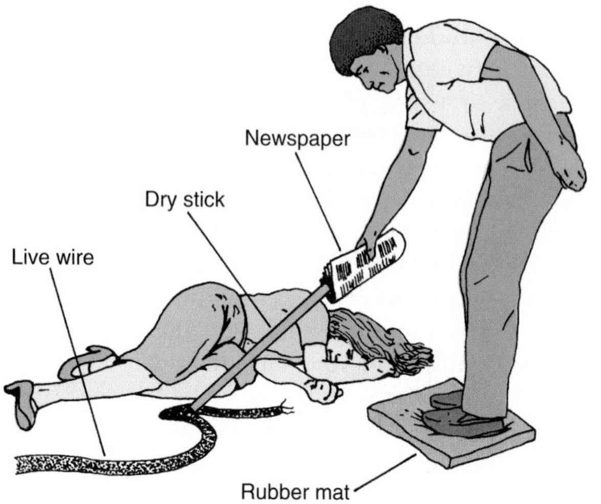

Fig. 45.5 Separating a victim from a live electrical wire while avoiding similar shock.

> **Safety Alert**
>
> **Lightning**
>
> There are no safe locations outside during a lightning storm. The National Weather Service's slogan is "When thunder roars, go indoors." When camping or participating in other outdoor activities, plan ahead for shelter. If no safe shelter is available, avoid water, high ground, open spaces, and metal objects. Do not seek shelter under canopies, small picnic or rain shelters, or trees. If out in the open, do not lie down but keep moving toward shelter. If inside, avoid plumbing fixtures and electrical appliances, including computers and cord phones. If in the car, do not touch surfaces that readily conduct electricity (National Oceanic and Atmospheric Administration, *National Weather Service Lightning Safety*, n.d.).

CHEMICAL INJURY

Strong chemicals capable of burning the skin and mucous membranes will continue to destroy tissue unless they are diluted and removed immediately. For this reason, any area burned by chemicals must be quickly flushed with large amounts of water (with some exceptions) until all traces of the chemical have been removed; the burned area is then covered with a dressing.

Water is not used for burns caused by dry lime or phenol. Dry lime should be brushed from the skin and clothing unless there is enough water to remove *all* traces of the powder. Small amounts of water will react chemically with the lime to produce a highly **corrosive** (destroys gradually) substance. Phenol (carbolic acid) is not water soluble. The phenol is first removed by alcohol, and the burned area is then rinsed with water. **If a corrosive chemical has been ingested, the poison control center should be contacted for instructions and proper dosage of an antidote.** Vomiting should *not* be induced or encouraged. No attempt should be made to neutralize an ingested chemical substance because this can cause further damage to the esophagus and stomach.

Patients with chemical burns should be transported to a hospital as soon as possible. If possible, the treating health care provider should be informed about (1) the offending agent, physical form, and concentration; (2) the route and volume of exposure; (3) the timing and extent of irrigation; and (4) any coexisting injuries. See Chapter 43 for burn injury management.

CHOKING EMERGENCIES

Obstructed airway is the seventh leading cause of accidental death. Adults as well as children can become choking victims and need immediate intervention to prevent death from asphyxiation. Both partial and complete airway obstruction should be treated promptly; even a partial obstruction can result in inadequate airflow. **If the person is conscious and able to cough or speak, they may not need assistance in expelling the object from their throat.** In this situation, they should be encouraged to cough vigorously and breathe as deeply as they can. Their coughing efforts are more effective than outside intervention; others present should stay with them and call for help as needed. When the choking victim cannot speak, cough, or independently expel the foreign object, abdominal thrusts are used to force the object up and out (see Chapter 13).

? Think Critically

You are dining in a restaurant and observe someone at another table apparently choking. What steps would you take to assist?

CARDIOPULMONARY RESUSCITATION

Many phenomena cause sudden cessation of breathing and circulation, from electrical shock to drowning to cardiac arrest. **CPR is indicated when the person shows (1) absence of response to stimuli, (2) absence of respirations, and (3) absence of a carotid pulse.** When a person stops breathing spontaneously and their heart stops beating, "clinical death" has occurred. Within 4 to 6 minutes, the cells of the brain, which are most sensitive to lack of oxygen, begin to deteriorate. If the oxygen supply is not restored immediately, the patient suffers irreversible brain damage and "biological death" occurs.

The American Heart Association (AHA) Guidelines for CPR are revised every 5 years to reflect the most current research and consensus by international experts. The 2010 guidelines implemented the **C-A-B (chest compressions, airway, breathing)** sequence, and that is still the sequence in the current protocol. The guidelines emphasize the importance of high-quality CPR. To help ensure high-quality CPR, effective January 1, 2019, all CPR training facilities must use an instrumented directive feedback device or manikin when teaching adult CPR skills. These devices measure depth and rate of compressions and give verbal and/or visual feedback on how the individual is meeting the standard (American Heart Association, 2017). The guidelines are based on research that indicates that the highest survival rates for cardiac arrest among adults occurs for witnessed ventricular fibrillation (VF) or pulseless ventricular tachycardia in which the critical interventions of chest compressions and defibrillation are implemented. There should be minimal delay or interruption to chest compressions for pulse checks or any other action. The AHA recommends **hands-only CPR** for the lay rescuer. The idea of hands-only CPR for lay rescuers is intended to encourage bystanders to intervene only with chest compressions and to **push hard, push fast** at a rate of at least 100 compressions per minute. Beyond the fear of contagion, it was determined that positioning the head and delivering initial breaths was delaying the delivery of chest compressions. In the health care setting, high-quality CPR means that the chest compressions must be delivered with the correct depth and rate with adequate recoil and that any pauses for ventilation, pulse checks, or switching rescuer positions or procedures such as application of equipment or defibrillation must be kept to the absolute minimum.

Health care providers are held to a higher standard of care, and intervention must be based on assessment of the patient and tailored to address the most likely cause. For example, if you witness a sudden collapse of a patient in the hospital, VF would be a likely assumption. The sequence would be to establish unresponsiveness and breathlessness, activate the response team, check the pulse in 10 seconds or less, start compressions, defibrillate with the **automated external defibrillator (AED)** as soon as it is available, and ventilate with an Ambu bag. Adapt and delegate as personnel and equipment arrive at the scene.

In the community, the use of the AED combined with activation of the EMS response system and CPR gives a victim of VF the best chance for survival. AEDs are now located in most public buildings, health clubs, airlines, malls, and sporting venues. As soon as the AED is brought to the scene, the device must be turned on; it will audibly give step-by-step instructions. When the AED indicates that it is analyzing the rhythm, all CPR and any direct contact with the victim must stop. If the AED identifies a shockable rhythm, it will either automatically charge or give instructions to charge the device. Once the AED is charged, the instructions will state to "stand clear" of the victim. To prevent being shocked, everyone must avoid touching the victim when the charge is delivered. If indicated, a single shock is delivered, and CPR is resumed immediately.

Table 45.2 presents current techniques of CPR. For the most up-to-date science, refer to a current CPR handbook. Recertification is generally required every 2 years; however, studies show that skills are not retained for that length of time unless reviewed.

SHOCK

Shock is a condition that starts at the cellular level and gradually spreads to produce clinical signs and symptoms. The hallmark of shock is lack of adequate **perfusion** (blood supply) to tissues, which results in lack of oxygen and nutrients. This deficit causes anaerobic metabolism and the production of lactic acid and organ dysfunction. Conditions of low circulating volume (hypovolemic shock), decreased cardiac output (cardiogenic shock), impairment of circulation (obstructive shock), or maldistribution of volume (neurogenic, anaphylactic, or septic shock) cause decreased perfusion (Table 45.3). Perfusion requires adequate blood volume; the blood

Table 45.2 Cardiopulmonary Resuscitation for Adults

COMPONENT	ACTION FOR LAY RESCUER	ACTION FOR HEALTH CARE PROVIDER
Recognize symptoms and need for assistance	If victim is unresponsive or is not breathing or gasping only. Call for help.	The sudden collapse of an adult is likely to be cardiac in origin; call for help, start CPR, and defibrillate as soon as the AED is available. Any adult that is unresponsive or has breathing issues needs EMS care. The sooner the call is placed, the sooner help will arrive.
Pulse check	Lay rescuers are not taught this step.	≤10 seconds, carotid. While checking the pulse assess for signs of breathing.
CPR sequence	C-A-B.	C-A-B.
Compression rate	At least 100–120/min. Pushing hard, pushing fast, and allowing for the chest to recoil between compressions has been found to be most effective.	At least 100–120/min. Pushing hard, pushing fast, and allowing for the chest to recoil between compressions has been found to be most effective. Consider using an automated chest compression device for consistent high-quality chest compressions.
Compression depth	At least 2 inches (differs for children and infants).[a]	At least 2 inches (differs for children and infants).[a]
Compression interruption	Minimize interruptions in chest compressions.	Limit interruptions to less than 10 seconds (i.e., rotating compressors, delivering shock, pulse check). Rescuers should change compressors every 2 min to prevent fatigue and decreased efficiency of compressions.
Airway	Untrained lay rescuers should not delay compressions to perform airway maneuvers.	Head tilt–chin lift; use jaw thrust if cervical injury is suspected.
Compression ratio to rescue breathing (no advanced airway placed)	Compressions only for untrained lay rescuers.	30:2 for one or two health care rescuers. Use one-way valve for mouth to mask ventilations. Use bag valve mask as soon as available.
AED use	Use as soon as possible.	Use as soon as possible. For an out-of-hospital, unwitnessed cardiac arrest, EMS may initiate 1.5 to 3 min of CPR before attempting defibrillation.

[a]Consult a pediatrics text and the American Heart Association guidelines for additional data that are specific to children and infants.
AED, Automated external defibrillator; *C-A-B,* chest compressions, airway, breathing; *CPR,* cardiopulmonary resuscitation; *EMS,* emergency medical services.

vessels must be intact, without obstruction to flow, and the pump (the heart) must be working correctly.

SIGNS AND SYMPTOMS

Early recognition and treatment of impending shock results in better outcomes. Compensated shock occurs when the body is able to maintain blood pressure and perfusion by increasing heart rate and vasoconstriction of peripheral vessels. The only clinical signs at this point may be increased heart rate and cool skin. The clinical symptoms associated with the second stage of shock reflect lack of oxygen to essential organs; this is decompensated shock. Signs and symptoms reflect decreased cardiac output, such as confusion, restlessness, diaphoresis, rapid thready pulse, increased respiratory rate, cold clammy skin, decreased blood pressure, and diminishing urinary output to less than 20 mL/h (Fig. 45.6). Decompensated shock can quickly move to the third stage, which is irreversible shock from which recovery is impossible.

HYPOVOLEMIC SHOCK

Hypovolemic shock is the most common form of shock. A blood loss of even 500 mL in a fragile adult may cause hypovolemic shock. Table 45.4 shows the amount of blood loss and consequent clinical manifestations. Any significant loss of fluid volume can result in hypovolemic shock (Fig. 45.7). Blood loss from trauma or gastrointestinal (GI) bleeding, plasma leaking from a burn, severe vomiting and diarrhea, and internal bleeding from pancreatitis are examples of conditions that may lead to hypovolemia.

Older Adult Care Points

Older adults may develop shock with smaller blood loss because of decreased vascular tone and impaired cardiac function. Many are on antihypertensive medications that impair the vasoconstrictive ability of vessels.

Table 45.3 Comparison Chart of Shock

TYPE	CAUSE	CLINICAL SIGNS AND SYMPTOMS	MANAGEMENT
Hypovolemic	External blood loss Trauma GI losses Burns Internal bleeding	↓ BP ↑ HR Tachypnea Oliguria Cool, pale skin Altered mentation	Stop fluid loss Replace lost volume
Cardiogenic	Myocardial infarction Cardiomyopathy Valve dysfunction	↓ BP ↑ HR Dysrhythmias Oliguria Cool, pale skin Altered mentation Chest pain	Improve contractility with medications Mechanical support as needed Prevent or treat dysrhythmias
Obstructive	Cardiac tamponade Tension pneumothorax Pulmonary embolism Aortic stenosis	↓ BP ↑ HR dysrhythmias Oliguria Cool, pale skin Altered mentation Chest pain JVD	Eliminate the source of obstruction or compression
Distributive			
Neurogenic	Cervical spinal cord injury Spinal anesthesia	↓ BP ↓ HR Hypothermia Warm, dry, flushed skin Oliguria Altered mentation	Eliminate and treat the cause Maintain BP with IV fluids
Anaphylactic	Chemicals (latex, perfume, soap) Drugs (antibiotics, contrast media, blood products) Food (peanuts, shellfish, eggs, wheat, nuts, milk) Bites or stings (wasps, bees, spiders, fire ants)	↓ BP ↑ HR dysrhythmias Tachypnea Chest pain Warm, dry, flushed skin Oliguria Dyspnea, cough stridor	Remove offending agent or slow absorption Maintain airway Modify or block effects of mediators: epinephrine, antihistamines, steroids
Septic	Bacteria Immunosuppression Malnutrition Invasive procedures and devices Traumatic wounds or burns Infection elsewhere in the body (urinary tract, peritoneum, respiratory tract)	↓ BP ↑ HR Oliguria Cool, pale skin Altered mentation Hyperthermia	Identify source of infection Antibiotic therapy Medical asepsis Support BP with fluids and pressors if needed Avoid NPO status; initiate and maintain nutrition Control hyperthermia

Adapted from Sole ML, Klein DG, Moseley MJ: *Introduction to critical care nursing,* ed 7, St. Louis, 2017, Elsevier.
BP, Blood pressure; *GI,* gastrointestinal; *HR,* heart rate; *IV,* intravenous; *JVD,* jugular venous distention; *NPO,* nothing by mouth.

Treatment

The primary interventions for **hypovolemia** are to stop the fluid loss, if possible, and to replace fluids. **In all situations of hypovolemic shock, volume replacement is essential.** To infuse large volumes of fluid and/or blood products, adequate IV access is extremely important. Two large-bore peripheral IV sites or placement of a central line with multiple lumens is needed. If IV access cannot be obtained, intraosseous access may be implemented. If large volumes of fluid are required for fluid resuscitation, warming the fluids can help prevent hypothermia. If hemorrhage is present, crystalloids (i.e., normal saline or lactated Ringer solution) or colloids (e.g., albumin or hetastarch) will be infused until blood products are available for transfusion. Packed red blood cells are given to replenish cell volume. Units of packed cells contain citrate as an anticoagulant. If multiple units of blood are rapidly infused, the citrate can bind with ionized calcium, decreasing the amount of circulating calcium. This can depress cardiac function and alter coagulation; therefore in massive transfusions, IV calcium is also given. If a large volume of blood is lost,

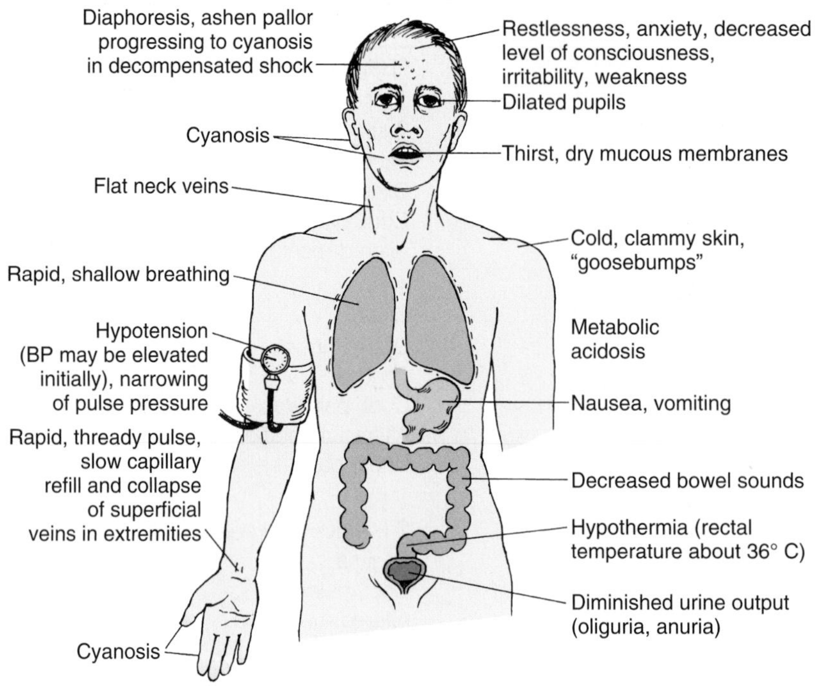

Fig. 45.6 Clinical signs of shock. *BP,* Blood pressure.

Table 45.4 Clinical Manifestations of Blood Loss

VOLUME LOST	CLINICAL MANIFESTATIONS
10%	None
20%	At rest, no signs or symptoms; slight postural hypotension when standing; tachycardia with exercise
30%	Blood pressure and pulse normal when supine; postural hypotension and tachycardia with exercise
40%	Below-normal blood pressure, central venous pressure, and cardiac output at rest; rapid, thready pulse and cold, clammy skin
50%	Shock and potential death

Adapted from Lewis SL, Heitkemper MM, Bucher L, et al.: *Medical-surgical nursing: assessment and management of clinical problems,* ed 10, St. Louis, 2017, Elsevier.

clotting factors will also need to be replaced. Fresh frozen plasma is given for replacement of clotting factors. Platelets may also be given.

If fluid loss is from GI sources, isotonic solutions will be used to replenish the fluid and electrolytes. Burn patients require replacement of lost plasma, which is rich in protein. Crystalloids containing salt and colloids, such as albumin, will be administered to rehydrate burn victims (see Chapter 43). Monitoring of vital signs, level of consciousness, and urine output helps assess response to therapy.

CARDIOGENIC SHOCK

Cardiogenic shock occurs when the heart is incapable of pumping enough blood to meet the needs of the body because of a primary cardiac injury or dysfunction. MI is the primary cause of coronary cardiogenic shock because of the direct damage of the heart muscle from a heart attack. The heart also can be rendered ineffective as a pump by noncoronary causes, such as cardiomyopathy or valvular dysfunction.

> **Clinical Cues**
>
> Oxygen should always be administered to patients in shock or suspected shock.

> **Think Critically**
>
> You are caring for a patient who has vomited large amounts of blood. You expect to see a compensatory increase in pulse, but in fact the pulse rate remains between 50 and 60 beats per minute. Why would you want to double-check this patient's medication history?

Treatment

In cardiogenic shock, the first-line treatment is to restore myocardial function if possible. Myocardial ischemia resulting from acute coronary syndromes is the primary cause of cardiogenic shock. Percutaneous coronary intervention or coronary artery bypass grafting can help restore oxygen to the myocardium, improving function. Chemical and mechanical treatments are used with the goal of supporting the impaired heart muscle without increasing the workload of the heart. Vasopressor agents (e.g., norepinephrine and dopamine), inotropic agents (e.g., dobutamine), or phosphodiesterase inhibitors (e.g., inamrinone) are used to increase the contractility of

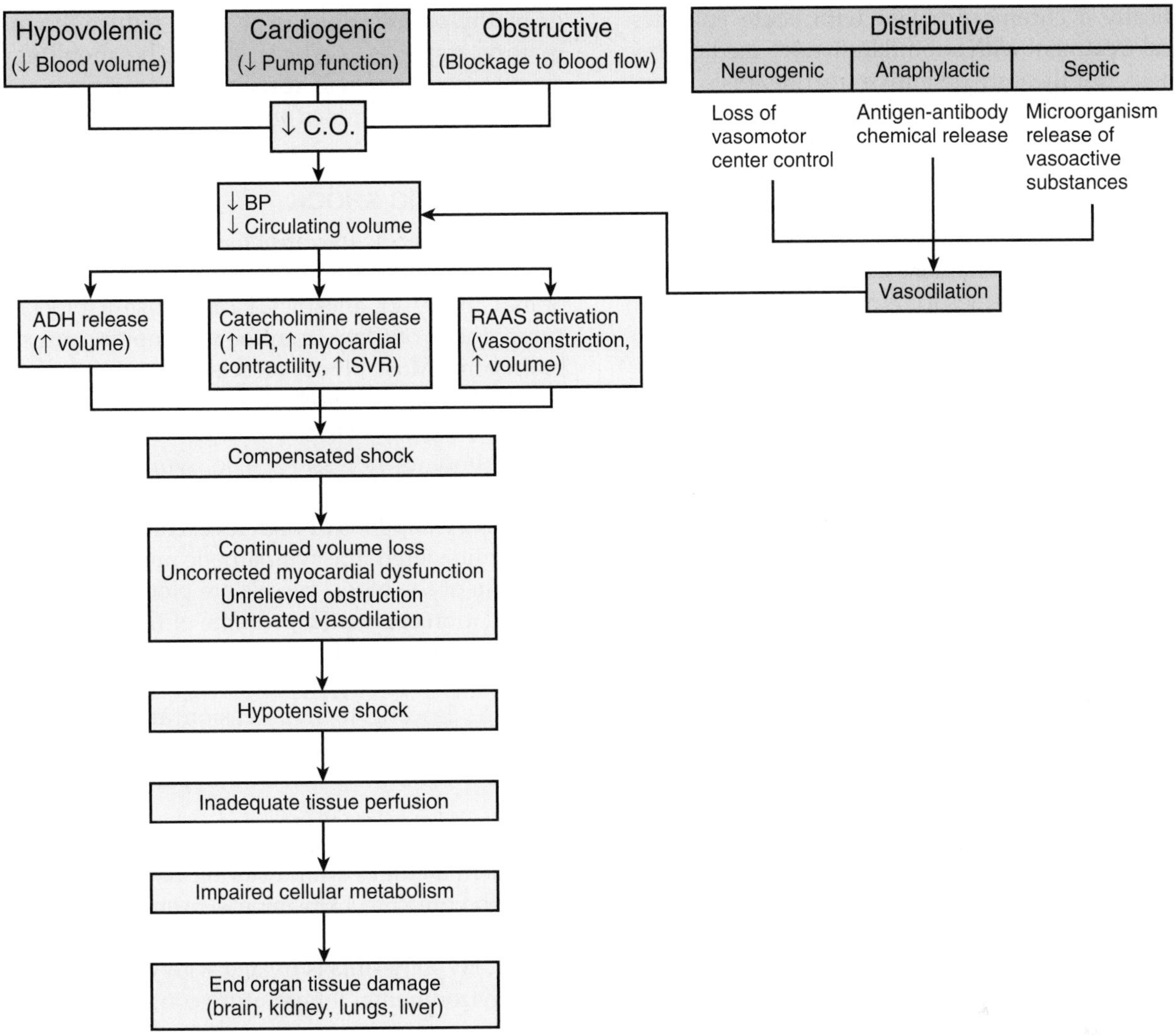

Fig. 45.7 Pathophysiology of shock. *ADH,* Antidiuretic hormone; *BP,* blood pressure; *C.O.,* cardiac output; *HR,* heart rate; *RAAS,* renin-angiotensin-aldosterone system; *SVR,* systemic vascular resistance.

cardiac muscle (positive inotropy) (Ren, 2017). However, as the heart works harder, it requires more oxygen. If the heart is already damaged, pushing it to do more will only worsen the inadequate circulation.

In conjunction with the positive inotropes, vasodilators (e.g., nitroglycerin or nitroprusside) are judiciously used to decrease cardiac workload by decreasing afterload. When the heart ejects blood into the systemic circulation, it must overcome the pressure of the closed aortic valve and the resistance of the peripheral blood vessels. The blood vessels constrict as part of the compensatory mechanisms, similar to an adjustable nozzle on a hose: as the nozzle opening is enlarged, less pressure is required than if the nozzle is turned to the smallest setting. Similarly, if the blood vessels are dilated, the heart does not have to work as hard to expel the blood. Diminished workload lessens the oxygen demand of the cardiac muscle. Vasodilators must be used cautiously to enhance cardiac performance without compromising blood pressure. The intra-aortic balloon pump (IABP) is a mechanical left ventricular assist device that supports cardiac function; the IABP is used in critical care units (see Chapter 19, Fig. 19.3).

OBSTRUCTIVE SHOCK

Tissue perfusion can be impaired when there is a mechanical obstruction to blood flow. In conditions such as pericardial tamponade, tension pneumothorax, or constrictive pericarditis, there is a physical obstruction that prevents adequate filling or emptying of the heart. In conditions such as aortic dissection or massive pulmonary embolus, there is a problem in the blood vessels that prevents forward flow of blood.

Treatment

Pericardial tamponade is treated by inserting a needle into the pericardial sac and removing the fluid that is compressing the heart. Tension pneumothorax is also treated by needle decompression. A needle or thoracostomy tube is inserted to release the air trapped in the chest that is putting pressure on the heart. Constrictive pericarditis does not usually have a sudden onset. It is typically a chronic problem with acute episodes. Medical treatment with antiinflammatory medications may help, but the only definitive treatment is surgery. Aortic dissection is one of many causes of chest pain, and diagnosis can be difficult, but the patient must be taken immediately to the operating room for repair of the vessel. Massive pulmonary embolus (PE) is usually fatal. A less severe PE will be treated with heparin to prevent further clot formation. Thrombolytic therapy or interventional techniques to remove the clot or infuse thrombolytics directly are all available for use in specific circumstances.

DISTRIBUTIVE SHOCK (MALDISTRIBUTION OF FLUIDS)

Distributive shock involves a maldistribution of the fluid within the vascular system. If the vessels dilate and the volume of fluid stays the same, the pressure decreases (vasogenic shock). All forms of distributive shock involve vasodilation of blood vessels, resulting in a "relative hypovolemia." There is no actual volume loss, but physiologically the patient appears to be hypovolemic.

ANAPHYLACTIC SHOCK

Acute allergic reactions can result in life-threatening anaphylactic shock. Classic anaphylaxis is a massive immune response set up by a previous exposure to the antigen. However, the body can respond to substances without prior exposure, causing the same clinical signs and symptoms. In anaphylactic shock, the antigen-antibody reaction that occurs releases **vasoactive** substances that cause massive vasodilation as well as increased capillary permeability. This combination of factors results in hypotension. These mediators can also cause bronchoconstriction and **angioedema** of the laryngeal tissue, causing an acute airway emergency. Other signs and symptoms may include skin rash and generalized flushing, headache, or lightheadedness.

Treatment

If possible, the antigen should be removed immediately. With a bee sting, prompt removal of the stinger may help. If the anaphylaxis results from an ingested or inhaled substance, removal may not be possible, so treatment begins immediately. Treatment of anaphylactic shock includes airway management, including intubation when necessary, and administration of epinephrine intramuscularly in the vastus lateralis (thigh). Epinephrine helps maintain blood pressure, counteracts the effects of the released mediators, and inhibits further release of mediators from mast cells and basophils. Bronchodilators may also be administered.

Administration of fluid is also needed. Although the actual circulating volume reduction from leaking capillaries is not enough to cause hypotension, vasodilation is more than enough to cause a significant drop in blood pressure. An antihistamine such as diphenhydramine (Benadryl) is given; dexamethasone or methylprednisolone is given to reduce the inflammatory response. Patients should be monitored for several hours even if response to treatment is good because antihistamines and epinephrine will wear off (Mustafa, 2018).

NEUROGENIC SHOCK

Neurogenic shock, the rarest form of shock, has a triad of symptoms: hypotension, bradycardia, and hypothermia. Spinal injury or anesthesia can cause a blockage in sympathetic outflow from the vasomotor center of the brainstem. Most blood vessels are never completely constricted or completely dilated. This in-between state is known as *vascular tone* and allows for constriction or dilation as necessary. The sympathetic nervous system maintains this state of readiness. When spinal cord injury happens or high levels of spinal anesthesia are administered, the sympathetic impulses regulating the state of the blood vessels are blocked, and passive vasodilation occurs. The volume of fluid circulating in the blood vessels is the same, but the space within the blood vessels enlarges. This results in a lower blood pressure, leading to hypotension and a shock state. Proper stabilization of spinal injuries can prevent or minimize conditions that lead to neurogenic shock.

Treatment

Treatment includes administering crystalloids to maintain blood pressure. Dopamine is given for a combination of hypotension, bradycardia, and decreased cardiac output. Hypothermia is treated with warming blankets and environmental temperature control.

SYSTEMIC INFLAMMATORY RESPONSE SYNDROME, SEPSIS, AND SEPTIC SHOCK

The inflammatory response is part of the cascade of events that comprise the body's immune response. Once the threat has been dealt with, feedback mechanisms inhibit the release of chemicals, and the immune system goes back into a state of readiness. In some situations, this does not happen, and the substances that cause inflammation continue to be released. This clinical picture is known as **systemic inflammatory response syndrome (SIRS)**. **SIRS can occur because of an infection or from noninfectious conditions.**

SIRS is the first part of a continuum that leads to sepsis, then severe sepsis, and ultimately **multisystem organ dysfunction syndrome (MODS)**, defined as two or more organ systems showing signs of dysfunction. The usual clinical progression starts with symptoms indicating SIRS, moving into sepsis, then severe sepsis and MODS complicated by disseminated intravascular coagulation (DIC). If this sequence of events continues, mortality rates range from 28% to 80%. The wide range is affected by multiple variables such as age, preexisting illnesses, and access to treatment. Early recognition and effective treatment of this cascade of events are the most significant factors in reducing mortality risk.

A patient presenting with two or more of the following is diagnosed with SIRS:

1. Temperature greater than 102.2° F (39° C) or less than 96.8° F (36° C)
2. Heart rate greater than 90 beats per minute
3. Respiratory rate greater than 20 breaths per minute or $PaCO_2$ less than 32 mm Hg
4. White blood cell count greater than 12,000 cells/mm^3 or less than 4000 cells/mm^3 or more than 10% bands

Many hospitalized patients meet these criteria (Kaplan, 2018). Not all patients meeting the SIRS criteria progress to sepsis, and septic patients do not always display two or more of the SIRS criteria. SIRS is now considered a dysregulated inflammation syndrome and not used in the sepsis definition. The score in current use is the Sequential Organ Failure Assessment (SOFA), which is a predictor of mortality based on how well the different organ systems are functioning. The quick SOFA or qSOFA is used at the bedside and consists of evaluating whether the patient has an altered mental status, systolic blood pressure of 100 mm Hg or less, or respiratory rate of 22 breaths per minute or more. If two or more of these are present in a patient with an infection, sepsis is diagnosed (Singer et al., 2016).

Septic shock is diagnosed when a patient with sepsis is hypotensive, requiring vasopressor medications to maintain a mean arterial blood pressure of 65 mm Hg or more, and a serum lactate level greater than 2 mmol/L despite fluid volume replacement. Symptoms of septic shock that reflect the hypotensive state include altered mental status, hypoxemia, oliguria, ileus, and decreased capillary refill.

During septic shock, the inflammatory process, in addition to causing clotting and activation of the immune system, releases chemicals that cause vasodilation and increased capillary permeability. The vasodilation, as with the other forms of distributive shock, causes blood pressure to fall. The leaking capillaries cause fluid loss, which increases the severity of the hypotension. The infecting organism secretes toxins from the cell wall that also react with the blood vessels and cell membranes, causing further increased capillary permeability and further loss of fluid from the vascular space, cellular injury, and greatly increased cellular metabolic rate.

Bacteria are the organisms most commonly associated with infections leading to sepsis and septic shock. Gram-negative bacteria such as *Pseudomonas aeruginosa*, *Escherichia coli*, and *Klebsiella pneumoniae* and gram-positive bacteria such as *Staphylococcus* and *Streptococcus* are normally present in the environment. Health care–associated infections can lead to sepsis, with deadly outcomes. Meticulous care must be taken with IV sites, Foley catheters, and other devices that disrupt the body's protective mechanisms.

Treatment and Nursing Management

In 2003, 11 international organizations launched the Surviving Sepsis Campaign. Since then the recommendations have been revised several times to reflect current research. The most recent changes made by the international committee were in 2016. Recommendations include initiation of a sepsis resuscitation bundle as soon as hypoperfusion is recognized. Early detection of sepsis is a cornerstone to successful outcomes; thus the importance of good nursing assessment and prompt reporting of findings is underscored. When a patient is at risk for sepsis, you should monitor for slight changes in condition: warm, dry, flushed skin; full, bounding pulse; normal to high blood pressure; and elevated urine output. The temperature may be normal or slightly elevated. Some patients do experience a high temperature with sepsis; however, older adults or others may experience hypothermia when septic.

When sepsis is identified, be vigilant for signs of septic shock. **If hourly urine output begins to decrease, the health care provider should be notified.** Monitor breath sounds for crackles; check for an increasing heart rate; and assess for increased fatigue, feelings of anxiety, and changes in mental status. Dependent edema may develop. If shock occurs, the skin will become cool and clammy and the peripheral pulses will be weak and thready. Blood pressure will fall as hypovolemia becomes more pronounced.

Once sepsis is suspected, appropriate treatment begins immediately. This includes fluid resuscitation with crystalloids or colloids to maintain blood pressure and oxygenation; intubation and mechanical ventilation may be required. Blood cultures are obtained, and broad-spectrum antibiotic therapy is started within 1 hour of diagnosis of septic shock. Norepinephrine or epinephrine may be ordered to maintain blood pressure. Dobutamine may be used if the blood pressure and cardiac output do not respond to fluid challenge or vasopressors (Levy, Evans, & Rhodes, 2018).

When the immune system initiates the inflammatory response, it also initiates the clotting cascade. The body is responding to an unknown threat and prepares to fight off foreign organisms and/or to stop bleeding, so both systems are activated. In sepsis, the heightened coagulant state of the body leads to multiple small clots forming in the microcirculation, which is known as *disseminated intravascular coagulation (DIC)*. These small clots clog up the circulation to organs. This clotting leads to organ damage throughout the body.

The extensive clotting that occurs throughout the body in DIC uses up most of the clotting factors in the blood. As a result, bleeding occurs easily. Patients may ooze blood from previously dry wounds, from their gums, and around IV catheters and may bruise very easily. The clinical sign most noticeable is bleeding from any break in the skin.

If an event occurs that triggers clotting, normally the process to dissolve the clot is also activated. This allows the clot to stop the bleeding and then be reabsorbed when no longer needed, conserving the clotting factors for reuse. In DIC this process is altered. To restore the normal sequence, anticoagulants are given to stop the clotting factors from being used up. Although it may seem contradictory to give a medication that will prevent clots when the patient is bleeding, the clots that have formed in the small blood vessels are harming the patient by blocking blood flow to vital organs. The clotting factors are being used for clots that are harmful while not being available in the areas they are needed.

NURSING MANAGEMENT

You must be vigilant in identifying patients who are at risk for developing shock. For example, postsurgical patients are always at risk for hemorrhage, which could lead to hypovolemic shock or infection, potentially causing sepsis and septic shock. Maintaining adequate fluid volume and blood pressure are key components in adequately managing shock.

ASSESSMENT (DATA COLLECTION)

Ongoing evaluation of the patient's level of consciousness, vital signs (including temperature), skin signs, and urine output is essential to the recognition and management of shock. Serial assessment data are compared with the previous data and with the baseline assessment. **Watching for changes and trends in physical and laboratory findings is extremely important.** This information must be reported to the health care provider so they can make treatment decisions. In accordance with National Patient Safety Goals, recognition of and response to changes in a patient's condition are particularly applicable to the prognosis of shock. The Joint Commission requires the availability of rapid response teams to help with the assessment and management of patients who are unstable. Early activation of appropriate help can save lives.

NURSING DIAGNOSIS, PLANNING, AND IMPLEMENTATION

The primary problem for a patient in shock is altered tissue perfusion. The planning of care for a patient in shock should include measures to monitor and maintain a patent airway, tissue perfusion, body temperature, and skin integrity (Nursing Care Plan 45.1).

The treatment goals for shock are to restore circulating volume and to treat the underlying cause, if possible. In most types of shock, blood pressure responds to administration of IV fluids. The exception to this is cardiogenic shock, in which the pump cannot manage the fluids that are already present and pump support is needed. If an IV is not in place, volume can be redistributed to the central circulation by laying the patient flat and elevating the legs 10 to 12 inches.

Nursing Care Plan 45.1 Care of a Patient Exhibiting Symptoms of Shock

SCENARIO

Bob Jones, a 22-year-old, was involved in a motor vehicle accident and sustained a blunt force abdominal injury and multiple extremity fractures.

PROBLEM STATEMENT/NURSING DIAGNOSIS

Fluid volume deficit related to blood loss.

SUPPORTING ASSESSMENT DATA

Objective: BP 90/40, P 150, skin pale and clammy. Patient alert and oriented with complaints of 10/10 pain.

Goals/Expected Outcomes	Nursing Interventions	Selected Rationale	Evaluation
Patient will have adequate BP to maintain vital organ perfusion as evidenced by remaining alert and oriented, urine output ≥30 cc/h, cap refill <3 seconds.	Monitor vital signs, central venous pressure (when used) q5min to q1h as indicated by patient condition. Monitor urine output q1h.	Maintain a high index of suspicion for hypovolemia and shock. Early detection and treatment of shock prevents complications.	BP is maintained at >90 mm Hg systolic and urine output is ≥30 mL/h.
	Maintain patent IV sites. Administer fluids as ordered.	Volume replacement is essential and requires adequate access.	IV fluid bolus of 500 mL given. IV fluids infusing at 150 mL/h via peripheral IV sites in both forearms (total of 300 mL/h).
	Note quality and strength of peripheral pulses with vital signs.	Weak, thready pulses indicate decreased cardiac output.	Pulses are weak and thready.
	Monitor laboratory and radiography results.	Evaluate patient's response to therapy.	Laboratory and radiograph results are pending.

PROBLEM STATEMENT/NURSING DIAGNOSIS

Potential for altered gas exchange related to altered blood flow.

Nursing Care Plan 45.1 Care of a Patient Exhibiting Symptoms of Shock—cont'd

SUPPORTING ASSESSMENT DATA

Objective: BP 80/40, blood loss secondary to trauma, respiratory rate 32/min.

Goals/Expected Outcomes	Nursing Interventions	Selected Rationale	Evaluation
Pulse oximetry maintained at ≥95%	Maintain patent airway. Elevate head of bed if tolerated by BP and spinal fracture is ruled out.	Enhances lung expansion.	Patient breathing is rapid, but not labored at 32/min. Supine position maintained for BP 90/40.
	Administer oxygen to keep Spo_2 ≥95%. Monitor pulse oximetry.	Maximizes the oxygen-carrying capacity of the available hemoglobin.	Pulse oximetry reading is 99% with patient on nonrebreather mask.
	Auscultate breath sounds q2-4h.	The patient is at risk for ARDS.	Lung sounds clear or changes are identified and reported promptly.
	Investigate alterations in level of consciousness.	Decreased levels of oxygen can cause alterations in sensorium.	No change in level of consciousness. Is alert, talkative, and seems anxious.

PROBLEM STATEMENT/NURSING DIAGNOSIS

Fear of possible death related to presence of a life-threatening situation.

SUPPORTING ASSESSMENT DATA

Subjective: Patient states that he is scared and wants to know if he will live.

Goals/Expected Outcomes	Nursing Interventions	Selected Rationale	Evaluation
Patient and family will express that fear is reduced.	Maintain a calm and reassuring presence.	This will reduce anxiety and the patient's oxygen need.	Patient and family is reassured when the nurse is present.
	Explain activities, medications, treatments, and equipment simply and honestly.	Information facilitates cooperation and increases feelings of control.	The patient and family states that all of their questions were answered.
	Demonstrate concern and respect for patient and family.	Extending an attitude of concern makes it easier for patients and families to discuss concerns.	The patient and family discussed concerns with the health care team.
	Offer to call spiritual or religious leader or support.	People with spiritual belief systems find comfort in visits by others of the same beliefs.	Family states they are from out of town and would like the hospital chaplain to visit.

CRITICAL THINKING QUESTIONS

1. What complications is this patient at risk for developing?
2. If this patient were 72 years old instead of 22 years old, how would that change your care?

ARDS, Acute respiratory distress syndrome; *BP*, blood pressure; *IV*, intravenous; *P*, pulse.

◆ EVALUATION

If interventions are effective, there should be improvement in tissue perfusion. This can be evaluated by monitoring blood pressure, urine output, and level of consciousness. These are key indicators of adequacy of blood flow to vital organs. Other indicators to monitor include capillary refill, color and temperature of the skin, and the amplitude of pulses in the extremities. With adequate fluid and medication administration, systolic blood pressure should be maintained above 90 mm Hg. This should provide enough blood flow to the kidneys to generate 20 to 30 mL of urine output per hour. If there are no preexisting neurologic problems, the patient should return to previous level of consciousness.

Get Ready for the Nclex® Examination!

Key Points

- Good Samaritan laws protect medical personnel from liability when offering emergency medical care for victims of accidental injury.
- Signs and symptoms that usually precede aggression or attack include increasing agitation or resistance, aggressive behavior, pacing, frowning, hyperalertness, increasing demands, or glaring.
- Victims of intimate partner or domestic abuse and violence may be reluctant to voluntarily reveal abuse or identify the abuser.
- Three elements that emergency nurses use for clinical decisions are (1) events or incidents that preceded the emergency visit, (2) mechanism of injury, and (3) index of suspicion.
- Triage is the process of setting priorities for treatment.
- Neck or spinal injury is suspected in multiple injuries, falls, or blunt force impact.
- Flail chest occurs when three or more ribs are broken in two or more places; flail chest compromises respirations because the chest wall is unstable. Treatment includes intubation and mechanical ventilation.
- Symptoms of pneumothorax or hemothorax include labored, shallow respirations; lack of movement on one side of the chest when the person inhales and exhales; and chest pain.
- Penetrating abdominal trauma is frequently associated with gun or knife wounds. Patients with blunt trauma to the abdomen should have serial assessments to identify slow hemorrhage or occult injury.
- Poison control centers need the following information to assist in diagnosis and treatment: patient's age, weight, medical and medication history, and allergies; what, when, and why the substance was taken; current signs and symptoms, with vital signs and laboratory results; and any treatment rendered.
- Bite wounds should be cleaned immediately with soap and warm running water for 5 to 10 minutes.
- Chemical burns should be flushed with large amounts of water (with some exceptions) until all traces of the chemical have been removed.
- The American Heart Association guidelines emphasize C-A-B (chest compressions, airway, breathing) and the importance of high-quality CPR and recommend hands-only CPR for the lay rescuer.
- Treatment of shock generally includes infusion of large volumes of IV fluid.
- Blood pressure support in cardiogenic shock involves support for the pump (the heart) rather than adding volume.

Additional Learning Resources

SG Go to your Study Guide for additional learning activities to help you master this chapter content.

Go to your Evolve website (http://evolve.elsevier.com/deWit/medsurg) for the following FREE learning resources:

- Animations, audio, and video
- Answers and rationales for questions and activities
- Glossary with pronunciations in English and Spanish
- Interactive Review Questions and more!

Review Questions for the NCLEX® Examination

1. To control a gushing bleed of the lower leg, what should you do initially?
  1. Apply direct pressure to the wound.
  2. Compress the artery above the wound.
  3. Check the circulation to the foot.
  4. Snugly secure a bulky dressing.

  NCLEX Client Need: Physiological Integrity: Physiological Adaptation

2. In the event of any type of poisoning that occurs in the home setting, what is the initial course of action?
  1. Save the poison container and contents.
  2. Save a sample of vomitus for analysis.
  3. Call poison control.
  4. Induce vomiting.

  NCLEX Client Need: Safe and Effective Care Environment: Safety and Infection Control

3. A teenager—alert, oriented, and in no apparent distress—is brought to the ED by EMS on a backboard with spine immobilization in place. He reports diving into a lake and bumping his head. Based on the mechanism of injury, which assessment are you most likely to initiate?
  1. Assessment of water safety behavior
  2. Serial abdominal assessments with hematocrit
  3. Frequent vital signs to monitor for shock
  4. Peripheral motion and sensation with mental status checks

  NCLEX Client Need: Physiological Integrity: Reduction of Risk Potential

4. You make a home visit to a 70-year-old patient on a cold winter day. On your arrival, the patient demonstrates excessive coughing, shortness of breath, drowsiness, and confusion. Mucous membranes are cherry red. What is your first action?
  1. Question the patient about recent food or fluid consumption.
  2. Call for emergency help and open the windows.
  3. Search the house for evidence of poisons and then call poison control.
  4. Locate the source of odors or try to get the patient to walk out of the house.

  NCLEX Client Need: Physiological Integrity: Physiological Adaptation

5. You are talking to a community group about strategies to prevent heat-related illness. What advice is appropriate to give to the group? *(Select all that apply.)*
  1. Drink fluids that are nonalcoholic, noncaffeinated, and low in sugar content.

2. When you are thirsty, drink fluids and avoid eating salty foods.
3. Stay indoors with cooling systems.
4. In the heat, wear lightweight, light-colored, loose-fitting clothing.
5. Limit outdoor activities to spring or fall when the weather is cooler.
6. Use sun protection such as wide-brimmed hats, sunglasses, and sunscreen.

NCLEX Client Need: Health Promotion and Maintenance

6. A 24-year-old man is brought to the ED with respiratory distress after being stung by a bee. Which order from the health care provider should you anticipate as a priority intervention?
   1. Administer racemic epinephrine by inhalation.
   2. Establish peripheral IV access.
   3. Give 0.5 mg of epinephrine intramuscularly in the lateral thigh.
   4. Draw blood for laboratory tests.

   NCLEX Client Need: Physiological Integrity: Pharmacological Therapies
7. A patient is brought to the ED with severe gastrointestinal bleeding and hypovolemic shock. What is the priority intervention for this patient?
   1. Insert a nasogastric tube and attach it to low wall suction.
   2. Draw a blood sample for a type and crossmatch.
   3. Measure the amount of emesis and check for blood.
   4. Establish two large-bore peripheral IV sites.

   NCLEX Client Need: Safe and Effective Care Environment: Coordinated Care
8. When taking care of a patient with sepsis, what is the first sign that would signal impending septic shock?
   1. Increasing urine output
   2. Decreasing heart rate
   3. Decreasing blood pressure
   4. Change in mental status

   NCLEX Client Need: Physiological Integrity: Physiological Adaptation
9. A patient is 6 hours postoperative with signs of deficient fluid volume. The health care provider orders a fluid challenge of 400 mL lactated Ringer solution stat over 20 minutes. What would be considered a desirable response to the treatment?
   1. Decrease in blood pressure
   2. Increase in urinary output
   3. Increase in body weight
   4. Increase in pulse rate

   NCLEX Client Need: Physiological Integrity: Pharmacological Therapies
10. A patient was bitten by a stray dog and rushed to the ED. Which measure must be done first?
   1. Apply antibiotic ointment on affected sites.
   2. Cover with a clean bandage and immobilize.
   3. Rinse wound with soap and warm running water for 5 to 10 minutes.
   4. Give tetanus booster shot if patient has not had one in the past 5 years.

   NCLEX Client Need: Safe and Effective Care Environment: Coordinated Care

Critical Thinking Questions

Scenario A

While watching a sporting event from the stands, you notice that the person sitting in front of you has slumped over. You touch her shoulder and ask if she is all right. There is no response, and you see no signs of breathing.

1. What is the most likely explanation for this witnessed event of sudden unconsciousness?
2. What should you do first?
3. An AED is on scene. What is your role in the use of this equipment?
4. How do Good Samaritan laws affect you and any interventions you may perform on this woman?

Scenario B

You are on your way home from work and you see a car hit a teenage boy on a bicycle. You stop to help the cyclist. He is unconscious, has a large scalp laceration that is bleeding profusely, and has an obviously fractured left leg.

1. If you need to open his airway, what method should you use?
2. What should you do about the scalp laceration and broken leg?
3. What is your legal obligation in this setting?

Scenario C

While working as a student nurse in the hospital's emergency unit, you notice that patients who have been injured or are very ill sometimes become hostile and combative. Some try to assault members of the emergency team, and others use abusive and threatening language.

1. Discuss with your classmates some reasons why patients may behave in these ways when they are injured or very ill.
2. What are some ways in which violent patients who are not mentally ill can be handled to prevent assault and encourage cooperation with the emergency staff?
3. What resources are available to help manage combative patients?
4. What patient history or information might help clarify aggressive behavior?

Scenario D

Your 80-year-old male patient, admitted yesterday for pneumonia, has become confused, hypotensive, oliguric, clammy, and pale.

1. What are the possible explanations for his clinical signs and symptoms?
2. What are your priorities for his care?
3. Discuss what treatment is indicated.
4. How will you know if your treatment has been effective?

46 Care of Patients With Cognitive Function Disorders

http://evolve.elsevier.com/deWit/medsurg

Objectives

Theory

1. Discuss common cognitive disorders and nursing interventions for each.
2. Compare and contrast the etiology and symptoms of **delirium** (acute cognitive disorder) and **dementia** (chronic cognitive disorder).
3. Examine the incidence and significance of cognitive disorders in the older adult population.

Clinical Practice

4. Create a plan of care for a patient with Alzheimer disease.

Key Terms

Alzheimer disease (ĂWLTZ-hī-mĕr dĭ-ZĒZ, p. 1074)
biomarker (BĪ-ō-măr-kĕr, p. 1077)
cognition (kŏg-NĬ-shŭn, p. 1074)
confabulation (kŏn-făb-u-LĀ-shŭn, p. 1076)
delirium (dĕ-LĬR-ē-ŭm, p. 1074)
delusion (dĕ-LŪ-shŭn, p. 1075)
dementia (dē-MĔN-shē-ă, p. 1074)
global amnesia (GLŌ-băl ăm-NĒ-zhē-ă, p. 1084)
hallucinations (hă-lū-sĭ-NĀ-shŭnz, p. 1075)
illusions (ĭ-LŪ-shŭnz, p. 1075)
sundown syndrome (SŬN-doun-ĭng, p. 1082)
vascular dementia (VĂS-kū-lăr dē-MĔN-shē-ă, p. 1074)

Concepts Covered in This Chapter

- Sensory Perception
- Cognition
- Family Dynamics
- Safety
- Care Coordination

OVERVIEW OF COGNITIVE DISORDERS

Cognition refers to mental processes of perception, memory, judgment, and reasoning. It includes the ability to perceive and process information. **A *cognitive disorder* is diagnosed when there is a significant change in cognition from a previous level of functioning.** Cognitive disorders greatly affect the quality of life for affected individuals, families, and friends. Although cognitive disorders do occur across the life span, they are often linked to the neurobiological changes that accompany aging. Cognitive disorders have become increasingly common with the aging of the population. Disorders of cognition include delirium and dementia.

Delirium (acute confusion) is characterized by a change in overall cognition and level of consciousness over a short time. **Dementia** is characterized by several cognitive deficits, to memory in particular, and tends to be more chronic. Both conditions are classified according to cause or origin of disease. For example, delirium can be related to sepsis. Dementia may be caused by multiple small blood clots that cause brain tissue damage (known as **vascular dementia**) or arises from an unknown origin such as with **Alzheimer disease**. The difference between the two conditions is that delirium is an *acute* condition that requires immediate treatment and is reversible, whereas dementia is a chronic condition that is irreversible. It also is important to note that delirium can coexist with dementia. If delirium is recognized and promptly treated, a patient with preexisting dementia should be restored to a previous level of functioning.

DELIRIUM

Many conditions or physiologic alterations can cause delirium. Some examples include cerebrovascular accident; drug overdose, toxicity, or withdrawal; tumors; systemic infections; anesthesia; fluid and electrolyte imbalances; and malnutrition. The onset of delirium is sudden. The patient may be alert or lethargic, depending on the cause of the delirium, or may appear very confused. The attention span changes, and overall awareness of the environment is decreased. Orientation and recent and immediate memory are impaired. Speech may be incoherent, and overall thinking can be disorganized and distorted. The patient will not be able to communicate thoughts in a meaningful way. The patient may experience **illusions** (misinterpretations of reality). For example, a pen may appear to be a knife, or a shadow on the floor may appear to be a menacing monster. If a patient appears to be talking to someone who is not there, it is likely that they are experiencing **hallucinations** (seeing or hearing things that are not there). If the patient insists that a nurse is an angel of death, this is an example of a **delusion** (belief in a false idea).

Clinical Cues

Assessment for and treatment of the underlying cause of delirium is essential. Physical restraints should be avoided. Reorientation, a calm environment and reduction of sound, explanations of proceedings, and calm reassurance are first-line interventions. An antipsychotic medication may be used to prevent harm to the patient or others if needed.

Problem-solving ability and judgment may be diminished but not completely absent. Consequently, the patient may not make good decisions, or may become combative or hostile if you or a family member attempts to intervene. Treatment is always based on the underlying cause for delirium.

Older Adult Care Points

It is not unusual to see a hospitalized older adult with dementia who has been previously conscious become drowsy, disoriented, combative, and unable to recognize family and friends. You should suspect delirium or acute confusion. An important evaluation is to note medications given and the response to these. Anticholinergic medications have potent central nervous system effects and can cause a sudden episode of confusion. Consider whether the dose is too high for age and physiologic functioning. Question whether there is a cumulative effect, or if medications are interacting. Delirium and dementia can coexist, and the acute condition needs to be recognized and treated, not merely dismissed as part of the preexisting condition of dementia.

Clinical Cues

Does your patient have depression, dementia, or delirium? Listen closely to the patient's words. A depressed patient may speak very little, but the speech is generally logical and will contain sad and negative thoughts and feelings of hopelessness. A patient with dementia may confabulate or will have difficulty finding words. A patient with delirium is more likely to be incoherent or loud when talking.

SUBSTANCE-INDUCED DELIRIUM

Substance-induced delirium can be caused by withdrawal from a substance, intoxication with a substance, or side effects from a medication (see Chapter 48). Many classes of medications can produce symptoms of delirium. Common examples include anesthetics, analgesics, sedative-hypnotics, any products with anticholinergic activity (tricyclic antidepressants, antihistamines, theophylline derivatives, and antipsychotics), and histamine (H_2)-receptor blockers (e.g., famotidine, cimetidine, and ranitidine). Commonly prescribed beta blockers and nonsteroidal antiinflammatory drugs (NSAIDs) can also cause symptoms of delirium.

Clinical Cues

In cases of delirium or acute confusion, you must assess the patient's medication history, look for any signs of infection, and assess current fluid and electrolyte status. Also, if you have reason to suspect that the patient may have sustained a fall, assess for head trauma.

Diagnosis and treatment depend on taking a thorough history. Early recognition can facilitate a faster recovery. If the patient is unable to give a history, caregivers may be able to help. Ask about whether the patient takes over-the-counter medications or supplements; these can be responsible for interactions with prescribed medication. If medications accumulate over several days, elimination of the substance from the body takes much longer and places the patient in even greater danger.

Older Adult Care Points

Older adults have a high risk for substance-induced delirium because of overall decreased metabolism and reduction in liver and kidney function. A general principle that health care providers generally follow when prescribing medications to older adults is to give the smallest amount possible and increase the amount only as symptoms indicate. Therefore you must carefully observe and report subtle changes in behavior, vital signs, and laboratory results.

DEMENTIA

There are several different types of dementia, and these conditions are also classified according to the underlying cause. The *Diagnostic and Statistical Manual of Mental Disorders,* 5th edition (DSM-5) classifies types such as neurocognitive disorder due to Alzheimer disease; vascular neurocognitive disorder (for which prompt treatment of hypertension and vascular disease is necessary to prevent long-term complications); neurocognitive disorder with Lewy bodies; and neurocognitive disorder due to Parkinson disease, among other conditions (American Psychiatric Association, 2013). The key to understanding care of patients with dementia is that regardless of the underlying cause of the disorder, nursing care is very similar.

The onset for dementia is slow, and the condition may progress over months to years. The patient is generally alert in the mild stage, yet alertness may decline over time. Orientation to person, place, and time and recent memory may be impaired. In later stages of dementia, patients lose remote memory as well. Patients with dementia have difficulty with abstracting thoughts and have a poverty of thoughts. **Confabulation** (making up words or experiences to fill conversational gaps) and impaired judgment are common. Often there is a noticeable change in personality. These patients experience fragmented sleep rather than a reversed cycle.

> **Complementary and Alternative Therapies**
>
> **Herbs With Sedative Effects**
>
> Herbs that have a sedative effect include chamomile, hops, and valerian. These can be used in a tea or taken in capsules. A popular method of promoting sleep is to place a few drops of lavender onto the pillowcase. If your patient is using herbs or alternative therapies, advise them to inform their health care provider because of potential drug-herb interactions or contraindications because of medical conditions.

ALZHEIMER DISEASE

Etiology and Pathophysiology

AD is the most common degenerative disease of the brain. More than 5.7 million Americans have AD (Alzheimer's Association, 2018b), and there is no known cause or cure. In AD, there is a loss of neurons in the frontal and temporal lobes. The atrophy in these areas accounts for the patient's inability to process and integrate new information and to retrieve memories. Brain biopsies of patients with AD have revealed nerve cells that are tangled and twisted and an abnormal buildup of proteins. Production of neurotransmitters (e.g., acetylcholine, serotonin) is relatively decreased for these patients. Although the cause of AD is not fully understood, certain identifiable risk factors have been determined. These include:

- Age
- Family history
- Genetics
- Ethnicity
- History of head injury
- History of heart health

AD typically affects people older than 65 years but can also strike younger people. The age group of 85 years and older is currently the fastest-growing age group in the United States (Alzheimer's Association, 2018c). It is estimated that one third of this age group have AD (Alzheimer's Association, 2018c). People who have a parent or sibling with AD or who have risk or deterministic genes for AD are at higher risk for developing this condition than others (Alzheimer's Association, 2018c). Individuals with a history of head injury or poor heart health are at increased risk for developing AD (Alzheimer's Association, 2018c). Older adults who are Latino or African American have a higher likelihood of developing AD than older adults of other ethnicities (Alzheimer's Association, 2018c).

> **Health Promotion**
>
> **Diet and Memory**
>
> Studies show that fish and omega-3 polyunsaturated fats, fruits and vegetables, curcumin (curry spice), and a traditional Mediterranean diet may lower the risk for loss of cognitive function and/or AD.

> **Health Promotion**
>
> **Exercise for the Brain**
>
> Longitudinal studies have shown that challenging intellectual activity is associated with a decreased risk for dementia. Playing "brain games" by using computerized apps can be an effective way of exercising the brain (Anderson & Grossberg, 2014). Regular exercise and social interaction also can help maintain a healthy brain.

Signs and Symptoms

AD has a slow onset and variable rate of progression. Eventually, it is fatal. Although the Alzheimer's Association divides behavioral patterns and symptoms into seven stages, other sources divide the disease progression into three stages: mild cognitive decline, moderate cognitive decline, and severe or late cognitive decline. The early signs and symptoms of beginning mental deterioration include forgetfulness; recent memory loss; difficulty learning and remembering; inability to concentrate; and a decline in personal hygiene, appearance, and inhibitions. Later, the patient becomes quite confused and unable to make judgments, has difficulty communicating, suffers losses in motor function, and becomes dependent on others. Behavioral manifestations can also be categorized into three stages (Box 46.1).

> **Complementary and Alternative Therapies**
>
> **Pet Therapy**
>
> Pet therapy may help patients to improve memory (e.g., calling the therapy dog's name), coordination (e.g., throwing a ball for the dog), object identification (e.g., directing the dog to get the ball), language (e.g., talking to the dog), and attention (e.g., caring for the dog). Research shows that canine-assisted therapies have been beneficial in providing occupational and environmental support to individuals with dementia, which has increased their overall well-being, engagement, and function (Wood et al., 2017).

> **Think Critically**
>
> Some patients with dementia may act in a sexually inappropriate way because of loss of social reserve. How do you address a patient's behavior, given these circumstances?

Diagnosis

In making a diagnosis of AD, the health care provider uses a detailed medical and family history and conducts a thorough physical, neurologic, and functional assessment.

The benefits of early diagnosis include being able to include the patient in the planning for the future, to ensure safety, and to provide the family with understanding of the disease process. This can be especially effective if preclinical AD is diagnosed (Dubois et al., 2016), which involves identifying the diagnosis before clinical symptoms are apparent.

Box 46.1 Behavioral Patterns in Mild, Moderate, and Severe Alzheimer Disease

MILD
- Progressive short-term memory loss
- Slow, progressive loss of intellectual ability
- Difficulty in learning new things
- Small but noticeable changes in ability to perform at work or socially
- Decline in ability to plan ahead
- Decreased ability to perform usual activities of daily living (ADLs)
- Variable mood; depression is common and worsens symptoms
- Noticeable personality change
- Social withdrawal

MODERATE TOWARD SEVERE
- Aware of deficits; may confabulate to cover memory lapses
- Needs repeated instructions for simple tasks
- Needs day care or constant home care—can be very burdensome for the family
- Wanders away
- May have beginning incontinence
- Experiences outbursts of anger, hostility, paranoia

SEVERE
- Unable to speak or ambulate
- Profound memory loss; no recognition of family
- Difficulty swallowing
- Weight loss
- Bedridden
- Fetal position
- End-stage consequences of poor nutritional state and bedridden status: pressure injuries, respiratory failure, contractures, pneumonia

Treatment

Researchers continue to seek to create a vaccine to prevent AD (Marciani, 2018). Recent research shows that patients with obstructive sleep apnea share fluid **biomarker** links to Alzheimer disease and vascular dementia, suggesting that these conditions may have common underlying mechanisms (Baril et al., 2018). As research continues, this finding may help health care providers identify patients with obstructive sleep apnea who are at risk for development of dementia, allowing time for therapeutic intervention (Baril et al., 2018). Currently medications are used that may improve intellectual functioning and slow the progression of the disease, yet these do not provide a cure. The evidence indicates that the benefit of these drugs is modest. Table 46.1 describes medications used to treat cognitive disorders and their nursing implications. Behavioral interventions include (1) identifying the triggering situation, (2) having medical evaluations to determine contributing causes, (3) using nondrug and drug approaches to manage behavior, and (4) using coping mechanisms (Alzheimer's Association, 2018d).

❖ NURSING MANAGEMENT

◆ ASSESSMENT (DATA COLLECTION)

Nurses are often the first health care professionals who encounter a patient in the early stages of AD. Know and be vigilant for the 10 early signs and symptoms associated with AD (Alzheimer's Association, 2018a) (Box 46.2). For example, the family may tell you, "We think Dad is having problems with his memory. He keeps misplacing things and sometimes can't remember that we've visited him." Ask the patient and the family questions about memory, ability to perform activities

Table 46.1 Drugs Commonly Used to Treat Cognitive Disorders

MEDICATION	ACTION	PATIENT EDUCATION	NURSING IMPLICATIONS
Donepezil (Aricept) Galantamine (Razadyne) Memantine (Namenda) Rivastigmine (Exelon; transdermal patch available)	Causes elevated acetylcholine levels in the brain and slows progression of Alzheimer disease symptoms.	Take oral medication with food to decrease GI distress. Report any skin reactions if using the transdermal patch. Slows progression of symptoms but is not a cure. Take frequent drinks of cool liquids or use sugarless gum or candy for dry mouth. Increase fiber and fluids to prevent constipation. Common side effects (nausea, vomiting, headaches and dizziness, GI bleeding, urinary frequency, anorexia) should be reported to health care provider.	Be alert for abdominal pain, fatigue, hypotension, and agitation. Monitor CBC, liver, and renal function tests. Signs of overdose include severe nausea and vomiting, bradycardia, hypotension, convulsions, or severe muscle weakness. Rivastigmine patch: first patch should be applied on the day after the last oral dose, then rotate sites; replace every 24 h.

CBC, Complete blood cell count; *GI*, gastrointestinal.

of daily living (ADLs), and any subtle changes in personality by giving specific common examples (e.g., "Does your loved one forget to turn off the stove or to lock the doors?"). These patients should be referred to the health care provider because they need an in-depth assessment and an extensive physical examination. Assessment should include the necessary data to plan interventions to protect the patient.

Box 46.2 Ten Early Signs and Symptoms of Alzheimer Disease

1. Memory loss that disrupts daily life
2. Challenges in planning or solving problems
3. Difficulty completing familiar tasks at home, at work, or at leisure
4. Confusion with time or place
5. Trouble understanding visual images and spatial relationships
6. New problems with words in speaking or writing
7. Misplacing things with inability to retrace steps
8. Decreased or poor judgment
9. Withdrawal from work or social activities
10. Changes in mood or personality

From Alzheimer's Association: *10 early signs and symptoms of Alzheimer's* (website): www.alz.org/alzheimers-dementia/10_signs

Clinical Cues

Before you begin to assess an older adult patient, consider the changes that normal healthy older adults might be experiencing because of aging. For example, it is normal to have some very minor decline in memory; however, a healthy older adult should be able to create new memories, act purposefully, and accomplish ADLs independently.

◆ NURSING DIAGNOSIS AND PLANNING

Nursing problems are identified to maximize safety and to minimize complications resulting from loss of cognitive function. For example, you will consider the patient's potential for injury, the ability to provide self-care, and the caregiver burden associated with the diagnosis of AD when planning care. You will consider the stage of the disease, and the caregiver should be encouraged from the beginning to participate in developing the long-term goals (Nursing Care Plan 46.1) since the patient will sustain losses in every area of function as the disease progresses.

◆ IMPLEMENTATION AND EVALUATION

Patients with AD need interventions that enhance memory, such as holiday decorations that are appropriate to the season or photos of family and friends to help them reminisce. Reminiscence therapy can also include

Nursing Care Plan 46.1 Care of a Patient With Dementia

SCENARIO

Mrs. Whitt, an 85-year-old with dementia, has been living with her daughter. The daughter works full time and occasionally takes business trips for up to a week in duration. Recently the daughter began to seek alternate, supervised living arrangements for her mother, yet at this time Mrs. Whitt still resides with her daughter. "Mom is confused and withdrawn most of the time. She needs reminders to eat and coaching to go to the bathroom. I try my best, but I am overwhelmed with Mom and work. I have a brother, but he lives in another state and can't help much." The daughter appears tired but is very patient with her mother. You observe Mrs. Whitt wandering alone and trying to go outside. You redirect her several times, and she mistakes you for one of her children.

PROBLEM STATEMENT

Confusion due to cognitive impairment.

SUPPORTING ASSESSMENT DATA

Subjective: Per daughter, patient is "confused most of the time."
Objective: Mistakes you for her child.

Goals/Expected Outcomes	Nursing Interventions	Selected Rationale	Evaluation
Patient will function at an optimal level for the degree of cognitive losses at this time.	Identify and re-identify self.	Patient may not recognize people previously introduced.	Patient repeatedly mistakes nurses for one of her children.
Patient will follow concrete instructions.	Speak clearly and calmly while directly facing the patient, using short phrases. Repeat as needed.	Facilitates communication. Stimulation of two senses (visual and auditory) facilitates understanding.	Speaking clearly and calmly, and repeating as needed, helps patient understand.
	Do not approach patient from behind.	Surprises and scares the patient.	Letting the patient see you prevents an anxious reaction.
	Use pictures to communicate.	Pictures are more easily understood than oral words.	Use of pictures can be easier to process than the written word.

Nursing Care Plan 46.1 Care of a Patient With Dementia—cont'd

Goals/Expected Outcomes	Nursing Interventions	Selected Rationale	Evaluation
	Be consistent in approach, assign the same staff as much as possible, and maintain daily structure and routine.	Familiar faces and repetitive patterns decrease additional confusion.	Patient functioned well this morning when A.M. routine was followed and primary caregivers were assigned.
	Break down all tasks into simple steps and encourage completion of one step at a time.	Single steps are less complex and easier to achieve.	Today patient was able to brush own teeth as instructed, step by step.
	Encourage reminiscing about the past.	Remote memory is more likely to be intact than recent memory.	Appears to enjoy talking about her cat from the 1990s.

PROBLEM STATEMENT

Altered self-care ability due to cognitive impairment.

SUPPORTING ASSESSMENT DATA

Subjective: Per daughter, "needs reminders to eat and coaching to go to the bathroom."

Objective: Needs repetitive verbal prompting to eat and go to the bathroom.

Goals/Expected Outcomes	Nursing Interventions	Selected Rationale	Evaluation
Patient will perform ADLs independently or with minimal assistance from caregivers.	Assess the patient's ability to perform ADLs independently or with minimal assistance.	Provides baseline for daily planning (abilities may wax and wane on different days and at different times of day).	Is able to physically perform most ADLs but needs verbal coaching for each step.
	Encourage patient to maintain independence in performing ADLs.	Maintain maximal independence for as long as possible to increase self-esteem and stimulate cognitive processes.	Daughter reports that "it is really faster just to do everything for her" yet acknowledges the benefit of promoting the patient's independence.
	Allow patient to wear own clothes.	Familiar objects decrease confusion.	Usually recognizes own clothing but needs coaching for dressing; can manipulate Velcro fasteners.
	Use clothing with zippers and Velcro.	Ease of equipment decreases frustration.	
	Praise for any and all accomplishments.	Reinforces desired behavior.	Appears to enjoy interaction and feedback.
	Use simple, direct explanations when demonstrating the specific behavior patient is to complete.	Verbal and visual cues help decrease confusion.	Follows instructions, does not ask for help.
	Maintain regular toileting schedule.	Bowel and bladder routine decreases incidences of incontinence.	Toileting schedule q4h; patient usually continent.
	Encourage the use of finger foods.	Simplifies eating while maintaining intake.	Eats all food if encouraged and if food is pre-cut into bites.

PROBLEM STATEMENT/NURSING DIAGNOSIS

Social isolation due to cognitive changes.

SUPPORTING ASSESSMENT DATA

Subjective: Per daughter, confused or withdrawn most of the time.

Objective: Walking alone; does not ask for help or interact spontaneously without prompts.

Goals/Expected Outcomes	Nursing Interventions	Selected Rationale	Evaluation
Patient will participate in group activities.	Assess preferred patterns of social activity from earlier years.	Ideally, current socialization should mimic past patterns to reinforce familiarity.	Social contact usually limited to family. Occasionally went to church.

Continued

Nursing Care Plan 46.1 Care of a Patient With Dementia—cont'd

Goals/Expected Outcomes	Nursing Interventions	Selected Rationale	Evaluation
Patient will demonstrate socially acceptable behavior.	Provide group activities that are simple, such as singing or simple crafts.	Simple activities decrease frustration and serve as a means to communicate.	Appears to enjoy movies and musical groups.
	Stay with the patient during social activities as needed.	Provides support and reassurance.	Does not initiate conversation with others but will respond if spoken to.
	Do not force patient to participate in any social activity.	Socialization can be stressful and forcing activity is nontherapeutic and counterproductive.	Readily agreed to go to all activities today.
	Gradually increase social interaction with other staff and patients.	Gradual exposure increases comfort level and familiarity.	Will sit with others but does not initiate interaction. Will speak to other patients if they speak to her.

PROBLEM STATEMENT

Potential for caregiver burnout due to emotional and physical demands of providing ongoing care to mother.

SUPPORTING ASSESSMENT DATA

Subjective: "I try my best, but I am overwhelmed with Mom and work."

Objective: Caregiver works full time at a job requiring business trips; appears tired but is very patient with her mother.

Goals/Expected Outcomes	Nursing Interventions	Selected Rationale	Evaluation
Caregiver will verbalize ways to perform the caregiver role without becoming overwhelmed. Caregiver will openly express feelings.	Assess caregiver's ability to meet the needs of the patient while maintaining self-care.	Provides a baseline for planning.	Caregiver expresses willingness to care for her mother but does work full time and must be away at times.
	Actively listen to caregiver's fears and concerns.	Allowing expression helps to build trust and rapport; also helps caregiver and nurse to clarify issues.	Fears for mother's safety; is concerned about wandering.
	Educate the caregiver about dementia and its expected course and the patient's specific cognitive deficits.	Providing accurate information allows caregiver to have realistic expectations.	Written information given, and discussion of dementia provided to caregiver.
	Help caregiver understand realistic prognosis for their loved one.	Understanding prognosis helps the caregiver to begin the process of anticipatory grieving.	Caregiver appears unsure about the future, verbalizes understanding that her mother is going to get worse.
	Make caregiver aware of community resources such as respite care.	Community support groups and resources are available to provide care, education, and support.	Referred to support group for caregivers of patients with dementia.
	Encourage caregiver's participation in support groups.	Sharing with people who are experiencing similar problems decreases feelings of alienation and allows sharing of information.	
	Will refer to an online support group. Support caregiver in taking steps to maintain own health.	Daughter must be healthy to continue supporting her mother.	Daughter discussed respite care and plans to take occasional breaks.

Nursing Care Plan 46.1 Care of a Patient With Dementia—cont'd

PROBLEM STATEMENT
Wandering due to cognitive impairment.

SUPPORTING ASSESSMENT DATA
Subjective: Per daughter, "Mom is confused."
Objective: Wandering by herself and trying to get outside despite repetitive redirection.

Goals/Expected Outcomes	Nursing Interventions	Selected Rationale	Evaluation
Patient will remain within the boundaries of the center (or the family property) unless accompanied by others.	Place in a limited-access unit. Put complex locks on the doors. Allow access to fenced yard.	Securing the environment allows the patient to roam safely but without restraints.	Patient remained safe in secure unit. Went out to grounds with nursing student in the A.M.
	Use identification bracelets or sew ID labels on clothes.	ID methods facilitate location and return if the patient gets lost.	Discussed sewing labels into clothes with daughter.
	Label all rooms and doors.	Patient may be wandering because she cannot find the bathroom, cafeteria, etc.	Arrows to bathroom appear especially useful.
	Remove visual cues that trigger wandering (e.g., car keys).	Visual cues such as car keys can trigger a past familiar behavior (e.g., driving to work).	Asked for keys; redirected into common area.
	Check on patient at frequent designated intervals.	Removing these helps promote safety.	Has not been wandering.
	Notify police and neighbors to be on the alert.	Police and neighbors can quickly contact caregiver if patient is noted to be wandering.	Discussed with daughter about notifying neighbors and police.

Critical Thinking Questions
1. How would you react if Mrs. Whitt's daughter stated that she was afraid her mother would not get proper care if she were placed in a nursing home?
2. What interventions could you initiate to protect patients like Mrs. Whitt from physical injury related to confusion?

ADLs, Activities of daily living; *ID*, identification.

Clinical Cues

When caring for confused patients, evidence-based practice supports the need for careful observation and documentation of patterns of behavior. This process, which is part of a systems approach to care, is called **dementia care mapping** (Surr, Griffiths, & Kelley, 2018). For example, you observe that your confused patient consistently tries to get out of bed on the right side, despite the facts that the safety devices are on the left and that there is more room on the left side. This suggests that the patient has an automatic habit of getting out of bed on the right side; these data can now be shared within the interprofessional team to adapt the room and increase patient safety.

creating a life-story book that helps the patient review accomplishments and increase self-esteem. Although safety is a primary concern, restraints are rarely appropriate for patients with AD; creative interventions that are specific to the individual and family can ensure safety while preserving dignity. For example, placement of a pleasant musical bell on the front door can prevent a confused older adult from leaving the house undetected. Placing written name tags on commonly used household objects, such as the bathroom door or the patient's room door, seems to help the patient function better within the home setting. Visual cues such as a picture of a toilet on the bathroom door are helpful as the disease progresses. Supporting the family will be a priority, particularly if the patient is being cared for at home. Help the family create realistic expectations and refer them to respite care and support groups.

Clinical Cues

If a patient becomes resistant or agitated when asked to do something or when trying to accomplish a task, redirect the patient to something else and return to the desired task later.

Patients with AD may seem to require very infrequent evaluation because the disease can progress very slowly and obvious changes in behavior or success in meeting goals may seem very gradual. However, vigilant evaluation will help you detect subtle changes in behavior that may signal delirium or progression of the disease. Also, any small successes can and should be shared with the family (see Nursing Care Plan 46.1).

NURSING MANAGEMENT

ASSESSMENT (DATA COLLECTION)

On admission, an extensive mental status examination should be conducted by the health care provider and

Cultural Considerations

Race Factors

Research shows that older adults who are Latino or African American have a higher likelihood of developing AD than older adults who are Caucasian (Alzheimer's Association, 2018c).

the registered nurse (RN) to obtain a baseline for the patient's thought content, intellectual functioning, mood, affect, and judgment. After the baseline is established, the Mini-Mental State Examination (MMSE) can be used for ongoing assessment. The MMSE is a popular shortened version of the mental status examination that was developed by Folstein and colleagues in 1975. It can be used for patients who have cognitive thought disorders to assess orientation, memory, and ability to follow commands. It consists of 11 easily scored items and should take about 5 to 10 minutes to administer. Examples of items would include "What day is it? What city is this? What am I holding (common objects such as a pen or paper clip)?" Administration should be done without the patient feeling it is a "test." The Montreal Cognitive Assessment (MoCA) is another screening tool that has been shown to be very effective when screening for dementia and its progression (Roalf et al., 2017).

Think Critically

Think of one or two ways you can assess immediate, recent, and remote memory. How would you know whether the patient's memory is accurate?

Complementary and Alternative Therapies

Agitated Patient

Music, recordings of soft ocean sounds, therapeutic touch (avoid touching if the patient is violent or angry), or aromatherapy may help calm an agitated patient with **sundown syndrome**. Having your patient sit by a light box in the early morning may also help, particularly if the patient has depression.

Think Critically

How would you conduct a pain assessment for a patient with dementia?

◆ PROBLEM STATEMENTS

Nursing problem statements for patients with cognitive disorders include the following:

- Acute confusion due to delirium induced by infection
- Chronic confusion due to progressive memory loss
- Social isolation due to inability to recognize friends and family
- Altered self-care ability due to decreased psychomotor abilities
- Potential for injury due to faulty judgment
- Sleep disturbances due to age-related changes
- Wandering due to disorientation to time and place
- Potential for caregiver burden due to prolonged 24-hour responsibility of caregiving

◆ PLANNING

Expected outcomes are written for the problems identified from assessment data. For these problems, they might include the following:

- (For patients with delirium) Patient will demonstrate orientation to person, place, and time within 24 to 48 hours after starting antibiotic therapy.
- Patient will recognize self and primary caregiver (e.g., daughter) during hospital stay.
- Patient will interact with family and friends during weekly visits.
- Patient will perform ADLs with assistance as needed during this shift.
- Patient will remain safe and free from harm during this shift.
- Patient will rest and sleep for at least 6 hours every 24-hour period.
- Patient will remain on unit or within fenced grounds during this shift.
- Family will identify signs and symptoms of caregiver burden during counseling session at the end of the week.

◆ IMPLEMENTATION

In accordance with National Patient Safety Goals, nurses must identify patients who have safety risks; this includes patients with cognitive disorders. Planning care for a patient with delirium involves accurately assessing the acute condition, stabilizing the patient, reducing environmental stimuli, providing reality orientation, and assisting the health care provider in determining the cause. Planning care for a patient with dementia frequently involves the caregivers and should be done with long-term goals in mind. Patients in the early stages of AD may be experiencing difficulties with ADLs; however, they may attempt to hide their condition. Forgetting to turn off the stove or to lock the doors is not uncommon. Regardless of the cause, the loss of cognition is devastating, and it is important to maintain the patient's dignity, provide for safety and optimal level of functioning, and promote quality of life. Interventions to provide safety and minimize anxiety for patients with dementia and delirium are similar. **However, when caring for a patient whose sudden change in behavior may be caused by delirium, time is of the essence.** Assess the patient frequently, document your findings, and be certain that the health care provider is notified. Because the level of consciousness may be clouded, reduce distractions in the environment. It may be necessary to medicate patients with anxiolytics for severe anxiety or with antipsychotics if the misinterpretation of the environment causes them to be aggressive.

Safety Alert

Antipsychotic Drugs

You should be aware that atypical antipsychotics such as olanzapine (Zyprexa), quetiapine (Seroquel), and risperidone (Risperdal) are approved for use in schizophrenia but are not approved for use with older patients who display behavioral changes related to dementia, as there is risk of death in this population with use of these drugs.

Patients may be able to remember their own name but be confused about place and time. A patient who is experiencing acute confusion or delirium will benefit from repeated orientation to person, place, and time. It is not adequate to repeat this information once or twice. It must be repeated frequently and in a calm, soothing manner. Your calm attitude is very important in reducing the patient's anxiety. Box 46.3 lists guidelines to conduct reality orientation for confused patients.

Assignment Considerations

Reality Orientation

Nursing assistants (NAs) can be instrumental in the ongoing orientation of confused patients. First, identify those patients who would benefit from reality orientation. Then give the NA specific instructions about how to orient to person, place, and time (e.g., "Hi, Mrs. Gonzalez. I am Sam, the nursing assistant at Sunshine Care Center. It is 8 A.M. on Tuesday, June 28. It's a nice, warm summer day today."). Teach the NA how to use visual cues to orient patients (e.g., "Mrs. Gonzalez, this calendar will help you remember the day, month, and year.").

Box 46.3 Guidelines for Reality Orientation

WHAT IS REALITY ORIENTATION?

- Reality orientation is a therapeutic program consistently implemented by all nursing staff to orient a patient to person, place, and time. This method includes the use of verbal communication techniques as well as written signs indicating the current date, month, or room identification (Camargo, Justus, & Retzlaff, 2015). Clocks with large numbers are included to help the patient know the correct time.
- Special group sessions are also used to orient patients. These sessions focus on person, place, and time as well as certain holiday events. These groups improve orientation and provide opportunities for social interaction.

WHEN TO USE REALITY ORIENTATION

- The use of reality orientation is appropriate when a patient is experiencing acute confusion or delirium. A sudden episode of confusion is very frightening, and orienting the patient is a way to allay fear and anxiety.
- Patients experiencing global amnesia do not benefit from repeated verbal reality orientation.
- For patients with dementia, gentle reminders of the day or time need to be repeated often and without the expectation that the patient will remember something that was said 5 minutes ago.
- All aspects of reality orientation are helpful for all patients with cognitive disorders. When used with patients experiencing acute confusion, the expectation is that the patient will become completely oriented and return to a previous level of functioning. When used with patients with chronic confusion, the goal is to preserve dignity and maintain optimum function.

EXAMPLES OF WAYS TO IMPLEMENT REALITY ORIENTATION AND REDUCE CONFUSION

- Under no circumstances should you ever chastise or become frustrated when a patient cannot remember. This would be inappropriate and nontherapeutic.
- Verbalize to patients in a consistent and caring manner who you are, where they are, and the date and time: "Good morning, Mrs. Singh. I am your nurse, Chris, at the Harmony Nursing Care Center. It is 8 A.M. on Wednesday, October 25, and it is time for breakfast."
- Look directly at the patient when you are speaking.
- Ask only one simple question at a time.
- Ask questions that can be answered with a "yes" or "no": "Would you like to eat in the dining room?"
- Eliminate environmental distractions when talking to a patient.
- Break down tasks such as dressing into simple one-step tasks.
- Ask the patient to do only one task at a time.
- Use therapeutic touch, when appropriate, to convey acceptance.
- When possible, schedule caregivers who are familiar to the patient.
- Provide general orientation to the calendar year by using holiday decorations.
- Decrease the noise level in the environment by decreasing the use of overhead paging systems and ringing or buzzing call lights.
- Label photos of people familiar to the patient with the names of the people who are in the photos.
- Limit visitors to one or two at a time.
- Place the patient's name in large block letters in the room and on clothing.
- Use symbols rather than words on signs indicating the location of the dining room or bathroom.
- When misperceptions are present, clarify them for the patient: "No, Mr. Lee, I am not your daughter; I am your nurse, Shawn. Your daughter will be here after you eat lunch."
- When special low-stimulus units designed for patients with chronic confusion are not available, use yellow tape to mark specific boundaries for the patient.
- Give frequent reassurances.
- Keep the patient's room well lit.
- Encourage the use of hearing aids and prescription glasses.
- Have clocks, calendars, and personal items in clear view of the patient.
- Encourage reminiscing about happy times in life.

A patient experiencing acute confusion may become combative or may attempt to climb out of bed or remove therapeutic equipment. If restraints are used as a last resort, the patient may be at risk for physical problems such as immobility, strangulation, or asphyxiation or for psychological issues such as anger, humiliation, loss of autonomy, and decreased functioning.

Legal and Ethical Considerations

Use of Restraints

Remember, having to restrain a patient for behavior problems is considered an unusual circumstance that requires clear documentation on the events leading to the need for restraints, **all alternatives tried before restraint,** the type of restraint, strict accounting for time in and out of restraints, and the assessment and care given to the patient while in restraints. Offer and document bathroom breaks, fluid and food, and skin care with each 1- to 2-hour check. The total number of hours in restraints or seclusion must be noted, with supporting documentation. Box 46.4 presents guidelines on the use of restraints and alternatives to restraints.

An individual with chronic confusion in the late stages of dementia will not benefit from repetitive information. If **global amnesia** (generalized loss of memory) is present, the patient will not be able to remember family, friends, or events, regardless of how many times you repeat the information. Moreover, expecting the patient to remember leads to frustration. Use of pictures or symbols, such as arrows pointing to the bathroom, can facilitate daily tasks and clarify communication. Creative therapies such as video histories, use of familiar songs, pet therapy, and aromatherapy may enrich the quality of life for these individuals.

Complementary and Alternative Therapies

Smell

The limbic system or "old brain" is associated with the sense of smell. Use of familiar smells reinforces remote memories. For example, the smell of pine or fir can trigger memories of happy Christmases spent with family and friends. Rosemary and clary sage have been found to be helpful. Aromatherapy, if not contraindicated for other medical reasons, can be administered by inhalation, bathing, massage, or topically.

Box 46.4 Alternatives to and Guidelines for the Use of Restraints

ALTERNATIVES TO RESTRAINTS

Acute Care Settings

- Encourage family members and friends to stay with the patient.
- Assign a sitter for one-on-one observation.
- Encourage oral feedings instead of intravenous or nasogastric feedings. (Avoid inserting tubes that can be pulled out.)
- Remove catheters and drains as soon as possible.
- Decrease glaring lighting, reduce noise, and minimize stimulation.
- Keep the patient close to the nurses' station.
- Be certain the call button is within easy reach.
- Place the bed in the lowest setting and use three side rails to keep the patient from rolling out. A bed alarm may also be helpful, if permitted per agency policy.
- Check on the patient frequently to offer nutrition, fluids, pain relief, and toileting assistance as appropriate.

Long-Term Care Facilities

- Place the mattress on the floor to prevent the patient from falling out of bed.
- Talk to the patient, even when the patient is not responding to you or is responding in an inappropriate way.
- Incorporate relaxation techniques, such as back massage and hydrotherapy, into the plan of care.
- Use therapeutic communication techniques to encourage the patient to verbalize feelings.
- Encourage ambulation, recreational, physical, and occupational therapy when possible.
- Encourage participation in as many ADLs as possible.
- Initiate diversional activities, such as listening to radio, television, and music.
- Maintain a regular schedule for toileting.

GUIDELINES FOR THE SAFE USE OF RESTRAINTS

- Document *all* efforts to assist the patient without physical restraints and the outcomes.
- Restraints must never be used to punish or control the patient and should be used for the shortest time possible.
- All restraints must have a health care provider's order.
- Clearly document in the electronic health record or paper chart the reason for the restraint, the type selected, and the time frame for use.
- Use the least restrictive type of restraint that will accomplish the objective.
- Obtain informed consent from the patient or the patient's family before using restraints.
- Have a written institutional policy on restraints available for the patient and family.
- Make certain that all staff have adequate in-service training on the use of restraints.
- Use hand mitts for patients who are receiving IV therapy or who have catheters or nasogastric tubes.
- If hand mitts do not work, consider wrist restraints.
- Apply restraints snugly, ensuring that circulation is not impeded.
- Check the area distal to the restraint every 2 hours (or according to agency policy) for circulation and function.
- Remove the restraints and change the patient's position at least every 2 hours.
- Apply active or passive ROM to the affected joints and muscles.
- Secure restraints to the bed frames, not the side rails.
- Tie restraints with quick-release knots.
- Document the care given to the patient while in restraints.

ADLs, Activities of daily living; *IV*, intravenous; *ROM*, range of motion.

Complementary and Alternative Therapies

Massage

Head and face massage have been used to reduce agitation in patients with AD (Keshavarz, 2018). Additional benefits include meeting the human need for nurturing touch, decreasing mild depression, reducing mental stress, improving circulation, and relieving muscle tension and stiffness.

Think Critically

Is it always necessary to encourage a patient to see and acknowledge reality? What about older adult patients who have severe dementia and believe they are living in their own homes, even though they are in a nursing home?

Nurses who care for patients with dementia need to be aware of the importance of maintaining the dignity of the patient and family. In the later stages of dementia, patients experience numerous deficits in self-care, such as grooming and toileting. It is very important to treat both patients and families with respect. Call the patient by name, provide for privacy, and individualize your care for this patient based on culture and history.

Clinical Cues

Pull the curtain or close the door and drape the patient appropriately to provide privacy and protect dignity for toileting or when performing procedures, whether the patient is cognizant.

Older Adult Care Points

When working with older adults, do not confuse clear and supportive communication with "elderspeak." Elderspeak is a style of speech that includes baby talk, exaggerated tones and slow speed, elevated pitch and volume, and simplified vocabulary. Being overly nurturing ("Come on, sweetie, let's eat now.") or overly controlling ("Sit down and finish your food!") is perceived as patronizing and demeaning and does not promote communication.

Assessment of Interventions for the Family

The family should also be assessed for their knowledge and ability to relate to the illness and care of a family member with dementia. The goal of treatment is preservation of function, and this should be clarified when working with the family. For example, if the patient lives at home, the family will need to understand that a person with dementia responds much better if there are daily routines and a structured environment. Assist the family to develop a schedule that includes adequate time for hygiene care, meals, medications, and activities such as walking. Home care nurses can help the family create a safe environment after fully assessing the home.

If a patient tends to wander or get lost, the family will live in a constant state of hypervigilance to ensure the safety of their loved one. Help family members recognize potential wandering behaviors: looking for keys, preparing to go to somewhere, restlessness and pacing, getting lost going to the bathroom or to the bedroom, or performing a task without actually accomplishing anything (e.g., moving dirty dishes from place to place without actually washing them). You can make practical suggestions such as sewing identification labels into clothing, using a bell that signals when an exit door is opened, or wearing a bracelet with a GPS chip. Box 46.5 presents additional tips for families.

Families should also be assessed for signs of caregiver role strain. Observe and assist family members to recognize when they themselves experience denial, irritability, anxiety, sleeplessness, and anger—and note that these signs suggest that the illness of the older adult is taking its toll on the caregivers. Family members often are exhausted from the daily requirements of providing round-the-clock care. Families who receive intensive support and counseling may be able to manage the care of a patient with AD in the home for longer periods of time.

Box 46.5 Suggestions for Families Caring for a Person With Alzheimer Disease

- Make and keep a copy of the daily schedule and stick to the schedule as closely as possible.
- Orient the person as necessary to maintain safety and promote maximum functioning.
- Minimize the number of caregivers.
- Simplify the environment to minimize confusion.
- Keep the environment as quiet as possible.
- Schedule rest breaks throughout the day for yourself and your loved one.
- Change your expectations; forcing thought and interaction causes frustration.
- Offer the person help when needed and distraction as necessary.
- Always supervise the use of medications.
- Always approach the person from the front before touching.
- Use distraction if agitated. Walking, gardening, rocking in a rocking chair, sanding wood, and folding laundry are good examples of distraction.
- Apply many of the safeguards used for young children, such as storing cleaning solutions, pesticides, medications, and nonedible items in locked cabinets.
- Put protective caps on all unused electrical outlets.
- Remove all sharp objects.
- Remove all throw rugs and keep hallways and stairs free of clutter.
- Keep the house well lit.
- Attach safety grab bars in the bathroom.
- Protect windows and doors with Plexiglas.
- Rather than restrict the person from wandering, provide a safe area in which to wander.
- Establish and maintain bedtime rituals.

Encourage caregivers to consider day care or respite care. These options give the family members a much-needed psychological and physical rest. In addition, families should be encouraged to use support groups such as the Alzheimer's Association.

Think Critically

How would you help a family member recognize and acknowledge the need for respite care?

Families also need to be encouraged to talk openly and frankly about quality of life and about end-of-life issues such as advance directives. Preferably these talks should be completed when the patient still has adequate cognitive functioning. If not, it can be difficult for families to determine who becomes the spokesperson and needs to be encouraged to get a power of attorney and a living will for the patient. Families need considerable support in these matters. Refer to Nursing Care Plan 46.1 for additional nursing management information.

◆ EVALUATION

Because confusion is present in all cognitive disorders, keeping the patient free of injury is of primary importance. Evaluate whether the patient is returning to or moving toward a previous level of cognitive and psychomotor functioning and whether the cause of acute delirium has been determined or eliminated. An additional expected outcome, particularly for patients with dementia, is that the patient and family will be able to verbalize the stages of illness and maintain realistic expectations for their loved one.

COMMUNITY CARE

If patients with dementia or delirium are hospitalized, the inpatient stay will typically be for a short time and usually related to a medical cause. Patients with AD are not placed in psychiatric hospitals because antipsychotic medications or psychotherapy does not work for these patients. For a variety of financial and personal reasons, many families are choosing to keep their older adults at home. Nurses who make home visits will often encounter families attempting to care for a relative who is experiencing dementia. Teaching must be done about the stages of dementia and about strategies that will make the living arrangement more acceptable (see Box 46.5).

In the later stage of dementia, placement in an extended care facility sometimes is necessary. Many nursing homes have special units dedicated to patients with dementia. In these units, safety precautions are a primary concern. Entrance and exit doors have special codes so that patients cannot wander off the unit. "Wandering pathways" are created using corridors, walkways, or outdoor spaces that allow for walking and roaming with security and safety. Nurses in these units spend considerable time educating families about the stages of AD and helping families with the inevitable grieving process.

Get Ready for the NCLEX® Examination!

Key Points

- Cognition includes the mental processes of perception, memory, judgment, and reasoning.
- Delirium is characterized by acute confusion; signs and symptoms may include a shortened attention span; disorientation; impairment in recent and remote memory; incoherent speech; disorganized thinking; and possible presence of delusions, hallucinations, and illusions.
- Dementia is chronic confusion that has slow onset (months to years); signs and symptoms include impairments in memory, poverty of thoughts, difficulties with abstract thoughts and judgments, confabulation, and changes in personality.
- AD is the most common degenerative disease of the brain and usually affects people older than 65 years; it has three or more stages.
- Goals of treatment for cognitive disorders include achieving an optimal level of functioning, ensuring safety, educating caregivers, and preserving the dignity of the patient and family.
- Nursing interventions for AD depend on the stage of illness. General interventions include maintaining a calm and soothing manner, ensuring environmental safety, using appropriate reality orientation, and monitoring the effects of medications.
- Families commonly choose to care for older adults at home; teach the family about cognitive disorders and provide practical information about safety in the home environment.
- Observation for caregiver strain of the family members caring for a cognitively impaired patient at home is needed.

Additional Learning Resources

SG Go to your Study Guide for additional learning activities to help you master this chapter content.

Go to your Evolve website (http://evolve.elsevier.com/deWit/medsurg) for the following FREE learning resources:

- Animations, audio, and video
- Answers and rationales for questions and activities
- Glossary with pronunciations in English and Spanish
- Interactive Review Questions and more!

Review Questions for the NCLEX® Examination

1. Alzheimer disease has a greater impact on society than delirium because: *(Select all that apply.)*
   1. memory deficits become progressive.
   2. it often improves with correction of the underlying cause.
   3. it causes mental decline and the need for ongoing, more involved care.
   4. the expense of care for dementia patients is a drain on society and families.
   5. a family member may have to leave the workforce to care for the patient.

   NCLEX Client Need: Psychosocial Integrity
2. You recognize which of the following as symptoms associated with delirium?
   1. Fading short-term memory, withdrawn behavior, and depression
   2. Inattention to hygiene, sad countenance, little verbal expression
   3. Confusion, incoherent speech, sudden onset of symptoms
   4. Inability to recognize familiar objects, angry outbursts, confusion

   NCLEX Client Need: Physiological Integrity: Reduction of Risk Potential
3. You identify which patient behavior as indicative of mild Alzheimer disease?
   1. Has difficulty swallowing during meals
   2. Needs repeated instructions for simple tasks
   3. Has difficulty learning new things
   4. Cannot recognize familiar people

   NCLEX Client Need: Physiological Integrity: Physiological Adaptation
4. Which nursing interventions are appropriate for a caregiver of a patient with Alzheimer disease? *(Select all that apply.)*
   1. Encourage verbalization of feelings.
   2. Refer the caregiver to respite care or day care programs.
   3. Remind the caregiver to maintain composure.
   4. Assess for alternative family support and resources.
   5. Reassure the caregiver that everything will be okay.
   6. Encourage consideration of admission to a nursing home.
   7. Tell the caregiver to focus on past happy times with the client.

   NCLEX Client Need: Psychosocial Integrity
5. The caregiver of a patient with dementia tells you, "I just can't do this anymore. I am physically and emotionally exhausted." What is the appropriate initial response?
   1. "Have you considered use of respite care?"
   2. "I am so sorry that you are experiencing this."
   3. "Do you have other family members who can help?"
   4. "Community resources are available that may be helpful."

   NCLEX Client Need: Psychosocial Integrity
6. The long-term care nurse notices that a resident with chronic dementia is uncharacteristically drowsy and lethargic. What is the appropriate nursing intervention?
   1. Allow the resident to go to sleep.
   2. Include the resident in a social group for stimulation.
   3. Perform a mental status examination and obtain vital signs.
   4. Call the health care provider to report a change in mental status.

   NCLEX Client Need: Physiological Integrity: Physiological Adaptation
7. Which interventions will you teach to the caregivers of a patient with Alzheimer disease? *(Select all that apply.)*
   1. Place door locks up high on the doors.
   2. Redirect to another activity when the patient becomes confused.
   3. Keep lights low in the evening to decrease stimulation.
   4. Offer finger foods to increase caloric intake when restless.
   5. Provide lively activity in the late afternoon to prevent sundown syndrome.
   6. Use clothing with Velcro or other easy fasteners.

   NCLEX Client Need: Psychosocial Integrity
8. Which alternative to restraints will you select for an older adult patient on a medical-surgical unit who is confused and trying to get out of bed?
   1. Raise four side rails of the bed.
   2. Put the patient's mattress on the floor.
   3. Keep the patient in a wheelchair close to the nurses' station.
   4. Use hand mitts and a soft vest with Velcro fasteners.

   NCLEX Client Need: Safe and Effective Care Environment: Safety and Infection Control
9. Which caregiver statement regarding donepezil (Aricept) indicates a need for further nursing teaching?
   1. "I should give this drug with food to minimize gastric distress."
   2. "Aricept is rarely used because it causes liver problems."
   3. "I must increase fiber and fluid in my loved one's diet."
   4. "Providing frequent sips of cool liquids is helpful."

   NCLEX Client Need: Physiological Integrity: Pharmacological Therapies
10. You observe that a patient with mild dementia has difficulty buttoning a shirt. Which nursing intervention is appropriate?
    1. Verbally coach the patient using simple directions.
    2. Leave the patient alone and give extra time and privacy.
    3. Have the nursing assistant help the patient get dressed.
    4. Give the patient a shirt with Velcro fasteners.

    NCLEX Client Need: Psychosocial Integrity

Critical Thinking Questions

Scenario A

Mr. Sanchez is a 75-year-old patient who has been diagnosed with dementia. The life partner of Mr. Sanchez tells you that he is worried about taking care of Mr. Sanchez at home "when the dementia gets really bad."

1. What are some questions you could ask Mr. Sanchez's partner to further assess his fears?
2. What teaching could you provide to the partner at this time to help prepare him to care for Mr. Sanchez throughout the course of this diagnosis?

Scenario B

You are caring for an 85-year-old patient who has been residing in a nursing home for the past 3 years. The nurse's aide reports to you that when assisting with her bath, the patient seemed disoriented and became uncharacteristically combative.

1. Describe what you will assess when you enter the patient's room.
2. What would your initial nursing interventions be?
3. How might you explain the patient's sudden change in behavior?

Scenario C

During a routine wellness visit for Jessie, a 41-year-old patient, you learned that her father has been diagnosed with vascular dementia recently and that she is terrified that this will happen to her.

1. How would you initially respond to Jessie?
2. What type of preventive education might be helpful to share with her?

Scenario D

You are caring for an older adult patient with dementia who has been attempting to pull out a feeding tube and an intravenous line for most of the evening. The patient is easily agitated and strikes out at caregivers when trying to get out of bed.

1. What assessments would you make before calling the health care provider for a restraint order?
2. What interventions will you try before using restraints?
3. If restraints are ordered, describe what you must document.

Care of Patients With Anxiety, Mood, and Eating Disorders

47

http://evolve.elsevier.com/deWit/medsurg

Objectives

Theory

1. Discuss common anxiety disorders and nursing interventions for each.
2. Explain common mood disorders and nursing interventions for each.
3. Distinguish common eating disorders and nursing interventions for each.

Clinical Practice

4. Create a plan of care for a patient with suicidal ideation.

Key Terms

affect (ĂF-ĕkt, p. 1099)
anorexia nervosa (ăn-ŏ-RĔK-sē-ă nĕr-VŌ-să, p. 1103)
bipolar disorder (bī-PŌ-lăr dĭs-ŎR-dĕr, p. 1098)
bulimia nervosa (bū-LĒ-mē-ă nĕr-VŌ-să, p. 1103)
dysthymia (dĭs-THĪ-mē-ă, p. 1094)
electroconvulsive therapy (ECT) (ĕ-LĔK-trō-kŏn-VŬL-sĭv THĔR-ă-pē, p. 1095)
flight of ideas (flīt ŭv ī-DĒ-ŭz, p. 1098)
generalized anxiety disorder (GAD) (jĕn-ĕr-ăl-ĪZD ăng-ZĪ-ĭ-tē dĭs-ŎR-dĕr, p. 1090)
hypersomnia (hī-pĕr-SŎM-nē-ă, p. 1099)
hypomania (hī-pō-MĂN-ē-ă, p. 1098)
insomnia (ĭn-SŎM-nē-ă, p. 1099)
lanugo (lă-NŪ-gō, p. 1104)
major depressive disorder (MĀ-jŏr dĕ-PRĔ-sĭv dĭs-ŎR-dĕr, p. 1094)
mania (MĀ-nē-ă, p. 1098)
obsessive-compulsive disorder (OCD) (ŏb-SĔS-ĭv cŏm-PŬL-sĭv dĭs-ŎR-dĕr, p. 1091)
phobia (FŌ-bē-ŭ, p. 1090)
post-traumatic stress disorder (PTSD) (pōst-trăw-MĂT-ĭk strĕs dĭs-ŎR-dĕr, p. 1091)
pressured speech (PRĔ-shĕrd spēch, p. 1098)
psychomotor retardation (sī-kō-MŌ-tĕr rē-tăr-DĀ-shŭn, p. 1094)

Concepts Covered in This Chapter

- Anxiety
- Coping
- Mood and Affect
- Stress

ANXIETY AND RELATED DISORDERS

Anxiety is an expected, common emotion that is considered normal and healthy unless it becomes debilitating and impairs a person from functioning to their fullest extent in everyday life. Abnormal or debilitating anxiety is intense and feels life threatening to the individual. There is a 30% heritability associated with generalized anxiety disorder (Gottschalk, 2017). All patients are at risk for anxiety disorders because of physical, psychosocial, developmental, cultural, and spiritual implications that affect lives. Patients with anxiety disorders may have another mental health issue such as major depressive disorder or substance abuse.

Anxiety is often self-limiting and alleviated without intervention. However, intervention may be necessary to prevent potential harm toward self or aggression toward others. You can be instrumental in helping a patient recover from a panic level of anxiety. Table 47.1 describes the various levels of anxiety and their nursing management, and Fig. 47.1 depicts the relationship among stress, anxiety, and related behaviors. By remaining calm and supportive, you provide a safety net for the patient. Panic-level anxiety is challenging and may require medication. Patients with increased anxiety need teaching about how to manage attacks and prevent or mitigate further attacks. They need to be taught how to relax and should attempt to determine the underlying cause of their anxiety. Anxiety can recur at a greater level of severity; therefore early intervention is important.

Think Critically

Recall a time when you felt very anxious. What were your feelings and behaviors? What strategies did you use to manage your own anxiety?

Table 47.1 Nursing Management for Levels of Anxiety

LEVEL OF ANXIETY	ASSESSMENT	NURSING GOAL	NURSING MANAGEMENT
Mild	Increased alertness, motivation, and attentiveness.	To assist patient to tolerate mild level of anxiety	Help patient identify and describe feelings. Help patient develop the capacity to tolerate mild anxiety and use the anxiety conscientiously and constructively.
Moderate	Perception narrowed, selective inattention, physical discomforts.	To reduce anxiety; long-term goal directed toward helping patient understand cause of anxiety and healthy ways of coping with it	Provide outlet for tension such as walking, crying, working at simple, concrete tasks. Encourage patient to discuss feelings.
Severe	Behavior becomes automatic; connections between details are not seen; senses are drastically reduced.	To assist in channeling anxiety	Recognize own level of anxiety. Link patient's behavior with feelings. Protect defenses and coping mechanisms. Identify and modify anxiety-provoking situations.
Panic	Overwhelmed; inability to function or communicate; possible bodily harm to self and others; loss of rational thought.	To be supportive and protective	Provide nonstimulating, calm, structured environment. Avoid touching. Stay with patient. Administer medications as ordered, if necessary.

Adapted from Zerwekh J, Garneau A: *Illustrated study guide for the NCLEX-PN exam,* ed 8, Chandler, Ariz., 2017, Nursing Education Consultants, Inc.

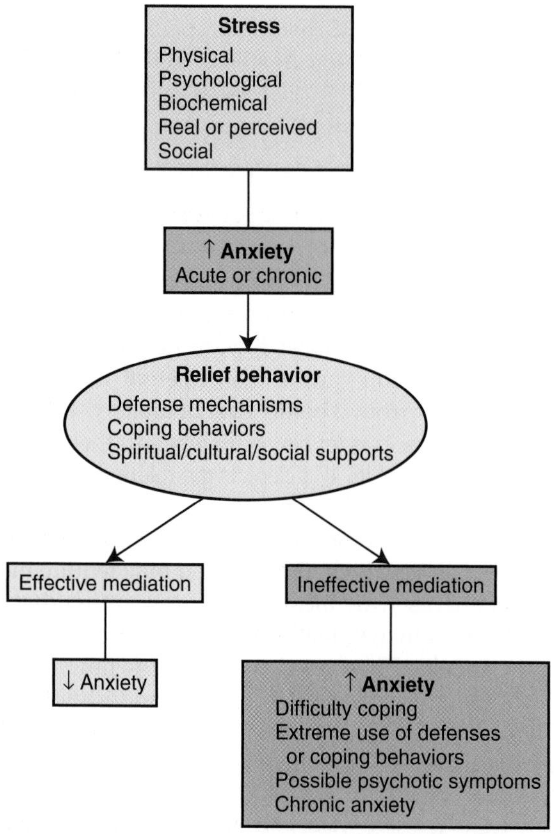

Fig. 47.1 Stress, anxiety, and behavioral effects.

GENERALIZED ANXIETY DISORDER

A person who experiences persistent, unrealistic, or excessive worry about two or more life circumstances for 6 months or longer is exhibiting symptoms associated with **generalized anxiety disorder (GAD)**. GAD usually develops slowly and is chronic in nature. Patients with GAD worry more than what is considered average. They often worry about multiple concerns at a time, instead of feeling anxious about one particular issue or circumstance. For example, a person may worry about taking an upcoming test, and then once the test is over and the grade is posted, the anxiety diminishes or disappears. An individual with GAD may worry not only about the test, but also about whether passing the test will result in a failing grade, which could culminate in being dismissed from college. In addition to worrying about the test in this capacity, the individual with GAD may also experience anxiety about other things such as whether they are a good friend, if they are smart enough to perform in the classroom or at a certain job, and what other people think of them. Despite there being no actual problems, individuals with GAD have difficulty stopping the cycle of worrying.

Physiologic symptoms associated with GAD include tachycardia, restlessness, sweating, fatigue, muscular tension, shortness of breath, and difficulty concentrating.

PHOBIAS

A person with a **phobia** experiences excessive, irrational fear of a specific activity, situation, or object. This fear can lead to avoidance or extreme anxiety that interferes with normal responsibilities and routines. Common phobias include fear of heights (acrophobia), spiders (arachnophobia), and enclosed spaces like elevators (claustrophobia). Phobias are thought to run in families.

OBSESSIVE-COMPULSIVE DISORDER

A person with **obsessive-compulsive disorder (OCD)** experiences an **obsession,** recurrent or intrusive thoughts that they cannot stop thinking about, and these thoughts create anxiety. A **compulsive act** is an act that the person feels compelled to perform. For example, a person may experience extreme anxiety and begins performing repetitive handwashing in an attempt to reduce that anxiety. Time spent in these thoughts and rituals can become overwhelming to the point of interfering with normal life.

POST-TRAUMATIC STRESS DISORDER

Post-traumatic stress disorder (PTSD) is characterized by a previous event that involved threatened death or serious injury to self or others during which the individual experienced intense fear, helplessness, or horror. The remembrance of such events produces feelings of intense distress along with anxiety, nightmares, and/or flashbacks (dissociative experience in which the event is relived) that are recurrent. PTSD can occur after any traumatic event that was outside of usual experience, including a cumulative experience such as immigration. Military combat; detention as a prisoner of war; and exposure to natural disasters, plane or train accidents, assault, and rape are examples of situational traumatic experiences that may cause PTSD. Symptoms typically begin within 3 months of the trauma, but onset may not occur until months or years later. The person experiencing PTSD may feel as if the traumatic event is happening now, even though it happened in the past. There is generally avoidance of any stimuli associated with the trauma, which may include talking about it or participating in activities that are reminders of the event. The person with PTSD may have difficulty sleeping, be very irritable, have difficulty concentrating, and be hypervigilant. Difficulty with relationships often accompanies PTSD because the person often feels detached from others. Substance use may occur in an effort to relieve anxiety.

Cultural Considerations

Post-Traumatic Stress Disorder and Military Personnel

Some veterans who served in combat zones develop PTSD, particularly those who were injured, were present when fellow soldiers were killed or seriously injured, or were involved in fighting where many civilians were killed. Research shows that a number of factors increase the risk for development of PTSD in military members: what role the member was assigned, what the politics were surrounding the event, where wars were fought, and the type of enemy faced (National Center for PTSD, 2017).

Cultural Considerations

Post-Traumatic Stress Disorder and Immigrant Patients

It is important to assess all patients for possible PTSD, as circumstances that cause this condition are varied. Research shows that immigration places individuals at risk for PTSD, not because of one specific event but because of the cumulative process that can contribute to the condition (de Arellano et al., 2017).

Because PTSD is often associated with military experience, the following websites provide screening tools and other resources to help veterans with this condition:

- www.ptsd.va.gov/professional/assessment/overview/index.asp
- www.maketheconnection.net
- www.ptsd.va.gov/public/treatment/therapy-med/va-ptsd-treatment-programs.asp
- www.realwarriors.net/ptsd

Desensitization; support groups; exercise regimens; eye movement desensitization and reprocessing (EMDR); and medications such as sleep aids, antidepressants, and anxiolytics can be very helpful.

EMDR involves a process in which the patient is asked to think about the distressing event and shift their gaze from one side to the other. As unpleasant feelings are uncovered, the therapist redirects the eye movements using EMDR, thus helping the patient to release the emotions. This form of psychotherapy has been shown to be very helpful in treating patients with PTSD (Wilson et al., 2018).

DIAGNOSIS OF ANXIETY DISORDERS

To help health care providers define and diagnose behavioral disorders more consistently, the American Psychiatric Association (2013) publishes a manual that establishes guidelines for how diagnoses are made. The *Diagnostic and Statistical Manual of Mental Disorders,* Fifth edition, text revision (DSM-5), provides a set of diagnostic criteria (specific behaviors) and a specific time frame for each mental health disorder.

TREATMENT OF ANXIETY DISORDERS

Patients with anxiety disorders can be treated with supportive therapy and **anxiolytic** (antianxiety) medications. Supportive therapies include individual therapy, education about relaxation techniques, and stress management. These patients benefit from a nonjudgmental nurse who exercises good listening skills and use of therapeutic communication. Evidence-based practice shows that a variety of psychotherapeutic approaches are effective in treating anxiety disorders; the health care provider can work with the patient to agree on the best approach (Box 47.1).

Benzodiazepines are prescribed situationally for anxiety disorders. These can be very effective in the short term to help patients manage anxiety while they

Box 47.1 Advanced Practice Psychotherapeutic Interventions

- *Psychodynamic therapy:* Therapist helps the patient link a past event to current feelings. This insight is believed to help patients modify feelings and behavior.
- *Cognitive-behavioral therapy:* Therapist helps the patient identify unhealthy thoughts or undesirable responses that occur because of a situation or event, and then the patient is assisted to change ways of thinking about an event and therefore to change emotional response and behavior.
- *Motivational interviewing:* Therapist enhances motivation for change by matching the patient's ability to problem solve with specific strategies. Principles include expressing empathy, developing discrepancy, supporting self-efficacy, and working with resistance.
- *Interpersonal therapy:* Therapist helps the patient identify the problem, then selects a strategy to address the problem. The goal is to eliminate symptoms by improving social relationships.
- *Group therapy:* Therapist leads group sessions of 5 to 10 patients who have similar needs or problems. Patients share feelings, thoughts, ideas, and experiences; they realize, "I am not alone in my experience."
- *Behavioral therapy:* Therapist assists the patient to change behavior by using rewards, punishment, repetition, imitation, or exposure to stimuli—but understanding of the underlying cause is not essential. There are four types of behavioral therapy: modeling, operant conditioning, systematic desensitization, and aversion therapy.

Clinical Cues

Your patient may benefit from further education on stress management. Basic stress management techniques include talking to a friend, listening to music, taking a warm bath or shower, or going for a walk.

are working to develop new coping skills. Drugs from this category are alprazolam (Xanax), chlordiazepoxide (Librium), oxazepam, lorazepam (Ativan), and diazepam (Valium). Patients taking these drugs must be advised to use medications with caution because **tolerance** (the need for an increased dosage to achieve the desired effect) and physical and psychological dependency can occur. Health care providers will often work with patients to taper them off benzodiazepines if they have been taking them for an extended period.

Safety Alert

Sensitivity to Benzodiazepines

Older adults are very sensitive to benzodiazepines, and health care providers are very cautious about their use and dosage in this population. Lorazepam (Ativan) and alprazolam (Xanax) can cause confusion, oversedation, or disinhibition.

Buspirone (BuSpar), an anxiolytic, takes 3 to 4 weeks to reach therapeutic efficacy. The advantage of buspirone is less sedation with a decreased risk of dependency. Selective serotonin reuptake inhibitors (SSRIs), such as citalopram (Celexa) and sertraline (Zoloft), are often used to treat anxiety because they have fewer adverse effects. Table 47.2 presents a list of common medications used to treat anxiety.

Safety Alert

Use of SSRIs tends to pose a low to moderate risk for upper gastrointestinal (GI) bleeding (Anglin et al., 2014; Laursen et al., 2017). Observe gums and stool for signs of bleeding and check other medications the patient is receiving that may also have this side effect.

NURSING MANAGEMENT OF ANXIETY DISORDERS

ASSESSMENT (DATA COLLECTION)

Patients with an anxiety disorder should be assessed for subjective feelings of fear, apprehension, isolation, or the need for increased space. Physical symptoms may include trembling, feeling shaky, increased muscle tension, muscle soreness, easy fatigability, difficulty concentrating or making decisions, and restlessness. Patients may be hypervigilant, have difficulty sleeping, and be irritable. The autonomic nervous system response can cause an increase in blood pressure, dyspnea, palpitations, dry mouth, dizziness, and nausea.

Evidence-based guidelines suggest that screening tools can be used by *any* health care worker if an older adult is showing signs of an anxiety disorder. Examples of these assessment tools are the Mini-Mental State Examination, Geriatric Anxiety Inventory, Short Anxiety Screening Test, Hospital Anxiety and Depression Scale, Trauma Screening Questionnaire, and Rating Anxiety in Dementia Scale. After initial screening, the health care provider should be notified to further assess and determine the diagnosis.

Clinical Cues

When a short-acting anxiolytic is administered, observe the patient for signs of relief of anxiety, which should include a calmer demeanor and cessation of hand-wringing, pacing, or restlessness. The patient should voice lessened feeling of apprehension and an increased ability to focus or concentrate, if the medication is effective.

Older Adult Care Points

Older adults may have strong spiritual beliefs that assist in coping with anxiety. Friendships, social contacts, and activities associated with spiritual organizations also play a large part in achieving positive mental health. Evidence suggests that older adults benefit from individualized interventions that incorporate personal spiritual beliefs (MacKinlay & Burns, 2017).

Table 47.2 Drugs Commonly Used to Treat Anxiety

CLASSIFICATION	ACTION	NURSING IMPLICATIONS	PATIENT EDUCATION
Benzodiazepines			
Alprazolam (Xanax) Chlordiazepoxide (Librium) Diazepam (Valium) Lorazepam (Ativan) Oxazepam Clorazepate (Tranxene)	Have depressant action on CNS and inhibit stimulation of the brain Used for anxiety disorders and insomnia Depress the CNS	Watch for signs of orthostatic hypotension. Monitor for side effects: drowsiness, confusion, palpitations, dry mouth, nausea and vomiting, and occasional nightmares. Older adults may have significantly increased risk for falls.	Warn to not take any other CNS depressants, including alcohol. Potentially addictive; use only as prescribed. Can cause drowsiness and lethargy. Advise not to stop taking these medications abruptly.
Nonbenzodiazapine			
Buspirone (BuSpar)	Interacts with serotonin receptors Used for anxiety and sleep disorders	Always a scheduled medication, never PRN. May cause headaches, dizziness, or drowsiness but much less so compared with the benzodiazepines.	Takes 7–10 days for symptoms to subside and several weeks for optimal results. No evidence of tolerance or physical dependence. Advise not to stop taking this medication abruptly.
Dual-Action Reuptake Inhibitors (Serotonin and Norepinephrine) (SNRIs)			
Duloxetine (Cymbalta) approved for GAD	Increases activity of serotonin and norepinephrine	Most common side effects are nausea, dry mouth, sleepiness, and constipation.	Advise that driving or operating machinery could be dangerous.
Venlafaxine (Effexor)	Inhibits reuptake of serotonin and norepinephrine	Side effects include nausea, drowsiness, headache, dry mouth, constipation, anorexia.	Teach to take with food and not to stop drug abruptly. Advise to avoid tasks requiring motor skills and alertness until response to drug is known.
SSRIs (See Table 47.3)			

CNS, Central nervous system; *GAD*, generalized anxiety disorder; *PRN*, as needed; *SNRIs*, serotonin-norepinephrine reuptake inhibitors; *SSRIs*, selective serotonin reuptake inhibitors.

◆ NURSING DIAGNOSIS

Problem statements for anxiety include the following:

- Anxiety due to threat to self-concept
- Fear due to environmental threat
- Social impairment due to extreme anxiety in social situations
- Coping deficit due to panic attack
- Role performance confusion due to inability to carry out work responsibilities
- Feelings of powerlessness due to inability to cope when facing a specific phobic object (e.g., a spider)
- Grief due to exposure to trauma and loss
- Distress due to an overwhelming life-threatening event

◆ PLANNING

Expected outcomes are written for each problem. For the problems mentioned, expected outcomes might include the following:

- Patient will demonstrate decreased symptoms of anxiety (e.g., pacing, crying) within 3 days.
- Patient will verbalize feelings of safety before discharge.
- Patient will attend group meeting today accompanied by primary nurse.
- Patient will practice three coping strategies to use during a panic attack before discharge.
- Patient will identify three tasks at which they excel at work, during this shift.
- Patient will verbalize increased feelings of control when encountering phobic object within 1 month.
- Patient will express grief and loss related to trauma and loss before discharge.
- Patient will experience fewer nightmares related to traumatic event within 3 months.

Planning care for a patient with an anxiety disorder involves promoting a physically and psychologically safe environment. For example, a quiet, clean, and noncluttered environment and verbal reassurance should be provided. Remind the patient that they are safe and the staff is here to help. Methods to reduce the symptoms of anxiety include therapeutic communication, such as active listening, being physically present, offering emotional reassurance, giving clear and concise instructions, and administering prescribed medications. As the acute anxiety passes, the focus of care is to help the patient develop healthy coping mechanisms.

Complementary and Alternative Therapies

Essential Oils

Essential oils like lavender have been shown to have a calming and soothing effect. These oils can be used in a variety of ways, such as diffusing.

Complementary and Alternative Therapies

Reduce Stress to Decrease Anxiety

Research has demonstrated that massage reduces cortisol levels with "stress-alleviating" effects and increases serotonin and dopamine with "activating" effects. Yoga has been shown to potentially reduce anxiety and depression, although its mechanism of action is not yet fully understood (Pascoe & Bauer, 2015).

Nutrition Considerations

Promoting Relaxation

Advise your patient that stimulants such as coffee and colas should be avoided, as these can contribute to restlessness. Consumption of raw nuts and seeds, whole grains, and fresh fruits and vegetables helps build the body's reserve and strength. Bananas, rice, milk, turkey, and pasta contain tryptophan, which may help induce relaxation.

Older Adult Care Points

Older adults often express somatic concerns rather than openly verbalizing emotional distress. You may observe an older adult with anxiety who reports an upset stomach, inability to sleep, or headache. Medications (e.g., levothyroxine [Synthroid], or theophylline) that the older adult is taking may increase feelings of anxiety. Certain medical conditions, such as problems with the thyroid or cardiac system, and altered blood sugar can also mimic anxiety disorders.

◆ IMPLEMENTATION

When intervening with a patient who is experiencing extreme levels of anxiety, maintain a calm and reassuring attitude. Stay with the patient and attend to physical needs as necessary. Decrease stimuli by dimming the lights, turning off the television or radio, and limiting the number of people in the area. Be sure to use clear, simple statements and repeat them as necessary. When extreme levels of anxiety resolve, additional interventions are used to help the patient learn to cope more effectively with anxiety-provoking stimuli (see Table 47.1).

Clinical Cues

Anxiety can be contagious, spreading rapidly from person to person until a large number of people are affected. Use therapeutic communication skills to help the patient de-escalate. Maintain a calm voice and a relaxed body position and convey confidence in your own ability to maintain control of personal anxiety. Self-control exhibited by you helps the patient mimic calm behavior and control anxiety.

When the anxiety is under control, assist in helping the patient to use problem-solving strategies. The long process of determining root causes of the anxiety can take years of therapy, but you can make referrals as needed and provide support in the moment.

◆ EVALUATION

Evaluate the status of the patient with an anxiety disorder before discharge from the hospital, clinic, or emergency department. Carefully document whether outcome criteria were met and if symptoms were relieved. **If symptoms are not totally resolved, clearly document that the patient's level of anxiety is not a threat to self or others at the time of discharge.** Also include a plan for follow-up care and a plan to obtain emergency care if needed.

DEPRESSIVE DISORDERS

Mood disorders are common. Individuals experiencing clinical depression are more than just sad; they often feel a sense of hopelessness and despair that cannot be alleviated by usual means. This hopelessness can lead to thoughts of suicide. Specific types of depression vary in presentation and length of duration. For example, persistent depressive disorder (**dysthymia**) refers to a condition that results in a depressed mood for most of the day, for more days than not, for at least 2 years (American Psychiatric Association, 2013). Disruptive mood dysregulation disorder is characterized by severe recurrent temper outbursts that occur three or more times weekly and are accompanied by an irritable mood for most of the day, nearly every day (American Psychiatric Association, 2013). Substance use—especially of alcohol—often produces symptoms that may be diagnosed as substance/medication-induced depressive disorder. The most common disorder in this overarching category is major depressive disorder.

MAJOR DEPRESSIVE DISORDER

Major depressive disorder is diagnosed when at least five symptoms characteristic of depression have been present for at least 2 weeks. These symptoms include an overwhelming feeling of sadness, inability to feel pleasure or experience interest in daily activities, weight gain or loss not attributed to diet, sleep disturbances, fatigue or loss of energy, feelings of worthlessness, difficulty in making decisions or concentrating, and suicidal thoughts (American Psychiatric Association, 2013). Patients with depression may have **psychomotor retardation** in which speech, movements, and thought processes are slowed. However, it is not uncommon to see agitation and irritability in a depressed person. These symptoms may be **subjective** (described by the patient) or **objective** (observable by others).

Before making a diagnosis of depression, the health care provider must be certain that there are no medical conditions present that could mimic depression, such as hypothyroidism. Patients who have suffered a stroke or myocardial infarction, have cancer, or are newly diagnosed with a chronic disease such as diabetes need to be screened for depression because major illness can lead to this condition. A pharmacologic type of depression may be induced by many medications, including antihypertensives, sedatives, anxiolytics, antipsychotics, steroids, and hormones.

Think Critically

How would you differentiate symptoms of depression and hypersomnia from a possible medication side effect?

There is increasing evidence that major depressive disorder is caused by a biochemical imbalance. It is also thought that there could be genetic and environmental influences. What is not fully understood is how these elements interact to precipitate an episode of major mental illness. Whereas the signs and symptoms of mild depression usually subside, research findings indicate that major depression is very likely to recur with even greater severity; therefore regardless of the cause, symptoms of depression need to be addressed.

Older Adult Care Points

Although older adults have many risk factors for depression that increase with age (such as loss of friends and body changes), development of major depression is not a normal part of the aging process. Research shows that most older adults are not depressed most of the time. Older adults want to enjoy good mental health, but cost and access to mental health services may be barriers for those who wish to seek treatment for symptoms.

Treatment

Patients who are depressed respond best to a combination of antidepressant medication and psychotherapy.

Complementary and Alternative Therapies

St. John's Wort

Herbal remedies such as St. John's wort have been used for mild to moderate depression and anxiety; however, patients should be advised that taking monoamine oxidase inhibitors (MAOIs) or SSRIs with St. John's wort can cause adverse drug-herb interactions. Many medications can interact with St. John's wort.

Complementary and Alternative Therapies

Music Therapy for Depression

Evidence-based practice suggests that people with major depression are receptive to music therapy and show improvement in mood (Raglio et al, 2015).

Hospitalization may be necessary if the patient has a high potential for suicide. Since the 1960s, medications have made a great difference in the lives of people who are depressed. The first-line medications used to treat depression are SSRIs and serotonin-norepinephrine reuptake inhibitors (SNRIs). Tricyclic antidepressants or MAOIs may also be considered. Drugs are very effective in treating depressive symptoms; however, they can cause some serious side effects (Table 47.3).

Evidence-based practice indicates that medications should be started at the lowest dose and increased gradually; however, it is also important that the patient receives a sufficient dose for an appropriate length of time. If the patient experiences medication failure, adherence may be more difficult to achieve.

Safety Alert

Serotonin Syndrome

SSRIs have the potential to cause serotonin syndrome. This is a potentially life-threatening condition that could start 30 minutes to 48 hours after taking the medication. Symptoms include change of mental status, increase in pulse and fluctuation in blood pressure, loss of muscular coordination, and hyperthermia. Treatment includes stopping the medication, administering intravenous (IV) fluids, and decreasing the patient's temperature.

Electroconvulsive therapy (ECT) is the oldest form of brain stimulation therapy used for severe depression. After exhausting medication therapy options, or if the patient is severely depressed or actively suicidal, ECT may be considered. ECT consists of an electrical shock delivered to the brain via electrodes applied to the temples. This shock artificially induces a grand mal seizure lasting 30 to 90 seconds. The patient typically receives 8 to 12 treatments spread over several weeks. ECT is typically done on an outpatient basis in the early morning.

The potential risks associated with the procedure include increased intracranial pressure, increased blood pressure (especially for those with essential hypertension), and cardiac dysrhythmias. Short-term memory loss, occasional headaches, and confusion are expected but usually resolve in minutes to hours after the procedure. This should be explained to the patient and family before treatment. Preprocedure teaching includes taking nothing by mouth for 6 to 8 hours before the procedure; obtaining a signed consent; and removing dentures, jewelry, hairpins, contact lenses, and hearing aids. The patient will receive a preoperative medication such as atropine sulfate and a short-acting general anesthetic. After the procedure is completed, vital signs are monitored, and the patient is reoriented. Before discharge, the patient is fed, and the caregivers are reminded about the expected short-term memory loss.

Other forms of brain stimulation therapy have shown promise. Repetitive transcranial magnetic stimulation (rTMS) and magnetic seizure therapy (MST) are noninvasive methods; a magnet is placed on the skull, then areas of the brain are stimulated by pulsations. Vagus

Table 47.3 Drugs Commonly Used to Treat Depression

CLASSIFICATION	ACTION	NURSING IMPLICATIONS	PATIENT TEACHING
Tricyclics			
Amitriptyline (Elavil) Clomipramine (Anafranil) Imipramine (Tofranil) Maprotiline (Ludiomil) Nortriptyline (Pamelor) Desipramine (Norpramin) Doxepin Protriptyline (Vivactil) Trimipramine (Surmontil)	Inhibit the reuptake of neurotransmitters (serotonin and norepinephrine). Used to treat depression.	Monitor for side effects: dry mouth, blurred vision, tachycardia, cardiac dysrhythmias, postural hypotension, constipation, urinary retention, and esophageal reflux. Usually taken at bedtime. Monitor patient for suicidal ideation. An overdose of these medications could be fatal.	Mood elevation may take 7–28 days. Full recovery from major depression may take 6–8 wk or longer. Instruct to avoid alcohol and working around machines and heavy equipment. Drowsiness, dizziness, and hypotension will usually subside after the first few weeks. Warn not to stop taking these medications abruptly.
MAO Inhibitors (MAOIs)			
Isocarboxazid (Marplan) Phenelzine (Nardil) Tranylcypromine (Parnate) Selegiline (Eldepryl)	Inhibits the MAO enzyme, thereby preventing breakdown of dopamine, norepinephrine, and serotonin.	Monitor for common side effects: weight gain, postural hypotension, edema, change in cardiac rate and rhythm, urinary retention, constipation, insomnia, weakness, and fatigue. Monitor blood pressure very closely during the first few weeks of treatment. Take a medication history to identify use of medications that increase the heart rate, such as ephedrine, stimulants, alcohol, narcotics, TCAs, or antihypertensives; report findings to health care provider.	Instruct to avoid foods high in tyramine, such as turkey, aged cheeses; red wine, sherry, and beer; pickled or smoked fish; fermented meats; and artificial sweeteners because drug-food interactions can cause a life-threatening hypertensive crisis. If the medication is discontinued for any reason, dietary restrictions should continue for at least 14 days. Teach to go to the ED immediately for headaches.
Selective Serotonin Reuptake Inhibitors (SSRIs)			
Citalopram (Celexa) Escitalopram (Lexapro) Fluoxetine (Prozac) Paroxetine (Paxil) Sertraline (Zoloft) Fluvoxamine (Luvox)	Block the reuptake of serotonin. Used for depression, anxiety disorders, and bulimia.	These medications elevate mood faster than the TCAs or MAOIs. They are not as sedating and do not have the anticholinergic side effects of TCAs or MAOIs. Monitor for common side effects such as nausea, nervousness, insomnia, anxiety, and sexual dysfunction.	Take with food if GI distress occurs. Take drug in the morning for optimal effects. Full therapeutic effects may take 4 wk or more. Decreased libido or impotence may occur; check with health care provider for guidance. Do not stop medications abruptly.
Atypical Antidepressants			
Trazodone	Blocks the reuptake of norepinephrine, serotonin, and dopamine.	Side effects are similar to the SSRIs.	Instruct to immediately contact health care provider if **priapism** (a painful, prolonged erection of the penis) occurs.
Bupropion (Wellbutrin)	—	In doses >450 mg/day, can cause seizures: assess for history of head trauma or seizure disorder. Used to treat depression in patients who are not responding to other antidepressants.	Instruct to immediately contact health care provider if seizures occur.

Table 47.3 Drugs Commonly Used to Treat Depression—cont'd

CLASSIFICATION	ACTION	NURSING IMPLICATIONS	PATIENT TEACHING
Nefazodone	—	Can cause liver failure.	Teach to report yellowing of the skin or sclera, anorexia, or malaise.
Mirtazapine (Remeron)	—	Can cause agranulocytosis.	Warn to immediately report sore throat, fever, or other infection signs.
Venlafaxine (Effexor)	—	In doses >300 mg/day, potentiates risk of sustained hypertension; assess for history of hypertension.	Instruct to continue taking BP medications as prescribed.
Duloxetine (Cymbalta)	—	Side effects are similar to the SSRIs.	Monitor for hypoglycemia.
Desvenlafaxine (Pristiq)	—	Common side effects: dizziness, fatigue, headaches, nausea, dry mouth, diarrhea, constipation, and decreased appetite.	Instruct patient and family to report suicidal ideations.

BP, Blood pressure; *ED*, emergency department; *GI*, gastrointestinal; *MAO*, monoamine oxidase; *TCAs*, tricyclic antidepressants.

nerve stimulation (VNS) and deep brain stimulation (DBS) use a surgically implanted pacemaker to stimulate nerve tissue that is used in the treatment of epilepsy. DBS is still undergoing trials as it relates to treatment for depression.

NURSING MANAGEMENT OF DEPRESSIVE DISORDERS

ASSESSMENT (DATA COLLECTION)

Collect information about feelings of sadness, hopelessness, and a loss of interest in usual activities. Identify whether the patient is at risk for suicide. Assess the patient for changes in ability to fulfill family, social, or occupational obligations, as well as appetite, recent weight loss or gain, and changes in normal eating pattern. A person with a depressive disorder may also have somatic concerns, such as headache, stomachache, dizziness, nausea, indigestion, constipation, and change in sexual responsiveness. The inability to concentrate and indecisiveness are also often associated with mood disorders.

NURSING DIAGNOSIS

Common problem statements for patients experiencing depression include the following:

- Altered activity tolerance due to psychomotor retardation
- Decreased hope due to inability to achieve career goals
- Spiritual disconnection due to questioning the meaning of life
- Grief due to loss (e.g., divorce)
- Decreased self-esteem due to past failures
- Altered self-care ability due to lack of motivation
- Potential for violence due to repressed anger and grief

PLANNING

For these problems, expected outcomes might include the following:

- Patient will participate in at least one unit of activity today and gradually increase participation as activity tolerance improves.
- Patient will identify two short-term goals that would contribute to achieving overall long-term career goals by the end of shift.
- Patient will verbalize renewal of faith in a higher power after two or three visits from hospital clergy.
- Patient will express feelings of loss and sadness about divorce within 1 month.
- Patient will relate at least one "success story" about self every day for 1 week.
- Patient will participate with assistance (e.g., verbal coaching) in activities of daily living (ADLs) (e.g., brush own teeth) for 1 week and gradually increase independent completion of ADLs before discharge.
- Patient will refrain from harming self or others during this shift.

Planning care for a patient with depression involves promoting safety, adequate nutrition, and rest. Initially the patient may require assistance in performing ADLs until the severe depression subsides. People experiencing a depressive episode may not have the mental energy necessary to concentrate on work or relationships. As their energy level improves, help the patient begin to set small goals such as meeting personal hygienic needs and gradually work toward the greater goal of reentry into the community.

IMPLEMENTATION

The priority nursing intervention for a patient with a depressive disorder is to protect the patient from acting on impulses to harm themselves. Medications used to treat depression often are indicated. Help the patient understand that sometimes pharmacologic intervention is necessary to combat depression at the biochemical level; reversing depression is not merely a matter of thinking happy or pleasant thoughts. Comparing the need for medication to that for a condition such as diabetes or a heart problem may help the patient feel less stigmatized. **Once the antidepressant medications begin to take effect, the risk for self-harm increases because the patient now has sufficient energy to complete the act.** It is critical to continue monitoring the patient as the medication reaches a therapeutic level. Genuine caring and concern and close monitoring are very important.

Clinical Cues

When you spend a lot of time caring for a patient with a depressive disorder, you may find that you feel very tired, subdued, or even personally somewhat depressed. Share this experience with your clinical instructor or a classmate, and remember that to give excellent patient care, identifying your feelings and protecting your own mental health are essential.

Think Critically

What types of goals are suitable for a 22-year-old nursing student who has been diagnosed with major depressive disorder? The patient has been prescribed sertraline but still reports feeling overwhelmed with life.

◆ EVALUATION

Daily evaluation of the patient's condition includes determining whether the outcome criteria for physical and emotional needs were met. These include safety and issues related to decreased energy levels, such as helping with ADLs. Also evaluate the patient's ability to participate in social activities and to express feelings. Part of this overall assessment includes determining the effectiveness of medications. Sometimes it takes several different trials of a combination of drugs to achieve the desired effect. It is also important to remember that many medications used to treat depressive disorders take 2 to 6 weeks to become effective.

BIPOLAR DISORDER

A diagnosis of bipolar disorder is considered when a patient experiences episodes of extreme sadness, hopelessness, and helplessness interspersed with periods of extreme elation and hyperactivity. Bipolar I disorder is characterized by episodes of major depression with at least one episode of manic or hypomanic behavior. **Mania** is an elevation in mood that includes increased grandiosity or irritability that is present for at least 1 week; it is present in bipolar disorder. A manic person may exhibit **pressured speech**, which is talking that is loud, rapid, and difficult to interrupt, or **flight of ideas**, in which the speaker goes from topic to topic with little or no connection between them. There is an inability to concentrate; a decreased need for sleep or nutrients; and an increase in goal-directed activity, impulsive spending, and hypersexuality. Unstable and frequently changing, or **labile,** behavior is often seen in manic patients; a mood of frivolity and joking can rapidly change to agitation and extreme paranoia. **The agitation and irritability seen in manic patients can lead to aggressive behavior.** Manic individuals may require hospitalization for an inability to eat or sleep for days that leads to complete physical and mental exhaustion and aggressive behavior. Sometimes individuals will rapidly switch from being extremely depressed to being euphoric and manic.

Bipolar II disorder is characterized by one or more depressive episodes with at least one episode of **hypomania**, a hyperinflated or irritable mood lasting for at least 4 days that does not involve psychosis. Patients with cyclothymic disorder exhibit hypomanic episodes alternating with minor depressive episodes. Substance/medication-induced bipolar and related disorder may be considered when a patient has a marked mood change that is elevated, expansive, or irritable and that can clearly be connected to development during or soon after substance intoxication or withdrawal from a medication (American Psychiatric Association, 2013). Unspecified bipolar and related applies to conditions with bipolar features that do not meet the criteria for the other specified disorders.

Treatment

Lithium and mood stabilizers are the most effective pharmaceutical treatments for bipolar disorder. Lithium carbonate has been the drug of choice used to stabilize manic behavior for decades. Lithium has a narrow therapeutic range, so serum lithium levels must be determined 8 to 12 hours after the first dose, then two or three times per week for the first month, and then weekly to monthly. See Table 47.4 for nursing implications for patients taking lithium. Because it may take 2 to 3 weeks for lithium to become effective, currently anticonvulsant drugs such as divalproex sodium (Depakote) and carbamazepine (Tegretol) are used in the treatment of mania along with quetiapine (Seroquel), an atypical antipsychotic, and BuSpar or another antianxiety drug. Lamotrigine (Lamictal) is effective for the depressive episodes. Risperidone (Risperdal), aripiprazole (Abilify), and ziprasidone HCl (Geodon) are also approved for treatment of bipolar disorder. All of these can be used safely in combination with lithium. In addition to stabilizing patients with medication, it is sometimes necessary to hospitalize patients with manic symptoms, particularly if they are a danger to themselves or others or are suffering from exhaustion caused by extreme hyperactivity. Ketamine has been shown to be effective in relieving depression and suicidal thoughts associated with bipolar disorder (Kraus et al., 2017); however, long-term side effects are not known and require further study.

Table 47.4 Nursing Implications for Patients Taking Lithium

CLASSIFICATION	ACTION	NURSING IMPLICATIONS	PATIENT TEACHING
Antimanic agent	Alters the release, synthesis, and reuptake of neurotransmitters in the brain (i.e., dopamine, norepinephrine, serotonin). Does not cure bipolar disorder but helps decrease the manic behavior.	Takes 7–14 days to reach therapeutic level (10.6–1.2 mEq/L) (Stahl, 2018). Blood levels should be drawn 8–12 h after the first dose, then two or three times per week for the first month, and then weekly to monthly until a maintenance level is reached. Sodium depletion or dehydration could cause toxicity; therefore monitor fluid intake and dietary sodium. Diuretics should be avoided. Monitor renal and thyroid function periodically.	Encourage normal salt intake. Teach to drink 2500–3000 mL fluids per day. Advise to take with meals to decrease gastric distress and to avoid caffeinated drinks because of diuretic effects. Instruct to immediately report diarrhea, vomiting, tremors, or lack of coordination.

NURSING MANAGEMENT OF BIPOLAR DISORDER

ASSESSMENT (DATA COLLECTION)

Assessing patients with bipolar disorder requires observing mood, affect, and physical signs and symptoms. Mood is assessed by asking the patient questions about feelings and observing facial expression and body language. **Affect** is a term used to describe a person's external expression of emotion. A person with a flat or blunted affect may report feeling fine, but their facial expression and overall demeanor convey sadness. The sadness described by depressed individuals is intense and creates feelings of worthlessness and hopelessness. Conversely, the mood of a patient with mania is one of grandiosity. In a manic episode, the patient may feel invincible and recklessly engage in extremely dangerous behavior.

Assess how the patient has been resting. A patient in the depressive stage of bipolar disorder may report sleeping all the time (**hypersomnia**) or falling asleep easily but then waking up after 2 to 3 hours and being unable to get back to sleep (**insomnia**), whereas patients who are manic are unable to sleep. It is not unusual for them to report that they have not slept for days.

NURSING DIAGNOSIS

Typical problem statements for mania may include the following:

- Altered nutrition due to shortened attention span while trying to eat and weight loss
- Potential for self-harm or harm to others due to labile emotional state
- Sleep disturbances due to hyperactivity or hypersomnia
- Communication barriers due to flight of ideas and pressured speech
- Role performance disturbances due to inability to perform child care duties
- Nonadherence with treatment plan due to refusal to take medications during manic phase

PLANNING

For these problems, expected outcomes include the following:

- Patient will consume at least 1500 calories during a 24-hour period.
- Patient will refrain from hurting self during this shift.
- Patient will sleep and rest at least 6 hours within a 24-hour period.
- Patient will demonstrate a decrease in pressured speech and flight of ideas before discharge.
- Patient and family will identify and use substitutes and resources for child care until the patient is able to resume family responsibilities.
- Patient will identify two methods of ensuring medication adherence before discharge.

Planning care for a patient with bipolar disorder involves intervention to promote safety, adequate nutrition, and sleep. Patients in a manic state can be a source of danger to others on the unit. Manic patients can quickly escalate in behavior from good-natured humor into active aggression. It is often necessary to assign a sitter to stay with the patient until the medications have reduced agitation and hyperactivity.

Assignment Considerations

Hygienic Care of Manic Patients

On a medical-surgical unit, you may delegate hygienic care to nursing assistants (NAs). When caring for a patient with mania, teach the NA that the patient may have a shortened attention span; therefore the hygienic care may have to be accomplished in small steps over the course of the day.

IMPLEMENTATION

Nursing interventions for a patient with bipolar disorder include keeping the patient safe, providing a high calorie intake, administering mood stabilizer medications, and providing for a restful sleep. Patients with mania may be malnourished. Small, frequent, high-calorie meals and finger foods can be helpful when the patient may not sit down long enough to eat. Close observation and documentation of mood, verbalizations, and behavior are very important. It may be necessary to redirect a patient experiencing mania in a quiet area away from others to decrease environmental stimulation.

When communicating with a patient experiencing mania, it is essential to maintain a calm demeanor. Until the medications are effective, therapeutic communication consists of setting limits. When setting limits, clearly state the initial expectations of the patient's behavior. For example, you might say, "Mr. Smith, I am talking to Ms. Jones right now, so please stop interrupting us and wait for me in the dayroom. I will be with you as soon as we are finished." The consequences for noncompliance should be stated with the request; consistent follow-through on consequences is essential. "If you interrupt us one more time, I cannot help you with your project today and you will have to wait until tomorrow." To avoid being manipulated or triangulated by the patient, it is important that all staff members be consistent. Sometimes, because of the severity of the mania, the patient is unable to comply with simple requests. In these instances, it is necessary to distract or redirect the patient rather than attempt to use reason.

When the patient is stabilized, provide information about medications and the rationale for their long-term use, even when the patient feels better. Adherence is important because it is not unusual for the patient to stop taking medications once the manic symptoms subside (Nursing Care Plan 47.1).

◆ EVALUATION

Determine whether the outcome criteria for the patient's physical needs—such as safety, nutrition, and rest—and

Nursing Care Plan 47.1 Care of a Patient With Bipolar Disorder (Manic Phase)

SCENARIO

A 27-year-old male patient has been newly diagnosed with bipolar disorder. He is currently euphoric, grandiose, loud, and very talkative. Although he can be charming, he is currently argumentative and intrusive and is verbally aggressive toward other patients. He states, "I'm going to get in your face whenever I feel like it!" He is continuously walking around the unit and has trouble sitting still for meals or conversation. He reports to you, "I haven't slept well or eaten much for the past 3 days."

PROBLEM STATEMENT

Potential for violence directed at others due to manic state.

SUPPORTING ASSESSMENT DATA

Subjective: "I'm going to get in your face whenever I feel like it!"

Objective: Argumentative, intrusive, and verbally aggressive toward others.

Goals/Expected Outcomes	Nursing Interventions	Selected Rationale	Evaluation
Patient and others on unit will remain free from harm during this shift.	Observe patient's behavior frequently (q15min).	Changes in behavior can signal impending violence toward self or others.	Patient pacing and talking loudly; checked q15min × 3.
	Redirect or distract patient (e.g., walk outside, make bed, talk to nurse).	Helps control impulses and channel excess energy.	Patient easily redirected with verbal suggestions; likes to talk to nursing staff and mental health assistant.
	Move patient away from others as necessary.	Agitated and aggressive behavior is contagious and escalates in proximity to others.	Patient was verbally directed to go to room. Patient was observed for 1 h on a 1:1 basis by mental health assistant.
	Administer medications as prescribed and monitor effectiveness.	Chemical restraints may be necessary if patient cannot control behavior.	Administered PO lorazepam. Patient continues to be hypervigilant and loud but able to sit for 5–6 min without pacing, 45 min after given lorazepam. Use this opportunity to teach patient to adhere to outpatient medication regimen to keep symptoms under control on a regular basis. Patient and others remain free from harm.

Nursing Care Plan 47.1 Care of a Patient With Bipolar Disorder (Manic Phase)—cont'd

PROBLEM STATEMENT/NURSING DIAGNOSIS

Altered nutrition due to inability to sit long enough to eat.

SUPPORTING ASSESSMENT DATA

Subjective: "I haven't … eaten much for the past 3 days."

Objective: Patient observed continuously moving and not eating meals.

Goals/Expected Outcomes	Nursing Interventions	Selected Rationale	Evaluation
Patient will assume regular eating habits within 1 wk.	Weigh daily.	Provides objective information about nutritional status.	Patient's current weight is 160 lb (normal weight is 170 lb).
	Record food intake and calculate calorie counts.	To determine whether nutritional intake is adequate.	Patient ate sandwich (300 calories) and drank a glass of milk (120 calories).
Determine food likes and dislikes.	Ask patient what foods are his favorite.	Increases likelihood that he will eat if given favorite food.	Patient will eat any type of food but needs constant reminders to finish food.
	Offer small, frequent, high-calorie meals and finger foods.	To meet nutritional needs "on the run."	Patient was offered eggs, toast, bacon, and orange juice for breakfast. Patient was able to eat bacon, orange juice, and toast "on the run" but refused eggs.
	Stay with patient during meals.	Provides support and encouragement to eat as much as possible.	Patient able to eat meals but requires less coaching if given PRN lorazepam 30 min before meals.
	Administer vitamin and mineral supplements.	Replaces some dietary deficiencies.	Patient agrees to take supplements for duration of hospitalization. Patient eating three meals per day but requires monitoring and lorazepam.

PROBLEM STATEMENT/NURSING DIAGNOSIS

Disturbed sleep pattern due to manic activity.

SUPPORTING ASSESSMENT DATA

Subjective: "I haven't slept well … for the past 3 days."

Objective: Observed continuously walking and has not rested last night nor today.

Goals/Expected Outcomes	Nursing Interventions	Selected Rationale	Evaluation
Patient will return to normal patterns of rest and sleep within 3 days.	Provide a quiet environment with low stimuli.	Quiet environment is conducive to rest and sleep.	Patient placed in private room; however, quiet environment was not helpful last night.
	Monitor and record sleeping patterns.	Determines whether rest is adequate and normal pattern is resuming.	Patient slept 2 h last night and 6 h after lunch.
	Before bedtime provide comfort measures such as warm shower and relaxing music.	Teaches habits that signal bedtime and helps with relaxation.	Patient having difficulty with sleeping; warm milk offered. Suggested resting in bed even if not sleepy, but patient continued to be restless, rising frequently to come to nurses' station last night.
	Prohibit intake of caffeine-containing foods in the evening hours.	CNS stimulants can cause restlessness.	Patient agrees to stop drinking coffee for duration of hospitalization, "but it won't make any difference."
	Administer sedative medications as prescribed.	Potentiates sedation at the biochemical level.	Temazepam (Restoril) offered for sleep but refused. Patient is sleeping 2–3 h at night but has not been able to reestablish normal cycle.

CRITICAL THINKING QUESTIONS

1. How will you respond to the patient's intrusiveness and need for attention?
2. Why is the patient at risk for injury to self if he is not hospitalized during the manic phase?

CNS, Central nervous system; *PO*, oral; *PRN*, as needed.

psychosocial needs were met. Document whether the symptoms are resolving or fully resolved. Note whether the patient can communicate effectively and resume social and occupational roles. Evaluate teaching regarding whether the patient and caregivers have a plan to maintain medication adherence and follow-up appointments.

PATIENTS WITH SUICIDAL IDEATION

Clinical Cues

The Centers for Disease Control and Prevention (CDC, 2018) reported that there were approximately 45,000 suicides in the United States in 2016. This number represents a rise of 30% in half of the states since 1999 (CDC, 2018).

NURSING MANAGEMENT OF PATIENTS WITH SUICIDAL IDEATION

ASSESSMENT (DATA COLLECTION)

Risk factors for suicide include family history of suicide; history of a previous attempt; terminal illness; addiction to drugs or alcohol; diagnosis of borderline personality disorder, major depressive disorder, or bipolar disorder; and excessive stress. Suicide assessment includes determining the level of risk (low, moderate, or high) for accomplishing the act of suicide, the presence of a distinct plan, and means of acting on the plan. Be caring and nonjudgmental in your approach; however, do not hesitate to be direct. You cannot cause a patient to commit suicide by asking questions, nor will you be bringing up something that a patient with suicidal ideation hasn't already thought about. Quite importantly, the patient is likely to feel relieved that you are not afraid to hear about suicide and that you can talk openly about this difficult subject in a professional and nonjudgmental way.

Clinical Cues

If you identify a patient with signs of suicidal thoughts or behaviors, first ensure patient safety and then immediately report these behaviors to the health care provider. Depending on the setting, the patient may need a psychiatric consultation, transfer to a medical-psychiatric unit (if they are currently hospitalized), initiation of intensive suicide precautions (i.e., one-on-one observation), and/or referral to a crisis worker.

The probability of a completed suicide attempt increases with male gender, weapon availability (guns or knives), poor support system, social isolation, and the influence of mood-altering chemicals. However, all suicide threats and gestures should be taken seriously.

NURSING DIAGNOSIS

Common problem statements for patients at risk for suicide include the following:

- Potential for self-harm due to overwhelming feelings and/or previous suicide attempt

Focused Assessment

Questions to Ask a Patient With Suicidal Ideation

- Are you feeling suicidal?
- Do you have a plan to take your life?
- Can you think of any event that may have caused you to feel this way?
- Do you have (means to take a life) in your possession? (e.g., this might be a stash of medication, a rope, or a lethal weapon such as a firearm)
- Who is a part of your support system?
- Do you drink or use drugs on a regular basis?
- Has anyone in your family made a previous suicide attempt?
- Are you currently taking antidepressants?
- Have you experienced a major loss recently?
- What is your history with past close relationships?
- Have you given away any of your possessions recently?

Think Critically

Women are two times more likely to attempt suicide, but men are four times more likely to complete the suicide act (American Foundation for Suicide Prevention, 2018). Why might older adult white men have the highest rate for completed suicide?

- Decreased power due to dependency in relationships
- Decreased hope due to viewing the future as bleak and grim
- Spiritual disconnection due to loss of belief in higher power or purpose
- Altered coping ability due to use of avoidance of problems
- Altered self-esteem due to unmet dependency needs

PLANNING

For the problems mentioned, expected outcomes might include the following:

- Patient will refrain from injuring self during this shift.
- Patient will identify three examples of dependency in relationships and describe how this dependency affects their life during group therapy sessions.
- Patient will verbalize one or two future events to look forward to and enjoy.
- Patient will demonstrate renewal of usual spiritual activities (e.g., attending church, meditating) within 2 months.
- Patient will identify at least two coping mechanisms by the end of the week.
- Patient will list at least two ways to meet personal needs during this shift.

Planning care for a patient at risk for suicide involves ensuring a safe environment by determining the level of risk and initiating the appropriate suicide precautions.

As the risk for suicide decreases, the focus of nursing care shifts to assisting the patient to develop alternative methods to cope and solve problems.

Legal and Ethical Considerations

Safe Environment for a Patient With Suicidal Ideation

Although patients have the right to bring and keep personal items, health care agencies have the legal responsibility to maintain a safe environment for a patient with suicidal ideation. Belts, shoelaces, hairdryers or curling irons with long cords, and even undergarments such as a bra could be used in a self-strangulation attempt and should be taken away as necessary.

◆ IMPLEMENTATION

Protecting a patient with suicidal ideation from self-harm is the priority nursing intervention. Suicide precautions for a high level of risk may consist of placing the patient in a seclusion room with one-to-one (1:1) observation, where one caregiver is assigned to be with the patient continuously. A health care provider's order is required for 1:1 seclusion; however, in some agencies a 1:1 measure can be initiated temporarily by the nursing staff until the health care provider is notified. The observer may have to remain close enough (arm's length) to immediately intervene if the patient attempts self-harm. As the level of risk decreases, the patient is allowed to have more personal space; for example, 1:1 may continue in the dayroom, but visual contact must be maintained at all times. In addition, all items with a potential for self-harm must be removed, such as sharp or pointed objects, glass objects, or pills. Observe the patient for "cheeking," which is a behavior to avoid taking medication by holding the pill in the cheek pouch rather than swallowing it. Patients with suicidal ideation may attempt to hoard medication to use in an overdose attempt.

Active listening and a caring attitude are necessary to build a trusting relationship with a patient who is severely depressed and has suicidal ideation. Even if the patient is unwilling to talk, indicate to the patient both verbally and nonverbally that you care and are available to listen. Your attention and presence convey respect and help the patient build self-esteem and a sense of self-worth.

◆ EVALUATION

Patients with suicidal ideation need to be reassessed and evaluated frequently (i.e., every 15 minutes), and the plan of care should be adjusted accordingly to ensure safety and prevent self-harm. As the patient stabilizes and the level of risk decreases, add outcomes related to gaining new coping skills, renewing hope and a sense of purpose, improving communication skills, and preparing to resume life in a community setting. The status of the patient just before discharge should be carefully documented to reflect the absence of suicidal ideations and the implementation of a follow-up plan with a specific method to access emergency care if suicidal feelings return. According to The Joint Commission's Core Measures, when patients are discharged from a facility, the plan of care should be communicated to the health care provider who assumes the care of the patient. This is particularly important for patients who have attempted suicide or expressed suicidal thoughts.

EATING DISORDERS

ANOREXIA NERVOSA

Anorexia nervosa is characterized by the patient's refusal to maintain minimal body weight or eat adequate quantities of food. Patients with this disorder experience a disturbance in the perception of body shape and size and an extreme fear of becoming fat. The patient may strive for perfection and control by controlling caloric intake. Intricate food rituals (e.g., shifting food around the plate, collecting recipes, and making elaborate meals for others) may develop, and the patient may have superstitions about food (e.g., eating ice cream immediately reflects a weight gain in the hips). Excessive exercise is commonly used as another means of staying thin. In many cultures, the emphasis on a slim body has influenced young people's body image. This disorder has been historically associated with female patients, yet anorexia nervosa affects all ages and genders (National Association of Anorexia Nervosa and Associated Disorders, n.d.). Individuals who have anorexia nervosa often have coexisting psychiatric conditions.

Diagnostic criteria include the following (American Psychiatric Association, 2013):

- Energy intake restriction less than body requirements
- Intense fear of gaining weight or becoming fat, even though underweight
- Disturbance in the way in which one perceives their own body weight or shape, or persistent denial of this problem

Anorexia nervosa subtypes include the following:

- The restricting subtype (a patient restricts food, yet there is an absence of self-induced vomiting or misuse of laxatives, diuretics, or enemas)
- The binge eating/purging subtype (there is a presence of regular binge eating and purging during an episode of anorexia nervosa)

? Think Critically

How does culture influence people's body image?

BULIMIA NERVOSA

Patients with **bulimia nervosa** induce vomiting after consuming large quantities of food. This binge eating occurs usually during a stressful situation and in secrecy, and generally involves consumption of high-calorie, non-nutritious foods. After the episode, the patient experiences feelings of shame, guilt, and self-criticism. Laxatives, enemas, or diuretics may be taken to purge the system after the binge, or the patient may self-induce vomiting. Weight may remain stable; often patients with bulimia nervosa maintain an average weight. Bulimia and anorexia nervosa can occur simultaneously in some patients, and both require intense intervention and therapy.

TREATMENT OF EATING DISORDERS

The goal of treatment in eating disorders is to restore nutritional health and a normal body weight. If there is a rapid weight loss of 30% and the patient with anorexia nervosa is medically unstable, the first step is hospitalization to correct fluid and electrolyte imbalances and severe weight loss. After the medical condition is stabilized, behavior modification is the focus of treatment, whether the patient has anorexia nervosa or bulimia. Therapy is long term and may require years to fully address the disorder. Both inpatient treatment and outpatient treatment are available with services to meet the needs of the individual and family unit. Support groups can provide opportunities for growth and sharing of feelings and information. The long-term goal is for the patient to achieve a sense of self-worth and self-acceptance that is not exclusively based on appearance.

NURSING MANAGEMENT OF PATIENTS WITH AN EATING DISORDER

ASSESSMENT (DATA COLLECTION)

Collect information about compulsive dieting, severe weight loss, excessive exercise, binging, purging, restricting, or an unrealistic body image. The patient may be in denial. Amenorrhea, muscle wasting, dry skin, constipation, and development of **lanugo** (downy hair covering the body) can occur with anorexia nervosa. Cardiac dysrhythmias, hypotension, and hypothermia can be life threatening. Fluid and electrolyte imbalances can occur in patients with anorexia nervosa as well as in patients with bulimia.

Individuals with bulimia nervosa may maintain a normal weight. Assess for binge eating behaviors, tooth marks or callouses on the knuckles from repeated attempts to induce vomiting, and dental caries from exposure to stomach acid. Other signs and symptoms include heartburn, vomiting of blood, or constipation from dehydration.

NURSING DIAGNOSIS

Common priority problems for patients with eating disorders include the following:

- Nutrition alteration due to refusal to eat or purging behaviors
- Potential for electrolyte imbalance due to limited intake or self-induced vomiting
- Altered body image due to sociocultural and media influence
- self-esteem due to repeated negative feedback from others
- Limited coping ability due to using maladaptive dietary practices to cope with stress
- Altered family functioning due to the eating disorder of the patient

> **Clinical Cues**
>
> A patient with an eating disorder is attempting to gain a sense of control by controlling dietary intake; therefore it is important to avoid power struggles over food. Use a matter-of-fact approach and help the patient experience control in non–food-related areas.

PLANNING

For the problems mentioned, expected outcomes might include the following:

- Patient will take in at least _____ calories per day for 1 week and gradually increase caloric consumption to regain 85% of ideal body weight within _____ months.
- Patient will refrain from self-induced vomiting during this shift.
- Patient will discuss four or five ways in which culture and media influence self-image.
- Patient will identify examples of negative feedback from others and discuss how that feedback personally affects them.
- Patient will identify three alternative coping strategies to replace maladaptive dietary practices before discharge.
- Patient and family will identify three family activities (non–food related and non–exercise related) that provide support to the adolescent (e.g., discussing a homework assignment).

Planning care for a patient with an eating disorder involves ensuring a safe environment, helping to restore weight (in the case of anorexia nervosa), creating adaptive behaviors, and correcting nutritional deficiencies. As the physical needs are met, the focus of nursing care shifts to assisting the patient to develop a realistic body image, increase self-esteem, increase feelings of control, and practice new coping skills.

IMPLEMENTATION

The initial interventions for eating disorders are targeted toward physical health and safety. Suicide precautions are initiated if necessary, and fluid and electrolyte imbalances are corrected. Nutritional status, weight gain, and behaviors such as excessive exercise or self-induced vomiting are monitored. Use a supportive, nonjudgmental approach to assist the patient in building self-esteem, assertiveness, a realistic body image, and age-appropriate peer relationships. Power struggles and discussions of food should be avoided.

EVALUATION

In the acute phase, patients with eating disorders need evaluation of outcome criteria that ensure safety, nutritional, and electrolyte and fluid balance needs. Changing beliefs about food or body image, building self-esteem, learning new coping skills, and restructuring eating habits may take months or even years to achieve;

therefore small goals are reasonable and achievement of these goals should be carefully documented. Evaluate the patient's readiness to resume life in a community setting with healthier eating habits and the family's ability to support the patient's efforts.

COMMUNITY CARE

As hospital stays become shorter, many patients with anxiety, depressive, or eating disorders will be hospitalized only long enough to stabilize life-threatening symptoms. They will then be seen in outpatient clinics, in long-term care, at home, or in day programs. Medication adherence is a key place where you can teach and support the patient. Once a patient feels better and the crisis is over, there may be a tendency to stop taking medications. Regular visits to the health care provider and social support systems are essential.

Get Ready for the NCLEX® Examination!

Key Points

- The four levels of anxiety are mild, moderate, severe, and panic.
- Examples of anxiety and related disorders include generalized anxiety disorder, phobic disorder, obsessive-compulsive disorder, and post-traumatic stress disorder.
- Assess for physical symptoms of anxiety: increased blood pressure, pulse, respirations, and urinary output; dry mouth; nausea; diarrhea; trembling; muscular tension; restlessness; hypervigilance; and insomnia.
- Assess for the psychological symptoms of anxiety: feelings of impending doom, fear, guilt, anger, helplessness, irritability, and low self-esteem.
- Interventions for patients with anxiety disorders include remaining calm, decreasing environmental stimuli, teaching relaxation techniques and stress management, medicating with anxiolytics as necessary, and determining root causes of anxiety as indicated.
- PTSD may occur after any extremely traumatic event and occurs both in combat veterans and in civilians who have experienced such an event. It often appears within 3 months of the event but may not occur until months or years later.
- Assess for physical indicators of a depressive disorder: weight loss or weight gain, sleep disturbances, fatigue or loss of energy, and psychomotor retardation.
- Assess for psychological indicators of a depressive disorder: feelings of sadness, worthlessness, hopelessness, or excessive guilt; inability to feel pleasure or disinterest in daily activities; difficulty in making decisions or concentrating; and recurrent thoughts of death or suicide.
- Interventions for patients with a depressive disorder include active listening, assessing for suicidal ideations, attending to physical needs, administering and monitoring the effectiveness of antidepressant medications, assisting in goal setting, and educating about medications and ECT.
- Bipolar I disorder is characterized by episodes of extreme sadness, hopelessness, and helplessness alternating with periods of extreme elation and hyperactivity.
- Assess for physical indicators of bipolar I disorder: hypersomnia or insomnia; change in appetite; and somatic concerns such as headache, stomachache, dizziness, nausea, indigestion, and change in sexual responsiveness.
- Assess for psychological indicators of bipolar I disorder: irritability, grandiosity, delusions, labile emotions, flat affect, sadness, indecisiveness, and inability to concentrate.
- Interventions for patients in a manic phase include ensuring the safety of the patient and others, providing a high-calorie diet and finger foods, setting limits on behavior, administering and monitoring the effectiveness of antimanic medications, and encouraging rest and sleep.
- Assess for a suicide plan, including lethality level and means to act on the plan.
- Interventions for patients with suicidal ideation include developing a trusting relationship, one-on-one observation, removing dangerous objects, and talking openly about the patient's suicidal thoughts.
- Anorexia nervosa involves restriction of caloric intake, the extreme fear of becoming fat, and a disturbance in perception of body size.
- Bulimia nervosa is characterized by the practice of inducing vomiting, often after binge eating.
- Assess for physical symptoms of an eating disorder: amenorrhea, electrolyte imbalances, dry skin, constipation, muscle wasting, facial puffiness, lanugo, dysrhythmias, hypotension, hypothermia, and dental caries (related to self-induced vomiting).
- Assess for psychological and behavioral symptoms of an eating disorder: denial of problem, compulsive dieting, preoccupation with food, unrealistic body image, low self-esteem, and shame (related to binge eating).
- Interventions for patients with eating disorders include monitoring nutritional intake and weight, monitoring behaviors such as excessive exercise and self-induced vomiting, and assisting to build self-esteem and assertiveness.

Additional Learning Resources

SG Go to your Study Guide for additional learning activities to help you master this chapter content.

Go to your Evolve website (http://evolve.elsevier.com/deWit/medsurg) for the following FREE learning resources:

- Animations, audio, and video
- Answers and rationales for questions and activities
- Glossary with pronunciations in English and Spanish
- Interactive Review Questions more!

Review Questions for the NCLEX® Examination

1. A patient is irritable, pacing, crying, and becoming increasingly agitated. Which is the appropriate nursing intervention?
   1. Discussing suicide openly
   2. Administering an ordered antidepressant medication
   3. Staying with the patient while making the surroundings less stimulating
   4. Offering small nourishing meals and finger foods to sustain nutrition

   NCLEX Client Need: Psychosocial Integrity
2. A 53-year-old female is diagnosed with generalized anxiety disorder. Which behavior do you anticipate?
   1. Runs out of the room when she notices a spider in the corner
   2. Continuously checks to see if doors are shut and locked
   3. Has difficulty concentrating and excessively worries about her family
   4. Wakes at night screaming because of recurrent nightmares

   NCLEX Client Need: Psychosocial Integrity
3. You are caring for four patients with major depressive disorder. Which patient do you identify as at highest risk for suicide?
   1. 23-year-old African American female
   2. 37-year-old Hispanic male
   3. 42-year-old Asian American female
   4. 57-year-old Caucasian male

   NCLEX Client Need: Physiological Integrity: Reduction of Risk Potential
4. A patient is taking lithium. For which symptoms will you monitor?
   1. Hypertension and headache
   2. Diarrhea and slurred speech
   3. Confusion and blurred vision
   4. Convulsion and polyuria

   NCLEX Client Need: Physiological Integrity: Pharmacological Therapies
5. A patient verbalizes an overwhelming feeling of worthlessness, difficulty in making decisions or concentrating, and suicidal thoughts. You determine the suicide risk by asking which questions? *(Select all that apply.)*
   1. "Are you feeling suicidal?"
   2. "Do you have a plan for taking your life?"
   3. "Why do you want to commit suicide?"
   4. "What would you accomplish by killing yourself?"
   5. "Do you drink or use drugs on a regular basis?"
   6. "Have you considered how your family would feel?"
   7. "Have you recently given away any of your belongings?"

   NCLEX Client Need: Psychosocial Integrity
6. A patient who is disheveled and disinterested in hygiene reports overwhelming feelings of sadness and loss of energy. Which nursing interventions are appropriate? *(Select all that apply.)*
   1. Explain the importance of hygiene to health and appearance.
   2. Encourage the patient to "look good and feel good."
   3. Plan extra time to help the patient complete hygiene ADLs.
   4. Instruct the nursing assistant to do partial hygiene.
   5. Encourage participation in performing ADLs.
   6. Do everything for the patient until they have recovered.
   7. Have the same caregiver assist daily if possible.

   NCLEX Client Need: Physiological Integrity: Basic Care and Comfort
7. A patient taking an SSRI suddenly develops a rapid pulse, fluctuating blood pressure, fever, loss of muscle coordination, and mental status changes. You prepare for which intervention?
   1. Infuse IV fluids and administer an antipyretic.
   2. Obtain an electrocardiogram and start oxygen through a nasal cannula.
   3. Administer an antidote and encourage oral fluids.
   4. Monitor the patient closely and continue the medication.

   NCLEX Client Need: Physiological Integrity: Pharmacological Therapies
8. You are admitting a young adult with a tentative diagnosis of bulimia. Which behavior do you anticipate?
   1. Vomiting after eating large quantities of food
   2. Obsessing over exercising constantly
   3. Stating suicidal thoughts to others
   4. Cutting food on the plate into tiny bites

   NCLEX Client Need: Psychosocial Integrity

9. You are caring for an 18-year-old patient who is diagnosed with anorexia nervosa. What is an appropriate expected outcome for the patient?
   1. Consume 35% or more of meals.
   2. Develop improved eating behaviors.
   3. Verbalize the importance of eating.
   4. Identify barriers to eating.

   NCLEX Client Need: Safe and Effective Care Environment: Coordinated Care
10. A patient with flight of ideas and easy distractibility cannot sit through mealtime. Which nursing intervention is appropriate?
    1. Give three high-calorie meals on a regular schedule.
    2. Offer finger foods such as a meat and cheese sandwich.
    3. Provide a pleasant, odor-free environment.
    4. Encourage family meals and socialization while eating.

    NCLEX Client Need: Physiological Integrity: Reduction of Risk Potential

Critical Thinking Questions

Scenario A

You are working in a pediatrician's office and the mother of a child who was recently diagnosed with cancer becomes hysterical. You briefly assess her and find that she is at a panic level of anxiety.

1. Explain why closed questions (questions that can be answered with a yes or no or with very specific answers) and short, simple sentences delivered in a clear, kind tone would be effective when talking with the mother.
2. What signs and behaviors would indicate that your interventions are successfully helping this mother to reduce her anxiety?

Scenario B

You are a home health nurse caring for an older adult who had a stroke 6 months ago. One day his wife takes you aside and tells you that she is concerned because he is not sleeping or eating well, and he has told her that he wants to "end it all."

1. What questions would you ask the patient?
2. What questions would you ask the wife?
3. What type of community support is available for this couple?

Scenario C

A 44-year-old patient arrives at the emergency department after a high-speed chase with the police. The patient is using profane language, is unable to sit down even for a few minutes, and switches rapidly from being fun-loving and humorous to angry and aggressive. The health care provider diagnoses the patient with bipolar disorder and orders a calming intramuscular injection.

1. How would you approach the patient to administer the injection?
2. What are the major safety concerns for this patient while in the emergency department?
3. What nursing interventions are necessary at this time?

Scenario D

You are assigned to care for a 21-year-old who has been admitted for treatment of anorexia nervosa. She tells you she would like to delay breakfast to take a walk around the unit. You kindly but firmly tell her that she cannot delay breakfast. After an hour of sitting in the dining area, her breakfast is still untouched. She tells you she really cannot eat this morning because she feels so fat.

1. How will you respond to the patient?
2. How will you ensure that the patient receives nutrition this morning?
3. What can you do to help the patient gain a more realistic body image?

Scenario E

You are caring for an older adult with major depression. Several regimens of medication were tried without success, and the psychiatrist has recommended ECT.

1. Explain ECT to another nursing student.
2. What are the most common side effects of ECT?
3. What are the risks associated with the procedure?
4. Outline the preprocedural and postprocedural care for a patient undergoing ECT.

48 Care of Patients With Substance-Related and Addictive Disorders

http://evolve.elsevier.com/deWit/medsurg

Objectives

Theory

1. Discuss common substance-related and addictive disorders and nursing interventions for each.
2. Examine the significance of denial and rationalization in substance-related and addictive disorders.
3. Describe the effects of a patient's substance-related or addictive disorder on family.
4. Identify the primary physiologic effects of each disorder.
5. Discuss the medical use of opioids, addiction, and overdose epidemic.
6. Determine appropriate interventions for a patient recovering from addiction.

Clinical Practice

7. Create a plan of care for a patient with alcohol use disorder.
8. Assist with the care of a patient undergoing alcohol withdrawal.

Key Terms

abuse (ăb-ūz, p. 1109)
addiction (ă-DĬK-shŭn, p. 1115)
codependent (KŌ-dĭ-PĔN-dĕnt, p. 1111)
confabulation (kŏn-făb-ū-LĀ-shŭn, p. 1114)
denial (dĕ-NĪ-ăl, p. 1109)
dependency (dĭ-PĔN-dĕn-sē, p. 1109)
detoxification (dĕ-tŏk-sĭ-fĭ-KĀ-shŭn, p. 1112)
dual diagnosis (dūl dī-ĭg-NŌ-sĭs, p. 1109)
enabling (ĕn-Ā-blĭng, p. 1110)
Korsakoff syndrome (KŌR-să-kŏf SĬN-drōm, p. 1113)
"meth" (mĕth, p. 1116)
psychoactive substances (sī-kō-ĂK-tĭv SŬBZ -tăn-sĕz, p. 1109)
rationalization (ră-shŭn-ăl-ī-ZĀ-shŭn, p. 1109)
substance use disorder (SŬBZ -tănz ūz dĭs-ŌR-dĕr, p. 1108)
tolerance (TŎL-ŭr-ŭns, p. 1109)
Wernicke encephalopathy (VĔR-nĭ-kē ĕn-sĕf-ă-LŎP-ă-thē, p. 1113)
withdrawal (with-DRŎ-ĕl, p. 1109)

Concepts Covered in This Chapter

- Family Dynamics
- Self-Management
- Nutrition
- Gas Exchange
- Sensory Perception
- Mood and Affect
- Addiction
- Health Promotion
- Safety

SUBSTANCE USE DISORDER AND ALCOHOL USE DISORDER

Substance use disorders, a cluster of cognitive, behavioral, and physiologic symptoms that contributes to an individual's continual use of a substance, have the potential for causing medical problems and death (American Psychiatric Association, 2013). They also have the potential to create many emotional and physical problems for family, coworkers, and friends. There are many theories about the cause of substance and alcohol abuse. In 1956 alcoholism was recognized by the American Medical Association as a medical disease rather than a personal shortcoming (Bettinardi-Angres & Angres, 2010). There are still stigmas associated with alcoholism and the abuse of other substances, although society has made progress in attempting to redirect people toward understanding the disease process associated with substance use. Research suggests that there is a genetic link for approximately 50% of the risk for alcohol use disorder. Although other neurobiologic, social, and psychological theories exist, substance use is still not fully understood. Those at higher risk for substance use disorder include those who (SAMHSA, 2018):

- Have parents who use or used drugs and alcohol
- Have psychiatric disorders
- Live in areas of poverty and violence
- Have easy access to substances

Think Critically

What personal experiences have you or someone you've known had with substance use, and how might such experiences affect your care of a patient who has a substance use disorder?

Box 48.1 Common Terms Used to Describe Substance Use Disorders

- *Abuse:* Use of a psychoactive substance in a nontherapeutic manner or illicit use of prescription drugs.
- *Dependency:* Presence of physical and psychological symptoms of addiction.
- *Psychological dependence:* Craves or feels compelled to use a substance to feel good.
- *Addiction or physical dependence:* Needs the substance to prevent symptoms of withdrawal, not merely to sustain the feeling of euphoria that was present with early use of the drug.
- **Tolerance***:* Need for increased amounts of substances to achieve the desired effect.
- **Withdrawal***:* Stopping the drug results in a group of symptoms.

A substance use disorder may be diagnosed when individuals have problems with one of ten specific substances (American Psychiatric Association, 2013):

- Alcohol
- Caffeine
- Cannabis
- Hallucinogens
- Inhalants
- Opioids
- Sedatives, hypnotics, and anxiolytics
- Stimulants
- Tobacco
- Other (or unknown) substances

The term *substance use disorder* implies that there is a recognizable set of signs and symptoms related to the ingestion of a psychoactive substance. **Psychoactive substances** are any mind-altering agents capable of changing a person's mood, behavior, cognition, level of consciousness, or perceptions. **Abuse** of substances is considered maladaptive and nontherapeutic, and manifestation of psychological or physical symptoms implies a **dependency** on substances. Box 48.1 lists common terms associated with substance use. The *Diagnostic and Statistical Manual of Mental Disorders,* Fifth edition (DSM-5) outlines diagnostic criteria. A substance use disorder is considered if, within a 12-month period, the individual repeatedly demonstrates symptoms such as failure to meet usual obligations, creates danger to self or others, has legal problems, or has poor interpersonal relationships because of substance use (American Psychiatric Association, 2013). Mild substance use disorder requires two to three symptoms. Substance abuse and dependency are considered one disorder. **Dual diagnosis** indicates that a patient has been diagnosed with a substance use problem as well as a mental health disorder.

SIGNS AND SYMPTOMS

Symptoms of substance abuse vary greatly, depending on the substance taken, the duration of use, and the tolerance that may have developed. The patient should be observed for physical, behavioral, and psychological symptoms (Fig. 48.1). Problems with fine motor control may be observed when the individual is trying to perform simple tasks such as walking or eating. Observe the skin for needle tracks, bruises, excessive perspiration, excoriation, or poor condition that suggests malnutrition. Behavioral symptoms should be compared with baseline, if possible; other conditions such as dementia, delirium, and metabolic or psychiatric disorders must be considered if behavioral changes are noted. **Denial** and **rationalization** are the most common defense mechanisms used by individuals who are substance users. For example, a patient who drinks two 12-packs of beer every weekend may exhibit denial by saying, "I only drink a couple of cans of beer every now and then." The same patient who rationalizes may say, "I just have a couple of beers to relax." Remember that people who abuse substances may not seek help voluntarily. Denial and rationalization become entrenched behaviors and are difficult to eradicate. A review of defense mechanisms is presented in Table 48.1.

Think Critically

Treating patients with a **dual diagnosis** can be challenging. Imagine that you are caring for a patient with schizophrenia who admits to drinking alcohol and using "lots of drugs all of the time." What additional challenges need to be considered when this patient is discharged to a community setting?

Legal and Ethical Considerations

Substance Use Among Health Care Workers

People who work in the health care field are particularly vulnerable to substance abuse because of the availability of drugs and the tendency to care for others while ignoring personal problems. The prevalence of nurses who use substances is similar to that in the general population, meaning that this is not an uncommon problem (Kunyk, 2015). Most states have established confidential programs to assist health care professionals in obtaining help for the problem rather than immediately forfeiting their professional license. Signs and symptoms of substance use include frequently calling in sick or always working (to have access to drugs), performing inadequate patient care, frequently leaving for breaks, offering to give pain medications, and a trend of patients reporting no relief after receiving pain medications.

EFFECTS OF SUBSTANCE USE ON FAMILY AND FRIENDS

Anyone living in proximity to a person who uses substances will be affected. People who are abusing substances may be unavailable for emotional intimacy because life becomes centered on the substance of choice rather than on relationships or responsibilities. Family members may experience a multitude of feelings, including anger, rage, embarrassment, guilt, shame,

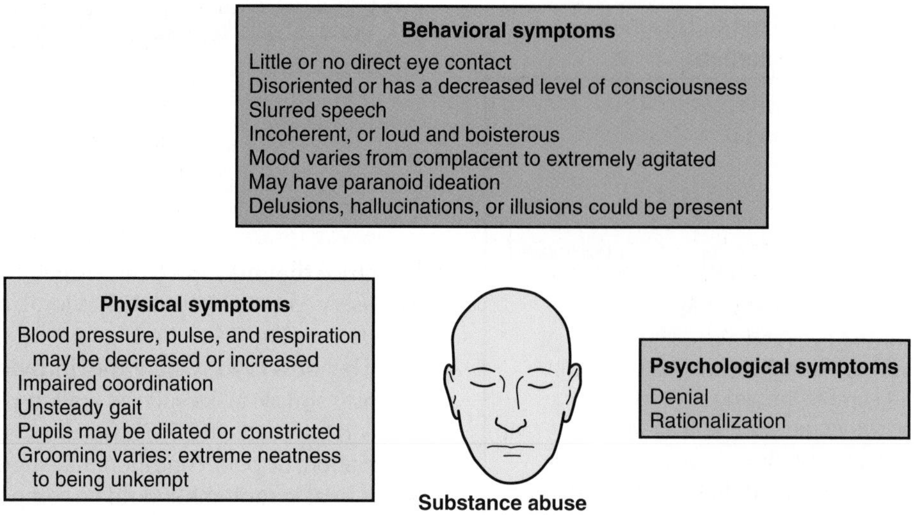
Behavioral symptoms
Little or no direct eye contact
Disoriented or has a decreased level of consciousness
Slurred speech
Incoherent, or loud and boisterous
Mood varies from complacent to extremely agitated
May have paranoid ideation
Delusions, hallucinations, or illusions could be present
Physical symptoms
Blood pressure, pulse, and respiration may be decreased or increased
Impaired coordination
Unsteady gait
Pupils may be dilated or constricted
Grooming varies: extreme neatness to being unkempt
Psychological symptoms
Denial
Rationalization
Substance abuse

Fig. 48.1 Signs and symptoms of substance abuse.

Table 48.1 Common Defense Mechanisms

DEFENSE MECHANISMS	CHARACTERISTICS	EXAMPLE
Denial	Ignoring reality and refusing to be swayed by evidence.	A person with alcohol use disorder states, "I do not have a problem with alcohol. I never drink before 5 P.M."
Rationalization	Justifying a behavior or action by making an excuse or an explanation.	A student states, "I failed the class because the teacher didn't like me."
Displacement	Discharging intense feelings for one person onto another object or person who is less threatening.	A person has an argument with a coworker and goes home and yells at a child.
Identification	Modeling behavior after someone else.	A student starts dressing and talking like a popular peer.
Intellectualization	Using excessive reasoning and logic to counter emotional distress.	A nursing student is upset by the death of a patient but instead talks at length about the equipment on the code cart.
Reaction-formation	Unknowingly acting out an intense feeling in an opposite manner.	A person treats someone whom they unconsciously dislike in an overly friendly manner.
Regression	Returning to an earlier level of behavior when severely threatened.	A 7-year-old resumes bedwetting and thumb sucking during the first few days of hospitalization.
Repression	Unconsciously blocking an unwanted thought or memory from open expression.	A person does not remember what happened during a sexual assault.
Splitting	Viewing people or situations as all good or all bad.	A patient praises a nurse one day, then hates and scorns the same nurse the next day.
Sublimation	Rechanneling an impulse into a more socially desirable acceptable activity.	A person has angry feelings about work and takes up kickboxing.

and hopelessness. The family may also use denial and rationalization to cope.

Family or friends of a person who uses substances may engage in *enabling* or may be *codependent*. **Enabling** involves allowing a person to continue in the behavior of using substances by lessening consequences for the behavior. Often a person who enables thinks they are "helping" the person; unfortunately, exempting the user from consequences only encourages the same continued behavior.

In maintaining their own denial about the situation, those who engage in enabling cover up for their troubled loved one and attempt to maintain a status quo. Calling in sick for the person using substances is a common example of enabling behavior. Enabling keeps the substance-dependent person from facing consequences, which ultimately supports continued denial. Those who enable often have a difficult time understanding that their behavior is counterproductive to the health and well-being of the loved one who uses substances.

Think Critically

How might a family enable their loved one? Is enabling ever helpful?

Codependency is another behavior that occurs in circumstances of substance abuse. A person who is **codependent** overcompensates and tries to "fix the situation" or to control the person who uses substances. For example, a teenager may repeatedly go to the bar and retrieve a parent who is drunk, and then assume all household and child care duties until the parent can function. Because overcompensating does not work, people who are codependent feel powerless and attempt to control even more. A vicious, self-destructive cycle that is difficult to break is established. The overcompensating also keeps the person who uses substances from facing reality objectively.

DISORDERS ASSOCIATED WITH SUBSTANCE-RELATED AND ADDICTIVE DISORDERS

ALCOHOL USE DISORDER

Alcohol is a central nervous system (CNS) depressant and is a commonly abused substance. It is widely available, legally sanctioned, and relatively inexpensive. Abuse of this substance is found at all socioeconomic levels.

Alcoholism is a major health problem and is a factor in many other instances of death and morbidity. Health complications include **cirrhosis** (liver damage), cardiomyopathy, **gastrointestinal bleeding**, pancreatitis, hypertension, stroke, sleep disturbances, malnutrition, peripheral neuropathies, cognitive impairment, **leukopenia** (decreased white blood cells), **thrombocytopenia** (decreased platelets), and chronic infection. Alcohol is also frequently associated with traffic accidents, domestic abuse, and suicide. Concurrent abuse of other substances **(polysubstance abuse)** is common. Until alcoholism reaches advanced stages, it is often easy to conceal the problem. The Joint Commission (2017) requires an admission screening for substance use and alcohol use in the past 12 months, including type, amount, use frequency, and problems with use, during the first 3 days of a hospital admission (The Joint Commission, 2016).

ALCOHOL INTOXICATION AND ALCOHOL WITHDRAWAL

A 12-oz bottle of beer, a 6-oz glass of wine, and a 1.5-oz single shot of whiskey contain the same amount of alcohol. It takes approximately 1 hour for the body to metabolize one standard drink. A person is intoxicated when the amount of alcohol ingested creates physical or mental impairment. A number of factors can affect intoxication, such as the type of alcohol consumed, the quantity and speed of ingestion, whether food was consumed concurrently, the person's history of alcohol use (e.g., heavy drinker, novice drinker, social drinker), general health status, and concurrent use of other drugs or substances that depress the CNS. Early symptoms of intoxication include drowsiness, slurred speech, loss of coordination, loss of inhibition, euphoria, and mild impairment of judgment. If drinking continues, motor function worsens, confusion progresses, and increasingly stronger stimuli are required to arouse the drinker. Later signs of excessive ingestion that can indicate alcohol poisoning include mental confusion or stupor, inability to be roused, coma, seizures, slow or irregular breathing, hypothermia, and bluing of the skin (National Institute on Alcohol Abuse and Alcoholism, n.d.)

Alcohol withdrawal occurs when a person with a physical dependence on alcohol stops drinking. Early symptoms of withdrawal may manifest within 6 to 12 hours after the last drink; these include anxiety, irritability, and agitation. Progressive symptoms include increased blood pressure and pulse, tremors, nausea and vomiting, diaphoresis, delirium tremens ("DTs"), hallucinations, and seizures. Major withdrawal symptoms can occur 2 to 3 days after the last drink and may last for 3 to 5 days.

Older Adult Care Points

Older adults are at risk for alcohol and substance abuse. Drinking may be an attempt to alleviate depression, pain, or loneliness. The function of vital organs (especially the liver and kidneys) diminishes with age; loss of body mass and decrease in body fluids result in a higher concentration of ingested substances. With decreased liver and kidney function, the by-products of alcohol are not cleared from the body as efficiently. Organ damage or failure and neuropsychiatric effects can occur. Older adults may be at higher risk for complications if they also take alcohol-interactive medications (Barry & Blow, 2016).

Diagnosis

To establish a diagnosis of alcohol use disorder, the health care provider will consider symptoms such as presence of withdrawal, significant impairment in family relationships, impact on occupational productivity, presence of **blackouts** (a temporary loss of recent memory that occurs while drinking), drinking despite serious personal and professional consequences, and evidence of tolerance.

It can be challenging to get the patient to acknowledge that there is a problem. Unless there is **self-diagnosis** ("I am an alcoholic"), treatment will be for the benefit of caregivers but will not foster long-term recovery for the patient.

Think Critically

You are caring for a patient with a history of alcohol use disorder who has been admitted for alcohol withdrawal. After a visitor leaves, you notice the smell of alcohol on the patient's breath. What will you do?

Treatment for Alcohol Withdrawal

Withdrawal can be life threatening, especially withdrawal from alcohol and certain anxiolytics, such as benzodiazepines. Withdrawal treatment consists of two phases. Initial priorities focus on detoxifying and stabilizing the patient. **Detoxification** refers to the process of ridding the body of the abused substance, without causing harmful ill effects. Treatment decisions may be based on assessment scales such as the Clinical Institute Withdrawal Scale for Alcohol, Revised (CIWA-Ar) (Sullivan, Schneiderman, Naranjo, & Sellers, 1989). CIWA-Ar is a largely subjective tool that indicates the severity of the withdrawal and suggests whether admission to the hospital is warranted or outpatient treatment is adequate. Chlordiazepoxide (Librium), diazepam (Valium), or oxazepam is given in titrated doses. Phenytoin (Dilantin) and magnesium sulfate (if magnesium levels are low) may be given to prevent seizures. Promethazine (Phenergan), prochlorperazine, ibuprofen (Motrin), or dicyclomine (Bentyl) may be given for the symptoms of nausea, vomiting, pain, or cramps. Intravenous (IV) fluids are used to correct dehydration. Some agencies use a "banana bag," which includes normal saline, magnesium sulfate, folic acid, and multivitamins. More recent literature suggests that a combination of 200 to 500 mg IV thiamine every 8 hours, 64 mg/kg of magnesium sulfate (approximately 4 to 5 g for most adult patients), and 400 to 1000 mcg IV folate be given as supplementation on the first day of admission (Flannery, Adkins, & Cook, 2016).

Table 48.2 lists the medications used to treat substance use.

Once the patient is stable and able to participate in a treatment program, therapy consists of confronting the patient's denial and encouraging self-diagnosis. Disulfiram (Antabuse) is a drug that causes unpleasant reactions if the patient decides to return to drinking any time after starting the drug and including 14 days after stopping it. Even small quantities of alcohol that might be inhaled from aftershave could trigger serious reactions such as chest pain, nausea and vomiting, hypotension, weakness, blurred vision, and confusion. Naltrexone can be used to block the craving for alcohol

Table 48.2 Drugs Commonly Used to Treat Substance Abuse

CLASSIFICATION	ACTION	NURSING IMPLICATIONS
Drugs Used to Discourage Relapse		
Naltrexone (Vivitrol)	Competitively binds to opiate receptors to prevent narcotic's effects. Used for alcohol rehabilitation.	Advise patient about side effects of naltrexone: dizziness, fatigue, headache, nausea, nervousness, sleeplessness, and vomiting. Screen for history of liver problems. Vivitrol is a nonaddictive, once-monthly injection. Caution that concurrent use of heroin can cause withdrawal symptoms or even death.
Acamprosate calcium (Campral)	Similar to naltrexone.	Advise patient about side effects: diarrhea, fatigue, nausea, and flatulence.
Nalmefene (Revex)	Similar to naltrexone.	Must be administered IM or IV. Side effects include nausea, vomiting, tachycardia, and hypertension.
Drugs Used to Treat Heroin Abuse or Discourage Relapse		
Opioid Analgesic Methadone Buprenorphine (Suboxone)	Produces mild euphoria; used as a heroin substitute in rehabilitation programs.	Extreme caution with use in older adults; debilitated patients; or patients with renal or hepatic impairment, hypothyroidism, Addison disease, head injury, urethral stricture, enlarged prostate, or respiratory conditions. Advise patient about side effects of dizziness or drowsiness. Monitor for constipation and encourage fluids and fiber. Methadone tablets should be dissolved in orange juice. Buprenorphine is taken sublingually.
Drug Used to Treat Heroin Overdose		
Narcotic Antagonist Naloxone (Narcan)	Competes with opioid receptors and blocks (or reverses) the action of narcotics. Used for patients who have narcotics overdose.	Abrupt reversal of CNS depression may cause nausea, vomiting, and increased pulse and blood pressure. Short half-life; watch for recurrent respiratory depression. May have to give repeated doses q2–3 min or an IV infusion.

Table 48.2 Drugs Commonly Used to Treat Substance Abuse—cont'd

CLASSIFICATION	ACTION	NURSING IMPLICATIONS
Drugs Used to Treat Nicotine Addiction		
Nicotine polacrilex (Nicorette) Nicotine transdermal (Nicotrol)	Delivers lower doses of nicotine. Used in smoking or tobacco cessation programs.	*Patch:* Apply patch immediately after opening to prevent evaporation. Do not cut or fold patch. Advise patient that patch should not be used longer than 3 mo. If no benefit within 4 wk, unlikely that continued use will produce desired effects; consult health care provider. *Gum:* Instruct patient to chew gum slowly for about 30 min. Advise patient about gradual withdrawal from gum after 3 mo; not recommended for use longer than 6 mo. *Lozenges:* Advise patient to suck on lozenge until dissolved; no chewing, biting, or swallowing. Do not eat or drink for 15 min after finishing lozenge.
Bupropion (Zyban)	Weakly blocks reuptake of serotonin, epinephrine, and dopamine. At lower doses, used in smoking cessation programs. (At higher doses is used as an antidepressant.)	Advise patient that drug may cause insomnia; do not take at bedtime. Do not chew, divide, or crush tablets. Treatment usually lasts 7–12 wk. May not notice therapeutic effect for 1 wk. Instruct to avoid alcohol while taking this drug.
Varenicline (Chantix)	Blocks nicotine from binding at the receptor sites.	Teach patient to begin taking Chantix 1 wk before stop date. Side effects include nausea or decreased appetite, headaches, insomnia, or vivid dreams. Use cautiously in renal impairment. May cause suicidal tendency; report suicidal thoughts to health care provider immediately.

CNS, Central nervous system; *IM,* intramuscular; *IV,* intravenous.

and to prevent relapse in the recovery phase. Vivitrol is a once-monthly injectable form of naltrexone.

Group therapy helps break through denial and gives the patient a new sense of belonging and identity. Behavioral therapy helps with self-discipline and discourages impulsive behavior. Limit setting is one of the foundations of behavioral therapy, and it is essential that all members of the behavioral team participate and completely agree about the limits. Brief interventions have been shown to reduce alcohol intake in hazardous or harmful drinkers (Kaner et al., 2018). The acronym FRAMES defines the brief approach: **F**eedback about personal status, **R**esponsibility to change, **A**dvice for change, **M**enu for options, **E**mpathy in counseling, and **S**elf-efficacy for changes (Miller & Sanchez, 1993). In accordance with *Healthy People 2030* patients treated in the emergency room for alcohol or other substance use related problem should be referred for follow up care.

Referral to a 12-step program, such as Alcoholics Anonymous (AA), is also integral to most treatment plans. AA has been in existence since 1935 and is the primary approach to alcoholism rehabilitation in the United States; although there is no "cure" for alcoholism, there is hope for ongoing recovery. Evidence-based practice shows that continued active participation in AA results in decreased alcohol consumption. Health care providers and nurses can assist by helping the patient make the first call for AA information, locating local sites, and asking about meetings. Box 48.2 lists the 12 steps of AA.

Think Critically

The adult child of an 80-year-old patient insists that the patient be admitted to a detox (detoxification) program. The patient states, "At my age, with my health problems, my fixed income, and everything else I have to worry about, having a drink or two is the least of my problems." Discuss your personal reactions and your professional responsibilities in dealing with this patient and family member.

Complications

Wernicke encephalopathy is a life-threatening yet reversible medical emergency that arises from thiamine deficiency, with symptoms that include confusion, gait ataxia, and abnormal involuntary eye movements (Alzheimer's Association, 2018). **Korsakoff syndrome** is

Box 48.2 The Twelve Steps of Alcoholics Anonymous

1. We admitted we were powerless over alcohol—that our lives had become unmanageable.
2. Came to believe that a Power greater than ourselves could restore us to sanity.
3. Made a decision to turn our will and our lives over to the care of God *as we understood Him.*
4. Made a searching and fearless moral inventory of ourselves.
5. Admitted to God, to ourselves, and to another human being the exact nature of our wrongs.
6. Were entirely ready to have God remove all these defects of character.
7. Humbly asked Him to remove our shortcomings.
8. Made a list of all persons we had harmed and became willing to make amends to them all.
9. Made direct amends to such people wherever possible, except when to do so would injure them or others.
10. Continued to take personal inventory and when we were wrong, promptly admitted it.
11. Sought through prayer and meditation to improve our conscious contact with God, *as we understood Him,* praying only for knowledge of His will for us and the power to carry that out.
12. Having had a spiritual awakening as the result of these steps, we tried to carry this message to alcoholics, and to practice these principles in all our affairs.

From Alcoholics Anonymous: *The big book online,* ed 4, New York, 2005, AA World Services, Inc. The Twelve Steps and Twelve Traditions are reprinted with permission of Alcoholics Anonymous World Services, Inc. ("AAWS"). Permission to reprint the Twelve Steps and Twelve Traditions does not mean that AAWS has reviewed or approved the contents of this publication, or that A.A. necessarily agrees with the views expressed herein. A.A. is a program of recovery from alcoholism *only*—use of the Twelve Steps and Twelve Traditions in connection with programs and activities which are patterned after A.A., but which address other problems, or in any other non-A.A. context, does not imply otherwise.

a chronic, irreversible, memory disorder that arises after a severe lack of thiamine (vitamin B_1) (Alzheimer's Association, 2018). Treatment involves large doses of thiamine (vitamin B_1) and abstinence from alcohol. Thiamine acts as a nerve insulator in the body and is absent in the diets of most individuals with chronic alcohol use disorder.

Clinical Cues

Thiamine should always be given before glucose to prevent triggering Wernicke encephalopathy (So, 2016).

An individual with Korsakoff syndrome has grossly impaired memory and gait disturbance. **Confabulation** (fabrication or distortion of memories) commonly is seen as an attempt to communicate. A brain scan will show brain atrophy; currently there is no treatment to totally reverse this condition, but long-term administration of thiamine, other vitamins, and magnesium may improve symptoms.

USE OF OTHER CENTRAL NERVOUS SYSTEM DEPRESSANTS

Other CNS depressants subject to inappropriate use and dependence include barbiturates and anxiolytics, including benzodiazepines. Sometimes these drugs are mixed with alcohol use, which can be fatal. Drugs in this category are often initially prescribed by a health care provider for insomnia or anxiety. They can also be purchased illegally. There has been an increase in nonmedical use of prescription drugs, specifically for opioid misuse, which has led to today's "opioid overdose crisis" that costs the United States more than $78 billion annually (National Institute on Drug Abuse, 2018). The increase in abuse of prescription drugs suggests that policy and practice changes continue to be required. Health care provider education initiatives have been helpful in decreasing the number of prescribed opioids; universal use of prescription monitoring programs, routine monitoring of insurance claims information, and increased vigilance for signs of abuse continue to be implemented and needed.

Benzodiazepines (e.g., clonazepam [Klonopin], lorazepam [Ativan], oxazepam, temazepam [Restoril]) have similar side effects: drowsiness, hypotension, relaxation, and slurred speech. A chronic user may display lack of motivation, memory loss, poor concentration, irritability, aggression, and anxiety. When an individual who has been abusing drugs that depress the CNS goes through withdrawal, symptoms may include an elevated pulse and blood pressure, nervousness, and heightened anxiety. Flunitrazepam (Rohypnol) is classified as a benzodiazepine and may look like a packaged prescription medication because it is produced and used in some countries for insomnia; however, it is illegal in the United States. Rohypnol has been informally known as the "date-rape drug" because of publicized reports of people using it to taint the drink of a victim. It produces **anterograde amnesia** (inability to remember events that happened while under the influence of a substance), along with muscle relaxation, drowsiness, and slowed motor performance.

Older Adult Care Points

Insomnia is not atypical in older adults. Great care must be taken when prescribing sedatives and hypnotics for this population, and careful patient teaching must be provided. Benzodiazepines have a long half-life and are not excreted readily by the body. Decreased liver and renal function can quickly lead to toxicity and dependence, so individuals with slowed liver and renal function may experience a cumulative effect and toxic side effects.

Treatment

A patient who is addicted to benzodiazepines may be given a drug from a similar category in titrated doses. With the long half-life of benzodiazepines, the initial symptoms of withdrawal may not appear for 3 to 5 days.

The amount prescribed during the withdrawal period depends on the severity of the addiction. Table 48.3 presents the symptoms of intoxication with and withdrawal from CNS depressants. Patients benefit from individual psychotherapy and referral to a 12-step program (i.e., Narcotics Anonymous), as well as from teaching on alternative ways to induce sleep and relieve anxiety.

OPIATE USE

Opiate analgesics can also be obtained legally or illegally. Opioid misuse is one of the United States' largest current crises (National Institute on Drug Abuse, 2018). The process of **addiction** may begin with a drug prescribed lawfully for severe pain. If patients rely solely on narcotics to relieve chronic pain, addiction may occur. With continued opioid use comes increased tolerance and possible physical dependence. These can be treated by slowly decreasing dosages of the opiates. For symptoms of use, withdrawal, and overdose, see Table 48.3.

Complementary and Alternative Therapies

Pain

Assist patients to explore adjunctive therapies to alleviate pain. These include meditation, visualization, biofeedback, hypnosis, and acupuncture. Aromatherapy with fragrant oils such as jasmine or patchouli can stimulate endorphins (natural painkillers produced by our bodies).

Table 48.3 Characteristics of Commonly Abused Substances

SUBSTANCE	USUAL METHODS OF ADMINISTRATION	SYMPTOMS ASSOCIATED WITH USAGE	EFFECTS OF OVERDOSE	WITHDRAWAL SYNDROME
Alcohol	Oral	Drowsiness, ataxia, initial euphoria and aggressive or belligerent behavior, muscular incoordination. At higher alcohol levels, slurred speech, marked ataxia and muscular incoordination, marked cognitive impairment.	Amnesia, tremors, hypothermia, seizures, respiratory failure, coma, death.	Nausea, vomiting, anorexia, agitation, hallucinations, seizures, increased body temperature, increased blood pressure and heart and respiratory rate, possibly death.
Opiates (narcotic analgesics)	Oral, inhalation, IV	Euphoria, drowsiness, decreased respirations, constricted pupils.	Decreased respirations, shallow breathing, clammy skin, seizures, possibly death.	Watery eyes, runny nose, yawning, anorexia, irritability, tremors, panic, cramps, nausea, chills, sweating.
CNS stimulants (cocaine, amphetamines, "bath salts")	Inhalation, oral, IV, smoked	Increased alertness, excitation, euphoria, increased pulse and blood pressure, insomnia, anorexia.	Agitation, hyperthermia, hallucinations, convulsions, cardiac dysrhythmias, possibly death. Bath salts may cause paranoia, violence, and suicide.	Apathy, long periods of sleep, irritability, depression, disorientation.
CNS depressants (anxiolytics and barbiturates)	Oral	Slurred speech, disorientation, drunken behavior without odor of alcohol.	Shallow respiration, clammy skin, dilated pupils, weak and rapid pulse, coma, possibly death.	Anxiety, insomnia, tremors, delirium, convulsions, possibly death.
Cannabis (marijuana)	Inhaled, oral	Euphoria, relaxed inhibitions, increased appetite, disoriented behavior.	Fatigue, paranoia, psychosis.	None.
Hallucinogens (LSD, PCP)	Oral	Illusions, hallucinations, impaired perception.	Effects are increased and intensified; psychosis, flashbacks, possibly death.	In some patients, drug cravings, headache, and sweating occur (National Institutes of Health: National Institute on Drug Abuse, 2018).

CNS, Central nervous system; *IV,* intravenous; *LSD,* lysergic acid diethylamide; *PCP,* phencyclidine.

Treatment

The greatest danger associated with opiate use is overdose, which can result in respiratory depression and death. Treatment for an overdose usually consists of administration of a narcotic antagonist, such as naloxone (Narcan).

Clinical Cues

Administration of IV naloxone (Narcan) can produce dramatic and rapid results. A patient who has overdosed may arouse very suddenly with nausea, vomiting, tachycardia, and increased blood pressure. **Do *not* assume that the danger is over; continue monitoring closely.** The half-life of Narcan is short; the opiate action will resume and can cause respiratory depression. The health care provider will determine if subsequent doses of naloxone (Narcan) are indicated.

Clinical Cues

Withdrawal from opiates is not life threatening, but it can be very difficult and uncomfortable for patients who experience abdominal cramps, irritability, profuse sweating, muscle aches, fever and chills, and cravings. Treatment involves helping the individual successfully withdraw from the drug. Methadone maintenance programs are successful in helping patients who have a heroin addiction. Buprenorphine (Suboxone) is used for opiate substitute therapy; this drug can be given at a health care provider's office and comes in a sublingual form. There are restrictions on who can prescribe this medication and on the number of patients the health care provider can treat at one time. This represents a significant barrier to treatment, considering that current estimates for the United States indicate that 984,000 million people use heroin and 2.1 million people used prescription drugs nonmedically for the first time in the past year (Substance Abuse Center for Behavioral Health Statistics and Quality, 2017). See Table 48.2 for nursing implications related to medications to treat opiate overdose and recovery.

For street drugs such as heroin, a relatively cheap illicit drug compared to cocaine, rehabilitation can be difficult unless the environmental and social factors (e.g., breaking off relationships with friends who abuse substances) are also changed. It is not unusual for an individual addicted to heroin to require an elongated period in some type of supervised alternative living program. Group, individual, and behavioral therapy and participation in a 12-step program (i.e., Narcotics Anonymous) are also essential to success. Other interventions such as exercise therapy can be beneficial due to the mental boost that people experience (Neale, Nettleton, & Pickering, 2012).

Support groups are useful to any individual who is trying to make a major life change or to someone who has experienced a major life-changing event. Individuals who misuse substances but who are trying to change to a totally different lifestyle can also benefit from this extra support. The purpose of support groups is to help promote healthy relationships, learn and practice new coping skills, and reduce stress and anxiety. Support groups borrow from the principles of group therapy: universality (we have similar experiences), cohesiveness (we have a feeling of belonging), catharsis (expressing feelings makes us feel better), altruism (you help me, I'll help you), information giving (this worked for me, it might help you), improved social skills (you can say this in group, now say it to your family), and intrapersonal learning (Yalom & Leszcz, 2005). Nurses should refer patients and encourage them to use this valuable resource.

Think Critically

Why might some people feel threatened by the idea of participating in a support group? What are your personal feelings about disclosing information in a group?

STIMULANT USE

Three common categories of CNS stimulants are amphetamines, cocaine, and "bath salts." Amphetamines can cause an increase in pulse rate and blood pressure, excitation, anorexia, and hyperactive reflexes; they can also produce life-threatening conditions such as cardiac dysrhythmias, seizures, or hyperthermia.

Misuse can range from consumption of small and infrequent amounts to ingestion of large amounts, which causes prolonged sleeplessness and anorexia. Sleep deprivation of this magnitude can lead to extreme agitation, hostility, and transient psychosis and can be fatal. People who are withdrawing from stimulants experience drowsiness, headache, lethargy, nausea, alterations in eating and sleeping patterns, and sometimes cravings.

Methamphetamine, known as "speed," **"meth,"** "crank," or "crystal," is injected or smoked (Fig. 48.2). "Meth" is highly addictive, and users often end up taking progressively larger doses to get the same effect. "Meth labs" are unfortunately easy to establish in an average household, garage, trailer, or similar structure; common household chemicals or over-the-counter medications

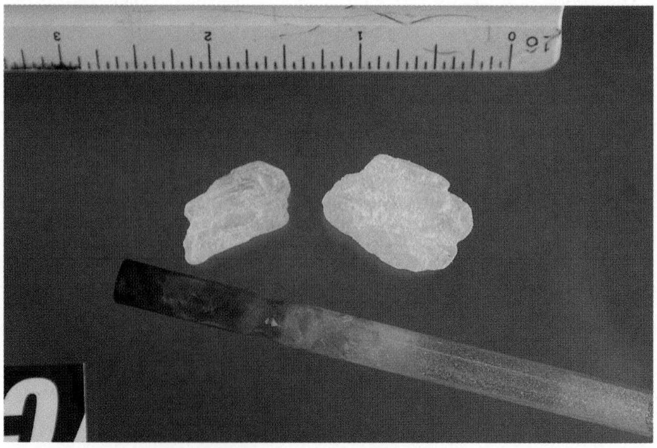

Fig. 48.2 Methamphetamine. (Courtesy U.S. Drug Enforcement Administration.)

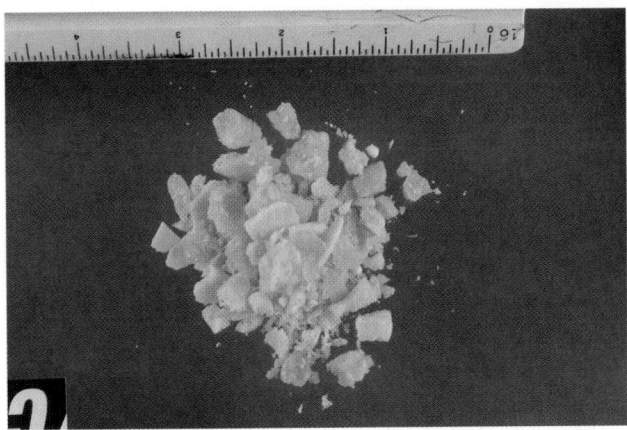

Fig. 48.3 Crack cocaine. (Courtesy U.S. Drug Enforcement Administration.)

are "cooked," creating a harmful residue that lingers on the walls and in the air well after the cooking process is finished. Chronic users may develop toxic psychosis and experience paranoia, hallucinations, and delusions. "Meth" use functionally and structurally alters the brain. Weight loss, poor nutrition, skin sores, and serious tooth decay are common effects of methamphetamine use.

Cocaine, also known as "coke," "snow," "blow," and "nose candy," is an expensive, highly addictive drug that can cause death, even in small doses. Cocaine is a short-acting substance and is more commonly used for binges. It produces euphoria, increased energy, and a sense of well-being. The stimulating effects are very fast acting and energizing. However, the effects after the "high" are equally intense, and users are subject to severe emotional lows. The powder is either "snorted" (intranasal administration) or dissolved and taken intravenously. "Crack," a purified form of cocaine, is smoked by placing it in a pipe or smoking it with marijuana or tobacco (Fig. 48.3). This "freebasing" of cocaine reduces it to its purest form. This is the most dangerous type of administration; it produces an immediate rush and accounts for many overdoses and lethal reactions.

"Bath salts" or "plant food" is a powder that is inhaled, injected, ingested, or smoked to produce an effect close to that of cocaine or amphetamine. It is available over the internet and is popular among nightclub patrons. These drugs are derived from cathinone, a Schedule I controlled substance. There are many varieties in varying chemical combinations, and they are highly addictive. High doses bring a risk of violence, paranoid psychoses, and suicide.

Treatment

Treatment for abuse of CNS stimulants is similar to treatment for alcohol abuse. Initially the treatment protocol is symptom specific and managed by medications. Anxiolytics or antipsychotics may be used for agitation or aggressive behavior, and antidepressants may be used for depressive symptoms. Contingency management has been shown to be the most effective behavioral intervention to discourage cocaine use (Stotts et al., 2015). Patients who abuse CNS stimulants must also be taught ways to cope with the psychological craving that often leads to relapse. Therapeutic communities or residential programs are other options. The recovering addict stays for 6 to 12 months while undergoing behavioral therapies.

NICOTINE USE

Nicotine is highly addictive and causes increased respiration, decreased pulmonary function, and a chronic cough. Use of tobacco is related to more than 480,000 deaths per year (Centers for Disease Control and Prevention, 2018) and contributes to development of lung cancer and other lung diseases, such as emphysema. Pipe smokers and people who chew tobacco are more prone to oral cancer. Smoking has been implicated in many other health conditions, including heart disease, stroke, many cancers, hypertension, premature wrinkling of the skin, bad breath, and discoloration of the fingernails. In addition, deaths from secondhand smoke inhalation total more than 41,000 annually (Centers for Disease Control and Prevention, 2018). Withdrawal symptoms can begin as soon as 24 hours after the cessation of smoking and include irritability, tension, decreased heart rate, and insomnia. Cigarettes are legal and accessible, and the craving continues long after the patient quits smoking; therefore resumption of the habit is common. Electronic cigarettes used with flavoring, once touted by manufacturers as a safe alternative to cigarette smoking, have been shown to cause "popcorn lung," a condition similar to chronic obstructive pulmonary disease (COPD) that results in scarring of the air sacs in the lungs and narrowing of the airways (American Lung Association, 2018).

Cultural Considerations

New Consumer Markets

There has been a decrease in cigarette smoking in the United States since 2005 (Centers for Disease Control and Prevention, 2016). In 1966 the U.S. Surgeon General's health warnings were placed on all cigarette packages. Since then, similar warnings have been put on other tobacco products. Television and radio advertising for cigarettes was banned in 1971. Education and an increase in cigarette taxes, along with restrictions on smoking in public places, have also contributed to the decrease.

Treatment

Nicotine replacement therapy (NRT) is available in patches, lozenges, gum, sublingual tablets, inhalant, and nasal spray. Self-help groups, hypnosis, and acupuncture are among the treatments available for nicotine addiction. Bupropion (Zyban) and varenicline (Chantix) are approved in the United States as medications to help patients stop smoking. Smoking cessation programs support the *Healthy People 2030* goals and emphasize the positive effects of quitting, such as better overall health for the individual and the family, an increased sense of smell and taste, and saving money. Evidence-based practice suggests that nursing teaching helps patients stop smoking (Rice, Heath, Livingstone-Banks, & Hartman-Boyce, 2017). Multicomponent interventions for smoking cessation that include an onsite visit, follow-up phone calls, enhanced education about NRT, and motivational interviewing are effective. The most useful aspects of counseling are helping the patient develop a plan and identifying barriers to quitting. Resources such as a "quit plan," available through www.smokefree.gov, can help patients get organized. The quit plan can include setting a stop date, asking friends and family for help, anticipating how to combat cravings, and removing all tobacco products and accessories from the house, car, and workplace.

Clinical Cues

The Agency for Healthcare Research and Quality (AHRQ, 2012) recommends the "five *As*" approach for helping patients to quit using tobacco: (1) *Ask* about tobacco use, (2) *Advise* to quit, (3) *Assess* willingness to quit, (4) *Assist* to quit, and (5) *Arrange* follow-up.

Legal and Ethical Considerations

Do As I Say, Not As I Do

Nurses who use tobacco may be much less effective in helping patients with smoking cessation interventions; possibly they have the same misconceptions and difficulties in quitting that patients have. To be more effective in helping patients to quit, health care workers who are using tobacco should actively participate in their own smoking cessation efforts.

CANNABIS USE

The leaves and flowering tops of the *Cannabis sativa* (marijuana) plant are dried, loosely rolled in cigarette paper, and smoked. It is commonly used as a "gateway substance" (substance that leads the way or opens the gate to more dangerous and serious substance use) by individuals. The active ingredient in marijuana is effective in controlling nausea in patients who are receiving chemotherapy and helping to relieve some types of chronic pain. Medical marijuana is legally sold in 31 states, the District of Columbia, Guam, and Puerto Rico (National Conference of State Legislatures, 2018); recreational marijuana is legal in 9 states.

Marijuana is typically smoked, but it can also be ingested. It acts quickly (15 minutes), and the effects last for up to 4 hours. General effects are a mild euphoria; increased appetite; and increased sensitivity to sound, colors, and other environmental elements. Impaired coordination, decreased mental concentration, and altered judgment are also present. In large doses, the person may experience psychotic symptoms. Marijuana is believed not to be physically addictive, but it may lead to psychological dependence and a lack of motivation and ambition. There is no particular withdrawal syndrome for cannabis, so treatment must focus on issues related to the general dangers of substance abuse.

HALLUCINOGEN AND INHALANT USE

Two common drugs that cause hallucinations are lysergic acid diethylamide (LSD) and phencyclidine hydrochloride (PCP, or angel dust). These hallucinogens are believed to be somewhat less physiologically addictive compared with other psychoactive substances; however, there are extremely unpredictable effects. Hallucinogens cause distortion of the senses, an inability to separate fact from fantasy, impaired sense of time, and severely impaired judgment. Users never know whether they will have a good "trip" or a bad one. Uncontrolled **flashbacks** (feelings and sensations associated with use, despite being drug-free) can occur. This group of drugs is very dangerous because use is known to cause panic, paranoia, and death from extremely impaired judgment.

Inhalants are psychologically and physiologically addictive. Commonly abused inhalants include glue, nail polish remover, aerosol-packaged products (e.g., deodorants), paint thinner, and other types of solvents. Symptoms of use include acute confusion, excitability, and sometimes hallucinations. Prolonged use of inhalants causes permanent damage to all body organs and a psychological dependence. Inhalants are most commonly used by teenagers and children because they are inexpensive and easily accessible.

Think Critically

You are caring for a 14-year-old who discloses experimentation with glue sniffing. The patient reports stopping this behavior and asks you not to share this information with their parents. How will you handle this situation? Who can you consult to clarify your legal and ethical obligations?

Treatment

Treatment for hallucinogen and inhalant use includes provision of safety for the individual who may be experiencing a "bad trip." Emergency measures may be necessary to provide respiratory support for an individual who has impaired gas exchange as a result of inhalants.

NURSING MANAGEMENT

ASSESSMENT FOR SUBSTANCE ABUSE (DATA COLLECTION)

A general physical assessment, including vital signs, is necessary. Any life-threatening physical problems must be quickly identified and treated. For example, patients can and do die of cardiac dysrhythmias associated with stimulant abuse, whereas patients who have overdosed on heroin are at risk for respiratory arrest.

Any patient who enters the health care system should be screened for substance abuse so that early intervention can prevent the immediate and long-term consequences of substance misuse. Obtain a substance and alcohol history that includes the type of substance used, the amount taken, and the duration and pattern of use. For patients scheduled for surgery, a thorough preoperative history is essential because a patient who normally drinks can return from surgery to a busy surgical unit and develop symptoms of alcohol withdrawal. An event of this type can complicate postoperative recovery and can be fatal.

Focused Assessment

Data Collection for Substance and Alcohol Use

Ask the following questions during history taking to determine past and present substance and/or alcohol use:

- Have you ever had a drinking or substance abuse problem?
- When did you last drink or use drugs of any kind?
- What substances (alcohol, tobacco, or illicit substances) are you currently using?
- What other types of drugs (prescription and nonprescription) do you routinely take?
- How much do you drink or how much do you use?
- How often do you drink or use substances?
- Have you ever tried to cut down or control your substance use or drinking?
- Have you noticed that now it takes more of the substance or drink to get the same effect you got several months ago?
- Have you noticed any withdrawal symptoms?
- Have you ever been treated for liver disease, hepatitis, heart disease, anemia, or overdose?
- Have you had any recent falls, accidents, or injuries?
- Have you ever stopped drinking or using drugs for a period?
- Have you ever been in treatment for substance abuse?
- Is there a family history of alcoholism or substance abuse?
- What is your relationship status? If in a relationship, is it a happy one?
- Have you ever been in trouble with the law?
- What is your occupation? Are you experiencing any difficulties at work?

A quick and simple assessment tool for alcohol abuse is the CAGE questionnaire, which includes four questions regarding the patient's feelings about their drinking and specific habits. A "yes" answer to two or more of the four questions has a 90% correlation with alcohol abuse. Also, obtain information about past and current function in family, social, and occupational roles. Remember that denial is a primary defense mechanism used in these disorders. Therefore it often is necessary to ask the family to describe their perception of the user's problem and the extent of substance use. At the appropriate time, assess the effects of the user's behavior on the family and explore the presence of codependent or enabling behaviors.

◆ NURSING DIAGNOSIS

Problem statements for substance use disorders include the following:

- Confusion due to excessive or chronic alcohol consumption
- Denial of physical and psychological dependence on a substance
- Altered family functioning due to substance addiction
- Potential for injury due to impaired judgment
- Altered role performance due to inability to complete assigned work duties
- Nonadherence with the treatment plan with substance abstinence

Clinical Cues

Patients enter the health care system with medical concerns or injuries but may also have unidentified substance use problems. When taking a routine admission history, ask about the use of substances. This information is needed to evaluate drug-drug interactions and any potential toxic effects on the body organs (i.e., heart, kidneys, liver). Use an objective approach and tone of voice when you ask: "Do you smoke or drink alcohol? What kind of prescription, over-the-counter, or illicit (street) drugs do you use?" In accordance with National Patient Safety Goals, your findings contribute to a complete list of medications. This medication reconciliation list should be communicated to the health care team, sent to other facilities if the patient is transferred, and provided to the patient when discharged.

◆ PLANNING

Expected outcomes chosen to resolve the patient's problems are created for the specific problems. For the problems mentioned, expected outcomes may include the following:

- Patient will demonstrate less confusion after receiving thiamine and abstaining from alcohol before discharge.
- Patient will discuss how reliance on substances is affecting quality of life during today's group therapy session.
- During weekly sessions with social service counselor, the patient and family will communicate needs and identify sources of support to sustain the family.
- Patient will remain safe from harm or injury during this shift.
- Patient will resume job duties within _____ months.
- Patient will participate in a 12-step program at least three times per week.

Older Adult Care Points

When working with older adults, assess for substance use disorders; this group is at high risk because of loneliness, multiple losses, and limited resources. Do not overlook the potential for inappropriate substance use in older adults by automatically attributing behaviors to aging, depression, or dementia.

Collaborative goal setting is very important when working with an individual who is addicted to a substance. In addition to working with the patient, it is necessary that you collaborate with the family. Setting goals with the patient and excluding the family or friends often lead to failure or relapse. Planning care for a patient with a substance use disorder includes promoting physical and psychological safety, providing a safe withdrawal from the substance, and ensuring adequate nutrition and sleep. To prevent relapse, education about substance abuse becomes a priority goal. The education may be started in a treatment center but needs to be continued after discharge for at least 1 year. People who abuse substances need opportunities to learn and practice new coping skills in a supportive environment.

Think Critically

Do you have any habits such as smoking, drinking too much alcohol, or consuming excess quantities of caffeine? How does your personal behavior affect what you will say to your patients about making changes for a healthier lifestyle?

◆ IMPLEMENTATION

Nursing intervention depends on the severity of the substance use disorder. Initial interventions for the patient focus on physical recovery. For example, cardiac monitoring, pulse oximetry, IV access, and other emergency measures may be indicated. Potentially fatal effects of drugs and/or alcohol use, such as cardiac dysrhythmias, hypotension, and respiratory depression, must receive priority attention. If the patient is intoxicated, orienting to person, place, and time and providing for physical safety are essential. You may need to advocate that the patient remains in a protected environment until judgment and coordination return. Ensuring adequate sleep and a balanced diet high in proteins and multivitamins are also part of early intervention.

If the patient is having symptoms of withdrawal, detoxification must be medically managed by giving antianxiety agents, such as chlordiazepoxide (Librium). Close monitoring of vital signs is important because signs of alcohol withdrawal include an increase in blood pressure and heart rate. Preventing the patient from experiencing a seizure or delirium tremens is an essential part of the detoxification process.

Clinical Cues

When monitoring and reporting changes in blood pressure, keep several factors in mind: patient's baseline, trends (if available), and medications (last dose and type). Also assess for accompanying subjective symptoms such as dizziness or lightheadedness (hypotension), headache, or blurred vision (hypertension).

Once the substance is cleared from the body, nursing intervention is directed toward helping the patient lead a drug-free life. This includes alleviating the symptoms and confronting denial. You must also observe for signs of suicide. Patients who are addicted often feel they cannot live without the euphoria and consolation of the substance experience.

Assignment Considerations

One-to-One Observation

A certified nursing assistant (CNA) or unlicensed assistive personnel (UAP) is frequently assigned to sit with a patient who needs one-to-one (1 : 1) supervision. Before assigning personnel to this task, clarify with the health care provider or registered nurse (RN) the purpose of 1 : 1 observation and the stability of the patient. For example, recall that opioid withdrawal is not life threatening, but that due to the discomfort of this process, the patient may be temporarily placed on 1 : 1 observation to prevent **elopement** (leaving) to seek drugs to satisfy the intense craving. It would be appropriate to assign a CNA or UAP to prevent elopement. In contrast, an agitated patient who is withdrawing from alcohol is not physically stable, and this care should be managed by an RN.

Patients who are in the early recovery process from substance abuse benefit greatly from therapeutic conversations, and a caring, concerned attitude is very important. Patients must grieve the loss of the substance, and they also feel guilt and shame for acts that were committed while under the influence. To help the patient "work through" these feelings, be an active listener and offer support and validation as necessary. Mandating a patient to stop using substances is not an effective intervention; however, you should support the patient's decision to stop and teach that the physical symptoms of withdrawal will not last forever. The craving will last longer than the withdrawal symptoms but is manageable if the patient has a strong motivation to change toward a healthy lifestyle. You can assist these patients to identify ways to cope with the craving, such as helping them make a list of activities that could be used to distract attention from the craving, such as calling a friend, taking a brisk walk, cleaning the house, or eating a nutritious snack. You can help the patient identify settings, circumstances, or relationships that contributed to the substance abuse pattern, then identify alternative settings and relationships that are now part of the new lifestyle. For example, polysubstance use might routinely occur in a bar or lounge with friends after having a few beers but is less likely to occur in a movie theater with friends who are eating popcorn.

If the patient is addicted to heroin, the recovery process will be lengthy because of the lifestyle changes that are necessary. With heroin addiction, there may have been some illegal actions and maladaptive coping. The patient needs to be educated about the disease process and needs to learn new coping methods (Nursing Care Plan 48.1).

Intervening With the Family

A trusting relationship must be developed with the family, or they may continue to focus on the patient

Nursing Care Plan 48.1 Care of a Patient With a Substance Use Disorder

SCENARIO

Jack Walters is a 47-year-old man brought in by his supervisor for admission to a "detox" unit. The supervisor states that he last saw Mr. Walters drinking about 10 hours ago. He states that Jack is a good worker but could lose his job if he doesn't get help. Mr. Walters jokingly replies, "My boss is a worrier. I'm just a social drinker. My wife and kids know I'm okay." The supervisor states that Mr. Walters's wife frequently makes excuses for Jack's absences but seems unaware of the depth of the problem. Mr. Walters seems slightly anxious and irritable. He appears thin and malnourished.

PROBLEM STATEMENT

Potential for injury due to effects of substance and complications of withdrawal.

SUPPORTING ASSESSMENT DATA

Objective: Slightly anxious and irritable; last known drink 10 hours ago.

Goals/Expected Outcomes	Nursing Interventions	Selected Rationale	Evaluation
Patient will remain free from any injury this shift. Patient will withdraw from alcohol without any dangerous effects.	Assess for early symptoms of withdrawal (e.g., agitation, irritability, anxiety) and notify health care provider or RN of first signs.	Early detection of withdrawal allows for prompt intervention to prevent life-threatening complications.	Is anxious and irritable.
	Administer medications (e.g., chlordiazepoxide [Librium]) as prescribed by provider.	Decreases neurologic irritability at the biochemical level.	30 min after administration of medication, patient appears more relaxed.
	Remain with patient during times of confusion and disorientation.	Provides support and decreases agitation.	Currently alert and oriented.
	Restrain and/or place in seclusion as ordered if the patient becomes a danger to self or others.	May temporarily be unable to control aggressive or self-harm impulses. May attempt to leave.	Is verbally hostile and denies substance abuse problems but shows no signs of physical aggression.
	Ensure safe environment (i.e., call bell within reach, bed in lowest position).	Safety is a priority, and patient judgment and coordination may be temporarily impaired.	Did not sustain any injury during the shift.

PROBLEM STATEMENT

Denial due to minimization of the symptoms of addiction.

SUPPORTING ASSESSMENT DATA

Subjective: States, "My boss is a worrier. I'm just a social drinker."

Objective: Supervisor's report and Mr. Walters's perception of problem are incongruent.

Goals/Expected Outcomes	Nursing Interventions	Selected Rationale	Evaluation
Patient will acknowledge the abuse of substances and the unhealthy effects on his life.	Approach the patient in a nonjudgmental manner.	Helps to build trust and rapport.	Is agreeable to talking but is unable to disclose feelings.
	Gently confront the denial as you gain the trust of the patient.	Breaking through denial is essential to recovery.	Denial continues.
Patient will openly acknowledge the need for substance use disorder treatment.	Help the patient see the need for treatment and abstinence.	May be unaware of or is ignoring the long-term consequences of substance use.	Denies need for treatment.
	Inform the patient about the negative aspects of addictive processes.	Helps the patient make an informed decision.	Verbally acknowledges that substances are harmful for others, "but I don't drink that much."
	Encourage patient to list the harmful effects he has experienced.	Increases insight and facilitates self-diagnosis.	Denies that substances are harming him.
Patient will agree to attend ninety 12-step meetings in 90 days.	Encourage attendance at a 12-step program to help break through the denial.	Provides support by others who have experienced the same condition.	Agrees to go to a 12-step program but thinks it is unnecessary.

Continued

Nursing Care Plan 48.1 Care of a Patient With a Substance Use Disorder—cont'd

PROBLEM STATEMENT/NURSING DIAGNOSIS

Altered family functioning due to patient's use of alcohol.

SUPPORTING ASSESSMENT DATA

Subjective: Per supervisor, wife frequently makes excuses but seems unaware of the problem.
Objective: Wife is absent; supervisor is advocating for treatment.

Goals/Expected Outcomes	Nursing Interventions	Selected Rationale	Evaluation
Family will be able to identify and share feelings.	Invite family to participate.	Family may be unaware or need assistance to break through their denial.	Wife and children did come in to talk with provider and social worker about patient's condition.
	Assess for presence of denial, shame, or guilt.	Feelings of denial, shame, and guilt are expected but may be repressed.	Family members expressed support for patient but are unable to disclose personal feelings.
	Encourage expression of genuine feelings.	Opportunity for expression of feelings helps build trust and rapport.	Trust and rapport are being established, but communication between family members continues to be ineffective.
	Teach how to recognize feelings and safe ways to express them (e.g., "I love you, but I am not going to stay here while you drink.").	New communication methods are needed to help the family break old patterns.	Currently family is not openly acknowledging how patient's behavior affects each member, but they agree to attend group therapy.
	Educate the family about the altered roles present in addictive families (e.g., wife overcompensating for husband).	Family members may be unaware of how the illness is affecting role function.	Family is not identifying dysfunctional roles but appears open to exploring the family situation.
	Define the term *enabling* for family members.	Identifying and defining enabling help family to recognize this behavior.	Entire family appears to be in denial at this time; denies enabling behaviors.
	Encourage family members to state at least one time when they engaged in enabling behavior.	Increases insight into own behavior.	
	Offer family members alternative choices to enabling behavior (e.g., telling the patient that he must call in sick for himself).	Family needs new ways to cope with old problems.	Family open to learning more about disease process and how to cope with patient's behavior.
	Have family members practice and role play alternative responses to enabling behavior.	Practice in a safe environment allows family to test new skills.	Family having difficulty with role play.
Family will agree to attend at least six 12-step meetings in the next 12 days.	Encourage family members to attend a 12-step support meeting.	Provides support by sharing with others who are experiencing the same problem.	Family agrees to go to a 12-step group this weekend.

PROBLEM STATEMENT/NURSING DIAGNOSIS

Altered nutrition due to poor food intake, inadequate absorption of nutrients, poor appetite.

SUPPORTING ASSESSMENT DATA

Objective: Appears thin and malnourished.

Goals/Expected Outcomes	Nursing Interventions	Selected Rationale	Evaluation
Patient will self-select a nutritious diet.	Assess ability to feed self.	May have impairment in fine motor coordination.	Able to independently feed self; shows some fine tremors in hands.

Nursing Care Plan 48.1 Care of a Patient With a Substance Use Disorder—cont'd

Goals/Expected Outcomes	Nursing Interventions	Selected Rationale	Evaluation
Patient will gain 5 lb within 1 mo; signs of peripheral neuropathy (numbness and tingling) will disappear.	Watch for nausea, vomiting, diarrhea. Administer antacids, antiemetics, and IV fluids as ordered.	Alcohol can cause gastritis and alterations in absorption.	Currently no nausea or vomiting.
	Document intake and output and food intake. Weigh patient.	To monitor nutritional status and progress toward goal.	Weighs 140 lb (ideal body weight 165 lb). Finishes all food trays.
	Collaborate with patient to determine food preferences.	Increases likelihood of consumption.	Eats all types of food.
	Encourage small, frequent meals, high in proteins with 50% carbohydrates.	Small meals are easier to tolerate, and foods rich in nutrition will replace loss due to poor dietary practices.	States that he sometimes forgets to eat but knows he should gain some weight ("Will try harder").
	Administer multivitamins, especially thiamine (vitamin B_1) and niacin, as ordered.	Patient is at risk for Wernicke encephalopathy.	Agrees that supplements are a good idea and will continue to take them after discharge.
	Consult nutritionist.	Collaboration with specialist ensures best plan.	Consultation with nutritionist will help patient understand healthy food choices he can make after discharge.

CRITICAL THINKING QUESTIONS

1. What are some questions that would be appropriate to ask Mrs. Walters since she was willing to come in and meet with the health care team?
2. Mr. Walters is currently far from being ready to acknowledge his condition. What are some things that might signal that he is breaking through the denial?

IV, Intravenous; *RN*, registered nurse.

rather than on their own recovery. Families need to learn in what manner they might have been enabling their loved one, and they need time to practice new behaviors that will require the patient to take responsibility. Family members should be encouraged to express how the crisis is affecting them. There may be a need to refer families to legal or social services if the person is abusing illegal drugs or if there was an arrest for driving while intoxicated. The family often feels shame and guilt and shares the stigma associated with substance use. Encourage them to seek support from groups such as Nar-Anon, Al-Anon, or Alateen. Family members may consider substance misuse a moral weakness rather than a disease. Educating them about the neurobiological theories may help them reconsider their attitudes and relieve some guilt. To be effective in working with patients who use substances, you must examine your own attitudes and make certain that patients and families are treated with respect.

Think Critically

A patient discloses social drinking, but the patient's partner and children tell you that the patient drinks to the point of intoxication at least three times a week. What would you say to the family? What would you say to the patient?

◆ EVALUATION

Recovery from a substance use disorder is a lengthy process. Ridding the body of substances can take weeks, particularly if there is coexisting liver damage. Often the patient is malnourished, physically exhausted, and in poor general health. Return to an optimum healthy state may take 6 months to 1 year. Recovery of psychological or emotional health takes even longer. If the patient started misusing drugs at a very young age, emotional development may have been stunted. Coping mechanisms to deal with anxiety or emotional pain may have never properly developed if the individual used substances instead.

Consequently, nurses working in the hospital may see only early physical recovery. Evaluating overall effectiveness of substance use treatment is measured in years rather than weeks. Admitting a patient to a hospital and guiding them safely though detoxification are necessary, even though these are small, beginning steps in the overall process of recovery.

COMMUNITY CARE

Nurses who work in emergency departments and busy outpatient clinics often see individuals who have medical problems related to substance use. *Healthy People 2030* goals include a proactive approach to use these incidental contacts to screen for substance use and appropriately refer these patients right away to prevent costly long-term complications.

Inpatient hospital stays for individuals with addiction are usually short. If the patient has some type of insurance, it is not unusual for the insurance company to pay only for medical detoxification. Any further treatment that is necessary would be performed on an outpatient basis.

Deciding to become sober and/or substance free typically requires lifestyle changes. Changes of this magnitude are not made overnight. Individuals who are addicted to substances may need ongoing medical support, as well as support from the recovery community. Encourage patients who are attempting recovery to seek help and make the recovery process a priority. You can be instrumental in facilitating public awareness and in educating patients about the responsible use, and ultimate hazards, of mood-altering substances. Nurses should also be politically attuned to legislation that regulates product availability and marketing of substances.

Get Ready for the NCLEX® Examination!

Key Points

- Substance use disorder is diagnosed when ingestion of psychoactive substances such as alcohol, drugs, or other substances results in recognizable signs and symptoms.
- Psychoactive substances are mind-altering agents capable of changing or altering a person's mood, behavior, cognition, arousal level, level of consciousness, and perceptions.
- Abuse implies use of a psychoactive substance in a nontherapeutic manner or the illicit use of prescription drugs.
- Dependence implies the presence of physical or psychological symptoms of addiction; when the substance use is stopped, withdrawal symptoms appear.
- Withdrawal symptoms occur when there is an attempt to stop using a substance.
- Symptoms of withdrawal from CNS depressants include increased blood pressure and pulse, nervousness, and heightened anxiety.
- Symptoms of withdrawal from CNS stimulants include drowsiness, headache, lethargy, nausea, alterations in eating and sleeping patterns, and cravings.
- Medical conditions related to alcohol use disorder include liver damage, cardiomyopathy, hypertension, gastrointestinal bleeding, stroke, sleep disturbances, malnutrition, peripheral neuropathies, chronic infection, cognitive impairment, Wernicke's encephalopathy, and Korsakoff syndrome.
- Assess for physical, psychological, and behavioral symptoms of abuse or withdrawal.
- Take a history from the patient and the family to determine type, amount, and pattern of use.
- General nursing interventions when caring for patients with substance use disorders include observing for life-threatening conditions, safely managing detoxification, orienting the patient to reality, providing a balanced diet high in protein and multivitamins, setting limits, confronting denial, identifying enabling behaviors and teaching new coping mechanisms, and referring to a 12-step program.
- Denial and rationalization are primary defense mechanisms used by the patient who uses substances and by the family.
- Enabling behaviors ("helping" a person so that the consequences of unhealthy behavior are less severe) or codependency (occurs when a family member or friend attempts to control the behaviors of the person who uses substances) further inhibit recovery.
- Older adults may drink to alleviate depression and loneliness. Decreased liver and renal function can quickly lead to toxicity and dependence.

Additional Learning Resources

SG Go to your Study Guide for additional learning activities to help you master this chapter content.

Go to your Evolve website (http://evolve.elsevier.com/deWit/medsurg) for the following FREE learning resources:

- Animations, audio, and video
- Answers and rationales for questions and activities
- Glossary with pronunciations in English and Spanish
- Interactive Review Questions and more!

Review Questions for the NCLEX® Examination

1. You are taking a history for a patient who needs emergency surgery and who freely admits to using marijuana, alcohol, cocaine, and hallucinogens. Which is the appropriate nursing question?
   1. "Does your partner know that you are using drugs?"
   2. "When was the last time you drank or took a substance?"
   3. "How frequently are you using these drugs and alcohol?"
   4. "Have you ever tried to get treatment for your substance use?"

   NCLEX Client Need: Physiological Integrity: Reduction of Risk Potential

2. Which patient response indicates that large doses of vitamin B_1 for treatment of Wernicke encephalopathy are working?
   1. No seizure activity
   2. Less confusion and improvement of memory
   3. Decreased urge to drink alcohol
   4. No tremors, nausea, or vomiting

   NCLEX Client Need: Physiological Integrity: Pharmacological Therapies
3. Which patient statement indicates a positive step in the recovery from alcohol use disorder?
   1. "I do think my job is at the root of my alcohol consumption."
   2. "I don't have any power over the effects alcohol has on me."
   3. "I don't ever want to use alcohol again."
   4. "To stay sober I will increase my exercise and eat healthy foods."

   NCLEX Client Need: Psychosocial Integrity
4. The spouse of a patient with alcohol use disorder makes excuses to their children when the patient fails to do things that were promised. What is the priority problem?
   1. Limited coping ability
   2. Altered family functioning
   3. Absence of compliance
   4. Decreased self-esteem

   NCLEX Client Need: Psychosocial Integrity
5. The usage of "bath salts" is a societal problem because it: *(Select all that apply.)*
   1. is illegal in all states under federal law.
   2. is the most addictive of all abused substances.
   3. is easily obtained over the internet and in many stores.
   4. potentially causes violence, paranoia, and suicide.
   5. causes lung cancer if smoked excessively.

   NCLEX Client Need: Health Promotion and Maintenance
6. A postoperative patient who also has alcohol use disorder was given chlordiazepoxide for increased blood pressure, increased pulse, tremors, nausea and vomiting, and diaphoresis. What is the rationale for use of this medication?
   1. Prevention of postoperative clot formation
   2. Reduction of symptoms of alcohol withdrawal
   3. Control of blood pressure
   4. Relief of postoperative nausea and vomiting

   NCLEX Client Need: Physiological Integrity: Pharmacological Therapies
7. What is the appropriate nursing response when a patient with alcohol use disorder asks, "What is the purpose of Antabuse"?
   1. "It blocks the craving for alcohol."
   2. "The medication causes unpleasant symptoms when you drink."
   3. "The drug keeps you from having seizures."
   4. "It controls symptoms of nausea, vomiting, pain, or cramps."

   NCLEX Client Need: Physiological Integrity: Pharmacological Therapies
8. The wife of a patient suggests that the patient may have a problem with substance use. Which assessment questions should you ask the patient? *(Select all that apply.)*
   1. "What substances are you currently using?"
   2. "How often do you drink or use illicit substances?"
   3. "When did you last drink or use drugs of any kind?"
   4. "How do you feel about people who use substances?"
   5. "Why does your wife think you have a substance abuse problem?"
   6. "Is there a family history of alcoholism or substance abuse?"

   NCLEX Client Need: Psychosocial Integrity
9. Which patient do you anticipate may have a dual diagnosis? The patient with:
   1. bipolar disorder and anxiety
   2. alcohol use disorder and alcohol intoxication
   3. schizophrenia and cannabis use disorder
   4. major depressive disorder and PTSD.

   NCLEX Client Need: Psychosocial Integrity
10. A patient is in the early recovery process and is attempting to lead a drug-free life. Which nursing intervention is the most appropriate?
    1. Remind the patient of the discomfort and pain that occurred during detoxification.
    2. Tell the patient that there is no need to feel guilty or ashamed.
    3. Help the patient to identify relationships that were part of the substance use pattern.
    4. Advise the patient that stopping forever is the only choice for a drug-free life.

    NCLEX Client Need: Psychosocial Integrity

Critical Thinking Questions

Scenario A

Mrs. Gordon was recently widowed and misses her spouse very much. As she enters the health care provider's office, she is noted to be stumbling. She has slurred speech and an alcohol-like smell to her breath. When you approach her, Mrs. Gordon begins to cry and says she doesn't want to see the provider; she is going to drive home.

1. What type of assessment will you perform on this patient?
2. How will you ensure Mrs. Gordon's safety?

Scenario B

Ms. Suter, age 25 years, is a patient in an outpatient health care provider's office. She admits to a history of illicit substance abuse and states that she has been drug free for the past year. You notice that she leaves the treatment room to use the bathroom; when she returns her coordination is slightly impaired and she seems inappropriately euphoric and giddy. You observe her hiding a plastic bag in her purse.

1. How would you handle this situation?
2. What types of documentation should you perform?

Scenario C

Mr. Fischer, a 44-year-old construction worker, was admitted for emergency orthopedic surgery yesterday evening after falling from a roof. He begins yelling profanity and is irritable and argumentative. He seems to have difficulty concentrating on your questions. His wife states that Mr. Fischer must not have told the surgeon that he drinks 12 beers nightly.

1. What do you anticipate is happening to Mr. Fischer?
2. What other signs and symptoms would you assess for at this time?
3. Provide appropriate nursing interventions, given Mr. Fischer's condition.

Scenario D

Mr. Dubois is a 25-year-old patient. His father states that the family frequently argues over Mr. Dubois's drinking. The father feels that his son is "weak," yet the mother and Mr. Dubois state that his drinking is "not a big deal."

1. Discuss emotional and psychological responses that are common among patients and families when there is a substance use problem.
2. What could you say to the father to help him understand that substance use disorder is a physical and psychological problem that can be treated?
3. How could you help the mother understand that she may be enabling her son's behavior?

Care of Patients With Thought and Personality Disorders

49

http://evolve.elsevier.com/deWit/medsurg

Objectives

Theory

1. Discuss common thought and personality disorders.
2. Choose effective communication tactics for a patient experiencing psychosis.
3. Identify effective teaching strategies for a patient with a personality disorder.
4. Determine appropriate nursing interventions for a patient with schizophrenia.
5. Explore how to modify personal feelings of bias when caring for a patient with manipulative behaviors.
6. Discuss the role of medications in treatment of thought and personality disorders.

Clinical Practice

7. Care for a medical surgical patient who also has a thought and personality disorder diagnosis.
8. Create a plan of care for a patient with borderline personality disorder.

Key Terms

akathisia (ă-kă-THĒ-zhă, p. 1130)
alogia (ă-LŌ-jyă, p. 1129)
anhedonia (ăn-hĕ-DŌ-nyă, p. 1129)
atypical antipsychotics (ā-tĭ-pĭ-kăl ăn-tē-sī-KŎT-ĭks, p. 1131)
avolition (ă-vō-LĬ-shŭn, p. 1129)
borderline personality disorder (BPD) (BŎR-dĕr-līn pĕr-sŏ-NĂL-ĭ-tē dĭs-ŌR-dĕr, p. 1138)
command hallucinations (KŎM-mănd hă-lū-sĭ-NĀ-shŭns, p. 1131)
delusions (dĕ-LŪ-zhŭn, p. 1127)
dystonic reaction (dĭs-TŎN-ĭk rē-ĂK-shŭn, p. 1130)
first-generation antipsychotics (fĕrst jĕ-nĕ-RĀ-shŭn ăn-tē-sī-KŌ-tĭks, p. 1130)
hallucinations (hă-lū-sĭ-NĀ-shŭn, p. 1127)
illusion (ĭ-LŪ-zhŭn, p. 1128)
loose associations (lūs u-sō-sē-Ā-shĕnz, p. 1131)
milieu therapy (mēl-yū THĔR-ă-pē, p. 1139)
negative symptoms (NĔG-ă-tĭv, p. 1129)
neologisms (NĒ-ō-lō-jĭzm, p. 1131)
oculogyric crisis (ŏk-ū-lō-JĪ-rĭk KRĪ-sĭs, p. 1130)
personality disorders (pĕr-sŏ-NĂL-ĭ-tē dĭs-ŌR-dĕrz, p. 1134)
positive symptoms (PŎ-zĭ-tĭv SĬMP-tŭm, p. 1128)
psychotherapy (sī-kō-THĔR-ă-pē, p. 1139)
psychotic features (sī-KŎ-tĭk, p. 1127)
schizophrenia (skĭt-sō-FRĒ-nē-ă, p. 1127)
splitting (SPLĬ-tĭng, p. 1138)
tardive dyskinesia (TĂR-dīv dĭs-kĭ-NĒ-zhē-ă, p. 1130)
therapeutic alliance (thĕr-ŭ-PYŪ-tĭk U-LĪ-ĕns, p. 1134)
thought disorders (thŏt dĭs-ŌR-dĕr, p. 1127)
word salad (wĕrd SĂ-lĕd, p. 1131)

Concepts Covered in This Chapter

- Self-Management
- Mood and Affect
- Cognition
- Psychosis
- Communication
- Safety

OVERVIEW OF THOUGHT DISORDERS

The *Diagnostic and Statistical Manual of Mental Disorders*, Fifth edition (DSM-5) (American Psychiatric Association, 2013) defines **thought disorders** by the presence of psychotic symptoms. **Schizophrenia** is the most common thought disorder. Examples of **psychotic features** include **hallucinations** (hearing, seeing, smelling, tasting, or feeling something that is not there), **delusions** (false fixed ideas), and disorganized speech and/or behavior.

It is estimated that 1.1% of the general population is affected with schizophrenia; this represents 3.5 million Americans (Schizophrenia and Related Disorders Alliance of America, 2018).

SCHIZOPHRENIA

Etiology and Pathophysiology

The exact cause of schizophrenia is unknown, but several types of theories exist: genetic, neurobiological, brain structure abnormalities, and influences from psychological and environmental factors. Evidence suggests that several genes on several different chromosomes may play a role. Neurobiologically, structural differences and abnormality of the amount of the neurotransmitter dopamine are believed to contribute to the disorder. Neurotransmitters are chemical messengers that are produced and stored in the nerve terminal **(axon)**

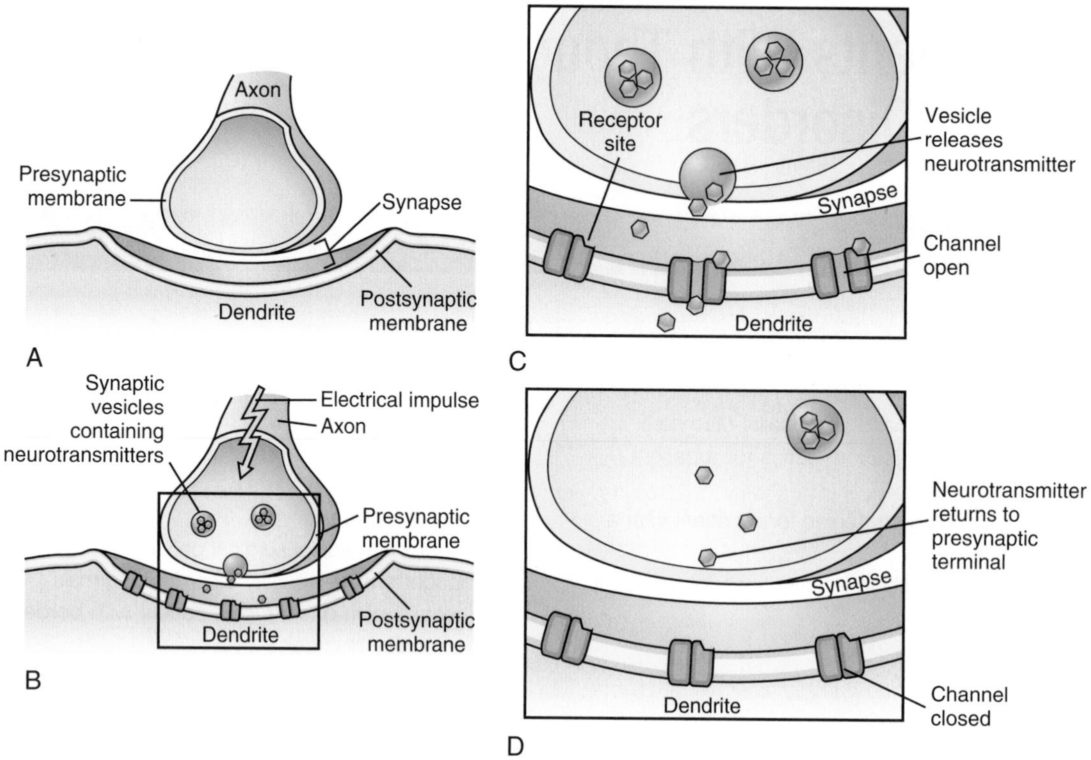

Fig. 49.1 Neurotransmitters. **A,** Axon with stored neurotransmitters and dendrite with receptor sites. **B** and **C,** Electrical impulse causes release of neurotransmitter. **D,** Receptor sites close and neurotransmitter returns to storage.

(Fig. 49.1). Low dopamine activity in the cortex of the cingulate gyrus contributes to the negative symptoms of schizophrenia, and higher than usual dopamine activity in the limbic system contributes to the positive symptoms. Other neurotransmitters such as serotonin, norepinephrine, and gamma-aminobutyric acid (GABA) also interact in the disorder, although this process it not fully understood. Glutamate continues to be researched as another contributory factor (Howes, McCutcheon, & Stone, 2015). Brain structure abnormalities in individuals with schizophrenia have been identified and include enlargement of the lateral cerebral ventricles; reduced cortical, frontal lobe, and hippocampus volume; and increased fissure size on the surface of the brain.

Prenatal stressors such as birth complications, prenatal viral infection, poor maternal nutrition, and exposure to toxins have been studied as contributory factors to the development of schizophrenia. Psychological stress appears to precipitate the disease when other factors are present in people who appear to be susceptible. Environmental factors such as exposure to chronic poverty or a high-crime environment also have an effect. Schizophrenia usually develops between the ages of 15 and 25 years (Halter, 2018).

Patients with schizophrenia often experience cognitive impairment such as difficulty with memory, judgment, problem solving, and decision making. Coexisting mental health problems such as anxiety and depression can also occur. Overall, the individual's quality of life is affected by schizophrenia, making it challenging for many of these patients to function independently in society.

Complementary and Alternative Therapies

Omega-3 Fatty Acids

A study by Qiao and colleagues (2018) found that patients with schizophrenia who exhibited violent behavior demonstrated less violent behaviors when treated with fish oil (360 mg docosahexaenoic acid [DHA] and 540 mg eicosapentaenoic acid [EPA]); however, it is important to note that this treatment did not change the presence of negative and positive symptoms.

Signs and Symptoms

Signs and symptoms associated with schizophrenia are divided into positive (present) and negative (absent) symptoms (Fig. 49.2). **Positive symptoms** of schizophrenia are those that should *not* be there. Examples include hallucinations, delusions, disordered thinking or loose associations between thoughts, and hearing voices **(auditory hallucinations)** that tell the person what to do.

Delusions can be either grandiose or persecutory. An individual who believes he is a king is having **delusions of grandeur.** Individuals with **delusions of persecution** believe that they are being persecuted by agencies, by other people, or by supernatural beings. An **illusion** is a misinterpretation of something that really exists. For example, an electrical cord appears to be a snake, or a pencil is misinterpreted to be a knife blade. When **ideas of reference** occur, the individual believes that events or situations are occurring because of—or specifically for—them. A common idea of reference is to believe that people on the television are sending

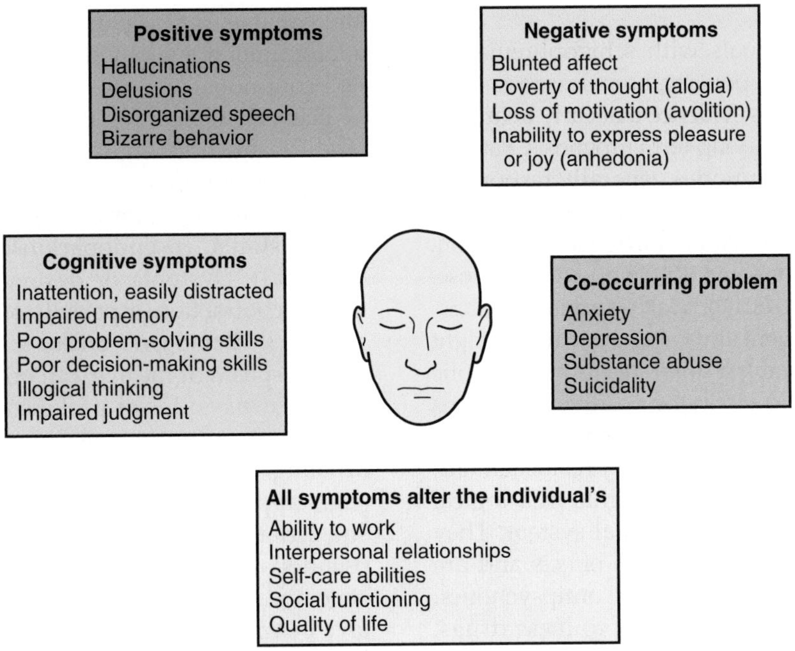

Positive symptoms
Hallucinations
Delusions
Disorganized speech
Bizarre behavior
Negative symptoms
Blunted affect
Poverty of thought (alogia)
Loss of motivation (avolition)
Inability to express pleasure or joy (anhedonia)
Cognitive symptoms
Inattention, easily distracted
Impaired memory
Poor problem-solving skills
Poor decision-making skills
Illogical thinking
Impaired judgment
Co-occurring problem
Anxiety
Depression
Substance abuse
Suicidality
All symptoms alter the individual's
Ability to work
Interpersonal relationships
Self-care abilities
Social functioning
Quality of life

Fig. 49.2 Signs and symptoms of schizophrenia.

special telepathic messages. Positive symptoms are much more responsive to medication therapy compared with negative symptoms; however, some patients will tell you that "the voices are always there, but if I take my medications the voices are less intrusive."

Negative symptoms are abilities or personal characteristics that are **absent** or lost to the patient with schizophrenia. Think of elements of personality that make people motivated, socially outgoing, happy, and active in daily life, and then take those away. The results are negative symptoms: apathy, social withdrawal, psychomotor retardation, flat affect (obvious absence of emotional expression), poverty of thoughts (**alogia**), lack of motivation (**avolition**), and inability to experience pleasure or joy (**anhedonia**). These symptoms are notoriously more difficult to treat because the patient often does not seek help.

Think Critically

Why might friends and family fail to recognize that there is a problem when schizophrenia first develops in a teenager or young adult? Describe how you might feel, and how it would change your life, if someone you love developed schizophrenia as a teenager or as a young adult.

Safety Alert

Be Cautious, Not Fearful

Having a dual diagnosis of substance abuse and schizophrenia is the greatest predictor of potential violence in a patient with schizophrenia (Rund, 2018). Be mindful of symptoms of escalation, such as pacing, rolling fingers or making fists, or speaking increasingly harshly or loudly. Use strategies to de-escalate the patient's behaviors, always being mindful to keep yourself and others safe.

Table 49.1 Types of Behaviors Associated With Schizophrenia

BEHAVIORAL TYPE	BEHAVIORS MANIFESTED
Paranoia	Exhibits extreme suspiciousness, delusions of grandeur, and delusions of persecution. Can be hostile and aggressive. Auditory hallucinations are common.
Catatonia	Exhibits a stuporous condition associated with rigidity, unusual posturing, and waxy flexibility (maintains a limb in one position for a long time). Also demonstrates echopraxia (imitating the motions of others) and echolalia (involuntary repetition of words spoken by others). Exhibits unpredictable behavior because behavior is controlled by delusions and hallucinations.
Disorganization	Exhibits flat affect, silliness, and incoherence. Has gross thought disturbances, including word salad and neologisms. Delusions and hallucinations are common.

Diagnosis

Diagnosis is based on criteria found within the DSM-5 (American Psychiatric Association, 2013). Although schizophrenia is a single diagnosis under DSM-5 criteria, behaviors such as paranoia, catatonia, and disorganization are associated with this disorder (Table 49.1). Note that many patients with schizophrenia have other mental illness problems and may have a dual diagnosis.

Treatment

If left untreated, individuals with schizophrenia are particularly vulnerable to poverty, homelessness, drug abuse, and suicide. There is evidence that early treatment for schizophrenia improves long-term prognosis. Patients who are treated for first episodes generally respond to the therapeutic effects and require lower doses of antipsychotic medications. After starting a medication, the patient should be monitored for therapeutic response. The onset of different medications takes varying amounts of time, so teach the patient and caregivers that it might take several weeks to notice a difference. Antipsychotic medications (neuroleptics) treat the positive symptoms of schizophrenia (Box 49.1). **First-generation antipsychotics** are very effective in stopping auditory hallucinations, enabling the patient to connect thoughts in a logical manner, and eliminating the delusional system. They do cause serious and unpleasant side effects and are less commonly prescribed than atypical antipsychotics. However, some patients respond well to these drugs, and particularly for patients who have taken them for a long time, it is likely that a successful drug regimen will continue.

The side effects for these medications include the familiar anticholinergic effects of dry mouth, flushing, urinary retention, and constipation. These drugs also can cause **extrapyramidal side effects** (EPSs), including dystonia, pseudoparkinsonism, and akathisia (Fig. 49.3). Dystonia or **dystonic reaction** is an acute muscle contraction, especially of the tongue, face, neck, and back. **Oculogyric crisis**, a fixed upward gaze or muscle spasm of the eye, can occur. **Pseudoparkinsonism,** or drug-induced parkinsonism, consists of poor balance, flat affect, slowed movements, tremors, and drooling. **Akathisia** presents as motor restlessness (e.g., tapping a foot, rocking, pacing) or apprehension and irritability. Treatment for akathisia, dystonia, or pseudoparkinsonism is to lower the dosage of the first-generation antipsychotic or change the medication and give benztropine (Cogentin).

Tardive dyskinesia is a primary concern because symptoms are irreversible once they have developed if not caught early. Symptoms include tongue protrusion; lip smacking; sucking; chewing; blinking; lateral jaw movements; grimacing; shoulder shrugging; pelvic thrusting; wrist and ankle flexion or rotation; foot tapping and toe movements; and rapid, purposeless, and irregular movements. Movements are often described as writhing and wormlike. Monitor for signs of tardive dyskinesia, particularly in patients who have been taking a first-generation antipsychotic medication for longer than 6 to 12 months. The Abnormal Involuntary Movement Scale (AIMS) is an effective tool to measure symptoms associated with tardive dyskinesia.

Other adverse effects associated with the use of antipsychotic medications include blurred vision; bone

Box 49.1 Drugs Used to Treat Schizophrenia

CONVENTIONAL DRUGS	ATYPICAL DRUGS[a]
Chlorpromazine	Clozapine (Clozaril)[b]
Fluphenazine hydrochloride	Aripiprazole (Abilify)
Haloperidol (Haldol)	Olanzapine (Zyprexa)
Loxapine	Quetiapine (Seroquel)
Molindone	Risperidone (Risperdal)
Perphenazine	Ziprasidone (Geodon)
Thioridazine	Paliperidone (Invega)
Trifluoperazine	Iloperidone (Fanapt)
	Asenapine (Saphris)

[a]These drugs have fewer side effects than the conventional medications.
[b]First atypical antipsychotic; only prescribed with caution because of potential agranulocytosis. Frequent monitoring of white blood cell count is necessary.

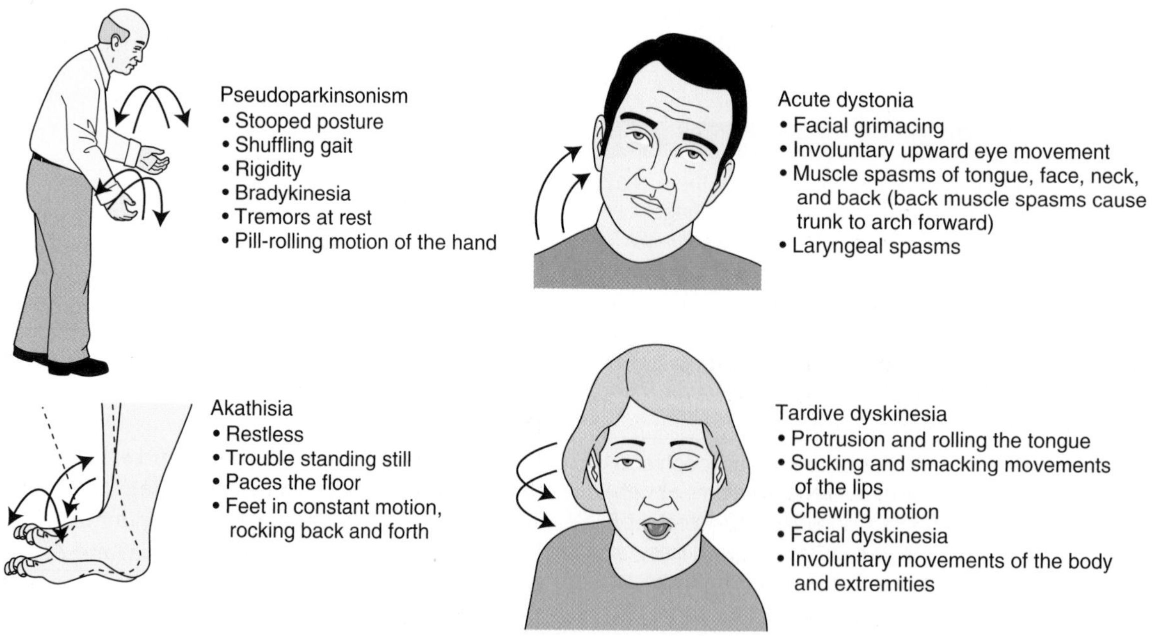

Pseudoparkinsonism
• Stooped posture
• Shuffling gait
• Rigidity
• Bradykinesia
• Tremors at rest
• Pill-rolling motion of the hand
Acute dystonia
• Facial grimacing
• Involuntary upward eye movement
• Muscle spasms of tongue, face, neck, and back (back muscle spasms cause trunk to arch forward)
• Laryngeal spasms
Akathisia
• Restless
• Trouble standing still
• Paces the floor
• Feet in constant motion, rocking back and forth
Tardive dyskinesia
• Protrusion and rolling the tongue
• Sucking and smacking movements of the lips
• Chewing motion
• Facial dyskinesia
• Involuntary movements of the body and extremities

Fig. 49.3 Characteristics of pseudoparkinsonism, acute dystonia, akathisia, and tardive dyskinesia.

marrow suppression; cardiac dysrhythmias; endocrine changes such as elevation of blood sugar, weight gain, and breast enlargement; and **hepatotoxicity** (liver injury and jaundice). **Neuroleptic malignant syndrome** is a rare reaction; however, it is life threatening, and the patient typically will be transferred to the intensive care unit. Symptoms include high fever, increased pulse, muscle rigidity, stupor, incontinence, elevated white blood cell count, hyperkalemia, and renal failure.

Older Adult Care Points

Older adults who are taking antipsychotic medications are at a higher than usual risk for developing serious side effects. Baseline cardiac, renal, hepatic, and hematologic studies need to be done before initiating psychotropic drugs. The beginning dosages should be one half to one third of the normal adult dosage. Older adults need to be watched very closely for difficulty swallowing, constipation and fecal impaction, weight gain, memory impairment, and orthostatic hypotension.

Atypical antipsychotics (see Box 49.1) have the advantages of fewer side effects, particularly tardive dyskinesia, than first-generation antipsychotics and offer some success with treating negative symptoms. Olanzapine comes in a quickly dissolving oral form that is a potential alternative to an injection. This form is more expensive; however, it eliminates the risk of needle-stick injury if the patient is combative, and it discourages "cheeking" (attempts to avoid swallowing by holding the pill in the cheek pouch). Aripiprazole (Abilify) is a medication called a dopamine system stabilizer. Medications approved for schizophrenia include paliperidone (Invega), iloperidone (Fanapt), and asenapine (Saphris). Table 49.2 presents medication side effects and nursing implications for drugs used to treat thought disorders.

Clinical Cues

Clozapine (Clozaril) is significantly more effective than the other atypical antipsychotics but is less frequently prescribed because of the very slim risk of developing **agranulocytosis** (decreased white blood cells). Patients on this drug must have frequent blood tests.

Negative symptoms are treated with medication, a therapeutic environment that includes therapeutic relationships with nurses, and education about basic living skills. Historically, individuals with schizophrenia were shunned and stigmatized because of unusual and bizarre behavior. Evidence-based practice indicates that with early intervention, many individuals can manage symptoms and maintain independent and productive lives outside of an institution, as long as they adhere to the therapeutic regime. Programs such as the Program of Assertive Community Treatment (PACT) and assertive community treatment (ACT) provide elements of patient and family support, education about disease management, and skills training.

Dialogue therapy has been identified as a possible intervention to improve symptoms and function in patients with schizophrenia, although further research is needed to confirm this preliminary finding (Haram et al., 2018).

Older Adult Care Points

Because of the negative symptoms of social withdrawal, apathy, and sometimes paranoia, older adults with schizophrenia may not be as likely to seek help. They may ignore physical problems and may not report pain associated with physical ailments. This can present unique challenges for nurses who work in long-term care.

Legal and Ethical Considerations

Rights of Psychiatric Patients

Patients with psychiatric conditions, just like all patients, have the right to refuse medication and other therapies. Denial, paranoia, stigmatization, and lack of insight into illness may contribute to the decision to refuse treatment. In emergency situations, such as when the patient may pose harm to self or others, the health care provider can order administration of involuntary medications and/or place the patient on an involuntary hold. For routine ongoing treatment, the patient must be deemed incompetent, and a court order must be obtained if the staff are to override the patient's right to refuse therapy.

Clinical Cues

Patients with schizophrenia may have trouble answering questions, conversing coherently, or expressing feelings. It may be challenging to understand the patient because of **neologisms** (making up new words), **word salad** (disorganized mix of words, phrases, and fragments), or **loose associations** (expression of ideas that do not logically connect). Remember to offer yourself ("Mr. Gardner, if you would like to talk or walk around the unit, I can spend some time with you today.") and attempt to understand ("Mr. Gardner, I am having a little difficulty understanding what you are saying, but I can tell you are trying to say something important."). Spending even small amounts of time with a patient with schizophrenia can build trust and rapport. This therapeutic nursing intervention also allows the patient to practice social skills.

NURSING MANAGEMENT

ASSESSMENT (DATA COLLECTION)

When collecting information from patients who have thought disorders, the interview may need to be brief. It may be difficult for the individual to remain focused for very long. Mental status assessment tools, such as the Mini-Mental State Examination (MMSE) (see Chapter 21), are useful in evaluating thinking processes. Observe the patient's ability to think logically and assess for the presence of psychotic features. Assessing the content and themes of hallucinations and delusions is important to ensure safety. For example, **command hallucinations**

Table 49.2 Nursing Implications for Antipsychotic Drugs Used to Treat Thought Disorders

COMMON SIDE EFFECTS	NURSING IMPLICATIONS
Anticholinergic Side Effects	
Dry mouth	Provide adequate fluids. Suggest sugarless hard candy or gum and good oral care.
Urinary retention and hesitancy	Monitor voiding and elimination patterns.
Constipation	Administer stool softener as ordered. Encourage water and high-fiber foods.
Blurred vision	Remind patient that blurred vision will cease once the body becomes accustomed to the drug.
Photophobia	Remind patient to wear sunglasses and a hat when in the sun.
Sexual dysfunction	Remind patient to alert treatment team about sexual difficulties.
Common Extrapyramidal Side Effects	
Pseudoparkinsonism: Masklike facies, stiff and stooped posture, shuffling gait, drooling, fine tremors, and pill-rolling movement.	May need to switch to a different antipsychotic. Administer anticholinergic medications such as benztropine (Cogentin).
Akathisia: Characterized by pacing and motor restlessness.	Notify health care provider. Antipsychotic medication may need to be changed or an anticholinergic added to the drug regimen. Symptoms disappear when the drug is discontinued.
Other Adverse Neuromuscular Effects	
Tardive dyskinesia: May start after several months or several years of taking antipsychotic medication. It is characterized by tongue protrusion, lip smacking, sucking, chewing, blinking, lateral jaw movements, grimacing, shoulder shrugging, pelvic thrusting, wrist and ankle flexion or rotation, foot tapping and toe movements, and rapid, purposeless, and irregular movements.	Prevention by assessment; encourage checkups every 3 mo. Discontinuing the drug does not always relieve symptoms. No specific treatment other than discontinuing the drug. Give soft foods. Have patient wear soft shoes or slippers.
Neuroleptic malignant syndrome: A rare but potentially fatal reaction to antipsychotic medications. It is characterized by high fever, increased pulse, muscle rigidity, stupor, diaphoresis, hyperkalemia, incontinence, elevated white blood cell count, and renal failure.	Early detection increases survival rate. Stop all medications. Give supportive, symptomatic care. Decrease body temperature. Hydrate (oral and IV). Correct electrolyte imbalance. Medicate for dysrhythmias as ordered. Renal dialysis is indicated for renal failure.
Cardiovascular Side Effects	
Orthostatic hypotension Tachycardia Paliperidone (Invega) can cause cardiac dysrhythmias (i.e., QT prolongation)	Report to health care provider or RN any history of cardiac disease before starting the medication. Check blood pressure and pulse before giving medications. Inform patient to sit at edge of bed and dangle feet before rising to prevent falls. Inform patient that tolerance will develop in several weeks. Increase fluid intake to expand vascular volume as ordered.
Miscellaneous Side Effects	
Sleepiness and fatigue	Inform patient that tolerance to the dosage will develop in 1–2 wk.
Photosensitivity	Administer medication at bedtime. Avoid direct sunlight. Wear protective clothing and sunscreen when outside.
Weight gain	Monitor food intake and make healthy food choices.
Hives and contact dermatitis	Notify health care provider if there is a rash; may need to discontinue or change the drug.

IV, Intravenous; *RN*, registered nurse.

are voices that the patient hears that direct them to harm self or others. Your patient may be experiencing delusions of persecution and be suspicious of staff and therefore refuse to eat. Observe for stressors that seem to trigger or exacerbate disorganized behavior.

Patients with thought disorders may have difficulty verbalizing physical symptoms, and routine physical assessment should be performed to identify or monitor potential health problems. An initial and ongoing assessment of functionality, including activities of daily living (ADLs) and social skills, should be conducted. For example, the patient may have a disheveled appearance; dress strangely with clothing worn in layers, backward, or inside out; or wear seasonally inappropriate items. The patient may disrobe at inappropriate times. A nursing goal would be to help the patient recognize and adopt socially and seasonally appropriate attire that is worn as indicated.

◆ NURSING DIAGNOSIS

Typical problem statements for thought disorders may include the following:

- Confusion due to extreme anxiety and delusional thoughts
- Altered sensory perception (hallucinations) due to biochemical imbalance
- Limited coping ability in work or social situations due to impaired thought processes
- Altered communication ability due to disorganized thoughts
- Social isolation due to paranoia
- Altered self-care ability due to cognitive deficits
- Absence of adherence due to medication regimen
- Potential for violence due to command hallucinations

◆ PLANNING

Sample outcomes for the listed problem statements might include the following:

- Patient will verbally acknowledge that delusional thinking and beliefs increase during times of intense anxiety.
- Patient will spend decreased time attending to hallucinations before discharge.
- Patient will develop skills to adapt to a small social group within 6 months.
- Patient will communicate basic needs more clearly within 1 week.
- Patient will attend the community meeting for 30 minutes today.
- Patient will wash face and hands with supervision this morning.
- Patient will identify three methods that will increase adherence to medication regimen (after discharge) at first follow-up appointment.
- Patient will refrain from hurting self or others during this shift.

Planning care for a patient with a thought disorder involves promoting safety, monitoring medications intended to relieve agitation or psychosis, observing for signs of medication side effects, promoting social skills, and ensuring adequate nutrition and sleep. Care for patients with thought disorders is ongoing, with intermittent situational treatment for acute episodes. Patients need to be educated about the medications and coping skills necessary to function outside of a hospital setting. It is not unusual for a patient to stop taking medications because the voices returned and said that medications are unnecessary or harmful. For patients who are nonadherent to treatment, long-acting injectable forms of medication may be prescribed to prevent relapse.

Clinical Cues

Monitor your professional appearance and clothing when working with patients who have thought disorders. Be a role model who wears clean, matching, and appropriate clothing. Avoid flashy and dangling jewelry because patients are easily distracted by such objects. Do not place items like necklaces, lanyards, scarves, ties, or stethoscopes around your neck, as patients who are agitated can easily grab these and induce choking.

Think Critically

How can you help a patient with schizophrenia adhere to the medication regimen?

◆ IMPLEMENTATION

Priority nursing interventions when caring for patients with schizophrenia include administering antipsychotic medications, monitoring effectiveness, and identifying adverse effects. Antipsychotics have many serious side effects, some of which can be life threatening.

Patient Teaching

Antipsychotic Medications

Patients taking antipsychotic medications should be advised not to use alcohol. Combining alcohol and antipsychotic medications may impair judgment, thinking, and coordination because of the additional central nervous system depression.

Clinical Cues

In accordance with National Patient Safety Goals, two forms of identity must be checked before giving medication or blood products or taking blood samples. When patients are not able to state their correct legal name (because of confusion or psychosis), an alternative method is to have two health care providers verify the patient's identity.

When dealing with a patient who is experiencing active psychosis, use a calm and caring approach. Do not touch the patient without warning or permission, especially if agitation or paranoia is present. During active hallucinations, provide reorientation. "Mr. Gardner, you seem to be listening to something. I am not hearing any voices. Come and talk to me." Strategies for helping patients to manage persistent auditory hallucinations include monitoring what triggers the hallucinations, talking with someone, listening to music, watching TV, saying "stop," using earplugs, doing deep-breathing or relaxation exercises, and engaging in a favorite activity.

Cultural Considerations

Language

Use therapeutic communication and be attentive, respond to the underlying feelings, and gently verbalize concern. "Mr. Gardner, you seem really anxious to tell me something. I am trying to understand." During times of stress, it is natural for a patient to revert to a first language. If your patient speaks English as a second language, obtain the assistance of a translator if you are having difficulty understanding them. The interpreter can translate, and you can then determine whether the patient is having disturbances in communication or whether the verbalizations that sound like word salad are actually a mixture of English and another language. It is important to remember that a translator should be used at all times for a patient who is unable to speak or understand English.

Think Critically

You are caring for a patient who does not trust you. How will you establish trust and rapport with this patient?

Nursing interventions for patients with thought disorders include establishing trust and teaching the patient and family how to manage the signs and symptoms of the disorder. An attitude of acceptance is necessary to promote trust. Begin by offering yourself and being available to the patient even if they initially reject your efforts to establish a therapeutic relationship. Model conventional social behaviors such as greeting the patient by name—"Good morning, Mr. Gardner"—and making friendly eye contact.

Cultural Considerations

Eye Contact

Lack of direct eye contact does not necessarily signal disinterest or an unwillingness to communicate. Direct eye contact may be considered a sign of disrespect by people from different cultural backgrounds.

Give patients positive feedback for making attempts to overcome negative symptoms: "You seemed very interested in the group discussion topic today." Do not make promises that you cannot keep, and if you make a promise, be sure to follow through.

Consistently invite the patient to join groups even if they reject the initial invitations: "Mr. Gardner, we are going to play cards. Would you like to join us?" Acknowledge and thank the patient for efforts to interact, even if those efforts are small or limited: "Thank you for talking to me today." Leave the door open for future interactions: "I understand if you don't want to talk today; maybe we can try tomorrow." Although these patients may have difficulty sustaining an interaction for even 1 or 2 minutes, persistent effort builds the **therapeutic alliance** (relationship between the patient and nurse) and increases the patient's self-esteem.

Complementary and Alternative Therapies

Music Therapy

Music therapy can be used with selected patients to treat positive and negative symptoms of schizophrenia. Participation in music groups increases socialization and stimulates interest. Encourage participants to express how the music makes them feel and to discuss their favorite kinds of music.

Nursing Care Plan 49.1 lists specific problem statements and interventions for individuals with thought disorders. Box 49.2 lists additional interventions for patients who are angry, hostile, aggressive, manipulative, or paranoid.

◆ EVALUATION

To evaluate the effectiveness of nursing interventions, it is necessary to monitor the patient's progress toward expected outcomes. Adherence to the treatment plan, which includes taking antipsychotic medications, should decrease hallucinations and delusions (positive symptoms) and improve sleep. It traditionally takes longer to achieve expected outcomes via treatment for the negative symptoms of schizophrenia than for the positive symptoms. Progress toward outcomes for the negative symptoms should include a decrease in psychomotor retardation, increase in self-care, improved affect, increase in motivation, more trusting behavior toward others, and decrease in social withdrawal.

OVERVIEW OF PERSONALITY DISORDERS

Personality disorders are enduring patterns of behavior in which there is no loss of contact with reality or impaired cognition. The patient with a personality disorder demonstrates an ongoing, inflexible pattern of behavior that is markedly different from others within the individual's culture.

Symptoms of personality disorders can be identified in childhood or are observed in adolescence and early adulthood. Four characteristics of personality disorders are:

1. Inflexible and maladaptive response to life events
2. Serious difficulty in areas of personal and work relationships
3. Tendency to evoke interpersonal conflict
4. Tendency to evoke a negative empathic response from others

Nursing Care Plan 49.1 Care of a Patient With Schizophrenia

SCENARIO

Evan Henry is a 30-year-old man who was diagnosed with schizophrenia 5 years ago. He was taken to the emergency department yesterday after being found by police, wandering in a shopping mall and approaching people to tell them that "they are being followed by demons." Evan was admitted to the psychiatric unit and is assessed to be disheveled with poor hygiene. He sits by himself and is reluctant to interact with staff or other patients on the unit. When his dietary tray arrives for lunch, he pushes it away and says, "I know the demons poisoned my food." When he finally speaks with you, he says, "I am Jesus. I am here to save you and to destroy the demons around you. I hear them talking to you."

PROBLEM STATEMENT/NURSING DIAGNOSIS

Confusion due to delusional thinking, loose associations, or neurobiochemical imbalances.

SUPPORTING ASSESSMENT DATA

Subjective: States that people "are being followed by demons."

Objective: Believes he is Jesus and that he is here to save people and destroy demons.

Goals/Expected Outcomes	Nursing Interventions	Selected Rationale	Evaluation
Patient will be able to talk for 5 min without discussing delusions. Patient will be able to distinguish between reality and nonreality before discharge.	Assess the themes of delusions. Assess for situations that trigger anxiety and stress.	Delusional themes suggest fears and safety issues. Anxiety and stress are theorized to increase delusions and disorganized behavior.	Has a belief that people are being followed by demons. Has a belief that he is Jesus. Currently very anxious and actively delusional; assessment for associated triggers continues.
	Reflect the underlying feelings. ("It's frightening if you feel there are bad presences around you or others.")	Acknowledging feelings validates the patient's experience without agreeing with the delusional content.	Appears suspicious and fearful.
	State reality as you perceive it. ("I believe that the hospital is a safe place.")	Corrects misperceptions without directly arguing against patient's perspective.	Reassured that the hospital is a safe place but continues to be fearful.
	Avoid arguing about the patient's delusional system.	Arguing causes patient to verbally defend own beliefs and potentially strengthens the delusional system.	Occasionally patient appears to recognize certain staff members but continues to be in a delusional state.
	Redirect discussions to real people and events.	Helps patient stay focused on reality.	Continues unwavering in his belief in demons. Does respond when called by name (Evan); however, continues to verbalize the belief that he is Jesus.
	Administer antipsychotic medications as ordered and monitor for effectiveness and side effects.	Counteracts psychosis at the biochemical level.	Agrees to take risperidone (Risperdal) if administered by certain nurses. Outcomes not met. Continue plan.

PROBLEM STATEMENT/NURSING DIAGNOSIS

Altered self-care ability due to cognitive impairment.

SUPPORTING ASSESSMENT DATA

Objective: Disheveled with poor hygiene.

Goals/Expected Outcomes	Nursing Interventions	Selected Rationale	Evaluation
Patient will independently perform self-care within 1 wk.	Encourage the patient to independently perform ADLs according to current level of ability.	Performing ADLs helps the patient focus on real tasks and decreases time spent in delusional thinking.	Is not initiating ADLs but will perform brief tasks (e.g., washing face) with coaching and supervision.

Continued

Nursing Care Plan 49.1 Care of a Patient With Schizophrenia—cont'd

Goals/Expected Outcomes	Nursing Interventions	Selected Rationale	Evaluation
Patient will dress appropriately and maintain appropriate hygiene before discharge.	Make available only the clothes the patient is to wear.	Limiting choices decreases confusion and indirectly suggests appropriate attire.	Is continuously changing clothes unless locked out of room.
	Intervene as necessary if patient is unable to complete daily care.	Initially the patient may not be able to complete ADLs because of impaired thought processes.	Unlicensed assistive personnel verbally directed patient to shower. Patient became verbally hostile; therefore shower deferred for today. Will try to have patient's brother assist him tomorrow.
	Offer positive reinforcement for any completed portion of ADLs.	Increases likelihood that desired behavior will be repeated.	Acknowledges feedback by looking up when spoken to.
	Assist the patient to make a structured plan for completing hygiene and ADLs.	Having a plan provides structure, goals, and ways to achieve goals, which helps the patient complete tasks.	Verbally advised that shower is deferred for today but that brother will help tomorrow. Agrees to wash hands and face today. Outcomes not met. Continue plan.

PROBLEM STATEMENT/NURSING DIAGNOSIS

Altered sensory perception due to neurobiochemical imbalance and anxiety.

SUPPORTING ASSESSMENT DATA

Subjective: Reports "hearing demons" around people.
Objective: Appears to be hearing voices.

Goals/Expected Outcomes	Nursing Interventions	Selected Rationale	Evaluation
Patient will verbalize three ways to cope with hallucinations this week and verbalize a decrease in hallucination frequency before discharge.	Observe behavior that suggests that hallucination is occurring (e.g., talking to self, listening intently).	Staff can interrupt the hallucination in progress.	Observed in listening position and talking to self. Is actively hallucinating today (more than yesterday), appears upset; reason unclear.
	Assess for theme of hallucinations, especially command hallucinations (e.g., voices that say, "Kill others.").	Knowing themes helps anticipate violent or unexpected behavior.	Hearing command hallucinations. ("I am here to save you.")
	Redirect when hallucinations occur (e.g., "Talk with me.").	Interrupts hallucination in progress.	Patient does attend to nurse when spoken to; although he appears fearful, he will stay engaged for 10-15 seconds if he is given adequate personal space (e.g., 5 feet circumference).
	Help patient recognize the feelings that are present before the hallucination.	Anxiety, fear, and stress are theorized to exacerbate hallucinations.	Unclear why patient is agitated today; he is unable to verbalize specific feelings.
	State reality (e.g., "I understand that you hear voices. I do not hear those voices.").	Helps patient recognize and stay focused on reality.	Patient is actively hallucinating; only able to attend to nurse's voice for a few seconds at a time.
	Teach patient to identify and use strategies to interrupt the hallucinations (e.g., seek out nursing staff, sing, listen to music).	Allows patient to cope with hallucinations. (Recognize that for some patients, hallucinations never completely resolve.)	Unable to identify or teach alternative coping methods. Appears less agitated if not approached by other patients.
	Administer antipsychotic medications and monitor effectiveness and side effects.	Counteracts psychosis at the biochemical level.	Agrees to take risperidone (Risperdal) if administered by certain nurses. Outcomes not met. Continue plan.

Nursing Care Plan 49.1 Care of a Patient With Schizophrenia—cont'd

PROBLEM STATEMENT/NURSING DIAGNOSIS

Social isolation due to mistrust, bizarre behavior, or cognitive impairment.

SUPPORTING ASSESSMENT DATA

Subjective: "… demons are following you."

Objective: Reluctant to interact with the staff or other patients.

Goals/Expected Outcomes	Nursing Interventions	Selected Rationale	Evaluation
Patient will engage in social interaction with others on the psychiatric unit by eating one meal, attending two outings, or participating in one group within 2 wk.	Convey a warm, accepting attitude.	Builds therapeutic relationship.	Has some trust toward selected nurses.
	Spend some structured time with the patient every day.	Encourages social interaction with a set time and purpose.	Able to tolerate 10–15 seconds of contact with nurses. Responds to his own name.
	Determine patient's interests.	Patient more likely to engage if interested in activities.	Family states that Evan is interested in baseball. Shows some interest in watching sports on television.
	Model social interaction and conversation.	Patient may be unaware of how to converse with others.	Does not initiate conversations. Was able to attend group meeting yesterday but only for 5 min.
	Create opportunities for socialization (e.g., card games).	Patient may not know how to independently engage others.	
	Acknowledge and thank patient for any efforts to interact and participate in groups.	More likely to repeat behavior if encouraged and acknowledged.	Unable to participate in any group interaction today.
	Encourage the patient to interact with others, even if only briefly.	Brief contacts allow for gradual trust and familiarity to decrease suspiciousness.	Declined going to group music class this afternoon. Appears more restless compared with yesterday. Patient unable to verbalize source of distress, no known event or trigger identified. Will continue to observe. Outcomes not met. Continue plan.

Critical Thinking Questions

1. Why is it important for a patient like Evan to have consistent social support after discharge?
2. What can you, as a nurse, do to help decrease the social stigma of chronic mental illnesses such as schizophrenia?

ADLs, Activities of daily living.

Box 49.2 Specific Nursing Interventions for Patients Who Are Angry, Hostile, Aggressive, Manipulative, or Paranoid

ANGRY, HOSTILE, AND AGGRESSIVE BEHAVIOR

- Continuously assess for nonverbal cues (pacing, fidgeting, and increase in verbalizations) and intervene early.
- Maintain a calm, self-assured attitude.
- Listen and acknowledge that you care and want to help.
- Be culturally aware of how your patient is interpreting eye contact.
- Allow the patient to have adequate personal space.
- Encourage the patient to find a quiet, safe place.
- Maintain your own safety—have adequate staff visually present in the background. However, only one person should attempt verbal de-escalation.
- Stand to the side or sideways to present yourself as a smaller target. Your hands should be relaxed at your sides or with the palms turned upward.
- Be aware of the exits and position yourself so that the patient is not blocking the exit.
- Ask for permission before touching. Defer therapeutic touching.
- Honestly verbalize the patient's options. For example, say, "You can stay in the dayroom if you can remain calm; otherwise it will be necessary for you to go to the quiet (seclusion) room."
- Set a time frame for verbal de-escalation. If progress is made within the time limit, continue. If not, remind the patient of the initial time limit.
- Offer appropriate PRN medications as ordered. If the patient continues to escalate and the behavior becomes aggressive, restraints may be necessary.
- Application of physical restraints requires a team approach by trained staff.
- Inform the patient of the staff's intentions and actions.
- Accurately document the entire episode, including all efforts to use all less restrictive measures before considering physical restraints.

Continued

Box 49.2 Specific Nursing Interventions for Patients Who Are Angry, Hostile, Aggressive, Manipulative, or Paranoid—cont'd

MANIPULATIVE BEHAVIOR
- Set clear and realistic limits on specific behaviors.
- Establish realistic and enforceable consequences.
- Make certain that all staff are informed of the limits and agree with them.
- Specific limits need to be documented in the electronic health record.
- The decision to discontinue limits should be made by the entire staff and should be made only when the patient has demonstrated consistent positive behavior.
- Be self-aware and establish clear boundaries.

PARANOID BEHAVIOR
- Assign only one or two staff members to the patient.
- Initially make brief contact with the patient, and do not make unnecessary demands.
- Increase credibility by being honest, adhering to a stated schedule, and following through on commitments.
- Do not touch a patient who is experiencing paranoia.
- Do not mix medications with food.
- Supply food in commercially wrapped packages if the patient is refusing to eat.

PRN, As needed.

An actual diagnosis may not be made until the person reaches early adulthood; by then the entrenched behaviors are quite evident. It is not uncommon to note that patients with a personality disorder have experienced failed marriages or relationships, have poor work histories, and have difficulty relating to others.

The DSM-5 describes 10 different personality disorder types. Depending on the descriptive characteristics, these disorders are clustered into three separate categories. Cluster A includes behaviors that are considered odd or eccentric (schizotypal, schizoid, and paranoid). Cluster B describes behaviors that are considered dramatic, emotional, and erratic (antisocial, borderline, histrionic, and narcissistic). Individuals with Cluster C behaviors appear anxious and fearful (avoidant, dependent, and obsessive-compulsive). A final type of personality disorder is personality disorder NOS (not otherwise specified), which can be used by the health care provider when a definitive personality disorder cannot be identified at the time of the encounter. Box 49.3 provides a brief description of each of these personality disorders. Many psychiatrists feel that a personality disorder cannot be diagnosed until a person is 18 years old because a child's personality evolves over the early years of life. This chapter discusses borderline personality disorder because of its dramatic presentation and recognizability (Halter, 2018).

Box 49.3 Description of Personality Disorders

CLUSTER A (ODD AND ECCENTRIC)
- *Schizotypal:* Exhibits difficulty with close relationships, distortions in thinking and feeling, and odd or eccentric behavior.
- *Schizoid:* Exhibits withdrawal from social relationships and a restricted affect.
- *Paranoid:* Exhibits distrust and suspiciousness of others and feels that others wish them harm or evil.

CLUSTER B (DRAMATIC, EMOTIONAL, AND ERRATIC)
- *Antisocial:* Exhibits disregard for and violation of the rights of others; lacks empathy.
- *Borderline:* Exhibits instability in interpersonal relationships and self-concept, labile emotions, and marked impulsivity.
- *Histrionic:* Exhibits pattern of extreme emotionality and attention-seeking behavior.
- *Narcissistic:* Exhibits grandiose behavior, intense need for admiration, and lack of empathy.

CLUSTER C (ANXIOUS AND FEARFUL)
- *Avoidant:* Exhibits social inhibition, feelings of inadequacy, and fear of rejection.
- *Dependent:* Exhibits behavior that is submissive and clinging; needy.
- *Obsessive-compulsive:* Exhibits behavior that is concerned with excessive orderliness, perfectionism, and need for control.

BORDERLINE PERSONALITY DISORDER

The main features of **borderline personality disorder (BPD)** include marked emotional and mood instability, self-image distortion, impulsivity, and difficulty in interpersonal relationships (Halter, 2018). Individuals with this disorder tend to attach quickly and easily to others and fear real or imagined abandonment. Emotions and relationships are experienced with heightened intensity. In response to potential abandonment from caregivers or significant others, it is not unusual for these patients to engage in self-mutilating behavior (e.g., cutting on arms or legs or placing cigarette burns on their body) or suicidal gestures. Therapeutic goals of treatment for patients who self-mutilate include acquiring positive coping methods, learning methods of better impulse and emotional control, and increasing self-awareness.

? Think Critically

You are a school nurse who enters a restroom that smells of smoke. At that moment, a student emerges from a stall and touches the hot ash of a burning cigarette to their wrist, sustaining a burn before you can stop them. What is your first action? What is your secondary action?

Splitting, a primitive defense mechanism, is the inability to see both the positive and the negative aspects of others (Halter, 2018). The patient with BPD sees people as either entirely good or entirely bad. Splitting often involves idealizing a person and then devaluing the same person when they do not meet the needs of a patient with BPD. For example, a patient with BPD may favor one nurse by stating, "You are the best nurse I have ever had. No one else understands me like you do." However, when the nurse has left the patient to care for others, or for a day off, the patient with BPD may then say, "I can't believe you just left me. I was so alone that I tried to cut my wrists, and it is all your fault." It is very important that staff decide on an approach to use with a particular patient to reduce the impact of splitting. To implement the plan properly, all team members must agree and be consistent in implementing the approach.

Impulsivity in at least two of the following areas also is characteristic of BPD: gambling, overeating, spending impulsively, abusing substances, engaging in unsafe sex, binge eating, or driving recklessly (American Psychiatric Association, 2013). The outcome of engaging in one or more of these impulsive behaviors is often the reason for hospital admission.

Treatment

Treatment for people with BPD involves long-term psychotherapy, such as individual counseling and group or family therapy. The purpose of **psychotherapy** is to help patients identify problem areas and work to change or modify behaviors, attitudes, and feelings. Dialectical behavior therapy (DBT) has been shown to be the most effective method of treatment for patients with BPD (May, Richardi, & Barth, 2016). This therapy includes individual counseling, telephone support, and skills training and has been shown to reduce self-destructive and impulsive episodes, anxiety, and hospitalization. In addition, DBT can be used to help the family members of patients. Patients with personality disorders can also benefit from milieu therapy. **Milieu therapy** uses the structured environment of a hospital or group home setting to help patients participate as active members of that community and practice social behaviors. Medications are not usually indicated for personality disorders, although they are sometimes prescribed when there is a concurrent psychiatric disorder.

NURSING MANAGEMENT

ASSESSMENT (DATA COLLECTION)

Collect information about how the individual views self and others. Obtain a history of former relationships and identify how the individual typically expresses feelings and manages stress. It is important to refrain from making hasty judgments about patients. For example, adolescents may impulsively act out by misusing substances. They may appear to have identity problems, yet these behaviors often accompany normal growth and development trends. As teens mature, these traits often disappear. It is important to remember to remain nonjudgmental and professional in your care, as a stigma exists that patients with BPD are difficult or undesirable. Box 49.4 lists examples of behaviors you may observe when assessing a patient with a personality disorder.

Box 49.4 Assessing Patients With a Personality Disorder

Assess for the following:
- Acting without thinking; impulsivity
- Anger and possible rage when others do not share the same point of view
- Consistent poor judgment in making decisions
- Constant seeking of praise and admiration
- Evidence of self-destructive behavior
- Excessive use of manipulation to get needs met
- Expression of a need to control others
- Extreme envy of others
- Low self-esteem
- Self-centeredness
- Treatment of others as objects, not people
- Unreliability

NURSING DIAGNOSIS

Typical problem statements for BPD may include the following:
- Social isolation due to immature and manipulative behavior
- Decreased self-esteem due to childhood abuse and neglect
- Limited coping ability due to emotional state outbursts
- Anxiety due to perceived threats of abandonment
- Potential for injury related to feelings of guilt and rejection

PLANNING

Sample outcomes for the listed problem statements include the following:
- Patient will discuss one example of how personal behavior alienates others by the end of the week.
- Patient will share two personal qualities that they like about themself in today's group meeting.
- Patient will identify three methods to cope with intense emotions (e.g., anger at staff or significant others) within 1 week.
- Patient will identify situations that provoke feelings of abandonment (e.g., favorite nurse is on vacation) and state two methods to reduce accompanying anxiety during this shift.
- Patient will substitute a safe behavior (e.g., talking to nurse, counting to 100) for self-mutilating behavior when experiencing feelings of anger, fear, guilt, or rejection during hospitalization.

Planning for the care of a patient with BPD requires involvement of the entire team to define goals and to prevent the patient's attempts at staff manipulation. Staff debriefing time helps members of the team to maintain a professional and optimistic focus when working with patients who have this condition.

Assignment Considerations

Interpersonal Skills

When planning care for patients, incorporate the strengths and interpersonal skills of your team members and delegate appropriately. For example, you need to delegate a nursing assistant to escort a 25-year-old female patient to group therapy on the unit. The patient has been observed attempting to manipulate male staff members; therefore consider assigning an experienced female nursing assistant who recognizes yet does not respond to manipulative behavior to carry out this task.

◆ IMPLEMENTATION

Setting limits for patients with BPD is a priority intervention. Individuals must be taught healthy and nonmanipulative ways to have their needs met. To work with patients who have BPD, the staff needs to maintain appropriate boundaries without being controlling, rigid, and inflexible. Patients with this disorder often ask you to "bend the rules" or grant special privileges. The staff needs to consistently set limits with caring and empathy, offer a rationale, and decline negotiation. If the patient views the limit setting as punitive, the behavior is certain to recur. This does not mean that the patient will always gladly accept the limit setting and be grateful for your concern. It does mean that you are assisting the patient in developing an internal sense of boundaries, which should drive subsequent changes in behavior.

It is also necessary to maintain a safe environment for patients with BPD because they can be impulsive and act with little internal locus of control. It may be necessary to initiate suicide precautions or help the patient who is self-mutilating to stop this behavior. See Chapter 47 for information on suicide precautions.

Patients with personality disorders have an ability to invoke strong feelings in caregivers. If you note a particularly intense reaction to a patient (excessive sympathy, empathy, anger, or frustration), it is important to talk about these feelings with a professional. Identify and express the feelings that the patient's behavior evokes. Awareness of your own feelings will help you modify your reactions and focus on the therapeutic aspects of your relationship with the patient.

◆ EVALUATION

Achievement of long-term outcomes is demonstrated by new, healthy coping strategies for handling stressors, verbalizing anger without acting out, increasing independent decision making, and decreasing manipulative behaviors to have needs met. It is expected that in times of stress, the patient may revert to previously learned behaviors. Remain with the patient and encourage implementation of new behaviors.

COMMUNITY CARE

At one time individuals with thought disorders were hospitalized indefinitely. Hospitalization is now reserved for stabilization; then patients are released to a less restrictive type of care.

Safety Alert

Be Alert for Suicidal Ideations

Many patients who have schizophrenia think about suicide sometime during their lifetime. Community health nurses are in a position to make regular contact with these patients, assess for suicide even if the patient does not raise the issue, clearly communicate the intention to see the patient again, and help the patient make a crisis response plan that includes hospitalization as needed. Evidence shows that community-based interventions may have a positive impact on functioning and in reducing hospital readmissions for patients with schizophrenia (Asher, Patel, & DiSilva, 2017).

Patients with personality disorders are not hospitalized unless they present an imminent danger to themselves via self-mutilation or suicidal gestures. You will encounter patients with personality disorders in a variety of settings outside a psychiatric hospital. Setting limits and appropriate boundaries continues to be an effective intervention, regardless of the setting.

Patients with chronic mental illnesses like schizophrenia or personality disorders are at high risk for social problems and may have limited encounters with health care professionals. In accordance with *Healthy People 2030* goals, a greater percentage of people who are homeless with mental health problems should receive mental health services.

Get Ready for the NCLEX® Examination!

Key Points

- Thought disorders are characterized by disorganized thoughts and behavior and hallucinations. Mood and interpersonal relationships are altered.
- Schizophrenia is the most commonly diagnosed thought disorder and usually is diagnosed between 15 and 25 years of age.
- The positive symptoms of schizophrenia (hallucinations, delusions, and disordered thinking) can be treated with antipsychotic medications.
- The negative symptoms of schizophrenia (apathy, social isolation, psychomotor retardation, blunted affect, poverty of thoughts, and lack of motivation) are responsive to some of the newer atypical medications but are more difficult to treat.

- Long-term social skills training and ongoing family and community support are essential for patients with schizophrenia.
- Older adults taking antipsychotics are at greater risk for developing extrapyramidal symptoms, tardive dyskinesia, and neuroleptic malignant syndrome. Beginning doses should be one half to one third of the normal adult dose.
- General nursing management includes establishing trust and rapport, encouraging social skills, administering medications and monitoring effects, and educating the patient and caregivers about the illness and the therapeutic regimen.
- Personality disorders are characterized by enduring traits.
- Borderline personality disorder is the most prevalent personality disorder. The hallmarks of personality disorders are inflexible and maladaptive response to life events, serious difficulty in personal and work relationships, a tendency to evoke interpersonal conflict, a tendency to evoke a negative empathic response from others, and impulsivity.
- For a patient with a personality disorder, assess the patient's view of self and others, expression of feelings, and behaviors that interfere with life and relationships.
- General nursing management of patients with personality disorders includes building trust, setting limits, teaching coping skills, preventing self-harm, and encouraging insight into behavior.

Additional Learning Resources

SG Go to your Study Guide for additional learning activities to help you master this chapter content.

Go to your Evolve website (http://evolve.elsevier.com/deWit/medsurg) for the following FREE learning resources:
- Animations, audio, and video
- Answers and rationales for questions and activities
- Glossary with pronunciations in English and Spanish
- Interactive Review Questions and more!

Review Questions for the NCLEX® Examination

1. A patient taking antipsychotic medications develops a flat affect with drooling, a shuffling gait, and tremors. You would look for a health care provider order in the MAR for which medication?
   1. Benztropine (Cogentin)
   2. Haloperidol (Haldol)
   3. Amantadine (Symmetrel)
   4. Trihexyphenidyl (Artane)

   NCLEX Client Need: Physiological Integrity: Pharmacological Therapies
2. You are administering medication to a familiar patient who has been on the unit for several weeks. When you ask, "What is your name?", the patient replies, "I am Jesus Christ, the son of God." What is the appropriate nursing action?
   1. Give the medication because you know the patient is confused.
   2. Document that the patient cannot verify identity and hold the medication.
   3. Hold the medication until the family can bring in a picture identification.
   4. Have a second nurse verify the patient's identity and document accordingly.

   NCLEX Client Need: Physiological Integrity: Pharmacological Therapies
3. Which patient statement regarding antipsychotic medication indicates a need for further teaching?
   1. "The medication helps me think more logically."
   2. "The medication makes my mouth dry."
   3. "The medication improves my mood."
   4. "The medication helps stop the voices."

   NCLEX Client Need: Physiological Integrity: Pharmacological Therapies
4. A patient reports taking chlorpromazine (Thorazine) for 4 months. Which symptom do you identify as a concern?
   1. Muscle rigidity
   2. Tongue protrusion
   3. Photophobia
   4. Dry eyes

   NCLEX Client Need: Physiological Integrity: Pharmacological Therapies
5. What is the priority action when you are caring for a patient with active hallucinations?
   1. Assess the content and themes of hallucinations.
   2. Give an antipsychotic medication.
   3. Take the patient to a secluded area.
   4. Set boundaries and explain rationale.

   NCLEX Client Need: Safe and Effective Care Environment: Coordinated Care
6. What is your therapeutic response to a patient who states, "The food service workers put poison in my food, and there is a bomb in bathroom"?
   1. "Who do you think is doing all these things?"
   2. "Let's go together and check the bathroom."
   3. "Tell me how you believe these things are happening."
   4. "I believe that the hospital is a safe place."

   NCLEX Client Need: Psychosocial Integrity
7. What trusting nursing interventions are appropriate when a patient demonstrates negative symptoms of apathy, social isolation, and lack of motivation? *(Select all that apply.)*
   1. Offer self and be available.
   2. Reorient to person, place, and time.
   3. Keep all promises.
   4. Invite the patient to join groups.
   5. Leave the door open for future interactions.
   6. Encourage independence in ADLs.

   NCLEX Client Need: Psychosocial Integrity

8. A patient with command hallucinations is readmitted for an acute psychotic episode. What priority problem do you identify?
   1. Altered sensory perception
   2. Potential for violence
   3. Anxiety
   4. Altered coping ability

   NCLEX Client Need: Psychosocial Integrity
9. You are caring for a patient with a personality disorder. Which statement made by you indicates a need for additional education on setting boundaries?
   1. "I can spend 20 minutes talking with you, and then I have to pass medications."
   2. "I understand that you are bored, but you have to complete the task."
   3. "If you promise not to cause trouble, I'll give you the magazine."
   4. "When someone is speaking in group, it is polite to listen while they speak."

   NCLEX Client Need: Psychosocial Integrity
10. What interventions should you use when a patient is becoming progressively louder and more aggressive? *(Select all that apply.)*
    1. Continuously assess for pacing, fidgeting, and increase in verbalizations.
    2. Maintain a calm, self-assured attitude, even if frightened.
    3. Listen and state, "I care and want to help."
    4. Move close to the patient to provide reassurance.
    5. Set strict limits on the patient's behavior.
    6. Stand to the side or sideways to present self as a smaller target.
    7. Explain the hospital policy and offer the patient a copy.

    NCLEX Client Need: Psychosocial Integrity

Critical Thinking Questions

Scenario A

You are caring for Mrs. Hawkins, a patient with a fixed delusional system with religious overtones who is pacing and becoming increasingly agitated. The patient begins to cry and yell that God is coming back, and no one will be saved.

1. How will you approach the patient and help her de-escalate?
2. What behaviors would cause you to consider implementing physical restraint?

Scenario B

A parent brings a 40-year-old patient to the health care provider's office, asking for a refill of antipsychotic medication. The parent states that the patient is not adherent to medication therapy.

1. How do you approach this scenario, recognizing Health Insurance Portability and Accountability Act (HIPAA) law?
2. What nursing interventions would you implement to address the patient?
3. What type of community referrals may be appropriate for this patient and parent?

Scenario C

A patient with schizophrenia is hospitalized on an inpatient psychiatric unit. The nurses find it difficult to understand the patient due to symptoms associated with thought disorders and manifestation of word salad, neologisms, and loose associations. The patient is not aggressive but cannot interact with others for more than a few seconds at a time.

1. What nursing interventions could be used to address the patient's inability to communicate?
2. Write a communication goal that would be appropriate for this patient.
3. Identify an activity that would increase socialization for this patient.

Scenario D

A 26-year-old female patient who is well known to the nurses in an emergency department comes to the ED with a superficial scratch on the wrist. She cries to you, "You are the best nurse here. You're always so kind and understanding. Would you call my boyfriend and tell him that I am here? I cut myself because we just broke up."

1. What behaviors suggest that this patient may have a personality disorder?
2. How would you respond to the patient's request to call her boyfriend?

appendix A

Most Common Laboratory Test Values

Table A.1 Reference Intervals for Hematology

TEST	CONVENTIONAL UNITS	SI UNITS
Cell Counts		
Erythrocytes (red blood cells)		
Males	4.7–6.1 million/mm^3	$4.7–6.1 \times 10^{12}$/L
Females	4.2–5.4 million/mm^3	$4.2–5.4 \times 10^{12}$/L
Children (varies with age)	4.0–6.0 million/mm^3	$4.0–6.0 \times 10^{12}$/L
Leukocytes, total	5000–10,000/mm^3	$5–10 \times 10^9$/L
Leukocytes, differential counts[a]		
Neutrophils	55%–70%	$2500–8000 \times 10^9$/L
Lymphocytes	20%–40%	$1000–4000 \times 10^9$/L
Monocytes	2%–8%	$2–8 \times 10^9$/L
Eosinophils	1%–4%	$1–4 \times 10^9$/L
Basophils	0.5%–1%	$0.5–1 \times 10^9$/L
Platelets	150,000–400,000/mm^3	$150–400 \times 10^9$/L
Reticulocytes	25,000–75,000/mm^3 (0.5%–1.5% of erythrocytes)	$25–75 \times 10^9$/L
Coagulation Tests		
Bleeding time (template)	1–9 min	1–9 min
D-Dimer	<0.5 mcg/mL	<0.5 mg/L
Factor VIII and other coagulation factors	50%–150% of normal	0.5–1.5 of normal
Fibrin split products (Thrombo-Wellcotest)	<10 mcg/mL	<10 mg/L
Fibrinogen	200–400 mg/dL	2.0–4.0 g/L
Partial thromboplastin time, activated (aPTT)	20–25 seconds	20–35 seconds
Prothrombin time (PT)	12.0–14.0 seconds	12.0–14.0 seconds
Reported as international normalized ratio (INR)	0.8–1.1	
Coombs test		
Direct	Negative	Negative
Indirect	Negative	Negative
Corpuscular Values of Erythrocytes		
Mean corpuscular hemoglobin (MCH)	27–31 pg/cell	27–31 pg/cell
Mean corpuscular volume (MCV)	80–95 fL	80–95 fL
Mean corpuscular hemoglobin concentration (MCHC)	32–36 g/dL	320–360 g/L
Haptoglobin	50–220 mg/dL	0.5–2.2 g/L
Hematocrit		
Males	42%–52% mL/dL	0.42–0.52 volume fraction
Females	37%–47% mL/dL	0.37–0.47 volume fraction
Newborns	44%–64% mL/dL	0.44–0.64 volume fraction
Children (varies with age)	32%–44% mL/dL	0.32–0.44 volume fraction

Continued

Table A.1 Reference Intervals for Hematology—cont'd

TEST	CONVENTIONAL UNITS	SI UNITS
Hemoglobin		
Males	14.0–18.0 g/dL	8.7–11.2 mmol/L
Females	12.0–16.0 g/dL	7.4–9.9 mmol/L
Newborns	14–24 g/dL	10.25–12.11 mmol/L
Children (varies with age)	9.5–15.5 g/dL	6.96–10.25 mmol/L
Hemoglobin A_{1C}	4%–5.9% of total	0.040–0.059 of total
Hemoglobin A_2	2.0%–3.0% of total	0.02–0.03 of total
Methemoglobin	0.06–0.24 g/dL	9.3–37.2 μmol/L
Erythrocyte Sedimentation Rate (ESR)		
Westergren		
Males	0–15 mm/h	0–15 mm/h
Females	0–20 mm/h	0–20 mm/h

[a]Conventional units are percentages; SI units are absolute cell counts.

Table A.2 Reference Intervals[a] for Clinical Chemistry (Blood, Serum, and Plasma)

ANALYTE	CONVENTIONAL UNITS	SI UNITS
Acid phosphatase, serum (prostatic acid phosphatase [PAP])	0.13–12.6 U/L	2.2–10.5 U/L
ACTH (see Corticotropin)		
Alanine aminotransferase (ALT), serum (SGPT)	4–36 U/L	4–36 U/L
Albumin, serum	3.5–5 g/dL	35–50 g/L
Aldosterone, plasma		
Standing	5–30 ng/dL	0.14–0.80 nmol/L
Recumbent	3–10 ng/dL	0.08–0.30 nmol/L
Alkaline, phosphatase (ALP), serum		
Adult	30–120 U/L	0.5–2.0 μkat/L
Adolescent	60–300 U/L	32.5–162.3 U/dL
Ammonia nitrogen, plasma	10–80 mcg/dL	6–47 μmol/L
Amylase, serum	60–120 Smogyi units/dL	30–220 U/L
Anion gap, serum calculated	12–20 mEq/L	12–20 mmol/L
Aspartate aminotransferase (AST), serum (SGOT)	1–35 U/L	0–0.58 μkat/L
Base excess, arterial blood, calculated	0 ± 2 mEq/L	0 ± 2 mmol/L
Bicarbonate		
Venous plasma	23–29 mEq/L	23–29 mmol/L
Arterial blood	21–28 mEq/L	21–28 mmol/L
Bilirubin, serum total	0.3–1.0 ng/dL	5.1–17 μmol/L
Direct (conjugated)	0.1–0.3 mg/dL	1.7–5.1 μmol/L
Indirect (unconjugated)	0.2–0.8 mg/dL	3.4–12.0 μmol/L
Calcium, serum	9.0–10.5 mg/dL	1.9–2.60 mmol/L
Calcium, ionized, serum	4.5–5.6 mg/dL	1.05–1.30 mmol/L
Carbon dioxide, total, serum or plasma	23–30 mEq/L	23–30 mmol/L
Carbon dioxide tension (P_{CO_2}), arterial blood	35–45 mm Hg	35–45 mm Hg
Ceruloplasmin, serum	23–50 mg/dL	230–500 mg/L
Chloride, serum or plasma	98–106 mEq/L	98–106 mmol/L
Cholesterol, serum or EDTA plasma		
Desirable range	<200 mg/dL	<5.20 mmol/L
Low-density lipoprotein (LDL) cholesterol	<130 mg/dL	<3.36 mmol/L
High-density lipoprotein (HDL) cholesterol	30–80 mg/dL	0.80–2.05 mmol/L
Males	>45 mg/dL	>0.75 mmol/L
Females	>55 mg/dL	>91 mmol/L

Table A.2 Reference Intervals[a] for Clinical Chemistry (Blood, Serum, and Plasma)—cont'd

ANALYTE	CONVENTIONAL UNITS	SI UNITS
Corticotropin (ACTH), plasma		
Males	7–69 pg/mL	7–69 ng/L
Females	6–58 pg/mL	6–58 ng/L
Cortisol, plasma		
8 A.M.	5–23 mcg/dL	138–635 nmol/L
4 P.M.	3–13 mcg/dL	83–359 nmol/L
Creatinine, serum		
Males	0.6–1.35 mg/dL	53–114.92 µmol/L
Females	0.5–1.2 mg/dL	44.2–106.08 µmol/L
Creatine kinase (CK), serum		
Males	55–170 U/L	55–170 U/L
Females	30–135 U/L	30–135 U/L
Creatinine kinase MB isoenzyme, serum	<5% of total CK activity <5% of ng/mL by immunoassay	<5% of total CK activity <5% of ng/mL by immunoassay
Estradiol, adult		
Males	10–50 pg/mL	35–183.5 pmol/L
Females		
Follicular	20–350 pg/mL	73–1284 pmol/L
Ovulatory	150–750 pg/mL	550–2752 pmol/L
Luteal	30–450 pg/mL	110–1651 pmol/L
Fibrinogen, plasma	200–400 mg/dL	2.0–4.0 g/L
Folate, serum	5–25 ng/mL	11–57 nmol/L
Follicle-stimulating hormone (FSH), plasma		
Males	1.42–15.4 mIU/mL	1.42–15.4 IU/L
Females, premenopausal (ovulatory peak)	6.17–17.2 mIU/mL	6.17–17.2 IU/L
Females, postmenopausal	19.3–100.6 mIU/mL	19.3–100.6 IU/L
Gamma-glutamyltransferase (GGT), serum	8–38 U/L	8–38 IU/L
Gastrin, fasting, serum	0–180 pg/mL	0–180 mg/L
Glucose, fasting, plasma or serum	74–106 mg/dL	4.1–5.9 nmol/L
Growth hormone (hGH), plasma, adult, fasting		
Males	<5 ng/mL	<5 mcg/L
Females	<10 ng/mL	<10 mcg/L
Haptoglobin, serum	50–220 mg/dL	0.5–2.2 g/L
Beta-hydroxybutyrate	0.3–2.8 mg/dL	20–280 µmol/L
Immunoglobulins, serum (see Table A.8)		
Iron, serum		
Males	80–180 mcg/dL	14.32–32.22 µmol/L
Females	60–160 mcg/dL	10.74–28.64 µmol/L
Iron-binding capacity, serum	250–460 mcg/dL	45–82 µmol/L
Transferrin	250–410 mcg/dL	45–73 µmol/L
Males	215–365 mg/dL	2.15–3.65 g/L
Females	250–380 mg/dL	2.50–3.80 g/L
Transferrin saturation		
Males	20%–50%	20%–50%
Females	15%–50%	15%–50%
Lactate		
Venous whole blood	5.0–20.0 mg/dL	0.6–2.2 mmol/L
Arterial whole blood	3–7 mg/dL	0.3–0.8 mmol/L
Lactate dehydrogenase (LD), serum	100–190 U/L	100–190 U/L
Lipase, serum	0–160 U/L	0–160 U/L

Continued

Table A.2 Reference Intervals[a] for Clinical Chemistry (Blood, Serum, and Plasma)—cont'd

ANALYTE	CONVENTIONAL UNITS	SI UNITS
Lutropin (LH), serum		
Males	1.24–7.8 U/L	1.24–7.8 IU/L
Females		
Follicular phase	1.68–15 U/L	1.68–15 IU/L
Midcycle peak	21.9–56.6 U/L	21.9–56.6 IU/L
Luteal phase	0.61–16.3 U/L	0.61–16.3 IU/L
Postmenopausal	14.2–52.3 U/L	14.2–52.3 IU/L
Magnesium, serum	1.3–2.1 mg/dL	0.65–1.05 mmol/L
Osmolality	285–295 mOsm/kg water	285–295 mmol/kg water
Oxygen, blood, arterial, room air		
Partial pressure (PaO_2)	80–100 mm Hg	80–100 mm Hg
Saturation (SaO_2)	95%–100%	95%–100%
pH, arterial blood	7.35–7.45	7.35–7.45
Phosphate, inorganic, serum		
Adult	3.0–4.5 mg/dL	1.0–1.5 mmol/L
Child	4.5–6.5 mg/dL	1.45–2.1 mmol/L
Potassium		
Serum	3.5–5.0 mEq/L	3.5–5.0 mmol/L
Plasma	3.5–4.5 mEq/L	3.5–4.5 mmol/L
Progesterone, serum, adult		
Males	10–50 ng/dL	31.80–159 nmol/L
Females		
Follicular phase	<50 ng/dL	<159 nmol/L
Luteal phase	300–2500 ng/dL	9.54–79.5 nmol/L
Prolactin, serum		
Males	3–13 ng/mL	3–13 μg/L
Females	3–27 ng/mL	3–27 μg/L
Protein, serum, electrophoresis		
Total	6.4–8.3 g/dL	64–83 g/L
Albumin	3.5–5.0 g/dL	35–50 g/L
Globulins		
$Alpha_1$	0.1–0.3 g/dL	1.0–3.0 g/L
$Alpha_2$	0.6–1.0 g/dL	6.0–10.0 g/L
Beta	0.7–1.1 g/dL	7.0–11.0 g/L
Globulin	2.3–3.4 g/dL	23–34 g/L
Rheumatoid factor	<60 U/mL	<60 kIU/L
Sodium, serum or plasma	135–145 mEq/L	135–145 mmol/L
Testosterone, plasma		
Males, adult	280–1080 ng/dL	9.7–37.5 nmol/L
Females, adult	<70 ng/dL	<2.43 nmol/L
Thyroglobulin	3–42 ng/mL	
Males	0.5–53.0 ng/mL	0.5–53.0 μg/L
Females	0.5–43.0 ng/mL	0.5–43.0 μg/L
Thyrotropin (hTSH), serum	0.3–5 μU/mL	0.35–5.0 mU/L
Thyrotropin-releasing hormone (TRH) stimulation test	<10 μU/mL	<10 mIU/L
Thyroxine (FT_4), free, serum	0.8–2.8 ng/dL	26–36 pmol/L
Thyroxine (T_4), serum total	4.5–12.0 mcg/mL	58–154 nmol/L
Thyroxine-binding globulin (TBG)	1.7–3.6 mg/dL	1.7–3.6 mg/L
Triglycerides, serum, after 12-h fast		
Males	40–160 mg/dL	0.4–1.6 g/L
Females	35–135 mg/dL	0.35–1.35 g/L
Triiodothyronine (T_3), serum	70–190 ng/dL	1.1–2.9 nmol/L
Troponin I	<0.03 ng/mL	<0.03 ng/mL

Table A.2 Reference Intervals[a] for Clinical Chemistry (Blood, Serum, and Plasma)—cont'd

ANALYTE	CONVENTIONAL UNITS	SI UNITS
Uric acid		
Males	4.0–8.5 mg/dL	0.24–0.51 mmol/L
Females	2.7–7.3 mg/dL	0.16–0.43 mmol/L
Urea, nitrogen, serum or plasma (blood urea nitrogen [BUN])	10–20 mg/dL	3.6–7.1 mmol/L
Vitamin B_{12}, serum	160–950 pg/mL	118–701 pmol/L

[a]Reference values may vary, depending on the method and sample source used.
ACTH, Adrenocorticotropic hormone; *EDTA,* ethylenediaminetetraacetic acid; *hTSH,* human thyroid-stimulating hormone; *kIU,* killiunit; *LH,* luteinizing hormone; *MB,* muscle/brain; *mIU,* microunit; *mU,* milliunit; *SGPT,* serum glutamic pyruvic transaminase.

Table A.3 Reference Intervals[a] for Therapeutic Drug Monitoring (Serum or Plasma)

ANALYTE	THERAPEUTIC RANGE	TOXIC CONCENTRATIONS	PROPRIETARY NAME(S)
Analgesics			
Acetaminophen	Varies	>25 mcg/mL	Tylenol, Datril
Salicylate	100–250 mcg/mL	>300 mcg/mL	Aspirin, Bufferin
Antibiotics			
Amikacin	15–25 mcg/mL	>250 mcg/mL	Amkin
Gentamicin	5–10 mcg/mL	>12 mcg/mL	Garamycin
Tobramycin	5–10 mcg/mL	>12 mcg/mL	Nebcin
Vancomycin	5–35 mcg/mL	Trough level >20 mcg/mL	Vancocin
Anticonvulsants			
Carbamazepine	5–12 mcg/mL	>12 mcg/mL	Tegretol
Ethosuximide	40–100 mcg/mL	>100 mcg/mL	Zarontin
Phenobarbital	10–30 mcg/mL	>40 mcg/mL	Luminal
Phenytoin	10–20 mcg/mL	>30 mcg/mL	Dilantin
Primidone	5–12 mcg/mL	>15 mcg/mL	Mysoline
Valproic acid	50–100 mcg/mL	>100 mcg/mL	Depakene
Antineoplastics and Immunosuppressives			
Cyclosporine	100–400 ng/mL	>400 ng/mL	Sandimmune
Methotrexate	>0.01 μmol	>10 μmol/24 h	
Tacrolimus	5–15 ng/mL	>20 ng/mL	Prograf
Bronchodilators and Respiratory Stimulants			
Caffeine	3–15 ng/mL	>30 ng/mL	Elixophyllin
Theophylline (aminophylline)	10–20 mcg/mL	>20 mcg/mL	Quibron
Cardiovascular Drugs			
Amiodarone (obtain specimen more than 8 h after last dose)	0.5–2.5 mcg/mL	>3.0 mcg/mL	Cordarone
Digoxin (obtain specimen more than 6 h after last dose)	0.8–2.0 ng/mL	>2.4 ng/mL	Lanoxin
Disopyramide	2–5 mcg/mL	>5 mcg/mL	Norpace
Lidocaine	1.5–5.0 mcg/mL	>5 mcg/mL	Xylocaine
Mexiletine	0.7–2.0 mcg/mL	>2 mcg/mL	Mexitil
Procainamide	4–10 mcg/mL	>16 mcg/mL	Pronestyl
Propranolol	50–100 ng/mL	>150 ng/mL	Inderal
Quinidine	2–5 mcg/mL	>10 mcg/mL	Cardioquin, Quinaglute

Continued

Table A.3 Reference Intervals[a] for Therapeutic Drug Monitoring (Serum or Plasma)—cont'd

ANALYTE	THERAPEUTIC RANGE	TOXIC CONCENTRATIONS	PROPRIETARY NAME(S)
Psychopharmacologic Drugs			
Amitriptyline	120–150 ng/mL	>500 ng/mL	Elavil, Triavil
Bupropion	25–100 ng/mL	Not applicable	Wellbutrin
Desipramine	150–300 ng/mL	>500 ng/mL	Norpramin
Imipramine	150–300 ng/mL	>500 ng/mL	Tofranil
Lithium (obtain specimen 12 h after last dose)	0.8–1.2 mEq/L	>2 mEq/L	Lithobid
Nortriptyline	50–150 ng/mL	>500 ng/mL	Aventyl, Pamelor

[a]Values may vary depending on the method and sample collection device used. Always consult the reference values provided by the laboratory performing the analysis.

Table A.4 Reference Intervals[a] for Clinical Chemistry (Urine)

ANALYTE	CONVENTIONAL UNITS	SI UNITS
Acetone and acetoacetate, qualitative	Negative	Negative
Albumin		
Qualitative	Negative	Negative
Quantitative	10–100 mg/24 h	0.15–1.5 μmol/day
Aldosterone	3–20 mcg/24 h	8.3–55 nmol/day
Amylase	<5000 Somogyi units/24 h	6.5–48.1 units/h
Amylase/creatinine clearance ratio	<2	<2
Bilirubin, qualitative	Negative	Negative
Chloride (varies with intake)	110–250 mEq/24 h	110–250 mmol/day
Cortisol, free	<100 mcg/24 h	<276 nmol/day
Cystine or cysteine	Negative	Negative
Delta-aminolevulinic acid	1.5–7.5 mg/24 h	11–57 μmol/24 h
Glucose	50–300 mg/24 h	0.3–1.7 mmol/day
Hemoglobin and myoglobin, qualitative	Negative	Negative
Homogentisic acid, qualitative	Negative	Negative
17-Hydroxycorticosteroids		
Males	3–10 mg/24 h	8.3–27.6 μmol/day
Females	2–8 mg/24 h	5.5–22.1 μmol/day
5-Hydroxyindoleacetic acid		
Qualitative	Negative	Negative
Quantitative	2–8 mg/24 h	10–40 μmol/day
17-Ketosteroids		
Males	6–20 mg/24 h	20–70 μmol/day
Females	6–17 mg/24 h	20–60 μmol/day
Osmolality	50–1200 mOsm/kg water	50–1200 mmol/kg water
pH	4.6–8.0	4.6–8.0
Phenylpyruvic acid, qualitative	Negative	Negative
Phosphate	0.4–1.3 g/24 h	13–42 mmol/day
Porphobilinogen		
Qualitative	Negative	Negative
Quantitative	<2 mg/24 h	<9 μmol/day
Porphyrins		
Males	8–149 mcg/24 h	10–160 nmol/day
Females	3–78 mcg/24 h	5–95 nmol/day
Potassium	25–100 mEq/24 h	25–100 mmol/day

Table A.4 Reference Intervals[a] for Clinical Chemistry (Urine)—cont'd

ANALYTE	CONVENTIONAL UNITS	SI UNITS
Pregnanediol		
Males	0.0–1.9 mg/24 h	0.0–6.0 µmol/day
Females		
Proliferative phase	0.0–2.6 mg/24 h	0.0–8.0 µmol/day
Luteal phase	2.6–10.6 mg/24 h	8–33 µmol/day
Postmenopausal	0.2–1.0 mg/24 h	0.6–3.1 µmol/day
Protein, total		
Qualitative	Negative	Negative
Quantitative	0–8 mg/dL	0–8 mg/dL
Sodium (regular diet)	60–260 mEq/24 h	60–260 mmol/day
Specific gravity		
Random specimen	1.003–1.030	1.003–1.030
24-h collection	1.015–1.025	1.015–1.025
Urate (regular diet)	250–750 mg/24 h	1.5–4.4 mmol/day
Urobilinogen	0.5–4.0 mg/24 h	0.6–6.8 µmol/day
Vanillylmandelic acid (VMA)	1.0–8.0 mg/24 h	5–40 µmol/day

[a]Values may vary, depending on the method used.

Table A.5 Reference Intervals for Toxic Substances

ANALYTE	CONVENTIONAL UNITS	SI UNITS
Arsenic, urine	Normal ≤50 mcg/L 24 h	<1.7 µmol/day
Bromides, serum, inorganic	<100 mg/dL	<10 mmol/L
Toxic symptoms	140–1000 mg/dL	14–100 mmol/L
Carboxyhemoglobin, blood	Saturation, percent	
Urban environment	<5%	<0.05
Smokers	<12%	<0.12
Symptoms		
Headache	>15%	>0.15
Nausea and vomiting	>25%	>0.25
Potentially lethal	>50%	>0.50
Ethanol, blood	<0.05 mg/dL <0.005%	<1.0 mmol/L
Intoxication	>100 mg/dL >0.1%	>22 mmol/L
Marked intoxication	300–400 mg/dL 0.3%–0.4%	65–87 mmol/L
Alcoholic stupor	400–500 mg/dL 0.4%–0.5%	87–109 mmol/L
Coma	>500 mg/dL 0.5%	>109 mmol/L
Lead, blood		
Adults	<20 mcg/dL	<1.0 µmol/L
Children	<10 mcg/dL	<0.5 µmol/L
Lead, urine	<80 mcg/24 h	<0.4 µmol/day
Mercury, urine	<10 mcg/24 h	<150 nmol/day

Table A.6 Reference Intervals for Tests Performed on Cerebrospinal Fluid

TEST	CONVENTIONAL UNITS	SI UNITS
Cells	<5 mm^3, all mononuclear	<5 × 10^6/L, all mononuclear
Protein electrophoresis	Albumin predominant	Albumin predominant
Glucose	50–75 mg/dL (20 mg/dL less than in serum)	2.8–4.2 mmol/L (1.1 mmol/L less than in serum)
Immunoglobulin G (IgG)		
Children <14 yr	<8% of total protein	<0.08 of total protein
Adults	<14% of total protein	<0.14 of total protein
IgG index	0.3–0.6	0.3–0.6
Oligoclonal banding on electrophoresis	Absent	Absent
Pressure, opening	<20 cm H_2O	<20 cm H_2O
Protein, total	15–45 mg/dL	150–450 mg/L

Table A.7 Reference Intervals for Tests of Gastrointestinal Function

TEST	CONVENTIONAL UNITS
Fecal fat estimation	
Qualitative	No fat globules seen by high-power microscope
Quantitative	2–7 g/24 h (>95% coefficient of fat absorption)
Gastric acid output	
Basal	
Males	0.0–10.5 mmol/h
Females	0.0–5.6 mmol/h
Maximum (after histamine or pentagastrin)	
Males	9.0–48.0 mmol/h
Females	6.0–31.0 mmol/h
Ratio: basal/maximum	
Males	0.0–0.31
Females	0.0–0.29
Secretin test, pancreatic fluid	
Volume	>1.8 mL/kg/h
Bicarbonate	>80 mEq/L
D-Xylose absorption test, urine	>20% of ingested dose excreted in 5 h

Table A.8 Reference Intervals for Tests of Immunologic Function

TEST	CONVENTIONAL UNITS	SI UNITS
Complement, serum		
C3	75–175 mg/dL	0.75–1.75 g/L
C4	22–45 mg/dL	220–450 mg/L
Total hemolytic (CH_{50})	150–250 U/mL	150–250 U/mL
Immunoglobulins, serum, adult		
IgG	640–1350 mg/dL	6.4–13.5 g/L
IgA	70–310 mg/dL	0.70–3.1 g/L
IgM	90–350 mg/dL	0.90–3.5 g/L
IgD	0.0–6.0 mg/dL	0.0–60 mg/L
IgE	0.0–430 ng/dL	0.0–430 mg/L
Autoantibodies, serum, adult		
Antinuclear antibody	<1:40	—
Anti-dsDNA antibody	0–40 U	0–40 U/mL
Anti-CCP	0–19 units	—
Rheumatoid factor	0–30 mg/dL	—

CCP, Cyclic citrullinated peptide; *dsDNA,* double-stranded deoxyribonucleic acid.

Table A.9 Lymphocyte Subsets, Whole Blood, Heparinized*

ANTIGEN(S) EXPRESSED	CELL TYPE	PERCENTAGE	ABSOLUTE CELL COUNT
CD3	Total T cells	56–77	860–1880
CD19	Total B cells	7–17	140–370
CD3 and CD4	Helper-inducer cells	32–54	550–1190
CD3 and CD8	Suppressor-cytotoxic cells	24–37	430–1060
CD3 and DR	Activated T cells	5–14	70–310
CD2	E rosette T cells	73–87	1040–2160
CD16 and CD56	Natural killer (NK) cells	8–22	130–500

*Gender, age, and ethnicity cause variations in reference ranges for lymphocytes.

appendix

B Standard Precautions*

Assume that every person is potentially infected or colonized with an organism that could be transmitted in the health care setting and apply the following infection control practices during the delivery of health care. *Category 1B/1C*

A. HAND HYGIENE

1. During the delivery of health care, avoid unnecessary touching of surfaces in close proximity to the patient to prevent (1) contamination of clean hands from environmental surfaces and (2) transmission of pathogens from contaminated hands to surfaces.
2. When your hands are visibly dirty, contaminated with proteinaceous material, or visibly soiled with blood or body fluids, wash your hands with either a non-antimicrobial soap and water or an antimicrobial soap and water. *Category 1A*
3. If your hands are not visibly soiled, or after removing visible material with non-antimicrobial soap and water, decontaminate your hands. The preferred method of hand decontamination is with an alcohol-based hand rub. Alternatively, hands may be washed with an antimicrobial soap and water. Frequent use of alcohol-based hand rub immediately after handwashing with non-antimicrobial soap may increase the frequency of dermatitis. *Category 1B*
   Perform hand hygiene:
   - Before having direct contact with patients
   - After contact with blood, body fluids or excretions, mucous membranes, nonintact skin, or wound dressings
   - After contact with a patient's intact skin (e.g., when taking a pulse or blood pressure or lifting a patient)
   - If your hands will be moving from a contaminated body site to a clean body site during patient care
   - After contact with inanimate objects (including medical equipment) in the immediate vicinity of the patient
   - After removing gloves
4. Wash your hands with non-antimicrobial soap and water or with antimicrobial soap and water if contact with spores (e.g., *Clostridium difficile* or *Bacillus anthracis*) is likely to have occurred. The physical action of washing and rinsing your hands under such circumstances is recommended because alcohols, chlorhexidine, iodophors, and other antiseptic agents have poor activity against spores. *Category 2*
5. Do not wear artificial fingernails or extenders if duties include direct contact with patients who are at high risk for infection and associated adverse outcomes (e.g., those in intensive care units [ICUs] or operating rooms). *Category 1A*
   - Develop an organizational policy on the wearing of non-natural nails by health care personnel who have direct contact with patients outside of the groups specified above.

B. PERSONAL PROTECTIVE EQUIPMENT (PPE)

Observe the following principles of use:

- Wear PPE when the nature of anticipated patient interaction indicates that contact with blood or body fluids may occur. *Category 1B/1C*
- Prevent contamination of clothing and skin during the process of removing PPE. *Category 2*
- Before leaving the patient's room or cubicle, remove and discard PPE. *Category 1B/1C*

GLOVES

Wear gloves when it can be reasonably anticipated that contact with blood or other potentially infectious materials, mucous membranes, nonintact skin, or potentially contaminated intact skin (e.g., of a patient incontinent of stool or urine) could occur. Wear gloves with fit and durability appropriate to the task. Wear disposable medical examination gloves for providing direct patient care. Wear disposable medical examination gloves or reusable utility gloves for cleaning the environment or medical equipment. Remove gloves after contact with a patient and/or the surrounding environment (including medical equipment) using proper technique to prevent hand contamination. Do not wear the same pair of gloves for the care of more than one patient. Do not wash gloves for the purpose of reuse because this practice has been associated with transmission of

---

*Sections pertinent to adult health care nursing extracted from Siegel JD, Rhinehart E, Jackson M, et al.: *Guideline for isolation precautions: preventing transmission of infectious agents in healthcare settings 2007*, Atlanta, 2007 (last update April 2019), Centers for Disease Control and Prevention.

pathogens. Change gloves during patient care if your hands move from a contaminated body site (e.g., perineal area) to a clean body site (e.g., face).

GOWNS

Wear a gown that is appropriate to the task to protect skin and prevent soiling or contamination of clothing during procedures and patient care activities when contact with blood, body fluids, secretions, or excretions is anticipated. Wear a gown for direct patient contact if the patient has uncontained secretions or excretions. Remove gown and perform hand hygiene before leaving the patient's environment. Do not reuse gowns, even for repeated contacts with the same patient. Routine donning of gowns on entrance into a high-risk unit (e.g., ICU, neonatal ICU [NICU]) is not indicated.

MOUTH, NOSE, AND EYE PROTECTION

Use PPE to protect the mucous membranes of your eyes, nose, and mouth during procedures and patient care activities that are likely to generate splashes or sprays of blood, body fluids, secretions, and excretions. Select masks, goggles, face shields, and combinations of each according to the need anticipated by the task performed. During aerosol-generating procedures (e.g., bronchoscopy, suctioning of the respiratory tract [if not using in-line suction catheters], endotracheal intubation) in patients who are not suspected of being infected with an agent for which respiratory protection is otherwise recommended (e.g., *Mycobacterium tuberculosis,* SARS, or hemorrhagic fever viruses), wear one of the following: a face shield that fully covers the front and sides of the face, a mask with attached shield, or a mask and goggles (in addition to gloves and gown).

PATIENT CARE EQUIPMENT AND INSTRUMENTS/DEVICES

Establish policies and procedures for containing, transporting, and handling patient care equipment and instruments/devices that may be contaminated with blood or body fluids. Remove organic material from critical and semicritical instruments/devices, using recommended cleaning agents before high-level disinfection and sterilization to enable effective disinfection and sterilization processes. Wear PPE (e.g., gloves, gown), according to the level of anticipated contamination when handling patient care equipment and instruments/devices that are visibly soiled or may have been in contact with blood or body fluids.

CARE OF THE ENVIRONMENT

Establish policies and procedures for routine and targeted cleaning of environmental surfaces as indicated by the level of patient contact and degree of soiling. Clean and disinfect surfaces that are likely to be contaminated with pathogens, including those that are in close proximity to the patient (e.g., bed rails, overbed tables) and frequently touched surfaces in the patient care environment (i.e., doorknobs, surfaces in and surrounding toilets in patients' rooms) on a more frequent schedule compared with that for other surfaces (e.g., horizontal surfaces in waiting rooms). Use Environmental Protection Agency (EPA)–registered disinfectants that have microbiocidal (i.e., killing) activity against the pathogens most likely to contaminate the patient care environment. Use in accordance with manufacturer's instructions. Review the efficacy of in-use disinfectants when evidence of continuing transmission of an infectious agent (e.g., rotavirus, *C. difficile,* norovirus) may indicate resistance to the in-use product and change to a more effective disinfectant as indicated.

TEXTILES AND LAUNDRY

Handle used textiles and fabrics with minimum agitation to prevent contamination of air, surfaces, and persons. If laundry chutes are used, ensure that they are properly designed, maintained, and used in a manner to minimize dispersion of aerosols from contaminated laundry.

SAFE INJECTION PRACTICES

The following recommendations apply to the use of needles, cannulas that replace needles, and, where applicable, intravenous delivery systems. Use aseptic technique to prevent contamination of sterile injection equipment. Do not administer medications from a syringe to multiple patients even if the needle or cannula of the syringe is changed. Needles, cannulas, and syringes are sterile, single-use items; they should not be reused for another patient or to access a medication or solution that might be used for a subsequent patient. Use fluid infusion and administration sets (i.e., intravenous bags, tubing, and connectors) for one patient only and dispose of appropriately after use. Consider a syringe or needle/cannula contaminated once it has been used to enter or connect to a patient's intravenous infusion bag or administration set. Use single-dose vials for parenteral medications whenever possible. Do not administer medications from single-dose vials or ampules to multiple patients or combine leftover contents for later use. If multidose vials must be used, both the needle or cannula and syringe used to access the multidose vial must be sterile. Do not keep multidose vials in the immediate patient treatment area, and store them in accordance with the manufacturer's recommendations; discard if sterility is compromised or questionable. Do not use bags or bottles of intravenous solution as a common source of supply for multiple patients.

Infection control practices for special lumbar puncture procedures indicate wearing a surgical mask when placing a catheter or injecting material into the spinal canal or subdural space (i.e., during myelograms, lumbar puncture, and spinal or epidural anesthesia).

WORKER SAFETY

Adhere to federal and state requirements for protection of health care personnel from exposure to blood-borne pathogens.

appendix

C Standard Steps for All Nursing Procedures

AT THE BEGINNING OF THE PROCEDURE

STEP A: PERFORM TASK ACCORDING TO PROTOCOL

- Mentally review the steps of the task beforehand. If you are uncertain how to do a task, ask your team leader, resource nurse, instructor, or charge nurse.
- Plan for efficiency of time and effort while delivering safe care.

STEP B: CHECK ORDERS, COLLECT EQUIPMENT AND SUPPLIES, AND PERFORM HAND HYGIENE

- Verify that the procedure is to be done for the patient.
- Check the agency's policies and procedures manual for the accepted method of performing the procedure.
- Process equipment and supply charges.
- Take all equipment and supplies to the patient's room.

STEP C: IDENTIFY AND PREPARE PATIENT

- Greet the patient, introduce yourself, and check the patient's identification band. Use two identifiers during the identification process.
- Explain what you are going to do in terms the patient can understand.
- Elicit questions and answer clearly.
- Provide necessary teaching related to the procedure to be performed.

STEP D: PROVIDE PRIVACY, INSTITUTE SAFETY PRECAUTIONS, AND ARRANGE SUPPLIES AND EQUIPMENT

- Close the door or curtains and drape the patient before beginning the procedure or discussing information the person might want kept confidential.
- Check equipment for breaks or wear and for safety.
- Set up the equipment and supplies in an orderly, methodical fashion.
- Raise the bed to an appropriate working height.
- Raise the side rail before turning the patient and be certain that the wheels are locked.
- Perform hand hygiene to prevent contaminating the patient with organisms from the computer keyboard, the nurses' station, and the supply room.

DURING THE PROCEDURE

STEP E: USE STANDARD PRECAUTIONS AND ASEPTIC TECHNIQUE AS APPROPRIATE

- Protect yourself from blood and body fluids by wearing gloves.
- If there is a danger of splashing blood or body fluids, wear protective glasses or goggles and an impermeable cover gown or apron.
- Be very careful with sharp instruments and needles so as not to nick your skin. (See Appendix B.)

AT THE END OF THE PROCEDURE

STEP X: REMOVE GLOVES AND OTHER PROTECTIVE EQUIPMENT

- After making certain the patient is clean and dry, dispose of used supplies, remove goggles and other protective equipment, and discard or store appropriately.
- To remove gloves without contaminating yourself, begin by pulling one glove off without touching your skin; hold the removed glove in the palm of the remaining gloved hand and then reach to the inside of the other glove and roll it down the hand.
- Dispose of the gloves in the trash.
- Perform hand hygiene immediately.

STEP Y: RESTORE UNIT

- Collect the used equipment; dispose of, clean, or store items in the proper places.
- Make the person comfortable, tidy the bed and unit, place the call light and personal items within reach, and provide for safety by lowering the bed.
- Remove used equipment.
- Place soiled linens in a soiled-linen hamper.
- Clean reusable items and return them to the storage or processing area (central supply). Discontinue use of the equipment on the computer so no further charges will be made.
- Remove unsightly, odorous, or potentially infectious trash from the room.
- Inquire if anything else is needed.
- Perform hand hygiene before leaving the room.

STEP Z: RECORD AND REPORT PROCEDURE

- Document assessment findings and the details of the procedure performed, or care given, in the chart. Include any problems encountered and the patient's response to the care or treatment. The recording should be accurate, specific, concise, and appropriate and should include the specific time the procedure was performed and how it was done.
- Report abnormalities encountered to the charge nurse or health care provider.

References

CHAPTER 1: CARING FOR MEDICAL-SURGICAL PATIENTS

QSEN Competencies: 2018. Retrieved from: http://qsen.org/competencies/pre-licensure-ksas/.

The American Hospital Association (AHA): *The Patient Care Partnership: Understanding Expectations, Rights and Responsibilities*, 2003.

Institute of Medicine (US) Committee on the Health Professions Education Summit: In Greiner Ann C., Knebel Elisa, editors: *Health professions education: a bridge to quality*, Washington (DC), 2003, National Academies Press (US). HYPERLINK: http://www.nap.edu/

The Joint Commission: *Sentinel alert event, 58*: 2017. Retrieved from: https://www.jointcommission.org/assets/1/18/SEA_58_Hand_off_Comms_9_6_17_FINAL_(1).pdf.

The Leapfrog Hospital Safety Grade: organization, 2017. Theleapfroggroup, Choosing the right hospital. Retrieved from: https://www.leapfroggroup.org/hospital-choice/choosing-right-hospital.

The National Council of State Boards of Nursing (NCSBN): *ANA and NCSBN Joint Statement on Delegation*, 2006, 2016. Retrieved from: https://www.ncsbn.org/Delegation_joint_statement_NCSBN-ANA.pdf.

CHAPTER 2: CRITICAL THINKING AND THE NURSING PROCESS

Alfaro-Lefevre R: *Critical thinking, clinical reasoning, and clinical judgment*, ed 6, St. Louis, 2017, Elsevier.

Knecht P: *Success in practical/vocational nursing: from student to leader*, ed 8, St. Louis, 2017, Elsevier.

Williams P: *deWit's fundamental concepts and skills for nursing*, ed 5, St. Louis, 2018, Elsevier.

CHAPTER 3: FLUIDS, ELECTROLYTES, ACID-BASE BALANCE, AND INTRAVENOUS THERAPY

Joint Commission: *Universal protocol*, 2019. Retrieved from: www.jointcommission.org/PatientSafety/UniversalProtocol.

CHAPTER 4: CARE OF PREOPERATIVE AND INTRAOPERATIVE SURGICAL PATIENTS

American Society of Anesthesiologists: *Standards for basic anesthetic monitoring*, 2015. Retrieved from: http://www.asahq.org/quality-and-practice-management/standards-guidelines-and-related-resources/standards-for-basic-anesthetic-monitoring.

American Society of Anesthesiologists: Practice guidelines for preoperative fasting and the use of pharmacologic agents to reduce the risk of pulmonary aspiration, *Anesthesiology* 126(3):376–393, 2017.

Berrios-Torres SI, Umscheid CA, Bratzler DW: Centers for disease control and prevention guideline for the precention of surgical site infection, 2017, *JAMA Surg* 152(8):784–791, 2017.

Flanagan DA, Kerin A: How is intraoperative music therapy beneficial to adult patients undergoing general anesthesia? A systematic review, *Anesthesia eJournal* 5(2):2017.

Smith FD: Caring for surgical patients with piercings, *AORN J* 136(6):583–596, 2016.

CHAPTER 5: CARE OF POSTOPERATIVE SURGICAL PATIENTS

Anderson DJ, Sexton DJ: *Overview of control measures for prevention of surgical site infection*, 2018. Retrieved from: https://www.uptodate.com/contents/overview-of-control-measures-for-prevention-of-surgical-site-infection-in-adults.

Gestring M: *Negative pressure wound therapy*, 2018. Retrieved from: https://www.uptodate.com/contents/negative-pressure-wound-therapy.

Gould MK, Garcia DA, Wren SM, et al: Prevention of VTE in nonorthopedic surgical patients: Antithrombotic therapy and prevention of thrombosis, 9 ed: American College of Chest Physicians Evidence-Based Clinical Practice Guidelines, *Chest* 141(2 Suppl):e227S–e277S, 2012.

IHI: 2013a.

Kalff JC, Wehner S, Litkouhi B: *Measures to prevent prolonged postoperative ileus*, 2018. Retrieved from: https://www.uptodate.com/contents/measures-to-prevent-prolonged-postoperative-ileus.

Litman RS: *Malignant hyperthermia: clinical diagnosis and management of acute crisis*, 2018. Available from: https://www.uptodate.com/contents/malignant-hyperthermia-clinical-diagnosis-and-management-of-acute-crisis.

The Joint Commission: *Quality and Core Measure Updates: Surgical Care Improvement Project*, 2017. Available from: https://www.jointcommission.org/venous_thromboembolism/.

CHAPTER 6: INFECTION PREVENTION AND CONTROL

Agency for Healthcare Research and Quality: *Health care-associated infections*, 2017. Available from: https://psnet.ahrq.gov/primers/primer/7/health-care-associated-infections.

Centers for Disease Control and Prevention: *Guide to infection prevention for outpatient settings: minimum expectations for safe care*. Available from: https://www.cdc.gov/hai/settings/outpatient/outpatient-care-guidelines.html.

Kelly CP, Lamont JT, Bakken JS: Clostridium difficile *infection in adults: treatment and prevention*, 2018. Available from: https://www.uptodate.com/contents/clostridium-difficile-infection-in-adults-treatment-and-prevention.

Liu Y-Z, Wang Y-X, Jiang C-L: Inflammation: the common pathway of stress-related diseases, *Front Hum Neurosci* 11:316, 2017.

Marschall J, Memel LA, Yoke DS, et al: Strategies to prevent central line-associated bloodstream infections in acute care hospitals: 2014 update, *Infectional control and hospital epidemiology* 35(7):753–771, 2014. Available from: http://www.jstor.org/stable/10.1086/676533.

Napolitano LM: Sepsis 2018: definitions and guideline changes, *Surg Infect (Larchmt)* 19(2):117–125, 2018.

The Joint Commission: *Hospital national patient safety goals*, 2018. Available from: https://www.jointcommission.org/assets/1/6/2018_HAP_NPSG_goals_final.pdf.

The Joint Commission: *Citing observations for hand hygiene compliance - update*, 2017. Available from: https://www.jointcommission.org/assets/1/18/Update_Citing_Observations_of_Hand_Hygiene_Noncompliance.pdf.

CHAPTER 7: CARE OF PATIENTS WITH PAIN

Ahn AC: *Acupuncture*, 2018. Retrieved from: https://www.uptodate.com/contents/acupuncture.

Arnold RM, Childers JW: *Management of acute pain in the patient chronically using opioids*, 2018. Retrieved from: https://www.uptodate.com/contents/management-of-acute-pain-in-the-patient-chronically-using-opioids.

Bonshtein U: Hypnosis for pain relief, *J Anest Inten Care Med* 5(2):555657, 2018.

Center for Disease Control: *Opioid overdose*, 2017. Retrieved from: https://www.cdc.gov/drugoverdose/epidemic/index.html.

Center for Medicare and Medicaid Services: *Requirements for hospital medication administration, particularly intravenous (IV) medications and post-operative care of patients receiving IV opioids*, 2014. Retrieved from: https://www.cms.gov/Medicare/Provider-Enrollment-and-Certification/SurveyCertificationGenInfo/Downloads/Survey-and-Cert-Letter-14-15.pdf.

Chaudhry SR, Bhimji SS: *Biochemistry, endorphin.* (updated 2018 Jan 20). In StatPearls (internet): StatPearls Publishing, Treasure Island, FL. Retrieved from: https://www.ncbi.nlm.nih.gov/books/NBK470306/.

Czarnecki ML, Turner HN: *Core curriculum for paint management nursing*, ed 3, St. Louis, 2018, Elsevier.

Health and Human Services: *Secretary Price announces HHS strategy for fighting opioid Crisis*, 2017. Retrieved from: https://www.hhs.gov/about/leadership/secretary/speeches/2017-speeches/secretary-price-announces-hhs-strategy-for-fighting-opioid-crisis/index.html

Institute for safe medication practices: *Worth Repeating ... Recent PCA by proxy event suggests reassessment of practices that may have fallen by the wayside*, 2016. Retrieved from: https://www.ismp.org/resources/worth-repeating-recent-pca-proxy-event-suggests-reassessment-practices-may-have-fallen.

Jackson V, Nabati L: *Ethical considerations in effective pain management at the end of life*, 2018. Retrieved from: https://www.uptodate.com/contents/ethical-considerations-in-effective-pain-management-at-the-end-of-life.

Kovac AL, Mehta N, Salerno S, et al: 446 peripheral nerve blocks for analgesia in burn unit patients: a retrospective study, *J Burn Care Res*, 39(Suppl 1): S195–S196, 2018.

Lewis S, Bucher L, Heitkemper M, et al: *Medical-surgical nursing*, ed 10, St. Louis, 2017, Elsevier.

Murphy N, Karlin-Zysman C, Anandan S: Management of chronic pain in the elderly: a review of current and upcoming novel therapeutics, *Am J Ther* 25(1): e36–e43, 2018.

Turk DC, Gatchel RJ: *Psychological approaches to pain management; a practitioner's handbook*, ed 3, New York, 2018, The Guilford Press.

CHAPTER 8: CARE OF PATIENTS WITH CANCER

American Cancer Society: *Cancer facts and statistics*, 2017. Retrieved from: https://www.cancer.org/research/cancer-facts-statistics.html.

Faherty S: *NIH complete in-depth genomic analysis of 33 cancer types*, 2018. Retrieved from: https://www.genome.gov/news/news-release/NIH-completes-in-depth-genomic-analysis-of-33-cancer-types.

Hooly RJ, Durand MA, Philpotts LE: Advances in digital breast tomosynthesis, *AJR Am J Roentgenol* 208(2):256–266, 2017. doi:10.2214/AJR.16.17127.

National Cancer Institute, 2015. Retrieved from: http://www.cancer.gov/clinicaltrials.

National cancer institute: *Hormone therapy for breast cancer*, 2017. Retrieved from: https://www.cancer.gov/types/breast/breast-hormone-therapy-fact-sheet.

Siegel RL, Miller KD, Jemal A: Cancer statistics, 2019, *CA Cancer J Clin* 69(1):7–34, 2019. https://doi.org/10.3322/caac.21551.

U.S. Department of Health and Human Services: *The Health Consequences of smoking - 50 years of progress*, 2014. Retrieved from: https://www.ncbi.nlm.nih.gov/books/NBK179276/pdf/Bookshelf_NBK179276.pdf.

CHAPTER 9: CHRONIC ILLNESS AND REHABILITATION

Alzheimer's Association: 2017 Alzheimer's disease facts and figures, *Alzheimers Dement* 13(4):325–373, 2017.

American Psychological Association: *Choosing words for talking about disability*, 2018. Retrieved from: http://www.apa.org/pi/disability/resources/choosing-words.aspx.

Andelic N, Howe EI, Hellstrom T, et al: *Centers for Disease Control*, 2018.

Armour BS, Courtney-Long EA, Fox MH, et al: Prevalence and causes of paralysis-United States, *Am J Public Health* 106(10):1855–1857, 2016.

Centers for Disease Control and Prevention: *Chronic disease prevention and health promotion*, 2018. Retrieved from: https://www.cdc.gov/chronicdisease/about/index.htm.

Edward K-L: Chronic illness and wellbeing: using nursing practice to foster resilience as resistance, *Chronic Illn* 22(13):741–746, 2013.

Hartford Institute for Geriatric Nursing: n.d. Retrieved from: https://consultgeri.org/gitt-2.0-toolkit.

National Center for Health Statistics. Health, United States: *2017: with special feature on mortality*, Maryland., 2018, Hyattsville.

Scales D: *Sundowning: Why hospital staffs dread nightfall, and how to help seniors avoid it*, 2015. Retrieved from: http://www.wbur.org/commonhealth/2015/11/20/sundowning-seniors-nightfall-delirium.

The Joint Commission: *Nursing Care Center: 2018 National Patient Safety Goals*, 2019.

Walker N, Scott T, Dissanayaka NN, et al: Persisting use of physical restraint: knowledge translation vs. attitudes, *Int J Clin* 2018.

World Health Organization: *Spinal cord injury; Fact sheet*. 2013. http://www.who.int/news-room/fact-sheets/detail/spinal-cord-injury.

Yevchak AM, Steis MR, Evans LK: Sundown syndrome: a systematic review of the literature, *Res Gerontol Nurs* 5(4):294–308, 2012.

CHAPTER 10: THE IMMUNE AND LYMPHATIC SYSTEMS

Centers for Disease Control and Prevention: *Vaccine information statements (VISs)*, 2018. Retrieved from: https://www.cdc.gov/vaccines/hcp/vis/about/required-use-instructions.html.

Centers for Disease Control and Prevention: *Immunization Schedules*, 2018. Retrieved from: https://www.cdc.gov/vaccines/schedules/hcp/adult.html#schedules.

Louveau A, Smirnov I, Keyes TJ, et al: Structural and functional features of central nervous system lymphatics, *Nature* 523(7560):337–341, 2015.

CHAPTER 11: CARE OF PATIENTS WITH IMMUNE AND LYMPHATIC DISORDERS

American Autoimmune Related Diseases Association (AARDA): *Autoimmune disease list*, 2018. Retrieved from: https://www.aarda.org/diseaselist/.

American Cancer Society: *What is Kaposi sarcoma?*, 2018. Retrieved from: www.cancer.org/cancer/kaposisarcoma/detailedguide/kaposi-sarcoma-what-is-kaposi-sarcoma.

American Cancer Society: *Hodgkin disease*, 2018. Retrieved from: http://www.cancer.org/acs/groups/cid/documents/webcontent/003105-pdf.pdf.

American Cancer Society: *Key statistics for non-Hodgkin lymphoma*, 2018. Retrieved from: https://www.cancer.org/cancer/hodgkin-lymphoma/about/key-statistics.html.

American Cancer Society: *Survival rate and factors that affect prognosis (Outlook) for Non-Hodgkin lymphoma*, 2016. Retrieved from: https://www.cancer.org/cancer/non-hodgkin-lymphoma/detection-diagnosis-staging/factors-prognosis.html.

American Red Cross: *Risks and complications*, 2018. Retrieved from: https://www.redcrossblood.org/donate-blood/blood

-donation-process/what-happens-to-donated-blood/blood-transfusions/risks-complications.html.

AVERT: *HIV strains and types*, 2018. Retrieved from: https://www.avert.org/professionals/hiv-science/types-strains.

Barouch DH, Tomaka FL, Wegmann F, et al: Evalution of a mosaic HIV-1 vaccine in a multiculture, randomized, double-blind, placebo-controlled, phase 1/2a clinical trial (APPROACH) and in rhesus monkeys (NHP 13-19), *Lancet* 2018. Retrieved from: http://dx.doi.org/10.1016/S0140-6736(18)31364-3.

Bloomfield SF, Rook GAW, Scott EA, et al: Time to abandon the hygiene hypothesis: new perspective on allergic disease, the human microbiome, infectious disease prevention and the role of targeted hygiene, *Perspect Public Health* 136(4):213–224, 2016.

Cancer.net: *Lymphoma – Non-Hodgkin: Statistics*, 2018. Retrieved from: https://www.cancer.net/cancer-types/lymphoma-non-hodgkin/statistics.

Centers for Disease Control and Prevention: *Basic statistics*, 2018. Retrieved from: https://www.cdc.gov/hiv/basics/statistics.html.

Centers for Disease Control and Prevention: *HIV/AIDS*, 2018. Retrieved from: https://www.cdc.gov/hiv/basics/index.html.

Centers for Disease Control and Prevention: *National Center for Health Statistics*. Retrieved from: https://www.cdc.gov/nchs/fastats/life-expectancy.htm.

Goldenberg DL: *Clinical manifestations and diagnosis of fibromyalgia in adults*, 2017. Retrieved from: https://www.uptodate.com/contents/clinical-manifestations-and-diagnosis-of-fibromyalgia-in-adults.

HIV.gov: *HIV treatment as prevention*, 2018. Retrieved from: https://www.hiv.gov/hiv-basics/hiv-prevention/using-hiv-medication-to-reduce-risk/hiv-treatment-as-prevention.

HIV.gov: *US statistics*, 2017. Retrieved from: https://www.hiv.gov/hiv-basics/overview/data-and-trends/statistics.

U.S. Department of Agriculture (USDA): *ChooseMyPlate*, 2018. Retrieved from: http://www.choosemyplate.gov.

CHAPTER 12: THE RESPIRATORY SYSTEM

Agency for Healthcare Research and Quality (AHRQ): *Treating tobacco use and dependence: 2008 update*, 2018. From: https://www.ahrq.gov/professionals/clinicians-providers/guidelines-recommendations/tobacco/index.html.

American Cancer Society: *Esophageal cancer risk factors*, 2017. Retrieved from: https://www.cancer.org/cancer/esophagus-cancer/causes-risks-prevention/risk-factors.html.

American Cancer Society: *What are the risk factors for laryngeal and hypopharyngeal cancers?*, 2017. Retrieved from: http://www.cancer.org/cancer/laryngealandhypopharyngealcancer/detailedguide/laryngeal-and-hypopharyngeal-cancer-risk-factors.

Centers for Disease Control and Prevention (CDC): *Tuberculosis*, 2017. Retrieved from: https://www.cdc.gov/tb/topic/testing/tbtesttypes.htm.

Centers for Disease Control and Prevention (CDC): *Guillain-Barre Syndrome (GBS)*, 2017. Retrieved from: http://www.cdc.gov/flu/protect/vaccine/guillainbarre.htm.

Healthy People 2020: 2018. Retrieved from:, https://www.healthypeople.gov/2020/topics-objectives.

The Joint Commission: *Accountability measure list*, 2018. Retrieved from: http://www.jointcommission.org/accountability_measures.aspx.

Schwartz RA: *Clubbing of the Nails*, 2017. Retrieved from: https://emedicine.medscape.com/article/1105946-overview#a4.

Sertel Şelale D, Uzun M: The value of microscopic-observation drug susceptibility assay in the diagnosis of tuberculosis and detection of multidrug resistance, *APMIS* 126(1):38–44, 2018.

CHAPTER 13: CARE OF PATIENTS WITH DISORDERS OF THE UPPER RESPIRATORY SYSTEM

American Cancer Society: *About laryngeal and hypopharyngeal cancer*, 2017. Retrieved from: https://www.cancer.org/cancer/laryngeal-and-hypopharyngeal-cancer/about.html.

American Heart Association: *Adult basic life support: 2015 AHA guidelines for cardiopulmonary resuscitation and emergency cardiovascular care*, Dallas, Texas, 2015, American Heart Association.

Centers for Disease Control and Prevention: *Multidrug-resistant organisms (MDRO) Management*. 2017. Retrieved from: https://www.cdc.gov/infectioncontrol/guidelines/mdro/index.html.

Hyzy R: *Overview of tracheostomy*, 2016. Retrieved from: https://www.uptodate.com/contents/overview-of-tracheostomy.

The Joint Commission: *New Joint Commission advisory on non-pharmacologic and non-opioid solutions for pain management*, 2018. Retrieved from: https://www.jointcommission.org/new_joint_commission_advisory_on_non-pharmacologic_and_non-opioid_solutions_for_pain_management/.

Shah UK: *Tonsillitis and Peritonsillar Abscess Treatment and Management*, 2018. Retrieved from: http://emedicine.medscape.com/article/871977-treatment#d11.

CHAPTER 14: CARE OF PATIENTS WITH DISORDERS OF THE LOWER RESPIRATORY SYSTEM

Aggarwal V, Nicolais CD, Lee A, et al: *Acute management of pulmonary embolism*, 2017. Retrieved from: https://www.acc.org/latest-in-cardiology/articles/2017/10/23/12/12/acute-management-of-pulmonary-embolism.

American Cancer Society: *Lung cancer*. Retrieved from: https://www.cancer.org/cancer/lung-cancer.html. 2018.

American Lung Association: *Lung Health & Diseases; Mesothelioma*, 2018. Retrieved from: http://www.lung.org/lung-health-and-diseases/lung-disease-lookup/mesothelioma/.

American Society for Microbiology: *Tuberculosis drugs work better with Vitamin C*, 2018. Retrieved from: https://www.asm.org/index.php/newsroom/item/7031-tuberculosis-drugs-work-better-with-vitamin-c.

Baylor College of Medicine: *Introduction to Infectious Diseases*, 2018. Retrieved from: https://www.bcm.edu/departments/molecular-virology-and-microbiology/emerging-infections-and-biodefense/introduction-to-infectious-diseases.

Berry J: *Breathing exercises for people with COPD*, 2017. Retrieved from: https://www.medicalnewstoday.com/articles/315044.php.

Centers for Disease Control and Prevention: *Causes of pneumonia*, 2018. Retrieved from: https://www.cdc.gov/pneumonia/causes.html.

Centers for Disease Control and Prevention: *Influenza (Flu): Disease burden of influenza*, 2018. Retrieved from: https://www.cdc.gov/flu/about/disease/burden.htm.

Cousins JL, Wark PAB, McDonald VM: Acute oxygen therapy:a review of prescribing and delivery practices, *Int J Chron Obstruct Pulmon Dis* 11:1067–1075, 2016.

Cystic Fibrosis Foundation: *FDA approves ivacaftor for 23 additional CFTR mutations*, 2017. Retrieved from: https://www.cff.org/News/News-Archive/2017/FDA-Approves-Ivacaftor-for-23-Additional-CFTR-Mutations/.

Drugbank: *Pretomanid*, 2018. Retrieved from: https://www.drugbank.ca/drugs/DB05154.

Food and drug administration: *Fluoroquinolone antibiotics: FDA requires labeling canges due to low blood sugar levels and mental health side effects*, 7/10/2018. Retrieved from: https://www.fda.gov/Safety/MedWatch/SafetyInformation/SafetyAlertsforHumanMedicalProducts/ucm612979.htm.

Grohskopf LA, Sokolow LZ, Broder KR, et al: Prevention and control of seasonal influenza with vaccines: recommendations of the Advisory Committee on Immunization Practices — United States, 2017–18 influenza season, *MMWR Recomm Rep* 66(RR–2):1–20, 2017. http://dx.doi.org/10.15585/mmwr.rr6602a1.

Houghton LA, Lee AS, Badri H, et al: Respiratory disease and the oesophagus: reflux, reflexes and microaspiration, *Nat Rev Gastroenterol Hepatol* 13:445, 2016. http://dx.doi.org/10.1038/nrgastro.2016.91. online.

National Institutes of Health Chronic Obstructive Pulmonary Disease (COPD) 2018. Retrieved from: https://report.nih.gov/nihfactsheets/ViewFactSheet.aspx?csid=77.

National Vital Statistics Reports: *Deaths: Final Data for 2015*, 66 (6), 2017. Retrieved from: https://www.cdc.gov/nchs/data/nvsr/nvsr66/nvsr66_06.pdf.

Ouellette DR: *Pulmonary embolism guidelines*, 2018. Retrieved from: https://emedicine.medscape.com/article/300901-guidelines#g2.

Rubin LJ, Hopkins W: *Classification and prognosis of pulmonary hypertension in adults*, 2018. Retrieved from: https://www.uptodate.com/contents/classification-and-prognosis-of-pulmonary-hypertension-in-adults.

Timsit J-F, Esaied W, Neuville M, et al: Update on ventilator-associated pneumonia, *F1000Res* 6:2061, 2017. http://doi.org/10.12688/f1000research.12222.1.

World Health Organization: *The top 10 causes of death*, 2018. Retrieved from: http://www.who.int/en/news-room/fact-sheets/detail/the-top-10-causes-of-death.

Zirk-Sadowski J, Masoli JA, Delgado J, et al: Proton-pump inhibitors and long-term risk of community-acquired pneumonia in older adults, *J Am Geriatr Soc* 66(7):2018. http://doi.org/10.1111/jgs.15385.

CHAPTER 15: THE HEMATOLOGIC SYSTEM

AWHONN: Quantification of blood loss: AWHONN practice brief number 1, *Nurs Womens Health* 19(1):96–98, 2015.

CHAPTER 16: CARE OF PATIENTS WITH HEMATOLOGIC DISORDERS

Center for Disease Control: *Hemophilia, Data & Statistics*, 2018. Retrieved from: https://www.cdc.gov/ncbddd/hemophilia/data.html.

FDA: *Information on Erythropoiesis-Stimulating agents (ESA) epoetin alfa (marketed as Procrit, Epogen), darbepoetin alfa (marketed as Aranesp)*, 2017. Retrieved from: https://www.fda.gov/Drugs/DrugSafety/ucm109375.htm.

Field JJ, Vichinsky EP, DeBaun MR: *Overview of the management and prognosis of sickle cell disease*, 2018. Retrieved from: https://www.uptodate.com/contents/overview-of-the-management-and-prognosis-of-sickle-cell-disease.

Gorski L, Hadaway L, Hagle ME, et al: Infusion therapy standards of practice, *J Infus Nurs* 39(1S):2016. ISSN 1533-1458.

Harper JL: *Iron deficiency anemia treatment and management*, 2018. Retrieved from: https://emedicine.medscape.com/article/202333-treatment#d7.

Kim S, Kim S, Park Y, et al: Nutritional intervention for a patient with acute lymphoblastic leukemia on allogenic peripheral blood stem cell transplantation, *Clin Nutr Res* 7(3):223–228, 2018.

Leung LLK: *Clinical features, diagnosis, and treatment of disseminated intravascular coagulation in adults*, 2018. Retrieved from: https://www.uptodate.com/contents/clinical-features-diagnosis-and-treatment-of-disseminated-intravascular-coagulation-in-adults.

Leukemia & Lymphoma Society: *Facts and statistics*, 2018. Retrieved from: https://www.lls.org/http%3A/llsorg.prod.acquia-sites.com/facts-and-statistics/facts-and-statistics-overview/facts-and-statistics.

Nihara Y, Miller ST, Kanter J, et al: A phase 3 trial of L-glutamine in sickle cell disease, *N Engl J Med* 379:226–235, 2018.

Ribeil JA, Hacein-Bey-Abina S, Payen E, et al: Gene therapy in a patient with sickle cell disease, *N Engl J Med* 376:848–855, 2017.

Rodgers GP, George A 2018. *Hydroxyurea use in sickle cell disease*. Retrieved from: https://www.uptodate.com/contents/hydroxyurea-use-in-sickle-cell-disease.

Schrier SL: *Treatment of iron deficiency anemia in adults*, 2018. Retrieved from: https://www.uptodate.com/contents/treatment-of-iron-deficiency-anemia-in-adults.

CHAPTER 17: THE CARDIOVASCULAR SYSTEMS

Benjamin EJ, Virani SS, Callaway CW, et al; on behalf of the American Heart Association Council on Epidemiology and Prevention Statistics Committee and Stroke Statistics Subcommittee: Heart disease and stroke statistics – 2018 update: a report from the American Heart Association, *Circulation* 137:e67–e492, 2018.

Harvard Medical School: *The genetics of heart disease: an update*, 2017. Retrieved from: https://www.health.harvard.edu/heart-health/the-genetics-of-heart-disease-an-update.

McCulloch DK: *Glycemic control and vascular complications in type 1 diabetes mellitus*, 2018. Retrieved from: https://www.uptodate.com/contents/glycemic-control-and-vascular-complications-in-type-1-diabetes-mellitus.

National Institute on Drug Abuse: *Health Consequences of drug misuse*, 2017. Retrieved from: https://www.drugabuse.gov/publications/health-consequences-drug-misuse/cardiovascular-effects.

Wang SS: *Metabolic syndrome*, 2017. Retrieved from: http://emedicine.medscape.com/article/165124-overview.

Whelton PK, Carey RM, Aronow WS, et al: 2017 ACC/AHA/AAPA/ABC/ACPM/AGS/APhA/ASH/ASPC/NMA/PCNA guideline for the prevention, detection, evaluation and management of high blood pressure in adults, *J Am Coll Cardiol* 71(19):e127–e248, 2018.

World Health Organization: *Mean systolic blood pressure*, 2018. Retrieved from: http://www.who.int/gho/ncd/risk_factors/blood_pressure_mean_text/en/.

Zafari AM: *Myocardial Infarction*, 2018. Retrieved from: http://emedicine.medscape.com/article/155919-overview.

CHAPTER 18: CARE OF PATIENTS WITH HYPERTENSION AND PERIPHERAL VASCULAR DISEASE

Alexander MR: *Hypertension*, 2018. Retrieved from: https://emedicine.medscape.com/article/241381-overview#aw2aab6b2b3aa.

Dominguez JA: *Peripheral arterial occlusive disease treatment and management*, 2018. Retrieved from: https://emedicine.medscape.com/article/460178-overview.

Lew WK: *Varicose Vein Surgery*, 2017. Retrieved from: http://emedicine.medscape.com/article/462579-overview.

Patel K: *Deep Venous Thrombosis Treatment and Management*, 2017. Retrieved from: http://emedicine.medscape.com/article/1911303-treatment.

Rahimi SA: *Abdominal Aortic Aneurysm*, 2017. Retrieved from: https://emedicine.medscape.com/article/463147-overview.

Rodriguez AL: *Atherosclerotic disease of the carotid artery*, 2017. Retrieved from: https://emedicine.medscape.com/article/1979501-overview.

Schonwald S: *Licorice poisoning*, 2017. Retrieved from: https://emedicine.medscape.com/article/817578-overview#a5.

Weiss R: *Venous insufficiency*, 2017. Retrieved from: http://emedicine.medscape.com/article/1085412-overview.

Young DR, Fischer H, Arterburn D, et al: Associations of overweight/obesity and socioeconomic status with hypertension prevalence across racial and ethnic groups, *J Clin Hypertens* 20:532–540, 2018.

CHAPTER 19: CARE OF PATIENTS WITH CARDIAC DISORDERS

AHA: *Know your fats*, 2017. Retrieved from: http://www.heart.org/HEARTORG/Conditions/Cholesterol/PreventionTreatmentofHighCholesterol/Know-Your-Fats_UCM_305628_Article.jsp.

Borlaug BA, Colucci WS: *Treatment and prognosis for heart failure with preserved ejection fraction*, 2018. Retrieved from: https://www.uptodate.com/contents/treatment-and-prognosis-of-heart-failure-with-preserved-ejection-fraction.

Center for Disease Control and Prevention. National Center for Chronic Disease Prevention and Health Promotion, 2018. Retrieved from: https://www.cdc.gov/chronicdisease/index.htm.

Centers for Medicare & Medicaid Services: *Core ser of adult health care quality measures for Medicaid*, 2018. Retrieved from: https://www.medicaid.gov/medicaid/quality-of-care/downloads/medicaid-adult-core-set-manual.pdf.

Nishimura RA, Otto CM, Bonow RO, et al: 2017 AHA/ACC focused update of the 2014 AHA/ACC Guideline for the Management of Patients With Valvular Heart Disease, *Circulation* 135(25):e1159–e1195, 2017.

Yancy CW, Jessup M, Bozkurt B, et al: 2017 ACC/AHA/HFSA focused update of the 2013 ACC/AHA guideline for the management of heart failure: a report of the American College of Cardiology/American Heart Association task force on clinical practice guidelines and the Heart Failure Society of America, *Circulation* 136(6):e136–e161, 2017. doi:10.1161/CIR.0000000000000509.

CHAPTER 20: CARE OF PATIENTS WITH CORONARY ARTERY DISEASE AND CARDIAC SURGERY

American Heart Association: *Coronary microvascular disease (MVD)*, 2017. Retrieved from: http://www.heart.org/HEARTORG/Conditions/HeartAttack/SymptomsDiagnosisofHeartAttack/Coronary-Microvascular-Disease-MVD_UCM_450320_Article.jsp#.W4R4quhKiUk.

Eisen HJ: *Patient Information: Heart transplantation (beyond the basics)*, 2018. Retrieved from: http://www.uptodate.com/contents/heart-transplantation-beyond-the-basics.

FDA: *Grapefruit juice and some drugs don't mix*, 2017. Retrieved from: https://www.fda.gov/ForConsumers/ConsumerUpdates/ucm292276.htm.

Fleming J, Aspry KE, Resnicow K, Etherton PM: *Translating the ACC/AHA lifestyle management guideline into practice: Advice for cardiologists from experts in nutrition behavioral medicine and cardiology*, 2016. Retrieved from: https://www.acc.org/latest-in-cardiology/articles/2015/12/31/10/12/translating-the-acc-aha-lifestyle-management-guideline-into-practice.

Rivera-Bou WL: *Thrombolytic Therapy*, 2017. Retrieved from: http://emedicine.medscape.com/article/811234-overview.

Wenger NK: *Efficacy of cardiac rehabilitation in patients with coronary disease*, 2018. Retrieved from: http://www.uptodate.com/contents/efficacy-of-cardiac-rehabilitation-in-patients-with-coronary-heart-disease.

Zafari AM: *Myocardial Infarction Clinical Presentation*, 2018. Retrieved from: https://emedicine.medscape.com/article/155919-overview. Chapter 21: The Neurologic System.

CHAPTER 21: THE NEUROLOGIC SYSTEM

Abrams GM, Wakasa M: *Chronic complications of spinal cord injury and disease*, 2018. Retrieved from: https://www.uptodate.com/contents/chronic-complications-of-spinal-cord-injury-and-disease.

Nair S, Surendran A, Prabhakar RB, et al: Comparison between FOUR score and GCS in assessing patients with traumatic head injury: a tertiary centre study, *Int Surg J* 4:656, 2017. doi:10.18203/2349-2902.isj20170209.

CHAPTER 22: CARE OF PATIENTS WITH HEAD AND SPINAL CORD INJURIES

Atlas SJ: *Taming the pain of sciatica:For most people, time heals and less is more*, 2017. Retrieved from: https://www.health.harvard.edu/blog/taming-pain-sciatica-people-time-heals-less-2017071212048.

Carney N, Totten A, O'Reilly, et al: *Guidelines for the management of severe traumatic brain injury 4th ed*. Retrieved from: https://braintrauma.org/uploads/03/12/Guidelines_for_Management_of_Severe_TBI_4th_Edition.pdf.

Drappatz J: *Management of vasogenic edema in patients with primary and metastatic brain tumors*, 2018. Retrieved from: https://www.uptodate.com/contents/management-of-vasogenic-edema-in-patients-with-primary-and-metastatic-brain-tumors#H2267496419.

Evans RW, Whitlow CT: *Acute mild traumatic brain injury (concussion) in adults*, 2018. Retrieved from: https://www.uptodate.com/contents/acute-mild-traumatic-brain-injury-concussion-in-adults.

Hansebout RR, Kachur E: *Acute traumatic spinal cord injury*, 2018. Retrieved from: https://www.uptodate.com/contents/acute-traumatic-spinal-cord-injury.

Howells T, Smielewski P, Donnelly J, et al: Optimal cerebral perfusion pressure in centers with different treatment protocols, *Crit Care Med* 46(3):e235–e241, 2018.

Lennon S, Ramdharry G, Verheyden G, editors: *Physical Management for neurological conditions*, ed 4, Traumatic Brain Injury, 2018, Elsevieres.

National Spinal Cord Injury Statistical Center [NSCISC]: *Spinal cord injury facts and figures at a glance*, 2018. Retrieved from: https://www.nscisc.uab.edu/Public/Facts%20and%20Figures%20-%202018.pdf.

Qaseem A, Wilt TJ, McLean RM, et al: 2017 Noninvasive treatments for acute, subacute and chronic low back pain: a clinical practice guideline from the American college of physicians, *Ann Intern Med* 166(7):514–530, 2017.

Rajajee V: *Traumatic brain injury: Epidemiology, classification and pathophysiology*, 2018. Retrieved from: https://www.uptodate.com/contents/traumatic-brain-injury-epidemiology-classification-and-pathophysiology.

ReWalk: *First and only exoskeleton cleared by the FDA*, 2018. Retrieved from: http://www.ReWalk.com.

Stephenson R: *Autonomic dysreflexia in spinal cord injury*, 2018. Retrieved from: https://emedicine.medscape.com/article/322809-overview#a3.

CHAPTER 23: CARE OF PATIENTS WITH BRAIN DISORDERS

American Brain Tumor Association [ABTA]: *Brain tumor FAQs*. Retrieved from: https://www.abta.org/about-brain-tumors/brain-tumor-faqs/

Bajwa ZH, Ho CC, Khan SA: *Trigeminal neuralgia*, 2018. Retrieved from: https://www.uptodate.com/contents/trigeminal-neuralgia.

Batchelor T: *Initial postoperative therapy for glioblastoma and anaplastic astrocytoma astrocytoma*, 2018. Retrieved from: https://www.uptodate.com/contents/initial-postoperative-therapy-for-glioblastoma-and-anaplastic-astrocytoma.

Blumenfeld AM: Botox for chronic migraine: tips and tricks. *Practical Neurology*, February 2018. Retrieved from: http://practicalneurology.com/2018/02/botox-for-chronic-migraine-tips-and-tricks/.

Centers for Disease Control and Prevention: *EpilepsyData and statistics*, 2018a. Retrieved from: https://www.cdc.gov/epilepsy/data/index.html.

Centers for Disease Control and Prevention: *Stroke, Conditions that increase risk for stroke*, 2018b. Retrieved from: https://www.cdc.gov/stroke/conditions.htm.

Centers for Disease Control and Prevention: *Stroke facts*, 2017. Retrieved from: http://www.cdc.gov/stroke/facts.htm.

Centers for Disease Control and Prevention: *Vaccines and preventable diseases*, 2017. Retreived from: https://www.cdc.gov/vaccines/vpd/mening/hcp/recommendations.html.

Furie KL, Ay H: *Definition, etiology, and clinical manifestations of transient ischemic attack*, 2018. Retrieved from: https://www.uptodate.com/contents/definition-etiology-and-clinical-manifestations-of-transient-ischemic-attack.

Glauser T, Shinnaer S, Gloss D, et al: Evidence-Based guideline: treatment of convulsive status epilepticus in children and adults: report of the guideline committee of the American epilepsy society, *Epilepsy Curr* 16(1):48–61, 2016.

Hasbun R: *Meningitis*, 2017. Retrieved from: http://emedicine.medscape.com/article/232915-treatment.

Loeffler JS: *Epidemiology, clinical manifestations and diagnosis of brain metastases*, 2018. Retrieved from: https://www.uptodate.com/contents/epidemiology-clinical-manifestations-and-diagnosis-of-brain-metastases.

National Institutes of Health, National Institute on Drug Abuse: *Health Consequences of drug misuse*, 2017. Retrieved from: https://www.drugabuse.gov/publications/health-consequences-drug-misuse/neurological-effects.

National Institute of neurological disorders and stroke [NINDS]: *Migraine information page, 2018, U.S. Department of Health and Human Service, Public Health Service, National Institutes of Health.* Retrieved from: https://www.ninds.nih.gov/Disorders/All-Disorders/Migraine-Information-Page.

Powers WJ, Rabinstein AA, Ackerson T, et al; on behalf of the American Heart Association Stroke Council: 2018 Guidelines for the early management of patients with acute ischemic stroke: a guideline for healthcare professionals from the American Heart Association/American Stroke Association, *Stroke* 49:e46–e99, 2018.

Puledda F, Shields K: Non-pharmacological approaches for migraine, *Neurother* 15(2):336–345, 2018.

Said S, Kang M: *Viral Encephalitis*, 2018. Retrieved from: https://www.ncbi.nlm.nih.gov/books/NBK470162/.

Taylor DC: *Bell Palsy*, 2018. Retrieved from: http://emedicine.medscape.com/article/1146903-overview.

The Joint Commission: *Acute Stroke Ready Inpatient (ASR-IP)*, 2018. Retrieved from: https://manual.jointcommission.org/releases/TJC2018A1/AcuteStrokeReadyInpatient.html.

Winstein CJ, Stein J, Arena R, et al: *Guidelines for adult stroke rehabilitation and recovery guideline for healthcare professionals from the American Heart World Health Organization, Epilepsy*, 2018. Retrieved from: http://www.who.int/news-room/fact-sheets/detail/epilepsy.

Winstein CJ, Stein J, Arena R, et al: Association/American stroke association, *Stroke* 47(6):e98–e169, 2016.

CHAPTER 24: CARE OF PATIENTS WITH PERIPHERAL NERVE AND DEGENERATIVE NEUROLOGIC DISORDERS

Andary MT: *Guillain-Barre Syndrome treatment & management*, 2018. Medscape Reference. Retrieved from: http://emedicine.medscape.com/article/315632-treatment.

Armon CA: *Amyotrophic lateral sclerosis*, 2018. Retrieved from: https://emedicine.medscape.com/article/1170097-overview#a1.

Carroll WM: 2017 McDonald MS diagnostic criteria: Evidence-based revisions, *Mult Scler* 24(2):92–95, 2018.

Food and Drug Administration (FDA) *Current and resolved drug shortages and discontinuations reported to FDA*, 2017. Retrieved from: https://www.accessdata.fda.gov/scripts/drugshortages/dsp_ActiveIngredientDetails.cfm?AI=Edrophonium+Chloride+%28ENLON%29+Injection%2C+USP&st=d&tab=tabs-2.

Harmon M: *Exercise as part of everyday life*, 2016. National Multiple Sclerosis Society. Retrieved from: https://www.nationalmssociety.org/NationalMSSociety/media/MSNationalFiles/Brochures/Brochure-Exercise-as-Part-of-Everyday-Life.pdf.

Hauser RA: *Parkinson Disease treatment & management*, 2018. Medscape Reference. Retrieved from: http://emedicine.medscape.com/article/1831191-treatment.

Jankovic J: *Etiology and pathogenesis of Parkinson Disease*, 2018. UpToDate: Wolters Kluwer. Retrieved from: http://www.uptodate.com/contents/etiology-and-pathogenesis-of-parkinson-disease.

Koskie B, Kim S: *Multiple sclerosis:Facts statistics, and You*, 2018. Retrieved from: https://www.healthline.com/health/multiple-sclerosis/facts-statistics-infographic#1.

Lakhan SE: *Alzheimer Disease*, 2018. Retrieved from: https://emedicine.medscape.com/article/1134817-overview.

NINDS (National Institute of Neurological Disorders and Stroke): *Deep brain stimulation for movement disorders fact sheet*, 2018a. Retrieved from: https://www.ninds.nih.gov/Disorders/Patient-Caregiver-Education/Fact-Sheets/Deep-Brain-Stimulation-Movement-Disorders-Fact.

NINDS (National Institute of Neurological Disorders and Stroke): *Guillain-Barre syndrome*, 2018b, Bethesda, Md., U.S. Department of Health and Human Services. Retrieved from: https://www.ninds.nih.gov/Disorders/All-Disorders/Guillain-Barr%C3%A9-Syndrome-Information-Page.

Ondo WG: *Clinical features and diagnosis of restless leg syndrome and periodic limb movement disorders in adults*, 2018. Retrieved from: https://www.uptodate.com/contents/clinical-features-and-diagnosis-of-restless-legs-syndrome-and-periodic-limb-movement-disorder-in-adults.

CHAPTER 25: THE SENSORY SYSTEM: EYE

AMD.org: *Research on AMD*, 2019. Retrieved from: http://www.ucirvineamd.org/research.html.

American Academy of Ophthalmology (AAO): *Frequency of Ocular Examinations*, 2015. Retrieved from: https://www.aao.org/clinical-statement/frequency-of-ocular-examinations.

American Foundation for the Blind: *Facts and Figures on Adults with Vision Loss*, 2018. Retrieved from: http://www.afb.org/info/blindness-statistics/adults/facts-and-figures/235#demographics.

American Optometric Association: *UV Protection*, 2018. Retrieved from: https://www.aoa.org/patients-and-public/caring-for-your-vision/uv-protection.

Arroyo JG: *Age-related macular degeneration: clinical presentation, etiology and diagnosis*, 2018. Retrieved from: https://www.uptodate.com/contents/age-related-macular-degeneration-clinical-presentation-etiology-and-diagnosis.

Baker-Schena L: *Expensive drugs. EyeNet Magazine*, 2017. Retrieved from: https://www.aao.org/eyenet/article/expensive-drugs.

Bashour M: *Corneal foreign body clinical presentation. Medscape Reference*, 2018. Retrieved from: http://emedicine.medscape.com/article/1195581-clinical.

Boyd K: *What is glaucoma?*, 2018. Retrieved from: https://www.aao.org/eye-health/diseases/what-is-glaucoma.

Brady CJ: *How to remove a foreign body from the eye*, 2018. Retrieved from: https://www.merckmanuals.com/professional/eye-disorders/how-to-do-eye-procedures/how-to-remove-a-foreign-body-from-the-eye.

Food and Drug Administration: *Eye cosmetic safety*, 2018. Retrieved from: https://www.fda.gov/Cosmetics/ProductsIngredients/Products/ucm137241.htm.

Foster CS: *Dry eye disease (keratoconjunctivitis sicca)*, 2017. Retrieved from: https://emedicine.medscape.com/article/1210417-treatment.

Glaucoma.org: *Five common glaucoma tests*, 2017. Retrieved from: http://www.glaucoma.org/glaucoma/diagnostic-tests.php.

Grant TA: *Marijuana and glaucoma*, 2018. Retrieved from: http://glaucomatoday.com/2018/04/marijuana-and-glaucoma/.

Ignotz KD: *Clinical trials scheduled for drug-eluting contact lens*, 2018. Retrieved from: https://www.healio.com/optometry/contact-lenses-eye-wear/news/online/%7B4b7663bf-9c1e-4cb4-a0de-88a7ee0fb2e0%7D/clinical-trials-scheduled-for-drug-eluting-contact-lens.

Isaacson A, Swioklo S, Connon CJ: 3D bioprinting of a corneal stroma equivalent. In *Expermental eye research*, vol 173, 2018, pp 188–193.

Lains I, Kelly RS, Miller JB, et al: Human plasma metabolomics study across all stages of age-related macular degeneration identifies potential lipid biomarkers, *Opthamalmology* 125(2):245–254, 2018.

Mayo Clinic: *Retinal Detachment*, 2018. Retrieved from: https://www.mayoclinic.org/diseases-conditions/retinal-detachment/diagnosis-treatment/drc-20351348.

McClure LA, Tannenbaum SL, Zheng DD, et al: Eye health knowledge and eye health information exposure among Hispanic/Latino individuals: results from the Hispanic Community Health Study/Study of Latinos, *JAMA Ophthalmol* 135(8):878–882, 2017.

National Eye Institute: *Eye Health Tips*, 2010. Retrieved from: https://nei.nih.gov/healthyeyes/eyehealthtips.

National Eye Institute: *What the Age-related eye disease studies mean for you*, 2018. Retrieved from: https://nei.nih.gov/areds2/PatientFAQ.

National Institutes of Health: *NIH discovery brings stem cell therapy for eye disease closer to the clinic*, 2018. Retrieved from: https://www.nih.gov/news-events/news-releases/nih-discovery-brings-stem-cell-therapy-eye-disease-closer-clinic.

Pazirandeh S, Burns DL: *Overview of vitamin A*, 2018. Retrieved from: https://www.uptodate.com/contents/overview-of-vitamin-a.

Shtein RM: *Dry eyes*, 2018. Retrieved from: https://www.uptodate.com/contents/dry-eyes.

Ventocilla M: *Ophthalmologic approach to chemical burns*. Medscape Reference, 2018. Retrieved from: http://emedicine.medscape.com/article/1215950-overview.

CHAPTER 26: THE SENSORY SYSTEM: EAR

Better Hearing Institute: *Addressing hearing loss sooner brings many benefits*, 2015. Retrieved from: http://www.betterhearing.org/news/addressing-hearing-loss-sooner-brings-many-benefits.

Dinces EA: *Treatment of tinnitus*, 2018. Retrieved from: https://www.uptodate.com/contents/treatment-of-tinnitus.

Furman JM: *Vestibular neuritis and labyrinthitis*, 2018. Retrieved from: https://www.uptodate.com/contents/vestibular-neuritis-and-labyrinthitis.

Moskowitz HS: *Meniere disease*, 2018. Retrieved from: https://www.uptodate.com/contents/meniere-disease2.

National Institute on Deafness and Other Communication Disorders: *Noise-Induced hearing loss*, 2017. Retrieved from: https://www.nidcd.nih.gov/health/noise-induced-hearing-loss.

Weber PC: *Evaluation of hearing loss in adults*, 2018. Retrieved from: https://www.uptodate.com/contents/evaluation-of-hearing-loss-in-adults.

CHAPTER 27: THE GASTROINTESTINAL SYSTEM

Afdhal NH, Zakko SF: *Gallstones: Epidemiology, risk factors and prevention*. 2018. Retrieved from: https://www.uptodate.com/contents/gallstones-epidemiology-risk-factors-and-prevention.

American College of Radiology: *Virtual colonoscopy can attract younger Americans to follow new ACS guidelines*, 2018. Retrieved from: https://www.acr.org/Media-Center/ACR-News-Releases/2018/Virtual-Colonoscopy-Can-Attract-Younger-Americans-to-Follow-New-ACS-Guidelines.

Chemmanur AT: *Biliary Disease*. 2018. Retrieved from: https://emedicine.medscape.com/article/171386-overview.

Clarke MM, Stanhewicz AE, Kenney LW: Commercial hydration beverages effectively prolong positive fluid balance in older adults compared to water, *Med Sci Sports Exerc* 50(5S):386, 2018.

Elhardello O, Macfie J: Bowel sounds: is it time for surgeons to hang up their stethocopes?, *World J Surg Res* 1:1066, 2018. Retrieved from: http://www.surgeryresearchjournal.com/pdfs_folder/wjssr-v1-id1066.pdf.

Gregorian T, Lewis J, Tsu L: Opioid induced constipation: clinical guidance and approved therapies, *US Pharm* 42(12):15–19, 2017.

Micozzi MS: *Fundamentals of complementary, alternative, and integrative medicine*, ed 6, St. Louis, 2019, Elsevier.

Murphy J: *Closing in on a hepatitis C vaccine*. 2018. Retrieved from: https://www.mdlinx.com/infectious-disease/article/1404.

Schwartz JM, Carithers RL: *Epidemiology and etiologic associations of hepatocellular carcinoma*, 2018. Retrieved from: https://www.uptodate.com/contents/epidemiology-and-etiologic-associations-of-hepatocellular-carcinoma.

WebMD: *Using probiotics for diarrhea*, 2018. Retrieved from: http://www.webmd.com/digestive-disorders/probiotics-diarrhea.

Wolf AMD, Fontham ETH, Church RT, et al: Colorectal cancer screening for averae-risk adults: 2018 guideline update from the American Cancer Society, *CA Cancer J Clin* 68(4):250–281, 2018.

CHAPTER 28: CARE OF PATIENTS WITH DISORDERS OF THE UPPER GASTROINTESTINAL SYSTEM

American Cancer Society: *Esophagus cancer*, 2018a. Retrieved from: http://www.cancer.org/cancer/esophaguscancer/detailedguide/esophagus-cancer-key-statistics?docSelected=esophagus-cancer-what-is-cancer-of-the-esophagus.

American Cancer Society: *Oral cavity and oropharyngeal cancer*, 2018b. Retrieved from: http://www.cancer.org/cancer/oral-cavityandoropharyngealcancer/detailedguide/oral-cavity-and-oropharyngeal-cancer-key-statistics.

American Cancer Society: *Palliative therapy for cancer of the esophagus*, 2017. Retrieved from: http://www.cancer.org/cancer/esophaguscancer/detailedguide/esophagus-cancer-treating-palliative-therapy.

American Cancer Society: *Stomach cancer*, 2018c. Retrieved from: http://www.cancer.org/cancer/stomachcancer/detailedguide/stomach-cancer-key-statistics.

Anand BS: *Peptic ulcer disease*, 2018. Retrieved from: https://emedicine.medscape.com/article/181753-overview.

Cook D, Guyatt G: Prophylaxis against upper gastrointestinal bleeding in hospitalized patients, *N Engl J Med* 378(26):2506–2516, 2018.

Garvey WT, Mechanick LI, Brett EM, et al: 2016 American association of clinical endocrinologists and American college of endocrinology comprehensive clinical practice guidelines for medical care of patients with obesity, *Endocr Pract* 22(Suppl 3):2016.

Harding SM: *Gastroesophageal reflux and asthma*, 2018. Retrieved from: https://www.uptodate.com/contents/gastroesophageal-reflux-and-asthma.

Masab M: *Esophageal cancer treatment & management*, 2018. Retrieved from: https://emedicine.medscape.com/article/277930-treatment.

Saltzman JR: *Approach to acute upper gastrointestinal bleeding in adults*, 2018. Retrieved from: http://www.uptodate.com/contents/approach-to-acute-upper-gastrointestinal-bleeding-in-adults.

Warren M, Beck S, Rayburn J: *The state of obesity: 2018. Robert Wood Johnson Foundation and Trust for America's Health*. Retrieved from: https://stateofobesity.org/wp-content/uploads/2018/09/stateofobesity2018.pdf.

Wolf MM: *Proton pump inhibitors: overview of use and adverse effects in the treatment of acid related disorders*, 2018. Retrieved from: https://www.uptodate.com/contents/proton-pump-inhibitors-overview-of-use-and-adverse-effects-in-the-treatment-of-acid-related-disorders.

CHAPTER 29: CARE OF PATIENTS WITH DISORDERS OF THE LOWER GASTROINTESTINAL SYSTEM

American Cancer Society: *Colorectal cancer facts and figures*, 2018. Retrieved from: http://www.cancer.org/cancer/colonandrectum cancer/detailedguide/colorectal-cancer-key-statistics.

American Cancer Society: *Colorectal cancer risk factors*, 2018a. Retrieved from: https://www.cancer.org/cancer/colon-rectal-cancer/causes-risks-prevention/risk-factors.html.

American Cancer Society: *Colorectal cancer signs and symptoms*, 2018b. Retrieved from: https://www.cancer.org/cancer/colon-rectal-cancer/detection-diagnosis-staging/signs-and-symptoms.html.

Black P: Cultural and religious beliefs in stoma care nursing, *Br J Nurs* 18(13):790–793, 2009.

Bordeianou L: *Overview of management of mechanical small bowel obstruction in adults*. Retrieved from: https://www.uptodate.com/contents/overview-of-management-of-mechanical-small-bowel-obstruction-in-adults.

Cagir B: *What vaccine is available for the prevention of rectal cancer?* 2018. Retrieved from: https://www.medscape.com/answers/281237-100613/what-vaccine-is-available-for-the-prevention-of-rectal-cancer.

Craig S: *Appendicitis Workup*, 2018. Retrieved from: http://emedicine.medscape.com/article/773895-workup#aw2aab6b5b9.

Ghoulam EM: *Diverticulitis*, 2018. Retrieved from: https://emedicine.medscape.com/article/173388-overview.

Halas-Liang M: *Peppermint and IBS*, 2018. Retrieved from: https://irritablebowelsyndrome.net/food/peppermint-ibs/.

Hooper J: *Clinical and lifestyle concerns with an ostomy*, 2017. Retrieved from: http://www.shieldhealthcare.com/community/wp-content/uploads/2015/11/Clinical-and-Lifestyle-Concerns-Handout.pdf.

Kalff JC, Wehner S, Litkouhi B: *Measures to prevent prolonged postoperative ileus*, 2018. Retrieved from: https://www.uptodate.com/contents/measures-to-prevent-prolonged-postoperative-ileus.

Lehrer JK: *Irritable bowel syndrome*, 2018. Retrieved from: http://emedicine.medscape.com/article/180389-overview.

Moreira TG, Horta LS, Games-Santos AC, et al: CLA-supplemented diet accelerates experimental colorectal cancer by inducing TGF- -producing macrophages and T cells, *Mucosal Immunol* 12(1):p188–p199, 2019. doi:10.1038/s41385-018-0090-8.

Peppercorn MA, Farrell RJ: *Management of severe ulcerative colitis*, 2018. Retrieved from: http://www.uptodate.com/contents/management-of-severe-ulcerative-colitisin-adults.

Rowe WA: *Inflammatory bowel disease treatment and management*, 2017. Retrieved from: http://emedicine.medscape.com/article/179037-treatment#aw2aab6b6b8.

Zheng Y, Yu T, … Lin L: *Efficacy and safety of 5-hydroxytryptamine 3 receptor antagonists in irritable bowel syndrome: a systematic review and meta-analysis of randomized controlled trials*, 2017. Retrieved from: https://journals.plos.org/plosone/article?id=10.1371/journal.pone.0172846 https://doi.org/10.1371/journal.pone.0172846.

CHAPTER 30: CARE OF PATIENTS WITH DISORDERS OF THE GALLBLADDER, LIVER, AND PANCREAS

American Cancer Society: *Pancreatic cancer risk factors*, 2016. Retrieved from: https://www.cancer.org/cancer/pancreatic-cancer/causes-risks-prevention/risk-factors.html.

American Cancer Society: *Key statistics for pancreatic cancer*, 2018. Retrieved from: https://www.cancer.org/cancer/pancreatic-cancer/about/key-statistics.html.

Bloom AA: *Cholecystitis Medication*, 2014. Retrieved from: http://emedicine.medscape.com/article/171886-medication#3.

Carale J: *Portal Hypertension*, 2017. Retrieved from: https://emedicine.medscape.com/article/182098-overview.

Chopra S: *GB virus C (hepatitis G) infection*, 2018. Retrieved from: https://www.uptodate.com/contents/gb-virus-c-hepatitis-g-infection.

Chopra S: *Patient information: Nonalcoholic fatty liver disease (NAFLD), including nonalcoholic steatohepatitis (NASH)(Beyond the Basics)*, 2018. Retrieved from: http://www.uptodate.com/contents/nonalcoholic-fatty-liver-disease-nafld-including-nonalcoholic-steatohepatitis-nash-beyond-the-basics.

Cicalese L: *Hepatocellular Carcinoma Treatment and Management*, 2018. Retrieved from: http://emedicine.medscape.com/article/197319-treatment.

Goldberg E, Chopra S: *Cirrhosis in adults: Etiologies, clinical manifestation and diagnosis*, 2018. Retrieved from: https://www.uptodate.com/contents/cirrhosis-in-adults-etiologies-clinical-manifestations-and-diagnosis.

HHS.gov: *Hepatitis B basic information*, 2017. Retrieved from: https://www.hhs.gov/hepatitis/learn-about-viral-hepatitis/hepatitis-b-basics/index.html.

National Digestive Diseases Information Clearinghouse: *Gallstones*, 2017. Retrieved from: http://digestive.niddk.nih.gov/ddiseases/pubs/gallstones/definition-facts.

OPTN National Data: *Liver Kaplan-Meier graft survival rates for transplants performed: 2008-2015 Based on OPTN data as of Nov 9, 2018*. Retrieved from: https://optn.transplant.hrsa.gov/data/view-data-reports/national-data/#.

Rakel D: *Integrative medicine*, ed 4, Philadelphia, 2018, Elsevier.

Ryan DP, Mamon H: *Treatment for potentially resectable exocrine pancreatic cancer*, 2018. Retrieved from: https://www.uptodate.com/contents/treatment-for-potentially-resectable-exocrine-pancreatic-cancer.

Samji NS: *Viral Hepatitis*, 2017. Retrieved from: https://emedicine.medscape.com/article/775507-overview.

Shergill R, Syed W, Rizvi SA, et al: Nutritional support in chronic liver disease and cirrhotics, *World J Hepatol* 10(10):685–694, 2018.

Swaroop S: *Clinical manifestations and diagnosis of acute pancreatitis*, 2018. Retrieved from: https://www.uptodate.com/contents/clinical-manifestations-and-diagnosis-of-acute-pancreatitis.

Samji NS: *Viral hepatitis*, 2017. Retrieved from: https://emedicine.medscape.com/article/775507-overview.

University of Pittsburgh Schools of the Health Sciences: Colder, darker climates increase alcohol consumption and liver disease, *ScienceDaily*, 2018. Retrieved January 2, 2019 from: www.sciencedaily.com/releases/2018/11/181114080917.htm.

Uppal D: Pragmatic management of nutrition in severe acute pancreatitis, *Pract Gastroenterol* XLII(9):20–33, 2018.

Wolf DC: *Cirrhosis*, 2018. Retrieved from: https://emedicine.medscape.com/article/185856-overview#a1.

CHAPTER 31: THE MUSCULOSKELETAL SYSTEM

Centers for Disease Control: *Important facts about falls*, 2017. Retrieved from: http://www.cdc.gov/HomeandRecreatinalSafety/Falls/adutfalls.html.

Li F, Harmer P, Fitzgerald K, et al: Effectiveness of a therapeutic tai ji quan intervention vs a multimodal exercise intervention to prevent falls among older adults at high risk of falling, *JAMA Intern Med* 178(10):1301–1310, 2018.

Muscular Dystrophy Association: *Find a neuromuscular disease*, 2018. Retrieved from: https://www.mda.org/disease/list.

National Institute of Health, Medline Plus: *Using a Cane*, 2017. Retrieved from: http://www.nlm.nih.gov/medlineplus/ency/patientinstructions/000343.htm.

Starkebaum GA: *Calcium, vitamin D and your bones*, 2018. Retrieved from: https://medlineplus.gov/ency/patientinstructions/000490.htm.

CHAPTER 32: CARE OF PATIENTS WITH MUSCULOSKELETAL AND CONNECTIVE TISSUE DISORDERS

American Cancer Society: *Chemotherapy for Osteosarcoma*. Retrieved from http://www.cancer.org/cancer/osteosarcoma/detailedguide/osteosarcoma-treating-chemotherapy, 2018.

Ault A: *FDA warns on fracture risks with PPIs*, 2010. Retrieved from: http://www.researchgate.net/publication/251489620_FDA_Warns_on_Fracture_Risks_With_PPIs.

Bal BS: *Hip Resurfacing*, 2018. Retrieved from: https://emedicine.medscape.com/article/1358168-overview.

Berry J: *Home remedies for fast back pain relief*, 2018. Retrieved from: https://www.medicalnewstoday.com/articles/322582.php.

Bethel M: *Osteoporosis*, 2018. Retrieved from: https://emedicine.medscape.com/article/330598-overview.

Chicea L: AB1390Osteoporosis associated morbidity analysis can reveal targets for better disease diagnosis and management, *Ann Rheum Dis* 77:1779–1780, 2018.

Cohen S, Mikuls TR: *Initial treatment of rheumatoid arthritis in adults*, 2018. Retrieved from: https://www.uptodate.com/contents/initial-treatment-of-rheumatoid-arthritis-in-adults.

ConsumerLab.Com: *Recommended daily intakes and upper limits for vitamins and minerals*. Retrieved from: https://www.consumerlab.com/RDAs/.

DerSarkissian C: *Phantom limb pain*, 2017. Retrieved from: http://www.webmd.com/pain-managementguide/phantom-limb-pain.

Garcia-Rodriguez JA, Longino DL, Johnston I: Forearm volar slab splint, *Can Fam Physician* 64(8):581–583, 2018.

Liede A, Wade S, Lethen J, et al: An observational study of concomitant use of emerging therapies and denosumab or zoledronic acid in prostate cancer, *Clin Ther* 40(4):536–549.e3, 2018.

Lozada CJ: *Osteoarthritis*, 2018. Retrieved from: http://emedicine.medscape.com/article/330487-overview.

Mayo Clinic: *Phantom pain: Treatment and drugs*. Retrieved from http://www.mayoclinic.org/diseases-conditions/phantom-pain/basics/treatment/con-20023268, 2018.

Micozzi MS: *Fundamentals of complimentary, alternative and integrative medicine*, ed 6, St. Louis, 2019, Elsevier.

Nassar Y, Richter S: Proton-pump inhibitor use and fracture risk: an updated systematic review and Meta-analysis, *J Bone Metab* 25(3):141–151, 2018.

National Center for Complementary and Integrative Health Approaches: *Rheumatoid arthritis and complementary health approaches*, 2019. Retrieved from: https://nccih.nih.gov/health/RA/getthefacts.htm?lang=en.

National Institutes of Health (NIH): *Osteoporosis in men*, 2015. Retrieved from: www.niams.nih.gov/Health_Info/Bone/Osteoporosis/men.asp.

National Institutes of Health (NIH): *Osteoporosis in men*. Retrieved from www.niams.nih.gov/Health_Info/Bone/Osteoporosis/men.asp, 2015.

Ogura T, Bryant T, Minas T: Long term outcomes of autologous chondrocyte implantation in adolescent patients, *Am J Sports Med* 45(5):1066–1074, 2017.

Olseson CV: *Osteoporosis rehabilitation: a practical approach*, Switzerland, 2017, Springer.

Qaseem A, Forciea MA, McLean RM, et al., for the Clinical Guidelines Committee of the American College of Physicians: Treatment of low bone density or osteoporosis to prevent fractures in men and women: a clinical practice guideline update from the American College of Physicians, *Ann Intern Med* 166(11):818–839, 2017.

Rakel D: *Integrative medicine*, ed 4, Philadelphia, 2018, Elsevier.

Rosen HN: *Risks of bisphosphonate therapy in patients with osteoporosis*, 2018. Retrieved from: https://www.uptodate.com/contents/risks-of-bisphosphonate-therapy-in-patients-with-osteoporosis.

Tousun B, Aslan O, Servet T: Preoperative positon splint versus skin traction in patients with hip fracture: an experimental study, *Int J Orthop Trauma Nurs* 28:8–15, 2018.

U.S. National Library of Medicine: *Pin care*. Retrieved from http://www.nlm.nih.gov/medlineplus/ency/patientinstructions/000481.htm, 2018.

US Preventive Services Task Force: Screening for osteoporosis to prevent fractures: US Preventive Services Task Force Recommendation Statement, *JAMA* 319(24):2521–2531, 2018.

Venables PJW, O'Dell JR: *Diagnosis and differential diagnosis of rheumatoid arthritis*, 2018. Retrieved from: http://www.uptodate.com/contents/diagnosis-and-differential-diagnosis-of-rheumatoid-arthritis.

Vuurberg G, Hoorntje A, Wink L, et al: Diagnosis, treatment and prevention of ankle sprains: update of an evidence-based clinical guideline, *Br J Sports Med* 52(15):2018.

CHAPTER 33: THE URINARY SYSTEM

Abello A, Das AK: Electrical neuromodulation in the management of lower uriary tract dysfunction: evidence, experience and future prospects, *Ther Adv Urol* 10(5):165–173, 2018.

Centers for Disease Control and Prevention: *Data and Statistics: HAI Prevalence Survey*. Retrieved from www.cdc.gov/HAI/surveillance/index.html, 2018.

Inker LA, Perrone RD: *Assessment of kidney function*, 2018. Retrieved from: https://www.uptodate.com/contents/assessment-of-kidney-function.

Lukacz ES: *Evaluation of women with urinary incontinence*, 2018. Retrieved from: https://www.uptodate.com/contents/evaluation-of-women-with-urinary-incontinence.

O'Reilly N, Nelson HD, Conry JM, et al: Screening for urinary incontinence in women: a recommendation from the Women's preventive services initiative, *Ann Intern Med* 169(5):I-22, 2018.

Pagana KD, Pagana TJ: *Mosby's manual of diagnostic and laboratory tests*, ed 6, St. Louis, 2018, Elsevier.

Vasavada SP: *Urinary incontinence*, 2018. Retrieved from: https://emedicine.medscape.com/article/452289-overview.

CHAPTER 34: CARE OF PATIENTS WITH DISORDERS OF THE URINARY SYSTEM

American Cancer Society: *Key statistics for bladder cancer*, 2019. Available from: http://www.cancer.org/cancer/bladdercancer/detailedguide/bladder-cancer-key-statistics.

American Cancer Society: *Treatment of bladder cancer by stage*, 2017. Available from: https://www.cancer.org/cancer/bladder-cancer/treating/by-stage.html.

Bagalá N: *Dr. Anthony Atala – Wake Forest institute for regenerative medicine*, 2018. Available from: https://www.leafscience.org/dr-anthony-atala-wake-forest-institute-for-regenerative-medicine/.

Belton P: *"A new bladder made from my cells gave me my life back"*, 2018. Available from: https://www.bbc.com/news/business-45470799.

Dave CN: *Nephrolithiasis*, 2018. Available from: https://emedicine.medscape.com/article/437096-overview.

Golper RA: *Continuous renal replacement therapy in acute kidney injury*, 2018. Available from: https://www.uptodate.com/contents/continuous-renal-replacement-therapy-in-acute-kidney-injury.

Mattiucci M: *Dialysis indications*, 2018. Available from: https://step2.medbullets.com/renal/120688/dialysis-indications.

Rakel D: *Integrative medicine*, ed 4, Philadelphia, 2018, Elsevier.

Shariat SF, Bochner BH, Donahue TF, et al: *Urinary diversion and reconstruction following cystectomy*, 2018. Available from: https://www.uptodate.com/contents/urinary-diversion-and-reconstruction-following-cystectomy.

U.S. Department of Health & Human Services: *Organ Procurement and transplant network*, 2018. Available from: https://optn.transplant.hrsa.gov/governance/compliance/.

CHAPTER 35: THE ENDOCRINE SYSTEM

American Diabetes Association Diabetes Care: 2018 Jan; 41 (Supplement 1): S144-S151. https://doi.org/10.2337/dc18-S014.

Pagna KD, Pagna TJ: *Mosby's diagnostic and laboratory tests*, ed 6, St. Louis, 2018, Elsevier/Mosby.

CHAPTER 36: CARE OF PATIENTS WITH PITUITARY, THYROID, PARATHYROID, AND ADRENAL DISORDERS

Blake MA: *Pheochromocytoma*, 2018. Available from: http://emedicine.medscape.com/article/124059-overview.

Gonzalez-Campoy JM: *Hypoparathyroidism medication*, 2018. Available from: https://emedicine.medscape.com/article/122207-medication#4.

Griffing GT: *Addison Disease*, 2018. Available from: http://emedicine.medscape.com/article/116467-overview.

Ross DS: *Disorders that cause hyperthyroidism*, UpToDate, 2017. Available from: http://www.uptodate.com/contents/disorders-that-cause-hyperthyroidism.

Sharma PK: *Thyroid cancer*, 2018. Available from: http://emedicine.medscape.com/article/851968-overview.

Sterns RH: *Diuretics and calcium balance*. UpToDate, 2018. Available from: http://www.uptodate.com/contents/diuretics-and-calcium-balance.

Surks MI: *Iodine-induced thyroid dysfunction*, 2017. Available from: https://www.uptodate.com/contents/iodine-induced-thyroid-dysfunction.

CHAPTER 37: CARE OF PATIENTS WITH DIABETES AND HYPOGLYCEMIA

American Diabetes Association: Standards of medical care in diabetes—2018, *Diabetes Care* 41(Suppl 1):S13–S27, 2018.

Bhavsar AR: *Diabetic retinopathy treatment and management*, 2018. Available from: http://emedicine.medscape.com/article/1225122-treatment.

Jockers D: *Is the ketogenic diet acidic?* 2019. Available from: https://drjockers.com/ketogenic-diet-acidic/.

Klemm S: *Carbohydrates – part of a healthful diabetes diet*, 2019. Available from: https://www.eatright.org/health/diseases-and-conditions/diabetes/carbohydrates-part-of-a-healthful-diabetes-diet.

Murphy SL, Xu JQ, Kochanek KD, et al: *Mortality in the United States, 2017*, Hyattsville, MD, 2018, National Center for Health Statistics. NCHS Data Brief, no 328.

Peters AL: *Which CGM for which diabetes patient?* 2018. Available from: https://www.medscape.com/viewarticle/892267.

Pozzilli P, Pieralice S: Latent autoimmune diabetes in adults: current status and new horizons, *Endocrinol Metab (Seoul)* 33(2):147–159, 2018.

Richardson SJ, Morgan NG: Enteroviral infections in the pathogenesis of type 1 diabetes: new insights for therapeutic intervention, *Curr Opin Pharmacol* 43:11–19, 2018.

Thomas B: *Kidney-pancreas transplantation*, 2018. Available from: https://emedicine.medscape.com/article/1830202-overview.

Umpierrez GE, Klonoff DC: Diabetes technology update: use of insulin pumps and continuous glucose monitoring in the hospital, *Diabetes Care* 41:1579–1589, 2018.

CHAPTER 38: THE REPRODUCTIVE SYSTEM

American Cancer Society (ACS): *Breast cancer detailed guide*, Atlanta, 2017, Author.

American College of Obstetricians and Gynecologists: *Practice Bulletin on Emergency Contraception (2010; reaffirmed 2018)*, 2018. Retrieved from: https://www.acog.org/Clinical-Guidance-and-Publications/Practice-Bulletins/Committee-on-Practice-Bulletins-Gynecology/Emergency-Contraception#45.

Billings Life: *Billings Ovulation Method*, 2015. Retrieved from: https://billings.life/en/what-is-the-billings-ovulation-method/natural-signal-of-fertility-2.html.

Centers for Disease Control and Prevention: *Youth risk behavior surveillance, 2015*, 2016. Retrieved from: https://www.cdc.gov/healthyyouth/data/yrbs/pdf/2015/ss6506_updated.pdf.

Centers for Disease Control and Prevention: *Contraception*, 2017. Retrieved from: https://www.cdc.gov/reproductivehealth/contraception/index.htm.

Centers for Disease Control and Prevention: *A guide to taking a sexual history*, n.d. Retrieved from: https://www.cdc.gov/std/treatment/sexualhistory.pdf.

Dizon D, Katz A: *Overview of sexual dysfunction in male cancer survivors*, 2018. Retrieved from: www.uptodate.com.

Eliason M, Chinn P: *LGBTQ Cultures: what health care professionals need to know about sexual and gender diversity*, ed 3, Philadelphia, PA, 2018, Wolters Kluwer.

Kaunitz A: *Emergency contraception*, 2018. Retrieved from: www.uptodate.com.

Marquette University: *Natural family planning*, 2018. Retrieved from: https://nfp.marquette.edu/.

Martin K, Barbieri R: *Overview of the use of combination oral contraceptives*, 2018. Retrieved from: www.uptodate.com.

McCance K, Huether S: *Pathophysiology: the biologic basis for disease in adults and children*, ed 8, St. Louis, 2019, Elsevier.

Pagana K, Pagana TJ, Pagana TN: *Mosby's diagnostic & laboratory test reference*, ed 13, St. Louis, MO, 2017, Elsevier.

The Joint Commission: *Advancing effective communication, cultural competence, and patient- and family-centered care for the LGBT community: A field guide*, 2014. Retrieved from: https://www.jointcommission.org/assets/1/18/LGBTFieldGuide_WEB_LINKED_VER.pdf.

U.S. Food and Drug Administraiton: *Seasonale*, 2018. Retrieved from: https://www.accessdata.fda.gov/scripts/cder/daf/index.cfm?event=BasicSearch.process.

U.S. Preventative Services Task Force: *Draft recommendation statement: Cervical cancer screening*, 2017. Retrieved from: https://www.uspreventiveservicestaskforce.org/Page/Document/draft-recommendation-statement/cervical-cancer-screening2.

Ulipristal: Drug information: 2018. Retrieved from: www.uptodate.com.

CHAPTER 39: CARE OF WOMEN WITH REPRODUCTIVE DISORDERS

ACOG: *The Menopause years*, 2018. Retrieved from: https://www.acog.org/Patients/FAQs/The-Menopause-Years.

ACOG: *Cervical Cancer Screening*, 2017. Retrieved from: https://www.acog.org/Patients/FAQs/Cervical-Cancer-Screening.

ACOG: *ACOG revises breast cancer screening guidance: Ob-Gyns promote shared decision making*, 2017. Retrieved from: https://www.acog.org/About-ACOG/News-Room/News-Releases/2017/ACOG-Revises-Breast-Cancer-Screening-Guidance--ObGyns-Promote-Shared-Decision-Making.

American College of Obstetrics and gynecologists: *Hormone Therapy: Resource overview*, 2018. Retrieved from: https://www.acog.org/Womens-Health/Hormone-Therapy.

American Psychiatric Association: *Supplement to Diagnostic and statistical manual of mental disorders 3 ed*, 2017. Retrieved from: https://psychiatryonline.org/pb-assets/dsm/update/DSM5Update_October2017-1508425177203.pdf.

Balsamo R, Illiano E, Zucchi A, et al: Sacrocolpopexy with polyvinylidene fluoride mesh for pelvic organ prolapse: mid term caomarative outcomes with polypropylene mesh, *Eur J Obstet Gynecol Reprod Biol* 220:74–78, 2018.

Breastcancer.org: *Exposure to Chemical in cosmetics*, n.d. Retrieved from: https://www.breastcancer.org/risk/factors/cosmetics.

Carlson RH: Anastrozole, tamoxifen recurrence rates similar in DCIS, but with different side effects. *Oncology Times* 38(3):12–13, 2016.

Caspar RF, Yonkers KA: *Epidemiology and pathogenesis of premenstrual syndrome and premenstrual dysphoric disorder*, 2018. Retreived from: https://www.uptodate.com/contents/epidemiology-and-pathogenesis-of-premenstrual-syndrome-and-premenstrual-dysphoric-disorder.

Chu VH: *Staphylococcal toxic shock syndrome*, 2018. Retrived from: https://www.uptodate.com/contents/staphylococcal-toxic-shock-syndrome.

Ferrari F, Arrigoni F, Miccoli A, et al: Effectiveness of magnetic resonance-guided focused ultrasound surgery (MRgFUS) in the uterine adnomyosis treatment: technical approach and MRI evaluation, *Radiol Med* 121(2):153–161, 2016.

Food and Drug Administration: *Menopause*, 2018. Retrieved from: https://www.fda.gov/forconsumers/byaudience/forwomen/ucm117978.htm.

Food and Drug Administration: *Prolia® (denosumab)*, 2017. Retrieved from: https://www.accessdata.fda.gov/drugsatfda_docs/label/2017/125320s181lbl.pdf#page=27.

Goldberg T, Fidler B: Conjugated estrogens/bazedoxifene (Duavee): a novel agent for the treatment of moderate-to-severe vasomotor symptoms associated with menopause and the prevention of postmenopausal osteoporosis, *P T* 40(3):178, 2015.

Kaunitz A: *Hormonal contraception for prevention of menstruation*, 2017. Retrieved from: www.uptodate.com.

McCance K, Huether S: *Pathophysiology: the biologic basis for disease in adults and children*, ed 8, St. Louis, MO, 2019, Elsevier.

Mendiratta V: Primary and secondary dysmenorrhea, premenstrual syndrome, and premenstrual dysphoric disorder. In Lobo, et al, editors: *Comprehensive gynecology*, Philadelphia, PA, 2017, Elsevier., pp 815–828.

Mirhashemi SM, Sahmani M, Salehi B, et al: Metabolic response to omega-3 fatty acids and vitamin e co-supplementation in patients with fibrocystic breast disease: a randomized, double-blind, placebo-controlled trial, *Arch Iran Med* 20(8):466, 2017.

National Women's Health Network: *Hysterectomy*, 2018. Retrieved from: https://www.nwhn.org/hysterectomy/.

National Cancer Institute (NCI): Retrieved from: https://bcrisktool.cancer.gov/.

Nguyen TT, Hoskin TL, Habermann EB, et al: Breast cancer-related lymphedema risk is related to multidisciplinary treatment and not surgery alone: results from a large cohort study, *Ann Surg Oncol* 24(10):2972–2980, 2017.

Piccart-Gebhart M, Holmes E, Baselga J, et al: Adjuvant lapatinib and trastuzumab for early human epidermal growth factor receptor 2–positive breast cancer: results from the randomized phase III adjuvant lapatinib and/or trastuzumab treatment optimization trial, *J Clin Oncol* 34(10):1034, 2016.

Pru JK: Another link between exercise and relief from postmenopausal decline, *Menopause* 24(6):602–603, 2017.

Resolve.org: *Who has infertility*? 2018. Retrieved from: https://resolve.org/infertility-101/what-is-infertility/fast-facts/.

RxList: *Minivelle*, 2018. Retrieved from: https://www.rxlist.com/minivelle-drug.htm.

Saper R: *Overview of herbal medicine and dietary supplements*, 2018. Retrieved from: www.uptodate.com.

Sprout Pharmaceuticals: *Addyi*, 2018. Retrieved from: https://addyi.com/assets/pdf/Addyi_full_prescribing_info.pdf.

Tamoxifen: 2018. Retrieved from: https://www.uptodate.com/contents/tamoxifendruginformation?search=tamoxifen&source=search_result&selectedTitle=1~148&usage_type=default&display_rank=1.

Thorne JG, James PD, Reid RL: Heavy menstrual bleeding: is tranexamic acid a safe adjunct to combined hormonal contraception? *Contraception* 2018.

U.S. Preventive Services Task Force (USPSTF): 2018. Retrieved from: https://www.uspreventiveservicestaskforce.org/Page/Document/UpdateSummaryFinal/cervical-cancer-screening2.

Zhang X, Cook K, Warri A, et al: Lifetime genistein intake increases the response of mammary tumors to tamoxifen in rats, *Clin Cancer Res* 23(3):814–824, 2017.

CHAPTER 40: CARE OF MEN WITH REPRODUCTIVE DISORDERS

American Cancer Society: *Key statistics for prostate cancer*, 2018a. Retrieved from: https://www.cancer.org/cancer/prostate-cancer/about/key-statistics.html.

American Cancer Society: *Key statistics for testicular cancer*, 2018b. Retrieved from: https://www.cancer.org/cancer/testicular-cancer/about/key-statistics.html.

American Cancer Society: *Risk factors for penile cancer*, 2018c. Retrieved from: https://www.cancer.org/cancer/penile-cancer/causes-risks-prevention/risk-factors.html.

American Cancer Society: *Testicular cancer survival rates*, 2018d. Retrieved from: https://www.cancer.org/cancer/testicular-cancer/detection-diagnosis-staging/survival-rates.html.

American Cancer Society: *What's new in prostate cancer research?* 2018e. Retrieved from: https://www.cancer.org/cancer/prostate-cancer/about/new-research.html.

American Urological Association: *Management of benign prostatic hypertrophy*, 2010, confirmed 2014. Retrieved from: http://www.auanet.org/benign-prostatic-hyperplasia-(2010-reviewed-and-validity-confirmed-2014).

Centers for Disease Control and Prevention: *Mumps home: For healthcare providers*, 2018. Retrieved from: https://www.cdc.gov/mumps/hcp.html.

Cunningham C, Rosen R: *Overview of male sexual dysfunction*, 2018. Retrieved from: www.uptodate.com.

Drugs.com: *FDA Alert: 5-alpha reductase inhibitors (5-ARIs): Label Change—Increased Risk of Prostate Cancer*, 2014. Retrieved from Drugs.com.

Glaser JL: Examining Male Infertility; The Association Between Age, Environment, and Reproductive Success in Male Patients that have Participated in Assisted Reproductive Technology, 2015.

Ju XB, Gu XJ, Zhang ZY, et al: Efficacy and safety of Saw Palmetto Extract Capsules in the treatment of benign prostatic hyperplasia, *Zhonghua nan ke xue=National journal of andrology* 21(12):1098–1101, 2015.

Lim K: Epidemiology of clinical benign prostatic hypertrophy, *Asian Journal of Urology* 4(3):148–151, 2017.

Michaelson M, Oh W: *Epidemiology of and risk factors for testicular germ cell tumors*, 2018. Retrieved from: www.uptodate.com.

Mireille KP, Desire DDP, Pierre K: Male sexual disorders in patients with Parkinson disease: treatment with natural remedies, *Advances in Tissue Engineering and Regenerative Medicine* 3(2):00061, 2017.

Pettaway C: *Carcinoma of the penis: Epidemiology, risk factors, and pathology*, 2017. Retrieved from: www.uptodate.com.

Pinsky P, Prorok P, Kramer B: Prostate cancer screening – A perspective on the current state of the evidence, *N Engl J Med* 376:1285–1289, 2017.

Rees J, et al: Diagnosis and treatment of chronic bacterial prostatitis and chronic prostatitis/chronic pelvic pain syndrome: a consensus guideline, *BJU Int* 116(4):509–525, 2015.

Sartor A: *Risk factors for prostate cancer*, 2018. Retrieved from: www.uptodate.com.

United States Preventative Task Force: Screening for prostate cancer, *JAMA* 319(18):1901, 2018.

US Department of Health and Human Services: *How common is male infertility, and what are its causes?* 2016. Retrieved from: https://www.nichd.nih.gov/health/topics/menshealth/conditioninfo/infertility.

CHAPTER 41: CARE OF PATIENTS WITH SEXUALLY TRANSMITTED INFECTIONS

Centers for Disease Control & Prevention: *Trichomoniasis*, 2016. Retrieved from: https://www.cdc.gov/std/tg2015/trichomoniasis.htm.

Centers for Disease Control and Prevention: *Reported STDs in the United States, 2016*, 2017a. Retrieved from: https://www.cdc.gov/nchhstp/newsroom/docs/factsheets/STD-Trends-508.pdf.

Centers for Disease Control and Prevention: *Sexually transmitted diseases: Adolescents and young adults*, 2017b. Retrieved from: https://www.cdc.gov/std/life-stages-populations/adolescents-youngadults.htm.

Centers for Disease Control and Prevention: *2016 Sexually Transmitted Diseases Surveillance*, 2018a. Retrieved from: https://www.cdc.gov/std/stats16/default.htm.

Centers for Disease Control and Prevention: *HIV among people age 50 and older*, 2018b. Retrieved from: https://www.cdc.gov/hiv/group/age/olderamericans/index.html.

Centers for Disease Control and Prevention: *Recommended Immunization Schedule for Children and Adolescents Aged 18 Years or Younger, United States, 2018*, 2018c. Retrieved from: https://www.cdc.gov/vaccines/schedules/hcp/imz/child-adolescent.html#f14.

Centers for Disease Control and Prevention: *PEP*, 2018d. Retrieved from: https://www.cdc.gov/hiv/basics/pep.html.

Ross J: *Pelvic inflammatory disease: Pathogenesis, microbiology, and risk factors*, 2018. Retrieved from: www.uptodate.com.

Sobel J: *Bacterial vaginosis: Clinical manifestations and diagnosis*, 2017. Retrieved from: www.uptodate.com.

Swan A: Acute HIV infections in primary care, *Adv Nurse Pract* 17(9):49–54, 2009.

CHAPTER 42: THE INTEGUMENTARY SYSTEM

Alguire PC, Mathes BM: *Skin biopsy techniques*, 2017. Retrieved from: https://www.uptodate.com/contents/skin-biopsy-techniques.

CDC: *Indoor tanning is not safe*, 2018. Retrieved from: http://www.cdc.gov/cancer/skin/basic_info/indoor_tanning.htm.

Drezner MK: *Patient information: Vitamin D deficiency (beyond the basics). UpToDate*, 2019. Retrieved from: http://www.uptodate.com/contents/vitamin-d-deficiency-beyond-the-basics?view=print.

FDA: *Sunscreen*, 2018. Retrieved from: http://www.fda.gov/drugs/resourcesforyou/consumers/buyingusingmedicinesafely/understandingover-the-countermedicines/ucm239463.htm.

Giger JN: *Transcultural nursing: assessment and intervention*, ed 7, St. Louis, 2017, Elsevier.

Healthy People: 2020.

LeBlanc K, et al: Best practice recommendations for the prevention and management of skin tears in aged skin. *Wounds International*, 2018. Retrieved from: http://www.skintears.org/wp-content/uploads/2018/12/BEST-PRACTICE-DOCUMENT-2018-FOR-THE-PREVENTION-AND-MANAGEMENT-OF-SKIN-TEARS-IN-AGED-SKIN-WOUNDS-INTERNATIONAL.pdf.

Muro E, Ruiz G, Wise J, et al: *Basin glove: disposable wash basin liner in the prevention of HAIs*, 2018. Retrieved from: https://infectioncontrol.tips/2018/06/11/basin-glove-disposable-wash-basin-liner-prevention-hais/.

CHAPTER 43: CARE OF PATIENTS WITH INTEGUMENTARY DISORDERS AND BURNS

Agency for healthcare Research and Quality (AHRQ): *AHRQ's safety program for nursing homes: on-time prevention*, 2017. Retrieved from: https://www.ahrq.gov/professionals/systems/long-term-care/resources/ontime/index.html.

Ambardekar N: *Plastic surgery for burns and other wounds*, 2017. Retrieved from: https://www.webmd.com/skin-problems-and-treatments/plastic-surgery-burns#1.

American Burn Association: *Burn injury fact sheet*, 2017. Retrieved from: https://ameriburn.org/wp-content/uploads/2017/12/nbaw-factsheet_121417-1.pdf.

American Cancer Society: *Cancer Facts and Figures*, 2018. Retrieved from: https://www.cancer.org/content/dam/cancer-org/research/cancer-facts-and-statistics/annual-cancer-facts-and-figures/2018/cancer-facts-and-figures-2018.pdf.

Bader DL, Worsley PR: Technologies to monitor the health of loaded skin tissues, *Biomed Eng Online* 17(1):1, 2018.

Centers for Disease Control and Prevention: Chickenpox transmission. *Centers for Disease Control and Prevention*, 2018. Retrieved from: http://www.cdc.gov/chickenpox/about/transmission.html.

Centers for Disease Control and Prevention: Shingles overview. *Centers for Disease Control and Prevention*, 2018a. Retrieved from: http://www.cdc.gov/shingles/about/overview.html.

Chan CH, Yang SF, Yeh HW, et al: Risk of pneumonia in patients with burn injury: a population-based cohort study, *Clin Epidemiol* 10:1083–1091, 2018.

Cochran A: *Nutritional demands and enteral formulas for monderate-to-severe burn patients*, 2018. Retrieved from: https://www.uptodate.com/contents/nutritional-demands-and-enteral-formulas-for-moderate-to-severe-burn-patients.

Drugs.com: *Veltin*, 2018. Retrieved from: http://www.drugs.com/veltin.html.

Dummer R, Ascierto P, Gogas HJ, et al: Encorafenib plus binietinib versus vemurafenib or encorafenib in patients with BRAF-mutant melanoma (COLUMBUS): a multicnetre, open-label, randomized phase 3 trial, *Lancet Oncol* 19(5):603–615, 2018d.

Edsberg LE, Black JM, et al Revised national pressure ulcer advisory panel pressure injury staging system. *J Wound Ostomy Continence Nurs* 2016; 43(6): p 585–597.

FDA: *Isotretinoin (marketed as Accutane) capsule information*, 2018. Retrieved from: https://www.fda.gov/Drugs/DrugSafety/ucm094305.htm.

Gestring M: *Negative pressure wound therapy*, 2018. Retrieved from: http://www.uptodate.com/contents/negativ-pressure-wound-therapy#H3.

Guenther LC: *Pediculosis and pthiriasis (lice infestation)*, 2018. Retrieved from: https://emedicine.medscape.com/article/225013-overview.

Ho RTH, Wang C-W, Ng S-M, et al: The effect of T'ai Chi exercise on immunity and infections: a systematic review of controlled trials, *J Altern Complement Med* 19(2):1–8, 2013. doi:10.1089/acm.2011.0593.

Jones MW, Cooper JS: *Hyperbaric, wound healing*, 2019. Retrieved from: https://www.ncbi.nlm.nih.gov/books/NBK459172/.

Korman N: *Comorbid disease in psoriasis*. 2019. Retrieved from: https://www.uptodate.com/contents/comorbid-disease-in-psoriasis.

Micozzi MS: *Fundamentals of complementary, alternative and integrative medicine*, ed 6, St. Louis, 2019, Elsevier.

Nair HKR: Microcurrent as an adjunt therapy to accelerate chronic wound healing and reduce patient pain, *J Wound Care* 27(5):296–306, 2018.

National Pressure Ulcer Advisory Panel [NPUAP]: *Prevention and treatment of pressure ulcers: quick reference guide*, 2014. Retrieved from: https://www.npuap.org/wp-content/uploads/2014/08/Updated-10-16-14-Quick-Reference-Guide-DIGITAL-NPUAP-EPUAP-PPPIA-16Oct2014.pdf.

Nedelec B, LaSalle L: Postburn itch: A review of the literature, *Wounds* 30(1):10–16, 2018.

Rakel D: *Integrative medicine*, ed 4, Philadelphia, 2018, Elsevier.

Rice PL, Orgill DP: *Emergency care of moderate and severe thermal burns in adults*, 2018. Retrieved from: https://www.uptodate.com/contents/emergency-care-of-moderate-and-severe-thermal-burns-in-adults#H17.

Rondinelli J, Zuniga S, Kipnis P, et al: Hospital-acquired pressure injury, risk-adjusted comparisons in an integrated healthcare delivery system, *Nurs Res* 67(1):16–25, 2018.

Saghaleini SH, et al: Pressure ulcer nutrition. *Indian J Crit Care Med* 2018; 22(4): 283–289.

Scapin S, Echevarria-Guanillo ME, et al: Virtual reality in the treatment of burn patients: a systematic review, *Burns* 44(6):1403–1416, 2018.

Tenenhaus M, Rennekampff HO: *Topical agents and dressings for local burn wound care*, 2018. Retrieved from: https://www.uptodate.com/contents/topical-agents-and-dressings-for-local-burn-wound-care.

University of Michigan: *Efforts to prevent pressure ulcers in hospitals may not be making headway on the worst kind*, 2018. Retrieved from: https://medicalxpress.com/news/2018-11-efforts-pressure-ulcers-hospitals-headway.html.

University of Wisconsin-Madison: *It's not a shock: better bandage promotes powerful healing*. Retrieved from: https://www.sciencedaily.com/releases/2018/11/181129122445.htm.

Wiechman S, Sharar S: *Management of burn wound pain and itching*, 2018. Retrieved from: https://www.uptodate.com/contents/management-of-burn-wound-pain-and-itching.

CHAPTER 44: CARE OF PATIENTS DURING DISASTERS, BIOTERRORISM ATTACKS, AND PANDEMIC INFECTIONS

American Society for Microbiology: *Researchers engineer dual vaccine against anthrax and plague*, 2018. Retrieved from: https://medicalxpress.com/news/2018-10-dual-vaccine-anthrax-plague.html.

Centers for Disease Control and Prevention: *Disaster Mental Health Primer: Key principles, issues and questions*, 2018. Retrieved from: https://emergency.cdc.gov/coping/selfcare.asp.

Centers for Disease Control and Prevention: *Botulism*, 2019. Retrieved from: http://www.cdc.gov/nczved/divisions/dfbmd/diseases/botulism/#prevent.

Centers for Disease Control and Prevention: *Guidance on personal protective equipment to be used by healthcare workers during the management of patient with ebola virus disease in US hospitals, including procedures for putting on and removing*, 2018b. Retrieved from: http://www.cdc.gov/vhf/ebola/healthcare-us/ppe/guidance.html.

Centers for Disease Control and Prevention: *Emergency preparedness and response: bioterrorism agents/diseases*, 2017. Retrieved from: https://emergency.cdc.gov/agent/agentlist-category.asp.

Centers for Disease Control and Prevention: *Viral Hemorrhagic Fevers*, 2018c. Retrieved from: https://www.cdc.gov/vhf/virus-families/index.html.

Global Biodefense: *Mobile diagnostic: FDA authorizes use of first ebola fingerstick test with portable reader*. Retrieved from: https://globalbiodefense.com/2018/11/11/mobile-diagnostic-fda-authorizes-use-of-first-ebola-fingerstick-test-with-portable-reader/.

Institute of Medicine (IOM): *Crisis Standards of Care: a systems framework for catastrophic disaster response*, Washington, DC, 2012, The National Academies Press. Retrieved from: http://www.nap.edu/openbook.php?record_id=13351.

Labrague LJ, Hammand K, Gloe DS, et al: Disaster preparedness among nurses: a systematic review of literature, *Int Nurs Rev* 65(1):41–53, 2018.

Madsen JM: *Chemical terrorism: rapid recognition and initial medical management*, 2018. Retrieved from: https://www.uptodate.com/contents/chemical-terrorism-rapid-recognition-and-initial-medical-management.

Pae JS: *CBRNE-Radiation Emergencies*, 2018. Retrieved from: http://emedicine.medscape.com/article/834015-overview#a8.

Radiation Emergency Medical Management: *Personal Protective Equipment (PPE) in a Radiation Emergency*, 2018. Retrieved from: http://www.remm.nlm.gov/radiation_ppe.htm.

TRACIE: *Topic collection: hospital sure capacity and immediate bed availability*, 2019. Retrieved from: https://asprtracie.hhs.gov/technical-resources/58/hospital-surge-capacity-and-immediate-bed-availability/56.

TRACIE: *Topic collection: Pre-hospital patient decontamination*, 2019a. Retrieved from: https://asprtracie.hhs.gov/technical-resources/39/pre-hospital-patient-decontamination/37.

Williams M, Sizemore DC: *Biologic, chemical and radiation terrorism review*, 2018. Retrieved from: https://www.ncbi.nlm.nih.gov/books/NBK493217/.

World Nuclear Association: *Nuclear radiation and health effects*, 2018. Retrieved from: http://www.world-nuclear.org/info/Safety-and-Security/Radiation-and-Health/Nuclear-Radiation-and-Health-Effects/.

CHAPTER 45: CARE OF PATIENTS WITH EMERGENCIES, TRAUMA, AND SHOCK

American College of Surgeons: *Poor access to trauma center linked to higher death rates in more than half of US states*, 2018. Retrieved from: https://medicalxpress.com/news/2018-10-poor-access-trauma-center-linked.html.

American Heart Association: *Frequently asked questions: AHA requirement on use of feedback devices in adult CPR training*, 2017. Retrieved from: http://ahainstructornetwork.americanheart.org/idc/groups/ahaecc-public/@wcm/@ecc/documents/downloadable/ucm_495655.pdf.

American Red Cross: *Spinal backboarding procedure*, 2012. Retrieved from: https://con2.classes.redcross.org/learningcontent/PHSS/Lifeguarding/Lifeguarding_032112/media/pdf/LG_PM_CH11_Skill_Sheet_SPINAL_BACKBOARDING_PROCEDURE_SHALLOW_WATER.pdf.

Barrett J: *Human Bites*, 2018. Retrieved from: http://emedicine.medscape.com/article/218901-overview.

Centers for Disease Control and Prevention: *Extreme Heat*, 2018. Retrieved from: http://www.cdc.gov/extremeheat/index.html.

Centers for Disease Control and Prevention: *Unintentional Drowning: Get the facts*, 2016a. Retrieved from: http://www.cdc.gov/HomeandRecreationalSafety/Water-Safety/waterinjuries-factsheet.html.

Centers for Disease Control and Prevention: *Motor vehicle crash deaths*, 2016. https://www.cdc.gov/vitalsigns/motor-vehicle-safety/#overview.

Centers for Disease Control and Prevention: *Unintentional Drowning: Get the facts*, 2016. Retrieved from: http://www.cdc.gov/HomeandRecreationalSafety/Water-Safety/waterinjuries-factsheet.html.

Centers for Disease Control and Prevention: *Prescription Drug Overdose in the United States: Fact Sheet*, 2018b. Retrieved from: http://www.cdc.gov/drugoverdose/index.html.

Centers for Disease Control and Prevention: *Tick Removal*, 2019. Retrieved from: http://www.cdc.gov/ticks/removing_a_tick.html.

Daley BJ: *Snakebite*, 2018. Retrieved from: http://emedicine.medscape.com/article/168828-overview.

de Campos J, White TW: Chest wall stabilization in trauma patients: why, when, and how?, *J Thorac Dis* 10(Suppl 8):S951–S962, 2018.

Doud Galli SK: *Animal Bites*, 2018. Retrieved from: http://emedicine.medscape.com/article/881171-overview.

Dowell M: *These are the leading causes of death in the US*, 2018. Retrieved from: https://www.cheatsheet.com/health-fitness/these-are-the-leading-causes-of-death-in-the-u-s.html/.

Fischer PE, Perina DG, Delbridge TR, et al: Spinal motion restriction in the trauma patient – a joint position statement, *Prehosp Emerg Care* 22(6):659–661, 2018.

Helman RS: *Heatstroke*, 2018. Retrieved from: http://emedicine.medscape.com/article/166320-overview.

Huecker MR, Smock W: Domestic violence. In *StatPearls [Internet]*, Treasure Island (FL), 2019, StatPearls Publishing. Available from: https://www.ncbi.nlm.nih.gov/books/NBK499891/. [Updated 2019 May 2].

Kaplan LJ: *Systemic Inflammatory Response Syndrome*, 2018. Retrieved from: http://emedicine.medscape.com/article/168943-overview.

Kardon EM: *Caustic Ingestions*, 2018. Retrieved from: http://emedicine.medscape.com/article/813772-overview.

Ladika S. *Violence against nurse: casualties of caring*. Retrieved from: https://www.managedcaremag.com/archives/2018/5/violence-against-nurses-casualties-caring.

Legome EL: *Blunt Abdominal Trauma*, 2019. Retrieved from: http://emedicine.medscape.com/article/1980980-overview.

Levy MM, Evans LE, Rhodes A: The surviving sepsis campaign bundle: 2018 update, *Crit Care Med* 46(6):997–1000, 2018.

Mustafa SS: *Anaphylaxis*, 2018. Retrieved from: http://emedicine.medscape.com/article/135065-overview.

Nursing Home Abuse Center: *Elder abuse statistics*, 2018. Retrieved from: https://www.nursinghomeabusecenter.com/elder-abuse/statistics/.

Offner P: *Penetrating Abdominal Trauma*, 2017. Retrieved from: http://emedicine.medscape.com/article/2036859-overview.

Perrone M: *Drug epidemic ensnares 25-year old pill for nerve pain*, 2018. Retrieved from: https://apnews.com/70e49b15a082431db4938c5a324df677.

Ren X: *Cardiogenic Shock*, 2017. Retrieved from: http://emedicine.medscape.com/article/152191-overview#aw2aab6b2b3.

Shochat GN: *Carbon Monoxide Toxicity*, 2018. Retrieved from: http://emedicine.medscape.com/article/819987-overview.

Singer M, Deutschman CS, Seymour CW, et al: The Third International Consensus Definitions for Sepsis and Septic Shock (Sepsis-3), *JAMA* 315(8):801–810, 2016.

The Joint Commission: *Specifications manual for national hospital quality measures*, 2018. Retrieved from: https://www.jointcommission.org/specifications_manual_for_national_hospital_inpatient_quality_measures.aspx.

Zafren K, Mechem CC: *Frostbite*, 2018. Retrieved from: https://www.uptodate.com/contents/frostbite.

Zonnoor B: *Frostbite*, 2018. Retrieved from: https://emedicine.medscape.com/article/926249-overview.

CHAPTER 46: CARE OF PATIENTS WITH COGNITIVE DISORDERS

Alzheimer's Association: *10 early signs and symptoms of Alzheimer's*, 2018a. Retrieved from: https://www.alz.org/alzheimers-dementia/10_signs.

Alzheimer's Association: *Fact and figures*, 2018b. Retrieved from: https://www.alz.org/alzheimers-dementia/facts-figures.

Alzheimer's Association: *Risk factors*, 2018c. Retrieved from: https://www.alz.org/alzheimers-dementia/what-is-alzheimers/risk-factors.

Alzheimer's Association: *Treatments for behavior*, 2018d. Retrieved from: https://www.alz.org/alzheimers-dementia/treatments/treatments-for-behavior.

American Psychiatric Association: *Diagnostic and statistical manual of mental disorders*, ed 5, Washington, DC, 2013, Author.

American Psychiatric Association: *Diagnostic and statistical manual of mental disorders*, ed 5, Arlington, VA, 2013, Author.

Anderson K, Grossberg GT: Brain games to slow cognitive decline in Alzheimer's disease, *J Am Med Dir Assoc* 15(8):536–537, 2014.

Baril AA, Carrier J, Lafrenière A, et al: Biomarkers of dementia in obstructive sleep apnea, *Sleep Med Rev* 2018.

Camargo CHF, Justus FF, Retzlaff G: The effectiveness of reality orientation in the treatment of Alzheimer's disease, *Am J Alzheimers Dis Other Demen* 30(5):527–532, 2015.

Dubois B: Preclinical Alzheimer's disease: Definition, natural history, and diagnostic criteria, *Alzheimers Dement* 12(3):292–323, 2016.

Keshavarz S, Mirzaei T, Ravari A: Effect of Head and Face Massage on Agitation in Elderly Alzheimer's Disease Patients, *Evid Based Care* 7(4):46–54, 2018.

Marciani DJ: Development of an Effective Alzheimer's Vaccine. In *Immunology*, 2018, pp 149–169.

Roalf DR, Moore TM, Mechanic-Hamiliton D, et al: Bridging cognitive screening tests in neurological disorders: a cross-walk between the s-MoCA and MMSE, *Alzheimers Dement* 13(8):947–952, 2017.

Surr CA, Griffiths AW, Kelley R: Implementing Dementia Care Mapping as a practice development tool in dementia care services: a systematic review, *Clin interv Aging* 13:165, 2018.

Wood W, Fields B, Rose M, et al: Animal-assisted therapies and dementia: a systematic mapping review using the Lived Environment Life Quality (LELQ) Model, *Am J Occup Ther* 71(5):7105190030p1–7105190030p10, 2017.

CHAPTER 47: CARE OF PATIENTS WITH ANXIETY, MOOD, AND EATING DISORDERS

American Foundation for Suicide Prevention: *Suicide statistics*, 2018. Retrieved from: https://afsp.org/about-suicide/suicide-statistics/.

American Psychiatric Association: *Diagnostic and statistical manual of mental disorders*, ed 5, Arlington, VA, 2013, Author.

Anglin R, et al: Risk of upper gastrointestinal bleeding with selective serotonin reuptake inhibitors without concurrent nonsteroidal anti-inflammatory use: a systematic review, *Am J Gastroenterol* 109(6):811–819, 2014.

Centers for Disease Control and Prevention: *Suicide rising across the U.S.*, 2018. Retrieved from: https://www.cdc.gov/vitalsigns/suicide/index.html.

de Arellano MA, Andrews AR III, Reid-Quiñones K, et al: *Immigration trauma among Hispanic youth: missed by trauma assessments and predictive of depression and PTSD symptoms*, 2017.

Gottschalk M: Genetics of generalized anxiety disorder and related traits, *Dialogues Clin Neurosci* 19(2):158–169, 2017.

Kraus C, et al: Administration of ketamine for unipolar and bipolar depression, *Int J Psychiatry Clin Pract* 21(1):2–12, 2017.

Laursen SB, Leontiadis GI, Stanley AJ, et al: The use of selective serotonin receptor inhibitors (SSRI s) is not associated with increased risk of endoscopy-refractory bleeding, rebleeding or mortality in peptic ulcer bleeding, *Aliment Pharmacol Ther* 46(3):355–363, 2017.

MacKinlay E, Burns R: Spirituality promotes better health outcomes and lowers anxiety about aging: the importance of spiritual dimensions for baby boomers as they enter older adulthood, *J Relig Spiritual Aging* 29(4):248–265, 2017.

National Association of Anorexia Nervosa and Associated Disorders: *Eating disorder statistics*. n.d. Retrieved from: http://www.anad.org/get-information/about-eating-disorders/eating-disorders-statistics/.

National Center for PTSD: *How common is PTSD?* 2017. Retrieved from: https://www.ptsd.va.gov/public/PTSD-overview/basics/how-common-is-ptsd.asp.

Pascoe MC, Bauer IE: A systematic review of randomised control trials on the effects of yoga on stress measures and mood, *J Psychiatr Res* 68:270–282, 2015.

Raglio A, Attardo L, Gontero G, et al: Effects of music and music therapy on mood in neurological patients, *World J Psychiatry* 5(1):68, 2015.

Stahl S: *Stahl's essential psychopharmacology prescriber's guide*, ed 6, Cambridge, UK, 2018, University Printing House.

Wilson G, Farrell D, Barron I, et al: The use of eye-movement desensitization reprocessing (EMDR) therapy in treating post-traumatic stress disorder—a systematic narrative review, *Front Psychol* 9:2018.

CHAPTER 48: CARE OF PATIENTS WITH SUBSTANCE-RELATED AND ADDICTIVE DISORDERS

Alzheimer's Association: *Korsakoff syndrome*, 2018. Retrieved from: https://www.alz.org/alzheimers-dementia/what-is-dementia/types-of-dementia/korsakoff-syndrome.

American Lung Association: *Popcorn lung: A dangerous risk to e-flavored cigarettes*, 2018. Retrieved from: http://www.lung.org/about-us/blog/2016/07/popcorn-lung-risk-ecigs.html.

American Psychiatric Association: *Diagnostic and statistical manual of mental disorders*, ed 5, Washington, DC, 2013, Author.

Barry KL, Blow FC: Drinking over the lifespan: focus on older adults, *Alcohol Res* 38(1):115, 2016.

Bettinardi-Angres K, Andgres D: Understanding the disease of addiction, *J Nurs Regul* 1(20):13–17, 2010.

Centers for Disease Control and Prevention: Current cigarette smoking among Adults—United States, 2016, *Morb Mortal Wkly Rep* 67(2):53–59, 2018.

Centers for Disease Control and Prevention: *Diseases and death*, 2018. Retrieved from: https://www.cdc.gov/tobacco/data_statistics/fact_sheets/fast_facts/index.htm.

Flannery A, Adkins D, Cook A: Unpeeling the evidence for the banana bag: Evidence-based recommendations for the management of alcohol-associated vitamin and electrolyte deficiencies in the ICU, *Crit Care Med* 44(8):1545–1552, 2016.

Kaner EF, Beyer FR, Muirhead C, et al: Effectiveness of brief alcohol interventions in primary care populations, *Cochrane Database Syst Rev* (2):2018.

Kunyk D: Substance use disorders among registered nurses: prevalence, risks and perceptions in a disciplinary jurisdiction, *J Nurs Manag* 23(1):54–64, 2015.

*Miller WR, Sanchez VC: Motivating young adults for treatment and lifestyle change. In Howard G, editor: *Issues in Alcohol Use and Misuse in Young Adults*, Notre Dame, IN, 1993, University of Notre Dame Press.

National Conference of State Legislatures: *State medical marijuana laws*, 2018. Retrieved from: http://www.ncsl.org/research/health/state-medical-marijuana-laws.aspx.

National Institutes of Health: National Institute on Drug Abuse: *What are hallucinogens?* 2016.Retrieved from: https://www.drugabuse.gov/publications/drugfacts/hallucinogens.

National Institute on Drug Abuse: *Opioid overdose crisis*, 2018. Retrieved from: https://www.drugabuse.gov/drugs-abuse/opioids/opioid-overdose-crisis.

Neale J, Nettleton S, Pickering L: Heroin users' views and experiences of physical activity, sport, and exercise, *Int J Drug Policy* 23(2):120–127, 2012.

Rice V, Health L, Livingstone-Banks J, et al: Nursing interventions for smoking cessation, *Cochrane Database Syst Rev* (12):Art. No.: CD001188, 2017. doi:10.1002/14651858.CD001188.pub5.

SAMHSA: *Risk and protective factors*, 2018. Retrieved from: https://www.samhsa.gov/capt/practicing-effective-prevention/prevention-behavioral-health/risk-protective-factors.

So Y: *Wernicke encephalopathy*, 2016. Retrieved from: www.uptodate.com.

Stotts AL, Vujanovic A, Heads A, et al: The role of avoidance and inflexibility in characterizing response to contingency management for cocaine use disorders: a secondary profile analysis, *Psychol Addict Behav* 29(2):408, 2015.

Substance Abuse Center for Behavioral Health Statistics and Quality: *Results from the 2016 National Survey on Drug Use and Health: Detailed Tables. SAMHSA.* https://www.samhsa.gov/data/sites/default/files/NSDUH-DetTabs-2016/NSDUH-DetTabs-2016.htm. Published September 7, 2017.

*Sullivan J, Schneiderman K, Naranjo C, et al: Assessment of alcohol withdrawal: the revised Clinical Institute Withdrawal Assessment for Alcohol Scale (CIWA-Ar), *Br J Addict* 84(11):1353–1357, 1989.

The Joint Commission: *Specifications manual for Joint Commission national quality measures (v2016A): Substance use*, 2016. Retrieved from: https://manual.jointcommission.org/releases/TJC2016A/DataElem0155.html.

*Yalom I, Leszcz M: *The theory and practice of group psychotherapy*, ed 5, New York, NY, 2005, Basic Books.

*Indicates a classic reference

CHAPTER 49: CARE OF PATIENTS WITH THOUGHT AND PERSONALITY DISORDERS

American Psychiatric Association: *Diagnostic and statistical manual of mental Disorders*, ed 5, Arlington, VA, 2013, Author.

Asher L, Patel V, De Silva MJ: Community-based psychosocial interventions for people with schizophrenia in low and middle-income countries: systematic review and meta-analysis, *BMC Psychiatry* 17(1):355, 2017.

Halter M: *Varcarolis' foundations of psychiatric-mental health nursing: a clinical Approach*, ed 8, St. Louis, 2018, Elsevier.

Haram A, Jonsbu E, Fosse R, et al: Psychotherapy in schizophrenia: a retrospective controlled study, *Psychosis* 10(2):110–121, 2018.

Howes O, McCutcheon R, Stone J: Glutamate and dopamine in schizophrenia: an update for the 21st century, *J Psychopharmacol (Oxford)* 29(2):97–115, 2015.

May J, Richardi T, Barth K: Dialectical behavior therapy as treatment for borderline personality disorder, *Ment Health Clin* 6(2):62–67, 2016.

Qiao Y, Mei Y, Han H, et al: Effects of omega-3 in the treatment of violent schizophrenia patients, *Schizophr Res* 195:283–285, 2018.

Rund BR: The association between schizophrenia and violence, *Schizophr Res* 199:39–40, 2018.

Schizophrenia and Related Disorders Alliance of America: *About schizophrenia*, 2018. Retrieved from: https://sardaa.org/resources/about-schizophrenia/.

Bibliography

CHAPTER 1: CARING FOR MEDICAL-SURGICAL PATIENTS

About Healthy People. 2018. Retrieved from: https://www.healthypeople.gov/2020/About-Healthy-People.

Centers for Medicare Services (CMS): *Hospital-Acquired Conditions*. Retrieved from: http://www.cms.gov/Medicare/Medicare-General-Information/MedicareGenInfo/index.html 2016.

Errors, Injuries, Accident, Infections. 2017. Retrieved from: http://www.hospitalsafetygrade.org/what-is-patient-safety/errors-injuries-accidents-infections.

Health and Human Services. 2017. *Strategic Plan 2014-2018*. Retrieved from: https://www.hhs.gov/about/strategic-plan/strategic-goal-1/index.html?language=es.

Medicare.gov: *The official US government site for Medicare: What Medicare covers*. 2018. Retrieved from: http://www.medicare.gov.

Knecht P: *Success in practical/vocational nursing*, ed 8, Philadelphia, 2017, Elsevier.

Starmer AJ, Schnock KO, Lyons A, et al: Effects of the I-PASS Nursing Handoff Bundle on communication quality and workflow, *BMJ Qual Saf* 26:949–957, 2017.

CHAPTER 3: FLUIDS, ELECTROLYTES, ACID-BASE BALANCE, AND INTRAVENOUS THERAPY

Ansel B, Boyce M, Embree J: Extending short peripheral catheter dwell time: a best practice discussion, *J Infus Nurs* 40(3):143–146, 2017.

Boron WF, Boulpaep EL: *Medical physiology*, ed 3, Philadelphia, 2017, Elsevier.

CDC: *Healthcare-associated infections, Central line-associated bloodstream infection (CLABSI)*, 2016. Retrieved from: https://www.cdc.gov/hai/bsi/bsi.html.

CDC: *Infection control, Intravascular catheter related infection*, 2017. Retrieved from: https://www.cdc.gov/infectioncontrol/guidelines/bsi/recommendations.html.

Emmett M: *Serum anion gap in conditions other than metabolic acidosis*, 2018. Retrieved from: https://www.uptodate.com/contents/serum-anion-gap-in-conditions-other-than-metabolic-acidosis.

Hubert RJ, VanMeter KC: *Gould's pathophysiology for health professions*, ed 6, St. Louis, 2018, Elsevier.

Ignatavicius DD, Workman ML: *Medical-surgical nursing: critical thinking for collaborative care*, ed 8, St. Louis, 2016, Elsevier.

Jarvis C: *Physical examination and health assessment*, ed 7, St. Louis, 2016, Elsevier.

Lewis SL, Bucher L, Heitkemper MM, et al: *Medical-surgical nursing: assessment and management of clinical problems*, ed 10, St. Louis, 2017, Elsevier.

Sole ML, Goldenberg Klein D, Moseley MJ: *Introduction to critical care nursing*, ed 7, St Louis, 2017, Elsevier.

United States Geological Services: *The water in you*, 2018. Retrieved from: http://water.usgs.gov/edu/propertyyou.html.

CHAPTER 4: CARE OF PREOPERATIVE AND INTRAOPERATIVE SURGICAL PATIENTS

Adler AC: *General anesthesia*, 2018. Retrieved from: https://emedicine.medscape.com/article/1271543-overview.

American Association of Nurse Anesthetists (AANA): Vaping 'no better' than smoking when surgery is needed. *ScienceDaily*, 2017, November 15. Retrieved from: www.sciencedaily.com/releases/2017/11/171115175653.htm.

Cowperthwaite L, Holm RL: Guideline implementation: preoperative patient skin antisepsis, *AORN J* 101(1):71–80, 2015.

Crookston KP: *The approach to the patient who refuses blood transfusion*, 2018. Retrieved from: https://www.uptodate.com/contents/the-approach-to-the-patient-who-refuses-blood-transfusion.

Deverick JA, Sexton DJ: *Antimicrobial prophylaxis for prevention of surgical site infection in adults*, 2018. Retrieved from: https://www.uptodate.com/contents/antimicrobial-prophylaxis-for-prevention-of-surgical-site-infection-in-adults.

Graff V: Role of music in the perioperative setting, *ASRA News* 17(2):27–29, 2017.

Wechter DG: *Smoking and surgery*, 2018. Retrieved from: https://medlineplus.gov/ency/patientinstructions/000437.htm.

CHAPTER 5: CARE OF POSTOPERATIVE SURGICAL PATIENTS

Berrios-Torres SI, Umscheid CA, Bratzler DW, et al: Center for disease control and prevention guideline for the prevention of surgical site infection, 2017, *JAMA Surg* 152(8):784–791, 2017.

Menaka P, Douketis JD: *Prevention of venous thromboembolic disease in adult no orthopedic surgical patients*, 2018. Retrieved from: https://www.uptodate.com/contents/prevention-of-venous-thromboembolic-disease-in-adult-nonorthopedic-surgical-patients.

CHAPTER 6: INFECTION PREVENTION AND CONTROL

Applegate E: *The anatomy and physiology learning system*, ed 4, Philadelphia, 2010, Saunders.

Bozena P, Tunbridge A, Hall S, et al: A unified personal protective equipment ensemble for clinical reponse to possible high consequence infectious disease: a consensus document on behalf of the HCID programme, *J Infect* 77(6):496–502, 2018.

Burchum J, Rosenthal L: *Lehne's Pharmacology for nursing care*, ed 10, St. Louis, 2019, Elsevier.

Ignatavicius DD, Workman ML, Rebar C, et al: *Medical-surgical nursing: patient centered collaborative care*, ed 9, St. Louis, 2018, Elsevier.

Munford RS: Sepsis. In Mandell GL, Bennett JE, Dolin R, editors: *Mandell, Douglas, and Bennett's principles and practice of infectious disease*, ed 8, Philadelphia, 2015, Elsevier Saunders, pp 906–926.

Patton K, editor: *Anatomy & physiology*, ed 10, St. Louis, 2019, Elsevier.

RutSkidmore-Roth L: *Mosby's nursing drug reference*, ed 32, St. Louis, 2019, Elsevier.

Williams P, editor: *deWit's Fundamental concepts and skills for nursing*, ed 5, Philadelphia, 2018, Elsevier Saunders.

CHAPTER 7: CARE OF PATIENTS WITH PAIN

Benzon H, Raja SN, Fishman SM, et al: *Essentials of pain medicine*, ed 4, St. Louis, 2018, Elsevier.

Dahlen L, Oakes JM: A review of Physiology and Pharmacology related to acute perioperative pain management, *AANA J* 85(4):300–308, 2017.

Institute for Chronic Pain: *What is the Neuromatrix of Pain?* 2017. Retrieved from: http://www.instituteforchronicpain.org/understanding-chronic-pain/what-is-chronic-pain/neuromatrix-of-pain.

National Institute on Drug Abuse: *Marijuana as Medicine*, 2018. Retrieved from: https://www.drugabuse.gov/publications/drugfacts/marijuana-medicine.

Strada EA, Portenoy RK: *Psychological, rehabilitative and integrative therapies for cancer pain*, 2018. Retrieved from: https://www.uptodate.com/contents/psychological-rehabilitative-and-integrative-therapies-for-cancer-pain.

CHAPTER 8: CARE OF PATIENTS WITH CANCER

Anderson JA, et al: Red and processed meat consumption and breast cancer: UK biobank cohort study and meta-analysis, *Eur J Cancer* 90:73–82, 2018.

Chikara S, et al: Oxdative stress and dietary phytochemicals: role in cancer chemoprevention and treatment, *Cancer Lett* 413:122–134, 2018.

Del Fabbro E, Orr TA, Stella SM: Practical approaches to managing cancer patients with weight loss, *Curr Opin Support Palliat Care* 11(4):272–277, 2017.

Hilfiker R, Meichtry A, Eicher M, et al: Exercise and other non-pharmacological interventions for cancer-related fatigue in patients during or after cancer treatment: a systematic review incorporating an indirect-comparisons meta-analysis, *Br J Sports Med* 2017. doi:10.1136/bjsports-2016-096422. [Epub ahead of print]. pii: bjsports-2016-096422.

Komen MMC, et al: Patient-reported outcome and objective evaluation of chemotherapy-induced alopecia, *Eur J Oncol Nurs* 33:49–55, 2018.

Kruse M, Abraham J: Management of chemotherapy-induced alopecia with scalp cooling, *J Oncol Pract* 14(3):149–154, 2018.

Mattox TW: Cancer cachexia: cause, diagnosis, and treatment, *Nutr Clin Pract* 32(15):599–606, 2017.

Mirrakhimov AE: Hypercalcemia of malignancy: an update on pathogenesis and management, *N Am J Med Sci* 7(11):483–493, 2015.

Moryl N, et al: Patient-reported outcomes and opioid use by outpatient cancer patients, *J Pain* 19(3):278–290, 2018.

Mustian KM, et al: Comparison of pharmaceutical, psychological, and exercise treatments for cancer-related fatigue: a meta-analysis, *JAMA Oncol* 3(7):961–968, 2017.

Ozgul E, Unsar S, Yacan L, et al: Pain experiences of patients with advanced cancer: a qualitative descriptive study, *Eur J Oncol Nurs* 33:28–34, 2018.

Paice JA: Cancer pain management and the opioid crisis in America: how to preserve hard-earned gains in improving quality of cancer pain management, *Cancer* 2018. doi:10.1002/cncr.31303. [Epub ahead of print]. Review.

Ramazan A, et al: Opioid use in gynecologic oncology in the age of the opioid epidemic: part II- Balancing safety and accessibility, *Gynecol Oncol* 2018. doi:10.1016/j.ygyno.2018.02.008. [Epub ahead of print]. pii: S0090-8258(18)30127-6.

Tonia T, et al: Erythropoietin or darbepoetin for patients with cancer, *Cochrane Database Syst Rev* (12):CD003407, 2012.

Vernieri C, et al: Diet and supplements in cancer prevention and treatment: clinical evidences and future perspectives, *Crit Rev Oncol Hematol* 123:57–73, 2018.

Yasunaga JI, Matsuoka M: Onoclogic spiral by infectious pathogens: cooperation of multiple factors in cancer development, *Cancer Sci* 109:24–32, 2017.

Zheng J, et al: Obesity-associated digestive cancers: a review of mechanisms and interventions, *Tumour Biol* 39(3):1–11, 2017.

CHAPTER 9: CHRONIC ILLNESS AND REHABILITATION

Angulo Sevilla D, Carreras Rodriguez MT, Heredia Rodriguez P, et al: Is There a Characteristic Clinical Profile for Patients with Dementia and Sundown Syndrome?, *J Alzheimers Dis* 62(1):335–346, 2018.

Canevelli M, Valletta M, Trebbastoni A, et al: Sundowning in Dementia: Clinical Relevance, Pathophysiological Determinants, and Therapeutic Approaches, *Front Med (Lausanne)* 3:73, 2016.

Cotter VT, Evans LK: *Avoiding Restraints in Hospitalized Older Adults with Dementia. Try this: Best Practices in Nursing Care to Older Adults with dementia*. 2018; https://consultgeri.org/try-this/dementia/issue-d1.

Disability and quality of life 20 years after traumatic brain injury Brain and Behavior. Retrieved from: https://onlinelibrary.wiley.com/doi/full/10.1002/brb3.1018.

Fletcher K: *Nursing Standard of Practice Protocol: Recognition and Management of Dementia. ConsultGeri*. 2012; https://consultgeri.org/geriatric-topics/dementia.

Francis-Coad J, Haines T, Etherton-Beer C, et al: Evaluating the impact of operating a falls prevention community of practice on falls in a residential aged care setting, *Journal of Clinical Gerontology and Geriatrics* 9(1):5–12, 2018.

Gray-Mitchell D, Quigley PA: *Nursing standard of practice protocol: Fall Prevention*. 2012. https://consultgeri.org/geriatric-topics/falls.

Kane R, Ouslander JG, Resnick B, et al: Immobility. In *Essentials of Clinical Geriatrics*, ed 8, 2018, McGraw-Hill Education LLC.

Kresevic DM: *Nursing Standard of Practice Protocol: Assessment of Physical Function. ConsultGeri*. 2012; https://consultgeri.org/geriatric-topics/function.

Larsen PD: Chronicity. In Larsen PD, editor: *Lubkin's chronic illness: impact and intervention*, ed 10, Burlington, MA, 2019, Jones & Bartlett Learning.

Larsen PD: The Illness Experience. In Larsen PD, editor: *Lubkin's chronic illness: impact and intervention*, ed 10, Burlington, MA, 2019.

Mauk K: *Gerontological Nursing: Competencies for Care*, ed 4, Burlington, MA, 2018, Jones & Bartlette Learning.

Nada A, Howe EI, Torgeir H, et al: Disability and quality of life 20 years after traumatic brain injury, *Brain Behav* 8(7):e01018, 2018.

Quigley P, Bulat T, Kurtzman E, et al: Fall Prevention and Injury Protection for Nursing Home Residents, *J Am Med Dir Assoc* 11(4):284–293, 2010.

Shih YH, Pai MC, Huang YC, et al: Sundown Syndrome, Sleep Quality, and Walking Among Community-Dwelling People with Alzheimer Disease, *J Am Med Dir Assoc* 18(5):396–401, 2017.

Silva MWB, Sousa-Munoz RL, Frade HC, et al: Sundown syndrome and symptoms of anxiety and depression in hospitalized elderly, *Dement Neuropsychol* 11(2):154–161, 2017.

Tullman DF, Fletcher K, Foreman MD: *Nursing Standard of Practice Protocol: Delirium*. 2012.

Vlaeyen E, Coussement J, Leysens G, et al: Characteristics and effectiveness of fall prevention programs in nursing homes: A systematic review and meta-analysis of randomized controlled trials, *J Am Geriatr Soc* 63(2):211–221, 2015.

Walker N, Scott T, Dissanayaka NN, et al: Persisting use of physical restraint: Knowledge Translation vs. Attitudes, *IJCNMH* 5:1, 2018. doi: https://doi.org/10.21035/ijcnmh.2018.5.1.

CHAPTER 10: THE IMMUNE AND LYMPHATIC SYSTEMS

Applegate E: *The anatomy and physiology learning system*, ed 4, Philadelphia, 2010, Elsevier Saunders.

Centers for Disease Control and Prevention: *Vaccine Excipient & Media Summary*. Retrieved from: https://www.cdc.gov/vaccines/pubs/pinkbook/downloads/appendices/B/excipient-table-2.pdf.

Herlihy B: *The human body in health and illness*, ed 6, St. Louis, 2018, Elsevier.

Huether SE, McCance KL: *Understanding pathophysiology*, ed 6, St. Louis, 2017, Elsevier.
Hubert RJ, VanMeter KC: *Gould's pathophysiology for the health professions 6e*, St. Louis, 2018, Elsevier.
Itkin M: *Techniques in vascular and interventional radiology*. 19(4). 2016. Retrieved from: https://www.techvir.com/article/S1089-2516(16)30043-9/fulltext.
Van Meter KC, Hubert RJ: *Gould's pathophysiology for the health professions*, ed 6, St. Louis, 2018, Elsevier.
Weed HG, Baddour LM: *Postoperative fever*, 2018. Retrieved from: https://www.uptodate.com/contents/postoperative-fever.

CHAPTER 11: CARE OF PATIENTS WITH IMMUNE AND LYMPHATIC DISORDERS

Abbas AK, Lichtman AH, Pillai S: *Basic immunology: function and disorders of the immune system*, ed 5, St. Louis, 2016, Elsevier.
Centers for Disease Control and Prevention: *Terms, definitions and calculations used in CDC HIV surveillance publications*, 2016. Retrieved from: https://www.cdc.gov/hiv/statistics/surveillance/terms.html.
Centers for Disease Control and Prevention: *2018 quick reference guide: Recommended laboratory HIV testing algorithm for serum or plasma specimens*, 2018. Retrieved from: https://stacks.cdc.gov/view/cdc/50872.
Centers for Disease Control and Prevention: *Lupus, Lupus Detailed Fact Sheet*, 2018. Retrieved from: https://www.cdc.gov/lupus/facts/detailed.html.
US Department of Health and Human Services: *AIDSinfo, HIV Treatment*, 2018. Retrieved from: https://aidsinfo.nih.gov/understanding-hiv-aids/fact-sheets/21/58/fda-approved-hiv-medicines/.
US Department of Health and Human Services: *Health resources and servcies administration. Guide for HIV/AIDS Clinical Care*, 2018. Retrived from: https://stacks.cdc.gov/view/cdc/23447.
Wallace DJ: *Overview of the management and prognosis of systemic lupus erythematosus in adults*, 2018. Retrieved from: https://www.uptodate.com/contents/overview-of-the-management-and-prognosis-of-systemic-lupus-erythematosus-in-adults.

CHAPTER 12: THE RESPIRATORY SYSTEM

Healthy People 2030: *Topics and objectives: Tobacco use*, 2019. Retrieved from: http://www.healthypeople.gov/2020/topicsobjectives2020/overview.aspx?topicid=41.
National Cancer Institute: *Head and Neck Cancers*, 2017. Retrieved from: http://www.cancer.gov/cancertopics/factsheet/Sites-Types/head-and-neck.

CHAPTER 13: CARE OF PATIENTS WITH DISORDERS OF THE UPPER RESPIRATORY SYSTEM

Hemila H, Chalker E: The effectiveness of high dose zinc acetate lozenges on carious common cold symptoms: a meta-analysis, *BMC Fam Pract* 16(1):24, 2015.
National Reye's Syndrome Foundation: *What is the Role of Aspirin in Triggering Reye's?* Retrieved from: http://www.reyessyndrome.org/aspirin.html.

CHAPTER 14: CARE OF PATIENTS WITH DISORDERS OF THE LOWER RESPIRATORY SYSTEM

Cairo JM: *Mosby's respiratory care equipment*, ed 10, St. Louis, 2018, Elsevier.
Caronia JR: *Restrictive lung disease*, 2018. Retrieved from: http://emedicine.medscape.com/article/301760-overview#a0104.
Centers for Disease Control and Prevention: *Influenza (Flu): Diagnosing flu*, 2018a. Retrieved from: https://www.cdc.gov/flu/about/qa/testing.htm.
Centers for Disease Control and Prevention: *Pneumonia can be prevented—vaccines can help*, 2018b. Retrieved from: http://www.cdc.gov/Features/Pneumonia/.
Centers for Disease Control and Prevention: *Tuberculosis*, 2018c. Retrieved from: https://www.cdc.gov/tb/default.htm.
Global Initiative for Asthma: *Global Strategy for Asthma Management and Prevention*, 2018. Retrieved from: www.ginasthma.org.
Tan WW: *Non-Small Cell Lung Cancer Treatment and Management*, 2018. Retrieved from: http://emedicine.medscape.com/article/279960-treatment#aw2aab6b6b5.

CHAPTER 15: THE HEMATOLOGIC SYSTEM

Dhule S, Gawali S: Platelet aggregation and clotting time in type II diabetic males, *Natl J Physiol Pharm Pharmacol* 4(2):121–123, 2013.
Gauer RL, Braun MM: Thrombocytopenia, *Am Fam Physician* 85(6):611–622, 2012.
Hooper M, Hudson P, Porter F, et al: Patient journeys: diagnosis and treatment of pernicious anaemia, *Br J Nurs* 23(7):376–381, 2014.
Lieew G, Wang JJ, Rochtchina E, et al: Complete blood count and retinal vessel calibers, *PLoS ONE* 9(7):e102230, 2014.
Lilly KJ, Pirundini PA, Fox AA, et al: Restoration of the coagulation cascade: a case report, *Perfusion* 29(3):272–274, 2014.
Madjid M, Fatemi O: Components of the complete blood count as risk predictors for coronary heart disease, *Tex Heart Inst J* 40(1):17–29, 2013.
Nasciemento T, Andrade M, Oliveira R, et al: Neutropenia occurrence and management in women with breast cancer receiving chemotherapy, *Rev Lat Am Enfermagem* 22(2):301–308, 2014.
Oakley R, Tharakan B: Vascular hyperpermeability and aging, *Aging Dis* 5(2):114–125, 2014.
Tong H, Liu Z, Lu C, et al: Clinical and laboratory features of adult biphenotypic acute leukemia, *Asia Pac J Clin Oncol* 9:146–154, 2013.

CHAPTER 16: CARE OF PATIENTS WITH HEMATOLOGIC DISORDERS

Besa E: *Chronic myeologenous leukemia*, 2018. Retrieved from: http://emedicine.medscape.com/article/199425-overview.
Kessler CM: *Immune Thrombocytopenic Purpura*, 2018. Retrieved from: https://emedicine.medscape.com/article/202158-overview.
Levi MM: *Disseminated Intravascular Coagulation treatment and management*, 2018. Retrieved from: http://emedicine.medscape.com/article/199627-treatment.
Sandler SG: *Transfusion Reactions*, 2017. Medscape. Retreived from: https://emedicine.medscape.com/article/206885-overview.
Schrier SL: *Treatment of aplastic anemia in adults*, 2018. Retrieved from: https://www.uptodate.com/contents/treatment-of-aplastic-anemia-in-adults.
Shah D: *Multiple Myeloma*, 2018. Retrieved from: https://emedicine.medscape.com/article/204369-overview.

CHAPTER 17: THE CARDIOVASCULAR SYSTEMS

Agency for Health Care Research and Quality: n.d. At: http://www.ahrq.gov/patients-consumers/prevention/lifestyle/index.html.
CDC: *Division for heart disease and stroke prevention, Women and heart disease fact sheet*. 2017. Retrieved from: https://www.cdc.gov/dhdsp/data_statistics/fact_sheets/fs_women_heart.htm.
Centers for Disease Control and Prevention: *Division for heart disease and stroke prevention; women and heart disease fact sheet*, 2017. Retrieved from: http://www.cdc.gov/dhdsp/data_statistics/fact_sheets/fs_women_heart.htm.

CHAPTER 18: CARE OF PATIENTS WITH HYPERTENSION AND PERIPHERAL VASCULAR DISEASE

Elliott WJ, Varon J: Evaluation and treatment of hypertensive emergencies in adults. *UpToDate*, 2018. Retrieved from: ww.uptodate.com/contents/evaluation-and-treatment-of-hypertensive-emergencies-in-adults.

Kahn SR, Shapiro S, Wells PS, et al; for the SOX trial investigators: Compression stockings to prevent post-thrombotic syndrome: a randomized placebo-controlled trial, *Lancet* 383(9920):880–888, 2014.

CHAPTER 19: CARE OF PATIENTS WITH CARDIAC DISORDERS

Brusch JL: *Infective endocarditis*, 2019. Retrieved from: http://emedicine.medscape.com/article/216650-overview.

FDA: *Grapefruit juice and some drugs don't mix*, 2017. Retrieved from: https://www.fda.gov/ForConsumers/ConsumerUpdates/ucm292276.htm.

Fleming J, Aspry KE, Resnicow K, et al: *Translating the ACC/AHA lifestyle management guideline into practice: Advice for cardiologists from experts in nutrition behavioral medicine and cardiology*, 2016. Retrieved from: https://www.acc.org/latest-in-cardiology/articles/2015/12/31/10/12/translating-the-acc-aha-lifestyle-management-guideline-into-practice.

Masoudi FA, Calkins H, Kavinsky CJ, et al: 2015 ACC/HRS/SCAI left atrial appendage occlusion device societal overview: a professional society overview from the American College of Cardiology, Heart Rhythm Society, and the Society for Cardiovascular Angiography and Interventions, *J Am Coll Cardiol* 2015. Retreived from: www.scai.org/Assets/57c179eb.../scai-2015-06-29-laaocclusion-expertconsensus-pdf.

Zafari AM: *Myocardial Infarction Clinical Presentation*, 2018. Retrieved from: https://emedicine.medscape.com/article/155919-overview.

CHAPTER 20: CARE OF PATIENTS WITH CORORNARY ARTERY DISEASE AND CARDIAC SURGERY

Kalyanasyndaram A: *Comparison of revascularization procedures in coronary artery disease*, 2014. Retrieved from: http://emedicine.medscape.com/article/164682-overview.

CHAPTER 21: THE NEUROLOGIC SYSTEM

Alexander MS, Marson L: The neurologic control of arousal and orgasm with specific attention to spinal cord lesions: integrating preclinical and clinical sciences, *Auton Neurosci* 209(2018):90–99, 2018.

Betts JG, Desaix P, Johnson E, et al: *Anatomy and Physiology*. 2018. Retrieved from: https://opentextbc.ca/anatomyandphysiology/.

CHAPTER 22: CARE OF PATIENTS WITH HEAD AND SPINAL CORD INJURIES

Chin LS, Kopell BH: *Spinal cord injuries treatment & management*. Medscape, 2018. Retrieved from: http://emedicine.medscape.com/article/793582-treatment#aw2aab6b6b4.

Frieden TR, Houry D, Baldwin G: *Report to Congress: Traumatic brain injury in the United States: Epidemiology and Rehabilitation, CDC*. Retrieved from: https://www.cdc.gov/traumaticbraininjury/pdf/tbi_report_to_congress_epi_and_rehab-a.pdf.

Prevention of venous thromboembolism in individuals with spinal cord injury: clinical practice guidelines for health care providers, 3rd ed., *Top Spinal Cord Inj Rehabil* 22(3):209–240, 2016.

Rajajee V: *Management of acute severe traumatic brain injury*, 2018. Retrieved from: https://www.uptodate.com/contents/management-of-acute-severe-traumatic-brain-injury#H13.

CHAPTER 23: CARE OF PATIENTS WITH BRAIN DISORDERS

Kumar YK, Mehta SB, Ramachandra M: Computer simulation of Cerebral Arteriovenous Malformation-validation analysis of hemodynamics parameters, *Peer J* 5:e2724, 2017.

Nanda A: *Transient ischemic attack*, 2017. Retrieved from: https://emedicine.medscape.com/article/1910519-overview#a5.

Schachter SC: *Vagus nerve stimulation therapy for the treatment of epilepsy*, 2018. Retrieved from: https://www.uptodate.com/contents/vagus-nerve-stimulation-therapy-for-the-treatment-of-epilepsy.

CHAPTER 24: CARE OF PATIENTS WITH PERIPHERAL NERVE AND DEGENERATIVE NEUROLOGIC DISORDERS

Crystal H: *Alzheimer's disease causes, stages, and symptoms*, 2018. Retrieved from: http://www.medicinenet.com/alzheimers_disease_causes_stages_and_symptoms/article.htm.

Davis CP: *Myasthenia Gravis facts*, 2018. Retrieved from: http://www.medicinenet.com/script/main/art.asp?articlekey=425.

Luzzio C: *Multiple Sclerosis*, 2018. Retrieved from: https://emedicine.medscape.com/article/1146199-overview.

Slavin KV: *Deep brain stimulation for Parkinson disease*, 2017. Retrieved from: https://emedicine.medscape.com/article/1965354-overview, www.nationalmssociety.org or by writing to the National Multiple Sclerosis Society, 733 Third Avenue, 3rd Floor, New York, NY, 10017.

Tarsy D: *Pharmacologic treatment of Parkinson diseas*, 2018. Retrieved from: https://www.uptodate.com/contents/pharmacologic-treatment-of-parkinson-disease.

WebMD: *Planning daily activities with Parkinson's Disease*, 2018. Retrieved from: http://www.webmd.com/parkinsons-disease/guide/parkinsons-daily-activities.

CHAPTER 25: THE SENSORY SYSTEM: EYE

Dahl AA: *Toxic/Nutritional optic neuropathy clinical presentation*, 2018. Retrieved from: https://emedicine.medscape.com/article/1217661-clinical.

Rosenbaum JT: *Uveitis: etiology, clinical manifestations and diagnosis*, 2018. Retrieved from: https://www.uptodate.com/contents/uveitis-etiology-clinical-manifestations-and-diagnosis.

CHAPTER 26: THE SENSORY SYSTEM: EAR

Li JC: *Meniere Disease (Idiopathic endolymphatic hydrops)*. Medscape Reference, 2018. Retrieved from: http://emedicine.medscape.com/article/1159069-overview.

Limb CJ, Lustig LR, Durand ML: *Acute otitis media in adults*, 2018. Retrieved from: https://www.uptodate.com/contents/acute-otitis-media-in-adults.

Megerian CA: *Cochlear implant surgery*, 2018. Retrieved from: https://emedicine.medscape.com/article/857242-overview.

National Institute on Deafness and Other Communication Disorders: *Quick Statistics*, 2016. Retrieved from: https://www.nidcd.nih.gov/health/statistics/quick-statistics-hearing.

Park JK, Vernick DM, Ramakrishna N: *Vestibular schwannoma (acoustic neuroma)*, 2018. Retrieved from: https://www.uptodate.com/contents/vestibular-schwannoma-acoustic-neuroma.

Shah RK: *Hearing impairment workup*, 2017. Retrieved from: https://emedicine.medscape.com/article/994159-workup#c8.

Shohet JA: *Otosclerosis*, 2018. Retrieved from: https://emedicine.medscape.com/article/859760-overview.

Waltzman AA: *Otitis externa treatment and management*, 2018. Retrieved from: https://emedicine.medscape.com/article/994550-treatment#d7.

Weber PC: *Hearing amplification in adults*, 2018. Retrieved from: https://www.uptodate.com/contents/hearing-amplification-in-adults.

CHAPTER 27: THE GASTROINTESTINAL SYSTEM

Mehta N: *Drug-induced hepatotoxicity*, 2016. Retrieved from: http://emedicine.medscape.com/article/a69814-overview.

National Institute of Health: *Gallstones*, 2017. Retrieved from: http://digestive.niddk.nih.gov/ddiseases/pubs/gallstones/#4.

Björnsson ES: Hepatotoxicity by drugs: the most common implicated agents, *Int J Mol Sci* 17(2):224, 2016.

Chan WW: *Ambulatory pH monitoring*. 2017. Retrieved from: https://www.merckmanuals.com/professional/gastrointestinal-disorders/diagnostic-and-therapeutic-gi-procedures/ambulatory-ph-monitoring.

CHAPTER 28: CARE OF PATIENTS WITH DISORDERS OF THE UPPER GASTROINTESTINAL SYSTEM

Jensen PJ: *Acute hemorrhagic erosive gastropathy and reactive gastropathy*, 2018. Retrieved from: https://www.uptodate.com/contents/acute-hemorrhagic-erosive-gastropathy-and-reactive-gastropathy.

Mansfield PF: *Surgical management of invasive gastric cancer*, 2018. Retrieved from: https://www.uptodate.com/contents/surgical-management-of-invasive-gastric-cancer.

National Digestive Diseases Information Clearing House: *Barrett's esophagus*, 2017. Retrieved from: http://digestive.niddk.nih.gov/ddiseases/pubs/barretts/.

Qureshi WA: *Hiatal hernia treatment and management*, 2016. Retrieved from: https://emedicine.medscape.com/article/178393-treatment#d8.

Rockey D: *A randomized controlled trial of nasogastric tube placement in patients with upper gastrointestinal bleeding, Digestive Disease Week, 2014 (abstract 1035)*, 2014. Retrieved from: http://www.medpagetoday.com/MeetingCoverage/DDW/45641.

Sandhu DS, Fass R. Current trends in the management of gastroesophageal reflux disease. *Gut Liver* 2018; 12(1): 7–16.

CHAPTER 29: CARE OF PATIENTS WITH DISORDERS OF THE LOWER GASTROINTESTINAL SYSTEM

Brooks DC: *Overview of abdominal wall hernias in adults*, 2018. Retrieved from: https://www.uptodate.com/contents/overview-of-abdominal-wall-hernias-in-adults.

Pemberton JH: *Acute colonic diverticulitis: surgical treatment*, 2018. Retrieved from: https://www.uptodate.com/contents/acute-colonic-diverticulitis-surgical-management.

Pemberton JH: *Acute colonic diverticulitis: medical management*, 2018 Retrieved from: https://www.uptodate.com/contents/acute-colonic-diverticulitis-medical-management.

Scemons D: The ins and outs of ostomy management, *Nursing Made Incredibly Easy* 11(5):32–41, 2013.

Smink D, Soybel DI: *Management of acute appendicitis in adults*, 2018. Retrieved from: https://www.uptodate.com/contents/management-of-acute-appendicitis-in-adults.

Wald A: *Clinical manifestations and diagnosis of irritable bowel syndrome in adults*, 2018. Retrieved from: https://www.uptodate.com/contents/clinical-manifestations-and-diagnosis-of-irritable-bowel-syndrome-in-adults.

CHAPTER 30: CARE OF PATIENTS WITH DISORDERS OF THE GALLBLADDER, LIVER, AND PANCREAS

Freedman SD: *Overview of the complications of chronic pancreatitis*, 2018. Retrieved from: https://www.uptodate.com/contents/overview-of-the-complications-of-chronic-pancreatitis.

National Digestive Diseases Information Clearinghouse: *ERCP (Endoscopic Retrograde Cholangiopancreatography)*, 2016. Retrieved from: http://digestive.niddk.nih.gov/ddiseases/pubs/ercp/.

Sood GK: *Acute liver failure*, 2017. Retrieved from: http://emedicine.medscape.com/article/177354-overview.

Steel PAD: *Acute Cholecystitis and Biliary Colic*, 2017. Retrieved from: http://emedicine.medscape.com/article/1950020-overview#a1.

CHAPTER 31: THE MUSCULOSKELETAL SYSTEM

AL-Bashaireh AM, Haddad LG, Weaver M, et al: The effect of tobacco smoking on musculoskeletal health: a systematic review, *J Environ Public Health* 2018:106, 4184190, 2018. https://doi.org/10.1155/2018/4184190.

CHAPTER 32: CARE OF PATIENTS WITH MUSCULOSKELETAL AND CONNECTIVE TISSUE DISORDERS

American Cancer Society: *Chemotherapy for Osteosarcoma*, 2018. Retrieved from: http://www.cancer.org/cancer/osteosarcoma/detailedguide/osteosarcoma-treating-chemotherapy.

Mayo Clinic: *Phantom pain: Treatment and drugs*, 2018. Retrieved from: http://www.mayoclinic.org/diseases-conditions/phantom-pain/basics/treatment/con-20023268.

U. S. National Library of Medicine: *Pin care*, 2018. Retrieved from: http://www.nlm.nih.gov/medlineplus/ency/patientinstructions/000481.htm.

WebMD: *Vitamin and mineral supplements: Glucosamine*, 2018. Retrieved from: http://www.webmd.com/vitamins-and-supplements/lifestyle-guide-11/supplement-guide-glucosamine.

CHAPTER 33: THE URINARY SYSTEM

Centers for Disease Control and Prevention: *Data and Statistics: HAI Prevalence Survey*, 2018. Retrieved from: www.cdc.gov/HAI/surveillance/index.html.

Pagana KD, Pagana TJ: *Mosby's manual of diagnostic and laboratory tests*, ed 6, St. Louis, 2018, Elsevier.

CHAPTER 34: CARE OF PATIENTS WITH DISORDERS OF THE URINARY SYSTEM

American Cancer Society: *Kidney cancer treatment: targeted therapies*, 2018. Available from: https://www.cancer.org/cancer/kidney-cancer/treating/targeted-therapy.html.

Journal of Community Nursing: The provision of adequate hydration in community patients, *J Commun Nurs* 28(1):73, 2014.

Fulop T: *Acute Pyelonephritis*, 2018. Available from: https://emedicine.medscape.com/article/245559-overview.

Parmar MS: *Acute glomerulonephritis*, 2018. Available from: https://emedicine.medscape.com/article/239278-overview.

Pirkle JL: *Evaluating patients for chronic peritoneal dialysis and selection of modality*, 2018. Available from: https://www.uptodate.com/contents/evaluating-patients-for-chronic-peritoneal-dialysis-and-selection-of-modality.

Preminger GM: *Options in the management of renal and ureteral stones in adults*, 2018. Available from: https://www.uptodate.com/contents/options-in-the-management-of-renal-and-ureteral-stones-in-adults.

Sachdeva K: *Renal cell carcinoma treatment & management*, 2018. Available from: https://emedicine.medscape.com/article/281340-treatment#d11.

CHAPTER 35: THE ENDOCRINE SYSTEM

Dorion D: *Thyroid Anatomy*, 2017. Retrieved from: http://reference.medscape.com/article/835535-overview.

Kerkelä R, Ulvila J, Magga J: Natriuretic peptides in the regulation of cardiovascular physiology and metabolic events, *J Am Heart Assoc* 4:2015. e002423.

Medline Plus: *Radioactive iodine uptake*, 2017. Retrived from: http://reference.medscape.com/article/835535-overview.

Nieman LK: *Establishing the diagnosis of Cushing's syndrome*, 2017. Retrieved from: https://www.uptodate.com/contents/establishing-the-diagnosis-of-cushings-syndrome.

Schreiber D: *Natriuretic peptides in congestive heart failure*, 2018. Retrieved from: https://emedicine.medscape.com/article/761722-overview.

CHAPTER 36: CARE OF PATIENTS WITH PITUITARY, THYROID, PARATHYROID, AND ADRENAL DISORDERS

American Diabetic Association: Standards of medical care in diabetes—2018, *Diabetes Care* 41(Suppl 1):S13-S27, 2018.

Corenblum B: *Hypopituitarism (Panhypopituitarism)*, 2018. Available from: http://emedicine.medscape.com/article/122287-overview.

Diaz-Thomas A: *Gigantism and Acromegaly treatment and management*, 2017. Available from: http://emedicine.medscape.com/article/925446-treatment.

Goyal N: *Thyroidectomy*, 2018. Available from: http://emedicine.medscape.com/article/1891109-overview#a1.

Hoffman RP: *Thyroiditis*, 2018. Available from: https://emedicine.medscape.com/article/925249-overview.

Kattah JC: *Pituitary Tumors*, 2018. Available from: http://emedicine.medscape.com/article/1157189-overview#a0104.

Khardori R: *Diabetes Insipidus*, 2018. Available from: http://emedicine.medscape.com/article/117648-overview.

Orlander PR: *Hypothyroidism*, 2018. Available from: http://emedicine.medscape.com/article/122393-overview.

Pagana KD, Pagana TJ, Pagana TN: *Mosby's manual of diagnostic and laboratory tests*, ed. 6, St. Louis, 2018, Elsevier/Mosby.

CHAPTER 37: CARE OF PATIENTS WITH DIABETES AND HYPOGLYCEMIA

American Diabetes Association: *Statistics about diabetes*, 2018a. Available from: http://www.diabetes.org/diabetes-basics/statistics/.

Avichal D: *Hyperosmolar hyperglycemic state*, 2019. Available from: https://emedicine.medscape.com/article/1914705-overview.

Kaufman DB: *Pancreas transplantation*, 2018. Available from: http://emedicine.medscape.com/article/429408-overview.

CHAPTER 38: THE REPRODUCTIVE SYSTEM

About FemCap: 2017. Retrieved from: https://femcap.com/about-the-femcap/.

Merck: *What is Nexplanon?* 2018. Retrieved from: https://www.nexplanon.com/what-is-nexplanon/.

Planned Parenthood: *How effective are female condoms*. 2017. Retrieved from: https://www.plannedparenthood.org/learn/birth-control/female-condom/how-effective-are-female-condoms.

Planned Parenthood: *Birth control pill*. 2018. Retrieved from: https://www.plannedparenthood.org/learn/birth-control/birth-control-pill.

Planned Parenthood: *Birth control ring*. 2018. Retrieved from: https://www.plannedparenthood.org/learn/birth-control/birth-control-vaginal-ring-nuvaring.

Planned Parenthood: *Birth control shot*. 2018. Retrieved from: https://www.plannedparenthood.org/learn/birth-control/birth-control-shot.

Planned Parenthood: *Birth control sponge*. 2018. Retrieved from: https://www.plannedparenthood.org/learn/birth-control/birth-control-sponge.

Planned Parenthood: *Diaphragm*. 2018. Retrieved from: https://www.plannedparenthood.org/learn/birth-control/diaphragm.

Planned Parenthood: *Skin patch*. 2018. Retrieved from: https://www.plannedparenthood.org/learn/birth-control/birth-control-patch.

Planned Parenthood: *Spermicide*. 2018. Retrieved from: https://www.plannedparenthood.org/learn/birth-control/spermicide.

Planned Parenthood: *Tubal ligation*. 2018. Retrieved from: https://www.plannedparenthood.org/learn/birth-control/sterilization.

Planned Parenthood: *Vasectomy*. 2018. Retrieved from: https://www.plannedparenthood.org/learn/birth-control/vasectomy.

CHAPTER 43: CARE OF PATIENTS WITH INTEGUMENTARY DISORDERS AND BURNS

Ayoade FO: *Herpes simplex*, 2018. Retrieved from: https://emedicine.medscape.com/article/218580-overview.

Foster K: Clinical guidelines in the management of burn injury: A review and recommendations from the organization and delivery of burn care committee, *J Burn Care Res* 35(4):271–283, 2014.

Habashy J: *Psoriasis*, 2019. Retrieved from: https://emedicine.medscape.com/article/1943419-overview.

Janniger CK: *Herpes Zoster (Shingles)*, 2019. Retrieved from: https://emedicine.medscape.com/article/1132465-overview.

Scapin et al: 2018.

WebMD: *Plastic surgery for burns and other wounds*. Retrieved from: http://www.webmd.com/skin-problems-and-treatments/plastic-surgery-burns, 2017.

CHAPTER 44: CARE OF PATIENTS DURING DISASTERS, BIOTERRORISM ATTACKS, AND PANDEMIC INFECTIONS

Association of Public Health Nurses: *The role of the public health nurse in disaster preparedness, response and recovery*, 2013. Retrieved from: http://www.achne.org/files/public/APHN_RoleOfPHNinDisasterPRR_FINALJan14.pdf.

Cennimo DJ: *Anthrax*, 2018. Retrieved from: https://emedicine.medscape.com/article/212127-overview.

Centers for Disease Control and Prevention: *Smallpox*, 2019a. Retrieved from: https://www.cdc.gov/smallpox/index.html.

Ciottone GR: *CBRNE-Chemical warfare agents*, 2019. Retrieved from: http://emedicine.medscape.com/article/829454-overview#a1.

Dufel SE: *CBRNE—Plague*, 2017. Retrieved from: http://emedicine.medscape.com/article/829233-overview.

Federal Interagency Committee on Emergency Medical Services: *National implementation of the model uniform core criteria for mass casualty incident triage*, 2013. Retrieved from: http://www.ems.gov/nemsac/dec2013/FICEMS-MUCC-Implementation-Plan.pdf.

FEMA – Homeland Security: *Nation Preparedness Report*, 2013. Retrieved from: https://training.fema.gov/emiweb/edu/highref/National%20Preparedness%20Report-March%2030.2013-natprep-2013.pdf.

Hooker E: *Biological Warfare*, 2019. Retrieved from: http://www.emedicinehealth.com/biological_warfare/article_em.htm#history_of_biological_warfare.

CHAPTER 45: CARE OF PATIENTS WITH EMERGENCIES, TRAUMA, AND SHOCK

Culleiton A, Simko LM: Caring for patients with burn injuries, *Nursing* 43(8):26–34, 2013.

Kalil A: *Septic Shock*. 2019. Retrieved from: http://emedicine.medscape.com/article/168402-overview.

Mancini MC: *Blunt Chest Trauma*. 2018. Retrieved from: http://emedicine.medscape.com/article/428723-overview.

Shahani R: *Penetrating Chest Trauma*. 2017. Retrieved from: http://emedicine.medscape.com/article/425698-overview.

Society of Critical Care Medicine: *Surviving Sepsis Campaign Bundles*. 2016. Retrieved from: http://www.survivingsepsis.org/guidelines/Pages/default.aspx.

National Oceanic and Atmospheric Administration National Weather Service Lightning Safety. Retrieved from: https://www.weather.gov/safety/lightning-safety.

CHAPTER 46: CARE OF PATIENTS WITH COGNITIVE DISORDERS

American Foundation for Suicide Prevention: *Suicide statistics*, 2018. Retrieved from: https://afsp.org/about-suicide/suicide-statistics/.

Anglin R, et al: Risk of upper gastrointestinal bleeding with selective serotonin reuptake inhibitors without concurrent nonsteroidal anti-inflammatory use: A systematic review, *Am J Gastroenterol* 109(6):811–819, 2014.

Centers for Disease Control and Prevention: *Suicide rising across the U.S*, 2018. Retrieved from: https://www.cdc.gov/vitalsigns/suicide/index.html.

de Arellano MA, Andrews III AR, Reid-Quiñones K, et al: *Immigration trauma among Hispanic youth: Missed by trauma assessments and predictive of depression and PTSD symptoms*. 2017.

Gottschalk M: Genetics of generalized anxiety disorder and related traits, *Dialogues Clin Neurosci* 19(2):158–169, 2017.

Halter M: *Varcarolis' Foundations of Psychiatric-Mental Health Nursing: A Clinical Approach*, ed 8, St. Louis, MO, 2018, Elsevier.

Kraus C, et al: Administration of ketamine for unipolar and bipolar depression, *Int J Psychiatry Clin Pract* 21(1):2–12, 2017.

Laursen SB, Leontiadis GI, Stanley AJ, et al: The use of selective serotonin receptor inhibitors (SSRI s) is not associated with increased risk of endoscopy-refractory bleeding, rebleeding or mortality in peptic ulcer bleeding, *Aliment Pharmacol Ther* 46(3):355–363, 2017.

MacKinlay E, Burns R: Spirituality promotes better health outcomes and lowers anxiety about aging: The importance of spiritual dimensions for baby boomers as they enter older adulthood, *J Relig Spiritual Aging* 29(4):248–265, 2017.

National Association of Anorexia Nervosa and Associated Disorders: *Eating disorder statistics*, n.d. Retrieved from: http://www.anad.org/get-information/about-eating-disorders/eating-disorders-statistics/.

National Center for PTSD: *How common is PTSD?* 2017. Retrieved from: https://www.ptsd.va.gov/public/PTSD-overview/basics/how-common-is-ptsd.asp.

Pascoe MC, Bauer IE: A systematic review of randomised control trials on the effects of yoga on stress measures and mood, *J Psychiatr Res* 68:270–282, 2015.

Raglio A, Attardo L, Gontero G, et al: Effects of music and music therapy on mood in neurological patients, *World J Psychiatry* 5(1):68, 2015.

Stahl S: *Stahl's Essential Psychopharmacology Prescriber's Guide*, ed 6, Cambridge, UK, 2018, University Printing House.

Wilson G, Farrell D, Barron I, et al: The Use of Eye-Movement Desensitization Reprocessing (EMDR) Therapy in Treating Post-traumatic Stress Disorder—A Systematic Narrative Review, *Front Psychol* 9:2018.

CHAPTER 47: CARE OF PATIENTS WITH ANXIETY, MOOD, AND EATING DISORDERS

Halter M: *Varcarolis' foundations of psychiatric-mental health nursing: a clinical approach*, ed 8, St. Louis, MO, 2018, Elsevier.

CHAPTER 48: CARE OF PATIENTS WITH SUBSTANCE-RELATED AND ADDICTIVE DISORDERS

*Agency for Healthcare Research and Quality: *Five major steps to intervention (The "5 A's")*. 2012. Retrieved from: https://www.ahrq.gov/professionals/clinicians-providers/guidelines-recommendations/tobacco/5steps.html.

National Institute on Alcohol Abuse and Alcoholism: *A word about alcohol poisoning*. n.d. Retrieved from: https://www.niaaa.nih.gov/alcohol-poisoning.

*Indicates a classic reference

CHAPTER 49: CARE OF PATIENTS WITH THOUGHT AND PERSONALITY DISORDERS

Guy W: *ECDEU assessment manual for psychopharmacology: revised (DHEW publication number ADM 76-338). Rockville, MD, US Department of Health, Education and Welfare, Public Health Service, Alcohol, Drug Abuse and Mental Health Administration, NIMH Psychopharmacology Research Branch, Division of Extramural Research Programs*, 1976, pp 534–537.

May J, Richardi T, Barth K: Dialectical behavior therapy as treatment for borderline personality disorder, *Mental Health Clinician* 6(2):62–67, 2016.

Glossary

A

abduction Movement away from the midline of the body.
ablation The removal of a part, as by incision; eradication.
ablation therapy Removing or destroying tissue causing abnormal function such as treatment for hyperthyroidism using radioactive iodine (^{131}I).
abrasion A wound caused by rubbing or scraping the skin or mucous membrane.
absorption The passage of liquids or other substances through a body surface and into its tissues and fluids, as in absorption of the end products of digestion into the intestinal villi.
abuse Misuse; excessive or improper use.
acceptance Admission of reality, as in the reality of death; the final stage in the process of dealing with dying and death.
accommodation Adjustment, especially of the ocular lens for seeing objects at varying distances.
achlorhydria The absence of hydrochloric acid from maximally stimulated gastric secretions.
acid A substance that yields hydrogen ions in solution.
acid-base balance A normal condition in which the narrow range of normal pH and the normal ratio of carbonic acid to bicarbonate ions are maintained.
acidosis A condition in which the pH of body fluids is below normal range because of either a loss of base bicarbonate or an accumulation of acid.
acquired Occurring from factors outside the organism, as in response to the environment.
acquired immunity Immunity involving the functioning of the immune system acquired by natural infection or vaccination (active immunity) or by transfer of antibody from an immune donor (passive immunity).
acquired immunodeficiency syndrome (AIDS) A group of symptoms believed to be caused by a virus (HIV) that infects and destroys T lymphocytes.
acromegaly A chronic disease of adults caused by hypersecretion of the pituitary growth hormone and characterized by enlargement of many parts of the skeleton.
active immunity Immunity acquired by producing one's own antibody.
active listening Listening with concentration and focused energy.
active transport Movement of substances from an area of lower concentration to an area of higher concentration, requiring energy to accomplish.
acuity The degree of seriousness of illness or injury.
acupressure The application of digital pressure on a part of the body to relieve pain or produce anesthesia.
acupuncture A technique for treating certain painful conditions and for producing regional anesthesia by passing long, thin needles through the skin to specific points.
acute kidney injury Occurs suddenly as a result of physical injury usually secondary to hypoperfusion, infection, inflammation, or damage from toxic chemicals.
acute myocardial infarction Ischemic necrosis of an area of the heart muscle resulting from sudden occlusion of blood flow through one or more branches of the coronary arteries.
acute pain Sharp, severe pain of short duration.
acute renal failure Sudden loss of kidney function. Older term, now called *acute kidney injury.*
addiction A psychological craving for alcohol or drugs with the presence of withdrawal symptoms if the substance cannot be obtained.
Addisonian crisis Sudden insufficiency of the glucocorticoid cortisol that can lead to shock.
adduction Movement toward the midline of the body.
adenohypophysis The anterior lobe of the pituitary gland.
adhesion A fibrous band that binds together two parts that are normally separated; often occurs after surgery in the abdomen.
adjuvant That which assists, such as a drug added to a prescription that enhances the action of the principal ingredient.
adrenergic Having action that mimics that of the sympathetic nervous system.
adrenocortical Indicating the cortex of the adrenal gland.
adrenocorticotropic hormone (ACTH) A "tropic" hormone of the anterior pituitary gland that acts on the adrenal cortex causing the release of cortisol.
adulthood A stage of life at which an individual has reached biological maturity, usually at age 20 years in humans.
advance directive A document prepared while an individual is alive and competent that contains instructions for future health care.
adventitious Acquired; arising sporadically; nonnative.
advocate Supporting, protecting and speaking out for the rights of the patient.
aerobe A microorganism that requires oxygen for survival.
aerobic Requiring oxygen to live.
aerosol A suspension of a drug or other substance that is dispensed in a cloud or mist.
affect The external expression; mood.
afferent Carries impulses to the CNS.
ageism Prejudice against aging and elderly people.
agent A party authorized to act on behalf of another.
agglutination One type of antigen-antibody reaction in which a solid antigen clumps together with a soluble antibody.
agnosia The loss of the power to recognize the significance of sensory stimuli.
agranulocytosis A condition of deficiency, or absolute lack, of granulocytic white blood cells.
airway The passage by which air enters and leaves the lungs; also, a device used to secure unobstructed respiration.
akathisia A condition of motor restlessness; a common extrapyramidal side effect of neuroleptic drugs.
albumin, serum A plasma protein formed principally in the liver and constituting about 60% of the protein concentration in the plasma.
aldosterone A mineralocorticoid steroid hormone produced by the adrenal cortex. Works in the renal tubules to retain sodium and conserve water by reabsorption; increases urinary potassium excretion.
alkalosis A condition in which the pH of body fluids is above normal because of either a loss of acid or an accumulation of base bicarbonate.
allergen(s) Any substance capable of triggering an exaggerated immune response.
allergy (allergies) An abnormal and individual hypersensitivity to a particular allergen; acquired by exposure to the allergen and manifested after reexposure.

alleviate To relieve; to make easier to bear.
alliance An agreement to cooperate made between a free-standing independent facility and a hospital.
allogeneic Having a different genetic constitution but belonging to the same species.
allograft Transplant tissue obtained from the same species.
alogia A psychiatric term meaning poverty of thoughts.
alopecia Baldness or loss of hair.
Alzheimer disease (AD) The most common degenerative disease of the brain, with no known cause or cure. The disease causes loss of neurons in the frontal and temporal lobes and primarily affects people older than 65 years but can also occur in younger people.
amenorrhea The absence of menstruation.
anabolic Constructive in nature; the opposite of catabolic.
anabolism The building up of the body substance; the constructive phase of metabolism.
anaerobe An organism that lives in an oxygen-free environment.
anaerobic Able to live in an oxygen-free environment.
analgesia The absence of normal sense of pain.
analgesic(s) A pain reliever.
anaphylaxis An unusual or exaggerated allergic reaction.
anasarca Generalized massive edema resulting from severe depletion of albumin.
anastomosis A communication between two tubular organs; also, surgical, traumatic, or pathologic formation of a connection between two normally distinct structures.
androgen(s) Any steroid hormone that promotes male characteristics.
anemia(s) A condition in which there are too few functioning red blood cells to meet the oxygen needs of tissues.
anesthesia The loss of feeling or sensation.
aneurysm A sac formed by localized dilation of the wall of a blood vessel or the heart.
anger A feeling of hostility and bitterness against a situation or person; the second stage in acceptance of death.
angina pectoris Exertional chest pain caused by ischemia of the heart muscle and increased demand for oxygen.
angioedema A vascular reaction representing localized edema under the deepest layer of the skin and the development of urticaria.
angiography Radiographic studies of the arteries, veins, or lymph vessels of the body.
anhedonia Inability to experience pleasure or joy.
animate Alive.
anion A negatively charged atomic particle.
anion gap The difference between the negative ions and the primary measured positive ions.
ankylosis Abnormal immobility and consolidation and obliteration of a joint.
anorexia A lack or loss of appetite for food.
anorexia nervosa An eating disorder in which there is an aberration of eating patterns, severe weight loss, and malnutrition.
anosmia The absence of the sense of smell; also called *anosphresia* and *olfactory anesthesia.*
anovulation Failure of the ovary to produce or release mature eggs.
antibiotic An agent that is capable of either killing or inhibiting the growth of microorganisms.
antibody (antibodies) An immune globulin molecule capable of adhering to and interacting only with the antigen that induced its synthesis.
anticoagulants Substances that suppress, delay, or nullify the coagulation of blood.
antidiuretic hormone A hormone that decreases the production of urine by increasing the reabsorption of water by the renal tubules. It is secreted by the hypothalamus and stored in the posterior lobe of the pituitary gland.
antidysrhythmic agents Substances that help return the heart rate and rhythm to more normal values and restore the origin of the heart's electrical activity to its natural pacemaker.
antiemetic An agent that prevents or relieves nausea and vomiting.
antifungal(s) An agent that is destructive to or inhibitive of the growth of fungi.
antigen(s) Any substance that can produce an antagonist.
antigen-antibody reaction An immune response that occurs when an antibody comes into contact with the specific antigen for which it was formed. In a transfusion reaction, the response is a clumping together, or agglutination, of the red blood cells carrying the antigens.
antihistamine An agent that counteracts the effects of histamine; used to relieve the symptoms of an allergic reaction.
antihypertensive A medication to prevent or control high blood pressure.
antimicrobial agent A substance capable of either killing or suppressing the multiplication and growth of microorganisms.
antineoplastic agent A substance that inhibits the maturation and proliferation of malignant cells.
antiseptic(s) Any substance that inhibits the growth of bacteria outside the body; in contrast, a germicide kills the bacteria outright.
antitoxin A specific kind of antibody produced in response to the presence of a toxin.
antitussive An agent that inhibits the cough reflex in the cough center in the brain.
antivenin A substance used to neutralize the venom of a poisonous animal.
anuria Diminished or absent production of urine by the kidney.
apathetic thyrotoxicosis Milder hyperthyroidism signs and symptoms seen in older adult patients compared with symptoms seen in the typical adult patient.
aphakic eye An eye without a lens, as after a cataract extraction.
aphasia A defect in or loss of the power of expression by speech, writing, or signs or in the comprehension of spoken or written language.
aphonia The loss of the voice.
apical Pertaining to the apex of a structure, particularly the heart.
aplastic Having deficient or arrested development.
aplastic anemia Deficient red cell production caused by a bone marrow disorder.
apnea Temporary cessation of breathing.
apoptosis The process of programmed cell death that occurs naturally when cells are old, damaged, or unhealthy.
apraxia The loss or impairment of acquired motor skills due to brain dysfunction.
arrhythmia (also dysrhythmia) Variation from the normal rhythm, especially of the heartbeat.
arteriosclerosis A group of diseases characterized by thickening and loss of elasticity of the arterial walls.
arthritis Inflammation of a joint.
arthrocentesis The surgical puncture of a joint cavity for aspiration of synovial fluid.
arthroplasty Surgery performed on a joint to increase mobility or decrease pain.
arthroscopy Endoscopic examination of the interior of a joint.
ascites The accumulation of edematous fluid within the peritoneal cavity.
asepsis, medical The destruction and containment of infectious agents by using antiseptic agents and techniques to limit their spread.
assessment, nursing Data-gathering activities for the purpose of collecting a complete, relevant database from which a nursing diagnosis or problem statement can be made.
asterixis A motor disturbance marked by intermittent tremor of the hand; a characteristic of hepatic coma. Also called "flapping tremor."

asthma A condition marked by recurrent attacks of paroxysmal dyspnea, with wheezing from spasmodic contraction of the bronchi.
astigmatism An error of refraction in which light rays are not sharply focused on the retina because of abnormal curvature of the cornea or lens.
ataxia Uncoordinated motor movements.
atelectasis The collapsed or airless state of the lung.
atherosclerosis A disease process in which fibrinous plaques are laid down within the walls of the arteries, thus narrowing the lumens of the vessels and predisposing them to the development of intravascular clots.
atopy The tendency to develop allergies.
atrial fibrillation Rapid, irregular, and ineffective contractions of the atria.
atrial natriuretic peptide A hormone involved in the regulation of renal and cardiovascular homeostasis. It is produced in the atrium and helps normalize blood pressure and volume by causing mild diuresis.
atrophy Wasting, or a decrease in size, from lack of use.
atypical antipsychotics Newer medications used for treating schizophrenia with fewer side effects.
audiometry The measurement of sound perception.
audit An official examination of the record of all aspects of patient care.
aura A peculiar sensation preceding the appearance of more definite symptoms, especially a sensation, that occurs immediately before an epileptic seizure.
aural Pertaining to the ear.
auscultation Listening for sounds produced within the body, usually with a stethoscope.
autograft A graft transferred from one part of a patient's body to another.
autoimmune disease A disease caused by the body's failure to recognize its own cells, thus rejecting them as it would a foreign substance.
autoimmune thyroiditis (Hashimoto thyroiditis) A condition in which the body produces antibodies against the thyroid, which in turn destroy the gland.
autoimmunity A defective cellular immune response in which antibodies are produced against normal tissues of the person's body.
autoinoculation Inoculation with microorganisms from one's own body.
autologous Indicating something that has its origin within an individual, as in transfusion with one's own blood.
automated external defibrillator (AED) A defibrillator found in many public places that is used to treat cardiac arrest.
automatisms Repetitive, automatic actions such as lip smacking.
autonomic dysreflexia Hyperreflexia, an uninhibited and exaggerated reflex response of the autonomic nervous system to some type of stimulation in patients with spinal cord injuries.
avolition A lack of motivation.
avulsion The tearing away of part or all of an organ or structure.
axon The projection, or process, of a neuron that transmits impulses away from the cell body.
azotemia Retention in the blood of urea, creatinine, and other nitrogenous protein metabolites that are normally eliminated in the urine.

B

Babinski reflex A reflex action elicited by stimulating the sole of the foot and characterized by dorsiflexion of the great toe and flaring of the smaller toes. A positive Babinski reflex indicates an abnormality in the motor control pathways of the nervous system.
bacteria Microscopically small organisms belonging to the plant kingdom, some of which can produce disease in humans.
bacterial vaginosis A bacterial disease of the vagina.
bactericidal Able to kill bacteria.
bacteriophage A virus that destroys bacteria by lysis. The virus is usually of a type specific for the kind of bacteria it attacks.
bacteriostatic Able to slow duplication of bacteria.
bargaining An attempt to make an arrangement whereby one gives something to gain something in return; the third stage in acceptance of death.
bariatrics The field of medicine that focuses on the treatment and control of obesity and diseases associated with obesity.
basal insulin Amount of insulin that would normally be produced by the pancreas, given as a long-acting insulin in diabetic patients.
base A substance that combines with acids to form salts.
basement membrane The noncellular layer that secures the overlying epithelium to the underlying tissue.
behavior The manner in which one conducts oneself in response to social stimuli, an inner need, or a combination of the two.
belief A currently held idea or value derived from culture and experience.
benign Not very harmful; nonmalignant.
benign pituitary adenoma A benign tumor of the pituitary gland that secretes excessive amounts of hormone. The hormone secreted can be any of those released by the pituitary gland.
bereaved Experiencing the reaction of grief and sadness on learning of the loss of a loved one.
biliary Pertaining to bile, the bile ducts, or the gallbladder.
biliary colic Acute pain resulting from obstruction of a bile duct, usually caused by cholelithiasis.
binder A broad bandage most commonly used as an encircling support of the abdomen or chest.
biofeedback A training program designed to develop one's ability to control the autonomic (involuntary) nervous system.
biological response modifier (BRM) An agent that manipulates the immune system in hopes of controlling or curing a malignancy.
biologic dressing Materials obtained from a patient's intact skin, cadavers, or animals that is used to treat burn victims.
biomarker A measurable substance that indicates the presence of disease, infection, or toxic exposure.
biomedicine Biological medicine; focuses on the biological aspects of medicine.
biopsy Removal of living cells for the purpose of examining them microscopically.
biosynthetic A biological substance created by chemical processes. A term used for artificial skin that can be used as a temporary measure for grafting in burn victims.
bioterrorism An attack that involves the deliberate release of microorganisms or toxins derived from living organisms that cause disease or death to humans, animals, or plants on which we depend for food.
bipolar disorder A mood disorder in which manic and depressive episodes occur.
bisexual An individual who is sexually attracted to others of either sex.
bivalve(d) Split through all layers of the material.
bladder, cord A dysfunction of the urinary bladder caused by damage to the spinal cord.
bladder, neurogenic A dysfunction of the urinary bladder caused by a lesion of the central or peripheral nervous system and characterized by lack of awareness of the need to void.
blepharitis An infection of the glands and lash follicles along the margin of the eyelid.
blood gases, arterial (ABGs) Arterial blood sample measuring the partial pressure exerted by oxygen and carbon dioxide. ABGs reflect the ability of the lungs to exchange these gases, the effectiveness of the kidneys to retain and eliminate bicarbonate, and the acid-base balance.

blood urea nitrogen Blood test measuring urea levels, indicating kidney function and fluid balance.
B-lymphocyte A sensitized lymphocyte that is responsible for antibody formation and the development of humoral immunity.
bolus dose A dose of short- or rapid-acting insulin that is used to manage elevations in blood glucose and bring the next blood glucose measurement into range.
borborygmi Gurgling, splashing sounds normally heard over the large intestine; rumbling in the bowels.
borderline personality disorder A mental disorder defined by the DSM-5 as "a pattern of instability in interpersonal relationships, self-image and affect, and marked impulsivity."
botulism Food poisoning caused by a neurotoxin produced by *Clostridium botulinum,* sometimes found in improperly canned or preserved foods.
brachytherapy Internal radiation therapy; involves introducing a radioactive element (isotope) into the body.
bradycardia An abnormally slow heart rate, usually fewer than 60 beats per minute.
bradykinesia Slow movement; a symptom seen with Parkinson disease.
bradypnea Abnormally slow breathing.
brain natriuretic peptide or B-type natriuretic peptide Hormone released by the ventricles of the heart that promotes loss of water and sodium ions from the kidney tubules and causes vasodilatation.
bronchiectasis Chronic dilation of the bronchi marked by fetid breath and paroxysmal coughing, with the expectoration of mucopurulent matter.
bronchodilator A drug that acts directly on the smooth muscles of the bronchi to relax them and relieve bronchospasm.
bronchogram A radiograph of the bronchial tree using a radiopaque substance that is introduced into the trachea.
bronchoscopy Insertion of an endoscope for diagnosis and treatment of disorders of the bronchi.
bruit An abnormal sound of venous or arterial origin heard on auscultation caused by turbulent blood flow over vascular structures.
buccal mucosa Mucous membrane lining the inside of the mouth.
bulimia nervosa A mental disorder that occurs predominantly in females characterized by episodes of binge eating that continue until terminated by abdominal pain, sleep, or self-induced vomiting.
bulla (bullae) A blister; a round, fluid-filled lesion of the skin, usually more than 5 mm in diameter.
burns, full-thickness Burns in which all of the epithelializing elements of the skin and those tissues lining the sweat glands, hair follicles, and sebaceous glands are destroyed.
burns, partial-thickness Burns in which the epithelializing elements remain intact.

C

C-A-B Chest compressions, airway, breathing.
cachexia A profound state of general ill health and malnutrition.
calculus (calculi) An abnormal concretion, usually of mineral salts, occurring mainly in hollow organs or their passages (e.g., renal calculus, or kidney stone).
callus A thickened area of the epidermis caused by pressure or friction.
caloric testing Testing to check the oculovestibular reflex. A patient's eye movements are observed while the external ear canal is irrigated with cold water. Absence of eye movement indicates a brainstem lesion.
candidiasis An infection with a fungus of the genus *Candida,* especially *C. albicans.* It is usually a superficial infection of the moist cutaneous areas of the body, although it becomes more severe in immunocompromised patients.
capitation A payment method wherein the health care provider is paid a monthly contracted rate for each member patient assigned regardless of the type or number of services provided.
capnography Measurement of inhaled and exhaled carbon dioxide as recorded on a capnogram.
caput medusa Dilated cutaneous veins around the umbilicus in patients who have cirrhosis of the liver.
carbuncles A collection of infected hair follicles. They most often occur on the back of the neck, the upper back, and the lateral thighs.
carcinogen Any substance or agent that produces or increases the risk of developing cancer in humans or lower animals.
carcinoma(s) A malignant growth made up of epithelial cells.
cardiac glycosides A group of compounds containing a carbohydrate molecule (e.g., digitalis) that affects the contractile force of the heart muscle.
cardiac output Stroke volume multiplied by the heart rate, calculating the amount of blood pumped by the heart in 1 minute.
cardiac tamponade Compression of the heart caused by collection of fluid in the pericardial sac.
cardiogenic shock A shock state caused by pump failure of the heart.
cardiomyopathy Disease of the myocardium, especially from primary disease of the heart muscle.
cardiomyoplasty A procedure in which the latissimus dorsi muscle is detached from its natural position, brought around to the front of the body, and wrapped around the heart. A pacemaker, connected to the heart and back muscle, helps boost the heart's pumping action.
cardiopulmonary resuscitation The reestablishment of heart and lung action after they have suddenly stopped.
cardiotonic(s) An agent that strengthens the contractions of the heart muscle.
cardioversion A mild electrical shock delivered to the heart at a specific time in the cardiac cycle to interrupt an abnormal rhythm and begin a new, normal rhythm of electrical impulse and contraction.
carpopedal spasm A spasm of the hand, thumbs, foot, or toes that accompanies tetany.
carriers People who harbor infectious organisms within their bodies without manifesting any outward symptoms of the infection.
cartilage A type of connective tissue in which fibers and cells are embedded in a semisolid gel material.
catabolic Destructive in nature; the opposite of anabolic.
catabolism The phase of metabolism in which larger molecules are broken down and energy is released; the destructive phase of metabolism.
cataract(s) An opacity of the lens of the eye.
catecholamines One of a group of biogenic amines that have a sympathomimetic action; examples are dopamine, norepinephrine, and epinephrine.
category-specific precautions A system of precautionary measures organized according to types of diseases (e.g., respiratory or enteric) and initiated to prevent the spread of disease.
cations Positively charged atomic particles.
cauterize To burn with a cautery, or to apply one.
CD lymphocyte A type of lymphocyte that is the master regulator of the human immune system. It is the primary site of replication for HIV.
cell(s) The basic structural unit of living organisms.
cell-mediated immunity Immunity resulting from activation of sensitized lymphocytes.
cellulitis Inflammation of cellular or connective tissue.
central hearing loss Impaired perception of sound caused by pathology above the junction of the eighth cranial nerve and the brainstem (in the brain).

cerumen Earwax.
chalazion An infection of the meibomian gland of the eye; an internal stye.
chancre A primary syphilis skin lesion that begins as a papule and develops into a red, bloodless, painless ulcer with a scooped-out appearance.
chemonucleolysis Treatment of a herniated intervertebral disk by dissolution of a portion of the nucleus pulposus by injection of a chemolytic agent.
chemotherapy Use of chemicals, especially drugs, in the treatment of such diseases as cancer, infection, and some mental illnesses.
cholecystectomy The removal of the gallbladder.
cholecystitis An inflammation of the gallbladder.
choledocholithiasis A condition in which gallstones lodge in the common bile duct.
cholelithiasis The presence of stones within the gallbladder or biliary tract.
cholinergic An agent that produces the effect of acetylcholine.
chorea Involuntary muscle twitching.
chronic illness Disease that lasts longer than 3 months and has no cure.
chronic pain Pain of long duration showing little change, or slowly progressive pain.
chronic renal failure A progressive loss of kidney function that develops over the course of many months or years.
chronologic Occurring in a natural time sequence.
Chvostek sign Low calcium level that manifests as muscle irritability when the facial nerve is gently tapped.
chyme The mixture of partly digested food and digestive secretions found in the stomach and small intestine during digestion of a meal.
cirrhosis A liver disease characterized by diffuse interlacing bands of fibrous tissue dividing the hepatic parenchyma into micronodular or macronodular areas.
cirrhosis of the liver A condition characterized by destruction of normal hepatic structures and their replacement with necrotic tissue and scarring.
claudication, intermittent A syndrome characterized by intensification of limb pain as exercise is increased; related to occlusion of arteries in the legs.
climacteric Endocrine, somatic, and psychic changes that occur at the end of the female reproductive period (menopause); also, normal diminution of testicular activity in the male.
clinical judgment Using clinical data obtained by observation, assessment, the EHR, and nursing knowledge to make decisions regarding patient care.
clinical pathway A tool used to track patient progress along a set path in a managed care system.
clonic Alternating contraction and relaxation of muscles.
clonus Abnormal neuromuscular activity, characterized by rapidly alternating involuntary contraction and relaxation of skeletal muscle; occurs with epileptic seizure.
coarctation Narrowing (of the aorta).
code of ethics A set of rules governing one's conduct.
codependency A behavior pattern in which a family member or friend of a substance abuser attempts to control the behavior of the dependent person.
cognition The mental processes of perception, memory, judgment, and reasoning.
coinsurance Insurance in which both the insurer and the patient pay the medical bill.
coitus Sexual intercourse.
colectomy The removal of part of the colon.
colic A spasm causing pain; may be biliary, renal, intestinal, or uterine.
collaboration The act of working or cooperating with another.
collaborator One who works cooperatively with another.
collagen A fibrous protein found in skin, bone, cartilage, and ligaments.
colonization The process in which a group of organisms, especially bacteria, live together and multiply.
colostomy (colostomies) The surgical creation of an opening in the colon to allow fecal material to pass outside.
colporrhaphy The operation of suturing the vagina.
colposcopy The visual examination of the vagina and cervix with a specially designed endoscope that allows the detection of malignant growths in their early stages.
comedo (comedones) A plug of keratin and sebum in an enlarged pore; a blackhead.
command hallucinations Voices the patient hears that direct the patient to harm self or others.
communicable Passed from one person to another directly, through touch, droplet or aerosolization, or indirectly, by using a contaminated object; contagious or able to be spread.
communicable disease A disease that may be transmitted directly or indirectly from one individual to another.
compartment syndrome External or internal pressure that seriously restricts circulation to the area.
complementary and alternative medicine (CAM) Types of treatments for medical disorders that do not rely on traditional medicine but frequently are combined with traditional medical treatment for a disorder.
complement system A complex series of enzymatic proteins that interact to combine with the antigen-antibody complex, producing lysis of intact antigen cells.
complement system of proteins A series of protective proteins that are activated in the inflammatory response.
complete blood cell count (CBC) The number of each kind of cell in a sample of blood.
compliance An expression of the ability of lung tissue to distend when filled with air.
computed tomography (CT) scan A computer-aided technique in which small sections of tissue within an organ can be visualized by radiograph.
concept(s) An idea, thought, or notion derived from experiences and information acquired from one's external environment.
concussion A closed head injury considered a mild TBI, in which the brain hits against the skull at the time of the blow, resulting in neurologic injury.
conductive hearing loss Impaired perception of sound caused by a dysfunction of either the external or the middle ear.
confabulation A behavioral reaction to memory loss in which the patient fills in memory gaps with made-up facts and experiences.
confusion The state of not being aware of or oriented to time, place, or self.
congenital Present at birth.
congestive heart failure The exhaustion of the heart muscle and a resultant engorgement of the heart's chambers and the blood vessels. Eventually, sluggish blood flow leads to retention of fluid and edema in the lungs and elsewhere in the body.
congruent Matches the feeling tone of what is said verbally.
conjugate Working in union; equally coupled.
conjunctivitis An inflammation of the membrane covering the eyeball and lining the eyelids.
consciousness Responsiveness of the mind to impressions made by the senses.
contactant A substance that produces an allergic or sensitivity response when in direct contact with the skin.
contamination The presence of a noxious agent, such as bacteria or radiation, in a place where it is not wanted.
contracture An adaptive shortening of skeletal muscle tissue that is not subjected to normal stretching and contraction.
contralateral On or affecting the opposite side of the body.
contusion A bruise; an injury of a part without a break in the skin.

conventional antipsychotics Neuroleptics used to treat the positive symptoms of schizophrenia. Cause serious and unpleasant side effects and are becoming less commonly prescribed.
convulsion A state of involuntary muscle contractions and relaxations.
copayment The amount a member of an HMO or other health care plan must pay for each visit to the health care provider.
COPD Chronic obstructive pulmonary disease.
coronary artery bypass graft (CABG) Surgery in which a blood vessel is grafted onto the coronary artery to improve blood flow.
coronary insufficiency Decreased or insufficient blood flow in the coronary arteries.
coronary occlusion The closing off of a coronary artery and interruption of its blood flow.
cor pulmonale Heart disease characterized by hypertrophy of the right ventricle because of pulmonary hypertension.
correction dose Short- or rapid-acting insulin used to manage elevations in blood glucose and bring the next blood glucose measurement into range.
corrosive Containing a destructive agent that produces disintegration or wearing away.
cost containment The need to hold costs to within fixed limits.
counter-regulatory hormones Hormones that act in the opposite way of another, such as growth hormone, glucagon, and epinephrine, which are released during the night and cause an increase in blood glucose. They act "counter" to insulin.
coup-contrecoup injury An injury that occurs when the head is moving rapidly and hits a stationary object. The contents within the cranium hit the inside of the skull (coup) and then bounce back and hit the opposite side, causing a second injury (contrecoup).
crackles An abnormal respiratory sound heard on auscultation during inspiration; can be a bubbling noise or a popping sound. Crackles do not clear with coughing.
creatinine A nonprotein substance that is formed in muscle in relatively small and constant amounts, passes into the bloodstream, and is eliminated by the kidneys. Urine creatinine levels are diminished and blood levels increased when glomerular filtration is impaired.
Credé technique Exerting downward pressure with the open hand over the suprapubic area to facilitate emptying of the urinary bladder.
cremasteric reflex The retraction of the testicles when the inner thigh is stroked. This reflex is absent with testicular torsion.
crepitation A sound like that of hair rubbed between the fingers; occurs when bone fragments rub together.
crepitus A crackling, crinkly or grating sound or feeling under the skin or in the joints.
cretinism A congenital condition caused by lack of thyroid secretion characterized by arrested physical and mental development, dystrophy of the bones and soft parts, and lowered basal metabolism.
criterion A standard for judging a condition or establishing a diagnosis.
critical thinking Purposeful, considered, organized cognitive processing used to examine a problem or situation or to evaluate the thinking of others.
crust An outer layer of solid matter formed by dried exudate or secretion.
cryoprecipitate Blood product derived from plasma that contains fibrinogen and clotting factors.
cryosurgery The destruction of tissue by application of extreme cold, as in removal of cataracts.
cryotherapy The therapeutic use of cold or freezing.
cryptorchidism (cryptorchism) The failure of one or both testes to descend into the scrotum during fetal life.
culdoscopy The direct inspection of the female viscera through an endoscope introduced into the pelvic cavity through the posterior vaginal fornix.
culture The propagation of microorganisms or living tissue cells in media conducive to their growth.
curettage Cleansing of a surface of an organ with a spoon-shaped instrument (curet).
Curling ulcer A type of ulcer caused by decreased perfusion to other organs, which causes changes in the gastric mucosa.
Cushing syndrome Manifestations of excess levels of the hormone cortisol from the adrenal cortex.
cyanosis A bluish tinge to the skin caused by lack of oxygen and accumulation of carbon dioxide in the blood.
cystitis An inflammation of the urinary bladder.
cystocele A protrusion or herniation of the bladder through the wall of the vagina.
cystogram A radiograph of the urinary bladder using a contrast medium.
cystoscopy Endoscopic examination of the interior of the bladder.
cytokine A low-molecular-weight protein secreted by various cell types and involved in cell-to-cell communication. It coordinates antibody and T cell immune interactions and augments immune reactivity.
cytology The study of cells and their origin, structure, function, and pathology.
cytotoxic Destructive to cells.

D

dactylitis An inflammation of a finger or toe.
database A collection of facts and figures for analysis from which conclusions may be drawn.
data collection The systematic collection of physical and psychosocial data for a patient who is having a problem. Part of assessment within the nursing process.
dawn phenomenon A condition sometimes encountered in type 1 diabetes characterized by increased blood glucose in the morning caused by release of hormones during the night.
deaf Partially or completely lacking the sense of hearing.
death(s) The cessation of all physical and chemical processes that invariably occurs in all living organisms. *See also* Dying.
debride Peel away dead tissue.
debridement The removal of all foreign material and dead tissues from or adjacent to a traumatic or infected lesion until healthy tissue is exposed.
debriefing Questioning of personnel involved and obtaining knowledge about event and problems that occurred (during a disaster).
decerebrate posturing *See* Extensor posturing.
decontamination The freeing of a person or an object of some contaminating substance such as radioactive material.
decorticate posturing *See* Flexor posturing.
decubitus ulcer(s) A breakdown in the skin and underlying tissues caused by long-standing pressure, ischemia, and damage to the underlying tissue.
deductible The yearly amount an insured person must spend out-of-pocket before a medical insurance plan begins to pay its share.
defecate To evacuate the bowels; to have a bowel movement.
defibrillation Stopping fibrillation of the heart with electrical current.
dehiscence The separation of all layers of a surgical wound.
dehydration Excessive loss of water from tissues of the body.
delegate To authorize and send another as one's representative (to carry out a task).
delegation Allocation of patient care activities to team members.
delirium An altered state of consciousness that is usually acute and of short duration.
delusion A false, fixed belief that cannot be changed with rational explanation.

dementia A broad impairment of intellectual function that usually is progressive.
demyelination (demyelinization) Destruction of the myelin sheath of nerve tissue.
dendrite Any of the threadlike extensions of the cytoplasm of a neuron.
denial A defense mechanism in which the existence of intolerable conditions is unconsciously rejected; the first stage in the acceptance of death.
denuded When the protective layer or covering is removed through surgery, trauma, or pathologic change.
deoxyribonucleic acid (DNA) The primary genetic material of all cellular organisms.
dependency The state of reliance on a substance; implies that there are physical and psychological symptoms of addiction. Term used to describe substance use disorder.
dependent (nursing action) Requiring an order from a health care provider.
dependent rubor A dusky-red color that dangling feet may take on after elevating the feet and legs above the heart for 1 to 2 minutes and that indicates arterial insufficiency.
depression A morbid sadness, dejection, or melancholy; a stage in the acceptance of death.
depression (of immune function) The decreased ability of the immune system to function normally.
dermabrasion Planing of the skin done by mechanical means to smooth the skin and remove scars.
dermatitis An inflammation of the skin.
dermatology The medical specialty concerned with diagnosing and treating skin disorders.
dermatome A nerve tract.
dermatophytosis Any superficial fungal infection caused by a dermatophyte and involving the stratum corneum of the skin, hair, and nails.
detoxification The process of ridding the body of a drug without causing harmful ill effects.
developmental task(s) A task that should be completed during a specific life period to ensure continuing psychosocial growth and maturity.
deviation Departure from normal.
diabetes insipidus (DI) Occurs as a result of decreased production of antidiuretic hormone (ADH) and is characterized by the production of copious amounts of dilute urine.
diabetic nephropathy Kidney disease secondary to chronic high blood glucose levels.
diabetic neuropathy A disorder of the peripheral nerves that is associated with diabetes mellitus and is characterized by sexual impotence in the male, neurogenic bladder, and pain or loss of feeling in the lower extremities.
diabetogenic Causing diabetes.
diagnosis, nursing A concise statement of a patient's actual or potential health problems that nurses, because of their education and experience, are able and licensed to treat.
diagnosis-related groups (DRGs) The classifications used to determine Medicare payments for patient care based on medical diagnoses.
dialysis The diffusion of solute molecules through a semipermeable membrane, with the molecules passing from the more concentrated solution to the less concentrated one.
dialysis, peritoneal The use of the peritoneum as a dialyzing membrane to remove waste products that have accumulated in the body as a result of renal failure.
diaphoresis Excessive perspiration.
diastole The phase of the cardiac cycle in which the heart muscle relaxes between contractions; during this phase the two ventricles are dilated by blood flowing through them and the coronary arteries are perfused.
diastolic blood pressure Arterial pressure during diastole, recorded as the bottom number in the pressure measurement.
diffusion The spontaneous mixing of the molecules or ions of two or more substances; the result of random thermal motion.
digital Pertaining to or resembling a finger or toe.
digitalization The initial administration of digitalis to build up a therapeutic blood level of the drug.
diplopia Double vision; seeing two images.
disability Difficulty in performing certain tasks because of impairment.
disaster A natural or human-caused (bioterrorism or nuclear) event that overwhelms the community's existing emergency resources.
disease An abnormal condition affecting the function or integrity of parts of the body not due to trauma.
disinfectant(s) An agent that destroys infection-producing organisms.
dislocation Stretching or tearing of ligaments around a joint with complete displacement of a bone.
disseminated Widespread.
disseminated intravascular coagulation (DIC) A disorder in which tissue damage causes widespread, excessive blood clotting in the microcirculation; subsequently, the body's blood clotting factors are depleted, and hemorrhage occurs.
distal In a position farthest from the point of reference.
distraction Diversion of attention from present experience (e.g., pain).
diuresis The excretion of excess fluid in the urine.
diuretic(s) An agent that promotes excretion of urine.
diurnal Happening during daylight hours.
diverticulitis The inflammation of the diverticula.
diverticulosis The presence of diverticula, in the absence of diverticulitis.
diverticulum (diverticula) A small blind pouch resulting from a protrusion of the mucosa of a hollow organ through weakened areas in the organ's muscle wall.
documentation The recording of significant information in a patient's medical record or chart.
dowager's hump An abnormal backward curve of the cervical spine as a result of osteoporosis and/or Cushing syndrome.
Down syndrome A congenital disorder characterized by physical malformations and some degree of mental retardation; also called *trisomy 21 syndrome* because it involves an extra copy of chromosome 21.
DRGs *See* Diagnosis-related groups.
drug-eluting stent A metal stent placed in the artery to help maintain patency of the vessel that emits a substance to prohibit cell growth over the stent.
drusen Yellow exudates found beneath the retinal pigment epithelium, representing extracellular debris.
dual diagnosis The diagnosis of a patient with a substance abuse problem and a mental health disorder.
dumping syndrome A group of symptoms caused by too-rapid passage of food through the upper gastrointestinal tract.
dying A stage of life; a process that, from a medical point of view, begins when a person has a disease that is untreatable and inevitably ends in death; the final stages of a fatal disease. *See also* Death(s).
dynamic Having vital force or inherent power.
dysarthria Slurring or indistinct speech articulation; difficulty speaking.
dyscrasia An imbalance of formed elements, as in blood dyscrasia.
dysfunctional uterine bleeding Uterine bleeding at times other than during normal menstruation.
dysmenorrhea Painful or difficult menstruation.
dyspareunia Difficult or painful coitus in women.
dyspepsia Impairment of the power or function of digestion; usually referring to epigastric discomfort after meals.
dysphagia Difficulty swallowing.
dysphasia Difficulty speaking; usually caused by a brain lesion.

dyspnea Labored or difficult breathing.
dysrhythmia A variation from the normal heart rhythm.
dysthymia A disturbance in mood that manifests in long-term mild depression.
dystonic reactions Acute contractures of the tongue, face, neck, and back.
dysuria Painful urination.

E

eccentric Departing from conventional custom or practice; differing conspicuously in behavior, appearance, or opinions.
ecchymosis (ecchymoses) An irregularly shaped, blue-black skin discoloration caused by bleeding beneath the skin.
ECG (also EKG) *See* Electrocardiogram.
ectopic Located away from normal position, as in ectopic pregnancy.
ectropion An outward turning of the eyelid.
edema An accumulation of fluid surrounding tissues or in body cavities.
edematous Pertaining to, or affected with, edema (abnormal fluid in the tissue).
EEG *See* Electroencephalogram.
efferent Carries impulses away from the CNS.
effleurage A massage technique with long, light, or firm strokes over the spine and back. May be circular strokes done with the fingertips.
effluent A discharge or outflow (e.g., the contents flowing out of an ileostomy or colostomy).
effusion An escape of fluid into a part or tissue, as an exudation or transudation.
ejaculation Ejection of the seminal fluid from the male urethra.
ejection fraction The percentage of blood that is ejected from the left ventricle during systole.
elastance The extent to which the lungs can return to their original position after being distended.
electrocardiogram The record produced by amplification of the electrical impulses normally generated by the heart.
electroconvulsive therapy (ECT) The oldest form of brain stimulation therapy used for severe depression. Considered after several unsuccessful regimens of medication. Consists of electric shock to the brain via electrodes applied to the scalp while the patient is under general anesthesia.
electroencephalogram A recording of changes in electric potentials in various areas of the brain.
electrolyte(s) A chemical substance that, when dissolved in water, dissociates into ions and thus can conduct an electric current.
electromyography The recording and study of intrinsic electrical properties of skeletal muscle; useful in diagnosing neuromuscular disorders.
elimination Discharge from the body of indigestible materials and waste products of metabolism.
embolism A sudden obstruction of arterial blood flow by a blood clot or a mass that has been brought to the site in the bloodstream.
embolus A clot or plug of material (usually from a thrombus) carried by blood flow that lodges in a vessel and obstructs blood flow.
emesis Substance produced by vomiting.
empathy The ability to recognize and share the emotions and states of mind of another; understanding another's behavior.
emphysema A chronic pulmonary disease characterized by increase beyond normal in the size of air spaces distal to the terminal bronchiole with destructive changes in their walls.
empyema The presence of infected and purulent exudate within the pleural cavity.
enabling Doing something for a substance-dependent person that keeps the person from facing consequences. Term used with substance abuse.
encapsulated Surrounded by a fibrous capsule.
encephalopathy Any dysfunction of the brain caused by a disease or condition.
endarterectomy The surgical removal of thickened atheromatous areas of the innermost layer of an artery.
endemic Present in a community at all times.
endocarditis An inflammation of the membrane lining the cavities of the heart, including the valves and connective structures.
endocrine Secreting internally directly into the bloodstream; refers to glandular function.
endogenous Coming from within.
endometriosis The presence of endometrial tissue in locations outside the uterus.
endorphin(s) Any of a group of opiate-like peptides naturally produced by the body.
endoscopy Examination with an endoscope that allows for direct visual inspection of the interior of hollow organs and body cavities.
endotoxin(s) A heat-stable toxin that is present in the intact bacterial cell wall, is pyrogenic, and can increase capillary permeability.
endotracheal intubation Airway management with a tube inserted through the mouth or nose into the trachea.
end-stage renal disease The final stage of chronic and irreversible renal failure requiring dialysis.
engraftment Successful establishment of the graft in bone marrow transplantation.
enteral feeding Feeding a patient by means of a tube passed into the stomach either from the nasal passage or through the abdominal wall.
enterocele A hernia containing intestines.
enterostomal Related to an abdominal stoma, or artificial opening of the intestine onto the surface of the body.
entropion Inversion of the eyelid margin.
enucleation Removal of an organ or other mass intact from a surrounding cover (e.g., the eyeball from the orbit).
environment All the physical and psychological factors that influence or affect the life or survival of an individual.
enzyme Any protein that acts as a catalyst, increasing the rate at which chemical reaction occurs.
epidemic(s) A disease that simultaneously attacks many people in a geographic area, is widely diffused, and spreads rapidly.
epidermophytosis A fungal infection that most often affects the feet, especially between the toes; also called *athlete's foot* or *dermophytosis.*
epididymis A small, oblong body resting on and beside the posterior surface of the testes that constitutes the first part of the excretory duct of each testis.
epidural Situated on or outside the dura mater.
epidural hematoma A hematoma that forms above the dura caused by rapid leakage of blood, usually from the middle meningeal artery, which quickly elevates intracranial pressure.
epigastric Pertaining to the region over the pit of the stomach.
epilepsy A group of neurologic disorders characterized by recurrent episodes of convulsive seizures, sensory disturbances, abnormal behaviors, loss of consciousness, or all of these.
epistaxis Nosebleed.
equilibrium Balance.
erectile dysfunction The inability to consistently achieve or maintain an erection that is firm enough for sexual intercourse; also called *impotence.*
erection The state of swelling, hardness, and stiffness observed in the penis of the male and to a lesser extent in the clitoris of the female.
erythema Redness of the skin.
erythrasma A chronic bacterial infection of the major skinfolds, marked by red or brownish patches on the skin.
erythrocyte sedimentation rate The rate at which red blood cells settle out of unclotted blood in 1 hour.

erythropoiesis Formation of red blood cells, or erythrocytes.
eschar A castoff of dead tissue, as from a burn, corrosive application, or gangrene.
escharotomy Surgical incision of a constricting eschar in a burn victim to permit the cut edges to separate and restore blood flow to unburned tissue.
esophageal varices Varicosities of branches of the azygous vein that connects with the portal vein in the lower esophagus; related to portal hypertension and cirrhosis of the liver.
estrogens The female sex hormones, including estradiol, estriol, and estrone.
etiology Study of the cause of disease; origin.
eustachian tube Connects the middle ear with the throat.
euthanasia An easy or painless death; active euthanasia, or mercy killing, is the deliberate ending of the life of a person who is incurably and terminally ill; passive euthanasia is the withholding of "heroic" measures and allowing the person to die.
euthymia A normal mood or feeling state.
evaluation, of outcome Appraisal of the patient's progress toward achievement of the goals and objectives stated in the nursing care plan.
evaluation, of process Appraisal of nursing activities and what has been done to assess, plan, and implement nursing care.
evaluation, of structure Appraisal of the physical facilities, equipment, staffing, and other characteristics of an agency that affect the quality of nursing care.
evisceration (1) extrusion of internal organs; (2) removal of the contents of the eyeball, leaving the sclera intact.
excess An amount beyond what is usual or necessary.
excoriation Abraded, chafed, or scraped skin; damage to the surface of the skin.
excursion Range of movement (of the lungs).
exercises, isometric Active exercises performed against stable resistance, without change in the length of the muscle.
exfoliate To separate or peel off in scales, layers, or flakes.
exocrine Secreting externally via a duct to a body cavity or structure.
exogenous Coming from outside.
exophthalmos Abnormal protrusion of the eyeball.
exotoxin A potent toxin formed and excreted by the bacterial cell.
Expanded Precautions Use of Standard Precaution techniques with additional protective actions specific to the organism and location involved.
expected outcomes Results expected to be achieved by the patient from health care provider actions.
expectorate To spit out saliva or materials coughed up from the air passageways leading to the lungs.
extension A movement that brings a limb into or toward a straight position by increasing the angle between the bones forming a joint; opposite of flexion.
extensor posturing Where the arms are stiffly extended and held close to the body, the wrists are flexed outward, and the legs are stiff with toes pointed downward (plantar flexion). Indicates damage to the midbrain or brainstem.
extracellular Outside of the cell.
extracellular fluids Body fluids outside the cell walls.
extracorporeal Outside the body.
exudate Fluid that contains dead cells, serum, phagocytes, bacteria, or pus.

F

fasciotomy Linear incisions in the fascia down the extremity.
fecal impaction The accumulation of putty-like or hardened feces in the rectum or sigmoid colon.
feedback The process of providing a system with information about its output.
feedback, negative A corrective action in which a system is informed that its output is not satisfactory and a change is needed.
feedback, positive Information that tells a system its output is satisfactory.
fee-for-service Fee paid for services provided; a type of medical practice.
fetor hepaticus Foul-smelling breath associated with severe liver disease.
fibroid A thickened vascular mass in the uterus.
fibroma A fibrous, encapsulated connective tissue tumor.
fibrosis Fibrous tissue formation.
filtration Passage of a gas or liquid through a filter to separate out unwanted matter.
first-generation antipsychotics Very effective medications in stopping auditory hallucinations, enabling the patient to connect thoughts in a logical manner, and eliminating the delusional system.
fistula(s) Any abnormal, tubelike passage within the body between two internal organs or leading from an internal organ to the body surface.
flaccid Limp, weak, or relaxed.
flail chest Occurs when three or more ribs are broken in two or more places.
flatus Gas in the digestive tract.
flexion A movement that brings a limb into or toward a bent position by decreasing the angle between the bones forming a joint; opposite of extension.
flexor posturing The extension and stiffening of the legs with plantar flexion, adduction of the arms with the forearms bent upward, and wrists and fingers flexed on the chest. Indicates damage to the cortex.
flight of ideas Going from topic to topic in conversation with little or no connection.
flora Plant life, as distinguished from animal life.
fluid(s) The water and substances dissolved in it that form the internal environment.
fluid balance Equilibrium between the amount of fluid taken into the body and that lost through urine, feces, the lungs, skin, and possibly vomiting and fistulas.
fluid deficit(s) A fluid imbalance in which there is not enough fluid in one or more of the body's fluid compartments as a result of either inadequate intake or excessive loss.
fluid excess A fluid imbalance in which too much fluid accumulates in one or more of the body's fluid compartments as a result of either excessive intake or inadequate loss. *See also* Edema.
fluids, transcellular Body fluids that pass through cellular structures and eventually are eliminated from the body.
focused assessment Performed at the beginning of the shift and directed to areas in which the patient is experiencing health problems.
follicular pharyngitis An inflammation of the pharynx accompanied by purulent infection.
fracture(s) Interruption in the continuity of a bone.
friction rub A high-pitched, scratchy sound heard with the diaphragm of the stethoscope placed at the lower left sternal border of the chest; a symptom of pericarditis.
fructosamine assay A test that may be used to monitor control of glucose over a period of 2 to 3 weeks.
fulguration Destruction by electric cautery.
functional disorder A disorder that affects the function but not the structure of the body or body part.
fungus (fungi) A member of a group of organisms (mushrooms, yeasts, molds, etc.) that thrive in a warm, moist climate. Can cause infections that are difficult to eradicate because fungi tend to reproduce by means of spores that are resistant to ordinary disinfectants and antiseptics.
furuncles Inflammations of hair follicles. Also called *boils.*

G

galactosemia A genetic disorder in which there is a lack of the enzyme necessary for proper metabolism of galactose.
gangrene A necrosis, or death, of tissue, usually caused by deficient or absent blood supply.
gastritis An inflammation of the mucous membrane lining the stomach.
gastrojejunostomy The surgical creation of an anastomosis between the stomach and jejunum.
gastroparesis Delayed gastric emptying.
gastrostomy The surgical creation of an opening into the stomach to administer food and liquids.
gate control theory The proposal that synapses in the dorsal horn of the spinal cord act as gates and that pain signals compete with signals of other kinds of stimuli for passage through the gate and transmission to the brain.
gene One of the self-reproducing biological units of heredity that make up segments of the DNA molecule that controls cellular reproduction and function.
generalized anxiety disorder A persistent, unrealistic, or excessive worry about two or more life circumstances.
genital Pertaining to the external reproductive organs.
geriatrics The medical treatment of diseases commonly associated with aging and elderly persons.
gerontology The study of the problems of aging in all its aspects.
gigantism Excessive size. Seen in children with excessive secretion of growth hormone.
gingivitis An inflammation of the gingivae.
glaucoma A group of diseases of the eye characterized by increased intraocular pressure that can produce blindness if not managed successfully.
global amnesia Irretrievable total loss of memory.
globulin(s) A general term for proteins; separated into five fractions by serum protein electrophoresis and classified in order of decreasing electrophoretic mobility. The fractions are $alpha_1$, $alpha_2$, $beta_1$, $beta_2$, and gamma globulins.
glomerular filtration rate (GFR) The amount of blood filtered by the glomeruli in a given time (average GFR is about 125 mL/min).
glomerulonephritis An immunologic problem caused by an antigen-antibody reaction in the kidney.
glucagon(s) A polypeptide hormone secreted by the alpha cells of the islets of Langerhans.
glucocorticoid Any hormone released from the adrenal cortex that increases glucogenesis and thus raises the level of liver glycogen and blood glucose.
glucogenesis The formation of glucose from glycogen.
glucometer Blood glucose–monitoring machine.
glucose intolerance The inability to properly metabolize glucose.
glucose tolerance test A test to detect abnormal glucose metabolism; assists in diagnosis of diabetes mellitus.
glycemic Referring to the amount of glucose present in a substance.
glycemic control Control of glucose in the blood.
glycosuria Glucose in the urine.
glycosylated hemoglobin (HbA_{1c}; A1C) Hemoglobin with glucose attached to it; periodic measurements of hemoglobin A_{1c} can help determine a diabetic patient's average blood glucose level over a period of 3 to 4 months.
goal(s) A broad statement describing what is to be accomplished over a specified period.
goiter An enlargement of the thyroid gland.
gonads Gamete-producing glands; the ovaries and testicles.
goniometry The measurement of range of motion in a joint.
graft An implant or transplant of tissue or an organ.
gram negative Having the pink color of the counterstain used in the Gram method of staining microorganisms.
gram positive Retaining the violet color of the stain used in the Gram method of staining microorganisms.
granulocyte A leukocyte containing abundant granules in its cytoplasm; granulocytes include neutrophils, eosinophils, and basophils.
Graves disease An immune disorder that causes overproduction of thyroid hormones. Also called *toxic goiter*.
gynecomastia The development of abnormally large mammary glands in the male.

H

hallucination A sensory perception (touching, tasting, feeling, hearing, seeing) that occurs without external stimulation.
hand hygiene The primary intervention any health care provider can use to control the spread of infection; performed with soap and water, if the hands are visibly soiled, or with an alcohol-based hand-sanitizing solution.
handicap A social disadvantage that exists because of a disability.
"Hands-Only CPR" Intended only for lay rescuers and only chest compressions are delivered; rescue breathing or mouth-to-mouth resuscitation is not included.
Haversian system A canal system that runs through the bones and contains the blood and lymph vessels.
health The ability to function well physically and mentally and to express the full range of one's potential.
health care–associated infection Formerly known as a *nosocomial infection.* Can occur when a patient is cared for in any kind of health care setting and develops an infection not previously present.
health care–associated pneumonia (HCAP) Pneumonia that results from conditions related to being in a health care facility or receiving health care.
health maintenance organization (HMO) A type of group health care practice that provides basic and supplemental health maintenance and treatment services to enrollees who prepay a fixed periodic fee that is set without regard to the amount or kind of services received.
Healthy People 2030 A federal government mandate with goals for improving the health of the American people, with particular attention to health concerns of people in underserved groups.
hearing loss Impaired perception of sound.
heat exhaustion A disorder resulting from overexposure to heat or to the sun; also called *heat prostration.* It is caused by excessive perspiration and loss of body water and salt.
heatstroke A life-threatening condition resulting from prolonged exposure to environmental heat; also called *sunstroke.*
Helicobacter pylori A species of gram-negative, microaerophilic bacteria of the family Spirillaceae that causes gastritis and pyloric ulcers in humans.
helping relationship A relationship in which at least one of the parties intends to promote growth, development, maturity, improved functioning, and improved coping in the life of the other.
hemarthrosis A collection of blood in the joint space.
hematemesis Vomiting of blood.
hematocrit The volume percentage of red blood cells in whole blood.
hematoma(s) A localized collection of blood, usually clotted, that has leaked from adjacent blood vessels into an organ, space, or tissue.
hematuria Blood in the urine.
hemianopsia Blindness for half of the field of vision in one or both eyes.
hemicolectomy Removal of part of the colon.
hemiparesis Weakness affecting only one side of the body.
hemiparesthesia Abnormal sensation on one side of the body.
hemiplegia Paralysis of one half, or one side, of the body.
hemodialysis The removal of nitrogenous wastes from the blood by circulating arterial blood through a dialysate and returning it to the venous circulation.

hemodynamics The study of the movements of blood and the pressures being exerted in the blood vessels and the chambers of the heart.
hemoglobin The protein found in red blood cells that transports molecular oxygen in the blood; oxygenated hemoglobin (oxyhemoglobin) is bright red; unoxygenated hemoglobin is darker.
hemoglobinuria The presence of free hemoglobin in the urine.
hemolysis The rupture of red blood cells with release of hemoglobin into the plasma.
hemolytic Pertaining to the breakdown of red blood cells.
hemophilia An inherited disorder in which there is deficiency of one or more specific clotting factors in the blood.
hemoptysis Coughing and spitting of blood that can originate in the lungs, larynx, or trachea.
hemorrhoid A varicosity of a vein of the rectum. It may be internal (inside the sphincter muscles of the anus) or external (outside the sphincter muscles).
hemorrhoidectomy The surgical removal of hemorrhoids.
hemothorax A collection of blood in the pleural cavity.
hepatic encephalopathy Degenerative changes in the brain associated with liver failure.
hepatitis An inflammation of the liver.
hernia The protrusion or projection of an organ or a part of an organ through the wall of the cavity that normally contains it.
hernioplasty The repair of a hernia.
herniorrhaphy The surgical repair of a hernia.
herpesvirus Any of a large group of DNA viruses found in many animal species. Type 1 herpes simplex virus (HSV) produces lesions that are primarily nongenital. Type 2 HSV lesions most often are genital.
heterosexual A person who is sexually attracted to people of the opposite sex.
hiatal hernia Protrusion of a portion of the stomach through the opening in the diaphragm through which the esophagus passes.
hierarchy The arrangement of objects, elements, or values in a graduated series.
hirsutism The excessive growth of hair on the body.
histamine A compound released in response to allergy or injury; causes dilation of small blood vessels, a pooling of blood, and release of fluid into tissues.
HIV The causative agent for AIDS; *see* Human immunodeficiency virus.
HLA Human leukocyte antigen.
HMO *See* Health maintenance organization.
holism The belief that each person is a unified whole.
holistic care Attention to the mental, social, spiritual, and physical aspects of health and illness.
Homans sign Pain on passive dorsiflexion of the foot; a sign of thrombosis of deep calf veins.
homeopathy A practice based on the theory that a substance that produces symptoms of a disease when given in large doses to a healthy individual will cure the same symptoms when administered in small amounts.
homeostasis A tendency of biological systems to maintain stability in the internal environment while continually adjusting to changes necessary for survival.
homonymous hemianopia Blindness or defective vision in the right or left halves of the visual fields of both eyes.
homosexual A person who is sexually attracted to people of the same sex.
homozygous Having inherited a genetic trait from both parents.
hordeolum An external stye.
hormone A chemical produced by the cells of the body and transported by the bloodstream to target cells and organs on which it has a regulatory effect.
hospice A program that provides a continuum of home and inpatient care for terminally ill individuals and their families.
hospital-acquired pneumonia (HAP) Pneumonia symptoms that occur more than 48 hours after admission.
host An organism in which another, parasitic organism is nourished and harbored.
human immunodeficiency virus (HIV) A retrovirus that integrates itself into the genetic material of the cell it infects, changing the DNA of the host cell and damaging the immune system.
human needs Basic needs for survival and personal growth shared by all humans.
human needs theory The proposal that basic human needs act as stimuli to human behavior; Maslow postulated five levels of human needs: physiologic, safety and security, love and belonging, esteem, and self-actualization.
humoral Pertaining to body fluids or substances contained in them.
humoral immunity Antibody-mediated immunity, the result of B-cell action and the production of antibodies.
hydrocephalus Increased cerebrospinal fluid in the ventricles of the brain.
hydronephrosis Distention of the renal pelvis and calices with urine that cannot flow through obstructed ureters.
hydrostatic pressure The pressure or force caused by the presence of a fluid.
hyperalgesia Heightened response to painful stimuli.
hyperalimentation Total parenteral nutrition.
hypercalcemia An excessive amount of calcium in the blood (i.e., more than 5.5 mEq/L or 11 mg/dL).
hypercapnia An excessive amount of carbon dioxide in the blood.
hyperchloremia An excessive amount of chloride in the blood.
hyperesthesia Abnormal sensitivity to stimuli.
hyperglycemia An above-normal level of blood sugar, as in diabetes.
hyperkalemia An excessive amount of potassium in the blood.
hyperlipidemia An excessive amount of lipids in the blood.
hypermagnesemia An excessive amount of magnesium in blood plasma.
hypernatremia An excessive amount of sodium in the blood.
hyperopia A visual defect in which parallel light rays reaching the eye focus behind the retina; farsightedness.
hyperphosphatemia An excessive amount of phosphates in the blood.
hyperplasia An increase in the number of cells of an organ; extra cell growth.
hyperpyrexia An extremely elevated temperature.
hypersecretion Oversecretion.
hypersensitivity reactions An exaggerated immune response to an agent perceived by the body to be foreign. *See also* Allergy (allergies).
hypersomnia Sleeping for long periods.
hypertension Persistently high blood pressure; in adults, a systolic pressure equal to or greater than 130 mm Hg and a diastolic pressure equal to or greater than 80 mm Hg.
hyperthermia Unusually high fever.
hypertonic Of greater concentration.
hypertonic solution A solution in which the osmotic pressure (concentration) is greater than that of body fluids.
hypertrophy An increase in size of a structure or organ.
hyperuricemia An excessive amount of uric acid in the urine.
hyperventilation An abnormal breathing pattern in which an above-normal amount of air is moved in and out of the lungs.
hypervolemia An abnormal increase in the volume of circulating blood.
hypesthesia A dysesthesia consisting of abnormally decreased sensitivity, particularly to touch. Also called *hypoesthesia.*
hypnosis A subconscious condition, usually artificially induced, in which there is a response to suggestions and commands made by the hypnotist.

hypoalbuminemia An abnormally low level of albumin in the blood.
hypocalcemia An abnormally low level of calcium in the blood (i.e., less than 4.5 mEq/L or 8.5 mg/dL).
hypocapnia An abnormally low level of carbon dioxide in the blood, resulting from hyperventilation.
hypochloremia An abnormally low level of chloride in the blood.
hypochromic Pertaining to a condition of the blood in which the red blood cells have a reduced hemoglobin content.
hypodermoclysis Injection of fluid into subcutaneous tissue via continuous infusion.
hypoesthesia *See* Hypesthesia.
hypogammaglobulinemia An immune deficiency characterized by abnormally low levels of generally all classes of serum gamma globulins with increased susceptibility to infectious diseases.
hypoglycemia An abnormally low level of blood sugar.
hypoglycemic agents Agents that lower the blood sugar level (i.e., oral medications that are used to treat some forms of diabetes mellitus).
hypokalemia An abnormally low level of potassium in the blood.
hypomagnesemia An abnormally low level of magnesium in the blood plasma.
hypomania Inflated or irritable mood for at least 4 days. Less severe than mania.
hyponatremia An abnormally low level of sodium in the blood.
hypophosphatemia An abnormally low level of phosphates in the blood.
hypophysectomy Excision of the hypophysis cerebri.
hyposecretion Undersecretion.
hyposensitization A treatment used in managing hypersensitivity to a known allergen; the program involves regular injections of minute quantities of selected antigens over an extended period.
hypothalamus That portion of the diencephalon that lies beneath the thalamus at the base of the cerebrum; it activates, controls, and integrates many of the body's vital functions (e.g., regulation of metabolism, volume of body fluids, electrolyte content, and release of hormones).
hypothermia A serious loss of body heat caused by prolonged exposure to cold.
hypothyroidism Deficient activity of the thyroid gland.
hypotonic Of lesser concentration.
hypotonic solution One in which the osmotic pressure (concentration) is less than that of body fluids.
hypotonic state Pertaining to abnormally decreased muscular tone or tension.
hypoventilation An abnormal breathing pattern in which insufficient amounts of air are inhaled into the lungs.
hypovolemia Diminished blood volume.
hypoxemia Insufficient oxygenation of the blood.
hypoxia Deficiency of oxygen.
hysterectomy Surgical removal of the uterus.

I

iatrogenic Caused by medical treatment or diagnostic procedure.
iatrogenic disorder An adverse condition induced by effects of treatment by a health care provider or surgeon.
icterus Bile pigmentation of the tissues, membranes, and secretions.
idiopathic Of unknown cause.
idiosyncrasy A special characteristic by which a person differs from others.
ileal conduit A surgically created passageway that uses a portion of the ileum to direct the flow of urine from the ureters to the outside of the body.
ileostomy (ileostomies) An artificial opening in the ileum, created surgically, to drain fecal material from the small intestine.
ileus Intestinal obstruction, especially failure of peristalsis.
illusion A misperception of an actual sensory perception; misinterpretation of reality.
imagery Imagination; the calling up of mental pictures or events.
immune deficiency A lack of immune bodies and resultant impairment of the immune response to foreign agents.
immunity Resistance to a specific disease.
immunity, active Immunity acquired by producing one's own antibody.
immunity, passive Immunity acquired from a source other than one's own body, such as by transfer of antibody or lymphocytes from an immune donor.
immunization The process of rendering an individual immune by passive immunity or of becoming immune by active immunity.
immunocompetence The capacity to develop an immune response after exposure to an antigen.
immunoglobulin(s) A protein of animal origin with known antibody activity and a major component of humoral immunity. *See also* Antibody (antibodies).
immunoscintigraphy A radioactive scan of the immune structures.
immunosuppression The inhibition of the immune system to respond to infection or perceived threat; it may be a result of disease or deliberately induced such as in transplantation to prevent rejection of the donor organ.
immunotherapy Activation of the immune system to fight disease, the administration of immunopotentiators and immunocompetent lymphoid tissue for cancer treatment.
impairment Dysfunction of a specific organ or body system.
impetigo An infection of the skin, usually by streptococci or staphylococci.
implementation A deliberate action performed to achieve a goal; carrying out of nursing interventions.
impotence Inability of the male to achieve or maintain an erection.
impulsive Acting in response to an impulse because the action brings emotional release or pleasure even though the action may be harmful to oneself or socially unacceptable.
inanimate Not alive; dull, lifeless.
incidence The rate at which certain events occur.
incontinence An alteration in the control of bowel or urinary elimination, or both.
incretin mimetics Agents that mimic the action of incretins, hormones released from the intestine.
incubation The interval between exposure to infection and the appearance of the first symptom.
index of suspicion Keen observation to detect problems that are not initially obvious but are suspected because of history or circumstances that underlie the patient's decision to seek care.
induration An abnormally hard spot or place.
infarct A localized area of necrosis produced by ischemia caused by obstructed arterial supply or inadequate venous drainage.
infarction Occurrence of a localized area of dead tissue produced by inadequate blood flow.
infection The invasion and multiplication of pathogenic microorganisms in body tissue.
inference A deduction or conclusion.
infertility The condition of inability to produce offspring.
inflammation An immediate cellular response to any kind of injury to the cells and tissues.
ingestants Any substances taken orally, such as food or drink.
ingestion The taking of any substance, such as food, drugs, water, or chemicals, by mouth or through the digestive system.
inhalants Medication or compounds suitable for inhaling.
initial The beginning of a thing or process; the first.
injectables Fluids capable of being injected.

innate Belonging to the essential nature of something; existing in or belonging at birth.
innate immunity A person's natural (inborn) immunity to certain diseases.
inotropic Pertaining to the force or energy of muscular contractions, particularly of the heart.
insensible Unconscious; without feeling or consciousness.
insomnia A sleep disorder; an inability to sleep.
inspection The process of visual examination.
insufficiency The condition of being inadequate for a given purpose.
insulin A naturally occurring hormone secreted by the beta cells of the islets of Langerhans in the pancreas in response to increased levels of glucose in the blood.
insulin-dependent diabetes mellitus Type 1 diabetes; a form of the disease that requires replacement of endogenous insulin with regular injections of exogenous insulin.
insulin resistance A situation in which insulin interaction with glucose becomes less efficient and fat metabolism is abnormal.
insulin-to-carbohydrate ratios Used to adjust insulin doses to match carbohydrate intake.
intention tremor A tremor that occurs on attempt at voluntary movement.
interdisciplinary (collaborative) care plan A care plan composed through the collaboration of all health care team members caring for a patient.
intermittent claudication Cramping pain in the muscles of the lower extremities brought on by exercise and relieved by rest. A common symptom of arterial insufficiency; pain usually occurs in the calves of the legs but also can affect the muscles of the thighs and buttocks.
interstitial Placed or lying between.
interstitial fluids Body fluids located in the tissue spaces around the cells. *See also* Edema.
intervention Nursing activities performed by the nurse to meet the specified goals of a nursing care plan.
intracellular Within cells.
intracellular fluids Body fluids that are within cell walls.
intracerebral hematoma Bleeding that occurs into the brain tissue and not within the meningeal layers. Because of its location within brain tissue, surgical removal is usually not possible.
intractable pain Hard-to-manage pain; pain not relieved by ordinary methods.
intraocular Within the eye.
intrathecal Injected into the subarachnoid space of the spinal cord via lumbar puncture.
intrathoracic Within the thoracic cavity.
intravascular fluids Body fluids within the blood vessels composed of plasma and the substances it transports.
intravenous therapy The administration of fluids through a vein.
intussusception Telescoping of one part of the bowel into another.
ions Atoms or groups of atoms that have an electrical charge through the gain or loss of an electron.
ipsilateral On or affecting the same side of the body.
iridectomy Excision of part of the iris.
ischemia A deficiency of an oxygenated blood supply to a part as a result of functional constriction of a blood vessel or of actual obstruction, as by a clot.
islets of Langerhans Pancreatic cells. Beta cells, which secrete insulin, are found in these cells.
isolation technique Special precautionary procedures used to set apart a patient with a communicable disease; the purpose is to prevent the spread of infectious agents from the patient to others.
isometric Having equal dimensions; maintaining the same length.
isometric exercises Exercises that involve generating tension between two opposing sets of muscles.
isotonic Of equal solute concentration.
isotonic contraction A contraction that occurs when tension is developed in a muscle.
isotonic solution A solution in which the osmotic pressure is the same as that of intracellular fluid (e.g., normal saline [0.9% concentration]).
isotope One of a series of chemical elements that have nearly identical chemical properties but differ in their atomic weight and electrical charge. Many isotopes are radioactive.

J

jaundice A yellowing of the skin and mucous membranes that reflects excessively high blood levels of bilirubin (bile pigment).

K

keloid Excessive, abnormal scar formation in the skin after trauma or surgical incision.
keratitis An inflammation of the cornea.
keratosis (keratoses) Any horny growth, such as a wart or callosity; usually either actinic keratosis or seborrheic keratosis.
ketoacidosis The accumulation of ketone bodies in the blood because of incomplete metabolism of fats, resulting in metabolic acidosis.
ketonuria The presence of acetone bodies in the urine.
ketosis The accumulation in the body of the ketone bodies: acetone, beta-hydroxybutyric acid, and acetoacetic acid.
kinetic motion The motion of material bodies and the forces and energy associated with it.
Korsakoff syndrome Substance-induced persisting dementia.
Kupffer cells Large, highly phagocytic cells in the liver; they form part of the reticuloendothelial system.
kyphosis An abnormally increased curvature of the thoracic spine, which gives a "hunchback" appearance.

L

labile Unsteady, not fixed; easily disarranged.
lability Condition of instability; continually changing.
labyrinthitis An inflammation of the internal ear, including the vestibule, cochlea, and semicircular canal.
lanugo Downy hair covering the body.
laparoscopy The examination of the peritoneal cavity with a fiberoptic instrument inserted through a small abdominal incision.
laryngectomy The partial or total removal of the larynx by surgical excision; the person who has had a laryngectomy is called a *laryngectomee.*
laryngitis An inflammation of the larynx.
laryngoscope Instrument used to examine the larynx, usually for the purpose of placing an endotracheal tube.
laryngoscopy Direct or indirect visual examination of the larynx.
laser Stands for *l*ight *a*mplification by *s*timulated *e*mission of *r*adiation; converts light wavelengths into one small, intense, unified beam of single-wavelength radiation; used for diagnosis and surgery.
latent Not obvious; hidden.
latent TB infection (LTBI) An infection with *Mycobacterium tuberculosis* without current active disease.
lesions A circumscribed area of pathologically altered tissue.
leukapheresis A process by which blood is withdrawn from a vein, white blood cells are removed, and the remaining blood is reinfused in the patient.
leukemia A malignant disease of the blood-forming organs, marked by abnormal proliferation and development of leukocytes and their precursors in the blood and bone marrow.

leukocyte A colorless blood cell whose chief function is to protect the body against pathogenic microorganisms; white blood cell.
leukocytosis An increase in the number of white blood cells, or leukocytes, in the blood.
leukopenia A reduction in the number of leukocytes in the blood to $5000/mm^3$ or less.
leukoplakia Patches of thickened, white tissue on mucous membrane; considered a precursor to cancer.
leukotrienes A class of biologically active compounds that occur naturally in leukocytes and produce allergic and inflammatory reactions similar to those of histamine.
level of consciousness (LOC) A standardized system to describe the state of consciousness (i.e., alert wakefulness, drowsiness, stupor, or coma).
Lhermitte sign An electrical shock–like sensation felt along the spine when the neck is flexed.
libido The conscious or unconscious sexual drive.
lifestyle habits Entrenched practices related to work, recreation, diet, exercise, and other activities of daily living.
ligament Connective tissue that joins the bones of a joint together.
ligate To tie or bind.
lipodystrophy A disturbance of or defect in fat metabolism.
lipoma A fatty tumor.
lipoprotein Any of the macromolecular complexes that are transported in the blood.
lithiasis The formation of stones.
lithotripsy The crushing of a calculus in the kidney, bladder, urethra, or gallbladder.
long-term care An umbrella term that describes a range of services and may provide varying levels of care. A long-term care facility is a residential skilled nursing setting.
loose associations Disordered thinking with little connection between thoughts.
lordosis An abnormal forward curvature of the spine.
lozenge(s) A medicated tablet or disk.
lucid Clear, especially applied to clarity of the mind.
lymphadenitis An inflammation of the lymph nodes.
lymphadenopathy A disease of the lymph nodes, often producing enlargement.
lymphangiography Radiography of lymphatic vessels after injection of a contrast medium.
lymphangitis An inflammation of the lymph vessels.
lymphatic system An accessory system by which fluids can flow from tissue spaces into the blood.
lymphedema The swelling of tissues drained by the lymphatic system.
lymph nodes Small bundles of lymphatic tissue containing lymphocytes, the functions of which are filtration and phagocytosis.
lymphocyte A mononuclear, nongranulous leukocyte that is chiefly a product of lymphoid tissue and is important in the development of immunity.
lymphocyte, sensitized A nongranular lymphocyte that has been processed by either the thymus (T lymphocyte) or an unknown processing area (B lymphocyte) and is responsible for either cellular or humoral immunity.
lymphocyte-transforming factor A protein mediator that causes transformation and clonal expansion of nonsensitized lymphocytes that produce a toxin destructive to antigen.
lymphoma Any neoplastic disorder of lymphoid tissue.
lyse To produce decomposition; to destroy.
lysis The act of destruction; the gradual decline of a fever or disease; the opposite of crisis.

M

macrophage(s) A large, mononuclear phagocyte derived from monocytes; macrophages are components of the reticuloendothelial system.
macrophage-activating factor A mediator released by sensitized lymphocytes on contact with an antigen, the function of which is to induce in macrophages an increased content of lysosomal enzymes, more aggressive phagocytosis, and increased mitosis.
macrophage chemotaxis factor A protein mediator released by sensitized lymphocytes on contact with antigen, the function of which is to attract macrophages to the antigen site.
macule (macula) A discolored spot on the skin that is not raised above the surface. *Macula* is also used for an area on the retina of the eye.
major depressive disorder A mental disorder in which at least five symptoms characteristic of depression have been present for at least 2 weeks. Some of these symptoms include an overwhelming feeling of sadness, inability to feel pleasure or interest in daily activities, weight gain or loss not attributed to dieting, sleep disturbances, fatigue, difficulty concentrating, and suicidal thoughts.
malignancy *See* Carcinoma.
malignant Becoming progressively worse; resisting treatment and resulting in death; having the properties of anaplasia, invasiveness, and metastasis.
malignant hyperthermia A rare but life-threatening complication of general anesthetic agents, including halothane, isoflurane, enflurane, and succinylcholine.
mammography The x-ray examination of the soft tissues of the breast.
mammoplasty Plastic surgery of the breast.
managed care Organization of health care delivery that coordinates care delivery by various health team members in a timely, cost-effective manner.
mania An elevation in mood characterized by feelings of elation, excitement, or extreme irritability.
mass casualties Casualties in such numbers that the normal health care system has difficulty providing adequate care.
mastication Chewing.
mean, mathematical An average (e.g., mean corpuscular hemoglobin concentration, which is the concentration of hemoglobin in the average erythrocyte; mean arterial pressure [MAP], which indicates the average pressure during one cardiac cycle).
measurable The ability to be expressed numerically or to be described as to the extent or quantity (of a substance, energy, or time).
mechanism of injury Refers to how the injury occurred.
mediastinum The mass of tissues and organs separating the sternum in front and the vertebral column behind.
mediate To accomplish by indirect means; to act between two parties or sides.
Medicaid A federally funded, state-operated program that provides medical assistance to eligible people with low incomes.
medical nutrition therapy A registered dietitian (RD) or a certified diabetes educator (CDE) performs an in-depth assessment of type of diabetes, height-to-weight ratio, usual dietary intake, food preferences, exercise level, and daily schedule. A range of interventions are considered when designing a plan that is individualized for the patient.
Medicare A federally funded national health insurance program in the United States for people older than 65 years.
meditation The act of contemplative thinking.
melanoma A malignant, darkly pigmented mole or tumor of the skin.
melena Black, tarry stools.
menarche The onset of menstruation.
Ménière disease A group of symptoms produced by an increase in fluid in the labyrinthine spaces with swelling and congestion of the mucosa of the cochlea.
menopause The span of time during which the menstrual cycle wanes and gradually stops; *see* Climacteric.

menorrhagia Excessive menstruation.
menses The onset of the menstrual cycle.
menstruation The shedding of the uterine lining.
mentate To think.
MET Metabolic equivalent of task, a measure of heat production by the body; a term used with cardiac rehabilitation patients.
metabolic acidosis A condition in which the pH of body fluids is below 7.35 because of either an excessive production of carbonic acid through the oxidation of fats or a loss of bicarbonate.
metabolic alkalosis A condition in which the pH of body fluids is above 7.45 because of an excessive loss of acid, an above-normal intake or retention of base, or a low level of potassium in the blood.
metabolic syndrome A group of risk factors leading to heart disease, diabetes, and stroke. Hypertension, insulin resistance, high triglycerides with low HDL, and abdominal obesity constitute metabolic syndrome.
metabolism The sum of the physical and chemical processes by which living tissue is formed and maintained and by which large molecules are disassembled to provide energy.
metastasis The movement of disease from one organ or body part to a distant location (e.g., the migration of microorganisms and of malignant cells).
methamphetamine (meth) Highly addictive stimulant that affects the central nervous system. Users may develop toxic psychosis and experience paranoia, hallucinations, and delusions; use functionally and structurally alters the brain.
metrorrhagia Uterine bleeding occurring at irregular intervals and sometimes for prolonged periods.
microalbuminuria Presence of albumin in the urine, which is suggestive of early kidney disease.
microcytic Pertaining to a smaller-than-normal cell.
micron A unit of linear measure; equal to 0.001 mm.
micturition The voiding of urine.
milieu therapy Therapy in a structured environment of a hospital or group home setting to help patients participate as active members of the milieu community and practice social behaviors.
milliequivalent One-thousandth of a chemical equivalent, expressed as mEq; the concentration of electrolytes in a certain volume of solution is usually expressed as milliequivalents per liter (mEq/L).
mineralocorticoids A group of hormones produced by the adrenal cortex that affect sodium, chloride, and potassium levels in extracellular fluid.
miotic A drug that constricts the pupil.
mitosis A type of cell division of somatic cells in which each daughter cell contains the same number of chromosomes as the parent cell. It is the process by which the body grows and by which somatic cells are replaced.
mittelschmerz A sharp pain in the right or left lower quadrant, sometimes felt at midcycle around the time of ovulation.
modulation To regulate or adjust. The fourth of four phases associated with nociceptive pain in which the brain sends signals back down the spinal cord by release of neurotransmitters.
monocytes Mononuclear phagocytic leukocytes.
monoparesis Weakness in one limb.
monoplegia Paralysis of one limb.
morphologic Related to the science of structures and forms without regard to function.
mortality The state of death. Being mortal.
mucolytic Dissolving or destroying mucus.
mucorrhea The free discharge of mucus.
mucositis An inflammation of a mucous membrane.
multidrug-resistant organism (MDRO) A pathogen that has mutated as a result of inadequate dosages or delays in administration of antimicrobial medication and is now resistant to many medications.
multisystem organ dysfunction syndrome (MODS) A syndrome in which there is concurrent dysfunction of two or more organs.
muscle tone The readiness of a muscle to contract and relax normally.
mutation An unusual change in a gene occurring spontaneously or by induction. Mutation can occur in pathogenic organisms.
mycosis (mycoses) Any disease caused by a fungus.
mydriatic Dilating the pupil.
myocardial infarction (MI) Necrosis of the myocardium as a result of interruption of the blood supply to the area.
myocarditis An inflammation of the heart muscle.
myomectomy Surgical removal of a tumor from the uterine wall, accomplished by use of an endoscope.
myopia The error of refraction in which parallel light rays focus in front of the retina; nearsightedness.
myringotomy An incision into the eardrum.
myxedema A condition in an adult in which there are low thyroid levels.
myxedema coma Loss of brain function due to lack of thyroid hormone; can be precipitated by abrupt withdrawal of thyroid therapy, acute illness, or other stressors.

N

nebulizer An atomizer; a device for delivering drugs or water to the respiratory tract by forcing air or oxygen through a solution.
necrosis The changes that occur as a result of death of cells; caused by enzymatic degradation.
necrotic Pertaining to death of a portion of tissue.
negative feedback In the endocrine system, if the hormonal need of a target tissue is being satisfied, production or secretion of the hormone will be inhibited.
negative symptoms One of the two divisions of signs and symptoms of schizophrenia; include apathy, social isolation, psychomotor retardation, and lack of motivation.
neologism(s) In psychiatry, an invented word whose meaning may be known only to the person using it and may be related to their conflicts.
neoplasm A tumor; any new and abnormal growth.
nephrectomy Surgical removal of the kidney.
nephritic syndrome Kidney inflammation damages the basement membrane of the glomerulus, allowing large molecules such as red blood cells and protein, which normally would be retained in the bloodstream, to pass through to the urine. Can occur as a result of the same conditions that cause glomerulonephritis.
nephron The structural and functional unit of the kidney, which consists of the renal corpuscle, the proximal convoluted tubule, limbs of the loop of Henle, the distal convoluted tubule, and the collecting tubule; each nephron is able to form urine independently.
nephrosclerosis Atherosclerotic disease of the small renal arteries related to hypertension and eventual destruction of renal cells.
nephrostomy Formation of an artificial opening into the renal pelvis of the kidney from the skin.
nephrostomy tubes Tubes inserted to drain the renal pelvis.
nephrotic syndrome Damage to the glomerular basement membrane allows protein to be released in the urine; characterized by extensive proteinuria, hyperlipidemia (elevated blood lipids), hypoalbuminemia (low blood albumin), and severe edema.
nephrotoxic Substances that can be toxic to the kidneys.
networking Meeting people, exchanging phone numbers, expressing interest in other people and what they are doing, and establishing a business relationship that might be mutually beneficial.
neuroglycopenia A shortage of glucose in the brain.

neuron Any of the conducting cells of the nervous system; consists of a cell body containing the nucleus and cytoplasm and the axon and dendrites.
neuropathic pain Pain associated with a dysfunction of the nervous system; specifically, an abnormality in the processing of sensations.
neuropathy Any disease of the nerves.
neutropenia An abnormal decrease in the number of neutrophils in the blood.
neutrophilia An increase in the number of neutrophils in the blood.
neutrophils Granular leukocytes; also called *polymorphonuclear leukocytes.*
nociceptive pain Pain associated with pain stimuli from either somatic or visceral structures.
nocturia Excessive urination during the night.
nodules Small masses of tissue that can be detected by touch.
noncommunicable Cannot be carried from one person to another.
non–insulin-dependent diabetes mellitus Type 2 diabetes; a form of diabetes in which levels of endogenous insulin are adequate and control can be managed by diet and exercise and perhaps by an oral hypoglycemic agent.
nonjudgmental Avoiding judgment based on one's personal standards.
nonunion Failure to heal.
normal flora Flora most often found on or in body systems that have some form of contact with the outside environment. This flora prevents most harmful microorganisms from colonizing the body.
normo- A combining form indicating normal or usual.
North American Nursing Diagnosis Association–International (NANDA-I) An organization that formulates and validates nursing diagnoses.
nosocomial Pertaining to or originating in a hospital.
nuchal rigidity Stiffness and pain in the neck from inflammation of the meninges.
nurse practice act A legal statute describing the parameters of nursing practice.
nursing The diagnosis and treatment of human responses to actual or potential health problems. *See also* Nursing process.
nursing care plans Written plans of care that serve to communicate to the nursing staff and others the specific nursing diagnoses and prescribed nursing orders for directing and evaluating the effectiveness of the care given.
nursing diagnosis A statement of a health problem or of a potential problem in the patient's health status that a nurse is licensed and competent to treat.
nursing interventions Acts by nurses that implement the nursing care plan.
nursing process A goal-directed series of activities in which the practice of nursing accomplishes its goal of alleviating, minimizing, or preventing real or potential health problems.
nystagmus Involuntary, rapid rhythmic movement of the eyeball.

O

objective data Information obtained through the senses or measured by instruments.
objectives Well-defined steps toward the accomplishment of a goal; they should be realistic, be stated in measurable terms, and include the conditions under which they will be accomplished.
observation The act of watching carefully and attentively.
obsessive Having ideas, thoughts, or impulses that are persistent to an excessive degree.
obsessive-compulsive disorder A mental disorder characterized by recurrent or intrusive thoughts and rituals that can become overwhelming to the point of interfering with normal life.
obturator A device that is placed into a large-bore cannula during insertion to prevent potential blockage by tissues.
occult Obscure; concealed; hidden.
occult blood Hidden blood.
oculogyric crisis A side effect of antipsychotic medication characterized by uncontrolled rolling back of the eyes.
olfaction The act of smelling.
oligomenorrhea Decreased menstruation. Usually refers to menstrual periods that occur at an interval of 45 days or longer.
oliguria A diminished amount of urine formation.
oncogene A gene in a virus that can induce a cell to become malignant.
oncology The study of tumors.
onychomycosis A fungal infection of the fingernail or toenail.
oophoritis An inflammation of an ovary; ovaritis.
open access plan An insurance plan in which the patient can see any health care provider.
ophthalmologist A health care provider who specializes in treating eye disorders.
ophthalmoscope An instrument for examining the eye. The direct ophthalmoscope is used to inspect the back portion of the interior of the eyeball; the indirect ophthalmoscope permits stereoscopic inspection of the interior of the eye.
opportunistic infections (OIs) Infections that develop in an individual with a depressed immune system from organisms commonly found in the environment that are usually harmless.
opportunistic pathogen A fungus or bacterium, usually harmless, that causes infection in a person with a depressed immune system.
optic chiasm The part of the hypothalamus formed by the decussation, or crossing, of the fibers of the optic nerve from the medial half of each retina.
optician A specialist in the making of optical apparatus (e.g., eyeglasses).
optometrist A professional person trained to examine the eyes and prescribe eyeglasses or contact lenses to correct irregularities of vision.
orchiectomy The excision of one or both testes.
orchitis An inflammation of the testes.
orthopedic Referring to the correction of deformities of the musculoskeletal system.
orthopnea The ability to breathe easily only in the upright position.
orthopneic position Sitting up in bed with two or three pillows behind the back.
orthoses Casts or braces and splints.
orthostatic hypotension A fall in blood pressure that occurs when standing up from a sitting or lying position or when standing in a fixed position; characterized by dizziness, syncope, and blurred vision.
oscilloscope An instrument that makes visible on a screen the nature of an electrical current.
osmolality The osmotic pressure of a solution, expressed in osmoles or milliosmoles (mOsm) per kilogram of water.
osmosis The passage of solvent from a solution of lesser concentration to one of greater concentration through a selectively permeable membrane.
osmotic pressure Pressure that develops when two solutions of different concentrations are separated by a semipermeable membrane.
ossification Formation of or conversion into bone or a bony substance.
osteogenesis Growth of bone cells.
osteomyelitis A bacterial infection of the bone.
osteopenia Low bone mass.
osteoporosis A porous condition of bone caused by demineralization associated with aging or steroid medication.

otalgia Pain in the ear.
OTC Over the counter; available without a prescription.
otitis media An inflammation of the middle ear.
otorrhea Discharge from the ear with purulent matter due to infection or CSF in head trauma.
otoscope An instrument for examining the ear canal and eardrum.
outcome The result of an action.
ovulation The periodic ripening and rupture of the mature Graafian follicle and the discharge of the ovum from the cortex of the ovary.
oxidation The process by which a substance combines with oxygen.

P

pacemaker A mechanical device that provides electrical stimulation when an anatomic pacemaker fails; a cardiac pacemaker provides electrical stimulation when the heart rate is not adequate.
pain A feeling of distress or suffering caused by stimulation of specialized nerve cells; considered to occur whenever a person says it is present.
pain threshold The point at which pain is perceived.
pain tolerance The length of time or intensity at which a person will endure pain before outwardly responding to it.
palliative Designed to relieve symptoms when a disease cannot be cured.
palliative care Care of patients with chronic illness with the goal of symptom relief to improve quality of life.
palliative surgery Surgery performed to make a patient more comfortable.
palmar erythema A persistent redness of the palms that may be seen in liver disease.
palpation A physical examination technique in which the texture, size, consistency, and location of body parts are felt with the hands.
palpitation A rapid, violent, or throbbing pulsation, as an abnormally rapid throbbing or fluttering of the heart.
pancreatitis An inflamed condition of the pancreas.
pandemic An international outbreak of disease.
panhysterectomy The surgical removal of the entire uterus.
papilledema Swelling of the optic disc.
papule A small, round, solid, elevated lesion of the skin.
paracentesis The surgical puncture of a cavity to aspirate fluid. Usually refers to the peritoneal cavity.
paradoxical respirations Respirations in which, on inhalation, the diaphragm moves upward rather than downward, opposite to its normal movement.
paralytic ileus The absence of peristalsis; paralysis of the intestines.
paranoia A mental disorder in which a person exhibits delusions of persecution or of grandeur or a combination of both.
paraplegia Paralysis of the lower extremities.
parathormone A hormone produced and secreted by the parathyroid gland. Another name for parathyroid hormone.
parenteral Administered by a route other than the digestive tract.
paresthesia A feeling of tingling or numbness.
passive immunity Immunity acquired by transfer of antibody or lymphocytes from an immune donor.
patch test Similar to the scratch test except the allergen is simply placed on the surface of the skin and covered with an airtight dressing (patch).
patent Wide open.
pathogen A microorganism or substance capable of producing a disease.
pathologic Caused by a disease.
patient advocate A person who will advocate on the patient's behalf with the hospital, insurance company, or health care personnel.
PCA Patient-controlled analgesia.
pediculosis An infestation with lice.
pelvic inflammatory disease Inflammation of the internal female reproductive organs, usually caused by a bacterial infection.
peptic ulcer The loss of tissue lining the lower esophagus, stomach, or duodenum.
perception The recognition and interpretation of sensory stimuli that serve as a basis for comprehending, learning, and knowing or for motivating a particular action or reaction. Also, the third of four phases associated with nociceptive pain, during which impulses reach the brain and pain is recognized.
percussion The physical examination technique of tapping the body surface with the fingertips or fist to evaluate the size, borders, and consistency of some of the internal organs or to detect the presence of fluid in a body cavity.
percutaneous Through the skin.
perforation A hole or break in the retaining walls or membranes of an organ, as in perforated ulcer and perforated eardrum.
perfusion Supplying tissues and organs with nutrients and oxygen by blood flow through the arteries.
pericardial effusion A collection of serous or purulent exudate in the pericardial cavity.
pericardiocentesis The surgical puncture of the pericardial cavity for aspiration of fluid.
pericardiotomy The surgical incision of the pericardium.
pericarditis An inflammation of the sac that encloses the heart and the roots of the great vessels.
periodontal Located around a tooth.
perioperative Pertaining to the period extending from the time of hospitalization for surgery to the time of discharge.
periorbital Surrounding the socket of the eye.
peripheral Pertaining to the area outside the central region or structure.
peristalsis Involuntary wavelike contraction of organs with both longitudinal and circular muscle fibers that passes along the organ and propels its contents, as in peristalsis of the digestive tract.
peristomal Pertaining to the area around a stoma.
peritoneal dialysis Filtration of blood across the peritoneal membrane by instilling dialysate solution into the peritoneal cavity.
peritonitis An inflammation of the serous sac that lines the abdominal cavity and encloses the abdominal organs.
permeable Permitting passage of a substance.
personality disorder A mental disorder characterized by inflexible and maladaptive responses to life events, serious difficulty in personal and work relationships, a tendency to evoke interpersonal conflict, and a tendency to evoke a negative empathic response from others.
personal protective equipment (PPE) Equipment that forms some type of barrier to protect a person from exposure to bloodborne pathogens, body fluids, or other potentially infectious materials (e.g., gloves, covering gowns, face masks).
pessary A hard rubber ring inserted in the vagina to help keep the pelvic organs in place.
petechiae Very small, nonraised, round, purplish spots, caused by intradermal or submucosal bleeding, that later turn blue or yellow.
pH The concentration of hydrogen (H) in a solution; the higher the concentration of hydrogen ions, the lower the pH of the solution.
phacoemulsification A technique of cataract extraction in which high-frequency vibrations are used to fragment the lens.
phagocytosis The engulfing of microorganisms and other foreign matter by phagocytes.
phantom pain A sensation of discomfort occurring where an extremity has been amputated.
pharyngitis An inflammation or infection of the pharynx that usually produces a sore throat.

phenylketonuria A genetic disorder in which there is a defect in the metabolism of phenylalanine resulting in the presence of this amino acid in the urine.
pheochromocytoma A rare tumor of the adrenal medulla that secretes catecholamines (epinephrine and norepinephrine).
phlebitis An inflammation of a vein.
phlebotomy The surgical opening of a vein to draw blood, often done with a needle.
phobic disorder Excessive fear of a situation or object.
photocoagulation The alteration of proteins in tissue using light energy in the form of ordinary light rays or a laser beam.
photodynamic therapy A type of chemotherapy in which the action of the drug is enhanced by exposure to light.
photophobia Difficulty tolerating light.
pilonidal Pertaining to, characterized by, or having a tuft of hairs.
pilonidal sinus A lesion located at the cleft of the buttocks in the sacrococcygeal region; also called *pilonidal cyst.*
placebo(s) A supposedly inactive substance or procedure that can have either positive or negative effects on the relief of symptoms and that is usually given under the guise of effective treatment or in clinical trials of new drugs.
planning A phase of the nursing process in which a plan is developed with the patient, family, or significant other to provide a blueprint for nursing intervention to achieve specified goals. *See also* Nursing care plans.
plaque A patch or flat area on the skin. A semisolid buildup of substances such as dental plaque or atherosclerotic plaque.
plasma The liquid portion of blood in which formed elements are suspended; it contains plasma proteins, inorganic salts, nutrients, gases, wastes from the cells, and various hormones and enzymes.
plasma cell A spherical or ellipsoidal cell involved in the synthesis, storage, and release of antibody.
plasmapheresis The separation of the cells and components of the blood.
platelets The smallest formed elements in the blood; important in coagulation and blood clotting.
plethora A general term denoting a red, florid complexion or an excess of blood.
pleurisy An inflammation of the pleura.
Pneumocystis jirovecii An opportunistic pathogen that produces infection of the lung associated with acquired immunodeficiency syndrome (AIDS); formerly *Pneumocystis carinii.*
pneumonectomy The excision of lung tissue, especially of an entire lung.
pneumonia An inflammation of the lungs with consolidation.
pneumothorax The accumulation of air or gas in the pleural cavity, resulting in partial or complete collapse of the lung on the affected side.
point-of-service (POS) option An option offered by some managed care plans in which a member pays an extra fee to see a desired health care provider outside of the care plan.
poison control center Resource for immediate free advice on management of toxin exposure.
polyarteritis Multiple sites of inflammatory and destructive lesions in the arterial system.
polycystic ovarian syndrome An endocrine disturbance characterized by anovulation, amenorrhea, hirsutism, and infertility.
polycythemia An elevation in the total number of blood cells.
polydipsia Excessive thirst that results in drinking large quantities of water.
polymorphonuclear leukocytes The fully developed cells of the granulocyte series, especially neutrophils, the nuclei of which contain three or more lobes.
polyphagia Increased hunger.
polyuria The production of an excessive amount of urine.
positive symptoms One of the two divisions of signs and symptoms seen with schizophrenia; includes hallucinations, delusions, and disordered thinking.
postictal state The condition of a person right after a seizure.
post-traumatic stress disorder A mental disorder characterized by recurrent symptoms of anxiety that some individuals may experience after encountering an extreme, life-threatening event. Nightmares or flashbacks may be part of the symptoms.
PPO *See* Preferred provider organization.
precancerous Term used to refer to a growth that is not yet but probably will become cancerous.
precipitate A deposit separated from a suspension or solution by precipitation; the reaction of a reagent that causes the deposit to fall to the bottom or float near the top.
preferred provider organization (PPO) An organization of health care providers, hospitals, and pharmacists whose members discount their services to subscriber patients.
premature ejaculation Occurs when the ejaculation reflex is not controlled and the release of semen occurs before release is desired. It is the most common ejaculation problem in men.
premenstrual syndrome A group of symptoms experienced by some women for several days before the onset of the menstrual period.
prepuce The foreskin or fold of skin over the glans penis in the male.
presbycusis Impairment of hearing in older adults.
presbyopia Farsightedness that occurs normally with aging.
pressor A substance that causes a rise in blood pressure. Norepinephrine is an example of a "pressor" hormone. Norepinephrine maintains blood pressure.
pressured speech Talking that is loud, rapid, and difficult to interrupt.
pressure ulcer A sore caused by pressure from a splint or other appliance or from the body itself when it has remained immobile in bed for extended periods.
preventive Hindering the occurrence of something, especially disease.
priapism A prolonged penile erection resulting in a large, hard, and painful penis unrelated to sexual desire or activity.
primary immune deficiency disorders Diseases that are acquired as a result of a genetic disorder that causes impairment or nonfunctioning of the immune system.
primary union The joining of two edges of a wound that are close together, resulting in a thin scar after healing; also called *healing by first intention.*
priority Preference established based on emergency or need.
priority setting Setting the sequence of actions according to importance or priority.
problem-oriented medical record (POMR) A system of documentation in which the information is arranged according to specific problems presented by the patient at the time of seeking health care. The four components are database, problem list, initial plan, and follow-up. *See also* Progress notes.
process A series of actions that move from one point to another on the way to completing a goal.
prodromal stage The early or very beginning stage of an illness.
prodrome An early sign of a developing condition or disease.
prognosis The predicted outcome of the course of a disease.
progress notes Entries in the medical record describing what has been done in the care of the patient and their response to the intervention.
prolapse The falling down or displacement of a part or all of an organ, as in prolapse of a stoma or prolapse of the uterus.
promoter(s) A type of epigenetic carcinogen that promotes neoplastic growth only after initiation by another substance; a cocarcinogen.
prophylactic Something done or used to prevent infection or disease.

prospective payment system A payment system for reimbursing hospitals for inpatient health care services in which a predetermined rate is set for treatment of specific illnesses.
prostaglandins A group of naturally occurring fatty acids that stimulate contraction of the uterine and other smooth-muscle tissue.
prostate-specific antigen (PSA) A protein produced by the prostate that is present in elevated levels in patients with cancer or other diseases of the prostate.
prosthesis An artificial substitute for a missing part, such as an eye, limb, or tooth, used for functional or cosmetic reasons, or both.
protease inhibitor A drug that works at the last stage of viral reproduction.
protective isolation Special precautionary procedures to minimize exposure to infectious agents in a patient who has an immune deficiency or who is otherwise susceptible to infection.
proteinuria An excess of serum proteins in the urine.
protocol The plan for a course of medical treatment.
protozoa A phylum comprising the unicellular organisms; most are free-living, but some lead commensalistic, mutualistic, or parasitic existences.
provider A person or an agency that provides health care services.
proximal Closest to a point of reference.
pruritus Itching.
PSA velocity A trend in PSA levels over time that may indicate a need for further tests to diagnose prostate cancer.
pseudocyst An abnormal or dilated cavity resembling a true cyst but not lined with epithelium. Also called *adventitious cyst* or *false cyst*.
psychoactive substances Mind-altering agents capable of changing or altering a person's mood, behavior, cognition, arousal level, level of consciousness, and perceptions.
psychomotor retardation A slowing of speech, movement, and thought process often seen in depressed patients.
psychotherapy A type of therapy that helps patients identify problem areas and work to change or modify behaviors, attitudes, and feelings.
psychotic features Hallucinations, delusions, and grossly disorganized behavior.
ptomaines Toxic substances produced by the action of putrefactive bacteria on proteins and amino acids.
ptosis Drooping of the upper eyelid so that it partially or completely covers the cornea.
pulmonary edema A diffuse accumulation of fluid in the tissues and air spaces of the lung.
pulmonary embolus A mass of clotted blood or other formed element in the lung that has traveled through the bloodstream from another location.
pulse deficit The difference between the radial and apical pulse rates.
pulsus paradoxus A drop in systolic blood pressure of greater than 10 mm Hg on inspiration.
purpura Purplish areas caused by bleeding into the skin or mucous membranes.
purulence The condition of producing or discharging pus.
purulent Full of pus.
pus A liquid product of inflammation composed of albuminous substances, a thin fluid, and leukocytes; generally yellow.
push hard, push fast CPR guidelines recommending at least 100 compressions per minute and a depth of at least 2 inches.
pustule A small, round, pus-filled lesion of the skin.
pyelogram A radiograph of the kidney and ureters after injection of a contrast medium that may be administered intravenously (IV pyelogram) or by way of the ureters (retrograde pyelogram).
pyelonephritis An inflammation of the kidney and renal pelvis.
pyrogen Any agent that causes fever.
pyuria Pus in the urine.

Q

quadriplegia Paralysis of all four extremities.
quadriplegic A person with paralysis of all four limbs.

R

rad Radiation absorbed dose; the unit used for measuring doses of radiation.
radiation therapy The use of radiant energy from radioactive materials or high-voltage x-rays to treat disease.
radioimmunoassay A laboratory method for measuring minute quantities of specific antibodies or any antigen, such as a hormone or drug, against which antibodies have been produced.
radionuclide A radioactive substance given to the patient before radiography or scanning.
radiopaque Not penetrable by x-rays; appears white on radiograph.
rales Older term for abnormal respiratory sounds heard on auscultation with a stethoscope indicating some pathologic condition. *See* Crackles.
range of motion The extent, measured in degrees of a circle, through which a joint can be extended and flexed.
rationalization A defense mechanism in which a patient finds logical reasons (justification) for their behavior while ignoring the real reasons.
realistic Attainable, based on the patient's condition and desire.
rectocele A protrusion of the rectum and posterior vaginal wall into the vagina.
recurrent Returning at intervals.
referred pain Pain felt in a part away from its point of origin.
reflex (reflexes) The sum of any autonomic (automatic) response mediated by the nervous system and not requiring conscious movement.
refraction The determination of refractive errors (inability to focus light rays on the retina) and their correction with eyeglasses.
regeneration The natural renewal of a structure.
regimen A prescribed scheme of diet, exercise, or activity to achieve certain ends.
rehabilitation The processes of treatment and education that help a disabled or deconditioned individual attain maximum function, a sense of well-being, and a personally satisfying level of independence.
relapse Recurrence of disease after a period of improvement.
remission Absence or reduction in disease symptoms; may be partial or complete, temporary or permanent.
remittent Having alternating periods of abating and returning, such as a fever that comes and goes.
renal stenosis Blockage or narrowing of the renal artery because of atherosclerosis or scarring.
replicate To duplicate, reproduce, or copy.
replication The process of duplicating or reproducing.
reservoir A passive host or carrier that harbors pathogenic organisms without harm to itself and is a source from which others can be infected.
residual urine Urine that remains in the bladder immediately after urination.
resorption The breakdown of tissue by body chemicals with assimilation of the component parts as in resorption of bone in osteoporosis.
respiration The taking in of oxygen, its use in the tissues, and the giving off of carbon dioxide.
respiratory acidosis A condition in which the pH of body fluids is below 7.35 because of failure of the lungs to exhale sufficient amounts of carbon dioxide.

respiratory alkalosis A condition in which the pH of body fluids is above 7.45 because of excessive removal of carbon dioxide by the lungs, as in hyperventilation.
resuscitation Revival after apparent death. Correction of essential physiologic disorders, fluid, cardiopulmonary.
reticuloendothelial system A network of cells and tissues found throughout the body, especially in the blood, connective tissue, spleen, liver, lungs, bone marrow, and lymph vessels; these cells play a role in blood cell formation and destruction and in inflammation and immunity.
retinopathy A pathologic condition of the retina associated with diabetes mellitus.
retrograde Moving backward; degenerating from a better to a worse state.
retrograde ejaculation Occurs when the semen travels toward the bladder rather than exiting the penis.
retrospective Dealing with the past.
retrospective payment system Medicare payment based on actual costs submitted to government; used before 1983.
retrovirus A type of virus that contains RNA.
reverse transcriptase An enzyme that is present in retroviruses.
rhinitis An inflammation of the mucous membrane of the nose.
rhinoplasty A plastic surgical operation on the nose, either reconstructive, restorative, or cosmetic.
rhizotomy A surgical procedure to sever a spinal nerve root.
rhonchi Coarse rattling sounds in the bronchial tubes caused by a partial obstruction.
rickettsia A genus of small, rod-shaped to round microorganisms found in tissue cells of lice, fleas, ticks, and mites and transmitted to humans by their bites.
rigor mortis The stiffness that occurs in dead bodies.
robotics The science of designing mechanical, computerized instruments for procedures.
Roux-en-Y Any Y-shaped anastomosis in which the small intestine is included.
rubor A dusky-red color seen in patients with arterial insufficiency.
rugae Ridges or folds on a mucous membrane.

S

safer sex Any sexual practice that is performed with the use of a barrier to prevent the exchange of body fluids.
salpingitis An inflammation of a fallopian or eustachian tube.
sarcoidosis A chronic, progressive, systemic granulomatous reticulosis of unknown etiology, involving almost any organ or tissue.
sarcoma A tumor, often highly malignant, composed of cells derived from connective tissue.
scabies An infestation with the mange mite.
scaling The shedding of small, thin, dry layers of skin.
scarring The replacement of damaged tissue with fibrous tissue.
schizophrenia A mental illness that causes unusual, bizarre behavior (hallucinations and delusions).
sclerotherapy The injection of a solution that causes the vessel to dry up and disintegrate.
scoliosis Lateral curvature of the spine.
scotoma An area of lost vision in the visual field.
scratch test A test in which the skin is pricked by a needle and a drop of the suspected allergen is applied to the area. A needle is then used to slightly scratch the skin just below the epidermis.
sebaceous Containing or pertaining to sebum, an oily, fatty matter secreted by the sebaceous glands.
secondary union The healing of a wound in which the edges are far apart and cannot be brought together; the wound fills with granulation tissue and heals from the edges inward.
sedative(s) An agent that calms nervousness, irritability, and excitement.
seizure(s) An attack of uncontrollable muscular contractions; a convulsion.
self-care The process by which one initiates and carries out certain health practices to maintain life, health, and personal well-being.
semen A thick, opalescent, viscid secretion discharged from the urethra of the male at the climax of sexual excitement (orgasm).
seminal Concerning the semen or seed.
senile lentigines Areas where melanocytes increase in production, producing brown age spots.
senile purpura Dark purplish-red ecchymoses occurring on the forearms and backs of the hands in the older adult.
sensitivity reaction An exaggerated response to agents perceived by the body as foreign.
sensorineural hearing loss Impaired perception of sound caused by a dysfunction in the inner ear or the eighth cranial nerve due to continued exposure to excessively high levels of sound.
sensory loss Impairment of acuity of sight, hearing, taste, touch, and/or smell.
sentinel infections Infections that may indicate an underlying immunosuppression.
sentinel node biopsy A biopsy of lymph nodes that receive drainage from the anatomic area of a tumor to determine spread of the disease.
sepsis The presence of specific signs and symptoms in the setting of a known or suspected infection.
septicemia Infective microorganisms circulating in the bloodstream.
sequelae An abnormal condition that follows and is the result of a disease.
seroconversion The point at which antibodies to specific antigens are detectable in the blood.
seroma A collection of serum forming a tumor-like mass.
serosanguineous Containing both serum and blood.
serum (sera) The clear, liquid portion of blood that does not contain fibrinogen or blood cells. Immune serum is blood serum from the bodies of people or animals that have produced antibody; inoculation with such serum produces passive immunity.
serum sickness A hypersensitivity reaction to a foreign serum or other antigen.
sexually transmitted infection An infection that is transmitted by direct sexual contact.
shearing action Superficial layers of tissue are pulled and stretched across deeper layers of tissue.
shedding Losing or casting off by a natural process.
Sheehan syndrome A rare but serious postpartum complication that involves infarction of the pituitary gland secondary to postpartum hemorrhage.
shock Acute circulatory failure caused by derangement of circulatory control, obstruction, pump failure, or loss of circulating fluid.
shunting Physiologically bypassing, as when blood flows past the alveoli but the membrane is thickened and gases cannot cross into or out of the blood.
sickle cell disease A genetic disorder in which sickle hemoglobin is found in the red blood cells.
slit lamp An instrument for examining the surface of the eye through a biomicroscopic lens.
smear A specimen for microscopic and cytologic study; the material is spread thinly and evenly across a slide with a swab or loop.
SOAP Acronym for *S*ubjective and *O*bjective data, *A*ssessment, and *P*lanning.
solute The substance that is dissolved in a solution.

Somogyi effect A blood glucose rebound phenomenon caused by overtreatment with insulin.
source-oriented record keeping A system of documentation in which information is arranged according to the person, department, or other source of information.
specific gravity The weight of a substance compared with the weight of an equal amount of another substance taken as a standard; for liquids, the standard usually is water (specific gravity of 1). Measures the concentration of urine in relation to water.
spermatogenesis The production of sperm.
spermatozoa The mature mobile sperm cells.
spider angioma A form of telangiectasis with a central elevated red dot the size of a pinhead from which small blood vessels radiate; often occurs with liver disease.
spirochete Any organism that is a member of the order Spirochaetales.
spirometer An instrument for measuring air taken into and expelled from the lungs.
splenomegaly Enlargement of the spleen.
splitting A personality trait that involves initial idealization of a caregiver or friend, followed by a devaluing of that same person.
spores Reproductive cells, usually unicellular, produced by plants and some protozoa.
sprain The wrenching or twisting of a joint with partial or complete tearing of the ligaments.
sputum A substance expelled by coughing or clearing the throat.
Standard Precautions Precautions designed to prevent the transmission of microorganisms from one patient to another as well as to protect health care workers from unnecessary exposure to infection.
stapedectomy The surgical removal of the stirrup of the middle ear and its replacement with a prosthetic device.
stasis Standing still; stagnation; usually refers to fluid.
status epilepticus A grave condition in which there is a rapid, unrelenting series of seizures without intervening periods of consciousness and with absence of respiration. Irreversible brain damage may occur if seizures are not controlled.
steatorrhea Stool that is bulky, frothy, and foul smelling and usually floats in the toilet because of the presence of excess fat.
stem cells Generalized mother cells, the descendants of which specialize, often in different functions; an example is an undifferentiated mesenchymal cell that is the progenitor of the blood and fixed-tissue cells of the bone marrow.
stenosis The narrowing or contraction of a passageway or opening.
stent A tubular device to give support to the interior of a vessel or tube, preventing its collapse.
stereotaxis A method of precisely locating areas in the brain.
stereotype(s) A simplification used to describe all members of a specific group without exception.
sterilization, microbe The process of rendering an article free of microorganisms and their pathogenic products.
Steri-Strips Small, reinforced, sterile adhesive strips placed over a healing incision to hold it together after sutures are removed.
STI Sexually transmitted infection.
stoma(s) A mouth-like opening, especially one that is created surgically for the elimination of urine or fecal material.
stomatitis A generalized inflammation of the oral mucosa.
strabismus A deviation of the eye that cannot be controlled voluntarily.
strain The pulling or tearing of either muscle or tendon, or both.
stress incontinence The loss of urine during a sneeze or cough.
stridor A harsh, high-pitched respiratory sound such as the inspiratory sound often heard in acute laryngeal obstruction.
stroke volume Equals the amount of blood ejected by a ventricle during one contraction.
stromal cells Connective tissue cells of the supporting tissue or matrix of an organ.
stye An infected swelling near the margin of the eyelid.
subcutaneous Beneath or to be introduced beneath the skin.
subcutaneous emphysema Interstitial emphysema characterized by the presence of air in the subcutaneous tissue, usually caused by intrathoracic injury.
subdural hematoma The accumulation of blood in the subdural space.
subjective data Data that the patient provides about a symptom that cannot be seen, felt, or heard by an examiner (e.g., pain).
subluxation A partial or incomplete dislocation of a bone from its place in a joint.
substance use disorder A problem with one or more substances causing health issues or interfering with life activities.
subsystem A system within a larger system.
"sucking" chest wound A wound in which the pleural cavity has been penetrated, allowing air and gas to enter the cavity and produce pneumothorax.
sundowning The phenomenon of becoming confused and disoriented at night, although oriented during the day.
suppression Inhibition, such as interfering with immune response.
suprasystem A highly complex system.
surge capacity The maximum services that a facility can offer when every resource is mobilized.
susceptible Being predisposed or sensitive to the effects of an infectious disease, allergen, or other pathogenic agent; lacking immunity or resistance.
sympathectomy A surgical excision or interruption in some portion of the sympathetic nerve pathways.
syncope Fainting.
syndrome A combination of signs and symptoms associated with a pathologic process or disease.
syndrome of inappropriate antidiuretic hormone (SIADH) ADH is produced even though normovolemia or hypervolemia is present, resulting in fluid retention.
synovial fluid The transparent viscid fluid found in joint cavities, bursae, and tendon sheaths.
synthesis The process or processes involved in the formation of a complex substance from simpler elements or compounds; opposite of decomposition.
synthesize To put together (data) into a logical whole.
system An organized whole composed of interacting parts.
systemic inflammatory response syndrome (SIRS) A condition in which the body's inflammatory response causes signs and symptoms (tachycardia, tachypnea, hypotension, oliguria, and fever) without a documented source of infection.
systole The phase of the cardiac cycle in which the ventricles contract and force blood into the aorta and pulmonary arteries; the systolic pressure is recorded as the top number in a blood pressure reading.
systolic blood pressure Arterial pressure during systole.

T

tachycardia A rapid heart rate, more than 100 beats per minute.
tachypnea Abnormal rapidity of respiration.
tamponade The stoppage of blood flow to an organ or part of the body by pressure.
tardive dyskinesia A common extrapyramidal side effect seen with antipsychotics; patients may exhibit lip-smacking, tongue protrusion, blinking, sucking, chewing, and lateral jaw movements.
target cells/tissues Cells and tissues that are affected by a specific hormone.

telangiectases Dilation of the capillaries causing small red or purple clusters; also called *spider veins.*
tendons Connective tissue that connects the muscles to the bones.
TENS Transcutaneous electrical nerve stimulation.
tertiary Third in order or stage.
testis The male gonad. One of two reproductive glands located in the scrotum that produce the male reproductive cells and the male hormone, testosterone.
tetany The continuous tonic spasm of a muscle; associated with calcium deficit, vitamin D deficiency, and alkalosis.
tetraplegia Another term for quadriplegia (paralysis of all four extremities).
thalamus Either of two large structures composed of gray matter and situated at the base of the cerebrum that act as a relay station for impulses traveling from the spinal cord and brainstem to the cerebral cortex.
thanatologist One who studies death.
thanatology The medicolegal study of the dying process and death.
theory (theories) A belief, policy, or principle proposed or followed as the basis of action.
therapeutic Having medicinal or healing properties.
therapeutic alliance Relationship between the patient and nurse established for the purpose of helping the patient to build trust and achieve therapeutic goals.
thermal Pertaining to heat.
thoracentesis The surgical puncture and drainage of the thoracic cavity.
thoracotomy The surgical incision of the wall of the chest.
thought disorder A mental disorder characterized by disorganized thought, behavior, and hallucinations. Mood and interpersonal relationships are altered.
thrombectomy The excision of a clot.
thrombocytopenia A decreased number of platelets.
thrombocytopenic purpura A bleeding disorder characterized by a marked decrease in the number of platelets, resulting in multiple bruises, petechiae, and hemorrhage into the tissues.
thrombolytic Dissolving or splitting up a thrombus.
thrombophlebitis An inflammation of a vein related to formation of a blood clot within the vessel.
thrombosis The formation, development, or presence of a blood clot within a blood vessel.
thrombus A stationary blood clot in the circulatory system.
thymus An endocrine gland that lies in the upper chest beneath the sternum and that, during fetal life, sensitizes certain stem cells that eventually become T lymphocytes.
thyrocalcitonin A hormone secreted by the thyroid gland.
thyroid crisis A sudden increase in the output of thyroxine and resultant extreme elevation of all body processes.
thyroid panel A group of tests performed to evaluate thyroid function.
thyroid storm *See* Thyroid crisis.
thyrotoxicosis A toxic condition that results from hyperactivity of the thyroid gland. *See* Thyroid crisis.
thyroxine (T_4) A hormone secreted by the thyroid gland. Four iodine molecules are attached to thyroid hormone (T_4), making it metabolically inactive. When one iodine is removed, it becomes the active form T_3. *See* Triiodothyronine.
time-referenced Measured by an educated guess as to how long it will take to attain the outcome.
tinea Ringworm; a name applied to many different fungal infections of the skin. The specific type usually is designated by a modifying term (e.g., tinea capitis, or ringworm of the scalp).
tinea pedis A fungal infection of the foot; also called *athlete's foot.*
tinnitus A ringing, buzzing, or other continuous noise in the ear.
T lymphocytes White blood cells destined to provide cellular immunity that have passed through the thymus and migrated to the lymph nodes.
tolerance Increased resistance to a drug or substance that occurs when there is a need for increased amounts of substances to achieve the desired effect. Term used with substance use disorder.
tonic A state of rigid contraction of the muscles.
tonometer An instrument for measuring tension or pressure, especially intraocular pressure.
tophus (tophi) A deposit of sodium biurate in tissues near a joint, in the ear, or in bone, as occurs in gout.
topical Pertaining to the surface of a part of the body, as in topical medications applied to an area of the skin.
torsion The act of twisting or condition of being twisted.
total parenteral nutrition Intravenous feeding to provide all nutritional needs over time.
tourniquet A device for compressing an artery or vein; its use as an emergency measure to relieve hemorrhage is generally recommended only if the victim's life is threatened and other measures fail to stop massive blood loss.
toxin A poisonous substance.
tracheostomy A surgical incision into the trachea to insert a tube through which the patient can breathe.
traction The exertion of a pulling force, as that applied to a fractured bone or dislocated joint, to maintain proper positioning.
tranquilizers A group of agents that provide calm and relief from anxiety.
transcellular Between cells, but within an epithelial membrane.
transcellular fluid Secretions and excretions that move through cell membranes and eventually leave the body.
transduction The first of four phases associated with nociceptive pain. Tissue damage stimulates the nociceptors and initiates pain sensation.
transfer factor A factor occurring in sensitized lymphocytes that recruits additional lymphocytes and transfers to them the ability to confer cell-mediated immunity.
transformation A change to another form.
transfusion The administration of whole blood or blood components directly into the bloodstream.
transmission The second of four phases associated with nociceptive pain. Involves movement of sensation to the spinal cord.
Transmission-Based Precautions Used in addition to Standard Precautions. Protective actions and equipment are implemented based on how the organism is spread rather than on the organism itself. Contact, airborne, and droplet transmission are the current modes requiring specific precautions.
triage The classification of casualties in an emergency department or location of a disaster by the gravity of the injury, urgency of treatment, and place for treatment.
triiodothyronine (T_3) A hormone secreted by the thyroid gland. Active form of thyroid hormone.
Trousseau sign Carpal spasm elicited by inflating a blood pressure cuff above the systolic blood pressure caused by low blood calcium.
tuberculin test An evaluation of sensitivity to the tubercle bacillus; an intradermal injection of a purified protein derivative of tuberculin (the Mantoux test) or a blood sample may be drawn for the testing; a positive reaction in either type of test indicates the need for further diagnostic procedures.
tuberculosis Any of the infectious diseases caused by species of *Mycobacterium* and characterized by the formation of tubercles and caseous necrosis in the tissues.
tumor A swelling or growth of a mass in the body due to abnormal tissue that can be benign or malignant.
tumor marker A blood test to detect biochemical substances synthesized and released into the bloodstream by tumor cells; used mainly to confirm a diagnosis of cancer or response to cancer therapy.

tumor-node-metastasis (TNM) staging system A system for classifying cancers according to the extent to which the malignancy has spread.
turgor Elasticity of the skin; helps determine hydration status.
tympanoplasty An operative procedure on the eardrum or ossicles of the middle ear to restore or improve hearing in patients with a conductive hearing loss.

U

ultrasonography An imaging technique in which deep anatomic structures are recorded by depicting the echoes of ultrasonic waves that have been directed into the tissues; the echoes (reflections) returning from the structures are converted into electrical impulses that are displayed on a screen, thus presenting a "picture" of the tissues being examined.
unlicensed assistive personnel (UAP) Nursing assistants, technicians, unit secretaries, and aides who do not hold a professional license to perform some aspects of health care delivery and are hired to perform specific repetitive tasks.
urea nitrogen A major protein metabolite that is not recycled by the body but is excreted in the urine; blood urea nitrogen levels indicate the ability of the kidney to filter and excrete waste products.
uremia Retention in the blood of urea, creatinine, and other nitrogenous wastes normally eliminated in the urine; more correctly called *azotemia*.
uremic syndrome Symptoms produced by uremia.
ureterostomy (ureterostomies) Surgical creation of a stoma to divert urine to the outside.
urethritis Inflammation of the urethra.
urinalysis Analysis of a sample of urine, most often done to detect protein, glucose, acetone, blood, pus, and casts.
urinary diversion Creation of an artificial opening (stoma) on the skin surface for elimination of urine from a pouch created from a segment of intestine as a urine reservoir.
urinary frequency Voiding more often than every 2 hours. This can be the result of inflammation, decreased bladder capacity, psychological disorders, pregnancy, or increased fluid intake.
urinary hesitancy A delay in starting the stream of urine; may be related to partial obstruction.
urinary incontinence Involuntary passing of urine.
urinary retention Retaining or holding urine in the bladder; inability to start the urine stream or to completely empty the bladder.
urodynamics Study of normal pressures in the bladder.
uroflowmetry Pressure flow studies of the bladder.
urticaria Hives.

V

vaccination The injection of a vaccine into the body to produce immunity to a specific disease.
vaccines Suspensions of attenuated or killed microorganisms administered to provide active immunity to infectious disease. Usually given by injection but may be intranasal, intradermal, or oral.
vagotomy The surgical interruption of impulses carried by the vagus nerve or nerves; may be done to reduce the production of gastric secretions and to inhibit gastric motility, as part of the treatment for peptic ulcer.
Valsalva maneuver An increase of thoracic pressure; may by induced by forcible exhalation against the closed glottis, as in straining at stool.
value A personal belief about the worth of something that is cherished or held dear.
valvuloplasty A procedure in which a balloon catheter is threaded via the circulatory system through the heart and into the valve. The balloon is inflated to break open a stenosed valve.
varices Twisted and swollen veins.
varicose veins Enlarged and tortuous veins in which the distorted shape is the result of accumulations of pooled blood.
vascular dementia A broad term used to describe any type of dementia caused by vessel disease.
vascular disorders An abnormal functioning of blood vessels, either arterial or venous. Peripheral arterial disorders are most commonly caused by atherosclerosis. Peripheral venous problems are caused by defective valvular function.
vasectomy Excision of the vas (ductus) deferens or a portion of it; bilateral vasectomy results in sterility.
vasoactive Tending to cause vasodilation or vasoconstriction.
vector(s) A carrier, usually one that transmits disease.
venereal Pertaining to or resulting from sexual intercourse.
ventilation The movement of air from the external environment to the gas exchange units of the lung.
ventilator-associated pneumonia (VAP) Pneumonia that occurs 48 to 72 hours after endotracheal intubation.
vertigo A sensation of movement of one's self or of one's surroundings; dizziness.
vesicant Blistering; causing or forming blisters.
vesicle A small sac containing a serous liquid; a small blister.
vesicostomy The formation of an opening into the urinary bladder through the abdominal wall.
viable Capable of living.
virulence The degree of ability of an organism to cause disease.
viscera The internal organs contained within a cavity.
viscous Sticky, gummy, gelatinous; thicker than usual.
vitrectomy The removal of the contents of the vitreous chamber.
voiding When urine passes from the bladder through the urethra during urination; to urinate.
volvulus A twisting of the bowel upon itself, causing obstruction.
vulvectomy The excision of the vulva.

W

wart An epidermal growth of viral origin.
Wernicke encephalopathy Damage to brain cells caused by chronic alcohol abuse.
wheal A localized area of edema on the body surface.
wheeze(s) A form of rhonchus characterized by a high-pitched or low-pitched musical quality caused by airflow through a narrowed airway.
withdrawal Symptoms that are caused by the sudden discontinuation of a substance to which an individual has become physiologically or psychologically dependent.
word salad A meaningless mixture of words and phrases characteristic of advanced schizophrenia.

X

xanthelasma A planar xanthoma involving the eyelid(s). Cholesterol deposits under the skin, identified by sharply demarcated yellow spots.
xanthoma A lipid deposit in the skin.
xenograft A surgical graft of tissue from an individual of one species to an individual of a different species.
xerostomia The lack of saliva; dry mouth.

Y

yeast A term for fungi that reproduce by budding.

Z

zygomatic Pertaining to the zygomatic bone that forms the zygomatic arch and part of the orbit for the eye.

Index

Page numbers followed by "*f*" indicate figures, "*t*" indicate tables, and "*b*" indicate boxes.

B

N

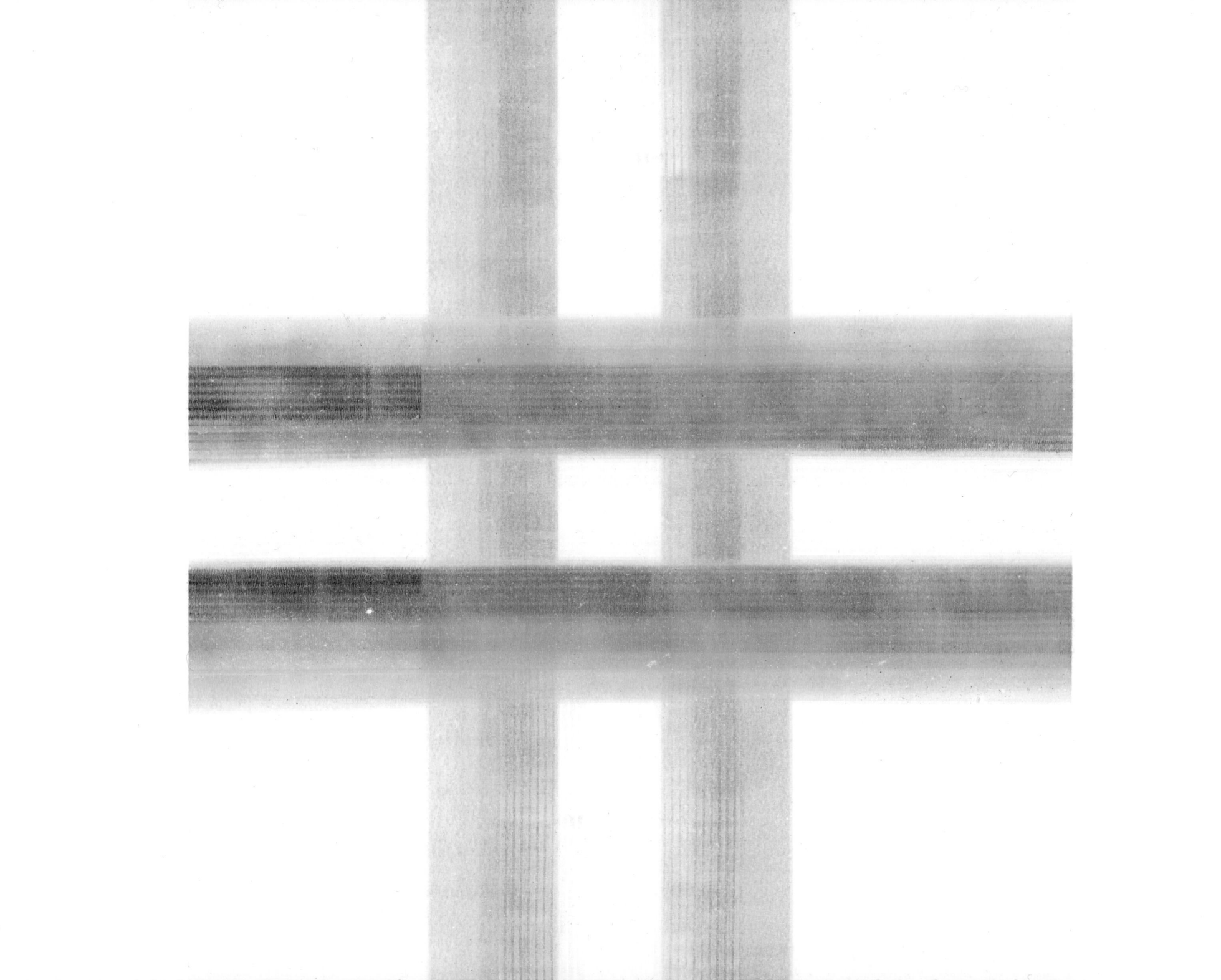

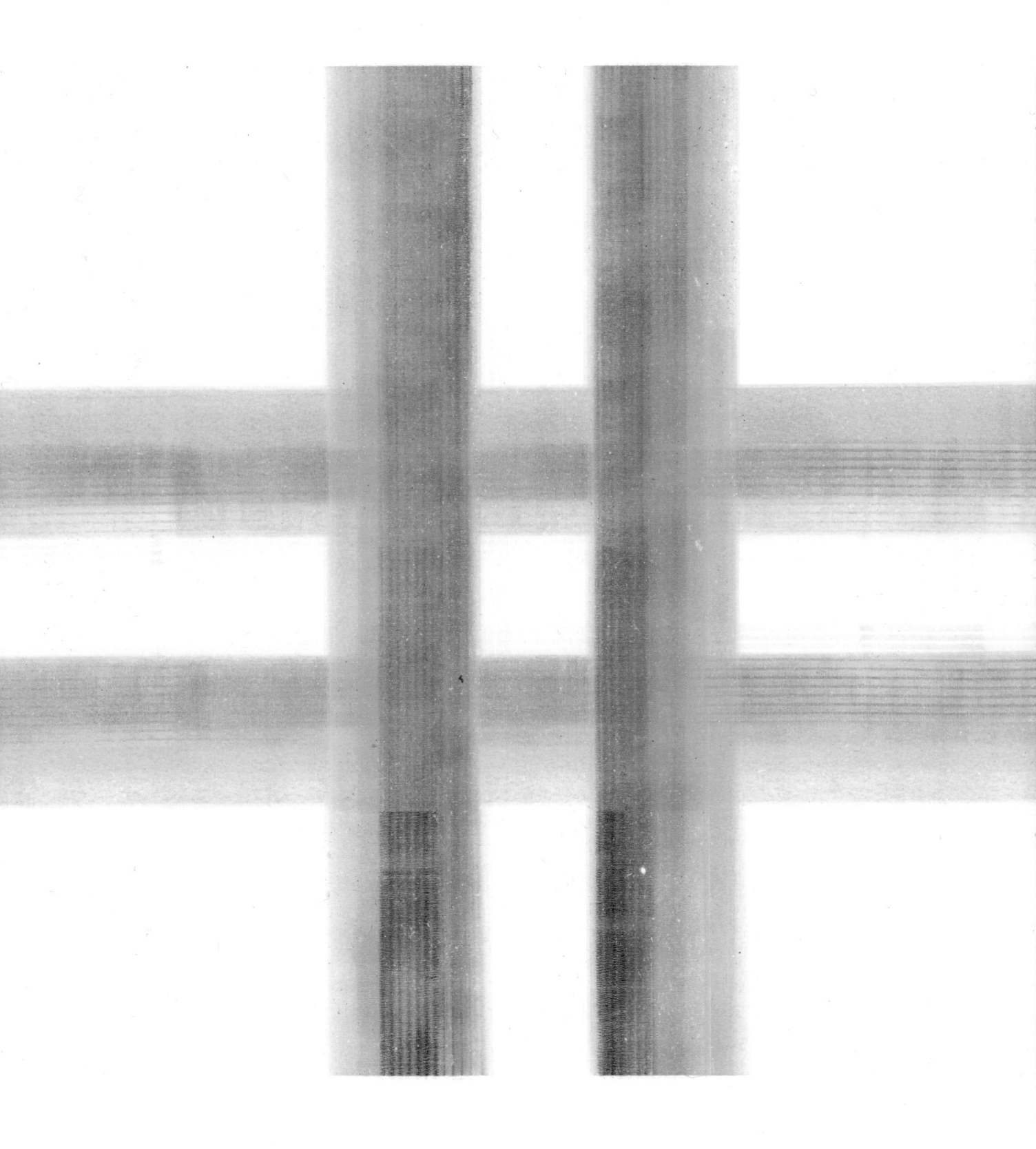